Foreword

The primary immunodeficiency diseases, the first of which were recognized over 50 years ago, are now generally appreciated as major health problems by affected patients, their families, physicians, and even the general public. In 1999, this book was the first comprehensive compendium devoted to primary immunodeficiency diseases. While most are relatively rare, some of these conditions, like IgA deficiency and common variable immunodeficiency, occur with a frequency that makes these patients likely to be seen by most physicians.

The study of patients with these genetically determined immune disorders in conjunction with the study of animal models has led to remarkable progress in our understanding of the interacting components of the complex immune system and how they function in humans. As a consequence, earlier recognition and better treatment options are provided for patients with primary immunodeficiency diseases, as well as for the even larger number of individuals with secondary immune deficiency conditions. This authoritative book, now in its second edition, contains a comprehensive account of currently available information. In the short years since the first publication, the number of known immunodeficiency genes has grown from less than 70 to well over 120, reflecting the tremendous expansion of knowledge in this field. The rich base of information contained in these pages makes it clear that there are few fields in medicine in which laboratory-based research and the study of diseases in patients have been so mutually complementary as for the primary immunodeficiency diseases.

The first immunodeficiency diseases to be identified, namely X-linked agammaglobulinemia, and the more clinically severe congenital lymphopenic syndromes were diseases that are now known to reflect compromised development in the effector limbs of the adaptive immune system. Experimental delineation of the developmentally distinct lineages of lymphocytes, the thymus-dependent population of T cells, and the bone marrow–derived B cells, made possible the recognition of their respective roles in cell-mediated and humoral immunity. Accordingly, the primary immunodeficiency diseases were found to belong to distinct classes, those primarily affecting T cell development, like the thymic underdevelopment seen in the DiGeorge syndrome, and those featuring impaired B cell development and antibody production, as seen in Bruton X-linked agammaglobulinemia. Severe combined immunodeficiency (SCID), recognized first by Glanzmann and Riniker, featured instead a developmental failure of both T and B cells. With the ensuing molecular biology revolution, the pace of the genetic analysis of the immunodeficiency diseases quickened remarkably. As more and more details have been learned about the life history of T and B lineage cells, many of the genetically determined defects in these differentiation pathways can now be identified quite precisely in genetic and molecular terms.

As is indicated in the contents of this book, we currently have sufficient information about the lymphocyte differentiation pathways to categorize primary immunodeficiency diseases into gene mutations that affect (1) DNA transcription factors; (2) rearrangement and expression of the T cell receptor (TCR) and immunoglobulin genes; (3) signal transducing components of the TCR and B cell receptor (BCR) complexes; (4) essential signaling pathway elements employed by TCR and BCR; (5) coreceptor molecules that are essential for normal function of T and B cells; (6) cytokines and cytokine receptors that promote T and B cell production, proliferation, and differentiation; and (7) cell surface molecules that are necessary for normal lymphocyte homing and intercellular interactions in the peripheral lymphoid tissues, including the spleen, lymph nodes, intestinal Peyer's patches, and appendix. It has also become increasingly evident that the normal function of the effector T and B cell populations depends on other types of cells as well. An especially important cell partner is the dendritic cell, because it responds to potential pathogens by presenting antigen to initiate the T cell response and, in turn, the B cell response. Although few primary immunodeficiency diseases have as yet been attributed to developmental flaws in this cell type, impaired dendritic cell function is an important component of the immunodeficiency caused by gene mutations that prevent CD40 expression or expression of the CD40 ligand on T cells.

The specific adaptive immune responses mediated by T and B cells and their collaborators, although essential, are only a part of the overall host defense strategy. There is an ever-growing awareness that innate immunity is equally important and complex. Disorders of the complement system, abnormal function of phagocytic cells, and deficiencies of the chemokines and chemokine receptors that influence lymphocyte–phagocytic cell interactions can all result in an impaired ability to eliminate pathogens. Natural killer cells with their diverse array of activating and inhibitory receptors are also beginning to be recognized as one of the dysfunctional cell types in some immunodeficiency disorders.

Infections are the major complications of the immunodeficiency diseases, and, as recognized by the late Robert Good, a true giant in the establishment of the field and author of the original forword to the first edition of this book, the types of infections differ according to the specific gaps in host defense. Primary antibody deficiency states predispose to serious bacterial infections, as do certain complement component and neutrophil deficiencies. Viral and fungal infections are particularly notable in patients with T cell dysfunction. Different infectious disease patterns are seen with other host defense defects. For example, mycobacterial and salmonella infections are common in patients who have mutations in the genes for IL-12 or the receptors for IL-12 and interferon-γ, because these signaling molecules are especially important for normal macrophage activation to kill intracellular pathogens. Characterization of the different patterns of infections has been significantly enhanced by the development of databanks devoted to patients with the relatively rare primary immunodeficiency diseases.

Treatment has advanced in parallel with improved diagnosis of immunodeficiency diseases, understanding of their cellular and molecular basis, and better definition of their clinical consequences. Prophylactic antibiotics can be helpful in reducing the frequency of certain types of infections. Immunoglobulin replacement, employed first by Bruton to treat a boy with congenital agammaglobulinemia, has been refined through the development of safe and efficient preparations of intravenous immunoglobulin. Better ways to perform bone marrow transplantation have made this life-saving mode of cellular engineering safer and

available to more patients with severe combined immunodeficiency disease. Enzyme replacement can benefit SCID patients with adenosine deaminase deficiency. Finally, gene therapy has proven effective for the cure of two types of SCID, albeit presently with an attendant risk of lymphoproliferative disease. For all too many patients with primary immunodeficiency diseases, however, a cure is still not yet possible and will come only with improved knowledge that must be gained through continued study. In the meantime, early diagnosis remains the key for a quality life for many patients with an immunodeficiency disease. Toward this end, this newly updated book provides a remarkably comprehensive and clinically useful source of information about this challenging group of disorders.

Max D. Cooper, M.D.
The University of Alabama at Birmingham
and the Howard Hughes Medical Institute
Birmingham, AL

Foreword to the First Edition

Modern immunology can be considered to have been launched in 1952, when Colonel Ogden Bruton described an 8-year old boy who, from 2 years of age, experienced recurrent, life-threatening infections including episodes of bacterial pneumonia and septicemia. Using the newly-introduced technique, serum electrophoresis, Bruton found the boy to be agammaglobulinemic. When challenged with antigens, he failed to produce specific antibodies. Upon treatment by passive immunization with large doses of intramuscularly-injected gammaglobulin, his susceptibility to infections was dramatically terminated. Detailed investigations of similar patients, by Charles Janeway in Boston and my group in Minneapolis, demonstrated many similarly affected children, and proved that agammaglobulinemia was often an X-linked, inherited disorder.

In the course of caring for agammaglobulinemic patients, we realized that they were especially susceptible to encapsulated bacterial pathogens, including *Streptococcus pneumoniae*, *Haemophilus influenzae*, *Streptococcus pyogenes*, *Pseudomonas aeruginosa*, and to a lesser extent, *Staphylococcus aureus*. In contrast however, they could impressively resist infections caused by fungi, coliforms, tuberculosis, bacillus Calmette-Guérin (BCG), and many viruses such as measles, chicken pox, rubella, and vaccinia. Thus, the susceptibility profile of agammaglobulinemic patients bisected the microbial universe. As an experiment of nature, patients with X-linked agammaglobulinemia (XLA) introduced us to additional, crucially important concepts concerning how plasma cells and lymph node germinal centers, which are lacking in agammaglobulinemic patients, must be the source of antibodies providing resistance to encapsulated bacterial pathogens. We reasoned that distinct mechanisms of defense that were intact in agammaglobulinemic patients must have been designed to protect against other types of infections. Lymphocytes in the deep paracortical regions of lymph nodes, which appeared normal in XLA patients, were found to mediate this second type of immune protection, cellular immunity, which was later shown to be dependent on the thymus. This conclusion was partially derived from the study of a different group of patients, those with DiGeorge syndrome, who had congenital absence of the thymus.

Thus, it was evident from the beginning that patients with immunodeficiencies, as experiments of nature, helped us to bisect not only the microbial universe, but also the universe of lymphoid cells and the universe of immunological responses. Further investigations throughout the 1960s, 1970s, and 1980s confirmed that this compartmentalization related to the fundamental lymphocyte dichotomy of B cells versus thymus-dependent T cells. Moreover, patients with different immunodeficiency syndromes helped define the nature and the role in immune responses of other components of the host defense system, such as phagocytes and complement, and to recognize the diseases that occur when these components are absent or not functional.

Over the last decade, advances in molecular biology have allowed for an even greater understanding of the immune system, and the multitude of molecular pathways that regulate growth, differentiation, communication, and effector functions within and between cells. In 1993, two groups of researchers, led by David Vetrie and Satoshi Tsukada, discovered that the difficulties of Bruton's patient and other patients with XLA were due to many different mutations of an X-linked gene that encodes a B-cell specific tyrosine kinase, Btk. In the few years since that discovery, the molecular genetic universe has expanded phenomenally, so that almost every month there is news of the identification of another immune disease gene.

The present volume, edited by Professors H. D. Ochs, C.I.E. Smith, and J. M. Puck, is the first comprehensive guide to this new molecular genetic universe. Herein, diseases of the immune system are presented and analyzed, both in terms of their clinical features and in the context of the impressive molecular and genetic definitions which can be put forward in 1998. Over 90 well-defined primary diseases of the human immune system are listed in the introductory chapter of this book; specific diseases are discussed in later chapters organized by syndrome (Part II). The current understanding of each disorder is outlined, including discussions of clinical issues and clinical presentation, infections, genetic mutations, protein function, cell biology, and management. Framing these discussions of individual diseases are two equally modern presentations—first, a section of seven chapters outlining the essential concepts of immunology and genetics needed to understand primary immunodeficiency diseases, and at the end, a section covering the most current approaches to assessment and treatment of patients with these conditions. Each authoritative chapter is written by a world leader in the field, or in many cases by a pair or group of immunological specialists with complementary perspectives, to present the most up-to-date and complete information available.

This book is an impressive demonstration of how far we have come. Recent studies of primary immunodeficiency diseases have, perhaps more than any other group of diseases, revealed the power of modern molecular genetics to define diseases in precise molecular terms. This approach has already suggested therapeutic possibilities which have proven successful; it has also set the stage for testing gene therapies meant to cure primary immunodeficiency diseases at the molecular level. Just how disruptions of Btk account for all of the morphological and immunological abnormalities and disease susceptibilities of patients with XLA has not yet been elucidated, but future work will show how this molecule interacts with other gene products in the B lymphocyte. Studying XLA will continue to reveal fundamental issues in lymphology and immunobiology.

The knowledge of primary immunodeficiency diseases reflected in this volume continues to grow, based on insights derived from the study of individuals with primary immunodeficiency exemplified by Bruton's original agammaglobulinemic patient. Analysis of each of the immune system diseases in its own way represents the molecular interpretation of an informative experiment of nature. In the aggregate, these analyses help us understand more deeply how man can exist free of infection while living in a veritable sea of microorganisms. This volume constitutes a milestone, marking where we now stand and indicating where we are heading, as we continue to interpret lessons in a most constructive fashion from the greatest teachers of modern immunology: patients with primary immunodeficiency diseases.

Robert A. Good, M.D., Ph.D., D.Sc.
All Children's Hospital
St. Petersburg, Florida
July 1998

Contents

Contributors

Mario Abinun, MD, MSc
Department of Pediatrics
Newcastle General Hospital
Newcastle upon Tyne, United Kingdom

Jan Andersson, MD
Department of Clinical-Biological Sciences (DKBW)
Developmental and Molecular Immunology
Center for Biomedicine
University of Basel
Basel, Switzerland

Andrew G. Aprikyan, PhD
Department of Medicine
University of Washington
Seattle, WA

Susannah Brydges, PhD
National Institute of Arthritis and Musculoskeletal
and Skin Diseases
National Institutes of Health
Bethesda, MD

Rebecca H. Buckley, MD
Department of Pediatrics
Duke University Medical Center
Durham, NC

Fabio Candotti, MD
Genetics and Molecular Biology Branch
National Human Genome Research Institute
National Institutes of Health
Bethesda, MD

Jean-Laurent Casanova, MD, PhD
University of Paris René Descartes-INSERM U 550
Hôpital Necker–Enfants Malades
Paris, France

Helen M. Chapel, MD
Department of Clinical Immunology
John Radcliffe Hospital
Oxford, United Kingdom

Talal A. Chatila, MD
Department of Pediatrics
David Geffen School of Medicine
University of California at Los Angeles
Los Angeles, CA

Krystyna H. Chrzanowska, MD, PhD
Department of Medical Genetics
The Children's Memorial Health Institute
Warsaw, Poland

Mary Ellen Conley, MD
Department of Immunology
St. Jude Children's Research Hospital
Memphis, TN

John T. Curnutte, MD, PhD
DNAX Research, Inc.
Palo Alto, CA

David C. Dale, MD
University of Washington
Seattle, WA

Anthony L. DeFranco, MD
Department of Microbiology & Immunology
University of California San Francisco
San Francisco, CA

Henri de la Salle, PhD
EFS-Alsace, Strasbourg
Université Louis-Pasteur
Strasbourg, France

Genevieve de Saint Basile, MD, PhD
INSERM U 429
Hôpital Necker–Enfants Malades
Paris, France

Jean-Pierre de Villartay, PhD
INSERM U429
Hôpital Necker Enfants-Malades
Paris, France

Martin Digweed
Institut für Humangenetik
Humboldt-Universität
Charite-Campus Virchow
Berlin, Germany

Lionel Donato, MD
Centre Hospilalier Régional Universitaire de Strasbourg
Hopital de Hautepierre
Pediadric Pneumology
Strasbourg, France

Deborah A. Driscoll, MD
Department of Obstetrics and Gynecology
University of Pennsylvania
Philadelphia, PA

Anne Durandy, MD, PhD
INSERM U 429
Hopital Necker–Enfantes Malades
Paris, France

Melissa E. Elder, MD, PhD
Department of Pediatrics
University of Florida
Gainesville, FL

Teresa Español, MD
Inmunología
Hospital Vall d'Hebron
Barcelona, Spain

Amos Etzioni, MD
Meyer Children's Hospital
Rappaport School of Medicine, Technion
Haifa, Israel

Alain Fischer, MD
Imserm U429
Hôpital Necker–Enfants Malades
Paris, France

Eleonora Gambineri, MD
Department of Pediatrics
"Anna Meyer" Children's Hospital
University of Florence
Florence, Italy

Raif S. Geha, MD
Division of Immunology
Children's Hospital
Harvard Medical School
Boston, MA

James J. German, MD
Department of Pediatrics
Weill Medical College of Cornell University
New York, NY

Ulf Grawunder, MD
Department of Clinical-Biological Sciences (DKBW)
Developmental and Molecular Immunology
Center for Biomedicine
University of Basel
Basel, Switzerland

Bodo Grimbacher, MD
Department of Medicine
Medizinische Universitätsklinik
Freiburg, Germany

Neetu Gupta, MD
Department of Microbiology & Immunology
University of California San Francisco
San Francisco, CA

Maria Halonen, MD
Department of Molecular Medicine
National Public Health Institute
Biomedicum Helsinki
Helsinki, Finland

Lennart Hammarström, MD, PhD
Department of Clinical Immunology
Karolinska University Hospital in Huddinge
Stockholm, Sweden

Daniel Hanau, MD, DSc
INSERM U 725
EFS-Alsace, Strasbourg
Université Louis-Pasteur
Strasbourg, France

R. Scott Hansen, PhD
Department of Medicine
Medical Genetics
University of Washington
Seattle, WA

John M. Harlan, MD
Department of Medicine
University of Washington
Seattle, WA

Markku Heikinheimo, MD
Children's Hospital
Biomedicum Helsinki
University of Helsinki
Helsinki, Finland

Harry R. Hill, MD
Departments of Pathology, Pediatrics, and Medicine
University of Utah
Salt Lake City, UT

Rochelle Hirschhorn, MD
Section of Medical Genetics
Departments of Medicine, Cell Biology and Pediatrics
New York University School of Medicine
New York City, NY

Steven M. Holland, MD
Chief, Laboratory of Clinical Infectious Diseases
National Institute of Allergy and infectious Diseases
National Institutes of Health
Bethesda, MD

Keith M. Hull, MD, PhD
National Institute of Arthritis and Musculoskeletal
*   and Skin Diseases*
National Institutes of Health
Bethesda, MD

Sirpa Jalkanen, MD, PhD
MediCity Research Lab
University of Turku
Turku, Finland

Ilkka Kaitila, MD, PhD
Clinical Genetics Research
Haartman Institute
University of Helsinki
Helsinki, Finland

Daniel L. Kastner, MD, PhD
Genetics and Genomics Section
National Institute of Arthritis and Musculoskeletal and Skin Diseases
National Institutes of Health
Bethesda, MD

Taco W. Kuijpers, MD, PhD
Emma Children's Hospital
Academic Medical Center
University of Amsterdam
Amsterdam, The Netherlands

Martin F. Lavin
Queensland Institute of Medical Research
The Bancroft Centre
Brisbane, Australia

Françoise Le Deist, MD
Departments of Pediatrics and Microbiology
University of Montreal
Hopital Sainte Justine
Montreal, Canada

Michael Levin, MD
Brighton and Sussex Medical School
University of Sussex
Brighton, United Kingdom

Barbara Lisowska-Grospierre, PhD
INSERM U 429
Université René Descartes
Hopital Necker–Enfants Malades
Paris, France

Tak W. Mak, MD
Campbell Family Institute for Breast
 Cancer Research
Princess Margaret Hospital
Toronto, Canada

Fritz Melchers, PhD
Max Planck Institute for Infection Biology
Berlin, Germany;
University of Basel
Biozentrum
Basel, Switzerland

Siraj Misbah, MSc
Department of Clinical Immunology
John Radcliffe Hospitals
Oxford, United Kingdom

Melanie J. Newport, PhD
Brighton and Sussex Medical School
University of Sussex
Brighton, United Kingdom

Luigi D. Notarangelo, MD
Department of Pediatrics
"Angelo Nocivelli" Institute for Molecular Medicine
University of Brescia
Brescia, Italy

Robert L. Nussbaum, MD
Department of Medicine and
 Institute for Human Genetics
University of California, San Francisco
San Francisco, CA

Hans D. Ochs, MD
Department of Pediatrics
University of Washington
Seattle, WA

Pamela S. Ohashi, PhD
Campbell Family Institute for Breast Cancer Research
Ontario Cancer Institute
University Health Network
Departments of Medical Biophysics and Immunology
University of Toronto
Toronto, Ontario, Canada

Leena Peltonen-Palotie, MD, PhD
Department of Medical Genetics, University of Helsinki
Department of Molecular Medicine, National
 Public Health Institute
Biomedicum
Helsinki, Finland

Jaakko Perheentupa, MD
Department of Pediatrics
University of Helsinki
Helsinki, Finland

Hilkka Piirilä, MSc
Institute of Medical Technology
University of Tampere
Tampere, Finland

Alessandro Plebani, MD
Department of Pediatrics
"Angelo Nocivelli" Institute for Molecular Medicine
University of Brescia
Brescia, Italy

Jennifer M. Puck, MD
Department of Pediatrics and Institute for Human Genetics
University of California, San Francisco
San Francisco, CA

Marianne Pusa, MSc
Institute of Medical Technology
University of Tampere
Tampere, Finland

Paul G. Quie, MD
International Medical Education
 and Research Program
University of Minnesota Medical School
Minneapolis, Minnesota

Jose R. Regueiro, MD
Inmunologia
Facultad de Medicina
Universidad Complutense
Madrid, Spain

Walter Reith, MD
Department of Pathology and Immunology
University of Geneva Medical School
Centre Medical Universitaire
Geneva, Switzerland

Patrick Revy, MD
INSERM U 429
Hôpital Necker–Enfants Malades
Paris, France

Frédéric Rieux-Laucat, PhD
INSERM U 429
Hôpital Necker–Enfants Malades
Paris, France

Chaim M. Roifman, MD
Division of Immunology and Allergy
The Hospital for Sick Children
Toronto, Canada

Antonius Rolink, MD, PhD
Developmental and Molecular Immunology
Center for Biomedicine
University of Basel
Basel, Switzerland

Dirk Roos, PhD
Department of Blood Cell Research
Sanquin Research and Landsteiner Laboratory
Academic Medical Center
University of Amsterdam
Amsterdam, The Netherlands

Fred S. Rosen
Department of Pediatrics and Center for Blood Research
Harvard Medical School
Boston, MA

Marko Salmi, MD, PhD
MediCity Research Laboratory
National Public Health Institute
University of Turku
Turku, Finland

Crina Samarghitean, MD
Institute of Medical Technology
University of Tampere
Tampere, Finland

Anne B. Satterthwaite, PhD
Department of Internal Medicine
University of Texas Southwestern Medical Center
at Dallas
Dallas, TX

Mary E. Saunders, PhD
Campbell Family Institute for Breast Cancer Research
Toronto, Ontario, Canada

Volker Schuster, MD
Department of Pediatrics
University of Leipzig
Leipzig, Germany

Klaus Schwarz, MD
Institute for Clinical Transfusion Medicine and
Immunogenetics
Department of Transfusion Medicine
University of Ulm
Ulm, Germany

Yosef Shiloh, PhD
Department of Human Genetics and Molecular
Medicine
Sackler School of Medicine
Tel Aviv University
Ramat Aviv, Israel

C. I. Edvard Smith, MD, PhD
Clinical Research Center
Karolinska Institutet at Novum-Huddinge
Stockholm, Sweden

Gerald J. Spangrude, PhD
Department of Hematology
University of Utah
Salt Lake City, UT

Richard A. Spritz, MD
Human Medical Genetics
University of Colorado Health Sciences
Center-Fitzsimons
Aurora, CO

E. Richard Stiehm, MD
Department of Pediatrics
Mattal Children's Hospital at UCLA
Los Angeles, CA

Stephen E. Straus, MD
Laboratory of Clinical Infectious Disease
National Institute of Allergy and Infectious Diseases
National Institutes of Health
Bethesda, MD

Markus Stumm, PhD
Institut für Humangenetik
Otto-von-Guericke-Universität
Magdeburg, Germany

Kathleen E. Sullivan, MD, PhD
Department of Pediatrics
University of Pennsylvania
School of Medicine
Philadelphia, PA

Cox Terhorst, PhD
Division of Immunology
Beth Israel Deaconess Medical Center
Harvard Medical School
Boston, MA

Troy R. Torgerson, MD, PhD
Department of Pediatrics
University of Washington
Seattle, WA

Jouni Väliaho, MSc
Institute of Medical Technology
University of Tampere
Tampere, Finland

Mauno Vihinen, PhD
Institute of Medical Technology
University of Tampere
Tampere, Finland

Anna Villa, MD, PhD
CNR-ITB
Segrate, Italy

A. David B. Webster, MD
Department of Clinical Immunology
Royal Free Hospital School of Medicine
London, United Kingdom

Corry Weemaes, PhD
Department of Pediatrics
University Hospital Nijmegen
Nijmegen, Netherlands

Rolf-Dieter Wegner, MD
Institut für Humangenetik
Humboldt-Universität
Charite–Campus Virchow
Berlin, Germany

Arthur Weiss, MD, PhD
Howard Hughes Medical Institute
University of California San Francisco
San Francisco, CA

Cisca Wijmenga, PhD
Complex Genetics Section
DBG-Department of Medical Genetics
University Medical Center Utrecht
Utrecht, Netherlands

Jerry A. Winkelstein, MD
Department of Pediatrics
Johns Hopkins University School of Medicine
Baltimore, MD

Owen N. Witte, MD
Howard Hughes Medical Institute
University of California Los Angeles
Los Angeles, CA

Kuender D. Yang, MD, PhD
Chang Gung Children's Hospital at
  Kaohsiung
Chang Gung University
Taiwan, Republic of China

Rae S. M. Yeung, MD, PhD
The Hospital for Sick Children
University of Toronto
Toronto, Ontario, Canada

Steven F. Ziegler, PhD
Department of Immunology
Benaroya Research Institute
Virginia Mason Medical Center
Seattle, WA

I

Overview

1

Genetically Determined Immunodeficiency Diseases: A Perspective

C. I. EDVARD SMITH, HANS D. OCHS, and JENNIFER M. PUCK

We are in an era of explosive growth in our understanding of the molecular and genetic basis of immune defects. In the early 1990s, only a handful of genes were known to be associated with these diseases, but now many are recognized and the process of discovering additional immunodeficiency genes is proceeding rapidly. Advances in basic research in immunology, combined with the availability of the DNA sequence of nearly the entire human and mouse genomes plus refined technologies for localizing disease traits, have led to the discovery of the precise molecular basis for 140 or more disorders of human host defenses. A recent example of novel approaches is the discovery of CD3δ deficiency through use of microarray technology (Dadi et al., 2003; Chapter 16). The ability to redefine genetic diseases of the immune system in molecular terms has made possible improved diagnosis, appreciation of the spectrum of clinical presentations that can be traced to a given disease gene, genetic counseling and testing, and, most exciting, new therapeutic strategies including gene therapy. Moreover, the discovery of each previously unknown disease gene feeds back into the pool of scientific knowledge of immunology, illuminating and strengthening our evolving models of immune pathways.

This volume contains accounts of gene identification, mutation detection, and clinical and research applications for a wide array of distinct genetic immune disorders. A summary of known inherited immunodeficiencies is provided in Table 1.1. The methods used to identify and understand these disorders constitute a survey of modern molecular genetics and human immunology. The first edition of this book in 1999 marked an historic turning point in the field of immunodeficiencies, demonstrating that many of primary disorders of the immune system could be understood at the molecular level. Seven years later, we are sure that new discoveries will continue to make this collection incomplete even as it is published, but we can also proudly document

an unanticipated fast pace of progress in dissecting the complex immunologic networks responsible for protecting individuals from a hostile environment.

Since the publication of the first edition, the rate of new discoveries in the field has not slowed down. Instead, a flurry of new disease entities has been defined and new treatment regimens have been introduced, the most notable being successful treatment by gene therapy for two genotypes of severe combined immunodeficiency (Chapter 48).

Of great interest is the new identification of human diseases caused by mutations affecting components of the innate immune system. Previously, defects in the complement system pathways (Chapter 42) and the interferon γ (IFN-γ) signaling pathway (Chapter 28) were recognized, and mouse models of innate immune mediators such as the Toll receptors were reported. However, the true function of innate immune pathways in humans could not be fully appreciated until naturally occurring loss-of-function mutations were identified and characterized in human patients. The recent report of patients with bacterial infections who lack the protein IRAK4, mediating signaling downstream from the Toll receptor, provides a new opening for learning the significance of the innate immune system in protecting humans from infections and cancer (Picard et al., 2003).

Important developments during the past 15 years have increased our understanding of disease processes. A majority of the novel primary immunodeficiency disease genes were identified by mapping a familial abnormality to a chromosomal region, followed by the analysis of candidate genes. In some cases the function of the identified gene product had already been studied in detail prior to identification of human disease-causing mutations, but frequently new insights, some quite surprising, have arisen from relating an immune system gene to a clinical phenotype. For example, even though the function of CD45 phosphatase was

Table 1.1. Primary Immunodeficiency Diseases

Designation and Gene Name*	Defective Protein, Pathogenesis	Inheritance	Locus	Reference or Book Chapter
A. Combined B and T Cell Immunodeficiencies				
1. Severe combined immunodeficiency (SCID) without T and B cells (T⁻B⁻)				
a. SCID with leukocyte deficiency. Reticular dysgenesis.	Stem cell defect affecting maturation of leukocytes, including all lymphocytes	AR	Unknown	de Waal and Seynhaeve, 1959
b. SCID with radiosensitivity. Artemis deficiency. *DCLRE1C*	DNA cross-link repair 1C protein/Artemis	AR	10p13	11
c. SCID with RAG1 deficiency *RAG1*	Recombinase-activating protein 1. Deficient rearrangement of B and T cell receptor genes (*RAG1* and *RAG2* are adjacent genes)	AR	11p13	11
d. SCID with RAG2 deficiency *RAG2*	Recombinase-activating protein 2. Deficient rearrangement of B and T cell receptor genes	AR	11p13	11
2. SCID with nonfunctional T and B cells				
a. Omenn syndrome with *RAG1* deficiency *RAG1*	Recombinase-activation protein 1, partially deficient rearrangement of B and T cell receptor genes	AR	11p13	11
b. Omenn syndrome with *RAG2* deficiency *RAG2*	Recombinase-activation protein 2 partially deficient rearrangement of B and T cell receptor genes	AR	11p13	11
c. Omenn syndrome with Artemis deficiency *DCLRE1C*	DNA cross-link repair 1C protein Artemis	AR	10p13	11
d. Omenn syndrome with IL-7Rα deficiency *IL-7R*	Interleukin-7 receptor α chain	AR	5p13	11
e. DNA ligase deficiency IV *LIG4*	Ligase IV, ATP-dependent	AR	13q33–34	11,30
f. SCID with microcephaly due to deficiency of non-homologous end-joining factor 1 *NHEJ1*	DNA repair factor (XRCC4-like factor, Cernunnos) involved in non-homologous end-joining	AR	2q35	11,30
3. SCID without T cells (T⁻B⁺)				
a. X-linked SCID (γc-chain deficiency) *IL2RG*	Common γ (γc) chain protein, a component of receptors for cytokines IL-2, -4, -7, -9, -15, and -21.	XL	Xq13.1–13.3	9
b. SCID with Jak3 (Janus kinase 3) deficiency *JAK3*	Janus-activating kinase 3 (Jak3), a cytoplasmic tyrosine kinase interacting with γc to transmit signals from IL-2, -4, -7, -9, -15, and -21	AR	19p13.1	10
c. SCID with IL-7Rα deficiency *IL7R*	Interleukin-7 receptor α chain	AR	5p13	11
d. SCID with CD45 deficiency *PTPRC*	Protein tyrosine phosphatase receptor type C	AR	1q31–q32	13
e. SCID with CD3 δ-chain deficiency *CD3D*	CD3δ component of CD3 antigen receptor complex	AR	11q23	16
f. Human Nude/SCID *FOXN1*	Forkhead box N1 protein, winged-helix-nude (*Whn*). Transcription factor required for thymus and hair follicle development	AR	17q11–q12	Frank et al., 1999
4. Deficiencies of purine metabolism				
a. SCID with ADA (adenosine deaminase) deficiency *ADA*	ADA is required for purine metabolism; elevated purine metabolites (primarily dATP) toxic to T and B cells	AR	20q13.2–q13.11	12
b. SCID with PNP (purine nucleoside phosphorylase) deficiency *NP*	PNP is required for purine metabolism; elevated purine metabolites (primarily dGTP) toxic to T and B cells	AR	14q13.1	12
5. MHC class II (major histocompatiblity complex class II) deficiency secondary to deficiencies of transcription factors for MHCII expression				
a. CIITA (MHCII transactivator) deficiency *MHC2TA*	MHCII transactivating protein, a non-DNA binding component of the MHCII promoter-binding complex; complementation group A	AR	16p13	17
b. RFXANK deficiency *RFXANK*	Regulatory factor X-associated ankyrin-containing protein, an MHCII promoter-binding protein; complementation group B	AR	19p12	17

(continued)

Table 1.1. (*continued*)

Designation and Gene Name*	Defective Protein, Pathogenesis	Inheritance	Locus	Reference or Book Chapter
c. RFX-5 deficiency *RFX5*	MHCII promoter X box regulatory factor 5, an MHCII promoter-binding protein; complementation group C	AR	1q21	17
d. RFXAP deficiency *RFXAP*	Regulatory factor X-associated protein, an MHCII promoter-binding protein; complementation group D	AR	13q	17
6. MHC class I deficiency				
a. TAP1 deficiency *TAP1*	Transporter protein associated with antigen presentation 1	AR	6q21.3	18
b. TAP2 deficiency *TAP2*	Transporter protein associated with antigen presentation 2	AR	6q21.3	18
c. Tapasin deficiency *TAPBP*	TAP binding protein (tapasin)	AR	6p21.3	18
7. Class-switch recombination defect (hyper-IgM syndromes) affecting both B and T cells; see also B.6.				
a. CD40L deficiency *TNFSF5*	CD40 ligand (CD154). Tumor necrosis factor superfamily member 5	XL	Xq26	19
b. CD40 deficiency *TNFRSF5*	CD40. Tumor necrosis factor receptor superfamily member 5	AR	20q12–q.13.2	19
8. Non-SCID CD3 deficiency due to absence of proteins forming the CD3 complex required for T cell receptor signaling See A.2.e for SCID with CD3δ deficiency				
a. CD3ε deficiency *CD3E*	CD3ε polypeptide	AR	11q23	16
b. CD3γ deficiency *CD3G*	CD3γ polypeptide	AR	11q23	16
c. *CD3Z*-deficiency	CD3ζ polypeptide (TiT3 complex)	AR	1q22–q25	Rieux-Laucat et al., 2006
9. CD8 deficiency *CD8A*	CD8 antigen, α polypeptide (p32)	AR	2p12	16
10. ZAP-70 deficiency *ZAP-70*	Cytoplasmic tyrosine kinase ZAP-70 (T-cell receptor ζ-chain associated protein kinase, 70kDa). Signaling from the T-cell receptor during T-lineage development	AR	2q12	14
11. IL-2 R α-chain deficiency *IL2RA*	IL-2 receptor α-chain is required for regulation and control of autoreactive T cells	AR	10p14–p15	15
12. p56 Lck deficiency *LCK*	Lymphocyte-specific protein tyrosine kinase. Required for T cell maturation in the thymus	AR	1p34.3	14

B. Deficiencies Predominantly Affecting Antibody Production

1. Agammaglobulinemia				
a. XLA (X-linked agammaglobulinemia) *BTK*	Btk (Bruton agammaglobulinemia tyrosine kinase) required for intracellular signaling in B cell development	XL	Xq21.3	21
b. X-linked hypogammaglobulinemia with growth hormone deficiency	Btk not affected; unknown	XL	X	21
c. μ heavy-chain deficiency *IGHM*	μ heavy-chain. Required for development of B cells from B lineage progenitors	AR	14q32.3	22
d. λ5 surrogate light-chain deficiency *IGLL1*	λ5 surrogate light-chain. Part of receptor complex on pre-B cells required for B lineage differentiation	AR	22q11.22	22
e. Igα deficiency *CD79A*	Ig-associated α chain signaling component of pre-B and B cell receptor complex required for B lineage differentiation and B cell signaling	AR	19q13.2	22
f. BLNK deficiency *BLNK*	B-cell linker/SLP-65/BASH. B cell signaling protein	AR	10q23.2–q23.33	22
g. *LRRC8* deficiency	Leucine rich repeat containing 8 transmembrane protein	AD	9q34.2	Sawada et al., 2003
2. Selective deficiency of Ig isotypes/subclasses due to isolated or combined deficiencies				
a. IgA deficiency	Failure of IgA B cell differentiation	Complex	—	23
b. α1 subclass deficiency *IGHA1*	IgA1 is the major IgA subclass	AR	14q32.33	23
c. α2 subclass deficiency *IGHA2*	IgA2 is mainly found in the gastrointestinal tract	AR	14q32.33	23

(*continued*)

Table 1.1. (*continued*)

Designation and Gene Name*	Defective Protein, Pathogenesis	Inheritance	Locus	Reference or Book Chapter
d. γ1 subclass deficiency *IGHG1*	IgG1 constitutes 65% of serum IgG	AR	14q32.33	23
e. γ2 subclass deficiency *IGHG2*	IgG2 constitutes 25% of serum IgG	AR	14q32.33	23
f. γ3 subclass deficiency (partial) *IGHG3*	IgG3 constitutes 8% of serum IgG. Partial IgG3 deficiency is associated with the 'g' allotype and caused by reduced isotype switching	AR	14q32.33	Yount et al., 1967
g. γ4 subclass deficiency *IGHG4*	IgG4 constitutes 4% of serum IgG	AR	14q32.33	23
h. IgG subclass deficiency with or without IgA deficiency	Defect in differentiation of a B lymphocyte subset or in expression of IgG	Unknown	—	23
i. ε isotype deficiency *IGHE*	IgE is encoded by a single gene	AR	14q32.33	23
3. Light-chain deficiency				
a. κ light-chain deficiency *IGKC*	κ light chain binds to a heavy chain to form immunoglobulins	AR	2p11	Stavnezer-Nordgren et al., 1985
4. Common variable immunodeficiency (for WHIM see F8)				
a. Common variable immunodeficiency of unknown origin	Serum IgG low, IgA low or absent, IgM variable. Variable impairment of T cell function	Complex	—	23
b. ICOS (inducible costimulator) deficiency *ICOS*	ICOS is expressed by activated T cells and interacts with ICOSL (B7RP-1). Deficiency results in late-onset B cell loss	AR	2q33	23
c. CD19 deficiency *CD19*	CD19 antigen expressed by B cells	AR	16p11.2	23
d. TACI deficiency *TNFRSF13B*	Tumor necrosis factor receptor super family member 13B	AD, AR	17p11.2	23
e. BAFF receptor deficiency *TNFRSF13C*	Tumor necrosis factor receptor super family member 13C	AR	22q13.1–q13.3	23
5. Other antibody deficiencies				
a. Antibody deficiency with normal immunoglobulin levels	Defective antigen-specific antibody production	Unknown	—	43
b. Transient hypogammaglobulinemia of infancy	Delayed maturation of T cell helper function	Unknown	—	Gitlin and Janeway, 1956; Tiller and Buckley, 1978; Kilic et al., 2000
6. Defects of class-switch recombination and somatic hypermutation (hyper-IgM syndromes) affecting B cells; see also A.7.				
a. AID deficiency *AICDA*	Activation-induced cytidine deaminase	AR	12p13	20
b. UNG deficiency *UNG*	Uracil-DNA glycosylase	AR	12	20
c. Selective deficiency in Ig class-switch recombination	Defect downstream of AID, normal somatic hypermutation	Unknown	—	20
C. Defects in Lymphocyte Apoptosis				
1. Autoimmune lymphoproliferative syndrome (ALPS); see also D.2.				
a. ALPS type Ia (defective CD95) *TNFRSF6*	Apoptosis mediator CD95 (Fas/APO-1) required for lymphocyte homeostasis Induces apoptosis via engagement of FasL	AD, AR	10q23–q24.1	24
b. ALPS type Ib (defective CD178) *TNFSF6*	Fas Ligand (FasL). Inducing apoptosis via engagement of Fas	AD	1q23	24
c. ALPS type IIa (caspase 10 deficiency) *CASP10*	Caspase 10; apoptosis-related cysteine protease	AR	2q33–q34	24
d. ALPS type IIb (caspase 8 deficiency) *CASP8*	Caspase 8; apoptosis-related cysteine protease *CASP8* and *CASP10* are adjacent genes	AR	2q33–q34	24
D. Other Well-Defined Immunodeficiency Syndromes				
1. Wiskott-Aldrich syndrome, X-linked thrombocytopenia and X-linked neutropenia *WASP*	Wiskott-Aldrich syndrome protein (WASP), especially important in platelets and T cells	XL	Xp11.22	31

(*continued*)

Table 1.1. (*continued*)

Designation and Gene Name*	Defective Protein, Pathogenesis	Inheritance	Locus	Reference or Book Chapter
2. Autoimmune disorders; see also C.1.				
a. APECED (autoimmune polyendocrinopathy with candidiasis and ectodermal dystrophy) *AIRE*	Autoimmune regulator-1 (AIRE-1) or APECED protein. Transcription factor expressed in the thymus	AR	21q22.3	25
b. IPEX (immune deficiency/dysregulation, polyendocrinopathy, enteropathy, X-linked) *FOXP3*	Forkhead box P3 transcription factor. Expressed by $CD4^+$ $CD25^+$ regulatory T cells (T reg)	XL	Xp11.23	26
3. X-linked lymphoproliferative syndrome (Duncan disease) *SH2D1A*	SH2 domain protein 1A (also called SLAM-associated protein, SAP). Involved in intra-cellular signaling of T and NK cells; protects against severe outcome of EBV infection	XL	Xq25–q26	32
4. DiGeorge/velo-cardio-facial syndrome. (22q11.2 deletion syndrome) *DGCR*	Multiple congenital anomalies most often due to deletion of *DGCR* (DiGeorge chromosomal region). Developmental defect of thymus. May be associated with congenital heart disease, hypoparathyroidism, and other congenital abnormalities	AD	22q11.2	33
5. CHH (cartilage-hair hypoplasia) *RMRP*	RNA component of mitochondrial RNA-processing endoribonuclease	AR	9p13	36
6. Hyper-IgE recurrent infection syndrome (Job syndrome)	Unknown	AD, AR, Sporadic	Some cases Chromosome 4	34
7. Chronic mucocutaneous candidiasis	Unknown	AR, AD	2p (AD)	Chilgren et al., 1967; Atkinson et al., 2001

E. Defects of Phagocyte Function

1. Chronic granulomatous disease caused by defective intracellular oxidative burst required for bacterial and fungal killing.

Designation and Gene Name*	Defective Protein, Pathogenesis	Inheritance	Locus	Reference or Book Chapter
a. X-linked CGD *CYBB*	Cytochrome phagocyte oxidase (phox) gp91phox. Cytochrome b-245 β-polypeptide	XL	Xp21.1	37
b. p22phox deficiency *CYBA*	Cytochrome oxidase p22phox	AR	16q24	37
c. p47phox deficiency *NFC1*	Cytochrome oxidase p47phox	AR	7q11.23	37
d. p67phox deficiency *NFC2*	Cytochrome oxidase p67phox	AR	1q25	37
2. Leukocyte adhesion defects (LAD)				
a. LAD1 *ITGB2*	CD18 cell surface protein. Cell surface adhesion complex (CD11a,b,c/CD18) requires integrin β2 (CD18) to be stably expressed	AR	21q22.3	38
b. LAD2 *NAALLAD2*	N-acetylated α-linked acidic dipeptidase2. Fucose transporter required for proper carbohydrate addition; patient cells lack sialyl-Lewis X	AR	11q14.3–q21	38
c. LAD3	Defect in G protein-coupled receptor (GPCR)-mediated stimulation of integrins at the endothelial contact. May affect Rap-1 regulation	AR	Unknown	38
d. LAD with RAC2 deficiency *RAC2*	RAS-related, RHO family small GTP-binding protein RAC2. Predominant in neutrophils, involved in O_2^- production, actin cytoskeleton	AR	22q12.13–q13.2	38
3. Chediak-Higashi syndrome *LYST*	Lysomal trafficking regulator. Required for formation of lysosomes and cytoplasmic granules	AR	1q42–q43	40
4. Griscelli syndrome				
a. Griscelli syndrome type 1 *MYO5A*	Myosin-VA (5A). Involved in organelle transport	AR	15q21	41

(*continued*)

Table 1.1. (*continued*)

Designation and Gene Name*	Defective Protein, Pathogenesis	Inheritance	Locus	Reference or Book Chapter
b. Griscelli syndrome type 2 *RAB27A*	Rab27A, GTP-binding protein. Regulates cytotoxic granule exocytosis associated with the accelerated phase of Griscelli syndrome. Myosin-VA (5A) and Rab27A are closely linked on chromosome 15q21	AR	15q21	41
5. Glucose 6-phosphate dehydrogenase deficiency *G6PD*	Granulocyte intracellular killing defect associated with complete absence of G6PD in phagocytes	XL	Xq28	37
6. Myeloperoxidase (MPO) deficiency *MPO*	MPO is required to convert H_2O_2 to hypohalous acid. Intracellular killing of fungi is impaired.	AR	17q23.1	Lehrer and Cline, 1969; Nauseef et al., 1994
7. Glycogen storage disease type 1b *SLC37A4*	Solute carrier family 37 (glycerol-6-phosphate transporter), member 4. Neutropenia, impaired neutrophil migration due to defective glucose 6-phosphate translocase	AR	11q23.3	Hiraiwa et al., 1999

8. Neutropenia
   a. Cyclic neutropenia and severe congenital neutropenias
    ELA2
	Neutrophil elastase 2. Includes Kostmann syndrome	AR (AD)	19p13.3	39

b. Congenital X-linked neutropenia *WASP*	Wiskott-Aldrich Syndrome Protein (WASP)—see D.1	XL	Xp11.22	31
9. Dyskeratosis congenita *DKC1*	Dyskeratosis congenita 1, dyskerin. Affected males have epithelial abnormalities, cancer predisposition, bone marrow failure	XL	Xq28	Heiss et al., 1998
10. Shwachman Bodian Diamond syndrome *SBDS*	Highly conserved protein of unknown function. Pancreatic insufficiency and bone marrow dysfunction, including neutropenia	AR	7q11	Boocock et al., 2003
11. Familial hemophagocytic lymphohistiocytosis (FHL)				
a. *FHL1*	Unknown	AR	9q22	41
b. FHL2 Perforin deficiency *PRF1*	Perforin 1 (pore forming protein)	AR	10q22	41
c. FHL3 *UNC13D*	Vesicle priming protein unc-13 homolog D (*C. elegans*)	AR	17q25.3	41

F. Defects of the Innate Immune System: Receptors and Signaling Components

1. Interferon-γ receptor deficiency. Cell surface receptors for IFNγ protect against salmonella and mycobacterial disease.

a. IFNγ receptor 1 deficiency *IFNGR1*	IFNγ-receptor 1 (or α-chain) is required for binding as well as signaling by associating with Jak1.	AR	6q23–24	28
b. IFNγ receptor 2 deficiency *IFNGR2*	IFNγ-receptor 2 (or β-chain) is required for signaling by associating with Jak2.	AR	21q22.1–q22.2	28
2. IL-12 p40 deficiency *ILI2B*	Interleukin-12 40 KD subunit. IL-12 is required for the production of IFN γ by T and NK cells	AR	5q31.1–q33.1	28
3. IL-12Rβ1 deficiency *ILI2RB*	Receptor β chain for interleukin-12	AR	19p13.1	28
4. STAT1 deficiency *STAT1*	Signal transducer and activator of transcription 1, 91 KDa.	AD, AR	2q12–q13.2	28
5. STAT5b deficiency *STAT5B*	Signal transducer and activator of transcription 56, 80 KDa. Immunodeficiency and growth hormone insensitivity	AR	17q21	Kofoed et al., 2003
6. IRAK-4 deficiency *IRAK4*	Interleukin-1 receptor-associated kinase 4	AR	12q12	Picard et al., 2003 Chapter 8
7. X-linked anhidrotic ectodermal dysplasia with immunodeficiency *IKKBG*	Inhibitor of κ light polypeptide gene enhancer in B cells, kinase γ. NF-κB essential modulator (NEMO)	XL	Xq28	36
8. Anhidrotic ectodermal dysplasia with T cell deficiency *NFKB1A*	Nuclear factor of κ light polypeptide gene enhancer in B cells, inhibitor α	AD	14q13	36
9. Warts, hypogammaglobulinemia, recurrent bacterial infections, and 'myelokathexis' (WHIM) *CXCR4*	Chemokine C-X-C motif receptor 4 (CXCR4)	AD	2q21	23

(continued)

Table 1.1. (*continued*)

Designation and Gene Name*	Defective Protein, Pathogenesis	Inheritance	Locus	Reference or Book Chapter
G. DNA Breakage-Associated and DNA Epigenetic Modification Syndromes (for Artemis, ligase IV, and NHEJ1 deficiency—see section A2)				
1. DNA breakage-associated syndromes				
a. Ataxia-telangiectasia (A-T) mutated *ATM*	Cell cycle check point ATM protein kinase	AR	11q22.3	29
b. Nibrin *NBS1*	Nijmegen breakage syndrome 1 protein nibrin. Participates in DNA repair together with RAD50 and MRE11	AR	8q21	30
c. Bloom syndrome *BLM*	DNA repair protein BLM	AR	15q26.1	30
d. A-T like disease (A-TLD) *MRE11A*	DNA damage-response protein	AR	11q21	30
e. DNA ligase deficiency I *LIG1*	Ligase I, DNA, ATP-dependent.	AR	19	30
2. Immunodeficiency, centromere instability and facial abnormalities syndrome (ICF) *DNMT3B*	DNA (cytosine-5)-methyltransferase 3b.	AR	20q11.2	35
H. Defects of the Classical Complement Cascade Proteins				
1. C1q deficiency				
a. *C1QA*	C1 α-polypeptide	AR	1p36.3–p.34.1	42
b. *C1QB*	C1 β-polypeptide	AR	1p36.3–p.34.1	42
c. *C1QG*	C1 γ-polypeptide	AR	1p36.3–p.34.1	42
2. C1r and C1s deficiency				
a. *C1R*	C1r subcomponent. Often combined with C1s defect	AR	12p13	42
b. *C1S*	C1s subcomponent. Often combined with C1r defect	AR	12p13	42
3. C2 deficiency *C2*	*C2* gene is encoded within the MHC cluster	AR	6p21.3	42
4. C3 deficiency *C3*	Major factor for both classical and alternative complement pathways	AR	19p.13.3	42
5. C4 deficiency				
a. *C4A*	C4A subunit	AR	6p21.3	42
b. *C4B*	C4B subunit. *C4A* and *C4B* are adjacent genes within the MHC cluster.	AR	6p21.3	42
6. C5 deficiency *C5*	C5 peptide. Initiates formation of the membrane attack complex (MAC)	AR	9q33–9q34.1	42
7. C6 deficiency *C6*	C6 peptide. Part of MAC	AR	5p13	42
8. C7 deficiency *C7*	C7 peptide. Part of MAC	AR	5p13	42
9. C8 deficiency				
a. *C8A*	C8α-polypeptide	AR	1p32	42
b. *C8B*	C8β-polypeptide	AR	1p32	42
c. *C8G*	C8γ-polypeptide, binds covalently to the C8α-chain; C8 is part of MAC.	AR	9q	42
10. C9 deficiency *C9*	C9 peptide. Part of MAC. *C6*, *C7*, and *C9* genes are clustered on chromosome 5p13.	AR	5p13	42
I. Defects of the Alternative Complement Pathway				
1. Factor B deficiency *BF*	Factor B serine protease. Interacts with factor D. The gene is encoded within the MHC cluster.	AR	6p21.3	42
2. Factor D deficiency *DF*	Factor D interacts with factor B.	AR	19p13.3	42
3. Factor H1 deficiency *HF1*	Factor H deficiency leads to uncontrolled activation of the alternative C′ pathway. A polymorphism (Y402H) is responsible for ~ 50% of age-related macular degeneration.	AR	1q32	42; Edwards et al., 2005; Haines et al., 2005; Klein et al., 2005
4. Properdin factor C deficiency *PFC*	Contributes to activation of C3 via the alternative pathway.	XL	Xp11.3–p11.23	42
J. Complement Regulatory Proteins				
1. C1 inhibitor deficiency *C1NH*	C1 inhibitor, a serine protease inhibitor. Haploinsufficiency results in hereditary angioedema	AD	11q11–q13.1	42

(*continued*)

Table 1.1. (*continued*)

Designation and Gene Name*	Defective Protein, Pathogenesis	Inheritance	Locus	Reference or Book Chapter
2. C4-binding protein deficiency	Presumed defect in C4 binding; dissociates and degrades C4 (classical C- pathway)			
a. *C4BPA*	C4 binding protein α	AR	1q32	42
b. *C4BPB*	C4 binding protein β	AR	1q32	42
3. Decay-accelerating factor (CD55) deficiency *DAF*	Glycosyl phosphatidylinositol (GPI)-anchored antigen. Impairs C′ killing by controlling both pathways	AR	1q32	42
4. Factor I deficiency *IF*	C3-inactivator	AR	4q25	42
5. CD59 (antigen P18-20) or protectin deficiency *CD59*	20 kDa GPI-anchored antigen. Inhibits lysis by classical C′ pathway	AR	11p13	42
6. Mannose-binding lectin deficiency				
a. Mannose-binding lectin deficiency *MBL2*	Mannose-binding lectin activates a distinct, antibody-independent complement pathway	AR and AD	10q11.2	42
b. Mannan-binding lectin-associated serine protease 2 deficiency *MASP2*	Mannan-binding serine protease 2. Activates complement pathway by cleaving mannose-binding lectin	AR	1p36.3–p36.2	42
K. Periodic Fever Syndromes				
1. Familial Mediterranean fever (FMF) *MEFV*	Pyrin (marenostrin)	AR	16p13.3	27
2. Hyperimmunoglobulinemia D with periodic fever syndrome, hyper-IgD syndrome *MVK*	Mevalonate kinase	AR	12q24	27
3. Tumor necrosis factor receptor-associated periodic syndrome (TRAPS) *TNFRSF1A*	TNF receptor 1 cytokine receptor (CD120a)	AD	12p13.2	27
4. Cold autoinflammatory syndrome 1				
a. Familial cold urticaria (FCU) and Muckle-Wells syndrome (MWS) *CIAS1*	Cryopyrin / NALP3/PYPAF1	AD	1q44	27
b. Chronic infantile neurological, cutaneous and articular syndrome CINCA syndrome *CIAS1*	Cyropyrin / NALP3/PYPAF1	AD	1q44	27
5. Granulomatous sinovitis with uveitis and cranial neuropathies (Blau syndrome) *CARD15*	Caspase recruitment domain (CARD) family, member 15. Intracellular sensor of bacterial peptidoglycan	AD	16q12	27
6. Crohn's disease *CARD15*	Caspase recruitment domain (CARD) family, member 15. Intracellular sensor of bacterial peptidoglycan. Mutated in a subset of Crohn's disease	Polygenic	16q12	27

AD, autosomal dominant; AR, autosomal recessive; EBV, Epstein-Barr virus; NK, natural killer; XL, X-linked.

*Gene names, in italics, according to the Human Genome Organization, http://www.gene.ucl.ac.uk/nomenclature/; Wain et al., 2002, and online Mendelian Inheritance in Man, http://www.nebi.nlm.nih.gov/omim/.

studied extensively over several years and known to be essential for lymphocyte activation, no one had predicted that CD45 deficiency would result in human severe combined immunodeficiency (SCID) (Chapter 13). In an even more unexpected development, the identification of a defective RNA component of an endoribonuclease as the cause of cartilage-hair hypoplasia was certainly not anticipated (Chapter 36).

Infections, Autoimmunity, and Cancer: Features of Genetic Immunodeficiencies

The hallmark of primary immunodeficiencies is an increased susceptibility to infections. However, both malignancies and autoimmune disorders are known to occur at high rates, compared to their incidence in control populations, in patients with certain immunodeficiency syndromes. In this book we have included diseases caused by genes encoding functionally important components of lymphocytes, phagocytes, and proteins in the innate immune system. This means that we have broadened the traditional meaning of the word *immunodeficiency*, which was introduced to describe the lack of a component protecting an individual from infections. The majority of leukocyte abnormalities indeed cause susceptibility to infections. In some diseases the defective component is only expressed in leukocytes, and the defect, therefore, is inherent to this lineage. In other abnormalities, such as ataxia telangiectasia (Chapter 29), Bloom syndrome (Chapter 30), and DiGeorge anomaly (Chapter 33), the gene is expressed outside the hematopoietic lineage and nonimmune features may even prevail. Among patients with most complement defects and periodic fevers, abnormal susceptibility to infection is less pronounced.

Autoimmunity is often a complex phenomenon involving dysregulation or imbalance in immune pathways and networks. However, discovery of apoptosis defects associated with autoimmunity, such as the mutations in the apoptosis mediator CD95 (Fas) in patients with autoimmune lymphoproliferative syndrome (ALPS), illustrates that mutations in a single gene can have an important effect (Chapter 24). This syndrome is often due to a dominant interfering mutation of CD95 that impairs physiologic apoptosis with the subsequent potential for accumulating self-reactive lymphocytes, which in turn mediate autoimmune responses. More generally, the observation was made many years ago that the incidence of autoimmune disorders is increased in certain primary immunodeficiency diseases, such as common variable immunodeficiency and immunoglobulin A (IgA) deficiency (Chapter 23) and Wiskott-Aldrich syndrome (Chapter 31).

Allergy is recognized as having a genetic component, but at present is not associated with a single-gene primary immunodeficiency. However, high levels of IgE are associated with hypomorphic mutations (i.e., with residual protein activity) in the genes, which cause Omenn syndrome (Chapter 11) and in patients with the Wiskott-Aldrich syndrome or immune dysregulation, polyendocrinopathy, enteropathy with X-linked inheritance (IPEX). In certain hyper-IgE syndromes, which can be inherited as an autosomal dominant or recessive trait, very high levels of IgE are found, but the molecular cause is not yet known (Chapter 34).

Enhanced tumor susceptibility is not a hallmark of all primary immunodeficiencies, but in certain disorders such as Wiskott-Aldrich syndrome (WAS) the frequency of malignancy, particularly lymphoma, is known to be high (Chapter 31). Malignancies in immunocompromised individuals may be secondary to chronic infections, which may induce overstimulation of the immune system and thus increase the risk of transforming mutations associated with cell division. Tumor development in patients with primary immunodeficiencies has also been attributed to defective

"immune surveillance" on the theory that the immune cells, particularly natural killer (NK) cells, are programmed to eliminate transformed cells. Another mechanism contributing to tumor development is impaired eradication of microorganisms with an oncogenic potential such as Epstein Barr virus (EBV); EBV lymphoproliferative disease is seen in several immunodeficiencies, particularly X-linked lymphoproliferative disease (Chapter 32). In some inherited immunodeficiencies with an increased incidence of tumors, however, such as Artemis deficiency and Bloom syndrome, the mutated gene encodes an enzyme affecting DNA breakage and rejoining (Chapters 11, 29, and 30).

Genetic Immunodeficiencies in the Spectrum of Host Defense Disorders

The immune system is part of the multifaceted general defense system evolved to protect higher organisms from harmful invasion of microorganisms. The first lines of defense against infections are anatomical, mechanical, and chemical barriers. When the skin or mucosa is breached—for instance, by a burn or abnormality involving the skin or respiratory tract (severe eczema, cystic fibrosis, or disorders of ciliary function in respiratory epithelium)—susceptibility to infections is readily apparent. Similarly, the normally low pH of the stomach or vagina and the action of secreted enzymes and antibacterial defensins discourage bacterial invasion. Because small numbers of potentially pathogenic organisms routinely get past these barrier defenses, the reticuloendothelial system, principally the spleen, serves to filter and neutralize invaders in the bloodstream. Thus splenic deficiency, most commonly due to sickling hemoglobinopathies, is a major cause of immune compromise. Phagocytes and lymphocytes and their humoral products constitute a highly specialized and coordinated network responsible for selective recognition and elimination of microorganisms that have passed through the body's outer barriers.

The most common causes of immunodeficiency worldwide are acquired. These are most often malnutrition and immunosup-

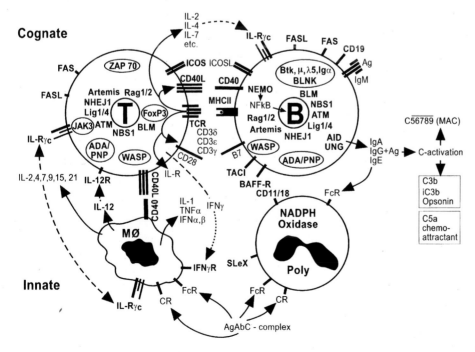

Figure 1.1. Simplified schematic diagram of mediators of leukocyte activation and interactions between T and B cells, macrophages, and neutrophils. Secreted, membrane-associated, and cytoplasmic proteins are labeled in boldface if primary immunodeficiency disorders are known to result when they are absent or defective. IL-Rc, common chain of IL-2, 4, 7, 9, and 15 receptors; IFN-R, interferon receptor; TCR, T cell receptor; SLeX, S-Lewis X receptor. For other abbreviations, see Table 1.1.

pression secondary to bacterial, fungal, parasitic, and particularly viral infections, not only with human immunodeficiency virus (HIV) but also with other viruses, such as measles and EBV. In developed countries, iatrogenic immunosuppression is also found in settings of cancer therapy, organ transplantation, and chronic steroid administration.

In contrast, diseases for which the primary cause is a heritable defect in an immune system gene are infrequent; the common estimate is around 1 per 10,000 births, but the true incidence is not known. Such rare events might be considered to have limited significance on the global scale. However, an understanding of rare, heritable immunodeficiencies at the molecular level helps physicians diagnose and treat individuals with acquired immune deficits. There is also a long list of additional inherited syndromes that appear related to immune deficiency (Ming et al., 1996). The recent appreciation of the interplay between different combinations of inherited and environmental factors promises to help investigators uncover the molecular etiology of more common disorders with complex inheritance, such as the majority of common variable immunodeficiency and IgA deficiency although also here single gene defects without any known environmental influence have been identified (Chapter 2). On the other hand, a certain genetic makeup may protect an individual from infections; for example, persons lacking the chemokine receptor CCR5 on the surface of their T cells are relatively protected from HIV infection, as this virus uses CCR5 as a coreceptor (Deng et al., 1996; Dragic et al., 1996; Biti et al., 1997).

Although this book's main focus is on the recognizable, single-gene primary immunodeficiency syndromes and their molecular defects, the advances in understanding of these diseases have furthered our knowledge of the normal development and function of each component of the immune system. New insights from primary immunodeficiency demonstrate that efficient protection against microorganisms depends not only on the performance of each individual component but, equally important, on a flawless interdigitation of the innate immune system, neutrophils, and activated T and B lymphocytes.

Figure 1.1 shows a simplified diagram of many major components of the immune system and of gene products that are critical for the development and regulation of immune responses. Each of the molecules highlighted in bold letters has been associated with a primary heritable immunodeficiency. Under normal circumstances, the costimulation of B cells by antigens, antigen-activated T cells, and lymphokines results in the production of antibodies of evolving isotypes from IgM to IgG and with increasingly high affinity. These antibodies form antigen–antibody complexes to opsonize microorganisms, neutralize viruses, and activate the complement cascade. Some of the complement subunits liberated during complement activation are potent chemotactic agents that attract neutrophils and macrophages. To emigrate from the vascular spaces, phagocytic cells need adhesion molecules and a cytoskeletal system that permits movement. To trap antigen for presentation to T cells, macrophages with Fc and complement receptors and also follicular dendritic cells and B cells are strategically distributed throughout the tissues. Before the T- and B-cell–specific responses to invasion can be mobilized, the innate immune system provides significant basic protection.

Evolution of the Classification of Genetic Immunodeficiencies

The first descriptions of immunodeficiency diseases grew out of clinical observations of patients with recurrent, severe, or unusual infections, the common denominator of most genetically determined primary immunodeficiency disorders. The types of pathogenic organisms, the course of the infections, and the effectiveness of available therapies were, over time, recognized to be correlated with the nature of the immune defect. These clinical observations remain the most important tools for suspecting and diagnosing patients with immunodeficiency (see Chapter 43). For example, recurrent sinopulmonary infections might suggest an antibody disorder, while bacterial, viral, and fungal infections, which fail to respond to conventional treatment, suggest T cell or combined defects.

As our appreciation of the different host defense mechanisms has progressed, new immunologic tests have evolved that have improved the diagnostic capability of physicians caring for patients with an abnormal predisposition to infection. From the discovery of agammaglobulinemia and its consequences by Bruton (1952) to the enumeration and phenotyping of B cells, T cells, and T-cell subsets and the functional testing of lymphocytes and phagocytes in vitro, we have come a long way in understanding normal immune processes and recognizing specific abnormalities in immunodeficient patients. Classification combining immunological tests and empirical observations has in turn led to improved therapeutic approaches, such as immunoglobulin replacement for patients with agammaglobulinemia.

Grouping of human immunodeficiencies into a series of syndromes by clinical presentation and laboratory findings has made it possible to recognize how dysfunction of each of the distinct branches of the immune system, and in some cases genetically distinct disease entities, can produce a particular pattern of infections and clinical presentations. Such a disease classification system has been composed and periodically updated by the World Health Organization Scientific Group on Primary Immunodeficiency Diseases (WHO Scientific Group, 1995, 1997; Chapel et al., 2003). As new syndromes have been discovered and their associated genes identified, the nomenclature describing primary immunodeficiency disorders has been modified and expanded (Wain et al., 2002, 2004).

Molecular disease classification is now being integrated with ever-more sophisticated and specific in vitro testing of immune cell functions. This new level of definition serves to refine further the clinical and laboratory classifications already established, making possible longitudinal clinical follow-up and tailoring of treatments for each genotype. In Table 1.1 a summary of currently recognized primary disorders of the immune system is given and each disorder associated with a known disease gene has the gene name listed along with the disease name. The logical extension of this type of classification is to gather information from large numbers of patients with each specific gene disorder into databases that include clinical presentation, molecular data including specific gene mutations, treatments, outcome, and long-term follow-up. Some attempts in this direction have already been made (Smith and Vihinen, 1996; Levy et al., 1997; Winkelstein et al., 2003); the rarity of each individual disorder dictates that databases of pooled patient information are necessary to provide unprecedented ability to analyze the immunodeficiency diseases.

Spectrum of Clinical Immunodeficiency Syndromes

How many mutated genes causing primary immunodeficiency diseases are there? Mutations interfering with expression may be irrelevant if the gene product is redundant or nonessential; mutations may escape detection by producing profound abnormalities

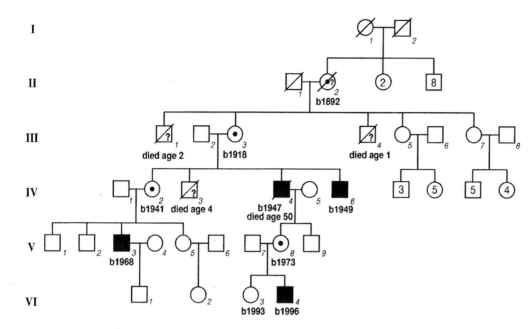

Figure 1.2. Pedigree of a family with X-linked agammaglobulinemia (XLA), illustrating medical progress in diagnosing and treating affected males. Males, squares; males diagnosed with XLA, filled squares. Females, circles; mutation carriers, circles with filled center. Slash, deceased. Individuals who may have had the XLA mutation are indicated with a question mark. Year of birth (b) and age of death are indicated for selected individuals. Individuals III-1, III-4, and IV-3 died of pneumonia. IV-4 died of pulmonary insufficiency, having suffered many bouts of pneumonia from early childhood until diagnosis at age 7.

incompatible with viability; or mutations may cause a heritable disease with a characteristic phenotype. The total number of genes in humans is estimated to be around 22,000. Estimates based on subtraction experiments suggest that the number of genes primarily involved in leukocyte development and function may be more than 1000. Allowing for some redundancy, somewhat fewer than 1000 single-gene primary immunodeficiencies might be possible, around seven times the number now recognized in Table 1.1.

The more common single-gene immunodeficiency diseases have been studied extensively, but their true frequencies in different populations are still only roughly estimated. The most frequently seen monogenic primary immunodeficiencies are X-linked, requiring only a single mutational event to be manifest. More than 2000 patients with one of five X-linked immunodeficiencies have recently been collectively registered and reported (see Chapter 45). There are far more immunodeficiency disorders that are inherited as autosomal recessive traits. However, because they require loss of function of both copies of a gene on homologous chromosomes, the incidence of these diseases is far lower. If one considers that an estimated number of genetically determined human diseases is around 5000 and over 2300 have been mapped on the human genome (Online Mendelian Inheritance in Man, 2005), it is clear that many potential primary immunodeficiency disorders have so far not been identified as distinct entities. If they have actually occurred, they may have presented as sporadic cases and not been recognized as genetically determined immune deficiencies.

Furthermore, mutations located in different regions of the same gene may cause diseases with different manifestations or phenotypes, referred to as *allelic heterogeneity* (see Chapter 2). This is exemplified by mutations of the *WAS* gene, some of which tend to present as full-blown WAS, whereas others are more regularly associated with X-linked thrombocytopenia and still others with isolated neutropenia (see Chapter 31).

Progress in Diagnosis and Treatment

Progress in immunology, genetics, and molecular biology has changed the way we diagnose and treat affected patients. This is illustrated by the histories of families with multiple generations

of affected members. Figure 1.2 represents a kindred now recognized to be carrying X-linked agammaglobulinemia (XLA) (Chapter 21). Inspection of the pedigree reveals that individual III-3, born in 1918, is an obligate carrier of this condition. It is interesting that she had two brothers who died early in life; although definitive information is lacking, they may have been affected with XLA. Her oldest son, IV-3, suffered from recurrent upper and lower respiratory tract infections and died of pneumonia in 1948 at the age of 4 years. Her two younger sons, IV-4 and IV-6, were able to receive the newly available antibiotic penicillin. They survived multiple episodes of pneumonia and were diagnosed with XLA in the mid-1950s, shortly after Bruton's discovery of agammaglobulinemia (Bruton, 1952). By the time intramuscular immunoglobulin treatment was instituted, both boys had developed chronic lung disease and bronchiectasis. IV-4 was one of the first patients treated with high doses of intravenous immunoglobulin (IVIG) for echovirus infection with dermatomyositis, fasciitis, and meningitis (Mease et al., 1981). He died of chronic respiratory failure at the age of 50.

The younger generations of this family have a much more hopeful prognosis. When individual V-3 developed his first pneumonia at the age of 2, he was referred to a university center, where the diagnosis of XLA was confirmed and treatment with immunoglobulin was initiated. He has remained healthy with regular immunoglobulin replacement and presently has a full-time job and no chronic disease. XLA was diagnosed in the youngest member of this kindred, VI-3, at the time of birth by documentation of absent B cells in cord blood. He was immediately started on immunoglobulin treatment and remains completely healthy.

Gene therapy has been pursued in primary immunodeficiencies since the early trials of gene replacement for adenosine deaminase (ADA) deficiency in 1990 (Chapter 48). However, only in 2000 was therapeutic benefit achieved, when patients with X-linked SCID became the first humans to have their disease reversed by gene therapy as their sole treatment (Cavazzana-Calvo et al., 2000). Recent reports of highly effective gene therapy protocols for both X-linked SCID, due to common γ-chain deficiency, and ADA SCID (Aiuti et al., 2003) demonstrate the promise of correction of known gene defects in hematopoietic stem cells, which can then be self-renewing and capable of differentiating into healthy and functional immune cells. However, the occurrence of a leukemia in three X-linked SCID patients due to insertion of the retroviral gene vector near a T-cell transcription factor, LMO-2 (Hacein-Bey-Abina et al., 2003), indicates that further research into gene therapy will be needed to improve its safety as well as efficacy.

Genetic Services for Families with Genetic Immunodeficiencies

With an incidence estimated at 1 per 10,000 births and heavy use of medical care services by affected patients, the impact of significant primary immunodeficiency diseases as a whole on health care is considerable. The incidence of immunodeficiencies is lower than that of cystic fibrosis in Caucasians or of congenital hypothyroidism (about 1 per 2500) but comparable to that of phenylketonuria (1 per 10,000) (Scriver et al., 2001). Because of the large number of specific immunodeficiency entities and their widely varying abnormalities, population screening has not yet been implemented for this group of diseases. Therefore, maintaining a high index of suspicion through education of physicians and the public is essential for timely diagnosis.

Precise genetic diagnosis conveys benefits to patients, their families, and the health care system. Because even patients with X-linked immunodeficiencies often have a negative family history, recognition that the condition is genetic is important. Prediction of recurrence risks, genetic counseling, and carrier and prenatal testing are now available for a large number of immunodeficiencies (Chapter 44).

Genetic Immunodeficiencies and Immunology

The pleiotropy of primary immunodeficiency diseases has become even more evident and reflects the complexity of the human immune system itself. The existence of multiple molecular defects underlying similar phenotypes has helped in elucidating critical immune system components. This is well illustrated by the recent discovery of several new genes (*AID, UNG, CD40*) related to failure to generate IgG, IgA, and IgE immunoglobulins while making normal or increased levels of IgM, originally named "hyper-IgM syndrome." In the most common form of this syndrome, the X-linked form, affected individuals carry mutations in the gene for CD40 ligand (*CD40L*) (Chapter 19). Identification of autosomal recessive forms of the syndrome has been crucial for our current understanding of the phenotypic variation among these patients. Thus, the former assembly of patients with "hyper-IgM" into one major group is outdated. Instead, disease-specific criteria have been redefined. In many patients an increased level of IgM is not found; furthermore, the spectrum of infections varies among individuals with mutations in different genes. Thus, in the defects for CD40 ligand and its receptor CD40, cellular immunity is impaired in addition to the humoral defect. Conversely, mutations in the *AID* and *UNG* genes are phenotypically restricted to the B cell lineage. The distinct gene abnormalities produce susceptibility to different classes of infections as well as having different histopathological changes in secondary lymphoid organs. Thus, basic immunology research receives critical clues from humans with immunodeficiencies that cannot always be appreciated, or may not even exist, in animal models.

References

Aiuti A, Ficara F, Cattaneo F, Roncarolo MG. Gene therapy for adenosine deaminase deficiency. Curr Opin Allergy Clin Immunol 3(6):461–466, 2003.

Atkinson TP, Schäffer AA, Grimbacher B, Schroeder HW Jr., Woellner C, Zerbe CS, Puck JM. An immune defect causing dominant chronic mucocutaneous candidiasis and thyroid disease maps to chromosome 2p in a single family. Am J Hum Genet 69:791–803, 2001.

Biti R, French R, Young J, Bennetts B, Stewart G. HIV-1 infection in an individual homozygous for the CCR5 deletion allele. Nat Med 3:252–253, 1997.

Boocock GRB, Morrison JA, Popovic M, Richards N, Ellis L, Durie PR, Rommens M. Mutations in *SBDS* are associated with Shwachman-Diamond syndrome. Nat Genet 33:97–101, 2003.

Bruton OC. Agammaglobulinemia. Pediatrics 9:722–727, 1952.

Buckley RH, Wray BB, Belmaker EZ. Extreme hyperimmunoglobulinemia E and undue susceptibility to infection. Pediatrics 49:59–70, 1972.

Cavazzana-Calvo M, Hacein-Bey S, de Saint Basile G, Gross F, Yvon E, Nusbaum P, Selz F, Hue C, Certain S, Casanova JL, Bousso P, Deist FL, Fisher A. Gene therapy of human severe combined immunodeficiency (SCID)-X1 disease. Science 288(5466):669–672, 2000.

Chapel H, Geha R, Rosen F (for the IUIS PID Classification Committee). Primary immunodeficiency diseases: an update. Clin Exp immunol 132:9–15, 2003.

Chilgren RA, Quie PG, Meuwissen HJ, Hong R. Chronic mucocutaneous candidiasis, deficiency of delayed hypersensitivity, and selective local antibody defect. Lancet 2:688–693, 1967.

Dadi HK, Simon AJ, Roifman CM. Effect of CD3delta deficiency on maturation of alpha/beta and gamma/delta T-cell lineages in severe combined immunodeficiency. N Engl J Med 349:1821–1828, 1993.

Deng, H, Liu R, Ellmeier W, Chou S, Unutmaz D, Burkhart M, Di Marzio P, Marmon S, Sutton RE, Hill CM, Davis CB, Peiper SC, Schall TJ, Littman DR, Landau NR. Identification of a major co-receptor for primary isolates of HIV-1. Nature 381:661–666, 1996.

de Waal OM, Seynhaeve V. Reticular dysgenesia. Lancet 2:1123–1125, 1959.

Dragic T, Litwin V, Allaway GP, Martin SR, Huang Y, Nagashima KA, Cayanan C, Maddon PJ, Koup RA, Moore JP, Paxton WA. HIV-1 entry into CD4 cells is mediated by the chemokine receptor CC-CKR-5. Nature 381:667–673, 1996.

Edwards AO, Ritter R 3rd, Abel KJ, Manning A, Panhuysen C, Farrer LA. Complement factor H polymorphism and age-related macular degeneration. Science 308:421–424, 2005.

Frank J, Pignata C, Panteleyev AA, Prowse DM, Baden H, Weiner L, Gaetaniello L, Ahmad W, Pozzi N, Caerhalmi-Friedman PB, Aita VM, Uyttendaele H, Gordon D, Ott J, Brissette JL. Christiano AM. Exposing the human nude phenotype. Nature 398:473–474, 1999.

Gitlin D, Janeway CA. Agammaglobulinemia. Congenital, acquired and transient forms. Prog Hematol 1:318–329, 1956.

Hacein-Bey-Abina S, Von Kalle C, Schmidt M, McCormack MP, Wulffraat N, Leboulch P, Lim A, Osborne CS, Pawliuk R, Morillon E, Sorensen R, Forster A, Fraser P, Cohen JI, de Saint Basile G, Alexander I, Wintergerst U, Frebourg T, Aurias A, Stoppa-Lyonnet D, Romana S, Radford-Weiss I, Gross F, Valensi F, Delabesse E, Macintyre E, Sigaux F, Soulier J, Leiva LE, Wissler M, Prinz C, Rabbitts TH, Le Deist F, Fischer A, Cavazzana-Calvo M. LMO2-associated clonal T cell proliferation in two patients after gene therapy for SCID-X1. Science 302(5644):400–401, 2003.

Haines JL, Hauser MA, Schmidt S, Scott WK, Olson LM, Gallins P, Spencer KL, Kwan SY, Noureddine M, Gilbert JR, Schnetz-Boutaud N, Agarwal A, Postel EA, Pericak-Vance MA. Complement factor H variant increases the risk of age-related macular degeneration. Science 308:419–421, 2005.

Heiss NS, Knight SW, Vulliamy TJ, Klauck SM, Wiemann S, Mason PJ, Poustka A, Dokal I. X-linked dyskeratosis congenita is caused by mutations in a highly conserved gene with putative nucleolar functions. Nat Genet 19:32–38, 1998.

Hiraiwa H, Pan CJ, Lin B, Moses SW, Chou JY. Inactivation of the glucose 6-phosphate transporter causes glycogen storage disease type 1b. J Biol Chem 274:5532–5536, 1999.

Kilic SS, Tezcan I, Sanal O, Metin A, Ersoy F. Transient hypogammaglobulinemia of infancy: clinical and immunologic features of 40 new cases. Pediatr Imt 42:647–650, 2000.

Klein RJ, Zeiss C, Chew EY, Tsai JY, Sackler RS, Haynes C, Henning AK, SanGiovanni JP, Mane SM, Mayne ST, Bracken MB, Ferris FL, Ott J, Barnstable C, Hoh J. Complement factor H polymorphism in age-related macular degeneration. Science 308:385–389, 2005.

Kofoed EM, Hwa V, Little B, Woods KA, Buckway CK, Tsubaki J, Pratt KL, Bezrodnik L, Jasper H, Tepper A, Heinrich JJ, Rosenfield FG. Growth hormone insensitivity associated with a STAT5b mutation. N Engl J Med 349:1139–1147, 2003.

Lehrer RI, Cline MJ. Leukocyte myeloperoxidase deficiency and disseminated candidiasis: the role of myeloperoxidase in resistance to *Candida* infection. J Clin Invest 48:1478–1488, 1969.

Levy J, Espanol-Boren T, Thomas C, Fischer A, Tovo P, Bordigoni P, Resnick I, Fasth A, Baer M, Gomez L, Sanders EAM, Tabone M-D, Plantaz D, Etzioni A, Monafo V, Abinun M, Hammarstrom L, Abrahamsen T, Jones A, Finn A, Klemola T, DeVries E, Sanal O, Peitsch MC, Notarangelo LD. Clinical spectrum of X-linked hyper-IgM syndrome. J Pediatr 131:47–54, 1997.

Mease PJ, Ochs HD, Wedgwood RJ. Successful treatment of echovirus meningoencephalitis and myositis-fasciitis with intravenous immune globulin therapy in a patient with X-linked agammaglobulinemia. N Engl J Med 304:1278–1281, 1981.

Ming JE, Stiehm ER, Graham JM Jr. Immunodeficiency as a component of recognizable syndromes. Am J Med Genet 60:378–398, 1996.

Nauseef W, Brigham S, Cogley M. Hereditary myeloperoxidase deficiency due to a missense mutation of arginine 569 to tryptophan. J Biol Chem 269:1212–1216, 1994.

Online Mendelian Inheritance in Man, OMIM (TM). McKusick-Nathans Institute for Genetic Medicine, Johns Hopkins University (Baltimore, MD) and National Center for Biotechnology Information, National Library of Medicine (Bethesda, MD), 2000. World Wide Web URL: http://www.ncbi.nlm.nih.gov/omim/

Picard C, Puel A, Bonnet M, Ku CL, Bustamante J, Yang K, Soudais C, Dupuis S, Feinberg J, Fieschi C, Elbim C, Hitchcock R, Lammas D, Davies G, Al-Ghonaium A, Al-Raves H, Al-Jumaah S, Al-Hajjar S, Al-Mohsen IZ, Frayha HH, Rucker R, Hawn TR, Aderem A, Tufenkeji H, Haraguchi S, Day NK, Good RA, Gougerot-Pocidalo MA, Ozinsky A, Casanova JL. Pyogenic bacterial infections in humans with IRAK-4 deficiency. Science 299(5615):2076–2079, 2003.

Rieux-Laucat F, Hivroz C, Lim A, Mateo V, Pellier I, Selz F, Fischer A, Le Deist F. Inherited and somatic CD3zeta mutations in a patient with T-cell deficiency. N Engl J Med 354:1913–1921, 2006.

Sawada A, Takihara Y, Kim JY, Matsuda-Hashii Y, Tokimasa S, Fujisaki H, Kubota K, Endo H, Onodera T, Ohta H, Ozono K, Hara J. A congenital mutation of the novel gene LRRC8 causes agammaglobulinemia in humans. J Clin Invest 112:1707–1713, 2003.

Scriver CR, Beaudet AL, Sly WS, Valle D, Stanbury JB, Wyngaarden JB, Fredrickson DS. The Metabolic and Molecular Basis of Inherited Disease, 8th ed. New York: McGraw-Hill, 2001.

Smith CIE, Vihinen M. Immunodeficiency mutation databases—a new research tool. Immunol Today 17:495–496, 1996.

Stavnezer-Nordgren J, Kekish O, Zegers BJ. Molecular defects in a human immunoglobulin kappa chain deficiency. Science 230:458–461, 1985.

Tiller TL Jr., Buckley RH. Transient hypogammaglobulinemia of infancy: review of the literature, clinical and immunologic features of 11 new cases, and long-term follow-up. J Pediatr 92:347–353, 1978.

Wain HM, Bruford EA, Lovering RC, Lush MJ, Wright MW, Povey S. Guidelines for human gene nomenclature. Genomics 79:464–470, 2002.

Wain HM, Lush MJ, Ducluzeau F, Khodiyar VK, Povey S. Genew: the Human Gene Nomenclature Database, 2004 updates. Nucl Acids Res 32(Database issue):D255–D257, 2004.

Winkelstein JA, Marino MC, Ochs H, Fuleihan R, Scholl PR, Geha R, Stiehm ER, Conley ME. The X-linked hyper-IgM syndrome: clinical and immunologic features of 79 patients. Medicine (Baltimore) 82(6):373–384, 2003.

WHO Scientific Group. Primary immunodeficiency diseases. Clin Exp Immunol 99:1–24, 1995.

WHO Scientific Group. Primary immunodeficiency diseases. Clin Exp Immunol 109(Suppl):1–28, 1997.

Yount, WJ, Kunkel HG, Litwin SD. Studies of the Vi (gamma-2c) subgroup of gamma-globulin. A relationship between concentration and genetic type among normal individuals. J Exp Med 125:177–190, 1967.

2

Genetic Principles and Technologies in the Study of Immune Disorders

JENNIFER M. PUCK and ROBERT L. NUSSBAUM

Medical genetics is the subspecialty of medicine concerned with the investigation, diagnosis, treatment, counseling, and management of patients and families with inherited disease. Research in medical genetics focuses on identifying the genes involved in human hereditary diseases and the changes in DNA sequence that cause or predispose to these diseases; elucidating disease pathogenesis, including both genetic and environmental factors; understanding the inheritance patterns of diseases in families; developing new treatments or cures for hereditary disorders; and helping patients and families make reproductive decisions and cope with the impact of genetic disorders on the health of family members. Although a complete discussion of medical genetics is beyond the scope of this book and can be reviewed in several texts (Vogel and Motulsky, 1996; Scriver et al., 2001; Nussbaum et al., 2006), it is essential to present here an overview of the terminology, concepts, and methods of modern molecular genetics. This introduction will outline the approaches that have led to the identification of the genes involved in over 140 specific disorders of the immune system. These findings should make possible further revolutionary changes, not only in the discovery of additional disease genes, but also in understanding the pathogenesis of defects in host defenses. Using this understanding, we may create effective new therapies.

The normal complement of 46 chromosomes in a human cell consists of 23 pairs of homologous chromosomes (Fig. 2.1). Twenty-two of the 23 pairs are *autosomes* and are the same in men and women; the remaining pair, the *sex chromosomes*, consist of two X chromosomes in females and one X and one Y (carrying the male-determining genes) in males. The two homologous chromosomes that make up any of the 22 pairs (23 pairs in females) are identical in size, centromere placement, and arrangement of genes.

It is customary in human genetics to refer to the location of a particular gene on a chromosome as the *locus* for that gene. The DNA sequence in and around a gene (such as in introns, flanking regions, or even within coding regions) may be variable among the individuals in the population. The term *allele* is used to describe different DNA sequence variants, and the particular pair of alleles an individual possesses for a given gene is called the *genotype*. Alleles can be rare, deleterious mutations that cause disease, or fairly frequent normal variants of no known clinical significance. If greater than 2% of the population has a DNA sequence that differs from the DNA sequence in other individuals, the variation is called a *polymorphism*. A group of polymorphic alleles at a set of loci close together in a row on a single chromosome is called a *haplotype*. Because the loci are close to each other, recombination between homologous chromosomes will occur only rarely in the region containing these loci and therefore the entire block of alleles contained in a particular haplotype tend to be inherited together.

Mechanisms of Inheritance

Mendelian vs. Complex Inheritance

Mendelian inheritance is a term used to describe the hereditary patterns seen in diseases caused by DNA mutations in single genes inherited from parents by their offspring. Thus, Mendelian disorders include most of the rare primary immunodeficiency diseases described in this book. An increasing awareness of a genetic contribution to other diseases has led to the designation *non-Mendelian* or *complex inheritance* to refer to instances in which an individual's genetic makeup has a more variable and more complex role in disease causation. Examples of complex

16

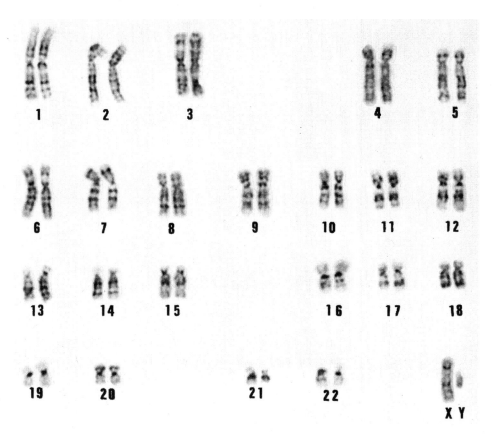

Figure 2.1. Normal human metaphase chromosomes from a male, aligned to show the 22 pairs of autosomes, plus one X and one Y. The banding pattern is revealed by Giemsa staining. Giemsa-light regions are particularly rich in genes. (Kindly provided by Amalia Dutra.)

diseases include multifactorial diseases in which one or more gene mutations must interact with each other and/or environmental factors in order for a disease to be manifest.

Autosomal Recessive Inheritance

In autosomal recessive inheritance (Fig. 2.2), disease usually results when a person inherits two defective copies of the same autosomal gene; the affected individual can be either a homozygote, if two identically defective copies of the same gene are inherited, or a compound heterozygote if there are two different deleterious mutations in the gene. The parents are unaffected heterozygotes who carry one normal copy and one abnormal copy of the gene. By definition, in recessive disease, heterozygous carriers of recessive disorders are not affected because the normal copy of the gene compensates for the defective copy. The typical familial inheritance pattern in autosomal recessive illness is for disease to occur in one or more full brothers and sisters, with both genders affected equally and both parents unaffected. Recessive disorders are seen with increased frequency in children of consanguineous marriages, in which the parents are related to each other (Fig. 2.2), and in genetically isolated populations, because both parents have a greater chance of carrying the same defective gene inherited from a single common ancestor. The genotypes of affected individuals in such instances are expected to show homozygous mutations. A lack of family history is not an argument against autosomal recessive inheritance because, with small sibship sizes typical of many contemporary families, a single affected child born to unaffected parents is the rule rather than the exception.

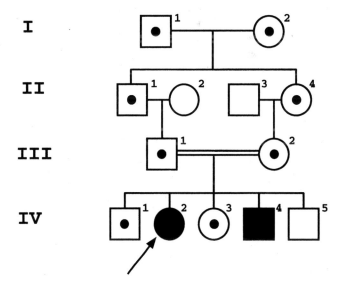

Figure 2.2. Autosomal recessive inheritance. Circles, females; squares, males; filled symbol, affected; symbol with dot, silent carrier. Roman numerals designate generations, with each individual within a generation identified by an integer. This pedigree demonstrates a consanguineous mating, double horizontal line, between cousins III-1 and III-2 (a typical, but not required characteristic of autosomal recessive disease pedigrees). An arrow marks the proband, the first person in the family to come to medical attention. For updated conventions for pedigree drawing, see Bennett et al. (1995).

Recessive illness usually results from loss of function of a gene whose product is normally present in excess so that even a half-normal amount of the gene product is adequate to prevent disease. For example, homozygotes with deletion of the first exon of the gene encoding adenosine deaminase (ADA) have a profound deficiency of the enzyme, resulting in early onset of severe combined immunodeficiency (SCID) (see Chapter 12). In contrast, heterozygotes, with one deleted and one functional copy of the gene, have an amount of enzyme activity intermediate between that found in normals and that in patients with ADA-deficient SCID; but even a small fraction of the normal activity is sufficient to protect them from expressing any immunological defect.

Autosomal Dominant Inheritance

In autosomal dominant inheritance (Fig. 2.3), an individual needs only one copy of a gene alteration for the disease to occur. The parent from whom the genetic alteration was inherited may himself or herself be affected, or may be a silent, or *nonpenetrant*, carrier. Alternatively, neither parent may harbor the alteration seen in the child if the child's mutation arose spontaneously in one of the two gametes, egg or sperm, from which the child was formed. The typical inheritance pattern in autosomal dominant illness is to see multiple affected individuals, both genders affected equally, with transmission of the disease from one generation to the next. A lack of family history is not a strong argument against autosomal dominant inheritance, however, because a nonpenetrant carrier parent or a new mutation will make the affected individual appear as a sporadic occurrence of the disease in the family.

If a dominantly inherited condition requires the presence of an alteration on only one chromosome, it would seem contradictory that some heterozygotes for the defective gene can show no evidence of the disease (lack of penetrance), as illustrated for individual II-4 in Figure 2.3. However, such lack of penetrance is a well-described phenomenon in autosomal dominant disorders. Incomplete penetrance is seen if the onset of the disorder is age-dependent or if an additional factor or factors, such as a second spontaneous somatic mutation or an environmental agent or influence, must be superimposed on the underlying genetic defect in order for the disease to become clinically evident.

Mutations can cause dominantly inherited diseases through a number of different mechanisms. In the most straightforward situation, abnormal amounts of the gene product may be inadequate or allow accumulation toxic metabolites. For example, deficiency of one copy of a gene or multiple genes contained within microdeletions of chromosome 22 is responsible for DiGeorge

syndrome (see Chapter 33). This model for dominant inheritance is called *haploinsufficiency*. In contrast, more than two copies of a gene may also cause disease inherited in an autosomal dominant manner, as is seen with duplication of the *PMP22* gene in Charcot-Marie-Tooth IA peripheral neuropathy (Boerkel et al., 2002) or triplication of the α-synuclein gene in familial Parkinson disease (Singleton et al., 2003).

In a second pathogenetic mechanism, a *gain of novel function*, a dominant mutation may cause a new or altered protein to be made that is endowed with a novel or toxic activity not found in the normal gene product. An example is the acute myeloid leukemia M4Eo subtype associated with a somatic (not germline, and thus not inherited from one generation to the next) inversion of chromosome 16 (Liu et al., 1993). This chromosomal rearrangement causes the apposition of the 5′ portion of the transcription factor gene *CBFB* with the 3′ end of the gene encoding myosin heavy chain, a structural protein of muscle. The result is a chimeric protein that interacts in an abnormal way with other transcription elements to interfere with the normal transcription program of myeloid progenitor cells.

A third type of mutation frequently causing dominant inheritance is *dominant negative* mutation, such as that seen in most patients with an autoimmune lymphoproliferative syndrome (see Chapter 24). Patients with heterozygous mutations in the gene encoding the apoptosis mediator CD95 or Fas have defective programmed cell death through the homotrimeric Fas receptor complex. In vitro studies of the mutated gene products show not only failure of the mutant protein to transmit a death signal itself but also interference by these altered Fas proteins with death signal transmission by coexpressed normal Fas (Fisher et al., 1995). The mutated Fas proteins may produce steric interference when incorporated into the normal trimeric Fas receptor complex.

Finally, a mechanism operating in some dominantly inherited cancer syndromes is that of a *two-hit* process (Knudson, 1971). The first hit is an inherited mutation that inactivates one allele of a tumor-suppressor gene, rendering an individual heterozygous for the mutated gene. One defective allele for this type of inheritance is not in itself sufficient to cause disease. However, an individual who carries only one normal copy of a tumor-suppressor gene is at markedly increased risk for developing cancer. All that is required is that a single somatic cell undergo a second mutation inactivating the remaining normal allele for that one cell to undergo pathologic, unregulated growth and produce a clonal cancer. Second hits are frequently genomic deletions in a single cell as it divides, resulting in *loss of heterozygosity* at the disease locus in the tumor cells.

X-Linked Inheritance

Mutations in X-linked genes have strikingly different consequences in males and females and cause diseases with a distinctive X-linked pattern of inheritance (Fig. 2.4). This is because of the different number of X chromosomes in males and females and the unique biological properties of the mammalian X chromosome. In a male carrying a defective X-linked gene, clinically apparent abnormality always occurs because his only copy of the gene is disrupted. Male hemizygosity for the X chromosome explains the large number of X-linked immunodeficiencies (Fig. 2.5) and the high proportion of males diagnosed with inherited immunodeficiency. In females with X-linked gene defects, the situation is more complex. In order to provide dosage compensation and to equalize gene expression for X-linked genes in males and females, one of the two X chromosomes in a female's somatic

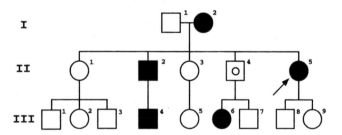

Figure 2.3. Autosomal dominant inheritance. Note male-to-male transmission from subject II-2 to III-4, strongly suggesting dominant inheritance. II-4 is a nonpenetrant carrier. Circles, females; squares, males; filled symbol, affected; symbol with circle, at risk but currently unaffected carrier; arrow, proband.

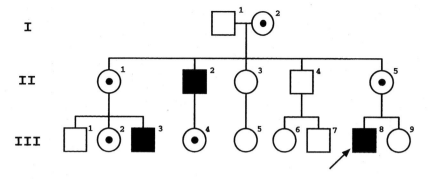

Figure 2.4. X-linked inheritance. Circles, females; squares, males; filled symbol, affected; symbol with dot, silent carrier. Male-to-male transmission is not present.

cells is chosen at random, early in embryonic life, to undergo a near total and irreversible inactivation (Lyon, 1966). Thus, in contrast to the situation with a heterozygote for an autosomal gene mutation, a female heterozygous for an X-linked gene mutation does not have a uniform population of cells, each of which expresses both the normal and abnormal gene. Instead, the somatic tissues of a female are made of a mixture of cells, some of which have an active X chromosome carrying the normal gene, while the rest have an active X carrying the abnormal gene. The relative proportion of cells with one or the other X chromosome active in any one tissue averages 50%, but may differ substantially depending on chance and the number of precursor cells for that tissue that were present in the embryo when X inactivation took place. The fraction of cells in a tissue that have an active X chromosome carrying the normal gene is usually sufficient for normal function of the tissue, so female heterozygotes for X-linked disorders are usually silent carriers. If, however, the cells that

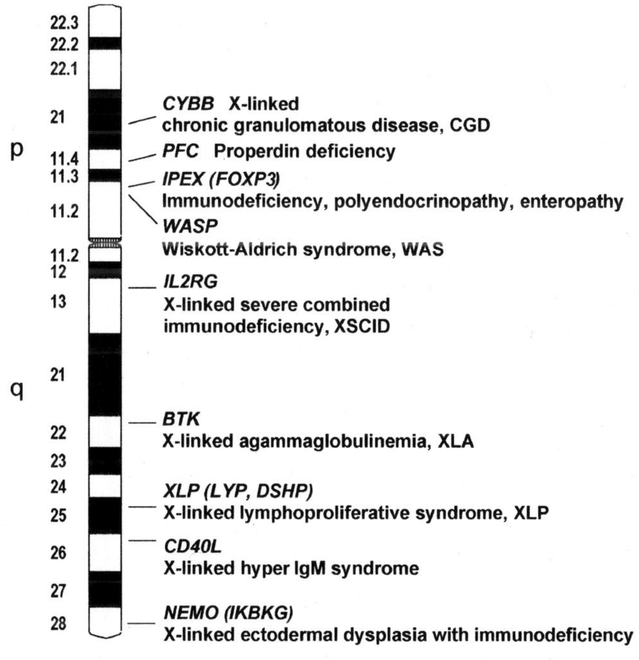

have inactivated the X chromosome carrying the normal gene predominate in a tissue, female heterozygotes may be symptomatic. Thus, the terms *dominant* and *recessive* as applied to autosomal disorders are not strictly applicable to X-linked diseases.

In female carriers of some X-linked conditions, such as X-linked SCID due to defects in the IL-2Rγ receptor (see Chapter 9) or X-linked agammaglobulinemia (XLA) due to defects in the Btk kinase (see Chapter 21), the expected random X inactivation in the lymphocyte population targeted by the gene defect is not seen (Puck, 1993). In these situations, a female carrier of X-linked SCID (or of XLA) will have no lymphocytes (or in the case of XLA no B cells) whose active X chromosome carries the mutation because the fraction of the lymphocyte precursors that have inactivated the X chromosome carrying the normal version of the gene cannot develop and differentiate normally. As a result, the target lymphocyte population for each disease will show marked "skewing" of X-inactivation. The abnormal X-inactivation pattern seen in X-linked immunodeficiencies is discussed in greater detail in the chapters related to specific diseases and in Chapter 44.

A typical X-linked inheritance pattern (Fig. 2.4) is characterized by multiple affected male siblings and cousins as well as affected males in additional generations, all affected members of the kindred being related through unaffected female relatives. However, a lack of family history does not rule out an X-linked inheritance mechanism for immune deficiency. As with autosomal dominant disorders, a spontaneous new mutation in an X-linked gene can cause the disease to appear in the family, either directly in a male, or by the creation of a silent female carrier who passes the mutation on to her male children. One-third of the cases of X-linked diseases severe enough to prevent reproduction by affected males are expected to be the first manifestation in their pedigree of a new mutation (Haldane, 1935). Because males donate a Y chromosome and not an X chromosome to their sons, documenting male-to-male transmission of any trait in any pedigree rules out X-linked inheritance.

22.3
22.2
22.1

21

p 11.4
11.3

11.2

CYBB X-linked
chronic granulomatous disease, CGD
PFC Properdin deficiency
IPEX (FOXP3)
Immunodeficiency, polyendocrinopathy, enteropathy
WASP
Wiskott-Aldrich syndrome, WAS

11.2
12

13

IL2RG
X-linked severe combined
immunodeficiency, XSCID

q 21

22
23

24
25

26

27

28

BTK
X-linked agammaglobulinemia, XLA

XLP (LYP, DSHP)
X-linked lymphoproliferative syndrome, XLP

CD40L
X-linked hyper IgM syndrome

NEMO (IKBKG)
X-linked ectodermal dysplasia with immunodeficiency

Figure 2.5. Idiogram of human chromosome X, illustrating the major Giemsa bands and conventional cytogenetic nomenclature, including p (short) arm and q (long) arm, integers denoting major bands increasing from centromere to telomere, and additional digits to the right of the decimal point denoting sub-bands. The loci on the X chromosome of known human immune disease genes are indicated.

Heterogeneity

Genetic heterogeneity is a broad term used to describe departures from the simple models of "one gene—one enzyme" or "one mutation—one disease." Diseases can show *allelic heterogeneity*, in which different mutations in the same gene cause disease, as is the rule in single-gene immunodeficiency diseases. *Locus heterogeneity* occurs in diseases such as SCID in which a similar phenotype of opportunistic infections from of lack of cellular and humoral immunity can arise from mutations in a number of different genes; the diseases caused by mutations at these different loci are termed *genocopies*. In contrast, a *phenocopy* is an acquired, not a genetic, disease that resembles genetic forms of the disease.

Still more complicated models of inheritance appear to be operating in disorders such as common variable immune deficiency and IgA deficiency (see Chapter 23) or atopic disease. In these disorders one can observe a clearly increased incidence within families; however, an obvious Mendelian pattern of inheritance is not seen. A genetic contribution to such diseases is suspected when there is greater concordance of the disease in monozygotic (identical) twins than in dizygotic (fraternal) twins and when there is an increased risk for the disease in relatives of affected patients compared to that in the population at large. The risk of a second affected individual in a family is greater the closer the blood relationship with the proband. Such complex inheritance patterns, well described in asthma and insulin-dependent diabetes mellitus, are the result of interactions between genes at different loci combined with unidentified, but substantial environmental effects.

How to Identify Disease Gene Loci

Abnormal Protein Products

The first disease genes to be recognized as mutated in immune disorders were identified by defining abnormalities in their protein products. Adenosine deaminase deficiency was originally identified as a purine metabolic defect, and subsequently the absence of ADA enzyme activity was noted in patients who lacked lymphocytes and had immune defects (see Chapter 12; Giblett et al., 1972). This approach was fruitful in ADA-deficient SCID because the enzyme encoded by the disease gene turned out to be a "housekeeping" gene, expressed in all normal cells. It was subsequently appreciated that the amount of ADA protein normally found in lymphocytes is far greater than that in other tissues and that T cells are exquisitely sensitive to elevated levels of its substrates, including deoxyadenosine. These facts help to explain why ADA deficiency is much more harmful to lymphocytes than to other cell types, although effects on organs such as the liver and central nervous system are recognized. The general method of first identifying protein abnormalities in immune disorders and then documenting gene lesions has been less successful for disease genes that have restricted tissue expression or are only active in an early stage of differentiation of the target cell type. For these, positional cloning and testing for mutations in candidate genes have been essential.

Cytogenetic Abnormalities

When clinical disorders are associated with abnormalities in the number or structure of an individual's chromosome complement, cytogenetic techniques can lead to the identification of disease genes. Metaphase chromosomes from dividing cells can be stained with Giemsa to reveal segmental banding patterns that uniquely characterize each human chromosome (Fig. 2.1). Cytogenetic analysis involves comparison of each chromosome to the standard karyotype idiogram, as illustrated for the X chromosome in Figure 2.1. Hybridization of labeled DNA probes to denatured chromosomes, known as fluorescent in situ hybridization, or FISH (Color Plate 2.1), can pinpoint much smaller regions of the genome to indicate the chromosomal location of a disease-associated microdeletion, duplication, or rearrangement. The example in Plate 2.1 shows hybridization of a fluorescent labeled cosmid containing the Fas-associated death domain (*FADD*) gene to identify its localization to human chromosome 11q13.3 (Kim et al., 1996).

Aneuploidy, or abnormal chromosome number, is associated with immune defects. Trisomy 21, or Down syndrome, the most common genetic cause of human mental retardation, is accompanied by depressed in vitro immune responses and by increased incidence of autoimmunity and infections, the leading cause of death in Down syndrome (Epstein, 2001).

At the subchromosomal level, *contiguous gene deletion syndromes* are collections of clinical manifestations resulting from consistently observed chromosomal deletions spanning multiple neighboring genes. An example is the chromosome 11p13 deletion syndrome associated with Wilms tumor, aniridia, genitourinary anomalies, and mental retardation (Haber, 2001; Schaffer et al., 2001). Larger deletions produce the complete phenotype, while smaller disruptions involving single genes within the region produce limited phenotypes, such as isolated aniridia. A contiguous gene deletion syndrome in the context of an immunodeficiency has been postulated, but not proven, in DiGeorge syndrome, which is associated with deletions of chromosome 22q11 (see Chapter 33; Schaffer et al., 2001).

Rare or unique chromosomal abnormalities are occasionally found in the context of primary genetic disorders. Coexistence of a chromosomal translocation, duplication, or deletion and an abnormal phenotype in a patient is very unlikely to be a coincidence; rather, the cytogenetic lesion provides direct evidence for the genetic localization of a disease. One of the best examples of chromosomal abnormality leading to gene identification is the contiguous gene deletion syndrome produced by interstitial deletion of chromosome Xp21 in male patients suffering from multiple disorders including chronic granulomatous disease as well as Duchenne muscular dystrophy, retinitis pigmentosa, and McLeod hemolytic anemia (see Chapter 37; Schaffer et al., 2001).

Disease Gene Localization by Linkage Mapping

DNA polymorphisms

Each child inherits one chromosome of each pair of homologous chromosomes from one parent and the other chromosome of the homologous pair from the other parent. The parent of origin of each chromosome in a pair can be identified by tracing the inheritance of *DNA polymorphisms*, small differences in DNA sequence between chromosomes. Polymorphic alleles for linkage analysis were originally detected by different lengths of the DNA segments seen on Southern blots of DNA digested with various restriction endonucleases (restriction fragment length polymorphisms, or RFLPs) (Drayna and White, 1985). By 1990, RFLPs were largely replaced by short tandem repeat polymorphisms (STRPs) composed of stretches of simple dinucleotide, trinucleotide, or tetranucleotide, repeats of variable length, such as CACACACA · · · · CA. The number of repeats in an STRP can vary tremendously, with as many as a dozen alleles or more found in populations of healthy subjects. STRPs occur frequently in the genome and can be assayed by the polymerase chain reaction (Litt and Luty, 1989; Weber and May, 1989). More recently, single nucleotide polymorphisms (SNPs) have begun to replace STRPs as useful polymorphisms (Sachidanandam et al., 2001; Holden, 2002). Although SNPs are comprised of only two alleles and, therefore, are less informative than STRPs, they can be analyzed much more inexpensively than STRPs by high-throughput technology. Because SNPs are far more frequent, occurring approximately every 1000 base pairs, SNP variants are dense enough to be used for association studies (see below). For more information on genetic marker loci, see Chapter 44.

Meiotic crossing-over

In the absence of abnormal cytogenetic findings to point to the chromosomal locus for a genetic disorder, mapping of a disease gene usually relies on *linkage analysis* in kindreds in which the disorder affects multiple individuals. Gene mapping by linkage analysis is made possible by the normal phenomenon of *meiotic recombination*, or crossing-over during gametogenesis. During the first meiotic division, each pair of homologous chromosomes lines up randomly on the spindle and then separates in the course of the first reduction division of meiosis I. This independent assortment of chromosomes during meiosis I is responsible for randomly distributing one member of each pair of homologous chromosomes into each gamete. It is also in meiosis I that homologous segments of two chromatids form a pair of homologous chromosomes that interchange their genetic material by crossing over at points of contact, known as *chiasmata* (Fig. 2.6). On average, between two and four chiasmata develop between every pair of homologous chromosomes during each meiosis.

Suppose two polymorphic loci are situated at locus 1 and locus 2 on the same chromosome, as shown in Figure 2.6, and there are polymorphic alleles A and a at locus 1 and alleles B and b at locus 2. Also suppose that a parent is heterozygous at both loci (genotype Aa Bb), and, in addition, allele A at locus 1 happens to be on the same chromosome (same DNA molecule) as allele B at locus 2, while alleles a and b are both on the other chromosome. If no crossing-over occurs in the interval between locus 1 and locus 2 during meiosis, each gamete will receive either the chromosome containing alleles A and B or the one carrying alleles a and b (*nonrecombinant*). If, however, a crossing-over event between the two loci in the Aa/Bb individual occurs, the resulting gametes will have a chromosome with a new (*recombinant*) combination of alleles, i.e., either alleles A and b or a and B. From a knowledge of the genotypes of parents and their offspring, one can count the number of offspring resulting from a gamete carrying a crossover between locus 1 and locus 2 and determine the observed *recombination frequency* with which crossing-over events happen between the two loci during gametogenesis.

If crossing-over occurs approximately uniformly along a chromosome, then the chance of a crossing-over event should reflect how far apart the two loci are on that chromosome. The further apart the loci are physically, the greater the chance that at least one crossover will occur between them; the closer they are to each other, the smaller the chance of crossing over. It is straightforward to show that if two loci are so far apart that at least one crossover will always occur in the chromosomal interval between locus 1 and 2 during gamete formation, then 50% of all the offspring will have the nonrecombinant and 50% the recombinant genotype (Nussbaum et al., 2006). At the other extreme, when two loci are so close together that crossovers almost never occur, the observed recombination frequency will approach zero. Between these two extremes are *linked* loci on a chromosome. These loci have less than 50% recombination in offspring since recombinants can arise only through a relatively rare crossing-over event that just happens to fall within the short segment of chromosome separating them. For such loci, the frequency of recombinant offspring will be somewhere between 0% and 50%. Thus, in principle one should be able to correlate recombination frequency with the actual distance between two loci. This is the case when two loci are reasonably close, with a recombination frequency less than 10%; recombination frequency then translates directly into a theoretical *genetic distance*, measured in units called *centiMorgans* (cM), where 1% recombination frequency is equal to 1 cM. This relationship does not hold when loci are loosely linked (recombination frequencies >10%–20%) because of the chance that two independent crossovers, rather than just one, will occur between the two loci. A double crossover will not be detected as a recombination between the two markers and, thus, the measured recombination frequency will always be less than the genetic distance in cM.

In physical terms, the average recombination rate across the entire genome is 1.2 cM per megabase (Mb) of DNA, which means that 1 cM of genetic distance represents approximately 830,000 base pairs of DNA (Kong et al., 2002). The correlation between genetic distance and molecular distance, however, can vary with the gender of the individual in whom the meiosis is occurring and the region of the chromosome being examined. Overall, across all 22 autosomes, the recombination rate in males is 0.9 cM per Mb whereas it is 1.5 cM per Mb in females, presumably because of biologic differences in meiosis I in female vs. male gametogenesis. As one looks at smaller and smaller segments of DNA, the average recombination frequency per DNA segment length becomes increasingly inhomogeneous. For example, telomeric regions have threefold higher recombination per unit length of DNA in males than do centromeric regions. At an even finer scale, recombination becomes very nonuniform, with some segments of a few thousand bases showing a 200 times higher recombination rate than that of neighboring segments of equal length (Jeffreys et al., 2001; Gabriel et al., 2002).

Model-based linkage analysis

Linkage analysis is used to map genes responsible for diseases inherited in a classical Mendelian pattern (Borecki and Suarez, 2001). Affected and unaffected members of families in which the

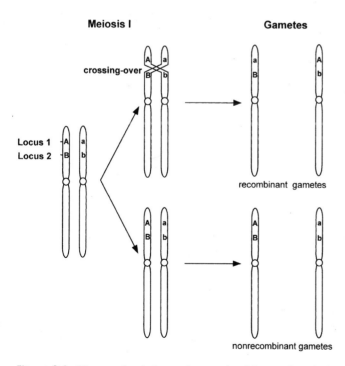

Figure 2.6. Diagram of meiotic crossing-over involving two hypothetical loci, 1 and 2. Alleles at locus 1 are A and a, alleles at locus 2 are B and b. Recombinant gametes are products of a crossover event between locus 1 and locus 2.

disease is being inherited are studied by determining their geno-types at a large number of polymorphic genetic marker loci whose positions are known along each chromosome. Recombination events between the disease locus and all of the genetic markers are counted. If the inheritance pattern is known by inspection of the pedigree (model-based analysis), one can score each affected and unaffected individual as either showing or not showing a crossover between the disease locus and each marker locus tested to determine the recombination frequency. For most of the markers, one expects a 50% recombination frequency because they are not linked to the disease locus; indeed, most markers are not even on the same chromosome as the disease locus. If a marker seems to show less than a 50% frequency of offspring carrying chromosomes with a recombination between the marker locus and the disease locus, this marker locus may be linked to the disease locus.

How is the recombination frequency between the disease and particular marker loci actually measured and the significance of any apparent reduced recombination frequency below 50% assessed in a statistically valid manner? The statistical method used to measure the recombination frequency between genetic loci is called the maximum *LOD* (for logarithm-of-odds) score method, and its features are summarized in Table 2.1. The result of a LOD score analysis consists of two parts. The first part, called θ_{max} by convention, is the best estimate (in a statistical sense) of the recombination frequency between the disease locus and a polymorphic marker locus in a set of families. The value of θ_{max} is, therefore, a measure of genetic distance between two loci. The second parameter, z_{max}, is a measure of how good that estimate of θ_{max} actually is. When z_{max} is greater than 1.5, linkage is strongly suggested. If z_{max} is larger than 3, the likelihood that the loci are linked is a thousand times (10^3) greater than the likelihood that the linkage data are purely the result of chance. Thus LOD scores with z_{max} of 3 or greater are taken as nearly definitive proof that two loci are linked.

LOD score analysis will demonstrate which polymorphic loci of known location are linked to the disease by finding the smallest value of θ_{max} with the largest z_{max}, preferably 3 or greater. Linkage of the disease gene to a marker of known location on a chromosome thereby places the disease gene in the same general location as the marker on that chromosome.

Affected relative analysis (model-free linkage analysis)

Model-based linkage works best when one or a few loci of reasonably high penetrance are responsible for a disease and thus demonstrate a Mendelian inheritance pattern in families. For many disease loci, no Mendelian pattern is discernible because there may be many loci of reduced penetrance as well as gene–gene and gene–environment interactions. In this situation, another approach to mapping disease genes is used, called the *affected-relative method*. This approach makes no assumption about the inheritance pattern of the disease (thus it is "model-free") but simply relies on the fact that two siblings share half of their alleles, having inherited them from their parents. Or in genetic terms, siblings are identical by descent at half the loci in their genomes. If a particular gene contributes to the development of disease, however, then pairs of siblings who are both affected by the disease will share the alleles at loci linked to the disease gene significantly more frequently than 50% of the time.

The affected-relative method is inherently less powerful than linkage analysis but is more suitable than conventional linkage analysis for detecting a genetic contribution to disease when the disease shows significant lack of penetrance or is inherited as a complex trait. The affected-relative approach has been applied to autoimmune diseases, diabetes, asthma, and atopic disease.

Association Studies

Model-based and model-free linkage analysis both depend on looking in families for linkage between a disease gene and markers distributed throughout the genome. In contrast, association studies are done in populations, not families (Borecki and Suarez, 2001). Suppose a disease-producing or predisposing gene originated many generations ago (Fig. 2.7), in a region of a chromosome with a particular haplotype defined by a particular set of alleles at nearby loci (Todd, 2001). An association between the disease-producing or predisposing gene and this haplotype is likely to be preserved through many generations because the loci containing the alleles that define the haplotype are so close to the disease locus that they are unlikely to recombine during the many meioses that occurred as the disease gene was passed down through the generations (Jorde, 2000). In this case, the disease-causing allele and the alleles making up the haplotype at closely linked markers remain together, a situation known as *linkage disequilibrium*. As a result, the haplotype on which the disease gene originated will be found with increased frequency among affected individuals compared to in the population in general. Such in-

Table 2.1. Characteristics of the LOD Score

1. The LOD score is a measure of the degree of linkage between two genetic markers.
2. The LOD score information comes in two parts:
   θ, the recombination fraction
   z, the logarithm of the odds that the markers are linked, rather than unlinked
3. θ measures how frequently recombination occurs between two genetic markers. It is a statistical average derived from observing how often a recombination is seen in actual families. *The smaller θ is, the closer two markers are to each other.*
4. z is a logarithmic measure of how good the estimate of θ really is. Every integer increase in z is a 10-fold improvement in certainty that θ "really" is what it has been measured to be. *The higher the z, the more significant the measurement of θ is.*

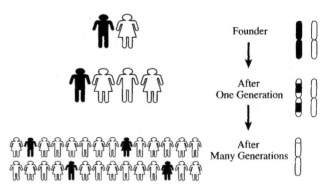

Figure 2.7. Linkage by descent in a hypothetical population in which a disease mutation can be traced to a founder. Marker alleles very close to the disease gene are unlikely to be separated by crossing over and constitute a disease-associated haplotype, which is preserved over many generations. (Kindly provided by Dennis Drayna.)

Table 2.2A. Relative Risk Ratio Analysis

	Disease Present	Disease Absent
Haplotype present	a	b
Haplotype absent	c	d

Relative risk (RR) ratio describes the risk of having a disease with vs. without a given genetic determinant. RR ratio = $[a/(a+b)]/[c/(c+d)]$.

creased frequency can be assessed using a case–control study design. An under- or overrepresentation of the haplotype among affected individuals is measured using the *relative risk ratio* (RR ratio) in a two-by-two table (Table 2.2A). The RR ratio is calculated as the proportion of individuals with disease among those with a given haplotype divided by the proportion of individuals with the disease who lack the haplotype. A RR ratio >1 indicates an association between the haplotype and the disease in the population whereas a ratio <1 suggests the haplotype is protective against the disease. The significance of any deviation from 1 must of course be assessed by an appropriate statistical test.

For example, there are mutant alleles of the gene encoding the mannose-binding lectin (MBL), a circulating opsonization factor, that reduce serum levels of this protein to <10% of normal in individuals homozygous for one of these alleles. A study of the frequency of MBL-deficient genotypes in invasive pneumococcal disease (Kronberg and Garred, 2002) revealed the data shown in Table 2.2B. The frequency of homozygotes among individuals with invasive disease was elevated with a RR ratio of 2.1. The elevation was statistically significant ($p < 0.0001$); 95% confidence limits placed the relative risk of invasive pneumococcal disease given an MBL deficient allele at 1.64- to 2.62-fold greater than the risk of healthy control subjects.

Association studies can be powerful tools for identifying alleles that appear to increase or decrease susceptibility to various diseases. However, an association by itself does not prove a causal relationship between the variant alleles and the disease phenotype. For example, all alleles in linkage disequilibrium with a variant found to be associated with a disease will also show an association without being directly causally related, although documentation of linkage of a risk factor to all such alleles (a risk-associated haplotype) would provide important information. For example, the iron-overload disease hemochromatosis and certain alleles at the HLA-A locus are closely associated, but the HLA-A alleles themselves do not actually cause hemochromatosis. Instead, there is significant linkage disequilibrium between particular HLA-A alleles and mutations at the closely linked *HFE* gene that is actually responsible for the disease (Gandon et al., 1996).

Association studies have not been as successful as one might wish, as evidenced by the frequent failure of many follow-up stud-

Table 2.2B. Alleles of *MBL* Gene Predispose to Invasive Pneumococcal Disease*

	Invasive Pneumococcal Disease	Healthy Controls
Homozygous for MBL deficiency alleles	48	61
Not homozygous for MBL deficiency alleles	329	1221

RR ratio = $[48/(48+61)]/[329/(329+1221)] = 2.075$.
*Kronberg and Garred (2002).

ies to replicate original reports of association (Hirschhorn et al., 2002). One particular difficulty arises from an artifact known as stratification. A population in which various ethnic subgroups do not freely intermarry is a stratified population. The frequency of particular haplotypes in different ethnic groups may vary because these groups have been geographically separated throughout many thousands of years of human history before they came together into a modern population. If an ethnic group in the population does not intermarry with the general population and happens to have a higher incidence of a particular disease for such historical reasons, any haplotypes whose frequencies in this subgroup differ from those in the general population will appear to be artifactually associated with the disease. Stratification can be managed by proper study design and careful selection of appropriate control groups (Pritchard and Rosenberg, 1999).

Positional Cloning

The methodologies outlined above provide the means for obtaining information about the location of many disease genes in the human genome. With the localization of disease genes, even prior to specific gene identification and finding mutations, carrier detection and prenatal diagnosis may become possible for the first time. Furthermore, knowing where a disease gene is located can be the first step in discovering what it is. Availability of the entire sequence of the human genome has revolutionized disease gene identification after linkage to a specific genetic region has been established.

Identification of Candidate Genes

Once a disease gene has been localized to a particular critical region of a chromosome, all the genes located in this region must be evaluated as candidates for alterations responsible for the disease phenotype. The entire complement of genes in any region of human DNA can now be readily ascertained by searching public databases containing the complete human genome sequence deposited by the Human Genome Project (Baxevanis, 2001). In addition to genomic sequence, mRNA sequences from all the expressed genes in a wide variety of tissues are also available (Riggins and Strausberg, 2001).

Evaluation of Candidate Genes to Define a Disease-causing Gene

Once the set of candidate genes in the critical region of linkage or association is obtained through mining genomic and mRNA sequence databases, candidates can be evaluated to determine which one is the disease gene. Northern blots are used to determine the full length of the transcript and tissue expression pattern and to test patients affected with the disease for alterations in mRNA size or quantity. Finally, sequence comparison must reveal deleterious mutations in the alleles of affected patients that are not present in alleles of healthy controls.

The changes in DNA responsible for causing deleterious mutations in genes are extremely heterogeneous. In some cases, deletion of part or all of the DNA encoding the gene has occurred, resulting in production of no mRNA or a defective mRNA transcript lacking important portions of the gene sequence. Small insertions or deletions of a few base pairs may alter the triplet reading frame and create mRNA carrying incorrect codons and, often, a premature termination downstream of the small insertion or deletion. In other cases, single point mutations can interfere with normal RNA processing, such as splicing of exons, resulting in mRNAs that either retain noncoding intronic sequences in the transcript or lack all or part of a coding exon. Some point mutations within coding regions change an amino acid codon into a stop codon (*nonsense mutation*), thereby inserting a premature termination into the mRNA. Still other point mutations may alter a codon from that of one amino acid to another (*missense mutation*). Regardless of which of the above mutation mechanisms has occurred, mutant mRNAs are frequently poorly transcribed or highly unstable; cells carrying such mutations may appear to lack mRNA entirely rather than producing abnormal mRNA.

Mutations that occur over and over again on independent genetic backgrounds are known as *hot-spot mutations*. The most frequent is the alteration of the dinucleotide cytosine-guanine (CG) to thymadine-guanine (TG) either on the coding or anticoding strand. It is believed that the cytosine within a CG dinucleotide is at high risk for undergoing C-to-T transition because such cytosines are frequently covalently modified by methylation at the 5 position of the pyrimidine ring. Spontaneous deamination of a methylcytosine results in a thymidine, which may not be repaired promptly by the cell because it is not recognized as an abnormal base within DNA. Hypotheses for the mechanisms of these mutations and data on their frequency, as well as a lexicon of mutations observed in human genetic disease, have been compiled by Cooper and Krawczak (1995).

The impact of any particular mutation depends on the effect that mutation has on the transcription of the gene into mRNA, the translation of the mRNA into a protein product, and the post-translational processing and stability of any mutant protein that is made. Moreover, functional consequences of mutations also depend on the physiological and environmental context of the cell, tissue, and individual carrying the mutation. In many diseases, a myriad of different mutations can lead to the same final common pathway: the loss of a functional gene product. In the inherited immune disorders as a rule, there are dozens of different mutations that can disrupt function of the gene product and bring about the disease. However, in certain types of genetic disease, a particular mutation may affect the function of a protein in a subtle and unique way and thereby cause a highly specific phenotype. For example, only a few, highly specific missense mutations in the β-globin gene result in a protein with the physicochemical properties that cause the hemoglobin to form crystals under low oxygen conditions, as seen in sickle-cell anemia. Thus the mutation repertoire for sickle-cell disease is severely restricted.

By means of positional cloning, human disease genes have been successfully identified solely on the basis of their genomic location, with little or no knowledge of the nature of the pathophysiological process responsible for the disease. These mutations overwhelmingly affect the coding portions of genes or occur at highly conserved regions of introns immediately adjacent to exons. The coding portions of genes, however, constitute only 4%–5% of sequence of a gene, and thus constitute a mere 1%–2% of the genome. With detailed information on the sequence of the human genome, we are likely to discover other alterations in noncoding regions that contribute to disease, perhaps in ways more subtle than are found with severe, deleterious mutations typical of Mendelian disorders with high penetrance. In such cases, linkage mapping is only the beginning of the study of pathogenesis of genetic disease and correlations between genotype and phenotype. Such variants may be in regulatory or intronic sequences and may alter expression or function only to a limited degree. Variants affecting levels of gene expression are not always adjoining the coding sequence; examples are known of locus control regions,

enhancers, and other sequences altering expression that are 10 to 100 or more kilobases distant from the coding sequences they influence. Finding such alterations and proving they are the cause of disease will be a major challenge to genetics research in the years to come.

Assets of the Human Genome Project

The Human Genome Project (HGP), first conceptualized in the mid-1980s and officially launched in 1990, had as its stated primary goal the determination of the complete sequence of human DNA. Along the way, the HGP set a number of intermediate goals aimed at developing new tools and biological reagents of outstanding utility and importance for medical genetics research (Green, 2001). An initial goal was creation of a genetic map with highly polymorphic markers spaced approximately every 2–5 cM for genetic mapping. This goal was more than realized, with the identification of nearly 7000 STRPs or microsatellite markers, highly variable DNA segments containing strings of two- to four-nucleotide units detectable by polymerase chain reaction. Microsatellite markers formed the foundation for the first dense genetic linkage map of human DNA that covered over 3600 cM of genetic distance at an average spacing less than 1 cM. Single nucleotide polymorphisms, which are far more frequent than STRPs, have been developed for high-throughput parallel linkage mapping.

As sequencing was scaled up and cost per nucleotide sequenced decreased, the HGP became a dynamic international scientific enterprise. By 2003, a virtually complete, highly accurate sequence of the human genome was freely available in databases accessible through the Internet (International Human Sequencing Consortium, 2001). We are now in an era when the information gained through the HGP is being brought to bear on many aspects of molecular biology, evolutionary studies, and medical practice (Collins et al., 2003). For example, the sequence has provided for the first time a near-complete catalog of human genes and revealed that there are an estimated 20,000 to 25,000 human genes, occupying about 40% of the genome. Such catalogs now form the basis of the powerful new technology known as *expression arrays* (Geschwind, 2003). Sequences corresponding to many or nearly all human transcripts are individually mounted in a two-dimensional array on a glass or silicon wafer. Messenger RNA from two sources (such as normal and cancerous cells from the same tissue) are labeled with two different fluorescent dyes, mixed together, and allowed to hybridize to the array. The intensity of fluorescence from each of the two dyes at each address on the array provides a measure of the relative amount of the transcript of each gene in the two sources from which the mRNA was isolated. The relative amounts of tens of thousands of transcripts can be compared simultaneously, providing a profile of the expression of transcripts in a diseased tissue compared to that in an unaffected standard tissue. Such profiles are not only useful as biomarkers but may also provide crucial insights into disease pathogenesis.

With completion of the human genome sequence, genetic variation can also be investigated in far more detail than before. A complete catalog of all human sequence variation can be compiled along with an assessment of which variants have functional consequences. As of 2003, millions of the estimated total of 10 million SNPs present in the aggregate over all human populations have been identified and catalogued (Sachidanandam et al., 2001; Holden, 2002). These SNPs form the basis for genome-wide population studies designed to identify particular haplotypes that harbor DNA variants that contribute to common, complex diseases.

Table 2.3. Internet Resources for Genetic Information

Name	Internet Address	Description
NCBI	www.ncbi.nlm.nih.gov	National Center for Biotechnology Information, a division of the National Library of Medicine. Repository for genomic sequence, cloned genes, expressed sequence tags, Unigene project data, SNPs, expression data, haplotype blocks, and more
UCSC Genome Bioinformatics	http://genome.ucsc.edu/	University of California, Santa Cruz. Annotated assembly of human and other genomes including genes, predicted genes, markers, and more
Ensembl Genome Browser	http://www.ensembl.org/	The Wellcome Trust, Sanger Institute genomic information site. Repository for genomic sequence, comparative species homologies, genes, predictions, and more
OMIM	http://www.ncbi.nlm.nih.gov:80/entrez/ query.fcgi?db=OMIM	Online Mendelian Inheritance in Man, an online, searchable "knowledge base" of human genetic disorders, including clinical description, genetic data, and molecular characterization of known disease genes
HUGO Mutation Database	http://wwwhgmd.cf.ac.uk/docs/oth_mut.html	Human Genome Organization site linking Web sites involved in describing and cataloguing the mutations responsible for human genetic disease
GeneTests	http://www.genetests.org/	Publicly funded medical genetics information resource listing clinical and research laboratories providing diagnostic testing for genetic diseases in North America
Immune Deficiency Foundation	http://www.primaryimmune.org/	U.S. national organization dedicated to research, education, and advocacy for primary immune deficiency diseases
Jeffrey Modell Foundation	http://www.jmfworld.com/	Foundation supporting and advocating research and education about primary immunodeficiency
European Society for Immunodeficiencies	http://www.esid.org/	Physician information, disease databases

Shown in Table 2.3 is an annotated list of some of the most important Web sites that hold genome and genetic data of crucial importance in medical genetics research and patient care.

Ethical Issues in Genetic Testing

There are numerous ethical issues surrounding human genetics as scientific knowledge and medical technology come to grips with the three central tenets of medical ethics: *beneficence* (doing good for the patient), *autonomy* (safeguarding the individual's rights to control his or her medical care and be free of coercion), and *equity* (ensuring that all individuals are treated equally and fairly). A full discussion of these issues is beyond the scope of this chapter, but a few examples arising in immunodeficiency diseases serve to illustrate some of these aspects of medical ethics and genetics.

As more and more genes are identified and found to be involved in human genetic disease, our ability to perform molecular diagnosis will continue to increase dramatically. An inescapable consequence of this rapidly accelerating knowledge is the time lag between acquiring the ability to diagnose genetic disease and developing effective interventions to prevent or treat diseases once they are diagnosed. For the immunodeficiency diseases, recent advances in therapy, from new antibiotics to immunoglobulin replacement to bone marrow transplantation and gene therapy, have placed clinical immunologists at the forefront of developing the tools to close the gap between diagnosis and treatment. How such tools are used and whether they are readily available to all who need them are clearly issues of fairness in the application of scientific knowledge.

An additional aspect of the growth of genetic knowledge is in the area of disease predisposition. Increasingly, molecular tools are allowing clinicians to identify individuals and relatives who are at risk for disease that may have an onset much later in life than when the molecular testing is being done. Testing healthy individuals for disease predispositions encoded in their genomes has obvious benefits in identifying people at risk who may be able to modify their lifestyles and/or begin appropriate preventive therapy; but it also carries the risk of serious adverse psychological damage, stigmatization in society, and discrimination in insurance and employment. Ethical problems with genetic testing are especially acute when the testing identifies a predisposition for a disorder for which current medical technology provides little or no treatment when clinical disease actually develops. Thus, the issue of beneficence becomes quite central to testing in this setting. Is knowing the result of a genetic test doing more good than harm, or more harm than good?

The ethics of genetic testing is also an acute issue when testing children for the carrier state of diseases, such as X-linked immunodeficiences that pose no threat to a female child's own health but identify a substantial risk for having affected offspring. The autonomy of children, including their right to make decisions for themselves about learning about their own genetic constitution, must be balanced against the desire of parents to obtain such information and transmit it to their children in the manner they believe best. As the power of genetic diagnoses increases, there is an increasingly greater need to educate health care providers, patients, their families, and society at large to make informed decisions about how to use genetic information wisely and for maximum benefit.

References

Baxevanis AD. Information retrieval from biological databases. Methods Biochem Anal 43:155–185, 2001.

Bennett RL, Steinhaus KA, Uhrich SB, O'Sullivan CK, Resta RG, Lochner-Doyle D, Markel DS, Vincent V, Hamanishi J. Recommendations for standardized human pedigree nomenclature. J Genet Counseling 4:267–279, 1995.

Boerkoel CF, Takashima H, Garcia CA, Olney RK, Johnson J, Berry K, Russo P, Kennedy S, Teebi AS, Scavina M, Williams LL, Mancias P, Butler IJ, Krajewski K, Shy M, Lupski JR. Charcot-Marie-Tooth disease and related neuropathies: mutation distribution and genotype–phenotype correlation. Ann Neurol 51:190–201, 2002.

Borecki IB, Suarez BK. Linkage and association: basic concepts. Adv Genet 42:45–66, 2001.

Collins FS, Green ED, Guttmacher AE, Guyer MS. A vision for the future of genetics research. Nature 422:835–847, 2003.

Cooper DN, Krawczak M. Human Gene Mutation. Oxford: Bios Scientific, 1995.

Drayna D, White R. The genetic linkage map of the human X chromosome. Science 15:753–758, 1985.

Epstein CJ. Down syndrome. In: Scriver CR, Beaudet AL, Sly WS, Valle D, eds. The Metabolic and Molecular Bases of Inherited Disease, 8th ed. New York: McGraw-Hill, pp. 1223–1256, 2001.

Fisher GH, Rosenberg FJ, Straus SE, Dale JK, Middelton LA, Lin AY, Strober W, Lenardo MJ, Puck JM. Dominant interfering *Fas* gene mutations impair apoptosis in a human autoimmune lymphoproliferative syndrome. Cell 81:935–946, 1995.

Gabriel SB, Schaffner SF, Nguyen H, et al. The structure of haplotype blocks in the human genome. Science 296:2225–2229, 2002.

Gandon G, Jouanolle AM, Chauvel B, et al. Linkage disequilibrium and extended haplotypes in the HLA-A to D6S105 region: implications for mapping the hemochromatosis gene (HFE). Hum Genet 97:103–113, 1996.

Geschwind DH. DNA microarrays: translation of the genome from laboratory to clinic. Lancet Neurol. 2:275–282, 2003.

Giblett ER, Anderson JE, Cohen F, Pollara B, Meuwissen HJ. Adenosine deaminase deficiency in two patients with severely impaired cellular immunity. Lancet 2:1067–1069, 1972.

Green ED. The Human Genome Project and its impact on the study of human disease. In: Scriver CR, Beaudet AL, Sly WS, Valle D, eds. The Metabolic and Molecular Bases of Inherited Disease, 8th ed. New York: McGraw-Hill, pp. 259–298, 2001.

Haber DA. Wilms tumor. In: Scriver CR, Beaudet AL, Sly WS, Valle D, eds. The Metabolic and Molecular Bases of Inherited Disease, 8th ed. New York: McGraw-Hill, pp. 865–876, 2001.

Haldane JBS. The rate of spontaneous mutation of a human gene. J Genet 31:317–326, 1935.

Hirschhorn JN, Lohmueller K, Byrne E, et al. A comprehensive review of genetic association studies. Genet Med 4:45–61, 2002.

Holden AL. The SNP consortium: summary of a private consortium effort to develop an applied map of the human genome. Biotechniques Suppl: 22–24, 26, 2002.

International Human Sequencing Consortium. The human genome: sequencing and initial analysis. Nature 409:860–921, 2001.

Jeffreys AJ, Kauppi L, Neumann R. Intensely punctate meiotic recombination in the class II region of the major histocompatibility complex. Nat Genet 29:217–222, 2001.

Jorde LB. Linkage disequilibrium and the search for complex disease genes. Genome Res 10:1435–1444, 2000.

Kim PKM, Dutra AS, Chandrasekharappa SC, Puck JM. Genomic structure and mapping of human FADD, an intracellular mediator of lymphocyte apoptosis. J Immunol 157:5461–5466, 1996.

Knudson AG Jr. Mutation and cancer: statistical study of retinoblastoma. Proc Natl Acad Sci USA 68:820–823, 1971.

Kong A, Gudbjartsson DF, Sainz J, Jonsdottir GM, Gudjonsson SA, Richardsson B, Sigurdardottir S, Barnard J, Hallbeck B, Masson G, et al. A high-resolution recombination map of the human genome. Nat Genet 31: 241–247, 2002.

Kronberg G, Garred P. Mannose-binding lectin genotype as a risk factor for invasive pneumococcal infection. Lancet 360:1176, 2002.

Litt M, Luty JA. A hypervariable microsatellite revealed by in vitro amplification of a dinucleotide repeat within the cardiac muscle actin gene. Am J Hum Genet 44:397–401, 1989.

Liu P, Tarle SA, Hajra A, Claxton DF, Marlton P, Freedman M, Siciliano MJ, Collins FS. Fusion between transcription factor CBF/PEBP2 and a myosin heavy chain in acute myeloid leukemia. Science 261:1041–1044, 1993.

Lyon MF. X-chromosome inactivation in mammals. Adv Teratol 1:25–54, 1966.

Nussbaum RL, McInnes RR, Willard HF. Genetics in Medicine, 7th ed. Philadelphia: Harcourt Health Sciences, 2006.

Pritchard JK, Rosenberg NA. Use of unlinked genetic markers to detect population stratification in association studies. Am J Hum Genet 65:220–228, 1999.

Puck JM. X-linked immunodeficiencies. In: Harris H, Hirschhorn K, eds. Advances in Human Genetics, vol. 21. New York: Plenum Press, pp. 107–144, 1993.

Riggins GJ, Strausberg RL. Genome and genetic resources from the Cancer Genome Anatomy Project. Hum Mol Genet 10:663–667, 2001.

Sachidanandam R, Weissman D, Schmidt SC, et al. A map of human genome sequence variation containing 1.42 million single nucleotide polymorphisms. Nature 409:928–933, 2001.

Schaffer LA, Ledbetter DH, Lupski JR. Molecular cytogenetics of contiguous gene syndromes: mechanisms and consequences of gene dosage imbalance. In: Scriver CR, Beaudet AL, Sly WS, Valle D, eds. The Metabolic and Molecular Bases of Inherited Disease, 8th ed. New York: McGraw-Hill, pp. 1291–1324, 2001.

Scriver CR, Beaudet AL, Sly WS, Valle D, eds. The Metabolic and Molecular Bases of Inherited Disease, 8th ed. New York: McGraw-Hill, 2001.

Singleton A, Farrer M, Johnson J, Singleton A, Hague S, et al. Triplication of the normal alpha-synuclein gene is a cause of hereditary Parkinson's disease. Science 302:841, 2003.

Todd JA. Multifactorial diseases: ancient gene polymorphism at quantitative trait loci and a legacy of survival during our evolution. In: Scriver CR, Beaudet AL, Sly WS, Valle D, eds. The Metabolic and Molecular Bases of Inherited Disease, 8th ed. New York: McGraw-Hill, pp. 193–202, 2001.

Vogel F, Motulsky AG. Human Genetics, 3rd ed. Berlin: Springer-Verlag, 1996.

Weber JL, May PE. Abundant class of human DNA polymorphisms which can be typed using the polymerase chain reaction. Am J Hum Genet 44: 388–396, 1989.

3

Mammalian Hematopoietic Development and Function

GERALD J. SPANGRUDE

The origins of the mammalian immune response are found in hematopoiesis. Most of the diseases discussed in this book are mediated by mutations in genes that function during the course of hematopoietic development at the level of the progenitors for specific cell lineages (severe combined immunodeficiencies) or at the level of the expression of signaling molecules that promote differentiation (MHCII deficiency), or at the level of the functional potential of mature effector cells (leukocyte adhesion deficiency, chronic granulomatous disease). The common theme throughout the diseases discussed in this volume is the origin of the cellular components of specific and nonspecific immunity, the hematopoietic stem cell (HSC). While specific mutations in particular genes can result in defects in highly specialized mature cell populations, the resulting immunodeficiencies are distinguished by the biochemical result of the disrupting mutation and not by the developmental origin of the defective cellular response. This presents both an opportunity and a caution in the design of therapies for some of these diseases.

Bone marrow transplantation is one avenue for treatment of some immunodeficiencies, but in the absence of a related, genetically matched donor, the risks inherent in allotransplantation often outweigh the potential benefits. Transplantation of gene-corrected autologous cells can theoretically overcome the allotransplantation issue. While many of the immunodeficiencies might be corrected by genetic therapy, it is important to recognize that alterations in gene expression directed at correcting one developmental defect may be accompanied by an equally disruptive alteration in hematopoietic function as a result of expressing the corrected gene in cell lineages where it is not normally found.

The challenges of genetic therapy for immunodeficiencies are great, and the global effect of correction aimed at one blood lineage on the entire blood-forming system must not be overlooked.

This chapter will give an overview of our current understanding of hematopoiesis, specifically focusing on the transplantable HSC, to provide a basis for considering the common origin of most immunodeficiencies and the prospects for bone marrow transplantation as a therapeutic intervention.

Overview of Hematopoietic Stem Cells

Because of the relatively short life span of most blood cells, a high rate of production is necessary throughout life to maintain normal numbers. In adult mammals, the major source of blood is the bone marrow. It is here that the HSC is found, represented at a frequency of fewer than 1 cell per 10^4 marrow cells (Neben et al., 1993).

The nature and identification of HSC remain somewhat controversial in that isolation of these cells is technically demanding and definitive assays for HSC function are lacking. The HSC is now known to comprise a heterogeneous mixture of cells with various degrees of functional activity in transplants and culture assays. Figure 3.1 depicts three levels of hematopoietic stem and progenitor cells, defined functionally as cells with the potential to differentiate into a variety of lineages of mature cell types. The most primitive of these three populations is the HSC, which is capable of differentiating along all hematopoietic lineages. In addition, this group of cells can be maintained in sufficient numbers to ensure lifelong blood production through a process known as *self-renewal*, which results in replacement of cells in this compartment when they are lost through differentiation.

Various lines of experimental evidence indicate that these primitive HSCs enter the cell cycle only infrequently (Bradford et al., 1997; Cheshier et al., 1999), and they are generally thought of as being metabolically quiescent (Hodgson and Bradley,

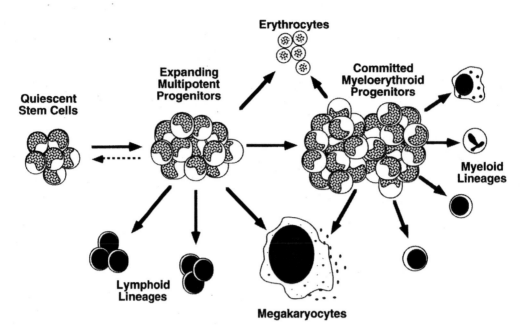

Figure 3.1. A model of the hierarchy of primitive hematopoietic stem (HSC) and progenitor cells. Quiescent stem cells are representative of the pluripotent HSC, with both self-renewing potential and the ability to differentiate as any type of blood cell. These HSCs occasionally enter the cell cycle and contribute to the expanding multipotent progenitor pool. Retrograde movement back into the quiescent state may explain the process of self-renewal. Once expansion is under way, the ability to self-renew is lost. The expanding multipotent pool can directly differentiate as lymphoid or myeloerythroid progeny. Commitment to the myeloerythroid lineages results in further expansion of these progenitors during differentiation, and subsequent restriction to specific lineages results in precursor cells with limited proliferative potential.

1984). When one of these cells enters a cycle of cell division, this member of the hematopoietic hierarchy can be thought of as entering the "expanding multipotent progenitor" pool (Fig. 3.1). Although the mechanism of self-renewal is not understood, one possibility is that retrograde movement of at least one daughter cell back into the quiescent pool is responsible for maintenance of adequate numbers of primitive HSCs. The pool of expanding multipotent progenitors retains developmental potential for all hematopoietic lineages but gradually loses the ability to self-renew. After an undefined number of cell divisions, these cells lose their ability to differentiate along the lymphoid lineages and enter the third pool depicted in Figure 3.1, the "committed myeloerythroid progenitors." These cells then are selected to differentiate as various types of mature cells, depending on the cytokines available in the specific areas of the marrow where they differentiate.

Embryology of Hematopoiesis

Blood cells develop in essentially the same manner in embryos of all mammals. Embryonic mammalian hematopoiesis can be divided into three distinct phases: mesoblastic, hepatic, and myeloid (Wintrobe, 1967). The *mesoblastic phase* (also known as the *vitelline phase* because of the predominance of morphologically recognizable hematopoietic cells in the yolk sac) persists for about 10 weeks in human embryos (about 12 days in the mouse). During this time, the predominant blood cell type observed morphologically is the primitive (nucleated) erythrocyte in the yolk sac, which can be detected as early as 18 days of gestation in humans. During the *hepatic period* (beginning at 6–8 gestational weeks in the human or 10–12 days in the mouse), the fetal liver assumes the major responsibility for blood formation and continues to be hematopoietic until shortly before birth. In humans, a transient period of splenic hematopoiesis precedes the *myeloid*

phase, which initiates in marrow cavities at 10–12 weeks of gestation (15–16 days in the mouse), and by 20 weeks the majority of blood formation in human embryos occurs in the bone marrow. While splenic hematopoiesis is only a transient stage during human development, the spleen remains hematopoietically active throughout the adult life of the mouse. In spite of this, the bone marrow remains the primary site of blood formation, as it contains at least 10-fold higher levels of assayable progenitors than those in spleen.

As discussed above, the primary anatomical site where hematopoiesis is first observed in mammalian embryos is extraembryonic, in the numerous blood islands of the yolk sac. The liver primordium is subsequently seeded by migrating HSCs and rapidly becomes the predominant site of embryonic blood production. Recent experimental evidence suggests that a separate origin of hematopoiesis is also present intraembryonically in mammals, as is the case in lower vertebrates. Intraembryonic hematopoiesis in mammals is localized in a specialized splanchnopleural region of mesoderm that includes the dorsal aorta and the mesonephros and genital ridge (AGM region, see Fig. 3.2; Muller et al., 1994). Although morphologically recognizable hematopoietic elements are present only in the yolk sac during early embryogenesis, progenitor assays can detect hematopoietic activity in the AGM region prior to the appearance of progenitors in the fetal liver (Medvinsky and Dzierzak, 1996). It is currently unclear whether the fetal liver is colonized by HSC deriving from the yolk sac, the AGM, or both. However, one series of experiments demonstrated lymphoid and multipotent myeloid generative activity in the region of the dorsal aorta prior to establishment of circulation in the mouse embryo (Cumano et al., 1996). Therefore, it seems clear that mammalian hematopoiesis initiates within the developing embryo as well as in the yolk sac (reviewed in Dzierzak and Medvinsky, 1995).

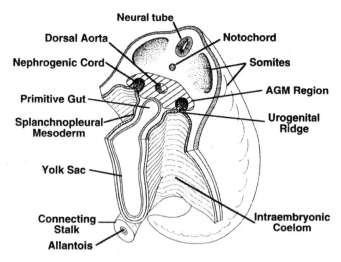

Figure 3.2. Morphology or early mammalian embryogenesis and the origins of the blood-forming cells. The embryo depicted here is human and at the beginning of the fourth week of gestation, just prior to differentiation of the mesonephros and genital ridge from the nephrogenic cord. While morphologically distinct blood cells are already present in the blood islands (not depicted here) of the yolk sac, no blood production is evident in the body of the embryo. Surgical dissection of the AGM region (hatched area in the figure) followed by specific assays for hematopoietic function has demonstrated that primitive hematopoietic stem and progenitor cells are also present in the AGM, even though no morphologically identifiable blood cells can be detected. Adapted from *Illustrated Human Embryology, Volume 1: Embryogenesis,* by Tuchmann-Duplessis et al. (translated by L.S. Hurley), Paris: Masson, 1975. Used with permission.

Transplantation of yolk sac cells into irradiated adult animals does not result in engraftment. However, HSC activity has been demonstrated in early (day 10) mouse yolk sac after transplantation into neonatal recipient animals, possibly because of an obligate localization of these cells in the hematopoietic liver for further maturation into HSCs prior to marrow colonization (Yoder and Hiatt, 1997). It is likely that the yolk sac promotes primarily primitive hematopoiesis (nucleated red cells that transiently function during embryogenesis) while the embryonic source of hematopoiesis is predominantly definitive (the stable, long-term source of hematopoiesis). However, after the onset of blood circulation both types of hematopoietic function are present in both anatomic locations during subsequent development.

The AGM and the yolk sac are both mesodermally derived. The primordial cells that initiate formation of the hematopoietic system migrate to the AGM and yolk sac from the caudal portion of the early primitive streak during gastrulation (Bloom, 1938). The proliferating cells of the blood islands differentiate along two distinct pathways: one to form the endothelial cell boundaries of the first blood vessels at the periphery of the blood islands, and the other to give rise to primitive blood cells in the center of the islands. Thus, the common mesenchymal ancestry of endothelium and blood cells can be traced to a relatively late period during their ontogeny. Within the mammalian embryo, clusters of hematopoietic cells are not observed in the AGM region but rather are seen intravascularly as clumps of cells attached to the aortic endothelium (Dzierzak and Medvinsky, 1995). In birds, the onset of intraembryonic hematopoiesis is morphologically obvious, and for many years this was generally felt to be a fundamental difference between mammalian hematopoiesis and that of lower vertebrates.

Microenviroments of Hematopoiesis

Bone Marrow and the Niche

Bone is a calcified extracellular matrix of collagen and glycosaminoglycans that is synthesized by osteoblasts—bone-forming cells. The medullary cavity of bone may be hematopoietically active and contain so-called red marrow, or it may be predominantly inactive and filled with fat cells (white marrow). During the process of aging in humans, the anatomical sites of medullary hematopoiesis are progressively limited, beginning at birth when hematopoietic activity was distributed throughout the skeleton. By 18 years of age, most hematopoietically active marrow is found in central locations such as the pelvis, sternum, and ribs (Amos and Gordon, 1995). The medullary cavity and haversian canals of bone, which house blood vessels, are lined with a membrane called the *endosteum.* Occasional osteoclasts, which destroy bone, are found in the walls of the medullary cavity and are associated with areas of bone resorption.

The endosteum and its associated osteoclasts are of particular interest because the most primitive HSCs for blood formation appear to be localized near the walls of the medullary cavity (Lord et al., 1975; Gong, 1978; Uchida et al., 1994). The process of hematopoiesis depends on HSC in an intimate association with nonhematopoietic tissue cells in the medullary cavity of bone and, in some rodents, in the spleen (reviewed in Testa and Dexter, 1990). These tissue cells are generally termed *stromal cells,* a generic term that may be applied to any of a wide variety of nonmobile cells (reviewed in Dorshkind, 1990). The matrix of the medullary cavity includes structural elements of the blood vascular system, nerve fibers, and a system of reticular cells and fibers. This matrix is established during embryogenesis before the initiation of hematopoiesis. Thus, it provides a specialized microenvironment that supports hematopoietic cells within the parenchyma.

The bone marrow microenvironment probably has several distinct functions with regard to hematopoiesis (Fig. 3.3). First, it must provide conditions to maintain pluripotent HSCs in a primitive state throughout an animal's lifetime, thus ensuring an adequate supply of the seeds of hematopoiesis. Second, it must provide appropriate inductive signals for primitive HSCs to direct regulated development of erythroid, myelomonocytic, and B-lymphoid lineages. The processes of maintenance and differentiation of HSCs must be balanced to sustain a regulated frequency of functionally mature blood cell populations without depleting the HSC pool. The role of regulating the maintenance and differentiation of HSCs is filled by the stromal-cell elements of the marrow microenvironment, although in the case of erythropoiesis the kidney is also intimately involved in an endocrine manner through the production of erythropoietin. In addition to producing cytokines, marrow stromal cells also mediate proliferation and differentiation of hematopoietic progenitors via direct cell–cell interactions, using both common and specialized cell adhesion molecules (Kincade, 1991; Long et al., 1992).

The distinct functions of HSCs and the microenvironments that support them are clearly seen in two mutant mouse strains that were selected after mutations at the "dominant spotting" (W) and "steel" (Sl) loci on chromosomes 5 and 10, respectively (Schultz and Sidman, 1987). The products of these two loci interact to result in normal hematopoietic development and function; the Sl gene product is expressed by the microenvironment, while the W gene product is expressed by the hematopoietic cells (reviewed in Witte, 1990).

Overview

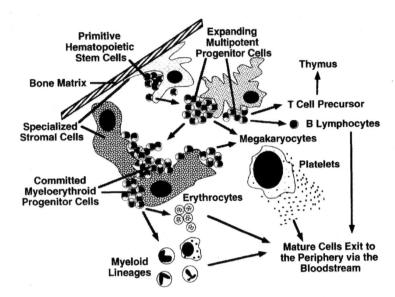

Figure 3.3. The bone marrow microenvironment includes a complex mixture of parenchymal cells that support mainte-nance and differentiation of hematopoietic cells by secretion of cytokines as well as via cell–cell interactions. The associations between developing hematopoietic cells and their supportive microenvironment are largely uncharacterized; this diagram is strictly a generalized representation of the notion that interac-tions with stromal cells are thought to regulate various stages of hematopoietic development in specific manners.

Over the last few years direct evidence for a bone marrow niche critical for HSC has accumulated (Suda et al., 2005). Thus, osteoblasts have been shown to be an integral part of a niche wherein the HSC is believed to reside (Calvi et al., 2003; Zhang et al., 2003). Moreover, the frequency of HCS seems to be de-pendent on the number of osteoblasts (Zhang et al., 2003; Visnjic et al., 2004) and parathyroid hormone was reported to increase hematopoiesis by inducing the synthesis of Jagged 1, which serves as a ligand for notch signaling (Calvi et al., 2003). Conversely, ostopontin serves as a negative regulator with defective mice showing increased jagged 1 and angiopoetin 1 expression (Stier et al., 2005). Of particular interest to the field of primary immun-odeficiencies, the ATM protein, defective in ataxia telangiectasia, was recently reported to regulate the reconstitutive capacity of HSCs (Ito et al., 2004).

Spleen

Another example of the importance of HSC–stromal cell interac-tions in regulating hematopoietic growth is provided by the mouse spleen; in mice hematopoietic activity is maintained in the spleen throughout adult life. Although both the bone marrow and spleen support erythropoiesis and granulopoiesis, the spleen is domi-nantly erythropoietic, whereas granulopoiesis exceeds erythro-poiesis in the bone marrow. Implantation of bone fragments into irradiated spleens allows the two types of microenvironments to exist in juxtaposition. In such cases, individual colonies of hematopoietic cells that arise at the border of the two microenvi-ronments are frequently granulocytic in the vicinity of the bone fragment and erythroid in the splenic area (Wolf and Trentin, 1968). Results from these experiments argue that microenviron-mental differences can dictate developmental pathways followed by individual multipotent cells.

Other examples of microenvironments that induce specialized hematopoietic growth include the B and T lymphocyte lineages, which develop predominantly in bone marrow and thymus, respec-tively. These observations are consistent with an "instructive" role for microenvironments in directing lineage commitment (Metcalf, 1998). An equally compelling case can be made for a stochastic model of hematopoietic differentiation (Enver et al., 1998), and it is likely that both mechanisms function in various lineages and stages of development.

Hematopoiesis in Culture

The establishment of long-term cultures of bone marrow stromal elements has provided further evidence that specialized stromal cells contribute to microenvironments that support hematopoiesis. In addition, culture systems have been developed that selectively support HSC maintenance with either myeloid and erythroid de-velopment (Dexter and Lajtha, 1974), B-cell development (Whit-lock and Witte, 1982), or T-cell development (Anderson et al., 1993). These culture systems involve the establishment in vitro of specialized stromal cell monolayers or reaggregation of stromal cells and progenitors into a three-dimensional structure to mimic organ culture of the intact thymus. Stromal cell monolayers may be heterogeneous, consisting of fibroblasts, endothelial cells, adi-pocytes, and mononuclear-derived macrophages and dendritic cells, or they may be established in vitro as cell lines of clonal ori-gin that have been screened and selected to optimally support hematopoietic development.

Early observations of the myeloid cultures developed by Dexter and colleagues indicated that adipocytes were most closely associ-ated with hematopoiesis in vitro. The subsequent development of stromal cell lines (Hunt et al., 1987; Kodama et al., 1992) has strengthened these findings; the stromal cell lines that support in vitro growth of early lymphoid and myeloid cells and maintain spleen colony-forming cells are adipocyte-like and resemble ad-ventitial reticular cells. These latter cells are fibroblastoid cells that form a cellular network, or reticulum, within the bone marrow cav-ity. They accumulate neutral lipid deposits under certain conditions and are secretory, producing collagen and other proteins (Hunt et al., 1987). The bone marrow and thymus culture systems prom-ise to provide clues that will clarify the roles of cell–cell interac-tions and of soluble growth factors in regulating hematopoiesis.

Isolating Mouse Hematopoietic Stem Cells

Because of the important biological and medical implications inherent in the concept of a rare population of primitive cells be-ing responsible for continuous replenishment of all circulating blood cells, efforts to identify and isolate HSCs date back to the first quantitative assays of hematopoietic development (re-viewed in Spangrude, 1989; Visser and Van Bekkum, 1990). Af-ter description of the in vivo spleen colony-forming assay (Till and McCulloch, 1961), development of an in vitro colony assay followed a few years later (Bradley and Metcalf, 1966). Although early efforts to enrich primitive hematopoietic cells relied on these assays, the limitations of the assays in reflecting the self-renewal potential of HSC was recognized early on. Velocity and equilibrium centrifugation studies demonstrated that bone marrow cells with an inherent capacity to produce splenic colonies could be separated from those capable of in vitro colony formation (Worton et al., 1969a, 1969b), and that self-renewal potential, as indicated by the content of splenic colony-forming units (CFU-S) within individual spleen colonies, could be separated from the bulk of the CFU-S in normal bone marrow (Worton et al., 1969a). These observations indicated that CFU-S activity might not directly correlate with self-renewal potential, a problem that has not been conclusively resolved. However, the early separation studies demonstrated that cell separation methods could indeed be applied to dissect the hierarchy of primitive hematopoietic cells.

Mouse HSC can be enriched from adult bone marrow by use of a number of methods. In one approach to the identification and enrichment of mouse HSCs, monoclonal antibodies specific for antigens that characterize cells belonging to specific mature and committed hematolymphoid lineages are used to identify these cells in bone marrow suspensions (Muller-Sieburg et al., 1986). The marked cells can be depleted by a solid-phase immunological method such as panning (Jordan et al., 1990) or use of immunomagnetic particles (Bertoncello et al., 1989; Ikuta et al., 1990). The remaining population of cells, termed *lineage-negative* (Lin⁻), contains approximately 5% of the initial number of bone marrow cells and consists of a mixed population of multipotent HSCs, early progenitors, and late progenitors. Lin⁻ cells can be further fractionated with specific monoclonal antibodies that recognize antigens expressed by a variety of hematopoietic and nonhematopoietic cells—for example, Thy-1 (Muller-Sieburg et al., 1986), Ly-6A/E (Spangrude and Brooks, 1992), c-kit (Okada et al., 1991a; de Vries et al., 1992), and major histocompatibility complex class I molecules (Mulder et al., 1984). The lectin wheat germ agglutinin has also been useful in discriminating multipotent HSCs from early- and late-stage progenitors as there is a relatively high number of binding sites for the lectin on multipotent HSCs compared to that on later-stage progenitors (Visser et al., 1984). When combined with a depletion of cells expressing high levels of lineage differentiation antigens, any one of these markers alone or in combination will identify a group of primitive hematopoietic cells in adult bone marrow or fetal liver. This multiparameter approach is necessary because no one cell-surface antigen has been identified that is expressed only by HSCs. Most currently defined HSC markers continue to be expressed as the cells differentiate and new, lineage-specific markers appear.

Heterogeneity of the Hematopoietic Stem Cell Compartment

Cell populations resulting from antibody selection techniques are heterogeneous in function, suggesting a complex organizational structure within the HSC compartment. The heterogeneity is mostly with respect to self-renewal potential, since a high frequency of cells isolated by antibody enrichment are multipotent for both lymphoid and myeloid lineages (Spangrude and Johnson, 1990). The subset of multipotent cells possessing extensive self-renewal potential is resistant to killing by 5-fluorouracil and other cell cycle–active agents (Hodgson and Bradley, 1979). This

finding suggests that these cells are metabolically quiescent or that they possess elevated levels of a multidrug resistance mechanism (Chaudhary and Roninson, 1991).

Several methods have been used to select for long-term repopulating cells from antibody-enriched HSC populations. The vital mitochondrial dye rhodamine-123 can be used to distinguish cell populations on the basis of metabolic activity, and self-renewing HSCs are predominantly recovered from the group of cells exhibiting low mitochondrial staining (Bertoncello et al., 1985). Rhodamine-123 is also a substrate for multidrug efflux pumps. However, it is likely that the discrimination between the self-renewing and non-self-renewing HSC subsets by rhodamine-123 is due to differences in mitochondrial content and activity (Kim et al., 1998). In a second strategy vital nucleic acid dyes such as Hoescht 33342 are used to identify cells not in cycle (Neben et al., 1991; Wolf et al., 1993).

Finally, specific combinations of antibody markers can select for self-renewing HSCs (Morrison and Weissman, 1994). The combination of cell-surface and metabolic markers allows the recovery of a population of cells capable of long-term repopulation of irradiated animals after transplantation of less than 10 cells (Wolf et al., 1993; Spangrude et al., 1995). In contrast, over 10^5 normal bone marrow cells are required to produce a similar level of reconstitution.

The published methods for enriching populations of HSCs from mouse bone marrow and fetal tissues have dramatically improved the ability of researchers to explore the early events in normal mammalian hematopoiesis. As more enriched populations have become available for experimental use, it has become possible to critically test these cells for their ability to respond to recombinant cytokines by proliferating (Li and Johnson, 1992; Sitnicka et al., 1996), to assess the developmental pathways that the cells will follow under defined conditions in vitro (de Vries et al., 1991), and to explore the ability of small numbers of cells to repopulate lethally irradiated animals over long periods of time (Spangrude et al., 1995).

Characteristics of Human Hematopoietic Stem Cells

The demonstration that the CD34 antigen is expressed by progenitor cells in human bone marrow (Civin et al., 1984) has allowed many investigators to explore the HSC compartment in humans. Applying the same general approach that was successful in the mouse, several groups have combined negative selection for lineage markers; positive selection for CD34 (Andrews et al., 1986), Thy-1 (Baum et al., 1992), or c-kit (Briddell et al., 1992); and selection for low staining with rhodamine-123 (Srour et al., 1991) to achieve high enrichments of human hematopoietic progenitor cells. Positive selection for CD34 alone has been used as a method to enrich for progenitors prior to bone marrow transplantation after chemotherapy for a number of malignancies (Berenson et al., 1991; Shpall et al., 1994). Highly purified CD34⁺ Thy⁺ Lin⁻ cells have also been used clinically for transplants after myeloablative chemotherapy (Archimbaud et al., 1996). In allograft transplants for treatment of immunodeficiencies, selection for HSCs by specific antigen expression may decrease the potential for graft-vs.-host disease (Flake et al., 1996). In addition, attempts to introduce normal counterparts of defective endogenous genes into the hematopoietic system for treatment of immunodeficiencies (Mulligan, 1993; Candotti et al., 1996) require that the target population be relatively enriched for self-renewing HSCs. However, in light of a pronounced genetic variability of HSC phenotype in mice (Spangrude and Brooks, 1992, 1993), caution should be exercised when making the assumption that most HSCs in most human individuals express CD34 or Thy-1. Recently, the existence of human stem cells that lack CD34 has been proposed (Nakauchi, 1998).

In recent years, a great deal of attention has been focused on augmentation and acceleration of engraftment in bone marrow transplant settings by cytokine therapy in the recovery phase, and on the use of peripheral blood-derived stem/progenitor cells as a source of hematopoietic stem cells for human transplantation. While hematopoietic progenitors are rarely found circulating in peripheral blood under normal circumstances (Micklem et al., 1975), cytotoxic drug treatment, the administration of hematopoietic cytokines (Bodine et al., 1993), or both treatments in sequence (Siena et al., 1989) induce a rapid peripheralization of hematopoietic stem/progenitor cells. These cells can be harvested by multiple leukophoresis sessions over several days, frozen for storage, and infused to mediate hematopoietic recovery following marrow ablative therapy. There is a significant effect of peripheral blood-derived stem and progenitor cells on the kinetics of recovery during the pancytopenic phase, when infection and hemorrhage can result in significant patient morbidity and mortality. A variety of studies have documented dramatic effects on both neutrophil and platelet recovery when peripheral blood stem cells, with or without supplemental cytokines, were used to mediate hematopoietic recovery following high-dose chemotherapy (Benjamin et al., 1995; Basser et al., 1996). Enrichment of HSCs from normal donor peripheralized blood progenitor products (Weaver et al., 1993; Murray et al., 1995) may enable efficient allotransplantation without graft-vs-host disease in the treatment of many immunodeficiencies (Flake et al., 1996).

Assays for Hematopoietic Stem Cells

A great deal of attention has been focused on the development of assay systems that specifically detect the activity of the most primitive of HSCs for hematopoiesis (Fig. 3.4). One approach to an in vivo clonal assay for long-term repopulation is limiting dilution competitive repopulation to derive a measure of competitive repopulating units (CRUs) (Szilvassy et al., 1990). In this assay, very small numbers of genetically marked cells are transferred into anemic W/Wv mice (Boggs et al., 1982) or irradiated animals. In the latter case, a radioprotective dose of normal marrow cells is also provided to mediate radioprotection, and the development of donor-derived populations is followed over long periods of time. This approach has been used to estimate the frequency of long-term repopulating cells in normal marrow suspensions (Boggs et al., 1982; Micklem et al., 1987). Enrichment of mouse HSCs from bone marrow resulted in repopulation of recipient animals after transfer of single injected cells (Smith et al., 1991; Spangrude et al., 1995).

Because it is very difficult to determine what the seeding efficiency of this assay is—that is, how frequently an intravenously injected cell seeds to a microenvironment such as the spleen or bone marrow where hematopoiesis is supported—it is not possible to know how frequent the long-term repopulating cell was in the original population; only a minimum frequency can be determined. Further, since there is ample evidence that long-term repopulation is usually quasiclonal in radiation-reconstitution models, the absence of progeny in the long term may indicate that the single injected HSC is one of many in a quiescent state, rather than supporting the idea that the cell was unable to self-renew and give rise to progeny over a long period of time (Van Zant et al., 1992).

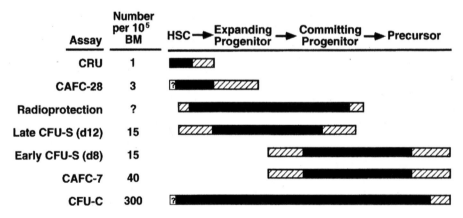

Figure 3.4. Assays that detect various members of the hematopoietic hierarchy. A number of assays currently used to detect hematopoietic stem and progenitor cells are listed along with the approximate frequency of the normal mouse bone marrow cells detected by these assays and a general indication of the level of the hematopoietic hierarchy detected by each assay. The black and shaped portions of the bars indicate strong and weak activity, respectively, in the indicated assay. The assays are abbreviated as follows: CRU, competitive repopulating unit, a transplantation assay that measures the clonal frequency of cells able to contribute long term to blood formation in a transplant recipient. CAFC, cobblestone- area–forming cell, a cell culture assay that measures the ability of stem and progenitor cells to form within 7–28 days a morphologically distinct colony of cells in association with a monolayer of cultured stromal cells; Radioprotection, the potential of transplanted stem and progenitor cells to mediate hematological rescue of lethally irradiated animals; CFU-S, colony-forming units (spleen), a transplant assay that measures formation of clonally derived colonies of proliferating hematopoietic cells in the spleens of irradiated animals 8 or 12 days after transplant; CFU-C, colony-forming units (culture), a culture assay that measures expansion of clones of cells in a semisolid culture medium in response to soluble growth factor stimulation. This assay can also be performed by seeding single cells into culture wells. The frequency of responding cells in each assay has been taken from Neben et al. (1993) and Szilvassy et al. (1996); these numbers will vary depending specific assay conditions and the age and strain of the donor mouse from which bone marrow cells are obtained.

Unknown seeding efficiencies and the quasiclonal repopulation problems compound the difficulty of measuring the frequency of long-term repopulating cells, even when a remarkable level of enrichment for the activity has been achieved.

Very soon after the description of the CFU-S assay by Till and McCulloch in 1961, the question of whether splenic colonies truly represent the proliferation of primitive HSCs became an important issue. Since the criteria for defining HSCs at that time included multilineage potential and a capacity for self-renewal, it naturally followed that one should be able to demonstrate the presence of new colony-forming cells within spleen colonies. This hypothesis was tested in a double transplant experiment by either excising individual spleen colonies (Siminovitch et al., 1963) or pooling the entire spleen from a CFU-S experiment (Siminovitch et al., 1964) for transplant into secondary irradiated recipients. The results revealed a broad heterogeneity in the ability of splenic colonies to initiate new splenic colonies. Also, when a longer period of time was allowed to elapse prior to harvesting spleen colonies for secondary transplant, the number of colonies containing secondary CFU-S increased. Many more colonies harvested 14 days after injection contained CFU-S compared to colonies harvested after 8 days. While a reasonable interpretation at the time invoked an extended time frame necessary for the self-renewal process within spleen colonies (Lewis and Trobaugh, 1964), later work revealed that the majority of early (day 8) CFU-S disappeared a few days later and that at least half of the late (days 11–13) colonies arose from a separate group of hematopoietic cells (Magli et al., 1982; Wolf and Priestley, 1986). These intrinsic differences in CFU-S hinted at the limited utility of the CFU-S assay to detect HSCs; only after a secondary transplant could one be assured of the self-renewing potential inherent in the original spleen colony.

Refinements in HSC characterization and enrichment have strengthened the concept that many types of hematopoietic cells that form spleen colonies lack the ability to reconstitute long-term hematopoiesis in irradiated animals (Ploemacher and Brons, 1988). Conversely, several groups have demonstrated long-term repopulating potential in the apparent absence of splenic colony-forming potential (Ploemacher and Brons, 1989; Jones et al., 1990; Wolf et al., 1993). While it is not yet clear whether inhibitory cytokines (Graham et al., 1990) or splenic seeding considerations (Spangrude and Johnson, 1990) may explain the failure of certain HSC preparations to form spleen colonies, it is very clear that spleen colony formation is not a unique characteristic of primitive HSCs (Hodgson and Bradley, 1979; Magli et al., 1982). Further, the inability to use such an assay in the investigation of human hematopoiesis, with the possible exception of chimeric human–mouse model systems (McCune et al., 1988), dictates the need to develop specific in vitro assays for HSCs.

Many recent attempts to develop specific in vitro assays for HSCs have relied on coculture of candidate HSC populations with feeder layers of bone marrow–derived stromal cells. A number of laboratories have used this approach to analyze hematopoiesis with mouse and human models (Ploemacher et al., 1989; Sutherland et al., 1990). In this assay there are two phases: an expansion phase in which the primitive HSC number is increased without a large degree of differentiation, and a detection phase when the products of the initial expansion are read out. In the expansion phase, self-renewal must be favored over differentiation, and the typical approach is to use a stromal cell feeder layer under the conditions originally defined by Dexter and colleagues (Dexter and Lajtha, 1974) to culture HSC populations. In most cases, the second phase of the assay involves harvesting the cells that differenti-

ate in the cultures and testing these progeny cells for the ability to produce macroscopic colonies in semisolid medium under the influence of a variety of cytokines (the culture colony-forming unit, or CFU-C assay). While the readout of colony formation is not an activity uniquely associated with HSCs, the differentiation of HSCs in these stromal cell cocultures is thought to result in the production and thus a net increase in the number of colony-forming cells. The results of such an assay are fairly quantitative, but the assay is not clonal because individual colonies in the second phase of the assay do not reflect single-input HSCs. However, if the coculture is initiated under limiting dilution conditions (Ploemacher et al., 1989; Sutherland et al., 1990), an estimate of the frequency of the HSCs in any given cell population is possible. Furthermore, a higher absolute number of colony-forming cells produced in any one culture is interpreted as an indicator of a more primitive initiating HSC. This culture system, and variants thereof, is usually termed the *long-term culture initiating cell* (LT-CIC) assay.

Cocultures of HSC and supportive bone marrow stroma evolve to generate unique associations between the two cell types. The mobile HSC interdigitates between and beneath the stromal monolayer, resulting in HSCs with a characteristic nonrefractile appearance by phase-contrast microscopy. These stromal-covered cells proliferate to form clusters of tightly packed cells that have been referred to as *cobblestone areas*, and the assay to detect such events is known as the *cobblestone area-forming cell* (CAFC) assay (Ploemacher et al., 1989; Neben et al., 1993). The frequency of formation of cobblestone areas can be correlated to hematopoietic repopulating activity in vivo, and the kinetics of cobblestone area formation reflects the relative maturation stage of the initiating cells, with more primitive cells requiring a longer period of time to establish a cobblestone area. These observations have been incorporated into the CAFC assay, which does not rely on a readout of CFU-C, but rather quantitates the frequency of cobblestone areas as a function of time (Ploemacher et al., 1991; Weilbaecher et al., 1991; Neben et al., 1993). There is currently no strong evidence that stromal cell systems effectively reproduce the bone marrow environment in terms of self-renewal of HSCs (Spooncer et al., 1985). The stromal cocultures can produce CFU-C from input HSCs over prolonged periods of time (van der Sluijs et al., 1990), but it is unclear to what extent HSCs can actually self-renew in these cultures relative to the in vivo environment.

While some correlation has been made between long-term reconstitution of lethally irradiated animals and some in vitro culture systems (Ploemacher et al., 1991), in fact the only definitive method available to define the self-renewing characteristics of HSCs is by transplantation in vivo (Orlic and Bodine, 1994). The availability of genetically defined strains of mice that allow easy identification of donor-derived cells in the peripheral blood of recipient animals in an otherwise syngeneic transplant (Harrison, 1980; Spangrude et al., 1988) provides a valuable model system for HSC function that has not yet been entirely duplicated by in vitro culture systems (van der Sluijs et al., 1993). The major limitation of the in vitro systems is that, in general, the development of only one or a few hematopoietic lineages is supported. Also, sole reliance on long-term culture initiation as an indicator of HSC function ignores the known capacity of mammalian cells to adapt to tissue culture conditions. Recently, immunodeficient strains of mice have been widely used as an in vivo model for engraftment of both normal and leukemic hematopoietic cells from human sources (Wang et al., 1998). Although not optimal for analysis of long-term hematopoiesis, this assay allows detailed study of stem cell homing to bone marrow and multilineage differentiation in the context of a normal microenvironment.

Colony Stimulating Factors and Hematopoietic Stem Cell Regulation

Although stromal cell cocultures have proved to be a useful model for studying the development of HSCs in vitro, ideally one would prefer to identify and characterize the stromal cell–derived cytokines responsible for driving each stage of hematopoiesis. Many hematopoietic cytokines have been identified and purified and have had their genes cloned (reviewed in Metcalf, 1989). However, as single agents, these molecules are primarily involved in later stages of myeloid and lymphoid differentiation. Early hematopoietic progenitors require as many as three cytokines to induce colony formation in vitro (Bartelmez et al., 1989), and it is not yet clear whether the most primitive HSCs respond to known cytokines at all (Fig. 3.4). Interleukin (IL)-1 and IL-3, in combination with colony-stimulating factor 1 (macrophage colony-stimulating factor, or M-CSF), are sufficient to drive in vitro colony formation by highly enriched populations of HSCs (Kriegler et al., 1990). A similar combination of cytokines, but not single cytokines, was shown to stimulate highly enriched HSCs at a clonal level to differentiate into osteoclasts as well as mature blood cells (Hagenaars et al., 1989). Leukemia inhibitory factor and IL-6 have both been identified as costimulators of primitive HSCs when used in combination with IL-3 (Okada et al., 1991b; Leary et al., 1990). The combination of IL-3 and IL-6 provides the stimulation necessary to achieve retroviral infection of primitive HSCs in vitro (Bodine et al., 1990). Finally, several cytokines such as steel factor (Lowry et al., 1992), Flt3 ligand (Shah et al., 1996), thrombopoietin (Broudy et al., 1995; Sitnicka et al., 1996), and basic fibroblast growth factor (Gabbianelli et al., 1990) have been shown to potentiate colony formation by highly enriched progenitors populations in combination with other cytokines. Taken together with numerous reports of negative regulatory influences mediated by macrophage inflammatory protein 1 (Graham et al., 1990), tumor necrosis factor (Rogers and Berman, 1994), and transforming growth factor (Jacobsen et al., 1995), these studies reinforce the concept of synergism and antagonism between the effects of colony-stimulating factors on primitive HSCs (Jacobsen et al., 1994).

Self-Renewal of Hematopoietic Stem Cells

A major advantage of using a mouse model system to define basic characteristics of the HSC is that, given the paucity of experimental methods, it can be used to demonstrate the most critical of HSC functions, self-renewal. The concept of self-renewal in hematopoiesis can be interpreted in several ways. One possibility is that self-renewal of HSCs occurs at each cell division, which requires that HSCs divide in the complete absence of differentiation. This leads to the conclusion that one HSC may contribute indefinitely to hematopoiesis, a critical assumption for the application of gene therapy protocols in immunodeficiencies. If, however, one envisions a heterogeneous compartment of HSCs, all of which share the ability to initiate development in multiple hematopoietic lineages but differ in ability to give rise to more multipotent cells, the conclusion is consistent with the clonal succession model as proposed by Kay (1965) and there is less optimism for prolonged correction of genetic defects by gene therapy. A supraoptimal number of non-self-renewing multipo-

tent cells, each possessing a high but finite intrinsic proliferative potential, would be adequate to ensure long-term hematopoiesis (Spangrude, 1992). An intermediate situation consisting of essential elements from both extremes produces a further variation.

It will be difficult to prove or disprove the proposal that one HSC can divide to produce progeny of identical proliferative and developmental potential; however, many experiments have demonstrated the reality of clonal succession and of the heterogeneous nature of the HSC compartment. Sequential activation of HSC clones leads to clonal or quasiclonal contributions to hematopoiesis, as demonstrated by transplantation experiments between animals differing at isoenzyme loci (Micklem et al., 1987; Abkowitz et al., 1995) or by transplants of bone marrow cells carrying unique retrovirally induced genetic markers (Jordan and Lemischka, 1990). Serial transplantation of bone marrow, which eventually leads to a loss of repopulating activity (Harrison et al., 1990), can demonstrate two distinct phases of engraftment in recipient animals. The first phase is unsustained, apparently because more committed members of the HSC compartment being unable to maintain hematopoiesis in the long term. The second phase is sustained and is due to very primitive HSCs (Jones et al., 1989). These observations are compatible with clonal succession and with the generation-age hypothesis (Rosendaal et al., 1976), which extends the clonal succession model to predict that the number of generations an HSC is removed from its initial progenitor is inversely proportional to its proliferation potential (and hence hematopoietic-repopulating potential) and directly proportional to its state of activation. This means that the ability of any individual HSC to self-renew is limited, but the compartment of multipotent cells possesses the self-renewing ability of the sum of all individual HSCs.

Application of transplantation pressure in hematopoiesis results in exhaustion of HSCs (Harrison et al., 1990). In a very intriguing study, allophenic chimeras, made by aggregating embryos of two inbred mouse strains, were used to show that HSC exhaustion can be observed under normal developmental pressure (Van Zant et al., 1990). In these experiments, one partner mouse strain (DBA/2) has spleen colony-forming cells, of which 24 are normally in cell cycle, whereas in the other partner strain (C57BL/6) only 2.6 of these cells are in cycle. In allophenic chimeras between these two strains, the DBA/2 HSC population predominated early in life, only to be overtaken and eventually eclipsed by the C57BL/6 population. A similar observation was made after bone marrow transplants from chimeras into irradiated F1 recipients. These experiments bear out basic predictions of the generation-age hypothesis and point to intrinsic differences in the HSC as a factor in the longevity of hematopoiesis and of life span. Do HSCs also self-renew at a cellular level? This question is critical to the concept of gene therapy as a permanent cure for immunodeficiencies. To answer this question definitively we will need more sophisticated techniques of cell culture and analysis.

Conclusions

The outcome of human bone marrow transplantation may be improved if enriched populations of early progenitors and HSCs are transplanted rather than whole bone marrow or pheresis products. This could be true in allogeneic transplants, where graft-vs.-host disease might be eliminated by T-cell depletion, and also in autotransplants, where residual tumor cells in the graft may contribute to relapse (Gazitt et al., 1995). Application of gene therapy to human immunodeficiency treatments via transplantation will also require HSC enrichment to improve the efficiency of targeting functional genes to the hematopoietic generative compartment. It is critical that we understand the biology of hematopoiesis and know how to maximize the self-renewing potential of transplanted HSCs. Researchers working in the human system must currently rely on assay systems for long-term repopulation that have not been thoroughly examined for their specific mechanism of detecting the critical (self-renewing) populations of cells. Unraveling of the mysteries of the HSC compartment has been complicated by the difficulty in obtaining native HSCs in any large quantity for classical cell biological studies. This problem is compounded by the observation that HSC biology (phenotype and function) varies among mouse strains, making concrete rules for early hematopoiesis difficult to formulate.

Several recent studies suggest that bone marrow–derived hematopoietic stem cells may have broader developmental potential than originally thought, as examples of differentiation into epithelium, hepatocytes, neurons, and muscle have been reported (Krause et al., 2001; Lagasse et al., 2000). The phenomenon of differentiation across lineage barriers is often referred to as *plasticity*. Furthermore, evidence suggests that multipotent cells capable of generating blood and other tissues exist in many adult tissues (Anderson et al., 2001). Although these new observations may open new avenues to treatment of genetic diseases, this field is still highly controversial, with reports describing both the existence and the essential lack of plasticity (Anderson et al., 2001; Wagers et al., 2002; Goodell, 2003; Raff, 2003; Theise and Wilmut, 2003; Wagers and Weissman, 2004). In some cases fusions between cells have been found as the underlying mechanism (Alvarez-Dolado et al., 2003; Vassilopoulos et al., 2003).

The marked propensity of HSCs to rapidly differentiate in most in vitro culture systems (Rebel et al., 1994) has hampered our ability to investigate under controlled, in vitro conditions the hierarchy of the HSC compartment and to approach the question of how to maintain the essential "stemness" of HSC populations. The possibility that self-renewal in the HSC compartment is limited to a finite number of cell divisions may indicate that even under the best conditions unlimited expansion of true HSCs is an impossible goal to attain. This possibility has an obvious impact on proposals for gene therapy of immunodeficiencies through transplantation, since self-renewal of transduced stem cells is the only vehicle by which this may be accomplished. At the present time, development of better clinical methods for management of the complications of allogeneic transplants may be a more expedient method by which to treat congenital immunodeficiencies.

References

Abkowitz JL, Persik MT, Shelton GH, Ott RL, Kiklevich JV, Catlin SN, Guttorp P. Behavior of hematopoietic stem cells in a large animal. Proc Natl Acad Sci USA 92:2031–2035, 1995.

Alvarez-Dolado M, Pardal R, Garcia-Verdugo JM, Fike JR, Lee HO, Pfeffer K, Lois C, Morrison SJ, Alvarez-Buylla A. Fusion of bone-marrow-derived cells with Purkinje neurons, cardiomyocytes and hepatocytes. Nature 425:968–973, 2003.

Amos TAS, Gordon MY. Sources of human hematopoietic stem cells for transplantation. Cell Transpl 4:547–569, 1995.

Anderson DJ, Gage FH, Weissman IL. Can stem cells cross lineage boundaries? Nat Med 7:393–395, 2001.

Anderson G, Jenkinson EJ, Moore NC, Owen JJ. MHC class II–positive epithelium and mesenchyme cells are both required for T-cell development in the thymus. Nature 362:70–73, 1993.

Andrews RG, Singer JW, Bernstein ID. Monoclonal antibody 12–8 recognizes a 115-kD molecule present on both unipotent and multipotent hematopoietic colony-forming cells and their precursors. Blood 67:842–845, 1986.

Archimbaud E, Philip I, Coiffier B, Michallet M, Salles G, Sebban C, Roubi N, Lopez F, Bessueille L, Mazars P, Juttner C, Atkinson K, Philip T.

CD34THY1Lin peripheral blood stem cells (PBSC) transplantation after high dose therapy for patients with multiple myeloma. Blood 88:595a, 1996.

Bartelmez SH, Bradley TR, Bertoncello I, Mochizuki DY, Tushinski RJ, Stanley ER, Hapel AJ, Young IG, Kriegler AB, Hodgson GS. Interleukin 1 plus interleukin 3 plus colony-stimulating factor 1 are essential for clonal proliferation of primitive myeloid bone marrow cells. Exp Hematol 17:240–245, 1989.

Basser RL, Rasko JE, Clarke K, Cebon J, Green MD, Hussein S, Alt C, Menchaca D, Tomita D, Marty J, Fox RM, Begley CG. Thrombopoietic effects of pegylated recombinant human megakaryocyte growth and development factor (PEG-rHuMGDF) in patients with advanced cancer. Lancet 348:1279–1281, 1996.

Baum CM, Weissman IL, Tsukamoto AS, Buckle A, Peault B. Isolation of a candidate human hematopoietic stem-cell population. Proc Natl Acad Sci USA 89:2804–2808, 1992.

Benjamin RJ, Linsley L, Axelrod JD, Churchill WH, Sieff C, Shulman LN, Elias A, Ayash L, Malachowski ME, Uhl L. The collection and evaluation of peripheral blood progenitor cells sufficient for repetitive cycles of high-dose chemotherapy support. Transfusion 35:837–844, 1995.

Berenson RJ, Bensinger WI, Hill RS, Andrews RG, Garcia-Lopez J, Kalamasz DF, Still BJ, Spitzer G, Buckner CD, Bernstein ID, Thomas ED. Engraftment after infusion of CD34 marrow cells in patients with breast cancer or neuroblastoma. Blood 77:1717–1722, 1991.

Bertoncello I, Bradley TR, Hodgson GS. The concentration and resolution of primitive hemopoietic cells from normal mouse bone marrow by negative selection using monoclonal antibodies and Dynabead monodisperse magnetic microspheres. Exp Hematol 17:171–176, 1989.

Bertoncello I, Hodgson GS, Bradley TR. Multiparameter analysis of transplantable hemopoietic stem cells: I. The separation and enrichment of stem cells homing to marrow and spleen on the basis of rhodamine-123 fluorescence. Exp Hematol 13:999–1006, 1985.

Bloom W. The embryogenesis of mammalian blood. In Downey H, ed. Handbook of Hematology. New York: Paul B Hoebar, pp. 863–922, 1938.

Bodine DM, Seidel N, Karlsson S, Nienhuis AW. The combination of IL-3 and IL-6 enhances retrovirus mediated gene transfer into hematopoietic stem cells. Prog Clin Biol Res 352:287–299, 1990.

Bodine DM, Seidel NE, Zsebo KM, Orlic D. In vivo administration of stem cell factor to mice increases the absolute number of pluripotent hematopoietic stem cells. Blood 82:445–455, 1993.

Boggs DR, Boggs SS, Saxe DF, Gress LA, Canfield DR. Hematopoietic stem cells with high proliferative potential. Assay of their concentration in marrow by the frequency and duration of cure of W/Wv mice. J Clin Invest 70:242–253, 1982.

Bradford GB, Williams B, Rossi R, Bertoncello I. Quiescence, cycling, and turnover in the primitive hematopoietic stem cell compartment. Exp Hematol 25:445–453, 1997.

Bradley TR, Metcalf D. The growth of mouse bone marrow cells in vitro. Aust J Exp Biol Med Sci 44:287–299, 1966.

Briddell RA, Broudy VC, Bruno E, Brandt JE, Srour EF, Hoffman R. Further phenotypic characterization and isolation of human hematopoietic progenitor cells using a monoclonal antibody to the c-kit receptor. Blood 79:3159–3167, 1992.

Broudy VC, Lin NL, Kaushansky K. Thrombopoietin (c-mpl ligand) acts synergistically with erythropoietin, stem cell factor, and interleukin-11 to enhance murine megakaryocyte colony growth and increases megakaryocyte ploidy in vitro. Blood 85:1719–1726, 1995.

Calvi LM, Adams GB, Weibrecht KW, Weber JM, Olson DP, Knight MC, Martin RP, Schipani E, Divieti P, Bringhurst FR, Milner LA, Kronenberg HM, Scadden DT. Osteoblastic cells regulate the haematopoietic stem cell niche. Nature 425:841–846, 2003.

Candotti F, Johnson JA, Puck JM, Sugamura K, O'Shea JJ, Blaese RM. Retroviral-mediated gene correction for X-linked severe combined immunodeficiency. Blood 87:3097–3102, 1996.

Chaudhary PM, Roninson IB. Expression and activity of P-glycoprotein, a multidrug efflux pump, in human hematopoietic stem cells. Cell 66:85–94, 1991.

Cheshier SH, Morrison SJ, Liao X, Weissman IL. In vivo proliferation and cell cycle kinetics of long-term self-renewing hematopoietic stem cells. Proc Natl Acad Sci USA 96:3120–3125, 1999.

Civin C, Strauss LC, Brovall C, Fackler MJ, Schwartz JF, Shaper JH. Antigenic analysis of hematopoiesis. III. A hematopoietic progenitor cell surface antigen defined by a monoclonal antibody raised against KG1a cells. J Immunol 133:157–165, 1984.

Cumano A, Dieterlen-Lievre F, Godin I. Lymphoid potential, probed before circulation in mouse, is restricted to caudal intraembryonic splanchnopleura. Cell 86:907–916, 1996.

de Vries P, Brasel KA, Eisenman JR, Alpert AR, Williams DE. The effect of recombinant mast cell growth factor on purified murine hematopoietic stem cells. J Exp Med 173:1205–1211, 1991.

de Vries P, Brasel KA, McKenna HJ, Williams DE, Watson JD. Thymus reconstitution by c-kit-expressing hematopoietic stem cells purified from adult mouse bone marrow. J Exp Med 176:1503–1509, 1992.

Dexter TM, Lajtha LG. Proliferation of haemopoietic stem cells in vitro. Br J Haematol 28:525–530, 1974.

Dorshkind K. Regulation of hemopoiesis by bone marrow stromal cells and their products. Annu Rev Immunol 8:111–137, 1990.

Dzierzak E, Medvinsky A. Mouse embryonic hematopoiesis. Trends Genet 11:359–366, 1995.

Enver T, Heyworth CM, Dexter TM. Do stem cells play dice? Blood 92:348–351, 1998.

Flake AW, Roncarolo MG, Puck JM, Almeida-Porada G, Evans MI, Johnson MP, Abella EM, Harrison DD, Zanjani ED. Treatment of X-linked severe combined immunodeficiency by in utero transplantation of paternal bone marrow. N Engl J Med 335:1806–1810, 1996.

Gabbianelli M, Sargiacomo M, Pelosi E, Testa U, Isacchi G, Peschle C. "Pure" human hematopoietic progenitors: permissive action of basic fibroblast growth factor. Science 249:1561–1564, 1990.

Gazitt Y, Reading CC, Hoffman R, Wickrema A, Vesole DH, Jagannath S, Condino J, Lee B, Barlogie B, Tricot G. Purified CD34 Lin Thy stem cells do not contain clonal myeloma cells. Blood 86:381–389, 1995.

Gong JK. Endosteal marrow: a rich source of hematopoietic stem cells. Science 199:1443–1445, 1978.

Goodell MA. Stem-cell "plasticity": befuddled by the muddle. Curr Opin Hematol 10:208–213, 2003.

Graham GJ, Wright EG, Hewick R, Wolpe SD, Wilkie NM, Donaldson D, Lorimore S, Pragnell IB. Identification and characterization of an inhibitor of haemopoietic stem cell proliferation. Nature 344:442–444, 1990.

Hagenaars CE, van der Kraan AAM, Kawilarang de Haas EWM, Visser JWM, Nijweide PJ. Osteoclast formation from cloned pluripotent hemopoietic stem cells. Bone Miner 6:179–189, 1989.

Harrison DE. Competitive repopulation: a new assay for long-term stem cell functional capacity. Blood 55:77–81, 1980.

Harrison DE, Stone M, Astle CM. Effects of transplantation on the primitive immunohematopoietic stem cell. J Exp Med 172:431–437, 1990.

Hodgson GS, Bradley TR. Properties of haematopoietic stem cells surviving 5-fluorouracil treatment: evidence for a pre-CFU-S cell? Nature 281:381–382, 1979.

Hodgson GS, Bradley TR. In vivo kinetic status of hematopoietic stem and progenitor cells as inferred from labeling with bromodeoxyuridine. Exp Hematol 12:683–687, 1984.

Hunt P, Robertson D, Weiss D, Rennick D, Lee F, Witte ON. A single bone marrow–derived stromal cell type supports the in vitro growth of early lymphoid and myeloid cells. Cell 48:997–1007, 1987.

Ikuta K, Kina T, MacNeil I, Uchida N, Peault B, Chien YH, Weissman IL. A developmental switch in thymic lymphocyte maturation potential occurs at the level of hematopoietic stem cells. Cell 62:863–874, 1990.

Ito K, Hirao A, Arai F, Matsuoka S, Takubo K, Hamaguchi I, Nomiyama K, Hosokawa K, Sakurada K, Nakagata N, Ikeda Y, Mak TW, Suda T. Regulation of oxidative stress by ATM is required for self-renewal of haematopoietic stem cells. Nature 431:997–1002, 2004.

Jacobsen FW, Stokke T, Jacobsen SEW. Transforming growth factor-beta potently inhibits the viability-promoting activity of stem cell factor and other cytokines and induces apoptosis of primitive murine hematopoietic progenitor cells. Blood 86:2957–2966, 1995.

Jacobsen SE, Ruscetti FW, Ortiz M, Gooya JM, Keller JR. The growth response of LinThy-1 hematopoietic progenitors to cytokines is determined by the balance between synergy of multiple stimulators and negative cooperation of multiple inhibitors. Exp Hematol 22:985–989, 1994.

Jones RJ, Celano P, Sharkis SJ, Sensenbrenner LL. Two phases of engraftment established by serial bone marrow transplantation in mice. Blood 73:397–401, 1989.

Jones RJ, Wagner JE, Celano P, Zicha MS, Sharkis SJ. Separation of pluripotent haematopoietic stem cells from spleen colony-forming cells. Nature 347:188–189, 1990.

Jordan CT, Lemischka IR. Clonal and systemic analysis of long-term hematopoiesis in the mouse. Genes Dev 4:220–232, 1990.

Jordan CT, McKearn JP, Lemischka IR. Cellular and developmental properties of fetal hematopoietic stem cells. Cell 61:953–963, 1990.

Kay HEM. How many cell generations? Lancet 2:418–419, 1965.

Kim MJ, Cooper DD, Hayes SF, Spangrude GJ. Rhodamine-123 staining in hematopoietic stem cells of young mice indicates mitochondrial activation rather than dye efflux. Blood 91:4106–4117, 1998.

Kincade PW. Molecular interactions between stromal cells and B lymphocyte precursors. Semin Immunol 3:379–390, 1991.

Kodama H, Nose M, Yamaguchi Y, Tsunoda J-I, Suda T, Nishikawa S, Nishikawa S-I. In vitro proliferation of primitive hemopoietic stem cells supported by stromal cells: evidence for the presence of a mechanism(s) other than that involving c-kit recepter and its ligand. J Exp Med 176: 351–361, 1992.

Krause DS, Theise ND, Collector MI, Henegariu O, Hwang S, Gardner R, Neutzel S, Sharkis SJ. Multi-organ, multi-lineage engraftment by a single bone marrow–derived stem cell. Cell 105:369–377, 2001.

Kriegler AB, Bradley TR, Bertoncello I, Hamilton JA, Hart PH, Piccoli DS, Hodgson GS. Progenitor cells in murine bone marrow stimulated by growth factors produced by the AF1–19T rat cell line. Exp Hematol 18: 372–378, 1990.

Lagasse E, Connors H, Al-Dhalimy M, Reitsma M, Dohse M, Osborne L, Wang X, Finegold M, Weissman IL, Grompe M. Purified hematopoietic stem cells can differentiate into hepatocytes in vivo. Nat Med 6:1229–1234, 2000.

Leary AG, Wong GG, Clark SC, Smith AG, Ogawa M. Leukemia inhibitory factor differentiation-inhibiting activity/human interleukin for DA cells augments proliferation of human hematopoietic stem cells. Blood 75: 1960–1964, 1990.

Lewis JP, Trobaugh FE Jr. Haematopoietic stem cells. Nature 204:589–590, 1964.

Li CL, Johnson GR. Rhodamine 123 reveals heterogeneity within murine Lin, Sca-1 hemopoietic stem cells. J Exp Med 175:1443–1447, 1992.

Long MW, Briddell R, Walter AW, Bruno E, Hoffman R. Human hematopoietic stem cell adherence to cytokines and matrix molecules. J Clin Invest 90:251–255, 1992.

Lord BI, Testa NG, Hendry JH. The relative spacial distributions of CFUs and CFUc in the normal mouse femur. Blood 46:65–72, 1975.

Lowry PA, Deacon D, Whitefield P, McGrath HE, Quesenberry PJ. Stem cell factor induction of in vitro murine hematopoietic colony formation by "subliminal" cytokine combinations: the role of "anchor factors". Blood 80:663–669, 1992.

Magli MC, Iscove NN, Odartchenko N. Transient nature of early haematopoietic spleen colonies. Nature 295:527–529, 1982.

McCune JM, Namikawa R, Kaneshima H, Shultz LD, Lieberman M, Weissman IL. The SCID-hu mouse: murine model for the analysis of human hematolymphoid differentiation and function. Science 241:1632–1639, 1988.

Medvinsky A, Dzierzak E. Definitive hematopoiesis is autonomously initiated by the AGM region. Cell 86:897–906, 1996.

Metcalf D. The molecular control of cell division, differentiation commitment and maturation in haemopoietic cells. Nature 339:27–30, 1989.

Metcalf D. Lineage commitment and maturation in hematopoietic cells: the case for extrinsic regulation. Blood 92:345–347, 1998.

Micklem HS, Anderson N, Ross E. Limited potential of circulating haemopoietic stem cells. Nature 256:41–43, 1975.

Micklem HS, Lennon JE, Ansell JD, Gray RA. Numbers and dispersion of repopulating hematopoietic cell clones in radiation chimeras as functions of injected cell dose. Exp Hematol 15:251–257, 1987.

Morrison SJ, Weissman IL. The long-term repopulating subset of hematopoietic stem cells is deterministic and isolatable by phenotype. Immunity 1:661–673, 1994.

Mulder AH, Bauman JG, Visser JWM, Boersma WJ, van den Engh GJ. Separation of spleen colony-forming units and prothymocytes by use of a monoclonal antibody detecting an H-2K determinant. Cell Immunol 88: 401–410, 1984.

Muller AM, Medvinsky A, Strouboulis J, Grosveld F, Dzierzak E. Development of hematopoietic stem cell activity in the mouse embryo. Immunity 1:291–301, 1994.

Muller-Sieburg CE, Whitlock CA, Weissman IL. Isolation of two early B lymphocyte progenitors from mouse marrow: a committed pre-pre-B cell and a clonogenic Thy-1-lo hematopoietic stem cell. Cell 44:653–662, 1986.

Mulligan RC. The basic science of gene therapy. Science 260:926–932, 1993.

Murray L, Chen B, Galy A, Chen S, Tushinski R, Uchida N, Negrin R, Tricot G, Jagannath S, Vesole D, Barlogie B, Hoffman R, Tsukamoto A. Enrichment of human hematopoietic stem cell activity in the CD34Thy-1Lin subpopulation from mobilized peripheral blood. Blood 85:368–378, 1995.

Nakauchi H. Hematopoietic stem cells: are they CD34-positive or CD34-negative? Nat Med 4:1009–1010, 1998.

Neben S, Anklesaria P, Greenberger J, Mauch P. Quantitation of murine hematopoietic stem cells in vitro by limiting dilution analysis of cobblestone area formation on a clonal stromal cell line. Exp Hematol 21: 438–443, 1993.

Neben S, Redfearn WJ, Parra M, Brecher G, Pallavicini MG. Short- and long-term repopulation of lethally irradiated mice by bone marrow stem cells enriched on the basis of light scatter and Hoechst 33342 fluorescence. Exp Hematol 19:958–967, 1991.

Okada S, Nakauchi H, Nagayoshi K, Nishikawa S, Miura Y, Suda T. Enrichment and characterization of murine hematopoietic stem cells that express c-kit molecule. Blood 78:1706–1712, 1991a.

Okada S, Suda T, Suda J, Tokuyama N, Nagayoshi K, Miura Y, Nakauchi H. Effects of interleukin 3, interleukin 6, and granulocyte colony-stimulating factor on sorted murine splenic progenitor cells. Exp Hematol 19:42–46, 1991b.

Orlic D, Bodine DM. What defines a pluripotent hematopoietic stem cell (PHSC): will the real PHSC please stand up! Blood 84:3991–3994, 1994.

Ploemacher RE, Brons NHC. In vivo proliferative and differential properties of murine bone marrow cells separated on the basis of rhodamine-123 retention. Exp Hematol 16:903–907, 1988.

Ploemacher RE, Brons RHC. Separation of CFU-S from primitive cells responsible for reconstitution of the bone marrow hemopoietic stem cell compartment following irradiation: evidence for a pre-CFU-S cell. Exp Hematol 17:263–266, 1989.

Ploemacher RE, van der Sluijs JP, van Beurden CAJ, Baert MRM, Chan PL. Use of limiting-dilution type long-term marrow cultures in frequency analysis of marrow-repopulating and spleen colony-forming hematopoietic stem cells in the mouse. Blood 78:2527–2533, 1991.

Ploemacher RE, van der Sluijs JP, Voerman JS, Brons NHC. An in vitro limiting-dilution assay of long-term repopulating hematopoietic stem cells in the mouse. Blood 74:2755–2763, 1989.

Raff M. Adult stem cell plasticity: fact or artifact? Annu Rev Cell Dev Biol 19:1–22, 2003.

Rebel VI, Dragowska W, Eaves CJ, Humphries RK, Lansdorp PM. Amplification of Sca-1LinWGA cells in serum-free cultures containing steel factor, interleukin-6, and erythropoietin with maintenance of cells with long-term in vivo reconstituting potential. Blood 83:128–136, 1994.

Rogers JA, Berman JW. TNF-alpha inhibits the further development of committed progenitors while stimulating multipotential progenitors in mouse long-term bone marrow cultures. J Immunol 153:4694–4703, 1994.

Rosendaal M, Hodgson GS, Bradley TR. Haemopoietic stem cells are organised for use on the basis of their generation-age. Nature 264:68–69, 1976.

Schultz LD, Sidman CL. Genetically determined murine models of immunodeficiency. Annu Rev Immunol 5:367–404, 1987.

Shah AJ, Smogorzewska EM, Hannum C, Crooks GM. Flt3 ligand induces proliferation of quiescent human bone marrow CD34CD38 cells and maintains progenitor cells in vitro. Blood 87:3563–3570, 1996.

Shpall EJ, Jones RB, Bearman SI, Purdy MH, Franklin WA, Heimfeld S, Berenson RJ. Transplantation of CD34 hematopoietic progenitor cells. J Hematother 3:145–147, 1994.

Siena S, Bregni M, Brando B, Ravagnani F, Bonadonna G, Gianni AM. Circulation of CD34 hematopoietic stem cells in the peripheral blood of high-dose cyclophoshamide-treated patients: enhancement by intravenous recombinant human granulocyte-macrophage colony-stimulating factor. Blood 74:1905–1914, 1989.

Siminovitch L, McCulloch EA, Till JE. The distribution of colony-forming cells among spleen colonies. J Cell Comp Physiol 62:327–336, 1963.

Siminovitch L, Till JE, McCulloch EA. Decline in colony-forming ability of marrow cells subjected to serial transplantation into irradiated mice. J Cell Comp Physiol 64:23–32, 1964.

Sitnicka E, Lin N, Priestley GV, Fox N, Broudy VC, Wolf NS, Kaushansky K. The effect of thrombopoietin on the proliferation and differentiation of murine hematopoietic stem cells. Blood 87:4998–5005, 1996.

Smith LG, Weissman IL, Heimfeld S. Clonal analysis of hematopoietic stem-cell differentiation in vivo. Proc Natl Acad Sci USA 88:2788–2792, 1991.

Spangrude GJ. Enrichment of murine haemopoietic stem cells: diverging roads. Immunol Today 10:344–350, 1989.

Spangrude GJ. Characteristics of the hematopoietic stem cell compartment in adult mice. Int J Cell Cloning 10:277–285, 1992.

Spangrude GJ, Brooks DM. Phenotypic analysis of mouse hematopoietic stem cells shows a Thy-1-snegative subset. Blood 80:1957–1964, 1992.

Spangrude GJ, Brooks DM. Mouse strain variability in the expression of the hematopoietic stem cell antigen Ly-6A/E by bone marrow cells. Blood 82:3327–3332, 1993.

Spangrude GJ, Brooks DM, Tumas DB. Long-term repopulation of irradiated mice with limiting numbers of purified hematopoietic stem cells: in vivo expansion of stem cell phenotype but not function. Blood 85:1006–1016, 1995.

Spangrude GJ, Heimfeld S, Weissman IL. Purification and characterization of mouse hematopoietic stem cells. Science 241:58–62, 1988.

Spangrude GJ, Johnson GR. Resting and activated subsets of mouse multipotent hematopoietic stem cells. Proc Natl Acad Sci USA 87:7433–7437, 1990.

Spooncer E, Lord BI, Dexter TM. Defective ability to self-renew in vitro of highly purified primitive haematopoietic cells. Nature 316:62–64, 1985.

Stier S, Ko Y, Forkert R, Lutz C, Neuhaus T, Grunewald E, Cheng T, Dombkowski D, Calvi LM, Rittling SR, Scadden DT. Osteopontin is a hematopoietic stem cell niche component that negatively regulates stem cell pool size. J Exp Med 201:1781–1791, 2005.

Srour EF, Leemhuis T, Brandt JE, vanBesien K, Hoffman R. Simultaneous use of rhodamine 123, phycoerythrin, Texas red, and allophycocyanin for the isolation of human hematopoietic progenitor cells. Cytometry 12:179–183, 1991.

Suda T, Arai F, Hirao A. Hematopoietic stem cells and their niche. Trends Immunol 2005 in press.

Sutherland HJ, Lansdorp PM, Henkelman DH, Eaves AC, Eaves CJ. Functional characterization of individual human hematopoietic stem cells cultured at limiting dilution on supportive marrow stromal layers. Proc Natl Acad Sci USA 87:3584–3588, 1990.

Szilvassy SJ, Humphries RK, Lansdorp PM, Eaves AC, Eaves CJ. Quantitative assay for totipotent reconstituting hematopoietic stem cells by a competitive repopulation strategy. Proc Natl Acad Sci USA 87:8736–8740, 1990.

Szilvassy SJ, Weller KP, Chen B, Juttner CA, Tsukamoto A, Hoffman R. Partially differentiated ex vivo expanded cells accelerate hematologic recovery in myeloablated mice transplanted with highly enriched long-term repopulating stem cells. Blood 88:3642–3653, 1996.

Testa NG, Dexter TM. Cell lineages in haemopoiesis: comments on their regulation. Semin Immunol 2:167–172, 1990.

Theise ND, Wilmut I. Cell plasticity: flexible arrangement. Nature 425:21, 2003.

Till JE, McCulloch EA. A direct measurement of the radiation sensitivity of normal mouse bone marrow cells. Radiat Res 14:213–222, 1961.

Tuchmann-Duplessis H, David G, Haegel P. Illustrated Human Embryology, Vol. 1: Embryogenesis (translated by L.S. Hurley). Paris: Masson, 1975.

Uchida N, Aguila HL, Fleming WH, Jerabek L, Weissman IL. Rapid and sustained hematopoietic recovery in lethally irradiated mice transplanted with purified Thy-1.1-lo LinSca-1 hematopoietic stem cells. Blood 83:3758–3779, 1994.

van der Sluijs JP, de Jong JP, Brons NHC, Ploemacher RE. Marrow repopulating cells, but not CFU-S, establish long-term in vitro hemopoiesis on a marrow-derived stromal layer. Exp Hematol 18:893–896, 1990.

van der Sluijs JP, van den Bos C, Baert MRM, van Beurden CAJ, Ploemacher RE. Loss of long-term repopulating ability in long-term bone-marrow culture. Leukemia 7:725–732, 1993.

Van Zant G, Holland BP, Eldridge PW, Chen JJ. Genotype-restricted growth and aging patterns in hematopoietic stem cell populations of allophenic mice. J Exp Med 171:1547–1565, 1990.

Van Zant G, Scott-Micus K, Thompson BP, Fleischman RA, Perkins S. Stem cell quiescence/activation is reversible by serial transplantation and is independent of stromal cell genotype in mouse aggregation chimeras. Exp Hematol 20:470–475, 1992.

Vassilopoulos G, Wang PR, Russell DW. Transplanted bone marrow regenerates liver by cell fusion. Nature 422:901–924, 2003.

Visnjic D, Kalajzic Z, Rowe DW, Katavic V, Lorenzo J, Aguila HL. Hematopoiesis is severely altered in mice with an induced osteoblast deficiency. Blood 103:3258–3264, 2004.

Visser JWM, Bauman JGJ, Mulder AH, Eliason JF, de Leeuw AM. Isolation of murine pluripotent hemopoietic stem cells. J Exp Med 159:1576–1590, 1984.

Visser JWM, Van Bekkum DW. Purification of pluripotent hemopoietic stem cells: past and present. Exp Hematol 18:248–256, 1990.

Wagers AJ, Sherwood RI, Christensen JL, Weissman IL. Little evidence for developmental plasticity of adult hematopoietic stem cells. Science 297:2256–2259, 2002.

Wagers AJ, Weissman IL. Plasticity of adult stem cells. Cell 116:639–648, 2004.

Wang JC, Lapidot T, Cashman JD, Doedens M, Addy L, Sutherland DR, Nayar R, Laraya P, Minden M, Keating A, Eaves AC, Eaves CJ, Dick JE. High level engraftment of NOD/SCID mice by primitive normal and leukemic hematopoietic cells from patients with chronic myeloid leukemia in chronic phase. Blood 91:2406–2414, 1998.

Weaver CH, Buckner CD, Longin K, Appelbaum FR, Rowley S, Lilleby K, Miser J, Storb R, Hansen JA, Bensinger W. Syngeneic transplantation with peripheral blood mononuclear cells collected after the administration of recombinant human granulocyte colony-stimulating factor. Blood 82: 1981–1984, 1993.

Weilbaecher K, Weissman I, Blume K, Heimfeld S. Culture of phenotypically defined hematopoietic stem cells and other progenitors at limiting dilution on Dexter monolayers. Blood 78:945–952, 1991.

Whitlock CA, Witte ON. Long-term culture of B lymphocytes and their precursors from murine bone marrow. Proc Natl Acad Sci USA 79:3608–3612, 1982.

Wintrobe MM. The origin and development of the cells of the blood in the embryo, infant, and adult. In: Clinical Hematology. Philadelphia: Lea and Febiger, pp. 1–62, 1967.

Witte ON. Steel locus defines new multipotent growth factor. Cell 63:5–6, 1990.

Wolf NS, Kone A, Priestley GV, Bartelmez SH. In vivo and in vitro characterization of long-term repopulating primitive hematopoietic cells isolated by sequential Hoechst 33342-rhodamine 123 FACS selection. Exp Hematol 21:614–622, 1993.

Wolf NS, Priestley GV. Kinetics of early and late spleen colony development. Exp Hematol 14:676–682, 1986.

Wolf NS, Trentin JJ. Hemopoietic colony studies. V. Effect of hemopoietic organ stroma on differentiation of pluripotent stem cells. J Exp Med 127: 205–214, 1968.

Worton RG, McCulloch EA, Till JE. Physical separation of hemopoietic stem cells differing in their capacity for self-renewal. J Exp Med 130:91–103, 1969a.

Worton RG, McCulloch EA, Till JE. Physical separation of hemopoietic stem cells from cells forming colonies in culture. J Cell Physiol 74:171–182, 1969b.

Yoder MC, Hiatt K. Engraftment of embryonic hematopoietic cells in conditioned newborn recipients. Blood 89:2176–2183, 1997.

Zhang J, Niu C, Ye L, Huang H, He X, Tong WG, Ross J, Haug J, Johnson T, Feng JQ, Harris S, Wiedemann LM, Mishina Y, Li L. Identification of the haematopoietic stem cell niche and control of the niche size. Nature 425: 836–841, 2003.

4

T Cell Development

RAE S. M. YEUNG, PAMELA S. OHASHI, MARY E. SAUNDERS, and TAK W. MAK

The purpose of this chapter is to give a broad overview of some of the complexities involved in T cell development. T cells are key regulators of specific immunity, and their function is determined by events that occur during an intricate developmental process in the thymus. An understanding of T cell development is thus fundamental to our understanding of immune responses. While a variety of different receptor–ligand interactions are important during T cell development, none are as crucial as those mediated via the T cell antigen receptor (TCR). Although the exact nature of the TCR was not elucidated until the early 1980s (Hedrick et al., 1984; Yanagi et al., 1984), experiments done in the 1970s led to the finding that T cell specificity is linked to proteins encoded by genes in the major histocompatibility complex (MHC) (Shearer, 1974; Zinkernagel and Doherty, 1974). The MHC is known as the H-2 complex in mice and as the HLA (human leukocyte antigen) complex in humans. Unlike B cells, T cells generally do not respond to whole protein or native antigens. Instead, T cells recognize peptide fragments of foreign or self-antigens complexed with MHC molecules. Furthermore, a given T cell recognizes only a particular peptide–MHC complex in a process referred to as *MHC restriction* (Zinkernagel and Doherty, 1979).

The interaction of a developing thymocyte's TCR with peptide presented on self-MHC in the thymus determines the fate of that thymocyte. Only some become the mature T cells that patrol the body's periphery and respond to foreign antigen. The molecular interactions that lead to the elimination of self-reactive thymocytes ("negative selection") and the survival of those that can potentially mount protective immune responses ("positive selection") are complex. Our understanding of thymic ontogeny has been greatly enhanced through the use of genetic tools, particularly mutant animal models. In this context, the use of *transgenic* and *gene-targeted* mice has been especially revealing. We begin

this chapter with a brief description of these technologies and their utility. We then give overviews of the TCR proteins and the genes encoding them, followed by a discussion of the coreceptors CD4 and CD8, which have enormous influence on T cell development. Finally, we describe the stages of T cell development in detail at both the cellular and molecular levels, noting where appropriate the various mutations that have helped to define each stage.

Transgenic and Gene Targeting Technology

T cell development consists of a sequence of well-coordinated processes in which immature progenitor cells enter the thymus, participate in a complex developmental process, and emerge as mature T cells able to function in host defence. In the past, it was difficult to dissect the unique roles of the multitude of genes involved in thymocyte maturation. Natural mouse mutants existed and furnished much information on immune system development but, in most cases, the identity of the genes mutated in these animals was unknown. With the advent of recombinant DNA technology in the 1970s, it became possible to splice different gene sequences and their control elements together. Subsequent refinements allowed the expression of exogenous genes in experimental animals, an investigative method called *transgenesis*. As is detailed throughout this chapter, the study of transgenic mice bearing genes of relevance to immune responses revealed much about their function (Cantrell, 2002). However, the expression of these genes was necessarily nonphysiologic, and researchers sought a means of eliminating the function of a specific endogenous gene to determine its effects. In 1989, *gene-targeting* technology was developed which allowed researchers to delete a single gene in a whole animal. The study of these genetically modified "knockout" mice has provided us with invaluable data on the functions of single genes in vivo (Mak et al., 2001). Immunologists readily embraced gene-targeting technology because the loss of many immunological genes is still compatible with normal embryonic development, meaning that a relatively healthy mutant animal can often be recovered and studied.

We will now give a short description of methodologies underlying transgenesis and gene targeting, and the related methodology of RAG complementation.

Transgenesis

Transgenesis is the expression of an exogenous gene of interest in a cell. By placing the transgene of interest under the control of a tissue-specific promoter, the effect of the gene on a specific cell type can be examined. The copy number and location of integration of the transgene in the host cell genome can affect its expression. When and where the transgene's promoter is operational are also relevant, as transgene expression may be activated at different times or at different locations in different cell types. Transgenes are useful for probing the relationship between structure and function of a molecule: the expression of a mutated version of a protein that has been engineered to lack a particular domain may reveal the importance of that domain or protein. Transgenes can also be used to rescue function in gene-deficient mice and thus assess the nature of the original defect. For example, if a mutant in which a developmental process is blocked can be rescued by the overexpression of a molecule known to promote cell survival, it is likely that the original mutation affected a protein with a role in survival. This protein may be quite distinct from the product of the transgene.

A *dominant negative* (D^{m}N) transgene can be used to interfere with the expression of an endogenous protein. Often the protein derived from a D^{m}N transgene is a catalytically inactive version of the molecule of interest, the theory being that large quantities of such a protein (5- to 10-fold excess) will compete with the endogenous protein for essential substrates or cofactors. It should be ensured that the promoter used to drive D^{m}N transgene expression is capable of achieving the necessary high level of expression. It is also essential to determine how much interference is required to completely inactivate the endogenous protein, and how specific an inhibitor the D^{m}N molecule truly is. It is not unusual for a D^{m}N inhibitor to sequester molecular intermediates needed by more than one endogenous enzyme or pathway. This latter characteristic can be an advantage when one wants to overcome redundancy of function and simultaneously disable all isoforms of a protein of interest.

Constitutively active transgenes can also be constructed to overcome natural control mechanisms within a cell. Mutations of residues in negative control sequences or enzymatic catalytic sites can result in constitutive activation of a protein. A difficulty with these types of mutants is that nonphysiological expression of the gene in question occurs by definition: the molecule is likely not produced at either the normal location, time, or concentration, forcing a guarded intepretation of results. Temporal control of transgenes can be exerted by placing them under the control of promoters engineered to be regulated by the addition of the antibiotic tetracycline (Gossen et al., 1995) or the synthetic estrogen tamoxifen (Littlewood et al., 1995). Transgenes encoding bacterial toxins are valuable tools because of their specificity and high potency at low concentration. For example, transgenes encoding the bacterial cholera, botulism, and pertussis toxins have been used as inhibitors to determine the roles of G proteins in various intracellular signaling pathways (Chaffin and Perlmutter, 1991; Henning et al., 1997).

With respect to studying T-cell development, transgenes have been placed under the control of various promoters that restrict expression of the genes they regulate primarily to the T lineage. Such promoters include the proximal promoter of the gene encoding the Src family protein tyrosine kinase p56^{Lck} (Lck) (Allan et al., 1992), the promoters of the genes encoding the CD4 and CD8 coreceptors (Ellmeier et al., 1999), and a modified CD2 promoter (Zhumabekov et al., 1995). These promoters are expressed both in thymocytes and in peripheral T cells but at different stages of development. For example, the expression of transgenes under the control of the Lck promoter can be detected in the earliest thymocytes, whereas the CD2 promoter is generally not activated until a later stage.

While "standard" trangenesis as described above is undeniably a powerful and useful technology, it has the disadvantage of random integration of the transgene. Knock-in technology rectifies this defect because the transgene is introduced into a precise location in the genome by homologous recombination—that is, the transgene is designed such that sequences flanking the gene of interest are homologous in sequence to the endogenous locus and thus ensure that the transgene integrates in its natural position. The natural transcription controls of the gene of interest are thus preserved (unlike standard transgenesis) and the danger of overexpression artefacts is reduced. Knock-in mutations can be used to introduce reporter constructs to facilitate detection of a hard-to-monitor gene, or regulatory constructs can be added to alter expression patterns. For example, to investigate control of IL-4 expression in vivo, a reporter gene was "knocked into" the IL-4 locus (Pannetier et al., 1999). This study led to the generation of much useful information on the regulation of effector T-cell differentiation (Hu-Li et al., 2001).

Gene Targeting

The basic principle of gene targeting is replacement of the gene of interest via homologous recombination between exogenous DNA (a targeting vector or knock-out construct) and its endogenous chromosomal homologue (Capecchi, 1989; reviewed in Koller and Smithies, 1992) (Fig. 4.1). The targeting vector contains flanking sequences that are identical to endogenous DNA sequences, ensuring that the endogenous gene is replaced with the mutated version. The homologous recombination event yields an insertion, replacement, or deletion of the targeted genomic locus, depending on the design of the knockout construct. It was shown in the early 1980s that multipotent embryonic stem (ES) cells from mouse embryos could be cultured and manipulated in vitro and then reintegrated back into a wild-type mouse blastocyst. When returned to the embryonic environment, the manipulated ES cells resumed normal development and contributed to all cell lineages including germ cells. By combining gene-targeting technology with the transfection and culture of murine ES cells, mice with mutations in a single gene can be generated. To create a knockout mouse, murine ES cells are injected in vitro with the targeting vector. To enrich for those rare ES cells that have undergone homologous recombination, a selectable marker gene, such as that encoding neomycin resistance, is usually included in the targeting construct. A negative selection marker (such as a toxic gene) may also be included in the flanking region of the construct to kill cells in which random integration of the targeting construct has occurred (Yagi et al., 1990; Hasty et al., 1991). Embryonic stem cells that have undergone homologous recombination are detected by polymerase chain reaction (PCR) assays and confirmed by genomic Southern blot analysis (Capecchi,

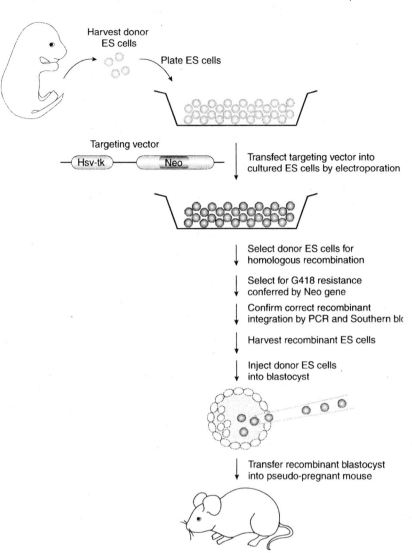

Figure 4.1. The classical approach to gene targeting in embryonic stem (ES) cells. Gene targeting is carried out in wild-type mouse ES cells cultured for manipulation. A targeting construct is engineered in which the gene of interest is disrupted by the insertion of the *neo* gene. The thymidine kinase *Hsv-tk* gene can be placed outside the target gene as a negative selection marker. The construct is transfected into the cultured ES cells, usually by electroporation. If homologous recombination occurs, only the *neo*/target gene sequences will be inserted into the chromosomal DNA of the ES cells. Selection with the neomycin-like drug G418 will kill any nonrecombinant ES cells. Selection with gancyclovir will kill any nonhomologous recombinants carrying the *Hsv-tk* gene. ES cells heterozygous for the targeted mutation as confirmed by polymerase chain reaction (PCR) and Southern blotting are injected into a mouse blastocyst. The chimeric blastocyst is then implanted into a pseudopregnant female. Homozygosity for the targeted mutation is achieved by subsequent breeding steps.

1989). The recombinant cells are microinjected into a mouse blastocyst which is then implanted into a pseudopregnant female. The resulting chimeric mice transmit the knockout genes to their offspring (Robertson et al., 1986). The progeny are analyzed for presence of the knockout mutation and interbred to achieve homozygosity. The phenotype of the null-mutant mouse is then assessed to obtain knowledge of the gene's function.

While gene knockouts are extremely useful for deducing the functions of many genes, there are some caveats to their use. Unanticipated alternative or aberrant splicing of exons or the synthesis of truncated translation products can complicate interpretation of the data. In addition, an engineered mutation in one gene may have an unexpected effect on a neighboring gene, making it difficult to distinguish the true source of the observed phenotype. Mutations that affect the architecture of an organ may indirectly influence the differentiation or behavior of the cells of interest within it. Genetic background can have a huge influence on expression of the phenotype of the mutant mouse, and redundancy in molecular systems may mean that the function of missing gene may be compensated for by the function of another gene. Finally, if the gene in question has a double function in the immune system and in embryonic development, embryonic or perinatal lethality may preclude analysis of the gene's function in adult tissues.

Some of these problems can be circumvented by the Cre-LoxP and FLP-FRT recombination systems that allow tissue- or stage-specific gene expression (Metzger and Chambon, 2001). In the former, Cre recombinase from bacteriophage P1 recognizes bacterial LoxP sequences flanking the mammalian genomic DNA to be deleted. Cre-mediated recombination of two loxP sites in *cis* orientation results in the deletion of all DNA between them (Sternberg et al., 1986). FLP-recombinase from yeast carries out the same function by recombining flanking FRT sequences (O'Gorman et al., 1991). Transgenic expression of Cre or FLP by use of a tissue-specific promoter thus allows the generation of tissue-specific knockouts. For example, constructs in which Cre expression is controlled by the T cell–specific promoter of the Lck gene can be used to induce the deletion of loxP-flanked genes only in T cells (Fig. 4.2). Inducible knockout of a gene can be achieved by placing Cre under the control of tetracycline transactivation systems, insect hormones, or analogues of mammalian steroid hormones (Kuhn et al., 1995; Rajewsky et al., 1996). A caveat with respect to the use of Cre recombinase (in particular) is that the efficiency of gene deletion in a tissue will depend on the efficiency of transgenic Cre expression in that tissue, a highly variable parameter.

A specific mutation of a gene of interest can also be generated using the knock-in approach. For example, a knock-in construct

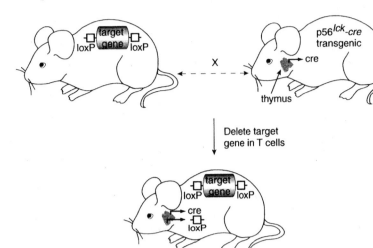

Figure 4.2. Cre/loxP-mediated gene targeting. Genetic manipulation of ES cells produces a mouse in which the gene of interest is "floxed," or flanked by two *loxP* sites. The floxed mouse is then crossed with a transgenic mouse expressing *Cre* recombinase under the control of a tissue-specific promoter; in this case, the p56^lck promoter which is active only in T cells. Cre expressed in the thymi of the double transgenic progeny of this cross recombines adjacent *loxP* sites and deletes the gene of interest only in T cells.

was created in which the dimerization domain of the key hematopoietic signaling phosphatase CD45 was disrupted by a point mutation. Analyses of transgenic animals expressing this mutated gene showed that CD45 activity was lost in the absence of the dimerization function and that control of lymphocyte proliferation was compromised (Majeti et al., 2000).

RAG Complementation

RAG complementation provides a system in which to test the role of a particular gene in lymphocyte development and function. The recombination activation genes (*Rag1* and *Rag2*) are essential for V(D)J rearrangement of the antigen receptor genes in B and T cells (Schatz et al., 1989). Mice lacking either RAG1 or RAG2 are viable but lack mature T and B cells (Shinkai et al., 1992, 1993; Mombaerts et al., 1992b). When ES cells homozygous for a knockout mutation are microinjected into blastocysts of RAG-deficient mice, all lymphocytes developing in these chimeric animals are necessarily derived from the RAG+ knockout ES cells (Chen et al., 1994) (Fig. 4.3). The effect of the knockout mutation on specific immunity can then be analyzed. RAG complementation is particularly useful when the homozygous knockout phenotype is embryonic lethal.

TCR/CD3 Complex

We now return to the T cell itself, first examining the structure of its antigen receptor. The TCR is responsible for the recognition of both foreign and self antigens, and thus is central to both T-cell development and the mounting of specific immune responses. Inability to recognize foreign antigen can lead to overwhelming infection, while inappropriate recognition of self-antigen can result in autoimmunity.

TCRs are heterodimeric proteins composed of either TCRα and β chains, or TCRγ and δ chains. Thymocytes and the majority of peripheral T cells bear αβ TCRs but about 5%–10% of all T cells bear γδ TCRs. All TCRαβ heterodimers recognize peptides complexed with MHC molecules, but some TCRγδ molecules recognize nonpeptide antigens either directly or bound to the MHC-like molecule CD1. For both αβ and γδ TCRs, recognition of the antigen depends on the binding site formed by portions of the αβ or γδ chains. However, surface expression of the TCR and antigen-specific T-cell signaling and activation depend on the association of the TCR with the CD3 complex. The CD3

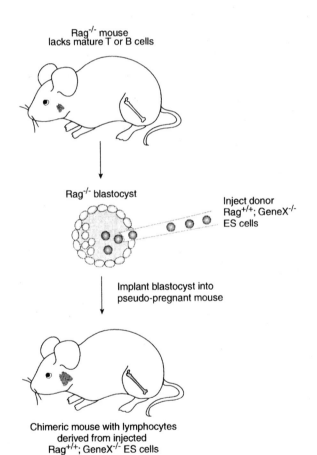

Figure 4.3. RAG-deficient blastocyst complementation. Mice deficient for either RAG1 or RAG2 are viable but lack mature T and B lymphocytes. To examine lymphocyte development and behavior in the absence of a gene of interest (gene X), wild-type embryonic stem (ES) cells homozygous for deletion of gene X (RAG+/+; gene X−/−) are injected into RAG-deficient blastocysts. The chimeric blastocysts are implanted in pseudopregnant females where they develop into pups in which any lymphocytes present are necessarily derived from the gene X−/− ES cells. Because the gene deletion in this system is somatic, RAG complementation is particularly useful for examining the function in lymphocyte development of genes that are embryonic lethal when deleted in the germ line.

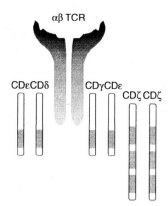

Figure 4.4. αβTCR/CD3 on the cell surface. Schematic drawing of the αβTCR/CD3 complex in the T-cell membrane. The TCRαβ heterodimer is associated with three other CD3 dimers: CD3εδ, CD3γε, and (most often) CD3ζζ. The CD3ε, δ, and γ chains each contain one immunoreceptor tyrosine-based activation motif (ITAM) sequence (black rectangles) important for signal transduction, while the CDζ chain contains three ITAMs. The TCRαβ heterodimer is responsible for antigen recognition, whereas the CD3 chains convey intracellular signals via activation of kinases associated with their cytoplasmic tails (see Fig. 4.6).

complex consists of at least five distinct membrane proteins, CD3γ, δ, ε, ζ, and η, which are noncovalently associated both with each other and the TCR heterodimer (Weiss and Littman, 1994). The CD3γ, δ, and ε chains are found as γε and δε subunits within the TCR/CD3 complex (Blumberg et al., 1990; Malissen and Malissen, 1996), whereas the ζ chain is found as a homodimer (in 90% of TCRs) or as a ζη heterodimer (~10% of TCRs). The CD3ζ and η chains are splice variants derived from the same gene. Other splice variants encoded by the CD3ζ gene have been described, such as CD3θ and CD3ι (Malissen and Malissen, 1996). The minimal stoichiometry of the most common αβ TCRs is TCRαβ: CD3γεCD3δεCD3ζζ (Fig. 4.4). All CD3 chains contain at least one of the tyrosine-rich immunoreceptor tyrosine-based activation motifs (ITAMs) essential for initiating intracellular signaling following antigen binding to the TCR.

TCR Genes

An αβ TCR binds to peptide–MHC via its variable (V) region located at the extracellular N-terminus of the heterodimer. The V region is linked to an invariable extracellular region, a transmembrane domain, and a short intracellular domain at the carboxyl terminus of the protein. These latter elements are encoded by the constant (C) region exons of the TCR loci (Davis and Bjorkman, 1988). The V regions of both component TCR chains contribute to the antigen binding site, and each chain's V region is encoded by a V exon. Analogous to the immunoglobulin (Ig) light-chain gene, the TCRα and γ V exons contain a V (variable) and a J (joining) gene segment, while, like the Ig heavy-chain gene, the TCRβ and δ V exons contain a V, a D (diversity), and a J gene segment. In each developing thymocyte, the V and J or V, D, and J gene segments forming the V exons are randomly chosen from the huge array of multiple V, D, and J gene segments present in germline TCR loci. In a process known as *somatic gene rearrangement*, the site-specific RAG1/2 recombinases initiate the joining of the chosen V, D, and J gene segments at the DNA level (Schatz et al., 1989; Chen et al., 1994). The double-stranded DNA protein kinase (dsDNA-PK) catalyzes the ligation of the rearranged gene segments to form a complete and

unique V exon for each TCR chain in each developing thymocyte (Kirchgessner et al., 1995). The V exon sequences are then joined to the C exon sequences by conventional RNA splicing prior to translation of both chains and heterodimer assembly. It is the random rearrangement of V(D)J gene segments that generates most of the enormous diversity of TCRs expressed on mature T cells (Toyonaga et al., 1985; Davis and Bjorkman, 1998). Additional diversity is introduced at V-D-J junctions through the introduction of template-independent (or N) nucleotides during V(D)J rearrangement. N-nucleotide addition is mediated by the enzyme terminal deoxynucleotidyl transferase (TdT) (Tonegawa, 1983).

The Coreceptors

While the TCR antigen binding site is responsible for the recognition of specific peptide in the binding groove of an MHC molecule, the CD8 and CD4 molecules function as coreceptors by binding to nonpolymorphic regions of the MHC class I and class II molecules, respectively. The coreceptors facilitate TCR signal transduction because the cytoplasmic domains of both CD4 and CD8 are physically associated (with differing stoichiometry) with Lck tyrosine kinase (see below; Veillette et al., 1988; Turner et al., 1990; Weiss and Littman, 1994). Both CD4 and CD8 have important roles in the ontogeny and selection of thymocytes and in the activation of mature T cells resident in peripheral lymphatic organs (Wallace et al., 1993).

CD8 and MHC Class I

CD8 is a cell surface glycoprotein expressed on MHC class I–restricted T cells. In mice, thymocytes and peripheral T cells generally express CD8 as heterodimers of CD8α (Lyt-2) and CD8β (Lyt-3). On human T cells, CD8 is composed of homodimers of a single subunit, the homologue of murine CD8α. The greatest sequence similarity between human and murine CD8α is located in the transmembrane (79%) and cytoplasmic (5%) domains (Littman, 1987). The MHC class I molecule to which CD8 binds is a heterodimer composed of an MHC class I α chain noncovalently associated with the invariant β2-microglobulin (β2M) chain. The corresponding gene symbol is *B2m*. β2M is crucial for the expression of the MHC class I molecule on the cell surface. The peptides associated with MHC class I molecules are generally derived from endogenous proteins degraded by proteasomes in the cytosol. The peptides are translocated into the endoplasmic reticulum (ER) by a heterodimeric transmembrane transporter complex with structural similarity to ATP binding cassette transporters (Spies and DeMars, 1991). The TAP1 (transporter associated with antigen processing-1) and TAP2 subunits of this transporter complex are encoded by the *Tap1* and *Tap2* genes which map to the MHC class II region (Deverson et al., 1990; Monaco et al., 1990). Once in the ER lumen, the endogenous peptides are immediately loaded into the binding grooves of newly synthesized MHC class I molecules (Androlewicz and Cresswell, 1996).

Since interaction with peptide-loaded MHC class I is required for CD8+ T-cell development, disruptions in either the *B2m* gene or the *Tap* genes have severe effects on the mature CD8+ T-cell population. For example, a drastic reduction in the number of CD8+ T cells is observed in gene-targeted β2M-deficient mice (Koller et al., 1990; Zijlstra et al., 1990), and a similar phenotype is observed in animals in which the *Tap1* gene has been deleted (Van Kaer et al., 1992). Cytotoxic T-cell functions are severely impaired in these mutant mouse strains because they lack CD8+

T cells; however, T-helper activities mediated by CD4+ lymphocytes are normal.

CD4 and MHC Class II

CD4 (L3T4 in the mouse) is a 55 kDa single-chain glycoprotein with four Ig-like extracellular domains (D1–D4), a transmembrane region, and a cytoplasmic domain (Littman, 1987). Comparison of the human and mouse CD4 amino acid sequences reveals 55% similarity, with the greatest homology shared between the cytoplasmic domains. CD4 molecules interact with MHC class II molecules in both functional studies and binding assays (Greenstein et al., 1984; Doyle and Strominger, 1987). The two most distal extracellular domains of CD4 bind to the nonpolymorphic β2 domain of MHC class II molecules. The intracellular domain of CD4 is associated with large quantities of Lck, making it particularly important for the initiation of the complex TCR signaling cascade (Glaichenhaus et al., 1991). The majority of T helper functions, which consist primarily of the secretion of cytokines required for the complete activation of B cells and cytotoxic T cells, are carried out by CD4+ T cells.

The MHC class II molecule to which CD4 binds is a heterodimer composed of an MHC class II α chain noncovalently associated with an MHC class II β chain. MHC class II molecules generally present peptides from exogenous sources. Because both MHC class I and II molecules are assembled in the ER, and both are capable of binding peptides, a mechanism must exist in the ER to protect the peptide-binding groove of class II molecules from occupancy with endogenous peptides (Neefjes and Ploegh, 1992). The invariant chain (Ii) is coordinately expressed with MHC class II in the ER and associates with newly synthesized MHC class II molecules such that the binding of peptide in the MHC class II groove is blocked. As the MHC class II–Ii complexes traverse the increasingly acidic intracellular antigen-processing compartments, Ii undergoes stepwise degradation by cathepsin-like proteases until only a fragment of Ii, called *CLIP* (class II–associated invariant chain peptide), remains in the binding groove (Roche, 1995). CLIP peptides were initially discovered by examination of mutant antigen-presenting cell (APC) lines that exhibited unstable MHC class II molecules (Mellins et al., 1990). These APCs were able to present exogenous peptide fragments but could not process whole protein antigens or present peptides derived from them to T cells. Further study showed that these mutant cell lines had mutations in the HLA-DM gene that maps to the class II region of MHC between HLA-DP and HLA-DQ (Fling et al., 1994; Morris et al., 1994). The murine homologue of HLA-DM is H2-M. Both HLA-DM and H2-M are heterodimers with low homology to conventional MHC class II proteins (Roche, 1995). HLA-DM/H-2M colocalizes with MHC class II molecules in an endolysosomal compartment called the *MHC class II compartment* (MIIC) (Roche, 1995) and functions as a peptide exchanger. HLA-DM/H-2M catalyzes the release of CLIP peptides from the MHC class II groove and the subsequent loading of processed exogenous peptides (Denzin and Cresswell, 1995; Sherman et al., 1995). Accordingly, HLA-DM/H-2M is most effective at pH 4.5–6, the pH range prevalent in later antigen-processing compartments. Once the MHC class II molecule is loaded with peptide, HLA-DM/H-2M is released and the peptide–MHC complex makes its way to the APC surface.

The functions of many molecules involved in the exogenous antigen processing pathway have been clarified through studies of knockout mice. The development and function of CD4+ T cells are disturbed in mice lacking Ii, confirming the crucial role of this protein in normal MHC class II antigen presentation (Viville et al., 1993). In H2-M-deficient mice, normal amounts of MHC class II molecules are present on the cell surface but the majority of them are associated with CLIP rather than exogenous peptide (Fung-Leung et al., 1996; Martin et al., 1996; Miyazaki et al., 1996). Unexpectedly, positive selection of MHC class II–restricted CD4+ T cells appeared intact in these animals and they possessed large numbers of CD4+ T cells that responded vigorously to antigens presented by normal APCs. However, APCs from H2-M-deficient mice were unable to stimulate syngeneic or allogeneic T lymphocytes to respond against self-antigens or foreign antigens (Fung-Leung et al., 1996). In MHC class II–deficient mice (Cosgrove et al., 1991; Grusby et al., 1991; Kontgen et al., 1993), thymocyte development is blocked at an early stage and CD4+ lymphocytes are virtually absent in peripheral lymphoid organs. However, the development and functions of peripheral CD8+ cytotoxic T cells are normal. Surprisingly, there were significant numbers of CD4+ T cells in the thymi of MHC class II–deficient mice, although these cells were not of a mature phenotype. A subset of these unusual CD4+ cells was found to be restricted to MHC class I–like CD1 molecules (Cardell et al., 1995).

Overview of T Cell Development and TCR Signaling

In this section, we present brief overviews of the stages of thymocyte development and introduce the signaling pathways vital to this process. It is hoped that the reader will then have a better understanding of the in-depth discussion of thymocyte selection processes that follows.

Stages of T Cell Development

T cell development takes place in the thymus in a well-defined process during which precursor thymocytes divide, rearrange their antigen receptor DNA, and express functional TCRs and coreceptors. Thymic ontogeny can be divided into three major stages distinguished by the expression of certain cell surface receptors (Sebzda et al., 1999) (Fig. 4.5). The first major stage is the triple negative (TN) stage, in which neither the TCR, CD4, nor CD8 is expressed. Some immunologists refer to this stage as the double negative (DN) or CD4−CD8− stage. It is during the third phase of this stage (DN3; see below) that rearrangement of the VDJ segments of the TCRβ (but not TCRα) locus commences. The TCRβ chain pairs with an invariant TCRα-like chain known as the pre-Tα chain (or the TCRVα chain or gp33) to form a pre-TCR complex on the cell surface. In the second major stage of development, thymocytes commence expression of both coreceptors and are known as double positive (DP) or CD4+CD8+ thymocytes. Rearrangement of the TCRα locus occurs, expression of pre-Tα is extinguished, and true TCRαβ heterodimers are expressed on the surfaces of DP thymocytes. It is at this point that positive and negative selection of DP thymocytes occur. In the third major stage of thymocyte development, DP cells that have been positively selected up-regulate expression of the TCR/CD3 complex. Recognition of MHC class I molecules by the TCR leads to the down-regulation of the expression of CD4 and the maturation of single positive (SP) CD8+ thymocytes. Conversely, the interaction of a TCR with MHC class II results in the cessation of CD8 expression and the maturation of SP CD4+ T thymocytes. Mature CD4+ and CD8+ T cells then emerge from the thymus and take up residence in the periphery, ready to detect foreign antigens.

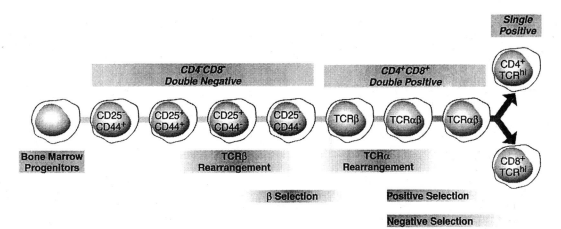

Figure 4.5. Overview of thymocyte development. Simplified scheme of thymocyte development based on the expression of the markers CD25 and CD44, the TCR, and the coreceptors CD4 and CD8. As bone marrow–derived hematopoietic progenitors differentiate, three broad stages of thymocyte development can be distinguished: the double negative (DN) stage (no expression of CD4 or CD8; also no expression of a mature TCR); the double positive (DP) stage (expression of both CD4 and CD8; eventual expression of a mature TCR); and the single positive (SP) stage (expression of either CD4 or CD8 and a mature TCR). During the DN stage, the TCRβ gene undergoes somatic recombination and thymocytes that express a functional TCRβ chain are allowed to mature fur-

ther. This process is called *β-selection*. During the DP stage, the TCRα gene undergoes somatic recombination to generate a functional TCRα chain that combines with the TCRβ chain to form a functional heterodimer. Double positive thymocytes expressing TCRαβ heterodimers are then subjected to negative selection to remove cells expressing TCRs that strongly recognize self-peptide/MHC complexes (potentially autoreactive cells), and positive selection to ensure the maturation of cells expressing TCRs that only weakly recognize self-peptide/MHC complexes. It is these latter cells that enter the SP stage and become mature CD4+ and CD8+ T cells capable of mounting immune responses to pathogens in the periphery.

Two major events occur during thymocyte development to ensure that an optimal T cell repertoire is generated. Negative thymic selection refers to the deletion by induced apoptosis of potentially self-reactive thymocytes—that is, those cells that strongly recognize self-peptide presented on self-MHC by thymic stromal cells *Positive selection* refers to the differentiation of thymocytes that only weakly recognize self-peptide presented on self-MHC (those cells that are more likely to recognize foreign peptide presented on self-MHC). Positive selection thus generates a T cell repertoire that is restricted to self-MHC (Bevan, 1977; Zinkernagel et al., 1978; Zinkernagel and Doherty, 1979), and negative selection ensures that that repertoire is self-tolerant (Kappler et al., 1987a, 1987b, 1988; MacDonald et al., 1988). Immunologists call the outcome of these processes the establishment of *central tolerance*. T cell clones that recognize self-antigens but escape deletion or inactivation in the thymus are functionally inactivated in the periphery by mechanisms of *peripheral tolerance*.

TCR Signaling Cascade

The binding of TCR/CD3 and a coreceptor to peptide-MHC triggers a signaling cascade that conveys information from the T cell surface to its nucleus. The transcription of a variety of new genes is induced while that of other genes is inhibited. Cellular responses are mediated through mobilization of the actin cytoskeleton, and a multimolecular structure called the *immunological synapse* (IS) or *supramolecular activation cluster* (SMAC) forms at the interface of the T cell and the APC (Bromley et al., 2001). Immunologists are still in the throes of elucidating all the players in this cascade, the means by which they interact with each other, and how their activities lead to T cell responses. Studies of the structure of SMACs in mature T cells and thymocytes have turned up some intriguing differences. In mature T cells activated by engagement of their TCRs by antigen, a central SMAC forms in which a ring of the adhesion binding partners LFA-1 and ICAM-1 surrounds

an inner cluster of TCR/peptide-MHC complexes (Monks et al., 1998). However, in thymocytes, a decentralized SMAC is formed in which multiple TCR/peptide-MHC complexes accumulate in areas of ICAM-1 exclusion (Hailman et al., 2002).

As noted above, the antigen binding subunits of the TCR cannot transduce signals themselves and depend on the ITAM-bearing CD3 chains for this function. The CD3 proteins do not possess intrinsic enzymatic activity but are coupled to cytoplasmic tyrosine kinases that interact with a host of other kinases, adaptor proteins, and transcription factors to bring about the downstream effects of antigen recognition (Hermiston et al., 2002) (Fig. 4.6). Among those membrane-bound kinases responsible for the earliest events in TCR-induced signal transduction are the Src family protein tyrosine kinases (PTKs) Lck and p59[fyn] (Fyn). Lck interacts noncovalently with cysteine residues in the cytoplasmic tails of both CD4 and CD8 (Yamaguchi and Hendrickson, 1996), whereas Fyn associates directly with the CD3 chains of the TCR/CD3 complex. In a resting cell, phosphorylation of regulatory C-terminal residues by p50[csk] kinase (Csk) renders Lck and Fyn catalytically inactive. Antigen receptor binding in both T and B lymphocytes activates CD45, a transmembrane phosphotyrosine phosphatase (PTPase) expressed in all nucleated hematopoietic cells. In T cells, the intracellular domain of CD45 dephosphorylates the negative regulatory tyrosine residues of Lck and Fyn, thereby up-regulating their activities.

Once activated by CD45 dephosphorylation, Lck and Fyn phosphorylate ITAMs found within the CD3 complex. Phosphorylated ITAMs in CD3ζ chains recruit the kinase ZAP70 to the TCR complex, and this enzyme in turn recruits and activates the molecular adaptor proteins SLP76, LAT, and GADS. These adaptors recruit additional mediators such as Vav1, Itk, and Grb2 and subsequently key mid-stream transducers such as Rho GTPases, phosphatidylinositol 3-kinase (PI3K), phospholipase C-γ1 (PLCγ1), and Ras. Vav1 is expressed in all hematopoietic cells, contains SH2 and SH3 signaling domains, and functions

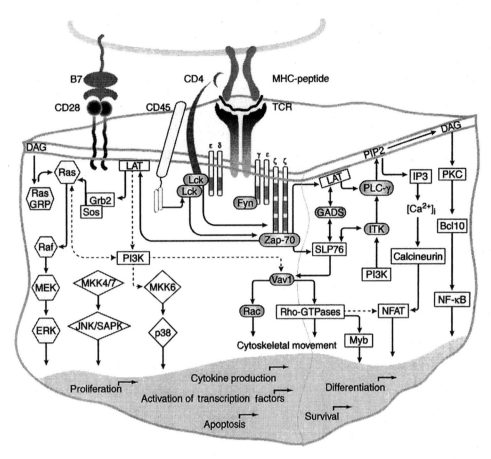

Figure 4.6. TCR signaling pathways. A schematic drawing of some of the signaling molecules involved in TCR signaling that influence thymocyte selection, based on gene targeting studies. See text for descriptions of molecular activities and interactions. $[Ca^{2+}]_i$, intracellular calcium; DAG, diacylglycerol; ERK, extracellular signal-regulated kinase; IP_3, inositol 1, 4, 5-triphosphate; LAT, linker for activation of T cells; MEK, mitogen-activated protein kinase (MAPK)/ERK kinase; MHC, major histocompatibility complex; MKK, MAPK kinase; PI3K, phosphatidylinositol 3-kinase; PIP2, phosphatidylinositol 4,5 bisphosphate; PKC, protein kinase C; PLC-γ, phospholipase Cγ; RasGRP, Ras guanyl-releasing protein; ZAP70, (CD3) zeta-associated kinase.

as a guanine nucleotide exchange factor for the Rac and Rho GT-Pases. These GTPases in turn promote thymocyte survival and differentiation as well as reorganization of the T cell actin cytoskeleton. Transgenic mice in which Rho function was genetically inactivated in the thymus showed a striking decrease in thymic cellularity and in levels of peripheral T cells that were due to a defect in thymocyte expansion (Henning et al., 1997). Studies of Vav1-deficient mice have confirmed that Vav1 is vital for the actin cap formation that supports SMAC assembly (Fischer et al., 1998; Holsinger et al., 1998; Wulfing, 2000). Actin cytoskeletion reorganization also requires the function of the Vav target gene *WASP*, which encodes the protein defective in Wiskott-Aldrich syndrome (Snapper et al., 1998; J. Zhang et al., 1999). In addition to cytoskeletal reorganization, Vav1-driven Rho family GTPases induce activation of the important transcription factor NFAT. Transcription of genes driven by NFAT is vital for the completion of T-cell activation and proliferation and cytokine production.

A second signaling pathway induced following ZAP70 activation depends on PLCγ1. PLCγ1 interacts with both LAT and Itk and mediates the hydrolysis of phosphatidylinositol 4,5 bisphosphate (PIP2) into diacylglycerol (DAG) and inositol 1,4,5-triphosphate (IP3). DAG production leads to activation of protein kinase C θ (PKCθ) and the recruitment of this isoform to the SMAC. PKCθ activation is also associated with the formation and recruitment of a protein complex containing the adaptors Bcl10 and MALT1. Bcl10 is specifically required for the activation of the transcription factor NF-κB following antigen receptor engagement (Rüland et al., 2001) but the precise role of MALT1 is not yet known. The second product of PLCγ1 action, IP3, induces an increase in the concentration of free cytoplasmic Ca^{2+} by binding to and opening insP3-regulated receptors in the ER

(Klausner and Samelson, 1991). This increase in intracellular calcium activates calcineurin, a serine/threonine phosphatase required for the activation of NFAT.

A third set of signaling pathways induced following TCR-mediated ZAP70 activation involves the MAPK (mitogen-activated protein kinase) family of signal transducers, particularly ERK (extracellular signal-regulated kinase). MAPK signaling cascades generally function in the proliferation and differentiation of hematopoietic cells (Rincon, 2001). Grb2, a molecule acting downstream of LAT, mediates the transduction of signals between the TCR and Sos, a guanine nucleotide exchange factor. Sos assists in Ras GTP exchange, resulting in the activation of Ras. Activated Ras in turn recruits the serine/threonine kinase Raf to the plasma membrane and activates it. Activated Raf phosphorylates MEK (MAPK/ERK kinase), which in turn phosphorylates ERK. Phosphorylated ERK induces transcription leading to the production of cytokines that support T cell differentiation. Other MAPK pathways are also triggered upon TCR engagement. Both the JNK/SAPK (jun kinase/stress-activated kinase) and p38 signaling pathways have been implicated in T cell activation and apoptosis. There is also extensive cross-talk between TCR signaling pathways. For example, DAG production can promote Ras activation because DAG interacts with the upstream Ras activator Ras guanyl-releasing protein (RasGRP).

Thymocyte Ontogeny

With this background in T cell development and TCR signaling molecules, we are ready to examine thymocyte ontogeny in detail. As we follow hematopoietic precursor cells on their journey from progenitors to thymocytes to mature T cells, we will discuss the effects on this process of various genes as demonstrated by the phenotypes of gene-targeted mice (Mak et al., 2001; Yeung et al., 1994). These animals have been of key importance in establishing that T cells mature through multiple genetic checkpoints (Fig. 4.7). For example, deletion of the TCRβ locus leads to a much earlier block in thymocyte development than the deletion of the TCRα locus (Mombaerts et al., 1992a). This unexpected result defined two distinct points at which TCR gene rearrangement takes place. Another surprise arose from the phenotype of Lck-deficient mice (Molina et al., 1992), which were found to have the same defects as TCRβ-deficient animals. Lck signaling function had not been expected to be important at so early a stage because it was generally assumed that the TCR was not expressed on early thymocytes. The door was thus opened to the discovery of the

pre-TCR signaling complex and a key checkpoint in T lymphopoiesis (reviewed in von Boehmer et al., 1999).

The Double Negative Stage

T Cell Development in the Bone Marrow

Hematopoietic cells originate in the fetal liver during embryonic development and in the bone marrow in adulthood. According to the most widely accepted model of murine hematopoiesis, a pluripotent hematopoietic stem cell (HSC) resident in the bone marrow differentiates into an HSC expressing the tyrosine kinase Flt3, and then into two early multipotent progenitors: the common myeloid progenitor (CMP) and the common lymphoid progenitor (CLP) (Borowski et al., 2002). Hematopoietic stem cells are capable of indefinite self-renewal in vivo and can reconstitute the complete spectrum of hematopoietic cells. Common myeloid progenitors and CLPs retain some self-renewal capacity and are able to differentiate into the full complement of either myeloid cells or lymphoid cells, respectively. It is still not entirely clear whether all CLPs remain in the bone marrow, or whether some can migrate to the thymus and differentiate into T cells in that location. In vitro experiments in adult mice have identified progeny of CMPs and CLPS that are more restricted in their potential. For example, cells giving rise only to neutrophils or monocytes have been isolated, as well as intermediates such as a B/T/natural killer (NK) precursor and an NK/T precursor, and still other cells limited to producing granulocytes, errthryocytes, monocytes, or macrophages.

Multiple growth factors, cytokines, and transcription factors play roles in initiating and maintaining lymphopoiesis (Berg and Kang, 2001). Function of the transcription factor PU.1 is essential for the development and maturation of both CLPs and CMPs. PU.1 controls the transcription of cytokine receptors needed to receive developmental signals such that PU.1$^{-/-}$ mice lack T cells, B cells, neutrophils, and macrophages. The level of PU.1 in a hematopoietic progenitor controls its destiny: low levels of PU.1 induce IL-7R expression and lymphoid development, whereas high levels of PU.1 suppress IL-7R expression and promote the expression of receptors for cytokines favoring myeloid development. IL-7, along with Flt3 ligand and c-kit ligand (growth factors derived from bone marrow stromal cells), is essential for the survival of the earliest committed T cell progenitors, and IL-7 is crucial for the maturation of these progenitors to lymphocytes. Mice with disruptions of the genes encoding either IL-7 or the IL-7R subunits have defects in cell cycle progression and thus exhibit impaired thymocyte development. If a transgene encoding the anti-apoptotic protein Bcl-2 is introduced into IL-7- or IL-7R-deficient mice, T cell development can be rescued (Akashi et al., 1997; Maraskovsky et al., 1997; von Freeden-Jeffry et al., 1997). This result implies that a primary function of IL-7 is to maintain thymocyte survival. Interestingly, signaling delivered through IL-7R is more important for γδ T-cell than for αβ T-cell development. IL-7R$^{-/-}$ mice have decreased numbers of αβ T cells but a complete absence of γδ T cells because of a failure in TCRγ locus rearrangement. Introduction of an already rearranged TCRγ transgene can rescue γδ T cell development in these animals (Kang et al., 1999). It is thought that signals initiated by IL-7 binding to IL-7R and transduced via the intermediaries Jak and STAT trigger changes to the accessibility of the TCRγ locus that are required for RAG recombinase binding (Schlissel et al., 2000).

Ikaros is a transcription factor acting slightly later than PU.1 that is also required for the development of CLP and its progeny (reviewed in Rothenberg and Anderson, 2002). Ikaros is thought

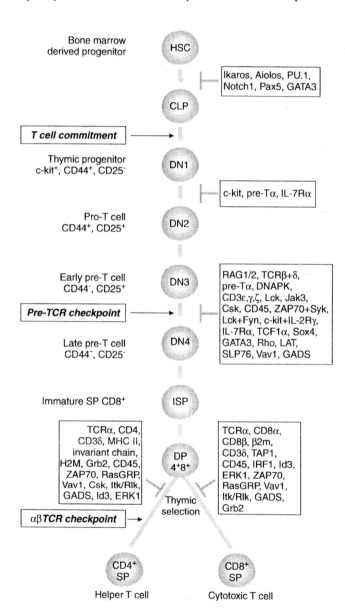

Figure 4.7. Checkpoints in thymocyte development as indicated by gene-targeting studies. Examination of the phenotypes of gene-targeted mice has allowed researchers to define specific genetic checkpoints during thymocyte development. Molecules whose functions are required at or around these checkpoints are indicated. See text for detailed descriptions of various stages. DN, double negative stage; DP, double positive stage; ISP, intermediate single positive stage; SP, single positive stage; +, double knockout mutant.

to repress the transcription of "lineage-inappropriate" genes by recruiting histone deacetylases that reduce the chromatin accessibility of a locus (Georgopolous, 2002). For example, CD19 (a B cell–specific gene) is repressed in T/B progenitors destined to become T cells, while CD4 and CD8 expression is repressed in those precursors destined to become B cells. A related transcription factor called Aiolos interacts with Ikaros to help establish T lineage commitment and thymocyte expansion. Mice with reduced levels of Ikaros or Aiolos fail to activate expression of the CD8α gene, leading to an apparent increase in immature T cells expressing CD4. Another important transcription factor involved in the divergence of T cell progenitors from B cell progenitors is GATA-3. GATA3$^{-/-}$ mice can produce B cells but not even the earliest of thymocyte populations.

There is now a considerable body of evidence that supports a role for the cell fate determination protein Notch-1 in T cell lineage commitment (Robey, 1999). The Notch proteins are a family of highly conserved transmembrane receptors that control binary cell fate decisions in diverse organisms. The Notch proteins regulate transcription directly by associating with nuclear factors (Artavanis-Tsakonas et al., 1999). Interaction between Notch-1 and one of its several ligands results in proteolytic cleavage of Notch-1 and the release of its intracellular domain (IC). The Notch-1 IC translocates to the nucleus and interacts with the CBF1 transcription factor, converting it from a repressor to an activator of genes involved in cell fate decisions (Hsieh et al., 1996; Struhl and Adachi, 1998). Among these are the HES genes, transcriptional repressors that act as downstream effectors in the Notch-1 signaling pathway. HES$^{-/-}$ mice either lack a thymus or have a small organ that is completely deficient in mature αβ and γδ T cells (B and NK cells are normal). Commitment to the T lineage results from the interaction of Notch-1 with Delta-1 (but not an alternative ligand, Jagged-1) (Jaleco et al., 2001). Indeed, in vitro, Delta-1 expressed ectopically by a bone marrow stromal cell line induces the differentiation of hematopoietic progenitors into both αβ and γδ T cells but not B cells (Schmitt and Zúñiga-Pflücker, 2002). The production of NK cells is independent of Delta-1 expression. This study thus shows that the lymphopoietic function of the thymic microenvironment, which had been difficult to replicate in vitro, is largely to supply ligands to induce Notch-1 signaling. In the absence of Notch signaling, V-to-DJ recombination in the TCRβ locus is impaired and thymocyte development is halted at this stage (Wolfer et al., 2002). Notch-1 also interferes with the activity of the E2A transcription factor that facilitates transcription of B cell–specific genes, blocking development down the B-cell path. Consistent with these findings, loss-of-function mutations of Notch-1 in newborn mice or in bone marrow stem cells result in a severe early block in T cell development and the appearance of ectopic B cells in the thymus (Radtke et al., 1999; Wilson et al., 2001). In addition, Notch-1 function can be manipulated to favor the development of B cells in the thymus (Koch et al., 2001; Izon et al., 2002). Conversely, expression of a constitutively active form of Notch-1 in bone marrow stem cells results in the ectopic development of precursor T cells outside the thymus (Pui et al., 1999; Allman et al., 2001).

Early lymphopoiesis is also influenced by signal transduction molecules. As mentioned above, Csk kinase negatively regulates Src family kinases in resting hematopoietic cells by phosphorylating specific tyrosine residues. Genetic disruption of the *Csk* gene causes multiple defects in organ development such that embryonic lethality occurs at days 9–10 of gestation (Imamoto and Soriano, 1993; Nada et al., 1993). Phosphorylation of the negative regulatory tyrosine residues of Fyn, Src, and p53/p56^{lyn} (Lyn, an-

other member of the Src family that is predominantly expressed in B cells) was greatly reduced, but not absent, in Csk$^{-/-}$ mice. Consequently, the catalytic activity of these Src family kinases was enhanced in in vitro assays, and various hyperphosphorylated proteins were detected in Csk$^{-/-}$ embryos. Studies of Csk$^{-/-}$ ES cells and Csk$^{-/-}$ RAG$^{-/-}$ reconstituted mice showed that Csk$^{-/-}$ hematopoietic precursors could colonize the bone marrow and thymus but that there was an early block in differentiation prior to the T-cell commitment stage (Gross et al., 1995). A conditional Csk knockout mutation specifically confined to the T lineage allowed the development of mature CD4^{+} T cells in a RAG-deficient background (Schmedt et al., 1998; Schmedt and Tarakhovsky, 2001).

T-Cell Development in the Thymus

The earliest precursor T cells that can be found within the thymus itself are the DN1 subset, characterized as HSA^{+} (heat-stable antigen; CD24) CD3^{-}CD4^{-}CD8^{-} and also c-kit^{+}CD44^{+}CD25^{-}. These cells, which constitute approximately 2%–5% of all thymocytes, have the ability to home directly to the thymus after intravenous transfer into a host animal (Shortman, 1992). DN1 cells subsequently up-regulate expression of CD25 to become DN2 or pro-T cells with a surface phenotype of CD44^{+}CD25^{+}. The pre-Tα chain is also expressed in these cells. When DN2 thymocytes become DN3 or early pre-T cells, they down-regulate expression of CD25 again to become CD44^{+}CD25^{-} cells. It is at this point that an obvious commitment to the αβ or γδ T lineage is made. Thymocytes at the DN3 stage commence somatic recombination in the TCRβ, γ, and δ loci, with rearrangement of the γ and δ gene segments preceding that of the β gene segments (Raulet et al., 1985). While only rearrangement of the TCRβ locus is required to initiate αβ T-cell maturation, both TCRγ and TCRδ must be productively rearranged to generate functional γδ T cells. Since the somatic recombinases RAG1/2 have been shown to be essential for the rearrangement of all TCR genes (Schatz et al., 1989), it is not surprising that mice deficient for either of these molecules have very early defects in lymphocyte development (Mombaerts et al., 1992b; Shinkai et al., 1992, 1993). The thymi of RAG1- or RAG2-deficient mice contain a decreased number of thymocytes (approximately 3×10^6 compared to about 1×10^8 thymocytes in normal mice) and T-cell development is arrested at the early DN2 stage. Similarly, mice with a natural mutation in the dsDNA-PK (*Prkdc*) gene show normal initiation of gene segment recombination but fail to ligate the segments together, resulting in a lack of mature T and B cells (Kirchgessner et al., 1995). In contrast, mice with a mutation in the *Tdt* gene responsible for N-nucleotide addition do not show altered T-cell development (Gilfillan et al., 1993; Komori et al., 1993).

The TCRα locus does not initiate rearrangement until considerably later than the other three loci. Instead, in thymocytes destined to become αβ T cells, newly synthesized TCRβ chains pair with pre-Tα chains to form pre-TCRs. Pre-TCRs undergo testing to determine whether the TCRβ chain can function in a signaling complex. Thus, disruption of the pre-Tα gene leads to an arrest in TCRαβ thymocyte development at a phenotypic stage similar to that in TCRβ-deficient mice (Fehling et al., 1995). Introduction of various transgenes encoding mutated versions of pre-Tα has demonstrated that the cytoplasmic domain of the pre-Tα chain is not required for pre-TCR function (Fehling et al., 1997) and that pre-TCR signaling does not require a ligand (Irving et al., 1998; Wiest et al., 1999). As long as the pre-Tα chain associates successfully with a functional TCRβ chain, exits the Golgi, and assembles with the CD3 complex in the plasma membrane microdomains, thymocyte development proceeds normally (O'Shea et al., 1997). Interestingly, pre-Tα-deficient mice exhibit normal development of γδ T cells, indicating that the γδ T lineage diverges from the αβ T lineage at the point of pre-TCR expression (Fehling et al., 1995; Malissen and Malissen, 1996). It is thought that pre-TCR signaling may "instruct" T precursors to divert down the αβ differentiation path. Indeed, the pre-TCR and γδ TCR differ in their signal initiation mechanisms. Unlike the pre-TCR, the γδ TCR does not associate with lipid microdomains in the plasma membrane and does not associate with CD3ε (Saint-Ruf et al., 2000). Further confirmation of this difference can be found in the phenotype of mice with a targeted disruption of the TCR Cδ exon. These animals have no detectable cell surface expression of any γδ TCR components but αβ T cell development is normal (Itohara et al., 1993). TCRδ knockout mice are also able to mount normal antibody responses after immunization with ovalbumin, indicating that αβ T helper cell function remains intact (Itohara et al., 1993). Conversely, development of γδ cells is unaffected by either *Tcra* or *Tcrb* mutations (Mombaerts et al., 1992a). Initial studies reported a role for Notch-1 in αβ/γδ T cell lineage commitment (Washburn et al., 1997), but it now appears that Notch-1 signaling supports the differentiation of both T-cell types (Schmitt and Zúñiga-Pflücker, 2002).

Only DN3 pre-T cells that have rearranged the TCRβ locus in-frame and have successfully combined it with the pre-Tα chain to form a functional pre-TCR on the thymocyte surface receive a signal permitting further development, a process called *β selection*. Pre-TCR signaling leads to activation of the transcription factor NF-κB, which controls the expression of numerous genes needed for survival and proliferation (Voll et al., 2000). Cells that have rearranged the TCRβ locus out-of-frame do not receive the survival signal and are induced to undergo apoptosis (Malissen and Malissen, 1996). As the β-selected thymocytes further evolve into DN4 or late pre-T cells, expression of CD44 is lost and the cells are phenotypically CD44⁻CD25⁻. These cells undergo a dramatic expansion that requires the activities of the transcription factors Tcf-1 and Sox4. Mice deficient for either of these molecules lack DP cells and have pre-T cells that fail to proliferate (Schilham and Clevers, 1998). DN4 cells that expand successfully pass through an immature single positive (ISP) stage in which CD8 is transiently expressed on the cell surface but a mature TCR is not yet present. The transition is then made to the DP stage in which both CD4 and CD8 are expressed, rearrangement of the TCRα locus occurs, and a complete TCRαβ heterodimer is finally expressed on the thymocyte surface. DP cells are then subjected to positive and negative thymic selection.

The importance of functional TCRβ chain rearrangement and pre-Tα/TCRβ expression for the transition from DN to DP thymocytes and for expansion of β-selected thymocytes is clearly demonstrated in the phenotype of TCRβ-deficient mice (Mombaerts et al., 1992a). These animals have a small thymus because of an early block in T cell development at the DN3 stage. The reduced numbers of cells making up the TCRβ⁻/⁻ thymus are present in equal proportions of DN and DP cells. Both these thymocyte populations lack detectable rearrangements of *Tcrb* genes and TCRαβ expression (Mombaerts et al., 1992a). However, recombination did occur at the TCRα locus, suggesting that TCRβ rearrangement and expression are not an absolute prerequisite for TCRα rearrangement.

Pre-TCR signaling also requires intact function of components of the CD3 complex, signal transduction molecules, and adaptor molecules further downstream. For example, CD3ε⁻/⁻ thymocytes, although still able to express rearranged TCRβ transcripts, are

blocked at the DN3 stage (Malissen et al., 1995). These findings imply that CD3ε expression is important for monitoring the productivity of TCRβ rearrangement by testing for pre-TCR signal transduction. Consistent with the association between pre-TCR signaling and αβ T commitment, rearrangements of TCRγ (*Tcrg*) and δ (*Tcrd*) gene segments are normal in CD3ε⁻/⁻ mice. Mice deficient for CD3ζ show a profound reduction in the amount of surface TCRs on DP cells as well as a reduced number of thymocytes (Liu et al., 1993; Love et al., 1993; Malissen et al., 1993; Ohno et al., 1993; Shores et al., 1998). In the peripheral lymphoid organs of double-mutant CD3ζη⁻/⁻ mice, unusual CD4⁺CD8⁻TCRαβ⁺ and CD4⁺CD8⁺TCRαβ⁺ cells were present that were positive for Thy-1 and CD44 surface expression but did not stain with anti-CD3ε or anti-HSA antibodies. Interestingly, the development of thymus-independent intestinal intraepithelial lymphocytes (IELs) occurred normally in these mice, and IELs expressed TCRs complexed with the FcεRIγ chain in the absence of CD3ζη (Love et al., 1993; Malissen et al., 1993).

Mice deficient for Lck kinase exhibit a small thymus because of an early block in the maturation of both TCRαβ and TCRγδ thymocytes (Molina et al., 1992). Mice transgenic for a dominant negative Lck mutation (Levin et al., 1993) have a phenotype similar to that of Lck⁻/⁻ mice. Conversely, a transgene encoding a constitutively active form of Lck can fully replace defective pre-TCR signaling in RAG1-deficient mice (Mombaerts et al., 1994). These results indicate that the catalytic activity of Lck is crucial for the maturation of all early thymocyte precursors. These results were confirmed using RAG complementation studies in which Lck was shown to be critical for signaling pathways activated by gamma-irradiation and CD3ε engagement in RAG-1⁻/⁻ immature thymocytes (Wu et al., 1996). The maturation of transgenic TCRγδ T cells was followed in Lck⁻/⁻ mice and found to be blocked at an early stage (Penninger et al., 1993). However, the development of these transgenic γδ T cells did not require the coexpression of CD4 or CD8, indicating that the Lck/CD4 and Lck/CD8 associations observed in normal T cells are not essential for thymocyte development (Penninger et al., 1993). Surprisingly, as was true for CD3ζη-deficient mice, intestinal TCRγδ T cells appeared to be unaffected by the Lck mutation (Penninger et al., 1993), indicating that Lck-mediated signal transduction may be differentially regulated in thymocytes, depending on the antigen recognized or the anatomical site of development.

Mice deficient for Fyn kinase do not display any overt phenotypic changes in T-cell development (Appleby et al., 1992; Stein et al., 1992), although they do display brain-associated defects (Grant et al., 1992; Stein et al., 1992). The proliferative responses of thymocytes and splenic T cells from Fyn-deficient mice were only slightly decreased after TCR/CD3 activation or stimulation with allogenic spleen cells, lectins, or bacterial superantigens. At the molecular level, a defect in Fyn expression resulted in altered patterns of tyrosine phosphorylation and decreased Ca²⁺ flux. However, double-mutant Lck/Fyn-deficient mice show a profound block at the DN3 stage of thymocyte differentiation that was more pronounced than that observed in Lck-deficient animals. These results indicate that Fyn can functionally compensate for Lck during early thymocyte development and pre-TCR signal transduction (Groves et al., 1996; van Oers, 1996).

Interestingly, mice lacking ZAP70 have a later block in thymopoiesis than that of Vav1-deficient mice, even though Vav1 functions downstream of ZAP70. It has been shown through RAG complementation that mice lacking Vav1 have only a small number of mature T cells because of a block at the DN3 stage. These mutant T cells proved to be hyporeactive to TCR/CD3 stimulation, and Ca^{2+} signaling was impaired (Fischer et al., 1995; Tarakhovsky et al., 1995; Zhang et al., 1995). In contrast, ZAP70-deficient mice have DP thymocytes but these cells do not progress to mature $CD4^+$ or $CD8^+$ SP cells. A block in positive and negative T-cell selection of DP thymocytes has been demonstrated in ZAP70$^{-/-}$ thymocytes (Negishi et al., 1995). Why the discrepancy between the phenotypes of Vav$^{-/-}$ and ZAP70$^{-/-}$ mice? SYK, a kinase related to ZAP70, is highly expressed in DP thymocytes (A.C. Chan et al., 1994). SYK$^{-/-}$ mice show impaired differentiation of B-lineage cells due to disruption of pre-BCR complex signaling but have no apparent block in the development of TCR$\alpha\beta$ thymocytes (Cheng et al., 1995; Turner et al., 1995). (These animals apparently do have a defect in the maturation of $\gamma\delta$ T cells.) However, double-mutant mice lacking both ZAP70 and SYK show a complete block in thymocyte development at the DN3 stage (just like Vav1-deficient mice), which implies that ZAP70 and SYK can compensate for each other's activity for pre-TCR signaling but not for thymic selection (Cheng et al., 1997).

Downstream of ZAP70, the molecular adaptors SLP-76 (Clements et al., 1998; Pivniouk et al., 1998), LAT (W. Zhang et al., 1999), and Gads (Yoder et al., 2001) are all essential for pre-TCR signaling and DN3 thymocyte maturation. Transgenic studies have shown that constitutively active Rac-1 can induce differentiation of pre-T cells but not proliferation (Gomez et al., 2000). In particular, constitutively active Rac-1 rescues functions missing in the absence of Vav and allows Vav1-deficient thymocytes to complete β-selection. A constitutively active Raf-1 transgene promotes thymocyte proliferation and differentiation but not allelic exclusion (Iritani et al., 1999). Other studies have suggested that allelic exclusion of the TCRβ locus requires SLP-76 (Aifantis et al., 1999) and PKCθ activity (Michie et al., 2001).

There have been some reports implicating Notch-1 in the DN-to-DP transition. Immature outer cortical DN thymocytes express high levels of Notch-1, whereas DP thymocytes express little or no Notch-1, and the most mature SP thymocytes express an intermediate level of Notch-1. It was proposed that Notch-1 down-regulation might be required for the maturation of cortical thymocytes (Hasserjian et al., 1996). Felli et al. (1999) further demonstrated a differential expression of different Notch isoforms (Notch-1, 2, and 3) and their ligands (Jagged-1 and 2) in the thymus, suggesting that thymocyte development is regulated by the interactions between different members of the Notch family and their cognate ligands in different thymic cell compartments.

The Double Positive Stage

The Coreceptors

$CD44^- CD25^+$ late pre-T cells (DN4) differentiate into $CD4^+ CD8^+$ DP thymocytes that rearrange the TCRα (*Tcra*) locus to generate a functional TCR$\alpha\beta$ heterodimer. Mice with a disruption in the *Tcra* locus consequently show a later block in development than do TCRβ-deficient mice. TCRα-deficient animals have a normal-sized thymus and a marked absence only of $CD4^+$ and $CD8^+$ SP cells (Mombaerts et al., 1992a; Philpott et al., 1992). Interestingly, normal numbers of both DN and DP thymocytes expressing TCRβ chains but not heterodimeric $\alpha\beta$ TCRs exist in TCR$\alpha^{-/-}$ animals. In older TCRα-deficient mice, an unusual $CD4^+ TCR\beta^{dull}$ lymphocyte population can be observed in the periphery that is even more apparent after the introduction of a TCRβ transgene (Philpott et al., 1992). These data indicate that,

while TCRα is not required for the DN-to-DP transition and the subsequent expansion of the DP thymocyte pool, its expression (along with that of TCRβ) is required for the DP-to-SP transition. The TCRα locus does not undergo allelic exclusion like the TCRβ locus and $V_\alpha J_\alpha$ rearrangements may continue within a given cell such that two TCRs containing different TCRα chains may be expressed on the surface (Heath et al., 1995). More recently, it has been noted that progression of $V_\alpha J_\alpha$ rearrangement is controlled by thymocyte survival in a way that regulates the T cell repertoire (Guo et al., 2002). It has been suggested that TCRs, like BCRs, may undergo secondary rearrangement in the form of receptor editing (McGargill et al., 2000).

As might be expected, the coreceptors CD4 and CD8 are crucial for DP thymocyte maturation. The CD8α chain is required for the surface expression of both CD8α and CD8β. Thus, in mice with a disrupted *Cd8a* gene there is a total absence of CD8 expression on T cell surface (Fung-Leung et al., 1991a, 1993). The vast majority of T cells in the periphery of these mutants are $CD4^+$ T cells whose maturation appears to be normal. Cytotoxic responses to alloantigens were partly impaired whereas cytotoxic responses to virus infections were severely inhibited. Studies of CD8$\alpha^{-/-}$ mice transgenic for a CD8α chain bearing point mutations of the Lck binding domain showed that the Lck-associative function of CD8 is not essential for thymic selection (I.T. Chan, 1993). Nevertheless, an absence of most of the CD8α cytoplasmic domain did have an inhibitory effect on the positive selection of cytotoxic cells (Fung-Leung et al., 1991b).

In mice with a disrupted *Cd8b* gene, the $CD8\alpha^+$ T-cell population in the thymus and in most peripheral lymphoid organs is reduced to 20%–30% of normal, and CD8α expression on thymocytes is decreased to approximately 50% of normal (Fung-Leung et al., 1994). This defect does not extend to IELs, cells that express a CD8$\alpha\alpha$ homodimer and develop extrathymically (Guy-Grand et al., 1991). Thus, CD8β is important only for thymically derived $CD8^+$ T cells. The absence of CD8β reduces but does not completely abolish thymic maturation of $CD8^+$ T cells. Moreover, peripheral T cells in CD8$\beta^{-/-}$ mice display effective cytotoxic activity against virus infections, a finding suggesting that CD8β is not essential for cytotoxic effector functions of $CD8^+$ T cells (Fung-Leung et al., 1994).

Mice with a disruption in the *Cd4* gene have markedly decreased T helper cell activity but normal development and function of $CD8^+$ T cells. These results indicate that expression of CD4 on progenitor cells and on DP thymocytes is not obligatory for the differentiation of $CD8^+$ cytotoxic effectors (Rahemtulla et al., 1991; Killeen et al., 1993). Curiously, CD4$^{-/-}$ mice are still able to mount detectable T-helper cell responses. This residual T helper activity has been attributed to a population of TCR$\alpha\beta^+ CD4^- 8^-$ T cells present in peripheral lymphatic organs (Locksley et al., 1993; Rahemtulla et al., 1994).

Mechanisms of Positive and Negative Thymic Selection

Positive selection of DP thymocytes results in the generation of mature $CD4^+$ TCR^{high} helper or $CD8^+$ TCR^{high} cytotoxic SP T cells that are able to react to non-self, whereas negative selection eliminates potentially harmful self-reactive T cells (von Boehmer et al., 1989b; Sebzda et al., 1999). The mechanisms governing positive and negative selection are dependent on physical interactions between the antigen-specific TCR expressed on developing thymocytes and peptide-MHC complexes expressed on surrounding thymic stromal cells. More than 80% of developing thymocytes express a TCR that does not recognize any self-peptide/self-MHC combination. These cells undergo apoptosis and are said to "die of neglect" or "die by non-selection default."

There were originally several models put forward to explain how the interaction of the TCR with thymic ligands could result in nonselection, positive selection, or negative selection. However, the preponderance of the most recent evidence gained from studies of animal models supports the "affinity/avidity model" of thymic selection (Sprent et al., 1988; Sebzda et al., 1999). This model proposes that the type of selection a thymocyte undergoes depends on the strength of the interaction between its TCR and its peptide-MHC thymic ligand (Fig. 4.8). According to this model, thymocytes with TCRs of low affinity or avidity for self-MHC do not receive any type of signal and undergo programmed cell death by default. However, thymocytes expressing TCRs with intermediate affinity or avidity for self-MHC receive a survival signal and are positively selected. These TCRs are those most likely to recognize foreign peptides presented in the context of self-MHC and thus may be useful in host defence against pathogen infections. In contrast, thymocytes expressing TCRs with high affinity or avidity for self-peptide/self-MHC receive a signal that induces them to undergo either clonal deletion or clonal inactivation. This negative selection of thymocyte clones removes potentially self-reactive cells. To test the affinity/avidity model, the outcome of thymic selection has been experimentally manipulated in fetal thymic organ cultures (FTOC) by titrating the density of specific peptide-MHC complexes. A low concentration of the peptide antigen recognized by a transgenic TCR resulted in positive selection, whereas a high concentration of the peptide antigen resulted in negative selection and immunological tolerance (Ashton-Rickardt et al., 1994; Hogquist et al., 1994; Sebzda et al., 1994). Bolstering the density hypothesis is the observation that negative selection is associated with maximal internalization of the engaged TCR, whereas fewer TCRs are internalized during positive selection (Mariathasan et al., 1998). As is discussed in more detail below, internalization

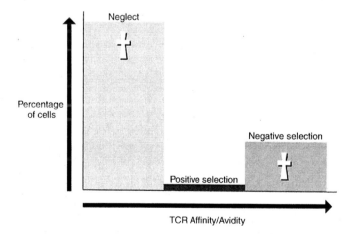

Figure 4.8. Affinity/avidity model of thymocyte selection. Schematic diagram of the relationship between the affinity and avidity of TCRs for peptide/self-MHC ligands (pMHC) presented in the thymus and the percentage of thymocytes directed toward the indicated cell fate. Thymocytes whose TCRs have low affinity or avidity (>80% of thymocytes) do not recognize pMHC and do not receive survival signals; they are not selected and die of neglect. Thymocytes with high affinity for pMHC ($\forall$18%) receive signals inducing apoptosis; these cells are negatively selected. Thymocytes with intermediate affinity for pMHC (<1%–2%) receive signals allowing them to survive, expand, and differentiate into mature T cells; these cells are positively selected.

of TCRs has been linked to modulation of downstream signal transduction.

Stromal Cell Involvement in Thymic Selection

Although it has been clear for some time that negative selection of autoreactive thymocytes occurs in the thymus (Ramsdell et al., 1989; Speiser et al., 1992), it has been less obvious which cell types are responsible for presenting the selecting ligands. Both bone marrow–derived cells and stromal cells in the thymus have been implicated, but comparatively few studies have been done to specifically identify the cell types involved. Peptides derived from ubiquitously expressed "housekeeping" proteins can be presented by thymic stromal cells and thus contribute to both positive and negative selection of thymocytes. However, until very recently, it was believed that T cells recognizing tissue-specific self-proteins were generally inactivated by peripheral tolerance mechanisms, since, by definition, tissue-specific proteins should not appear in the thymus. There was also some evidence that tissue-specific proteins shed into the circulation by the tissue in question could be taken up by recirculating APCs able to access the thymus (Heath and Carbone, 2001). However, despite sporadic reports that expression of tissue-specific proteins such as myelin and cytokeratin could be detected in the thymus itself (Heid et al., 1988; Jolicoeur et al., 1994; Pribyl et al., 1996; Smith et al., 1997), thymic expression of tissue-specific proteins was not fully appreciated (Hanahan, 1998). Experiments with transgenic mice expressing genes under the control of tissue-specific promoters often showed expression in the thymus as well as in the tissue of interest (Klein et al., 1995), but it remained possible that the promoters were displaying leaky expression because of their site of integration.

Recent studies have identified a population of medullary thymic epithelial cells (mTECs) located in the thymus that may play a key role in the establishment of central tolerance to tissue-specific proteins. Medullary TECs can transiently express a wide range of these molecules, allowing the deletion of reactive T-cell clones before their release to the periphery (Kyewski et al., 2002). Also, mTECs have been shown to express RNAs encoding hormones, secreted proteins, membrane proteins, and transcription factors, among other molecules. Experiments in transgenic and nontransgenic mice have confirmed that ectopic expression of a protein in mTECs leads to peripheral tolerance of that protein (Anderson et al., 2000; Klein et al., 2000; Derbinski et al., 2001). It has yet to be determined whether all mTEC clones can express all tissue-specific proteins or whether individual mTEC clones express different subsets of tissue-specific proteins. The latter situation would enable an individual mTEC cell to express a greater percentage of its cell surface proteins as the tissue-specific protein in question, increasing epitope density and the likelihood of a sufficiently strong TCR signal being delivered to the T cell to induce negative selection (Kyewski, 2002). Some have speculated that mTECs may also be involved in the differentiation of regulatory T cells that suppress autoimmune responses (Sakaguchi, 2000; Seddon and Mason, 2000).

It is not yet clear whether expression of tissue-specific genes in mTECs is the result of random derepression of transcription or a more directed activation process. Similarly, the influence of external factors on mTEC gene expression remains a mystery. However, new evidence has implicated a transcription factor called AIRE (autoimmune regulator) in mTEC-induced central tolerance (Anderson et al., 2002). Both humans and mice deficient for AIRE suffer from autoimmune symptoms that affect multiple organs (Bjorses et al., 1998; Anderson et al., 2002; Ramsey et al., 2002). (See Chapter 25). Analyses of transcription by cells of AIRE-deficient mice showed that mTEC expression of several tissue-specific proteins associated with various autoimmune symptoms was reduced in the absence of AIRE. Furthermore, although the highest levels of AIRE expression occurred in mTECs, AIRE was not required for the differentiation or antigen-presenting function of mTECs. Studies of chimeric animals in which AIRE expression was missing either from hematopoietic cells or from stromal cells showed that peripheral autoimmunity was present only in the latter situation. AIRE is known to interact with the transcriptional coactivator CREB-binding protein (Pitkanen et al., 2000), and it has been suggested that AIRE may participate in a multisubunit complex in mTECs that activates the transcription of multiple genes encoding tissue-specific proteins. Both AIRE-dependent and independent promiscuous expression of tissue-restricted self antigens in the thymus seems to occur (Derbinski et al., 2005). In the absence of AIRE, negative selection of T cells recognizing these proteins does not appear to occur, and tissue-reactive T cell clones escape to the periphery.

Several other molecules have been identified as being important for thymic stromal cell development and/or function. GHLF, Whn, Pax1, and Hox3a are all transcription or differentiation factors important for TEC development and the establishment of a normal thymic microenvironment (Nehls et al., 1994, 1996; Panigada et al., 1999; Su and Manley, 2000). "Sonic hedgehog" is a maturation factor produced by thymic stromal cells that acts on DN thymocytes to hold them at this stage of development (Outram et al., 2000). The transition to DP cells cannot occur until an unknown mechanism blocks sonic hedgehog signaling by thymic stromal cells.

Role of Signaling Molecules and Transcription Factors in Thymic Selection

Receptor proximal signaling elements such as components of the CD3 complex, CD45, Lck, and Vav influence thymic selection. While other CD3 chains are important for DN stages of thymocyte differentiation, CD3δ appears to act at a later stage such that γδ T cells are normal in Cd3δ-deficient mice (Dave et al., 1997). Analysis of these mutant animals has shown that they have specific defects in αβ DP positive selection, and point to CD3δ as the link between TCR engagement and ERK pathway activation during positive selection (Delgado et al., 2000; see below).

It is perhaps surprising that the phosphatase CD45, which functions to dephosphorylate Src family PTKs, is not essential for early thymocyte development. Strains of gene-targeted mice lacking the alternatively spliced exon 6 (Kishihara et al., 1993) or exon 9 (Byth et al., 1996) of CD45 have been generated. Myeloid lineage development is normal in these mutants, and B-cell development is normal until a stage of differentiation that correlates with BCR-dependent positive and negative selection (Cyster et al., 1996). Similarly, T cell development in CD45-deficient animals is blocked only at the transition of DP to mature CD4+ and CD8+ SP cells (Kishihara et al., 1993; Byth et al., 1996). Taken together, these results point to an important role for CD45 in T- and B-lymphocyte selection.

Lck and Vav1 have dual roles in thymocyte development. As well as being important for the DN-to-DP transition, Lck and Vav are required for the DP-to-SP transition. Genetic data have indicated that, although Lck is not required for superantigen-driven cell death of CD4+ T helper cells, it is involved in the proximal signaling pathways necessary for the TCR-mediated clonal deletion underlying negative selection (Penninger et al., 1996). Similar studies have shown that Vav1 regulates peptide-specific apoptosis in thymocytes and is required for both positive and negative selection (Turner et al., 1997; Kong et al., 1998).

Attempts have been made to find molecules and/or pathways that are exclusively involved in either positive or negative selection. For example, DᵐN transgenes have been used to inhibit various molecules within the MAPK pathways, including Ras and MEK (Alberola-Ila et al., 1995, 1996; Swan et al., 1995; O'Shea et al., 1996; Genot and Cantrell, 2000). Positive selection is blocked in these mutants and there are significant reductions in numbers of mature SP thymocytes. These results have been confirmed in mice genetically deficient for ERK1 (Pages et al., 1999) or its upstream mediator RasGRP (Dower et al., 2000). Other evidence suggests that the level of ERK signaling as induced by TCR affinity or avidity for the peptide-MHC complex in question determines positive vs. negative selection (Bommhardt et al., 2000; Mariathasan et al., 2000; Hogquist, 2001). In situations of negative thymocyte selection, ERK activation is vigorous but short-lived, while positive selection generates weak ERK signaling that is sustained (Werlen et al., 2000). It is speculated that ligands with low affinity for a TCR (positively selecting) do not trigger receptor internalization, allowing them to continue to trigger TCR signaling and to sustain moderate ERK activation. In contrast, high-affinity ligands (negatively selecting) induce vigorous ERK activation that is rapidly extinguished by TCR internalization. As mentioned above, ERK signaling leading to positive selection is also dependent on the extracellular transmembrane domain of CD3δ, which is required for association with LAT and the subsequent activation of other downstream transducers in the MAPK pathway (Delgado et al., 2000).

The Tec family kinases may also be involved in selection. Several members of the Tec family, including Itk and Rlk, have been shown to be important in setting the signaling thresholds for positive and negative selection (Liao and Littman, 1995; Schaeffer et al., 2000). Id3, a nuclear helix-loop-helix protein regulated by Itk, also appears to be involved in positive selection (Rivera et al., 2000; Bain et al., 2001). Genes specifically associated with negative selection have been harder to identify, although many have been implicated (reviewed in Sebzda et al., 1999). The engagement of costimulatory molecules such as CD28 by binding partners on thymic stromal APCs has been shown to promote negative selection (Page et al., 1993; Punt et al., 1994; Amsen and Kruisbeek, 1996). Interestingly, mice heterozygous for a null Grb2 mutation express subnormal levels of this adaptor and show impaired negative thymocyte selection (Gong et al., 2001). Positive selection is normal in these mutants. On the basis of the above findings, it has been proposed that negative selection may proceed to ERK activation via Grb2, but that positive selection takes a different route to ERK through Ras-GRP (Hogquist, 2001).

In contrast to the MAPK pathways, the phospholipid signaling pathway activated following TCR engagement does not appear to be important for thymic selection of DP cells. Analysis of mice deficient for PKCθ, the isoform of PKC that preferentially associates with the SMAC, has suggested that PKCθ does not play an essential role in either positive or negative selection (Sun et al., 2000a). It also remains controversial whether calcineurin is important for either positive or negative selection (Kane and Hedrick, 1996; Hayden-Martinez et al., 2000; Chan et al., 2002).

Interestingly, mice with a targeted disruption of the interferon regulatory factor-1 (IRF-1) gene have a block specifically in the development of DP cells into CD8 SP thymocytes as well as a profound reduction in mature CD8+ T cells (Matsuyama et al., 1993). The development of CD4+ T cells is normal. IRF-1 controls the expression of the *Tap* and other genes required for MHC class I loading, which explains part of the reduction in CD8+ T cells (White et al., 1996). However, there also appears to be a defect in selection that is intrinsic to CD8+ thymocytes (Penninger et al., 1997). IRF-2 binds the same promotor sequences as IRF-1 and acts as a transcriptional repressor. While IRF-2$^{-/-}$ mice have a defect in B-cell development, T-cell development is normal (Matsuyama et al., 1993).

Molecules that promote thymocyte survival can influence thymic selection in several ways. Without the induction and maintenance of thymocyte survival pathways, the window of opportunity for positive and negative selection would rapidly close. Studies of transgenic and knockout mice have shown that the genes encoding the antiapoptotic protein Bcl-X$_L$, RhoA GTPase, the transcription factors NFAT and c-Myb, the retinoid-related orphan receptor (RORγ), and members of the E family of regulatory proteins are important for DP thymocyte survival (Ma et al., 1995; Motoyama et al., 1995; Taylor et al., 1996; Oukka et al., 1998; Bain et al., 1999; Costello et al., 2000; Pearson and Weston, 2000; Sun et al., 2000b). Similarly, studies of mice transgenic for mutant NF-κB regulatory proteins that act as inhibitors have shown that this transcription factor is crucial for pre-T-cell survival and positive selection (Kuo and Leiden, 1999; Hettmann and Leiden, 2000; Voll et al., 2000). CD8+ T cells do not develop in the absence of NF-κB, whereas CD4+ T cells are more dependent on CREB.

The Single Positive Stage

The engagement of MHC class I or II during the positive selection of a DP thymocyte spurs it to proliferate and differentiate into mature CD8+ or CD4+ SP cells, respectively. This process is called *CD4/CD8 lineage commitment.*

Precisely how a DP cell determines that it should become a CD4+ SP or a CD8+ SP cell has yet to be completely elucidated. Models proposed to account for CD4/CD8 lineage commitment fall into two camps: those based on an instructive mechanism and those based on a stochastic (random choice) mechanism. The original instructive model proposed that differentiation into a CD4 or a CD8 cell was determined by engagement of the αβTCR plus CD4 or CD8 by either MHC class II or class I, respectively (von Boehmer et al., 1989a). In other words, thymocytes recognizing MHC class I were instructed to differentiate into CD8+T cells, while thymocytes expressing TCRs with affinity for MHC class II were instructed to become CD4+ T cells. Although initial results using TCR transgenic mice were consistent with this model, later analyses of various mutant mouse strains and of additional TCR transgenic mice favored a stochastic mechanism (Kaye et al., 1989; S.H. Chan et al., 1993; Davis et al., 1993; Itano et al., 1994; Robey et al., 1994; van Meerwijk et al., 1995; von Boehmer, 1996). Subsets of CD4+8^{lo} and CD4^{lo}8+ T cells expressing intermediate levels of CD4 and CD8 were identified in different MHC-deficient mutant mouse strains, consistent with the idea that DP thymocytes randomly down-regulate the expression of one or the other coreceptor as they move toward becoming mature CD4+8$^-$ and CD4$^-$8+ SP cells. This hypothesis was supported by findings that transgenic expression of

CD4 in thymocytes could mediate development of CD4$^-$8+ TCR transgenic cells in class I–deficient mice, and that transgenic expression of CD8 molecules could mediate development of CD4+8$^-$ TCR Tg cells in class II–deficient mice (Baron et al., 1994; S.H. Chan et al., 1994; Robey et al., 1994; van Meerwijk et al., 1995; von Boehmer, 1996).

More recent studies have continued to generate opposing bodies of evidence. Brugnera and colleagues have proposed a "coreceptor reversal" model that is at least partly instructive (Brugnera et al., 2000). This model posits that CD8 expression is first down-regulated in all DP thymocytes regardless of their MHC restriction, so that all thymocytes initially become CD4+ cells. Those thymocytes that subsequently receive both an IL-7 signal and a weak signal delivered by binding to MHC class I resume CD8 expression and down-regulate CD4 expression, effectively "reversing" their prior CD4+ phenotype to a CD8+ phenotype. However, those thymocytes that receive a signal through MHC class II maintain their CD4 expression and do not resume CD8 expression. The stochastic mechanism of CD4/CD8 commitment is supported by a study examining the deletion of a regulatory motif functioning as a silencer of CD4 expression (Leung et al., 2001). β2M-deficient mice, which usually have only very low numbers of CD8+ T cells, were transfected with a transgene conferring constant expression of CD4 due to the absence of the silencer. These mice contained mature T cells that expressed both CD4 and CD8 and exhibited MHC class II restriction. These cells developed into cytotoxic effectors after antigen stimulation.

Lck signaling has also been proposed as a mechanism of CD4/CD8 commitment because Lck associates with the cytoplasmic tails of both coreceptors (Turner et al., 1990). The model holds that strong Lck signaling favors the differentiation of DP cells into CD4+ SP cells, while little or no signaling results in CD8+ SP cells (Berg and Kang, 2001). The amount of Lck signaling is determined by the MHC restriction of the TCR: MHC class I–restricted TCRs bind to CD8, which is associated with low levels of Lck activity, whereas MHC class II–restricted TCRs bind to CD4, which is associated with about 20-fold higher levels of Lck activity. Experiments in which mutated CD8 molecules capable of binding different amounts of Lck were compared showed that the greater the amount of Lck bound to CD8, the more CD4+ T cells emerged from the DP population (Salmon et al., 1999). Yasutomo and colleagues (2000) devised an in vitro culture system that allowed them to monitor SP development following the binding of a TCR to either wild-type MHC class II (fully capable of binding Lck) or mutated MHC class II lacking the CD4 binding site (decreased Lck binding). In the absence of significant Lck binding, thymocyte differentiation was skewed to CD8+. The authors interpreted their data to mean that the duration of antigen signaling as transduced by Lck determines CD4/CD8 commitment. Additional evidence supporting a commitment model based on quantitative differences in Lck signaling has come out of transgenic studies in which constitutively active or D^{m}N mutants of Lck were used (Hernandez-Hoyos et al., 2000). Overexpression of Lck induced MHC class I–restricted thymocytes to develop into CD4+ T cells, whereas reduced levels of Lck drove MHC class II–restricted thymocytes down the CD8+ path. Confirmation of these results has been obtained by the introduction of a transgene specifying tetracycline-inducible Lck expression into Lck$^{-/-}$ cells (Legname et al., 2000). Induced expression of Lck resulted in high levels of Lck activity and the exclusive differentiation of CD4+ T cells.

There is some evidence supporting a role for ERK signaling in CD4/CD8 lineage commitment. In one study, high levels of ERK signaling appeared to favor CD4[+] over CD8[+] SP development. Transfection of mice with a transgene encoding a constitutively active form of ERK resulted in increased numbers of CD4[+] thymocytes but decreased numbers of CD8[+] cells (Sharp et al., 1997). Consistent with this result, CD4 maturation was blocked by inhibition of ERK signaling whereas CD8 development was enhanced (Bommhardt et al., 1999; Sharp and Hedrick, 1999). However, other studies have shown that CD8 differentiation can be blocked by deletion, inhibition, or interference with ERK activity (Alberola-Ila et al., 1995; Pages et al., 1999; Mariathasan et al., 2000).

Finally, some investigators have suggested that Notch-1 may contribute to CD4/CD8 lineage commitment, although its involvement is still the subject of much debate (Osborne and Miele, 1999; Robey, 1999; Deftos and Bevan, 2000; von Boehmer, 2001). Robey et al. demonstrated that expression of an active form of Notch-1 in developing T cells resulted in an increase in CD8[+] lineage cells and a decrease in CD4[+] lineage cells, even if MHC class I was absent (Robey et al., 1996; Robey, 1999). In addition, when Notch-1 signaling was blocked with antibodies, CD8[+] SP development was favored (Yasutomo et al., 2000). Complementary studies revealed that the CD4 silencer that prevents CD4 expression in DN and CD8 SP thymocytes has an HES-1 binding site (Kim and Siu, 1998), and HES genes are known to be regulated by Notch-1. However, other data have suggested that rather than promoting only the development of CD8[+] SP cells, Notch-1 signaling is involved in the maturation of both CD4 and CD8 SP thymocytes (Deftos et al., 1998, 2000). Still others believe that Notch-1 may exert its effect indirectly, by reducing the strength of signal delivered through the TCR (Anderson et al., 2001; Izon et al., 2001). Cells receiving high Notch-1 signals would have reduced signaling through the TCR and would consequently adopt the CD8 cell fate, whereas cells receiving lower Notch-1 signals would have stronger TCR signals and become CD4 cells.

Concluding Remarks

T cell development is coordinated by the concerted actions of a variety of surface receptors, signal transduction molecules, and transcription factors. Genetic engineering technology has provided valuable tools for the dissection of the complex multitude of genes and gene products involved in thymocyte ontogeny and T cell function. The use of mutant animals has been central to the identification of several important genetic checkpoints in thymic development. Overlapping gene functions have emphasized the enormous plasticity of the immune system, enabling the animal to adapt to changes and compensate for loss of key molecules. A greater understanding of T cell development will assist us in designing rational therapeutics for the treatment of cancer, autoimmunity, and chronic inflammatory diseases.

Acknowledgments

The authors would like to thank Maya Chaddah for expert rendering of the figures for this chapter.

References

Aifantis I, Pivniouk VI, Gartner F, Feinberg J, Swat W, Alt FW, von Boehmer H, Geha RS. Allelic exclusion of the T cell receptor beta locus requires the SH2 domain-containing leukocyte protein (SLP)-76 adaptor protein. J Exp Med 190:1093–1102, 1999.

Akashi K, Kondo M, von Freeden-Jeffry U, Murray R, Weissman IL. Bcl-2 rescues T lymphopoiesis in interleukin-7 receptor-deficient mice. Cell 89:1033–1041, 1997.

Alberola-Ila J, Forbush KA, Seger R, Krebs EG, Perlmutter RM. Selective requirement for MAP kinase activation in thymocyte differentiation. Nature 373:620–623, 1995.

Alberola-Ila J, Hogquist KA, Swan KA, Bevan MJ, Perlmutter RM. Positive and negative selection invoke distinct signaling pathways. J Exp Med 184:9–18, 1996.

Allan JM, Forbush KA, Permutter R. Functional dissection of the Lck proximal promoter. Mol Cell Biol 12:2758–2768, 1992.

Allman D, Karnell FG, Punt JA, Bakkour S, Xu L, Myung P, Koretzky GA, Pui JC, Aster JC, Pear WS. Separation of Notch-1 promoted lineage commitment and expansion/transformation in developing T cells. J Exp Med 194:99–106, 2001.

Amsen D, Kruisbeek AM. CD28-B7 interactions function to co-stimulate clonal deletion of double-positive thymocytes. Int Immunol 8:1927–1936, 1996.

Anderson AC, Nicholson LB, Legge KL, Turchin V, Zaghouani H, Kuchroo VK. High frequency of autoreactive myelin proteolipid protein-specific T cells in the periphery of naïve mice: mechanisms of selection of the self-reactive repertoire. J Exp Med 5:761–770, 2000.

Anderson AC, Robey EA, Huang YH. Notch signaling in lymphocyte development. Curr Opin Genet Dev 11:554–560, 2001.

Anderson MS, Venanzi ES, Klein L, Chen Z, Berzins SP, Turley SJ, von Boehmer H, Bronson R, Dierich A, Benoist C, Mathis D. Projection of an immunological self shadow within the thymus by the aire protein. Science 298:1395–1401, 2002.

Androlewicz MJ, Cresswell P. How selective is the transporter associated with antigen processing? Immunity 5:1–5, 1996.

Appleby MW, Gross JA, Cooke MP, Levin SD, Qian X, Perlmutter RM. Defective T cell receptor signaling in mice lacking the thymic isoform of p59fyn. Cell 70:751–763, 1992.

Artavanis-Tsakonas S, Rand MD, Lake RJ. Notch signaling: cell fate control and signal integration in development. Science 284:770–776, 1999.

Ashton-Rickardt PG, Bandeira A, Delaney JR, Van Kaer L, Pircher HP, Zinkernagel RM, Tonegawa S. Evidence for a differential avidity model of T cell selection in the thymus. Cell 76:651–663, 1994.

Bain G, Cravatt CB, Loomans C, Alberola-Ila J, Hedrick SM, Murre CF. Regulation of the helix-loop-helix proteins, E2A and Id3, by the Ras-ERK MAPK cascade. Nat Immunol 2:165–171, 2001.

Bain G, Quong MW, Soloff RS, Hedrick SM, Murre C. Thymocyte maturation is regulated by the activity of the helix-loop-helix protein, E47. J Exp Med 190:1605–1616, 1999.

Baron A, Hafen K, von Boehmer H. A human CD4 transgene rescues CD4-CD8+ cells in beta 2-microglobulin-deficient mice. Eur J Immunol 24: 1933–1936, 1994.

Berg LJ, Kang J. Molecular determinants of TCR expression and selection. Curr Opin Immunol 13:232–241, 2001.

Bevan MJ. In a radiation chimaera, host H-2 antigens determine immune responsiveness of donor cytotoxic cells. Nature 269:417–418, 1977.

Bjorses P, Aaltonen J, Horelli-Kuitunen N, Yaspo ML, Peltonen L. Gene defect behind APECED: a new clue to autoimmunity. Hum Mol Genet 7: 1547–1553, 1998.

Blumberg RS, Ley S, Sancho J, Lonberg N, Lacy E, McDermott F, Schad V, Greenstein JL, Terhorst C. Structure of the T-cell antigen receptor: evidence for two CD3 epsilon subunits in the T-cell receptor-CD3 complex. Proc Natl Acad Sci USA 87:7220–7224, 1990.

Bommhardt U, Basson MA, Krummrei U, Zamoyska R. Activation of the extracellular signal-related kinase/mitogen-activated protein kinase pathway discriminates CD4 versus CD8 lineage commitment in the thymus. J Immunol 163:715–722, 1999.

Bommhardt U, Scheuring Y, Bickel C, Zamoyska R, Hunig T. MEK activity regulates negative selection of immature CD4+CD8+ thymocytes. J Immunol 164:2326–2337, 2000.

Borowski C, Martin C, Gounari F, Haughn L, Aifantis I, Grassi F, von Boehmer H. On the brink of becoming a T cell. Curr Opin Immunol 14: 200–206, 2002.

Bromley SK, Iaboni A, Davis SJ, Whitty A, Green JM, Shaw AS, Weiss A, Dustin ML. The immunological synapse. Annu Rev Immunol 19:375–396, 2001.

Brugnera E, Bhandoola A, Cibotti R, Yu Q, Guinter TI, Yamashita Y, Sharrow SO, Singer A. Coreceptor reversal in the thymus: signaled CD4+CD8+ thymocytes initially terminate CD8 transcription even when differentiating into CD8+ T cells. Immunity 13:59–71, 2000.

Byth KF, Conroy LA, Howlett S, Smith AJ, May J, Alexander DR, Holmes N. CD45-null transgenic mice reveal a positive regulatory role for CD45 in early thymocyte development, in the selection of CD4+CD8+ thymocytes, and B cell maturation. J Exp Med 183:1707–1718, 1996.

Cantrell D. Transgenic analysis of thymocyte signal transduction. Nat Rev Immunol 2:20–27, 2002.

Capecchi MR. Altering the genome by homologous recombination. Science 244:1288–1292, 1989.

Cardell S, Tangri S, Chan S, Kronenberg M, Benoist C, Mathis D. CD1-restricted CD4+ T cells in major histocompatibility complex class II–deficient mice. J Exp Med 182:993–1004, 1995.

Chaffin KE, Perlmutter R. A pertussis toxin-sensitive process controls thymocyte emigration. Eur J Immunol 21:2565–2573, 1991.

Chan AC, Desai DM, Weiss A. The role of protein tyrosine kinases and protein tyrosine phosphatases in T cell antigen receptor signal transduction. Annu Rev Immunol 12:555–592, 1994.

Chan IT, Limmer A, Louie MC, Bullock ED, Fung-Leung W-P, Mak TW, Loh DY. Thymic selection of cytotoxic T cell independent of CD8α-Lck association. Science 261:1581–1584, 1993.

Chan SH, Cosgrove D, Waltzinger C, Benoist C, Mathis D. Another view of the selective model of thymocyte selection. Cell 73:225–236, 1993.

Chan SH, Waltzinger C, Baron A, Benoist C, Mathis D. Role of coreceptors in positive selection and lineage commitment. EMBO J 13:4482–4489, 1994.

Chan VSF, Wong C, Ohashi PS. Calcineurin Aα plays an exclusive role in TCR signaling in mature but not in immature T cells. Eur J Immunol 32:1223–1229, 2002.

Chen J, Shinkai Y, Young F, Alt FW. Probing immune functions in RAG-deficient mice. Curr Opin Immunol 6:313–319, 1994.

Cheng AM, Negishi I, Anderson SJ, Chan AC, Bolen J, Loh DY, Pawson T. The Syk and ZAP-70 SH2-containing tyrosine kinases are implicated in pre-T cell receptor signaling. Proc Natl Acad Sci USA 94:9797–9801, 1997.

Cheng AM, Rowley B, Pao W, Hayday A, Bolen JB, Pawson T. Syk tyrosine kinase required for mouse viability and B-cell development. Nature 378: 303–306, 1995.

Clements JL, Yang B, Ross-Barta SE, Eliason SL, Hrstka RF, Williamson RA, Koretzky GA. Requirement for the leukocyte-specific adapter protein SLP-76 for normal T cell development. Science 281:416–419, 1998.

Cosgrove D, Gray D, Dierich A, Kaufman J, Lemeur M, Benoist C, Mathis D. Mice lacking MHC class II molecules. Cell 66:1051–1066, 1991.

Costello PS, Cleverley SC, Galandrini R, Henning SW, Cantrell DA. The GTPase Rho controls a p53-dependent survival checkpoint during thymopoiesis. J Exp Med 192:77–85, 2000.

Cyster JG, Healy JI, Kishihara K, Mak TW, Thomas ML, Goodnow CC. Regulation of B-lymphocyte negative and positive selection by tyrosine phosphatase CD45 Nature 381:325–328, 1996.

Dave VP, Cao Z, Browne C, Alarcon B, Fernandez-Miguel G, Lafaille J, de la Hera A, Tonegawa S, Kappes DJ. CD3δ deficiency arrests development of the αβ but not γδ T cell lineage. EMBO J 16:1360–1370, 1997.

Davis CB, Killeen N, Crooks ME, Raulet D, Littman DR. Evidence for a stochastic mechanism in the differentiation of mature subsets of T lymphocytes. Cell 73:237–247, 1993.

Davis MM, Bjorkman PJ. T-cell antigen receptor genes and T-cell recognition. Nature 334:395–402, 1988.

Deftos ML, Bevan MJ. Notch signaling in T cell development. Curr Opin Immunol 12:166–172, 2000.

Deftos ML, He YW, Ojala EW, Bevan MJ. Correlating notch signaling with thymocyte maturation. Immunity 9:777–786, 1998.

Deftos ML, Huang E, Ojala EW, Forbush KA, Bevan MJ. Notch-1 signaling promotes the maturation of CD4 and CD8 SP thymocytes. Immunity 13: 73–84, 2000.

Delgado P, Fernandez E, Dave V, Kappes D, Alarcon B. CD3delta couples T-cell receptor signalling to ERK activation and thymocyte positive selection. Nature 406:426–430, 2000.

Denzin LK, Cresswell P. HLA-DM induces CLIP dissociation from MHC class II alpha beta dimers and facilitates peptide loading. Cell 82: 155–165, 1995.

Derbinsky J, Gabler J, Brors B, Tierling S, Jonnakuty S, Hergenhahn M, Peltonen L, Walter J, Kyewski B. Promiscuous gene expression in thymic epithelial cells is regulated at multiple levels. J Exp Med 202:33–45, 2005.

Derbinski J, Schulte A, Kyewski B, Klein L. Promiscuous gene expression in medullary epithelial cells mirrors the peripheral self. Nat Immunol 2: 1032–1039, 2001.

Deverson EV, Gow IR, Coadwell WJ, Monaco JJ, Butcher GW, Howard JC. MHC class II region encoding proteins related to the multidrug resistance family of transmembrane transporters. Nature 348:738–741, 1990.

Dower NA, Stang SL, Bottorff DA, Ebinu JO, Dickie P, Ostergaard HL, Stone JC. RasGRP is essential for mouse thymocyte differentiation and TCR signaling. Nat Immunol 1:317–321, 2000.

Doyle C, Strominger JL. Interaction between CD4 and class II MHC molecules mediates cell adhesion. Nature 330:256–259, 1987.

Ellmeier W, Sawada S, Littman DR. The regulation of CD4 and CD8 coreceptor gene expression during T cell development. Annu Rev Immunol 17:523–554, 1999.

Fehling HJ, Iritani BM, Krotkova A, Forbush KA, Laplace C, Perlmutter RM, von Boehmer H. Restoration of thymopoiesis in pTα–/– mice by anti-CD3ε antibody treatment or with transgenes enclding activated Lck or tailless pTα. Immunity 6:703–714, 1997.

Fehling HJ, Krotkova A, Saint-Ruf C, von Boehmer H. Crucial role of the pre-T-cell receptor alpha gene in development of alpha beta but not gamma delta T cells. Nature 375:795–798, 1995.

Felli MP, Maroder M, Mitsiadis TA, Campese AF, Bellavia D, Vacca A, Mann RS, Frati L, Lendahl U, Gulino A, Screpanti I. Expression pattern of Notch-1, 2 and 3 and Jagged-1 and 2 in lymphoid and stromal thymus components: distinct ligand–receptor interactions in intrathymic T cell development. Int Immunol 11:1017–1025, 1999.

Fischer KD, Kong YY, Nishina H, Tedford K, Marengere LE, Kozieradzki I, Sasaki T, Starr M, Chan G, Gardener S, Nghiem MP, Bouchard D, Barbacid M, Bernstein A, Penninger JM. Vav is a regulator of cytoskeletal reorganization mediated by the T-cell receptor. Curr Biol 8:554–562, 1998.

Fischer KD, Zmuldzinas A, Gardner S, Barbacid M, Bernstein A, Guidos C. Defective T-cell receptor signalling and positive selection of Vav-deficient CD4+ CD8+ thymocytes. Nature 374:474–477, 1995.

Fling SP, Arp B, Pious D. HLA-DMA and -DMB genes are both required for MHC class II/peptide complex formation in antigen-presenting cells. Nature 368:554–558, 1994.

Fung-Leung WP, Kundig TM, Ngo K, Panakos J, De Sousa-Hitzler J, Wang E, Ohashi PS, Mak TW, Lau CY. Reduced thymic maturation but normal effector function of CD8+ T cells in CD8 beta gene-targeted mice. J Exp Med 180:959–967, 1994.

Fung-Leung WP, Kundig TM, Zinkernagel RM, Mak TW. Immune response against lymphocytic choriomeningitis virus infection in mice without CD8 expression. J Exp Med 174:1425–1429, 1991a.

Fung-Leung WP, Schilham MW, Rahemtulla A, Kundig TM, Vollenweider M, Potter J, van Ewijk W, Mak TW. CD8 is needed for development of cytotoxic T cells but not helper T cells. Cell 65:443–449, 1991b.

Fung-Leung WP, Surh CD, Liljedahl M, Pang J, Leturcq D, Peterson PA, Webb SR, Karlsson L. Antigen presentation and T cell development in H2-M-deficient mice. Science 271:1278–1281, 1996.

Fung-Leung W-P, Wallace VA, Gray D, Sha WC, Pircher H, The HS, Loh DY, Mak TW. CD8 is needed for positive selection but differentially required for negative selection of T cell during thymic ontogeny. Eur J Immunol 23:212–216, 1993.

Genot E, Cantrell DA. Ras regulation and function in lymphocytes. Curr Opin Immunol 12:289–294, 2000.

Georgopolous K. Hematopoietic cell fate decisions, chromatin regulation and Ikaros. Nat Rev Immunol 2:162–174, 2002.

Gilfillan S, Dierich A, Lemeur M, Benoist C, Mathis D. Mice lacking TdT: mature animals with an immature lymphocyte repertoire. Science 261: 1175–1178, 1993.

Glaichenhaus N, Shastri N, Littman DR, Turner JM. Requirement for association of p56lck with CD4 in antigen-specific signal transduction in T cells. Cell 64:511–520, 1991.

Gomez M, Tybulewicz V, Cantrell DA. Control of pre-T cell proliferation and differentiation by the GTPase Rac-1. Nat Immunol 1:348–352, 2000.

Gong Q, Cheng AM, Akk AM, Alberola-Ila J, Gong G, Pawson T, Chan AC. Disruption of T cell signalling networks and development by Grb2 haploid insufficiency. Nat Immunol 2:29–35, 2001.

Gossen M, Freundlieb S, Bender G, Muller G, Hillen W, Bujard H. Transcriptional activation by tetracyclines in mammalian cells. Science 268: 1766–1769, 1995.

Gossler A, Doetschman T, Korn R, Serfling E, Kemler R. Transgenesis by means of blastocyst-derived embryonic stem cell lines. Proc Natl Acad Sci USA 83:9065–9069, 1986.

Grant SG, O'Dell TJ, Karl KA, Stein PL, Soriano P, Kandel ER. Impaired long-term potentiation, spatial learning, and hippocampal development in fyn mutant mice. Science 258:1903–1910, 1992.

Greenstein JL, Kappler J, Marrack P, Burakoff SJ. The role of L3T4 in recognition of Ia by a cytotoxic, H-2Dd-specific T cell hybridoma. J Exp Med 159:1213–1224, 1984.

Gross JA, Appleby MW, Chien S, Nada S, Bartelmez SH, Okada M, Aizawa S, Perlmutter RM. Control of lymphopoiesis by p50csk, a regulatory protein tyrosine kinase. J Exp Med 181:463–473, 1995.

Groves T, Smiley P, Cooke MP, Forbush K, Perlmutter RM, Guidos CJ. Fyn can partially substitute for Lck in T lymphocyte development. Immunity 5:417–428, 1996.

Grusby MJ, Johnson RS, Papaioannou VE, Glimcher LH. Depletion of CD4+ T cells in major histocompatibility complex class II–deficient mice. Science 253:1417–1420, 1991.

Guo J, Hawwari A, Hong L, Sun Z, Mahanta SK, Littman DR, Krangel MS, He Y-W. Regulation of the TCR repertoire by the survival window of CD4 + CD8 + thymocytes. Nat Immunol 3:469–476, 2002.

Guy-Grand D, Cerf-Bensussan N, Malissen B, Malassis-Seris M, Briottet C, Vassalli P. Two gut intraepithelial CD8+ lymphocyte populations with different T cell receptors: a role for the gut epithelium in T cell differentiation. J Exp Med 173:471–481, 1991.

Hailman E, Burack WR, Shaw AS, Dustin ML, Allen PM. Immature CD4+CD8+ thymocytes form a multifocal immunological synapse with sustained tyrosine phosphorylation. Immunity 16:839–848, 2002.

Hanahan D. Peripheral antigen-expressing cells in the thymic medulla: factors in self-tolerance and autoimmunity. Curr Opin Immunol 10:656–662, 1998.

Hasserjian RP, Aster JC, Davi F, Weinberg DS, Sklar J. Modulated expression of Notch-1 during thymocyte development. Blood 88:970–976, 1996.

Hasty P, Ramirez-Solis R, Krumlauf R, Bradley A. Introduction of a subtle mutation into the Hox-2.6 locus in embryonic stem cells. Nature 350:243–246, 1991.

Hayden-Martinez K, Kane LP, Hedrick SM. Effects of a constitutively active form of calcineurin on T cell activation and thymic selection. J Immunol 163:3713–3721, 2000.

Heath WR, Carbone FR. Cross-presentation, dendritic cells, tolerance and immunity. Annu Rev Immunol 19:47–64, 2001.

Heath WR, Carbone FR, Bertolino P, Kelly J, Cose S, Miller JF. Expression of two T cell receptor alpha chains on the surface of normal murine T cells. Eur J Immunol 25:1617–1623, 1995.

Hedrick SM, Cohen DI, Nielsen EA, Davis MM. Isolation of cDNA clones encoding T cell–specific membrane-associated proteins. Nature 308:149–153, 1984.

Heid HW, Moll I, Franke WW. Patterns of expression of trychocytic and epithelial cytokeratins in mammalian tissues. Differentiation 37:215–230, 1988.

Henning S, Galandrini R, Hall A, Cantrell DA. The GTPase Rho has a critical regulatory role in thymocyte development. EMBO J 16:2397–2407, 1997.

Hermiston ML, Xu Z, Majeti R, Weiss A. Reciprocal regulation of lymphocyte activation by tyrosine kinases and phosphatases. J Clin Invest 109:9–14, 2002.

Hernandez-Hoyos G, Sohn SJ, Rothenberg EV, Alberola-Ila J. Lck activity controls CD4/CD8 T cell lineage commitment. Immunity 12:313–322, 2000.

Hettmann T, Leiden JM. NF-κB is required for the positive selection of CD8+ thymocytes. J Immunol 165:5004–5010, 2000.

Hogquist K. Signal strength in thymic selection and lineage commitment. Curr Opin Immunol 13:225–231, 2001.

Hogquist KA, Jameson SC, Heath WR, Howard JL, Bevan MJ, Carbone FR. T cell receptor antagonist peptides induce positive selection. Cell 76:17–27, 1994.

Holsinger LJ, Graef IA, Swat W, Chi T, Bautista DM, Davidson L, Lewis RS, Alt FW, Crabtree GR. Defects in actin-cap formation in Vav-deficient mice implicate an actin requirement for lymphocyte signal transduction. Curr Biol 8:563–572, 1998.

Hsieh JJ, Henkel T, Salmon P, Robey E, Peterson MG, Hayward SD. Truncated mammalian Notch-1 activates CBF1/RBPJk-repressed genes by a mechanism resembling that of Epstein-Barr virus EBNA2. Mol Cell Biol 16:952–959, 1996.

Hu-Li J, Pannetier C, Guo L, Lohning M, Gu H, Watson C, Assenmacher M, Radbruch A, Paul WE. Regulation of expression of IL-4 alleles: analysis using a chimeric GFP/IL-4 gene. Immunity 14:1–11, 2001.

Imamoto A, Soriano P. Disruption of the csk gene, encoding a negative regulator of Src family tyrosine kinases, leads to neural tube defects and embryonic lethality in mice. Cell 7:1117–1124, 1993.

Iritani BM, Alberola-Ila J, Forbush KA, Perlmutter RM. Distinct signals mediate maturation and allelic exclusion in lymphocyte progenitors. Immunity 10:713–722, 1999.

Irving BA, Alt FW, Killeen N. Thymocyte development in the absence of pre-T cell receptor extracellular immunoglobulin domains. Science 280:905–908, 1998.

Itano A, Kioussis D, Robey E. Stochastic component to development of class I major histocompatibility complex–specific T cells. Proc Natl Acad Sci USA 91:220–224, 1994.

Itohara S, Mombaerts P, Lafaille J, Iacomini J, Nelson A, Clarke AR, Hooper ML, Farr A, Tonegawa S. T cell receptor delta gene mutant mice: independent generation of alpha beta T cells and programmed rearrangements of gamma delta TCR genes. Cell 72:337–348, 1993.

Izon DJ, Aster JC, He Y, Weng A, Karnell FG, Patriub V, Xu L, Bakkour S, Rodriguez C, Allman D, Pear WS. Deltex1 redirects lymphoid progenitors to the B cell lineage by antagonizing Notch-1. Immunity 16:231–243, 2002.

Izon DJ, Punt JA, Xu L, Karnell FG, Allman D, Myung PS, Boerth NJ, Pui JC, Koretzky GA, Pear WS. Notch-1 regulates maturation of CD4+ and CD8+ thymocytes by modulating TCR signal strength. Immunity 14:253–264, 2001.

Jaleco AC, Neves H, Hooijberg E, Gameiro P, Clode N, Haury M, Henrique D, Parreira L. Differential effects of Notch ligands Delta-1 and Jagged-1 in human lymphoid differentiation. J Exp Med 194:991–1002, 2001.

Jolicoeur C, Hanahan D, Smith KM. T-cell tolerance towards a transgenic β-cell antigen and transcription of endogenous pancreatic genes in thymus. Proc Natl Acad Sci USA 91:6707–6711, 1994.

Kane LP, Hedrick SM. A role for calcium influx in setting the threshold for CD4+CD8+ thymocyte negative selection. J Immunol 156:4594–4601, 1996.

Kang J, Coles M, Raulet DH. Defective development of gamma/delta T cells in interleukin 7 receptor-deficient mice is due to impaired expression of T cell receptor gamma genes. J Exp Med 190:973–982, 1999.

Kappler JW, Roehm N, Marrack P. T cell tolerance by clonal elimination in the thymus. Cell 49:273–280, 1987a.

Kappler JW, Staerz U, White J, Marrack PC. Self-tolerance eliminates T cells specific for Mls-modified products of the major histocompatibility complex. Nature 332:35–40, 1988.

Kappler JW, Wade T, White J, Kushnir E, Blackman M, Bill J, Roehm N, Marrack P. A T cell receptor V beta segment that imparts reactivity to a class II major histocompatibility complex product. Cell 49:263–271, 1987b.

Kaye J, Hsu ML, Sauron ME, Jameson SC, Gascoigne NR, Hedrick SM. Selective development of CD4+ T cells in transgenic mice expressing a class II MHC-restricted antigen receptor. Nature 341:746–749, 1989.

Killeen N, Sawada S, Littman DR. Regulated expression of human CD4 rescues helper T cell development in mice lacking expression of endogenous CD4. EMBO J 12:1547–1553, 1993.

Kim HK, Siu G. The notch pathway intermediate HES-1 silences CD4 gene expression. Mol Cell Biol 18:7166–7175, 1998.

Kirchgessner CU, Patil CK, Evans JW, Cuomo CA, Fried LM, Carter T, Oettinger MA, Brown JM. DNA-dependent kinase (p350) as a candidate gene for the murine SCID defect. Science 267:1178–1183, 1995.

Kishihara K, Penninger J, Wallace VA, Kundig TM, Kawai K, Wakeham A, Timms E, Pfeffer K, Ohashi PS, Thomas ML, et al. Normal B lymphocyte development but impaired T cell maturation in CD45-exon6 protein tyrosine phosphatase-deficient mice. Cell 74:143–156, 1993.

Klausner RD, Samelson LE. T cell antigen receptor activation pathways: the tyrosine kinase connection. Cell 64:875–878, 1991.

Klein L, Klugmann M, Nave KA, Tuohy VK, Kyewski B. Shaping of the autoreactive T-cell repertoire by a splice variant of self protein expressed in thymic epithelial cells. Nat Med 6:56–61, 2000.

Klein TC, Doffinger R, Pepys MB, Ruther U, Kyewski B. Tolerance and immunity to the inducible self antigen C-reactive protein in transgenic mice. Eur J Immunol 25:3489–3495, 1995.

Koch U, Lacombe TA, Holland D, Bowman JL, Cohen BL, Egan SE, Guidos CJ. Subversion of the T/B lineage decision in the thymus by lunatic fringe-mediated inhibition of Notch-1. Immunity 15:225–236, 2001.

Koller BH, Marrack P, Kappler JW, Smithies O. Normal development of mice deficient in beta 2M, MHC class I proteins, and CD8+ T cells. Science 248:1227–1230, 1990.

Koller BH, Smithies O. Altering genes in animals by gene targeting. Annu Rev Immunol 10:705–730, 1992.

Komori T, Okada A, Stewart V, Alt FW. Lack of N regions in antigen receptor variable region genes of TdT-deficient lymphocytes. Science 261:1171–1175, 1993.

Kong YY, Fischer KD, Bachmann MF, Mariathasan S, Kozieradzki I, Nghiem MP, Bouchard D, Bernstein A, Ohashi PS, Penninger JM. Vav regulates peptide-specific apoptosis in thymocytes. J Exp Med 188:2099–2111, 1998.

Kontgen F, Suss G, Stewart C, Steinmetz M, Bluethmann H. Targeted disruption of the MHC class II Aa gene in C57BL/6 mice. Int Immunol 5:957–964, 1993.

Kuhn R, Schwenk F, Aguet M, Rajewsky K. Inducible gene targeting in mice. Science 269:1427–1429, 1995.

Kuo CT, Leiden JM. Transcriptional regulation of T lymphocyte development and function. Annu Rev Immunol 17:149–187, 1999.

Kyewski B, Derbinski J, Gotter J, Klein L. Promiscuous gene expression and central T-cell tolerance: more than meets the eye. Trends Immunol 23:364–371, 2002.

Legname G, Seddon B, Lovatt M, Tomlinson P, Sarner N, Tolaini M, Williams K, Norton T, Kioussis D, Zamoyska R. Inducible expression of a p56Lck transgene reveals a central role for Lck in the differentiation of CD4 SP thymocytes. Immunity 12:537–546, 2000.

Leung RK, Thomson K, Gallimore A, Jones E, Van den Broek M, Sierro S, Alsheikhly AR, McMichael A, Rahemtulla A. Deletion of the CD4 silencer supports a stochastic mechanism of thymocyte lineage commitment. Nat Immunol 2:1167–1173, 2001.

Levin SD, Anderson SJ, Forbush KA, Perlmutter RM. A dominant-negative transgene defines a role for p56lck in thymopoiesis. EMBO J 12:1671–1680, 1993.

Liao XC, Littman DR. Altered T cell receptor signaling and disrupted T cell development in mice lacking Itk. Immunity 3:757–769, 1995.

Littlewood TD, Hancock DC, Danielian PS, Parker MG, Evan GI. A modified oestrogen receptor ligand-binding domain as an improved switch for the regulation of heterologous proteins. Nucl Acids Res 23:1686–1690, 1995.

Littman DR. The structure of the CD4 and CD8 genes. Annu Rev Immunol 5:561–584, 1987.

Liu CP, Ueda R, She J, Sancho J, Wang B, Weddell G, Loring J, Kurahara C, Dudley EC, Hayday A, et al. Abnormal T cell development in CD3-zeta–/– mutant mice and identification of a novel T cell population in the intestine. EMBO J 12:4863–4875, 1993.

Locksley RM, Reiner SL, Hatam F, Littman DR, Killeen N. Helper T cells without CD4: control of leishmaniasis in CD4-deficient mice. Science 261:1448–1451, 1993.

Love PE, Shores EW, Johnson MD, Tremblay ML, Lee EJ, Grinberg A, Huang SP, Singer A, Westphal H. T cell development in mice that lack the zeta chain of the T cell antigen receptor complex. Science 261:918–921, 1993.

Ma A, Pena JC, Chang B, Margosian E, Davidson L, Alt FW, Thompson CB. Bclx regulates the survival of double-positive thymocytes. Proc Natl Acad Sci USA 92:4763–4767, 1995.

MacDonald HR, Schneider R, Lees RK, Howe RC, Acha-Orbea H, Festenstein H, Zinkernagel RM, Hengartner H. T-cell receptor V beta use predicts reactivity and tolerance to Mlsa-encoded antigens. Nature 332:40–45, 1988.

Majeti R, Xu Z, Parslow TG, Olson JL, Daikh DI, Killeen N, Weiss A. An inactivating point mutation in the inhibitory wedge of CD45 causes lymphoproliferation and autoimmunity. Cell 103:1059–1070, 2000.

Mak T, Penninger J, Ohashi S. Knockout mice: a paradigm shift in modern immunology. Nat Rev Immunol 1:1–11, 2001.

Malissen B, Malissen M. Functions of TCR and pre-TCR subunits: lessons from gene ablation. Curr Opin Immunol 8:383–393, 1996.

Malissen M, Gillet A, Ardouin L, Bouvier G, Trucy J, Ferrier P, Vivier E, Malissen B. Altered T cell development in mice with a targeted mutation of the CD3-epsilon gene. EMBO J 14:4641–4653, 1995.

Malissen M, Gillet A, Rocha B, Trucy J, Vivier E, Boyer C, Kontgen F, Brun N, Mazza G, Spanopoulou E, et al. T cell development in mice lacking the CD3-zeta/eta gene. EMBO J 1:4347–4355, 1993.

Maraskovsky E, O'Reilly LA, Teepe M, Corcoran LM, Peschon JJ, Strasser A. Bcl-2 can rescue T lymphocyte development in interleukin-7 receptor-deficient mice but not in mutant Rag-1–/– mice. Cell 89:1011–1019, 1997.

Mariathasan S, Bachmann MF, Bouchard D, Ohteki T, Ohashi PS. Degree of TCR internalization and Ca^{2+} flux correlates with thymic selection. J Immunol 161:6030–6037, 1998.

Mariathasan S, Ho SS, Zakarian A, Ohashi PS. Degree of ERK activation influences both positive and negative thymocyte selection. Eur J Immunol 30:1060–1068, 2000.

Martin WD, Hicks GG, Mendiratta SK, Leva HI, Ruley HE, Van Kaer L. H2-M mutant mice are defective in the peptide loading of class II molecules, antigen presentation, and T cell repertoire selection. Cell 84:543–550, 1996.

Matsuyama T, Kimura T, Kitagawa M, Pfeffer K, Kawakami T, Watanabe N, Kundig TM, Amakawa R, Kishihara K, Wakeham A, et al. Targeted disruption of IRF-1 or IRF-2 results in abnormal type I IFN gene induction and aberrant lymphocyte development. Cell 75:83–97, 1993.

McGargill MA, Derbinski JM, Hogquist KA. Receptor editing in developing T cells. Nat Immunol 1:336–341, 2000.

Mellins E, Smith L, Arp B, Cotner T, Celis E, Pious D. Defective processing and presentation of exogenous antigens in mutants with normal HLA class II genes. Nature 343:71–74, 1990.

Metzger D, Chambon P. Site- and time-specific gene targeting in the mouse. Methods 24:71–80, 2001.

Michie AM, Soh JW, Hawley RG, Weinstein IB, Zuniga-Pflucker JC. Allelic exclusion and differentiation by protein kinase C–mediated signals in immature thymocytes. Proc Natl Acad Sci USA 98:609–614, 2001.

Miyazaki T, Wolf P, Tourne S, Waltzinger C, Dierich A, Barois N, Ploegh H, Benoist C, Mathis D. Mice lacking H2-M complexes, enigmatic elements of the MHC class II peptide-loading pathway. Cell 84:531–541, 1996.

Molina TJ, Kishihara K, Siderovski DP, van Ewijk W, Narendran A, Timms E, Wakeham A, Paige CJ, Hartmann KU, Veillette A, et al. Profound block in thymocyte development in mice lacking p56lck. Nature 357:161–164, 1992.

Mombaerts P, Anderson SJ, Perlmutter RM, Mak TW, Tonegawa S. An activated lck transgene promotes thymocyte development in RAG-1 mutant mice. Immunity 1:261–267, 1994.

Mombaerts P, Clarke AR, Rudnicki MA, Iacomini J, Itohara S, Lafaille JJ, Wang L, Ichikawa Y, Jaenisch R, Hooper ML, et al. Mutations in T-cell antigen receptor genes alpha and beta block thymocyte development at different stages. Nature 360:225–231, 1992a.

Mombaerts P, Iacomini J, Johnson RS, Herrup K, Tonegawa S, Papaioannou VE. RAG-1-deficient mice have no mature B and T lymphocytes. Cell 68:869–877, 1992b.

Monaco JJ, Cho S, Attaya M. Transport protein genes in the murine MHC: possible implications for antigen processing. Science 250:1723–1726, 1990.

Monks CR, Freiberg BA, Kupfer H, Sciaky N, Kupfer A. Three-dimensional segregation of supramolecular activation clusters in T cells. Nature 395:82–86, 1998.

Morris P, Shaman J, Attaya M, Amaya M, Goodman S, Bergman C, Monaco JJ, Mellins E. An essential role for HLA-DM in antigen presentation by class II major histocompatibility molecules. Nature 368:551–554, 1994.

Motoyama N, Wang F, Roth KA, Sawa H, Nakayama K, Nakayama K, Negishi I, Senju S, Zhang Q, Fujii S, et al. Massive cell death of immature hematopoietic cells and neurons in Bcl-x-deficient mice. Science 267:1506–1510, 1995.

Nada S, Yagi T, Takeda H, Tokunaga T, Nakagawa H, Ikawa Y, Okada M, Aizawa S. Constitutive activation of Src family kinases in mouse embryos that lack Csk. Cell 73:1125–1135, 1993.

Neefjes JJ, Ploegh HL. Intracellular transport of MHC class II molecules. Immunol Today 13:179–184, 1992.

Negishi I, Motoyama N, Nakayama K, Senju S, Hatakeyama S, Zhang Q, Chan AC, Loh DY. Essential role for ZAP-70 in both positive and negative selection of thymocytes. Nature 376:435–438, 1995.

Nehls M, Kyewski B, Messerle M, Waldschutz R, Schuddekopf K, Smith AJ, Boehm T. Two genetically separable steps I the differentiation of thymic epithelium. Science 272:886–889, 1996.

Nehls M, Pfeifer D, Schorpp M, Hedrich H, Boehm T. New member of the winged helix protein family disrupted in mouse and rat nude mutations. Nature 371:103–107, 1994.

O'Gorman S, Fox DT, Wahl GM. Recombinase-mediated gene activation and site-specific integration in mammalian cells. Science 251:1351–1355, 1991.

Ohno H, Aoe T, Taki S, Kitamura D, Ishida Y, Rajewsky K, Saito T. Developmental and functional impairment of T cells in mice lacking CD3 zeta chains. EMBO J 12:4357–4366, 1993.

Osborne B, Miele L. Notch and the immune system. Immunity 11:653–663, 1999.

O'Shea CC, Crompton T, Rosewell IR, Hayday AC, Owen MJ. Raf regulates positive selection. Eur J Immunol 26:2350–2355, 1996.

O'Shea CC, Thornell AP, Rosewell IR, Hayes B, Owen MJ. Exit of the pre-TCR from the ER/cisGolgi is necessary for signaling, differentiation, proliferation and allelic exclusion in immature thymocytes. Immunity 7:591–599, 1997.

Oukka M, Ho IC, de la Brousse FC, Hoey T, Grusby MJ, Glimcher LH. The transcription factor NFAT4 is involved in the generation and survival of T cells. Immunity 9:295–304, 1998.

Outram SV, Varas A, Pepicelli CV, Crompton T. Hedgehog signaling regulates differentiation from double-negative to double-positive thymocyte. Immunity 13:187–197, 2000.

Page DM, Kane LP, Allison JP, Hedrick SM. Two signals are required for negative selection of CD4+CD8+ thymocytes. J Immunol 151:1868–1880, 1993.

Pages G, Guerin S, Grall D, Bonino F, Smith A, Anjuere F, Auberger P, Pouyssegur J. Defective thymocyte maturation in p44 MAP kinase (ERK 1) knockout mice. Science 286:1374–1377, 1999.

Panigada M, Porcellini S, Sutti F, Doneda L, Pozzoli O, Consalez GG, Guttinger M, Grassi F. GKLF in thymus epithelium as a developmentally regulated element of thymocyte-stroma cross-talk. Mech Dev 81:103–113, 1999.

Pannetier C, Hu-Li J, Paul WE. Bias in the expression of IL-4 alleles: the use of T cell from a GFP knock-in mouse. Cold Spring Harbor Symp Quant Biol 64:599–602, 1999.

Pearson R, Weston K. c-Myb regulates the proliferation of immature thymocytes following β-selection. EMBO J 19:6112–6120, 2000.

Penninger J, Kishihara K, Molina T, Wallace VA, Timms E, Hedrick SM, Mak TW. Requirement for tyrosine kinase p56lck for thymic development of transgenic gamma delta T cells. Science 260:358–361, 1993.

Penninger JM, Sirard C, Mittrucker HW, Chidgey A, Kozieradzki I, Nghiem M, Hakem A, Kimura T, Timms E, Boyd R, Taniguchi T, Matsuyama T, Mak TW. The interferon regulatory transcription factor IRF-1 controls positive and negative selection of CD8+ thymocytes. Immunity 7:243–254, 1997.

Penninger JM, Wallace VA, Molina T, Mak TW. Lineage-specific control of superantigen-induced cell death by the protein tyrosine kinase p56(lck). J Immunol 157:5359–5366, 1996.

Philpott KL, Viney JL, Kay G, Rastan S, Gardiner EM, Chae S, Hayday AC, Owen MJ. Lymphoid development in mice congenitally lacking T cell receptor alpha beta-expressing cells. Science 256:1448–1452, 1992.

Pitkanen J, Doucas V, Sternsdorf T, Nakajima T, Aratani S, Jensen K, Will H, Vahamurto P, Ollila J, Vihinen M, Scott HS, Antonarakis SE, Kudoh J, Shimizu N, Krohn K, Peterson P. The autoimmune regulator protein has transcriptional transactivating properties and interacts with the common co-activator CREB-binding protein. J Biol Chem 275:16802–16809, 2000.

Pivniouk V, Tsitsikov E, Swinton P, Rathbun G, Alt FW, Geha RS. Impaired viability and profound block in thymocyte development in mice lacking the adaptor protein SLP-76. Cell 94:229–238, 1998.

Pribyl TM, Campagnoni C, Kampf K, Handley VW, Campagnoni AT. The major myelin protein genes are expressed in the human thymus. J Neurosci Res 45:812–819, 1996.

Pui JC, Allman D, Xu L, DeRocco S, Karnell FG, Bakkour S, Lee JY, Kadesch T, Hardy RR, Aster JC, Pear WS. Notch-1 expression in early lymphopoiesis influences B versus T lineage determination. Immunity 11:299–308, 1999.

Punt JA, Osborne BA, Takahama Y, Sharrow SO, Singer A. Negative selection of CD4+CD8+ thymocytes by T cell receptor–induced apoptosis requires a costimulatory signal that can be provided by CD28. J Exp Med 179:709–713, 1994.

Radtke F, Wilson A, Stark G, Bauer M, van Meerwijk J, MacDonald HR, Aguet M. Deficient T cell fate specification in mice with an induced inactivation of Notch-1. Immunity 10:547–558, 1999.

Rahemtulla A, Fung-Leung WP, Schilham MW, Kundig TM, Sambhara SR, Narendran A, Arabian A, Wakeham A, Paige CJ, Zinkernagel RM, et al. Normal development and function of CD8+ cells but markedly decreased helper cell activity in mice lacking CD4. Nature 353:180–184, 1991.

Rahemtulla A, Kundig TM, Narendran A, Bachmann MF, Julius M, Paige CJ, Ohashi PS, Zinkernagel RM, Mak TW. Class II major histocompatibility complex–restricted T cell function in CD4-deficient mice. Eur J Immunol 24:2213–2218, 1994.

Rajewsky K, Gu H, Kuhn R, Betz UA, Muller W, Roes J, Schwenk F. Conditional gene targeting. J Clin Invest 98:600–603, 1996.

Ramsdell F, Lantz T, Fowlkes BJ. A nondeletional mechanism of thymic self tolerance. Science 246:1038–1041, 1989.

Ramsey C, Winqvist O, Pyuhakka L, Halonen M, Moro A, Kämpe O, Eskelin P, Pelto-Huikko M, Peltonen L. Aire-deficient mice develop multiple features of APECED phenotype and show altered immune response. Hum Mol Genet 11:397–409, 2002.

Raulet DH, Garman RD, Saito H, Tonegawa S. Developmental regulation of T-cell receptor gene expression. Nature 314:103–107, 1985.

Rincon M. Map-kinase signaling pathways in T cells. Curr Opin Immunol 13:339–345, 2001.

Rivera RR, Johns CP, Quan J, Johnson RS, Murre C. Thymocyte selection is regulated by the helix-loop-helix inhibitor protein, Id3. Immunity 12:17–26, 2000.

Robertson E, Bradley A, Kuehn M, Evans M. Germ-line transmission of genes introduced into cultured pluripotential cells by retroviral vector. Nature 323:445–448, 1986.

Robey E. Regulation of T cell fate by Notch. Annu Rev Immunol 17:283–295, 1999.

Robey E, Chang D, Itano A, Cado D, Alexander H, Lans D, Weinmaster G, Salmon P. An activated form of Notch influences the choice between CD4 and CD8 T cell lineages. Cell 87:483–492, 1996.

Robey E, Itano A, Fanslow WC, Fowlkes BJ. Constitutive CD8 expression allows inefficient maturation of CD4+ helper T cells in class II major histocompatibility complex mutant mice. J Exp Med 179:1997–2004, 1994.

Roche PA. HLA-DM: an in vivo facilitator of MHC class II peptide loading. Immunity 3:259–262, 1995.

Rothenberg EV, Anderson MK. Elements of transcription factor network design for T-lineage specification. Dev Biol 246:29–44, 2002.

Rüland J, Duncan GS, Elia A, del Barco Barrantes I, Nguyen L, Plyte S, Millar DG, Bouchard D, Wakeham A, Ohashi PS, Mak TW. Bcl10 is a positive regulator of antigen receptor-induced activation of NF-κB and neural tube closure. Cell 104:33–42, 2001.

Saint-Ruf C, Panigada M, Azogui O, Debey P, von Boehmer H, Grassi F. Different initiation of pre-TCR and γδTCR signaling. Nature 406:524–527, 2000.

Sakaguchi S. Animal models of autoimmunity and their relevance to human diseases. Curr Opin Immunol 12:684–690, 2000.

Salmon P, Mong M, Kang XJ, Cado D, Robey E. The role of CD8α in the CD4 versus CD8 lineage choice. J Immunol 163:5312–5318, 1999.

Samelson LE, Phillips AF, Luong ET, Klausner RD. Association of the fyn protein-tyrosine kinase with the T-cell antigen receptor. Proc Natl Acad Sci USA 87:4358–4362, 1990.

Schaeffer EM, Broussard C, Debnath J, Anderson S, McVicar DW, Schwartzberg PL. Tec family kinases modulate thresholds for thymocyte development and selection. J Exp Med 192:987–1000, 2000.

Schatz DG, Oettinger MA, Baltimore D. The V(D)J recombination activating gene, RAG-1. Cell 59:1035–1048, 1989.

Schilham MW, Clevers H. HMG box-containing transcription factors in lymphocyte differentiation. Semin Immunol 10:127–132, 1998.

Schlissel MS, Durum SD, Muegge K. The interleukin 7 receptor is required for T cell receptor γ locus accessibility to the V(D)J recombinase. J Exp Med 191:1045–1050, 2000.

Schmedt C, Saijo K, Niidome T, Kuhn R, Aizawa S, Tarakhovsky A. Csk controls antigen receptor-mediated development and selection of T-lineage cells. Nature 394:901–904, 1998.

Schmedt C, Tarakhovsky A. Autonomous maturation of alpha/beta T lineage cells in the absence of COOH-terminal Src kinase (Csk). J Exp Med 193:815–826, 2001.

Schmitt TM, Zúñiga-Pflücker JC. Induction of T cell development from hematopoietic progenitor cells by delta-like-1 in vitro. Cell 17:749–756, 2002.

Sebzda E, Mariathasan S, Ohteki T, Jones R, Bachmann MF, Ohashi PS. Selection of the T cell repertoire. Annu Rev Immunol 17:829–874, 1999.

Sebzda E, Wallace VA, Mayer J, Yeung RS, Mak TW, Ohashi PS. Positive and negative thymocyte selection induced by different concentrations of a single peptide. Science 263:1615–1618, 1994.

Seddon B, Mason D. The third function of the thymus. Immunol Today 21:95–99, 2000.

Sharp LL, Hedrick SM. Commitment to the CD4 lineage mediated by extracellular signal-related kinase mitogen-activated protein kinase and lck signaling. J Immunol 163:6598–6605, 1999.

Sharp LL, Schwarz DA, Bott CM, Marshall CJ, Hedrick SM. The influence of the MAPK pathway on T cell lineage commitment. Immunity 7:609–618, 1997.

Shearer GM. Cell-mediated cytotoxicity to trinitrophenyl-modified syngeneic lymphocytes. Eur J Immunol 4:527–533, 1974.

Sherman MA, Weber DA, Jensen PE. DM enhances peptide binding to class II MHC by release of invariant chain-derived peptide. Immunity 3:197–205, 1995.

Shinkai Y, Koyasu S, Nakayama K, Murphy KM, Loh DY, Reinherz EL, Alt FW. Restoration of T cell development in RAG-2-deficient mice by functional TCR transgenes. Science 259:822–825, 1993.

Shinkai Y, Rathbun G, Lam KP, Oltz EM, Stewart V, Mendelsohn M, Charron J, Datta M, Young F, Stall AM, et al. RAG-2-deficient mice lack mature lymphocytes owing to inability to initiate V(D)J rearrangement. Cell 68:855–867, 1992.

Shores EW, Ono M, Kawabe T, Sommers CL, Tran T, Lui K, Udey MC, Ravetch J, Love PE. T cell development in mice lacking all T cell receptor zeta family members (zeta, eta, and FcepsilonRIgamma). J Exp Med 187:1093–1101, 1998.

Shortman K. Cellular aspects of early T-cell development. Curr Opin Immunol 4:140–146, 1992.

Smith KM, Olson DC, Hirose R, Hanahan D. Pancreatic gene expression in rare cells of thymic medulla: evidence for functional contribution to T cell tolerance. Int Immunol 9:1355–1365, 1997.

Snapper SB, Rosen FS, Mizoguchi E, Cohen P, Khan W, Liu CH, Hagemann TL, Kwan SP, Ferrini R, Davidson L, Bhan AK, Alt FW. Wiskott-Aldrich syndrome protein-deficient mice reveal a role for WASP in T but not B cell activation. Immunity 9:81–91, 1998.

Speiser DE, Pircher H, Ohashi PS, Kyburz D, Hengartner H, Zinkernagel RM. Clonal deletion induced by either radioresistant thymic host cells or lymnphohemopoietic donor cells at different stages of class I–restricted T cell ontogeny. J Exp Med 175:1277–1283, 1992.

Spies T, DeMars R. Restored expression of major histocompatibility class I molecules by gene transfer of a putative peptide transporter. Nature 351: 323–324, 1991.

Sprent J, Lo D, Gao EK, Ron Y. T cell selection in the thymus. Immunol Rev 101:173–190, 1988.

Stein PL, Lee HM, Rich S, Soriano P. pp59fyn mutant mice display differential signaling in thymocytes and peripheral T cells. Cell 70:741–750, 1992.

Sternberg N, Sauer B, Hoess R, Abremski K. Bacteriophage P1 cre gene and its regulatory region. Evidence for multiple promoters and for regulation by DNA methylation. J Mol Biol 187:197–212, 1986.

Struhl G, Adachi A. Nuclear access and action of notch in vivo. Cell 93: 649–660, 1998.

Su DM, Manley NR. Hox3a and Pax1 transcription factors regulate the ability of fetal thymic epithelial cells to promote thymocyte development. J Immunol 164:5753–5760, 2000.

Sun Z, Arendt CW, Ellmeier W, Schaeffer EM, Sunshine MJ, Gandhi L, Annes J, Petrzilka D, Kupfer A, Schwartzberg PL, Littman DR. PKC-θ is required for TCR-induced NF-κB activation in mature but not immature T lymphocytes. Nature 404:402–407, 2000a.

Sun Z, Unutmaz D, Zou YR, Sunshine MJ, Pierani A, Brenner-Morton S, Mebius RE, Littman DR. Requirement for RORγ in thymocyte survival and lymphoid organ development. Science 288:2369–2373, 2000b.

Swan KA, Alberola-Ila J, Gross JA, Appleby MW, Forbush KA, Thomas JF, Perlmutter RM. Involvement of p21ras distinguishes positive and negative selection in thymocytes. EMBO J 14:276–285, 1995.

Tarakhovsky A, Turner M, Schaal S, Mee PJ, Duddy LP, Rajewsky K, Tybulewicz VL. Defective antigen receptor-mediated proliferation of B and T cells in the absence of Vav. Nature 374:467–470, 1995.

Taylor D, Badiani P, Weston K. A dominant interfering Myb mutant causes apoptosis in T cells. Genes Dev 10:2732–2744, 1996.

Tonegawa S. Somatic generation of antibody diversity. Nature 302:575–581, 1983.

Toyonaga B, Yoshikai Y, Vadasz V, Chin B, Mak TW. Organization and sequences of the diversity, joining, and constant region genes of the human T-cell receptor beta chain. Proc Natl Acad Sci USA 82:8624–8628, 1985.

Turner JM, Brodsky MH, Irving BA, Levin SD, Perlmutter RM, Littman DR. Interaction of the unique N-terminal region of tyrosine kinase p56lck with cytoplasmic domains of CD4 and CD8 is mediated by cysteine motifs. Cell 60:755–765, 1990.

Turner M, Mee PJ, Costello PS, Williams O, Price AA, Duddy LP, Furlong MT, Geahlen RL, Tybulewicz VL. Perinatal lethality and blocked B-cell development in mice lacking the tyrosine kinase Syk. Nature 378:298–302, 1995.

Turner M, Mee PJ, Walters AE, Quinn ME, Mellor AL, Zamoyska R, Tybulewicz VL. A requirement for the Rho-family GTP exchange factor Vav in positive and negative selection of thymocytes. Immunity 7:451–460, 1997.

Van Kaer L, Ashton-Rickardt PG, Ploegh HL, Tonegawa S. TAP1 mutant mice are deficient in antigen presentation, surface class I molecules, and CD4-8+ T cells. Cell 71:1205–1214, 1992.

van Meerwijk JP, O'Connell EM, Germain RN. Evidence for lineage commitment and initiation of positive selection by thymocytes with intermediate surface phenotypes. J Immunol 154:6314–6323, 1995.

van Oers NSC, Lowin-Kropf B, Finlay D, Connolly K, Weiss A. Alpha-beta T cell development is abolished in mice lacking both Lck and Fyn. Immunity 5:429–436, 1996.

Veillette A, Bookman MA, Horak EM, Bolen JB. The CD4 and CD8 T cell surface antigens are associated with the internal membrane tyrosine-protein kinase p56lck. Cell 55:301–308, 1988.

Viville S, Neefjes J, Lotteau V, Dierich A, Lemeur M, Ploegh H, Benoist C, Mathis D. Mice lacking the MHC class II-associated invariant chain. Cell 72:635–648, 1993.

Voll RE, Jimi E, Phillips RJ, Barber DF, Rincon M, Hayday AC, Flavell RA, Ghosh S. NF-κB activation by the pre-T cell receptor serves as a selective survival signal in T lymphocyte development. Immunity 13:677–689, 2000.

von Boehmer H. CD4/CD8 lineage commitment: back to instruction? J Exp Med 183:713, 1996.

von Boehmer H. Coming to grips with Notch. J Exp Med 194:F43–F46, 2001.

von Boehmer H, Aifantis I, Feinberg J, Lechner O, Saint-Ruf C, Walter U, Buer J, Azogui O. Pleiotropic changes controlled by the pre-T cell receptor. Curr Opin Immunol 11:135–142, 1999.

von Boehmer H, Kishi H, Borgulya P, Scott B, van Ewijk W, The HS, Kisielow P. Control of T-cell development by the TCR alpha beta for antigen. Cold Spring Harb Symp Quant Biol 54(Pt 1):111–118, 1989a.

von Boehmer H, Teh HS, Kisielow P. The thymus selects the useful, neglects the useless and destroys the harmful. Immunol Today 10:57–61, 1989b.

von Freeden-Jeffry U, Solvason N, Howard M, Murray R. The earliest T lineage-commited cells depend on IL-7 for Bcl-2 expression and normal cell cycle progression. Immunity 7:147–154, 1997.

Wallace VA, Penninger J, Mak TW. CD4, CD8 and tyrosine kinases in thymic selection. Curr Opin Immunol 5:235–240, 1993.

Washburn T, Schweighoffer E, Gridley T, Chang D, Fowlkes BJ, Cado D, Robey E. Notch activity influences the alphabeta versus gammadelta T cell lineage decision. Cell 88:833–843, 1997.

Weiss A, Littman DR. Signal transduction by lymphocyte antigen receptors. Cell 76:263–274, 1994.

Werlen G, Hausmann B, Palmer E. A motif in the αβ T cell receptor controls positive selection by modulating ERK activity. Nature 406:422–426, 2000.

White LC, Wright KL, Felix NJ, Ruffner H, Reis LF, Pine R, Ting JP. Regulation of LMP2 and TAP1 genes by IFR-1 explains the paucity of CD8+ T cells in IRF-1-/- mice. Immunity 5:365–376, 1996.

Wiest DL, Berger MA, Carleton M. Control of early thymocyte development by the pre-T cell receptor complex: a receptor without a ligand? Semin Immunol 11:251–262, 1999.

Wilson A, MacDonald HR, Radtke F. Notch 1-deficient common lymphoid precursors adopt a B cell fate in the thymus. J Exp Med 194:1003–1012, 2001.

Wolfer A, Wilson A, Nemir M, MacDonald HR, Radtke F. Inactivation of Notch-1 impairs VDJβ rearrangement and allows pre-TCR-independent survival of early α/β lineage thymocytes. Immunity 16:869–879, 2002.

Wu G, Danska JS, Guidos CJ. Lck dependence of signaling pathways activated by gamma-irradiation and CD3 epsilon engagement in RAG-1(-/-)-immature thymocytes. Int Immunol 8:1159–1164, 1996.

Wulfing C, Bauch A, Crabtree GR, Davis MM. The vav exchange factor is an essential regulator in actin-dependent receptor translocation to the lymphocyte-antigen-presenting cell interface. Proc Natl Acad Sci USA 97:10150–10155, 2000.

Yagi T, Ikawa Y, Yoshida K, Shigetani Y, Takeda N, Mabuchi I, Yamamoto T, Aizawa S. Homologous recombination at c-fyn locus of mouse embryonic stem cells with use of diphtheria toxin A-fragment gene in negative selection. Proc Natl Acad Sci USA 87:9918–9922, 1990.

Yamaguchi H, Hendrickson WA. Structural basis for activation of human lymphocyte kinase Lck upon tyrosine phosphorylation. Nature 384:484–489, 1996.

Yanagi Y, Yoshikai Y, Leggett K, Clark SP, Aleksander I, Mak TW. A human T cell–specific cDNA clone encodes a protein having extensive homology to immunoglobulin chains. Nature 308:145–149, 1984.

Yasutomo K, Doyle C, Miele L, Fuchs C, Germain RN. The duration of antigen receptor signalling determines CD4+ versus CD8+ T-cell lineage fate. Nature 404:506–510, 2000.

Yeung RS, Penninger J, Mak TW. T-cell development and function in gene-knockout mice. Curr Opin Immunol 6:298–307, 1994.

Yoder J, Pham C, Iizuka YM, Kanagawa O, Liu SK, McGlade J, Cheng AM. Requirement for the SLP-76 adaptor GADS in T cell development. Science 291:1987–1991, 2001.

Zhang R, Alt FW, Davidson L, Orkin SH, Swat W. Defective signalling through the T- and B-cell antigen receptors in lymphoid cells lacking the vav proto-oncogene. Nature 374:470–473, 1995.

Zhang J, Shehabeldin A, da Cruz LA, Butler J, Somani AK, McGavin M, Kozieradzki I, dos Santos AO, Nagy A, Grinstein S, Penninger JM, Siminovitch KA. Antigen receptor-induced activation and cytoskeletal rearrangement are impaired in Wiskott-Aldrich syndrome protein-deficient lymphocytes. J Exp Med 190:1329–1342, 1999.

Zhang W, Sommers CL, Burshtyn DN, Stebbins CC, DeJarnette JB, Trible RP, Grinberg A, Tsay HC, Jacobs HM, Kessler CM, Long EO, Love PE, Samelson LE. Essential role of LAT in T cell development. Immunity 10:323–332, 1999.

Zhumabekov T, Corbella P, Tolaini M, Kioussis D. Improved version of a human CD2 minigene based vector for T cell–specific expression in transgenic mice. J Immunol Methods 185:133–140, 1995.

Zijlstra M, Bix M, Simister NE, Loring JM, Raulet DH, Jaenisch R. Beta 2-microglobulin deficient mice lack CD4-8+ cytolytic T cells. Nature 344: 742–746, 1990.

Zinkernagel RM, Callahan GN, Althage A, Cooper S, Klein PA, Klein J. On the thymus in the differentiation of "H-2 self-recognition" by T cells: evidence for dual recognition? J Exp Med 147:882–896, 1978.

Zinkernagel RM, Doherty PC. Restriction of in vitro T cell–mediated cytotoxicity in lymphocytic choriomenigitis virus within a syngeneic or semi-allogeneic system. Nature 248:701–702, 1974.

Zinkernagel RM, Doherty PC. MHC-restricted cytotoxic T cells: studies on the biological role of polymorphic major transplantation antigens determining T-cell restriction-specificity, function, and responsiveness. Adv Immunol 27:51–177, 1979.

5

Molecular Mechanisms Guiding B Cell Development

ANTONIUS G. ROLINK, JAN ANDERSSON, ULF GRAWUNDER, and FRITZ MELCHERS

B lymphocytes develop from hematopoietic stem cells. In the mouse, B cell development takes place at different sites in the body during ontogeny, starting at day 8–8.5 of gestation in yolk sac and fetal aorta (Cumano et al., 1993; Godin et al., 1993, 1995; Cumano and Godin, 2001; Ling and Dzierzak, 2002). When circulation of blood begins at day 9 of gestation, B cell precursors can still be found in the yolk sac and fetal aorta, and later—around days 10–11—in the liver, spleen, and omentum (Ogawa et al., 1988; Rolink and Melchers, 1991; Solvason et al., 1992; Melchers and Rolink, 1999; Cumano and Godin, 2001). From days 15 to 16 of gestation, B cell precursors are also found in the bone marrow. After birth, the bone marrow becomes the major site for B lymphopoiesis (Hardy et al., 1991; Rolink and Melchers, 1991; Rolink et al., 1993, 1994; Osmond et al., 1998; Melchers and Rolink, 1999; Hardy and Hayakawa, 2001). B cell development in mouse and human bone marrow from progenitor (pro) and precursor (pre) B cells to immature and mature sIg-positive B cells is characterized by changes in (1) rearrangement of immunoglobulin (Ig) heavy (H) and light (L) chain genes; (2) the expression of surface-bound and intracellular markers; (3) cell cycle status; (4) in vitro growth properties; and (5) life expectancy in vivo.

In this chapter we will use this nomenclature for the different stages of B cell development. Table 5.1 provides a comparison with the widely used "Philadelphia" nomenclature (Hardy et al., 1991; Hardy and Hayakawa, 2001) for early B cell stages. The table also shows the Ig rearrangement status of various developmental stages. Figure 5.1 summarizes the different early stages of B cell development in mouse and the markers expressed at these various stages. In Figure 5.2 presents a similar summary of the late stages of B cell development in mouse.

We have described in detail normal B cell development elsewhere (Rolink and Melchers, 1991; Ghia et al., 1998; Osmond et al., 1998; Melchers and Rolink, 1999). Briefly, the first identifiable cell within the B cell lineage, the pro-B cell, expresses low levels of CD45R (B220) together with c-kit, Flt3/FLK-2, and CD43, but does not yet express the lineage-specific marker CD19 (Rolink et al., 1996; Ogawa et al., 2000; Hardy and Hayakawa, 2001). The Ig heavy (IgH) chain loci in these cells are predominantly in (nonrearranged) germ-line configuration.

pre-BI cells following the earlier pro-B stage carry both IgH chain alleles DJ rearranged, with the exception of those found in rearrangement-deficient or defective mice, such as RAG1$^{-/-}$, RAG2$^{-/-}$, severe combined immunodeficiency (SCID), or J$_H$–deficient mice (Bosma et al., 1988; Mombaerts et al., 1992; Shinkai et al., 1992; Chen et al., 1993). The pre-BI cells express CD45R (B220), CD19, CD43, and c-kit on their surface, whereas TdT, RAG1, and RAG2 are expressed intracellularly (Rolink et al., 1991a, 1991b, 1993, 1994; Grawunder et al., 1995). Moreover, pre-BI cells express the two components of the surrogate light (SL) chain, λ_5 and V$_{preB}$ (Karasuyama et al., 1993, 1996). They have lost Flt3/FLK-2 expression (Ogawa et al., 2000) and do not yet express CD25 (Rolink et al., 1994). About 30%–40% of pre-BI cells are in the S, G$_2$–M phase of the cell cycle. pre-BI cells can also proliferate long term on stromal cells in the presence of IL-7 in vitro (Rolink et al., 1991a).

Pre-B-II cells have VDJ–rearranged IgH chain loci and can be subdivided by expression of SL chain and size into three populations (Rolink et al., 1994; Grawunder et al., 1995; Ghia et al., 1998; Osmond et al., 1998; Melchers and Rolink, 1999). All pre-B-II cells have lost c-kit and TdT but gained CD25 (TAC) surface expression (Rolink et al., 1994). Moreover, μH chain expression in the cytoplasm can be detected in over 95% of these cells (Rolink et al., 1994), thus indicating that the pre-B-II compartment is selected for those cells that have undergone productive V$_H$D$_H$J$_H$ rearrangement. Pre-B-II cells express intermediate

Table 5.1. Nomenclature and Immunoglobulin Rearrangement Status of Early Stages of Mouse B Cell Development

	Pro-B	Pre-BI	Large pre-B-II type 1	Large pre-B-II type 2	Small pre-B-II	Immature B
Basel nomenclature	Pro-B	Pre-BI	Large pre-B-II type 1	Large pre-B-II type 2	Small pre-B-II	Immature B
Philadelphia nomenclature	Pre-pro-B (Fr A)	Pro-B (Fr B/C)	Early pre-B (Fr C′)	Part of late pre-B (Fr D)	Part of late pre-B (Fr D)	New B (Fr E)
gH locus	GL	DJ	VDJ	VDJ	VDJ	VDJ
gL locus	GL	GL	GL	GL	VJ	VJ

gH, immunoglobulin heavy chain; IgL, immunoglobulin light chain.

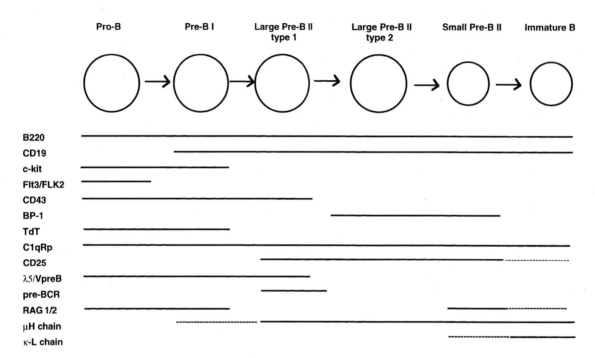

Figure 5.1. Markers used to identify early stages of mouse B cell development. Solid lines indicate that all cells express the marker, whereas broken lines indicate weak expression or only a fraction of the cells expressing the marker. Large circles represent cells that are cycling; small circles indicate resting cells.

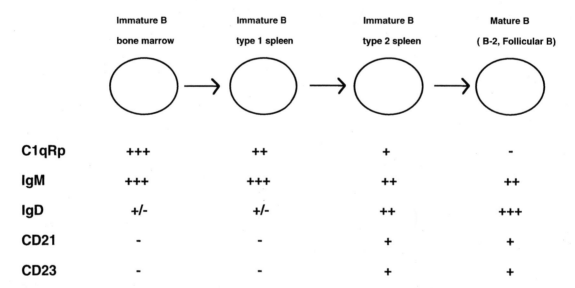

Figure 5.2. Markers used to identify late stages of mouse B cell development. Surface markers indicated are evaluated for staining intensities in FACS analyses.

levels of CD45R (B220) and CD19. All pre-B-II cells have lost the capacity to proliferate on stromal cells plus IL-7. About 15%–20% of pre-B-II cells are large, and 70%–80% of these are in the S, G_2–M phase of the cell cycle. Approximately 25% of these express the SL chain in complex with a μH chain on their surface (Rolink et al., 1994).

The noncycling, small pre-B-II population has also lost SL expression. Single-cell polymerase chain reaction (PCR) analysis (ten Boekel et al., 1995; Yamagami et al., 1999a, 1999b) has shown that these cells are in the process of L-chain rearrangement and are therefore the direct precursors of *immature* sIgM$^+$ sIgD$^-$ B cells. Some of the immature B cells formed in the bone marrow migrate to the spleen. Here they can be distinguished from their mature counterparts by expression of the C1qRp protein, recognized by the monoclonal antibodies (MAbs) 493 and AA4.1 (Rolink et al., 1998, 1999a, 2001; Norsworthy et al., 1999; Petrenko et al., 1999; Allman et al., 2001), and by their short life span (4 days vs. more than 6 weeks). The immature B cells in spleen can be subdivided into type 1 and type 2 (transitional cells), based on the differential expression of CD21, CD23, IgM, and IgD, as depicted in Figure 5.2 (Loder et al., 1999; Rolink et al., 2001). Both types of immature splenic B cells are very sensitive to anti-IgM–induced apoptosis in vitro.

In this chapter, we will summarize recent experimental evidence that further defines different cellular stages of B cell development. Special attention will be paid to mutant mice in which B cell development is impaired at various stages.

B Lineage Commitment

The differentiation of hematopoietic stem cells (HSCs) into the various hematopoietic lineages is usually pictured in a hierarchical fashion: these cells develop first into progenitors and then into precursors, with decreasing pluripotency and increasing commitment to single differentiation pathways (Weissman, 2000). Mice deficient for the basic helix-loop-helix proteins encoded by the *E2A* gene and early B cell factor (EBF) show an arrest of B cell development at the earliest stage prior to rearrangement of the IgH locus (Bain et al., 1994; Busslinger, 2004; Zhuang et al., 1994; Lin and Grosschedl, 1995; Matthias & Rolink, 2005). These findings, together with those showing that forced expression of E2A and EBF in hematopoietic precursors induce the transcription of several B lymphoid–specific genes (Kee and Murre, 1998; O'Riordan and Grosschedl, 1999; Romanow et al., 2000; Goebel et al., 2001), have implicated these two transcription factors in the control of B lineage commitment. However, this idea was recently challenged by findings made with mice deficient for the transcription factor Pax5.

Pax5-deficient mice exhibit a block in B cell development at the transition from $D_H J_H$–rearranged pre-BI to $V_H D_H J_H$–rearranged pre-B-II cells (Urbánek et al., 1994; Nutt et al., 1997). Pax5$^{-/-}$ pre-BI cells express various lymphoid and B cell–specific genes, including RAG-1, RAG-2, TdT, λ_5, V_{preB}, Igα, Igβ, E2A, and EBF, similar to wild-type pre-BI cells (Nutt et al., 1997, 1998; Schebesta et al., 2002). Moreover, like wild-type cells, Pax5$^{-/-}$ pre-B-1 cells have the long-term capacity to grow in vitro on stromal cells in the presence of IL-7 (Nutt et al., 1997, 1998; Schebesta et al., 2002). However, and in marked contrast to wild-type pre-BI cells, Pax5-deficient B cell precursors can under appropriate in vitro conditions develop into macrophages, granulocytes, osteoclasts, dendritic cells, and natural killer (NK) cells (Nutt et al., 1999; Schebesta et al., 2002; Busslinger, 2004).

Upon transplantation into an irradiated host, Pax5$^{-/-}$ pre-BI cells can differentiate into T cells, macrophages, granulocytes,

osteoclasts, dendritic cells, NK cells, and, in rare cases, even into erythrocytes (Nutt et al., 1999; Rolink et al., 1999b; Schebesta et al., 2002; Schaniel et al., 2002a). Furthermore, Pax5$^{-/-}$ pre-BI cells home to the bone marrow where they retain their phenotype and original differentiation state. These cells can then be recloned in vitro on stromal cells and IL-7. Upon retransplantation these cells again populate the bone marrow and also give rise to the various hematopoietic cells mentioned before (Rolink et al., 1999b; Schaniel et al., 2002b). Recently Schaniel et al. (2002b) showed that at least five serial transplantations can be performed with these Pax5$^{-/-}$ pre-BI cells without losing their hematopoietic multipotency and self-renewing capacity. Thus, Pax5$^{-/-}$ pre-BI cells exhibit features of pluripotent HSCs. Moreover, this unexpected in vitro and in vivo plasticity of Pax5$^{-/-}$ pre-BI cells in hematopoietic development strongly suggests that Pax5 expression determines B cell commitment.

Pax5 is known to both activate and repress transcription depending on the regulatory sequence context of the target gene (Nutt et al., 1999; Schebesta et al., 2002). This dual function of Pax5 is compatible with its role in B lineage commitment. On the one hand, Pax5 further activates B lymphoid–specific gene expression, as best illustrated by the induction of CD19 expression in Pax5$^{-/-}$ pre-BI cells after reconstitution with a Pax5-expressing recombinant retrovirus (Nutt et al., 1999). On the other hand, Pax5 represses the transcription of lineage-inappropriate genes, e.g., the macrophage colony-stimulating factor receptor (M-CSF-R) gene, thus rendering these pre-BI cells unresponsive to M-CSF and interfering with their capacity to differentiate into macrophages.

Pro-B Cells

The earliest fraction of B cell progenitors in the scheme of Hardy and colleagues (Hardy et al., 1991; Hardy and Hayakawa, 2001) is fraction A. The cells in this fraction are characterized by the expression of B220 and CD43 and the absence of heat-stable antigen (HSA) and BP-1. They constitute approximately 3% of the total nucleated bone marrow cells. It has been shown that, in contrast to all other stages of B cell development, these cells do not express CD19 (Rolink et al., 1996). In fact, it has been demonstrated that the vast majority of these cells do not belong to the B cell lineage. About 30% of these cells are precursors of NK cells: they express NK cell markers and, after stimulation with IL-2 in vitro, gain the ability to lyse NK cell targets very efficiently (Rolink et al., 1996). Another 30%–40% of the cells in this fraction coexpress CD4 at levels comparable to those found on T cells. However, these cells are not T lineage cells because they do not express components of the T cell receptor and are found in similar numbers in RAG1- and RAG2-deficient animals. Furthermore, these cells were unable to proliferate in an in vitro stromal cell/IL-7 culture system that enables the growth of pro- and pre-BI cells (Rolink et al., 1991a), thus these B220$^+$ CD4$^+$ cells are not progenitors of the B cell lineage. In addition, transplantation of these cells into RAG2$^{-/-}$ (gene name: *Rag2*) mice did not result in development of a detectable number of B cells or any other cell type of hematopoietic lineage. Several groups (Asselin-Paturel et al., 2001; Nakano et al., 2001; Nikolic et al., 2002) have recently indicated that these CD4$^+$ cells might be the murine counterparts of the so-called plasmacytoid dendritic cells of humans (Cella et al., 1999).

Within the population of B220$^+$, CD19$^-$, NK1.1$^-$, CD4$^-$ cells, a small subpopulation can be identified that expresses c-kit, Flt3/FLK-2, C1qRp, and λ_5 and exhibits B cell progenitor activity (Rolink et al., 1996; Ogawa et al., 2000). These cells can be grown on stromal cells in the presence of IL-7 and can differentiate into CD19$^+$ B lineage cells. However, whether these cells are already committed to the B cell lineage remains unknown. Transplantation of such cells grown for 2 weeks in vitro into RAG2-deficient mice results in the reconstitution of both B and T cell compartments (Rolink et al., unpublished observation).

pre-BI Cells

The next stage in B cell development relates to the so-called pre-BI cells. These cells have gained CD19 expression and lost Flt3/FLK-2 expression—i.e., they are B220$^+$, CD19$^+$, c-kit$^+$, CD43$^+$, SL$^+$, and C1qRp$^+$ and express TdT, RAG1, and RAG2 in the nucleus (Rolink et al., 1993, 1994, 1996; Ghia et al., 1998; Osmond et al., 1998; Ogawa et al., 2000). The L chain gene loci in these cells are in germ-line configuration and are transcriptionally still inactive (Grawunder et al., 1995; ten Boekel et al., 1995). Development at this stage is blocked in mice with deficiencies in the rearrangement machinery (Bosma et al., 1988; Mombaerts et al., 1992; Shinkai et al., 1992) and in mice harboring a deletion of the J$_H$ gene segment (Chen et al., 1993). This results in pre-BI cells with IgH chain loci in germ-line configuration. In contrast, the vast majority of pre-BI cells found in other strains of mice (rearrangement competent) have both IgH alleles DJ rearranged (Rolink et al., 1991a; ten Boekel et al., 1995).

A small segment (10%–20%) of the pre-BI cells have completed IgH chain rearrangements and express a μH chain in the cytoplasm (ten Boekel et al., 1997, 1998). Surprisingly, 50% of μH chains found in pre-BI cells are unable to pair with the SL components λ$_5$ and V$_{preB}$, and thus cannot make a precursor B cell antigen receptor (pre-BCR) (ten Boekel et al., 1997, 1998; see below). Also surprising was the finding that about 20% of these μH chains use the most D-proximal V$_H$ element V$_H$81X (ten Boekel et al., 1997). None of these V$_H$81X μH chains analyzed was able to form a pre-BCR. This might also explain why V$_H$81X μH chains are very rarely found in mature B cells (Decker et al., 1991; Carlsson et al., 1992; Huetz et al., 1993). The biological meaning of this biased V$_H$81X usage in pre-BI cells is still unclear.

In vitro, pre-BI cells can be propagated on stromal cells in the presence of IL-3, IL-7, or thymic stromal-derived lymphopoietin (TSLP) (Rolink et al., 1991a; Winkler et al., 1995a; Ray et al., 1996).

As mentioned above, an arrest in B cell development at the pre-BI stage is also found in Pax5$^{-/-}$ mice. However, the target genes of Pax5 that are responsible for this arrest have not yet been identified. Moreover, a block in B lymphopoiesis at this stage is also observed in animals that cannot form a pre-BCR—for example, mice deficient for λ$_5$ (Kitamura et al., 1992), V$_{preB1}$, and V$_{preB2}$ (Mundt et al., 2001), and membrane deposition of μH (μH$^{-/-}$ mice) (Kitamura et al., 1991) and Igβ (Gong and Nussenzweig, 1996). This block also occurs in mice that have a defect in pre-BCR signaling due to mutations of Syk (Cheng et al., 1995; Turner et al., 1995) and B cell linker protein (BLNK) (Jumaa et al., 1999; Pappu et al., 1999; Hayashi et al., 2000). A block at the pre-BI cell stage of development is also observed in IL-7- and IL-7R-deficient mice—i.e., IL-7$^{-/-}$, IL-7Rα$^{-/-}$, and IL-2Rγ$^{-/-}$ mice (Peschon et al., 1994; DiSanto et al., 1995; von Freeden-Jeffry et al., 1995). The block observed in membrane μH$^{-/-}$, Igβ$^{-/-}$, Igα$^{-/-}$, and Pax5$^{-/-}$ mice is absolute, whereas in other mice, later stages, including mature B cells, are found in the bone marrow and in peripheral lymphoid organs, although in far lower numbers than in wild-type mice.

Pre-B-II Cells

The next developmental stage along in B lineage is characterized by cytoplasmic μH chain expression, which defines the pre-B-II cell stage. These typical pre-B cells have lost the expression of c-kit and TdT, and most of them do not express CD43 (Rolink et al., 1994). In addition to μH chain expression, these cells have gained the expression of CD25 (Rolink et al., 1994).

The pre-B-II compartment can be subdivided into three different developmental subsets. The first stage contains large and actively cycling cells. On the surface, they express the pre-BCR consisting of the SL chain in association with the μH chain (Rolink et al., 1994; Winkler et al., 1995b; Karasuyama et al., 1996). These cells do not express RAG1 and RAG2 and carry their IgL chain loci still in germ-line configuration (Grawunder et al., 1995; ten Boekel et al., 1995). It is exactly at this stage of development that the allelic exclusion of the second H chain allele is likely to be established; a transient down-regulation of the VDJ rearrangement machinery might be involved in this process (Grawunder et al., 1995). At this stage the L chain loci are not yet transcriptionally active. The H chain locus might be rendered inaccessible for further rearrangements in ways that need to be clarified.

The importance of this stage, especially the membrane deposition of the pre-B receptor ensuring normal B cell development, is best illustrated in mutants unable to produce this receptor. In mice with a deletion in the transmembrane portion of their μH chain and mice with a deletion in the λ$_5$ part or the V$_{preB1}$ and V$_{preB2}$ part of the SL-encoding genes, large cycling pre-B-II cells are not detected. This results in a reduced number of small pre-B cells (Kitamura et al., 1991, 1992; Mundt et al., 2001). A similar phenotype is found in mice with a deletion in the genes encoding Igβ (Gong and Nussenzweig, 1996), indicating that the association between the pre-BCR and Igβ and Igα and consequent signaling via surface pre-BCR is required for the transition from pre-BI to pre-B-II cells.

In line with this, tyrosine kinase Syk–deficient mice and mice defective for the adapter protein BLNK display a block at this early stage of B cell development. This finding indicates a key role for Syk and BLNK in pre-BCR signaling (Cheng et al., 1995; Turner et al., 1995; Jumaa et al., 1999; Pappu et al., 1999; Hayashi et al., 2000).

The importance of the pre-BCR is also indicated in experiments in which RAG1$^{-/-}$ or RAG2$^{-/-}$ mice are supplemented with a transgenic μH chain (Rolink et al., 1994; Spanopoulou et al., 1994; Young et al., 1994). As discussed above, RAG1$^{-/-}$ and RAG2$^{-/-}$ mice are blocked at the pre-BI cell stage. However, supplementation with a rearranged μH gene, which allows them to express a pre-BCR, results in progression of B cell development in these mice up to the stage of small pre-B-II cells. Thus, expression of the pre-BCR ensures proliferative expansion that constitutes a positive selection for pre-B cells with a productive VDJ rearrangement that can lead to formation of a pre-BCR.

We have shown that this pre-BCR-mediated selection and expansion can be mimicked in vitro. Sorted pre-BI cells of wild-type mice cultured in plain medium (no cytokines added) expanded (Rolink et al., 2000) were selected for productive VDJ rearrangement. By day 5 of culture, 70%–80% of the cells recovered expressed IgM on their surface. No expansion and/or selection was observed in pre-BI cells of λ$_5$$^{-/-}$ mice—i.e., pre-BI cells that cannot form a pre-BCR. Single-cell experiments with wild-type pre-BI cells indicated that approximately 15% of them undergo this expansion and selection. Moreover, it was found that single ex vivo isolated pre-BI cells proliferate to different clone sizes in vitro. This finding may indicate that pre-BCRs with different fitness of pairing with the SL chain allow different numbers of divisions. Overall, these in vitro data suggest that pre-BCR exerts its function in a ligand-independent fashion. There is further evidence that IL-7 can enhance the efficiency of pre-BCR-mediated expansion (Stoddart et al., 2000).

It has been shown that the transmembrane form of the μH chain is necessary for IgH chain allelic exclusion. Thus, around 15% of the peripheral B cells expressing sIgM in F1 mice carrying a wild-type and a transmembrane-deficient μH chain allele express the deficient allele in the cytoplasm (Kitamura and Rajewsky, 1992). On the basis of this finding and the fact that pre-BCR expressing pre-B-II cells have down-modulated RAG1 and RAG2 expression (Grawunder et al., 1995), it has been suggested that the pre-BCR also mediates allelic exclusion. However, $\lambda_5^{-/-}$ and V_{preB1} and RAG2$^{-/-}$ mice that cannot form a pre-BCR still exhibit allelic exclusion, which indicates that a complete pre-BCR is not needed for this process (ten Boekel et al., 1997, 1998; Mundt et al., 2001).

In all likelihood, the next developmental stage following the pre-BCR-positive cells is the large, cycling pre-B-II cell stage, in which expression of the SL chain is lost (Rolink et al., 1994; Winkler et al., 1995b; Karasuyama et al., 1996). Unlike the pre-BCR-positive pre-B-II cells, the large, cycling pre-B-II cells express RAG1 and RAG2 at the RNA but not yet at the protein level (Grawunder et al., 1995). Moreover, sterile transcripts from the κL chain gene locus become detectable, although the L chain gene loci in these cells are still in germ-line configuration (ten Boekel et al., 1995). When the large, cycling pre-B-II cells become resting and small, a large proportion of the cells carry rearranged L chain genes (ten Boekel et al., 1995; Yamagami et al., 1999a, 1999b). Already at this stage, the κL and λL chain loci are rearranged in the characteristic 10:1 ratio. Experiments by Engel et al. (1999) and Goldmit et al. (2005) suggest that chromatin structural changes rendering Ig gene loci accessible for V(D)J recombination occur earlier within the κL chain gene locus than within the λL chain gene. This may explain the high frequency of κL chain–containing immunoglobulins in the mouse.

In wild-type mice, about half of the sIg$^+$ B cells have rearranged only one allele at the κL chain locus. Most of these cells show only a single rearrangement, preferentially to Jκ1, the most V proximal of the functional J segments. In marked contrast, small pre-B-II cells show a dramatically increased frequency of multiple κL chain rearrangements (Yamagami et al., 1999a, 1999b). Moreover, about 20% of small pre-B-II cells express a κL chain protein in the cytoplasm but not on the cell surface, although half of these cells have productively rearranged VκJκ segments. Although over 95% of all pre-B-II cells express μH chains in their cytoplasm, these μH-κL chain combinations are not expressed on the surface.

Two possible scenarios might account for the lack of surface expression of the μH-κL chain pairs. First, it is conceivable that certain μH-κL chain combinations may not be able to form an IgM molecule. Since the peripheral sIgM$^+$ B cell pool should contain only pairing combinations, the small pre-B-II pool may be enriched for those that do not fit together. Second, a given μH-κL chain combination may have paired properly and been deposited on the surface. However, if this IgM is autoreactive and encounters autoantigen in the bone marrow environment, this might lead to down-regulation of these autoreactive receptors from the cell surface. Both scenarios are by no means mutually exclusive.

Nemazee and colleagues (Tiegs et al., 1993; Nemazee, 2000) and Weigert and coworkers (Gay et al., 1993; Radic et al., 1993) have shown that recognition of autoantigen by immature B cells induces secondary rearrangements at the L chain loci and thus can change the cells' receptor specificity from self to non-self. In humans, a similar type of BCR editing has been observed (Dorner et al., 1998). Recently, Casellas et al. (2001) showed that the contribution of B cells that have undergone receptor editing to the total peripheral B cell repertoire is about 25%. However, mice deficient for the expression of κL chains due to a deletion of the constant κL region display patterns of κL chain gene rearrangements in small pre-B-II cells similar to those in wild-type mice. This finding would argue against the notion that most of the receptor editing is autoantigen recognition driven (Yamagami et al., 1999a, 1999b).

When autoreactive Ig transgenes are bred onto a rearrangement-deficient background—i.e., a situation where receptor editing is impossible—an absolute block at the transition from small, pre-B-II to immature B cells is observed (Andersson et al., 1995). For instance, RAG2$^{-/-}$ mice carrying the Sp6 anti-TNP IgM transgene display this absolute block in differentiation at the transition from small pre-B-II to immature B cells. It is assumed that this block in differentiation results from the cross-reaction of Sp6 anti-TNP IgM with dsDNA, an apparently abundant autoantigen in the bone marrow environment where extensive cell apoptosis occurs. However, injection of Sp6 transgenic RAG2$^{-/-}$ mice with the T cell–independent antigen TNP-Ficoll elicits a strong antibody response within 5 days. Hence, cross-reactive T cell–independent antigens might be able to overcome negative selection and clonal deletion of autoreactive B cells. This raises the possibility that T-independent antigens may be involved in the initiation of autoimmune diseases.

Immature B Cells

Osmond and colleagues (reviewed in Osmond, 1993) have determined that mice produce roughly 2×10^7 immature B cells per day in the bone marrow. These immature B cells then migrate through the terminal branches of central arterioles into the spleen. At this site, these immature B cells, which display life spans of about 4 days, differentiate into mature B cells with life spans of around 15 weeks (Rolink et al., 1998, 2001). In the spleen the immature B cells can be distinguished from their mature counterparts by the cell surface expression of the C1qRp protein recognized by MAbs 493 and AA4.1 (Rolink et al., 1998, 1999a, 2001; Petrenko et al., 1999). Based on the expression of CD21 and CD23, immature B cells in the spleen can be subdivided into two populations (transitional cells); CD21$^-$ CD23$^-$ and CD21$^+$ CD23$^+$ (Loder et al., 1999) (Fig. 5.2).

In the transition from bone marrow to the spleen, about 90% of immature B cells are lost. A large part of this loss can probably be explained by the deletion of autoreactive B cells in the bone marrow, and signaling through the BCR appears to play a key role for this process. Thus both Syk-deficient mice and mice expressing an Igα lacking the cytoplasmic tail (Igα$^{\Delta c/\Delta c}$) show a much more marked loss of B cells at this transition (Turner et al., 1995; Torres et al., 1996). Interestingly, immature B cells in Igα$^{\Delta c/\Delta c}$ mice have increased levels of tyrosine phosphorylation and expression of activation antigen (Torres and Hafen, 1999). This suggests that the intensity of signaling may be very critical for B cells passing this checkpoint. Similar findings were evident in Igα$^{\Delta c/\Delta c}$ mice carrying a soluble hen egg lysozyme (HEL) and an anti-HEL immunoglobulin transgene (Kraus et al., 1999). The finding that in CD45$^{-/-}$ mice more immature B cells enter the spleen might indicate that the phosphatase CD45 is critically involved in signaling thresholds (Rolink et al., 1999a, 2001).

Mice deficient for the transcriptional coactivator OBF (also called OCA-B or Bob-1) show a severe reduction of immature B cells in the spleen (Schubart et al., 1996). This reduction is even more dramatic in OBF/Oct-2 (Schubart et al., 2001) and OBF/Btk (Bruton's tyrosine kinase) (Schubart et al., 2000) double-mutant mice. The molecular mechanisms underlying these defects are still unclear. However, a Bcl-2 transgene expressed in the B lineage rescues this defect to a large extent in OBF/Btk double-mutant mice, a finding suggesting that life spans of immature B cells may play a role in this transition (A.G. Rolink, unpublished data).

Cross-linking of the BCR on the two immature B cell populations found in the spleen (Fig. 5.2) leads to the induction of apoptosis (Rolink et al., 1998; King and Monroe, 2000), which indicates that these cells are still sensitive for undergoing negative selection. Nevertheless, in wild-type mice, most immature splenic B cells enter the pool of long-lived mature B cells (Rolink et al., 1998). The finding that apoptosis induced by BCR cross-linking can be blocked by anti-CD40 and IL-4 (Rolink et al., 1998; King and Monroe, 2000) may indicate that these molecules are involved in the transition from immature to mature B cells. CD40- and IL-4-deficient mice, however, have normal numbers of mature B cells (Kopf et al., 1993; Kawabe et al., 1994).

Recently it has been shown that mice deficient for the tumor necrosis factor (TNF) family member BAFF (also termed TALL-1, THANK, Blys, and zTNF4 (Moore et al., 1999; Mukhopadhyay et al., 1999; Schneider et al., 1999; Shu et al., 1999; Gross et al., 2000) or its receptor BAFF-R (Thompson et al., 2001) are blocked in B cell development at the CD21$^-$ CD23$^-$ stage in the spleen—i.e., at the type 1 immature B cell stage (Fig. 5.2). Moreover, immature splenic B cells treated with BAFF in vitro acquire a mature phenotype and become resistant to BCR cross-linking-induced apoptosis (Batten et al., 2000; Rolink et al., 2002). Taken together, these findings strongly suggest that the interaction between BAFF and BAFF-R plays a crucial role in the transition from immature to mature B cells.

Other mutant mice with defects in the transition from immature to mature B cells have also been described. For instance, Btk-defective mice have normal numbers of immature splenic B cells; however, their number of mature B cells is reduced about fivefold. Because the life span of mature B cells in Btk$^{-/-}$ mice is indistinguishable from that found for wild-type B cells, the defect most probably reflects a reduced efficiency of Btk$^{-/-}$ immature splenic B cells in entering the mature compartment (Rolink et al., 1999a). The finding that a Bcl-2 transgene expressed in B cells can rescue this defect suggests that the Btk molecule might be involved in induction of survival.

Major histocompatibility complex (MHC) class II has also been implicated in the transition from immature to mature B cells in the spleen. Thus, mice deficient in the invariant chain (Ii$^{-/-}$) (Shachar and Flavell, 1996) and MHC class IIα$^{-/-}$ mice (Rolink et al., 1999a) display a severely reduced mature B cell compartment. In fact, the mature B cell pool is completely absent in Btk/Aα double-mutant mice. The defect in Aα$^{-/-}$ mice appears to be intrinsic to the B cells and may be due to a four- to fivefold reduced life span of mature B cells (Rolink et al., 1999a). The molecular mechanisms underlying these defects are still unclear. In particular, the finding that CTIIA$^{-/-}$ (Chang et al., 1996) and Aβ$^{-/-}$ (Cosgrove et al., 1991; Markowitz et al., 1993) mice, as

well as mice lacking all conventional MHC class II genes (Madsen et al., 1999), do not show such a defect makes the role of MHC class II in this transition very puzzling.

Mature B Cells

The peripheral mature B cell compartment can be subdivided into three subpopulations: B-1, B-2, and marginal zone B cells, which can be distinguished by the differential expression of various cell surface markers (Table 5.2). Thus, B-1 cells are characterized by the high expression of IgM and the low expression of IgD and B220. Moreover, these cells express CD11b/Mac-1 and part of them expresses CD5, but they do not express CD21 and CD23. B-2 cells express intermediate levels of IgM and high levels of IgD and B220. Moreover, these cells express intermediate levels of CD21 and CD23 and do not express CD11b/Mac-1 or CD5. Marginal zone (MZ) B cells, by contrast, express high levels of IgM and CD21 but no or very little IgD and CD23. B220 expression levels are intermediate, whereas CD11b/Mac-1 and CD5 expression cannot be detected in these cells.

In addition to their different surface marker phenotype, these three subpopulations of mature B cells preferentially localize in different parts of the body. Thus B-1 cells are primarily found in the peritoneal cavity and some in the spleen (Hardy and Hayakawa, 2001). B-2 cells are mainly found in the circulation and in the primary lymphoid follicles of secondary lymphoid organs. Marginal zone B cells localize in the spleen to a region that surrounds the primary lymphoid follicles (Dammers et al., 1999; Oliver et al., 1999; Martin et al., 2001).

B-1 cells have a self-renewing capacity and are mainly derived from fetal liver stem cells. These cells contribute to a large extent to T-independent antibody responses. Many B1 cells carry a BCR that has low affinity for self-antigens, and recent evidence shows that their development depends on BCR-derived positive selection signals (Hayakawa et al., 1999; for review see Hardy and Hayakawa, 2001).

Marginal zone B cells show an activated phenotype and respond better and faster than B-2 cells to low concentrations of mitogens such as lippopolysaccharide (LPS) (Oliver et al., 1999; Martin et al., 2001). These cells can rapidly differentiate into plasma cells when activated, primarily by T-independent antigens, although they may also respond to T-dependent antigens. Like B-1 cells, MZ B cells have been shown to be generated by a positive selection process (Martin and Kearney, 2000; Wellmann et al., 2001).

The vast majority of B2 cells in the mouse are small and resting, i.e., not activated. They are primarily responsible for T-dependent immune responses and thus are also the precursors of the memory B cell compartment. It is probable that, like B-1 and MZ B cells, the B-2 cell compartment is generated via positive

Table 5.2. Markers Used to Distinguish Different Mature B Cell Subpopulations

	B1	B2/follicular B	Marginal Zone B
IgM	+++	++	+++
IgD	+/-	+++	+/-
B220	+	+++	++
CD21	+/-	++	+++
CD23	+/-	++	+/-
CD5	+/-	-	-
CD11b/Mac-1	++	-	-

selection, although direct experimental evidence for this is not yet available.

It is now well established that the formation of all three mature B cell subpopulations requires the expression of a functional BCR (Lam et al., 1997)—i.e., a BCR with signaling properties. The numerous mutant mice created in the last couple of years, however, have indicated that the BCR signal strength needed for the formation of these three subpopulations might be different (for reviews see Hardy and Hayakawa, 2001; Cariappa and Pillai, 2002). These studies showed that mutations causing a weakening of the BCR signal strength affect formation of the B-1 compartment but not that of the B-2 and MZ B cell compartments. In addition to BCR signaling, non-BCR-related molecular interactions are also differentially required for the formation of the three mature B cell subpopulations.

In this respect, BAFF- and BAFF-R-deficient mice lack the B-2 and the MZ B cell compartment but display a normal B-1 compartment (Moore et al., 1999; Mukhopadhyay et al., 1999; Schneider et al., 1999; Shu et al., 1999; Gross et al., 2000; Thompson et al., 2001). In addition, mutations affecting the microarchitecture of secondary lymphoid organs, especially of the spleen, as well as those disturbing the migration and homing of cells can influence the generation of the different mature B cell compartments (Futterer et al., 1998; Guinamard et al., 2000; Lipp et al., 2000; Fukui et al., 2001; Girkontaite et al., 2001; Reif et al., 2002).

Human B Cell Development

B cell development in human bone marrow is very similar to that in the mouse, but the expression of various cell surface markers characterizing murine differentiation stages is different (Gougeon et al., 1990; Ghia et al., 1996). A summary of markers used to identify early stages of human B cell development is given in Table 5.3. Cells at the earliest stage of B cell development in human bone marrow corresponding to the mouse pro/pre-BI compartment are CD19[+] CD10[+] CD34[+]. They express TdT and RAG intracellularly, but not μH chains. On the surface these cells also express the SL chain. The proteins associated with the SL chain at this stage of differentiation have not yet been identified. Like their murine counterparts, these cells actively undergo cell division. However, in contrast to the murine system, it has not yet been possible to define conditions that allow long-term proliferation of human pre-B cells in vitro. At this point, we do not know whether the inability to grow these pro/pre-B cells is due to the lack of a proper stromal cell or to the appropriate cytokines not yet being identified. It is also noteworthy that IL-7 seems to be far less important in human than in mouse B cell development.

This is based on the finding that patients with an inactive IL-2Rγ chain (also called common γ-chain, which is part of the IL-7 receptor) appear to have normal B cell development (Gougeon et al., 1990; Noguchi et al., 1993), whereas IL-2Rγ[−/−] mice have a major block in B cell development during the transition from pre-BI to pre-B-II cells (DiSanto et al., 1995).

A human equivalent to the mouse pre-BCR-positive pre-B-II cells has been identified. These cells are characterized as CD19[+], CD10[+], CD34[−] TdT[−], RAG1[−], pre-B cell receptor-positive large, cycling cells. They carry productively $V_H D_H J_H$–rearranged IgH chain loci, while their L chain gene loci, as in the mouse, are still in germ-line configuration. Mutations inactivating the expression and/or signaling of the pre-BCR (Minegishi et al., 1998, 1999; Conley et al., 2000) indicate that this receptor plays a role in human B cell development similar to that in mice—namely, selection and proliferative expansion of VDJ in-frame rearranged pre-B cells. This assumption is based on the fact that the vast majority of precursor B cells in human bone marrow also express μH chains in the cytoplasm.

Analogous to B cell development in the mouse, the next B lineage differentiation stage is defined by pre-BCR-negative pre-B-II cells that are CD19[+], CD10[+], CD34[−], TdT[−], RAG1[+/−], cμ[+]. However, some minor differences between the phenotypes of these cells in mouse and humans are also apparent at this stage of differentiation. For instance, a small but significant number of the large pre-BCR-negative human pre-B-II have undergone L chain rearrangements. Furthermore, low levels of V_{preB} mRNA, but not of protein, are still detectable in these cells.

When the large and cycling pre-BCR-negative human pre-B-II cells become quiescent, they up-regulate RAG expression and lose the expression of V_{preB}. Single-cell PCR analysis has shown that most of these cells have rearranged their IgL chain loci. Therefore, these cells are comparable to small, resting pre-B-II cells in mouse.

Collectively, these results indicate that the different stages of B cell development in human bone marrow are very similar to those found in mouse. Their relative sizes of the different pre-B cell compartments in young mice and young humans are also comparable. The identification of patients with impaired B cell development at a certain stage of differentiation might help us to elucidate mouse/human parallels and differences in transcription factors, cell surface receptors, and signaling molecules in B cell development, to name a few important components.

Acknowledgments

A.G.R. is holds the Chair in Immunology, University of Basel, endowed by F. Hoffmann-La Roche Ltd., Basel.

Table 5.3. Markers Used to Identify Early Stages of Human B-Cell Development

Marker	Pro/pre-B-I	Large pre-B-II type 1	Large pre-B-II type 2	Small pre-B-II	Immature B
CD19	+	+	+	+	+
CD34	+	−	−	−	−
CD10	+	+	+	+	+
λ_5/V_{preB}	+	+	−	−	−
pre-BCR	−	+	−	−	−
TdT	+	−	−	−	−
μH chain	−	+	+	+	+
Rag 1	+	ND	ND	+	+

ND, not determined.

References

Allman D, Lindsley RC, DeMuth W, Rudd K, Shinton SA, Hardy RR. Resolution of three nonproliferative immature splenic B cell subsets reveals multiple selection points during peripheral B cell maturation. J Immunol 167:6834–6840, 2001.

Andersson J, Melchers F, Rolink A. Stimulation by T cell independent antigens can relieve the arrest of differentiation of immature autoreactive B cells in the bone marrow. Scand J Immunol 42:21–33, 1995.

Asselin-Paturel C, Boonstra A, Dalod M, Durand I, Yessaad N, Dezutter-Dambuyant C, Vicari A, O'Garra A, Biron C, Briere F, Trinchieri G. Mouse type I IFN-producing cells are immature APCs with plasmacytoid morphology. Nat Immunol 2:1144–1150, 2001.

Bain G, Maandag EC, Izon DJ, Amsen D, Kruisbeek AM, Weintraub BC, Krop I, Schlissel MS, Feeney AJ, van Roon M, et al. E2A proteins are required for proper B cell development and initiation of immunoglobulin gene rearrangements. Cell 79:885–892, 1994.

Batten M, Groom J, Cachero TG, Qian F, Schneider P, Tschopp J, Browning JL, Mackay F. BAFF mediates survival of peripheral immature B lymphocytes. J Exp Med 192:1453–1466, 2000.

Bosma M, Schuler W, Bosma G. The SCID mouse mutant. Curr Top Microbiol Immunol 137:197–202, 1988.

Busslinger M. Transcriptional control of early B cell development. Annu Rev Immunol 22:55–79, 2004.

Cariappa A, Pillai S. Antigen-dependent B-cell development. Curr Opin Immunol 14:241–249, 2002.

Carlsson L, Övermo C, Holmberg D. Developmentally controlled selection of antibody genes: characterization of individual V_H7183 genes and evidence for stage-specific somatic diversification. Eur J Immunol 22: 71–78, 1992.

Casellas R, Shih TA, Kleinewietfeld M, Rakonjac J, Nemazee D, Rajewsky K, Nussenzweig MC. Contribution of receptor editing to the antibody repertoire. Science 291:1541–1544, 2001.

Cella M, Jarrossay D, Facchetti F, Alebardi O, Nakajima H, Lanzavecchia A, Colonna M. Plasmacytoid monocytes migrate to inflamed lymph nodes and produce large amounts of type I interferon. Nat Med 5:919–923, 1999.

Chang CH, Guerder S, Hong SC, van Ewijk W, Flavell RA. Mice lacking the MHC class II transactivator (CIITA) show tissue- specific impairment of MHC class II expression. Immunity 4:167–178, 1996.

Chen J, Trounstine M, Alt FW, Young F, Kurahara C, Loring JF, Huszar D. Immunoglobulin gene rearrangement in B cell deficient mice generated by targeted deletion of the J_H locus. Int Immunol 5:647–656, 1993.

Cheng AM, Rowley B, Pao W, Hayday A, Bolen JB, Pawson T. Syk tyrosine kinase required for mouse viability and B-cell development. Nature 378: 303–306, 1995.

Conley ME, Rohrer J, Rapalus L, Boylin EC, Minegishi Y. Defects in early B-cell development: comparing the consequences of abnormalities in pre-BCR signaling in the human and the mouse. Immunol Rev 178:75–90, 2000.

Cosgrove D, Gray D, Dierich A, Kaufman J, Lemeur M, Benoist C, Mathis D. Mice lacking MHC class II molecules. Cell 66:1051–1066, 1991.

Cumano A, Furlonger C, Paige CJ. Differentiation and characterization of B-cell precursors detected in the yolk sac and embryo body of embryos beginning at the 10- to 12-somite stage. Proc Natl Acad Sci USA 90: 6429–6433, 1993.

Cumano A, Godin I. Pluripotent hematopoietic stem cell development during embryogenesis. Curr Opin Immunol 13:166–171, 2001.

Dammers PM, de Boer NK, Deenen GJ, Nieuwenhuis P, Kroese FG. The origin of marginal zone B cells in the rat. Eur J Immunol 29:1522–1531, 1999.

Decker DJ, Boyle NE, Klinman NR. Predominance off nonproductive rearrangements of V_H81X gene segments evidences a dependence of B cell clonal maturation on the structure of nascent H chains. J Immunol. 147:1406–1411, 1991.

DiSanto JP, Muller W, Guy-Grand D, Fischer A, Rajewsky K. Lymphoid development in mice with a targeted deletion of the interleukin 2 receptor gamma chain. Proc Natl Acad Sci USA 92:377–381, 1995.

Dorner T, Foster SJ, Farner NL, Lipsky PE. Immunoglobulin kappa chain receptor editing in systemic lupus erythematosus. J Clin Invest 102:688–694, 1998.

Engel H, Rolink A, Weiss S. B cells are programmed to activate kappa and lambda for rearrangement at consecutive developmental stages. Eur J Immunol 29:2167–2176, 1999.

Fukui Y, Hashimoto O, Sanui T, Oono T, Koga H, Abe M, Inayoshi A, Noda M, Oike M, Shirai T, Sasazuki T. Haematopoietic cell–specific CDM family protein DOCK2 is essential for lymphocyte migration. Nature 412: 826–831, 2001.

Futterer A, Mink K, Luz A, Kosco-Vilbois MH, Pfeffer K. The lymphotoxin beta receptor controls organogenesis and affinity maturation in peripheral lymphoid tissues. Immunity 9:59–70, 1998.

Gay D, Saunders T, Camper S, Weigert M. Receptor editing: an approach by autoreactive B cells to escape tolerance. J Exp Med 177:999–1008, 1993.

Ghia P, ten Boekel E, Rolink AG, Melchers F. B-cell development: a comparison between mouse and man. Immunol Today 19:480–485, 1998.

Ghia P, ten Boekel E, Sanz E, de la Hera A, Rolink A, Melchers F. Ordering of human bone marrow B lymphocyte precursors by single-cell polymerase chain reaction analyses of the rearrangement status of the immunoglobulin H and L chain gene loci. J Exp Med 184:2217–2229, 1996.

Girkontaite I, Missy K, Sakk V, Harenberg A, Tedford K, Potzel T, Pfeffer K, Fischer KD. Lsc is required for marginal zone B cells, regulation of lymphocyte motility and immune responses. Nat Immunol 2:855–862, 2001.

Godin I, Dieterlen-Lièvre F, Cumano A. Emergence of multipotent hemopoietic cells in the yolk sac and paraaortic splanchnopleura in mouse embryos, beginning at 8.5 days postcoitus. Proc Natl Acad Sci USA 92: 773–777, 1995.

Godin IE, Garcia-Porrero JA, Coutinho A, Dieterlen-Lievre F, Marcos MA. Para-aortic splanchnopleura from early mouse embryos contains B1a cell progenitors. Nature 364:67–70, 1993.

Goebel P, Janney N, Valenzuela JR, Romanow WJ, Murre C, Feeney AJ. Localized gene-specific induction of accessibility to V(D)J recombination induced by E2A and early B cell factor in nonlymphoid cells. J Exp Med 194:645–656, 2001.

Goldmit M, Ji Y, Skok Y, Roldan E, Jung S, Cedar H, Bergman Y. Epigenetic ontogeny of the igk locus during B cell development. Nat Immunol 6:198–203, 2005.

Gong S, Nussenzweig MC. Regulation of an early developmental checkpoint in the B cell pathway by Igβ. Science 272:411–414, 1996.

Gougeon ML, Drean G, Le Deist F, Dousseau M, Fevrier M, Diu A, Theze J, Griscelli C, Fischer A. Human severe combined immunodeficiency disease: phenotypic and functional characteristics of peripheral B lymphocytes. J Immunol 145:2873–2879, 1990.

Grawunder U, Leu TMJ, Schatz DG, Werner A, Rolink AG, Melchers F, Winkler TH. Down-regulation of *RAG-1* and *RAG-2* gene expression in preB cells after functional immunoglobulin heavy chain rearrangement. Immunity 3:601–608, 1995.

Gross JA, Johnston J, Mudri S, Enselman R, Dillon SR, Madden K, Xu W, Parrish-Novak J, Foster D, Lofton-Day C, Moore M, Littau A, Grossman A, Haugen H, Foley K, Blumberg H, Harrison K, Kindsvogel W, Clegg CH. TACI and BCMA are receptors for a TNF homologue implicated in B-cell autoimmune disease. Nature 404:995–999, 2000.

Guinamard R, Okigaki M, Schlessinger J, Ravetch JV. Absence of marginal zone B cells in Pyk-2-deficient mice defines their role in the humoral response. Nat Immunol 1:31–36, 2000.

Hardy RR, Carmack CE, Shinton SA, Kemp JD, Hayakawa K. Resolution and characterization of pro B and pre–pro B cell stages in normal mouse bone marrow. J Exp Med 173:1213–1225, 1991.

Hardy RR, Hayakawa K. B cell development pathways. Annu Rev Immunol 19:595–621, 2001.

Hayakawa K, Asano M, Shinton SA, Gui M, Allman D, Stewart CL, Silver J, Hardy RR. Positive selection of natural autoreactive B cells. Science 285:113–116, 1999.

Hayashi K, Nittono R, Okamoto N, Tsuji S, Hara Y, Goitsuka R, Kitamura D. The B cell–restricted adaptor BASH is required for normal development and antigen receptor-mediated activation of B cells. Proc Natl Acad Sci USA 97:2755–2760, 2000.

Huetz F, Carlsson L, Tornberg UC, Holmberg D. V-region directed selection in differentiating B lymphocytes. EMBO J 12:1819–1826, 1993.

Jumaa H, Wollscheid B, Mitterer M, Wienands J, Reth M, Nielsen PJ. Abnormal development and function of B lymphocytes in mice deficient for the signaling adaptor protein SLP-65. Immunity 11:547–554, 1999.

Karasuyama H, Melchers F, Rolink A. A complex of glycoproteins is associated with V_{preB}/λ_5 surrogate light chain on the surface of µ heavy chain–negative early precursor B cell lines. J Exp Med 178:469–478, 1993.

Karasuyama H, Rolink A, Melchers F. Surrogate light chain in B cell development. Adv Immunol 63:1–41, 1996.

Kawabe T, Naka T, Yoshida K, Tanaka T, Fujiwara H, Suematsu S, Yoshida N, Kishimoto T, Kikutani H. The immune responses in CD40-deficient mice: impaired immunoglobulin class switching and germinal center formation. Immunity 1:167–178, 1994.

Kee BL, Murre C. Induction of early B cell factor (EBF) and multiple B lineage genes by the basic helix-loop-helix transcription factor E12. J Exp Med 188:699–713, 1998.

King LB, Monroe JG. Immunobiology of the immature B cell: plasticity in the B-cell antigen receptor–induced response fine tunes negative selection. Immunol Rev 176:86–104, 2000.

Kitamura D, Kudo A, Schaal S, Müller W, Melchers F, Rajewsky K. A critical role of λ_5 in B cell development. Cell 69:823–831, 1992.

Kitamura D, Rajewsky K. Targeted disruption of μ chain membrane exon causes loss of heavy-chain allelic exclusion. Nature 356:154–156, 1992.

Kitamura D, Roes J, Kühn R, Rajewsky K. A B cell–deficient mouse by targeted disruption of the membrane exon of the immunoglobulin μ chain gene. Nature 350:423–426, 1991.

Kopf M, Le Gros G, Bachmann M, Lamers MC, Bluethmann H, Kohler G. Disruption of the murine IL-4 gene blocks Th2 cytokine responses. Nature 362:245–248, 1993.

Kraus M, Saijo K, Torres RM, Rajewsky K. Ig-alpha cytoplasmic truncation renders immature B cells more sensitive to antigen contact. Immunity 11:537–545, 1999.

Lam KP, Kuhn R, Rajewsky K. In vivo ablation of surface immunoglobulin on mature B cells by inducible gene targeting results in rapid cell death. Cell 90:1073–1083, 1997.

Lin H, Grosschedl R. Failure of B-cell differentiation in mice lacking the transcription factor EBF. Nature 376:263–267, 1995.

Ling KW, Dzierzak E. Ontogeny and genetics of the hemato/lymphopoietic system. Curr Opin Immunol 14:186–191, 2002.

Lipp M, Forster R, Schubel A, Burgstahler R, Muller G, Breitfeld D, Kremmer E, Wolf E. Functional organization of secondary lymphoid organs by homeostatic chemokines. Eur Cytokine Netw 11:504–505, 2000.

Loder F, Mutschler B, Ray RJ, Paige CJ, Sideras P, Torres R, Lamers MC, Carsetti R. B cell development in the spleen takes place in discrete steps and is determined by the quality of B cell receptor–derived signals. J Exp Med 190:75–89, 1999.

Madsen L, Labrecque N, Engberg J, Dierich A, Svejgaard A, Benoist C, Mathis D, Fugger L. Mice lacking all conventional MHC class II genes. Proc Natl Acad Sci USA 96:10338–10343, 1999.

Markowitz JS, Rogers PR, Grusby MJ, Parker DC, Glimcher LH. B lymphocyte development and activation independent of MHC class II expression. J Immunol 150:1223–1233, 1993.

Martin F, Kearney JF. Positive selection from newly formed to marginal zone B cells depends on the rate of clonal production, CD19, and Btk. Immunity 12:39–49, 2000.

Martin F, Oliver AM, Kearney JF. Marginal zone and B1 B cells unite in the early response against T-independent blood-borne particulate antigens. Immunity 14:617–629, 2001.

Matthias P, Rolink AG. Transcriptional networks in developing and mature B cells. Nat Rev Immunol 5:497–508, 2005.

Melchers F, Rolink A. B-lymphocyte development and biology. In: Paul WE, ed. Fundamental Immunology, 4th ed. Philadelphia: Lippincott-Raven, pp. 183–224, 1999.

Minegishi Y, Coustan-Smith E, Rapalus L, Ersoy F, Campana D, Conley ME. Mutations in Igalpha (CD79a) result in a complete block in B-cell development. J Clin Invest 104:1115–1121, 1999.

Minegishi Y, Coustan-Smith E, Wang YH, Cooper MD, Campana D, Conley ME. Mutations in the human lambda5/14.1 gene result in B cell deficiency and agammaglobulinemia. J Exp Med 187:71–77, 1998.

Mombaerts P, Iacomini J, Johnson RS, Herrup K, Tonegawa S, Papaioannou VE. RAG-1-deficient mice have no mature B and T lymphocytes. Cell 68:869–877, 1992.

Moore PA, Belvedere O, Orr A, Pieri K, LaFleur DW, Feng P, Soppet D, Charters M, Gentz R, Parmelee D, Li Y, Galperina O, Giri J, Roschke V, Nardelli B, Carrell J, Sosnovtseva S, Greenfield W, Ruben SM, Olsen HS, Fikes J, Hilbert DM. BLyS: member of the tumor necrosis factor family and B lymphocyte stimulator. Science 285:260–263, 1999.

Mukhopadhyay A, Ni J, Zhai Y, Yu GL, Aggarwal BB. Identification and characterization of a novel cytokine, THANK, a TNF homologue that activates apoptosis, nuclear factor-kappaB, and c-Jun NH2-terminal kinase. J Biol Chem 274:15978–15981, 1999.

Mundt C, Licence S, Shimizu T, Melchers F, Martensson IL. Loss of precursor B cell expansion but not allelic exclusion in VpreB1/VpreB2 double-deficient mice. J Exp Med 193:435–445, 2001.

Nakano H, Yanagita M, Gunn MD. CD11c(+)B220(+)Gr-1(+) cells in mouse lymph nodes and spleen display characteristics of plasmacytoid dendritic cells. J Exp Med 194:1171–1178, 2001.

Nemazee D. Receptor selection in B and T lymphocytes. Annu Rev Immunol 18:19–51, 2000.

Nikolic T, Dingjan GM, Leenen PJ, Hendriks RW. A subfraction of B220(+) cells in murine bone marrow and spleen does not belong to the B cell lineage but has dendritic cell characteristics. Eur J Immunol 32:686–692, 2002.

Noguchi M, Yi H, Rosenblatt HM, Filipovich AH, Adelstein S, Modi WS, McBride OW, Leonard WJ. Interleukin-2 receptor gamma chain mutation results in X-linked severe combined immunodeficiency in humans. Cell 73:147–157, 1993.

Norsworthy PJ, Taylor PR, Walport MJ, Botto M. Cloning of the mouse homolog of the 126-kDa human C1q/MBL/SP-A receptor, C1qR(p). Mamm Genome 10:789–793, 1999.

Nutt SL, Heavey B, Rolink AG, Busslinger M. Commitment to the B-lymphoid lineage depends on the transcription factor Pax5. Nature 401:556–562, 1999.

Nutt SL, Morrison AM, Dorfler P, Rolink A, Busslinger M. Identification of BSAP (Pax-5) target genes in early B-cell development by loss- and gain-of-function experiments. EMBO J 17:2319–2333, 1998.

Nutt SL, Urbanek P, Rolink A, Busslinger M. Essential functions of Pax5 (BSAP) in pro-B cell development: difference between fetal and adult B lymphopoiesis and reduced V-to-DJ recombination at the IgH locus. Genes Dev 11:476–491, 1997.

Ogawa M, Nishikawa S, Ikuta K, Yamamura F, Naito M, Takahashi K. B cell ontogeny in murine embryo studied by a culture system with the monolayer of a stromal cell clone, ST2: B cell progenitor develops first in the embryonal body rather than in the yolk sac. EMBO J 7:1337–1343, 1988.

Ogawa M, ten Boekel E, Melchers F. Identification of CD19(−)B220(+) c-Kit(+)Flt3/Flk-2(+)cells as early B lymphoid precursors before pre-BI cells in juvenile mouse bone marrow. Int Immunol 12:313–324, 2000.

Oliver AM, Martin F, Kearney JF. IgMhighCD21high lymphocytes enriched in the splenic marginal zone generate effector cells more rapidly than the bulk of follicular B cells. J Immunol 162:7198–7207, 1999.

O'Riordan M, Grosschedl R. Coordinate regulation of B cell differentiation by the transcription factors EBF and E2A. Immunity 11:21–31, 1999.

Osmond DG. The turnover of B-cell populations. Immunol Today 14:34–37, 1993.

Osmond DG, Rolink A, Melchers F. Murine B lymphopoiesis: towards a unified model. Immunol Today 19:65–68, 1998.

Pappu R, Cheng AM, Li B, Gong Q, Chiu C, Griffin N, White M, Sleckman BP, Chan AC. Requirement for B cell linker protein (BLNK) in B cell development. Science 286:1949–1954, 1999.

Peschon JJ, Morrissey PJ, Grabstein KH, Ramsdell FJ, Maraskovsky E, Gliniak BC, Park LS, Ziegler SF, Williams DE, Ware CB, et al. Early lymphocyte expansion is severely impaired in interleukin 7 receptor–deficient mice. J Exp Med 180:1955–1960, 1994.

Petrenko O, Beavis A, Klaine M, Kittappa R, Godin I, Lemischka IR. The molecular characterization of the fetal stem cell marker AA4. Immunity 10:691–700, 1999.

Radic MZ, Erikson J, Litwin S, Weigert M. B lymphocytes may escape tolerance by revising their antigen receptors. J Exp Med 177:1165–1173, 1993.

Ray RJ, Furlonger C, Williams DE, Paige CJ. Characterization of thymic stromal-derived lymphopoietin (TSLP) in murine B cell development in vitro. Eur J Immunol 26:10–16, 1996.

Reif K, Ekland EH, Ohl L, Nakano H, Lipp M, Forster R, Cyster JG. Balanced responsiveness to chemoattractants from adjacent zones determines B-cell position. Nature 416:94–99, 2002.

Rolink A, Grawunder U, Winkler TH, Karasuyama H, Melchers F. IL-2 receptor α chain (CD25,TAC) expression defines a crucial stage in preB cell development. Int Immunol 6:1257–1264, 1994.

Rolink A, Haasner D, Nishikawa SI, Melchers F. Changes in frequencies of clonable preB cells during life in different lymphoid organs of mice. Blood 81:2290–2300, 1993.

Rolink A, Kudo A, Karasuyama H, Kikuchi Y, Melchers F. Long-term proliferating early preB cell lines and clones with the potential to develop to surface-Ig positive mitogen-reactive B cells "in vitro" and "in vivo". EMBO J 10:327–336, 1991a.

Rolink A, Melchers F. Molecular and cellular origins of B lymphocyte diversity. Cell 66:1081–1094, 1991.

Rolink A, Streb M, Nishikawa SI, Melchers F. The c-kit encoded tyrosine kinase regulates the proliferation of early preB cells. Eur J Immunol 21:2609–2612, 1991b.

Rolink A, ten Boekel E, Melchers F, Fearon DT, Krop I, Andersson J. A subpopulation of B220+ cells in murine bone marrow does not express CD19 and contains natural killer cell progenitors. J Exp Med 183:187–194, 1996.

Rolink AG, Andersson J, Melchers F. Characterization of immature B cells by a novel monoclonal antibody, by turnover and by mitogen reactivity. Eur J Immunol 28:3738–3748, 1998.

Rolink AG, Brocker T, Bluethmann H, Kosco-Vilbois MH, Andersson J, Melchers F. Mutations affecting either generation or survival of cells influence the pool size of mature B cells. Immunity 10:619–628, 1999a.

Rolink AG, Nutt SL, Melchers F, Busslinger M. Long-term in vivo reconstitution of T-cell development by Pax5-deficient B-cell progenitors. Nature 401:603–606, 1999b.

Rolink AG, Schaniel C, Andersson J, Melchers F. Selection events operating at various stages in B cell development. Curr Opin Immunol 13:202–207, 2001.

Rolink AG, Tschopp J, Schneider P, Melchers F. BAFF is a survival and maturation factor for mouse B cells. Eur J Immunol 32:2004–2010, 2002.

Rolink AG, Winkler T, Melchers F, Andersson J. Precursor B cell receptor–dependent B cell proliferation and differentiation does not require the bone marrow or fetal liver environment. J Exp Med 191:23–32, 2000.

Romanow WJ, Langerak AW, Goebel P, Wolvers-Tettero IL, van Dongen JJ, Feeney AJ, Murre C. E2A and EBF act in synergy with the V(D)J recombinase to generate a diverse immunoglobulin repertoire in nonlymphoid cells. Mol Cell 5:343–353, 2000.

Schaniel C, Bruno L, Melchers F, Rolink AG. Multiple hematopoietic cell lineages develop in vivo from transplanted Pax5-deficient pre-B I–cell clones. Blood 99:472–478, 2002a.

Schaniel C, Gottar M, Roosnek E, Melchers F, Rolink AG. Extensive in vivo self-renewal, long-tem reconstitution capacity, and hematopoietic multipotency of Pax5-deficient precursor B-cell clones. Blood 99:472–478, 2002b.

Schebesta M, Heavey B, Busslinger M. Transcriptional control of B-cell development. Curr Opin Immunol 14:216–223, 2002.

Schneider P, MacKay F, Steiner V, Hofmann K, Bodmer JL, Holler N, Ambrose C, Lawton P, Bixler S, Acha-Orbea H, Valmori D, Romero P, Werner-Favre C, Zubler RH, Browning JL, Tschopp J. BAFF, a novel ligand of the tumor necrosis factor family, stimulates B cell growth. J Exp Med 189:1747–1756, 1999.

Schubart DB, Rolink A, Kosco-Vilbois MH, Botteri F, Matthias P. B-cell-specific coactivator OBF-1/OCA-B/Bob1 required for immune response and germinal centre formation. Nature 383:538–542, 1996.

Schubart DB, Rolink A, Schubart K, Matthias P. Cutting edge: lack of peripheral B cells and severe agammaglobulinemia in mice simultaneously lacking Bruton's tyrosine kinase and the B cell–specific transcriptional coactivator OBF-1. J Immunol 164:18–22, 2000.

Schubart K, Massa S, Schubart D, Corcoran LM, Rolink AG, Matthias P. B cell development and immunoglobulin gene transcription in the absence of Oct-2 and OBF-1. Nat Immunol 2:69–74, 2001.

Shachar I, Flavell RA. Requirement for invariant chain in B cell maturation and function. Science 274:106–108, 1996.

Shinkai Y, Rathbun G, Lam KP, Oltz EM, Stewart V, Mendelsohn M, Charron J, Datta M, Young F, Stall AM, Alt FW. RAG-2-deficient mice lack mature lymphocytes owing to inability to initiate V(D)J rearrangement. Cell 68:855–867, 1992.

Shu HB, Hu WH, Johnson H. TALL-1 is a novel member of the TNF family that is down-regulated by mitogens. J Leukoc Biol 65:680–683, 1999.

Solvason N, Chen X, Shu F, Kearney JF. The fetal omentum in mice and humans. A site enriched for precursors of CD5 B cells early in development. Ann NY Acad Sci 651:10–20, 1992.

Spanopoulou E, Roman CAJ, Corcoran LM, Schlissel MS, Silver DP, Nemazee D, Nussenzweig MC, Shinton SA, Hardy RR, Baltimore D. Functional immunoglobulin transgenes guide ordered B-cell differentiation in RAG-1 deficient mice. Genes Dev 8:1030–1042, 1994.

Stoddart A, Fleming HE, Paige CJ. The role of the preBCR, the interleukin-7 receptor, and homotypic interactions during B-cell development. Immunol Rev 175:47–58, 2000.

ten Boekel E, Melchers F, Rolink A. The status of Ig loci rearrangements in single cells from different stages of B cell development. Int Immunol 7:1013–1019, 1995.

ten Boekel E, Melchers F, Rolink AG. Changes in the V(H) gene repertoire of developing precursor B lymphocytes in mouse bone marrow mediated by the pre–B cell receptor. Immunity 7:357–368, 1997.

ten Boekel E, Melchers F, Rolink AG. Precursor B cells showing H chain allelic inclusion display allelic exclusion at the level of pre–B cell receptor surface expression. Immunity 8:199–207, 1998.

Thompson JS, Bixler SA, Qian F, Vora K, Scott ML, Cachero TG, Hession C, Schneider P, Sizing ID, Mullen C, Strauch K, Zafari M, Benjamin CD, Tschopp J, Browning JL, Ambrose C. BAFF-R, a newly identified TNF receptor that specifically interacts with BAFF. Science 293:2108–2111, 2001.

Tiegs SL, Russell DM, Nemazee D. Receptor editing in self-reactive bone marrow B cells. J Exp Med 177:1009–1020, 1993.

Torres RM, Flaswinkel H, Reth M, Rajewsky K. Aberrant B cell development and immune response in mice with a compromised BCR complex. Science 272:1802–1804, 1996.

Torres RM, Hafen K. A negative regulatory role for Ig-alpha during B cell development. Immunity 11:527–536, 1999.

Turner M, Mee PJ, Costello PS, Williams O, Price AA, Duddy LP, Furlong MT, Geahlen RL, Tybulewicz VL. Perinatal lethality and blocked B-cell development in mice lacking the tyrosine kinase Syk. Nature 378:298–302, 1995.

Urbánek P, Wang ZQ, Fetka I, Wagner EF, Busslinger M. Complete block of early B cell differentiation and altered patterning of the posterior midbrain in mice lacking Pax5/BSAP. Cell 79:901–912, 1994.

von Freeden-Jeffry U, Vieira P, Lucian LA, McNeil T, Burdach SEG, Murray R. Lymphopenia in interleukin (IL)-7 gene–deleted mice identifies IL-7 as a nonredundant cytokine. J Exp Med 181:1519–1526, 1995.

Weissman IL. Stem cells: units of development, units of regeneration, and units in evolution. Cell 100:157–168, 2000.

Wellmann U, Werner A, Winkler TH. Altered selection processes of B lymphocytes in autoimmune NZB/W mice, despite intact central tolerance against DNA. Eur J Immunol 31:2800–2810, 2001.

Winkler TH, Melchers F, Rolink AG. Interleukin-3 and interleukin-7 are alternative growth factors for the same B-cell precursors in the mouse. Blood 85:2045–2051, 1995a.

Winkler TH, Rolink A, Melchers F, Karasuyama H. Precursor B cells of mouse bone marrow express two different complexes with surrogate light chain on the surface. Eur J Immunol 25:446–450, 1995b.

Yamagami T, ten Boekel E, Andersson J, Rolink A, Melchers F. Frequencies of multiple IgL chain gene rearrangements in single normal or kappaL chain–deficient B lineage cells. Immunity 11:317–327, 1999a.

Yamagami T, ten Boekel E, Schaniel C, Andersson J, Rolink A, Melchers F. Four of five RAG-expressing JCkappa–/– small pre-BII cells have no L chain gene rearrangements: detection by high-efficiency single cell PCR. Immunity 11:309–316, 1999b.

Young F, Ardman B, Shinkai Y, Lansford R, Blackwell TK, Mendelsohn M, Rolink A, Melchers F, Alt FW. Influence of immunoglobulin heavy- and light-chain expression on B-cell differentiation. Genes Dev. 8:1043–1057, 1994.

Zhuang Y, Soriano P, Weintraub H. The helix-loop-helix gene E2A is required for B cell formation. Cell 79:875–884, 1994.

6

Signal Transduction by T and B Lymphocyte Antigen Receptors

NEETU GUPTA, ANTHONY L. DEFRANCO, and ARTHUR WEISS

Considerable progress has been made during the past several years toward our understanding of the processes by which T and B lymphocytes become activated. Antigen-specific activation of these quiescent cells involves the triggering of antigen receptors to induce signal transduction events that can lead to both the cell cycle progression and differentiation of T and B cells. A remarkable synergy has resulted from a convergence of studies of the most fundamental processes involved in T and B cell activation and those involving clinical and experimental immunodeficiency syndromes. Clinical and experimental immunodeficiency states often result when the functions of T and B cell antigen receptors (TCRs and BCRs) or critical components in the pathways regulated by these receptors are interrupted.

An increasing number of cell surface receptors on T and B cells contribute to the activation of these cells. However, the specificity of the response to antigen dictates that the antigen receptors on these cells play the central role. Although the forms of antigens recognized and the effector functions mediated by these two cell types are quite distinct, the mechanisms by which the antigen receptors transduce signals and the ensuing molecular events are remarkably similar. Stimulation of the TCR and BCR induces the protein tyrosine phosphorylation of a large number of proteins implicated in signal transduction processes that contribute to cellular activation. Here, we will focus on the means by which the TCR and BCR induce protein tyrosine phosphorylation and the consequences of these phosphorylation events.

Antigen Receptors on T and B Lymphocytes

The TCR and BCR are both oligomeric complexes that contain subunits responsible for antigen recognition and other subunits involved in signal transduction (Fig.6.1A). The repertoires of the clonally distributed ligand binding subunits of these receptors

are entrusted with the responsibility of recognizing the vast array of antigens or peptides that may be encountered through interactions with pathogens. In the case of the TCR, the antigen- or ligand-binding subunit consists of productively rearranged $\alpha\beta$ or $\gamma\delta$ heterodimers. The antigen-binding subunit of the BCR consists of the heavy and light chains of membrane immunoglobulin (Ig). Whereas these subunits have all of the information necessary for specific antigen recognition, their short cytoplasmic domains do not contain sufficient information to interact with cytoplasmic molecules involved in signal transduction.

In the case of the TCR, the $\alpha\beta$ or $\gamma\delta$ heterodimers assemble with the invariant CD3 γ, δ, and ϵ chains and a homo-or heterodimer of ζ and/or Fcγ chains. The precise stoichiometry of the assembly, which occurs in the endoplasmic reticulum, is not known, but there is evidence for CD3 ϵ chains forming noncovalent dimers with CD3δ or CD3γ (Blumberg et al., 1990; Kappes and Tonegawa, 1991). The assembly of all of the components is necessary for efficient expression on the plasma membrane. Human or murine immune deficiency syndromes characterized by T cell developmental arrests or functional defects and lower TCR expression have been associated with CD3γ or ϵ mutations (Perez-Aciego et al., 1991; Tanaka et al., 1995; see Chapter 16). Studies in T cell lines and heterologous cells show that most incomplete complexes are retained in the endoplasmic reticulum or golgi and shunted toward a degradative pathway (Klausner et al., 1990). Unusually placed transmembrane acidic and basic residues appear to play an important role in the interaction of these chains. The CD3 and ζ chain dimers are responsible for signal transduction function of the receptor.

Membrane Ig also assembles with invariant chains, Igα and Igβ involved in signal transduction. Like the CD3 chains, Igα and Igβ form heterodimers and each chain has a single extracellular Ig-like domain and intracellular domains with signaling

A.

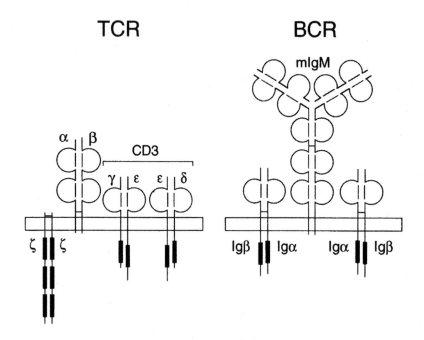

B.

hζ1	N Q L Y N E L N L G R R E E - Y D V L
hζ2	E G L Y N E L Q K D K M A E A Y S E I
hζ3	D G L Y Q G L S T A T K D T - Y D A L
hCD3γ	D Q L Y Q P L K D R E D D Q - Y S H L
hCD3ε	N P D Y E P I R K G Q R D L - Y S G L
hCD3δ	D Q V Y Q P L R D R D D A Q - Y S H L
rIgE FcR γ	D A V Y T G L N T R N Q E T - Y E T L
rIgE FcR β	D R L Y E E L - H V Y S P I - Y S A L
mIg α	E N L Y E G L N L D D C S M - Y E D I
mIg β	D H T Y E G L N I D Q T A T - Y E D I
BLV gp30	D S D Y Q A L L P S A P E I - Y S H L
EBV LMP-2	H S D Y Q P L G T Q D Q S L - Y L G L
SIV Nef	G D L Y E R L L R A R G E T - Y G R L
KSnV K1	L Q D Y Y S L H D L C T E D - Y T Q P
Consensus	D/E- - Y - - L - - - - - - - Y - - L

Figure 6.1. A. Schematic representation of the T cell antigen receptor (TCR) and B cell antigen receptor (BCR). B. Immunoreceptor tyrosine-based activation motifs present in hematopoietic receptors involved in antigen recognition and in viruses that infect T or B cells. h, human; r, rat; m, mouse; BLV, bovine leukemia virus; EBV, Epstein-Barr virus; SIV, simian immunodeficiency virus; KSHV, Kaposi's sarcoma–associated herpes virus.

function (Reth, 1992). The number of Igα/Igβ dimers associated with a membrane Ig tetramer unit has not been definitively established. Efficient cell surface expression of membrane Ig requires association with Igα and Igβ. Although charged amino acid residues are not present in the transmembrane domains of BCR subunits, these domains do interact with each other and this interaction is necessary for assembly (Venkitaraman et al., 1991). Thus, the BCR and TCR are both obligate multisubunit complexes in which antigen-binding functions and signal transduction functions are provided by distinct chains.

In addition to the antigen receptors found on mature lymphocytes, related receptors are found on pre-B cells in the bone marrow and on CD4⁻/CD8⁻ thymocytes (Roth and DeFranco, 1995; von Boehmer and Fehling, 1997). These receptors contain only one of the two antigen-binding chains, the one that is generated by recombination first during development of the cell, in combination with a surrogate for the second chain. In B cells, this "pre-BCR" contains the Ig μ heavy chain together with the λ_5 and V_{preB} proteins, each of which is thought to mimic one-half of the Ig light chain of the BCR. This pre-BCR also contains Igα/Igβ heterodimers. Similarly, the pre-TCR contains a complex of the TCRβ chain with an α chain surrogate called pre-Tα associated with CD3 and ζ chains. In both cases, these receptors play critical roles in allowing developing lymphocytes to sense the successful rearrangement of the first antigen receptor gene and pass through a developmental checkpoint, after which rearrangement at that locus ceases and rearrangement of the Ig light-chain gene or the TCRα gene increases.

The CD3 and ζ chains of the TCR and the Igα and Igβ chains of the BCR have substantial cytoplasmic domains containing sequences responsible for the signal transduction function of these receptors. These signal transduction functions were most definitively established through the use of chimeric receptors in which the cytoplasmic domains of several of these proteins were linked to the extracellular and transmembrane domains of heterologous proteins (Irving and Weiss, 1991; Romeo and Seed, 1991). Although these cytoplasmic domains do not encode enzymatic functions, they can confer TCR and BCR signal transduction functions to heterologous receptors. This signal transduction function is encoded in a sequence motif, termed *ITAM* (for immunoreceptor tyrosine-based activation motif), which is present as a single copy in all of the CD3 chains and the Igα and Igβ chains, and as three copies in the ζ chain (Fig. 6.1B). The ITAMs are also present and functionally active in the cytoplasmic domains of the nonligand-binding subunits of the high-affinity IgE Fc receptor, the phagocytic Fcγ receptors on macrophages, and the DAP-12 chain that associates with natural killer (NK) cell–activating receptors (Lanier, 2001). Interestingly, the ITAM sequence motif, D/ExxYxxL(x)6–8YxxL, in many of these chains is encoded by two exons with similar organization, suggesting a common evolutionary origin (Wegener et al., 1992). This also suggests that these antigen receptors use similar mechanisms to transduce signals. Mutagenesis studies have shown that both tyrosines and both leucines are critical for the ability of ITAMs to transfer signal transduction function to heterologous receptors (Sefton and Taddie, 1994). The residues surrounding the conserved tyrosines and leucines can be quite variable. A major question that arises and remains unsettled is whether ITAMs, which contain such variable sequences, have equivalent functions or whether part of their functions are distinctive. Some investigations have suggested that multiple ITAMs are present in TCRs and BCRs to recruit distinct signaling molecules (Frank et al., 1990; Clark et al., 1992; Siemasko and Clark, 2001). Others have suggested that the presence of multiple ITAMs may play a role in signal amplification (Irving et al., 1993; Law et al., 1993; Lin et al., 1996; Donnadieu et al., 2000; Love and Shores, 2000). In mouse experiments involving genetic deletion of all or part of the CD3ζ ITAMs, it was shown that the CD3γ, δ, ε subunits are sufficient for normal TCR signaling events and effector functions and that the CD3ζ ITAMs do not play any exclusive role (Ardouin et al., 1999). Mice containing mutations of the ITAM tyrosines in Igα did not exhibit any major defects in the development of B-2 cells, whereas there was a reduction in B-1 and marginal zone B cells. Combining the Igα mutation with a truncation in Igβ resulted in a dramatic arrest in B cell development at the pro-B cell stage demonstrating the requirement for functional ITAMs on at least one of the signal transducing chains of the BCR for progression through early development. Mice carrying a truncation in the cytoplasmic tail of Igβ alone progress to the immature stage and respond normally to BCR ligation; however, they are arrested at this stage in the bone marrow and die by apoptosis. These observations indicate that Igα and Igβ might have distinct biologic activities in vivo (Kraus et al., 2001; Reichlin et al., 2001).

As in other situations where pathogens have usurped or targeted normal cellular machinery to their benefit, at least four viruses that infect T or B cells encode ITAMs that appear to play an important role in their pathogenesis. The bovine leukemia virus, which can transform B cells, contains an ITAM in the cytoplasmic domain of the gp30 envelope glycoprotein that is critically important for viral infection and/or replication (Willems et al., 1995). An ITAM is also present in the latent membrane protein 2 (LMP2) of the Epstein Barr virus (EBV) and has been implicated in maintaining a state of viral latency in transformed B cell lines (Miller et al., 1995). Recent studies suggest that LMP2 serves to recruit E3 protein ubiquitin ligases that target BCR-activated protein kinases, thereby down-regulating BCR signaling (Winberg et al., 2000). In addition, SLP-65/BLNK, a signaling adaptor molecule that will be discussed later, was recently identified as a downstream effector of LMP2A. In EBV-infected B cells, one of the SLP-65 isoforms was found to be constitutively tyrosine phosphorylated, resulting in complex formation with CrkL and subsequent phosphorylation of Cbl and C3G (Engels et al., 2001a,b). In contrast, phospholipase C γ2 (PLCγ2) activation was completely blocked. Thus, during latent EBV infection, LMP2 has contrasting effects on SLP-65-regulated pathways. A rare mutation of the Nef protein of the simian immunodeficiency virus results in the creation of an ITAM sequence (Du et al., 1995). This mutation is associated with the unusual ability of this viral isolate to infect and replicate in primary resting T cells and cause a fulminant viral infection. Finally, human herpesvirus 8 (HHV8; also known as Kaposi's sarcoma [KS]-associated herpesvirus, or KSHV) which causes Kaposi's sarcoma, primary effusion lymphoma, and multicentric Castleman's disease, encodes the K1 gene product that contains an ITAM-like sequence in the C-terminal cytoplasmic tail. Expression of this protein leads to ligand-independent signaling in B cells that is abrogated upon mutation of the ITAMs (Lagunoff et al., 1999). Thus, the ITAM plays a critical role in normal T and B cell antigen receptor function and some pathogens have capitalized on this function.

ITAMs of T and B Cell Antigen Receptors Interact with Distinct Families of Protein Tyrosine Kinases

Stimulation of the TCR and BCR leads to the activation of protein tyrosine kinases (PTKs) that are critical for lymphocyte responses to antigen. Two families of cytoplasmic PTKs, members of the Src and Syk/ZAP-70 families, have been implicated in the most proximal signaling events induced by these receptors. Indeed, considerable evidence has accumulated to suggest a model in which the TCR and BCR ITAMs interact with these two families of PTKs in a sequential and coordinated manner (Fig. 6.2). Whereas the members of the families of the PTKs that are expressed in T and B cells differ, they appear to subserve similar functions.

In B cells and in T cell lines and T cell clones, the earliest event associated with antigen receptor stimulation is the tyrosine phosphorylation of ITAMs (Law et al., 1993; Iwashima et al., 1994). In contrast, in ex vivo T cells, phosphorylation of the ITAM tyrosines is present in the basal state (van Oers et al., 1993). Both the inducible and basal phosphorylation of ITAM tyrosines depends on members of the Src family (Iwashima et al., 1994; Richards et al., 1996; van Oers et al., 1996a). Src family kinases expressed in T cells are Lck, Fyn, and Yes and those expressed in B cells are primarily Lyn, Fyn, and Blk. These kinases are peripheral membrane proteins characterized by the following: (1) a unique N-terminal domain that is myristylated in all family

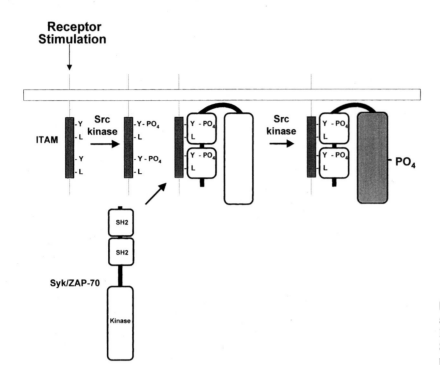

Figure 6.2. Model for sequential interaction of Src and Syk/ZAP-70 protein tyrosine kinases with an ITAM. Note that the subsequent interaction of the Src kinase, involving its SH2 domain, with the phosphorylated Syk or ZAP-70 kinase is not depicted.

members and also may be palmitoylated; (2) an SH3 domain involved in mediating protein–protein interactions by binding to proline-rich sequences; (3) an SH2 domain involved in mediating protein–protein interactions by binding phosphorylated tyrosine residues in the context of particular neighboring amino acid residues; (4) a catalytic domain; and, (5) a carboxy-terminal domain that contains a negative regulatory site of tyrosine phosphorylation.

In T cells, the functions of Lck and/or Fyn are critical for TCR signal transduction. Lck and Fyn both coimmunoprecipitate with the TCR complex and can interact with an ITAM (Samelson et al., 1990; Beyers et al., 1992), but genetic studies with cell lines and mice have indicated a more important role for Lck in the phosphorylation of the ITAMs (Iwashima et al., 1994; van Oers et al., 1996a). However, in the absence of Lck, or when Lck function might be limiting, Fyn may be able to play a compensatory role. This view is consistent with the developmental phenotypes seen in mice deficient in one or both of these kinases: mice deficient in Fyn have no developmental abnormality of conventional αβ T cells but they lack NK1.1+ T (NKT) cells (Appleby et al., 1992; Stein et al., 1992; Eberl et al., 1999), whereas the loss of Lck is associated with a severe but incomplete arrest in T cell development (Molina et al., 1992). The residual development seen in thymocytes lacking Lck is completely absent in thymocytes from mice deficient in both kinases (van Oers et al., 1996b). These thymocytes exhibit a complete developmental block at a stage where the function of the pre-TCR is important (Fehling et al., 1995). Presumably, this reflects the inability of the pre-TCR to transduce signals in the absence of Lck or Fyn.

A unique feature of Lck is the ability of its N-terminal region to associate with the cytoplasmic tails of the CD4 and CD8 coreceptors (Chow and Veillette, 1995). A primary role for Lck function in the initiation of TCR signaling is also consistent with its association with CD4 and CD8. The colocalization of CD4 or CD8 with the TCR during antigen recognition may serve to lo-

calize Lck in close proximity with the TCR, facilitating its participation in early signaling events.

In B cells the Src family kinases are also believed to be responsible for ITAM phosphorylation, although Syk may contribute as well. For example, in a chicken B cell line, DT-40, Lyn is apparently the only Src family kinase expressed. Disruption of the Lyn gene in these cells decreased anti–IgM–induced tyrosine phosphorylation of Igα and Igβ, but did not eliminate it (Takata et al., 1994). Moreover, subsequent signaling events were decreased but not eliminated. Conversely, when the BCR was expressed in the AtT-20 rat pituitary cell line following the introduction of cDNA expression vectors, BCR stimulation led to strong tyrosine phosphorylation of Igα and Igβ but minimal downstream signaling. These cells express Fyn but not Syk, Lyn, or Blk. Introduction of Syk restored some downstream signaling events and also boosted the stimulation-dependent phosphorylation of Igα and Igβ (Richards et al., 1996). In murine splenic B cells, Lyn is the most abundant Src family member present, although substantial amounts of Blk and Fyn are also detectable. B cells from mice rendered deficient in Lyn by targeted gene disruption exhibit significantly delayed tyrosine phosphorylation of Igα after BCR stimulation (Nishizumi et al., 1995; Chan et al., 1997), indicating that Lyn is important but not essential for Igα phosphorylation. Thus, the situation is a bit more complex than in T cells, but again, Src family kinases are primarily responsible for phosphorylation of Igα and Igβ ITAM tyrosines.

In the absence of coreceptor involvement, the low stoichiometry of the documented interactions of the Src family members with the TCR and BCR, as well as the apparent redundancy in some functions among these PTKs, raises questions about how TCR and BCR stimulation induces these kinases to phosphorylate the ITAMs. One point worth noting is that the stoichiometry of ITAM phosphorylation is low, even in systems where receptor stimulation is maximal. The basis for such interactions could be relatively nonspecific and involve ligand-induced association of receptors with membrane microdomains ("lipid rafts") where these Src kinases are concentrated. Alternatively, the association of the receptor and kinase could be based on an interaction between the SH2 domain of the Src family PTK and a small percentage of ITAMs that may be tyrosine phosphorylated in the basal state. The recruitment of Src family PTKs to phosphorylated ITAMs is attractive in view of studies suggesting that the tyrosine phosphorylated YEEI sequence, similar to the YXXL sequences in ITAMs, is a preferred binding site for the SH2 domains of Src kinases (Songyang et al., 1993). Most ITAMs have at least one negatively charged amino acid residue between the tyrosines and leucines (Fig. 6.1B). Indeed, cross-linking of chimeric transmembrane proteins with Igα or Igβ ITAMs leads to induced association of Lyn (Law et al., 1993). Moreover, the inducible phosphorylation of ζ chain ITAMs requires the function of the Lck SH2 domain (Straus et al., 1996). This could reflect a positive feedback loop whereby once a few ITAM tyrosines are phosphorylated, Lck binds and then phosphorylates other ITAMs of neighboring receptors aggregated by the triggering stimulus. While there are alternative explanations for the interactions of the Src PTKs with the TCR or BCR, receptor ligation does appear to increase the catalytic activity of these PTKs (Saouaf et al., 1994; Tsygankov et al., 1994).

Both tyrosines of an ITAM are necessary for its signal transduction function (Sefton and Taddie, 1994). The explanation for this dependency on both tyrosines is likely to reflect the requirement for tyrosine phosphorylation of both sites for high-affinity binding of a second type of PTK, ZAP-70 and/or Syk. ZAP-70 and Syk have a similar overall structure. They contain N-terminal tandem SH2 domains and a C-terminal catalytic domain. ZAP-70 is expressed exclusively in T cells and NK cells. Syk is more broadly expressed within the hematopoietic lineages. ZAP-70 and Syk bind to doubly phosphorylated ITAMs with relatively high affinity via an interaction that depends on both of their SH2 domains (Wange et al., 1993; Iwashima et al., 1994; Bu et al., 1995). The crystal structure of the ZAP-70 tandem SH2 domains bound to a doubly phosphorylated TCRζ ITAM peptide confirms that both SH2 domains interact with a single, doubly phosphorylated ITAM and helps explain their cooperative binding (Hatada et al., 1995). Similar data have been obtained for the crystal structure of Syk bound to an ITAM (Fütterer et al., 1998). Thus, inducible phosphorylation of ITAMs results in recruitment of ZAP-70 or Syk to the stimulated-receptor complex. If ITAMs are phosphorylated in the basal state, as has been observed in ex vivo thymocytes and peripheral T cells, ZAP-70 and/or Syk are bound and poised to respond to receptor stimulation (van Oers et al., 1994, 1996a).

The induction of PTK activity following Syk/ZAP-70 recruitment to the receptor complexes likely involves additional interactions between the Src and Syk/ZAP-70 PTKs. In vitro studies suggest that the binding of Syk, but not ZAP-70, to ITAMs can lead to its activation (Shiue et al., 1995). However, simple binding of Syk and ZAP-70 to ITAMs in vivo is probably not sufficient for stimulation of their kinase activity and subsequent signal transduction, since Syk and ZAP-70 bound to the ITAMs in ex vivo thymocytes are not activated (van Oers et al., 1994, 1996a). Rather, both Syk and ZAP-70 kinase activities are regulated primarily by phosphorylation of tyrosine residues within a regulatory loop of their catalytic domains (Chan et al., 1995; Wange et al., 1995). In the case of ZAP-70, this key phosphorylation event can be performed by Lck or Fyn but not by ZAP-70 itself (Chan et al., 1992, 1995; Wange et al., 1995). In contrast, Syk can activate itself, and this is seen in overexpression studies in Cos cells or upon cross-linking of a chimeric protein in which

Syk has been fused to the cytoplasmic domain of a transmembrane protein (Kolanus et al., 1993; Couture et al., 1994). Syk can probably also be activated by Src family PTKs such as Lyn. Thus, the Src kinases can play a critical role in Syk and ZAP-70 catalytic activation by phosphorylating the regulatory tyrosines. In addition to the tyrosines in the activation loop, there is evidence that other tyrosines are phosphorylated and are involved either in negative regulatory functions, i.e., Y292 in ZAP-70 (Chan et al., 1995; Wange et al., 1995; Kong et al., 1996; Zhao and Weiss, 1996; Magnan et al., 2001), or in positive regulatory functions, i.e., Y315 and Y319 in ZAP-70 (Gong et al., 2001b; Magnan et al., 2001). These phosphorylation sites are involved in recruitment of substrates that may contain SH2 domains with specificity for specifically phosphorylated sequence motifs, in a manner analogous to that observed with PTK growth factor receptors. Proteins that have been reported to bind to either Syk or ZAP-70 include Lck (Thome et al., 1995; Straus et al., 1996), Lyn (Law et al., 1996), Shc (Nagai et al., 1995), Vav (Katzav et al., 1994), PLCγ1 (Law et al., 1996), SHIP (an inositol 5-phosphatase) (Crowley et al., 1996), and Cbl (Fournel et al., 1996). The functions of some of these signaling components will be discussed in a later section.

A stable complex of Lck and ZAP-70 or Syk has been observed following TCR stimulation (Thome et al., 1995; Straus et al., 1996). The interaction appears to depend on the binding of the Lck SH2 domain to tyrosine phosphorylated residues in the interdomain B region of ZAP-70 (Y319) or Syk (Pelosi et al., 1999). A Y319F mutant of ZAP-70 retains full tyrosine kinase activity but is unable to reconstitute TCR-dependent Ca^{2+} mobilization, Ras activation, CD69 expression, and NFAT-dependent transcription in ZAP-70-deficient Jurkat cells. This functional defect may reflect the inability of the mutant ZAP-70 to interact with Lck, although other explanations are possible. For example, phosphorylation of Tyr319 also promotes the association of ZAP-70 with the SH2 domain of PLCγ1. Accordingly, ZAP-70-deficient cells reconstituted with Y319F mutant ZAP-70 show reduced tyrosine phosphorylation of PLCγ1 and the LAT adapter protein (Williams et al., 1998).

The relative contribution of the two families of PTKs toward phosphorylation of downstream substrates has not been clearly assessed. However, activation of Lck alone by cross-linking CD4 or CD8 fails to mimic TCR stimulation (Ledbetter et al., 1990). This suggests a critical function provided by Syk and ZAP-70 in later signal transduction events. Successful reconstitution of Syk-deficient B cells or ZAP-70-deficient T cells with ZAP-70 or Syk depends on the catalytic functions of these PTKs and the presence of the activating tyrosine of the kinase domain (Y518,Y519 for Syk, and Y493 for ZAP-70) (Kurosaki et al., 1995; Kong et al., 1996; Williams et al., 1998). Thus, a contribution of both Src and Syk/ZAP-70 kinases is likely to be important for effective downstream signaling events.

Both ZAP-70 and Syk play critical roles in lymphocyte development, presumably because signal transduction through immature and mature antigen receptors is critical for transition through certain developmental checkpoints. Mice and humans deficient in ZAP-70 exhibit distinct developmental arrests and marked impairment in TCR signal transduction function (Arpaia et al., 1994; Chan et al., 1994b; Elder et al., 1994; Negishi et al., 1995; see Chapter 14). A profound B cell developmental arrest and bleeding diathesis are the most prominent features of mice deficient in Syk (Cheng et al., 1995; Turner et al., 1995). Bleeding may be secondary to a collagen receptor signaling defect in platelets (Poole et al., 1997). The B cell developmental arrest in these mice occurs at the same stage as seen with mutations that prevent expression of the membrane-bound form of the Igμ heavy chain. Thus, it is thought that the developmental block results from impaired pre-BCR function. This interpretation is consistent with the impaired BCR signal transduction function observed in an avian B cell line deficient in Syk (Takata et al., 1994). Thus, the Syk and ZAP-70 PTKs play critically important roles in TCR and BCR signal transduction function.

In some systems it has been suggested that Syk and ZAP-70 may be interchangable (Gelfand et al., 1995; Kong et al., 1995). One clear difference is that Syk appears to be less dependent on interactions with Src kinases than is ZAP-70 (Kolanus et al., 1993; Chu et al., 1996). It is not yet clear whether Syk and ZAP-70 are completely functionally redundant with regard to activation of downstream signaling events. It is likely that these kinases do have unique functions in T cells. For instance, the αβ T cell lineage is primarily affected in mice made deficient in ZAP-70 (Negishi et al., 1995), whereas the γδ lineage of T cells in epithelial tissues is defective in Syk deficient mice (Mallick-Wood et al., 1996). Thus, many of the functions of these PTKs overlap, but they appear to have unique functions as well.

Regulation of Antigen Receptor Signal Transduction

Coreceptors on T Cells

The great sensitivity of the immune system has evolved to allow immune responses to be initiated early upon infection with pathogens. While receptors with high affinity exist within the derived repertoire of antigen receptors on T and B cells, the immune sytem has also developed mechanisms to increase the sensitivity of responsiveness until the clonal expansion of cells with high-affinity receptors can take place. T and B cells both have distinct coreceptor molecules that function in concert with antigen receptors to recognize antigen and induce signaling events. Here we will restrict our use of the term *coreceptors* to refer to molecules that recognize the molecular complex containing intact antigen or peptide antigen along with the antigen receptor.

The positive selection of most αβ thymocytes and the primary response of αβ T cells to antigen usually depend on the functional contributions of the coreceptors CD4 and CD8. The CD4 and CD8 molecules are integral membrane glycoproteins whose extracellular domains bind to the β2 domain of class II - major histocompatibility complex (MHC) molecules or the α3 domain of class I MHC molecules, respectively, on antigen-presenting cells (Janeway, 1992; Robey and Fowlkes, 1994). These interactions are of relatively low affinity and may depend on the simultaneous binding of the TCR as well. In fact, some evidence suggests that a TCR-initiated signaling event may be required for the recruitment and effective participation of the CD4 coreceptor (Xu and Littman, 1993). An alternative but not mutually exclusive view is that the CD4 or CD8 participation stabilizes the low-affinity TCR–MHC/peptide interaction and also potentiates TCR signal transduction by delivering Lck to the TCR complex (Fig. 6.3).

The cytoplasmic domains of CD4 and CD8 bind to the unique N-terminal region of Lck through a cysteine-containing motif shared by CD4 and CD8 (Chow and Veillette, 1995). This interaction is important but not absolutely essential for TCR signal transduction during development or at low antigen concentrations (Killeen and Littman, 1993). Several functional consequences may result from the interaction of Lck with the CD4 and CD8 coreceptors. In T cell clones or lines, if CD4 or CD8 delivers Lck to the TCR complex through colocalization driven by the interaction of the coreceptors with the MHC/peptide complex, the phosphorylation of ITAMs by Lck would be facilitated and subsequent interactions involving the phosphorylation and activation of ZAP-70 or Syk could be potentiated (Weiss, 1993). A similar interaction of the coreceptors of T cells in vivo would lead to the delivery of Lck into close proximity with ITAM-bound ZAP-70 or Syk, again potentiating their phosphorylation and activation. In addition to this initiating function of Lck in TCR signal transduction, Lck appears to contribute to T cell activation in a second way in which a CD4-bound Lck molecule binds to phosphorylated ZAP-70 or Syk via its SH2 domain, thereby stabilizing the interaction of the coreceptor with the TCR–MHC/peptide complex (Xu and Littman, 1993; Thome et al., 1995; Straus et al., 1996).

The ligation of coreceptors in the absence of TCR engagement has been reported to induce negative signals. Ligation of CD4 with anti-CD4 monoclonal antibodies primes the T cells for subsequent apoptosis when the TCR is stimulated (Newell et al., 1990). In vivo, this may be relevant to interactions of the HIV

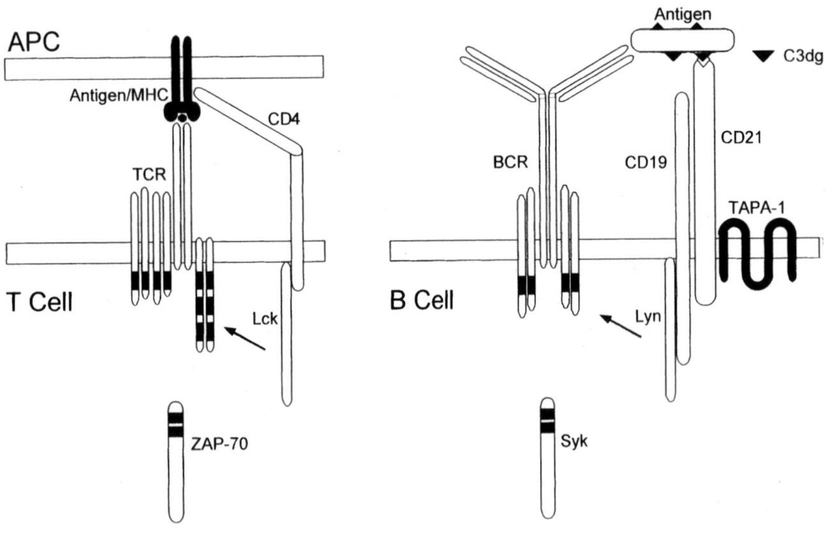

Figure 6.3. Models of coreceptor/antigen receptor engagement on T and B cells. APC, antigen-presenting cell; MHC, major histocompatibility complex.

gp120 protein with CD4, which can lead to apoptosis if the TCR is subsequently stimulated (Banda et al., 1992). The mechanisms underlying such coreceptor-induced inhibitory signals have not been clarified.

Mature CD4 or CD8 T cells are derived from thymocyte precursors that express both of these coreceptors. Evidence suggests that these two coreceptors play an active role in the decision process regarding lineage commitment (von Boehmer and Kisielow, 1993). Moreover, T cells that express CD4 or CD8, in addition to recognizing peptide antigens on distinct classes of MHC molecules, generally have distinct effector functions, helper or cytolytic functions, respectively. To explain this linkage of coreceptor expression to differentiated phenotype, it has been proposed that the engagement of the TCR with each of these coreceptors leads to distinct signaling events (Ratcliffe et al., 1992; von Boehmer and Kisielow, 1993; Itano et al., 1996). The identity of such specialized events remains unknown. Since the interaction of CD4 with Lck appears to be more avid than that of CD8 with Lck (Wiest et al., 1993), it is possible that there are quantitative and qualitative effects that should be considered.

Coreceptors on B Cells

The concept of coreceptors in B cell antigen recognition is a newly emerging concept, in part because a coreceptor involved in the recognition of native antigen is not often considered. However, recent studies suggest that complement fixed to soluble or particulate antigen may serve to colocalize complement receptors with the BCR and greatly potentiate BCR signaling and B cell activation (Fearon and Carter, 1995). Antigen/complement complexes or fusion proteins are much more potent inducers of B cells than native antigen. These observations suggest that coligation of the complement receptor and the BCR increases the sensitivity of the B cell response to antigen, analogous to the role of coreceptors in T cell activation.

The complement receptor that functions as coreceptor is CD21. It is part of a molecular complex formed by CD19, CD21 (complement receptor 2, CR2), and TAPA-1 (CD81) (Fig. 6.3). CD21 binds the complement proteolytic product C3dg. Ligands for CD19 and TAPA-1 have not been identified, although TAPA-1 serves as the receptor for infection by hepatitis C virus (Pileri et al., 1998). Coligation of CR2 or CD19 with the BCR lowers the effective concentration of anti-Ig required to induce early signal transduction events or B cell proliferation (Fearon and Carter, 1995). Similar observations have been made with a soluble antigen/complement fusion protein (Dempsey et al., 1996), suggesting that such synergy in coligation of these complexes is physiologically relevant. Interestingly, preligation of CD19 inhibits IgM-mediated B cell proliferation in a manner that is remarkably similar to the properties of the T cell coreceptors, CD4 and CD8.

The precise mechanism by which the CD19/CD21/TAPA-1 complex functions as a coreceptor is not clear. Stabilization of the extracellular ligand interactions is one possible mechanism. Src kinases, including Lyn, have been detected in CD19 immunoprecipitates (van Noesel et al., 1993), which suggests that the B cell coreceptor complex could bring these kinases into proximity of the BCR ITAMs or recruited kinases. In addition, the inducible phosphorylation of CD19 by BCR stimulation leads to the recruitment of a number of signaling molecules that could contribute to the initial events in BCR activation or could recruit potential substrates or signaling molecules (Fearon and Carter, 1995). The best-characterized interaction is with the p85

subunit of phosphatidylinositol 3-kinase (PI3K) (Tuveson et al., 1993). This results from the interaction of the p85 SH2 domains with phosphorylated CD19 residues containing the consensus motif YXXM. Activation of PI3K follows BCR stimulation and it participates in downstream signaling events as described later. CD19 also binds the signaling component Vav (see below) and this likely contributes to B cell activation as well. The positive role of CD19 in B cell activation is illustrated by the striking effects of altering CD19 expression genetically. B cells with elevated levels of CD19 are highly activated, whereas those with decreased levels are poorly stimulated by antigen (Sato et al., 1997).

Receptors with Inhibitory Functions

Recent studies have identified several receptors that appear to function in negatively regulating signal transduction by the TCR (the killer inhibitory receptors, KIRs; and CTLA-4) (Waterhouse et al., 1995; Yokoyama, 1995; Marengere et al., 1996) and the BCR (FcγRIIB, CD72, and PIR-B) (Brauweiler et al., 2000; Parnes and Pan, 2000; Takai and Ono, 2001). These receptors inhibit signal transduction by the TCR or BCR by recruiting from the cytoplasm inhibitory signaling proteins to the plasma membrane in close proximity to the stimulated antigen receptor. Among the proteins recruited to the membrane by these receptors are the cytoplasmic protein tyrosine phosphatases SHP-1 and SHP-2 and the inositol phosphatase SHIP-1. The mechanisms by which these proteins inhibit signal transduction by the TCR and BCR are beginning to be characterized.

The best characterized of these inhibitory receptors is FcγRIIB. Coligation of this receptor with the BCR inhibits B cell proliferative responses and promotes B cell apoptosis. Physiologically, coligation is likely to occur during the binding of antigen-antibody complexes to antigen-specific B cells. The presence of IgG bound to the antigen reflects the presence of specific antibody, so inhibition of further B cell activation is a mechanism for downregulating antibody production late in an immune response. Indeed, mice made deficient in FcγRIIB have heightened B cell responses to BCR stimulation (Takai et al., 1996). Coligation of the BCR with FcγRIIB leads to FcγRIIB tyrosine phosphorylation (Muta et al., 1994). The major inhibitory function of this receptor maps to a single tyrosine residue in its cytoplasmic domain that is in the context of an immunoreceptor tyrosine-based inhibitory motif (ITIM) with a consensus sequence I/L/VXYXXL. Phosphorylation of this tyrosine residue in the ITIM leads to the recruitment of the SHP-1 and SHP-2 protein tyrosine phosphatases (PTPs) and also the SHIP-1 inositol 5-phosphatase via their SH2 domains (D'Ambrosio et al., 1995; Chacko et al., 1996). The significance of SHP-1 and SHP-2 binding to FcγRIIB remains unclear. SHIP-1 is the primary effector of FcγRIIB and is thought to modulate its signaling function by hydrolysis of phosphatidylinositol 3,4,5 triphosphate (PIP$_3$), a key molecule involved in the translocation and assembly of a signaling complex consisting of PLCγ2 and Btk. These are required for PIP$_2$ hydrolysis and Ca^{2+} mobilization (see below; Gupta et al., 1997; Okada et al., 1998; Scharenberg et al., 1998; Hashimoto et al., 1999). FcγRIIB ligation also results in the inhibition of BCR-mediated Ras activation. In addition, SHIP forms a complex with another adaptor protein, p62^{dok}, which becomes strongly tyrosine phosphorylated upon BCR-FcγRIIB co-cross-linking and recruits RasGAP, a suppressor of Ras activity (Tamir et al., 2000; Yamanishi et al., 2000).

The related Ig superfamily members, paired immunoglobulin-like receptors (PIRs), have also been shown to modulate BCR signaling. These receptors are expressed not only on B cells but also macrophages, neutrophils, mast cells, and dendritic cells. These are type I transmembrane glycoproteins with six Ig-like domains related to human FcαR and bovine Fcγ2R, with the activating (PIR-A) and inhibitory (PIR-B) forms being expressed in a pairwise fashion. The ligand for these receptors is unknown, although co-cross-linking PIR-B with the BCR or the Fc receptor for IgE (FcεRI) results in inhibition of antigen receptor– or Fc receptor–mediated activation through the ITIMs present in the cytoplasmic tail. On B cells, PIR-B is constitutively tyrosine phosphorylated and associated with the tyrosine phosphatase SHP-1. PIR-A, by contrast, requires association with the Fc receptor common γ chain for its membrane expression and activation function (Kubagawa et al., 1999; Maeda et al., 1998, 1999). The functions of these proteins are not yet understood.

CD72 is the third receptor that negatively regulates B cell function. CD72 is a type II transmembrane protein belonging to the C-type lectin superfamily. It is expressed on the surface of B cells throughout their development and is thought to be a regulator of different stages of B cell development (Parnes and Pan, 2000; Kumanogoh and Kikutani, 2001). Absence of CD72 is associated with a significant increase in the number of IgM⁻IgD⁻ pre-B cells in the bone marrow whereas the mature IgM⁺IgD⁺ B cells are fewer in number. These findings indicate that CD72 may be required for the efficient transition from the pre-B cell to the immature B cell and/or from the immature to the mature B cell stage. CD72-deficient mice also have increased numbers of splenic B-1 cells and marginal zone B cells (Pan et al., 1999). This change in the relative distribution of B-1 and conventional B-2 cells has also been observed in mice that have been gene targeted for other negative regulators of BCR signaling—e.g., Lyn, SHP-1, and CD22. Interestingly, the cytoplasmic domain of CD72 contains two ITIMs, one of which has been shown to recruite SHP-1. Accordingly, the B cells from CD72-deficient mice are hyperresponsive to suboptimal doses of antigenic and mitogenic stimulation (Pan et al., 1999; Adachi et al., 2000).

Receptors with Dual Effects on Antigen Receptor Signaling

Another cell surface protein that influences the outcome of signaling via the BCR is CD22, a transmembrane glycoprotein that belongs to the family of Siglecs (sialic acid binding Ig-like lectins) and is expressed exclusively on B cells. The sialic acid binding activity of CD22 is largely undetectable in resting B cells; however, activation of the B cell results in CD22 binding to α2,6 sialylated

ligands, probably because of unmasking of the ligand binding domains (Nitschke et al., 2001). Upon BCR engagement, the cytoplasmic tail of CD22 is phosphorylated by the Src family kinase Lyn on six tyrosine residues. Three of these are in the context of ITIMs, which suggests a negative regulatory role for CD22. Lyn-deficient mice lack BCR-induced tyrosine phosphorylation of CD22, and this might contribute to the hyperactive state of B cells derived from these mice (Chan et al., 1998; Cornall et al., 1999).

There is also evidence that CD22 can signal positively. For example, the cytoplasmic tail of CD22 has been shown to recruit several signaling molecules including Lyn, Syk, PLCγ2, PI3K, Grb2, and Shc (Fearon and Carroll, 2000). In addition, B cells from CD22-deficient mice exhibit decreased overall tyrosine phosphorylation and proliferation, consistent with a positive signaling function of CD22. Further studies will be needed to better define the role of CD22 in B cell regulation. At the same time, CD22 also binds the tyrosine phosphatase SHP-1 and the inositol phosphatase SHIP, both of which are involved in the negative regulation of B cell activation. Accordingly, CD22-deficient B cells show augmented calcium responses which are regulated by membrane recruitment of SHP-1 and SHIP (Sato et al., 1996; Nitschke et al., 1997; Poe et al., 2000). Similarly, sequestering CD22 away from the BCR by preincubation with anti-CD22-coated beads leads to robust mitogen-activated protein kinase (MAPK) activation upon BCR stimulation, whereas coligating BCR with CD22 suppresses MAPK activation. It has been suggested that the *cis* binding of CD22 to the cell surface glycans could keep it sequestered away from the BCR and could thus prevent it from exerting a negative influence (Smith and Fearon, 2000).

Regulation by CD45 and Csk

The steady-state level of protein tyrosine phosphorylation is the result of a dynamic equilibrium involving the opposing actions of kinases and phosphatases. The function of Src PTKs is tightly regulated by tyrosine phosphorylation (Cooper and Howell, 1993). Phosphorylation of a tyrosine near the catalytic loop of the kinase domain is associated with the activated state of these kinases. In addition, the C-terminal regulatory region of the Src kinases contains a tyrosine residue whose phosphorylation negatively regulates their activity. In T and B cells, the phosphorylation of this negative regulatory site in Src PTKs appears to be regulated by the opposing actions of the transmembrane PTP CD45 and the cytoplasmic Csk PTK (Fig. 6.4) (Chan et al., 1994a; Chow and Veillette, 1995). The regulation of Lck in T cells by CD45 and Csk has been most thoroughly studied.

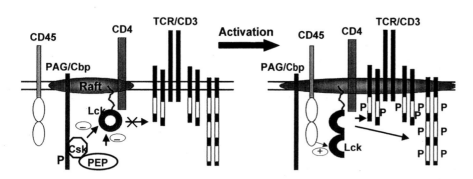

Figure 6.4. Dynamic regulation of Src family kinases by Csk and tyrosine phosphatases, CD45 and PEP, in plasma membrane microdomains (lipid rafts).

Various isoforms of CD45, derived by alternative splicing of exons 4–6, which encode portions of the extracellular domain, are expressed in a cell type– and activation-specific manner on all nucleated cells of the hematopoietic lineage (Trowbridge and Thomas, 1994). Although the regulated expression of specific isoforms of CD45 suggests that CD45 may be regulated by extracellular ligands, definitive identification of such ligands has not yet been achieved. It is also possible that the extracellular domain of CD45 interacts laterally with other molecules present in the same plasma membrane, thereby delivering the phosphatase domains to their targets. Some evidence of this has been obtained for interaction of the low–molecular weight isoforms of CD45 with CD4 and the TCR (Leitenberg et al., 1996). Like most transmembrane PTPases, CD45 contains two tandem PTP homology domains in its cytoplasmic domain. Only the membrane proximal PTP domain clearly has catalytic phosphatase function, although the membrane distal domain may play an important regulatory function as it appears to be necessary for PTP activity of CD45 (Johnson et al., 1992; Desai et al., 1994).

CD45 expression is required for normal T cell development in mice (Kishihara et al., 1993; Byth et al., 1996). Interestingly, B cell development is not dependent on CD45, although the B cells that do develop show functional defects. In peripheral mature T and B cells as well as cell lines and clones, CD45 is required for TCR- and BCR-induced signal transduction (Chan et al., 1994a; Trowbridge and Thomas, 1994). The PTP catalytic function of CD45 is required for TCR signal transduction (Desai et al., 1994). In its absence, the earliest phosphorylation of ITAMs or recruitment of ZAP-70 does not occur (Chu et al., 1996). In CD45-deficient T cell lines, although there is not an substantial increase in basal tyrosine phosphorylation of most proteins, the negative regulatory tyrosine phosphorylation sites of Lck and Fyn are hyperphosphorylated (Ostergaard et al., 1989; Hurley et al., 1993; McFarland et al., 1993; Desai et al., 1994). Phosphorylation of this site results in an inactive state of these PTKs because of a conformational constraint imposed by an intramolecular interaction between the C-terminal phosphotyrosine and the SH2 domain of the kinase (Sicheri and Kuriyan, 1997; Young et al., 2001). The observations made in CD45-deficient cells are consistent with the notion that the phosphotyrosine in the C-terminal region is a physiologic substrate of CD45 and the Lck and Fyn kinases are inactive in CD45-deficient cells. The greatly decreased activity of Lck and Fyn can account for the defect in TCR signal transduction function. Thus, in normal resting cells where these kinases are dephosphorylated at the C-terminal-negative regulatory sites, CD45 maintains the Src kinases in a TCR-responsive but not active state. Activation of Src family kinases involves the phosphorylation of a critical tyrosine within the regulatory loop of the kinase domain in addition to the lack of phosphorylation of the negative regulatory site.

Observations of isoform-specific effects of CD45 in reconstituted T cell hybridoma systems are suggestive of specific functions for the different isoforms (Novak et al., 1994; McKenney et al., 1995). Studies with an epidermal growth factor receptor-CD45 chimera suggest that ligand-induced dimerization may negatively regulate the phosphatase function of CD45 (Desai et al., 1993). Inactivation by dimerization of CD45 appears to be mediated by a putative wedge-like structure in the juxtamembrane region that blocks the catalytic site of the partner molecule during dimerzation (Majeti et al., 1998). Disruption of the wedge function in mice leads to lymphoproliferation and autoimmunity (Majeti et al., 2000). These studies strongly suggest that dimerization of CD45 regulates its activity and thereby restrains lymphocyte activation.

The PTK responsible for the phosphorylation of the negative regulatory sites of Src PTKs is Csk, a widely expressed PTK that contains SH2 and SH3 domains (Chow and Veillette, 1995). In the basal state, Csk and CD45 are presumably in equilibrium, maintaining the C-terminal tyrosines of Src family protein kinases primarily in the unphosphosphorylated form. Overexpression of Csk can inhibit TCR-induced protein tyrosine phosphorylation and interleukin-2 (IL-2) production, but does not lead to the hyperphosphorylation of the negative regulatory site in the basal state (Chow et al., 1993). Regulation of Csk occurs by its differential distribution between the cytosol and lipid raft fraction of the plasma membrane during lymphocyte activation (Fig. 6.4). The lipid raft resident transmembrane adaptor protein Cbp/PAG-85 was identified as a binding partner for Csk in resting T cells. Cbp is constitutively tyrosine phosphorylated in resting T cells and binds to Csk via the SH2 domain of the latter. According to one model, upon TCR cross-linking, Cbp is dephosphorylated by an unknown tyrosine phosphatase, thereby releasing Csk, which relocalizes to the cytosol, allowing the balance to be shifted in the favor of Src family kinase activation. Later, Cbp gets rephosphorylated and recruits Csk back to the lipid microdomains where it can exert its negative regulatory effect on Lck and Fyn once again (Peninger et al., 2001). In addition, an intracellular protein tyrosine phosphatase, proline-enriched phosphatase (PEP), which is expressed in hematopoeitic cells, has been found to associate with Csk via the SH3 domain of Csk. Substrate-trapping experiments using mutant PEP identified Zap-70 and FynT as two proximal targets of PEP-mediated inhibition and the site of dephosphorylation on FynT was mapped to the positive regulatory tyrosine 417. Thus, a complex of Csk-PEP acts synergistically to interfere with TCR signaling by phosphorylating the C-terminal negative regulatory tyrosine and dephosphorylating the activating tyrosine of Src family kinases (Cloutier and Veillette, 1999). In addition, two other members of the PEP family, PTP-PEST and PTP-HSCF, have been reported to cooperate with Csk in the regulation of antigen receptor signaling in T cells (Davidson and Veillette, 2001; Wang et al., 2001). Whether PEP, PTP-PEST, and PTP-HSCF all act redundantly or uniquely is currently unknown.

In Csk-deficient chicken B cells, Lyn was found to be highly phosphorylated at the autophosphorylation site and constitutively active. In addition, Syk was also constitutively activated, to an extent similar to that observed upon BCR stimulation. However, BCR cross-linking was still required for other cellular proteins to be tyrosine phosphorylated and for calcium mobilization and inositol 1,4,5-triphosphate (IP$_3$) generation (Hata et al., 1994). Homozygous mutant mice with a disruption in the Csk gene were found to have neural tube defects, were embryonic lethal, and died during gestation at days 9–10. The embryonic cells exhibited an increase in the activity of Src, Fyn, and Lyn kinases, which suggests that Csk regulates the activity of these kinases; this may be essential during embryogenesis (Imamoto and Soriano, 1993; Nada et al., 1993). The role of Csk in lymphocyte development was studied by conditionally inactivating Csk in immature thymocytes. Lack of Csk was found to override the requirement for pre-TCR, αβ TCR, and MHC class II for the development of CD4$^+$CD8$^+$ double-positive and CD4$^+$ single-positive thymocytes as well as peripheral CD4 αβ T-lineage cells (Schmedt el al., 1998). Thus, Csk and its substrates, the Src family kinases, mediate the effect of pre-TCR and αβ TCR on the development of αβ T cells. Triple knockout mice lacking Csk,

Lck, and Fyn show a block in the development of αβ T cells, indicating that Lck and Fyn are specific substrates for Csk during T cell development. Furthermore, Csk was shown to play a differential role in positive and negative selection during development (Schmedt and Tarakhovsky, 2001).

Signaling Pathways Activated by Antigen Receptor–Induced Tyrosine Phosphorylation

The stimulation of the TCR and BCR induces the tyrosine phosphorylation of many intracellular proteins and sets into motion a number of signaling pathways. A list of many of the proteins that are inducibly tyrosine phosphorylated is presented in Table 6.1. In the following sections, we will focus on some of the better-understood TCR- and BCR-regulated signaling pathways and discuss the involvement of some of these proteins in lymphocyte activation.

Role of Adaptor Proteins

Signal transduction via the TCR and BCR flows from the membrane proximal tyrosine kinases to downstream signaling reactions such as activation of Ras, MAPKs, actin rearrangement, and calcium-dependent pathways. The transmission of these signals requires the formation of multimolecular complexes consisting of adaptor proteins and signaling components (Table 6.1). The adaptor proteins lack enzymatic or transcriptional activity but are comprised of modular domains such as the SH2, SH3, PTB, PDZ, or PH domains or simply multiple tyrosines or prolines that can act as docking sites for some of the above domains (Pawson, 1995; Pawson and Nash, 2000).

Some adaptors are membrane proteins whereas others are cytosolic in unstimulated cells and are recruited to the plasma membrane by initial receptor signaling events. In the former category are the transmembrane adaptors LAT, which is required for TCR signaling, and CD19, which is a major coreceptor in B cells. Both proteins contain multiple tyrosine residues that are phosphorylated upon receptor ligation and form docking sites for

other downstream adaptors and signaling enzymes and therefore serve to nucleate the formation of multimeric signaling complexes, or "signalosomes." B cells likely contain an additional protein of this type as genetic ablation of CD19 decreases B cell activation but does not abolish it. In T cells, phosphorylated LAT recruits the cytosolic adaptor SLP-76 (Jackman et al., 1995) via the latter's C-terminal SH2 domain. SLP-76 also interacts with the adaptor Gads and with the signaling component Vav, whose function is described below. A close relative of SLP-76 expressed in B cells is B cell linker protein (BLNK) (Fu et al., 1998), also known as BASH (Goitsuka et al., 1998) or SLP-65 (Wienands et al., 1998). SLP-76 and BLNK have similar domain structures and recruit many of the same signaling molecules in T and B cells. Both SLP-76 and BLNK have a single C-terminal SH2 domain, acidic, basic, and proline-rich regions, and multiple tyrosines that get phosphorylated upon stimulation. They bind PLCγ, Nck, Vav, and Cbl (Jackman et al., 1995; Fu et al., 1998).

In cells lacking SLP76 or BLNK, proximal receptor engagement is uncoupled from distal events such as calcium flux and IL-2 activation (Clements et al., 1998; Yablonski et al., 1998; Pappu et al., 1999). Deficiency of SLP-76 or BLNK in mice leads to strong defects in T and B cell development, respectively (Clements et al., 1998; Pappu et al., 1999; Hayashi et al., 2000). However, despite the obvious parallels in the structure and function of SLP-76 and BLNK, B cells lacking BLNK could not be functionally complemented by SLP-76 alone. Reconstitution also required the addition of the adaptors LAT and Gads, which form a complex with SLP-76 (Ishiai et al., 2000). Presumably this reflects the formation of distinct but analogous complexes of adaptor proteins in B cells and T cells. The additional components of this complex in B cells are not yet defined. Recently, BLNK was shown to bind directly with the Igα chain of the BCR upon B cell stimulation. The interaction was mediated by the SH2 domain of BLNK and Y204 of Igα, which is located distal to and outside the ITAM (Engels et al., 2001b). Thus, it is possible that in B cells Igα plays a role similar to that of LAT in TCR signaling.

The Phosphatidylinositol Second Messenger Pathway

TCR or BCR stimulation results in the tyrosine phosphorylation and activation of PLCγ1 or PLCγ2 (Carter et al., 1991; Park et al., 1991; Weiss et al., 1991). PLCγ2 is preferentially expressed in B cells whereas PLCγ1 is preferentially expressed in T cells. The PLCγ isozymes are responsible for the hydrolysis of PI 4,5-bisphosphate yielding IP_3 and diacylglycerol (DAG), which lead to increases in cytoplasmic free calcium ($[Ca^{2+}]_i$) and activation of protein kinase C (PKC) isozymes, respectively (Majerus et al., 1990) (Fig. 6.5). The critical role of PLCγ in regulating these events in antigen receptor stimulation is supported by observations in an avian B cell line in which the PLCγ2 gene was inactivated (Takata et al., 1995) and PLCγ2 knockout mice (Hashimoto et al., 2000; Wang et al., 2000). The increase in $[Ca^{2+}]_i$ and activation of PKC have been shown to contribute to a variety of cellular responses in T and B cells.

Following TCR or BCR stimulation, PLCγ isozymes translocate to the membrane, where they become tyrosine phosphorylated on critical tyrosine residues (Todderud et al., 1990; DeBell et al., 1999; Rodriguez et al., 2001; Veri et al., 2001). This activates their catalytic activity (Nishibe et al., 1990). This translocation involves the recruitment of PLCγ isozymes via their SH2 domains to phosphorylated tyrosine residues on LAT in T cells and BLNK in B cells. In addition, some data suggest that the

Table 6.1. Antigen Receptor–Induced Tyrosine Phosphoproteins

	T Cells	B Cells
Plasma membrane proteins	TCR: CD3 δ, ε, γ	BCR: Igα
	ζ	Igβ
	CD5	CD19
	CD6	CD22
	LAT	FcγRIIB
Src kinases	Lck, Fyn	Lyn, Blk, Fyn
Syk/ZAP–70 kinases	ZAP–70, Syk	Syk
Downstream enzymes	MAP-kinases	MAP-kinases
	Vav	Vav
	PLC γ1	PLC γ2
	GAP (+/−)	GAP
		SHIP
Adaptors/others	Shc	Shc
	Cbl	Cbl
	SLP-76	BLNK
	Lnk	HS1
	Ezrin	Bam-32
	Valosin-containing	
	protein	BCAP
	Gads	p62dok
	HS1	Gab1

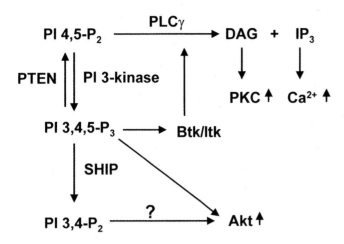

Figure 6.5. Critical signaling events involving phosphatidylinositol (PI)-containing lipids. Other abbreviations in text.

SH2 domain of PLCγ1 and γ2 may directly interact with tyrosine-phosphorylated Syk (Sillman and Monroe, 1995; Law et al., 1996). Moreover, the SH3 domain of PLCγ1 interacts with a proline-rich motif in SLP-76, which may explain the requirement of this adaptor for PLC activation (Yablonski et al., 1998, 2001). Whether the two PLCγ isozymes are differentially regulated remains to be determined.

Stimulation of the TCR and BCR results in a rapid and sustained increase in $[Ca^{2+}]_i$ (Gardner, 1989; Lewis and Cahalan, 1989). A requirement for this sustained increase for biological responses has often been observed (Goldsmith and Weiss, 1988). The immediate increase in $[Ca^{2+}]_i$ is the result of the release of intracellular stores of calcium through the action of IP_3 on the IP_3 receptor (Taylor and Marshall, 1992; Kurosaki et al., 2000). This release of the intracellular stores of calcium, however, results only in a transient rise in $[Ca^{2+}]_i$. The sustained increase requires an inward transmembrane flux of extracellular calcium, which occurs through mechanisms and channels that remain ill defined but may be a consequence of the emptying of the intracellular stores, a mechanism referred to as *capacitative calcium entry* (Bootman and Berridge, 1995). Both soluble mediators and tyrosine phosphorylation have been implicated in this capacitative flux of extracellular calcium (Parekh et al., 1993; Bootman and Berridge, 1995; Jayaraman et al., 1996).

The increase in $[Ca^{2+}]_i$ has effects on several downstream events, including the activation of calcium/calmodulin-dependent kinase II and calcineurin, a calcium/calmodulin-regulated protein serine/threonine phosphatase (also called PP2B). Although the activation of calcium/calmodulin-dependent kinase II has been implicated in T cell anergy (Nghlem et al., 1994), the regulation and function of calcineurin has received considerably greater attention. Calcineurin function has been implicated in T and B cell responses that depend on TCR and BCR functions in a wide variety of experimental systems. This connection was made possible through the use of the immunosuppressives cyclosporin A and FK506, which, when bound to their cellular receptors (cyclophilin and FKBP, respectively), function as specific inhibitors of calcineurin (Schreiber and Crabtree, 1992). Among the best examples illustrating the importance of calcineurin in lymphocyte responses are the studies of its role in the activation of a family of transcriptional factors, nuclear factor of activated T cells (NFAT), which plays an important role in the regulation of several lymphokine genes, including IL-2. Calcineurin catalytic function

has been shown to be required for the transformation of inactive cytoplasmic NFAT into active nuclear NFAT, where it interacts with AP-1 transcription factors (made up of Fos and Jun family members) at composite elements in the upstream IL-2 regulatory region (Flanagan et al., 1991). This requirement probably involves the dephosphorylation of the inactive cytoplasmic NFAT (Jain et al., 1993; Macian et al., 2001). In addition to its contribution to regulating transcriptional events, calcineurin has many other functions in response to antigen receptor activation, including a role in triggering the degranulation of cytolytic T cells.

The elevations of DAG following TCR or BCR stimulation of the phosphatidylinositol pathway results in the activation of PKC isozymes. There are several PKC isozymes expressed in T and B cells. Most are calcium- and phospholipid-dependent enzymes (PKCα, β1, and β2); some are calcium-independent (PKCε, δ, η, and θ) (Nishizuka, 1988). These isozymes can also be activated by phorbol esters as well as DAG. The functions of the individual isozymes are not clear. Approaches using activated forms of α, β, ε, and θ have suggested that all four isoforms may be able to regulate various transcription factors in T cells (i.e., AP-1 and NF-κB), but there may be some level of isozyme specificity on these factors (Genot et al., 1995). Inactivation of PKCθ results in defects of TCR-mediated activation of NF-κB (Sun et al., 2000). In contrast, inactivation of PKCβ has effects on B cell development that are reminiscent of Btk deficiency (Leitges et al., 1996). PKC activation has also been implicated in many other events, including CD4 and TCR down-regulation, Ras activation, and cytolytic granule exocytosis. These pleiomorphic effects suggest that PKC isozymes may be involved in many separate downstream events.

A remarkable synergy is observed in inducing T cell or B cell activation by the combined actions of calcium ionophores (to elevate $[Ca^{2+}]_i$) and phorbol esters (to activate PKC isozymes). This suggests that the pathways downstream of these events intersect at critical nodal points. These critical events are not established. However, there are candidates that would be responsive to both events, including calcium-dependent isozymes of PKC, an upstream regulator of the c-Jun N-terminal kinase (Su et al., 1994), or NFAT. The identification of molecules whose function depends on both of these events is likely to lead to critical new insights into the processes governing lymphocyte activation.

Ras Activation in T and B Cells

Ras proteins have been implicated in a wide variety of growth and differentiation responses (McCormick, 1993; Bar-Sagi and Hall, 2000). The activation of Ras proteins following antigen receptor stimulation has been shown to be a critical event in lymphocyte development and activation. The Ras proteins are a small family of 21 kDa GTP-binding proteins with GTPase activity. The activation state of Ras is determined by the form of guanine nucleotide bound to it: GTP-bound Ras is active and GDP-bound Ras is inactive. GDP-bound Ras becomes activated by interacting with guanine nucleotide exchange proteins (GEFs) which cause it to release GDP, allowing it to bind GTP. Conversely, GTP-bound Ras is inactivated by hydrolyzing the GTP to form GDP and PO_4, a reaction stimulated by GTPase activating proteins (GAPs). Thus, the activation of Ras could be a consequence of GEF stimulation, GAP inhibition, or a combination of both. The activation of Ras can lead to a variety of downstream events, including (1) the activation of the Erk MAPK pathway; (2) the activation of PI3K; and, (3) the activation of other small molecular–weight, GTP-binding proteins such as Rac and CDC42 (McCormick and Wittinghofer, 1996).

Initial studies of growth factor receptor PTKs in *Drosophila*, *C. elegans*, and mammalian fibroblasts identified an adaptor molecule called Drk, Sem 5, or Grb2, respectively, in the different species, that interacts with both the stimulated receptors and with a guanine nucleotide exchange factor called SOS (son of sevenless) (Schlessinger, 1993). Subsequently, in some systems another adaptor, called Shc, was found to function in linking Grb/SOS to the activated receptor PTKs. Genetic and biochemical studies indicate that Grb2/SOS proteins couple the stimulated PTK receptors to the activation of Ras. Currently it is thought that SOS action on Ras is primarily regulated by intracellular localization: receptor signaling induces a translocation of Grb2/SOS from the cytosol to the plasma membrane by virtue of the binding of Grb2 to tyrosine phosphorylated sites on the receptor itself or on adaptor proteins such as Shc (Aronheim et al., 1994). Shc phosphorylation and interaction with Grb2/SOS has been observed after TCR or BCR stimulation (Ravichandran et al., 1993; Saxton et al., 1994; Crowley et al., 1996), although its importance for activation of Ras in these cells is unclear.

The mechanisms by which antigen receptors activate Ras are not yet well established. Stimulation of the TCR and BCR induces activation of Ras (Downward et al., 1992) and the Erk MAPK. In lymphocytes, phorbol esters induce strong activation of Ras. This has generally been interpreted to reflect a role for PKC in the activation of Ras, but other interpretations are possible (see below). Initial studies of the mechanism by which phorbol esters activate Ras implicated a PKC-dependent inhibitory effect on GAP (Downward et al., 1990), but this has not been confirmed. GAP is tyrosine phosphorylated following BCR stimulation and to a lesser extent following TCR stimulation (Gold et al., 1993). In B cells, it is recruited to the membrane via the negative coreceptor FcγRIIB, SHIP, and the adaptor protein p62^{dok}, so it appears to function to limit Ras activation at least in this context.

Regulation of GEF function is probably more directly responsible for the positive activation of Ras by the TCR and BCR (Ravichandran et al., 1993). In some T cells, Grb2/SOS associate with the TCR-induced phosphorylated LAT, which would serve to translocate these complexes to the membrane and presumably stimulate Ras activation (Wange, 2000). Alternately, Ras activation may be a consequence of PLCγ1 activation. In this regard, the GEF RasGRP was recently identifed in T cells (Dower et al., 2000; Ebinu et al., 2000). This protein has calcium-binding EF hands and, more importantly, a DAG-binding domain. Thus, the activity of PLCγ1 may be directly translated into Ras activation through the recruitment of RasGRP. The EF hands may also bind phorbol esters, thereby explaining the ability of PMA to activate Ras (Izquierdo et al., 1992).

Some studies have implicated c-Cbl, an antigen receptor–inducible phosphoprotein, as a negative regulator of the interaction of Grb2 with SOS (Donovan et al., 1994; Yoon et al., 1995). Cbl also interacts with BLNK, a critical adaptor molecule required for the activation of PLCγ2, and exerts a negative regulatory effect on BCR signaling, possibly by inhibiting the binding of BLNK to PLCγ2. Accordingly, it was shown that BCR-mediated PLCγ2 activation is enhanced in DT40 cells deficient in Cbl (Yasuda et al., 2000). Clearly, these interactions are complex and much more needs to be learned about them.

Ras plays a critical role in lymphocyte activation. Dominant negative mutants of Ras can partially block IL-2 gene activation in T cells and completely block NFAT-based transcription (Cantrell,

1996). This is probably explained by the involvement of Ras in regulating the AP-1 components involved. An activated form of Ras, which cannot hydrolyze GTP, can synergize with calcium ionophores to induce NFAT-directed transcription. Similarly, BCR-induced transcription of the *egr-1* early response gene is mediated by Ras (McMahon and Monroe, 1995). Egr-1 appears to be important for BCR-induced up-regulation of ICAM-1 and CD44 expression (McMahon and Monroe, 1996). Ras also plays an important role in T cell development. For example, expression of activated Ras as a transgene can promote early T cell developmental transitions in recombinase activating gene (RAG)-deficient mice, which cannot express the pre-TCR (Swat et al., 1996). Similarly, blockade of the Ras pathway with inactivating mutants can interrupt normal thymic development (Alberola-lla et al., 1995; Crompton et al., 1996). Thus, a variety of observations position the activation of Ras as a critical event in antigen receptor signal transduction pathways.

As listed above, there are several reported downstream effectors of Ras. The effectors responsible for Ras function in different systems are not fully established and no single effector can usually substitute for the activated form of Ras in experimental models. The best-characterized Ras effector is the Raf-1 kinase. GTP-bound Ras interacts directly with the serine/threonine kinase Raf-1, translocating it to the membrane (Moodie et al., 1993; Van Aelst et al., 1993; Vojtek et al., 1993). The translocation of Raf-1 to the membrane can increase its activity, although other mechanisms have been implicated in Raf activation, including its tyrosine phosphorylation and transphosphorylation by dimerization (Marshall, 1996). The translocation to the membrane by Ras may simply concentrate Raf-1 there and allow it to dimerize and transphosphorylate. In any case, Raf-1 is activated in T and B cells in response to TCR and BCR stimulation or phorbol ester stimulation, corresponding to signals activating Ras (Cantrell, 1996). The activation of Raf-1 leads to its direct interaction and activation of a dual specific tyrosine/serine/threonine kinase, MEK-1, that in turn activates the Erk1/Erk2 MAP kinases.

MAP kinases have numerous functions including the phosphorylation and activation of transcription factors such as serum response factor, which can regulate c-fos and Egr-1 transcription. Thus, this antigen receptor–regulated cascade of events ending in MAP kinase activation can function to regulate transcriptional events leading to lymphocyte differentiation and activation. Specific inhibition of the Erk MAPK by using pharmacologic inhibitors of MEK1 and MEK2 blocked BCR-induced proliferation of mature B cells, but did not block apoptotic responses of immature B cells and an immature B cell line, indicating that Erk MAPK mediate some effects of BCR signaling but not others (Richards et al., 2001). Similarly, changes in activation of the three MAPK families, Erk, Jnk, and p38, were found to perturb development. Thus, genetically reduced expression of the adaptor protein Grb2 results in weaker Jnk and p38 activation but does not affect Erk, which, in turn, selectively decreases the ability of thymocytes to undergo negative but not positive selection (Gong et al., 2001a).

Vav Phosphorylation and Function in T and B Cells

Among the many TCR- and BCR-induced tyrosine phosphoproteins is the protooncogene *Vav* (Bustelo and Barbacid, 1992; Margolis et al., 1992). Vav is expressed exclusively in hematopoietic cells and trophoblasts, although two closely related family

Table 6.2. T and B Cell Defects in Vav-Deficient Mice

Event	Deficiency In:		
	Vav-1	Vav-2	Vav-1 and Vav-2
T cell development	↓ or ↓↓	Normal	↓↓
Thymocyte Ca^{2+} elevation	↓	Normal	ND
T cell proliferation	↓	Normal	ND
B cell development	Normal	Normal	↓
B1 cell development	↓↓	Normal	↓↓
B cell maturation in periphery	↓	Normal	↓
BCR-mediated proliferation	↓	↓	↓↓
BCR-mediated Ca^{2+} flux	↓	↓	↓↓
T-independent type 2 antibody response	Normal or ↓	↓	↓↓
T-dependent antibody response	↓	↓	ND

Results are based on data presented in (Turner, 1997; Fisher et al., 1998; Doody et al., 2001; Tedford et al., 2001). Entries with "or" reflect somewhat different results obtained in two different studies. ↓↓, more severe defect; ↓, moderate defect, especially upon suboptimal stimulation of TCR or BCR; ND, not determined.

members (Vav-2 and Vav-3) are now known and are expressed more widely. The original cellular Vav is now called Vav-1. It contains multiple distinct domains including a leucine-rich domain, a domain related to GEF domains of Rho-family GTPases, a pleckstrin homology (PH) domain, a zinc finger domain, two SH3 domains, and an SH2 domain. Deletion of the N-terminal 65 residues of Vav leads to a protein with transforming ability in NIH 3T3 fibroblasts (Katzav et al., 1991). Genetic experiments demonstrate that Vav plays an important role in antigen responses of T cells and B cells, but how it does so is not clear (DeFranco, 2001).

The importance of Vav in T cell signaling is underscored by the phenotype of Vav-1$^{-/-}$ mice, which are severely compromised in T cell function (Fischer et al., 1995; Tarakhovsky et al., 1995). These mice show defects in thymic cellularity, thymocyte positive and negative selection, peripheral T cell numbers, and peripheral T cell responses. While the deficiency of Vav-1 does not have any serious defects in the B cell compartment other than loss of the B-1 subtype of B cells, recent evidence from genetic knockouts of the Vav-2 gene alone or both Vav-1 and -2 together shows that Vav-1 and Vav-2 have both unique and redundant roles in BCR-mediated signaling (Doody et al., 2001; Tedford et al., 2001). The development of T and B cells in Vav-2-deficient mice is largely unaffected; however, these mice show a decrease in antibody responses to T-independent type 2 antigens and also a partial defect in T-dependent IgG production. Suboptimal stimulation of the BCR revealed defects in BCR responses such as calcium flux and proliferation in these mice. Vav-1 and Vav-2 double knockout mice, by contrast, had impaired B cell development and greatly diminished BCR responses, similar to the drastic effects of the Vav-1 knockout on T cells (Table 6.2).

Vav-1 appears to be a direct substrate for the ZAP-70, and possibly Syk, PTKs. Its SH2 domain has a consensus binding specificity for the sequence adjacent to Y315 (YESP) in ZAP-70 (Songyang et al., 1994). A homologous sequence is present in Syk. The binding of the SH2 domain of Vav-1 and Vav-1 tyrosine phosphorylation depends on this site in ZAP-70 (Wu et al., 1997). Moreover, the functional activity of ZAP-70 is markedly reduced by mutation of this site in a reconstitution system where NFAT activity is assessed. These results suggest that the interaction of ZAP-70 with Vav is an important event in antigen receptor signal transduction.

The function of Vav in TCR or BCR signaling pathways is not completely understood. On the basis of sequence homology and overexpression experiments in fibroblasts, it is likely that Vav regulates Rho, Rac, or Cdc 42 GTP-binding proteins (Adams et al., 1992; Bustelo et al., 1994). In one model system, overexpression of Vav in Jurkat T cells led to potentiation of TCR-mediated IL-2- and NFAT-regulated reporter constructs (Wu et al., 1995). This functional activity, which depends on TCR-specific signals, is also dependent on Ras, Lck, and calcineurin function. This suggests that Vav may function very proximally within the TCR pathway or in an alternate signaling pathway which, together with Ras and calcineurin regulated pathways, contributes to IL-2 gene expression. This is most likely to involve increased Rac and Cdc42 activity as evidenced by studies of Vav-deficient cells. The most prominent signaling defect in these cells is a failure of actin polymerization and antigen receptor clustering or cap formation (Fischer et al., 1998; Holsinger et al., 1998). As a consequence, there is inefficient immunological synapse formation (Wulfing et al., 2000). These effects suggest that the regulation of Rac and Cdc42 by Vav GEF function is a critical event in TCR signal transduction.

Surprisingly, biochemical defects in TCR signaling in Vav-1-deficient T cells include defects in phospholipase C tyrosine phosphorylation and Ca^{2+} mobilization (Fischer et al., 1995). This global effect of Vav deficiency suggests that Vav may have roles in T cell activation beyond Rac or Cdc42 activation. In this regard, it should be noted that Vav interacts with the TCR- and BCR-induced adaptors, SLP-76 (Jackman et al., 1995; Wu et al., 1996), and BLNK (Fu et al., 1998). The Vav SH2 domain is required for these interactions. As has been seen with Vav, overexpression of SLP-76 markedly potentiates TCR-mediated IL-2 promoter and NFAT-driven gene expression (Motto et al., 1996). Furthermore, overexpression of both Vav and SLP-76 synergistically induced basal and TCR-stimulated NFAT activity (Wu et al., 1996). These results suggest that a signaling complex containing Vav and SLP-76 plays an important but as yet undefined role in T lymphocyte activation. At least part of this function may be GEF-independent and may relate to an adaptor function of Vav (Kuhne et al., 2000).

Other Signaling Events

It is not our intention to be exhaustive in reviewing signaling events that occur following TCR and BCR stimulation, but two other events deserve brief mention. A prominent substrate of antigen receptor–induced tyrosine phosphorylation is the protein HS-1 (Kitamura et al., 1995). The function of HS-1 is not established, but lymphocyte antigen responses in mice deficient in HS-1 are partially defective (Taniuchi et al., 1995), demonstrating the importance of HS-1. Finally, antigen receptors also activate PI3K (Gold et al., 1992; Ward et al., 1992). The p85 subunit of PI3K is recruited to the membrane by binding of its SH2 domains to the consensus YXXM motif in the cytoplasmic tail of CD19 (Chalupny et al., 1995). Alternatively, it was shown that BCAP, an adaptor protein that is tyrosine phosphorylated by Syk and Btk, could recruit the p85 subunit of PI3K. DT40 B cells deficient in BCAP were unable to generate PIP_3 in response to BCR ligation and exhibited an impaired Akt response (Okada et al., 2000).

The main reaction catalyzed by PI3K is phosphorylation of PI 4,5-bisphosphate to generate PI 3,4,5-trisphosphate (see Fig. 6.5). This compound is a membrane-bound second messenger that recruits signaling molecules to the plasma membrane via their PH domains. Key signaling molecules attracted to the plasma membrane by PIP_3 are the Tec family of tyrosine kinases, Btk and Itk. These kinases have a PH domain followed by a Tec homology (TH), an SH3, an SH2, and a kinase domain (Smith et al. 2001). These molecules play an important role in phosphorylation and activation of PLCγ. Mutations in Btk are responsible for the pathogenesis of the heritable immunodeficiency disorder X-linked agammaglobulinemia (XLA) in humans and X-linked immunodeficiency (Xid) in mice (Chapter 21; for review see Conley et al., 2000; also Conley et al., 1994; Lindvall et al., 2005). The disease is characterized by a severe block in the transition of B cell progenitors into mature B lymphocytes, resulting in a complete absence of B and plasma cells and undetectable immunoglobulins (Vihinen et al., 2000). A similar phenotype was observed in mice lacking the p85α subunit, and its splice variants p55α and p50α. These mice had reduced peripheral mature B cell numbers and serum immunoglobulin corresponding to the somewhat less severe phenotype seen in mice with Btk deficiency (Fruman et al., 1999). Interestingly, PIP_3 is the substrate for SHIP, described above as one of the proteins that binds to FcγRIIB when it is co-engaged with the BCR. The product of the combined action of PI3K and SHIP is PI 3,4-bisphosphate. SHIP is tyrosine phosphorylated in BCR-stimulated B cells, but this is enhanced by co-engagement with FcγRIIB (Chacko et al., 1996). The relative amount of PI 3,4-bisphosphate may be controlled by FcγRIIB and possibly by other receptors on the B cell surface. Future studies may clarify the biological significance of these reactions.

In addition to SHIP, which removes the 5' phosphate from PIP_3 there is a second phosphatase that acts on PIP_3, PTEN, which removes the 3' phosphate (Fig. 6.5). PTEN is a prominent tumor suppressor and is frequently mutated in tumor cells (Maehama and Dixon, 1999). Interestingly, the Jurkat T cell line has a defective PTEN (Shan et al., 2000).

CD28 plays a critical costimulatory function in T cells by binding CD80 and CD86 (B7-1 and B7-2) on antigen-presenting cells. CD28 costimulation can lead to increased lymphokine production, enhanced proliferation, and diminished apoptosis in TCR-mediated responses (Salomon and Bluestone, 2001). CD28 has a consensus PI3K SH2 domain binding site and this site is phosphorylated following CD28 stimulation. The importance of CD28-mediated PI3K activation is at best controversial. Experiments in Jurkat cells often find a functional role of CD28 that is independent of the PI3K docking site. As mentioned above, Jurkat cells lack the PIP_3 phosphatase PTEN, so they may understate the importance of PIP_3 for CD28 function and emphasize the other signaling functions of CD28. In any case, at least one downstream effector of this pathway, the Akt serine/threonine kinase, can partially substitute for CD28 signals in T cell lines and in CD28-deficient T cells (Kane et al., 2001). Akt has a PH domain that binds PIP_3, which allows Akt to be recruited to the membrane in response to PIP_3 elevations—i.e., following CD28 stimulation. Once at the membrane, Akt is activated by a second kinase, PDK-1. The consequences of Akt activation are numerous and include antiapoptotic effects via Bad phosphorylation as well as transcriptional effects that may be mediated by Forkhead and NF-κB. Activation of Akt by CD28 has thus been linked to NF-κB pathways that regulate IL-2 and IFN-γ pathways. Akt is also activated in B cells following BCR ligation in a PI3K-dependent manner. This activity is inhibited upon BCR coligation with FcγRIIb1, a finding suggesting a functional role for SHIP-1 in this regulation and also explaining the increased apoptosis of B cells in these conditions (Aman et al., 1998; Gupta et al., 1999).

Compartmentalization of T and B Antigen Receptor Signaling

Signaling via the antigen receptors and recruitment of various signaling molecules into a "signalosome" is increasingly being viewed in the cell biological context. The spatial arrangement of various participants is seen as one of the key determinants in the regulation and outcome of signaling.

Formation of the Immunological Synapse

Efficient T cell activation requires sustained interaction between the TCR and MHCpeptide complex. Recent imaging studies of regions of contact between T cells and antigen-presenting cells have described the following sequence of events occurring at the plasma membrane: T cell polarization, initial adhesion, immunological synapse (IS) formation (early signaling), and IS maturation (sustained signaling). This involves the formation of a bull's-eye arrangement of molecules at the point of cell–cell contact with the TCR and MHCpeptide complexes clustering in the center (central supramolecular activation clusters, c-SMACs) and the adhesion molecules, LFA-1 and ICAM-1, forming a ring around the periphery (p-SMACs) (Fig. 6.6) (Bromley et al., 2001). Consistent with its role as a positive regulator of Src family kinase activation, CD45, which was initially thought to be excluded from the IS because of topological constraints, was recently shown to localize with the TCR in the c-SMAC. In addition, within the c-SMAC, CD45 was found to occupy a distinct subdomain separate from the TCR (Johnson et al., 2000). Recently, an IS similar to the one described above was reported to form between B cells and follicular dendritic cells (FDCs) (Batista et al., 2001). It was shown that the BCR could acquire intact antigen from the FDCs through the synapse and, after processing it, present the antigenic peptides to T cells expressing the specific TCR, thus resembling an "immunological relay race."

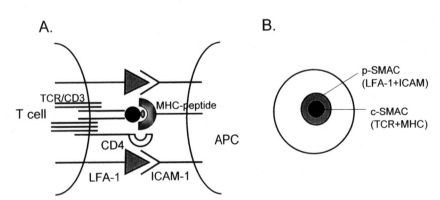

Figure 6.6. A. Schematic view of the critical elements forming the immunological synapse between a T cell and an antigen-presenting cell (APC). B. Bull's-eye arrangement of signaling molecules such as c-SMAC and p-SMAC.

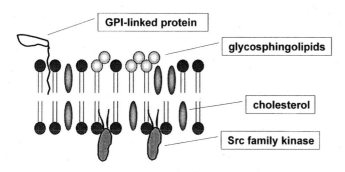

Figure 6.7. A schematic view of the organization of phospholipids and modified proteins in lipid rafts. GPI, glycosyl-phosphatidylinositol.

A Role for Plasma Membrane Microdomains in Signal Transduction

Another feature of the molecular reorganization that occurs upon antigen receptor ligation is the translocation of the TCR and BCR to membrane microdomains known as "lipid rafts" (Fig. 6.7). These are subdomains of the plasma membrane rich in cholesterol, sphingomyelin, and glycosphingolipids, that are resistant to extraction by nonionic detergents and can be biochemically purified on sucrose density gradients. Lipid rafts are home to glycosyl-phosphatidylinositol (GPI)-anchored proteins, members of the Src kinase family, heterotrimeric G proteins, and Ras family small G proteins, and contain bound actin (Harder and Simons, 1997; Brown and London, 1998). Several key participants of the antigen receptor signaling pathways are enriched in lipid rafts, including the coreceptors CD4 and CD8, the Src family kinases, Lck, Lyn, Fyn, the C-terminal Src-like kinase Csk, Cbp/PAG, and LAT (Cherukuri et al., 2001a). Cross-linking of the TCR and BCR induces association of these receptors with lipid rafts and also aggregation of lipid rafts into large patches on the cell surface, which may serve to hold multimolecular signaling complexes in close proximity for efficient signal transduction (Figs. 6.4 and 6.8) (Hoessli et al., 2000). In B cells, the raft components were demonstrated to internalize along with the receptor into the antigen-processing compartment (Cheng et al., 1999). Functional evidence for the significance of lipid rafts in antigen receptor signaling comes from experiments in which rafts were disrupted. Treatment of B or T cells with a variety of agents that disrupt rafts, such as methyl β-cyclodextrin, filipin, nystatin, or

polyunsaturated fatty acids, leads to loss of activation-induced calcium flux in both T and B cells. This finding suggests that the assembly of signaling molecules on lipid raft platforms is crucial for the outcome of activation (Aman et al., 2001; Awasthi-Kalia et al., 2001). In addition, the palmitoylation of LAT that directs its localization to lipid rafts is necessary for it to become efficiently tyrosine phosphorylated upon TCR engagement (Lin et al., 1999). Moreover, the presence of LAT in lipid rafts is absolutely required for coupling TCR engagement to activation of the Ras signaling pathway, increases in intracellular Ca^{2+}, and induction of the transcription factor NFAT (Finco et al., 1998; Zhang et al., 1998).

Interestingly, the developmental stage of B and T cells influences the ability of the BCR or TCR to enter lipid rafts and the outcome of signaling through the receptor. A fraction of the pre-BCR was found to be constitutively associated with lipid rafts, which may reflect constitutive signaling that promotes the developmental transition to the pre-B cell stage. Upon receptor cross-linking, additional pre-BCR molecules translocated to lipid rafts, where they were found to assemble a signaling complex consisting of tyrosine phosphorylated Lyn, Syk, Btk, PI3K, BLNK, Vav, and PLCγ2, all of which have been identified genetically as important for the cell to make the decision to progress to the next stage in its development (Guo et al., 2000). On the other hand, the BCR does not redistribute to lipid rafts upon receptor engagement in immature B cells, and this may contribute to the difference between the outcome of signaling in immature (deletion or anergy) and mature (activation) B cells (Sproul et al., 2000; Chung et al., 2001). Similarly, while the pre-TCR constitutively associates with lipid rafts, where it signals in a ligand-independent manner, the TCR in CD4+CD8+ immature thymocytes does not translocate to these domains upon ligation (Ebert et al., 2000).

Differences in BCR translocation to lipid rafts also correlate with the functional state of mature B cells. In this regard, tolerant B cells from double transgenic mice expressing both anti–hen egg lysozyme (HEL) Ig and soluble HEL failed to translocate their BCRs into a detergent-insoluble fraction compared to B cells from wild-type mice (Weintraub et al., 2000). Whether this reflects a defect in translocation to lipid rafts or a defect in attachment to the actin cytoskeleton is unclear. In addition, cross-linked BCR fails to enter lipid raft fractions in EBV-infected human B cells because of expression of the latent membrane protein LMP2A (Dykstra et al., 2001). These cells exhibit greatly

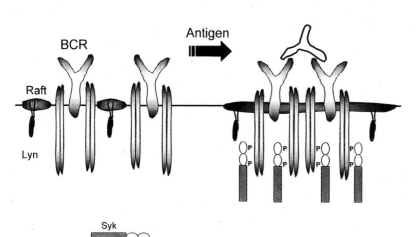

Figure 6.8. Proximal signaling events that occur in B cell lipid rafts upon antigen receptor ligation. Note that relative dimensions of BCR and lipid rafts are not to scale; however, antigen stimulation induces movement of the BCR into lipid rafts and congregation of the lipid rafts into larger structures.

diminished BCR signaling, although other mechanisms likely contribute to this functional effect. LMP2A causes degradation of Lyn and Syk via a E3 ubiquitin ligase mechanism. In contrast, CD19/CD21 coreceptors reduce the threshold for B cell activation, and this correlates with their ability to enhance the retention of the BCR in lipid rafts, thus retarding its internalization and degradation (Cherukuri et al., 2001a, b).

Lipid rafts may also form a link between the antigen receptors and the actin cytoskeleton. Cross-linking induces association of TCRζ to the cytoskeleton and this association is dependent on lipid raft integrity (Xavier et al., 1998). Actin-rich rings were found to organize around the contact area upon TCR ligation with coverslips coated with anti-TCR antibodies. Sustained contact required the presence of the lipid raft localized adaptor LAT (Bunnell et al., 2001). TCR-dependent actin remodeling is impaired by the inhibition of the binding between the Ena/VASP family of proteins and the fyb/SLAP adaptor protein. This result suggests that these proteins provide a crucial link between TCR signaling and the actin cytoskeleton (Krause et al., 2000). The motor forces that drive actin cytoskeletal rearrangement and lipid raft aggregation still remain largely unidentified.

Conclusions

Although T and B cells use distinct receptors to recognize completely different forms of antigens, the signal transduction machinery regulated by their antigen receptors functions remarkably similarly. This signaling machinery includes lymphocyte-specific components that interact with signaling components more ubiquitously expressed and used in a wide variety of systems. Lymphocyte function may be impaired by interruption of any of the critical components in these signaling cascades. However, discrete immune deficiency states are likely to affect the critical known and unknown components that are lymphoid-specific.

References

Adachi T, Wakabayashi C, Nakayama T, Yakura H, Tsubata T. CD72 negatively regulates signaling through the antigen receptor of B cells. J Immunol 164:1223–1229, 2000.

Adams JM, Houston H, Allen J, Lints T, and Harvey R. The hematopoietically expressed vav proto-oncogene shares homology with the *dbl* GDP-GTP exchange factor, the bcr gene and a yeast gene (CDC24) involved in cytoskeletal organization. Oncogene 7:611–618, 1992.

Alberola-lla J, Forbush KA, Seger R, Krebs EG, Perlmutter RM. Selective requirement for MAP kinase activation in thymocyte differentiation. Nature 373:620–623, 1995.

Aman MJ, Lamkin TD, Okada H, Kurosaki T, and Ravichandran KS. The inositol phosphatase SHIP inhibits Akt/PKB activation in B cells. J Biol Chem 273:33922–33928, 1998.

Aman MJ, Tosello-Trampont AC, Ravichandran K. Fc gamma RIIB1/SHIP-mediated inhibitory signaling in B cells involves lipid rafts. J Biol Chem 276:46371–46378, 2001.

Appleby MW, Gross JA, Cooke MP, Levin SD, Qian X, Perlmutter RM. Defective T cell receptor signaling in mice lacking the thymic isoform of p59^fyn. Cell 70:751–763, 1992.

Ardouin L, Boyer C, Gillet A, Trucy J, Bernard AM, Nunes J, Delon J, Trautmann A, He HT, Malissen B, Malissen M. Crippling of CD3-zeta ITAMs does not impair T cell receptor signaling. Immunity 10:409–420, 1999.

Aronheim A, Engelberg D, Li N, Al-Alawi N, Schlessinger J, Karin M. Membrane targeting of the nucleotide exchange factor Sos is sufficient for activating the Ras signaling pathway. Cell 78:949–961, 1994.

Arpaia E, Shahar M, Dadi H, Cohen A, Roifman CM. Defective T cell receptor signaling and CD8+ thymic selection in humans lacking ZAP-70 kinase. Cell 76:947–958, 1994.

Awasthi-Kalia M, Schnetkamp PP, Deans JP. Differential effects of filipin and methyl-β-cyclodextrin on B cell receptor signaling. Biochem Biophys Res Commun 287:77–82, 2001.

Banda NK, Bernier J, Kurahara DK, Kurrle R, Haigwood N, Sekaly R-P, Finkel TH. Crosslinking CD4 by human immunodeficiency virus gp120 primes T cells for activation-induced apoptosis. J Exp Med 176:1099–1106, 1992.

Bar-Sagi D, Hall A. Ras and Rho GTPases: a family reunion. Cell 103:227–238, 2000.

Batista FD, Iber D, Neuberger MS. B cells acquire antigen from target cells after synapse formation. Nature 411:489–494, 2001.

Beyers AD, Spruyt LL, Williams AF. Molecular associations between the T-lymphocyte antigen receptor complex and the surface antigens CD2, CD4, or CD8 and CD5. Proc Natl Acad Sci USA 89:2945–2949, 1992.

Blumberg R, Ley S, Sancho J, Lonberg N, Lacy E, McDermott F, Schad V, Greenstein J, Terhorst C. Structure of the T-cell antigen receptor: evidence for two CD3 ε subunits in the T-cell receptor–CD3 complex. Proc Natl Acad Sci USA 87:7220–7224, 1990.

Bootman MD, Berridge MJ. The elemental principles of calcium signaling. Cell 83:675–678, 1995.

Brauweiler AM, Tamir I, Cambier JC. Bilevel control of B-cell activation by the inositol 5-phosphatase SHIP. Immunol Rev 176:69–74, 2000.

Bromley SK, Burack WR, Johnson KG, Somersalo K, Sims TN, Sumen C, Davis MM, Shaw AS, Allen PM, Dustin ML. The immunological synapse. Annu Rev Immunol 19:375–396, 2001.

Brown DA, London E. Functions of lipid rafts in biological membranes. Annu Rev Cell Dev Biol 14:111–136, 1998.

Bu J-Y, Shaw AS, Chan AC. Analysis of the interaction of ZAP-70 and syk protein–tyrosine kinases with the T-cell antigen receptor by plasmon resonance. Proc Natl Acad Sci USA 92:5106–5110, 1995.

Bunnell SC, Kapoor V, Trible RP, Zhang W, Samelson LE. Dynamic actin polymerization drives T cell receptor–induced spreading: a role for the signal transduction adaptor LAT. Immunity 14:315–329, 2001.

Bustelo XR, Barbacid M. Tyrosine phosphorylation of the vav proto-oncogene product in activated B cells. Science 256:1196–1199, 1992.

Bustelo XR, Suen K,-L, Leftheris K, Meyers CA, Baracid M. Vav cooperates with Ras to transform rodent fibroblasts but is not a Ras GDP-GTP exchange factor. Oncogene 9:2405–2413, 1994.

Byth KF, Conroy LA, Howlett S, Smith AJH, May J, Alexander DR, Holmes N. CD45-null transgenic mice reveal a positive regulatory role for CD45 in early thymocyte development, in the selection of CD4+CD8+ thymocytes, and in B cell maturation. J Exp Med 183:1707–1718, 1996.

Cantrell D. T cell antigen receptor signal transduction pathways. Annu Rev Immunol 14:259–274, 1996.

Carter RH, Park DJ, Rhee SG, Fearon DT. Tyrosine phosphorylation of phospholipase C induced by membrane immunoglobulin in B lymphocytes. Proc Natl Acad Sci USA 88:2745–2749, 1991.

Chacko GW, Tridandapani S, Damen JE, Liu L, Krystal G, Coggeshall KM. Negative signaling in B lymphocytes induces tyrosine phosphorylation of the 145-kDa inositol polyphosphate 5-phosphatase, SHIP. J Immunol 157:2234–2238, 1996.

Chalupny NJ, Aruffo A, Esselstyn JM, Chan PY, Bajorath J, Blake J, Gilliland LK, Ledbetter JA, Tepper MA. Specific binding of Fyn and phosphatidylinositol 3-kinase to the B cell surface glycoprotein CD19 through their src homology 2 domains. Eur J Immunol 25:2978–2984, 1995.

Chan AC, Dalton M, Johnson R, Kong G-H, Wang T, Thoma R, Kurosaki T. Activation of ZAP-70 kinase activity by phosphorylation of tyrosine 493 is required for lymphocyte antigen receptor function. EMBO J 14:2499–2508, 1995a.

Chan AC, Desai DM, Weiss A. The role of protein tyrosine kinases and protein tyrosine phosphatases in T cell antigen receptor signal transduction. Annu Rev Immunol 12:555–592, 1994a.

Chan AC, Iwashima M, Turck CW, Weiss A. ZAP-70: a 70 kD protein tyrosine kinase that associates with the TCR ζ chain. Cell 71:649–662, 1992.

Chan AC, Kadlecek TA, Elder ME, Filipovich AH, Kuo W-L, Iwashima M, Parslow TG, Weiss A. ZAP-70 deficiency in an autosomal recessive form of severe combined immunodeficiency. Science 264:1599–1601, 1994b.

Chan VW, Lowell CA, DeFranco AL. Defective negative regulation of antigen receptor signaling in Lyn-deficient B lymphocytes. Curr Biol 8:545–553, 1998.

Chan VW, Meng F, Soriano P, DeFranco AL, Lowell CA. Characterization of the B lymphocyte populations in Lyn-deficient mice and the role of Lyn in signal initiation and down-regulation. Immunity 7:69–81, 1997.

Cheng AM, Rowley B, Pao W, Hayday A, Bolen JB, Pawson T. Syk tyrosine kinase required for mouse viability and B-cell development. Nature 378:303–306, 1995.

Cheng PC, Dykstra ML, Mitchell RN, Pierce SK. A role for lipid rafts in B cell antigen receptor signaling and antigen targeting. J Exp Med 190:1549–1560, 1999.

Cherukuri A, Cheng PC, Pierce SK. The role of the CD19/CD21 complex in B cell processing and presentation of complement-tagged antigens. J Immunol 167:163–172, 2001a.

Cherukuri A, Dykstra M, Pierce SK. Floating the raft hypothesis: lipid rafts play a role in immune cell activation. Immunity 14:657–660, 2001b.

Chow LML, Fournel M, Davidson D, Veillette A. Negative regulation of T-cell receptor signalling by tyrosine protein kinase p50^{csk}. Nature 365: 156–160, 1993.

Chow LML, Veillette A. The Src and Csk families of tyrosine protein kinases in hemopoietic cells. Semin. Immunol 7:207–226, 1995.

Chu DH, Spits H, Peyron J,-F, Rowley RB, Bolen JB, Weiss A. The Syk protein tyrosine kinase can function independently of CD45 and Lck in T cell antigen receptor signaling. EMBO J 15:6251–6261, 1996.

Chung JB, Baumeister MA, Monroe JG. Differential sequestration of plasma membrane-associated B cell antigen receptor in mature and immature B cells into glycosphingolipid-enriched domains. J Immunol 166:736–740, 2001.

Clark MR, Campbell KS, Kazlauskas A, Johnson SA, Hertz M, Potter TA, Pleiman C, Cambier JC. The B cell antigen receptor complex association of IG-α and Ig-β with distinct cytoplasmic effectors. Science 258:123–126, 1992.

Clements JL, Yang B, Ross-Barta SE, Eliason SL, Hrstka RF, Williamson RA, Koretzky GA. Requirement for the leukocyte-specific adapter protein SLP-76 for normal T cell development. Science 281:416–419, 1998.

Cloutier JF, Veillette A. Cooperative inhibition of T-cell antigen receptor signaling by a complex between a kinase and a phosphatase. J Exp Med 189: 111–121, 1999.

Conley ME, Parolini O, Rohrer J, Campana D. X-linked agammaglobulinemia: new approaches to old questions based on the identification of the defective gene. Immunol Rev 138:5–21. 1994.

Conley ME, Rohrer J, Rapalus L, Boylin EC, Minegishi Y. Defects in early B-cell development: comparing the consequences of abnormalities in pre-BCR signaling in the human and the mouse. Immunol Rev 178:75–90, 2000.

Cooper JA, Howell B. The when and how of Src regulation. Cell 73:1051–1054, 1993.

Cornall RJ, Goodnow CC, Cyster JG. Regulation of B cell antigen receptor signaling by the Lyn/CD22/SHP1 pathway. Curr Top Microbiol Immunol 244:57–68, 1999.

Couture C, Baier G, Oetken C, Williams S, Telford D, Marie-Cardine A, Baier-Bitterlich G, Fischer S, Burn P, Altman A, Mustelin T. Activation of p56^{lck} by p72^{syk} through physical association and N-terminal tyrosine phosphorylation. Mol Cell Biol 14:5249–5258, 1994.

Crompton T, Gilmour KC, Owen MJ. The MAP kinase pathway controls differentiation form double-negative to double-positive thymocyte. Cell 86:231–251, 1996.

Crowley MT, Harmer SL, DeFranco AL. Activation-induced association of a 145-kDa tyrosine phosphoprotein with Shc and Syk in B lymphocytes and macrophages. J Biol Chem 271:1145–1152, 1996.

D'Ambrosio D, Hippen KL, Minskoff SA, Mellman I, Pani G, Siminovitch KA, Cambier JC. Recruitment and activation of PTP1C in negative regulation of antigen receptor signaling by FcγR11B1. Science 268:293–297, 1995.

Davidson D, Veillette A. PTP-PEST, a scaffold protein tyrosine phosphatase, negatively regulates lymphocyte activation by targeting a unique set of substrates. EMBO J 20:3414–3426, 2001.

DeBell KE, Stoica BA, Veri MC, Di Baldassarre A, Miscia S, Graham LJ, Rellahan BL, Ishiai M, Kurosaki T, Bonvini E. Functional independence and interdependence of the Src homology domains of phospholipase C-gamma1 in B-cell receptor signal transduction. Mol Cell Biol 19:7388–7398, 1999.

DeFranco AL. Vav and the B cell signalosome. Nat Immunol 2:482–484. 2001.

Dempsey PW, Allison MED, Akkaraju S, Goodnow CC, Fearon DT. C3d of complement as a molecular adjuvant: bridging innate and acquired immunity. Science 271:348–350, 1996.

Desai DM, Sap J, Schlessinger J, Weiss A. Ligand-mediated negative regulation of a chimeric transmembrane receptor tyrosine phosphatase. Cell 73:541–554, 1993.

Desai DM, Sap J, Silvennoinen O, Schlessinger J, Weiss A. The catalytic activity of the CD45 membrane proximal phosphatase domain is required for TCR signaling and regulation. EMBO J 13:4002–4010, 1994.

Donnadieu E, Jouvin MH, Kinet JP. A second amplifier function for the allergy-associated FcεRI-β subunit. Immunity 12:515–523, 2000.

Donovan JA, Wange RL, Langdon WY, Samelson LE. The protein product of the c-cbl protooncogene is the 120-kDa tyrosine-phosphorylated protein in Jurkat cells activated via the T cell antigen receptor. J Biol Chem 269:22921–22924, 1994.

Doody GM, Bell SE, Vigorito E, Clayton E, McAdam S, Tooze R, Fernandez C, Lee IJ, Turner M. Signal transduction through Vav-2 participates in humoral immune responses and B cell maturation. Nat Immunol 2:542–547, 2001.

Dower NA, Stang SL, Bottorff DA, Ebinu JO, Dickie P, Ostergaard HL, Stone JC. RasGRP is essential for mouse thymocyte differentiation and TCR signaling. Nat Immunol 1:317–321, 2000.

Downward J, Graves J, Cantrell D. The regulation and function of p21ras in T cells. Immunol Today 13:89–92, 1992.

Downward J, Graves JD, Warne PH, Rayter S, Cantrell DA. Stimulation of p21^{ras} upon T-cell activation. Nature 346:719–723, 1990.

Du Z, Lang SM, Sasseville VG, Lackner AA, Ilyinskii PO, Daniel MD, Jung JU, Resrosiers RC. Identification of a nef allele that causes lymphocyte activations and acute disease in macaque monkeys. Cell 82:665–674, 1995.

Dykstra ML, Longnecker R, Pierce SK. Epstein-Barr virus coopts lipid rafts to block the signaling and antigen transport functions of the BCR. Immunity 14:57–67, 2001.

Eberl G, Lowin-Kropf B, MacDonald HR. NKT cell development is selectively impaired in Fyn-deficient mice. J Immunol 163:4091–4094, 1999.

Ebert PJ, Baker JF, Punt JA. Immature CD4$^+$CD8$^+$ thymocytes do not polarize lipid rafts in response to TCR-mediated signals. J Immunol 165: 5435–5442, 2000.

Ebinu JO, Stang SL, Teixeira C, Bottorff DA, Hooton J, Blumberg PM, Barry M, Bleakley RC, Ostergaard HL, Stone JC. RasGRP links T-cell receptor signaling to Ras. Blood 95:3199–3203, 2000.

Elder ME, Lin D, Clever J, Cahn AC, Hope TJ, Weiss A, Parslow TG. Human severe combined immunodeficiency due to a defect in ZAP-70, a T-cell tyrosine kinase. Science 264:1596–1599, 1994.

Engels N, Merchant M, Pappu R, Chan AC, Longnecker R, Wienands J. Epstein-Barr virus latent membrane protein 2A (LMP2A) employs the SLP-65 signaling module. J Exp Med 194:255–264, 2001a.

Engels N, Wollscheid B, Wienands J. Association of SLP-65/BLNK with the B cell antigen receptor through a non-ITAM tyrosine of Ig-α. Eur J Immunol 31:2126–2134, 2001b.

Fearon DT, Carroll MC. Regulation of B lymphocyte responses to foreign and self-antigens by the CD19/CD21 complex. Annu Rev Immunol 18: 393–422, 2000.

Fearon DT, Carter RH. The CD19/CR2/TAPA-1 complex of B lymphocytes: linking natural to acquired immunity. Annu Rev Immunol 13:127–149, 1995.

Fehling HJ, Krotkova A, Saint-Ruf C, von Boehmer H. Crucial role of the pre-T-cell receptor α gene in development of αβ but not γδT cells. Nature 375:795–798, 1995.

Finco TS, Kadlecek T, Zhang W, Samelson LE, Weiss A. LAT is required for TCR-mediated activation of PLCγ1 and the Ras pathway. Immunity 9: 617–626, 1998.

Fischer KD, Kong YY, Nishina H, Tedford K, Marengere LE, Kozieradzki I, Sasaki T, Starr M, Chan G, Gardener S, Nghiem MP, Bouchard D, Barbacid M, Bernstein A, Penninger JM. Vav is a regulator of cytoskeletal reorganization mediated by the T-cell receptor. Curr Biol 8:554–562, 1998.

Fischer K-D, Zmuldzinas A, Gardner S, Barbacid M, Bernstein A, Guidos C. Defective T-cell receptor signalling and positive selection of Vav-deficient CD4$^+$CD8$^+$ thymocytes. Nature 374:474–477, 1994.

Flanagan WM, Corthesy B, Bram, RJ, Crabtree GR. Nuclear association of a T-cell transcription factor blocked by FK-506 and cyclosporin A. Nature 352:803–807, 1991.

Fournel M, Davidson D, Weil R, Veillette A. Association of tyrosine protein kinase ZAP-70 with the protooncogene product p120^{cbl} in T lymphocytes. J Exp Med 183:301–306, 1996.

Frank S, Niklinska B, Orloff D, Mercep M, Ashwell J, Klausner R. Structural mutations of the T cell receptor zeta chain and its role in T cell activation. Science 249:174–177, 1990.

Fruman DA, Snapper SB, Yballe CM, Alt FW, Cantley LC. Phosphoinositide 3-kinase knockout mice: role of p85α in B cell development and proliferation. Biochem Soc Trans 27:624–629, 1999.

Fu C, Turck CW, Kurosaki T, Chan AC. BLNK: a central linker protein in B cell activation. Immunity 9:93–103, 1998.

Fütterer K, Wong J, Grucza RA, Chan AC, Waksman G. Structural basis for Syk tyrosine kinase ubiquity in signal transduction pathways revealed by the crystal structure of its regulatory SH2 domains bound to a dually phosphorylated ITAM peptide. J Mol Biol 281:523–537, 1998.

Gardner P. Calcium and T lymphocyte activation. Cell 59:15–20, 1989.

Gelfand EW, Weinberg K, Mazer BD, Kadlecek TA, Weiss A. Absence of ZAP-70 prevents signaling through the antigen receptor on peripheral blood T cells but not thymocytes. J Exp Med 182:1057–1066, 1995.

Genot EM, Parker PJ, Cantrell DA. Analysis of the role of protein kinase C-α, -ε, and -ζ in T cell activation. J Biol Chem 270:9833–9839, 1995.

Goitsuka, R, Fujmura Y, Mamada H, Umeda A, Morimura T, Uetsuka K, Doi K, Tsuji S, Kitamura D. BASH, a novel signaling molecule preferentially expressed in B cells of the bursa of Fabricius. J Immunol 161:5404–5408, 1998.

Gold MR, Chan VW-F, Turck CW, DeFranco AL. Membrane Ig cross-linking regulates phosphatidylinositol 3-kinases in B lymphocytes. J Immunol 148:2012–2022, 1992.

Gold MR, Crowley MT, Martin GA, McCormick F, DeFranco AL. Targets of B lymphocyte antigen receptor signal transduction include the p21ras GTPase-activating protein (GAP) and two GAP-associated proteins. J Immunol 150:377–386, 1993.

Goldsmith M, Weiss A. Early signal transduction by the antigen receptor without commitment to T cell activation. Science 240:1029–1031, 1988.

Gong Q, Cheng AM, Akk AM, Alberola-Ila J, Gong G, Pawson T, Chan AC. Disruption of T cell signaling networks and development by Grb2 haploid insufficiency. Nat Immunol 2:29–36, 2001a.

Gong Q, Jin X, Akk AM, Foger N, White M, Gong G, Wardenburg JB, Chan AC. Requirement for tyrosine residues 315 and 319 within ζ chain-associated protein 70 for T cell development. J Exp Med 194:507–518, 2001b.

Guo B, Kato RM, Garcia-Lloret M, Wahl MI, Rawlings DJ. Engagement of the human pre-B cell receptor generates a lipid raft-dependent calcium signaling complex. Immunity 13:243–253, 2000.

Gupta N, Scharenberg AM, Fruman DA, Cantley LC, Kinet JP, Long EO. The SH2 domain-containing inositol 5′-phosphatase (SHIP) recruits the p85 subunit of phosphoinositide 3-kinase during FcγRIIb1-mediated inhibition of B cell receptor signaling. J Biol Chem 274:7489–7494, 1999.

Gupta N, Scharenberg AM, Burshtyn DN, Wagtmann N, Lioubin MN, Rohrschneider LR, Kinet JP, Long EO. Negative signaling pathways of the killer cell inhibitory receptor and FcγRIIb1 require distinct phosphatases. J Exp Med 186:473–478, 1997.

Harder T, Simons K. Caveolae, DIGs, and the dynamics of sphingolipid-cholesterol microdomains. Curr Opin Cell Biol 9:534–542, 1997.

Hashimoto A, Hirose K, Okada H, Kurosaki T, Iino M. Inhibitory modulation of B cell receptor-mediated Ca²⁺ mobilization by Src homology 2 domain-containing inositol 5′-phosphatase (SHIP). J Biol Chem, 274:11203–11208, 1999.

Hashimoto A, Takeda K, Inaba M, Sekimata M, Kaisho T, Ikehara S, Homma Y, Akira S, Kurosaki T. Essential role of phospholipase C-γ2 in B cell development and function. J Immunol 165:1738–1742, 2000.

Hata A, Sabe H, Kurosaki T, Takata M, Hanafusa H. Functional analysis of Csk in signal transduction through the B-cell antigen receptor. Mol Cell Biol 14:7306–7313, 1994.

Hatada MH, Lu X, Laird ER, Green J, Morgenstern JP, Lou M, Marr CS, Phillips TB, Ram MK, Theriault K, Zoller MJ, Karas JL. Molecular basis for interaction of the protein tyrosine kinase ZAP-70 with the T-cell receptor. Nature 377:32–38, 1995.

Hayashi K, Nittono R, Okamoto N, Tsuji S, Hara Y, Goitsuka R, Kitamura D. The B cell–restricted adaptor BASH is required for normal development and antigen receptor–mediated activation of B cells. Proc Natl Acad Sci USA 97:2755–2760, 2000.

Hoessli DC, Ilangumaran S, Soltermann A, Robinson PJ, Borisch B, Nasir-Ud-Din. Signaling through sphingolipid microdomains of the plasma membrane: the concept of signaling platform. Glycoconj J 17:191–197, 2000.

Holsinger LJ, Graef IA, Swat W, Chi T, Bautista DM, Davidson L, Lewis RS, Alt FW, Crabtree GR. Defects in actin-cap formation in Vav-deficient mice implicate an actin requirement for lymphocyte signal transduction. Curr Biol 8:563–572, 1998.

Hurley TR, Hyman R, Sefton BM. Differential effects of expression of the CD45 tyrosine protein phosphatase on the tyrosine phosphorylation of the lck, fyn, and c-src tyrosine protein kinases. Mol Cell Biol 13:1651–1656, 1993.

Imamoto A, Soriano P. Disruption of the csk gene, encoding a negative regulator of Src family tyrosine kinases, leads to neural tube defects and embryonic lethality in mice. Cell 73:1117–1124, 1993.

Irving B, Weiss A. The cytoplasmic domain of the T cell receptor ζ chain is sufficient to couple to receptor-associated signal transduction pathways. Cell 64:891–901, 1991.

Irving BA, Chan AC, Weiss A. Functional characterization of a signal transducing motif present in the T cell receptor ζ chain. J Exp Med 177:1093–1103, 1993.

Ishiai M, Kurosaki M, Inabe K, Chan AC, Sugamura K, Kurosaki T. Involvement of LAT, Gads, and Grb2 in compartmentation of SLP-76 to the plasma membrane. J Exp Med 192:847–856, 2000.

Itano A, Salmon P, Kioussis D, Tolaini M, Corbella P, Robey E. The cytoplasmic domain of CD4 promotes the development of CD4 lineage T cells. J Exp Med 183:731, 1996.

Iwashima M, Irving BA, van Oers NSC, Chan AC, Weiss A. Sequential interactions of the TCR with two distinct cytoplasmic tyrosine kinases. Science 263:1136–1139, 1994.

Izquierdo M, Downward J, Graves JD, Cantrell DA. Role of protein kinase C in T-cell antigen receptor regulation of p21ras: evidence that two p21ras regulatory pathways coexist in T cells. Mol Cell Biol 12:3305–3312, 1992.

Jackman JK, Motto DG, Sun Q, Tanemoto M, Turck CW, Peltz GA, Koretzky GA, Findell PR. Molecular cloning of SLP-76, a 76-kDa tyrosine phosphoprotein associated with Grb2 in T cells. J Biol Chem 270:7029–7032, 1995.

Jain J, McCaffrey PG, Miner Z, Kerppola TK, Lambert JN, Verdine GL, Curran T, Rao A. The T-cell transcription factor NFATp is a substrate for calcineurin and interacts with Fos and Jun. Nature 365:352–355, 1993.

Janeway CA, Jr. The T cell receptor as a multicomponent signalling machine: CD4/CD8 coreceptors and CD45 in T cell activation. Annu Rev Immunol 10:645–674, 1992.

Jayaraman T, Ondrias K, Ondriasova E, Marks AR. Regulation of the inositol 1, 4, 5-triphosphate receptor by tyrosine phosphorylation. Science 272:1492–1494, 1996.

Johnson KG, Bromley SK, Dustin ML, Thomas ML. A supramolecular basis for CD45 tyrosine phosphatase regulation in sustained T cell activation. Proc Natl Acad Sci USA 97:10138–10143, 2000.

Johnson P, Ostergaard HL, Wasden C, Trowbridge IS. Mutational analysis of CD45: a leukocyte-specific protein tyrosine phosphatase. J Biol Chem 12:8035–8041, 1992.

Kane LP, Andres PG, Howland KC, Abbas AK, Weiss A. Akt provides the CD28 costimulatory signal for up-regulation of IL-2 and IFN-γ but not TH2 cytokines. Nat Immunol 2:37–44, 2001.

Kappes DJ, Tonegawa S. Suface expression of alternative forms of the TCR/CD3 complex. Proc Natl Acad Sci USA 88:10619–10623, 1991.

Katzav S, Cleveland JL, Heslop HE, Pulido D. Loss of the amino-terminal helix-loop-helix domain of the vav proto-oncogene activates its transforming potential. Mol Cell Biol 11:1912–1920, 1991.

Katzav S, Sutherland M, Packham G, Yi T, Weiss A. The protein tyrosine kinase ZAP-70 can associate with the SH2 domain of proto-Vav. J Biol Chem 269:32579–32585, 1994.

Killeen N, Littman DR. Helper T-cell development in the absence of CD4-p56lck association. Nature 364:729–732, 1993.

Kishihara K, Penninger J, Wallace VA, Kundig TM, Kawai K, Wakeham A, Timms E, Pfeffer K, Ohashi PS, Thomas ML, Furlonger C, Paige CJ, Mak TW. Normal B lymphocyte development but impaired T cell maturation in CD45-Exon6 protein tyrosine phosphatase-deficient mice. Cell 74:143–156, 1993.

Kitamura D, Kaneko H, Taniuchi I, Akagi K, Yamamura K, Watanabe T. Molecular cloning and characterization of mouse HS1. Biochem Biophys Res Commun 208:1137–1146, 1995.

Klausner RD, Lippincott-Schwartz J, Bonifacino JS. The T cell antigen receptor: insights into organelle biology. Annu Rev Cell Biol 6:403–431, 1990.

Kolanus W, Romeo C, Seed B. T cell activation by clustered tyrosine kinases. Cell 74:171–183, 1993.

Kong G, Dalton M, Wardenburg JB, Straus D, Kurosaki T, Chan AC. Distinct tyrosine phosphorylation sites in ZAP-70 mediate activation and negative regulation of antigen receptor function. Mol Cell Biol 16:5026–5035, 1996.

Kong G-H, Bu J-Y, Kurosaki T, Shaw AS, Chan AC. Reconstitution of Syk function by the ZAP-70 protein tyrosine kinase. Immunity 2:485–492, 1995.

Kraus M, Pao LI, Reichlin A, Hu Y, Canono B, Cambier JC, Nussenzweig MC, Rajewsky K. Interference with immunoglobulin (Ig) alpha immunoreceptor tyrosine-based activation motif (ITAM) phosphorylation modulates or blocks B cell development, depending on the availability of an Igbeta cytoplasmic tail. J Exp Med 194:455–469, 2001.

Krause M, Sechi AS, Konradt M, Monner D, Gertler FB, Wehland J. Fyn-binding protein (Fyb)/SLP-76-associated protein (SLAP), Ena/vasodilator-stimulated phosphoprotein (VASP) proteins and the Arp2/3 complex link T cell receptor (TCR) signaling to the actin cytoskeleton. J Cell Biol 149:181–194, 2000.

Kubagawa H, Cooper MD, Chen CC, Ho LH, Alley TL, Hurez V, Tun T, Uehara T, Shimada T, Burrows PD. Paired immunoglobulin-like receptors of activating and inhibitory types. Curr Top Microbiol Immunol 244:137–149, 1999.

Kuhne MR, Ku G, Weiss A. A guanine nucleotide exchange factor-independent function of Vav1 in transcriptional activation. J Biol Chem 275:2185–2190, 2000.

Kumanogoh A, Kikutani H. The CD100-CD72 interaction: a novel mechanism of immune regulation. Trends Immunol 22:670–676, 2001.

Kurosaki T, Johnson SA, Pao L, Sada K, Yamamura H, Cambier JC. Role of the Syk autophosphorylation site and SH2 domains in B cell antigen receptor signaling. J Exp Med 182:1815–1823, 1995.

Kurosaki T, Maeda A, Ishiai M, Hashimoto A, Inabe K, Takata M. Regulation of the phospholipase C-γ2 pathway in B cells. Immunol Rev 176:19–29, 2000.

Lagunoff M, Majeti R, Weiss A, Ganem D. Deregulated signal transduction by the K1 gene product of Kaposi's sarcoma–associated herpesvirus. Proc Natl Acad Sci USA 96:5704–5709, 1999.

Lanier LL. Face off—the interplay between activating and inhibitory immune receptors. Curr Opin Immunol 13:326–331, 2001.

Law CL, Chandran KA, Sidorenko SP, Clark EA. Phospholipase C-γ 1 interacts with conserved phosphotyrosyl residues in the linker region of Syk and is a substrate for Syk. Mol Cell Biol 16:1305–1315, 1996.

Law DA, Chan VW-F, Datta SK, DeFranco AL. B cell antigen receptor motifs have redundant signalling capabilities and bind the tyrosine kinases PTK72, Lyn and Fyn. Curr Biol 3:645–657, 1993.

Ledbetter JA, Gilliland LK, Schieven GA. The interaction of CD4 with CD3/Ti regulates tyrosine phosphorylation of substrates during T cell activation. Semin. Immunol 2:99–106, 1990.

Leitenberg D, Novak TJ, Farber D, Smith BR, Bottomly K. The extracellular domain of CD45 controls association with the CD4-T cell receptor complex and the response to antigen-specific stimulation. J Exp Med 183:249–259, 1996.

Leitges M, Schmedt C, Guinamard R, Davoust J, Schaal S, Stabel S, Tarakhovsky A. Immunodeficiency in protein kinase cβ-deficient mice. Science 273:788–791, 1996.

Lewis RS, Cahalan MD. Mitogen-induced oscillations of cytosolic Ca^{2+} and membrane Ca^{2+} current in human leukemic T cells. Cell Regul 1:99–112, 1989.

Lin J, Weiss A, Finco TS. Localization of LAT in glycolipid-enriched microdomains is required for T cell activation. J Biol Chem 274:28861–28864, 1999.

Lin S, Cicala C, Scharenberg AM, Kinet JP. The FcεRIβ subunit functions as an amplifier of FcεRIγ-mediated cell activation signals. Cell 85:985–995, 1996.

Lindvall JM, Blomberg KEM, Väliaho J, Vargas L, Heinonen JE, Berglöf A, Mohamed AJ, Nore BF, Vihinen M, Smith CIE. Bruton's tyrosine kinase: cell biology, sequence conservation, mutation spectrum, siRNA modifications and expression profiling. Immunol Rev 203:200–215, 2005.

Love PE, Shores EW. ITAM multiplicity and thymocyte selection: how low can you go? Immunity 12:591–597, 2000.

Macian F, Lopez-Rodriguez C, Rao A. Partners in transcription: NFAT and AP-1. Oncogene 20:2476–2489, 2001.

Maeda A, Kurosaki M, Kurosaki T. Paired immunoglobulin-like receptor (PIR)-A is involved in activating mast cells through its association with Fc receptor γ chain. J Exp Med 188:991–995, 1998.

Maeda A, Scharenberg AM, Tsukada S, Bolen JB, Kinet JP, Kurosaki T. Paired immunoglobulin-like receptor B (PIR-B) inhibits BCR-induced activation of Syk and Btk by SHP-1. Oncogene 18:2291–2297, 1999.

Maehama T, Dixon JE. PTEN: a tumour suppressor that functions as a phospholipid phosphatase. Trends Cell Biol 9:125–128, 1999.

Magnan A, Di Bartolo V, Mura AM, Boyer C, Richelme M, Lin YL, Roure A, Gillet A, Arrieumerlou C, Acuto O, Malissen B, Malissen M. T cell development and T cell responses in mice with mutations affecting tyrosines 292 or 315 of the ZAP-70 protein tyrosine kinase. J Exp Med 194:491–505, 2001.

Majerus PW, Ross TS, Cunningham TW, Caldwell KK, Jefferson AB, Bansal VS. Recent insights in phosphatidylinositol signaling. Cell 63:459–465, 1990.

Majeti R, Bilwes AM, Noel JP, Hunter T, Weiss A. Dimerization-induced inhibition of receptor protein tyrosine phosphatase function through an inhibitory wedge. Science 279:88–91, 1998.

Majeti R, Xu Z, Parslow TG, Olson JL, Daikh DI, Killeen N, Weiss A. An inactivating point mutation in the inhibitory wedge of CD45 causes lymphoproliferation and autoimmunity. Cell 103:1059–1070, 2000.

Mallick-Wood CA, Pao W, Cheng AM, Lewis JM, Kulkarni S, Bolen JB, Rowley B, Tigelaar RE, Pawson T, Hayday AC. Disruption of epithelial γδ T cell repertoires by mutation of the Syk tyrosine kinase. Proc Natl Acad Sci USA 93:9704–9709, 1996.

Marengere LEM, Waterhouse P, Duncan GS, Mittrucker H-W, Feng G-S, Mak T,W. Regulation of T cell receptor signaling by tyrosine phosphotase SYP association with CTLA-4. Science 272:1170–1173, 1996.

Margolis B, Hu P, Katzav S, Li W, Oliver JM, Ullrich A, Weiss A, Schlessinger J. Tyrosine phosphorylation of *vav* proto-oncogene product containing SH2 domain and transcription fctor motifs. Nature 356:71–74, 1992.

Marshall CJ. Raf gets it together. Nature 383:127–128, 1996.

McCormick F. How receptors turn Ras on. Nature 363:15–16, 1993.

McCormick F, Wittinghofer A. Interactions between Ras proteins and their effectors. Curr Opin Biotech 7:449–456, 1996.

McFarland EDC, Hurley TR, Pingel JT, Sefton BM, Shaw A, Thomas ML. Correlation between Src family member regulation by the protein-tyrosine-phosphatase CD45 and transmembrane signaling through the T-cell receptor. Proc Natl Acad Sci USA 90:1402–1406, 1993.

McKenney DW, Onodera H, Gorman L, Mimura T, Rothstein DM. Distinct isoforms of the CD45 protein-tyrosine phosphatase differentially regulate interleukin 2 secretion and activation signal pathways involving Vav in T cells. J Biol Chem 270:24949–24954, 1995.

McMahon SB, Monroe JG. Activation of the p21^{ras} pathway couples antigen receptors stimulation to induction of the primary response gene egr-1 in B lymphocytes. J Exp Med 181:417–422, 1995.

McMahon SB, Monroe JG. The role of early growth response gene 1 (egr-1) in regulation of the immune response. J Leukoc Biol 60:159–166, 1996.

Miller CL, Burkhardt AL, Lee JH, Stealey B, Longnecker R, Bolen JB, Kieff E. Integral membrane protein 2 of Epstein-Barr virus regulates reactivation from latency through dominant negative effects on protein-tyrosine kinases. Immunity 2:155–166, 1995.

Molina TJ, Kishihara K, Siderovski DP, van Ewijk W, Narendran A, Timms E, Wakeham A, Paige CJ, Hartmann K-U, Veillette A, Davidson D, Mak TW. Profound block in thymocyte development in mice lacking p56^{lck}. Nature 357:161–164, 1992.

Moodie SA, Willumsen BM, Weber MJ, Wolfman A. Complexes of Ras-GTP with Raf-1 and mitogen-activated protein kinase kinase. Science 260:1658–1661, 1993.

Motto DG, Ross EE, Wu J, Hendricks-Taylor LR, Koretzky GA. Implication of the GRB2-associated phosphoprotein SLP-76 in TCR-mediated IL-2 production. J Exp Med 183:1937–1943, 1996.

Muta T, Kuorsaki T, Misulovin Z, Sanchez M, Nussenzweig MC, Ravetch JV. A 13-amino-acid motif in the cytoplasmic domain of FcγR11B modulates B-cell receptor signalling. Nature 368:70-73, 1994.

Nada S, Yagi T, Takeda H, Tokunaga T, Nakagawa H, Ikawa Y, Okada M, Aizawa S. Constitutive activation of Src family kinases in mouse embryos that lack Csk. Cell 73:1125–1135, 1993.

Nagai K, Takata M, Yamamura H, Kurosaki T. Tyrosine phosphorylation of Shc is mediated through Lyn and Syk in B cell receptor signaling. J Biol Chem 270:6824–6829, 1995.

Negishi I, Motoyama N, Nakayama K-I, Nakayama K, Senju S, Hatakeyama S, Zhang Q, Chan AC, Loh DY. Essential role for ZAP-70 in both positive and negative selection of thymocytes. Nature 376:435–438, 1995.

Newell MK, Haughn LJ, Maroun CR, Julius MH. Death of mature T cells by separate ligation of CD4 and the T-cell receptor for antigen. Nature 347:286–289, 1990.

Nghlem P, Ollick T, Gardner P, Schulman H. Interleukin-2 transcriptional block by mukltifunctional Ca^{2+}/calmodulin kinase. Nature 371:347–350, 1994.

Nishibe S, Wahl MI, Hernandez-Sotomayor SM, Tonk NK, Rhee SG, Carpenter G. Increase of the catalytic activity of phospholipase C-γ1 by tyrosine phosphorylation. Science 250:1253–1256, 1990.

Nishizumi H, Taniuchi I, Yamanashi Y, Kitamura D, Ilic D, Mori S, Watanabe T, Yamamoto T. Impaired proliferation of peripheral B cells and indication of autoimmune disease in lyn-deficient mice. Immunity 3:549–560, 1995.

Nitschke L, Carsetti R, Ocker B, Kohler G, Lamers MC. CD22 is a negative regulator of B-cell receptor signaling. Curr Biol 7:133–143, 1997.

Nitschke L, Floyd H, Crocker PR. New functions for the sialic acid-binding adhesion molecule CD22, a member of the growing family of Siglecs. Scand J Immunol 53:227–234, 2001.

Novak TJ, Farber D, Leitenberg D, Hong SC, Johnson P, Bottomly K. Isoforms of the transmembrane tyrosine phosphatase CD45 differentially affect T cell recognition. Immunity 1:109–119, 1994.

Okada H, Bolland S, Hashimoto A, Kurosaki M, Kabuyama Y, Iino M, Ravetch JV, Kurosaki T. Role of the inositol phosphatase SHIP in B cell receptor–induced Ca^{2+} oscillatory response. J Immunol 161:5129–5132, 1998.

Okada T, Maeda A, Iwamatsu A, Gotoh K, Kurosaki T. BCAP: the tyrosine kinase substrate that connects B cell receptor to phosphoinositide 3-kinase activation. Immunity 13:817–827, 2000.

Ostergaard HL, Shackelford DA, Hurley TR, Johnson P, Hyman R, Sefton BM, Trowbridge IS. Expression of CD45 alters phosphorylation of the lck-encoded tyrosine protein kinase in murine lymphoma T-cell lines. Proc Natl Acad Sci USA 86:8959–8963, 1989.

Pan C, Baumgarth N, Parnes JR. CD72-deficient mice reveal nonredundant roles of CD72 in B cell development and activation. Immunity 11:495–506, 1999.

Pappu R, Cheng AM, Li B, Gong Q, Chiu C, Griffin N, White M, Sleckman BP, Chan AC. Requirement for B cell linker protein (BLNK) in B cell development. Science 286:1949–1954, 1999.

Parekh AB, Teriau H, Stuhmer W. Depletion of InsP3 stores activates a Ca2+ and K+ current by means of a phosphate and a diffusible messenger. Nature 364:814–818, 1993.

Park DJ, Rho HW, Rhee SG. CD3 stimulation causes phosphorylation of phospholipase C-γl on serine and tyrosine residues in a human T cell line. Proc Natl Acad Sci USA 88:5453–5456, 1991.

Parnes JR, Pan C. CD72, a negative regulator of B-cell responsiveness. Immunol Rev 176:75–85, 2000.

Pawson T. Protein modules and signalling networks. Nature 373:573–580, 1995.

Pawson T, Nash P. Protein-protein interactions define specificity in signal transduction. Genes Dev 14:1027–1047, 2000.

Pelosi M, Di Bartolo V, Mounier V, Mege D, Pascussi JM, Dufour E, Blondel A, Acuto O. Tyrosine 319 in the interdomain B of ZAP-70 is a binding site for the Src homology 2 domain of Lck. J Biol Chem 274:14229–14237, 1999.

Penninger JM, Irie-Sasaki J, Sasaki T, Oliveira-dos-Santos AJ. CD45: new jobs for an old acquaintance. Nat Immunol 2:389–396, 2001.

Perez-Aciego P, Alarcon B, Arnaiz-Villena A, Terhorst C, Timon M, Segurado OG, Regueiro JR. Expression and function of a variant T cell receptor complex lacking CD3-γ. J Exp Med 174:319–326, 1991.

Pileri P, Uematsu Y, Campagnoli S, Galli G, Falugi F, Petracca R, Weiner AJ, Houghton M, Rosa D, Grandi G, Abrignani S. Binding of hepatitis C virus to CD81. Science 282:938–941, 1998.

Poe JC, Fujimoto M, Jansen PJ, Miller AS, Tedder TF. CD22 forms a quaternary complex with SHIP, Grb2, and Shc. A pathway for regulation of B lymphocyte antigen receptor-induced calcium flux. J Biol Chem 275:17420–17427, 2000.

Poole A, Gibbins JM, Turner M, van Vugt MJ, van de Winkel JG, Saito T, Tybulewicz VL, Watson SP. The Fc receptor γ-chain and the tyrosine kinase Syk are essential for activation of mouse platelets by collagen. EMBO J 16:2333–2341, 1997.

Ratcliffe MJH, Coggeshall KM, Newell MK, Julius MH. T cell antigen receptor aggregation, but not dimerization, induces increased cytoplasmic calcium concentrations and reveals a lack of stable association between CD4 and the T cell receptor. J Immunol 148:1643–1651, 1992.

Ravichandran KS, Lee KK, Songyang A, Cantley LC, Burn P, Burakoff SJ. Interaction of Shc with the ζ chain of the T cell receptor upon T cell activation. Science 262:902–905, 1993.

Reichlin A, Hu Y, Meffre E, Nagaoka H, Gong S, Kraus M, Rajewsky K, Nussenzweig MC. B cell development is arrested at the immature B cell stage in mice carrying a mutation in the cytoplasmic domain of immunoglobulin β. J Exp Med 193:13–23, 2001.

Reth M. Antigen receptors on B lymphocytes. Annu Rev Immunol 10:97–121, 1992.

Richards JD, Dave SH, Chou CH, Mamchak AA, DeFranco AL. Inhibition of the MEK/ERK signaling pathway blocks a subset of B cell responses to antigen. J Immunol 166:3855–3864, 2001.

Richards JD, Gold MR, Hourihane SL, DeFranco AL, Matsuuchi L. Reconstitution of B cell antigen receptor–induced signaling events in a nonlymphoid cell line by expressing the Syk protein-tyrosine kinase. J Biol Chem 271:6458–6466, 1996.

Robey E, Fowlkes BJ. Selective events in T cell development. Annu Rev Immunol 12:675–705, 1994.

Rodriguez R, Matsuda M, Perisic O, Bravo J, Paul A, Jones NP, Light Y, Swann K, Williams RL, Katan M. Tyrosine residues in phospholipase Cγ2 essential for the enzyme function in B-cell signaling. J Biol Chem 276:47982–47992, 2001.

Romeo C, Seed B. Cellular immunity to HIV activated by CD4 fused to T cell or Fc receptor polypeptides. Cell 64:1037–1046, 1991.

Roth PE, DeFranco AL. Intrinsic checkpoints for lineage progression. Curr Biol 5:349–353, 1995.

Salomon B, Bluestone JA. Complexities of CD28/B7: CTLA-4 costimulatory pathways in autoimmunity and transplantation. Annu Rev Immunol 19:225–252, 2001.

Samelson LE, Phillips AF, Luong ET, Klausner RD. Association of the fyn protein-tyrosine kinase with the T-cell antigen receptor. Proc Natl Acad Sci USA 87:4358–4362, 1990.

Saouaf SJ, Mahajan S, Rowley RB, Kut SA, Fargnoli J, Burkhardt AL, Tsukada S, Witte ON, Bolen JB. Temporal differences in the activation of three classes of non-transmembrane protein tyrosine kinases following B-cell antigen receptor surface engagement. Proc Natl Acad Sci USA 91:9524–9528, 1994.

Sato S, Miller AS, Inaoki M, Bock CB, Jansen PJ, Tang ML, Tedder TF. CD22 is both a positive and negative regulator of B lymphocyte antigen receptor signal transduction: altered signaling in CD22-deficient mice. Immunity 5:551–562, 1996.

Sato S, Steeber DA, Jansen PJ, Tedder TF. CD19 expression levels regulate B lymphocyte development: human CD19 restores normal function in mice lacking endogenous CD19. J Immunol 158:4662–4669, 1997.

Saxton TM, van Oostveen I, Bowtell D, Aebersold R, Gold MR. B cell antigen receptor cross-linking induces phosphorylation of the p21ras oncoprotein activators SHC and mSOS1 as well as assembly of complexes containing SHC, GRB-2, mSOS1, and a 145-kDa tyrosine-phosphorylated protein. J Immunol 153:623–636, 1994.

Scharenberg AM, El-Hillal O, Fruman DA, Beitz LO, Li Z, Lin S, Gout I, Cantley LC, Rawlings DJ, Kinet JP. Phosphatidylinositol-3,4,5-trisphosphate (PtdIns-3,4,5-P3)/Tec kinase–dependent calcium signaling pathway: a target for SHIP-mediated inhibitory signals. EMBO J 17:1961–1972, 1998.

Schlessinger J. How receptor tyrosine kinases activate Ras. Trends Biochem Sci 18:273–275, 1993.

Schmedt C, Saijo K, Niidome T, Kuhn R, Aizawa S, Tarakhovsky A. Csk controls antigen receptor-mediated development and selection of T-lineage cells. Nature 394:901–904, 1998.

Schmedt C, Tarakhovsky A. Autonomous maturation of α/β T lineage cells in the absence of COOH-terminal Src kinase (Csk). J Exp Med 193:815–826, 2001.

Schreiber SL, Crabtree GR. The mechanism of action of cyclosporin A and FK506. Immunol Today 13:136–142, 1992.

Sefton BM, Taddie JA. Role of tyrosine kinases in lymphocyte activation. Curr Opin Immunol 6:372–379, 1994.

Shan X, Czar MJ, Bunnell SC, Liu P, Liu Y, Schwartzberg PL, Wange RL. Deficiency of PTEN in Jurkat T cells causes constitutive localization of Itk to the plasma membrane and hyperresponsiveness to CD3 stimulation. Mol Cell Biol 20:6945–6957, 2000.

Shiue L, Zoller MJ, Brugge JS. Syk is activated by phosphotyrosine-containing peptides representing the tyrosine-based activation motifs of the high affinity receptor for IgE. J Biol Chem 270:10498–10502, 1995.

Sicheri F, Kuriyan J. Structures of Src-family tyrosine kinases. Curr Opin Struct Biol 7:777–785, 1997.

Sieh M, Batzer A, Schlessinger J, Weiss A. GRB2 and phospholipase C-γl associate with a 36- to 38-kilodalton phosphotyrosine protein after T-cell receptor stimulation. Mol Cell Biol 14:4435–4442, 1994.

Siemasko K, Clark MR. The control and facilitation of MHC class II antigen processing by the BCR. Curr Opin Immunol 13:32–36, 2001.

Sillman AL, Monroe JG. Association of p72syk with the src homology-2 (SH2) domains of PLC γ 1 in B lymphocytes. J Biol Chem 270:11806–11811, 1995.

Smith CIE, Islam TC, Mattsson PT, Mohamed AJ, Nore BF, Vihinen M. The Tec family of cytoplasmic tyrosine kinases: mammalian Btk, Bmx, Itk, Tec, Txk and homologs in other species. Bioessays 23:436–446, 2001.

Smith KG, Fearon DT. Receptor modulators of B-cell receptor signalling—CD19/CD22. Curr Top Microbiol Immunol 245:195–212, 2000.

Songyang Z, Shoelson SE, Chaudhuri M, Gish G, Pawson T, Haser WG, King F, Roberts T, Ratnofsky S, Lechleider RJ, Neel BG, Birge RB, Fajardo JE, Chou MM, Hanafusa H, Schaffhausen B, Cantley LC. SH2 domains recognize specific phosphopeptide sequences. Cell 72:767–778, 1993.

Songyang Z, Shoelson SE, McGlade J, Olivier P, Pawson T, Bustelo XR, Barbacid M, Sabe H, Hanafusa H, Yi T, Ren R, Baltimore D, Ratnofsky S, Feldman RA, Cantley LC. Specific motifs recognized by the SH2 domains of Csk, 3BP2, fps/fes, GRB-2, HCP, SHC, Syk, and Vav. Mol Cell Biol 14:2777–2785, 1994.

Sproul TW, Malapati S, Kim J, Pierce SK. B cell antigen receptor signaling occurs outside lipid rafts in immature B cells. J Immunol 165:6020–6023, 2000.

Stein PL, Lee H-M, Rich S, Soriano P. pp59fyn mutant mice display differential signaling in thymocytes and peripheral T cells. Cell 70:741–750, 1992.

Straus DB, Chan AC, Patai B, Weiss A. SH2 domain function is essential for the role of the Lck tyrosine kinase in T cell receptor signal transduction. J Biol Chem 271:9976–9981, 1996.

Su B, Jacinto E, Hibi M, Kallunki T, Karin M, Ben-Neriah Y. JNK is involved in signal integration during costimulation in T lymphocytes. Cell 77:727–736, 1994.

Sun Z, Arendt CW, Ellmeier W, Schaeffer EM, Sunshine MJ, Gandhi L, Annes J, Petrzilka D, Kupfer A, Schwartzberg PL, Littman DR. PKC-θ is required for TCR-induced NF-κB activation in mature but not immature T lymphocytes. Nature 404:402–407, 2000.

Swat W, Shinkai Y, Cheng H-L, Davidson L, Alt FW. Activated Ras signals differentiation and expansion of CD4+8+ thymocytes. Proc Natl Acad Sci USA 93:4683–4687, 1996.

Takai T, Ono M. Activating and inhibitory nature of the murine paired immunoglobulin-like receptor family. Immunol Rev 181:215–222. 2001.

Takai T, Ono M, Hikida M, Ohmori H, Ravetch JV. Augmented humoral and anaphylactic responses in FcγRII-deficient mice. Nature 379:346–349, 1996.

Takata M, Homma Y, Kurosaki T. Requirement of phospholipase C-γ2 activation in surface immunoglobulin M-induced B cell apoptosis. J Exp Med 182:907–914, 1995.

Takata M, Sabe H, Hata A, Inazu T, Homma Y, Nukada T, Yamamura H, Kurosaki T. Tyrosine kinases Lyn and Syk regulate B cell receptor–coupled Ca2+ mobilization through distinct pathways. EMBO J 13:1341–1349, 1994.

Tamir I, Stolpa JC, Helgason CD, Nakamura K, Bruhns P, Daeron M, Cambier JC. The RasGAP-binding protein p62dok is a mediator of inhibitory FcγRIIB signals in B cells. Immunity 12:347–358, 2000.

Tanaka Y, Arbouin L, Gillet A, Lin S-Y, Magnan A, Malissen B, Malissen M. Early T-cell development in CD3-deficient mice. Immunol Rev 148:172–199, 1995.

Taniuchi I, Kitamura D, Maekawa Y, Fukuda T, Kishi H, Watanabe T. Antigen-receptor induced clonal expansion and deletion of lymphocytes is impaired in mice lacking HS1 protein, a substrate of the antigen-receptor-coupled tyrosine kinases. EMBO J 14:3664–3578, 1995.

Tarakhovsky A, Turner M, Schaal S, Mee PJ, Duddy LP, Rajewsky K, Tybulewicz VLJ. Defective antigen receptor–mediated proliferation of B and T cells in the absence of Vav. Nature 374:467–470, 1995.

Taylor CW, Marshall ICB. Calcium and inositol 1,4,5-trisphosphate receptors: a complex relationship. Trends Biochem Sci 17:403–407, 1992.

Tedford K, Nitschke L, Girkontaite I, Charlesworth A, Chan G, Sakk V, Barbacid M, Fischer KD. Compensation between Vav-1 and Vav-2 in B cell development and antigen receptor signaling. Nat Immunol 2:548–555, 2001.

Thome M, Duplay P, Guttinger M, Acuto O. Syk and ZAP-70 mediate recruitment of p56lck/CD4 to the activated T cell receptor/CD3/ζ complex. J Exp Med 181:1997–2006, 1995.

Todderud G, Wahl MJ, Rhee SG, Carpenter G. Stimulation of phospholipase C-γ1 membrane association by epidermal growth factor. Science 249:296–298, 1990.

Trowbridge IS, Thomas ML. CD45: an emerging role as a protein tyrosine phosphatase required for lymphocyte activation and development. Annu Rev Immunol 12:85–116, 1994.

Tsygankov AY, Spana C, Rowley RB, Penhallow RC, Burkardt AL, Bolen JS. Activation-dependent tyrosine phosphorylation of Fyn-associated proteins in T lymphocytes. J Biol Chem 269:7792–7800, 1994.

Turner M, Mee PJ, Costello PS, Williams O, Price AA, Duddy LP, Furlong MT, Geahlen RL, Tybulewicz VLJ. Perinatal lethality and blocked B-cell development in mice lacking the tyrosine kinase Syk. Nature 378:298–302, 1995.

Turner M, Mee PJ, Walters AE, Quinn ME, Mellor AL, Zamoyska R, Tybulewicz VL. A requirement for the Rho-family GTP exchange factor Vav in positive and negative selection of thymocytes. Immunity. 7:451–460, 1997.

Tuveson DA, Carter RH, Soltoff SP, Fearon DT. CD19 of B cells as a surrogate kinase insert region to bind phosphatidylinositol 3-kinase. Science 260:986–989, 1993.

Van Aelst L, Barr M, Marcus S, Polverino A, Wigler M. Complex formation between RAS and RAF and other protein kinases. Proc Natl Acad Sci USA 90:6213–6217, 1993.

van Noesel CJ, Lankester AC, van Schijndel GM, van Lier RA. The CR2/CD19 complex on human B cells contains the src-family kinase Lyn. Int Immunol 5:699–705, 1993.

van Oers NSC, Killeen N, Weiss A. ZAP-70 is constitutively associated with tyrosine phosphorylated TCR ζ in murine thymocytes and lymph node T cells. Immunity 1:675–685, 1994.

van Oers NSC, Killeen N, Weiss A. Lck regulates the tyrosine phosphorylation of the T cell receptor subunits and ZAP-70 in murine thymocytes. J Exp Med 183:1053–1062, 1996a.

van Oers NSC, Lowin-Kropf B, Finlay D, Connolly K, Weiss A. αβ T cell development is abolished in mice lacking both Lck and Fyn protein tyrosine kinases. Immunity 5:429–436, 1996b.

van Oers NSC, Tao W, Watts JD, Johnson P, Aebersold R, Teh H-S. Constitutive tyrosine phosphorylation of the T cell receptor (TCR) ζ subunit: regulation of TCR-associated protein kinase activity by TCR ζ. Mol Cell Biol 13:5771–5780, 1993.

Venkitaraman AR, Williams GT, Dariavach P, Neuberger MS. The B-cell antigen receptor of the five immunoglobulin classes. Nature 352:777–781, 1991.

Veri MC, DeBell KE, Seminario MC, DiBaldassarre A, Reischl I, Rawat R, Graham L, Noviello C, Rellahan BL, Miscia S, Wange RL, Bonvini E. Membrane raft-dependent regulation of phospholipase Cγ-1 activation in T lymphocytes. Mol Cell Biol 21:6939–6950, 2001.

Vihinen M, Mattsson PT, Smith CI. Bruton tyrosine kinase (BTK) in X-linked agammaglobulinemia (XLA). Front Biosci 5:D917–928, 2000.

Vojtek AB, Hollenberg SM, Cooper JA. Mammalian Ras interacts directly with the serine/threonine kinase Raf. Cell 74:205–214, 1993.

von Boehmer H, Fehling HJ. Structure and function of the pre-T cell receptor. Annu Rev Immunol 15:433–452, 1997.

von Boehmer H, Kisielow, P. Lymphocyte lineage commitment: instruction versus selection. Cell 73:207–208, 1993.

Wang B, Lemay S, Tsai S, Veillette A. SH2 domain-mediated interaction of inhibitory protein tyrosine kinase Csk with protein tyrosine phosphatase-HSCF. Mol Cell Biol 21:1077–1088, 2001.

Wang D, Feng J, Wen R, Marine JC, Sangster MY, Parganas E, Hoffmeyer A, Jackson CW, Cleveland JL, Murray PJ, Ihle JN. Phospholipase Cγ2 is essential in the functions of B cell and several Fc receptors. Immunity 13:25–35, 2000.

Wange RL. LAT, the linker for activation of T cells: a bridge between T cell–specific and general signaling pathways. Sci STKE 2000(63):RE1.

Wange RL, Guitian R, Isakov N, Watts JD, Aebersold R, Samelson LE. Activating and inhibitory mutations in adjacent tyrosines in the kinase domain of ZAP-70. J Biol Chem 270:18730–18733, 1995.

Wange RL, Malek SN, Desiderio S, Samelson LE. Tandem SH2 domains of ZAP-70 bind to T cell antigen receptor ζ and CD3ε from activated Jurkat T cells. J Biol Chem 268:19797–19801, 1993.

Ward SG, Reif K, Ley S, Fry MJ, Waterfield MD, Cantrell DA. Regulation of phosphoinositide kinases in T cells. J Biol Chem 267:23862–23869, 1992.

Waterhouse P, Penninger JM, Timms E, Wakeham A, Shahinian A, Lee KP, Thompson CB, Griesser H, Mak TW. Lymphoproliferative disorders with early lethality in mice deficient in Ctla-4. Science 270:985–988, 1995.

Wegener A-MK, Letourneur F, Hoeveler A, Brocker T, Luton F, Malissen B. The T cell receptor/CD3 complex is composed of at least two autonomous transduction modules. Cell 68:83–95, 1992.

Weintraub BC, Jun JE, Bishop AC, Shokat KM, Thomas ML, Goodnow, CC. Entry of B cell receptor into signaling domains is inhibited in tolerant B cells. J Exp Med 191:1443–1448, 2000.

Weiss A. T cell antigen receptor signal transduction: a tale of tails and cytoplasmic protein-tyrosine kinases. Cell 73:209–212, 1993.

Weiss A, Koretzky G, Schatzman R, Kadlecek T. Stimulation of the T cell antigen receptor induces tyrosine phosphorylation of phospholipase C γ1. Proc Natl Acad Sci USA 88:5484–5488, 1991.

Wienands J, Schweikert J, Wollscheid B, Jumaa H, Nielsen PJ, Reth M. SLP-65: a new signaling component in B lymphocytes which requires expression of the antigen receptor for phosphorylation. J Exp Med 188:791–795, 1998.

Wiest DL, Yuan L, Jefferson J, Benveniste P, Tsokos M, Klausner RD, Glimcher LH, Samelson LE, Singer A. Regulation of T cell receptor expression in immature CD4+CD8+ thymocytes by p56lck tyrosine kinase: basis for differential signaling by CD4 and CD8 in immature thymocytes expressing both coreceptor molecules. J Exp Med 178:1701–1712, 1993.

Willems L, Gatot JS, Mammerickx M, Portetelle D, Burny A, Kerkhofs P, Kettmann R. The YXXL signalling motifs of the bovine leukemia virus transmembrane protein are required for in vivo infection and maintenance of high viral loads. J Virol 69:4137–4141, 1995.

Williams BL, Schreiber KL, Zhang W, Wange RL, Samelson LE, Leibson PJ, Abraham RT. Genetic evidence for differential coupling of Syk family kinases to the T-cell receptor: reconstitution studies in a ZAP-70-deficient Jurkat T-cell line. Mol Cell Biol 18:1388–1399, 1998.

Winberg G, Matskova L, Chen F, Plant P, Rotin D, Gish G, Ingham R, Ernberg I, Pawson T. Latent membrane protein 2A of Epstein-Barr virus binds WW domain E3 protein-ubiquitin ligases that ubiquitinate B-cell tyrosine kinases. Mol Cell Biol 20:8526–8535, 2000.

Wu J, Katzav S, Weiss A. A functional T-cell receptor signaling pathway is required for p95^{vav} activity. Mol Cell Biol 15:4337–4346, 1995.

Wu J, Motto DG, Koretzky GA, Weiss A. Vav and SLP-76 interact and functionally cooperate in IL-2 gene activation. Immunity 4:593–602, 1996.

Wu J, Zhao Q, Kurosaki T, Weiss A. The Vav binding site (Y315) in ZAP-70 is critical for antigen receptor–mediated signal transduction. J Exp Med 185:1877–1882, 1997.

Wulfing C, Bauch A, Crabtree GR, Davis MM. The vav exchange factor is an essential regulator in actin-dependent receptor translocation to the lymphocyte-antigen-presenting cell interface. Proc Natl Acad Sci USA 97:10150–10155, 2000.

Xavier R, Brennan T, Li Q, McCormack C, Seed B. Membrane compartmentation is required for efficient T cell activation. Immunity 8:723–732, 1998.

Xu H, Littman DR. A kinase-independent function of lck in potentiating antigen-specific T cell activation. Cell 27:633–643, 1993.

Yablonski D, Kadlecek T, Weiss A. Identification of a phospholipase C-γ1 (PLC-γ1) SH3 domain-binding site in SLP-76 required for T-cell receptor-mediated activation of PLC-γ1 and NFAT. Mol Cell Biol 21:4208–4218, 2001.

Yablonski D, Kuhne MR, Kadlecek T, Weiss A. Uncoupling of nonreceptor tyrosine kinases from PLC-γ1 in an SLP-76-deficient T cell. Science 281:413–416, 1998.

Yamanishi Y, Tamura T, Kanamori T, Yamane H, Nariuchi H, Yamamoto T, Baltimore D. Role of the rasGAP-associated docking protein p62^{dok} in negative regulation of B cell receptor-mediated signaling. Genes Dev 14:11–16, 2000.

Yasuda T, Maeda A, Kurosaki M, Tezuka T, Hironaka K, Yamamoto T, Kurosaki T. Cbl suppresses B cell receptor-mediated phospholipase C (PLC)-γ2 activation by regulating B cell linker protein-PLC-γ2 binding. J Exp Med 191:641–650, 2000.

Yokoyama W. Right-side-up and up-side-down NK-cell receptors. Curr Biol 5:982–985, 1995.

Yoon CH, Lee J, Jongeward GD, Sternberg PW. Similarity of *sli-1*, a regulator of vulval development in *C. elegans*, to the mammalian proto-oncogene *c-cbl*. Science 269:1102–1105, 1995.

Young MA, Gonfloni S, Superti-Furga G, Roux B, Kurigan J. Dynamic coupling between the SH2 and SH3 domains of c-Src and Hck underlies their inactivation by C-terminal tyrosine phosphorylation. Cell 105:115–126, 2001.

Zhang W, Trible RP, Samelson LE. LAT palmitoylation: its essential role in membrane microdomain targeting and tyrosine phosphorylation during T cell activation. Immunity 9:239–246, 1998.

Zhao Q, Weiss. Enhancement of lymphocyte responsiveness by a gain-of-function mutation of ZAP-70. Mol Cell Biol 16:6765–6774, 1996.

7

Lymphoid Organ Development, Cell Trafficking, and Lymphocyte Responses

SIRPA JALKANEN and MARKO SALMI

A productive interaction between a lymphocyte and its cognate antigen is required to trigger an adequate immune response. Thus, it is not only the defects in the production and maturation of lymphocytes or in the activation machinery that can result in immunodeficiencies, but the same outcome can be seen if otherwise normal cells do not migrate properly within the body in search of foreign antigens. The best-known examples of this class of diseases are leukocyte adhesion deficiencies 1 and 2 (LAD1 and 2, see Chapter 38). The impact of proper lymphocyte recirculation between blood and different tissues and within the tissue stroma for eliciting an immune response already becomes evident by looking at the physical dimensions of our immune system.

Humans have approximately 10^{12} lymphocytes, each of which normally expresses receptors for only one antigen. Thus, for most antigens only some 100–1000 specific lymphocytes reside anywhere in the body. Moreover, at any moment only about 1% of these lymphocytes are in blood circulation whereas the rest are in tissues. The freely mobile cells in the blood travel at high velocity for their size. Even in small-caliber venules, where the extravasation takes place, an 8 μm–diameter cell moves about 500 μm/sec in the blood flow. Moreover, the total length of the circulatory tree has been estimated to exceed 100,000 km in an adult. These constraints make it very challenging for a specific cell to leave the blood at a desired site. At the same time, enormously large body surfaces are exposed to antigen invasion. The total area of the principal entry ports for antigens is about 2 m^2 in the skin, 400 m^2 in the gut, and 100 m^2 in the respiratory system. The antigens can be minute particles such as viruses or short foreign peptides. Thus it is clear that a highly efficient, adaptive immune response cannot rely on chance for random contact between the antigen and a specific lymphocyte anywhere in the body.

An elaborate system of lymphocyte recirculation has evolved to address these challenges (Carlos and Harlan, 1994; Springer,

1994; Butcher and Picker, 1996; Salmi and Jalkanen, 1997). Different functions of the immune system are compartmentalized to specific organs and tissues, and these units are then interconnected by lymphocyte trafficking via trees of vascular and lymphatic vessels (Fig. 7.1). Thus, primary lymphoid organs are specialized for production of huge numbers of lymphocytes. The specificity of a lymphocyte is also determined in these organs. The mature but antigenically inexperienced cells are then released into the circulation. These naive cells extravasate from the blood into secondary lymphoid organs (such as peripheral lymph nodes, Peyer's patches of gut). Simultaneously, antigens are concentrated into these very same organs from large epithelial surfaces (via an afferent lymphatic system to peripheral lymph nodes and via M cells into Peyer's patches). The secondary lymphoid organs are thus designed to collect and concentrate lymphocytes on the one hand and antigens on the other and to provide an optimal microenvironment for launching a productive immune response. Finally, the effector lymphocytes leave the secondary lymphoid organs, equipped with a capacity to migrate to the peripheral sites of inflammation. All the rest of the organs and tissues in the body can be regarded as tertiary immune tissues, which harbor significant numbers of lymphocytes only during an active immune response.

Lymphocyte Migration to Primary Lymphatic Organs

Lymphocyte trafficking first takes place during early ontogeny, when lymphoid precursor cells populate the lymphocyte-forming organs (Weissman, 2000). Initially, precursor cells from the yolk sac and/or aorta–gonad–mesonephros area migrate to fetal liver. Later, bone marrow becomes the main target for these precursor cells. After this stage the fate of B and T lymphocytes differs.

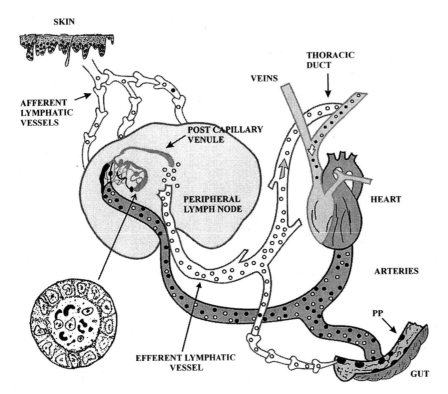

Figure 7.1. Lymphocytes recirculate between the blood and lymphoid organs. Most lymphocytes enter the peripheral lymph nodes or organized lymphoid tissues of the gut (Peyer's patches [PP] and appendix) via high endothelial venules. A low-level, continuous migration of lymphocytes from vascular beds such as skin to lymph nodes takes place via afferent lymphatics. The incoming lymphocytes migrate through the tissue parenchyma, enter the lymphatics, and are then carried within the efferent lymphatics back to the systemic blood circulation. Most of the venous circulation has been omitted for clarity. (Reproduced with permission from Salmi and Jalkanen, 1997).

B lymphocytes undergo their entire development in the cavity of bone marrow in contact with stromal cells. T cell precursors, by contrast, move further on to the thymus. They enter the thymus through cortical vessels and gradually migrate toward the medulla during the maturation processes. Finally, immunocompetent but naive B and T lymphocytes join the circulating pool of lymphocytes in the blood. Although these early migratory events are crucial for the development of the immune system, most of the molecular determinants involved in the trafficking remain to be elucidated.

Development of the lymphoid organs and their population of lymphocytes is regulated in a highly time-dependent manner (Bailey and Weiss, 1975; Bofill et al., 1985; Spencer et al., 1986; Campana et al., 1989). In humans, first CD3-positive thymocytes are found by week 10 of gestation. Anlage of secondary lymphoid organs have already started to develop earlier. Peripheral lymph nodes developing from a lymphatic plexus become recognizable around week 10, but development of high endothelial venule (HEV)-like vessels (the specialized vessels for lymphocyte recruitment, see below) and accumulation of early lymphocytes in these nodes can be seen only in 15- to 18-week old fetuses. In gut, mucosal villi appear around weeks 9–10 of gestation. By week 14, clusters of lymphocytes can be detected in the lamina propria and by 19 weeks well-organized Peyer's patches appear. The 12-week-old fetal spleen contains few lymphocytes, but at 14 weeks T and B cells are scattered throughout the organ. The early seeding of lymphocytes takes place in the absence of any external antigenic stimulation.

It is intriguing that the endothelial adhesion molecules, which govern lymphocyte trafficking in the adult, are expressed in a functional form very early during human development but in a remarkably different manner in terms of tissue specificity (Salmi et al., 2001). The gut addressin MAdCAM-1 (see below) is widely expressed in fetuses already at week 7. In fetuses, it is not only crucial for lymphocyte adhesion to vessels in gut, but it is also the most important determinant for lymphocyte binding to HEV in peripheral lymph nodes. Although the adult peripheral node addressin, PNAd (see below), is expressed in humans at week 15, it only gradually starts to dominate in mediating lymphocyte trafficking to peripheral lymph nodes during early childhood. On the basis of these findings it is likely that efficient lymphocyte recirculation takes place already in utero.

Trafficking of Lymphocytes to Secondary Lymphoid Organs

Peripheral lymph nodes, Peyer's patches, and spleen are the prime target organs for naive lymphocytes. In lymph nodes, a specialized vessel type called *high endothelial venule* (HEV), based on the characteristic cuboidal morphology of endothelial cells, allows efficient recruitment of blood-borne lymphocytes (Bjerknes et al., 1986; Kraal and Mebius, 1997). In these postcapillary venules, the shear stress is relatively low, and the endothelial surfaces protruding into the lumen of the vessels are rich in specific molecules needed for efficient adhesion. Moreover, the junctions between endothelial cells in these vessels are not typical tight junctions, rather, a flap-valve-like mechanism is operative at this site, which also facilitates cellular transmigration. Consequently, when the lymphocytes flow into HEV they undergo the different steps of the classical extravasation cascade very efficiently. It has been estimated that up to 50% of incoming lymphocytes make contacts with HEV lining in Peyer's patches and that even one cell in four can ultimately extravasate in these specialized organs (Bjerknes et al., 1986). On the basis of calculations in sheep, up to 15,000 lymphocytes can be expected to be transmigrating through HEV in a single lymph node every second (Girard and Springer, 1995).

Antigens are concentrated to lymph nodes through the other vessel system draining into these organs (Cella et al., 1997; Banchereau and Steinman, 1998). Free antigens or antigens taken up by dendritic cells enter lymph nodes from the periphery via afferent lymphatic vessels. These vessels empty into the subcapsular sinuses, from which cells and antigens can penetrate into the lymphoid areas while flowing through the fine lymphatic channels within the tissue. The dual vessel supply bringing in lymphocytes by blood and antigens by lymph maximizes the likelihood for lymphocyte–antigen contacts in lymph nodes.

When lymphocytes enter the lymphoid tissue they are further guided by chemotactic gradients into specific intraorgan locations. Most notably, different chemokines secreted by many cell types help to segregate lymphocytes into discrete T and B cell areas within the lymph node (Cyster, 1999; 2005). Thus B cells preferentially accumulate into cortical B cell follicles, whereas T cells are recruited into more diffuse subcortical T cell areas. While percolating through the tissue stroma the lymphocytes constantly search for their cognate antigens presented by different types of professional antigen-presenting cells also concentrated in lymph nodes. If they fail to find a specific antigen in the lymph node, they enter the lymphatic sinuses and leave the organ via efferent lymphatic vessels. These cells are then carried back to the blood system, since the main lymphatic trunks (such as ductus thoracicus) open into the major veins near the heart. Then these cells are free to move on in the circulation and to enter any other lymphoid tissue in the body during their continuous recirculation (Gowans and Knight, 1964). One cycle from the blood back to the blood takes about 1 day, hence any single lymphocyte has time to percolate through hundreds of lymph nodes until it dies. This patroling behavior of a lymphocyte is only interrupted and retargeted if it encounters its specific antigen within a lymphoid tissue (see below).

Lymphocyte recirculation through the spleen is profoundly different from that in the lymph nodes (Pabst, 1988). Notably, HEV are absent from the spleen and lymphocytes enter the white pulp via marginal zone sinuses, where macrophage-like cells surrounding the endothelial cells may be important for recruitment. In the splenic parenchyma, lymphocytes again migrate toward specific guidance molecules. However, here T cells migrate into confined T cell areas around the central arteriole, whereas B cells remain scattered in the corona. Splenic lymphocytes also seem to leave the organ via the splenic vein rather than via lymphatics. Although the spleen contains more lymphocytes than all the lymph nodes together, the migratory pathways in this organ specialized for concentrating blood-derived antigens remain rather poorly characterized.

Tissue-Selective Homing of Activated Lymphocytes

When a lymphocyte meets its cognate antigen in lymph nodes, its migratory properties change profoundly (Gowans and Knight, 1964; Watson and Bradley, 1998). The activated lymphocyte undergoes proliferation and differentiation in the lymph node. Thereafter, its progeny cells leave the node via the efferent lymphatics together with other naive lymphocytes. However, upon rearrival into the circulation, the antigen-activated effector cells no longer randomly recirculate to other lymph nodes. Instead, they have become imprinted so that they can preferentially traffic into the peripheral epithelial tissues through which the inciting antigen penetrated the body surfaces. This reprogramming involves at least changes in the expression profile of adhesion molecules and receptors for chemokines. These effector cells can leave the blood via the normal flat-walled postcapillary venules in the periphery and navigate into areas of microbial or other in-

flammatory stimuli. Hence, the effector cells are efficiently targeted to those locations where they can do the most good to defend the body.

A small population of effector cells ultimately turns into memory cells. These cells have the unique capacity to patrol the tertiary lymphoid tissues, mainly epithelial surfaces. Should the same antigenic exposure reoccur, the memory cells can evoke a rapid response against it. Again, the phenotypic changes in memory cells affect their recirculation potential. These cells (and effector lymphocytes) have profoundly decreased ability to immigrate into lymph nodes via HEV, thus they drain mainly into the local lymph nodes via the afferent lymphatics together with the antigen-presenting cells and antigens (Sallusto et al., 1999).

Under physiological conditions, two main recirculation routes for activated lymphocytes can be distinguished (Fig. 7.1) (reviewed in Carlos and Harlan, 1994; Springer, 1994; Butcher and Picker, 1996; Salmi and Jalkanen, 1997). Immunoblasts activated in peripheral lymph nodes preferentially migrate into the skin, whereas those responding to gut-derived antigens in Peyer's patches tend to return to the gut-associated lymphatic tissues (Butcher, 1999; Robert and Kupper, 1999). The gut-seeking immunoblasts enter mainly the intestine in the lamina propria, which is the body's largest nonorganized lymphoid tissue. These cells may also have the capacity to migrate into the respiratory and genitourinary tract, which have traditionally been included in the common gut-associated lymphoid system (Brandtzaeg et al., 1999). Thus, under normal conditions, the gut and nonmucosal lymphoid organs share the total pool of naive cells with all possible antigenic specificities, but upon activation, the subsequent migratory route sharpens the immune response into the affected tissue.

During pathologic inflammation there are characteristic changes in leukocyte trafficking (Carlos and Harlan, 1994; Springer, 1994; Butcher and Picker, 1996; Salmi and Jalkanen, 1997; Cines et al., 1998). First, in acute inflammation, polymorphonuclear leukocytes invade the affected site very rapidly, and only later are waves of monocyte and lymphocyte influx seen. In a primary challenge it takes about 3 days before antigen-specific immunoblasts enter the peripheral lesion, but during a secondary response the influx of memory-derived cells occurs much faster. Second, the exposure of flat-walled venules to proinflammatory mediators at a site of acute inflammation makes them much more adhesive toward different classes of leukocytes. Bathing of the affected tissue in inflammatory cytokines, microbial products, and other proadhesive compounds results in the rapid synthesis of many endothelial adhesion molecules that are absent from noninflamed vessels or only expressed at low levels. In chronic inflammation, even an HEV-like transformation of vessels in peripheral tissues is common and is quite often associated with notably lymphoid follicles in these nonlymphoid organs.

Different types of inflammation have typical features that also affect lymphocyte trafficking (Carlos and Harlan, 1994; Springer, 1994; Butcher and Picker, 1996; Salmi and Jalkanen, 1997; Butcher, 1999; Robert and Kupper, 1999). In general, both CD8 T-killer cells and CD4-positive Th1 and Th2 cells can infiltrate to sites of inflammation, but their relative proportions vary according to the underlying cause. The inflammatory stimulus and/or anatomic location results in a characteristic, although partially overlapping, pattern of expression and/or activation of adhesion molecules and chemotactic systems on both lymphocytes and endothelial cells, which translates into apparently tissue-selective migration patterns into inflamed tertiary sites.

For example, inflamed synovial membrane in rheumatitis displays features of lymphocyte homing, which are clearly distinct from those in peripheral lymph nodes, skin, and gut. In fact, restricted expression of homing-associated molecules on Th1 vs. Th2 CD4 lymphocytes may explain the preponderance of Th1 cells in certain inflammatory lesions (Syrbe et al., 1999; D'Ambrosio et al., 2000).

Molecular Mechanisms in Leukocyte Extravasation

The Multistep Adhesion Cascade

Lymphocytes and other leukocytes leave the blood in a multistep process that can be visualized both in vitro and in vivo as tethering, rolling, firm adhesion, and transmigration (Fig. 7.2) (Butcher, 1991; Springer, 1994; Carman and Springer, 2004). Tethering and rolling phases are mainly mediated by selectins and their sialomucin ligands. Transient and weak interactions between lymphocytes and endothelial cells formed by these molecular pairs lead to triggering of an activation step involving chemokines and their receptors. Activation is required for optimal adhesive behavior of leukocyte integrins that are inactive when cells are freely flowing in the bloodstream. However, engagement of other types of molecules, such as glycosyl-phosphatidylinositol (GPI)–linked proteins, on lymphocyte surface can result in integrin activation. During activation and firm adhesion, leukocytes change their shape and then start to transmigrate. Molecular mechanisms functioning at the transmigration step are poorly known but include metalloproteinases that help lymphocytes to penetrate the basement membrane. The path used by a transmigrating lymphocyte is rapidly closed by unknown repair mechanisms. Movement and final localization of a lymphocyte within the tissue is largely dependent on chemokine receptors and molecules binding to extracellular matrix proteins on its surface (Cyster, 1999; 2005).

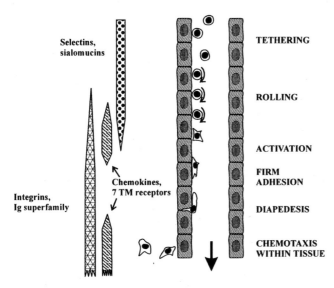

Figure 7.2. The multistep adhesion cascade of lymphocyte extravasation. The freely flowing, blood-borne lymphocyte starts the interaction with vascular endothelium by tethering and rolling that then proceeds to an activation step. Activation is followed by firm adhesion. Thereafter, the lymphocyte seeks an interendothelial junction, through which it penetrates into the tissue. The contribution of major molecular families at each step is illustrated.

The complexity of the multistep cascade functioning in leukocyte extravasation is comparable to blood clotting and complement-mediated killing, in which each step has to be executed correctly to achieve the goal. The extravasation cascade is made more complex by the fact that vascular beds in different organs and inflammatory conditions express some unique homing-associated molecules, and each leukocyte subset displays partially distinct homing-molecules on their surface. Because the lymphocyte can enter a particular tissue only if it is equipped by a set of molecules matching the ligands presented on vascular endothelium of this tissue, the composition of lymphocytic infiltration in each tissue is tightly controlled (Butcher, 1991; Springer, 1994; Salmi and Jalkanen, 1997).

The most relevant homing-related molecules (illustrated in Fig. 7.3) are presented below in more detail and in the order of their principal place in the adhesion cascade. It should be emphasized here, however, that functions of these molecules overlap in vivo and may depend on the characteristics of the vascular bed, where the interactions take place. For example, integrins are able to mediate rolling under low shear, and in narrow capillaries they may act without a clear preceding, selectin-mediated rolling phase (Springer, 1994; Salmi and Jalkanen, 1997).

Tethering and Rolling

Selectin and their sialomucin ligands

Selectins and their sialomucin ligands are the key players in tethering and rolling steps, because the lectin–carbohydrate bonds between these receptor–ligand pairs allow formation of rapid but transient and weak interactions typical of rolling behavior. There are three members of the selectin family that have been named, based on their main site of expression: L-selectin (CD62L) is present on different types of leukocytes, E-selectin (CD62E) is on endothelium, and P-selectin (CD62P) is on platelets and endothelium (Rosen, 1999; Vestweber and Blanks, 1999; Ley, 2001).

The common structural feature of these molecules is the N-terminal lectin domain, which is of fundamental importance in binding to sialyl Lewis X (sLeX) carbohydrate present on the sialomucin ligands of selectins (Fukuda et al., 1999; Rosen, 1999; Vestweber and Blanks, 1999; Ley, 2001). The ligand structures for L-selectin are presented by PNAd on HEV in peripheral lymph nodes, thus PNAd is fundamental to guiding L-selectin–positive lymphocytes into peripheral lymph nodes. PNAd consists of at least six different proteins, all decorated by a sulfated and fucosylated sLeX. Only four of them have been molecularly defined: glycosylation-dependent cell adhesion molecule-1 (GlyCAM-1), CD34, podocalyxin, and mucosal addressin cell adhesion molecule (MAdCAM-1). Interestingly, MAdCAM-1 has the proper glycosylation for L-selectin recognition only in organized lymphoid areas of the gut such as Peyer's patches but not in lamina propria vessels, allowing to a certain extent L-selectin–dependent entrance of cells to mucosal sites.

The importance of most homing-related molecules in vivo has been demonstrated by creating knockout mice (Table 7.1). Among the first were L-selectin–deficient mice that exhibit severely impaired lymphocyte homing to peripheral lymph nodes. In contrast, GlyCAM-1 knockout mice only have enlarged lymph nodes, a result suggesting a regulatory role for the soluble GlyCAM-1 molecule in lymphocyte homing. CD34 knockout mice are seemingly healthy despite defective eosinophil migration. Also, the genes important for proper post-translational modifications of the selectin ligands are disrupted. For example,

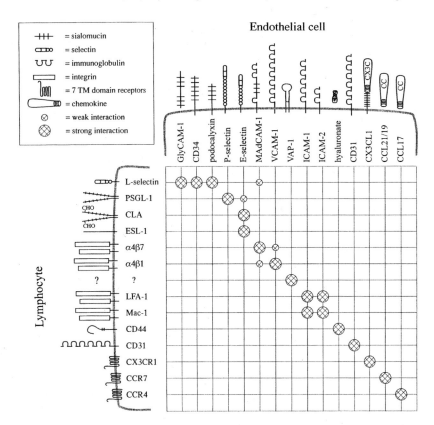

Figure 7.3. Homing-associated molecules involved in lymphocyte traffic. The most relevant lymphocyte surface molecules and their counter-receptors on vascular endothelium are depicted.

fucosyltransferase VII (Fuc-TVII)–deficient mice are not able to add the critical fucose moiety to the sLeX structure. Hence, they do not glycosylate L-selectin ligands properly and exhibit severe impairment in lymphocyte homing and leukocyte extravasation to sites of inflammation (Lowe, 1997). Lack of a highly HEV-specific sulfotransferase (GlcNAc6ST) leads to inefficient or absent sulfation of the sLeX motif, concomitant disappearance of L-selectin ligand activity, and decreased lymphocyte homing (Hemmerich et al., 2001).

Expression of both P- and E-selectin are induced at sites of inflammation. However, their expression kinetics differs remarkably. P-selectin is released within minutes from intracellular storage granules, Weibel-Palade bodies, and is translocated to the endothelial cell surface, whereas E-selectin requires new protein synthesis and its maximal expression is seen 4 hours after the induction of inflammation. The primary ligand for P-selectin is correctly tyrosine-sulfated P-selectin glycoprotein ligand-1 (PSGL), which is present on most leukocytes (McEver and Cummings, 1997). Depending on its glycosylation profile it can also bind to E-selectin, which has high affinity particularly toward cutaneous lymphocyte antigen (CLA), a specific glycoform of PSGL-1. CLA–E-selectin interaction appears to be important in directing lymphocytes to skin inflammations. In addition, E-selectin binds to a non-mucin-like E-selectin ligand-1 (ESL-1) on leukocytes (Vestweber and Blanks, 1999).

E-selectin knockout mice are apparently healthy, but their leukocytes roll faster than in normal mice, indicating that E-selectin is an important molecular brake at early steps of leukocyte–endothelial cell interactions. P-selectin–defective mice are also viable and fertile. They show neutrophilia due to a longer half-life of neutrophils. After induction of inflammation, leukocyte rolling is impaired for less than 2 hours in these mice. This finding suggests that P-selectin is indispensable only at early phases of inflammation (Frenette and Wagner, 1997). PSGL-1

knockout mice largely resemble P-selectin–deficient mice, thus confirming the importance of PSGL-1 at the rolling step (Yang et al., 1999). Mice deficient for both E- and P-selectin have also been generated. These mice exhibit much more profound defects than those of single knockouts, indicating that E- and P-selectin have overlapping functions and that they compensate each other (Frenette and Wagner, 1997). Furthermore, mice whose core 2β 1,6-*N*-acetylglucosaminyl transferase (C2-β-GlcNAcT) gene has been disrupted have a defect in the early step of branching of LeX oligosaccharide and therefore lose proper glycosylation of their E- and P-selectin ligands. These mice show normal lymphocyte homing to lymph nodes but their leukocytes cannot efficiently enter the sites of inflammation (Etzioni et al., 1999; Vestweber and Blanks, 1999). A human immunodeficiency disease, leukocyte adhesion defect 2 (LAD2), resembles characteristics of these knockout animals: LAD2 patients do not have functional selectin ligands because of a glycosylation defect. Leukocytes of these patients have decreased rolling capacity, although in static conditions leukocytes adhere efficiently to endothelial cells. Patients with LAD2 suffer from recurrent bacterial infections and also have other developmental abnormalities (Etzioni et al., 1999). This disease is presented in detail in Chapter 38.

CD43, CD44, and vascular adhesion protein-1

Other (nonselectin) molecules have also been shown to directly mediate rolling or tethering or to indirectly regulate this step. An example of a regulatory molecule is CD43, a long and negatively charged glycoprotein on lymphocytes that inhibits engagement of L-selectin, thus blocking the homing of lymphocytes. Its role is clearly demonstrated in CD43-deficient animals, which show enhanced lymphocyte homing to secondary lymphoid organs (Stockton et al., 1998). CD44 is a multifunctional member of the proteoglycan family that can mediate rolling of lymphocytes

Table 7.1. Phenotype of Gene-Targeted Mice Made Deficient for Individual Homing-Associated Molecule

Molecule	Main Abnormalities in Leukocyte Trafficking
L-selectin	Impaired lymphocyte homing to peripheral lymph nodes
E-selectin	Increased velocity of rolling leukocytes
P-selectin	Decreased leukocyte rolling at early stages of inflammation
GlyCAM-1	Enlarged lymph nodes
CD34	Impaired eosinophil accumulation in allergen-induced lung inflammation
PSGL-1	Decreased leukocyte rolling at early stages of inflammation
Fuc-TVII	Reduced leukocyte migration to sites of inflammation Reduced lymphocyte homing to peripheral lymph nodes
C2β GlcNAcT	Reduced leukocyte emigration to sites of inflammation
GlcNAc6ST	Decreased lymphocyte homing
ICAM-1	Impaired neutrophil migration to sites of inflammation
ICAM-2	Delayed easinophil accumulation in the airway lumen in allergy
VCAM-1	Embryonic lethal
CD31	Deficient migration through basement membrane
CD11a	Reduced lymphocyte trafficking to peripheral lymph nodes and to Peyer's patches Decreased leukocyte trafficking to sites of inflammation
CD11b	Decreased neutrophil emigration in ischemia/reperfusion injury
β2-integrin	No neutrophil emigration into the skin, normal emigration into inflamed peritoneum, and increased migration into inflamed lung
α4-integrin	Embryonic lethal, chimeric mice have reduced lymphocyte homing into Peyer's patches
β7-integrin	Impaired lymphocyte migration to Peyer's patches
CD43	Increased lymphocyte homing to secondary lymphoid organs
CD44	Decreased lymphocyte migration to peripheral lymph nodes and thymus
CCR4	No obvious defects in leukocyte trafficking
CCR7	Defective lymphocyte entry to lymph nodes and formation of T cell areas
CXCR5	Defect in formation of follicles in lymph nodes
CX3CL1	No obvious defects in leukocyte trafficking

on endothelial hyaluronan (Siegelman et al., 1999). In addition, triggering of CD44 activates lymphocyte function–associated antigen-1 (LFA-1), which may strengthen lymphocyte adhesion to endothelium. In vivo experiments using function-blocking antibodies suggest that CD44 is important in lymphocyte trafficking to sites of inflammation. Moreover, lymphocytes of CD44-deficient mice show impaired lymphocyte homing to peripheral lymph nodes and thymus (Protin et al., 1999).

Vascular adhesion protein-1 (VAP-1) is a unique member among the homing-related molecules, because in addition to its adhesive function at an early phase of the multistep cascade it possesses intrinsic enzymatic activity. The end products of the reaction catalyzed by this amine oxidase are aldehyde, ammonium, and hydrogen peroxide. All of them are potent compounds that may regulate the entire scene of inflammation by, for instance, aberrantly glycosylating endothelial proteins (aldehydes) or by up-regulating other adhesion proteins and metalloproteinases and inducing apoptosis (hydrogen peroxide). Regulation of VAP-1 function appears to involve its sequestration into intracellular granules, from which it is rapidly translocated to the endothelial surface upon induction of inflammation (Jalkanen and Salmi, 2001; Salmi and Jalkanen, 2001).

Activation

Chemokines and their receptors

Certain endothelial chemokines and their interaction with the seven pass transmembrane receptors on leukocytes are considered to be of fundamental importance at the activation step of the adhesion cascade. *Chemokines* are small molecules divided into the following families on the basis of their structural cysteine motifs: C, CC, CXC, and CX3C, where *C* is cysteine and *X* is any amino acid residue.

Chemokines are typically heparin-binding soluble molecules and many of them are not even produced by endothelial cells. How these molecules can exert their function at the luminal surface of endothelial cells where blood constantly flushes away any soluble gradients remains an enigma. The answer appears to be in the good diffusibility of these molecules, possibly via a specialized reticular conduit, through the lymph node to the abluminal side of the vessels. They can then be transcytosed to the luminal side of the endothelial cell, where they become immobilized by an avid binding to surface-expressed glycosaminoglycans. Chemokines injected subcutaneously can find their way to the luminal surface of HEV in the draining lymph nodes, and hence selectively enhance lymphocyte recruitment to the draining node (Middleton et al., 1997; Gretz et al., 2000). After chemokine binding, activation signals are transduced from the serpentine receptors via guanine nucleotide-binding (G) proteins via still poorly defined signaling routes that eventually result in affinity/avidity changes of leukocyte integrins (Mantovani, 1999; Zlotnik et al., 1999; Baggiolini, 2001; Gerard and Rollins, 2001; Mackay, 2001).

Different leukocyte subsets possess alternative sets of chemokine receptors that determine whether they are allowed to exit from the blood—for example, at HEV in peripheral lymph nodes or vasculature at sites of inflammation. For instance, T cells bearing CCR7 receptor become recruited to peripheral lymph nodes and mucosal sites where its ligand CCL21 (secondary lymphoid chemokine, SLC) is expressed on HEV. CCR7 also binds to CCL19 (EBV-induced molecule 1 ligand chemokine, ELC) present on HEV. B cells, by contrast, bind efficiently to areas of HEV devoid of CCL21 with a currently unknown receptor. They may also use CCL13 (B cell–attracting chemokine, BCA-1) in follicular vessels and directly enter the follicles using CXCR5 (Moser and Loetscher, 2001). CX3CL1 (Fractalkine) is structurally very different from other endothelial chemokines, because in addition to a soluble form it has a transmembrane form with a long stalk of sialomucin-like structure. CX3CL1 has a strong affinity toward T cells (Mackay, 2001). Tissue selectivity among chemokines has been demonstrated to exist at least in the skin, where endothelial CCL17 (thymus and activation-regulated chemokine, TARC) attracts CCR4-bearing lymphocytes (Campbell et al., 1999).

CCR7 knockout mice demonstrate the importance of this chemokine in lymphocyte trafficking, as these mice have defective T cell entry to lymph nodes (Cyster, 1999; 2005). In contrast, no obvious homing defects have been found in CX3CL1 and CCR4 knockout mice. The only abnormality discovered in CX3CL1–/– mice is the diminished number of cells belonging to the monocyte/macrophage lineage in the blood (Cook et al., 2001). The same population was diminished in CCR4–/– mice in the peritoneal cavity (Chvatchko et al., 2000), a finding suggesting that the function of these two chemokines can be compensated for by other molecules.

Other molecules

Engagement of several other leukocyte surface molecules can lead to activation of LFA-1, CD11a/CD18. However, only a few of them have been directly shown to result in increased leukocyte binding to endothelium. One of the molecules having this property is CD73, a GPI-linked molecule that has ectonucleotidase activity catalyzing conversion of extracellular AMP to adenosine (Resta et al., 1998; Airas et al., 2000). Adenosine regulates both E-selectin and integrin function and endothelial permeability (Cronstein and Weissmann, 1993; Cronstein, 1997). Interestingly, lack or diminished expression of CD73 is linked to a variety of immunodeficiency diseases, such as Wiskott-Aldrich syndrome, severe combined immunodeficiency, common variable immunodeficiency, primary hypogammaglobulinemia, selective IgA deficiency, and Omenn syndrome.

Firm Adhesion

Integrins and their immunoglobulin superfamily ligands

Certain integrins participate effectively in the arrest of leukocytes on endothelium through use of members belonging to the immunoglobulin superfamily as their vascular ligands. They can also function at the earlier steps of the cascade, even during rolling. Typical for integrins is that they are heterodimers consisting of α and β chains (Shimizu et al., 1999). Important integrins for leukocyte extravasation are $\alpha4\beta7$, LFA-1, and $\alpha4\beta1$. $\alpha4\beta7$ is a principal homing receptor for MAdCAM-1 and directs lymphocytes to mucosa-associated lymphatic tissues (Butcher, 1999). Its role as a mucosal homing receptor has been clearly demonstrated by $\beta7$ knockout animals. They have rudimentary Peyer's patches and their lymphocyte homing to mucosal sites is severely impaired. In contrast, lymphocyte homing to peripheral lymph nodes in these mice is intact (Wagner and Müller, 1998).

$\alpha4\beta1$, by contrast, exerts its role mainly at inflammatory sites, where it binds to its ligand, vascular cell adhesion molecule-1 (VCAM-1, CD106). Both VCAM-1 and $\alpha4$ knockout animals are embryonically lethal, indicating that besides homing they have more fundamental roles in embryonic development. Mice that are chimeric regarding the deletion of $\alpha4$ show diminished lymphocyte trafficking to Peyer's patches but not to other secondary lymphatic organs, a finding compatible with the phenotype of $\beta7$ knockouts (Wagner and Müller, 1998).

LFA-1 (CD11a/CD18) is a member of the group of four leukocyte integrins sharing the same β chain, $\beta2$ (CD18), while having unique α chains (CD11a, b, c, and d). LFA-1 is present on practically all leukocytes and mediates their binding to intercellular adhesion molecules 1 and 2 (ICAM-1 [CD54] and ICAM-2 [CD102]) in its active form (Wang and Springer, 1998; Shimizu et al., 1999; Hogg and Leitinger, 2001). Mac-1 (CD11b/CD18) also participates in leukocyte migration, but its role is heavily overshadowed by LFA-1. The role of leukocyte integrins in leukocyte trafficking is evident through the dramatic defects in leukocyte extravasation in patients suffering from LAD1 or its alternative form. These patients lack the normal $\beta2$ chain, consequently surface expression of all leukocyte α chains is prevented as well, or they express LFA-1 in a nonfunctional form (Etzioni et al., 1999). This deficiency is presented in more detail in Chapter 38 in this book.

Mice deficient in CD18 do not show as dramatic defects as those of LAD1 patients. Their neutrophils do not migrate into the skin but traffic normally to peritoneum and increased homing takes place in inflamed lung. CD11a−/− mice have impaired lymphocyte homing to both peripheral lymph nodes and Peyer's patches, a finding in keeping with the role of LFA-1 as a non–organ-specific homing molecule. In CD11b-negative mice, reduced neutrophil binding to endothelium is observed. Mice lacking ICAM-1 have a relatively mild phenotype compared to findings obtained from studies using function-blocking antibodies. These mice have decreased neutrophil migration to tissues in some inflammatory models. Lack of ICAM-2 normally constitutively present on endothelium does not cause any obvious defects in lymphocyte recirculation (Etzioni et al., 1999).

Transmigration

Transmigration is the least-analyzed phase in leukocyte extravasation process although recent progress has been made (Carman and Spring, 2004). Studies using function blocking antibodies have shown that CD31 is intimately involved in transmigration. CD31 belongs to the immunoglobulin superfamily and is expressed by several leukocyte subsets and continuous endothelium of all vessel types (Newman, 1997). On vascular endothelium its expression is concentrated on intercellular junctions. Unexpectedly, CD31-deficient mice show a normal overall transmigration capacity. However, the polymorphonuclear leukocytes are arrested between the endothelium and basement membrane, demonstrating that CD31 is needed in migration through the basement membrane (Duncan et al., 1999). Other molecules such as junctional adhesion molecule (JAM), LFA-1, and the ICAMs have been implicated in transmigration (Faveeuw et al., 2000; Dejana et al., 2001). Matrix metalloproteinase-2 (MMP-2), which is induced in T cells upon binding to endothelium, also plays a role in this invasive process.

Intraorgan Localization of Lymphocytes

Subsequent to entry into the lymphoid organs, lymphocytes start their voyage within the organs. For the migration, lymphocytes need balanced function of adhesion molecules capable of binding to extracellular matrix molecules (ECM), such as fibronectin, laminins, and collagens, and mechanisms to detach from the anchorage to ECM (Gretz et al., 1996). $\beta1$-integrins are essential for binding to various ECM, and lymphocytes can use CD44 to bind to fibronectin and collagens. Detaching mechanisms are poorly understood. Controlled and directional migration also needs proper chemokine receptors on the lymphocyte surface that respond to chemokines secreted by different cell types within the tissues. These interactions are important both in early phases of lymphocyte maturation, for example, in thymus and later during physiological lymphocyte recirculation and leukocyte movement at sites of inflammation (Mantovani, 1999; Zlotnik et al., 1999; Baggiolini, 2001; Gerard and Rollins, 2001; Mackay, 2001). During normal recirculation, CCL21 and CCL19 guide T cells to interfollicular areas within the nodes, whereas CCL13 produced by follicular dendritic cells attracts B cells expressing CXCR5 into the follicles (Fig. 7.4).

In addition to cell surface molecules mediating adhesion–de-adhesion steps in the intraorgan movement of lymphocytes, the pathways that transduce these surface signals into the locomotory machinery are important for proper localization (Sánchez-Madrid and del Pozo, 1999). Hence, specific receptors are clustered at the leading edge and trailing edge of the crawling lymphocyte. Via still incompletely understood mecha-

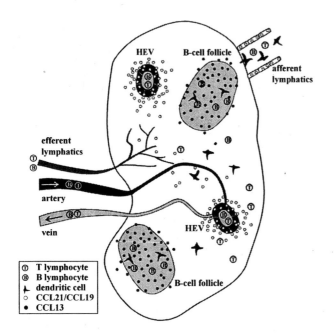

Figure 7.4. Chemokines contribute to both entrance and intraorgan localization of lymphocytes. CCL19 and CCL21 are involved in T lymphocyte entrance via high endothelial venules (HEV) into the node. They also guide T cells to the interfollicular areas in the lymph node. CCL13, by contrast, directs B lymphocytes into the follicles.

nisms, these molecules signal to the actomyosin and microtubuli networks within the cell, and translate the surface signals into polarized cell crawling. Just one example of the importance of these steps for proper immune defense is Wiskott-Aldrich syndrome, in which a defect in one of these effector signaling proteins leads to a severe immunodeficiency (Thrasher et al., 1998).

Dendritic cells entering the lymph nodes via afferent lymph and bringing antigens are key players in the immune response as antigen-presenting cells. CCL21 expressed in lymphatic endothelium assists dendritic cell entrance into the T cell areas allowing these two cell types to interact with each other. B cell collaboration with T cells is ensured by up-regulation of CXCR5 on a subset of T cells and CCR7 on B cells. This makes it possible for B and T cells to move to the boundary of the B and T cell zones and interact with each other. A spontaneously mutant mouse strain, *plt*, which has decreased expression of both CCL21 and CCL19, demonstrates the importance of these chemokines in intraorgan localization (and entry) of lymphocytes, as these mice have defective organization of T cell areas within lymph nodes. The phenotype of these mice is thus comparable to that of mice lacking the receptor for these chemokines (CCR7). In contrast, in CXCR5-negative mice development of B cell follicles is defective—again, in keeping with the function of this chemokine in B cell localization (Cyster, 1999).

Intraorgan localization also shows remarkable tissue specificity, best exemplified in the gut. Practically all lymphocytes in the small intestine have CCR9 whereas in the colon these cells are less frequent. Importantly, lymphocytes in several other tissues (excluding thymus) are CCR9 negative. The ligand for CCR9 is CCL25 (thymus-expressed chemokine, TECK), which is produced by gut epithelial cells and thus expected to guide CCR9-positive lymphocytes, especially to small intestine (Kunkel

et al., 2000). Whether CCL25–CCR9 interaction plays a role at the entrance phase to small intestine has not been directly demonstrated.

Conclusions

Optimal lymphocyte entry to primary lymphoid organs during development and to secondary lymphoid organs during recirculation, and efficient leukocyte trafficking to sites of inflammation are the key elements in adequate functioning of the immune system. Molecular mechanisms mediating lymphocyte contacts with the vascular wall are relatively well known. Knowledge of the network of chemokines and receptors needed for leukocyte entrance and intraorgan localization is increasing exponentially. In contrast, the mechanisms functioning during diapedesis through the vascular wall, leukocyte entry to afferent lymphatics at different vascular beds, and lymphocyte exit via efferent lymphatics within the lymphoid organs remain to be elucidated. The importance of leukocyte trafficking to the pathophysiology of human disease is reflected in the numerous attempts worldwide at manipulating the trafficking mechanisms of leukocytes to combat harmful inflammations.

Thus far, the number of patients diagnosed as having a defect in any of the molecules involved in leukocyte migration has been very small. One reason for this small number may be that many of the defects are not compatible with life. The tools for diagnosing patients who suffer from defective leukocyte trafficking are continuously being developed and may help to reveal many new disease entities. One example of recent advances is a study in which CXCR1 (receptor for IL-8) expression levels in neutrophils of normal and pyelonephritis-prone children were compared. Patients suffering from recurrent pyelonephritis had significantly lower CXCR1 levels than those of healthy controls, providing an explanation for these recurrences (Frendéus et al., 2000). Analogous findings can be expected to emerge from other disease groups in the near future.

Over the past few years, we have gained increasing insight into the salient molecular and physiological mechanisms guiding lymphocyte recirculation from the blood into the tissues and back to the circulation. In terms of our immune defense, this continuous patrolling process is important for guaranteeing maximal efficacy of a lymphocyte meeting its cognate antigen. Failure of this process inevitably leads to some form of immunodeficiency. Thus, a detailed understanding of the multifaceted extravasation cascade will help us to develop new strategies for guiding and redirecting lymphocyte trafficking into locations where lymphocytes are needed in immunodeficiency patients, where the system has gone awry for one reason or another.

References

Airas L, Niemelä J, Jalkanen S. CD73 engagement promotes lymphocyte binding to endothelial cells via a lymphocyte function-associated antigen-1-dependent mechanism. J Immunol 165:5411–5417, 2000.

Baggiolini M. Chemokines in pathology and medicine. J Intern Med 250: 91–104, 2001.

Bailey RP, Weiss L. Ontogeny of human fetal lymph nodes. Am J Anat 142: 15–27, 1975.

Banchereau J, Steinman RM. Dendritic cells and the control of immunity. Nature 392:245–252, 1998.

Bjerknes M, Cheng H, Ottaway CA. Dynamics of lymphocyte–endothelial interactions in vivo. Science 231:402–405, 1986.

Bofill M, Janossy G, Janossa M, Burford GD, Seymour GJ, Wernet P, Kelemen E. Human B cell development. II. Subpopulations in the human fetus. J Immunol 134:1531–1538, 1985.

Brandtzaeg P, Farstad IN, Haraldsen G. Regional specialization in the mucosal immune system: primed cells do not always home along the same track. Immunol Today 20:267–277, 1999.

Butcher EC. Leukocyte-endothelial cell recognition: three (or more) steps to specificity and diversity. Cell 67:1033–1036, 1991.

Butcher EC. Lymphocyte homing and intestinal immunity. In Ogra PL, Lamm ME, Bienenstock J, Mestecky J, Strober W, McGhee JR, eds. Mucosal Immunology. San Diego: Academic Press, pp. 507–522, 1999.

Butcher EC, Picker LJ. Lymphocyte homing and homeostasis. Science 272:60–66, 1996.

Campana D, Janossy G, Coustan-Smith E, Amlot PL, Tian W-T, Ip S, Wong L. The expression of T cell receptor-associated proteins during T cell ontogeny in man. J Immunol 142:57–66, 1989.

Campbell JJ, Haraldsen G, Pan J, Rottman J, Qin S, Ponath P, Andrew DP, Warnke R, Ruffing N, Kassam N, Wu L, Butcher EC. The chemokine receptor CCR4 in vascular recognition by cutaneous but not intestinal memory T cells. Nature 400:776–780, 1999.

Carlos TM, Harlan JM. Leukocyte-endothelial adhesion molecules. Blood 84:2068–2101, 1994.

Carman CV, Springer TA. A transmigratory cup in leukocyte diapedesis both through individual vascular endothelial cells and between them. J Cell Biol 167:377–388, 2004.

Cella M, Sallusto F, Lanzavecchia A. Origin, maturation and antigen presenting function of dendritic cells. Curr Opin Immunol 9:10–16, 1997.

Chvatchko Y, Hoogewerf AJ, Meyer A, Alouani S, Juillard P, Buser R, Conquet F, Proudfoot AE, Wells TN, Power CA. A key role for CC chemokine receptor 4 in lipopolysaccharide-induced endotoxic shock. J Exp Med 191:1755–1764, 2000.

Cines DB, Pollak ES, Buck CA, Loscalzo J, Zimmerman GA, McEver RP, Pober JS, Wick TM, Konkle BA, Schwartz BS, Barnathan ES, McCrae KR, Hug BA, Schmidt A-M, Stern DM. Endothelial cells in physiology and in the pathophysiology of vascular disorders. Blood 91:3527–3561, 1998.

Cook DN, Chen SC, Sullivan LM, Manfra DJ, Wiekowski MT, Prosser DM, Vassileva G, Lira SA. Generation and analysis of mice lacking the chemokine fractalkine. Mol Cell Biol 21:3159–3165, 2001.

Cronstein BN. The mechanism of action of methotrexate. Rheum Dis Clin North Am 23:739–755, 1997.

Cronstein BN, Weissmann G. The adhesion molecules of inflammation. Arthritis Rheum 36:147–157, 1993.

Cyster JG. Chemokines and cell migration in secondary lymphoid organs. Science 286:2098–2102, 1999.

Cyster JG. Chemokines, Sphingosine-1-phosphate, and cell migration in secondary lymphoid organs. Annu Rev Immunol 23:127–159, 2005.

D'Ambrosio D, Iellem A, Colantonio L, Clissi B, Pardi R, Sinigaglia F. Localization of Th-cell subsets in inflammation: differential thresholds for extravasation of Th1 and Th2 cells. Immunol Today 21:183–186, 2000.

Dejana E, Spagnuolo R, Bazzoni G. Interendothelial junctions and their role in the control of angiogenesis, vascular permeability and leukocyte transmigration. Thromb Haemost 86:308–315, 2001.

Duncan GS, Andrew DP, Takimoto H, Kaufman SA, Yoshida H, Spellberg J, Luis de la Pompa J, Elia A, Wakeham A, Karan-Tamir B, Muller WA, Senaldi G, Zukowski MM, Mak TW. Genetic evidence for functional redundancy of platelet/endothelial cell adhesion molecule-1 (PECAM-1): CD31-deficient mice reveal PECAM-1-dependent and PECAM-1-independent functions. J Immunol 162:3022–3030, 1999.

Etzioni A, Doerschuk CM, Harlan JM. Of man and mouse: leukocyte and endothelial adhesion molecule deficiencies. Blood 94:3281–3288, 1999.

Faveeuw C, Di Mauro ME, Price AA, Ager A. Roles of alpha(4) integrins/VCAM-1 and LFA-1/ICAM-1 in the binding and transendothelial migration of T lymphocytes and T lymphoblasts across high endothelial venules. Int Immunol 12:241–251, 2000.

Frendéus B, Godaly G, Hang L, Karpman D, Lundstedt A-C, Svanborg C. Interleukin 8 receptor deficiency confers susceptibility to acute experimental pyelonephritis and may have a human counterpart. J Exp Med 192:881–890, 2000.

Frenette PS, Wagner DD. Insights into selectin function from knockout mice. Thromb Haemost 78:60–64, 1997.

Fukuda M, Hiraoka N, Yeh JC. C-type lectins and sialyl Lewis X oligosaccharides. Versatile roles in cell–cell interaction. J Cell Biol 147:467–470, 1999.

Gerard C, Rollins BJ. Chemokines and disease. Nat Immunol 2:108–115, 2001.

Girard J-P, Springer TA. High endothelial venules (HEVs): specialized endothelium for lymphocyte migration. Immunol Today 16:449–457, 1995.

Gowans JL, Knight EJ. The route of re-circulation of lymphocytes in rat. Proc R Soc Lond Ser B 159:257–282, 1964.

Gretz JE, Kaldjian EP, Anderson AO, Shaw S. Sophisticated strategies for information encounter in the lymph node: the reticular network as a conduit of soluble information and a highway for cell traffic. J Immunol 157:495–499, 1996.

Gretz JE, Norbury CC, Anderson AO, Proudfoot AEI, Shaw S. Lymph-borne chemokines and other low molecular weight molecules reach high endothelial venules via specialized conduits while a functional barrier limits access to the lymphocyte microenvironments in lymph node cortex. J Exp Med 192:1425–1440, 2000.

Hemmerich S, Bistrup A, Singer MS, van Zante A, Lee JK, Tsay D, Peters M, Carminati JL, Brennan TJ, Carver-Moore K, Leviten M, Fuentes ME, Ruddle NH, Rosen SD. Sulfation of L-selectin ligands by an HEV-restricted sulfotransferase regulates lymphocyte homing to lymph nodes. Immunity 15:237–247, 2001.

Hogg N, Leitinger B. Shape and shift changes related to the function of leukocyte integrins LFA-1 and Mac-1. J Leukoc Biol 69:893–898, 2001.

Jalkanen S, Salmi M. Cell surface monoamine oxidases: enzymes in search of a function. EMBO J 20:3893–3901, 2001.

Kraal G, Mebius RE. High endothelial venules: lymphocyte traffic control and controlled traffic. Adv Immunol 65:347–395, 1997.

Kunkel EJ, Campbell JJ, Haraldsen G, Pan J, Boisvert J, Roberts AI, Ebert EC, Vierra MA, Goodman SB, Genovese MC, Wardlaw AJ, Greenberg HB, Parker CM, Butcher EC, Andrew DP, Agace WW. Lymphocyte CC chemokine receptor 9 and epithelial thymus-expressed chemokine (TECK) expression distinguish the small intestinal immune compartment: epithelial expression of tissue-specific chemokines as an organizing principle in regional immunity. J Exp Med 192:761–768, 2000.

Ley K. Functions of selectins. Results Probl Cell Differ 33:177–200, 2001.

Lowe JB. Selectin ligands, leukocyte trafficking, and fucosyltransferase genes. Kidney Int 51:1418–1426, 1997.

Mackay CR. Chemokines: immunology's high impact factors. Nat Immunol 2:95–101, 2001.

Mantovani A. The chemokine system: redundancy for robust outputs. Immunol Today 20:254–257, 1999.

McEver RP, Cummings RD. Cell adhesion in vascular biology. Role of PSGL-1 binding to selectins in leukocyte recruitment. J Clin Invest 100:485–491, 1997.

Middleton J, Neil S, Wintle J, Clark-Lewis I, Moore H, Lam C, Auer M, Hub E, Rot A. Transcytosis and surface presentation of IL-8 by venular endothelial cells. Cell 91:385–395, 1997.

Moser B, Loetscher P. Lymphocyte traffic control by chemokines. Nat Immunol 2:123–128, 2001.

Newman PJ. The biology of PECAM-1. J Clin Invest 99:3–7, 1997.

Pabst R. The spleen in lymphocyte migration. Immunol Today 9:43–45, 1988.

Protin U, Schweighoffer T, Jochum W, Hilberg F. CD44-deficient mice develop normally with changes in subpopulations and recirculation of lymphocyte subsets. J Immunol 163:4917–4923, 1999.

Resta R, Yamashita Y, Thompson LF. Ecto-enzyme and signaling functions of lymphocyte CD73. Immunol Rev 161:95–109, 1998.

Robert C, Kupper TS. Inflammatory skin diseases, T cells, and immune surveillance. N Engl J Med 341:1817–1828, 1999.

Rosen SD. Endothelial ligands for L-selectin: from lymphocyte recirculation to allograft rejection. Am J Pathol 155:1013–1020, 1999.

Sallusto F, Lenig D, Forster R, Lipp M, Lanzavecchia A. Two subsets of memory T lymphocytes with distinct homing potentials and effector functions. Nature 401:708–712, 1999.

Salmi M, Alanen K, Grenman S, Briskin M, Butcher EC, Jalkanen S. Immune cell trafficking in utero and early life is dominated by the mucosal addressin MAdCAM-1 in man. Gastroenterology, 121:853–864, 2001.

Salmi M, Jalkanen S. How do lymphocytes know where to go: current concepts and enigmas of lymphocyte homing. Adv Immunol 64:139–218, 1997.

Salmi M, Jalkanen S. VAP-1: an adhesin and an enzyme. Trends Immunol 22:211–216, 2001.

Sánchez-Madrid F, del Pozo MA. Leukocyte polarization in cell migration and immune interactions. EMBO J 18:501–511, 1999.

Shimizu Y, Rose DM, Ginsberg MH. Integrins in the immune system. Adv Immunol 72:325–380, 1999.

Siegelman MH, DeGrendele HC, Estess P. Activation and interaction of CD44 and hyaluronan in immunological systems. J Leukoc Biol 66:315–321, 1999.

Spencer J, MacDonald TT, Finn T, Isaacson PG. The development of gut associated lymphoid tissue in the terminal ileum of fetal human intestine. Clin Exp Immunol 64:536–543, 1986.

Springer TA. Traffic signals for lymphocyte recirculation and leukocyte emigration: the multistep paradigm. Cell 76:301–314, 1994.

Stockton BM, Cheng G, Manjunath N, Ardman B, von Andrian UH. Negative regulation of T cell homing by CD43. Immunity 8:373–381, 1998.

Syrbe U, Siveke J, Hamann A. Th1/Th2 subsets: distinct differences in homing and chemokine receptor expression? Springer Semin Immunopathol 21:263–285, 1999.

Thrasher AJ, Jones GE, Kinnon C, Brickell PM, Katz DR. Is Wiskott-Aldrich syndrome a cell trafficking disorder? Immunol Today 19:537–539, 1998.

Vestweber D, Blanks JE. Mechanisms that regulate the function of the selectins and their ligands. Physiol Rev 79:181–213, 1999.

Wagner N, Müller W. Functions of α4- and β7-integrins in hematopoiesis, lymphocyte trafficking and organ development. Curr Top Microbiol Immunol 231:23–32, 1998.

Wang J, Springer TA. Structural specializations of immunoglobulin superfamily members for adhesion to integrins and viruses. Immunol Rev 163:197–215, 1998.

Watson SR, Bradley LM. The recirculation of naive and memory lymphocytes. Cell Adhes Commun 6:105–110, 1998.

Weissman IL. Translating stem and progenitor cell biology to the clinic: barriers and opportunities. Science 287:1442–1446, 2000.

Yang J, Hirata T, Croce K, Merrill-Skoloff G, Tchernychev B, Williams E, Flaumenhaft R, Furie BC, Furie B. Targeted gene disruption demonstrates that P-selectin glycoprotein ligand 1 (PSGL-1) is required for P-selectin-mediated but not E-selectin-mediated neutrophil rolling and migration. J Exp Med 190:1769–1782, 1999.

Zlotnik A, Morales J, Hedrick JA. Recent advances in chemokines and chemokine receptors. Crit Rev Immunol 19:1–47, 1999.

8

Phagocytic System

KUENDER D. YANG, PAUL G. QUIE, and HARRY R. HILL

Phagocytes were initially thought to be harmful to the host, contributing to the untoward consequences of infection and inflammation. In 1898, Metchnikoff first suggested that "the essential and primary element in typical inflammation consists in a reaction of the phagocyte against a harmful agent." After establishing that phagocytes were helpful in defense against bacteria, Metchnikoff predicted that defects in phagocyte function might predispose the host to increased numbers and severity of infections due to microorganisms. Patients with decreased phagocyte counts or with phagocyte functional defects do, in fact, have recurrent or even fatal infections as well as impaired wound healing. Moreover, evidence has also accumulated demonstrating that aberrant phagocyte activation can contribute to untoward complications of inflammation. Functional defects in phagocytes can lead to recurrent cutaneous abscesses, periodontitis, paronychia, pneumonitis, osteomyelitis, and occasionally life-threatening sepsis. Aberrant phagocyte activation may result in the adult respiratory distress syndrome (ARDS), disseminated intravascular coagulation (DIC), and reperfusion injury. The kinetics of phagocyte production as well as the activation and function of phagocytes has been elucidated for the most part. Upon stimulation by colony-stimulating factors including stem cell factor (SCF), granulocyte-monocyte colony–stimulating factor (GM-CSF), granulocyte colony–stimulating factor (G-CSF), or interleukin-3 (IL-3), phagocyte precursors proliferate and differentiate under the control of certain transcription factors such as purine-rich DNA sequence binding protein (PU.1) and CAAT enhancer binding protein, α isoform (C/EBPα), for granulocytic differentiation, as well as PU.1 and mammary cell–activating factor B (c-MafB), for monocytic differentiation in the bone marrow (Tian et al., 1996). Corticosteroids, complement fragments (C3e, C3dg), and adrenergic neurotransmitters (epinephrine, norepinephrine) accelerate the release of mature phagocytes into the peripheral blood where they circulate and marginate along capillary endothelial surfaces. Adhesive glycoproteins including selectins such as P-selectin, L-selectin, and E-selectin as well as integrins such as fibronectin and complement receptors (CR3 and CR4) promote phagocyte adhesion. Selectins are involved in granulocyte rolling in the blood circulation, while integrins mediate adhesiveness and phagocyte extravasation. In response to chemoattractants such as C5a, IL-8, monocyte chemotactic factor, leukotrienes, and bacterial formylated peptides, phagocytes mobilize and enter tissues and inflammatory sites where they interact with and ingest target organisms, especially if these are coated with immunoglobulin and/or complement. This interaction of phagocytes with microbes is followed by ingestion, degranulation, and respiratory burst activity resulting in extracellular and intracellular killing of the target as well as inflammatory changes in the tissues. Monocytic phagocytes can also differentiate into dendritic cells that present antigens and secrete cytokines to promote optimal T lymphocyte differentiation and activation. Defects or unregulated activation in any aspect of the above phagocytic responses may result in immunodeficiency diseases with associated infections or serious inflammatory disorders. A variety of in vivo, ex vivo, and in vitro studies have resulted in the definition of these disorders and, in some cases, in the development of effective therapeutic regimens. As progress in the characterization of phagocyte activation pathways and function is made, immunopharmacological intervention, bone marrow transplantation, and potential gene therapy may offer hope to many of these patients. Prenatal diagnoses employing restriction fragment length polymorphism, polymerase chain reaction techniques, analysis of X-chromosome inactivation, measurement of gene products, and assessment of granulocyte function in fetal blood make these diseases potentially identifiable and/or treatable in utero or shortly after birth.

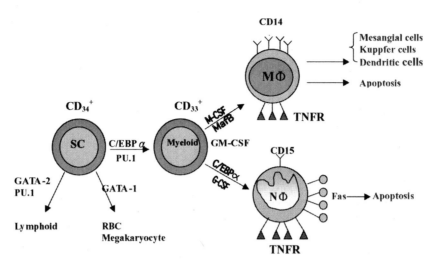

Figure 8.1. Differentiation of granulocytes and monocytes from myeloid progenitors. Myeloid progenitors derived from CD34+ stem cells (SC) display CD33+ under the influence of certain nuclear transcription factors. C/EBPα (CAAT enhancer binding protein, α isoform) and PU.1 (purine-rich DNA sequence binding protein) are the key transcription factors for myeloid cell lineage differentiation. Monocyte differentiation is further controlled by macrophage colony–stimulating factor (M-CSF) and expression of mammary cell-activating factor B (c-MafB), whereas granulocyte differentiation is influenced by C/EBPα expression and granulocyte colony–stimulating factor (G-CSF) stimulation. In contrast, differentiation of lymphocytes is mainly affected by GATA-2 expression and differentiation of red blood cells (RBC) is mainly affected by GATA-1 expression. MΦ, resident macrophages; NΦ, resident neutrophils; TNFR, tumor necrosis factor receptor.

Development and Distribution of Phagocytic System

There is evidence that human myelopoiesis occurs early in fetal life, as early as 6–8 weeks of gestational age (Rosenthal et al., 1983). Phagocyte progenitor cells arise from pluripotential hematopoietic stem cells in the bone marrow or in vitro agar culture systems. Bone marrow progenitor cells have been shown to grow into different colonies known as colony-forming units (CFU) granulocyte-monocyte (CFU-GM), granulocyte (CFU-G), and eosinophil (CFU-Eo) (Iscove et al., 1971; Clark and Kamen, 1987). These precursors can give rise to mature phagocytes, including polymorphonuclear granulocytes and mononuclear phagocytes, under the influence of colony stimulation factors (CSFs) such as SCF, GM-CSF, G-CSF, and IL-3. These growth and differentiation factors are derived mostly from the stromal cells in the bone marrow, while some are produced by myeloid cells in the reticuloendothelial system (reviewed by Yang and Hill, 1991, 2001). The differentiation of myeloid progenitors into mature phagocytes probably results in part from the acquisition of specific factor receptors on the cells at different phases of differentiation and maturation. Interaction of lectins on the stromal cells with receptors on phagocyte precursors may be involved in the process of growth and differentiation (Aizawa and Tavassoli, 1987; Nangia-Makker et al., 1993). A number of suppressing mechanisms, by contrast, including endocrine factors such as corticosteroids, erythropoietin levels, and cytokines from lymphoid and myeloid cells, have been shown to provide negative feedback signals. These endocrine factors and paracrine cytokines apparently play a central role in the bone marrow in keeping appropriate homeostasis and cellularity at a myeloid/erythroid (M/E) ratio between 1:3 and 1:4. The molecular mechanism to explain the commitment to different lineages has been recently deciphered. The concept that transcription factors rather than cytokine receptor signals are the early determinants of lineage commitment has been emphasized (Ward et al., 2000). As shown in Figure 8.1, transcriptional factors PU.1 and C/EBPα promote G-CSF receptor expression and induce terminal differentiation of granulocytes (Smith et al., 1996; Keeshan et al., 2003), whereas PU.1 and c-MafB promote monocytic differentiation (Hegde et al., 1999; Ward et al., 2000; McIvor et al., 2003). Moreover, the switch of stem cells to a myeloid-committed lineage is also mediated by the interaction between these transcriptional factors. Zhang et al. (1999) showed that GATA-1 repressed PU.1 expression and induced erythroid differentiation, but not myeloid differentiation. Similarly, the interaction of GATA-1 with C/EBPs specifically regulates eosinophil lineage differentiation (McNagny et al., 1998).

Phagocytes from a 20-week gestational-age fetus were found to have active phagocytic and respiratory burst activity. Phagocytes from full-term newborns, however, do not have complete functional activity. Neonatal granulocytes and monocytes have defects in bone marrow storage pools, cellular activation, and chemotaxis (Christensen et al., 1980, 1986; Marodi et al., 1984; Sacchi and Hill, 1984; Newton et al., 1989; Hill et al., 1991). Studies with adult phagocytes have indicated that a variety of cytokines and glycoproteins can modulate phagocyte functions. These results suggest that intact phagocyte function is due to intrinsic maturation but also modulated by environmental factors that alter the biochemical and physiological status of phagocytes. It is often necessary, therefore, to differentiate developmental defects from abnormalities due to extrinsic environmental factors.

Distribution of Granulocytes

Granulocytes are produced in the bone marrow and released into the blood and tissues where they act as the first line of defense in host resistance and wound healing. The total granulocyte pool is divided into two compartments: the bone marrow and the circulating pools. The bone marrow provides the environment for the proliferation of myeloblasts, promyelocytes, and myelocytes as well as maturation of metamyelocytes and band form granulocytes. The latter two populations represent the main marrow storage pool of granulocyte precursors containing $6–8 \times 10^9$ cells/kg bodyweight. The recycling and the proliferation and maturation phases of granulocytes in bone marrow require 2–3 days and 7–10 days, respectively (Yang and Hill, 1993). In the blood, granulocytes are in the circulating $(0.3–0.4 \times 10^9$ cells/kg) and marginating pools $(0.4 \times 10^9$ cells/kg). Endotoxin, corticosteroids, and complement fragments (C3e, C3d,g) cause accelerated release of mature granulocytes from bone marrow into the blood. Adrenergic neurotransmitters such as epinephrine and norepinephrine can promote blood granulocyte mobilization from the marginating pool into the circulatory pool. Granulocytes in the circulation have a short life span with a half-life of 6–8 hours. In spite of this short half-life, granulocyte numbers in the blood are normally maintained between 3000 and 6000 cells/mm^3.

Distribution of Monocytes and Macrophages

Monoblasts are the first recognizable cells of the monocyte series in the bone marrow. There are, however, few monoblasts found in the bone marrow since their storage pool is relatively small. The transit time from a monoblast to a monocyte takes approximately 6 days (Groopman and Golde, 1981). Promonocytes are the prominent cells of the monocyte series in the bone marrow and comprise a major storage pool containing 6×10^8 cells/kg (Johnston, 1988). Promonocytes mature into monocytes in the bone marrow and are released into the blood within 2 days. Circulating monocytes in the blood make up 3%–6% of the total leukocytes or about 300–600 cells/mm^3 $(0.3–0.6 \times 10^9$ cells/L), while three to four times as many monocytes mobilize in the marginating pool. These monocytes leave the circulation with a half-life of 1–3 days (Groopman and Golde, 1981; Johnston, 1988; Yang and Hill, 1993). Approximately 10^8 monocytes are released into the blood and randomly leave for the tissues every day. These monocytes may differentiate into dendritic cells in the blood and tissues in the presence of cytokines such as GM-CSF and IL-4 (Hashimoto et al., 2000). Monocytes can develop into myeloid dendritic cells bearing CD11c and CD14, different from plasmacytoid dendritic cells with a unique marker CD123 (Facchetti and Vermi, 2002; Doni et al., 2003). Myeloid dendritic cells and plasmacytoid dendritic cells not only display different cell surface markers but also produce individual mediators for priming T lymphocyte differentiation (Langenkamp et al., 2003). They can also transform into a variety of tissue macrophages, depending on dif-

ferent conditions in the tissues. The monocyte–macrophage system is widely distributed to a number of organs: microglial cells in the brain, Kupffer cells in the liver, osteoclasts in the bone marrow, Langerhans cells in the skin, mesangial cells in the kidney, and resident macrophages in lungs, spleen, thymus, lymph nodes, pleural and peritoneal cavities, and joint spaces. Macrophages may stay in tissues for a few months or even years. During acute inflammation, the transit time of monocytes from the bone marrow to the inflammatory tissue may be shortened from 2 days to 6–8 hours. In contrast to granulocytes, which do not replicate in the circulation or tissues, both circulating monocytes and tissue macrophages are able to replicate rapidly. In chronic inflammation, especially in a variety of granulomatous disorders, tissue macrophages may transform into giant cells or epithelioid cells in the presence of tumor necrosis factor alpha (TNF-α) and interferon gamma (IFN-γ) (Groopman and Golde, 1981; Johnston, 1988).

Activation and Function of Granulocytes

Granulocyte Activation

Granulocytes respond to a variety of solid and soluble stimuli via nonspecific and specific interactions. Nonspecific interactions including hydrogen bonds, van der Waals, hydrostatic and hydrophobic forces between cells, which along with soluble stimuli, may induce changes in membrane conformation. Specific ligation of ligands to specific receptors on granulocytes can also cause conformational changes in the plasma membrane that consequently mediates signal transduction, resulting in cytoskeleton reorganization, adhesion, respiratory burst activity, degranulation, movement, and phagocytosis. The kinetics of signal transduction is organized as shown in Figure 8.2. Ligation of chemokine or complement receptors (e.g., CXCR, C5aR) or Fc receptors (FcRIII, CD16) on the surface of granulocytes activates a pertussis toxin (PT)-sensitive G protein that directly or indirectly induces cytoskeleton (microfilament and microtubule) reorganization and stimulates phospholipase C (PLC) activation, resulting in hydrolysis of phosphatidylinositol (PI) into inositol 1,4,5-trisphosphate (IP$_3$) and 1,3-diacylglycerol (DAG) in a few seconds (Sandborg and Smolen, 1988). IP$_3$ elicits intracellular calcium mobilization that can promote respiratory burst activity and cell degranulation. DAG activates protein kinase C (PKC) to induce cellular activation through the phosphorylation of enzymes or regulatory proteins, which control cell adhesion and

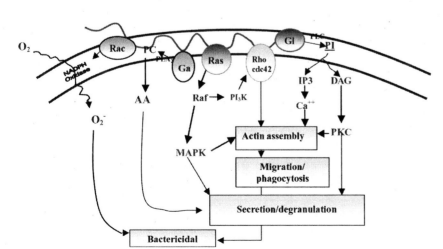

Figure 8.2. Activation and function of granulocytes. Granulocyte cell surface receptors such as chemokine (CXCR), complement (C5aR), and antibody Fc (FcRIII) receptors transduce signals for cell mobilization, phagocytosis, degranulation, and bactericidal activity upon activation. For details, see text. AA, arachidonic acid; DAG, diacylglycerol; Gi, GTP binding protein; IP3, inositol triphosphate; MAPK, mitogen-activated protein kinases; PC, phosphatidylcholine; PI, phosphatidylinositol; PI3K, phosphoinositol 3 kinase; PKC, protein kinase C; PLA2, phospholipase A2; PLC, phospholipase C; Ras, Raf, Rac, Rho, and Cdc42 are small GTP binding proteins.

locomotion. Several lines of evidence, however, indicate that stimulus–response transduction of signal may be mediated by systems other than the PT-sensitive G protein system. For instance, we have found that fibronectin-induced actin organization was also mediated by a PT-sensitive G protein pathway (Yang et al., 1994), whereas Southwick and coworkers (1989a) showed that leukocyte adhesion–induced actin polymerization was mediated by a PT-insensitive pathway. In addition, evidence suggests that hydrolysis of arachidonic acid (AA) and platelet-activating factor (PAF) from membrane phosphatidylcholine (PC) upon granulocyte activation is associated with activation of phospholipase A2 (PLA2), but not PT-sensitive G protein–mediated PLC (Sandborg and Smolen, 1988). Guanine nucleotide–stimulated NADPH oxidase activity is not sensitive to pertussis or cholera toxin (Gabig et al., 1987). A small GTP binding protein, p21 Rac, has been shown to be involved in the NADPH oxidase activation (Wientjes et al., 1996). Similarly, other small G proteins such as Rho and Ras-related Cdc42 GTP binding protein (Cdc42) are also involved in leukocyte adhesion and cytoskeleton organization (Dash et al., 1995; Nobes and Hall, 1995; Hildebrand et al., 1996). These data indicate that there are at least five different G proteins involved in the receptor–response transduction of signal for granulocyte activation and several secondary messengers coupled to these G proteins for signal regulation. Thus, it seems likely that granulocytes are specifically regulated in a variety of inflammatory reactions via different signal transduction pathways. In summary, activation of granulocytes requires several integrated signal pathways. A small G protein, Rac2, is specifically involved in triggering respiratory burst activity (Wientjes et al., 1996). A GTPase, Cdc42, together with Wiskott-Aldrich syndrome protein (WASP) activates actin assembly (Higgs and Pollard, 2000). Another small G protein, Ras, regulates phosphatidylinositol-3-kinase (PI3K) activities for coordination of granulocyte migration (Knall et al., 1997). Moreover, different G proteins can be coupled to different receptors and mediate the degranulation of granulocytes (Cokcroft and Sutchfield, 1989). The differentiation and activation of granulocytes are also regulated by mitogen-activated protein kinases (MAPKs) such as p38 and MEK signaling (Kim and Rikihisa, 2002; Miranda et al., 2002). Further exploration of granulocyte activation will likely contribute to the development of pharmacological intervention in treating certain inflammatory disorders.

Granulocyte Recognition and Adhesion

Generally, granulocytes function as scavengers in the blood circulation and tissues (reviewed by Yang and Hill, 1993, 2001). Adhesive glycoproteins on granulocytes including selectins, such as L-selectin and P-selectin, as well as integrins, such as fibronectin receptors and complement receptors (CR3 and CR4), direct granulocytes to specific locations and promote granulocyte adhesion and subsequent migration (see Chapter 38). Selectins are involved in granulocyte rolling in the blood circulation, whereas integrins mediate firm adhesion and granulocyte extravasation (Springer, 1990; Long, 1992). Environmental factors can affect the expression of integrin molecules on endothelial cells, promoting adhesion of granulocytes to endothelium, which is a prerequisite for granulocyte diapedesis and emigration into tissues. These factors include GM-CSF, IFN-γ, endotoxin, TNF-α, IL-1, IL-8, leukotriene B4 (LTB4), PAF, bacterial formylated peptides, such as formyl Met-Leu-Phe (fMLP) and C5a.

Granulocyte Migration

Granulocytes are capable of movement in a stimulated, random fashion called *chemokinesis* and in a directional migration pattern called *chemotaxis*. Following exposure to soluble or solid stimuli, the cytoskeleton of granulocytes is reoriented to regulate cell locomotion (Valerius et al., 1981). The cytoskeleton network in granulocytes, which is somewhat similar to that of muscle cells, is composed of actin and myosin as well as the structural protein tubulin, which makes up microtubules (Valerius et al., 1981; Oliver and Berlin, 1983). Assembly and disassembly of the cytoskeleton in granulocytes modulate cell locomotion in an exchangeable dynamic "gel sol" reaction. This gel sol reaction is affected by the interaction of ligands with receptors and regulated by receptor-signaling systems. A series of small G proteins such as Rho, Rac, and Cdc42 are known to mediate changes in the cytoskeleton and cell motility (Nobes and Hall, 1995). The Cdc42 that possesses GTPase activity promotes actin polymerization, whereas WASP is the effector for the Cdc42 GTPase and acts as a link between Cdc42 and the cytoskeleton (see Chapter 31; Kolluri et al., 1996; Symons et al., 1996). Mutation of WASP may impair cytoskeleton structure, resulting in dysfunction of leukocyte migration seen in patients with Wiskott-Aldrich syndrome reviewed by Ochs and Notarangelo 2005; see Chapter 31). In response to chemoattractants such as C5a, IL-8, PAF, leukotrienes, and fMLP, granulocytes reorganize their cytoskeleton and migrate into tissues and inflammatory sites where they interact with target organisms. This is followed by phagocytosis, respiratory burst activity, and degranulation.

Phagocytosis

The mechanism by which phagocytes ingest microorganisms involves two distinct stages: adhesion (attachment) and internalization. Attachment is mediated by specific ligand–receptor interactions and nonspecific bonds due to hydrophilic and hydrophobic interactions. Internalization results from a zippering process in which circumferential attachment of phagocyte receptors to the target forms an engulfed pouch that is subsequently fused to phagocytic granules. Attachment may be indistinguishable from engulfment when examined by light microscope. Experimental evidence has shown, however, that attachment and ingestion can be separated. When opsonins are not present, attachment may not be followed by ingestion. In addition, different types as well as the status of surface receptors on the phagocytes affect the efficiency of ingestion. Complement receptors (CR1, CR3) and IgG antibody receptors (FcγR) on granulocytes are the major receptors responsible for phagocytosis. FcγRs mediate phagocytosis but different classes of FcγRs (FcγR, I, II, III) may have different efficiencies. Certain FcγRs even play an inhibitory function on phagocyte activation and inflammatory regulation (Dietrich et al., 2000). Granulocytes may also take up microbes via nonspecific intercellular interactions (surface phagocytosis) that help humans survive exposure to invasive microorganisms before they develop specific antibodies.

Respiratory Burst Activity

During membrane perturbation or phagocytosis, granulocytes are activated to induce respiratory burst activity in which reactive oxygen intermediates are formed, resulting in oxygen-dependent bactericidal activities and killing of extracellular and intracellular organisms (see Chapter 37). The respiratory burst is triggered

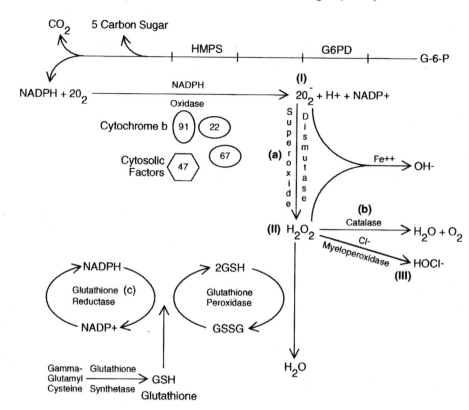

Figure 8.3. Respiratory burst pathways and recycling mechanisms in the phagocyte system. Upon phagocyte activation, cytosolic factors such as p47phox and p67phox are translocated into the plasma membrane in association with the membrane-bound flavocytochrome b_{558} involving a p91 heavy chain and a p22 light chain to transport electrons from NADPH to O_2, resulting of O^- production followed by H_2O_2 and OH^- formation. (I), (II), and (III) represent major respiratory burst activation pathways in phagocytes, whereas (a), (b), and (c) represent major antioxidative recycling pathways. GSH, reduced glutathione; GSSG, oxidized glutathione; G-6-P, glucose-6-phosphate; G6PD, glucose 6-phosphate dehydrogenase; HMP, hexose monophosphate shunt. (Derived with permission from Yang and Hill, J Pediatr 119:343, 1991.)

by activation of an NADPH oxidase coupled to a respiratory chain on the cell surface after translocation of cytosolic factors (Bjerrum and Borregaard, 1989). Respiratory burst activity associated with phagocyte activation is elicited by NADPH oxidase, which is composed of a flavocytochrome b_{558} associated with a gp91phox heavy chain and a p22phox light chain in the plasma membrane as well as cytosolic proteins, including p40phox, p47phox, p67phox, and a small G protein, p21 Rac (Wientjes et al., 1996). The membrane-bound flavocytochrome b_{558}, in conjunction with certain cytosolic factors after activation, serves to transport an electron from NADPH to O_2, resulting in O_2 (superoxide) formation (Fig. 8.3). Reactive oxygen intermediates including O_2^-, H_2O_2, and OH are produced, resulting in intracellular microbial killing. These oxygen radicals can also result in auto-oxidation and damage to the granulocyte itself and the surrounding tissues. Granulocytes, however, have several scavenger systems—superoxide dismutase (SOD), catalase, and glutathione reductase—to protect themselves from the oxidative injury. An imbalance between free radicals and endogenous scavengers has been implicated in many harmful processes associated with infections (Baehner et al., 1972; Cooper et al., 1972), endothelial damage (McCord et al., 1994; Bratt and Gyllenhammer, 1995), autoimmune diseases (Lefkowitz et al., 1995), and reperfusion injury (Siminiak et al., 1995). Thus, exogenous scavengers such as β-carotene, *N*-acetylcysteine, and vitamins A, C, and E have been suggested to prevent these disorders (Boxer et al., 1979; Jain et al., 1994; Pejaver and Watson, 1994). In addition to oxygen radicals, nitric oxide (NO) production has also been implicated in the function of granulocytes (Larfars and Gyllenhammer, 1998). However, the biologic role of NO production in human macrophages has been questioned (Harvey, 2000). Mouse macrophages appear to kill intracellular organisms such as *Mycobacterium tuberculosis* with NO. In contrast, human macrophages do not appear to use this mechanism, but use

another unknown mechanism mediated by a toll-like receptor (Thoma-Uszynski et al., 2001).

Degranulation

In addition to oxygen-dependent bactericidal activity, granulocytes undergo degranulation, which contributes to oxygen-independent bactericidal activity and modulation of tissue inflammation. Release of azurophilic granule contents such as myeloperoxidase, cationic protein, and acid hydrolases can potentiate the digestive and microbicidal activities of phagocytes, called *oxygen-independent cytotoxicity* (Spitznagel and Shafer, 1985). A cationic protein of approximately 55 kDa designated *bacterial/permeability-increasing protein* (BPI) contributes to killing of gram-negative bacteria but also binds to endotoxin, resulting in inhibition of inflammation (Froon et al., 1995). Secretion of secondary granules containing lysozyme (also found in azurophilic granules), collagenase, and lactoferrin also helps to regulate inflammation (Sandborg and Smolen, 1988; Yang and Hill, 1993). In addition, degranulation of tertiary granules is usually concomitantly associated with translocation of fresh receptors (CR1, CR3, fMLP, and laminin receptors), NADPH oxidase, and cytochrome b_{558} into the plasma membrane (Borregaard and Tauber, 1984; Miller et al., 1987; Sandborg, and Smolen 1988; Bjerrum and Borregaard, 1989). Membrane translocation of these receptors modulates granulocyte adhesion, movement, phagocytosis, and respiratory burst activity. The mechanism by which granulocytes undergo degranulation is closely related to ionic mobilization, microfilament rearrangement (Boyles and Bainton, 1979), and microtubule assembly (Oliver and Berlin, 1983). Factors that can affect membrane perturbation, signal transduction, and metabolic activity regulate the degranulation process. On the other hand, self-protection and prevention of tissue damage from the destructive granular contents may also result from antiprotease activities in the plasma and from protease inhibitors produced by other leukocytes (Kloczko et al., 1990; van de Winkel et al., 1990; Mohacsi et al., 1992; Allen and Tracy, 1995).

Granulocyte Apoptosis

Granulocytes tend to have a short half-life in blood circulation. Granulocyte cell death is mediated by the paracrine interaction of the programed death ligand Fas (FasL) with the death receptor Fas on the cell surface, leading to granulocyte apoptosis (Liles et al., 1996). Soluble FasL or cytokines that bind or regulate Fas expression on the cell surface may also cause granulocytes to either survive or undergo apoptosis (Villunger et al., 2000; see Chapter 24). Briefly, the granulocyte death program starts with ligand–receptor interaction, which is coupled to a signal cascade related to mitochondrial function. This is accompanied by cytochrome-c leakage, resulting in caspase-3 activation and irreversible nuclear condensation and DNA fragmentation (Susin et al., 1999). Promotion or inhibition of granulocyte apoptosis might be used as a potential strategy to modulate granulocytopoiesis and treat infectious or inflammatory diseases in the future.

Granulocyte Modulation of Inflammatory Reactions

There is also evidence that granulocytes have an important role in inflammatory and degenerative reactions resulting from tissue injury, tumor invasion, viral infection, autoimmune disorders, aging, and atherosclerosis. Enhancement of granulocyte adhesiveness to endothelium may result from thermal injury, hypoxia, bacterial sepsis, and immune complex disorders. Upon traumatic injury, platelets adhere and aggregate on the vascular endothelium and subsequently release chemotactic factors such as LTB4, transforming growth factor-β (TGF-β), and platelet-derived growth factors. This results in a rapid recruitment of granulocytes and fibroblasts that have a central role in tissue inflammation and wound healing (De Gaetano et al., 1989; Tsjugi et al., 1994). Thermal injury, hypoxia, and bacterial sepsis may cause adult respiratory distress syndrome, which likely results from enhanced and sustained granulocyte adhesiveness and release of toxic granulocyte-derived mediators (Dale, 1975; McCord et al., 1994). Immune complexes, either alone or associated with complement activation, may also promote granulocyte influx, adhesiveness, respiratory burst activity, and degranulation, and contribute to vasculitis and autoimmune inflammatory reactions (Bratt and Gyllenhammer, 1995; Lefkowitz et al., 1995). Cationic proteins released during degranulation are also implicated in bactericidal and cellular cytotoxicity. Furthermore, granulocytes have been shown to have antiviral properties (Roberts et al., 1994) and to mediate antibody-dependent cellular cytotoxicity (ADCC) against tumors (Vaickus et al., 1990; Kushner and Cheung, 1991), especially in the presence of cytokines such as the interferons and GM-CSF. Defects or abnormal activation in any aspect of the above granulocyte responses may result in immunodeficiency diseases or serious inflammatory disorders.

Activation and Function of Monocytes and Macrophages

Monocytes develop into tissue macrophages, possessing diverse morphology and functions dependent on environment and immunologic factors. Mononuclear phagocytes, similar to polymorphonuclear granulocytes, can move toward foreign invaders and denatured tissues and destroy them by ingestion, degranulation, and respiratory burst activity. Upon maturation into macrophages, cells of the monocyte series show increases in size, adhesiveness, and functional receptors (e.g., CR1, CR3, FcRI, and FcRII), resulting in enhancement of phagocytosis (Johnston, 1988; Newman et al., 1991). Some evidence indicates that cells of the monocyte series have relatively low microbicidal activity in comparison to granulocytes (Mathy-Hartert et al., 1996). These macrophages lose their myeloperoxidase (MPO), which mediates a potent microbicidal activity by catalyzing halides into halous acid. Loss of MPO may be a differential milestone by which harmless contact between cells of the monocyte series and other immune cells occurs. Lectin-like receptors as well as receptors for lipoproteins are mainly found on macrophages but not monocytes (Nangia-Makker et al., 1993; Watanabe et al., 1994). Defects in the former receptors may impair nonimmunologically mediated reticuloendothelial clearance, while dysregulation of lipoprotein uptake by macrophages may give rise to atherosclerosis.

In addition to the professional function of phagocytosis, cells of the monocyte series have a central role in the modulation of inflammation and tissue repair (De Gaetano et al., 1989; Tsuji et al., 1994). Upon activation, monocytes ingest particles, produce reactive oxygen molecules, release procoagulant factors, cytokines, and granules, and express adhesive molecules and Ia antigens. One of the most potent macrophage activators is IFN-γ. Deficiency of IFN-γ receptors or a defect in IFN-γ production due to IL-12 or IL-12 receptor deficiency can compromise intracellular mycobacterial killing by macrophages (Altare et al., 1998; Jouanguy et al., 1999; see chapter 28). Procoagulant factors from monocytes or macrophages are involved in coagulation and homeostasis (Carson et al., 1991; Spillert and Lazaro, 1991). Granules from the monocyte series contain lysozymes, proteases, elastase, and collagenase that may augment tissue damage. In contrast, granules containing $α_1$-protease inhibitor, $β_2$-macroglobulin, and IL-1 receptor antagonists from monocytes may provide a mechanism to protect tissues from damage (Kloczko et al., 1990; van de Winkel et al., 1990; Mohacsi et al., 1992; Allen and Tracy, 1995). Cytokines of the monocyte series act in an endocrine (affecting distant cells after bloodstream transportation), paracrine (affecting adjacent cells), and autocrine (affecting themselves) fashion. For instance, IL-1 can act in an endocrine fashion on the regulation of body temperature and sleep patterns in the hypothalamus. Paracrine cytokines of monocyte series include CSFs (GM-CSF, G-CSF, M-CSF, erythropoietin [EPO]), IL-12, TNF-α, and TGF-β, which are all known to be involved in immune regulation (Chehimi and Trinchieri, 1994; Matsumoto, 1995). Some of the cytokines also act in an autocrine manner on cells of the monocyte series themselves. For example, ligation of M-CSF to its receptor (a c-fms proto-oncogene product) on monocytes induces monocyte differentiation, activation, and proliferation (Horiguchi et al., 1986). Furthermore, cells of the monocyte series are the only cell population in the phagocyte series to express both major histocompatibility complex (MHC) class I and class II antigens (Ia antigens). Antigens are taken up by the monocyte/macrophage series and processed via biochemical and physical reactions. Dendritic cells derived from monocytes or other lineage cells are particularly effective on the antigen presentation to T cells (Facchetti et al., 2002; Doni et al., 2003). They are termed *professional antigen-presenting cells* (Cao et al., 2000). The antigens are presented as peptides associated with MHC molecules that lymphocyte antigen receptors recognize. Cells of the monocyte series bearing antigen/MHC class I complexes can be recognized and killed by cytotoxic T cells, whereas those bearing antigen/MHC class II molecules interact with helper T cells, resulting in clonal expansion of lymphocytes. Cytokines such as IL-2, IL-4, IL-5, IL-10, and IFN-γ produced by lymphocytes may act in an autocrine or paracrine fashion to amplify or suppress proliferation of lymphocyte subpopulations. Eicosanoids such as prostaglandin E2 (PGE2), cytokines (e.g., IL-12, TNF-α, TGF-β), and β2-macroglobulin from the monocyte series also have immunomodulating functions (van de Winkel et al., 1990; Chu et al., 1991; Hayes et al., 1995; Raab et al., 1995). Dysregulation in the antigen-presenting process may cause immunodeficiency and autoimmune diseases. Abnormal regulation of osteoclast differentiation and activation in the bone marrow by osteoprotegrin (Simonet et al., 1997), TNF-related activation-induced cytokine (TRANCE) (Wang et al., 1999), receptor activator of NFκB ligand (RANKL) (Koga et al., 2004), and osteopodin (Ishijima et al., 2001) have been implicated in osteopetrosis and osteoporosis.

Integration and Interaction of Phagocytes in Host Defense

There are two major pathways involved in host defense by leukocytes against exogenous microorganisms and endogenous debris or transformed tissues and cells (Fig. 8.4). In response to microbial invasion or tissue damage, granulocytes are attracted into areas by bacterial peptides, complement fragments such as C5a, or platelet-derived chemoattractants such as PAF and LTB4. Infiltration of granulocytes may result in clearance of microbes and tissue debris. If granulocytes fail to clear the infection or the tissue debris, activated granulocytes release monocyte chemotactic factors including fibronectin (Kreis et al., 1989) and monocyte

chemoattractant protein1 (MCP-1) (Wuyts et al., 1994), also called CC chemokine ligand-2 (CCL2), to attract monocytes (Doherty et al., 1990). Monocytes recruited into the area are able to release monokines such as IL-1, IL-10, IL-12, TGF-β and TNF-α to enhance lymphocyte infiltration and present antigens to lymphocytes for specific lymphocyte transformation (Chehimi and Trinchieri, 1994; Hayes et al., 1995; Matsumoto, 1995). Monocytes and their derived dendritic cells bearing toll-like receptors (TLRs) are responsible for bacterial and viral recognition and signal transduction for a link between innate and adaptive lymphocyte differentiation and activation (Coccia et al., 2004; Kim et al., 2004; Netea et al., 2004). Lymphocyte differentiation and activation may result in a cell-mediated immune reaction (Th1 reaction) and/or T-dependent humoral reactions (Th2 reaction). Th1, Th2, and regulatory T cells (Treg) can regulate one another through a cytokine network in which Th1 cytokines IFNγ and TNFβ promote cell-mediated immunity and suppress humoral immunity, Th2 cytokines IL-4 and IL-13 promote humoral immunity and suppress Th1 reaction, and Treg cytokines IL-10 and TGFβ regulate and terminate Th1 and Th2 reactions. Chemokines, including CC chemokine ligands (CCLs) and CXC chemokine ligand (CXCLs), from these specific immune reactions regulate phagocyte and lymphocyte functions (Fig. 8.4). The other phagocyte-mediated defense pathway is primarily mediated by resident macrophages in certain organs or in peritoneal and pleural spaces in which macrophages reside and circulate. In response to microbial invasion or endogenous and exogenous insults, resident macrophages release chemotactic factors such as CXCLs and CCLs to attract granulocytes and lymphocytes, respectively. Resident macrophages together with granulocytes act as scavengers to clear microbes or tissue debris; in addition, resident macrophages interact with lymphocytes to mediate specific lymphocyte transformation by which specific cell-mediated and humoral immune reactions are elicited and regulated (Fig. 8.4).

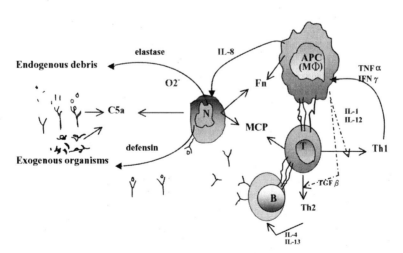

Figure 8.4. In the blood and interstitial tissues, neutrophils (N) act as the first line of host defense in clearance of exogenous organisms and endogenous debris through phagocytosis (via Fc receptors [FcR] and complement receptors [CR], etc.) and degranulation (elastase and defensin, etc.), and release monocyte chemotactic factors such as fibronectin (Fn) and CC chemokine ligands (CCLs) through which lymphocytes and antigen-presenting cells (APC) are attracted. The APC present antigen(s) to T cells, resulting in appropriate cellular (Th1), humoral (Th2), and regulatory T (T reg) cell reactions. Th1, Th2, and T reg cells can regulate one another through a cytokine network in which Th1 cytokines IFNγ and

TNFβ can promote cellular immunity and suppress humoral immunity. Th2 cytokines IL-4 and IL-13 can promote humoral immunity and suppress Th1 reaction, and Treg cytokines IL-10 and TGFβ can regulate and terminate Th1 and Th2 reactions. In tissues or in the pleural and peritoneal spaces, dendritic cells, monocytes, resident macrophages (MΦ), and APC play a central role in promotion of immune reaction via recognition of microorganisms and altered tissue antigens via receptors such as toll-like receptors (TLRs), and release chemoattractants such as CXC chemokine ligands (CXCLs) and CCLs to attract granulocytes and lymphocytes for both innate and adaptive immune responses.

Granulocyte Function Disorders

Historical Background

Kostmann (1956) first identified an autosomal recessive quantitative phagocyte disorder, congenital granulocytopenia. Patients with Kostmann disease (also called infantile agranulocytosis) usually develop severe, chronic, and eventually fatal bacterial infections early in life (see Chapter 39). Some cases may either be transmitted by an autosomal dominant trait or be sporadic. The first qualitative defect in phagocytes was identified later than Kostmann disease. This disorder, now called chronic granulomatous disease (CGD), frequently caused fatal infections in childhood (Bridges et al., 1959). It most frequently occurred in boys, suggesting an X-linked mode of inheritance (Carson et al., 1965; see Chapter 37). Quie and coworkers (1967) provided the first evidence of an inborn error of qualitative phagocyte function that resulted in CGD. These investigators discovered that granulocytes obtained from patients with CGD were able to ingest bacteria normally but unable to kill the ingested organisms. Of additional interest was the observation that granulocytes from the affected boys' mothers, presumed carriers in an X-linked disorder, were intermediate in their bactericidal capacity. Not only did these

observations establish the first intrinsic defect of phagocyte function, but the intermediate bactericidal defect in maternal granulocytes was consistent with the Lyon hypothesis. These results indicated that phagocyte bactericidal activity could be controlled by a specific gene, which is different from other phagocyte functions such as adhesion, movement, and ingestion. This suggested that other phagocyte defects might also be individually controlled by specific genes, contributing to recurrent infections.

Over the past 30 years, this hypothesis has been proven true. As shown in Table 8.1, an entire spectrum of phagocyte disorders involving adhesion, mobilization, respiratory burst activity, and degranulation defects has been recognized, and most are genetically determined. Serious phagocyte function defects such as the leukocyte adhesion disorders and CGD occur in approximately 2 in 100,000 people and represent one-fifth of the total congenital immunodeficiency patients. Other minor phagocyte defects such as myeloperoxidase (MPO) deficiency have a higher incidence of approximately 1 in 4000 to 1 in 2000 (Lehrer and Cline, 1969). As shown in Table 8.1, prenatal diagnoses, immunopharmacological correction, bone marrow or stem cell transplantation, and gene therapy may be available for certain phagocyte disorders, based on recent progress in the genetics, biochemistry, and physiology of phagocytes.

Table 8.1. Pathogenesis and Therapeutic Approaches of Phagocyte Function Disorders

Disease	Inheritance (Chromosome No.)	Defect	Therapy
Congenital granulocytopenia	AR, AD or XL	Differentiation arrest	G-CSF, GM-CSF/IL-3.
		Mutation in G-CSF receptor; neutrophil elastase; WASP	BMT
Cyclic granulocytopenia	AD (19p13.3)	Mutation of neutrophil elastase	G-CSF
Isoimmune granulocytopenia	AR (1q13.4)	Maternal antibody to CD16	IVIG
Leukocyte adhesion defect (LAD1)	AR (21q22.3)	Deficiency of surface adhesion molecule (CD18) with delayed separation of umbilical cord, lack of pus formation	BMT Antibiotics Hygienic precautions
LAD2	AR (11q14.3–isaQ921)	Selecting binding ligands (SLx) defect in fucosylation	BMT Antibiotics Fucose (oral)
X-linked CGD	XL (Xp22.1)	Cytochrome b_{558} heavy-chain gp91phox defect	Iconazole IFN-γ, BMT Trimethoprim Sulfamethroxazole
Autosomal CGD	AR (1q25; 7q11.23; 16q24)	Cytosolic p67phox, p47phox and membrane p22phox defects	Trimethoprim Sulfamethroxazole IFN-γ, Iconazole, BMT
Myeloperoxidase deficiency	AR (17q23.1)	Peroxidase deficiency	Fluconazole for candidiasis
Glutathione synthetase deficiency	AR (20q11.2)	NADPH regeneration defect, hemolysis and infections	Vitamin E
G6PD deficiency	XL (Xq28)	NADPH production defect in affected leukocytes	Symptomatic T_x
Job syndrome (4q?) Hyper IgE syndrome	Sporadic or AD (4q?)	Staph abscesses, fungal infections, elevated IgE; defective PMN chemotaxis	IFN-γ, prophylactic antibiotics, antifungal Vitamin C
Specific granule deficiency	AR	Recurrent infection with defects in chemotaxis and phagocytosis	Symptomatic T_x
Actin dysfunction	AR	Recurrent infections with defects in chemotaxis and phagocytosis	Symptomatic T_x
Chediak-Higashi syndrome	AR (1q42–43)	Mutation of LYST, partial albinism, giant granules in phagocytes and neurons	BMT
Griscelli syndrome	AR (15q211 both genes)	Myosin 5A deficiency RAB27A deficiency	BMT (for RAB27 deficiency)
IFN-γ receptors, type 1; type 2	AR (6q23–24) AR (21q21–22)	Infections with BCG, atypical TB, salmonellosis	Antibiotics (anti-TB)

AD, autosomal dominant; AR, autosomal recessive; BCG, bacille Calmette-Guérin; BMT, bone marrow transplantation; CGD, chronic granulomatous disease; G6PD, glucose-6-phosphate dehydrogenase; gp 91, glycoprotein 91; IVIG, intravenous immunoglobulin; TB, tubucerlosis; WASP, Wiskott-Aldrich syndrome protein; XL, X-chromosome linked.

Quantitative Phagocyte Defects

A blood granulocyte level of less than 1500/mm^3 is defined as *granulocytopenia*. Granulocytopenia may result from a decrease in bone marrow production or an increase in peripheral destruction of granulocytes by autoantibodies or the reticuloendothelial system. Congenital granulocytopenias are due to a decrease in bone marrow production resulting from defects in growth and differentiation of granulocytes (Weetman and Boxer, 1980). Several kinds of primary quantitative phagocyte deficiencies have been identified. Genetic agranulocytosis (Kostmann syndrome) was first identified as an autosomal recessive disease by Kostmann (1956). A mutation of the G-CSF receptor has been proposed (Deshpande et al., 1999) or, more recently, mutations of neutrophil elastase (Dale et al., 2000; see Chapter 39). Reticular dysgenesis is due to failure of bone marrow production of blood stem cells, resulting in pancytopenia (De Vaal and Seynhaeve, 1959; Church and Schlegel, 1985). Shwachman syndrome is characterized by granulocytopenia, pancreatic insufficiency, and failure to thrive (Shwachman et al., 1964). This syndrome appears to be an autosomal recessive trait; its gene may be located on the long arm of chromosome 6 or 12, as patients with this syndrome may demonstrate t(6; 12) translocations (Masuno et al., 1995). Cyclic granulocytopenia occurs in cycles with periods of normal granulocyte counts of approximately 3 weeks followed by granulocytopenia, secondary to a failure of maturation, which lasts approximately 1 week (Weetman and Boxer, 1980). The disease can be transmitted in an autosomal dominant fashion with mutations of a gene that has been mapped to chromosome 19p13.3 and identified as neutrophil elastase (Dale et al., 2000; see Chapter 39). Other forms of neutropenia in infancy are due to autoantibody (Bux et al., 1998) or maternal isoantibodies directed against CD16 (De Haas et al., 1995). A point mutation within the Cdc42 binding domain of WASP (L270P) that interferes with the self-inhibition of WASP and results in constant activation of Arp2/3 and actin polymerization has recently been shown to cause X-linked congenital neutropenia (Devriendt et al., 2001, see Chapter 31). It appears that a variety of genes that regulate granulocyte growth and differentiation at different levels can affect production of mature granulocytes, although specific gene defects have not always been identified. Patients with congenital granulocytopenia frequently get recurrent infections including omphalitis, septicemia, and abscess formation early in life. Bone marrow transplantation from matched or a T cell–depleted haploidentical donor may be able to rescue these patients if the diagnosis is established early in life. Patients living into childhood with progressive periodontitis and recurrent infections may be given colony growth factors such as GM-CSF, G-CSF, or a chimeric protein conjugating IL-3 with GM-CSF, which may benefit some patients. Transfusion of irradiated granulocytes may aid patients with overwhelming infections. In addition, early intervention with antibacterial and antifungal treatment and prophylaxis are important because patients with granulocytopenia are more susceptible to extracellular bacteria and fungi. To differentiate congenital granulocytopenia from acquired peripheral granulocyte destruction, bone marrow examination and antineutrophil antibody assessment is required (Yang and Hill, 1996).

Qualitative Phagocyte Defects

Qualitative phagocyte function defects may be divided into defects involving adhesion, movement, respiratory burst-dependent bactericidal activity, and degranulation. Many intrinsic and extrinsic factors contribute to defects in phagocyte function at different stages, resulting in recurrent infections and delayed wound healing.

Phagocyte adhesion deficiency

Three leukocyte adhesion disorders (LAD1, LAD2, and LAD3) have been identified (see Chapter 38). Most of the affected patients have LAD1 with deficiency of a family of surface glycoproteins, CD11/CD18. The CD11/CD18 family of glycoproteins share an identical β chain (CD18, gp 95 Kda) and separate α chains—CD11a (gp 180 Kda), CD11b (gp 165 Kda), and CD11c (gp 150 Kda)—which contribute to promotion of leukocyte adhesion, cell migration, phagocytosis, antigen presentation, and ADCC (Crowley et al., 1980; Anderson et al., 1985; Schmalstieg, 1988). Patients with LAD1 frequently show delayed separation of the umbilical cord, perirectal cellulitis, and staphylococcal and gram-negative bacterial infections. Patients surviving infancy often have progressive periodontitis and gingivitis. The gene responsible for LAD1 codes for the synthesis of CD18 and has been mapped to 21q22.3 (Marlin et al., 1986). The clinical manifestations of LAD2 are similar to those seen in LAD1, except that LAD2 patients are severely mentally retarded and deficient in expression of sialyl Lewis X, a carbohydrate ligand for E-selectin on endothelial cells (Etzioni et al., 1993; Phillips et al., 1995). The molecular defect of LAD3 is presently unknown; affected patients have symptoms similar to those observed in LAD1; in addition, they have a bleeding tendency. CD18 is normal but activation of integrins is defective (Kinashi et al., 2004).

Phagocyte movement (Chemotaxis) defects

Phagocyte mobilization involves an integated ligand–receptor signal coupling response. Defects at different levels of the response can affect granulocyte locomotion and migration (Table 8.2),

Table 8.2. Categories of Granulocyte Chemotaxis Disorders

Category	Disease	Defect (Inheritance)
Ligand deficiencies	C5 dysfunction	Congenital or developmental group A
	C5 degradation	or B streptococcal infections
Adhesion molecule defect	LAD1	CD18 deficiency (AR)
	LAD2	Selectin binding ligand (AR)
	Localized periodontitis	Adhesion molecule gp 108 (AD?)
Cytoskeleton assembly deficiency	Actin dysfunction	Retarded actin assembly (AR)
Membrane transportation defects	Chediak-Higashi syndrome	CHS protein (*LYST*) defect (AR)
	Griscelli syndrome	Myosin 5A defect (AR)
	Oculocutaneous albinism	Granule transportation defect
Extrinsic suppressing factors	Hyper-IgE syndrome	Defective chemotaxis (AD, sporadic)
	IgA paraproteins	Myeloma protein

AD, autosomal dominant; AR, autosomal recessive; CHS protein; Chediack-Higashi syndrome protein; LAD: leukocyte adhesion defect.

which explains the extensive heterogeneity existing among these disorders. No single clinical or laboratory finding is consistently abnormal within this group of disorders. Patients with phagocyte chemotactic deficiency can be classified into five different categories based on defects at different levels.

Defects at the ligand level.   Patients with congenital deficiency of complement components—C1, C4, C2, properdin, C3, and C5—may be unable to produce adequate amounts of C5a, resulting in a defect of chemotaxis (see Chapter 42). C5 functional deficiency has been reported in Leiner disease, which is characterized by seborrheic dermatitis, recurrent gram-negative bacterial infections, intractable diarrhea, and failure to thrive (Leiner, 1908). Patients with this syndrome are reported to have normal C5 levels, but C5 dysfunction associated with a humoral chemotactic and opsonic defect (Miller et al., 1970). The disease was described in two sequential infants in a family, and each died after an illness of several weeks, thus a genetic mechanism was proposed by Miller and Koblenzer (1972). The validity of these observations of C5 functional deficiency in patients with Leiner disease was challenged by the lack of a similar opsonic defect in patients with total absence of C5.

Defects at the receptor level.   Granulocytes with adhesive-glycoprotein deficiencies as in CD18 (LAD1) or sialyl Lewis X (LAD2) deficiency are unable to adhere to endothelium or interstitial tissue (see Chapter 38) and as a consequence show poor chemotaxis in vivo and in vitro. Juvenile periodontitis usually occurs in adolescents who have impaired chemotaxis and localized periodontitis (Van Dyke et al., 1981; Van Dyke, 1985). Limited evidence suggests that this syndrome is due to a missing cell surface glycoprotein (gp110) (Van Dyke et al., 1987).

Defects in mechanic organization.   Granulocyte cytoskeleton organization defect has been observed in patients with actin dysfunction syndrome (Boxer et al., 1974). One of the initial cases reported was subsequently diagnosed as leukocyte adhesion deficiency on the basis of intermediate levels of CD11b on neutrophils from surviving family members. Southwick et al. (1988) have shown that actin dysfunction is not usually present in leukocyte adhesion deficiency but, in rare patients with this disorder, actin polymerization may be abnormal. This may reflect a link between cell surface integrins and the actin cytoskeleton (Southwick et al., 1989a, 1989b).

Defects in receptor recycling.   Granulocytes with specific granule deficiency have been reported to have a chemotactic receptor recycling defect (Gallin et al., 1982). Granulocytes from patients with the Chediak-Higashi syndrome (see Chapter 40) have a chemotactic defect due to altered microtubular assembly and abnormal signal transduction (Oliver, 1978). This disease is transmitted by autosomal recessive inheritance; the defective gene is likely located on chromosome 1q42–q41 (Fukai et al., 1996). Another granule transport defect called Griscelli syndrome (Chapter 41), which includes albinism and granulocytopenia, is due to a myosin defect, encoded in chromosome 15q21, resulting in an abnormality of granule transport (Pastural et al., 2000).

Defects due to extrinsic suppressive or lack of enhancing factors. Many extrinsic suppressive factors such as immune complexes (Hanlon et al., 1980), steroids, and IgA paraproteins (Miller, 1975) can interfere with phagocyte chemotaxis. The hyper-IgE syndrome (Job syndrome, see Chapter 34), which has been associated with a granulocyte chemotaxis defect, is characterized by high levels of IgE, altered T cell activity (Geha et al., 1981), or release of allergic mediators (Hill, 1980). Alternatively, the increased concentration of IgE and defective neutrophil chemotaxis may result from abnormal IFN-γ production in response to patients' main pathogens, *Staphylococcus aureus* and *Candida albicans* (Borges et al., 2000). This disorder has been shown to be an autosomal dominant trait in certain families with incomplete penetrance (van Scoy et al., 1975; Hill et al., 1997), although most of the patients showed sporadic occurrence (Jacobs and Norman, 1977). In a subgroup of patients with hyper-IgE syndrome, the gene was mapped to chromosome 4q (Grimbacher et al., 1999). The disease has also been reported in association with osteogenesis imperfecta (Brestel et al., 1982; Hill, 1982).

Treatment of chemotactic disorders.   Patients with chemotactic disorders, like those with other phagocyte defects, frequently suffer recurrent cutaneous abscesses, mucocutaneous candidiasis, pneumonia, and otitis media. These disorders could be assessed with an in vivo Rebuck skin window test (Rebuck and Crowley, 1955) or by in vitro Boyden chamber chemotaxis (Hill, 1980). Although complete correction of granulocyte chemotactic defects is not possible, partial correction for certain patients has been achieved, as shown in Table 8.1. C5 dysfunction may be corrected by replacement with fresh plasma that contains normal C5. Vitamin C has been shown to enhance chemotaxis of granulocytes obtained from patients with Chediak-Higashi syndrome (Boxer et al., 1976). Studies from our laboratory have shown that IFN-γ can enhance in vitro chemotaxis of granulocytes obtained from patients with hyper-IgE syndrome (Jeppson et al., 1991; Petrak et al., 1994). For palliative treatment, histamine (H$_2$) antagonists have been reported to reduce the frequency of infection in patients with hyper-IgE syndrome (Thompson, 1988). High doses of vitamin C or E have also been reported to be beneficial in some patients. Prophylactic antimicrobial therapy with trimethoprim sulfamethoxazole or dicloxacillin is also often useful in decreasing the incidence of infections in many of these patients.

Disorders of phagocytic uptake

Primary defects in phagocytic uptake are rare; most are secondary to infections, drugs, or systemic disease. Patients with leukocyte adhesion deficiency show defects in particulate-mediated phagocytosis (Anderson et al., 1985). Another disorder resulting in phagocytic uptake deficiency is actin dysfunction syndrome. Granulocytes from a patient with actin dysfunction failed to polymerize actin, resulting in phagocytic defects (Boxer et al., 1974; Southwick et al., 1988). To differentiate an intrinsic phagocytic defect from secondary defects, one should cross over autologous and heterologous serum with the patient's and a control's granulocytes in a phagocytosis assay. Employing fluorescein (FITC)-labeled techniques, phagocytosis can be simply assessed with a flow cytometer (Yang and Hill, 1996). Studies of normal granulocytes demonstrated that several cytokines and glycoproteins enhance motility and phagocytic uptake (Gresham et al., 1986; Yang et al., 1988; Salyer et al., 1990). Such cytokines and glycoproteins may be candidates for the treatment of these phagocytic disorders. Patients with phagocytic defects due to opsonic deficiencies in antibody, complement, or fibronectin may be treated by infusion with the deficient component. For those with transient cytokine (e.g., IFN-γ) deficiency, treatment with a recombinant cytokine may reverse the immune dysfunction (Jeppson et al., 1991; Petrak et al., 1994; Wallis and Ellner, 1994).

Disorders of granulocyte respiratory burst activity

Granulocytes with defects in respiratory burst activity usually have normal or increased adhesion, chemotaxis, and phagocytic uptake but abnormal intracellular microbicidal activity. These disorders include CGD, glucose-6-phosphate dehydrogenase (G6PD) deficiency, MPO deficiency, and glutathione synthetase deficiency. Defects involving any component of the oxidase system seen in patients with CGD as well as defects associated with the generation of the cofactor for NADPH activation, seen in severe leukocyte G6PD deficiency, or impaired NADPH regeneration, seen in glutathione synthetase deficiency, may result in a deficiency in oxygen-dependent microbicidal activity. Chapter 37 of this text is devoted to chronic granulomatous disease. The gene coding for cytochrome b_{558} heavy-chain gp91phox (*CYBB*) is located on the short arm of the X chromosome whereas the gene coding for cytochrome b_{558} light-chain gp22phox (*CYBA*) is located on chromosome 16. Studies indicate that superoxide production requires the participation of both membrane-bound NADPH oxidase and cytosolic factors (Borregaard and Tauber, 1984). The genes coding for the cytosolic factors p47phox (*NFC1*) and p67phox (*NFC2*) are located on chromosomes 7 and 1, respectively (Smith and Curnutte, 1991). Severe forms of G6PD deficiency may present with a CGD-like clinical picture. Cooper et al. (1972) described a 52-year-old Caucasian female with hemolytic anemia, a leukemoid reaction, and fatal *Escherichia coli* sepsis whose leukocytes could not kill *Staphylococcus aureus*, *E. coli*, or *Serratia marcesens* but could kill H_2O_2-producing *Streptococcus faecalis*. Intraleukocyte reduction of nitroblue tetrazolium (NBT) dye did not occur, nor was H_2O_2 generated and the hexose monophosphate shunt stimulated. There was complete absence of leukocyte G6PD in the patient. Subsequently, Gray and colleagues (1973) reported three male siblings with a syndrome of chronic nonspherocytic hemolytic anemia and neutrophil dysfunction. Each had strikingly elevated reticulocyte counts, less than 1% NBT dye reduction under conditions in which 90% of control neutrophils reduced the dye, and undetectable concentrations of erythrocyte and leukocyte G6PD activity. The oldest boy had 13 episodes of right- or left-sided cervical lymphadenitis associated with mild anemia, slight jaundice, and low-grade fever before 10 years of age. Cultures were either negative or revealed coagulase-positive *S. aureus*. The second male sibling had neonatal jaundice for 6 weeks and several episodes of anemia and jaundice associated with upper respiratory tract infections; he also suffered two episodes of erythema nodosum and one episode of cervical lymphadenitis. The third sibling had neonatal jaundice but had no hemolytic episodes or increased susceptibility to infection. The parents were both healthy, but the mother had persistently elevated reticulocyte counts and 60%–70% of control values for erythrocyte and leukocyte G6PD. Profound deficiency of G6PD leads to a defect in NADPH production, causing impaired respiratory burst activity. The gene coding for G6PD is located on the X chromosome and has a widely variant polymorphism in different populations in the world. Studies in blacks and Caucasians have shown that Caucasians with G6PD deficiency more frequently have affected leukocytes (Ramot et al., 1959; Cooper et al., 1972; Gray et al., 1973; Owusu, 1973). The G6PD enzyme in leukocytes is encoded by the same gene as those in erythrocyte precursors and other tissues. G6PD activity in leukocytes is usually higher than in erythrocytes, so patients with G6PD deficiency–mediated hemolytic anemia usually have normal leukocyte function. Only when leukocytes have less than 5% of normal G6PD activity does abnormal bactericidal activity appear (Baehner et al., 1972). There may be other unknown factors in leukocytes from different races, which could affect G6PD activities, since patients with G6PD deficiency associated with CGD-like syndrome have been reported in Caucasians but not in blacks or Asians.

Glutathione levels are modulated by NADPH, glutathione reductase, and glutathione synthetase (Fig. 8.3). Granulocytes with glutathione reductase or glutathione synthetase deficiency show normal early respiratory burst activity. However, the continuous production of toxic oxygen products, which are normally handled by glutathione, results in auto-oxidative damage and defective microbicidal activity (Mohler et al., 1970; Jain et al., 1994). Both glutathione reductase and glutathione synthetase deficiencies are transmitted by autosomal recessive inheritance. Patients with glutathione reductase deficiency may have hemolytic crises but have normal phagocyte bactericidal activity, although the granulocyte respiratory burst activity stops abruptly within a few minutes of phagocytosis of bacteria. In contrast, patients with glutathione synthetase deficiency show abnormal bactericidal activity in addition to hemolysis of erythrocytes. Granulocytes with MPO deficiency have normal production of superoxide but defective generation of hypochlorite ion. Patients with this disorder are not uncommon (1 in 2000 to 1 in 4000 of the general population) but are frequently asymptomatic or at most have delayed granulocyte killing activity and recurrent candida infections (Parry et al., 1981). The MPO gene has been cloned and located on chromosome 17 (Weil et al., 1987).

The cellular and molecular bases of disorders related to oxidative microbicidal activity have been extensively explored and pharmacological approaches to treat such patients have been tried for three decades. Most of these therapies have been unsuccessful or controversial (Gonzalez and Hill, 1988). Recent studies have shown, however, that recombinant IFN-γ in a low dose ($50 \mu g/m^2$) given subcutaneously three times a week significantly reduces serious infections in patients with CGD (Ezekowitz et al., 1988; Sechler et al., 1988; International Chronic Granulomatous Disease Cooperative Study Group, 1991; Weening et al., 1995). Bone marrow transplantation in CGD patients has been reported to result in long-term chimeric engraftment with improvement in infectious complication (Kamani et al., 1988; Horwitz et al., 2001; Seger et al., 2002; Del Giudice et al., 2003). Identification of the genes responsible for both X-linked and autosomal recessive forms of CGD (Dinauer et al., 1987; Teahan et al., 1987) makes gene therapy for patients with CGD a future possibility (Zentilin et al., 1996). Indeed, during the 2004 European Society for Immunodeficiencies meeting in Versailles, successful gene therapy of two CGD patients with mutations of gp91phox was reported by a German–Swiss consortium. (Ott, et al., 2004). Glutathione synthetase deficiency can be partially corrected by administration of vitamin E (Boxer et al., 1979). Patients with MPO deficiency are usually asymptomatic; however, for those developing chronic candidiasis, ketaconazole or fluconazole are indicated (Table 8.1). Some very preliminary in vitro and in vivo studies suggest that IFN-γ may have some benefit in the treatment of hyper-IgE syndrome (Jeppson et al., 1991; Petrak et al., 1994).

Disorders of granulocyte degranulation

Specific granule deficiency. Oxygen-independent microbicidal defects can arise from absence of granules or from defective degranulation. Several patients lacking specific granules have been described. Studies of granule-deficient granulocytes show impaired bactericidal activity in addition to impaired chemotaxis (Gallin et al., 1982). The reason for granulocyte dysfunction in these patients is the failure of granule constituents to fuse into the phagosome, resulting in a decrease in oxygen-independent bactericidal activity and a decrease in expression of adhesion molecules and chemotactic receptors on the cell surface. Although it appears that patients with specific granule deficiency have an autosomal recessive inheritance, the gene responsible for the disorder has not yet been identified. Heterozygous siblings or parents are usually healthy and have normal phagocyte function. The diagnosis of granule deficiency is primarily based on the family history and clinical manifestations as well as the granulocyte morphology with an absence of specific granules (Gallin et al., 1982). Furthermore, granulocytes from patients with specific granule deficiency do not release certain constituents from specific granules and show a defect in membrane recycling of adhesion molecules and chemotactic receptors. The constituents inside specific granules such as transferrin and vitamin B12 binding protein can be detected by enzyme-linked immunosorbent assay (ELISA) and radioimmunoussay (RIA), respectively (Yang and Hill, 1996).

Granule-transporting defect. Chediak-Higashi syndrome, a granule-releasing deficiency disorder and its murine equivalent, the beige mouse, have in common a defect affecting all granule-containing cells such as melanocytes, neurons, and granulocytes (Blume and Wolff, 1972; Fukai et al., 1996). This syndrome, transmitted by autosomal recessive inheritance, is characterized by partial albinism, granulocytopenia, neurologic deficits, recurrent infections, and neoplastic transformation, especially lymphomas (see Chapter 40). The gene for the Chediak-Higashi syndrome (*LYST* or *CHS1*) has been identified and relevant mutations have been recognized (Barbosa et al., 1996; Nagle et al., 1996; Introne et al., 1999). The diagnosis of Chediak-Higashi is based on the characteristic clinical features and the laboratory findings of altered membrane fusion associated with giant azurophilic granules, defective chemotaxis, degranulation, and bactericidal activity of granulocytes (Boxer et al., 1976). Bactericidal defects in Chediak-Higashi syndrome have been reported to improve after administration of large doses of vitamin C. This may reduce the intracellular cyclic adenosine monophosphate (cAMP) level, resulting in improvement of chemotaxis and bactericidal activity (Boxer et al., 1976). Administration of G-CSF can partially correct Chediak-Higashi syndrome–associated granulocytopenia, chemotaxis, and phagocytosis in an animal model (Colgan et al., 1992). Bone marrow transplantation is the only option for curing patients with this syndrome (Vossen, 1988). Another form of granule transportation defect, Griscelli syndrome, characterized by albinism, granulocytopenia (see Chapter 41), and infections, is due to Myosin 5A or RAB27A deficiency (Pastural et al., 2000; Sanal et al., 2002).

Monocyte and macrophage function disorders

Monocytes and macrophages share the same ancestors with granulocytes, so most of the defects present in granulocyte function disorders occur in monocytes and macrophages, including the leukocyte adhesion disorders, phagocyte actin dysfunction, respiratory burst defects such as CGD, degranulation defects such as Chediak-Higashi syndrome, and specific granule deficiency. Primary macrophage function defects are relatively rare, as most of the macrophage function defects are secondary. Monocyte and macrophage function can be compromised by environmental agents, drugs, infections, and metabolic disorders,

resulting in immunodeficiency. For instance, smoke particles, asbestos, silica, hyperbaric oxygen, and air pollution can impair monocyte and macrophage function. In addition, monocytes and macrophages can be seriously impaired in patients with AIDS. Differential induction of cytokine profiles may contribute to resistance or susceptibility of macrophages to infection with intracellular organisms (Wallis and Eliner, 1994). Monokine enhancement of HIV infections and compromise of the antigen presentation by monocytes have been implicated in patients with both AIDS and tuberculosis. Monocytes obtained from patients with chronic mucocutaneous candidiasis may have impaired chemotactic activity (Snyderman et al., 1973), and monocytes obtained from a patient with common variable immunodeficiency were shown to have impaired antigen presentation to T cells (Eibl et al., 1982). Currently, four primary macrophage function defects have been identified: osteopetrosis, toll-like receptor signaling deficiency, IFN-γ receptor deficiency, and familial lysosomal storage diseases.

Osteopetrosis. This heterogenious hereditary disorder, due to dysfunction of osteoclasts (specialized macrophages), is the result of enhanced resorption of mineralized cartilage and bony remodeling (Reeves et al., 1979). This syndrome is commonly seen in offspring from consanguineous parents, which suggests an autosomal recessive trait (Sobacci et al., 2001). Some cases are reported to be mediated by an autosomal dominant trait, especially those found in the adult type of osteopetrosis (Grodum et al., 1995; Felix et al., 1996; Frattini et al., 2003). Some of the genes responsible for osteopetrosis have been identified (Sobacchi et al., 2001; Frattini et al., 2003). Heterozygous carriers have completely normal immune function, so carrier detection is not currently available, except for those with a known gene defect. Abnormal encroachment of sclerotic bone can compromise nerve foramen and bone marrow spaces, resulting in neurologic and hematopoietic defects. Prenatal diagnosis by fetal sonography may be made through recognition of sclerotic, dense, and radiopaque bones (Sen et al., 1995). Patients with osteopetrosis are usually characterized by a generalized increase in bone density, failure to thrive, hypocalcemia with low serum phosphate due to impaired bony resorption, and a variable degree of anemia, thrombocytopenia, and leukopenia. Although monocytes from osteopetrosis patients show normal or minimally impaired phagocyte function, bone marrow transplantation can rapidly reverse abnormal osteosclerotic changes and reconstitute immune function. This finding suggests that a selective macrophage (osteoclast) defect may be present in this disease (Reeves et al., 1979; Taylor et al., 1995; Felix et al., 1996; Sobacchi et al., 2001; Frattini et al., 2003).

Toll-like receptor signaling deficiency. There are at least 10 TLRs identified on monocytes and dendritic cells (Hornung et al., 2002; Doni et al., 2003; Coccia et al., 2004). Different TLRs can recognize different microorganisms and mediate signals for innate host defenses and adaptive T cell differentiation (Doni et al., 2003; Coccia et al., 2004; Netea et al., 2004). As a result, patients with defects in different TLRs may be susceptible to certain infections. Recently, a primary defect in TLR signaling has been reported that results in recurrent pneumococcal infections (Currie et al., 2004). Mutations in the interleukin receptor–associated kinase (IRAK-4) have been associated with pyogenic gram-positive bacterial infections and failure to sustain antibody responses (Picard et al., 2003; Day et al., 2004). The infections began early in life but became less frequent and milder with age.

Interferon gamma receptor deficiency. Two components of the IFN-γ receptor have been identified; they map to C6q23–q24 and C21q21–q22, respectively (Newport et al., 1996; Dorman et al., 1998). IFN-γ receptor deficiencies are autosomal recessive diseases that result in a defect in TNF-γ production and defective intracellular bactericidal activity. As a consequence, patients suffer disseminated atypical mycobacterial infections and salmonellosis (Jouanguy et al., 1999; Casanova and Abel, 2002). The disorders cannot be differentiated clinically from those with IL-12 or IL-12 receptor deficiencies (Altare et al., 1998), since IL-12 and IFN-γ are the major cytokines mediating intracellular bactericidal activity in macrophages (see Chapter 28).

Lysosomal storage diseases. Although macrophages may not be the only cell involved, accumulation of lipids or polysaccharides in macrophages may lead to the formation of foam cells and result in defective catabolic function. The fact that several storage diseases such as Gaucher disease, Fabry disease, and Hurler syndrome have been successfully treated by bone marrow transplantation (O'Reilly et al., 1984; Imaizumi, 1995; Krivit et al., 1995) further supports the concept that macrophage catabolic defects play a critical role in the pathogenesis of these diseases. The diagnosis of patients with lysosomal enzyme deficiency–associated lipidoses and mucopolysaccharidoses is usually based on clinical features showing characteristic dysmorphisms including those of the face, chest, and extremities as well as mental retardation and hepatosplenomegaly. The presence of urinary mucopolysaccharides is sometimes characteristic. A definitive diagnosis should be based on specific enzyme assays employing cultured fibroblasts or leukocytes. Heterozygous carriers in some of these storage diseases can be detected by showing one-half the amount of the normal lysosomal enzyme activity in cultured fibroblasts or leukocytes.

Most of the primary macrophage function defects can be effectively treated by bone marrow transplantation, which provides normally functioning macrophages. In some diseases, exogenous replacement with the normal enzyme may be useful. For instance, Hurler syndrome is associated with deficiency of iduronidase and can be partially corrected by replacement with the enzyme. In an animal study, Takahashi et al. (1994) showed that mutant mice with osteopetrosis lacked functional M-CSF activity; exogenous M-CSF could partially correct the defect. The M-CSF gene is mapped to C1p21 in human beings, but is apparently not the disease-causing gene in patients with osteopetrosis (Van Hul et al., 1997). Whether correction of cytokine or stromal cell factor defects in the bone marrow can reverse specific macrophage function defects remains to be determined.

Prevention and Treatment of Phagocyte Function Disorders

Primary Prevention

As demonstrated in Table 8.1, most of the phagocyte function disorders exhibit X-linked or autosomal recessive inheritance. Primary prevention for X-linked and autosomal recessive disorders is based on carrier detection (McCabe et al., 1989). Phagocyte disorders for which carrier detection is currently available include CGD (Newburger et al., 1979; Chapter 37), IL-12 receptor β1 deficiency (Chapter 28), leukocyte adhesion dysfunction (Chapter 38), and Wiskott-Aldrich syndrome (Chapter 31). Heterozygotes that carry a defective lysosomal enzyme gene encoding for macrophage storage disease can be detected by quantitating enzyme activity in cultured fibroblasts and leukocytes.

Prenatal Diagnosis

Early diagnosis of phagocyte function disorders can be made employing prenatal chromosome analysis, restriction fragment length polymorphism (RFLP), biochemical analysis, gene product determination, and phagocyte function assays. Chorionic villus sampling at 9–10 weeks of gestational age and fetal blood sampling at 16–20 weeks of gestational age (Perignon et al., 1987; Lau and Levinsky, 1988; Villa et al., 2000) can be carried out. Employing the NBT dye reduction test, CGD can be diagnosed prenatally at approximately 16–20 weeks of gestational age (Newburger et al., 1979). The polymerase chain reaction (PCR) may require only a tiny skin sample or amniotic fluid containing 10 to 100 cells and may replace chorion or fetal cord blood sampling for prenatal diagnosis, thereby resulting in lower risk to the pregnancy. Prenatal diagnosis of X-linked CGD by identification of the polymorphism (CA/GT)n repeats in gp91phox gene can be achieved in hours (Gorlin, 1998). If the mutation in a given CGD family is known, the analysis of fetal DNA can identify the status of the fetus. Patients with Chediak-Higashi syndrome have giant lysosomal granules in phagocytes and skin melanocytes. The characteristic morphology of these granules can be used to detect the syndrome in fetal cord blood samples at 18–20 weeks of gestational age. Similarly, fetal cord blood sampling may provide the diagnosis of disease or carrier detection in the leukocyte adhesion deficiency disorders as well as the IL-12 receptor β1 deficiency. Cord blood leukocytes or amniotic cells can be cultured to detect metabolic storage diseases by measuring suspected lysosomal enzyme activity. Prenatally detected phagocyte function disorders may be managed by termination of pregnancy or by early bone marrow or stem cell transplantation (see Chapter 47).

Management of Disease Complications

Patients with phagocyte function disorders should receive psychosocial and rehabilitative support. Appropriate administration of antibiotic prophylaxis, chest physiotherapy, and surgical drainage may decrease sequelae. Regular visits to a dentist familiar with the problems suffered by patients with phagocyte function disorders are essential, especially for leukocyte adhesion deficiency. Patients with phagocyte abnormalities who suffer from recurrent infections starting in infancy usually develop psychologic problems secondary to physical changes (skin scarring, coarse face, hearing loss, dental decay, and/or pulmonary dysfunction), loss of schooling, or the recurring need for hospitalization or intravenous antimicrobial therapy. Progress in bone marrow and stem cell transplantation and gene therapy will have a major impact on the long-term prognosis in these patients by providing techniques to permanently correct these disorders in the future.

References

Aizawa S, Tavassoli M. Interaction of murine granulocyte-macrophage progenitors and supporting stroma involves a recognition mechanism with galactosyl and mannosyl specificities. J Clin Invest 80:1698–1705, 1987.

Allen DH, Tracy PB. Human coagulation factor V is activated to the functional cofactor by elastase and cathepsin G expressed at the monocyte surface. J Biol Chem 270:1408–1415, 1995.

Altare F, Lammas D, Revy P, Jouanguy E, Doffinger R, Lamhamedi S, Drysdale P, Scheel-Toellner D, Girdlestone J, Darbyshire P, Wadhwa M, Dockrell H, Salmon M, Fischer A, Durandy A, Casanova JL, Kumararatne DS. Inherited interleukin 12 deficiency in a child with bacilli Calmette-Guerin and *Salmonella enteritidis* disseminated infection. J Clin Invest 102:2035–2040, 1998.

Anderson DC, Schmalstieg FC, Finegold MJ. The severe and moderate phenotypes of inheritable Mac-1, LFA-1 deficiency: their quantitative definition and relation to leukocyte dysfunction and clinical features. J Infect Dis 152:668–689, 1985.

Baehner RL, Johnston RB, Jr, Nathan DG. Comparative study of the metabolic and bactericidal characteristics of severely glucose-6-phosphate dehydrogenase-deficient polymorphonuclear leukocytes and leukocytes from children with chronic granulomatous disease. J Reticuloendothelial Soc 12:150–169, 1972.

Barbosa MD, Nguyen QA, Tchernev VT, Ashley JA, Detter IC, Blaydes SM, Brandt SJ, Chotai D, Hodgman C, Solari RCE, Lovett M, Kingsmore SF. Identification of the homologous beige and Chediak-Higashi syndrome genes. Nature 382:262–265, 1996.

Bjerrum OW, Borregaard N. Dual granule localization of the dormant NADPH oxidase and cytochrome b559 in human neutrophils. Eur J Haematol 43:67–77, 1989.

Blume RS, Wolff SM. The Chediak-Higashi syndrome: studies in four patients and a review of the literature. Medicine 51:247–280, 1972.

Borges WG, Augustine NH, Hill HR. Defective interleukin-12/interferon-gamma pathway in patients with hyperimmunoglobulinemia E syndrome. J Pediatr 136:176–180, 2000.

Borregaard N, Tauber M. Subcellular localization of human neutrophil NADPH oxidase, b-cytochrome and associated flavoprotein. J Biol Chem 259:47–52, 1984.

Boxer LA, Hedley-Whyte ET, Stossel TP. Neutrophil actin dysfunction and abnormal neutrophil behavior. N Engl J Med 291:1093–1099, 1974.

Boxer LA, Oliver JM, Spielberg SP, Allen JM, Schulman JD. Protection of granulocytes by vitamin E in glutathione synthetase deficiency. N Engl J Med 301:901–905, 1979.

Boxer LA, Watanabe AM, Rister M. Correction of leukocyte function in Chediak-Higashi syndrome by ascorbate. N Engl J Med 293:1041–1045, 1976.

Boyles S, Bainton DF. Changing patterns of plasma membrane-associated filaments during the initial phases of polymorphonuclear leukocyte adherence. J Cell Biol 82:347–368, 1979.

Bratt J, Gyllenhammar H. The role of nitric oxide in lipoxin A4-induced polymorphonuclear neutrophil-dependent cytotoxicity to human vascular endothelium in vitro. Arthritis Rheum 38:768–776, 1995.

Brestel EP, Klingberg WG, Veltri RW, Dorn JS. Osteogenesis imperfecta tarda in a child with hyper-IgE syndrome. Am J Dis Child 136:774–776, 1982.

Bridges RA, Berendes H, Good RA. A fatal granulomatous disease of childhood. Am J Dis Child 97:387–408, 1959.

Bux J, Behrens G, Jaeger G, Welte K. Diagnosis and clinical course of autoimmune neutropenia in infancy: analysis of 240 cases. Blood 91:181–186, 1998.

Cao H, Verge V, Baron C, Martinache C, Leon A, Scholl S, Gorin NC, Salamero J, Assari S, Bernard J, Lopez M. In vitro generation of dendritic cells from human blood monocytes in experimental conditions compatible for in vivo cell therapy. J Hematother Stem Cell Res 9:183–194, 2000.

Carson MJ, Chadwick DL, Brubaker CA, Cleland RS, Landing BH. Thirteen boys with progressive septic granulomatosis. Pediatrics 35:405–412, 1965.

Carson SD, Haire WD, Broze GJ, Jr, Novotny WF, Pirrucello SJ, Duggan MJ. Lipoprotein associated coagulation inhibitor, factor VII, antithrombin III, and monocyte tissue factor following surgery. Thromb Haemost 66:534–539, 1991.

Casanova JL, Abel L. Genetic dissection of immunity to mycobacteria: the human model. Annu Rev Immunol 20:581–620, 2002.

Chehimi J, Trinchieri G. Interleukin-12: a bridge between innate resistance and adaptive immunity with a role in infection and acquired immunodeficiency. J Clin Immunol 14:149–161, 1994.

Christensen RD, Harper TE, Rothstein G. Granulocyte-macrophage progenitor cells in term and preterm neonates. J Pediatr 109:1047–1051, 1986.

Christensen RD, Shigeoka AO, Hill HR, Rothstein G. Neutropenia and bone marrow exhaustion in human and experimental neonatal sepsis. Pediatr Res 14:806–808, 1980.

Chu CQ, Field M, Abney E, Zheng RQ, Allard S, Feldmann M, Maini RN. Transforming growth factor-beta 1 in rheumatoid synovial membrane and cartilage/pannus junction. Clin Exp Immunol 86:380–386, 1991.

Church JA, Schlegel RJ. Immune deficiency disorders. In Bellanti JA, ed. Immunology III. Philadelphia: WB Saunders, pp. 471–507, 1985.

Clark SC, Kamen R. The human hematopoietic colony-stimulating factors. Science 236:1229–1237, 1987.

Coccia EM, Severa M, Giacomini E, Monneron D, Remoli ME, Julkunen I, Cella M, Lande R, Uze G. Viral infection and Toll-like receptor agonists induce a differential expression of type I and lambda interferons in human plasmacytoid and monocyte-derived dendritic cells. Eur J Immunol 34:796–805, 2004.

Cockcroft S, Stutchfield J. The receptors for ATP and fMetLeuPhe are independently coupled to phospholipases C and A2 via G-protein(s). Biochem J 263:715–723, 1989.

Colgan SP, Gasper PW, Thrall MA, Boone TC, Blaricquaert AM, Bruyninckx WJ. Neutrophil function in normal and Chediak-Higashi syndrome cats following administration of recombinant canine granulocyte colony-stimulating factors. Exp Hematol 20:1229–1234, 1992.

Cooper MR, DeChatelet LR, McCall CE, LaVia MF, Spurr CL, Baehner RL. Complete deficiency of leukocyte glucose-6-phosphate dehydrogenase with defective bactericidal activity. J Clin Invest 51:769–778, 1972.

Crowley CA, Curnutte JT, Rosin RE, Andre-Schwartz J, Gallin JI, Klempner M, Snyderman R. Southwick FS, Stossel TP, Babior BM. An inherited abnormality of neutrophil adhesion: its genetic transmission and its association with a missing protein. N Engl J Med 302:1163–1168, 1980.

Currie AJ, Davidson DJ, Reid GS, Bharya S, MacDonald KL, Devon RS, Speert DP. Primary immunodeficiency to pneumococcal infection due to a defect in Toll-like receptor signaling. J Pediatr 144:512–518, 2004.

Dale DC. Comparison of agents producing a neutrophil leukocytosis in man: hydrocortisone, prednisolone, endotoxin and etiocholanolone. J Clin Invest 56:808–813, 1975.

Dale DC, Person RE, Bolyard AA, Aprikyan AG, Bos C, Bonilla MA, Boxer LA, Kannourakis G, Zeidler C, Welte K, Benson KF, Horwitz M. Mutations in the gene encoding neutrophil elastase in congenital cyclic neutropenia. Blood 97:2185–2186, 2000.

Dash D, Aepfelbacher M, Siess W. Integrin alpha IIb beta III-mediated translocation of cdc42Hs to the cytoskeleton in stimulated human platelets. J Biol Chem 270:17321–17326, 1995.

Day N, Tangsinmankong N, Ochs H, Rucker R, Picard C, Casanova JL, Haraguchi S, Good R. Interleukin receptor-associated kinase (IRAK-4) deficiency associated with bacterial infections and failure to sustain antibody responses. J Pediatr 144:524–526, 2004.

De Gaetano G, Cerletti C, Nanni-Coata MP, Poggi A. The blood platelet as an inflammatory cell. Eur Respir J 6:441s–445s, 1989.

De Haas M, Kleijer M, van Zwieten R, Roos D, von dem Borne AE. Neutrophil Fc gamma IIIb deficiency, nature, and clinical consequences: a study of 21 individuals from 14 families. Blood 86:2403–2413, 1995.

Del Giudice I, Iori AP, Mengarella A, Testi AM, Romano A, Cerrett R, Macri F, Iacobini M, Arcese W. Allogeneic stem cell transplant from HLA-identical sibling for chronic granulomatous disease and review of the literature. Ann Hematol 82:189–192, 2003.

Deshpande RV, Lalezari P, Pergolizzi RG, Moore MA. Structural abnormalities in the G-CSF receptor in severe congenital neutropenia. J Hematother Stem Cell Res 8:411–420, 1999.

De Vaal OM, Seynhaeve V. Reticular dysgenesis. Lancet 2:1123–1125, 1959.

Devriendt K, Kim AS, Mathijs G, Frints SG, Schwartz M, Van Den Oord JJ, Verhoef GE, Boogaerts MA, Fryns JP, You D, Rosen MK, Vandenberghe P. Constitutively activating mutation in WASP causes X-linked severe congenital neutropenia. Nat Genet 27:313–317, 2001.

Dietrich J, Nakajima H, Colonna M. Human inhibitory and activating Ig-like receptors which modulate the function of myeloid cells. Microb Infect 2:323–329, 2000.

Dinauer MC, Orkin SH, Brown R, Jesaitis AJ, Parkos CA. The glycoprotein encoded by the X-linked chronic granulomatous disease locus is a component of the neutrophil cytochrome b complex. Nature 327:717–720, 1987.

Doherty DE, Henson PM, Clark RA. Fibronectin fragments containing the RGDS cell binding domain mediate monocyte migration into the rabbit lung. A potential mechanism for C5 fragment-induced monocyte lung accumulation. J Clin Invest 86:1065–1075, 1990.

Doni A, Peri G, Chieppa M, Allavena P, Pasqualini F, Vago L, Romani L, Garlanda C, Mantovani A. Production of the soluble pattern recognition receptor PTX3 by myeloid, but not plasmacytoid, dendritic cells. Eur J Immunol 33:2886–2893, 2003.

Dorman SE, Holland SM. Mutation in the signal-transducing chain of the interferon gamma receptor and susceptibility to mycobacterial infection. J Clin Invest 101:2364–2369, 1998.

Eibl MM, Mannhalter JW, Zlabinger G, Mayr WR, Tilz GP, Ahinad R, Zielinski CC. Defective macrophage function in a patient with common variable immunodeficiency. N Engl J Med 307:803–806, 1982.

Etzioni A, Harlan JM, Pollack S, Phillips LM, Gershoni-Baruch R, Paulson JC. Leukocyte adhesion deficiency (LAD) II: a new adhesion defect due to absence of sialyl Lewis X, the ligand for selectins. Immunodeficiency 4:307–308, 1993.

Ezekowitz RAB, Dinauer MC, Jaffe HS, Orkin SH, Newburger PE. Partial correction of the phagocyte defect in patients with X-linked chronic granulomatous disease by subcutaneous interferon gamma. N Engl J Med 319:146–151, 1988.

Facchetti F, Vermi W. Plasmacytoid monocytes and plasmacytoid dendritic cells. Immune system cells linking innate and acquired immunity. Pathologica 94:163–175, 2002.

Felix R, Hofstetter W, Cecchini MG. Recent developments in the understanding of the pathophysiology of osteopetrosis. Eur J Endocrinol 134:143–156, 1996.

Frattini A, Pangrazio A, Susani L, Sobacchi C, Mirolo M, Abinum M, Andolina M, Flanagan A, Horwitz EM, Mihci E, Notarangelo LD, Rame U, Teti A, Van Hove J, Vujic D, Young T, Albertini A, Orchard PJ, Vezzoni P, Villa A. Chloride channel CICN7 mutations are responsible for severe recessive, dominant, and intermediate osteopetrosis. J Bone Miner Res 18:1740–1747, 2003.

Froon AH, Dentener MA, Greve JW, Ramsay G, Buurman WA. Lipopolysaccharide toxicity-regulating proteins in bacteremia. J Infect Dis 171:1250–1257, 1995.

Fukai K, Oh J, Karim MA, Moore KJ, Kandil HH, Ito H, Burger J, Spritz RA. Homozygosity mapping of the gene for Chediak-Higashi syndrome to chromosome 1q42–q44 in a segment of conserved synteny that induces the mouse beige locus (bg). Am J Hum Genet 59:620–624, 1996.

Gabig TO, English D, Akard L, Schell MJ. Regulation of neutrophil NADPH oxidase activation in a cell-free system by guanine nucleotides and fluoride. Evidence for participation of a pertussis and cholera toxin-insensitive G protein. J Biol Chem 262:1685–1690, 1987.

Gallin JI, Fletcher MP, Seligmann BE, Hoffstein S, Cehrs K, Mounessa N. Human neutrophil-specific granule deficiency: a model to assess the role of neutrophil-specific granules in the evolution of the inflammatory response. Blood 59:1317–1329, 1982.

Geha RS, Reinherz E, Leung D, McKee KJ, Jr. Deficiency of suppressor T cells in the hyperimmunoglobulin E syndrome. J Clin Invest 68:783–791, 1981.

Gonzalez LA, Hill HR. Advantages and disadvantages of antimicrobial prophylaxis in chronic granulomatous disease of childhood. Pediatr Infect Dis J 7:83–85, 1988.

Gorlin JB. Identification of (CA/GT)n polymorphisms within the X-linked chronic granulomatous disease (X-CGD) gene: utility for prenatal diagnosis. J Pediatr Hematol/Oncol 20:112–119, 1998.

Gray GR, Stamatoyannopoulos G, Naiman SC, Kliman MR, Klebanoff SJ, Austin T, Yoshida A, Robinson GC. Neutrophil dysfunction, chronic granulomatous disease, and non-spherocytic haemolytic anaemia caused by complete deficiency of glucose-6-phosphate dehydrogenase. Lancet 2:530–534, 1973.

Gresham HD, Clement LT, Lehmeyer JE, Griffin FM, Volanskis JE. Stimulation of human neutrophil Fc receptor–mediated phagocytosis by a low molecular weight cytokine. J Immunol 137:868–875, 1986.

Grimbacher B, Schaffer AA, Holland SM, Davis J, Gallin JI, Malech HL, Atkinson TP, Belohradsky BH, Buckley RH, Cossu F, Espanol T, Garty BZ, Matamoros N, Myers LA, Nelson RP, Ochs HD, Renner ED, Wellinghausen N, Puck JM. Genetic linkage of hyper-IgE syndrome to chromosome 4. Am J Human Genet 65:735–744, 1999.

Grodum E, Gram J, Brixen K, Bollerslev J. Autosomal dominant osteopetrosis: bone mineral measurements of the entire skeleton of adults in two different subtypes. Bone 16:431–434, 1995.

Groopman JE, Golde DW. The histiocytic disorders: a pathophysiologic analysis. Ann Intern Med 94:95–107, 1981.

Hanlon SM, Panayi GS, Laurent R. Defective polymorphonuclear leukocyte chemotaxis in rheumatoid arthritis associated with a serum inhibitor. Ann Rheumatol Dis 39:68–74, 1980.

Harvey BH. Acid-dependent dismutation of nitrogen oxides may be a critical source of nitric oxide in human macrophages. Med Hypotheses 54:829–831, 2000.

Hashimoto SI, Suzuki T, Nagai S, Yamashita T, Toyoda N, Matsushima K. Identification of genes specifically expressed in human activated and mature dendritic cells through serial analysis of gene expression. Blood 96:2206–2214, 2000.

Hayes MP, Wang J, Norcross MA. Regulation of interleukin-12 expression in human monocytes: selective priming by interferon-gamma of lipopolysaccharide-inducible p35 and p40 genes. Blood 86:646–650, 1995.

Hegde SP, Zhao J, Ashmun RA, Shapiro LH. c-Maf induces monocytic differentiation and apoptosis in bipotent myeloid progenitors. Blood 94:1578–1589, 1999.

Higgs HN, Pollard TD. Activation by Cdc42 and PIP(2) of Wiskott-Aldrich syndrome protein (WASp) stimulates actin nucleation by Arp2/3 complex. J Cell Biol. 150:F117–120, 2000.

Hildebrand JD, Taylor JM, Parsons JT. An SH3 domain-containing GTPase-activating protein for Rho and Cdc42 associates with focal adhesion kinase. Mol Cell Biol 16:3169–3178, 1996.

Hill HR. Laboratory aspects of immune deficiency in children. Pediatr Clin North Am 27:805–830, 1980.

Hill HR. The syndrome of hyperimmunoglobulinemia E and recurrent infections. Am J Dis Child 136:767–771, 1982.

Hill HR, Augustine NH, Alexander G, Carey JC, Ochs HD, Wedgwood RJ, Faville RJ, Quie PG, Leppert MF. Familial occurrence of Job's syndrome of hyper-IgE and recurrent infections. J Allergy Clin Immunol 995:395, 1997.

Hill HR, Augustine NH, Jaffe HS. Human recombinant interferon gamma enhances neonatal PMN activation and movement and increases free intracellular calcium. J Exp Med 173:767–770, 1991.

Horiguchi J, Warren MK, Ralph P, Kufe D. Expression of the macrophage specific colony-stimulating factor (CSF-1) during human monocytic differentiation. Biochem Biophys Res Commun 141:924–930, 1986.

Hornung V, Rothenfusser S, Britsch S, Krug A, Jahrsdorfer B, Giese T, Endres S, Hartmann G. Quantitative expression of toll-like receptor 1–10 mRNA in cellular subsets of human peripheral blood mononuclear cells and sensitivity to CpG oligodeoxynucleotides. J Immunol 168:4531–4537, 2002.

Horwitz ME, Barrett AJ, Brown MR, Carter CS, Childs R, Gallin JI, Holland SM, Linton GF, Miller JA, Leitman SF, Read EJ, Malech HL. Treatment of chronic granulomatous disease with nonmyeloablative conditioning and a T-cell-depleted hematopoietic allograft 344:926–927, 2001.

Imaizumi M. Bone marrow transplantation for lysosomal storage diseases. Jpn J Clin Med 53:3083–3088, 1995.

International Chronic Granulomatous Disease Cooperative Study Group. A controlled trial of interferon gamma to prevent infection in chronic granulomatous disease. N Engl J Med 324:509–516, 1991.

Introne W, Boissy RE, Gahl WA. Clinical, molecular, and cell biological aspects of Chediak-Higashi syndrome. Mol Genet Metab 68:283–303, 1999.

Iscove NN, Senn JE, Till JE, McCulloch EA. Colony formation by normal and leukemic human marrow cells in culture. Blood 37:1–5, 1971.

Ishijima M, Rittling SR, Yamashita T, Tsuji K, Kurosawa H, Nifuji A. Denhardt DT, Noda M. Enhancement of osteoclastic bone resorption and suppression of osteoblastic bone formation in response to reduced mechanical stress do not occur in the absence of osteopontin. J Exp Med 193:399–404, 2001.

Jacobs JC, Norman ME. A familiar defect of neutrophil chemotaxis with asthma, eczema, and recurrent infections. Pediatr Res 11:732–736, 1977.

Jain A, Buist NR, Kennaway NG, Powell BR, Auld PA, Martensson J. Effect of ascorbate or N-acetylcysteine treatment in a patient withhereditary glutathione synthetase deficiency. J Pediatr 124:229–233, 1994.

Jeppson JD, Jaffe HW, Hill HR. Use of recombinant human interferon gamma to enhance neutrophil chemotactic responses in Job syndrome of hyperimmunoglobulin E and recurrent infections. J Pediatr 118:383–387, 1991.

Johnston RB. Monocytes and macrophages. N Engl J Med 318:747–752, 1988.

Jouanguy E, Lamhamedi-Cherradi S, Lammas D, Dorman SE, Fondaneche MC, Dupuis S, Doffinger R. A human IFNλR1 small deletion hot spot associated with dominant susceptibility to mycobacterial infection. Nat Genet 21:370–378, 1999.

Kamani N, August CS, Campbell DE, Hassen NF, Douglas SD. Marrow transplantation in granulomatous disease. An update, with 6-year follow-up. J Pediatr 113:697–700, 1988.

Keeshan K, Santilli G, Corradini F, Perrotti D, Calabretta B. Transcription activation function of C/EBPalpha is required for induction of granulocytic differentiation. Blood 102:1267–1675, 2003.

Kim HY, Rikihisa Y. Roles of p38 mitogen-activated protein kinase, NF-kappaB, and protein kinase C in proinflammatory cytokine mRNA expression by human peripheral blood leukocytes, monocytes, and neutrophils in response to Anaplasma phagocytophila. Infect Immun 70:4132–4141, 2002.

Kim S, McAuliffe WJ, Zaritskaya LS, Moore PA, Zhang L, Nardelli B. Selective induction of tumor necrosis receptor factor 6/decoy receptor 3 release by bacterial antigens in human monocytes and myeloid dendritic cells. Infect Immun 72:89–93, 2004.

Kinashi T, Aker M, Sokolovsky-Eisenberg M, Grabovsky V, Tanaka C, Shamri R, Reigelson S, Etzioni A, Alon R. LAD-III, a leukocyte adhesion deficiency syndrome associated with defective Rap1 activation and impaired stabilization of integrin bonds. Blood 103:1033–1036, 2004.

Kloczko J, Bielawiec M, Giedrojc J, Radzwon P, Galar M. Human monocytes release plasma serine protease inhibitors in vitro. Haemostasis 20:229–232, 1990.

Knall C, Worthen GS, Johnson GL. Interleukin 8-stimulated phosphatidylinositol-3-kinase activity regulates the migration of human neutrophils independent of extracellular signal-regulated kinase and p38 mitogen-activated protein kinases. Proc Natl Acad Sci USA 94:3052–3057, 1997.

Koga T, Inui M, Inoue K, Kim S, Suematsu A, Kobayashi E, Iwata T, Ohnishi H, Matozaki T, Kodama T, Taniguchi T, Takayanagi H, Takai T. Costimulatory signals mediated by the ITAM motif cooperate with RANKL for bone homeostasis. Nature 428:758–763, 2004.

Kolluri R, Tolias KF, Carpenter CL, Rosen FS, Kirchhausen T. Direct interaction of the Wiskott-Aldrich syndrome protein with GTPase Cdc42. Proc Natl Acad Sci USA 93:5615–5618, 1996.

Kostmann R. Infantile genetic agranulocytopenia: new recessive lethal disease in man. Acta Paediatr Scand 45 (Suppl 105):1–78, 1956.

Kreis C, Fleur M, Menard C, Paquin R, Beaulieu AD. Thrombospondin and fibronectin are synthesized by neutrophils in human inflammatory joint disease and in a rabbit model of in vivo neutrophil activation. J Immunol 143:1961–1968, 1989.

Krivit W, Sung JH, Shapiro EG, Lockman LA. Microglia: the effector cell for reconstitution of the central nervous system following bone marrow transplantation for lysosomal and perisomal storage diseases. Cell Transplant 4:385–392, 1995.

Kushner BH, Cheung NK. Clinically effective monoclonal antibody 3F8 mediates nonoxidative lysis of human neuroectodermal tumor cells by polymorphonuclear leukocytes. Cancer Res 51:4865–4870, 1991.

Langenkamp A, Nagata K, Murphy K, Wu L, Lanzavecchia A, Sallusto F. Kinetics and expression patterns of chemokine receptors in human CD4+ T lymphocytes primed by myeloid or plasmacytoid dendritic cells. Eur J Immunol 33:474–482, 2003.

Larfars G, Gyllenhammar H. Stimulus-dependent transduction mechanisms for nitric oxide release in human polymorphonuclear neutrophil leukocytes. J Lab Clin Med 132:54–60, 1998.

Lau YL, Levinsky RJ. Prenatal diagnosis and carrier detection in primary immunodeficiency disorders. Arch Dis Child 63:758–764, 1988.

Lefkowitz DL, Mills K, Lefkowitz SS, Bollen A, Moguilevsky N. Neutrophil–macrophage interaction: a paradigm for chronic inflammation. Med Hypotheses 44:58–62, 1995.

Lehrer RI, Cline MJ. Leukocyte myeloperoxidase deficiency and disseminated candidiasis: the role of myeloperoxidase in resistance to Candida infection. J Clin Invest 48:1478–1488, 1969.

Leiner C. Erythrodermia desquamativa. Br J Child Dis 5:244–251, 1908.

Liles WC, Kiener PA, Ledbetter JA, Aruffo A, Klebanoff SJ. Differential expression of Fas(CD95) and Fas ligand on normal human phagocytes: implications for the regulation of apoptosis in neutrophils. J Exp Med 184:429–440, 1996.

Long MW. Blood cell cytoadhesion molecules. Exp Hematol 20:288–301, 1992.

Marlin SD, Morton CC, Anderson DC. LFA-1 immunodeficiency disease: definition of the genetic defect and chromosomal mapping of alpha and beta subunits of the lymphocyte function-associated antigen 1 (LFA-1) by complementation in hybrid cells. J Exp Med 164:855–867, 1986.

Marodi L, Leijh PCJ, van Furth R. Characteristics and functional capacities of human cord blood granulocytes and monocytes. Pediatr Res 18:1127–1131, 1984.

Masuno M, Imaizumi K, Nishimura G, Nakamura M, Saito I, Akagi K, Kuroki Y. Shwachman syndrome associated with de novo reciprocal translocation t(6)(q16.21.2). J Med Genet 32:894–895, 1995.

Mathy-Hartert M, Deby-Dupont G, Melin P, Lamy M, Deby C. Bactericidal activity against Pseudomonas aeruginosa is acquired by cultured human monocyte-derived macrophages after uptake of myeloperoxidase. Experimentia 52:167–174, 1996.

Matsumoto K. Decreased release of IL-10 by monocytes from patients with lipoid nephrosis. Clin Exp Immunol 102:603–607, 1995.

McCabe ERB, Leonard CO, Medici FN, Weiss L. Prenatal diagnosis for pediatricians. Pediatrics 84:741–744, 1989.

McCord JM, Gao B, Leff J, Flores SC. Neutrophil-generated free radicals: possible mechanisms of injury in adult respiratory distress syndrome. Environ Health Perspect 102 (Suppl 10):57–60, 1994.

McIvor Z, Hein S, Fiegler H, Schroeder T, Stocking C, Just U, Cross M. Transient expression of PU.1 commits multipotent progenitors to a myeloid fate whereas continued expression favors macrophage over granulocyte differentiation. Exp Hematol 31:39–47, 2003.

McNagny KM, Sieweke MH, Doderlein G, Graf T, Nerlow C. Regulation of eosinophil-specific gene expression by a C/EBP-Ets complex and GATA-1. EMBO J 17:3669–3680, 1998.

Metchnikoff E. 1898 Lectures on comparative pathology of inflammation, translated by FA Starling and EH Starling. London: Kegan Paul, Trench (cited in Abramson S L. Phagocyte deficiencies.) In Rich RR, ed. Clinical Immunology, Principles and Practice. St Louis: Mosby-Year Book, pp. 677–693, 1996.

Miller LJ, Bainton DF, Borregaard N, Springer TA. Stimulated mobilization of monocyte Mac-1 and p150.95 adhesion proteins from an intracellular vesicular compartment to the cell surface. J Clin Invest 80:535–544, 1987.

Miller ME. Pathology of chemotaxis and random mobility. Semin Hematol 12:59–82, 1975.

Miller ME, Koblenzer PJ. Leiner's disease and deficiency of C5. J Pediatr 80:879–880, 1972.

Miller ME, Nilsson UR, Myers KA. A familial deficiency of the phagocytosis-enhancing activity of serum related to a dysfunction of the fifth component of complement (C5). N Engl J Med 282:354–358, 1970.

Miranda MB, McGuire TF, Johnson DE. Importance of MEK-1/-2 signaling in monocytic and granulocytic differentiation of myeloid cell lines. Leukemia 16:683–692, 2002.

Mohacsi A, Fulop T, Jr, Kozlovszky B, Hauck M, Kiss I, Leovey A. Sera and leukocyte elastase-type protease and antiprotease activity in healthy and atherosclerotic subjects of various ages. J Gerontol 47:B154–158, 1992.

Mohler DN, Majerus PW, Minuch V, Hess CE, Garrick MD. Glutathione synthetase deficiency as a cause ofhereditary hemolytic disease. N Engl J Med 283:1253–1257, 1970.

Nagle DL, Karim MA, Woolf EA, Holmgren L, Bork P, Misumi DJ, McGrail SH, Dussault BJ, Jr, Perou CM, Boissy RE, Duyk GM, Spritz RA, Moore KJ. Identification and mutation analysis of the complete gene for Chediak-Higashi syndrome. Nat Genet 14:307–311, 1996.

Nangia-Makker P, Ochieng J, Christman JK, Raz A. Regulation of the expression of galactoside-binding lectin during human monocytic differentiation. Cancer Res 53:5033–5037, 1993.

Netea MG, Sutmuller R, Hermann C, Van der Graaf CA, Van der Meer JW, van Krieken JH, Hartung T, Adema G, Kullberg BJ. Toll-like receptor 2 suppresses immunity against Candida albicans through induction of IL-10 and regulatory T cells. J Immunol 172:3712–3718, 2004.

Newburger PE, Cohen HJ, Rothchild SB, Hobbin JC, Malawista SE, Mahoney JM. Prenatal diagnosis of chronic granulomatous disease. N Engl J Med 300:178–181, 1979.

Newman SL, Mikus LK, Tucci MA. Differential requirements for cellular cytoskeleton in human macrophage complement receptor-and Fc receptor–mediated phagocytosis. J Immunol 146:967–974, 1991.

Newport MJ, Huxley CM, Huston S, Hawrylowicz CM, Oostra BA, Williamson R, Levin M. A mutation in the interferon-γ-receptor gene and susceptibility to mycobacterial infection. N Engl J Med 335:1941–1949, 1996.

Newton JA, Augustine NH, Yang KD, Ashwood ER, Hill HR. Effect of pentoxifylline on developmental abnormalities in neutrophil cell surface receptor motility and membrane fluidity. J Cell Physiol 140:427–431, 1989.

Nobes CD, Hall A. Rho, rac and cdc42 GTPases: regulators of actin structure, cell adhesion, and motility. Biochem Soc Trans 23:456–459, 1995.

Ochs HD, Notarangelo LD. Structure and function of the Wiskott Aldrich syndrome protein (WASP). Current opinion in Hematology 12:284–291, 2005.

Oliver JM. Cell biology of leukocyte abnormalities—membrane and cytoskeletal function in normal and defective cells: a review. Am J Pathol 93:221–270, 1978.

Oliver JM, Berlin RD. Surface and cytoskeletal events regulating leukocyte membrane tcpography. Semin Hematol 20:282–304, 1983.

O'Reilly RJ, Brochstein J, Dinsmore R, Kirkpatrick D. Marrow transplantation for congenital disorders. Semin Hematol 21:188–221, 1984.

Ott GM. Stein S, Koehl U, Kunkel H, Siler U, Schilz A, Kuhlckek Schmidt M, von Kalli C, Hassan M, Hoelzer D, Seger R, Grez M, [abstract E.9]. Gene Therapy for X-linked Chronic Granulomatous Disease. Presented at the XI meeting of the European Society for Immunodeficiencies, Versailles, October 2004. Abstract E9, p97.

Owusu SK. Complete deficiency of glucose-6-phosphate dehydrogenase and neutrophil dysfunction. Lancet (ii): 796, 1973.

Parry MF, Root RK, Metcalf JA, Belaney KK, Kaglow LS, Richar WJ. Myeloperoxidase deficiency: prevalence and clinical significance. Ann Intern Med 95:293–301, 1981.

Pastural E, Ersoy F, Yalman N, Wulffraat N, Grillo E, Ozkinay F, Tezcan I, Gedikoglu G, Phipippe N, Fischer A, de Saint Basile G. Two genes are responsible for Griscelli syndrome at the same 15q21 locus. Genomics 63:299–306, 2000.

Pejaver RK, Watson AH. High-dose vitamin E therapy in glutathione synthetase deficiency. J Inherit Metab Dis 17:749–705, 1994.

Perignon JL, Durandy A, Peter MO, Freycon F, Dumez Y, Griscelli C. Early prenatal diagnosis of inherited severe immunodeficiencies linked to enzyme deficiencies. J Pediatr 111:595–598, 1987.

Petrak BA, Augustine NH, Hill HR. Recombinant human interferon gamma treatment of patients with Job syndrome of hyperimmunoglobulinemia E and recurrent infections. Clin Res 42:1A, 1994.

Phillips ML, Schwartz BR, Etzioni A, Bayer R, Ochs HD, Paulson JC, Harlan JM. Neutrophil adhesion in leukocyte adhesion deficiency syndrome type 2. J Clin Invest 96:2898–2906, 1995.

Picard C, Puel A, Bonnet M, Ku CL, Bustamante J, Yang K, Soudais C, Dupuis S, Feinberg J, Fieschi C, Elbim C, Hitchcock R, Lammas D, Davies G, Al-Ghonaium A, Al-Rayes H, Al-Jumaah S, Al-Hajjar S, Al-Mohsen IZ, Frayha HH, Rucker R, Hawn TR, Aderem A, Tufenkeji H, Haraguchi S, Day NK, Good RA, Gougerot-Pocidalo MA, Ozinsky A, Casanova JL. Pyogenic bacterial infections in humans with IRAK-4 deficiency. Science 299(5615)2076–2079, 2003.

Quie PG, White JO, Holmes B, Good RA. In vitro bactericidal capacity of human polymorphonuclear leukocytes: diminished activity in chronic granulomatous disease of childhood. J Clin Invest 46:668–679, 1967.

Raab Y, Sundberg C, Hallgren R, Knutson L, Gerdin B. Mucosal synthesis and release of prostaglandin E2 from activated eosinophils and macrophages in ulcerative colitis. Am J Gastroenterol 90:614–620, 1995.

Ramot B, Fisher S, Szeinbrug A, Adam A, Sheba C, Gafii D. A study of subject with erythrocyte glucose-6-phosphate dehydrogenase deficiency. II. Investigation of leukocyte enzyme. J Clin Invest 38:2234–2237, 1959.

Rebuck JW, Crowley JH. A method of studying leukocyte functions in vivo Ann NY Acad Sci 59:757–801, 1955.

Reeves JD, August CS, Humbert JR, Weston WL. Host defense in infantile osteopetrosis. Pediatrics 64:202–206, 1979.

Roberts RL, Ank BJ, Stiehm ER. Antiviral properties of neonatal and adult human neutrophils. Pediatr Res 36:792–798, 1994.

Rosenthal P, Rimin I, Umiel T. Ontogeny of human hemopoietic cells; analysis using monoclonal antibodies. J Immunol 31:232–237, 1983.

Sacchi F, Hill HR. Defective membrane potential changes in neutrophils from human neonates. J Exp Med 160:1247–1252, 1984.

Salyer JL, Bohnsack JF, Knape WA, Shigeoka AO, Ashwood ER, Hill HR. Mechanisms of tumor necrosis factor-alpha alteration of PMN adhesion and migration. Am J Pathol 136:831–841, 1990.

Sanal O, Ersoy F, Tezcan I, Metin A, Yel L, Manasche G, Gurgey A, Gurgey A, Berkel I, de Saint Basile G. Griscelli disease: genotype–phenotype correlation in an array of clinical heterogeneity. J Clin Immunol 22:237–243, 2002.

Sandborg RR, Smolen JE. Biology of disease: early biochemical events in leukocyte activation. Lab Invest 59:300–320, 1988.

Schmalstieg FC. Leukocyte adherence defect. Pediatr Infect Dis J 7: 867–872, 1988.

Sechler JMG, Malech HL, White CJ, Gallin JI. Recombinant human interferon-reconstitutes defective phagocyte function in patients with chronic granulomatous disease of childhood. Proc Natl Acad Sci USA 85:4874–4878, 1988.

Seger RA, Gungor T, Belohradsky BH, Blanche S, Bordigoni P, Di Bartolomeo P, Flood T, Landais P, Muller S, Ozsahin H, Passwell JH, Porta F, Slavin S, Wulffraat N, Zintl F, Nagler A, Cant A, Fischer A. Treatment of chronic granulomatous disease with myeloablative conditioning and an unmodified hemopoietic allorgraft: a survey of the European experience, 1985–2000. Blood 1000:4344–4350, 2002.

Sen C, Madazli R, Aksoy F, Ocak V. Antenatal diagnosis of lethal osteopetrosis. Ultrasound Obstet Gynecol 5:278–280, 1995.

Shwachman H, Diamond LK, Oski FA, Khaw K-T. The syndrome of pancreatic insufficiency and bone marrow dysfunction. J Pediatr 65:645–663, 1964.

Siminiak T, O'Gorman DJ, Shahi M, Hackett D, Sheridan DJ. Plasma mediated neutrophil stimulation during coronary angioplasty: autocrine effect of platelet activating factor. Br Heart J 74:625–630, 1995.

Simonet WS, Lacey DL, Dunstan CR, Kelley M, Chang MS, Luthy R, Nguyen HQ, Wooden S, Bennett L, Boone T, Shimamoto G, DeRose M, Elliott R, Colombero A, Tan HL, Trail G, Sullivan J, Davy E, Bucay N, Renshaw-Gegg L, Hughes TM, Hill D, Pattison W, Campbell P, Boyle WJ. Osteoprotegrin: a novel secreted protein involved in the regulation of bone density. Cell 89:309–319, 1997.

Smith LT, Hohaus S, Gonzalez DA, Dziennis SE, Tenen DG. PU.1 (Spi-1) and C/EBP alpha regulate the granulocyte colony-stimulating factor receptor promoter in myeloid cells. Blood 88:1234–1247, 1996.

Smith RM, Curnutte JT. Molecular basis of chronic granulomatous disease. Blood 77:673–686, 1991.

Snyderman R, Altman LC, Frankel A, Blaese RM. Defective mononuclear leukocyte chemotaxis: a previously unrecognized immune dysfunction. Studies in a patient with chronic mucocutaneous candidiasis. Ann Intern Med 78:509–513, 1973.

Sobacchi C, Frattini A, Orchard P, Porras O, Tezcan I, Andolina M, Babul-Hirji R, Baric L, Canham N, Citayat D, Dupuis-Girod S, Ellis I, Etzioni A, Fasth A, Fisher A, Gerritsen B, Gulino V, Horwitz E, Klamroth V, Lanino E, Mirolo M, Musio A, Matthijs G, Nonomaya S, Notarangelo LD, Ochs HD, Superti Furga A, Valiaho J, van Hove JL, Vihinen M, Vujic D, Vezzoni P, Villa A. The mutational spectrum of human malignant autosomal recessive osteopetrosis. Hum Mol Genet 10:1767–1773, 2001.

Southwick FS, Dabiri GA, Paschetto M, Zigmond SH. Polymorphonuclear leukocyte adherence induces actin polymerization by a transduction pathway which differs from that used by chemoattractants. J Cell Biol 109: 1561–1569, 1989a.

Southwick FS, Dabiri GA, Stossel TP. Neutrophil actin dysfunction is a genetic disorder associated with partial impairment of neutrophil actin assembly in three family members. J Clin Invest 82:1525–1531,1988.

Southwick FS, Howard TH, Holbrook T, Anderson DC, Stossel TP, Arnaout MA. The relationship between CR3 deficiency and neutrophil actin assembly. Blood 73:1973–1979, 1989b.

Spillert CR, Lazaro EJ. Contribution of the monocyte to thrombotic potential. Agents Actions 34:28–29, 1991.

Spitznagel JK, Shafer WM. Neutrophil killing of bacteria by oxygen-independent mechanisms: a historical summary. Rev Infect Dis 7:398–403, 1985.

Springer TA. Adhesion receptors of the immune system. Nature 346: 425–434, 1990.

Susin SA, Lorenzo HK, Zamzami N, Marzo I, Snow BE, Brothers GM, Mangion J, Macotot E, Costantini P, Loeffler M, Larochette N, Goodlett DR, Aebersold R, Siderovski DP, Penninger JM, Kroemer G. Molecular characterization of mitochondrial apoptosis-inducing factor. Nature 397: 441–446, 1999.

Symons M, Derry JM, Karlak B, Jiang S, Lemahieu V, Mccormick F, Francke U, Abo A. Wiskott-Aldrich syndrome protein, a novel effector for the GTPase CDC42Hs, is implicated in actin polymerization. Cell 84:723–734, 1996.

Takahashi K, Umeda S, Shultz LD, Hayashi S, Nishikawa S. Effects of macrophage colony-stimulating factor (M-CSF) on the development, differentiation, and maturation of marginal metallophilic macrophages and marginal zone macrophages in the spleen of osteopetrosis (op) mutant mice lacking functional M-CSF activity. J Leukoc Biol 55:581–588, 1994.

Taylor GM, Dearden SP, Will AM, Evans DI, Stevens RF, Simon S, Super M, Morrell G, Fergusson WD, Brown IH. Infantile osteopetrosis: bone marrow transplantation from a cousin donor. Arch Dis Child 73:453–454, 1995.

Teahan C, Rowe P, Parker P, Totty N, Segal AW. The X-linked chronic granulomatous disease gene codes for the β-chain of cytochrome b-245. Nature 327:720–721, 1987.

Thoma-Uszynski S, Stenger S, Takeuchi O, Ochoa MT, Engele M, Sieling PA, Barnes PF, Rollinghoff M, Bolcskei PL, Wagner M, Shizuo A, Norgard MV, Belisle JT, Godowski PJ, Bloom BR, Modlin RL. Induction of direct antimicrobial activity through mammalian toll-like receptors. Science 291:1544–1547, 2001.

Thompson RA. Immunodeficiency due to defects of polymorphonuclear leukocyte function. Immunol Invest 17:85–92, 1988.

Tian S-S, Tapley P, Sincich C, Stein RB, Rosen J, Lamb P. Multiple signaling pathways induced by granulocyte colony-stimulating factor involving activation of JAKs, STAT5, and/or STAT3 are required for regulation of three distinct classes of immediate early genes. Blood 88:4435–4444, 1996.

Tsuji T, Nagata K, Koike J, Todoroki N, Irimura T. Induction of superoxide anion production from monocytes and neutrophils by activated platelets through the P-selectin-sialyl Lewis X interaction. J Leukoc Biol 56: 583–587, 1994.

Vaickus L, Biddle W, Cemerlic D, Foon KA. Interferon gamma augments Lym-1-dependent, granulocyte-mediated tumor cell lysis. Blood 75: 2408–2416, 1990.

Valerius NH, Stendahi O, Hartwig JH, Stossel TP. Distribution of actin-binding protein and myosin in polymorphonuclear leukocytes during locomotion and phagocytosis. Cell 24:195–202, 1981.

Van de Winkel JG, Jansze M, Capel PJ. Effect of protease inhibitors on human monocyte IgG Fc receptor II. Evidence that serine esterase activity is essential for Fc gamma RII-mediated binding. J Immunol 145:1890–1896, 1990.

Van Dyke TE. Role of the neutrophil in oral disease. Receptor deficiency in leukocytes from patients with juvenile periodontitis. Rev Infect Dis 7: 419–425, 1985.

Van Dyke TE, Levine MJ, Tabak LA, Genco RJ. Reduced chemotactic peptide binding in juvenile periodontitis: a model for neutrophil function. Biochem Biophys Res Commun 100:1278–1284, 1981.

Van Dyke TE, Wilson-Burrows C, Offenbacher S, Henson P. Association of an abnormality of neutrophil chemotaxis in human periodontal disease with a cell surface protein. Infect Immun 55:2262–2267, 1987.

Van Hul W, Bollerslev J, Gram J, Van Hul E, Wuyts W, Benichou O, Vanhoenacker F, Willems PJ. Localization of a gene for autosomal dominant osteopetrosis (Albers-Schonberg disease) to chromosome 1p21. Am J Hum Genet 61:363–369, 1997.

Van Scoy RE, Hill HR, Ritts RE, Quie PG. Familiar neutrophil chemotaxis defect, recurrent bacterial infections, mucocutaneous candidiasis, and hyperimmunoglobulinemia E. Ann Intern Med 82:766–771, 1975.

Villa A, Bozzi F, Sobacchi C, Strina D, Fasth A, Pasic S, Notarangelo LD, Vezzoni P. Prenatal diagnosis of RAG-deficient Omenn syndrome. Prenat Diagn 20:56–59, 2000.

Villunger A, O'Reilly LA, Holler N, Adams J, Strasser A. Fas ligand, Bcl-2, granulocyte colony-stimulating factor, and p38 mitogen-activated protein kinase: regulators of distinct cell death and survival pathways in granulocytes. J Exp Med 192:647–658, 2000.

Vossen JM. Bone marrow transplantation in the treatment of severe immunodeficiencies: possibilities and problems. Immunol Invest 17:135–146, 1988.

Wallis RS, Eliner JJ. Cytokines and tuberculosis. J Leuk Biol 55:676–681, 1994.

Wang BR, Josien R, Choi Y. TRANCE is a TNF family member that regulates dentritic cell and osteoclast function. J Leukoc Biol 65:715–724, 1999.

Ward AC, Loeb DM, Soede-Bobok AA, Touw IP, Friedman AD. Regulation of granulopoiesis by transcription factors and cytokine signals. Leukemia 14:973–990, 2000.

Watanabe Y, Inaba T, Shimano H, Gotoda T, Yamamoto K, Mokuno H, Sato H, Yazaki Y, Yamada N. Induction of LDL receptor-related protein during the differentiation of monocyte-macrophages. Possible involvement in the atherosclerotic process. Arterioscler Thromb 14:1000–1006, 1994.

Weening RS, Leitz GJ, Seger RA. Recombinant human interferon-gamma in patients with chronic granulomatous disease—European follow-up study. Eur J Pediatr 154:295–298, 1995.

Weetman RM, Boxer LA. Childhood neutropenia. Pediatr Clin North Am 27:361–401, 1980.

Weil SC, Rosner GL, Reid MS, Chisholm RL, Farber NM, Spitznagel JK, Swanson MS. cDNA cloning of human myeloperoxidase: decrease in myeloperoxidase mRNA upon induction of HL-60 cells. Proc Natl Acad Sci USA 84:2057–2061, 1987.

Wientjes FB, Panayotou G, Reeves E, Segal AW. Interactions between cytosolic components of the NADPH oxidase: p40 phox interacts with both p67 phox and p47 phox. Biochem J 317:919–924, 1996.

Wuyts A, Proost P, Put W, Lenaerts JP, Paemen L, van Damme J. Leukocyte recruitment by monocyte chemotactic proteins (MCPs) secreted by human phagocytes. J Immunol Method 174:237–247, 1994.

Yang KD, Augustine NH, Gonzalez LA, Augustine NH, Hill HR. Effects of fibronectin on the interaction of polymorphonuclear leukocytes with unopsonized and antibody-opsonized bacteria. J Infect Dis 158:823–830, 1988.

Yang KD, Augustine NH, Shaio M, Bohnsack JF, Hill HR. Effects of fibronectin on actin organization and respiratory burst activity in neutrophils, monocytes, and macrophages. J Cell Physiol 158:347–353, 1994.

Yang KD, Hill HR. Neutrophil function disorders: pathophysiology, prevention, and therapy. J Pediatr 119:343–354, 1991.

Yang KD, Hill HR. Functional biology of the granulocyte-monocyte series. In Bick RL, ed. Hematology: Clinical and Laboratory Practice. Philadelphia: Mosby, pp. 1077–1092, 1993.

Yang KD, Hill HR. Assessment of neutrophil function. In Rich RB, ed. Clinical Immunology: Principles and Practice. St. Louis: Mosby-Year Book, pp. 2148–2156, 1996.

Yang KD, Hill HR. Granulocyte function disorders: aspects of development, genetics and management. Pediatr Infect Dis J 20:889–900, 2001.

Zentilin L, Tafuro S, Grassi G, Garcia R, Ventura A, Baralle F, Falaschi A, Giacca M. Functional reconstitution of oxidase activity in X-linked chronic granulomatous disease by retrovirus-mediated gene transfer. Exp Cell Res 225:257–267, 1996.

Zhang P, Behre G, Pan J, Iwama A, Wara-Aswapati N, Radomska HS, Auron PE, Tenen DG, Sun Z. Negative cross-talk between hematopoietic regulators; GATA proteins repress PU.1. Proc Natl Acad Sci USA 96:8705–8710, 1999.

II

Syndromes

9

X-Linked Severe Combined Immunodeficiency

JENNIFER M. PUCK

Severe combined immunodeficiency (SCID) comprises a collection of genetic defects that involve both humoral and cellular immunity. A profound lack of immune function leads to infections that are generally fatal in infancy unless the immune system can be reconstituted. X-linked SCID (XSCID, SCIDX1, MIM #300400) is caused by defects in *IL2RG* (MIM *308380), the gene encoding the interleukin-2 (IL-2) receptor γ chain (Online Mendelian Inheritance in Man [OMIM], 2000), also known as the common γ chain. XSCID is the most frequent genetic form of SCID. Its incidence is unknown, although it has been estimated to occur in at least 1 per 100,000 births. Males, who have a single X chromosome, are affected with XSCID. Female carriers, who have a mutated copy of the gene on one of their two X chromosomes and a normal copy on the other, remain healthy. However, carrier females can pass on the disease to their male offspring and the carrier state to their female offspring. XSCID appears to occur equally in all ethnic groups.

Both a striking male predominance of SCID in all published series and recognition of pedigrees with multiple affected males related through maternal lineages first suggested that XSCID would turn out to be the major form of SCID. When the XSCID genetic locus in Xq13.1 was identified so that mutation diagnosis could be performed, this prediction was directly confirmed (Buckley et al., 1997; Puck et al., 1997b). XSCID accounts for approximately half of all cases of SCID, although there is perhaps a larger proportion in the United States than in European populations (Buckley et al., 1997; Antoine et al., 2003; Buckley, 2004).

History and Variety of Genetic Forms

The first descriptions of a fatal congenital deficiency of lymphocytes date from the 1950s in Switzerland. Glanzmann and Riniker

(1950) described an idiopathic lymphocyte wasting syndrome with fatal *Candida albicans* infection. Following the discovery of agammaglobulinemia by Bruton (1952), Hitzig and Willi (1961) reported familial alymphocytosis combined with agammaglobulinemia that had a fatal outcome in infancy. No distinction between recessive and X-linked inheritance patterns was made in these early reports. The term "Swiss-type agammaglobulinemia," originally used to distinguish infants with fungal infections, lymphopenia, and early death, from less severely affected children with agammaglobulinemia alone, has been a source of confusion, in part because the "Swiss-type" label was subsequently applied to patients in kindreds in which SCID was X-linked. With improved immunological tools to characterize immune defects plus the ongoing identification of additional genes associated with specific forms of many immunodeficiencies, disease designations have become more precise.

Failure to recognize immunodeficiency as the underlying cause of recurrent diarrhea, pneumonia, septicemia, fungal infections, or failure to thrive is evident in family histories of many large kindreds in which several generations of male infants have died. Often in the past, these patients were mistakenly diagnosed as having dietary intolerances or cystic fibrosis because of diarrhea, poor weight gain, and pulmonary infections. Some were given diagnoses such as scarlet fever (from the rash of spontaneous graft vs. host disease [GVHD] from maternally derived lymphocytes) or diphtheria (when thrush extending down the throat was thought to represent a diphtheritic membrane). Even today, SCID is frequently not suspected upon presentation to primary physicians or even referral centers. In countries where newborns are routinely vaccinated against tuberculosis with the live attenuated mycobacterial organism bacillus Calmette-Guérin (BCG), infants with SCID may develop fatal, disseminated BCG infection. For these reasons, pediatric immunologists believe that the true incidence of SCID is greater than the 1 per 100,000 estimate based on diagnosed cases.

Prior to 1968, patients with XSCID almost always died within the first year of life. However, the achievement of immune reconstitution following bone marrow transplantation (BMT) from a human leukocyte antigen (HLA)-identical sibling marked the beginning of successful treatment (Gatti et al., 1968). The unavailability of histocompatible donors for the majority of XSCID patients led to the use of isolation in a germ-free environment for David, the Bubble Boy, a famous Texas patient who came to represent SCID to the general public. Although David succumbed to complications of Epstein-Barr virus (EBV) lymphoproliferation after a BMT at age 12 from a sibling (Shearer et al., 1985), the technique of T cell–depleted haploidentical BMT has now been successfully adopted for treatment of infants with XSCID (see Chapter 47). Early diagnosis, better antibiotics, and intensive supportive care have also contributed to the evolution of XSCID from a fatal to a treatable disease. Currently it is estimated that over 80%–90% of infants with XSCID can be saved by transplantation treatment (Antoine et al., 2003; Buckley, 2004).

Table 9.1 summarizes currently known SCID genotypes and cellular phenotypes and gives a rough breakdown of the relative percentage of cases caused by defects in each gene. Enumeration of T and B lymphocytes and, more recently, natural killer (NK) cells has provided useful correlations of lymphocyte phenotype with genotype. While all patients with SCID have very few T cells, over half have detectable or even increased numbers of B cells that are nonfunctional (T−B+ SCID) (Stephan et al., 1993; Buckley et al., 1997). Most of these patients are males, but from the existence of females with T−B+ SCID it is clear that both autosomal recessive and X-linked gene defects can produce this phenotype. T−B+ SCID is now associated with defects in any of several genes, including *JAK3*, encoding the signaling kinase that interacts intracellularly with the common γ chain; *IL7R*, encoding the α chain of the receptor for IL-7 (both discussed in Chapter 10); *CD45*, encoding the cell surface coreceptor CD45 (Chapter 13); the p51 tyrosine kinase *lck* gene (Chapter 14); and *TCRD*, encoding the δ chain of the CD3 complex (Chapter 16). In addition, humans with defects in the *FOXN1* transcription factor that is defective in athymic nude mice have autosomal recessive T−B+ SCID in addition to alopecia totalis (Frank et al., 1999). While most patients with T−B+ SCID lack NK cells, those with *IL7R* mutations and other defects specifically related to signaling through the T cell receptor generally have intact NK cell development (Table 9.1).

Patients with no T or B cells (T−B− SCID) have a more even ratio of males to females, a pattern suggesting autosomal recessive inheritance. Autosomal recessive T−B− SCID can be caused by complete deficiency of adenosine deaminase (Chapter 12) and also by defects in the proteins involved in the DNA rearrangement of T cell and B cell receptor genes (Chapter 11). Despite rapid progress in new SCID gene discovery in the past decade, documented in Table 9.1, there are still SCID patients whose molecular diagnosis remains unknown, and many additional SCID gene defects are likely to be found.

The discovery of the XSCID disease gene, *IL2RG* (Noguchi et al., 1993b; Puck et al., 1993b), has led to increased appreciation of the immunologic characteristics of this form of SCID,

Table 9.1. Genotypes Associated with Severe Combined Immunodeficiency

Gene Defect	Molecular Pathogenesis	Percent of SCID Cases*	Characteristic Lymphoctye Subpopulations		
			T Cells†	B Cells	Natural Killer Cells
IL2RG (X-linked)	Failure of signaling through common γ chain receptors for cytokines IL-2, -4, -7, -9, -15, -21 (Chapter 9)	46%	Low/absent	Present	Absent
ADA	Adenosine deaminase deficiency (Chapter 12)	16%	Low/absent	Absent	Absent
IL7R	Failure of signaling through IL-7 receptor (Chapter 10)	9%	Low/absent	Present	Present
JAK3	Failure of Janus kinase 3 activation by common γ chain (Chapter 10)	6%	Low/absent	Present	Absent
RAG1	Failure of T and B cell antigen receptor rearrangement (Chapter 11)	<2%	Absent	Absent	Present
RAG2	Failure of T and B cell antigen receptor rearrangement (Chapter 11)	<2%	Absent	Absent	Present
DCLRE1C	Failure of T and B cell antigen receptor rearrangement (Chapter 11)	<5%	Absent	Absent	Present
CD45	Lack of cell surface protein tyrosine phosphatase receptor, PTPRC, required for T and B cell activation by antigen (Chapter 13)	Rare	Low/absent	Present	Low, maybe variable
TCRD	CD3δ deficiency with lack of T cell development (Chapter 16)	Very rare	Low/absent	Present	Present
LCK	Lack of lymphocyte tyrosine kinase p56lck, required for T cell development and activation (Chapter 14)	Very rare	Low/absent	Present	Present
FOXN1	Lack of forkhead box N1 transcription factor, required for thymus and hair follicle development (ortholog of nude mouse) (Frank et al., 1999)	Very rare	Low/absent	Present	Present
RMRP	Lack of RNA component of mitochondrial RNA–processing endoribonuclease, causing cartilage-hair hypoplasia (CHH); variable immunodeficiency, in some cases severe (Chapter 36)	Very rare	Low/very low	Present	Maybe low
Complete DiGeorge syndrome	Aplasia of the thymus, most often with chromosome 22q11 deletion (Chapter 33)	Rare	Absent	Variable	Present
Currently unknown	Unknown, including reticular dysgenesis and congenital anomaly syndromes with SCID‡	Each one rare	Low/absent	Variable	Variable

*Based on Buckley (2004), Antoine et al. (2003), and unpublished estimates (J. Puck).

†Some patients have substantial numbers of maternally derived T cells at time of diagnosis.

‡For example, SCID with multiple intestinal atresia (Gilroy et al., 2004), SCID with musculoskeletal abnormalities (Tangsinmankong et al., 1999).

elucidation of molecular responses of lymphocytes to cytokines, and availability of carrier and prenatal diagnosis by direct detection of mutations. Furthermore, XSCID has become the first disease in humans to be successfully treated by gene therapy (Chapter 48).

Clinical and Pathologic Manifestations

Male infants with XSCID appear normal at birth. Presenting complaints are highly variable, as summarized in Table 9.2, and are generally not distinguishable from those of patients with autosomal forms of SCID except that female patients are assumed to have autosomal SCID. Although a family history can lead to laboratory confirmation of XSCID before or at the time of birth, over 50% of patients have no maternal male relatives with diagnosed immunodeficiency or early death consistent with XSCID. Whether due to chance and small sibship sizes or to newly arising mutations (see Strategies for Diagnosis of XSCID, below), the most common presentation of XSCID—and also the most common presentation of SCID of any genotype—is a sporadic affected male (Conley et al., 1990; Buckley et al., 1997). As transplacentally transferred maternal IgG wanes, infants with XSCID develop infections that bring them to medical attention generally by 3 to 6 months of age. Thrush or respiratory and gastrointestinal infections may at first seem routine, but they do not respond to the usual medical management. For example, otitis may not resolve despite several courses of oral antibiotics; respiratory syncytial virus (RSV) may be continuously present in pulmonary secretions for several months; and diarrhea leads to failure to gain weight, or even weight loss. Rashes, either erythematous or maculopapular, have been associated with GVHD, either from maternal cells transferred to the infant during birth or from transfusion of nonirradiated blood products prior to recognition of the immunodeficiency.

Table 9.2. Clinical Features of X-linked Severe Combined Immunodeficiency (XSCID)

Universal Features

Male gender
Presentation in first year, usually by age 6 months
Failure to thrive
Oral thrush, candida diaper rash
Absent tonsils
Persistence of infections despite conventional treatment

Common Features

Family history of similarly affected maternal male relatives
Chronic diarrhea
Respiratory congestion, cough
Fevers
Pneumonia, especially with *Pneumocystis jiroveci*
Sepsis, severe bacterial infections
Viral infections, including cytomegalovirus, adenovirus, Epstein-Barr virus, enteric viruses, varicella, herpes, and respiratory syncitial virus
Infections with opportunistic pathogens

Less Common Features

Erythematous skin rash (often with hepatomegaly and even lymphadenopathy) from spontaneous or transfusion-related graft vs. host disease
Recurrent bacterial meningitis
Disseminated infections (salmonella, varicella, Bacillus Calmette-Guérin; rarely, vaccine strain [live] poliovirus)

Table 9.3. Pathologic Findings in X-linked Severe Combined Immunodeficiency

Primary Absence of T Cell Precursors

Markedly small thymus gland
Vestigial thymic stroma present
Absence of lymphocytes in thymus
No Hassall's corpuscles in thymus
No corticomedullary distinction

Evidence of Infections Secondary to Immunodeficiency

Candida pharyngitis, esophagitis
Pneumonia or pulmonary infiltration with
  Candida, other fungi
  Pseudomonas, other gram-negative bacteria
  Pneumocystis carinii
  Cytomegalovirus

Evidence of Graft vs. Host Disease

Lymphocytic infiltration of skin, liver, other organs

Eventually, a clinical decompensation, diagnosis of an opportunistic pathogen, such as *Pneumocystis jiroveci* (formerly *P. carinii*), or a high index of suspicion leads to consideration of an immune disorder. Decompensating events include bacterial sepsis, meningitis, or deep-seated infections, as well as bacterial, fungal, or viral pneumonias. Three series of SCID patients in France (Stephan et al., 1993) and the United States (Bortin and Rimm, 1977; Buckley et al., 1997) reported a similar large range of infectious agents at presentation, primarily *Candida albicans*; *P. jiroveci*; *Pseudomonas, Salmonella*, and other gram-negative bacteria; gram-positive bacteria; respiratory viruses and viruses of the herpes family; and fungi. Infants with SCID who have received BCG vaccination may develop disseminated infection with this organism. Live polio vaccination has uncommonly caused poliomyelitis and carditis, but most infants have protective transplacentally acquired maternal antipoliovirus antibodies.

The hallmark of XSCID immunopathology (Table 9.3) is an extremely small thymus gland almost devoid of lymphocytes. Thymic stroma is present, but not well differentiated. There are no Hassall's corpuscles and no corticomedullary distinction. Thymic dendritic and epithelial cells are abnormal (Hale et al., 2004). Analysis of T cell receptor β chain rearrangement in thymic tissue from infants with XSCID has shown that the initial Dβ-to-Jβ recombination can occur, but subsequent VDJ rearrangement is blocked (Sleasman et al., 1994). Similarly, in extrathymic lymphoid organs, lymph nodes are small and poorly developed, and T lymphocytes cannot be found. Tonsils are absent. Other pathological findings in infants with XSCID who do not survive include manifestations of their terminal infections and, in some patients, lymphocytic infiltration of skin, liver, and other organs as a result of GVHD.

Unless treated by BMT, infants with XSCID generally succumb to infections before 1 year of age, but in rare cases the diagnosis of XSCID has been made in infants beyond their second birthday. A sheltered home environment may be a factor in late presentation. A mild clinical course has also been associated with particular mutational profiles of *IL2RG*, as discussed below.

Laboratory Findings

Laboratory values that are useful to diagnose all types of SCID are summarized in Table 9.4. A helpful clue from a simple laboratory test is a low absolute lymphocyte count, compared to values for age-matched normal infants. While not universal, this

Syndromes

Table 9.4. Laboratory Abnormalities in Infants with X-linked Severe Combined Immunodeficiency*

	XSCID Patients	Proportion with Low Numbers	Control Value Range, First Year*,†
Lymphocyte Counts			
Total lymphocytes/μl	<2000	90%	3400–9000
T cells/μl	200 (0–800)	100%	2500–5600
B cells/μl	1300 (0–3000)	5%	300–3000
NK cells/μl	<100	88%	170–1100
T Cell Receptor Excision Circles (TRECs)			
	Absent	100%	1 per 10 T cells
Antibody Concentrations†			
IgA, IgM	Extremely low		
IgG	Maternal levels at birth, low by age 3 months		
Lymphocyte Function†			
Mitogen responses	Very poor		
Mixed lymphocyte response	Very poor		
NK cytotoxicity	Usually very poor; occasionally normal		
Specific antibody	Very poor production		
Other Laboratory Tests			
Absent thymic shadow	Universal on chest radiogram		

*Adapted from Buckley et al. (1993, 1997); Chan and Puck (2005); Conley et al. (1990); Fischer (1992); Kalman et al. (2004); Schönland et al. (2003); Shearer et al. (2003); Stephan et al. (1993); Stiehm et al. (2004).

†Control ranges are approximate and age-dependent, and they may vary between laboratories. One should consult the immunology laboratory performing the test for best interpretation.

indicator should raise the suspicion of a congenital immunodeficiency in an infant with a significant infection. Because of arrested development of T cells, infants with SCID lack T cell receptor excision circles, or TRECs (Chan and Puck, 2005). TRECs are the episomal DNA circles formed by end-joining of genomic DNA segments removed during T cell receptor gene rearrangement; a quantitative polymerase chain reaction (PCR) across the joined ends is used to measure TREC number (Douek et al., 2000; Schönland et al. 2003).

Typically, but not always, the small numbers of lymphocytes found in patients with XSCID are predominantly or entirely B cells, which may be present in normal or even elevated numbers. Thus XSCID is the major disease accounting for T−B+ SCID. Mutation-proven XSCID patients reported by Buckley et al. (1997, 1999) have a lymphocyte profile to similar to that of the T−B+ patients (not all genotyped, but predominantly males) reported by Antoine et al., from Europe (2003).

The B cells found in infants with XSCID are immature and resemble the naive B cell population of normal cord blood in their expression of cell surface markers and in vitro antibody production restricted to immunoglobulin (Ig)M (Small et al., 1989). Sequence analysis of XSCID B cell immunoglobulin heavy chains has demonstrated normal VDJ rearrangement (Minegishi et al., 1994). However, there is overutilization of J_H3 segments, as seen in fetal and neonatal B cells, and a total lack of somatic hypermutation. In XSCID infants whose maternally acquired IgG antibodies have waned, specific responses to vaccines or infectious agents are severely impaired or absent. Other distinguishing characteristics of XSCID are low numbers of cells that bear NK cell markers and poor NK cell cytotoxicity.

Despite the utility of these generalizations, lymphocyte numbers and function are not uniform in all patients and may be subject to modification by genetic factors other than *IL2RG* mutation and by environmental factors. For example, patients with *IL2RG* mutations occasionally have low, rather than the typical normal to high, numbers of B cells. Also, patients with proven *IL2RG* defects have been reported who have NK cells and NK cytotoxicity (Pepper et al., 1995).

Spontaneous engraftment of maternal lymphocytes in males with XSCID can be detected by finding XX karyotypes on cytogenetic analysis, by HLA typing, or by using DNA polymorphic markers (Pollack et al., 1982; Conley et al., 1984; Puck et al., 2001). Maternal cells can be found in almost all XSCID patients if sensitive methods are used. Although there may be no discernible consequences of maternal engraftment, the maternal cells may elevate the lymphocyte counts of an infant with XSCID. When sufficient numbers of maternal cells are activated to respond to the infant's paternally derived histocompatibility antigens, an XSCID patient may have eosinophilia and circulating maternal, activated, DR+ T cells. In patients who have iatrogenic GVHD from transfusion of nonirradiated blood products, these abnormalities can become pronounced, and florid, acute GVHD can occur, including gatroenteritis, hepatitis, and lymphocytic infiltrates in skin, liver, and other organs.

Molecular Basis: The Disease Gene, *IL2RG*

X-linked SCID was mapped by linkage to the proximal long arm of the X chromosome by De Saint Basile et al. (1987). Gene mapping studies were hampered by the early lethality of XSCID in males and the lack of any clinical or immunologic abnormalities to distinguish carrier females. However, Puck et al. (1987) noted that in contrast to the expected random X chromosome inactivation in female tissues, obligate female carriers of XSCID had only

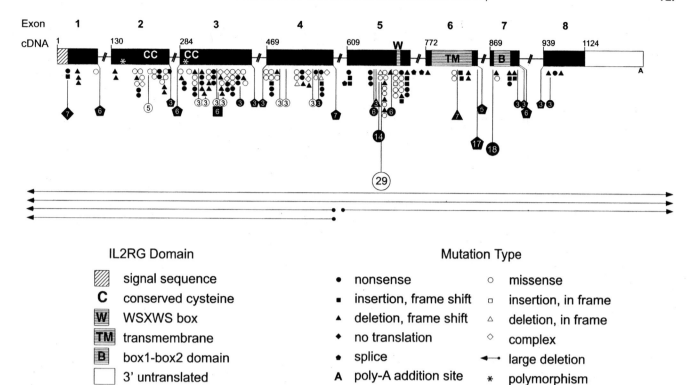

IL2RG Domain

▨	signal sequence
C	conserved cysteine
W	WSXWS box
TM	transmembrane
B	box1-box2 domain
☐	3' untranslated

Mutation Type

●	nonsense	○	missense
■	insertion, frame shift	□	insertion, in frame
▲	deletion, frame shift	△	deletion, in frame
◆	no translation	◇	complex
●	splice	←→	large deletion
A	poly-A addition site	*	polymorphism

Figure 9.1. Structure of *IL2RG* and mutations found in patients with X-linked SCID, both published and reported to IL2RGbase (http://www.genome.gov/DIR/GMBB/SCID; Puck et al., 1996); Genbank accession number L19546. At sites where multiple mutation events have occurred, mutation symbols are enlarged and number of unrelated subjects with mutation indicated.

the nonmutated X chromosome as the active X in their lymphocytes. This nonrandom X inactivation reflected a selective disadvantage in proliferation, differentiation, or survival of lymphocyte progenitors lacking a normal gene product at the SCIDX1 locus. Nonrandom X inactivation is found in T cells, B cells, and NK cells of XSCID carriers. In contrast, random X inactivation patterns are seen in their granulocytes, monocytes, and other tissues (Puck et al., 1987; Conley et al., 1988; Wengler et al., 1993). Thus the SCIDX1 gene product is necessary for the development of lymphoid but not myeloid cells from bone marrow stem cells.

Nonrandom X inactivation in lymphocytes was also used to assign the carrier status of female relatives of XSCID patients, increasing the number of informative individuals for genetic linkage in XSCID pedigrees. Further narrowing of the SCIDX1 region was made possible by the study of males with choroideremia and deafness, but not immunodeficiency, who had interstitial deletions below Xq13, (Puck et al., 1993a). Until this time, no genes related to the immune system were known to reside in the region defined by mapping studies. However, in 1993, two groups (Noguchi et al., 1993b; Puck et al., 1993b) realized that the γ chain of the receptor for IL-2, cloned the previous year (Takeshita et al., 1992), was located in the region where SCIDX1 had been placed. Deleterious mutations in *IL2RG*, the gene encoding this receptor, were found in XSCID patients, proving that *IL2RG* is the XSCID disease gene.

IL2RG encodes the γ chain of the IL-2 receptor; the gene product is now called the common γ chain, γc. Two chains of the IL-2 receptor were known to exist before the γ chain was identified. The β chain, constituitively expressed on T cells, has intermediate affinity for IL-2 by itself; and the α chain, expressed after T cell activation, boosts the affinity for IL-2 of the receptor

complex 100-fold. The existence of a γ chain was postulated when transfection of the α and β chains of IL-2 receptor into epithelial cell lines failed to produce a receptor that could transmit a signal. A third chain was co-immunoprecipitated with the β chain and subsequently purified by two-dimensional gel electrophoresis (Takeshita et al., 1992). Determination of the amino-terminal sequence led to isolation of full-length cDNA for *IL2RG*. The gene, depicted in Figure 9.1, spans 4.5 kb of genomic DNA in Xq13.1. The coding sequence of 1124 nucleotides is divided into eight exons. *IL2RG*, a type I protein, is a member of the cytokine receptor gene family. It encodes a 5' signal sequence of 22 amino acids, which is cleaved off while targeting the protein for cell surface expression. Four conserved cysteine residues are found at the extracellular amino-terminal end; the juxtamembrane extracellular motif encoded in exon 5, the WSXWS box, is a hallmark of all cytokine receptors; the highly hyrdophobic transmembrane domain of 29 amino acids occupies most of exon 6; and the proximal intracellular domain in exon 7 contains a Box1/Box2 signaling sequence homologous to SH2 subdomains of Src-related tyrosine kinases.

The three-dimensional structure of the γc protein has been characterized (Wang et al., 2005), and the exact spatial arrangement and interaction between γc and its extracellular contacts explains how IL-2 signaling is initiated at the extracellular surface (Stauber et al., 2006). The α chain binds IL-2 and delivers it to the β chain, following which the γ chain addition to the quaternary complex creates a highly stable signaling structure.

Function of γc, the *IL2RG* Gene Product

The first report of γc by Takeshita et al. (1992) established its expression in lymphocytes and cell lines of both T and B cell

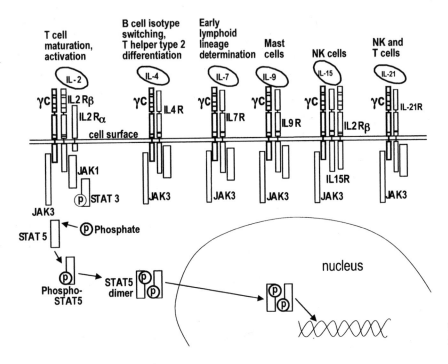

Figure 9.2. Role of the XSCID gene product γc in receptor complexes for multiple cytokines.

lineages. It is not expressed in liver or epithelial cells. Subsequent studies have shown expression in EBV-transformed B cell lines from normal individuals and and in mouse hematopoietic progenitor cells, from the earliest stem cell–enriched populations throughout development of myeloid and lymphoid lineages (Orlic et al., 1997). Expression of γc on murine thymocytes increases as they mature from CD4−/CD8− to double-positive to single-positive T cells, and further up-regulation occurs after lymphocyte activation (DiSanto et al., 1994a; Nakarai et al., 1994; Sugamura et al., 1996).

Recognition that γc was a component of the IL-2 receptor explained why mitogen responses are poor in infants with XSCID. DiSanto et al. (1994b) showed absence of both binding and internalization of IL-2 in B cell lines from XSCID patients. However, a mouse knockout of the gene for IL-2 did not have a SCID phenotype, but manifested immune dysregulation by developing autoimmune hemolytic anemia and inflammatory bowel disease (Schorle et al., 1991; Schimpl et al., 1994). This apparent paradox could be explained if γc were to have additional roles. Indeed, as shown in Figure 9.2, several groups subsequently demonstrated that the XSCID gene product is part of the receptor complexes for multiple cytokines: IL-4 (Kondo et al., 1993; Russell et al., 1993), IL-7 (Noguchi et al., 1993a), IL-9 (Russell et al., 1994), IL-15 (Giri et al., 1994a), and IL-21 (Habib et al., 2002, 2003).

Data from additional mouse knockout experiments and cellular cytokine activation studies suggest that the interaction between IL-7 and the IL-7 receptor complex, which contains γc, is an important signal for development of lymphocyte progenitors from undifferentiated hematopoietic stem cells. IL-7 receptor mRNA expression is coordinated with hematopoietic cell commitment to the lymphoid differentiation pathway (Orlic et al., 1997). Mice lacking either IL-7 or the IL-7 receptor α chain have a SCID phenotype with impaired lymphocyte development (DiSanto et al., 1995a), and IL-7 can induce rearrangement of the T cell receptor β locus in vitro by promoting expression of the recombinase genes *RAG1* and *RAG2* (Muegge et al., 1993).

The importance of IL-4, particularly acting through γc, for lymphocyte development and function is less clear. IL-4-deficient mice have T and B cells, although T helper function, particularly in induction of B cell isotype switching to IgE, is defective (Kuhn et al., 1991; Seder and Paul, 1994). Although IL-4 receptor complexes containing γc mediate optimal signaling from IL-4, γc-defective human XSCID B cell lines exhibit some IL-4 activation through IL-4 receptors without γc (Matthews et al., 1995; Taylor et al., 1997). Similarly, the physiologic significance of γc within the receptor complex for IL-9 is not yet clear. IL-15 activation of XSCID cell lines does not occur, and IL-15 signals are required for NK cell development (Kumaki et al., 1995; Matthews et al., 1995). IL-21 signaling is important for both innate and adaptive immune responses, not only enhancing NK cell effector functions and interferon-gamma (IFN-γ) production, but also augmenting T and B cell responses to specific antigens (Habib et al., 2003).

After interaction with any one of the above cytokines on the surface of a cell, γc trasmits an activation signal intracellularly by means of its association with JAK3, a member of the cytoplasmic Janus family of tyrosine kinases (Johnston et al., 1994; Miyazaki et al., 1994; Russell et al., 1994; Ihle, 1995). Specific tyrosine residues of JAK3 becomes phosphorylated and in turn relay the activation signal to one or more of the signal transducers and activators of transcription, or STAT proteins, which form dimers and migrate into the cell nucleus to alter the cellular transcription program (Fig. 9.2). There is a one-to-one correspondence between cytokine binding to γc and phosphorylation of JAK3: only γc appears to have the specificity to pass activation signals through JAK3. This fact is demonstrated not only by the lack of JAK3 phosphorylation, noted by several investigators to be a property of XSCID patient B cell lines (Russel et al., 1994; Candotti et al., 1996), but also by the recognition that lack of JAK3 causes SCID that, other than its autosomal recessive inheritance pattern, is indistinguishable from XSCID (Macchi et al., 1995; Russell et al., 1995). For a detailed discussion of JAK3 signaling and SCID, see Chapter 10.

Mutation Analysis in XSCID

IL2RG mutations have been reported in patients with XSCID from every racial group. A database of published and verified mutations, IL2RGbase (Puck et al., 1996), can be accessed on the World Wide Web at http://www.genome.gov/DIR/GMBB/SCID. The first 344 unrelated patients had 198 distinct mutations, of which all but 6 were changes in only one or a few nucleotides (Fig. 9.1). The mutations are assigned to the exons and surrounding splice sites in which they are located. XSCID-causing *IL2RG* mutations are not evenly distributed. Exon 5 is the site of 27% of all the mutations, followed by exon 3 with 21%, exon 4 with 14%, and exons 6 and 7 with 10% each. Only three mutations have been found in exon 8.

Hot spots for mutation in *IL2RG*

Recurrent mutations have been noted at several positions, or "hot spots" in *IL2RG*. In several instances, the new origin of a mutation has been proven by finding only the normal gene sequence in DNA from parents of female carriers or from mothers of affected males. Five hot spots for mutation involve the well-recognized mechanism of cytosine methylation and deamination to thymidine within a CpG dinucleotide (Cooper and Krawczak, 1993). The region of cDNA 666–691 of *IL2RG*, just 5′ to the WSEWS motif in exon 5, contains six CpG dinucleotides, the last of which has been the site of 29 independent missense mutations (Pepper et al., 1995). These mutations are both 690C → T, changing arginine 226 to cysteine (R226C), and 691G → A, reflecting a C-to-T mutation on the anticoding strand and changing the same arginine to a histidine (R226H). Just six nucleotides 5′ to this hot spot, the mutation 684C → T, causing a nonconservative missense mutation from arginine to tryptophan, R224W, has been reported 14 times in unrelated patients.

Two other hot-spot mutation sites are 879C → T, causing a premature termination, occurring 16 times (Pepper et al., 1995); and 868G → A, producing a R285Q missense mutation in the last nucleotide of exon 6, seen 14 times. A fifth CpG hot spot at cDNA 717, producing premature termination, has been noted six times, and interestingly was only recognized after collection of the mutations of multiple investigators into the database (Puck et al., 1996; see Chapter 45). Unfortunately, from the point of view of ease of molecular diagnostic testing, the above hot-spot mutations combined account for less than one-quarter of the XSCID-causing mutations. Unique mutations continue to be found as more patients are studied.

Point mutations in *IL2RG*

Single nucleotide changes, found in 57% of all XSCID probands, have produced 35 different termination codons (nonsense mutations, shown as filled circles in Fig. 9.1) and 62 different amino acid substitutions (missense mutations, open circles). It is important to assess the significance of missense mutations. Some are predicted to disrupt known essential elements, such as the first methionine that signals initiation of translation, the four conserved extracellular cysteine residues, the WSEWS motif conserved in all members of the cytokine receptor gene family, or the hydrophobic transmembrane domain. Functional significance is likely for mutations at sites that are conserved not only among mammals, such as human, mouse, rat, and dog, but also between human and more distant species, such as chicken or trout, or between *IL2RG* and other members of the cytokine gene family (Pepper et al., 1995). Amino acid substitutions repeatedly found to be the only change associated with XSCID in unrelated

kindreds are more likely to be pathogenic than to be incidental polymorphisms. Direct proof that a missense mutation is harmful requires testing a cell line from the affected patient for expression of IL2RG mRNA and determining whether γc protein is expressed at the cell surface, whether expressed γc can bind IL-2, and whether downstream targets such as JAK3 and STAT5 become phosphorylated (Puck et al., 1997b). Rare or private polymorphisms have been found in *IL2RG*, but none that are common in control populations.

Insertion and deletion mutations and splice mutations

Insertions (square symbols in Fig. 9.1) and deletions (triangles) account for 19% of XSCID mutations. The great majority of them produce frame shifts, predicted to encode variable numbers of missense amino acids before coming to a new termination codon. Similarly, 19% of XSCID mutations alter the conserved splice signals preceding and following each exon (pentagons, Fig. 9.1). One particularly subtle splice mutation, which has been found in six unrelated XSCID families, changes the attacking, or branch, point, adenosine, at position −15 in front of exon 3 (Tassara et al., 1995). The resulting mRNA is unstable because of the inability to form the lariat structure that is a necessary intermediate in mRNA processing. Because exons 2 through 7 of *IL2RG* contain numbers of nucleotides not divisible by 3, all splice mutations that produce exon skipping are predicted to cause frame shifts.

Expression of mRNA and mutated γc protein

B cells from XSCID patients can be transformed with EBV to make permanent cell lines for functional study. B cell lines from control individuals invariably express IL2RG mRNA and γc protein, detectable with a fluorescent-labeled anti-γc antibody (Ishii et al., 1994; Puck et al., 1993b, 1997b). Absent mRNA, demonstrable for all mutations that produce terminations throughout the first five *IL2RG* exons, is sufficient to prove that a patient with SCID has an *IL2RG* defect. However, studies by Puck et al. (1997b) showed that many *IL2RG* mutations are associated with normal mRNA quantity and size. Because such mutations include the frequently mutated hot-spot sites, as many as two-thirds of all XSCID patients may express some mRNA and abnormal γc protein. Similarly, many XSCID patients have detectable cell surface γc protein, specifically those with mutations in the intracellular domains encoded by *IL2RG* exons 7 and 8, with certain extracellular missense mutations or with in-frame insertions or deletions (Puck et al., 1997b). Direct testing of γc expression and function in peripheral blood from infants with SCID, as suggested by Gilmour et al. (2001), can be combined with sequence-based confirmation of molecular diagnosis but may be inadequate because of small samples available from lymphopenic infants, and inaccurate because of nonmutated maternal lympocytes that may be present in an affected infant's peripheral blood.

Genotype-phenotype correlation of XSCID mutations

The expression of functional γc is severely compromised by all but a handful of the mutations reported; exceptional cases with atypically mild disease, late presentation, or normal numbers of T cells have revealed important aspects of the moleulcar biology of γc. In affected males in a family from France, initially normal T cell numbers declined with time and T cell receptor diversity was limited by an *IL2RG* substitution of an A residue for the almost invariant G nucleotide at the end of exon 1 (129G → A). While the missense mutation in γc encoded by this change, D39N, appeared not to impair IL-2 binding, the loss of a G-terminal nucleotide in exon 1 caused most of the mRNA to be incorrectly spliced (DiSanto et al., 1994c).

In another mildly affected kindred from Galveston, Texas, many males with recurrent respiratory and viral infections had reduced but not absent T cells; an intracellular *IL2RG* point mutation L293Q within the Box-1/Box-2 intracellular portion of γc caused decreased interaction with JAK3, helping to prove the importance of JAK3 in the γc signaling pathway (Russell et al., 1994; Schmalstieg et al., 1995; Goldman et al., 2001).

Another XSCID patient was inexplicably mildly affected despite having inherited an *IL2RG* missense mutation that eliminated the fourth conserved cysteine residue (C115R), required for proper disulfide bond formation and normal configuration of all members of the cytokine receptor family (Stephan et al., 1996; Bousso et al., 2000). Investigations revealed reversion to wild-type sequence, probably at the level of a T lymphocyte progenitor, allowing production of functional T cells with normal γc. This case illustrated the powerful selective advantage of gene-corrected cells in XSCID, an argument in favor of retroviral gene therapy for this disease (see below).

Two unrelated patients had XSCID with normal numbers of poorly functioning T cells and shared the missense mutation R222C; one of these had a thymus biopsy demonstrating relatively normal histology with preservation of cortical and medullary regions (Scharfe et al., 1997; Mella et al., 2000). However, four other instances of this mutation have been associated with typical SCID (Clark et al., 1995; J. Puck, unpublished report), as have 14 instances of the missense mutation R224W at the same amino position. A patient with missense mutation L162R (Mella et al., 2000) and one with a defect in the poly-A addition site of IL2RG mRNA (Hsu et al., 2000) have also been reported. In addition to having more T cells than those of typical XSCID patients, these individuals survived for over a decade without successful allogeneic transplantation, exhibited activated, DR+ T cells, and suffered from growth delay and chronic pulmonary disease. Taken together, these natural experiments in mutagenesis indicate that low levels of normal γc or mutated γc with residual function can allow some T cell development to occur. Additional male patients with combined immunodeficiency less severe than typical SCID may have *IL2RG* mutations.

Strategies for Diagnosis

Once the clinical suspicion of a combined T and B cell immunodeficiency has been raised, whether by family history, low lymphocyte count, or recurrent or opportunistic infections, the diagnosis of SCID must be made by lymphocyte phenotyping and functional tests. X-linked SCID due to *IL2RG* mutation should then be considered in any male patient, although females with Turner syndrome (45 X0 chromosome complement instead of 46 XX) and rare females with constitutionally unbalanced X chromosome inactivation patterns are theoretically also at risk. A clear X-linked family history is sufficient to confirm XSCID with presumed *IL2RG* mutation, but the lack of such a family history does not rule out XSCID. New mutations in *IL2RG* are frequent. Indeed, only 33 of 87 genotype-proven XSCID cases (38%) in a large study had family pedigrees demonstrating X-linked inheritance (Puck et al., 1997b).

Further clues as to the specific XSCID genotype can be gleaned from immunological tests, but atypical values cannot rule out X-linked disease. Males with very few T cells, high proportions of B cells, and absent NK cells are quite likely to have

IL2RG defects, although autosomal recessive JAK3 mutations have an identical clinical and immunologic profile. Lymphocyte phenotyping can be misleading in the face of maternal T cell engraftment, transfusion of nonirradiated blood products, and/or infectious agents. The availability of an anti-γc monoclonal antibody makes it possible to evaluate patient peripheral blood lymphocytes for γc expression (Ishii et al., 1994; Puck et al., 1997b). If γc is clearly absent from patient cells as compared to controls, XSCID can be diagnosed. However, presence of γc may indicate that the patient's *IL2RG* gene is encoding an expressed but nonfunctional protein, or that maternal or other foreign cells in the infant's peripheral blood are positive for anti-γc staining.

Molecular testing for XSCID involves methods discussed in more detail in Chapter 44. Two indirect methods, linkage and maternal lymphocyte X chromosome inactivation, were used before identification of *IL2RG* as the XSCID disease gene. Linkage analysis for diagnosis is a valuable aid, but can only be applied in cases with a clear X-linked family history and available DNA from affected or obligate carrier family members. X chromosome inactivation was originally assayed in mothers of SCID patients by creating a large panel of independent human lymphocyte/hamster fibroblast hybrid cell lines grown in selective medium to ensure retention of the active human X chromosome. DNA from these hybrid clones was then genotyped with a polymorphic marker to identify which of the two X chromosomes was retained in each hybrid cell line (Puck et al., 1992). With the advent of PCR technology, a new assay was developed on the basis of digestion of a polymorphic segment of the androgen receptor gene, *AR*, with methylase-sensitive restriction enzymes. Selective methylation of the inactive *AR* allele, detected as preservation of only a single allele after digestion, suggested skewed X inactivation (Allen et al., 1992). Indirect methods are complex, expensive, time consuming, and not always interpretable, thus they have generally been used only in research laboratories. Although critically important for the gene hunt that identified *IL2RG*, they are now largely replaced by DNA sequence–based analysis.

Definition of the intron–exon boundaries of *IL2RG* and development of primers for PCR amplification of each exon plus flanking regulatory sequences has made mutation screening possible. Single-strand conformation polymorphism (SSCP), carried out by electrophoresis of single exon segments in nondenaturing conditions, was shown to have 83% sensitivity in identifying mutations in *IL2RG* (Puck et al., 1995, 1997a). A modification of this technique, dideoxy fingerprinting (ddF) (Sarkar al., 1992), had much better sensitivity as a clinical test and detected all of 87 mutations in the series of Puck et al. (1997a, 1997b). Direct sequence analysis of PCR-amplified DNA must be performed to determine the specific mutation observed by a screening technique. A nonpathogenic polymorphism would otherwise not be distinguishable from a deleterious mutation. DNA from females at risk of carrying a mutation known from studying other family members can be analyzed by a proven screening method for that mutation, such as SSCP or ddF, by sequencing, or by digestion with a restriction enzyme that can differentiate wild-type and mutant alleles (Puck et al., 1997a).

Carrier Detection and Prenatal Diagnosis

Females who carry an *IL2RG* mutation on one of their X chromosomes are immunologically indistinguishable from controls. However, they can be identified by nonrandom X chromosome inactivation, which is seen in their lymphocytes but not in their granulocytes or nonlymphoid cells (Conley et al., 1988; Puck et al., 1992). This skewed X inactivation is a result of the selective disadvantage of lymphocyte precursors that have inactivated the X chromosome with an intact *IL2RG* gene. When the identity of the mutation in a male proband is known, direct detection of the mutation in the heterozygous state in at-risk female relatives is possible as described above. It is also possible to identify *IL2RG* mutations in potential female carriers when no sample from an affected male is available (Puck et al, 1997a). Females carrying a pathogenic *IL2RG* mutation have a 50% risk of XSCID for each male pregnancy and a 50% risk that each female pregnancy will also carry the mutation. However, as expected with X-linked lethal disorders, new mutations are common and predictions based on testing maternal blood may be inaccurate. Female germ-line mosaicism has been documented in XSCID (Puck et al., 1995), and women have been identified whose blood lymphocytes had no mutation and random X inactivation but who passed an *IL2RG* mutation on to multiple affected offspring (Puck et al., 1995; O'Marcaigh et al., 1997). In 13% of 85 mothers of sons with proven XSCID mutations, the mutations were not present in maternal blood samples (Puck et al., 1997b). Because the mutations in such cases may have existed in only a single maternal oocyte or may represent extensive maternal mosaicism, the recurrence risk for these mothers must be given as between 0 and 50% for a subsequent male pregnancy.

Prenatal diagnosis can be performed by several methods, depending on the amount of information available about the genotype of the family requesting it. If a specific mutation is known, or if the inheritance pattern of SCID is known to be X-linked, analysis of linked polymorphic markers or specific mutation detection can be performed using chorionic villus sample (CVS) or amniocyte DNA prepared directly or obtained from cultured cells (Puck et al., 1990, 1997a). When the genotype of a deceased SCID proband is not known, fetal blood sampling has also been used. Although this procedure must be done later in pregnancy and entails more risk than CVS or amniocentesis, lymphocytopenia, low numbers of T cells, and poor T cell blastogenic responses to mitogens can be definitively demonstrated in affected fetuses by week 17 of gestation (Durandy et al., 1986).

No carrier or prenatal testing should take place without genetic counseling. In considering prenatal diagnosis, the diagnostic options should be weighed against testing at birth for families who would not terminate an affected pregnancy. Regardless of whether prenatal testing is undertaken, education and counseling can clarify the potential benefit of early BMT for affected infants. Many relatives of XSCID patients who did not survive in the past are not aware of the medical advances in transplantation therapy.

Puck et al. (1997a) studied prenatal diagnosis for X-linked SCID in clinical settings. The great majority of families at risk for having an affected pregnancy desired prenatal testing, regardless of whether termination of pregnancy was a consideration. In fact, in only 2 instances out of 13 predicted affected male fetuses did families terminate a pregnancy. To prepare for optimal treatment of an affected newborn, families and their medical providers selected BMT centers, undertook HLA testing of family members, and even began a search for a matched, unrelated bone marrow donor. One family chose an experimental in utero BMT, which was successful (Flake et al., 1996; see below).

Treatment and Prognosis

XSCID is generally fatal unless an immune system can be reconstituted, either by allogeneic transplantation or correction of autologous hematopoietic cells by gene therapy. Infants receiving allogeneic BMT soon after birth are less likely to have serious pretransplant infections or failure to thrive. They also appear to have more rapid engraftment, fewer post-transplant infections, less GVHD, and shorter hospitalizations than those whose transplants are delayed (Stephan et al., 1993; Giri et al., 1994b; Meyers et al., 2002; Antoine et al., 2003; Buckley, 2004). Supportive care and management of infections from the time of diagnosis through the transplantation period are essential. Intensive monitoring, parenteral nutrition, immunoglobulin replacement, and antibiotics including antifungal and antiviral agents have dramatically improved the survival of infants with XSCID. Patients should be isolated from exposure to infectious agents in the environment and should not receive live vaccinations. Attempts to maintain a totally aseptic "bubble" environment are not indicated; instead, prompt immune reconstitution should be the goal.

The best current treatment for XSCID is BMT from an HLA-matched, related donor. Unfortunately, most patients lack a matched sibling donor. Haploidentical, T cell–depleted BMT has proven successful (see Chapter 47). Transplantation protocols using matched unrelated bone marrow or cord blood stem cells have also become available. The techniques for eliminating mature T cells from the donor cell population and enriching for stem cells vary between centers and are evolving over time. Similarly, different centers have had different approaches regarding pretransplant chemotherapy for XSCID patients. The potential advantages of controlling GVHD from donor immunocompetent cells and clearing out host bone marrow in the hope of improving B cell engraftment must be weighed against the risks of cytotoxic treatment.

Previously, there were few useful data to compare the regimens used. But now, increased numbers of treated patients and specific mutation diagnosis for most infants with SCID allow these questions to be addressed. Nevertheless, it is not possible to predict which patients may develop GVHD, fail to make adequate antibodies, and require long-term immunoglobulin replacement, or eventually develop T cell dysregulation or decreased T cell function. Some of the oldest surviving individuals with XSCID received HLA-matched related BMT and are now in their 30s and in excellent health. As larger numbers of children are now growing up after transplantation for XSCID, long-term outcome data are becoming available (Antoine et al., 2003; Buckley, 2004). While some subjects remain healthy with full immune reconstitution, others continue to require immunoglobulin replacement, and some eventually experience declines in thymic output, decreased naive T cell numbers, and diminished T cell receptor diversity (Patel et al., 2000; Antoine et al., 2003; Sarzotti et al., 2003; Buckley et al., 2004).

The concept of prenatal treatment for XSCID has been controversial because of the risk of invasive procedures during pregnancy. Advantages of in utero treatment include early reconstitution, a protected intrauterine environment, and the possibility of introducing normal bone marrow stem cells at the gestational age when fetal hematopoiesis is shifting from fetal liver to bone marrow. Early attempts at human in utero BMT were severely compromised by technological limitations, septic complications, and GVHD. In at least two patients with XSCID, these difficulties have been overcome (Flake et al., 1996; Wengler et al., 1996). Fetuses between 17 and 20 weeks of gestation shown by molecular diagnosis to be affected with XSCID were infused intraperitoneally with haploidentical, T cell–depleted, CD34+ positively selected paternal bone marrow cells. In each of these two cases, infants were born with engrafted, functional T cells from

Table 9.5. Advantages and Disadvantages of Gene Therapy for XSCID

Advantages

Hematopoietic stem cells can be transduced ex vivo and then reinfused.

Graft-vs.-host disease is unlikely because gene-corrected cells are autologous.

Immune reaction against gene-corrected cells is unlikely in immunodeficiency.

The XSCID gene product γc is normally widely expressed in blood lineages. Overexpression of γc is apparently not harmful.

An in vivo selective advantage for γc⁺ cells favors expansion of corrected lymphocytes.

Gene therapy in XSCID animal models has been successful.

Human gene therapy trials have provided full reconstitution to XSCID infants.

Disadvantages

It is impossible to predict or direct where retroviral genes integrate in host DNA.

Retroviral insertion may inappropriately activate or inactivate host genes.

Leukemic proliferations of transduced cells have occurred in three of 10 gene therapy recipients in the French trial.

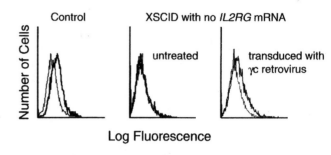

Figure 9.3. Expression of γc in B cell lines from a healthy control (left) and from an XSCID patient with undetectable *IL2RG* mRNA, before (middle) and after (right) transduction with a retrovirus containing *IL2RG* cDNA under control of the Maloney leukemia virus LTR.

their donors, whereas the XSCID mutation could still be confirmed in the infants' granulocytes. In follow-up both children were reported to have fully reconstituted immunity without requiring immunoglobulin supplementation (Bartolomé et al., 2002; Beggs et al., 2003).

New Therapies for XSCID

XSCID has recently been successfully treated by gene transfer therapy to hematopoietic stem cells, but serious adverse events have also occurred. Advantages of XSCID as a pilot disease for gene therapy as well as disadvantages that have come to light since initial positive results are summarized in Table 9.5 and discussed in detail in Chapter 48.

Advantages of gene therapy for immunodeficiencies include the safety of ex vivo transduction protocols; avoidance of GVHD often seen in BMT treatment; and the fact that patients lacking normal immunity will be unlikely to generate an immune response against a newly expressed protein. Specific features that favor XSCID as a pilot disease for gene therapy are ubiquitous expression of *IL2RG* mRNA in hematopoeitic cells (Orlic et al., 1997); apparent absence of toxicity of high levels of γc in hematopoietic lineages, suggesting that expression directed by strong retroviral promoters would not be harmful; and, most important, the natural selective advantage for survival and expansion of lymphocytes expressing wild-type γc, as previously demonstrated by the skewed X chromosome inactivation in lymphocyte lineages of female carriers (Puck et al., 1987, 1992) and somatic reversion to normal of a SCID-causing *IL2RG* mutation (Stephan et al., 1996). Substantial preclinical evidence of effectiveness of *IL2RG* gene therapy was available. Transduction with *IL2RG* retroviruses conferred new expression of normal γc upon B cell lines from XSCID patients (Fig. 9.3). The same treatment corrected the cytokine signaling defects in these cells, restoring their ability to phosphorylate JAK3 in response to IL-2 and IL-4 (Fig. 9.4) (Candotti et al., 1996; Hacein-Bey et al., 1996; Taylor et al., 1996). Isolated CD34⁺ cells from XSCID patients developed into T and B cells in a chimeric sheep model only after transduction with retroviruses encoding *IL2RG* (Tsai et al., 2002).

The first clinical trials of human XSCID gene therapy at the Necker Hospital in Paris by Cavazzana-Calvo et al. (2000) enrolled infants with no available HLA-matched donor. Bone marrow from the affected patients was aspirated, enriched for stem cells by positive selection with the cell surface marker CD34, cultured in activating cytokines, exposed to a retrovirus encoding a correct copy of *IL2RG* cDNA, and reinfused into the patients, who received no myelosuppressive treatment (Cavazzana-Calvo et al., 2000; Hacien-Bey-Abina et al., 2002). Of the first five patients treated, four became fully reconstituted with T cells and also developed the ability to make antibody responses (Hacien-Bey-Abina et al., 2002). The remaining infant suffered from disseminated BCG infection and received less than 1 million corrected cells per kg. He later received a successful haploidentical BMT. Further clinical trials in France and England (Thrasher et al., 2005) have proven that gene therapy for XSCID can be successful (see Chapter 48).

An unanticipated adverse event, leukemic proliferations of T cell clones bearing *IL2RG* retroviral insertion near a T cell oncogene, developed in three of 10 treated infants in the French trial, two of whom were the youngest at treatment, 1 and 3 months of age (Hacien-Bey-Abina et al., 2003). Both of these patients had experienced rapid and complete immune reconstitution, but developed leukemia at around 30 months after gene therapy. In each case, the leukemic cells had an insertion of the *IL2RG* retroviral vector near the 5' end of the *LMO2* gene, and one patient died of his leukemia. The second and third leukemia cases have entered continuous remission following treatment, and their immune reconstitution was preserved.

As of this writing at least 18 patients with XSCID have undergone attempts at gene therapy, including infants who have received gene therapy as primary treatment and older children after failure of attempted BMT (Hacein-Bey-Abina et al., 2003; Gaspar et al., 2004; Chinen et al., 2004; and J. Puck, personal communication). Further trials of gene therapy are proceeding with caution in view of new information on risks and benefits (Chinen and Puck, 2004). As part of the informed consent process, potential participants are warned about retroviral insertional mutagenesis, and methods for monitoring retroviral insertion sites have been instituted so that clonal proliferations can be detected at an early stage (see Chapter 48).

Animal Models

Mice rendered deficient in γc by gene targeting have been created and studied by several investigators (Cao et al., 1995; DiSanto el al., 1995b; Ohbo et al., 1996). Like humans with

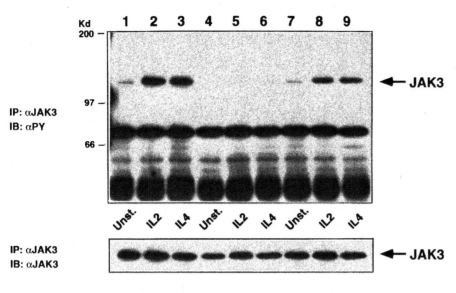

Figure 9.4. Phosphorylation of JAK3 induced by IL-2 and IL-4 in B cell lines from a healthy control (lanes 1–3) and from an XSCID patient before (lanes 4–6) and after (lanes 7–9) transduction with an *IL2RG* retrovirus (Candotti et al., 1996). After no stimulation or exposure to IL-2 or IL-4, cell lysates were immunoprecipitated (IP) with anti-JAK3 antiserum (αJAK3) and immunoblotted (IB) with antiphosphotyrosine (αPY), top, or αJAK3, bottom.

XSCID, γc-deficient mice have low numbers of T cells and NK cells. Unlike humans, however, γc knockout mice also lack B cells, but develop peripheral T cells with CD4+ surface phenotype over time. A mouse expressing a truncated, nonfunctional form of γc also had increased numbers of monocytes and hematopoietic progenitor cells bearing c-kit, Sca-1, and CD34 (Ohbo et al., 1996). Differences between the phenotypes of the different γc-deficient mice may reflect variation in background genes or environmental conditions, as humans with null mutations vs. truncated γc protein are not clinically or immunologically distinguishable. In humans IL-2 can bind to γc complexed with IL-2 receptor β chain, whereas IL-2 binding in the mouse depends on those two chains plus the IL-2 receptor α chain (Sugamura et al., 1996). The effect on XSCID phenotype of this and other interspecies differences in cytokine pathways involving γc remains to be clarified.

Another animal model for XSCID is the γc-deficient dog (Henthorn et al., 1994; Somberg et al., 1994, 1996; Felsburg et al., 2003). Originally diagnosed in a basset hound, the gene defect was bred into a large colony. *IL2RG* null mutations were identified in both this original model and in a second kindred of corgi dogs. The phenotype of these animals is similar to human XSCID in that affected dogs have growth failure, opportunistic and invasive infections, hypogammaglobulinemia, elevated numbers of B cells, and absent T cell mitogen responses. Failure of canine XSCID T cells to respond to IL-2 was noted even before the identification of *IL2RG* as the disease gene. Most affected dogs develop low numbers of peripheral blood T cells after several weeks of age, but these cells are poorly functional. Successful BMT has been performed in XSCID dogs, and gene transfer studies are under way. This large animal model may assist the development of new therapeutic approaches for human XSCID patients, such as cytokine administration to accelerate immune reconstitution after BMT.

Concluding Remarks

The dramatic turnaround in outlook for patients with XSCID and their families over the past generation is one of the most striking in modern medicine. A previously uniformly fatal disease is now treatable, the cause and pathogenesis of the disease are known, specific gene defects can be identified and traced in patients and

at-risk family members, and prenatal diagnosis opens up potential new avenues for effective treatment options. XSCID has become the first human disease to be treated successfully by gene therapy, although the tragic complication of leukemia in three gene therapy recipients must be further studied and understood. Defining which SCID-affected patients have *IL2RG* defects makes possible further studies of genotype-specific management, both in the process of immune reconstitution and in the late posttransplant follow-up period. Families with SCID are communicating with each other on the World Wide Web (for example, a SCID homepage at http://scid.net) and becoming advocates for newborn screening. Parents, physicians, and researchers have thus formed alliances to educate physicians and the public and to learn how to diagnose and manage XSCID even more effectively in the future.

References

Allen RC, Zoghbi HY, Moseley AB, Rosenblatt HM, Belmont JW. Methylation of HpaII and HhaI sites near the polymorphic CAG repeat in the human androgen-receptor gene correlates with X chromosome inactivation. Am J Hum Genet 51:1229–1233, 1992.

Antoine C, Muller S, Cant A, et al. Long-term survival and transplantation of haemopoietic stem cells for immunodeficiencies: report of the European experience 1968–99. Lancet 361:553–560, 2003.

Bartolomé J, Porta F, Lafranchi A, Rodrígues-Molina JJ, Cela E, Cantalejo A, et al. B cell function after haploidentical in utero bone marrow transplantation in a patient with severe combined immunodeficiency. Bone Marrow Transplant 29:625–628, 2002.

Beggs J, Campagnoli C, Sullivan KE, Johnson MP, Puck JM, Zanjani ED, Flake AW. Eight years later: T and B-cell function in a patient transplanted in utero for X-linked severe combined immunodeficiency. Blood 102(Suppl 2):480b, 2003.

Bortin MM, Rimm AA. Severe combined immunodeficiency disease: characterization of the disease and results of transplantation. JAMA 238: 591–600, 1977.

Bousso P, Wahn V, Douagl I, Horneff G, Pannetler C, Le Deist F, et al. Diversity, functionality, and stability of the T cell repertoire derived in vivo from a single human T cell precursor. Proc Natl Acad Sci USA 97: 274–278, 2000.

Bruton OC. Agammaglobulinemia. Pediatrics 9:722–727, 1952.

Buckley RH. Molecular defects in human severe combined immunodeficiency and approaches to reconstitution. Annu Rev Immunol 22:625–655, 2004.

Buckley RH, Schiff RI, Schiff SE, Markert LM, Williams LW, Harville TO, Roberts JL, Puck JM. Human severe combined immunodeficiency (SCID): genetic, phenotypic and functional diversity in 108 infants. J Pediatr 130: 378–387, 1997.

Buckley RH, Schiff SE, Schiff RI, Roberts JL, Markert L, Peters W, Williams LW, Ward FE. Haploidentical bone marrow stem cell transplantation in human severe combined immunodeficiency. Semin Hematol 30(Suppl 4): 92–104, 1993.

Buckley RH, Schiff SE, Schiff RI, et al. Hematopoietic stem-cell transplantation for the treatment of severe combined immunodeficiency. N Engl J Med 340:508–516, 1999.

Candotti F, Johnston JA, Puck JM, Sugamura K, O'Shea JJ, Blaese RM. Retroviral-mediated gene correction for X-linked severe combined immunodeficiency (XSCID). Blood 87:3097–3102, 1996.

Cao X, Shores EW, Hu-Li J, Anver MR, Kelsall BL, Russel SM, Drago J, Noguchi M, Grinberg A, Bloom ET, Paul WE, Katz SI, Love PE, Leonard WJ. Defective lymphoid development in mice lacking expression of the common cytokine receptor γ chain. Immunity 2:223–238, 1995.

Cavazzana-Calvo M, Hacein-Bey S, de Saint Basile G, Gross F, Yvon E, Nusbaum P, et al. Gene therapy of human severe combined immunodeficiency (SCID)-X1 disease. Science 288:669–672, 2000.

Chan K, Puck JM. Development of population-based newborn screening for severe combined immunodeficiency. J Allergy Clin Immunol 115:391–398, 2005.

Chinen J, Puck JM. Successes and risks of gene therapy in primary immunodeficiencies. J Allergy Clin Immunol 113:595–603, 2004.

Chinen J, Puck JM, Davis J, Linton G, Whiting-Theobald N, Woltz P, Buckley RH, Malech H. Ex vivo gene therapy of a preadolescent with X-linked severe combined immunodeficiency. Blood 104:410, 2004.

Clark PA, Lester T, Genet S, Jones AM, Hendriks R, Kevinsky RJ, Kinnon C. Screening for mutations causing X-linked severe combined immunodeficiency in the IL-2R gamma chain gene by single-strand conformation polymorphism analysis. Hum Genet 96:427–432, 1995.

Conley ME, Hong R, Buckley RH, Guerra-Hanson C, Roifman CM, Brockstein JA, Pahwa S, Puck JM. X-linked severe combined immunodeficiency: diagnosis in males with sporadic severe combined immunodeficiency and clarification of clinical findings. J Clin Invest 85:1548–1554, 1990.

Conley ME, Lavoie A, Briggs C, Guerra C, Puck JM. Non-random X chromosome inactivation in B cells from carriers of X-linked severe combined immunodeficiency. Proc Natl Acad Sci USA 85:3090–3094, 1988.

Conley ME, Nowell PC, Henle G, Douglas SD. XX T cells and XY B cells in two patients with severe combined immunodeficiency. Clin Immunol Immunopathol 31:87–95, 1984.

Cooper DN, Krawczak, M: Human Gene Mutation. Oxford, UK: Bios Scientific Publishers, 1993.

De Saint Basile G, Arveiler B, Oberlé J, Malcolm S, Levinsky R, Lau Y, Hofker M, Debre M, Fischer A, Griscelli C, Mandel, J-L. Close linkage of the locus for X chromosome-linked SCID to polymorpic markers in Xq11–q13. Proc Natl Acad Sci USA 84:7576–7579, 1987.

DiSanto JP, Certain S, Wilson A, MacDonald HR, Avner P, Fischer A, De Saint Basile G. The murine interleukin-2 receptor γ chian gene: organization, chromosomal localization and expression in the adult thymus. Eur J Immunol 24:3014–3018, 1994a.

DiSanto JP, Dautry-Varsat A, Certain S, Fischer A, de Saint Basile G: Interleukin-2 (IL-2) receptor γ chain mutations in X-linked severe combined immunodeficiency disease result in the loss of high-affinity IL-2 receptor binding. Eur J Immunol 24:475–479, 1994b.

DiSanto JP, Kuhn R, Muller W. Common cytokine receptor γ chain (γc)-dependent cytokines: understanding in vivo functions by gene targeting. Immunol Rev 148:19–34, 1995a.

DiSanto JP, Muller W, Guy-Grand D, Fischer A, Rajewsky K. Lymphoid development in mice with a targeted deletion of the interleukin 2 receptor γ chain. Proc Natl Acad Sci USA 92:377–381, 1995b.

DiSanto JP, Rieux-Laucat F, Dautry-Varsat A, Fischer A, De Saint Basile G. Defective human interleukin 2 receptor γ chain in an atypical X chromosome-linked severe combined immunodeficiency with peripheral T cells. Proc Natl Acad Sci USA 91, 9466–9470, 1994c.

Douek DC, Vescio RA, Betts MR, Brenchley JM, Hill BJ, Zhang L, et al. Assessment of thymic output in adults after haematopoietic stem cell transplant and prediction of T cell reconstitution. Lancet 355:1875–1881, 2000.

Durandy A, Dumez Y, Griscelli C. Prenatal diagnosis of severe inherited immunodeficiencies: a five year experience. In: Vossen J, Griscelli C, eds. Progress in Immunodeficiency Research and Therapy, Vol. 2. Amsterdam: Elsiever, pp. 323–327, 1986.

Felsburg PJ, Harnett BJ, Gouthro TA, Henthhorn PS. Thymopoeisis and T cell development in common gamma chain-deficient dogs. Immunol Res 27:235–245, 2003.

Fischer A. Severe combined immunodeficiencies. Immunodef Rev 3:83–100, 1992.

Flake AW, Almeida-Porada G, Puck JM, Roncarolo M-G, Evans MI, Johnson MP, Abella EM, Harrison DD, Zanjani ED. Treatment of X-linked SCID by the in utero transplantation of CD34 enriched bone marrow. N Engl J Med 355:1806–1810, 1996.

Frank J, Pignata C, Panteleyev AA, Prowse DM, Baden H, Weiner L, Taetaniello L, et al. Exposing the nude phenotype. Nature 398:473–474, 1999.

Gaspar HB, Parsley KL, Howe S, King D, Gilmore KC, et al. Gene therapy of X-linked severe combined immunodeficiency by use of a pseudotyped gammaretroviral vector. Lancet 364:2181–2187, 2004.

Gatti RA, Allen HD, Meuwissen HJ, Hong R, Good RA. Immunological reconstitution of sex-linked lymphopenic immunological deficiency. Lancet 2:1366–1368, 1968.

Gilmour KC, Cranston T, Loughlin S, Gwyther J, Lester T, Espanol T, et al. Rapid protein-based assays for the diagnosis of T⁻B⁺ severe combined immunodeficiency. Br J Haematol 112:671–676, 2001.

Gilroy RK, Coccia PF, Talmadge JE, Hatcher LI, Pirruccello SJ, Shaw BW Jr, et al. Donor immune reconstitution after liver–small bowel transplantation for multiple intestinal atresia with immunodeficiency. Blood 103: 1171–1174, 2004.

Giri JG, Ahdieh M, Eisenman J, Shanebeck K, Grabstein K, Kumaki S, Namen A, Park LS, Cosman D, Anderson D. Utilization of the beta and gamma chains of the IL-2 receptor by the novel cytokine IL-15. EMBO J 13:2822–2830, 1994a.

Giri N, Vowels M, Ziegler JB, Ford D, Lam-Po-Tang R. HLA non-identical T-cell-depleted bone marrow transplantation for primary immunodeficiency diseases. Aust N Z J Med 24:26–30, 1994b.

Glanzmann E, Riniker P. Essentielle Lymphocytophthose. Ein neues Krankeitsbild aus der Säuglingspathologie. Ann Paediat 174:1–5, 1950.

Goldman AS, Palkowetz KH, Rudloff HE, Dallas DV, Schmalstieg FC. Genesis of progressive T-cell deficiency owing to a single missense mutation in the common gamma chain gene. Scand J Immunol 54:582–592, 2001.

Habib T, Nelson A, Kaushansky K. IL-21: a novel IL-2-family lymphokine that modulates B, T, and natural killer cell responses. J Allergy Clin Immunol 112:1033–1045, 2003.

Habib T, Senadheera S, Weinberg K, Kaushansky K. The common gamma chain (gamma c) is a required signaling component of the IL-21 receptor and supports IL-21-induced cell proliferation via JAK3. Biochemistry 41:8725–8731, 2002.

Hacein-Bey H, Cavazzana-Calvo M, Le Deist F, Dautry-Varsat A, Hivroz C, Riviere I, Danos O, Heard JM, Sugamura K, Fischer A, De Saint Basile G. Gamma-c gene transfer into SCID X1 patients' B-cell lines restores normal high-affinity interleukin-2 receptor expression and function. Blood 87:3108–3116, 1996.

Hacein-Bey-Abina S, Le Deist F, Carlier F, Bouneaud C, Hue C, De Villartay JP, et al. Sustained correction of X-linked severe combined immunodeficiency by ex-vivo gene therapy. N Engl J Med 346:1185–1193, 2002.

Hacein-Bey-Abina S, Von Kalle C, Schmidt M, McCormack MP, Wulffraat N, Leboulch P, et al. LMO2-associated clonal T cell proliferation in two patients after gene therapy for SCID-X1. Science 302:415–419, 2003.

Hale LP, Buckley RH, Puck JM, Patel DD. Abnormal development of thymic dendritic and epithelial cells in human X-linked severe combined immunodeficiency. Clin Immunol 110:63–70, 2004.

Henthorn PS, Somberg RL, Fimiani V, Puck JM, Patterson DF, Felsburg PJ. IL-2Rγ gene microdeletion demonstrates that canine X-linked severe combined immunodeficiency is a homologue of the human disease. Genomics 23:69–74, 1994.

Hitzig WH, Willi H. Hereditary lymphoplasmocytic dysgenesis ("Alymphocytose mit Agammaglobulinämia"). Schweiz Med Wochenschr 91:1625–1633, 1961.

Hsu AP, Tsai EJ, Anderson SM, Fischer RE, Malech H, Buckley RH, Puck JM. Unusual X-linked SCID phenotype due to mutation of the poly-A addition signal of IL2RG. Am J Hum Genet 67(Suppl 2):A50, 2000.

Ihle JN. Cytokine receptor signaling. Nature 377:591–594, 1995.

Ishii N, Takeshita T, Kimura Y, Tada K, Kondo M, Nakamura M, Sugamura K. Expression of the interleukin-2 (IL-2) receptor γ chain on various populations in human peripheral blood. Int Immunol 6:1273–1277, 1994.

Johnston JA, Kawamura M, Kirken RA, Chen Y-Q, Blake TB, Shibuya K, Ortaldo JR, McVicar DW, O'Shea JJ. Phosphorylation and activation of the Jak-3 Janus kinase in response to interleukin-2. Nature 370:151–153, 1994.

Kalman L, Lindegren ML, Kobrynski L, Vogt R, Hannon H, Howard JT, Buckley RH. Mutations in genes required for T-cell development: IL7R, CD45, IL2RG, JAK3, RAG1, RAG2, ARTEMIS, and ADA and severe combined immunodeficiency: HuGE review. Genet Med 6:16–26, 2004.

Kondo M, Takeshita T, Ishii N, Nakamura M, Watanabe S, Arai K, Sugamura K. Sharing of the interleukin-2 (IL-2) receptor gamma chain between receptors for IL-2 and IL-4. Science 262:1874–1877, 1993.

Kuhn R, Rajewsky K, Muller W. Generation and analysis of interleukin-4 deficient mice. Science 254:707–709, 1991.

Kumaki S, Ochs HD, Timour M, Schooley K, Ahdieh M, Hill H, Sugamura K, Anderson D, Zhu Q, Cosman K, Giri JG. Characterization of B-cell lines established from two X-linked severe combined immunodeficiency patients: interleukin-15 binds to the B cells but is not internalized efficiently. Blood 86:1438–1436, 1995.

Macchi P, Villa A, Giliani S, Sacco MG, Frattini A, Porta F, Ugazio AG, Johnston JA, Candotti F, O'Shea JJ, Vezzoni P, Notarangelo LD. Mutations of Jak-3 gene in patients with autosomal severe combined immune deficiency (SCID). Nature 377:65–68, 1995.

Matthews DJ, Clark PA, Herbert J, Morgan G, Armitage RJ, Kinnon C, Minty A, Grabstein KH, Caput D, Ferrara P, Callard R. Function of the interleukin-2 (IL-2) receptor γ-chain in biologic responses of X-linked severe combined immunodeficient B cells to IL-2, IL-4, IL-13, and IL-15. Blood 85:38–42, 1995.

Mella P, Imberti L, Brugnoni D, Pirovano S, Candotti F, Mazzolari E, et al. Development of autologous T lymphocytes in two males with X-linked severe combined immune deficiency: molecular and cellular characterization. Clin Immunol 95:39–50, 2000.

Minegishi Y, Okawa H, Sugamura K, Yata J. Preferential utilization of the immature J_H segment and absence of somatic mutation in the CDR3 junction of the Ig H chain gene in three X-linked severe combined immunodeficiency patients. Int Immunol 6:1709–1715, 1994.

Miyazaki T, Kawahara A, Fujii H, Nakagawa Y, Minami Y, Liu Z-J, Oishi I, Silvennoinen O, Witthuhn BA, Ihle JN, Taniguchi T. Functional activation of JAK1 and JAK3 by selective association with IL-2 receptor subunits. Science 266:1045–1047, 1994.

Muegge K, Vila MP, Durum SK. Interleukin-7: a cofactor for V(D)J rearrangement of the T cell receptor b gene. Science 261:93–95, 1993.

Myers LA, Patel, DD, Puck JM, Buckley RH. Hematopoietic stem cell transplantation for SCID in the neonatal period leads to superior thymic output and improved survival. Blood 99:872–878, 2002.

Nakarai T, Robertson MJ, Streuli M, Wu, Z, Ciardelli TL, Smith KA, Ritz J. Interleukin 2 receptor g chain expression on resting and activated lymphoid cells. J Exp Med 180:241–251, 1994.

Noguchi M, Nakamura Y, Russell SM, Ziegler SF, Tsang M, Cao X, Leonard WJ. Interleukin-2 receptor γ chain: a functional component of the interleukin-7 receptor. Science 262:1877–1880, 1993a.

Noguchi M, Yi H, Rosenblatt HM, Filipovitch AH, Adelstein S, Modi WS, McBride OW, Leonard WJ. Interleukin 2 receptor g chain mutation results in X-linked severe combined immunodeficiency in humans. Cell 73:147–157, 1993b.

Ohbo K, Suda T, Hashiyama M, Mantani A, Ikebe M, Miyakawa K, Moriyama M, Nakamura M, Katsuki M, Takahashi K, Yamamura K, Sugamura K. Modulation of hematopoiesis in mice with a truncated mutant of the interleukin-2 receptor gamma chain. Blood 87:956–967, 1996.

O'Marcaigh AE, Puck JM, Pepper AE, Cowan MJ. Maternal germline mosaicism for an IL2RG mutation causing X-linked SCID in a Navajo kindred. J Clin Immunol 17:29–33, 1997.

Online Mendelian Inheritance in Man, OMIM (TM). McKusick-Nathans Institute for Genetic Medicine, Johns Hopkins University (Baltimore, MD) and National Center for Biotechnology Information, National Library of Medicine (Bethesda, MD), 2000. World Wide Web URL: http://www.ncbi.nlm.nih.gov/Omim/.

Orlic D, Girard L, Lee D, Anderson S, Puck JM, Bodine DM. Interleukin-7Rα and interleukin-2Rα mRNA expression increase as stem cells differentiate to T and B lymphocyte progentiors: implications for X-linked SCID. Exp Hematol 25:217–222, 1997.

Patel D, Gooding ME, Parrott RE, Curtis KM, Haynes BF, Buckley RH. Thymic function after hametopoietic stem-cell transplantation for the treatment of severe combined immunodeficiency. N Engl J Med 342:1325–1332, 2000.

Pepper AE, Buckley RH, Small TN, Puck JM. Two CpG mutational hot spots in the interleukin-2 receptor γ chain gene causing human X-linked severe combined immunodeficiency. Am J Hum Genet 57:564–571, 1995.

Pollack MS, Kirkpatrick D, Kapoor N, O'Reilly RJ. Identification by HLA typing of intrauterine derived maternal T cells in four patients with SCID. N Engl J Med 307:662–666, 1982.

Puck JM, Conley ME, Bailey LC. Refinement of localization of human X-linked severe combined immunodeficiency (SCIDX1) in Xq13. Am J Hum Genet 53:176–184, 1993a.

Puck JM, Deschenes SM, Porter JC, Dutra AS, Brown CJ, Willard HF, Henthorn PS. The interleukin-2 receptor gamma chain maps to Xq13.1 and is mutated in X-linked severe combined immunodeficiency, SCIDX1. Hum Mol Genet 2:1099–1104, 1993b.

Puck JM, de Saint Basile G, Schwarz K, Fugmann S, Fischer RE. IL2RGbase: a database of γc-chain defects causing human X-SCID. Immunol Today 17:507–511, 1996.

Puck JM, Hsu A, Tsai EJ, Buckley RH, Malech HL. XSCID due to poly-A site mutation has unique phenotype amenable to gene therapy. Mol Ther 3(Part 2):S242, 2001.

Puck JM, Krauss C, Puck SM, Buckley R, Conley ME. Prenatal test for X-linked severe combined immunodeficiency by analysis of maternal X-chromosome inactivation and linkage analysis. N Engl J Med 322:1063–1066, 1990.

Puck JM, Middelton LA, Pepper AE. Carrier and prenatal diagnosis of X-linked severe combined immunodeficiency: mutation detection methods and utilization. Hum Genet 99:628–633, 1997a.

Puck JM, Nussbaum RL, Conley ME. Carrier detection in X-linked severe combined immunodeficiency based on patterns of X chromosome inactivation. J Clin Invest 79:1395–1400, 1987.

Puck JM, Pepper AE, Bédard P-M, Laframboise R. Female germ line mosaicism as the origin of a unique IL-2 receptor γ-chain mutation causing X-linked severe combined immunodeficiency. J Clin Invest 95:895–899, 1995.

Puck JM, Pepper AE, Henthorn PS, Candotti F, Isakov J, Whitwam T, Conley ME, Fischer RE, Rosenblatt HM, Small TN, Buckley RH. Mutation analysis of IL2RG in human X-linked severe combined immunodeficiency. Blood 89:1968–1977, 1997b.

Puck JM, Stewart CC, Nussbaum RL. Maximum likelihood analysis of human T-cell X chromosome inactivation patterns: normal women versus carriers of X-linked severe combined immunodeficiency. Am J Hum Genet 50:742–748, 1992.

Russell SM, Johnston JA, Noguchi M, Kawamura M, Bacon CM, Friedmann M, Berg M, McVicar DW, Witthuhn BA, Silvennoinen O, Goldman AS, Schmalstieg FC, Ihle JN, O'Shea JJ, Leonard WJ. Interaction of IL-2Rb and gc chains with Jak1 and Jak3: implications for XSCID and XCID. Science 266:1042–1045, 1994.

Russell SM, Keegan AD, Harada N, Nakamura Y, Noguchi M, Leland P, Friedmann MC, Miyajima A, Puri RK, Paul WE, Leonard WJ. Interleukin-2 receptor gamma chain: a functional component of the interleukin-4 receptor. Science 262:1880–1883, 1993.

Russell SM, Tayebi N, Nakajima H, Riedy MC, Roberts JL, Aman MJ, Migone T-S, Noguchi M, Markert ML, Buckley RH, O'Shea JJ, Leonard WJ. Mutation of Jak3 in a patient with SCID: essential role of Jak3 in lymphoid development. Science 270:797–800, 1995.

Sarkar G, Yoon H, Sommer SS. Dideoxy fingerprinting (DDF): a rapid and efficient screen for the presence of mutations. Genomics 13:441–444, 1992.

Sarzotti M, Patel DD, Li X, Ozaki DA, Cao S, Langdon S, et al. T cell repertoire development in humans with SCID after nonablative allogeneic marrow transplantation. J Immunol 170:2711–2718, 2003.

Scharfe N, Shahar M, Roifman CM. An interleukin-2 receptor γ chain mutation with normal thymus morphology. J Clin Invest 100:3036–3043, 1997.

Schimpl A, Hunig T, Elbe A, Berberich I, Kraemer S, Merz H, Feller AC, Sadlack B, Schorle H, Horak I. Development and function of the immune system in mice with targeted disruption of the interleukin 2 gene. In: Bluethmann H, Ohashi P, eds. Transgenesis and Targeted Mutagenesis in Immunology. San Diego: Adacemic Press, p. 191, 1994.

Schmalstieg FC, Leonard WJ, Noguchi M, Berg M, Rudloff HE, Denney RM, Dave SK, Brooks EG, Goldman AS. Missense mutation in exon 7 of the common gamma chain gene causes a moderate form of X-linked combined immunodeficiency. J Clin Invest 95:1169–1173, 1995.

Schönland SO, Zimmer JK, Lopez-Benitez CM, Widmann T, Ramin KD, Goronzy JJ, et al. Homeostatic control of T-cell generation in neonates. Blood 102:1428–1434, 2003.

Schorle H, Holtschke T, Hunig T, Schimpl A, Horak I. Development and function of T cells in mice rendered interleukin-2 deficient by gene targeting. Nature 352:621–624, 1991.

Seder RA, Paul WE. Acquision of lymphokine-producing phenotype by CD4+ T cells. Annu Rev Immunol 12:635–673, 1994.

Shearer WT, Ritz J, Finegold MJ, Guerra IC, Rosenblatt HM, Lewis DL, Pollack MS, Taber LH, Sumaya CV, Grumet C, Cleary ML, Warnke R, Sklar J. Epstein-Barr virus–assocaited B-cell proliferations of diverse clonal origins after bone marrow transplantation in a 12-year-old patient with severe combined immunodeficiency. N Engl J Med 312:1151–1159, 1985.

Shearer WT, Rosenblatt HM, Gelman RS, Oyomopito R, Plaeger S, Stiehm ER, Wara DW, Douglas SD, Luzuriaga K, McFarland EJ, Yogev R, Rathore MH, Levy W, Graham BL, Spector SA. Lymphocyte subsets in healthy children from birth through 18 years of age: the Pediatric AIDS

Clinical Trials Group P1009 Study. J Allergy Clin Immunol 112:973–80, 2003.

Sleasman JW, Harville TO, White GB, George JF, Barrett DJ, Goodenow MM. Arrested rearrangement of TCR Vβ genes in thymocytes from children with X-linked severe combined immunodeficiency disease. J Immunol 153:442–448, 1994.

Small TN, Keever C, Collins N, Dupont B, O'Reilly RJ, Flomenberg N. Characterization of B cells in severe combined immunodeficincy disease. Hum Immunol 25:181–193, 1989.

Somberg RL, Robinson JP, Felsburg PJ. T lymphocyte development and function in dogs with X-linked severe combined immunodeficiency. J Immunol 153:4006–4012, 1994.

Somberg RL, Tipold A, Harnett BJ, Moore PF, Henthorn PS, Felsburg PJ. Postnatal development of T cells in dogs with X-linked severe combined immunodeficiency. J Immunol 156:1431–1435, 1996.

Stauber DJ, Debler EW, Horton PA, Smith KA, Wilson IA. Crystal structure of the IL-2 signaling complex: Paradigm for a heterodimeric cytokine receptor. Proc Natl Acad Sci USA [Epub ahead of print] PM ID 16477002, 2006.

Stephan JL, Vlekova V, Le Deist F, Blanche S, Donadieu J, De Saint-Basile G, Durandy A, Griscelli C, Fischer A. Severe combined immunodeficiency: a retrospective single-center study of clinical presentation and outcome in 117 patients. J Pediatr 123:564–724, 1993.

Stephan V, Wahn V, Le Deist F, Dirksen U, Broker B, Muller-Fleckenstein I, Horneff G, Schroten H, Fischer A, de Saint Basile G. Atypical X-linked severe combined immunodeficiency due to possible spontaneous reversion of the genetic defect in T cells. N Engl J Med 335:1563–157, 1996.

Stiehm RE, Ochs HD, Winkelstein JA, eds. Immunologic Disorders in Infants and Children, 5th ed. Philadelphia: Elsevier Saunders, 2004.

Sugamura K, Asao H, Kondo M, Tanaka N, Ishii N, Ohbo K, Nakamura M, Takeshita T. The interleukin-2 receptor γ chain: its role in the multiple cytokine receptor complexes and T cell development in XSCID. Annu Rev Immunol 14:179–205, 1996.

Takeshita T, Asao H, Ohtani K, Ishii N, Kumaki S, Tanaka N, Munakata H, Nakamura M, Sugamura K. Cloning of the gamma chain of the human IL-2 receptor. Science 257:379–382, 1992.

Tangsinmankong N, Day NK, Nelson RP Jr, Puck J, Good RA. Severe combined immunodeficiency in an infant with multiple congenital abnormalities. J Allergy Clin Immunol 103:1222–1223, 1999.

Tassara C, Pepper AE, Puck JM. Intron point mutation in IL-2 receptor γ chain causing X-linked severe combined immunodeficiency. Hum Mol Genet 4:1693–1695, 1995.

Taylor N, Candotti F, Smith S, Oakes SA, Jahn T, Isakov J, Puck JM, O'Shea JJ, Weinberg K, Johnston JA. Interleukin-4 signaling in B lymphocytes from patients with X-linked severe combined immunodeficiency. J Biol Chem 272:7314–7319, 1997.

Taylor N, Uribe L, Smith S, Jahn T, Kohn DB, Weinberg K. Correction of interleukin-2 receptor function in X-SCID lymphoblastoid cells by retrovirally mediated transfer of the gamma-c gene. Blood 87:3103–3107, 1996.

Thrasher AJ. Immune recovery following retroviral mediated common gamma chain gene therapy for X-linked severe combined immunodeficiency. In: American Society of Gene Therapy's Six Annual Meeting Executive Summaries, Vol 36, 2003.

Tsai EJ, Malech HL, Kirby MR, Hsu AP, Seidel NE, Porada CD, et al. Retroviral transduction of ILRG into CD34 from XSCID patients permits human T and B cell development in sheep chimeras. Blood 100:72–79, 2002.

Wang X, Rickert M, Garcia KC. Structure of the quaternary complex of interleukin-Z with its alpha, beta, and gamma_c receptors. Science 310: 1159–1163, 2005.

Wengler GS, Allen RC, Parolini O, Smith H, Conley ME. Nonrandom X chromosome inactivation in natural killer cells from obligate carriers of X-linked severe combined immunodeficiency. J Immunol 150:700–704, 1993.

Wengler GS, Lanfranchi A, Frusca T, Verardi R, Neva A, Brugnoni D, Giliani S, Fiorini M, Mella P, Guandalini F, Mazzolari E, Pecorelli S, Notarangelo LD, Porta F, Ugazio AG. In-utero transplantation of parental CD34 haematopoietic progenitor cells in a patient with X-linked severe combined immunodeficiency (SCIDXI). Lancet 348(9040):1484–1487, 1996.

10

Autosomal Recessive Severe Combined Immunodeficiency Due to Defects in Cytokine Signaling Pathways

FABIO CANDOTTI and LUIGI NOTARANGELO

Immunophenotypic and functional analysis of circulating lymphoid cells allows classification of severe combined immunodeficiency (SCID) into distinct subgroups (Fischer, 2001): (1) reticular dysgenesis; (2) adenosine deaminase deficiency; (3) SCID with a low number of circulating T and B cells and presence of natural killer (NK) cells (T−B− NK+ SCID); (4) SCID with a low number of circulating T lymphocytes and NK cells, but normal to increased number of B cells (T−B+ NK− SCID); (5) SCID with a low number of circulating T lymphocytes, but normal to increased number of B lymphocytes and presence of NK cells (T−B+ NK+ SCID); and (6) SCID characterized by severe functional defects. The subgroups of SCID with B lymphocytes (B+ SCID) account for at least 50% of all cases of SCID (Fischer et al., 1990; Stephan et al., 1993; Haddad et al., 1998; Bertrand et al., 1999; Buckley, 2000b, 2004; Antoine et al., 2003). Many are due to known molecular defects that interfere with signaling of a series of critical hematopoietic cytokines. Most patients with B+ SCID are males, a pattern reflecting the occurrence of X-linked SCID (see Chapter 9). This disorder is due to mutations at the *IL2RG* locus (Noguchi et al., 1993; Puck et al., 1993), which encodes the common γ chain (γc) shared by cytokine receptors for interleukin-2 (IL-2), IL-4, IL-7, IL-9, IL-15, and IL-21 (Leonard, 1996; Sugamura et al., 1996; Asao et al., 2001). The existence of autosomal recessive (AR) B+ SCID is indicated by the demonstration that B+ SCID may also occur in females, and in infants born to consanguineous parents (Stephan et al., 1993). Neither immunological nor clinical features can be used to distinguish between X-linked and AR B+ SCID (Stephan et al., 1993).

The finding that cytokine receptors that use the γc always associate with the intracellular Janus-associated tyrosine kinase (JAK) designated JAK3 (Fig. 10.1) and the discovery that the major cytokine receptor transducing subunit binds to another JAK kinase, JAK1 (Miyazaki et al., 1994; Russell et al., 1994), provided clues to the molecular basis of AR B+ SCID. A mild form of X-linked SCID in humans was shown to result from a point mutation in the cytoplasmic tail of γc, diminishing but not completely abolishing its interaction with JAK3 (Russell et al., 1994). On the basis this information, it was hypothesized that AR B+ SCID in humans could be caused by defects in JAK3. This hypothesis was proved correct by two groups of investigators who reported markedly reduced expression of JAK3 protein due to mutations in the *JAK3* gene in unrelated infants with B+ SCID (MIM *600173, #600802) (Macchi et al., 1995; Russell et al., 1995; Candotti et al., 1997; Online Mendelian Inheritance in Man, 2000).

The critical role of JAK3 for lymphoid development and function has been further illustrated by the generation of Jak3-deficient mice, using homologous recombination and gene disruption (Nosaka et al., 1995; Park et al., 1995; Thomis et al., 1995). The immunologic phenotype of Jak3 knockout mice is very similar to that of γc knockout mice (Cao et al., 1995; DiSanto et al., 1995; Ohbo et al., 1996), thus substantiating the notion that the γc and Jak3 proteins act together in the same signaling pathway.

Mice with targeted genetic disruption of the genes encoding IL-7 or the IL-7 receptor α chain (IL-7Rα) also have profound defects in T cell development that are similar to those of γc and Jak3 knockout animals (Peschon et al., 1994; von Freeden-Jeffry et al., 1995). This observation led to the additional hypothesis that mutations specifically affecting IL-7 signaling could result in SCID in humans. The search for such patients ultimately demonstrated that *IL7R* mutations can cause AR B+ SCID and that such patients have residual development of NK cells (Puel et al., 1998). Thus, AR B+ SCID patients provide additional evidence of the integral importance of cytokine signaling in the development of the immune system.

137

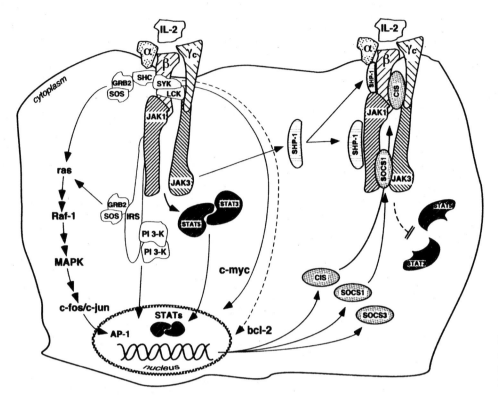

Figure 10.1. Schematic representation of the IL-2-mediated JAK–STAT signaling pathway and its negative regulation.

Biology of the JAK–STAT Signaling Pathway

The biological effects of cytokines are mediated through interaction with specific receptors; this leads to phosphorylation of intracellular proteins. Members of the cytokine receptor superfamily do not have intrinsic kinase activity, but recruit intracellular protein kinases following interaction with their ligands (Ihle, 1995; Taniguchi, 1995; Leonard and O'Shea, 1998). The tyrosine kinases that couple extracellular cytokine binding to intracellular phosphorylation of protein substrates, and eventually to cell growth and differentiation, are members of the Janus-associated kinase (JAK) family. The JAK kinases were originally cloned while searching for novel protein tyrosine kinases through a polymerase chain reaction (PCR)-based approach (Wilks, 1989), and their functional role was first demonstrated in response to interferons (Muller et al., 1993; Watling et al., 1993). Thus far, four distinct members of the JAK family are known in humans: JAK1, JAK2, JAK3, and Tyk2.

The JAK family members share a similar structure (Ihle, 1995; Taniguchi, 1995; Leonard and O'Shea, 1998), with a C-terminal kinase domain (termed JAK homology 1, JH1), a more proximal kinase-like domain (JH2) whose function is not completely defined, and five other N-terminal regions of homology (JH3–JH7). The JH2 domain lacks highly conserved critical residues found in other typical kinase domains; when expressed in a recombinant form, JH2 is in fact devoid of kinase activity, but instead has important regulatory functions perhaps through binding to the kinase domain and sequestering substrates until the kinase domain is activated by extracellular signals (Gurniak and Berg, 1996). The N-terminus of the JAKs has homology to another conserved domain defined in a superfamily of proteins called the FERM proteins (named for band 4.1, ezrin, radixin, and moesin). FERM domains were originally implicated in cross-linking of the cytoplasmic tails of transmembrane proteins to underlying structural and regulatory elements, but they may also mediate interactions with transmembrane receptor chains independent of cytoskeletal binding (Zhou et al., 2001).

The *JAK3* and *TYK2* genes are located near each other on human chromosome 19p13.1. The *JAK3* cDNA is composed of 4,064 nucleotides and contains an open reading frame that encodes 1,124 amino acids (Kawamura et al., 1994). Immunoprecipitation studies, using specific antisera, suggest a molecular weight of approximately 125 kDa (Kawamura et al., 1994). While JAK1, JAK2, and TYK2 are broadly expressed, JAK3 is largely restricted to the hematopoietic system (Kawamura et al., 1994). The cDNA of JAK3 (originally designated L-JAK) was identified in NK cells and NK-like cell lines, but not in resting T lymphocytes, although expression could be induced following in vitro T cell activation (Johnston et al., 1994; Kawamura et al., 1994). In B cells, JAK3 expression is increased following in vitro activation and is high in B cell malignancies (Tortolani et al., 1995). A splice variant, devoid of kinase activity, has also been identified in epithelial cells (Lai et al., 1995). Studies of murine Jak3 have revealed high levels of expression in fetal and adult thymus and somewhat lower levels in fetal liver, adult bone marrow, lymph nodes, spleen, and CD4+CD8+ thymocytes (Gurniak and Berg, 1996). These data imply a crucial functional role of the Jak3 protein in lymphoid differentiation.

The intracellular signaling mediated by JAKs has been extensively investigated. Members of the IL-2R superfamily (i.e., IL-2R, IL-4R, IL-7R, IL-9R, IL-15R, IL-21R) physically associate with JAK1 and JAK3 (Miyazaki et al., 1994; Russell et al., 1994; Foxwell et al., 1995; Johnston et al., 1995b; Malabarba et al., 1995; Pernis et al., 1995; Yin et al., 1995b). The observation that distinct cytokines signal through the same set of kinases indicates that JAKs are not directly involved in controlling the specificity of the signal. In the IL-2R, JAK1 interacts with the serine region of IL-2Rβ, whereas the 48 C-terminal residues of the γc chain are required to bind JAK3 (Miyazaki et al., 1994). Both regions of the IL-2R chains are critical for JAK activation and signal transduction (Johnston et al., 1994; Miyazaki et al., 1994; Witthuhn et al., 1994). Following cytokine–cytokine receptor interaction and dimerization of the cytoplasmic tails of the cytokine receptor chains, the JAKs are brought into close proximity and may cross-phosphorylate each other. Activation of JAK3 in response to IL-2, IL-4, and IL-7 is more pronounced than that of JAK1 (Witthuhn et al., 1994; Foxwell et al., 1995; Johnston et al., 1995b; Malabarba et al., 1995; Sharfe et al., 1995). In addition, JAKs phosphorylate the intracellular portions of cytokine receptor chains, thus generating docking sites for SH2-containing proteins (Ihle et al., 1994; Ivashkiv, 1995; Taniguchi, 1995).

Several signaling pathways are elicited by JAK1/JAK3 activation in members of the IL-2R cytokine receptors superfamily (Fig. 10.1). First, the phosphorylated cytokine receptor may associate with the adaptor SHC (Egan et al., 1993; Karnitz and Abraham, 1995), which is itself phosphorylated and binds to Grb2. Grb2 may thus anchor to Sos, the Ras guanine nucleotide exchanging factor (Li et al., 1993; Holsinger et al., 1995; Karnitz and Abraham, 1995). Membrane translocation of the Grb2/Sos complex catalyzes the conversion of inactive, GDP-bound Ras to the active, GTP-bound state. This results in the activation of raf-1, mitogen-activated protein kinase (MAPK), and eventually in the induction of immediate-early genes (c-*fos*, c-*jun*) (Blumer and Johnson, 1994). This signaling pathway, however, is apparently not used by all γc receptor complexes, and in particular is not triggered by IL-4 (Welham et al., 1994).

Second, JAKs may bind and phosphorylate insulin receptor substrates (IRSs) (Johnston et al., 1995b; Keegan et al., 1995; Sharfe et al., 1995; Yin et al., 1995a). JAK activation by IL-2, IL-4, IL-7, IL-9, and IL-15 results in phosphorylation of IRS-1, whereas evidence of JAK-dependent tyrosine phosphorylation of IRS-2/4PS (which is strictly homologous to IRS-1) has so far been obtained only for IL-2, IL-4, and IL-15 (Johnston et al., 1995b; Keegan et al., 1995). The ability to phosphorylate IRS substrates is restricted to proliferating cells, as IL-4-dependent proliferative responses are not obtained with IL-4R mutants that are unable to recruit IRS-1 (Keegan et al., 1994). Once activated, IRS may bind the SH2 domain of the p85 subunit of phosphatidylinositol-3-kinase (PI3K) (Myers et al., 1992; Sun et al., 1995), and the catalytic activity of the p110 subunit of PI3K is eventually elicited. In addition to promoting PI3K activation, tyrosine phosphorylated IRS may recruit Grb2 and thus amplify the Ras/raf-1 signaling pathway (White and Kahn, 1994).

A third essential component of the JAK signaling pathway is phosphorylation of the class of transcription factors known as signal transducers and activators of transcription (STATs) (Taniguchi, 1995; Ihle, 1996; Leonard and O'Shea, 1998). The STATs contain a tyrosine residue that may undergo JAK-mediated phosphorylation, and they also contain SH2 and SH3 domains. Following cytokine interaction with receptor and triggering of the JAK-mediated signaling pathway, STATs may interact with the cytokine receptor complex by binding via their SH2 domain to the phosphotyrosine of the cytokine receptor chain. In addition, following STAT phosphorylation, STAT–STAT homo- or heterodimerization occurs, with the SH2 domain of one STAT molecule binding to the phosphotyrosine of the second STAT. Six different classes of STATs have been reported; furthermore, two different forms of STAT5 (STAT5a and STAT5b) have been characterized at the molecular level (Lin et al., 1996). The specificity of the response to cytokines is largely dependent on the particular combination of STATs recruited by the different signal-transducing chains of the cytokine receptor (Fenghao et al., 1995; Foxwell et al., 1995; Gilmour et al., 1995; Hou et al.,

1995; Johnston et al., 1995a; Taniguchi, 1995; Ihle, 1996). The differences in the STAT binding residues of the various cytokine receptors result in recruitment of specific STATs. However, three crucial lymphocyte growth factors, IL-2, IL-7, and IL-15, all activate STAT3 and STAT5 (Fenghao et al., 1995; Foxwell et al., 1995; Gilmour et al., 1995; Hou et al., 1995). STAT5 is the predominant protein induced by IL-2 in phytohemagglutinin (PHA)-stimulated lymphocytes (Hou et al., 1995).

Following dimerization, STATs translocate to the nucleus, where they bind to consensus sequences in the enhancer elements of the promoter regions of target genes and favor gene transcription (Ihle, 1996). Gene accessibility to STAT binding is another mechanism through which specific responses to distinct cytokines are obtained. It has been suggested that JAK-dependent STAT activation is more crucial to cell differentiation than to proliferation. In fact, deletion of the C-terminal H domain of IL-2Rβ abolishes IL-2-induced STAT5 activation but not JAK1 and JAK3 activation; nor does it affect cell proliferation (Fujii et al., 1995). However, IL-4-induced thymocyte proliferation is somewhat diminished in STAT6 knockout mice, which suggests that STAT activation contributes to cytokine-induced growth-promoting activity (Kaplan et al., 1996; Shimoda et al., 1996; Takeda et al., 1996).

Additional possibly JAK-independent signaling pathways elicited following cytokine–cytokine receptor interaction include activation of src-related kinases (e.g., of lck, lyn, and fyn in response to IL-2) (Taniguchi and Minami, 1993), through their association with the acidic domain of IL-2Rβ. Deletion of this domain abolishes IL-2-induced lck activation yet does not affect IL-2-regulated cell growth, implying that activation of src-related kinases may not be crucial for cell proliferation. Finally, induction of Syk, c-myc and bcl-2 requires the S region of IL-2Rβ (Minami and Taniguchi, 1995). JAK3 mutants devoid of the JH1 kinase domain cause markedly diminished induction of c-myc, but intact induction of bcl-2. This finding indicates that these are independent signaling pathways and that JAK3 may be involved in c-myc transcription (Kawahara et al., 1995).

The need for JAK3 in IL-2-induced cell proliferation has been illustrated by the observation that in the NIH3T3αβγ cell line (which expresses the α, β, and γ chains of the IL-2 receptor, as well as JAK1 and JAK2, but not JAK3), IL-2 does not promote cell proliferation; however, proliferative response to IL-2 is restored after JAK3 is transfected into and expressed by these cells (Miyazaki et al., 1994). Furthermore, the requirement for integrity of the structure of JAKs in regulating cell growth and differentiation has been indicated by the fact that JAK3 mutants that lack the JH3–JH7 domains, but not the JH1 protein tyrosine kinase domain, are unable to interact with γc (Taniguchi, 1995), whereas mutants that lack the JH1 kinase domain may bind to γc, but are unable to transduce activation signals (cell growth, induction of c-*fos* and c-*myc*) in response to IL-2 (Taniguchi, 1995). Finally, overexpression of JAK3 mutants that lack the JH1 kinase domain may inhibit the IL-2-induced phosphorylation of JAK1 and JAK3 (Kawahara et al., 1995). Similar experiments with JAK2 mutants suggest that multiple JH domains are required for functional interaction with the cytokine receptor and target cytoplasmic substrates (Tanner et al., 1995).

A number of mechanisms serve to terminate the activity initiated by cytokine signals (Fig. 10.1). SH2 domain–containing protein tyrosine phosphatases SHP-1 and SHP-2 are important inhibitors of signaling events and are thought to dephosphorylate receptor chains and JAK molecules through SH2–phosphotyrosine interaction (Migone et al., 1998; You et al., 1999). Other mechanisms for attenuation of cytokine signaling involve the members of the suppressor of cytokine signaling (SOCS) family of proteins. These proteins are induced by cytokine stimulation following a classic feedback mechanism. Eight members of this family are known (CIS, SOCS1–7) (Yoshimura et al., 1995; Endo et al., 1997; Naka et al., 1997; Starr et al., 1997; Hilton et al., 1998). Although their function is incompletely understood, SOCS proteins appear to inhibit cytokine signaling through a variety of mechanisms, including competition with STATs for the phosphorylated docking sites on receptor chains and inhibition of kinase activities.

Severe Combined Immunodeficiency Due to Mutations of JAK3

Clinical Features

Mutations in the *IL2RG* gene encoding γc (see Chapter 9) are responsible for X-linked SCID in humans, who typically present with T⁻B⁺NK⁻ SCID. The recognition of the crucial role of JAK3 in signaling through γc-containing receptors led to the hypothesis that *JAK3* defects might account for autosomal forms of SCID in humans (Russell et al., 1994). In the original reports, three SCID patients with *JAK3* mutations were described (Macchi et al., 1995; Russell et al., 1995), and many other similar patients have subsequently been observed (Candotti et al., 1997; Bozzi et al., 1998; Buckley et al., 1999; Schumacher et al., 2000; Frucht et al., 2001; Mella et al., 2001; Roberts et al., 2004).

The clinical features of the first series JAK3-deficient patients who have been described in some detail are summarized in Table 10.1 and are indistinguishable from the features commonly observed in infants with X-linked SCID. In two cases, the diagnosis of SCID was established immediately after birth, either because of family history of SCID or because of fortuitous recognition of markedly reduced circulating T cells. Most patients, however, were diagnosed following development of upper and lower respiratory tract infections, variably associated with chronic diarrhea, central nervous system involvement, and failure to thrive during the first few months of life. In all cases, peripheral lymph nodes were undetectable. Although splice variants of *JAK3* mRNA have been identified in nonhematopoietic human tissues (Lai et al., 1995), no unique manifestations of primary organ dysfunction unrelated to immune deficiency have been detected in JAK3-deficient infants. Parental consanguinity was documented for 10 infants, 2 of whom were siblings.

Laboratory Findings

The immunologic phenotype of JAK3-deficient patients is very consistent (Table 10.1) and similar to that observed in infants with X-linked SCID. In the first series of 27 JAK3-deficient SCID patients, the proportion of CD3 lymphocytes was most often markedly reduced (0.2%–2%), while that of CD19 B cells was increased (74%–96%). Occasionally, as for patient 1 in Table 10.1, the proportion of circulating T cells may appear normal or near normal, due to the presence of maternally derived T lymphocytes. The augmented number of B lymphocytes often results in normal absolute lymphocyte counts (Table 10.1) and almost always in a less profound lymphopenia than that in patients with B⁻ SCID. An interesting feature of JAK3 deficiency, also typically shared by X-linked SCID, is the severely reduced number of NK cells; NK cytolytic activity is consequently absent or severely depressed (Macchi et al., 1995; Russell et al., 1995; Bozzi et al., 1998; Candotti et al., 1997; Buckley et al., 1999; Schumacher et al., 2000; Frucht et al., 2001; Mella et al., 2001).

Because JAK3 is constitutively expressed in NK cells (Kawamura et al., 1994) and carrier females of X-linked SCID have nonrandom inactivation of the mutated X chromosome in not only T and B cells but also in NK cells (Wengler et al., 1993), it appears that integrity of the γc/JAK3 signaling pathway is essential to development of NK cells.

In addition to being severely reduced in number, T cells from JAK3-deficient infants are also functionally impaired. The proliferative responses to mitogens, antigens, and alloantigens are abolished or severely reduced. Despite the increased proportion of circulating B cells, immunoglobulin serum levels are markedly decreased (with the possible exceptions of IgG that is maternally derived during the early months of life and IgM), and no antibody responses are elicited following antigen stimulation. Failure to generate antibody responses is partly due to lack of effective helper T cell activity, but it also reflects an intrinsic B cell defect. In fact, defective induction of STAT activation has been reported following cytokine stimulation in Epstein-Barr virus (EBV)-transformed B cells from these patients (Russell et al., 1995; Candotti et al., 1996; Oakes et al., 1996; Frucht et al., 2001).

The recent report of the immunological phenotype of a series of seven JAK3-deficient patients described by Roberts et al. (2004) has confirmed earlier findings in these patients. Interestingly, however, the typical immunologic phenotype, lack of circulating T cells, and increased proportion of B cells may change during the course of the disease. We observed a rapid appearance of T cells (up to 41% of total circulating lymphocytes) in the peripheral blood of patient 7, who had a typical T⁻B⁺NK⁻ phenotype during the first month of life (Table 10.1). The late-developing T cells were phenotypically and functionally abnormal. They were all CD4⁺ and coexpressed the activation markers CD45R0 and DR; in addition, they were found to be oligoclonal (Brugnoni et al., 1998), and they failed to respond to PHA and to CD3 stimulation alone, but showed some response to the combination of anti-CD3 and IL-2. At the same time that these T cells were found, the patient developed markedly elevated levels of serum IgE (1000 IU/ml, with normal levels being <100 IU/ml). Interestingly, this phenotype of partial preservation of the responsiveness to IL-2 by activated T cells correlated with *JAK3* gene mutations (A1537G and deletion exons 10–12) that permitted residual protein expression and function (Candotti et al., 1997). The contributory role of residual functional activity of JAK3 is less clear, however, if one considers that Jak3 knockout mice develop activated CD4 T cells (see below). It is therefore possible that the T cell differentiation defect imposed by JAK3 deficiency allows changes of the immunologic phenotype with time or that some degree of T cell development is possible independent from JAK3. Our recent observation of patients 22a and 22b (Table 10.1) add complexity to these considerations. One child of this kindred died of *Pneumocystis* pneumonia before any laboratory analysis could be performed; a second child (patient 22a) developed severe lymphoproliferative disease and an additional sibling (patient 22b) was clinically nearly normal, but had lymphopenia with oligoclonal T cell expansion and increased numbers of activated and memory T cells. These cells also had poor expression of the pro-apoptotic molecule, Fas ligand, which is typically up-regulated by IL-2; thus these cells were reminiscent of the T cells that develop in mice that are deficient in either γc or Jak3 (Frucht et al., 2001). These findings suggest that all patients with immunodeficiency and residual T cell function should probably be evaluated for possible JAK3 (and, if male, γc) mutations.

Table 10.1. Clinical and Immunological Features of 27 Patients with SCID due to *JAK3* Deficiency

Patient	Age at Diagnosis (months)	Lymphocytes/ μl	CD3 (%)	CD4 (%)	CD8 (%)	CD19 (%)	CD16 (%)	Response to PHA	IgG (g/L)	IgA (g/L)	IgM (g/L)	Failure to Thrive	Interstitial Pneumonia	Chronic Diarrhea	Other Features
1	5	4332	53*	53a**	1.5	23	1	Absent	0.4	0.3	0.4	−	−	+	Skin rash
2	10	2520	11	7	2	70	2	Absent	ND	0.1	1.2	+	−	−	
3	4	612	18	1	8	28	34	Absent	0.7	Undet.	0.1	−	−	−	
4	1		<3			92						+	+	−	
5	2	2304	<1	<1	<1	93	1	Absent	2.2	Undet.	0.4	−	−	−	Skin rash
6	3	1364	<1	<1	<1	77	<1	Absent	1.3	Undet.	0.2	+	+	+	
7	1.5	3000	2	1	2	74	13	Absent	8.6	Undet.	1.2	+	+	+	
8	9	792	<1	1		86	1	Absent	<0.5	Undet.	Undet.				
9		700	1			96	1	Absent							
10															
11a‡	7	2074	1	1	0	94	1	Absent	0.5	Undet.	0.6	+	−	−	Meningitis
11b‡	Birth	916	0.5	1	1	87	<1	Absent	1.6	Undet.	0.1	−	−	−	
12	7	3104	0	0.5	0.5	92	0.5	Absent	1.5	0.2	0.5	−	−	+	Skin rash
13	3	3210	8	0	0	97	0.5	Minimal	6.1†	0.7	2.3				
14	19	1630	2	4	5	91	0.3	Absent	16.7†	2.6	1.7	−	−	+	
15	4	3470	2	0	0	94		Minimal	<0.1	Undet.	0.1				
16	3	5640	48	18	35	45	1	Absent		0.2	0.9				
17	5	1020	0	0	0	26	1	Absent	14	2.6	5.7				
18	Birth	1020	1	0	0	96	3	Minimal		Undet.	0.3				
19	3		0	0	0	66	2	Absent							
20	6	970	31	12	20	83	1	Minimal	Undet.						
21		3000	7	7	2	24	42	Minimal			0.5				
22a‡	72	770	60	21	44	73	9	Weak	11.5	6.8	0.9				
22b‡	7	820	17	5	9	93	1	Weak	2.9	0.3	1.5				
23	6	1815	2	1	<1	75	2	Absent	0.1	Undet.	0.2	+	+	+	
24	4	1095	17	6	7	96		Minimal	7.8†	Undet.	0.6	+	+	+	
25	4	3340	1	<1	<1	96	0	Absent	0.1	Undet.	0.6	+	+	+	
Controls		1300−8500	67±7	44±11	23±9	12±5	10±3		2.2−8.4	0.1−0.6	0.2−0.7				

ND, not determined; PHA, phytohemagglutinin; Undet., undetectable.

*Maternal T cell engraftment documented.

†On intravenous immunoglobulins.

‡Patients 11a and 11b, as well as 22a and 22b, represent siblings.

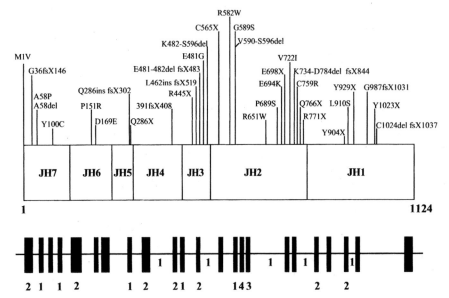

Figure 10.2. Schematic representation of organization of the human JAK3 protein and *JAK3* gene organization. In the upper panel, the boxes represent the JAK homology domains (JH1–JH7). Location and predicted protein effect of known *JAK3* mutations is indicated although not all mutant alleles give rise to stable mRNA or protein. The lower panel shows exons and introns of the *JAK3* gene (in scale) with the number of mutations found in each exon (solid boxes) and intron (connecting lines).

It is also well recognized that JAK3 is expressed in myelomonocytic cells, including human monocytes (Witthuhn et al., 1994; Musso et al., 1995), in vitro stimulation with lipopolysaccharide (LPS) and interferon increases JAK3 expression in monocytes (Musso et al., 1995). Furthermore, IL-2 and IL-4 (i.e., two cytokines that signal through γc-bearing receptors) have profound effects on cells of the monocyte–macrophage lineage (Fenton et al., 1992; Vannier et al., 1992; de Waal Malefyt et al., 1993) and induce tyrosine phosphorylation and activation of JAK3 in these cells (Witthuhn et al., 1994; Musso et al., 1995). The possibility that mutations of the *JAK3* gene might affect the differentiation and/or function of the myelomonocytic lineage has been considered. However, monocyte numbers are normal in JAK3-deficient SCID infants (Villa et al., 1996; L. Notarangelo, unpublished results) and monocytes from one JAK3-deficient patient showed normal responses to IL-2 (measured as release of tumor necrosis factor and IL-8) and to IL-4 (release of IL-1R antagonist) (Villa et al., 1996), indicating that JAK3 is dispensable for monocyte differentiation and responsiveness to cytokines that interact with γc receptors.

Molecular Basis of JAK3 Deficiency

JAK3 mutations identified in the published series of patients are reported in Figure 10.2. A total of 34 unique mutations affecting all seven structural JH domains have been identified. Many mutations are clustered in the JH2 and JH3 domains.

While there are no obvious mutational hot spots, five mutations (D169E, R445X, C565X, R651W, and V722I) have been described in two unrelated families each. The types of the 34 unique mutations identified in unrelated families (Fig. 10.2), include 14 missense, 9 nonsense, 5 splice site (2 of which resulted in deletion and frameshift at the mRNA level), 4 genomic deletion, and 2 insertion.

Functional Aspects

Most *JAK3* mutations drastically reduce the expression of the protein; however, a number of missense or small in-frame deletions have been identified that permit near-normal levels of protein

expression (Notarangelo et al., 2001; Roberts et al., 2004). The analysis of the effect of these mutations has provided important insights into the function of the different JAK3 domains.

Not unexpectedly, mutations of the kinase domain (JH1) can affect phosphorylation of JAK3 and its substrates IL-2Rβ and STAT5, as demonstrated in patients with nonsense and frameshift mutations (Notarangelo and Candotti, 2000; Schumacher et al., 2000). More interesting have been the consequences of the frequent mutations in the pseudokinase domain (JH2). Constitutive phosphorylation of JAK3 was detectable in a patient with a C759R missense mutation in the JH2 domain, yet IL-2 stimulation did not result in up-regulation of JAK3 phosphorylation, nor did it induce STAT5 phosphorylation. In other patients with missense or deletion mutations in the JH2 domain, no JAK3 or STAT5 phosphorylation occurred in response to IL-2 (Candotti et al., 1997). The functional effects of these mutations have also been evaluated with heterologous systems. Mutant JAK3s were normally expressed after cDNA transfection, but their kinase activity was undetectable in vitro (Chen et al., 2000). Moreover, JAK3 mutants were unresponsive to IL-2 stimulation, even though they could normally bind to γc. Surprisingly, however, the mutated JAK3 appeared in some cases to be hypertyrosine phosphorylated compared with wild-type JAK3. This finding suggests that the physiological role of the JH2 pseudokinase domain is to regulate kinase activity and therefore substrate phosphorylation by directly interacting with the JH1 kinase domain. To confirm this relationship, it was shown that, in contrast to the wild-type JAK3 pseudokinase domain, which modestly inhibits the JAK3-mediated signaling pathway, JAK3 with the mutated JH2 pseudokinase domains from the two patients studied had an increased capacity to inhibit kinase activity. Thus kinase dysregulation in these patients appeared to have contributed to their disease pathogenesis (Chen et al., 2000). Also in the JH2 domain, the R582W substitution was found to result in two different products: one had normal length but was not phosphorylated, and the other, with a 71 amino acid deletion in the downstream JH2 domain, was also expressed and could be phosphorylated, but was insufficient for signal transduction (Bozzi et al., 1998).

Mutations in the JH3 domain are also compatible with JAK3 expression, as was the case of a patient who carried one missense mutation (E481G) and one deletion (K482–S596del) in this domain. These are predicted to result in both a normal-sized and a low–molecular weight mutant JAK3 product. In EBV B cells from this patient, IL-2 induced some residual phosphorylation of the normal-sized mutant JAK3 product. Furthermore, STAT5 phosphorylation was also detected (although at reduced levels), indicating that the glutamic acid–to–glycine substitution at codon 481 in the JH3 domain does not completely abrogate JAK3 function. Interestingly, the immunological phenotype of this patient was atypical; he developed a substantial number of autologous T cells (although with abnormal phenotype and function) and NK lymphocytes (Candotti et al., 1997; Brugnoni et al., 1998).

Mutations in the N terminus of JAK3 have indicated the important role that this portion of the protein plays for receptor interaction. Cells from patients with single amino acid substitution or deletion in the JH7 domain express JAK3 protein with severely decreased interaction with γc. (Cacalano et al., 1999) and with abrogated in vitro catalytic activity (Zhou et al., 2001). Similar results can be observed in the presence of missense mutations affecting the JH2 domain (Roberts et al., 2004). A detailed molecular analysis with constructs carrying the SCID-associated FERM mutation has shown that the JAK3 FERM and kinase domains associate and reciprocally influence each other's function and structure (Zhou et al., 2001). Thus, in SCID patients with FERM mutations, two mechanisms contribute to the disease pathogenesis: impaired γc/JAK3 association and inactivation of catalytic activity.

Strategies for Diagnosis: From Disease Confirmation to Prenatal Diagnosis

From the published literature, JAK3 deficiency appears to account for ~6% of all cases of SCID in the United States, thus occupying a less prominent role than X-linked SCID and adenosine deaminase (ADA) deficiency (Roberts et al., 2004). Until more SCID patients are analyzed for JAK3 mutations, the prevalence of this defect within the heterogeneous group of SCID disorders cannot be firmly established.

In the single-center experience of the Department of Pediatrics, University of Brescia, 14 cases of JAK3 deficiency were identified in a cohort of 96 consecutive patients with SCID, giving an overall figure of 14.3%. However, because JAK3 deficiency is usually characterized by a consistent B+ phenotype, the proportion of JAK3 deficiency among infants with B+ SCID is higher (37.8% in the Brescia series). It is possible that this rather elevated figure reflects the high frequency of consanguineous marriages in some parts of Italy. In any case, it appears that after mutations at the IL2RG locus, mutations of the JAK3 gene are the second-most frequently reported molecular cause of B+ SCID in the Mediterranean region.

To date, the diagnostic identification of a JAK3 defect is through Western blotting and functional assays, once γc defects have been ruled out; in fact, all patients identified thus far had undetectable or severely reduced levels of JAK3 protein. Furthermore, EBV-transformed cell lines from these patients show striking defects in JAK3 and STAT5 phosphorylation upon stimulation with IL-2. The advent of fluorescence-activated cell sorter (FACS) analysis of STAT phoshorylation provides the opportunity for early functional analysis after EBV immortalization (Roberts et al., 2004). However, functional assays are presently highly specialized research tests and require availability of appropriate cell lines. Because of the low levels of expression

of the JAK3 protein in circulating B cells, generation of lymphoblastoid cell lines has been necessary for reproducible Western blot analysis, although protein assays on peripheral blood mononuclear cells (PBMCs) have also been successfully performed (Gilmour et al., 2001a). Regardless, molecular testing, based on identification of JAK3 mutations at the genomic level, remains the most reliable assay for the diagnosis of JAK3 deficiency. Analysis of JAK3 mutations has been facilitated by elucidation of the genomic structure (Riedy et al., 1996; Villa et al., 1996; Schumacher et al., 2000). From these data it is now known that the human JAK3 gene is organized into 23 exons and 22 introns. The complete definition of the intron–exon boundaries has allowed development of screening assays based on single-strand conformation polymorphisms (SSCP) techniques. This is particularly important for the evaluation of historical deceased cases of SCID when only DNA is available, as well as for patients fully reconstituted following bone marrow transplantation, in whom JAK3 mutations can be determined only by analyzing DNA from nonhematopoietic tissues. The characterization of the JAK3 genomic structure, for example, has allowed demonstration of splice-site mutations (Villa et al., 1996) and made possible the first prenatal diagnosis through SSCP-analysis on chorionic villi DNA (Schumacher et al., 1999). Because the JAK3 gene is not expressed in chorionic villi, prenatal diagnosis was based on genomic analysis.

Treatment and Prognosis

The prognosis for JAK3-deficient SCID patients is the same as for all cases of B+ SCID; unless treated by successful bone marrow transplantation, SCID due to JAK3 deficiency is a lethal disorder. Optimal results (up to 95% survival rate) have been obtained with bone marrow transplantation (BMT) from human leukocyte antigen (HLA)-matched siblings, whereas the survival rate is lower (~70%) when HLA-mismatched related donors are used. Furthermore, particularly when no conditioning regimen is given, engraftment of donor-derived T cells is associated with persistence of autologous B cells (Buckley, 2000a; Antoine et al., 2003), making post-transplantation treatment with infusion of immunoglobulins necessary on a chronic basis. Use of pretransplant conditioning has been claimed to favor the engraftment of donor-derived B cells (Wijnaendts et al., 1989; Dror et al., 1993; van Leeuwen et al., 1994; Haddad et al., 1998). However, it will be important to validate this assumption through prospective analysis of the outcome of bone marrow transplant in mutation-proven JAK3-deficient infants. In the Brescia series, of 13 Jak3-deficient patients who were treated with BMT, 9 received T-depleted marrow from haploidentical parents, 3 received T-depleted marrow from a matched unrelated donor (MUD), and only 1 had an HLA-identical sibling donor. In 12 of the 13 patients, engraftment of donor-derived T cells was achieved, whereas engraftment of donor-derived B cells was observed following HLA-matched and MUD transplantation, but less so following haploidentical transplantation. One patient who underwent haploidentical BMT died from infectious complications early after transplant, and one additional patient has severe neurological impairment due to pretransplant encephalitis. All of the four patients who received HLA-matched transplantation (three from a matched unrelated donor, and one from an HLA-identical sibling) are alive and well with full engraftment of both T and B lymphocytes of donor origin.

In a series of 10 JAK3-deficient patients who underwent BMT at Duke University Medical Center in North Carolina, 2 received

HLA-identical sibling marrow and 8 received maternal haploidentical transplantation without pretransplant cytoreductive chemotherapy. Among the latter patients, one died and a subsequent transplantation of cord blood (preceded by chemoablation) was necessary in one patient (Roberts et al., 2004). The nine surviving patients showed development of normal T cell immunity. Donor B cells, however, were detected only in the patient who received chemoablation, and six patients continued to require intravenous immunoglobulin (IVIG) therapy. Natural killer cell activity was not reconstituted in seven of the nine survivors (Roberts et al., 2004).

Because of the phenotypic and biological similarities between JAK3 deficiency and γc deficiency, and in light of the early success of gene therapy in the latter condition (Cavazzana-Calvo et al., 2000; Hacein-Bey-Abina et al., 2002), genetic correction of JAK3 deficiency may also result in clinical benefit. Preclinical experiments in vitro (Candotti et al., 1996; Oakes et al., 1996) and in vivo in a murine model (Bunting et al., 1998, 1999, 2000) have illustrated the potential benefit of gene therapy for JAK3 deficiency. Retroviral-mediated *JAK3* gene transfer was able to correct the biological abnormalities of JAK3-deficient human B cell lines, leading to reconstitution of IL-2 signaling as assessed by IL-2-induced phosphorylation of IL-2Rβ, JAK1, JAK3, and STAT5, as well as IL-2-mediated cell proliferation (Candotti et al., 1996; Oakes et al., 1996).

A compelling series of in vivo mouse experiments has also shown that ex vivo retroviral-mediated *JAK3* gene transfer into hematopoietic progenitors from JAK3 knockout mice was able to restore specific T and B cell functions in Jak3 knockout mice transplanted with gene-corrected cells. Treated mice developed T lymphocytes able to respond to mitogens and make specific cytotoxic responses. In addition, good reconstitution of humoral immunity was achieved following the procedure; experimental animals developed increased numbers of B lymphocytes and antibody production. More important, the same mice generated specific antibody responses upon immunization, and survived exposure to influenza virus (Bunting et al., 1998, 1999). Another crucial finding of these experiments was that myeloablation was not necessary to achieve these significant improvements (Bunting et al., 2000). The strong selective advantage of JAK3-corrected lymphoid cells over unmodified autologous counterparts, illustrated by these results, seems to indicate that preparative conditioning may not be needed for *JAK3* gene therapy in humans.

One potential concern of using current "gene addition" approaches is that the expression of the transferred gene is liberated from the physiologic cellular mechanisms of regulation, being constitutively expressed under the influence of strong viral promoters. Because of the important role of JAK3 in cell proliferation (Miyazaki et al., 1994; Oakes et al., 1996), deregulated JAK3 expression could potentially result in uncontrolled cell division and cause malignancy.

In the animal experiments above, however, adverse events were not observed, supporting development of a clinical trial that recently enrolled a single JAK3-deficient patient who had failed BMT treatment. The results of this human trial have not been published. However, the occurrence of leukemia in two children treated with gene therapy for X-linked SCID has caused this trial to be placed on clinical hold and prevented the accrual of additional patients. Analysis of the monoclonal leukemic cell populations in the X-linked SCID trial has shown that the retroviral vector was integrated in or near the *LMO2* gene locus, resulting in aberrant expression of this transcript (Hacein-Bey-Abina et al., 2003) (see Chapters 9 and 48).

Activation of LMO2 by translocation is found in some forms of childhood acute T lymphoblastic leukemias. The proliferation advantage given by the expression of γc to the cells containing the LMO2 integrants seems to explain the development of leukemia and it is reasonable to assume that expression of JAK3 could have similar consequences. For these reasons, in February 2005, the FDA Biological Response Modifiers Advisory Committee made the recommendation that, until more information is acquired, gene therapy for X-linked SCID and JAK3-SCID in the United States should be performed only in patients for whom alternative therapies are not available or have already failed.

Murine Models of JAK3 Deficiency

The crucial role of JAK3 in lymphoid differentiation and function has been assessed through animal models. In 1995, three groups reported studies of mice with targeted disruptions of *Jak3* (Nosaka et al., 1995; Park et al., 1995; Thomis et al., 1995). Viable homozygous Jak3 knockout mice of normal growth and size were generated in the expected proportion indicating that Jak3 is not crucial to fetal development and survival.

Pathologic examination of the thymus in Jak3 knockout mice revealed markedly reduced cellularity with a very low number of early lymphoid precursors (lin⁻/c-kit⁺), indicating abnormal seeding of lymphoid precursors into the thymus (Park et al., 1995). However, thymocyte differentiation stages were discernible, and CD4⁺ and CD8⁺ single-positive thymocyte subsets were identified. An excess of CD4⁺ over CD8⁺ single-positive cells developed with time, suggesting that cytokine signaling through γc/Jak3 is more crucial for the maturation and/or survival of the murine CD8 lineage than of CD4 thymocytes. The proliferative response of thymocytes to various combinations of mitogens was severely reduced and was not increased by addition of exogenous IL-2. Interestingly, intermediate responses to phorbol myristate acetate (PMA) or concanavalin A (Con A) and cytokines have been recorded with thymocytes from heterozygous mice (Park et al., 1995).

Although the spleen in Jak3-deficient mice was generally smaller than that in controls, its cellularity was less severely affected than that of the thymus. However, a sharp reduction of mature B220⁺sIgM⁺ B cells (around 1% of normal) was observed, associated with a profound defect of B cell differentiation in the bone marrow, where a reduced transition from pro-B (B220⁻CD43⁺) to pre-B (B220⁺CD43⁺) cells was documented (Park et al., 1995; Thomis et al., 1995). In the T cell compartment of the spleen, a progressive appearance of CD4⁺ T cells was observed; furthermore, these cells expressed activation antigens CD44 and CD69, but showed greatly diminished in vitro proliferation and little IL-2 production in response to mitogen stimulation (Thomis et al., 1995; Thomis and Berg, 1997). These abnormalities, also observed in γc knockout mice, may reflect anergy of splenic T cells, possibly as a result of prior stimulation through the T cell antigen receptor in the absence of Jak3. This would be consistent with the observation that activation of Jak3 is associated with prevention of anergy (Boussiotis et al., 1994). Indeed, peripheral expression of Jak3 is required to maintain T lymphocyte function. In transgenic mice that express Jak3 in the thymus but not in the periphery, T cell development in the thymus is restored, but progressive accumulation of activated and anergic T cells is observed in the spleen (Thomis and Berg, 1997).

In Jak3 knockout mice, self-reactive T cells are not deleted in the thymus and periphery; furthermore, the activated, anergic T cells that accumulate in the spleen contain self-reactive lymphocytes (Saijo et al., 1997). These data indicate that Jak3 expression is essential to the process of negative selection. Peripheral lymph nodes are nearly undetectable in Jak3 knockout mice. These mice also lack NK cells, T lymphocytes, dendritic epidermal T cells, and intestinal intraepithelial lymphocytes (Park et al., 1995).

The proportion of early hematopoietic precursors (lin$^-$/c-kit$^+$/Sca-1$^+$) in the bone marrow is normal, as are the numbers of monocytes, macrophages, and myeloid and erythroid lineage cells. However, myeloid lineages in these mice are also affected by the loss of Jak3. Splenomegaly is common in these mice by 4 months of age and increased numbers of neutrophils and cells of the monocytic lineage are present in the peripheral blood. If Jak3 knockout mice are crossed with a transgenic mouse expressing Jak3 in the T and NK cell compartments, the splenomegaly and myeloid expansion are accentuated, while no splenomegaly or myeloid expansion is apparent when Jak3 knockout mice are crossed with Rag1-deficient animals that lack T lymphocytes. These findings suggest that the absence of Jak3 in the T cell compartment is responsible for the dysregulated myelopoiesis in Jak3 knockout mice (Grossman et al., 1999). As mentioned above, no overt anomalies of the myeloid compartment are detectable in JAK3-deficient humans.

On the whole, the immunological abnormalities in Jak3 knockout mice are similar to those of γc knockout mice (Cao et al., 1995; DiSanto et al., 1995; Ohbo et al., 1996). Both knockouts share a profound defect in B cell differentiation but allow some T cell maturation (particularly of CD4$^+$ T cells). Furthermore, a similar phenotype (with disturbed differentiation of T and B lymphocytes) has been observed in IL-7R knockout (Peschon et al., 1994) and IL-7 knockout (von Freeden-Jeffry et al., 1995) mice, consistent with the notion that IL-7/IL-7R interaction and signaling through the γc/Jak3 axis is a nonredundant function in lymphoid development.

In contrast to what has been observed in mice, JAK3 and γc deficiencies in humans are not characterized by severe defects in B cell differentiation. This finding suggests that IL-7 is an essential pre-B cell growth factor in mice but not in humans.

Severe Combined Immunodeficiency Due to Mutations of IL-7 Receptor α Chain

Clinical Features

Patients with IL-7Rα deficiency present with classical signs and symptoms of SCID. The original report (Puel et al., 1998) described two patients with T$^-$B$^+$NK$^+$ SCID characterized by failure to thrive, recurrent otitis, viral infections, candidiasis, diarrhea, and fever. A subsequent report described an additional family with extensive consanguinity and three subjects affected with T$^-$B$^+$NK$^+$ SCID having persistent oral thrush and failure to thrive. Absence of palpable lymph nodes and thymus shadow on chest radiograph were also described. Three infants from the same family had died from failure to thrive, diarrhea, and fungal and bacterial infections (Roifman et al., 2000). In a series of 169 SCID cases diagnosesd at Duke University Medical Center, 16 patients (9.5%) were found to have IL-7Rα deficiency, thus making this disorder the third-most common case of SCID in that series, after X-linked SCID and ADA deficiency (Buckley, 2004).

Laboratory Findings

Lymphopenia with elevated numbers of B cells, greatly diminished CD3$^+$ T lymphocytes, and normal or elevated numbers of CD16$^+$ NK cells have been described as characteristic signs of

IL-7Rα deficiency. Proliferation to mitogens and allogeneic cells is defective, but NK cell killing of K562 target cells is normal. Patients have defective production of immunoglobilins and fail to respond to vaccinations (Puel et al., 1998; Roifman et al., 2000).

Molecular Basis of IL-7Rα Deficiency

IL-7Rα (CD127) is a type 1 cytokine receptor chain devoid of intrinsic tyrosine kinase activity. This 460 amino acid–long chain can bind IL-7 with consequent dimerization with γc, which in turn results in JAK3-mediated phosphorylation of IL-7Rα and recruitment of JAK2 and STAT5 transcription factors. The *IL7R* gene, located on chromosome 5p13 in humans, is organized into eight exons and seven introns, with exons 1–5 encoding the extracellular portion of the receptor, and exon 6 and exons 7–8 encoding the transmembrane region and the intracellular tail, respectively (MIM *146661, #608971) (Online Mendelian Inheritance in Man, 2000). The *IL7R* cDNA is 1,380 nucleotides long and encodes a protein of the estimated molecular weight of ~90 kDa. The expression of *IL7R* mRNA can be detected in the earliest stages of lymphocyte differentiation (CD4$^-$CD8$^-$ double-negative thymocytes and c-kit$^+$B220$^+$ B cell progenitors) (Sudo et al., 1993; Orlic et al., 1997).

Although the cases reported in the literature are still limited, mutations of *IL7R* seem heterogeneous; missense, nonsense, and splice mutations have all been found. These mutations resulted in compound heterozygosity for two missense mutations (Thr66Ile in exon 2 and Ile138Val in exon 4) or for a nonsense (Trp217stop in exon 5) and a splice mutation at the acceptor site of intron 4, respectively, in the first two patients described (Puel et al., 1998), and in homozygosity for a missense mutation (Pro132Ser in exon 4) in a consanguineous family (Roifman et al., 2000).

Functional Aspects

The mechanism leading to SCID for the Thr66Ile and Ile138Val missense mutations remains unclear. When expressed in heterologous systems, these mutants are able to bind IL-7 and induce STAT5 activation (Puel et al., 1998). However, these alleles were not expressed by the heterozygous parents of the proband, a finding suggesting that decreased mRNA expression or stability could account for the SCID phenotype in this patient. The Trp217stop and the −1 G>A mutations at the acceptor site of intron 4 are predicted to prevent expression of functional IL-7Rα (Puel et al., 1998). Interestingly, the Pro132Ser missense mutation interfered with IL-7 binding and signal transduction and thus caused disease in one family (Roifman et al., 2000).

Strategies for Diagnosis

It has been proposed that the T$^-$B$^+$NK$^+$ SCID immunophenotype is characteristic of IL-7Rα deficiency, although patients affected with other forms of B$^+$ SCID can also have considerable numbers of NK cells (Candotti et al., 1997; Brugnoni et al., 1998). Studies of IL-7Rα mRNA and/or protein expression (Western blot, flow cytometry) can be informative and be performed on fresh PBMCs (IL-7Rα is expressed on immature B and T cells, mature T and NK cells, and macrophages) or EBV-transformed lymphoblastoid B cells. The definitive diagnosis is provided by detection of pathogenic mutations in affected subjects and their parents. The available information about intron–exon boundaries of the IL-7Rα gene facilitates genomic DNA analysis for this disease.

Treatment and Prognosis

Allogeneic BMT can provide full immune reconstitution for IL-7Rα deficiency (Buckley et al., 1999; Roifman et al., 2000) and is the treatment of choice. Similar to other forms of B⁺ SCID, early diagnosis and prevention of infections are associated with better outcome of the transplantation procedure and ultimate prognosis for affected patients. Because it affects the same signaling pathway as that in XSCID and JAK3 deficiency, IL-7Rα deficiency may be a good candidate for gene therapy, with similar prospects of risks and success.

Murine Models of IL-7Rα Deficiency

IL-7Rα participates with both the IL-7 and thymic stromal lymphopoietin (TSLP) cellular receptors, in association with γc and TSLPR, respectively, a receptor chain with 24% homology to γc (Pandey et al., 2000; Park et al., 2000). IL-7Rα knockout mice, therefore, lack both IL-7 and TSLP signaling. These mice are viable and fertile and retain normal proportions of all major thymocyte populations during fetal life (Crompton et al., 1998). Adult IL-7Rα-deficient mice, however, present with ~20-fold reduction of thymic precursors and decreased peripheral lymphocyte numbers (Peschon et al., 1994). Thymocyte development is arrested at the CD4⁻CD8⁻ double-negative stage, before the occurrence of T cell receptor (TCR) gene rearrangement (Maki et al., 1996a; Candeias et al., 1997; Crompton et al., 1997; Perumal et al., 1997). The reduced numbers of T cells that populate the periphery are dysfunctional and characterized by impaired survival and reduced proliferation to mitogens and alloantigens (Maraskovsky et al., 1996). Development of γδ T cells is also blocked in IL-7Rα-deficient mice, whereas NK cells develop normally (He and Malek, 1996; Maki et al., 1996b; Kang et al., 1999). Interestingly, thymocyte development can be restored by introduction of a transgenic TCR, which suggests that IL-7Rα is needed to initiate TCR gene rearrangement (Crompton et al., 1997). T lymphopoiesis is also restored in IL-7Rα-deficient mice by the transgenic expression of the anti-apoptotic molecule bcl-2 and ameliorated by the concomitant absence of the pro-apoptotic protein Bax. These data indicate that the critical consequence of engagement of IL-7Rα in T cell development may be the integration of cell survival signals (Akashi et al., 1997; Maraskovsky et al., 1997; Khaled et al., 2002).

IL-7Rα-deficient mice also show an incomplete block of B cell development at the transition from the pro-B to pre-B cell stage, which results in a 10-fold reduction in precursor B cells and severely decreased numbers of mature, peripheral B lymphocytes expressing surface immunoglobulin (Peschon et al., 1994). This defect is not corrected by transgenic expression of Bcl-2 (Maraskovsky et al., 1998) and is characterized by normal D-J segment joining but impaired recombination of antibody heavy-chain V segments (Corcoran et al., 1998). The reduction of B lymphocyte numbers in IL-7Rα-deficient mice does not parallel the human phenotype, perhaps because the essential role of TSLP in maturation of pre-B cells in mice (Friend et al., 1994; Levin et al., 1999) is not conserved in humans (Reche et al., 2001; Soumelis et al., 2002).

IL-2 Receptorβ and IL-15 Receptorβ Chain Deficiency

IL-2 and IL-15 signal through cellular receptors that share both γc (CD132) and IL-2Rβ/IL-15Rβ chain (CD122), the latter encoded by the *IL2Rβ* gene (MIM *146710) on chromosome 22q11.2-q13 in humans (Online Mendelian Inheritance in Man, 2000). Their receptors are distinguished by their ligand-specific subunits, IL-2Rα (CD25) and IL-15Rα, respectively. IL-2 is predominantly produced by activated T cells and plays an essential role in control of peripheral self-tolerance (Nelson, 2002) through activation-induced cell death (Frucht et al., 2001), thymic selection (Bassiri and Carding, 2001), and maintenance of regulatory T cells (Shevach, 2000; McHugh et al., 2001; Shevach et al., 2001). After binding to its receptor, IL-2 activates JAK1, JAK3, and STAT5.

Despite shared receptor usage with IL-2, IL-15 has a quite distinct function. This cytokine is essential for the maintenance of CD8⁺ memory T cells that gradually decline after viral infections in the absence of IL-15 (Becker et al., 2002; Goldrath et al., 2002; Schluns et al., 2002). IL-15 is also important for the development of NK cells, as illustrated by the lack of NK cells in IL-15 knockout and IL-15Rα knockout mice (Mohamadzadeh et al., 2001; Becker et al., 2002; Goldrath et al., 2002). Thus, the NK cell deficiency observed in X-linked SCID and JAK3-deficient patients is thought to be due to lack of IL-15 signaling.

One recently described patient with T^low^B⁺NK⁻ SCID presented with undetectable expression of the β chain of the cellular receptor used by both IL-2 and IL-15 (Gilmour et al., 2001b). The infant, born to nonconsanguineous parents, had a history of severe infections including respiratory syncytial virus bronchiolitis, *Candida* enteritis, and meningoencephalitis. He had failure to thrive, hepatomegaly, and moderate lymphopenia. Immunophenotype analysis showed markedly reduced T cell numbers and absent NK cells, with B lymphocytes within normal range values. Serum immunoglobulin levels were normal, although the patient failed to produce specific antibodies following immunization with tetanus toxoid and *Hemophilus influenzae* vaccines. The patient underwent allogeneic BMT from an unrelated donor and had good immune reconstitution and resolution of clinical symptoms.

Flow cytometry and Western blot analyses showed significant decrease of IL-2Rβ/IL-15Rβ chain expression in the patient's PBMCs. Similarly, Northern blot analysis showed a marked reduction of *IL15R* mRNA expression in the proband's cells. No abnormalities of *IL15R* were demonstrated; whether this clinical presentation was due to undetected mutations of *IL15R* or a defect that prevented transcription of *IL15R* remains unclear.

It is interesting to note that mice lacking IL-2Rβ/IL-15Rβ show defective NK cell development, a phenotype observed in this patient. In contrast, T cells of IL-2Rβ/IL-15Rβ-deficient mice are abnormally activated, resulting in dysregulated differentiation of B cells into plasma cells and consequent high levels of serum immunoglobulins. Autoantibodies are also produced that cause hemolytic anemia (Suzuki et al., 1995).

Lck Deficiency

Lck (p56lck) is an intracellular protein tyrosine kinase that is critically involved in TCR-mediated signaling. Its N-terminal region associates with the cytoplasmic tail of the CD4 and CD8 coreceptors (Chow and Veillette, 1995), thus bringing Lck into close proximity with the TCR. Lck is known to contribute to tyrosine phosphorylation of the immunoreceptor tyrosine-based activation motifs (ITAMs) of the TCR complex (Iwashima et al., 1994; van Oers et al., 1996). In keeping with the role played by Lck in early steps of TCR-mediated signaling, targeting of the

Lck gene (Molina et al., 1992) or expression of a dominant negative Lck transgene (Levin et al., 1993) results in a severe T cell developmental defect, with profound thymic atrophy, a dramatic reduction in the number of double-positive thymocytes, and only few circulating mature T cells.

One infant with a putative Lck defect has been reported to date (Goldman et al., 1998). The patient presented with chronic diarrhea and failure to thrive at 1 month of age, and developed *Enterobacter cloacae* sepsis, cytomegalovirus infection, and persistent oral candidiasis. Laboratory investigation disclosed panhypogammaglobulinemia, lymphopenia with a low proportion (9%–22%) of CD4[+] T cells, and a progressive decline in T cell proliferation to mitogens and anti-CD3 monoclonal antibody. CD8[+] T cells, if activated with anti-CD3, failed to express the activation marker CD69, whereas activation with phorbol esthers and ionomycin resulted in normal CD69 expression, indicating a TCR signaling defect proximal to protein kinase C activation. A marked reduction in the level of Lck protein and an improperly spliced mRNA transcript of the *LCK* gene on chromosome lp35-34.3 (MIM *153390) lacking the exon 7 coding domain were demonstrated (Online Mendelian Inheritance in Man, 2000). The molecular basis for this abnormal finding remains unclear. The milder immunologic phenotype observed in the patient compared with gene-targeted *Lck* knockout mice could be explained by residual, although low, expression of Lck or species differences in redundancy of related signaling kinases. The clinical course of the infant was typical for SCID; he ultimately required BMT, which was reportedly curative.

Short Stature and Immunodeficiency Due to Mutations of STAT5b

Clinical Features

A single patient has recently been reported who had STAT5b deficiency resulting in postnatal growth failure, facial dysmorphism, and immunodeficiency (Kofoed et al., 2003; Rosenfeld et al., 2004). This daughter of consanguineous healthy parents of normal stature had severe growth failure with growth hormone insensitivity. By the age of 16.5 years she was the height of an average 6.5-year-old. She also suffered from chronic diarrhea, generalized eczema, and respiratory ailments, periodically requiring oxygen supplementation. A lung biopsy indicated lymphoid interstitial pneumonia for which the patient was treated with oral steroids. At age 8 she developed severe hemorrhagic varicella, followed by multiple episodes of herpes zoster. At age 10, progressive worsening of her pulmonary function occasioned a repeat lung biopsy in which *Pneumocystis jiroveci* and *Rodococcus equis* were isolated. Institution of appropriate treatment and chronic management of combined immunodeficiency have resulted in an improved quality of life.

Laboratory Findings

High levels of endogenous growth hormone, low insulin-like growth factor, normal growth hormone binding protein, and normal growth hormone receptor (GHR) coding sequence pointed to an intracellular defect distal to the GHR, a member of the cytokine receptor gene superfamily that acts through phosphorylation of STAT5b. Indeed, expression of STAT5b was only poorly detectable in patient fibroblasts, which failed to show phosphorylation of the protein in response to GH. STAT5a expression and phosphorylation were normal. Details about the patient's lymphocyte profile and immune functional studies have not been published in detail.

Molecular Basis of STAT5b Deficiency

This patient was found to be homozygous for the missense mutation in the *STAT5B* (MIM *604260) gene, which is located adjacent to STAT3 and STAT5A on human chromosome 17q11.2 (Online Mendelian Inheritance in Man, 2000). The mutation is due to the substitution of C for the G nucleotide at cDNA 2057 in the alanine 630 codon, changing alanine to proline (A630P). The mutation lies in the highly conserved SH2 domain of STAT5b. Although protein is produced (but poorly recognized by some monoclonal antibodies), it is unable to be phosphorylated, preventing dimerization, translation to the nucleus, and activation of transcription.

Functional Aspects and Animal Model of STAT5b Deficiency

STAT5a and STAT5b are transcription factors that are 96% homologous to each other and are located adjacent to one another in head-to-head orientation in both human and mouse, suggesting that these genes arose by gene duplication. The precise role of each of the two *STAT5* genes is not completely worked out in humans or in mice. Murine knockouts of STAT5a show impaired prolactin-dependent mammary gland development (Liu et al., 1997), while STAT5b knockout mice have a phenotype similar to that observed in GHR-deficient mice (Udy et al., 1997). Deletion of both STAT5a and STAT5b results in a phenotype closely resembling that observed in prolactin receptor–deficient mice, including decreased body size in males, anemia, and impaired mammary gland development in females. These features reflect the role of STAT5 proteins as intracellular transducers of signals from growth hormone, erythropoietin, and prolactin receptors. In addition, STAT5a and STAT5b double-knockout mice show a profound T cell proliferation defect similar to that observed in IL-2Rβ-deficient mice (Teglund et al., 1998). Partial T cell defects can be observed in both STAT5a and STAT5b single-knockout mice (Nakajima et al., 1997; Imada et al., 1998), indicating that the two STAT5 proteins play critical, redundant roles in mouse peripheral T cell activation and proliferation.

Diagnosis, Treatment, and Prognosis

The coexistence of extreme short stature and combined immunodeficiency may suggest STAT5b deficiency, particularly in a consanguineous family. Because only a single patient has been described to date, the clinical spectrum of disease severity is not known. The multiple roles of STAT5b in many tissues indicate that bone marrow transplantation would not be expected to correct the entire phenotype.

Concluding Remarks

The recent identification of patients with JAK3 deficiency and IL-7Rα deficiency has greatly contributed to our understanding of biological and clinical aspects of B[+] SCID. In a series of 96 children with SCID in Europe, JAK3 deficiency was found to be responsible for ~40% of the B[+] SCID patients, making JAK3 SCID nearly as common as X-linked SCID. This finding is in contrast to recent reports from the United States, where fewer than 10% of B[+] SCID patients with known genetic cause have defects in JAK3 (Buckley, 2000b). This discrepancy may reflect a real variability in the incidence of the disease in different gene pools, but it may also be due in part to an ascertainment bias. Autosomal recessive SCID is less likely to have a positive family history than X-linked SCID, and infants presenting with serious infections may die before referral to immunology centers for diagnosis. In addition, we have shown that several patients with *JAK3* defects express substantial amounts of JAK3 protein, indicating that specialized functional assays and DNA sequence determination are the only reliable tools for unequivocal identification of patients with SCID due to *JAK3* mutations. On the other hand, the development of molecular and biochemical assays to identify JAK3 (and γc) defects demonstrated that not all T⁻B⁺ SCID patients have abnormal JAK3 or γc and opened the way to the identification of *IL7R* and *IL2Rβ* defects (Puel et al., 1998; Gilmour et al., 2001b).

Longitudinal observation of patients with mutations in genes responsible for B⁺ SCID has clearly established the gradual appearance of circulating T lymphocytes with abnormal activation markers and low proliferative responses to mitogens (South et al., 1977; Morelon et al., 1996; Mella et al., 2000; Frucht et al., 2001). There is no clear explanation for these findings at present; however, in light of the progressive appearance and accumulation of activated and anergic T cells described in *Jak3* knockout mice, it is tempting to speculate that the occurrence of circulating T lymphocytes in these patients may reflect the natural history of *JAK3* deficiency as well as other immunodeficiencies caused by disorders of cytokine signaling. If this hypothesis proves to be correct, the clinical and immunological spectrum of these forms of combined immunodeficiencies may be broader than currently appreciated. Patients now classified as having combined immunodeficiency with residual T cell function could, in fact, carry mutations in genes of cytokine signaling molecules.

References

Akashi K, Kondo M, von Freeden-Jeffry U, Murray R, Weissman IL. Bcl-2 rescues T lymphopoiesis in interleukin-7 receptor-deficient mice. Cell 89:1033–1041, 1997.

Antoine C, Muller S, Cant A, Cavazzana-Calvo M, Veys P, Vossen J, Fasth A, Heilmann C, Wulffraat N, Seger R, Blanche S, Friedrich W, Abinun M, Davies G, Bredius R, Schulz A, Landais P, Fischer A. Long-term survival and transplantation of haemopoietic stem cells for immunodeficiencies: report of the European experience 1968–99. Lancet 361:553–560, 2003.

Asao H, Okuyama C, Kumaki S, Ishii N, Tsuchiya S, Foster D, Sugamura K. Cutting edge: the common gamma-chain is an indispensable subunit of the IL-21 receptor complex. J Immunol 167:1–5, 2001.

Bassiri H, Carding SR. A requirement for IL-2/IL-2 receptor signaling in intrathymic negative selection. J Immunol 166:5945–5954, 2001.

Becker TC, Wherry EJ, Boone D, Murali-Krishna K, Antia R, Ma A, Ahmed R. Interleukin 15 is required for proliferative renewal of virus-specific memory CD8 T cells. J Exp Med 195:1541–1548, 2002.

Bertrand Y, Landais P, Friedrich W, Gerritsen B, Morgan G, Fasth A, Cavazzana-Calvo M, Porta F, Cant A, Espanol T, Muller S, Veys P, Vossen J, Haddad E, Fischer A. Influence of severe combined immunodeficiency phenotype on the outcome of HLA non-identical, T-cell-depleted bone marrow transplantation: a retrospective European survey from the European Group for Bone Marrow Transplantation and the European Society for Immunodeficiency. J Pediatr 134:740–748, 1999.

Blumer KJ, Johnson GL. Diversity in function and regulation of MAP kinase pathways. Trends Biochem Sci 19:236–240, 1994.

Boussiotis VA, Barber DL, Nakarai T, Freeman GJ, Gribben JG, Bernstein GM, D'Andrea AD, Ritz J, Nadler LM. Prevention of T cell anergy by signaling through the gamma c chain of the IL-2 receptor. Science 266: 1039–1042, 1994.

Bozzi F, Lefranc G, Villa A, Badolato R, Schumacher RF, Khalil G, Loiselet J, Bresciani S, O'Shea JJ, Vezzoni P, Notarangelo LD, Candotti F. Molecular and biochemical characterization of JAK3 deficiency in a patient with severe combined immunodeficiency over 20 years after bone marrow

transplantation: implications for treatment. Br J Haematol 102:1363–1366, 1998.

Brugnoni D, Notarangelo LD, Sottini A, Airò P, Pennacchio M, Mazzolari E, Signorini S, Candotti F, Villa A, Mella P, Vezzoni P, Cattaneo R, Ugazio AG, Imberti L. Development of autologous, oligoclonal, poorly functioning T lymphocytes in a patient with autosomal recessive severe combined immunodeficiency due to defects of the Jak3 tyrosine kinase. Blood 91: 949–955, 1998.

Buckley RH. Advances in the understanding and treatment of human severe combined immunodeficiency. Immunol Res 22:237–251, 2000a.

Buckley RH. Primary immunodeficiency diseases due to defects in lymphocytes. N Engl J Med 343:1313–1324, 2000b.

Buckley RH. Molecular defects in human severe combined immunodeficiency and approaches to immune reconstitution. Annu Rev Immunol 22: 625–655, 2004.

Buckley RH, Schiff SE, Schiff RI, Markert L, Williams LW, Roberts JL, Myers LA, Ward FE. Hematopoietic stem-cell transplantation for the treatment of severe combined immunodeficiency. N Engl J Med 340: 508–516, 1999.

Bunting KD, Flynn KJ, Riberdy JM, Doherty PC, Sorrentino BP. Virus-specific immunity after gene therapy in a murine model of severe combined immunodeficiency. Proc Natl Acad Sci USA 96:232–237, 1999.

Bunting KD, Lu T, Kelly PF, Sorrentino BP. Self-selection by genetically modified committed lymphocyte precursors reverses the phenotype of JAK3-deficient mice without myeloablation. Hum Gene Ther 11:2353–2364, 2000.

Bunting KD, Sangster MY, Ihle JN, Sorrentino BP. Restoration of lymphocyte function in Janus kinase 3–deficient mice by retroviral-mediated gene transfer. Nat Med 4:58–64, 1998.

Cacalano NA, Migone TS, Bazan F, Hanson EP, Chen M, Candotti F, O'Shea JJ, Johnston JA. Autosomal SCID caused by a point mutation in the N-terminus of Jak3: mapping of the Jak3-receptor interaction domain. EMBO J 18:1549–1558, 1999.

Candeias S, Peschon JJ, Muegge K, Durum SK. Defective T-cell receptor gamma gene rearrangement in interleukin-7 receptor knockout mice. Immunol Lett 57:9–14, 1997.

Candotti F, Oakes SA, Johnston JA, Giliani S, Schumacher RF, Mella P, Fiorini M, Ugazio AG, Badolato R, Notarangelo LD, Bozzi F, Macchi P, Strina D, Vezzoni P, Blaese RM, O'Shea JJ, Villa A. Structural and functional basis for JAK3-deficient severe combined immunodeficiency. Blood 90: 3996–4003, 1997.

Candotti F, Oakes S, Johnston JA, Notarangelo LD, O'Shea JJ, Blaese RM. In vitro correction of JAK3-deficient severe combined immunodeficiency by retroviral-mediated gene transduction. J Exp Med 183:2687–2692, 1996.

Cao X, Shores EW, Hu-Li J, Anver MR, Kelsall BL, Russell SM, Drago J, Noguchi M, Grinberg A, Bloom ET, Paul WE, Katz SI, Love PE, Leonard WJ. Defective lymphoid development in mice lacking expression of the common cytokine receptor gamma chain. Immunity 2:223–238, 1995.

Cavazzana-Calvo M, Hacein-Bey S, de Saint Basile G, Gross F, Yvon E, Nusbaum P, Selz F, Hue C, Certain S, Casanova JL, Bousso P, Deist FL, Fischer A. Gene therapy of human severe combined immunodeficiency (SCID)-X1 disease. Science 288:669–672, 2000.

Chen M, Cheng A, Candotti F, Zhou YJ, Hymel A, Fasth A, Notarangelo LD, O'Shea JJ. Complex effects of naturally occurring mutations in the JAK3 pseudokinase domain: evidence for interactions between the kinase and pseudokinase domains. Mol Cell Biol 20:947–956, 2000.

Chow LM, Veillette A. The Src and Csk families of tyrosine protein kinases in hemopoietic cells. Semin Immunol 7:207–226, 1995.

Corcoran AE, Riddell A, Krooshoop D, Venkitaraman AR. Impaired immunoglobulin gene rearrangement in mice lacking the IL-7 receptor. Nature 391:904–907, 1998.

Crompton T, Outram SV, Buckland J, Owen MJ. A transgenic T cell receptor restores thymocyte differentiation in interleukin-7 receptor alpha chain-deficient mice. Eur J Immunol 27:100–104, 1997.

Crompton T, Outram SV, Buckland J, Owen MJ. Distinct roles of the interleukin-7 receptor alpha chain in fetal and adult thymocyte development revealed by analysis of interleukin-7 receptor alpha-deficient mice. Eur J Immunol 28:1859–1866, 1998.

de Waal Malefyt R, Figdor CG, Huijbens R, Mohan-Peterson S, Bennett B, Culpepper J, Dang W, Zurawski G, de Vries JE. Effects of IL-13 on phenotype, cytokine production, and cytotoxic function of human monocytes. Comparison with IL-4 and modulation by IFN-gamma or IL-10. J Immunol 151:6370–6381, 1993.

DiSanto JP, Muller W, Guy-Grand D, Fischer A, Rajewsky K. Lymphoid development in mice with a targeted deletion of the interleukin 2 receptor gamma chain. Proc Natl Acad Sci USA 92:377–381, 1995.

Dror Y, Gallagher R, Wara DW, Colombe BW, Merino A, Benkerrou M, Cowan MJ. Immune reconstitution in severe combined immunodeficiency disease after lectin-treated, T-cell-depleted haplocompatible bone marrow transplantation. Blood 81:2021–2030, 1993.

Egan SE, Giddings BW, Brooks MW, Buday L, Sizeland AM, Weinberg RA. Association of Sos Ras exchange protein with Grb2 is implicated in tyrosine kinase signal transduction and transformation. Nature 363:45–51, 1993.

Endo TA, Masuhara M, Yokouchi M, Suzuki R, Sakamoto H, Mitsui K, Matsumoto A, Tanimura S, Ohtsubo M, Misawa H, Miyazaki T, Leonor N, Taniguchi T, Fujita T, Kanakura Y, Komiya S, Yoshimura A. A new protein containing an SH2 domain that inhibits JAK kinases. Nature 387:921–924, 1997.

Fenghao X, Saxon A, Nguyen A, Ke Z, Diaz-Sanchez D, Nel A. Interleukin 4 activates a signal transducer and activator of transcription (Stat) protein which interacts with an interferon-gamma activation site-like sequence upstream of the I epsilon exon in a human B cell line. Evidence for the involvement of Janus kinase 3 and interleukin-4 Stat. J Clin Invest 96:907–914, 1995.

Fenton MJ, Buras JA, Donnelly RP. IL-4 reciprocally regulates IL-1 and IL-1 receptor antagonist expression in human monocytes. J Immunol 149:1283–1288, 1992.

Fischer A. Primary immunodeficiency diseases: an experimental model for molecular medicine. Lancet 357:1863–1869, 2001.

Fischer A, Landais P, Friedrich W, Morgan G, Gerritsen B, Fasth A, Porta F, Griscelli C, Goldman SF, Levinsky R, Vossen J. European experience of bone-marrow transplantation for severe combined immunodeficiency. Lancet 336:850–854, 1990.

Foxwell BM, Beadling C, Guschin D, Kerr I, Cantrell D. Interleukin-7 can induce the activation of Jak 1, Jak 3 and STAT 5 proteins in murine T cells. Eur J Immunol 25:3041–3046, 1995.

Friend SL, Hosier S, Nelson A, Foxworthe D, Williams DE, Farr A. A thymic stromal cell line supports in vitro development of surface IgM+ B cells and produces a novel growth factor affecting B and T lineage cells. Exp Hematol 22:321–328, 1994.

Frucht DM, Gadina M, Jagadeesh GJ, Aksentijevich I, Takada K, Bleesing JJH, Nelson J, Muul LM, Perham G, Morgan G, Gerritsen EJA, Schumacher RF, Mella P, Veys PA, Fleisher TA, Kaminski ER, Notarangelo LD, O'Shea JJ, Candotti F. Unexpected and variable phenotypes in a family with JAK3 deficiency. Genes Immunity 2:422–432, 2001.

Fujii H, Nakagawa Y, Schindler U, Kawahara A, Mori H, Gouilleux F, Groner B, Ihle JN, Minami Y, Miyazaki T, et al. Activation of Stat5 by interleukin 2 requires a carboxyl-terminal region of the interleukin 2 receptor beta chain but is not essential for the proliferative signal transmission. Proc Natl Acad Sci USA 92:5482–5486, 1995.

Gilmour KC, Cranston T, Loughlin S, Gwyther J, Lester T, Espanol T, Hernandez A, Savoldi G, Davies EG, Abinun M, Kinnon C, Jones A, Gaspar HB. Rapid protein-based assays for the diagnosis of T⁻ B⁺ severe combined immunodeficiency. Br J Haematol 112:671–676, 2001.

Gilmour KC, Fujii H, Cranston T, Davies EG, Kinnon C, Gaspar HB. Defective expression of the interleukin-2/interleukin-15 receptor beta subunit leads to a natural killer cell-deficient form of severe combined immunodeficiency. Blood 98:877–879, 2001b.

Gilmour KC, Pine R, Reich NC. Interleukin 2 activates STAT5 transcription factor (mammary gland factor) and specific gene expression in T lymphocytes. Proc Natl Acad Sci USA 92:10772–10776, 1995.

Goldman FD, Ballas ZK, Schutte BC, Kemp J, Hollenback C, Noraz N, Taylor N. Defective expression of p56lck in an infant with severe combined immunodeficiency. J Clin Invest 102:421–429, 1998.

Goldrath AW, Sivakumar PV, Glaccum M, Kennedy MK, Bevan MJ, Benoist C, Mathis D, Butz EA. Cytokine requirements for acute and basal homeostatic proliferation of naive and memory CD8⁺ T cells. J Exp Med 195:1515–1522, 2002.

Grossman WJ, Verbsky JW, Yang L, Berg LJ, Fields LE, Chaplin DD, Ratner L. Dysregulated myelopoiesis in mice lacking Jak3. Blood 94:932–939, 1999.

Gurniak CB, Berg LJ. Murine JAK3 is preferentially expressed in hematopoietic tissues and lymphocyte precursor cells. Blood 87:3151–3160, 1996.

Hacein-Bey-Abina S, Le Deist F, Carlier F, Bouneaud C, Hue C, De Villartay JP, Thrasher AJ, Wulffraat N, Sorensen R, Dupuis-Girod S, Fischer A, Davies EG, Kuis W, Leiva L, Cavazzana-Calvo M. Sustained correction of X-linked severe combined immunodeficiency by ex vivo gene therapy. N Engl J Med 346:1185–1193, 2002.

Hacein-Bey-Abina S, von Kalle C, Schmidt M, Le Deist F, Wulffraat N, McIntyre E, Radford I, Villeval JL, Fraser CC, Cavazzana-Calvo M, Fischer A. A serious adverse event after successful gene therapy for X-linked severe combined immunodeficiency. N Engl J Med 348:255–256, 2003.

Haddad E, Landais P, Friedrich W, Gerritsen B, Cavazzana-Calvo M, Morgan G, Bertrand Y, Fasth A, Porta F, Cant A, Espanol T, Muller S, Veys P, Vossen J, Fischer A. Long-term immune reconstitution and outcome after HLA-nonidentical T-cell-depleted bone marrow transplantation for severe combined immunodeficiency: a European retrospective study of 116 patients. Blood 91:3646–3653, 1998.

He YW, Malek TR. Interleukin-7 receptor alpha is essential for the development of gamma delta + T cells, but not natural killer cells. J Exp Med 184:289–293, 1996.

Hilton DJ, Richardson RT, Alexander WS, Viney EM, Willson TA, Sprigg NS, Starr R, Nicholson SE, Metcalf D, Nicola NA. Twenty proteins containing a C-terminal SOCS box form five structural classes. Proc Natl Acad Sci USA 95:114–119, 1998.

Holsinger LJ, Spencer DM, Austin DJ, Schreiber SL, Crabtree GR. Signal transduction in T lymphocytes using a conditional allele of Sos. Proc Natl Acad Sci USA 92:9810–9814, 1995.

Hou J, Schindler U, Henzel WJ, Wong SC, McKnight SL. Identification and purification of human Stat proteins activated in response to interleukin-2. Immunity 2:321–329, 1995.

Ihle JN. Cytokine receptor signalling. Nature 377:591–594, 1995.

Ihle JN. STATs: signal transducers and activators of transcription. Cell 84:1996.

Ihle JN, Witthuhn BA, Quelle FW, Yamamoto K, Thierfelder WE, Kreider B, Silvennoinen O. Signaling by the cytokine receptor superfamily: JAKs and STATs. Trends Biochem Sci 19:222–227, 1994.

Imada K, Bloom ET, Nakajima H, Horvath-Arcidiacono JA, Udy GB, Davey HW, Leonard WJ. Stat5b is essential for natural killer cell–mediated proliferation and cytolytic activity. J Exp Med 188:2067–2074, 1998.

Ivashkiv LB. Cytokines and STATs: how can signals achieve specificity? Immunity 3:1–4, 1995.

Iwashima M, Irving BA, van Oers NS, Chan AC, Weiss A. Sequential interactions of the TCR with two distinct cytoplasmic tyrosine kinases. Science 263:1136–1139, 1994.

Johnston JA, Bacon CM, Finbloom DS, Rees RC, Kaplan D, Shibuya K, Ortaldo JR, Gupta S, Chen YQ, Giri JD, et al. Tyrosine phosphorylation and activation of STAT5, STAT3, and Janus kinases by interleukins 2 and 15. Proc Natl Acad Sci USA 92:8705–8709, 1995a.

Johnston JA, Kawamura M, Kirken RA, Chen YQ, Blake TB, Shibuya K, Ortaldo JR, McVicar DW, O'Shea JJ. Phosphorylation and activation of the Jak-3 Janus kinase in response to interleukin-2. Nature 370:151–153, 1994.

Johnston JA, Wang LM, Hanson EP, Sun XJ, White MF, Oakes SA, Pierce JH, O'Shea JJ. Interleukins 2, 4, 7, and 15 stimulate tyrosine phosphorylation of insulin receptor substrates 1 and 2 in T cells. Potential role of JAK kinases. J Biol Chem 270:28527–28530, 1995b.

Kang J, Coles M, Raulet DH. Defective development of gamma/delta T cells in interleukin 7 receptor-deficient mice is due to impaired expression of T cell receptor gamma genes. J Exp Med 190:973–982, 1999.

Kaplan MH, Schindler U, Smiley ST, Grusby MJ. Stat6 is required for mediating responses to IL-4 and for development of Th2 cells. Immunity 4:313–319, 1996.

Karnitz LM, Abraham RT. Cytokine receptor signaling mechanisms. Curr Opin Immunol 7:320–326, 1995.

Kawahara A, Minami Y, Miyazaki T, Ihle JN, Taniguchi T. Critical role of the interleukin 2 (IL-2) receptor gamma-chain-associated Jak3 in the IL-2-induced c-fos and c-myc, but not bcl-2, gene induction. Proc Natl Acad Sci USA 92:8724–8728, 1995.

Kawamura M, McVicar DW, Johnston JA, Blake TB, Chen YQ, Lal BK, Lloyd AR, Kelvin DJ, Staples JE, Ortaldo JR, O'Shea JJ. Molecular cloning of L-JAK, a Janus family protein-tyrosine kinase expressed in natural killer cells and activated leukocytes. Proc Natl Acad Sci USA 91:6374–6378, 1994.

Keegan AD, Johnston JA, Tortolani PJ, McReynolds LJ, Kinzer C, O'Shea JJ, Paul WE. Similarities and differences in signal transduction by interleukin 4 and interleukin 13: analysis of Janus kinase activation. Proc Natl Acad Sci USA 92:7681–7685, 1995.

Keegan AD, Nelms K, White M, Wang LM, Pierce JH, Paul WE. An IL-4 receptor region containing an insulin receptor motif is important for IL-4-mediated IRS-1 phosphorylation and cell growth. Cell 76:811–820, 1994.

Khaled AR, Li WQ, Huang J, Fry TJ, Khaled AS, Mackall CL, Muegge K, Young HA, Durum SK. Bax deficiency partially corrects interleukin-7 receptor alpha deficiency. Immunity 17:561–573, 2002.

Kofoed EM, Hwa V, Little B, Woods KA, Buckway CK, Tsubaki J, Pratt KL, Bezrodnik L, Jasper H, Tepper A, Heinrich JJ, Rosenfeld RG. Growth hormone insensitivity associated with a STAT5b mutation. N Engl J Med 349:1139–1147, 2003.

Lai KS, Jin Y, Graham DK, Witthuhn BA, Ihle JN, Liu ET. A kinase-deficient splice variant of the human JAK3 is expressed in hematopoietic and epithelial cancer cells. J Biol Chem 270:25028–25036, 1995.

Leonard WJ. The molecular basis of X-linked severe combined immunodeficiency: defective cytokine receptor signaling. Annu Rev Med 47:229–239, 1996.

Leonard WJ, O'Shea JJ. Jaks and STATs: biological implications. Annu Rev Immunol 16:293–322, 1998.

Levin SD, Anderson SJ, Forbush KA, Perlmutter RM. A dominant-negative transgene defines a role for p56lck in thymopoiesis. EMBO J 12:1671–1680, 1993.

Levin SD, Koelling RM, Friend SL, Isaksen DE, Ziegler SF, Perlmutter RM, Farr AG. Thymic stromal lymphopoietin: a cytokine that promotes the development of IgM+ B cells in vitro and signals via a novel mechanism. J Immunol 162:677–683, 1999.

Li N, Batzer A, Daly R, Yajnik V, Skolnik E, Chardin P, Bar-Sagi D, Margolis B, Schlessinger J. Guanine-nucleotide-releasing factor hSos1 binds to Grb2 and links receptor tyrosine kinases to Ras signalling. Nature 363: 85–88, 1993.

Lin JX, Mietz J, Modi WS, John S, Leonard WJ. Cloning of human Stat5B. Reconstitution of interleukin-2-induced Stat5A and Stat5B DNA binding activity in COS-7 cells. J Biol Chem 271:10738–10744, 1996.

Liu X, Robinson GW, Wagner KU, Garrett L, Wynshaw-Boris A, Hennighausen L. Stat5a is mandatory for adult mammary gland development and lactogenesis. Genes Dev 11:179–186, 1997.

Macchi P, Villa A, Giliani S, Sacco MG, Frattini A, Porta F, Ugazio AG, Johnston JA, Candotti F, O'Shea JJ, Vezzoni P, Notarangelo LD. Mutations of Jak-3 gene in patients with autosomal severe combined immune deficiency (SCID). Nature 377:65–68, 1995.

Maki K, Sunaga S, Ikuta K. The V-J recombination of T cell receptor-gamma genes is blocked in interleukin-7 receptor-deficient mice. J Exp Med 184: 2423–2427, 1996a.

Maki K, Sunaga S, Komagata Y, Kodaira Y, Mabuchi A, Karasuyama H, Yokomuro K, Miyazaki JI, Ikuta K. Interleukin 7 receptor-deficient mice lack gamma/delta T cells. Proc Natl Acad Sci USA 93:7172, 1996b.

Malabarba MG, Kirken RA, Rui H, Koettnitz K, Kawamura M, O'Shea JJ, Kalthoff FS, Farrar WL. Activation of JAK3, but not JAK1, is critical to interleukin-4 (IL4) stimulated proliferation and requires a membrane-proximal region of IL4 receptor alpha. J Biol Chem 270:9630–9637, 1995.

Maraskovsky E, O'Reilly LA, Teepe M, Corcoran LM, Peschon JJ, Strasser A. Bcl-2 can rescue T lymphocyte development in interleukin-7 receptor-deficient mice but not in mutant rag-1-/- mice. Cell 89:1011–1019, 1997.

Maraskovsky E, Peschon JJ, McKenna H, Teepe M, Strasser A. Overexpression of Bcl-2 does not rescue impaired B lymphopoiesis in IL-7 receptor–deficient mice but can enhance survival of mature B cells. Int Immunol 10:1367–1375, 1998.

Maraskovsky E, Teepe M, Morrissey PJ, Braddy S, Miller RE, Lynch DH, Peschon JJ. Impaired survival and proliferation in IL-7 receptor-deficient peripheral T cells. J Immunol 157:5315–5323, 1996.

McHugh RS, Shevach EM, Thornton AM. Control of organ-specific autoimmunity by immunoregulatory CD4(+)CD25(+) T cells. Microbes Infect 3:919–927, 2001.

Mella P, Imberti L, Brugnoni D, Pirovano S, Candotti F, Mazzolari E, Bettinardi A, Fiorini M, De Mattia D, Martire B, Plebani A, Notarangelo LD, Giliani S. Development of autologous T lymphocytes in two males with X-linked severe combined immune deficiency: molecular and cellular characterization. Clin Immunol 95:39–50, 2000.

Mella P, Schumacher RF, Cranston T, de Saint Basile G, Savoldi G, Notarangelo LD. Eleven novel JAK3 mutations in patients with severe combined immunodeficiency-including the first patients with mutations in the kinase domain. Hum Mutat 18:355–356, 2001.

Migone TS, Cacalano NA, Taylor N, Yi T, Waldmann TA, Johnston JA. Recruitment of SH2-containing protein tyrosine phosphatase SHP-1 to the interleukin 2 receptor; loss of SHP-1 expression in human T-lymphotropic virus type I-transformed T cells. Proc Natl Acad Sci USA 95: 3845–3850, 1998.

Minami Y, Taniguchi T. IL-2 signaling: recruitment and activation of multiple protein tyrosine kinases by the components of the IL-2 receptor. Curr Opin Cell Biol 7:156–162, 1995.

Miyazaki T, Kawahara A, Fujii H, Nakagawa Y, Minami Y, Liu ZJ, Oishi I, Silvennoinen O, Witthuhn BA, Ihle JN, Taniguchi T. Functional activation of Jak1 and Jak3 by selective association with IL-2 receptor subunits. Science 266:1045–1047, 1994.

Mohamadzadeh M, Berard F, Essert G, Chalouni C, Pulendran B, Davoust J, Bridges G, Palucka AK, Bancherau J. Interleukin 15 skews monocyte differentiation into dendritic cells with features of Langerhans cells. J Exp Med 194:1013–1020, 2001.

Molina TJ, Kishihara K, Siderovski DP, van Ewijk W, Narendran A, Timms E, Wakeham A, Paige CJ, Hartmann KU, Veillette A, et al. Profound block in thymocyte development in mice lacking p56lck. Nature 357:161–164, 1992.

Morelon E, Dautry-Varsat A, Le Deist F, Hacein-Bay S, Fischer A, de Saint Basile G. T-lymphocyte differentiation and proliferation in the absence of the cytoplasmic tail of the common cytokine receptor gc chain in a severe combined immune deficiency X1 patient. Blood 89:1708, 1996.

Muller M, Briscoe J, Laxton C, Guschin D, Ziemiecki A, Silvennoinen O, Harpur AG, Barbieri G, Witthuhn BA, Schindler C, et al. The protein tyrosine kinase JAK1 complements defects in interferon-alpha/beta and -gamma signal transduction. Nature 366:129–135, 1993.

Musso T, Johnston JA, Linnekin D, Varesio L, Rowe TK, O'Shea JJ, McVicar DW. Regulation of JAK3 expression in human monocytes: phosphorylation in response to interleukins 2, 4, and 7. J Exp Med 181:1425–1431, 1995.

Myers MG Jr, Backer JM, Sun XJ, Shoelson S, Hu P, Schlessinger J, Yoakim M, Schaffhausen B, White MF. IRS-1 activates phosphatidylinositol 3'-kinase by associating with src homology 2 domains of p85. Proc Natl Acad Sci USA 89:10350–10354, 1992.

Naka T, Narazaki M, Hirata M, Matsumoto T, Minamoto S, Aono A, Nishimoto N, Kajita T, Taga T, Yoshizaki K, Akira S, Kishimoto T. Structure and function of a new STAT-induced STAT inhibitor. Nature 387:924–929, 1997.

Nakajima H, Liu XW, Wynshaw-Boris A, Rosenthal LA, Imada K, Finbloom DS, Hennighausen L, Leonard WJ. An indirect effect of Stat5a in IL-2-induced proliferation: a critical role for Stat5a in IL-2-mediated IL-2 receptor alpha chain induction. Immunity 7:691–701, 1997.

Nelson BH. Interleukin-2 signaling and the maintenance of self-tolerance. Curr Dir Autoimmun 5:92–112, 2002.

Noguchi M, Yi H, Rosenblatt HM, Filipovich AH, Adelstein S, Modi WS, McBride OW, Leonard WJ. Interleukin-2 receptor gamma chain mutation results in X-linked severe combined immunodeficiency in humans. Cell 73: 147–157, 1993.

Nosaka T, van Deursen JM, Tripp RA, Thierfelder WE, Witthuhn BA, McMickle AP, Doherty PC, Grosveld GC, Ihle JN. Defective lymphoid development in mice lacking Jak3. Science 270:800–802, 1995.

Notarangelo LD, Candotti F. JAK3-deficient severe combined immunodeficiency. Immunol Allergy Clin North Am 20:97–111, 2000.

Notarangelo LD, Mella P, Jones A, de Saint Basile G, Savoldi G, Cranston T, Vihinen M, Schumacher RF. Mutations in severe combined immune deficiency (SCID) due to JAK3 deficiency. Hum Mutat 18:255–263, 2001.

Oakes SA, Candotti F, Johnston JA, Chen Y-Q, Ryan JJ, Taylor N, Liu X, Hennighausen L, Notarangelo LD, Paul WE, Blaese RM, O'Shea JJ. Signaling via IL-2 and IL-4 in JAK3-deficient severe combined immunodeficiency lymphocytes: JAK3-dependent and -independent pathways. Immunity 5:605–615, 1996.

Ohbo K, Suda T, Hashiyama M, Mantani A, Ikebe M, Miyakawa K, Moriyama M, Nakamura M, Katsuki M, Takahashi K, Yamamura K, Sugamura K. Modulation of hematopoiesis in mice with a truncated mutant of the interleukin-2 receptor gamma chain. Blood 87:956–967, 1996.

Online Mendelian Inheritance in Man, OMIM (TM). McKusick-Nathans Institute for Genetic Medicine, Johns Hopkins University (Baltimore, MD) and National Center for Biotechnology Information, National Library of Medicine (Bethesda, MD), 2000. World Wide Web URL: http://www.ncbi.nlm.nih.gov/Omim/.

Orlic D, Girard LJ, Lee D, Anderson SM, Puck JM, Bodine DM. Interleukin-7R alpha mRNA expression increases as stem cells differentiate into T and B lymphocyte progenitors. Exp Hematol 25:217–222, 1997.

Pandey A, Ozaki K, Baumann H, Levin SD, Puel A, Farr AG, Ziegler SF, Leonard WJ, Lodish HF. Cloning of a receptor subunit required for signaling by thymic stromal lymphopoietin. Nat Immunol 1:59–64, 2000.

Park LS, Martin U, Garka K, Gliniak B, DiSanto JP, Muller W, Largaespada DA, Copeland NG, Jenkins NA, Farr AG, Ziegler SF, Morrissey PJ, Paxton R, Sims JE. Cloning of the murine thymic stromal lymphopoietin (TSLP) receptor: formation of a functional heteromeric complex requires interleukin 7 receptor. J Exp Med 192:659–670, 2000.

Park SJ, Saijo K, Takahashi TMO, Arase H, Hirayama N, Miyake K, Nakauchi H, Shirasawa T, Saito T. Developmental defects of lymphoid cells in JAK3 kinase-deficient mice. Immunity 3:771–782, 1995.

Pernis A, Gupta S, Yopp J, Garfein E, Kashleva H, Schindler C, Rothman P. Gamma chain-associated cytokine receptors signal through distinct transducing factors. J Biol Chem 270:14517–14522, 1995.

Perumal NB, Kenniston TW Jr, Tweardy DJ, Dyer KF, Hoffman R, Peschon J, Appasamy PM. TCR-gamma genes are rearranged but not transcribed in IL-7R alpha–deficient mice. J Immunol 158:5744–5750, 1997.

Peschon JJ, Morrissey PJ, Grabstein KH, Ramsdell FJ, Maraskovsky E, Gliniak BC, Park LS, Ziegler SF, Williams DE, Ware CB. Early lymphocyte expansion is severely impaired in interleukin 7 receptor-deficient mice. J Exp Med 180:1955, 1994.

Puck JM, Deschenes SM, Porter JC, Dutra AS, Brown CJ, Willard HF, Henthorn PS. The interleukin-2 receptor gamma chain maps to Xq13.1 and is mutated in X-linked severe combined immunodeficiency, SCIDX1. Hum Mol Genet 2:1099–1104, 1993.

Puel A, Ziegler SF, Buckley RH, Leonard WJ. Defective IL7R expression in T(–)B(+)NK(+) severe combined immunodeficiency. Nat Genet 20:394–397, 1998.

Reche PA, Soumelis V, Gorman DM, Clifford T, Liu M, Travis M, Zurawski SM, Johnston J, Liu YJ, Spits H, de Waal Malefyt R, Kastelein RA, Bazan JF. Human thymic stromal lymphopoietin preferentially stimulates myeloid cells. J Immunol 167:336–343, 2001.

Riedy MC, Dutra AS, Blake TB, Modi W, Lal BK, Davis J, Bosse A, O'Shea JJ, Johnston JA. Genomic sequence, organization and chromosomal organization of human Jak3. Genomics 37:57, 1996.

Roberts JL, Lengi A, Brown SM, Chen M, Zhou YJ, O'Shea JJ, Buckley RH. Janus kinase 3 (JAK3) deficiency: clinical, immunologic, and molecular analyses of 10 patients and outcomes of stem cell transplantation. Blood 103:2009–2018, 2004.

Roifman CM, Zhang J, Chitayat D, Sharfe N. A partial deficiency of interleukin-7R alpha is sufficient to abrogate T-cell development and cause severe combined immunodeficiency. Blood 96:2803–2807, 2000.

Rosenfeld RG, Kofoed E, Little B, Woods K, Buckway C, Pratt K, Hwa V. Growth hormone insensitivity resulting from post-GH receptor defects. Growth Horm IGF Res 14(Suppl A):S35–38, 2004.

Russell SM, Johnston JA, Noguchi M, Kawamura M, Bacon CM, Friedmann M, Berg M, McVicar DW, Witthuhn BA, Silvennoinen O, Goldman AS, Schmalstieg FC, Ihle JN, O'Shea JJ, Leonard WJ. Interaction of IL-2R beta and gamma c chains with Jak1 and Jak3: implications for XSCID and XCID. Science 266:1042–1045, 1994.

Russell SM, Tayebi N, Nakajima H, Riedy MC, Roberts JL, Aman MJ, Migone TS, Noguchi M, Markert ML, Buckley RH, O'Shea JJ, Leonard WJ. Mutation of Jak3 in a patient with SCID: essential role of Jak3 in lymphoid development. Science 270:797–800, 1995.

Saijo K, Park SY, Ishida Y, Arase H, Saito T. Crucial role of Jak3 in negative selection of self-reactive T cells. J Exp Med 185:351–356, 1997.

Schluns KS, Williams K, Ma A, Zheng XX, Lefrancois L. Cutting edge: requirement for IL-15 in the generation of primary and memory antigen-specific CD8 T cells. J Immunol 168:4827–4831, 2002.

Schmalstieg FC, Leonard WJ, Noguchi M, Berg M, Rudloff HE, Denney RM, Dave SK, Brooks EG, Goldman AS. Missense mutation in exon 7 of the common gamma chain gene causes a moderate form of X-linked combined immunodeficiency. J Clin Invest 95:1169–1173, 1995.

Schumacher RF, Mella P, Badolato R, Fiorini M, Savoldi G, Giliani S, Villa A, Candotti F, Tampalini A, O'Shea JJ, Notarangelo LD. Complete genomic organization of the human JAK3 gene and mutation analysis in severe combined immunodeficiency by single-strand conformation polymorphism. Hum Genet 106:73–79, 2000.

Schumacher RF, Mella P, Lalatta F, Fiorini M, Giliani S, Villa A, Candotti F, Notarangelo LD. Prenatal diagnosis of JAK3 deficient SCID. Prenat Diagn 19:653–656, 1999.

Sharfe N, Dadi HK, Roifman CM. JAK3 protein tyrosine kinase mediates interleukin-7-induced activation of phosphatidylinositol-3' kinase. Blood 86:2077–2085, 1995.

Shevach EM. Regulatory T cells in autoimmunity. Annu Rev Immunol 18:423–449, 2000.

Shevach EM, McHugh RS, Thornton AM, Piccirillo C, Natarajan K, Margulies DH. Control of autoimmunity by regulatory T cells. Adv Exp Med Biol 490:21–32, 2001.

Shimoda K, van Deursen J, Sangster MY, Sarawar SR, Carson RT, Tripp RA, Chu C, Quelle FW, Nosaka T, Vignali DA, Doherty PC, Grosveld G, Paul WE, Ihle JN. Lack of IL-4-induced Th2 response and IgE class switching in mice with disrupted Stat6 gene. Nature 380:630–633, 1996.

Soumelis V, Reche PA, Kanzler H, Yuan W, Edward G, Homey B, Gilliet M, Ho S, Antonenko S, Lauerma A, Smith K, Gorman D, Zurawski S, Abrams J, Menon S, McClanahan T, de Waal-Malefyt Rd R, Bazan F, Kastelein RA, Liu YJ. Human epithelial cells trigger dendritic cell mediated allergic inflammation by producing TSLP. Nat Immunol 3:673–680, 2002.

South MA, Montgomery JR, Richie E, Mukhopadhyay N, Criwell BS, Mackler BF, De Fazio SR, Bealmear P, Helm TR, Trentin JJ, Dressman

GR, O'Neill P. A special report: four-year study of a boy with combined immune deficiency maintained in strict reverse isolation from birth. IV. Immunological studies. Pediatr Res 11:71–78, 1977.

Starr R, Willson TA, Viney EM, Murray LJ, Rayner JR, Jenkins BJ, Gonda TJ, Alexander WS, Metcalf D, Nicola NA, Hilton DJ. A family of cytokine-inducible inhibitors of signalling. Nature 387:917–921, 1997.

Stephan JL, Vlekova V, Le Deist F, Blanche S, Donadieu J, De Saint-Basile G, Durandy A, Griscelli C, Fischer A. Severe combined immunodeficiency: a retrospective single-center study of clinical presentation and outcome in 117 patients. J Pediatr 123:564–572, 1993.

Sudo T, Nishikawa S, Ohno N, Akiyama N, Tamakoshi M, Yoshida H. Expression and function of the interleukin 7 receptor in murine lymphocytes. Proc Natl Acad Sci USA 90:9125–9129, 1993.

Sugamura K, Asao H, Kondo M, Tanaka N, Ishii N, Ohbo K, Nakamura M, Takeshita T. The interleukin 2 receptor gamma chain. Its role in the multiple cytokine receptor comlexes and T cell development in XSCID. Annu Rev Immunol 14:179–205, 1996.

Sun XJ, Wang LM, Zhang Y, Yenush L, Myers MG Jr, Glasheen E, Lane WS, Pierce JH, White MF. Role of IRS-2 in insulin and cytokine signalling. Nature 377:173–177, 1995.

Suzuki H, Kundig TM, Furlonger C, Wakeham A, Timms E, Matsuyama T, Schmits R, Simard JJ, Ohashi PS, Griesser H, et al. Deregulated T cell activation and autoimmunity in mice lacking interleukin-2 receptor beta. Science 268:1472–1476, 1995.

Takeda K, Tanaka T, Shi W, Matsumoto M, Minami M, Kashiwamura S, Nakanishi K, Yoshida N, Kishimoto T, Akira S. Essential role of Stat6 in IL-4 signalling. Nature 380:627–630, 1996.

Taniguchi T. Cytokine signaling through nonreceptor protein tyrosine kinases. Science 268:251–255, 1995.

Taniguchi T, Minami Y. The IL-2/IL-2 receptor system: a current overview. Cell 73:5–8, 1993.

Tanner JW, Chen W, Young RL, Longmore GD, Shaw AS. The conserved box 1 motif of cytokine receptors is required for association with JAK kinases. J Biol Chem 270:6523–6530, 1995.

Teglund S, McKay C, Schuetz E, van Deursen JM, Stravopodis D, Wang D, Brown M, Bodner S, Grosveld G, Ihle JN. Stat5a and Stat5b proteins have essential and nonessential, or redundant, roles in cytokine responses. Cell 93:841–850, 1998.

Thomis DC, Berg LJ. Peripheral expression of Jak3 is required to maintain T lymphocyte function. J Exp Med 185:197–206, 1997.

Thomis DC, Gurniak CB, Tivol E, Sharpe AH, Berg LJ. Defects in B lymphocyte maturation and T lymphocyte activation in mice lacking Jak3. Science 270:794–797, 1995.

Tortolani PJ, Lal BK, Riva A, Johnston JA, Chen YQ, Reaman GH, Beckwith M, Longo D, Ortaldo JR, Bhatia K, et al. Regulation of JAK3 expression and activation in human B cells and B cell malignancies. J Immunol 155:5220–5226, 1995.

Udy GB, Towers RP, Snell RG, Wilkins RJ, Park SH, Ram PA, Waxman DJ, Davey HW. Requirement of STAT5b for sexual dimorphism of body growth rates and liver gene expression. Proc Natl Acad Sci USA 94:7239–7244, 1997.

van Leeuwen JE, van Tol MJ, Joosten AM, Schellekens PT, van den Bergh RL, Waaijer JL, Oudeman-Gruber NJ, van der Weijden-Ragas CP, Roos MT, Gerritsen EJ, van den Berg H, Haraldsson A, Meera Kahn P, Vossen JM. Relationship between patterns of engraftment in peripheral blood and immune reconstitution after allogeneic bone marrow transplantation for (severe) combined immunodeficiency. Blood 84:3936–3947, 1994.

van Oers NS, Killeen N, Weiss A. Lck regulates the tyrosine phosphorylation of the T cell receptor subunits and ZAP-70 in murine thymocytes. J Exp Med 183:1053–1062, 1996.

Vannier E, Miller LC, Dinarello CA. Coordinated antiinflammatory effects of interleukin 4: interleukin 4 suppresses interleukin 1 production but upregulates gene expression and synthesis of interleukin 1 receptor antagonist. Proc Natl Acad Sci USA 89:4076–4080, 1992.

Villa A, Sironi M, Macchi P, Matteucci C, Notarangelo LD, Vezzoni P, Mantovani A. Monocyte function in a severe combined immunodeficient patient with a donor splice site mutation in the JAK3 gene. Blood 88:817–823, 1996.

von Freeden-Jeffry U, Vieira P, Lucian L, McNeil T, Burdach S, Murray R. Lymphopenia in interleukin (IL)-7 gene deleted mice identifies IL-7 as a nonredundant cytokine. J Exp Med 181:1519, 1995.

Watling D, Guschin D, Muller M, Silvennoinen O, Witthuhn BA, Quelle FW, Rogers NC, Schindler C, Stark GR, Ihle JN, et al. Complementation by the protein tyrosine kinase JAK2 of a mutant cell line defective in the interferon-gamma signal transduction pathway. Nature 366:166–170, 1993.

Welham MJ, Duronio V, Schrader JW. Interleukin-4-dependent proliferation dissociates p44erk-1, p42erk-2, and p21ras activation from cell growth. J Biol Chem 269:5865–5873, 1994.

Wengler GS, Allen RC, Parolini O, Smith H, Conley ME. Nonrandom X chromosome inactivation in natural killer cells from obligate carriers of X-linked severe combined immunodeficiency. J Immunol 150:700–704, 1993.

White MF, Kahn CR. The insulin signaling system. J Biol Chem 269:1–4, 1994.

Wijnaendts L, Le Deist F, Griscelli C, Fischer A. Development of immunologic functions after bone marrow transplantation in 33 patients with severe combined immunodeficiency. Blood 74:2212–2219, 1989.

Wilks AF. Two putative protein-tyrosine kinases identified by application of the polymerase chain reaction. Proc Natl Acad Sci USA 86:1603–1607, 1989.

Witthuhn BA, Silvennoinen O, Miura O, Lai KS, Cwik C, Liu ET, Ihle JN. Involvement of the Jak-3 Janus kinase in signalling by interleukins 2 and 4 in lymphoid and myeloid cells. Nature 370:153–157, 1994.

Yin T, Keller SR, Quelle FW, Witthuhn BA, Tsang ML, Lienhard GE, Ihle JN, Yang YC. Interleukin-9 induces tyrosine phosphorylation of insulin receptor substrate-1 via JAK tyrosine kinases. J Biol Chem 270: 20497–20502, 1995a.

Yin T, Yang L, Yang YC. Tyrosine phosphorylation and activation of JAK family tyrosine kinases by interleukin-9 in MO7E cells. Blood 85: 3101–3106, 1995b.

Yoshimura A, Ohkubo T, Kiguchi T, Jenkins NA, Gilbert DJ, Copeland NG, Hara T, Miyajima A. A novel cytokine-inducible gene CIS encodes an SH2-containing protein that binds to tyrosine-phosphorylated interleukin 3 and erythropoietin receptors. EMBO J 14:2816–2826, 1995.

You M, Yu DH, Feng GS. Shp-2 tyrosine phosphatase functions as a negative regulator of the interferon-stimulated Jak/STAT pathway. Mol Cell Biol 19:2416–2424, 1999.

Zhou YJ, Chen M, Cusack NA, Kimmel LH, Magnuson KS, Boyd JG, Lin W, Roberts JL, Lengi A, Buckley RH, Geahlen RL, Candotti F, Gadina M, Changelian PS, O'Shea JJ. Unexpected effects of FERM domain mutations on catalytic activity of Jak3: structural implication for Janus kinases. Mol Cell 8:959–969, 2001.

11

V(D)J Recombination Defects

JEAN-PIERRE DE VILLARTAY, KLAUS SCHWARZ, and ANNA VILLA

The vertebrate cognate immune system recognizes and responds to a virtually infinite number of foreign antigens via antigen-specific immunoglobulin (Ig) or T cell receptor (TCR) molecules expressed on the cell surface of B and T lymphocytes, respectively. While the Ig receptor of B cells binds to soluble antigens, the TCR receptor recognizes peptide antigens presented by human leukocyte antigen (HLA) molecules. In general, allelic exclusion prevents expression by a single lymphocyte of two different receptors encoded by homologous alleles. The expression of each distinct receptor is maintained in the clonal progeny of a lymphocyte.

V(D)J Recombination

Immunoglobulin and TCR chains consist of two structural domains: the constant regions mediate effector functions, while the variable part of the receptor chains forms the antigen-binding pocket. A site-specific recombination event (VDJ recombination) leads to generation of the variable domains of mature antigen receptor genes from a set of subgenic segments classified as variable (V), diversity (D), and joining (J) elements (for review see Schlissel and Stanhope-Baker, 1997; Nemazee 2000). In principle, each of the V elements can join to any of the D and J modules, thus a finite number of subgenes can establish the enormous antigen receptor diversity.

Seven gene loci encoding the Ig heavy (IgH) and light chains as well as the TCR α, β, γ, and δ chains can potentially undergo somatic DNA recombination during lymphocyte development. The loci share a similar conserved overall organization (Color Plate 11.IA); however, the precise number of subgenic segments and their organization vary between different loci and species (Litman et al., 1993).

The principle of V(D)J recombination is a simple cut-and-paste mechanism, fusing in each step two subgenic DNA segments (Color Plate 11.IB) (Lewis, 1994). This reaction is based on a universal tag for all V, (D), and J modules. These gene segments are flanked by recombination signal sequences (RSS) (Color Plate 11.IA), which consist of a conserved heptamer and an AT-rich nonamer nucleotide motif, separated by a 12 ± 1 bp or 23 ± 1 bp spacer (Ramsden et al., 1994). Spacer length, therefore, defines two types of RSSs, termed 12-RSS and 23-RSS, and efficient recombination occurs only between a 12-RSS and a 23-RSS, a restriction called the *12/23 rule*. Additional regulatory effects of RSS sequence on recombination have been recently described (Bassing et al., 2000).

The V(D)J recombination reaction can be divided into two main steps involving several different subreactions (Table 11.1). The first part of the recombination process is lymphocyte-specific and results through an endonucleolytic cut in DNA double-strand breaks (DSB) at the border between the RSS heptamer and the flanking coding segment. In vivo, in a single V(D)J recombination reaction, four DNA ends are generated simultaneously through the synchronous cut at two distinct gene segments: two blunt, phosphorylated signal ends and two hairpin-sealed coding ends. The second part of the V(D)J rearrangement involves the processing of the signal and coding ends, in which, ultimately, factors of a ubiquitous DNA double-strand repair pathway are recruited to link the signal and coding ends.

The standard products of V(D)J recombination result from ligation of the two coding elements (coding joints) and of the two heptamers of the RSS (signal joints). Depending on the orientation of the two RSSs to each other, the rearrangement process leads to a DNA deletion or inversion (Color Plate 11.IC). Most rearrangement events stem from a deletion of the DNA connecting the recombined V(D)J elements and produce an extrachromosomal DNA circle with a signal joint (Fujimoto and Yamagishi, 1987; Okazaki et al., 1987). At the TCRβ, TCRδ, and

153

Table 11.1. Mechanistic Steps in V(D)J Recombination and Proteins Involved*

Steps	Proteins
Lymphocytes-Specific Steps	
1. Locus accessibility	?
2. RSS recognition and nicking	RAG1 + RAG2
3. Synapsis of RSS	RAG1 + RAG2 + ?
4. Hairpin formation	RAG1 + RAG2
General DNA Double-Strand Break Repair Steps	
5. Hairpin opening	RAG1 + RAG2 and Artemis
6. Modification of coding ends	TdT + exonuclease(s)?
7. Recognition of DNA double strand	
Disassembly of synaptic complex	DNA-PKcs + Artemis
8. Ligation	XRCC4 + ligase IV

RSS, recombination signal sequence; TdT, terminal deoxynucleotidyl transferase.
*Alternative models suggest that steps 2 and 3 are interchangeable and that step 7 may precede steps 5 and 6.

Table 11.2. Constinents of the Recombinase Machinery

	Human Gene Locus	Human Disease	Animal Model	Cell Lines
RAG1	11p13	SCID	KO mouse	AMuLV-transformed pre-B cells
RAG2	11p13	SCID	KO mouse	AMuLV-transformed pre-B cells
TdT	10q23–24	—	KO mouse	—
Ku80	2q33–35	—	KO mouse	XRCC5 cells (xrs5, 6, XR-V9B, XR-V15B, sxi-1, -2, -3, etc.)
Ku70	22q13	—	KO mouse	XRCC6
DNA-PKcs	8q11	—	Murine *scid*	XRCC7 Equine *scid*
XRCC4	5q13	—	KO mouse	XRCC4
Ligase IV	13q33–34	Leaky SCID	KO mouse	Human fibroblast
Artemis	10p13	RS-SCID	KO mouse	Human fibroblast

AMuLV, Abelson murine leukemia virus; DNA-PKcs, DNA-protein kinase–dependent catalytic subunit; KO, knockout.

Igα loci, inversions have been noticed (Feddersen and van Ness, 1985; Malissen et al., 1986; Korman et al., 1989), with a slight preference of deletions over inversions (Hesse et al., 1987).

V(D)J recombination can result in alternative products such as "hybrid" or "open-and-shut" junctions (Plate 11.IC). *Hybrid joints* arise through the ligation of one coding end to the signal end of the other. In an *open-and-shut joint*, which is less common, the signal and coding ends created by site-specific cleavage are modified prior to their religation (Lewis, 1994). These alternative products are rare events, but they obey the rules of V(D)J recombination and are indicative of the notion that four open DNA ends are intermediates in the rearrangement process.

The signal ends are usually ligated without modification of the DNA (Lieber et al., 1988). In contrast, joining of coding ends is generally imprecise, with base losses and/or additions (N and P nucleotides) of approximately 10 to 15 nucleotides. This process helps to diversify the receptor repertoire but includes the risk of creating nonfunctional genes because of out-of-frame joining and/or introduction of premature stop codons. The enzyme terminal deoxynucleotidyl transferase (TdT) adds random, GC-enriched nucleotides (N nucleotides) to coding ends by a template-independent polymerization. P nucleotides represent short, palindromic repeats of coding end DNA. They are thought to be generated when the "hairpin," a coding end intermediate of the V(D)J recombination reaction (Color Plate 11.II), is resolved through an endonucleolytic attack, not at the tip of the covalently closed termini but within the coding element. Other mechanisms contributing to junctional diversity are erosion of a small and variable number of bases at coding ends by exo- or endonucleases, and homology joining through short-sequence homologies at free DNA ends (for review see Fugmann et al., 2000).

The "recombinase" machinery, a multiprotein complex, is responsible for the V(D)J recombination. At present, it is unclear if all of the recombinase constituents interact physically at a single time point or if single functions of the machinery follow each other in an ordered fashion. Nine proteins have been identified thus far as participating in the various phases of the V(D)J recombination reaction (Table 11.1). The recombination activating genes 1 and 2 (*RAG1* and *RAG2*) are necessary and sufficient to initiate V(D)J recombination on an accessible antigen receptor gene locus (McBlane et al., 1996). The second phase of this reaction requires Artemis in addition to *RAG1/RAG2* for the process

of the coding end intermediates. The template-independent DNA polymerase TdT adds N nucleotides and contributes substantially to receptor diversity. The DNA-dependent protein kinase (DNA-PK), with its DNA binding constituents KU70 and KU80 and its catalytic subunit DNA-PKcs, recognizes open DNA ends. *XRCC4* (the gene responsible for the defect present in cells of group 4 of X-ray cross-complementing cell lines) seems to interact with ligase IV in the ligation step of DNA DSB repair. Despite the recent cloning of Artemis, many different factors of the recombinase machinery (*trans*-acting factors for locus accessibility and exo- and endonucleases) are still unknown. Of the identified factors, only the *RAG1*, *RAG2*, ligase IV, and Artemis genes have been implicated in an inborn immunodeficiency (Table 11.2) (Schwarz et al., 1996; Villa et al., 1998; Corneo et al., 2000; Moshous et al., 2001; O'Driscoll et al., 2001). Lastly, a human severe combined immunodeficiency (SCID) condition with V(D)J recombination deficiency caused by an undescribed gene has recently been reported (Dai et al., 2003).

Complete *RAG1* and *RAG2* Deficieny (B⁻T⁻ SCID)

History

Siblings with diarrhea, candidiasis, lymphopenia, and diminished lymphoid tissue were first described by Glanzman and Riniker (1950). Thymic dysplasia and hypogammaglobulinemia were subsequently analyzed in new cases (Cottier, 1958; Hitzig et al., 1958). Knowledge of the antigen receptor gene structures and their processing allowed the definition of recombinase defective patients (Schwarz et al., 1991; Abe et al., 1994). A subgroup of patients with defective V(D)J recombination exhibited *RAG1/2* mutations (Schwarz et al., 1996).

Definition

The functional failure of one of the constituents of the V(D)J recombinase machinery, such as RAG1 or RAG2, results in a SCID without B and T cells (B⁻T⁻ SCID), MIM (Mendelian Inheritance in Man) numbers 179615 and 179616, respectively.

Clinical Manifestation

Severe combined immunodeficiency has an estimated incidence of approximately 1 per 100,000 live births (Stephan et al., 1993). In the original report, six patients of 30 SCID cases analyzed exhibited a RAG1/2 defect, thus the RAG deficiency may account for a substantial proportion of human SCID cases (Schwarz et al., 1996). In a recent large series about 20% of SCID cases were RAG-dependent (Villa et al., 2001).

The clinical presentation is relatively uniform. As a rule, no symptoms are detected during pregnancy or birth or within the first few weeks of life. In most cases, the symptoms start within the second or third month after birth. Infectious complications are the hallmark of the disease, with a high preponderance of opportunistic infections (e.g., *Pneumocystis carinii* infection). The clinical signs are characterized by chronic, persistent disease of the airways, recurrent acute pneumonia, therapy-resistant mucocutaneous candidiasis, eczematous dermatitis, and local as well as systemic bacterial infections (otitis, mastoiditis, purulent rhinitis and conjunctivitis, septic disease, meningitis, arthritis, and local abscesses). The recurrent infections in addition to chronic enteritis lead to therapy-resistant growth failure. Furthermore, intracellular parasites (*Listeria, Legionella*) as well as viruses (Epstein-Barr virus [EBV] and cytomegalovirus [CMV]) may cause lethal complications.

Noninfectious clinical manifestations may result from graft-vs.-host disease (GVHD). Because of the immunodeficiency, patients cannot reject allogeneic cells. Allogeneic cells are introduced into patients either through maternofetal transfusion or as supportive, nonirradiated blood products. While GVHD due to maternal lymphocytes is usually relatively mild with erythrodermia, eosinophila, enteritis, and hepatitis, GVHD following transfusion is frequently lethal. Vaccination with living organisms such as application of the bacillus Calmette-Guerin (BCG) strain may cause fatal consequences. All SCID children die within a few months if they are not provided with hematopoietic stem cells.

Physical examination of completely RAG-deficient patients reveals unusual infections and a characteristic absence of lymphatic organs. In most cases cervical lymph nodes and tonsils are undetectable.

Laboratory Findings

Patients exhibit no B and T cells of their own in the peripheral blood (B⁻T⁻ SCID) (Table 11.3). Maternal T lymphocytes have been detectable in more than 50 cases and functional natural killer (NK) cells are present. After loss of the initially present maternally transfused immunoglobulins, no antibodies circulate in the peripheral blood of *RAG*-deficient patients. In vivo and in vitro functional lymphocyte tests are not informative because of the lack of the respective cells.

The RAG1 and RAG2 deficiency is an autosomal recessive disease. Both genes are located on chromosome 11p13 (Oettinger et al., 1992; Schwarz et al., 1994). Carriers of the mutant genes are healthy without any immunologic disturbances and are therefore only detected through molecular identification of the mutation in question. A B⁻T⁻ SCID immunophenotype in umbilical cord blood may suggest, among others, a *RAG* defect that must be confirmed by molecular analysis.

Table 11.3. Laboratory Findings in Peripheral Blood of Recombination-Deficient Patients

	RAG-SCID	Omenn Syndrome	Artemis RS-SCID
B cells	−	−	−
T cells	−ᵃ*	+ (oligoclonal)	−
NK cells	+	+	+
Immunoglobulin	−	− (or low)	−
Function (in vivo and in vitro)			
B cells	NA	− very low	NA
T cells	NA	− (or low)	NA
NK cells	+	+	+
Radiosensitivity	−	−	+

NA, not applicable; NK, natural killer.

*After exclusion of maternally transfused T cells, which can be detected in more than 50% of the cases.

RAG Gene Structure and Function

The murine *Rag1* and *Rag2* genes were initially identified and cloned on the basis of their ability to rearrange an integrated artificial recombination substrate in a cell line (Schatz et al., 1989; Oettinger et al., 1990). The two complementing genes show a unique organization. Their 3′ ends face each other and are separated in human DNA by 15–18 kb. The coding sequences and the 3′ untranslated region (UTR) of both genes are located on one exon (Ichihara et al., 1992). *RAG1* possesses one extra 5′ UTR exon, whereas in the *RAG2* locus at least two 5′ UTR exons have been identified (Lauring and Schlissel, 1985). The amino acid sequence and the overall genomic organization are highly conserved throughout evolution from zebrafish to humans (Bernstein et al., 1994; Wienholds et al., 2002). No homologues have been found in lower organisms. The human *RAG1* gene codes for 1403 amino acids; the *RAG2* gene, for 527 amino acids.

RAG1 and RAG2 protein sequences are not related to each other. A sequence comparison of RAG1 with other proteins shows that RAG1 possesses five basic regions that are necessary for nuclear localization (binding sites for nuclear protein SRP1 and RCH1), a region with homology to bacterial invertases and homeodomain proteins, zinc finger domains, and a zinc binding dimerization motif (Color Plate 11.III) (Silver et al., 1993; Difilippantonio et al., 1996; Rodgers et al., 1996; Spanopoulou et al., 1996). More recently, extensive mutagenesis of acidic amino acids in RAG1 identified three catalytic residues (D600, D708, and E962, DDE motif) critical for both nicking and hairpin formation (Landree et al., 1999); two of these (D600 and D708) coordinate catalytic divalent metal ions (Kim et al., 1999; Landree et al., 1999; Fugmann et al., 2000b). These residues are located in a region that displays marked conservation in predicted secondary structure with the catalytic cores of other transposases (Fugmann et al., 2000b). Further insight into RAG1 activities has been derived from mutants blocking the hairpin formation, which are all in the vicinity of D600 (Kale et al., 2001). Recent studies have demonstrated that two regions of RAG1, the nonamer binding domain and the carboxy-terminal domain, contact DNA containing the coding flank at the cleavage site (Mo et al., 2001).

The molecular roles of RAG2 in V(D)J recombination are less known. The presence of RAG2 is required for all catalytic steps and helps to form the RAGRSS complex. Secondary structure prediction and mutagenesis studies have suggested that

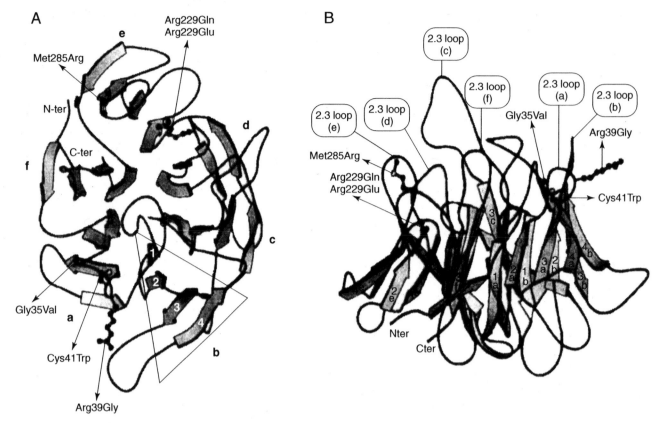

Figure 11.1. (A) Beta-propeller structure of RAG2. Each blade of the propeller consists of a four-stranded beta sheet. (B) Beta-propeller structure viewed along the perpendicular axis. Mutated amino acids are indicated.

RAG2 adopts a six-bladed β-propeller fold (Fig. 11.1) (Callebaut and Mornon, 1998; Corneo et al., 2000; Gomez et al., 2000), a structural motif found in many proteins of diverse function (Adams et al., 2000). Biochemical analysis of the recombinant RAG2 proteins has allowed the identification of a number of basic residues mutants defective in catalysis in vitro and V(D)J recombination in vivo, supporting the direct involvement of RAG2 in DNA binding during all steps of the cleavage reaction. According to these experiments, Schatz proposed a model for the interaction of RAG2 with DNA in which two amino acids (K119 and K283) directly contact DNA (Fugmann and Schatz, 2001). The C-terminal region of RAG2 (from aa 417 to 484) shows homology with the plant homology domain (PHD), a motif that has been identified in chromatin remodeling proteins. In line with a potential role in chromatin remodeling, this region has been implicated in facilitating the ordered rearrangement of IgH chains (Kirch et al., 1998) and in binding to the core histone proteins (West et al., 2005).

Another role of *RAG* genes is the ability to catalyze in vitro transpositional insertion which suggests that this process could be a source of genomic instability in vivo (Agrawal et al., 1998; Hiom et al., 1998). Recent work has shown that RAG transposase forms productive complexes with target DNA both before and after RSS cleavage and, these show a preference for transposition into nearby targets, such as Ig and TCR loci. This could bias transposition toward relatively safe regions in the genome (Neiditch et al., 2001). In addition, the transposition events are stimulated and targeted by the presence of distorted DNA structures such as hairpins (Lee et al., 2002). Because there are no evidence that RAG-mediated transposition occurs in vivo, it is

likely that regulatory mechanisms could limit the frequency of transposition events in lymphocytes. During lymphocyte development in adults, the *RAG* genes are convergently transcribed in thymic and bone marrow cells with a capability for V(D)J recombination (Schatz et al., 1989; Oettinger et al., 1990; Turka et al., 1991). Mature RAG proteins are localized to the nucleus (Silver et al., 1993; Leu and Schatz, 1995). In developing thymocytes, RAG expression is first detected in committed T cell precursors that are double negative (DN), whereas the first B cells expressing RAG1 and RAG2 are AA.4.1[+]HSA[−]B220[+]CD4[+] CD43[+] even at very low levels. The RAG expression increases as B cells mature. Following the proliferative expansion of pre-B and pre-T cells, a second wave of RAG expression is initiated in CD25[+] pre-BII cells and CD4[+] and CD8[+] (DP)T cells. This second expression has been shown to be regulated by elements at the 5′ end of RAG2 promoter (Yu et al., 1999). RAGs are not expressed in mature T cells. Immunohistochemical analysis detected RAG expression in germinal centers in the mouse (Han et al., 1996; Hikida et al., 1996); however, transgenic indicator and gene-targeted indicator lines have shown that the small number of cells expressing RAG are immature B cells (reviewed in Nagaoka et al., 2000).

The minimal promoter of RAG1 has been mapped (nucleotides 111 to 97 relative to the position of the major transcriptional start site) (Brown et al.,1997; Zarrin et al., 1997). The promoter exhibits neither the presence of an initiator motif nor a functional TATA box. Several potential recognition sites for the E2A-, Ikaros-, and ETS-family transcription factors are present within the RAG1 promoter. In addition, consensus PEPB2/CBF and Y-box/CCAAT sequence motifs are detectable.

Nuclear factor-Y (NF-Y) binds to the RAG1 Y-box motif. A mutation of the Y-box motif abolishes the binding of NF-Y transcription factor and significantly reduces RAG1 promoter activity (Brown et al., 1997). Through in vivo investigation with bacterial artificial chromosome transgenes containing a fluorescent indicator, the coordinate expression of RAG1 and RAG2 in B and T cells was found to be regulated by distinct genetic elements mapping on the 5′ side of the *RAG2* gene (Yu et al., 1999). Recently a new element, named Erag, which seems to have a role in RAG transcription in B cells, has been identified (Hsu et al., 2003).

Mutation Analysis

Mutagenesis experiments have defined core regions for RAG1 and RAG2 that are necessary and sufficient to recombine extrachromosomal V(D)J recombination substrates. The RAG1 core spans from amino acids 392 to 1011, whereas the RAG2 core extends from amino acids 1 to 382 (Sadofsky et al., 1993, 1994; Silver et al., 1993; Cuomo and Oettinger, 1994). Mutation analysis through single-strand conformation polymorphism (SSCP) assays in 14 T⁻B⁻ SCID patients detected six SCID cases with RAG defects (Table 11.4) (Schwarz et al., 1996). After sequencing the respective *RAG* genes, five missense and three nonsense mutations and one deletional mutation were detected (Table 11.4). All of the mutations were inherited. All human RAG1 substitutional mutations map to phylogenetically conserved residues within the RAG1 core region, whereas the Cys (478)-to-Tyr mutation of RAG2 is located outside the RAG2 core region. No functionally relevant RAG mutation was detected in healthy subjects or B SCID patients. After the first description of T⁻B⁻ SCID cases, many other mutations have been detected in RAG1 and RAG2 (Corneo et al., 2000, 2001; Gomez et al., 2000; Villa et al., 2001). Mutation analysis of RAG1 and RAG2 (http://bioinf.uta.fi/RAG1base and http://bioinf.uta.fi/RAG2 base) indicates that most of them are null mutations (nonsense or frameshift). In addition, although some patients with classical

Table 11.4. Structure and Mutational Analysis of *RAG1* and *RAG2* Genes

Patient (gender)	Allele[†]	Mutation[‡]	Amino Acid Change
RAG1			
P1 (m)	m	G 2276 to A	Glu 722 Lys
	p	G 2432 to T	Glu 774 Stop
P2 (f)	m	T 2926 to G	Tyr 938 Stop
	p	T 2926 to G	Tyr 938 Stop
P3 (m)**	m	C 579 to T	Ala 156 Val
	p	del	—
P4 (m)	m	C 2801 to T	Arg 897 Stop
	p	G 1983 to A	Arg 624 His
RAG2			
P5 (f)	m	G 2634 to A	Cys 478 Tyr
and P6 (m)	p	G 2634 to A	Cys 478 Tyr
P3 (m)ᶜ	m	G 1887 to A	Arg 229 Gln
	p	del	—

RAG1 and *RAG2* Mutations in B⁻ SCID Patients.

[†]Maternal (m) or paternal (p) alleles.

[‡]Nucleotide numbering according to Schatz et al. (1989) for *RAG1* and according to Ichihara et al. (1992) for *RAG2*.

**The paternal deletion encompassed the total *RAG1* and *RAG2* genes.

T⁻B⁻SCID bear missense mutations, biochemical studies have shown that these amino acid changes completely abrogate recombination ability and therefore represent null alleles (Schwarz et al., 1996; Corneo et al., 2000; Gomez et al., 2000). In transient transfection assays with artificial extrachromosomal rearrangement substrates, the mutants derived from completely RAG-deficient SCID patients show only residual recombination values that are typically 0.1–1 of wild type for both coding and signal joint formation. Although the mutant RAGs result in a marked decrease in recombination efficiency, rare signal and coding joints occur that are qualitatively indistinguishable from wild type, indicating that the enzymatic machinery following the initial DNA DSB induced by the RAG protein is unaffected by these mutations.

Pre-B and pre-T cells do not survive during lymphocyte development if they do not obtain a survival signal from their respective pre-B and pre-T cell receptors. The heavy chain of the IgM molecule and the TCR chain are necessary constituents of the respective receptors. In case of a complete RAG deficiency, V(D)J recombination cannot be initiated; thus IgM and TCR chains are not synthesized and are not available for a pre-B or pre-T cell receptor. The precursor lymphocytes receive no survival signal and die, hence the alymphocytosis in patients with complete RAG1 and RAG2 deficiency.

Diagnosis

At present, no simple functional test exists to reveal a V(D)J recombinase defect in general or a specific RAG defect. Protein analysis is not a practical alternative because the relevant recombining cells are a minority within the bone marrow cell population or are amenable to analysis only after thymic biopsy. Thus, only a direct or indirect genetic analysis of the *RAG* genes on genomic DNA can be carried out in B⁻T⁻ SCID cases.

Treatment

Treatment of RAG-defective children consists of a combination of supportive measures (see Chapter 46) and curative therapy of bone marrow or peripheral stem cell transplantation (see Chapter 47). An HLA-identical donor is no longer a prerequisite for reconstitutive hematopoietic stem cell transplantation, since depletion of T cells from a nonidentical graft omits or greatly reduces the risk of GVHD. When indicated, patients may be transplanted without a prior conditioning regimen because their immunodeficiency renders a reduced frequency of graft rejection. Survival after transplantation procedures in the small RAG-deficient group is 65%. In utero bone marrow transplantation (BMT) has also been performed in selected patients (F. Porta, personal communication).

An alternative therapeutic approach is gene therapy (Cavazzano-Calvo et al., 2000; Fisher et al., 2002). Although there have been no studies of RAG gene therapy in humans, experiments of retrovirally mediated *Rag2* gene transfer in hematopoietic stem cells of Rag2 knockout mice showed good results, opening the door to clinical application (Yates et al., 2002).

Animal Models of RAG1/2 Deficiency

Mice with homozygous deletions of either *Rag1* or *Rag2* have been created by gene targeting (Mombaerts et al., 1992; Shinkai et al., 1992). Both mouse strains exhibit an identical phenotype to that of each other or that of human RAG-deficient patients. The animals cannot initiate V(D)J recombination, thus lacking B and T cells and their immunological functions. During lymphocyte development, RAG1- and RAG2-deficient thymocytes accumulate as quiescent cells with a heat-stable antigen (HSA)-positive, CD25, CD4, c-kit-low phenotype resembling normal cells just prior to functional TCR chain expression. B cell development is halted at the pre-B cell stage (Mombaerts et al., 1992; Shinkai et al., 1992; Diamond et al., 1997). Functional defects other than the immunological ones are not known in Rag-deficient mice. There is only one report in the literature showing that Rag1 knockout mice exhibiting increased locomotor activity and reduced levels of fearfulness (Cushman et al., 2003).

Recently, Rag2 mice were generated replacing the endogenous Rag2 locus with core Rag2, thus generating mice lacking the "dispensable" C-terminal domain. These mice display a reduction in the total number of B and T cells, reflecting impaired lymphocyte development at the progenitor stage associated with reduced chromosomal V(D)J recombination (Liang et al., 2002; Akamatsu et al., 2003). This finding demonstrates that the C-terminal domain, which is dispensable for V(D)J recombination in vitro, has relevant functions in vivo. This is also true for the "dispensable" Rag1 N-terminal domain (see below).

Partial *RAG1* and *RAG2* Deficiency (Omenn Syndrome)

Omenn syndrome (OS) is a rare disorder that has been an enigma for pediatricians and immunologists for a long time. First defined in 1965 (Omenn, 1965), OS is a rare autosomal recessive disease characterized by symptoms of SCID associated with other findings including erythrodermia, eosinophilla, hepatosplenomegaly, lymphadenopathy, and elevated serum IgE levels, suggesting a defect in the activation and/or regulation of T cell proliferation (MIM 267700). The identification of specific mutations of *RAG* genes in OS patients has now made it clear that the underlying defect of this particular syndrome affects the maturation of both T and B lymphocytes and that the activation of the T cell subset is secondary to a partially defective V(D)J recombination process (Villa et al., 1998). However, the occurrence of the same mutation responsible for partial V(D)J activity in patients with T⁻B⁻ SCID and those with OS raises the possibility that additional factors such as epigenetic factors are required for the development of the Omenn phenotype (Corneo et al., 2001; Villa et al., 2001).

Clinical and Pathological Manifestations

Patients with OS present with early-onset generalized erythrodermia (Color Plate 11.IV), lymphadenopathy, hepatosplenomegaly, fever, protracted diarrhea, and failure to thrive. Protein loss due to diarrhea and exudative erythrodermia often leads to generalized edema. The presence of a massive inflammatory infiltrate gives the skin a unique appearance and consistency (pachydermia). Alopecia is a frequent finding (Aleman et al., 2001).

Despite the presence of reactive lymph nodes and variable, often elevated, numbers of circulating T lymphocytes, OS patients are severely immunodeficient and thus highly susceptible to bacterial, viral, and fungal infections. Unless treated by BMT the disease is invariably fatal. Infections and severe malnutrition are the main causes of death (Gomez et al., 1995). Septicemia, often arising from skin infections, is common.

The clinical hallmarks of the disease (summarized in Table 11.5) are reminiscent of GVHD. Indeed, in some cases the

Table 11.5. Diagnosis of Omenn Syndrome: Clinical and Laboratory Hallmarks

Clinical Features

Early onset, generalized erythrodermia
Failure to thrive
Protracted diarrhea
Edema
Lymphadenopathy
Hepatosplenomegaly
Severe infections (pneumonia, sepsis)

Laboratory Features

Hypoproteinemia
Frequent anemia, thrombocytopenia
Remarkable eosinophilia (usually >1000/μl)
Very low IgG, IgA, and IgM, but usually increased IgE
Very low or absent circulating B cells
Variable (often elevated) number of activated (CD45R0⁺, DR⁺) circulating T cells
Very low in vitro proliferative responses to antigens, variable response to PHA
Low, IgM-restricted, antibody responses

occurrence of maternal T cell engraftment in infants with SCID may result in clinically overt GVHD and mimic OS (Pollack et al., 1982; Le Deist et al., 1987). Furthermore, transfusion of unirradiated blood products into SCID babies also results in severe GVHD that resembles OS (Anderson and Weinstein, 1990). Because of the similarities in clinical presentation, these cases are also referred to as Omenn-like syndrome. For a diagnosis of OS, it is therefore essential that, in addition to typical clinical and laboratory findings, maternal T cell engraftment and transfusion-associated GVHD be excluded. The similarity of OS to GVHD is further reinforced by the pathologic features of OS. Skin biopsies reveal lymphocytic infiltrates in the upper dermis, with occasional histiocytes and eosinophils (Dyke et al., 1991). Immunohistochemical analysis shows that the lymphocytic infiltrate is composed of activated (CD45RO, DR) T cells, many of which coexpress CD30, a surface molecule predominantly expressed by lymphocytes producing Th2-type cytokines (Chilosi et al., 1996b). The differential diagnosis of OS includes severe atopic dermatitis, GVHD, and histiocytosis X, known as Letterer Siwe syndrome (Aleman et al., 2001).

Lymph node enlargement, typically observed in OS, is in contrast to the paucity of peripheral lymphoid tissue usually detected in patients with combined immune deficiencies. However, the lymph node architecture is severely altered in OS, as shown by a lack of follicles, depletion of the normal lymphocytic population, and increased proportion of interdigitating reticulum cells and eosinophils (Omenn, 1965; Barth et al., 1972; Dyke et al., 1991; Martin et al., 1995). On the basis of these findings, the disease was originally also named *familial reticuloendotheliosis with eosinophilia* (Omenn, 1965), or *combined immunodeficiency and reticuloendotheliosis with eosinophilia* (Ochs et al., 1974). Immunohistochemistry indicates that the lymphocytic component in the lymph nodes is due to activated T cells (CD3, CD45RO, DR) that often coexpress CD30 and/or CD25 (Chilosi et al., 1996a, 1996b; Brugnoni et al., 1997). In contrast, staining for B cells is typically negative. The splenic white pulp, Peyer's patches, and lamina propria of the gut are also markedly depleted of lymphocytes. Severe abnormalities have also been reported in the thymus, which is profoundly hypoplastic, with a noticeable depletion of the lymphoid components and often lack of Hassal's bodies (Barth et al., 1972; Businco et al., 1987).

Laboratory Findings

As summarized in Table 11.5, the main laboratory findings in OS consist of eosinophilia, hypogammaglobulinemia with increased serum IgE, presence of activated circulating T lymphocytes, in contrast to the usual lack of peripheral blood B cells, and a poor in vitro proliferative response of T lymphocytes to specific antigens (with variable responses to mitogens). Additional laboratory findings include the frequent occurrence of anemia (and sometimes of thrombocytopenia) and of severe hypoproteinemia due to protein loss through the stools and the skin.

In contrast to most forms of combined immunodeficiency, the total number of circulating T cells is variable but often elevated (Table 11.3). Distribution of the main T cell subsets (i.e., CD4 vs. CD8) is frequently imbalanced (Karol et al., 1983; Le Deist et al., 1985; Businco et al., 1987; Brugnoni et al., 1997). In a few cases, circulating T cells that express the form of the T cell antigen receptor (TCR) predominate over TCR T cells (Brugnoni et al., 1997). An extreme example of the variability in T cell number in OS (which has offered a crucial clue to the definition of the molecular basis of the disease) is represented by a pedigree in which one patient had typical OS with an increased number of circulating T cells, whereas one of his younger brothers died with B⁻T⁻ SCID (de Saint Basile et al., 1991).

Many of the immunological hallmarks of the disease reflect the presence of activated T cells that are skewed to a Th2 phenotype. Similar to what has been observed in the skin and lymph nodes, circulating T cells coexpress activation markers (CD45R0, DR, CD25, CD95, CD30). These activated T cells secrete predominantly Th2-type cytokines (IL-4, IL-5) upon in vitro activation. Accordingly, serum levels of IL-4 and IL-5 are increased. In contrast, the in vitro production of IL-2 and IFN-γ is reduced, as are their serum levels (Schandene et al., 1993; Chilosi et al., 1996a; Brugnoni et al., 1997). The abnormal production of IL-4 and IL-5 is supposed to be responsible for the increased production of IgE and eosinophilia, respectively.

The serum levels of IgG, IgA, and IgM are markedly reduced, yet in vivo antibody production is severely but not completely impaired (Le Deist et al., 1985), as indicated by a measurable although low and IgM-restricted antibody response to immunization with bacteriophage x174 (Ochs et al., 1974). Hypogammaglobulinemia is partially due to protein loss but also reflects defective B cell differentiation, with a very low or absent number of circulating B cells. Because B lymphocytes are usually undetectable in the lymph nodes and the gut, it remains unknown where the IgE secretion occurs.

Although T lymphocytes are consistently present and show an activated phenotype, they are functionally defective, with reduced proliferative responses to antigens and occasionally to mitogens as well (Le Deist et al., 1985; Businco et al., 1987; Brugnoni et al., 1997; Harville et al., 1997). Contributing to this T cell defect is increased cell death through two distinct mechanisms. Reduced expression of antiapoptotic molecules (e.g., bcl-2) and poor production of IL-2 (a growth-promoting cytokine) have been observed (Schandene et al., 1993; Brugnoni et al., 1997), both contributing to increased programmed cell death. Furthermore, it has been shown that T lymphocytes from OS patients are highly susceptible to activation-induced cell death (AICD), particularly through CD95 signaling (Brugnoni

et al., 1997). This susceptibility to CD95-dependent AICD likely reflects chronic antigenic stimulation in vivo. The observation that occasionally patients with OS have an expansion of TCR, double-negative (CD4⁻CD8⁻) T cells (Wirt et al., 1989) could reflect an attempt to overcome chronic in vivo activation, similar to what has been reported in patients with autoimmune lymphoproliferative disease (CD95 deficiency). Oligoclonality of circulating T cells has been consistently described in OS (Wirt et al., 1989; de Saint Basile et al., 1991; Harville et al., 1997; Rieux-Laucat et al., 1998; Villa et al., 1998). Although the use of distinct variable (V) gene segments is not particularly biased, few clones are expanded within each population of T cells that express specific V genes, as demonstrated by sequence analysis showing sets of identical V(D)J sequences (Harville et al., 1997; Villa et al., 1998). It has been hypothesized that restriction of the TCR repertoire could arise in the periphery or in the thymus, leading to the inability to properly accomplish all the steps required for intrathymic maturation. By analyzing T cells from both thymus and peripheral blood from a deceased patient, it has been demonstrated that the TCRβ repertoire is already restricted in the thymus, although further selection occurs in the periphery (Signorini et al., 1999; Pirovano et al., 2003).

Mutation Analysis in Patients with Omenn Syndrome

Because of the rarity of the disorder, analysis of OS by positional cloning has not been possible; for a long time the search for the responsible gene has been elusive. For this reason, most investigators have relied on the candidate gene approach to try to identify the molecular defect of OS. This strategy is particularly useful in genetic diseases affecting the immune system, as much information has been gathered over the past years on the various steps in the differentiation of lymphoid cells and on the genes involved in this maturation process.

As mentioned above, the clinical picture of OS is atypical and there were few reasons to suspect that *RAG* mutations could be responsible for this disease. However, one hint came from descriptions of the occurrence of OS and SCID within members of the same family (de Saint Basile et al., 1991). The issue was also complicated by the similarities between OS and SCID with maternal engraftment. Nevertheless, the analysis of *RAG* genes showed mutations in typical OS patients (Villa et al., 1998, Corneo et al., 2001). To explain why a defect in the same genes can give rise to such different phenotypes, factors such as genetic background, modifier genes, and epigenetic events are often called into question. However, it is now clear that mutations in different domains of *RAG* genes can affect the protein structure to various extents, leading either to null alleles in which the gene is completely inactivated or to hypomorphic alleles retaining variable degrees of function. This phenomenon is not unprecedented: among immunodeficiency diseases, one of the best examples is the Wiskott-Aldrich syndrome (WAS), X-linked thrombocytopenia (XLT), and X-linked neutropenia. Once thought to be separate entities, these disorders are now known to have abnormalities in the same gene, the WASP gene (Derry et al., 1994; Villa et al., 1995, Devriendt et al., 2001).

Careful analysis of the OS mutations support the hypothesis that while SCID represents "null" RAG alleles, the OS phenotype is caused by hypomorphic RAG alleles that retain a partial V(D)J recombination activity. According to this view, OS is a "leaky" SCID, allowing some degree of maturation along the

T cell lineage to occur. In contrast to the mutations noted in T⁻B⁻ SCID patients, Omenn patients show predominantly missense mutations, with at least one missense mutation being present in every patient. This finding, together with the presence of oligoclonal cells in the periphery, led us to suggest that limited V(D)J recombination events occur in these patients. Biochemical assays analyzing the capacity to mediate full V(D)J recombination events, *SCC* formation, and the introduction of double-strand breaks reveal that the proteins containing missense mutations have a reduced but still detectable activity. Hence, in general, SCID patients have two entirely defective alleles, whereas OS patients have at least one allele that is partially functional and capable of establishing the restricted receptor repertoire seen in OS. The view of the Omenn and SCID phenotypes as being dependent on the severity of the genotypic lesion in *RAG* genes is supported by analysis of the 56 OS patients described thus far in the literature (Villa et al., 1998; Wada et al., 2000; Corneo et al., 2001; Kumaki et al., 2001; Villa et al., 2001; Noordzij et al., 2002). Particularly interesting is the description of Omenn cases with alleles carrying nucleotide deletions in the N-terminal domain (Noordzji, 2000; Santagata et al., 2000; see also below).

The biochemical analysis of both null and hypomorphic mutations in *RAG1* and *RAG2* have provided valuable insights into the biology of the RAG1/RAG2 recombinase. The importance of the NBD has been reinforced by the finding that over 30% of *RAG1* mutations identified in Omenn patients result in amino acid substitutions in the NBD, a region spanning only 4% of the molecule. Furthermore, three different substitutions have been identified in the GGRPR motif of RAG1 at position R396 (to C, H, and L) in multiple Omenn patients. This "hot-spot residue" corresponds to R393 of mouse Rag1, located in a region that had previously been identified by homology to the Hin homeodomain and that, if mutated to R393L, retains 30% of wild-type activity. In addition, the capacity of Rag1 to form broad contacts outside of the nonamer is indirectly supported by the preponderance of substitutions in positively charged arginines throughout the molecule. This finding suggests that Rag1 uses a broad, positive-charged surface for interacting with the DNA.

The structural model of Rag2 as a six-bladed β-propeller molecule with a C-terminal PHD finger has been supported by functional data from a number of identified Omenn and SCID mutations. Amino acid substitutions in three SCID patients were localized to the second β strand of the first, second and fourth kelch repeats of RAG2 and were shown to abrogate the V(D)J recombination activity of the altered proteins (Corneo et al., 2000; Gomez et al., 2000). These β strands are highly conserved between and within kelch repeat-containing proteins, where they appear to form the hydrophobic structural core of the molecule. Site-directed mutagenesis targeting many residues in the second β strand revealed that nearly all of the mutant proteins were devoid of recombination activity, further confirming the importance of these conserved regions (Gomez et al., 2000). Moreover, many of the null and hypomorphic RAG2-active core mutations have a spatial clustering on one face of the predicted β propeller, thereby defining a potentially critical surface for interaction with RAG1 (Corneo et al., 2000). Indeed, two of the mutations, C41W and M285R, have been shown to reduce the interaction between RAG2 and RAG1 in coprecipitation assays (Villa et al., 1998). Further support of the structural model of RAG2 has been provided by the identification of four mutations leading to amino acid substitutions in the C-terminal PHD finger (C423Y, W453R, N474S, and C478Y). The W453R substitution was identified in an Omenn patient and has residual levels of recombination activity (Gomez et al., 2000), while the other three substitutions were found in T⁻B⁻ SCID patients and are likely inactive for recombination. Two of the altered amino acids, C423 and C478 (Schwarz et al., 1996, A. Villa et al., unpublished results), are predicted to coordinate zinc ion and are therefore entirely conserved in all known PHD fingers.

The in vivo importance of the RAG1 N terminus is supported by a novel class of frameshift mutations identified in a group of Omenn patients (Santagata et al., 2000). We have described seven Omenn patients with either one (A887) or two (AA368-9) nucleotides deleted in the 5′ coding region of RAG1, resulting in a frameshift and the predicted production of severely truncated and inactive forms of RAG1. In two cases the patients are homozygous for the allele harboring the frameshift deletion and in the remaining five cases the frameshift deletion alleles are coupled with alleles generating proteins that are fully inactive for recombination. Hence, the recombination activity responsible for generating the partial immune repertoire in these patients must be provided by the frameshift alleles. In fact, an N-terminus-truncated active RAG1 protein is generated from these alleles by reinitiation from internal in-frame methionine residues downstream of the deletion. Using a cell culture–based recombination assay, we observed a deficiency in both inversional and deletional recombination capacity of these mutants. While multiple in vitro assays of RAG function can be efficiently performed in the absence of the RAG1 N terminus, the immunodeficiency observed in these patients, coupled with work demonstrating the importance of the N terminus for recombination of endogenous immunoglobulin loci, provides compelling in vivo evidence for a critical role of the N terminus of RAG1 in the recombination reaction. Noordzij and colleagues have reported a similar T⁺/B⁻ Omenn patient homozygous for an allele with a single nucleotide deletion (T631) that also demonstrates partial recombination capacity and appears to result in the formation of a partially restricted receptor repertoire (Noordzij et al., 2000).

To gain further insight into the cellular defect resulting from loss of the initial amino acids of the N-terminal domain of RAG1, we analyzed the fluorescence localization in transfected cells of both wild-type and deleted forms of RAG1 fused in-frame to GFP protein. Interestingly, fluorescence was observed in cells transfected with both fusion constructs. Wild-type RAG1/GFP localized to the nucleus as expected, whereas the GFP fusion to Δ368A/369A-RAG1 had an aberrant pattern of localization with most of the fluorescence located in the cytoplasm. These data implicate a defective ability to properly migrate into the nucleus as a component of the pathogenesis associated with Δ368A/369A. This interpretation is strengthened by the identification, in another OS patient, of a frameshift mutation at nt 887, in which translation occurred at an internal methionine, showing similar aberrant cellular localization.

Mutation Analysis in Atypical SCID Patients

The analysis of a large series of immunodeficient patients with RAG defects has enabled the identification of a new group of patients with some, but not all, of the clinical and immunologic features of OS, a condition we call "atypical SCID/OS." In terms of the molecular basis this category seems to be more like OS than classic SCID because all of these patients carry at least one missense mutation, some of which are shared with those of OS patients. This finding supports the idea that in these patients, partial RAG activity is responsible for the development of a low number of T and possibly B lymphocytes. A third phenotype for mutations in recombination activating gene 1 (*RAG1*), in addition to the already known phenotypes of SCID and Omenn syndrome has been described (de Villartay et al., 2005; Ehl et al., 2005). The presence of partial RAG activity may be a prerequisite for OS but other epigenetic factors are needed to understand the disease (Corneo et al., 2001; Villa et al., 2001). Alternatively, it is possible that individual differences such as early or delayed medical treatment could contribute to clinical and immunological heterogeneity, particularly because some patients undergo to BMT very early in the course of the disease and this treatment could prevent the development of typical OS symptoms.

Treatment

Unless treated by BMT, OS is invariably fatal because of infections and/or malnutrition. The clinical presentation is usually so severe that supportive treatment is warranted, even before a diagnosis of OS is formally established (see Chapter 46).

Despite this broad supportive treatment, the clinical status of OS patients waiting for BMT often remains critical, mainly because of cutaneous and intestinal problems directly related to deranged T cell activation. As an attempt to overcome the activation of Th2 cells and to achieve better control of disease activity, different strategies have been used. The daily use of IFN-γ (the rationale being to restore the balance between Th1- and Th2-type cytokines) succeeded in the amelioration of clinical conditions in one infant, concurrently with a decrease in eosinophil count and increase in lymphocyte proliferation to mitogens (Schandene et al., 1993). Other groups have tried to block T cell activation using immunosuppressive drugs. Steroids have proven ineffective or only partially effective (Omenn, 1965; Barth et al., 1972; Ochs et al., 1974; Le Deist et al., 1985). Somewhat better results have been obtained with cyclosporine A (Wirt et al., 1989; Brugnoni et al., 1997). However, the potential beneficial effect of immunosuppressive drugs and IFN-γ is of limited duration, and ultimate treatment is still based on BMT. Because of the specific features of OS, the overall results of BMT in these children are less satisfactory than in other forms of combined immunodeficiencies. The first attempts reported in the literature were disappointing, as only 7 of 26 patients who received BMT were cured (Barth et al., 1972; Junker et al., 1988; Fischer et al., 1990, 1994; Bruckmann et al., 1991; Heyderman et al., 1991; Schofer et al., 1991; Loechelt et al., 1995). A high frequency of graft failure was observed, reflecting the presence of activated T cells that prevent engraftment of donor-derived hematopoietic stem cells. Aggressive conditioning with myeloablative and immune-suppressive drugs is needed to circumvent this problem. More recently, the use of appropriate supportive treatment and prophylaxis of infection, together with tailored conditioning regimens, has resulted in a better outcome for BMT. Taking advantage of these advances, Gomez et al. (1995) reported the cure of OS by BMT in six of nine patients; similarly, another group achieved successful treatment in four of five OS patients (Chilosi et al., 1996a; Brugnoni et al., 1997). The successful engraftment of donor-derived hematopoietic stem cells is associated with the development of normal numbers and functions of both T and B lymphocytes, with full clinical and immunological recovery.

Questions for Future Research

In light of these results, the pathogenesis of OS lies in a defect of the V(D)J recombination system that allows the occurrence of some rearrangements. For this reason, some T cells with bona fide

TCR rearrangements can exit the thymus, expand either in the thymus itself or in the periphery, and produce Th2-type cytokines, which in turn are responsible for some features of the characteristic phenotype of OS patients, such as hypereosinophilia and hyper-IgE.

Although the identification of a defect in V(D)J recombination has given an elegant unifying explanation for OS, several aspects have not yet been clarified. First, the reasons for the apparent expansion of the Th2 subset are not clear. Selective expansion of certain TCR clones may be a consequence of either intrathymic selection of specific rearrangements or peripheral expansion in response to infections or perhaps autoantigens. It has been suggested that given the extreme disorganization of the thymic microenvironment in OS, negative selection of autoreactive clones may be inoperative, and a few residual T cell clones may expand in the periphery because of their autoreactive character (Fischer and Malissen, 1998).

Another unexplained phenomenon is the fact that RAG proteins direct recombination in both B and T cells, yet B cells are absent in peripheral blood of OS patients. In view of the constant presence of elevated IgE levels in OS patients, it is clear that somewhere, perhaps in the gastrointestinal tract, B cells, which perform Ig loci rearrangements and switch to IgE production, do exist. It is noteworthy that V(D)J recombination deficiencies that lead to low-to-normal numbers of T cells in the absence of mature B cells is a recurring theme. When the differentiation defect in Rag-deficient or *scid* mice is rescued by DNA-damaging agents or by genetic manipulation such as by p53 or poly(ADP-ribose) polymerase (PARP) inactivation, the T cell, but not the B cell compartment, is restored (Danska et al., 1994; Guidos et al., 1995, 1996; Nacht et al., 1996; Livak et al., 1996; Bogue et al., 1997; Morrison et al., 1997). The mechanisms underlying these differences between B and T cell development remain to be defined.

Another point that must be clarified is the role of environmental factors in the pathogenesis of the Th2 expansion and the resulting clinical features. As observed in other cases, immune-deficient individuals have by definition a more intense antigen exposure and a defect in antigen clearance that results in persistent high antigen load. If, as in OS, the genetic defect is permissive and allows the development of limited clones of mature T cells, the antigen overload favors prolonged T cell activation that has been associated with increased IL-4 secretion and polarization toward a Th2 phenotype (Hsieh et al., 1993; Hosken et al., 1995). Re-creation of missense mutations in mice via homologous recombination could solve this problem by comparing mutant mice kept in germ-free facilities to those kept in a normal environment.

The Link between V(D)J Recombination and DNA Double-Strand Break Repair

V(D)J recombination is initiated by lymphoid-specific RAG1 and RAG2 proteins, which introduce DSBs precisely between Ig and TCR coding gene segments and flanking. RAG-mediated cleavage generates four broken-end intermediates: two blunt signal ends and two covalently closed (hairpin) coding ends. The subsequent resolution of V(D)J ends into coding and signal joints requires ubiquitously expressed factors playing a role in the DNA repair. The nonlymphoid-restricted components identified thus far are the DNA-PK–dependent catalytic subunit (DNA-PKcs), Ku70, Ku80, XRCC4, ligase IV, and, very recently, Artemis; all of these proteins play a role in DNA DSB repair as well as in V(D)J recombination. At least two other nonlymphoid-specific components are involved in the VDJ process, HMG1 and HMG2, although their role is not clear (reviewed in Bassing et al., 2002; Gellert, 2002). After the RSS cleavage, performed by RAG proteins, the RAG complex remains bound with the resulting 5′ phosphorylated blunt signal end and hairpin coding end (postcleavage complex). At this stage, the generation of junctional diversity is initiated by the opening of hairpin coding ends. The molecule responsible for hairpin opening is not known with certainty, although both RAG complex and MRE11 can mediate the hydrolysis of hairpin in vitro (Besmer et al., 1998; Shockett and Schatz, 1999; Fugmann et al., 2000). Recently it has been proposed that Artemis, after phosphorylation by DNA-PKcs, can play a key role in hairpin cleavage (Ma et al., 2002).

While the RAG proteins are specifically expressed in lymphoid cells, the rejoining steps require other actors of the DNA nonhomologous end-joining (NHEJ) machinery. NHEJ requires the heterodimeric Ku protein (Ku70 and Ku80) and a large protein DNA-PKcs, which associates with Ku to form the DNA-PK complex. DNA ligase IV and Xrcc4 are successively required for the rejoining steps. All the animal models carrying a defective gene of either one of the known V(D)J recombination/DNA repair factors, either natural (murine and equine *scid*) or engineered through homologous recombination, exhibit a profound defect in the lymphoid developmental program owing to an arrest of the B and T cell maturation at early stages (Nussenzweig et al., 1996; Zhu et al., 1996; Jhappan et al., 1997; Shin et al., 1997; Barnes et al., 1998; Frank et al., 1998; Gao et al., 1998a, 1998b; Taccioli et al., 1998). Mutants lacking Ku or Xrcc4/DNA ligase IV complex show pronounced defects in the rejoining of both blunt signal and hairpin coding ends, whereas mutants lacking DNA-PKcs show a marked impairment in coding join formation.

Radiosensitive B⁻T⁻ SCID

Definition

Some B⁻T⁻ SCID patients do not have a mutation in either the *RAG1* or *RAG2* genes, despite having the very same clinical presentation as that with typical RAG defects (Table 11.3). The alymphocytosis in these patients is accompanied by an increased cellular sensitivity to ionizing radiation (RS-SCID, MIM 602450 and 605988), a situation highly reminiscent of the murine *scid* condition, leading to the hypothesis that a general defect in the DNA repair machinery is responsible for this deficit. The RS-SCID phenotype is also found with high incidence among Athabascan-speaking Native American Indians (1 in 2000 live births among Navajo Indians) (Hu et al., 1988).

Laboratory Findings

Patients with RS-SCID are characterized by an increase sensitivity to ionizing radiation of bone marrow cells (CFU-GM) and primary skin fibroblasts (Cavazzana-Calvo et al., 1993), as well as a defect in V(D)J recombination in vitro, in fibroblasts (Nicolas et al., 1998). Although this condition suggests that RS-SCID could have a general DNA repair defect reminiscent of the murine *scid* condition, DNA-PK activity is normal in these patients and the implication of the DNA-PKcs gene has been unequivocally ruled out by genetic means in several consanguineous families (Nicolas et al., 1996). A role for all the other known genes involved in V(D)J recombination and DNA repair was equally excluded (Nicolas et al., 1996, 1998). V(D)J recombination analysis

in fibroblasts from Athabascan SCID patients suggested a common molecular defect (Moshous et al., 2000) and, therefore, the existence of a gene coding for a new factor of the V(D)J recombination. The disease-related locus in both situations was assigned to the short arm of human chromosome 10 (Li et al., 1998; Moshous et al., 2000).

The Artemis Factor

Given the location of the RS-SCID gene on human chromosome 10, an in silico strategy was adopted for its identification. Genomic DNA sequences released by the Sanger Center, which covered this chromosomal region, were systematically analyzed using two computer programs, FGENESH and GENESCAN, aimed at identifying putative genes in large genomic sequences. On the basis of a putative peptide proposed by these programs, a full-length cDNA coding for a new factor called *Artemis* was isolated (Moshous et al., 2001). Functional complementation studies and mutation analyses certified that Artemis was indeed the gene defective in RS-SCID (see below). As expected, because of the ubiquitous increase of cellular radiosensitivity in RS-SCIDs, the expression of Artemis was detected in every tissue tested. Although Artemis does not have any global homologues in the databases, BLAST search analyses revealed some interesting features of this new protein. Significant similarities to several proteins, including the yeast PSO2 and murine SNM1 proteins, were found over the first 360 amino acids of Artemis. Subsequent iterations with the PSI-BLAST program highlighted significant similarities of the first 150 amino acids to well-established members of the metallo-β-lactamase superfamily. The metallo-β-lactamase fold, first described for the *Bacillus cereus* β-lactamase (Carfi et al., 1995), is adopted by various metallo-enzymes with a widespread distribution and substrate specificity (Aravind, 1997). It consists of a four-layered β sandwich with two mixed β sheets flanked by α helices, with the metal-binding sites located at one edge of the β sandwich (Color Plate 11.V). Sequence analysis and secondary structure prediction for Artemis clearly indicated the conservation of motifs typical of the metallo-β-lactamase fold, participating in the metal-binding pocket and representing the catalytic site of the metallo-β-lactamases. Altogether, this analysis indicated that Artemis not only probably adopted the β-lactamase fold, but may also have conserved an associated catalytic activity, in contrast to several other proteins having lost many of the catalytic residues (Aravind, 1997).

Mutation Analysis

The first indication that Artemis was indeed the gene involved in the RS-SCID came from the identification of mutations in several patients (Color Plate 11.VI); 8 different alterations of the gene were found in 11 families. Although some of the mutations were recurrent, it was not possible to draw any clear correlation with the geographical origins of the patients. Several interesting features arose from the analysis of these mutations. First, three of the identified modifications involved genomic deletions spanning several exons, leading to frameshift and appearance of premature terminations in two cases and in-frame deletion of 216 amino acids in one case. This finding indicates that the Artemis gene may represent a hot spot for gene deletion. Second, none of the mutations consisted of simple nucleotide substitutions generating amino acid changes, and only one, the C279T modification, created a nonsense mutation. The other nucleotide changes affected splice donor sequences leading to either frameshifts in three cases or to in-frame deletion of part of the protein in one case. Another interesting feature is that in three patients the genomic deletion comprised exons 1 to 4, which resulted in a complete absence of Artemis, encoded cDNA. This deletion, which can be considered as resulting in a null allele, demonstrated that Artemis is not an essential protein for viability, in contrast to XRCC4 and DNA-ligase-IV, for example (Barnes et al., 1998; Frank et al., 1998; Gao et al., 1998a), or that it is partly redundant. Finally, the implication of Artemis in the RS-SCID condition was unequivocally established by complementation of the V(D)J recombination defect in patients' fibroblasts upon transfection of a wt Artemis cDNA. Other mutations of the Artemis gene, including amino acid substitutions, were subsequently described (Li et al., 2002; Kobayashi et al., 2003; Noordzij et al., 2003). Hypomorphic Artemis mutations have been described in a patient affected by Omenn syndrome. The clinical presentation as well as the immunophenotype of this OS is indistinguishable from that caused by hypomorphic mutations found in Rag1 and Rag2 mutations. (Ege et al., 2005). Artemis knockout mice are viable and recapitulate the phenotype seen in human RS-SCID patients, with one noticeable and interesting difference (Rooney et al., 2002). Significant numbers of bona fide mature T lymphocytes, mostly CD4+, are detected in the periphery of certain mice. Artemis deficiency in mice results in chromosomal fragments, fusion, and detached centromers in both embryonic stem cells and murine embryonic fibroblasts (Rooney et al., 2002, 2003). These findings strongly suggest that Artemis has an important role in genome stability and may be considered a genomic caretaker similar to other factors of the V(D)J recombination/DNA repair machinery. Indeed, hypomorphic mutations of Artemis in humans that allow the emergence of a few B and T lymphocytes are accompanied by the development of EBV-associated B-cell lymphomas in a general context of genomic instability (Moshous et al., 2003). This result is reminiscent of the pro-B cell lymphomas that emerge in NHEJ-deficient mice when crossed onto a cell-cycle checkpoint defect such as p53$^{-/-}$ (Ferguson et al., 2001).

Structure and Function

The repeated search for a global ortholog of both human and murine Artemis in other species in protein databases has failed to provide a strong candidate, and we are left with the similarity of Artemis to the various members of the metallo-β-lactamase family, including both murine SNM1 and yeast PSO2. However, Artemis is clearly not the human ortholog of either of these two proteins, for several reasons. First, despite their SNM1 similarity regions, the three proteins differ in their associated domains. In particular, the 331 amino acids composing the C-terminal region of Artemis are not present in SNM1/PSO2 and do not share any obvious similarities with any other known protein. Second, while murine and yeast SNM1/PSO2 mutants demonstrate a strong defect in the repair of DNA damages caused by DNA interstrand cross-linking agents (Henriques and Moustacchi, 1980; Dronkert et al., 2000), they do not display elevated sensitivity to ionizing radiations, indicating that these two proteins are probably not directly involved in the repair of DNA DSB. This is in sharp contrast to the phenotype of RS-SCID patients, whose primary molecular defect is indeed the absence of DNA DSB repair, illustrated by the lack of coding joint formation in the course of V(D)J recombination and the increased sensitivity of bone marrow and fibroblast cells to γ rays (Cavazzana-Calvo et al., 1993; Nicolas et al., 1998). Interestingly, Artemis, murine SNM1, and

yeast PSO2 share a domain adopting a metallo-β-lactamase fold (Aravind, 1997) and possibly its associated enzymatic activity, given the presence of nearly all the critical catalytic residues. However, there is no obvious consensus on the nature of the various metallo-β-lactamase substrates, outside of a general negatively charged composition. Sequence analysis revealed the existence of a conserved region that accompanies the metallo-β-lactamase domain in members of the Artemis/SNM1/PSO2 subfamily, including various other sequences related to nucleic acid metabolism such as two subunits of the cleavage and polyadenylation specificity factor (CPSF). We named this domain βCASP, for metallo-β-lactamase–associated CPSF Artemis SNM1/PSO2 domain (Callebaut et al., 2002). This domain harbors several conserved residues, which could play a role in the reaction catalyzed by members of this subfamily. It is tempting to speculate that this domain could contribute to substrate binding, in a way similar to the α-helical domain of glyoxalase, another member of the β-lactamase family (Cameron et al., 1999).

DNA DSB can be repaired either by homologous recombination (HR) or by the NHEJ (reviewed in Haber, 2000). Whereas HR is the predominant repair pathway in yeast, NHEJ is mostly used in higher eukaryotes and represents the DNA repair pathway followed during V(D)J recombination. At least two protein complexes are thought to act in concert or sequentially at the site of the RAG1/2-derived DSB. The Ku70-80 complex is probably recruited first at the site of the lesion, followed by the addition of the DNA-PKcs subunit. This initial complex is considered the primary DNA damage sensor that will activate the DNA repair machinery. The XRCC4/DNA-ligase IV complex represents the best candidate to actually repair the gap. Careful analysis of the various phenotypes among the different V(D)J recombination deficient models, including RS-SCID, has provided some hypotheses regarding the possible role of Artemis during V(D)J recombination. Two major differences exist between the RS-SCID condition and that of XRCC4 and DNA-ligaseIV knockout mice. First, a complete null allele of Artemis does not lead to embryonic lethality in humans. This observation, therefore, does not support an implication of Artemis in this phase of NHEJ. Second, the rejoining of linearized DNA constructs introduced in RS-SCID fibroblasts is not altered (J.P. de Villartay, unpublished observations), whereas this assay, when defective, is highly diagnostic of abnormal NHEJ in yeast (Teo and Jackson, 1997; Wilson et al., 1997). Perhaps the most evident link between Artemis and NHEJ is found in regard to the Ku/DNA-PK complex. Indeed, human RS-SCID patients and *scid* mice, which harbor a mutation in the DNA-PKcs encoding gene, are the only two known conditions in which a V(D)J recombination–associated DNA repair defect affects uniquely the formation of the coding joints, leaving signal joint formation unaltered. This is in striking contrast to all the other known V(D)J recombination/DNA repair deficiency settings. Hairpin-sealed coding ends represent the unprocessed V(D)J recombination intermediates that accumulate in murine *scid* lymphoid cells. Although recent data have indicated that RAG1 and RAG2 are capable of opening these hairpin structures in vitro, the situation of the murine *scid* strongly suggests that DNA repair factors such as DNA-PK may be required for this process in vivo. This observation suggests that Artemis, through its putative hydrolase activity, may participate in opening the hairpin at the coding ends in vivo. Artemis does indeed possess an intrinsic exonuclease activity in vitro that can be redirected to an endonuclease activity capable of resolving Rag1/2-generated hairpins in vitro when Artemis is complexed to and phosphorylated by DNA-PKcs (Ma et al., 2002). The catalytic core of Artemis is carried by the metallo-β-lactamase/βCASP domain (J.P. de Villartay, upublished observations). The accumulation of hairpin-sealed coding ends in thymocytes from Artemis knockout mice and scid/DNA-PKcs KO mice strongly support this function (Rooney et al., 2002).

DNA-Ligase IV Defects

As previously described, DNA ligase IV forms a complex with XRCC4, which is essential for NHEJ and for the V(D)J recombination process (Critchlow et al., 1997; Grawunder et al., 1997). The inactivation of both alleles of DNA ligase IV in a human pre-B cell line confers high radiosensibility and abrogates the V(D)J recombination activity (Grawunder et al., 1998a). Riballo and coworkers (1999) identified a patient with a defect in NHEJ bearing a missense mutation in the gene encoding DNA ligase IV. This patient did not show any immunodeficiency; however, he developed leukemia at age 14 and overresponded to radiotherapy (Riballo et al., 2001). More recently, the finding of LIG4 mutations in four patients diagnosed as having Nijmegen breakage syndrome (NBS) at clinical presentation but who were normal for NBS1 led to the identification of a new syndrome, designated *LIG4 syndrome*. This disorder is characterized by developmental delay, chromosomal instability, and immunodeficiency (O'Driscoll et al., 2001).

The clinical features of these patients resemble those of NBS but the cellular phenotype is distinct. Although cells from both syndromes show radiosensitivity, LIG4 cell lines have normal checkpoint function and are defective in DSB repair. The analysis of chromosome breakage in pheripheral blood lymphocytes obtained from LIG4 patients did not show any translocations or inversions involving chromosomes 7 and 14, which are typical of ataxia-telangiectasia and NBS.

Many of the features of patients with LIG4 syndrome resemble a particular form of dwarfism named *Seckel syndrome*, recently found to be due to AT and Rad3-related protien defects (O'Driscoll et al., 2003). Patients had microcephaly and one of them had a typical bird-like face. Pancytopenia is a common feature in these patients, but they do not develop a SCID phenotype, consistent with the hypothesis that the mutations impair but not abolish the VDJ activity. Another clinical feature is the occurrence of skin alteration (plantar warts, psoriasis, and photosensitivity). None of these patients developed cancer, although two of four patient showed hypothyroidism and hypogonadism.

Mutations

The first patient described by Riballo and coworkers (1999) who developed leukemia had a missense R278H mutation mapping to the ligase IV active site. The same mutation was also present in one of four patients, even though the clinical features were completely different. This discrepancy suggests that epigenetic factors may influence the onset of the disease. Two of the mutations identified in the other patients were stop mutations (R580X–R814X) leading to protein truncation in the BRCT region, which is supposed to interact with XRCC4 (Grawunder et al., 1998b). The fourth mutation, G469E, was an amino acid change located on a surface loop important for DNA binding. It is noteworthy that LIG4-null mutations in mice result in embryonic lethality. This finding suggests the hypothesis that the mutations found in these patients could be hypomorphic, thus explaining the mild phenotype of the immunodeficiency. However, the R580X stop mutation is not easily reconciled with this hypothesis.

Acknowledgments

We thank A. Jacobs for excellent secretarial assistance, S. Fugmann for helping in design of the figures, and L. Doostar, F. Radecke, and H.D. Ochs for review of the manuscript. This work was supported by a grant from Sonderforschungsbereich 322 of the Deutsche Forschungsgemeinschaft (K.S.), by BMBF grant IZKF.C05 (K.S.), by National Institutes of Health (NIH) grants A140181 (E.S.), and by grants from AFM/Telethon GAT0203 (A.V.). In addition, this work was supported by the Genoma 2000/IBTA project, funded by CARIPLO, Italy, and grant RBNE019J9W from MIUR-FIRB to A.V. This work was also supported by institutional grants from INSERM (J.P.V.) and grants from ARC (J.P.V.) and CEA (J.P.V.).

References

Abe T, Tsuge J, Kamachi Y, Torii S, Utsumi K, Akahori Y, Ichihara Y, Kurosawa Y, Matsuoka H. Evidence for defects in V(D)J rearrangements in patients with severe combined immunodeficiency. J Immunol 152:5504–5513, 1994.

Adams J, Kelso R, Cooler L. The kelch repeat superfamily of proteins: propeller of cell function. Trends Cell Biol 10:17–24, 2000.

Agrawal A, Eastman QM, Schatz DG. Transposition mediated by RAG1 and RAG2 and its implications for the evolution of the immune system. Nature 394:744–751, 1998.

Akamatsu Y, Monroe R, Dudley DD, Elkin SK, Gartner F, Talukder SR, Takahama Y, Alt FW, Bassing CH, Oettinger MA. Deletion of the RAG2 C terminus leads to impaired lymphoid development in mice. Proc Natl Acad Sci USA 100:1209–1214, 2003.

Aleman K, Noordzij JG, de Groot R, van Dogen JJ, Harrtwig NG. Reviewing Omenn syndrome. Eur J Pediatr 160:718–725, 2001.

Anderson KC, Weinstein HJ. Transfusion-assocaited graft-versus-host disease. N Engl J Med 323:315–321, 1990.

Aravind L. An evolutionary classification of the matallo-β-lactamase fold. In Silico Biology 1:69–91, 1997.

Barnes DE, Stamp G, Rosewell I, Denzel A, Lindahl T. Targeted disruption of the gene encoding DNA ligase IV leads to lethality in embryonic mice. Curr Biol 31:1395–1398, 1998.

Barth RF, Vergara G, Khurana SK, Lowman JT, Beckwith JB. Rapidly fatal familial histiocytosis associated with eosinophilia and primary immunological deficiency. Lancet ii:503–506, 1972.

Bassing CH, Alt FW, Hughes MM, D'Auteuil M, Wehrly TD, Woodman BB, Gartner F, White JM, Davidson L, Sleckamn BP. Recombination signal sequences restrict chromosomal VDJ recombination beyond the 12/23 rule. Nature 405:583–586, 2000.

Bassing CH, Swat W, Alt FW. The mechanism and regulation of chromosomal V(D)J recombination. Cell 109 (Suppl):S45–55, 2002.

Bernstein RM, Schluchter SF, Lake DF, Marchalonis JJ. Evolutionary conservation and molecular cloning of the recombinase activating gene 1. Biochem Biophys Res Commun 205:687–692, 1994.

Besmer E, Mansilla-Soto J, Cassard S, Sawchuk DJ, Brown G, Sadofsky M, Lewis SM, Nussenzweig MC, Cortes P. Hairpin coding end opening is mediated by RAG1 and RAG2 proteins. Mol Cell 2:817–828, 1998.

Bogue MA, Wang C, Zhu C, Roth DB. V(D)J recombination in Ku86-deficient mice: distinct effects on coding, signal and hybrid joint formation. Immunity 7:37–47, 1997.

Brandt VL, Roth DB. A recombinase diversified: new functions of the RAG proteins. Curr Opin Immunol 14:224–229, 2002.

Brown ST, Miranda GA, Galic Z, Hartmann JZ, Lyon CL, Aguilera RJ. Regulation of the RAG-1 promoter by the NF-Y transcription factor. J Immunol 158:5071–5074, 1997.

Bruckmann C, Lindner W, Roos R, Permanetter W, Haas, RJ, Haworth SG, Belohradsky BH. Severe pulmonary vascular occlusive disease following bone marrow transplantation in Omenn syndrome. Eur J Pediatr 150: 242–245, 1991.

Brugnoni D, Airo P, Facchetti F, Blanzuoli L, Ugazio AG, Cattaneo R, Notarangelo LD. In vitro cell death of activated lymphocytes in Omenn's syndrome. Eur J Immunol 27:2765–2773, 1997.

Businco L, Di Fazio A, Ziruolo MG, Boner A, Valletta EA, Ruco LP, Vitolo D, Ensoli B, Paganelli R. Clinical and immunological findings in four infants with Omenn's syndrome: a form of severe combined immunodeficiency with phenotypically normal T cells, elevated IgE, and eosinophilia. Clin Immunol Immunopathol 44:123–133, 1987.

Callebaut I, Mornon JP. The VDJ recombination activating protein RAG2 consists of a six bladed propeller and a PHD fingerlike domain, as revealed by sequence analysis. Cell Mol Life Sci 54:880–891, 1998.

Callebaut I, Moshous D, Mornon JP, and De Villartay JP. Metallo-β-lactamase fold within nucleic acids processing enzymes: the β-CASP family. Nucl Acids Res 30:3592–3601, 2002.

Cameron AD, Ridderstrom M, Olin B, Mannervik B. Crystal structure of human glyoxalase II and its complex with a glutathione thiolester substrate analogue. Structure Fold Des 7:1067–1078, 1999.

Carfi A, Pares S, Duee E, Galleni M, Duez C, Frere JM, Dideberg O. The 3-D structure of a zinc metallo-beta-lactamase from *Bacillus cereus* reveals a new type of protein fold. EMBO J 14:4914–4921, 1995.

Cavazzana-Calvo M, Hacein-Bey S, de Saint Basile G, Gross F, Yvon E, Nusbaum P, Selz F, Hue C, Certain S, Casanova JL, Bousso P, Deist FL, Fischer A. Gene therapy of human severe combined immunodeficiency (SCID)-X1 disease. Science 288:669–672, 2000.

Cavazzana-Calvo M, Le Deist F, de Saint Basile G, Papadopoulo D, de Villartay JP, Fischer A. Increased radiosensitivity of granulocyte macrophage colony–forming units and skin fibroblasts in human autosomal recessive severe combined immunodeficiency. J Clin Invest 91:1214–1218, 1993.

Chilosi M, Facchetti F, Notarangelo LD, Romagnani S, Del Prete G, Almerigogna F, De Carli M, Pizzolo G. CD30 cell expression and abnormal soluble CD30 serum accumulation in Omenn's syndrome: evidence for a T helper 2-mediated condition. Eur J Immunol 26:329–334, 1996a.

Chilosi M, Pizzolo G, Facchetti F, Notarangelo LD, Romagnani S, Del Prete G, Almerigogna F, De Carli M. The pathology of Omenn's syndrome. Am J Surg Pathol 20:773–774, 1996b.

Corneo B, Moshous D, Callebaut I, de Chasseval R, Fischer A, de Villartay JP. 3D clustering of human RAG2 gene mutations in severe combined immune deficiency (SCID). J Biol Chem 275:12672–12675, 2000.

Corneo B, Moshous D, Gungor T, Wulffrat N, Philippet P, Le Deist F, Fischer A, de Villartay JP. Identical mutations in RAG1 and RAG2 genes leading to defective V(D)Jrecombinase activity can cause either T-B- severe combined immune deficiency or Omenn syndrome. Blood 97:2772–2776, 2001.

Cottier H. Zur Histopathologie des Antikorpermangel-Syndroms. Transaction of 6th Congress of the European Society for Haematology, Copenhagen 1957. Basel: S. Karger, 1958.

Critchlow SE, Bowater RP, Jackson SP. Mammalian DNA double strand break repair protein XRCC4 interacts with DNA ligase IV. Curr Biol 7:588–598, 1997.

Cuomo CA, Oettinger MA. Analysis of regions of RAG-2 important for V(D)J recombination. Nucl Acids Res 22:1810–1814, 1994.

Cushman J, Lo J, Huang Z, Wasserfall C, Petitto JM. Neurobehavioral changes resulting from recombinase activation gene 1 deletion. Clin Diagn Lab Immunol 10:13–18, 2003.

Dai Y, Kysela B, Hanakahi LA, Manolis K, Riballo E, Stumm M, Harville TO, West SC, Oettinger MA, Jeggo PA. Nonhomologous end joining and V(D)J recombination require an additional factor. Proc Natl Acad Sci USA 100:2462–2467, 2003.

Danska JS, Pflumio F, Williams CJ, Huner O, Dick JE, Guidos CJ. Rescue of T cell–specific V(D)J recombination in scid mice by DNA damaging agents. Science 266:450–454, 1994.

Derry J, Ochs HD, Francke U. Isolation of a novel gene mutated in Wiskott-Aldrich syndrome. Cell 78:635–644, 1994.

de Saint-Basile G, Le Deist F, de Villartay JP, Cerf-Bensussan N, Journet O, Brousse N, Griscelli C, Fischer A. Restricted heterogeneity of T lymphocytes in combined immunodeficiency with hypereosinophilia (Omenn's syndrome). J Clin Invest 87:1352–1359, 1991.

de Villartay JP, Lim A, Al-Mousa H, Dupont S, Dechanet-Merville J, Coumau-Gatbois E, Gougeon ML, Lemainque A, Eidenschenk C, Jouanguy E, Abel L, Casanova JL, Fischer A, Le Deist F. A novel immunodeficiency associated with hypomorphic RAG1 mutations and CMV infection. J Clin Invest 115:3291–3299, 2005.

Devriendt K, Kim AS, Mathijs G, Frints SGM, Schwartz M, Van den Oord JJ, Verhoef GE, Boogaerts MA, Fryns JP, You D, Rosen MK, Vandenberghe P. Constitutively activating mutation in WASP causes X-linked severe congenital neutropenia. Nat Genet 27:313–317, 2001.

Diamond RA, Ward SB, Owada-Makabe K, Wang H, Rothenberg EV. Different developmental arrest points in RAG-2$^{-/-}$ and SCID thymocytes on two genetic backgrounds. J Immunol 158:4052–4064, 1997.

Difilippantonio MJ, McMahen CJ, Eastman QM, Spanopoulou E, Schatz D. RAG1 mediates signal sequence recognition and recruitment of RAG2 in V(D)J recombination. Cell 87:253–262, 1996.

Dronkert ML, de Wit J, Boeve M, Vasconcelos ML, van Steeg H, Tan TL, Hoeijmakers JH, Kanaar R. Disruption of mouse SNM1 causes increased sensitivity to the DNA interstrand cross-linking agent mitomycin C. Mol Cell Biol 20:4553–4561, 2000.

Dyke MP, Marlow N, Berry PJ. Omenn's disease. Arch Dis Child 6:1247–1248, 1991.

Ege M, Ma Y, Manfras B, Kalwak K, Lu H, Lieber MR, Schwarz K, Pannicke U. Omenn syndrome due to Artemis mutations. Blood 105:4179–4186, 2005.

Ehl S, Schwarz K, Enders A, Duffner U, Pannicke U, Kuhr J, Mascart F, Schmitt-Graeff A, Niemeyer C, Fisch P. A variant of SCID with specific immune responses and predominance of gammadelta T cells. J Clin Invest 115:3140–3148, 2005.

Feddersen RM, van Ness BG. Double recombination of a single immunoglobulin-chain allele: implications for the mechanism of rearrangement. Proc Natl Acad Sci USA 82:4793–4797, 1985.

Ferguson DO, Alt FW. DNA double strand break repair and chromosomal translocation: lessons from animal models. Oncogene 20:5572–5579, 2001.

Fischer A, Hacein-Bey S, Cavazzano-Calvo M. Gene therapy of severe combined immunodeficiency. Nat Rev Immunol 2:615–621, 2002.

Fischer A, Landais P, Friedrich W, Gerritsen B, Fasth A, Porta F, Vellodi A, Benkerrou M, Jais JP, Cavazzana-Calvo M, Souillet G, Bordigoni P, Morgan G, Van Dijken P, Vossen J, Locatelli F, di Bartolomeo P. Bone marrow transplantation (BMT) in Europe for primary immunodeficiencies other than severe combined immunodeficiency: a report from the European Group for Bone Marrow Transplantation and the European Group for Immunodeficiency. Blood 83:1149–1154, 1994.

Fischer A, Landais P, Friedrich W, Morgan G, Gerritsen B, Fasth A, Porta F, Griscelli C, Goldman SF, Levinsky R, Vossen J. European experience of bone-marrow transplantation for severe combined immunodeficiency. Lancet 336(8719):850–854, 1990.

Fischer A, Malissen B. Natural and engineered disorders of lymphocyte development. Science 280:237–243, 1998.

Frank KM, Sekiguchi JM, Seidl KJ, Swat W, Rathbun GA, Cheng HL, Davidson L, Kangaloo L, Alt FW. Late embryonic lethality and impaired V(D)J recombination in mice lacking DNA ligase IV. Nature 396:173–177, 1998.

Fugmann SD, Lee AI, Schockett PE, Villey IJ, Schatz DG. The RAG proteins and VDJ recombination: complexes, ends and transposition. Annu Rev Immunol 18:495–527, 2000a.

Fugmann SD, Schatz DG. Identification of basic residues in RAG2 critical for DNA binding by the RAG1–RAG2 complex. Mol Cell 899–910, 2001.

Fugmann SD, Villey U, Ptaszek LM, Schatz DG. Identification of two catalytic residues in RAG1 that define a single active site within the RAG1/RAG2 protein complex. Mol Cell 5:97–107, 2000b.

Fujimoto S, Yamagishi H. Isolation of an excision product of T-cell receptor α-chain gene rearrangements. Nature 327:242–243, 1987.

Gao Y, Chaudhuri J, Zhu C, Davidson L, Weaver DT, Alt FW. A targeted DNA-PKcs-null mutation reveals DNA-PK-independent functions for KU in V(D)J recombination. Immunity 9:367–376, 1998a.

Gao Y, Sun Y, Frank KM, Dikkes P, Fujiwara Y, Seidl KJ, Sekiguchi JM, Rathbun GA, Swat W, Wang J, Bronson RT, Malynn BA, Bryans M, Zhu C, Chaudhuri J, Davidson L, Ferrini R, Stamato T, Orkin SH, Greenberg ME, Alt FW. A critical role for DNA end-joining proteins in both lymphogenesis and neurogenesis. Cell 95:891–902, 1998b.

Gellert M. V(D)J recombination: RAG proteins, repair factors and regulation. Annu Rev Biochem 71:101–132, 2002.

Glanzmann E, Riniker P. Essentielle Lymphocytophtise. Ein neues Krankheitsbild aus der Sauglingspathologie. Ann Paediatr (Basel) 175:1–32, 1950.

Gomez CA, Ptaszek LM, Villa A, Bozzi Fm Sobacchi C, Brooks EG, Notarangelo LD, Spanopoulou E, Pan ZQ, Vezzoni P. Mutations in conserved regions of the predicted RAG2 kelch repeats block initiation of VDJ recombination and result in primary immunodeficiencies. Mol Cell Biol 20:5653–5664, 2000.

Gomez L, Le Deist F, Blanche S, Cavazzana-Calvo M, Griscelli C, Fischer A. Treatment of Omenn syndrome by bone marrow transplantation. J Pediatr 127:76–81, 1995.

Grawunder U, Wilm M, Wu X, Kulesza P, Wilson TE, Mann M, Lieber MR. Activity of DNA ligase IV stimulated by complex formation with XRCC4 protein in mammalian cells. Nature 388:492–495, 1997.

Grawunder U, Zimmer D, Fugmann S, Schwarz K, Lieber MR. DNA ligase IV is essential for V(D)J recombination and DNA double-strand break repair in human precursor lymphocytes. Mol Cell 2:477–484, 1998a.

Grawunder U, Zimmer D, Lieber MR. DNA ligase IV binds to XRCC4 via a motif located between rather than within its BRCT domains. Curr Biol 8:873–876, 1998b.

Guidos CJ, Williams CJ, Grandal I, Knowles G, Huang MTF, Danska JS. V(D)J recombination activates a p53-dependent DNA damage checkpoint in scid lymphocyte precursor. Genes Dev 10:2038–2054, 1996.

Guidos CJ, Williams CJ, Wu GE, Paige CJ, Danska JS. Development of CD4, CD8 thymocytes in RAG-deficient mice through a T cell receptor beta chain-independent pathway. J Exp Med 181:1187–1195, 1995.

Haber JE. Partners and pathways repairing a double-strand break. Trends Genet 16:259–264, 2000.

Han S, Zheng B, Schatz DG, Spanopoulou E, Kelsoe E. Neoteny in lymphocytes: Rag1 and Rag2 expression in germinal center B cells. Science 274:2094–2097, 1996.

Harville TO, Adams DM, Howard TA, Ware RE. Oligoclonal expansion of CD45R0 T lymphocytes in Omenn syndrome. J Clin Immunol 17:322–332, 1997.

Henriques JA, Moustacchi E. Isolation and characterization of pso mutants sensitive to photo-addition of psoralen derivatives in *Saccharomyces cerevisiae*. Genetics 95:273–288, 1980.

Heyderman RS, Morgan G, Levinsky RJ, Strobel S. Successful bone marrow transplantation and treatment of BCG infection in two patients with severe combined immunodeficiency. Eur J Pediatr 150:477–480, 1991.

Hesse JE, Lieber MR, Gellert M, Mizuuchi K. Extrachromosomal DNA substrates in pre-B cells undergo inversion or deletion at immunoglobulin V-(D)-J joining signals. Cell 49:775–783, 1987.

Hikida M, Mori M, Takai T, Tomochika K, Hamatani K, Ohmori H. Re-expression of RAG-1 and RAG-2 genes in activated mature mouse B cells. Science 274:2092–2094, 1996.

Hiom K, Melek M, Gellert M. DNA transposition by the RAG1 and RAG2 proteins: a possible source of oncogenic translocations. Cell 94:463–470, 1998.

Hitzig WH, Biro Z, Bosch H, Huser HJ. Agammaglobulinamie und Alymphozytose mit Schwund des lymphatischen Gewebes. Helv Padiatr Acta 13:551–585, 1958.

Hosken NA, Shibuya K, Heath AW, Murphy KM, O'Garra A. The effect of antigen dose on CD4 T helper cell phenotype development in a T cell receptor-alpha and -beta transgenic model. J Exp Med 182:1579–1584, 1995.

Hsieh CS, Macatonia SE, Tripp CS, Wolf SF, O'Garra A, Murphy KM. Development of TH1 CD4 cells through IL-12 produced by *Listeria*-induced macrophages. Science 260:547–549, 1993.

Hsu LY, Lauring J, Liang HE, Greenbaum S, Cado D, Zhuang Y, Schlissel MS. A conserved transcriptional enhancer regulates RAG gene expression in developing B cells. Immunity 19:105–117, 2003.

Hu DC, Gahagan S, Wara DW, Hayward A, Cowan MJ. Congenital severe combined immunodeficiency disease (SCID) in American Indians. Pediatr Res 24:239, 1988.

Ichihara Y, Hirai M, Kurosawa Y. Sequence and chromosome assignment to 11p13–p12 of human RAG genes. Immunol Lett 33:277–284, 1992.

Jhappan C, Morse HC, Fleischmann RD, Gottesman MM, Merlino G. DNA-PKcs: a Tcell tumour suppressor encoded at the mouse scid locus. Nat Genet 17:483–486, 1997.

Junker AK, Chan KW, Massing BG. Clinical and immune recovery from Omenn syndrome after bone marrow transplantation. J Pediatr 114:596–600, 1988.

Kale SB, Landree MA, Roth DB. Conditional RAG1 mutants block the hairpin formation block the hairpin formation step of VDJ recombination. Mol Cell Biol 21:459–466, 2001.

Karol RA, Eng J, Cooper JB, Dennison DK, Sawyer MK, Lawrence EC, Marcus DM, Shearer WT. Imbalances in subsets of T-lymphocytes in an inbred pedigree with Omenn syndrome. Clin Immunol Immunopathol 27:412–427, 1983.

Kim DR, Dai Y, Mundy CL, Yang W, Oettinger MA. Mutations of acidic residues in RAG1 define the active site of the V(D)J recombinase. Genes Dev 13:3070–3080, 1999.

Kirch SA, Rathbun GA, Oettinger MA. Dual role of RAG2 in V(D)J recombination: catalysis and regulation of ordered Ig gene assembly. EMBO J 17:4881–4886, 1998.

Kobayashi N, Agematsu K, Sugita K, Sako M, Nonoyama S, Yachie A, Kumaki S, Tsuchiya S, Ochs HD, Fukushima Y, Komiyama A. Novel Artemis gene mutations of radiosensitive severe combined immunodeficiency in Japanese families. Hum Genet 112:348–352, 2003.

Komori T, Okada A, Stewart V, Alt FW. Lack of N regions in antigen receptor variable region genes of TdT-deficient lymphocytes. Science 261:1171–1175, 1993.

Korman AJ, Mauyama J, Raulet DH. Rearrangement by inversion of a T-cell receptor variable region gene located 3 of the constant region gene. Proc Natl Acad Sci USA 86:267–271, 1989.

Kumaki S, Villa A, Asada H, Kawai S, Ohashi Y, Takahashi M, Hakozaki I, Nitanai E, Minegishi M, Tsuchiya S. Identification of anti-herpes simplex virus antibody-producing B cells in a patient with an atypical RAG1 immunodeficiency. Blood 98:1464–1468, 2001.

Landree MA, Wibbenmeyer JA, Roth DB. Mutational analysis of RAG1 and RAG2 identifies three active site amino acids in RAG1 critical for both cleavage steps of V(D)J recombination. Genes Dev 13:3059–3069, 1999.

Lauring J, Schlissel MS. Distinct factors regulate the murine RAG2 promoter in B and T cell lines. Mol Cell Biol 19:2601–2612, 1999.

Le Deist F, Fischer A, Durandy A, Arnaud-Battandier F, Nezelof C, Hamet M, De Proust Y, Griscelli C. Deficit immunitaire mixtre et grave avec hypereosinophilie. Arch Fr Pediatr 42:11–16, 1985.

Le Deist F, Raffoux C, Griscelli C, Fischer A. Graft vs graft reaction resulting in the elimination of maternal cells in a SCID patient with maternofetal GVHD after an HLA identical bone marrow transplantation. J Immunol 138:423–427, 1987.

Lee GS, Neiditch MB, Sinden RR, Roth DB. Targeted transposition by the V(D)J recombinase. Mol Cell Biol 22:2068–2077, 2002.

Leu TMJ, Schatz DG. Rag-1 and Rag-2 are components of a high molecular–weight complex, and association of rag-2 with this complex is rag-1 dependent. Mol Cell Biol 15:5657–5670, 1995.

Lewis SM. The mechanisms of V(D)J joining: lessons from molecular, immunological, and comparative analyses. Adv Immunol 56:127–150, 1994.

Li L, Drayna D, Hu D, Hayward A, Gahagan S, Pabst H, Cowan MJ. The gene for severe combined immunodeficiency disease in Athabascan-speaking Native Americans is located on chromosome 10p. Am J Hum Genet 62:136–144, 1998.

Li L, Moshous D, Zhou Y, Wang J, Xie G, Salido E, Hu D, de Villartay JP, Cowan MJ. A founder mutation in Artemis, an SNM1-like protein, causes SCID in Athabascan-speaking Native Americans. J Immunol 168:6323–6329, 2002.

Liang HE, Hsu LY, Cado D, Cowell LG, Kelsoe G, Schlissel MS. The "dispensable" portion of RAG2 is necessary for efficient V-to-DJ rearrangement during B and T cell development. Immunity 17:639–651, 2002.

Lieber MR, Hesse JE, Mizuuchi K, Gellert M. Lymphoid V(D)J recombination: nucleotide insertion at signal joints as well as coding joints. Proc Natl Acad Sci USA 85:8588–8592, 1988.

Litman GW, Rast JP, Shamblott MJ, Haire RN, Hulst M, Roess W, Litman RT, Hinds-Frey KR, Zilch A, Amemiya CT. Phylogenetic diversification of immunglobulin genes and the antibody repertoire. Mol Biol Evol 10:60–72, 1993.

Livak F, Welsh SC, Guidos CJ, Crispe IN, Danska JS, Schatz DG. Transient restoration of gene rearrangement at a multiple T cell receptor loci in gamma-irradiated scid mice. J Exp Med 184:419–428, 1996.

Loechelt BJ, Shapiro RS, Jyonouchi H, Filipovich AH. Mismatched bone marrow transplantation for Omenn syndrome: a variant of severe combined immunodeficiency. Bone Marrow Transplant 16:381–385, 1995.

Ma Y, Pannicke U, Schwarz K, Lieber MR. Hairpin opening and overhang by an Artemis/DNA dependent protein kinase complex in nonhomologous end joining and VDJ recombination. Cell 108:781–784, 2002.

Malissen M, McCoy C, Blanc D, Trucy J, Devaux C, Schmitt-Verhulst AM, Fitch F, Hood L, Malissen B. Direct evidence for chromosomal inversion during T-cell receptor β-gene rearrangement. Nature 319:28–33, 1986.

Martin JV, Willoughby PB, Giusti V, Price G, Cerezo L. The lymph node pathology of Omenn's syndrome. Am J Surg Pathol 19:1082–1087, 1995.

McBlane JF, Van Gent DC, Ramsden DA, Romeo C, Cuomo CA, Gellert M, Oettinger MA. Cleavage at a V(D)J recombination signal requires only RAG1 and RAG2 proteins and occurs in two steps. Cell 83:387–395, 1996.

Mo X, Bailin T, Sadofsky MJ. A C-terminal region of RAG1 contacts the coding DNA during V(D)J recombination. Mol Cell Biol 21:2038–2047, 2001.

Mombaerts P, Iacomini J, Johnson RS, Herrup K, Tonegawa S, Papaioannou V. RAG-1 deficient mice have no mature B and T lymphocytes. Cell 68:869–877, 1992.

Morrison C, Smith GCM, Stingl L, Jackson SP, Wagner E, Wang ZQ. Genetic interaction between PARP and DNA-PK in V(D)J recombination and tumorigenesis. Nat Genet 17:479–482, 1997.

Moshous D, Callebaut I, de Chasseval R, Corneo B, Cavazzana-Calvo M, Le Deist F, Tezcan I, Sanal O, Bertrand Y, Philippe N, Fischer A, de Villartay JP. Artemis, a novel DNA double-strand break repair/V(D)J recombination protein, is mutated in human severe combined immune deficiency. Cell 105:177–186, 2001.

Moshous D, Li L, de Chasseval R, Philippe N, Jabado N, Cowan MJ, Fischer A, de Villartay JP. A new gene involved in DNA double-strand break repair and V(D)J recombination is located on human chromosome 10p. Hum Mol Genet 9:583–588, 2000.

Moshous D, Pannetier C, Chasseval Rd R, Deist Fl F, Cavazzana-Calvo M, Romana S, Macintyre E, Canioni D, Brousse N, Fischer A, Casanova JL,

Villartay JP. Partial T and B lymphocyte immunodeficiency and predisposition to lymphoma in patients with hypomorphic mutations in Artemis. J Clin Invest 111:381–387, 2003.

Nacht M, Strasser A, Chan YR, Harris AW, Schlissel M, Bronson RT, Jacks T. Mutations in the p53 and SCID genes cooperate in tumorigenesis. Genes Dev 10:2055–2066, 1996.

Nagaoka H, Yu W, Nussenzweig MC. Regulation of RAG expression in developing lymphocytes. Curr Opin Immunol 12:187–190, 2000.

Neiditch MB, Lee GS, Landree MA, Roth DB. RAG transposase can capture and commit to target DNA before or after donor cleavage. Mol Cell Biol 21:4302–4310, 2001.

Nemazee D. Receptor selection in B and T lymphocytes. Annu Rev Immunol 18:19–51, 2000.

Nicolas N, Finnie NJ, Cavazzana-Calvo M, Papadopoulo D, Le Deist F, Fischer A, Jackson SP, de Villartay JP. Lack of detectable defect in DNA double-strand break repair and DNA-dependant protein kinase activity in radiosesitive human severe combined immunodeficiency fibroblasts. Eur J Immunol 26:1118–1122, 1996.

Nicolas N, Moshous D, Papadopoulo D, Cavazzana-Calvo M, de Chasseval R, le Deist F, Fischer A, de Villartay JP. A human SCID condition with increased sensitivity to ionizing radiations and impaired V(D)J rearrangements defines a new DNA recombination/repair deficiency. J Exp Med 188:627–634, 1998.

Noordzij JG, de Bruin-Versteeg S, Verkaik NS, Vossen J, de Groot R, Bernatowska E, Langerak AW, van Gent DC, van Dogen JJM. The immunophenotypic and immunogenotypic B cell differentiation arrest in bone marrow of RAG deficient patients corresponds to residual recombination activities of mutated RAG proteins. Blood 100:2145–2152, 2002.

Noordzij JG, Verkaik NS, van der Burg M, van Veelen LR, de Bruin-Versteeg S, Wiegant W, Vossen JM, Weemaes CM, de Groot R, Zdzienicka MZ, van Gent DC, and van Dongen, JJ. Radiosensitive SCID patients with Artemis gene mutations show a complete B-cell differentiation arrest at the pre-B-cell receptor checkpoint in bone marrow. Blood 101:1446–1452, 2003.

Nussenzweig A, Chen C, da Costa Soares V, Sanchez M, Sokol K, Nussenzweig MC, Li GC. Requirement for Ku80 in growth and immunoglobulin V(D)J recombination. Nature 382:551–555, 1996.

Ochs HD, David SD, Michelson E, Lerner KG, Wedgwood RJ. Combined immunodeficiency and reticuloendotheliosis with eosinophilia. J Pediatr 85:463–465, 1974.

O'Driscoll M, Cerosaletti KM, Girard PM, Dai Y, Stumm M, Kysela B, Hirsch B, Gennery A, Palmer SE, Seidel J, Gatti RA, Varon R, Oettinger MA, Neitzel H, Jeggo PA, Concannon P. DNA ligase IV mutations identified in patients exhibiting developmental delay and immunodeficiency. Mol Cell 8:1175–1185, 2001.

O'Driscoll M, Ruiz-Perez VL, Woods CG, Jeggo PA, Goodship JA. A splicing mutation affecting expression of ataxia-telangiectasia and Rad3-related protein (ATR) results in Seckel syndrome. Nat Genet 33:497–501, 2003.

Oettinger MA, Schatz DG, Gorka C, Baltimore D. RAG-1 and RAG-2, adjacent genes that synergitically activate V(D)J recombination. Science 248:1517–1523, 1990.

Oettinger MA, Stanger B, Schatz DG, Glaser T, Call K, Housman D, Baltimore D. The recombination activating genes, RAG1 and RAG2, are on chromosome 11p in humans and chromosome 2p in mice. Immunogenetics 35:97–101, 1992.

Okazaki K, Davis DD, Sakano H. T cell receptor gene sequences in the circular DNA of thymocyte nuclei: direct evidence for intramolecular DNA deletion in V-D-J joining. Cell 49:477–485, 1987.

Omenn GS. Familial reticuloendotheliosis with eosinophilia. N Engl J Med 273:427–432, 1965.

Pirovano S, Mazzolari E, Pasic S, Albertini A, Notarangelo LD, Imberti L. Impaired thymic output and restricted T cell repertoire in two infants with immunodeficiency and early onset generalized dermatitis. Immunol Lett 86:93–97, 2003.

Pollack MS, Kirkpatrick D, Kapoor N, Dupont B, O'Reilly RJ. Identification by HLA typing of intrauterine-derived maternal T cells in four patients with severe combined immunodeficiency. N Engl J Med 307:662–666, 1982.

Ramsden DA, Baetz K, Wu GE. Conservation of sequence in recombination signal sequence spacers. Nucl Acids Res 22:1785–1796, 1994.

Riballo E, Critchlow SE, Teo SH, Doherty AJ, Priestley A, Broughton B, Kysela B, Beamish H, Plowman N, Arlett CF, Lehmann AR, Jackson SP, Jeggo PA. Identification of a defect in DNA ligase IV in a radiosensitive leukemia in patient. Curr Biol 699–702, 1999.

Riballo E, Doherty AJ, Dai Y, Stiff T, Oettinger MA, Jeggo PA, Kysela B. Cellular and biochemical impact of a mutation in DNA ligase IV conferring clinical radiosensitivity. J Biol Chem 276:31124–31132, 2001.

Rieux-Laucat F, Bahadoran P, Brousse N, Selz F, Fischer A, Le Deist F, de Villartay JP. Highly restricted human T-cell repertoire beta (TCRB) chain diversity in peripheral blood and tissue-infiltrating lymphocytes in Omenn's syndrome (severe combined immunodeficiency with hypereosinophilia). J Clin Invest 102:312–321, 1998.

Rodgers KK, Bu Z, Fleming KH, Schatz DG, Engelman DM, Coleman JE. A unique zinc-binding dimerization motif domain in RAG-1 includes the C3HC4 motif. J Mol Biol 260:70–84, 1996.

Rooney S, Alt FW, Lombard D, Whitlow S, Eckersdorff M, Fleming J, Fugmann S, Ferguson DO, Schatz DG, Sekiguchi J. Defective DNA repair and increased genomic instability in Artemis-deficient murine cells. J Exp Med 197:553–565, 2003.

Rooney S, Sekiguchi J, Zhu C, Cheng HL, Manis J, Whitlow S, DeVido J, Foy D, Chaudhuri J, Lombard D, Alt FW. Leaky Scid phenotype associated with defective V(D)J coding end processing in Artemis-deficient mice Mol Cell 10:1379–1390, 2002.

Sadofsky MJ, Hesse JE, Gellert M. Definition of a core region of RAG-2 that is functional in V(D)J recombination. Nucl Acids Res 22:1805–1809, 1994.

Sadofsky MJ, Hesse JE, McBlane JF, Gellert M. Expression and V(D)J recombination activity of mutated RAG-1 proteins. Nucl Acids Res 21:5644–5650, 1993.

Santagata S, Gomez CA, Sobacchi C, Bozzi F, Abinun M, Pasic S, Cortes P, Vezzoni P, Villa A. N-terminal RAG1 frameshift mutations in Omenn's syndrome: internal methionine usage leads to partial V(D)J recombination activity and reveals a fundamental role in vivo for the N-terminal domains. Proc Natl Acad Sci USA 97:14572–14577, 2000.

Schandene L, Ferster A, Mascart-Lemone F, Crusiaux A, Grard C, Marchant A, Lybin M, Velu T, Sariban E, Goldman M. T helper type 2-like cells and therapeutic effects of interferon-gamma in combined immunodeficiency with hypereosinophilia (Omenn's syndrome). Eur J Immunol 23:56–60, 1993.

Schatz DG, Oettinger MA, Baltimore D. The V(D)J recombination activating gene, RAG-1. Cell 59:1035–1048, 1989.

Schlissel MS, Stanhope-Baker P. Accessibility and the developmental regulation of V(D)J recombination. Semin Immunol 9:161–170, 1997.

Shockett PE, Schatz DG. DNA hairpin opening mediated by the RAG1 and RAG2 proteins. Mol Cell Biol 19:4159–4166, 1999.

Schofer O, Blaha I, Mannhardt W, Zepp F, Stallmach T, Spranger J. Omenn phenotype with short-limbed dwarfism. J Pediatr 118:86–89, 1991.

Schwarz K, Gaus GH, Ludwig L, Pannicke U, Li Z, Lindner D, Friedrich W, Seger RA, Hansen-Hagge TE, Desiderio S, Lieber MR, Bartram CR. RAG mutations in human B cell-negative SCID. Science 274:97–99, 1996.

Schwarz K, Hameister H, Gessler M, Grzeschik KH, Hansen-Hagge TE, Bartram CR. Confirmation of the localization of the human recombination activating gene 1 (RAG1) to chromosome 11p13. Hum Genet 93:215–217, 1994.

Schwarz K, Hansen-Hagge TE, Knobloch C, Friedrich W, Kleihauer E, Bartram CR. Severe combined immunodeficiency (SCID) in man: B-cell-negative (B) SCID patients exhibit an irregular recombination pattern at the JH locus. J Exp Med 174:1039–1048, 1991.

Shin EK, Perryman LE, Meek K. A kinase negative mutation of DNA-PKcs in equine SCID results in defective coding and signal joint formation. J Immunol 158:3565–3569, 1997.

Shinkai Y, Rathbun G, Lam K-P, Oltz EM, Stewart V, Mendelsohn M, Charron J, Datta M, Young F, Stall AM, Alt FW. RAG-2-deficient mice lack mature lymphocytes owing to inability to initiate V(D)J rearrangement. Cell 68:855–867, 1992.

Signorini S, Imberti L, Pirovano S, Villa A, Facchetti F, Ungari M, Bozzi F, Albertini A, Ugazio AG, Vezzoni P, Notarangelo LD. Intrathymic restriction and peripheral expansion of the T cell repertoire in Omenn syndrome. Blood 94:3468–3478, 1999.

Silver DP, Spanopoulou E, Mulligan RC, Baltimore D. Dispensable sequence motifs in the RAG-1 and RAG-2 genes for plasmid V(D)J recombination. Proc Natl Acad Sci USA 90:6100–6104, 1993.

Spanopoulou E, Zaitseva F, Wang F-H, Santagata S, Baltimore D, Panayotou G. The homeodomain region of RAG-1 reveals the parallel mechanisms of bacterial and V(D)J recombination. Cell 87:263–276, 1996.

Stephan JL, Vlekova V, Le Deist F, Blanche S, Donadieu J, De Saint Basile G, Durandy A, Griscelli C, Fischer A. Severe combined immunodeficiency: a retrospective single-center study of clinical presentation and outcome in 117 cases. J Pediatr 123:5047–5072, 1993.

Taccioli GE, Amatucci AG, Beamish HJ, Gell D, Xiang XH, Torres Arzayus MI, Priestley A, Jackson SP, Marshak Rothstein A, Jeggo PA, Herrera VL. Targeted disruption of the catalytic subunit of the DNA-PK gene in mice confers severe combined immunodeficiency and radiosensitivity. Immunity 9:355–366, 1998.

Teo SH, Jackson SP. Identification of *Saccharomyces cerevisiae* DNA ligase 4. Involvement in DNA double-strand break repair. EMBO 16:4788–4795, 1997.

Villa A, Notarangelo L, Macchi P, Mantuano E, Cavagni G, Brugnoni D, Strina D, Patrosso MC, Ramenghi U, Sacco MG, Ugazio A, Vezzoni P. X-linked thrombocytopenia and Wiskott-Aldrich syndrome are allelic diseases with mutations in the WASP gene. Nat Genet 9:414–417, 1995.

Villa A, Santagata S, Bozzi F, Frattini A, Imberti L, Benerini Gatta L, Ochs HD, Schwarz K, Notarangelo LD, Vezzoni P, Spanopoulou E. Partial V(D)J recombination activity leads to Omenn syndrome. Cell 93: 885–896, 1998.

Villa A, Sobacchi C, Notarangelo LD, Bozzi F, Abinun M, Abrahamsen TG. Arkwright PD, Baniyash M, Brooks EG, Conley ME, Cortes P, Duse M, Schwarz K. VDJ recombination defects in lymphocytes due to *RAG* mutations: severe immunodeficiency with a spectrum of clinical presentations. Blood 97:81–88, 2001.

Wada T, Takei K, Kudo M, Shimura S, Kasahara Y, Koizumi S, Kawa-Ha K, Ishida Y, Imashuku S, Seki H, Yachie A. Characterization of immune function and analysis of *RAG* gene mutations in Omenn syndrome and related disorders. Clin Exp Immunol 119:148–155, 2000.

West KL, Singha NC, De Ioannes P, Lacomis L, Erdjument-Bromage H, Tempst P, Cortes P. A direct interaction between the RAG2 C terminus and the core histones is required for efficient V(D)J recombination. Immunity 23:203–212, 2005.

Wienholds E, Schulte-Merker S, Walderich B, Plasterk RH. Target-selected inactivation of the zebrafish rag1 gene. Science 297:99–102, 2002.

Wilson TE, Grawunder U, Lieber MR. Yeast DNA ligase IV mediates nonhomologous DNA end joining. Nature 338:495–498, 1997.

Wirt DP, Brooks EG, Vaidya S, Klimpel GR, Waldmann TA, Goldblum RM. Novel T-lymphocyte population in combined immunodeficiency with features of graft-versus-host disease. N Engl J Med 321:370–374, 1989.

Yates F, Malassis-Seris M, Stockholm D, Bouneaud C, Larousserie F, Noguiez-Hellin P, Danos O, Kohn DB, Fischer A, de Villartay JP, Cavazzana-Calvo M. Gene therapy of RAG-2$^{-/-}$ mice: sustained correction of the immunodeficiency. Blood 3942–3949, 2002.

Yu W, Misulovin Z, Suh H, Hardy RR, Jankovic M, Yannoutsos N, Nussenzweig MC. Coordinate regulation of RAG1 and RAG2 by cell type–specific DNA elements 5′ of RAG2. Science 285:1080–1084, 1999.

Zarrin AA, Fong I, Malkin L, Marsden PA, Berinstein Nl. Cloning and characterization of the human recombination activating gene1 (RAG1) and RAG2 promoter regions. J Immunol 159:4382–4394, 1997.

Zhu C, Bogue MA, Lim DS, Hasty P, Roth DB. Ku86-deficient mice exhibit severe combined immunodeficiency and defective processing of V(D)J recombination intermediates. Cell 86:379–389, 1996.

12

Immunodeficiency Due to Defects of Purine Metabolism

ROCHELLE HIRSCHHORN and FABIO CANDOTTI

Genetic deficiency of the purine salvage enzyme adenosine deaminase (ADA) provides the molecular basis for approximately 40% of autosomal recessive cases of severe combined immunodeficiency (SCID) and therefore approximately 20% of all cases of SCID (Hirschhorn, 1979b; Bertrand et al., 1999; Buckley, 2000). The identification, over two decades ago, of deficiency of ADA as the basis for immunodeficiency (MIM #102700) was serendipitous and unexpected (Giblett et al., 1972). By contrast, immunodeficiency due to genetic deficiency of purine nucleoside phosphorylase (PNP), the next enzyme in the purine salvage pathway, was identified by specific screening for deficiency of enzymes in this pathway in immunodeficient patients (Giblett et al., 1975). PNP immunodeficiency (MIM +164050) is even rarer than ADA deficiency, having been reported in fewer than 30 unrelated families (Markert, 1991; Carpenter et al., 1996; Markert et al., 1997; Sasaki et al., 1998; Dalal et al., 2001; Baguette et al., 2002; Moallem et al., 2002; Tsuda et al., 2002; Tabarki et al., 2003; Grunebaum et al., 2004). Study of patients with these two disorders has shed light on the significance of the purine salvage pathway for lymphoid cells as well as on the potential for development of new antileukemic agents (Hirschhorn, 1993; Markert, 1994; Suetsugu et al., 1999; Hershfield and Mitchell, 2001; Dillman, 2004).

Both ADA and PNP are ubiquitous, "housekeeping" enzymes whose deficiency essentially results in "metabolic poisoning," with the most deleterious effects manifested in lymphoid cells. As a result, both are diseases characterized by increasing attrition in immune function over time and by blocks at specific steps of differentiation of lymphoid cells. Because the toxic metabolites that accumulate on account of the enzyme defect derive primarily from dying cells, it is not surprising that clinical histories, particularly of later-onset patients, are consistent with the hypothesis that each infection results in additional attrition of immune cells and function.

Since the first edition of this book, several important advances concerning ADA and PNP deficiency have been made that include both clinical and basic science of these disorders. ADA deficiency continues to be diagnosed in ~20% of patents with SCID and therefore in ~40% of autosomal recessive patients. Interestingly, however, only two novel mutations have been reported in recent years (Ariga et al., 2001a), suggesting that this disease may be inherited from a restricted number of ancestors or founders in the populations studied or that only specific locations of the ADA gene are susceptible to the effects of genetic mutations. Additional cases of reversion of inherited ADA mutations have been described (Hirschhorn et al., 1996; Ariga et al., 2001b), reflecting the recent observations of somatic mosaicism, due to in vivo reversion to normal, of inherited mutations in several different immunolgic and nonimmunologic disorders (reviewed in Hirschhorn, 2003). On the clinical side, renewed interest has been devoted to the pathophysiology of previously described neurologic findings (Hirschhorn et al., 1980a) and of more recently described sensorial and cognitive function of ADA-deficient patients who do not seem to respond to hematopoietic cell transplantation (Tanaka et al., 1996; Rogers et al., 2001; Albuquerque and Gaspar, 2004). The report of severe mental retardation without immunodeficiency resulting from genetic deficiency of S-adenosylhomocysteine (SAH) hydrolase (Baric et al., 2004) raises the possible role of the secondary decrease of SAH hydrolase found in ADA deficiency in bringing about neurologic abnormalities. Finally, from a therapeutic perspective, results of a recent European survey indicate that haploidentical transplantation off allogeneic bone marrow has a poor prognosis in ADA deficiency (~25% survival at 3 years after the procedure) (Antoine et al., 2003). These findings coincide with reports of the first true successes of gene therapy for ADA deficiency (Aiuti et al., 2002a).

In the PNP field, the high-resolution crystal structure of PNP has been recently determined, allowing a more precise analysis of the active site of the enzyme and generating a more reliable model for substrate binding and for the design of PNP inhibitors (de Azevedo et al., 2003). Another development is the generation of a PNP "null" mouse model that has provided a new hypothesis as to the possible biochemical mechanisms leading to immunodeficiency (Arpaia et al., 2000). Finally, recent clinical observations have reinforced the notion that PNP-deficient patients often present with marked neurodevelopmental delay that clearly precedes the onset of immunodeficiency (Baguette et al., 2002; Tsuda et al., 2002), thus suggesting particular vulnerability of the nervous to PNP deficiency.

Clinical and Pathologic Manifestations

ADA Deficiency—Clinical Spectrum of Immunodeficiency

Early-onset disease

The early descriptions of clinical and pathologic manifestations in ADA-deficient SCID patients were based on retrospective studies of children diagnosed as having classical SCID with marked developmental delay and failure to thrive (Meuwissen et al., 1975; Hirschhorn, 1979a). Because of the original means of identifying patients to be tested for ADA deficiency, over 95% of the initial cases were clinically and immunologically virtually indistinguishable from patients with other forms of classical SCID. These ADA-deficient patients had neonatal-onset disease with lymphopenia, absence of both cellular and humoral immune function, failure to thrive, and a rapidly fatal course due to infections with fungal, viral, and opportunistic agents (Meuwissen et al., 1975; Hirschhorn, 1979a). Many of these early-onset cases lacked B cells as well as T cells and would now be classified as T^-B^- SCID. However, in addition to immunological defects, a distinguishing feature in approximately 50% of this group of patients was a skeletal abnormality of the costochondral junctions, best visualized by X-ray on a lateral exposure of the chest as cupping and flaring, and having a unique histological appearance (Cederbaum et al., 1976). A small percentage of cases, including the first two cases described, exhibited a somewhat delayed onset of disease, with diagnosis as late as the second year of life. In such patients there was transient retention of the capability to produce autologous immunoglobulins, although both patients produced essentially no specific antibodies (Table 12.1).

Delayed and late-onset disease

It is now apparent that the clinical spectrum resulting from ADA deficiency is much broader than that of classical SCID. Testing for ADA deficiency in a range of individuals with abnormal immune function has already broadened the spectrum considerably, not only in age of onset but also in immunologic abnormality. Initially patients with somewhat delayed onset were recognized in the first 2 years of life to have retention of immunoglobulins, similar to the first two described patients. An increasing number of patients are now being described with late-onset ADA deficiency, diagnosed from 3 to 15 years of age and even in adulthood, rather than only during infancy (see Table 12.1) (Geffner et al., 1986; Morgan et al., 1987; Levy et al., 1988; Hirschhorn et al., 1993b, 1996; Shovlin et al., 1993; Ozsahin et al., 1997; Hershfield, 1998; Antony et al., 2002). These late-onset patients will have significant immunodeficiency, but variable clinical

Table 12.1. Clinical Phenotypes in ADA Deficiency

1. Neonatal/infantile onset—severe combined immunodeficiency	Clinically indistinguishable from other forms of SCID, except for bony abnormality in 50% of patients. Progressive attrition of immunity.
2. Delayed or late onset—combined immunodeficiency	May present with recurrent bacterial sinopulmonary infections; lymphopenia, hyper-IgE, eosinophilia, autoimmunity. May be diagnosed in adulthood because of persistent viral warts, herpes zoster, immune-mediated thrombocytopenic purpura, lymphopenia.
3. ADA deficiency without immunodeficiency ("partial")	Identification by population screening or analysis of relatives of affected individuals. No confirmed immunodeficiency to date
4. Somatic mosaicism ("de novo" or "revertant" mutations)	May show improvement over time without therapy, lower than expected metabolite levels and residual ADA enzyme activity

manifestations, including an initial clinical history of recurrent sinopulmonary bacterial infections, primarily pneumonia frequently due to *Streptococcus pneumoniae*, and septicemia. After infection or immunization these children typically fail to produce antibody to some antigens such as *S. pneumoniae* polysaccharides. They may lack IgG2, but have markedly elevated IgE and/or eosinophilia. Immune dysregulation may be manifested by autoimmunity including autoimmune hypothyroidism, diabetes mellitus, hemolytic anemia, and idiopathic thrombocytopenia. All patients have had lymphopenia.

Similar to the late-onset patients, the small number of adult patients who have been diagnosed with ADA deficiency have had variety of infections and autoimmune clinical presentations, including recurrent sinopulmonary bacterial infections, pneumonia and septicemia. Persistent viral warts, recurrent herpes zoster infections, asthma, autoimmune hypothyroidism, hemolytic anemia, and idiopathic thrombocytopenia have been described. Initial immunologic investigations have revealed absence of IgG2, failure to produce antibody to pnemococcal antigens, elevated IgE, eosinophilia, and autoantibodies. Diagnosis of ADA-deficient immunodeficiency states in adulthood can be complicated by effects of administration of immunosuppresive medications for autoimmune disorders. The autoimmune phenomena probably reflect abnormal regulation of immune responses, as described for other forms of immunodeficiency. In all three cases described, lymphopenia was present prior to diagnosis of immunodeficiency (Shovlin et al., 1993; Ozsahin et al., 1997).

The first described cases of ADA deficiency with immunodeficiency diagnosed in adulthood were in two siblings, who in retrospect had the onset of immunologic abnormalities during late adolescence (Shovlin et al., 1993; Antony et al., 2002) and had recalcitrant warts as a major manifestation. One the sibs died with severe lung disease in her late 30s, despite enzyme replacement therapy (PEG-ADA, see Treatment and Prognosis). The surviving sib improved substantially with PEG-ADA but then developed an antibody response to the enzyme sufficient to preclude continued therapy for control of the severe dermatologic manifestations. One additional patient was diagnosed at the age of 39 after a long history of multiple infections and leukopenia in childhood. In adult life she was well until septicemia followed a caesarian section. She also exhibited hepatic granulomas of unknown etiology and pulmonary tuberculosis as well as asthma and elevated IgE (Ozsahin et al., 1997).

It is likely that these adult patients with ADA defects constitute one subset of patients currently classified as common variable immunodeficiency (CVID, see Chapter 23), although a screening of 44 unselected CVID patients failed to identify any individuals with ADA or PNP deficiency (Fleischman et al., 1998), suggesting that ADA deficients do not comprise a large subset of CVID. Perhaps selection for such markers as early lymphopenia, hyper-IgE, eosinophilia, asthma, and persistent warts might be informative.

ADA deficiency with normal clinical phenotype ("Partial" ADA deficiency)

An additional group of individuals with absence of ADA activity in erythrocytes has been identified by screening of normal populations or among healthy relatives of affected patients. Most of these individuals were identified as newborns through a screening program directed at early detection of ADA-deficient SCID patients. These patients were initially termed "partially deficient" because while they showed absent ADA activity in red blood cells (RBCs), they retained 5%–80% of normal ADA enzyme activity in nonerythroid cells (Hirschhorn et al., 1979a, 1983, 1989, 1990, 1997; Borkowsky et al., 1980; Hirschhorn and Ellenbogen, 1986). These children had dATP levels only marginally elevated and insignificant relative to values observed in immunodeficient patients. Although these children were healthy in early childhood, and one subject (homozygous for Ala215Thr mutations) as late as 18 years of age, their eventual outcomes are unknown. One of these children, lost to follow-up, carried a partial mutation heterozygous with a "null" similar to that of adult-onset patients (Shovlin et al., 1993).

A number of healthy relatives in families with a proband with SCID were found to carry additional ADA mutations and to exhibit very low levels of ADA activity in blood cells (Ozsahin et al., 1997; Ariga et al., 2001a).

ADA Deficiency—Nonimmunologic Abnormalities

Several abnormalities have been described in only a few patients and therefore could reflect effects of infectious agents rather than primary defects due to ADA deficiency. These include renal and adrenal abnormalities, neurologic abnormalities similar to those seen in PNP deficiency (see below), pyloric stenosis, and hepatic disease (Hirschhorn, 1979a; Ratech et al., 1985, 1989; Bollinger et al., 1996; Hershfield and Mitchell, 2001; R. Hirschhorn, unpublished results). Abnormal platelet aggregation has also been described (Schwartz et al., 1978). Although it is difficult to prove that neurological abnormalities are not secondary to viral encephalitis, we have suggested that these abnormalities might reflect interaction of high concentrations of adenosine with known adenosine A1 receptors in nervous tissue. This hypothesis was based on our finding of amelioration of neurologic manifestations concomitant with therapeutic measures that resulted in a lowering of metabolites that otherwise accumulate in ADA deficiency (Hirschhorn et al., 1980a). Lymphoma, often associated with cells bearing Epstein-Barr virus (EBV) genomes, has occurred in several patients (see Pathology section, below).

Recent observations have demonstrated that ADA deficiency can frequently be accompanied by cognitive and behavioral abnormalities, as well as neurosensorial deafness, that appear not to be shared by patients affected with other forms of SCID (Tanaka et al., 1996; Rogers et al., 2001; Albuquerque and Gaspar, 2004).

PNP Deficiency—Clinical Spectrum of Immunodeficiency

Purine nucleoside phosphorylase deficiency is a rare combined immunodeficiency disorder with autosomal recessive inheritance. Although the most characteristic immune abnormality is a profound T cell defect, abnormal B cell function, including defective antibody production, is common and in part due to abnormal T cell help (Giblett et al., 1975; Markert, 1991; Hershfield and Mitchell, 2001). In some patients clinical findings are compatible with the diagnosis of SCID and most patients present with failure to thrive; lymph nodes are small, the thymus is absent, and splenomegaly may be present in those patients with autoimmune disease. Additional patients have been described who did not present with clinically apparent immunodeficiency until later in childhood (Fox et al., 1977). It has been estimated that approximately 4% of patients with symptoms of SCID have PNP deficiency (Markert, 1991).

To date, patients with PNP deficiency from approximately 30 families have been identified and reported (Markert, 1991; Andrews and Markert, 1992; Aust et al., 1992; Tam and Leshner, 1995; Broome et al., 1996; Carpenter et al., 1996; Pannicke et al., 1996; Banzhoff et al., 1997; Markert et al., 1997; Sasaki et al., 1998; Yamamoto et al., 1999; Classen et al., 2001; Dalal et al., 2001; Baguette et al., 2002; Moallem et al., 2002; Tsuda et al., 2002; Dror et al., 2004; Grunebaum et al., 2004). The most common presenting complaint to clinical immunologists and/or infectious disease specialists is recurrent infections of the upper and lower respiratory tract due to common bacterial pathogens, viruses, or opportunistic infections such as *Candida albicans* and *Pneumocystis jiroveci*. These infections usually begin during the first year of life; however, the onset of symptoms may vary, with patients reported to be asymptomatic, in rare instances, until several years of age. Infections most commonly observed include pneumonia, otitis media, sinusitis, and urinary tract infections, usually caused by common bacterial pathogens. However, because of the profound T cell abnormality, disseminated vaccinia as a result of small pox vaccination, disseminated varicella, and persistent herpes simplex infection have been severe or even fatal. One patient developed chronic meningoencephalitis due to echovirus infection (Markert, 1991), a complication more often seen in patients with X-linked agammaglobulinemia. One single case of fatal pneumonia due to *Pneumocystis jiroveci* and *Legionella* infection has been observed (McGinniss et al., 1985). In contrast, PNP-deficient patients receiving *Bacillus* Calmette-Guérin (BCG) immunization have not developed disseminated disease (Markert, 1991).

PNP Deficiency—Nonimmunologic Abnormalities

Neurologic abnormalities develop in more than one-half of PNP-deficient children, a complication rarely observed in other types of SCID. These neurologic problems include spastic diplegia or tetraparesis, ataxia, tremor, retarded motor development, hyper- or hypotonia, behavioral difficulties, and varying degrees of mental retardation (Markert, 1991). Neurologic deficits have been observed in some patients prior to the onset of infection. The association of SCID and nervous system manifestations strongly suggests the diagnosis of PNP deficiency. Autoimmunity is another common finding in PNP deficiency. Thirteen of 34 patients had one or more autoimmune disorders, including autoimmune hemolytic anemia, idiopathic thrombocytopenia, autoimmune neutropenia, lupus, and central nervous vasculitis (Markert, 1991; Carpenter et al., 1996). Four of those patients had developed lymphoma or lymphosarcoma and one had a pharyngeal tumor.

Pathology

Examination of tissues at autopsy has been reported only in ADA-deficient patients with early-onset "classical" SCID. Abnormalities in spleen, lymph nodes, gut, and thymus reflect primarily an absence of cells of the lymphoid system (Hirschhorn, 1979b; Ratech et al., 1985, 1989). Thymic pathology, examined by biopsy as well as autopsy, demonstrates an absent or small dysplastic organ with absent or sparse lymphocytes, as seen in most SCID and not specific for ADA deficiency. Although florid pathology in this group of patients is predominantly limited to the immune system, some nonlymphoid organs also show unusual features (Simmonds et al., 1978; Hirschhorn et al., 1982; Mills et al., 1982). Thus, approximately 50% of early-onset ADA-deficient SCID patients exhibit a radiologically detectable bony lesion accompanied by a histologic appearance unique to ADA deficiency (Cederbaum et al., 1976). While the lesion may be pathognomonic histologically, we have shown that the radiologic abnormality is not specific for ADA-deficient SCID and can be seen in other disorders as well (Hirschhorn et al., 1979b). Nonetheless, the correct diagnosis of ADA-deficient SCID has not infrequently been suggested by the characteristic appearance of flared costochondral junctions on routine chest X-ray, best appreciated on a lateral view, as well as by the physical finding of a "rachitic rosary." Abnormalities of renal function have been noted in some patients, and we have described an unusual mesangial sclerosis in autopsy material from six of eight patients (Ratech et al., 1985). Renal abnormalities have also been described in the murine model for ADA deficiency, suggesting that this abnormality is due to the disease itself. Additionally, we have described in these same patients an unusual form of adrenal cortical fibrosis. However, in view of the overwhelming and multiple infections in these children, the significance of the renal and adrenal lesions remains to be evaluated by comparison with autopsy material from SCID patients who were not ADA deficient. In a single patient with neonatal onset of disease, hepatic pathology, with early giant-cell transformation, enlarged foamy hepatocytes, and portal and lobular eosinophilic infiltrates, has been reported (Bollinger et al., 1996). Again, despite the exclusion of known pathogens, it is difficult to consider this abnormality a primary result of ADA deficiency since these striking abnormalities were not appreciated in autopsies of the above eight patients with similar disease onset.

Both histologic and clinical evidence for graft-vs.-host disease (GVHD) have been commonly reported at the time of diagnosis because of maternal T cell engraftment or the administration of unirradiated blood products containing human leukocyte antigen (HLA)-incompatible lymphocytes that attacked the patient's tissues. Graft-vs.-host reactions are fortunately now a rare complication of transfusions, but they can still be observed after transplantation therapy.

The characteristic finding at autopsy of PNP-deficient patients is the marked depletion of lymphoid tissues (Markert, 1991). The thymus is absent or small and contains poorly formed Hassall's corpuscles. Tonsils are atrophic and germinal centers cannot be identified. Lymph nodes lack paracortical regions. The spleen shows lymphocytic depletion in the perivascular sheaths. In contrast, plasma cells can be identified in spleen, lymph nodes, and in the lamina propria of the intestines. Anatomic abnormalities associated with the neurologic deficits have not been investigated.

Laboratory Findings

Immunological Findings

Immunodeficient individuals with ADA deficiency

Lymphopenia and attrition of immune function over time are the two findings common to all presentations of immunodeficiency due to ADA deficiency (Table 12.2). Lymphopenia as well as elevation of toxic metabolites, such as deoxy-ATP (dATP) in RBCs, is already present prenatally and at birth, as has been demonstrated in affected pregnancies of families with prior children with early-onset ADA deficiency (Hirschhorn et al., 1980b; Linch et al., 1984). In early-onset patients, there is essentially a complete absence of lymphocytes and of both cellular and humoral immune function. Isoagglutinins are generally absent; immunoglobulins, particularly IgA and IgM, are low to absent, although absence of IgG, and occasionally other isotypes, is not easily evaluated because of maternally derived IgG and variable amounts of immunoglobulins transiently produced in infants. Antibody responses to T-dependent antigens are severely depressed. In ADA-deficient patients with delayed presentation, B cells and antibodies may be found, but eventually all functional antibodies are lost, and an oligoclonal distribution of immunoglobulin may be detected. Abnormal laboratory results seen in autoimmune states are another feature of late-onset patients.

Immunodeficiency in individuals with PNP deficiency

Deficiency in PNP has a profound effect on T cell function. Most patients are severely lymphopenic (<500 lymphocytes/mm^3) with a markedly depressed T lymphocytes (1%–3% of lymphocytes). Mitogen-induced lymphocyte proliferation is also severely impaired, and lymphocytes from most patients respond poorly in mixed lymphocyte reaction. However, several patients with normal responses to mitogens during infancy have subsequently progressed to nonresponsiveness. Although early reports suggested that B cell function in PNP deficiency may be normal, more recent studies clearly demonstrated abnormal B cell function. In some patients, a decline in antibody production was observed over time. Isohemagglutinins may be present or absent. Two patients with PNP deficiency were immunized with the T cell–dependent antigen, bacteriophage ΦX174, and responded with markedly depressed antibody titers, poor amplification, and complete inability to switch from IgM to IgG, a response that is almost identical to that of patients with ADA deficiency. These abnormal responses, characteristic for defective T and B cell interaction, are very similar to those observed in patients with X-linked hyper-IgM syndrome, whose defect is due to a primary T cell abnormality (Nonoyama et al., 1993). A possible explanation for a predominant T cell defect in PNP deficiency is discussed below. However, an intrinsic defect in B cell function has not been excluded.

Table 12.2. Commonly Found Abnormalities in Laboratory Tests of ADA-Deficient Individuals with Immunodeficiency

	Clinical Presentation Subtype		
Test	*Infantile Onset*	*Late Onset*	*Adult Onset*
ADA Enzyme Activity			
In erythrocytes	<1%	<1%	≤1%
In lymphocytes	0.5%	0.5%–3%	3%–?%
SAH hydrolase, erythrocytes	10%	10%	?
*Metabolites**			
Erythrocyte dATP[†]	327–2248	174–247	100–150
Lymphocyte dATP[‡]	1150	?	?
Urinary dAdo**	442–1500	54–270	
Urinary Ado**			
Plasma dAdo (μM)	0.6–2		
Plasma Ado (μM)	1–6		
Immunologic Tests			
Lymphopenia	++++	++	++
CD3 lymphocytes	Absent to trace	Markedly diminished	Markedly diminished
CD4/CD8 ratio	Too few cells to test	Often reversed	Reversed
Eosinophilia	Rare	Frequent	Frequent
Proliferation to PHA	Absent to markedly reduced	Absent to markedly reduced	Absent to markedly reduced
MLR	Reduced		
Antigen response	Absent to trace	Trace	Trace
Immunoglobulins	Maternal IgG	Low to absent (IgG2)	Normal; (low IgG2)
Specific antibody responses	Absent	Absent to very low	?
High IgE	Not reported	Frequent	Frequent
Infections	Predominantly viral, fungal, and opportunistic; also bacterial sepsis	Increasing proportion of bacterial sinopulmonary	Bacterial sinopulmonary; herpes zoster, herpes simplex; candida
Other clinical abnormalities	50% costochondral junction abnormality	Autoimmunity; possibly increased asthma incidence	Autoimmunity; possibly increased asthma incidence

Ado, adenosine; dAdo, deoxyadenosine; dATP, deoxyadenosine triphosphate; MLR, mixed lymphocyte reaction; PHA, phytohemagglutinin.

*Metabolite concentrations are based on R. Hirschhorn (published and unpublished data; see references in Hirschhorn et al., 1997, and Morgan et al., 1987).

[†]nmol/ml packed erythrocytes.

[‡]pmol/10[6] cells (Hirschhorn et al., 1992).

**nmol/g creatinine.

Biochemical Findings

Protein expression and enzymatic activity

Adenosine deaminase enzyme activity in cells from patients with classic ADA-deficient SCID is essentially undetectable (Table 12.2). The reported activity must take into account the minor activity of a nonrelevant isozyme that exhibits ADA activity but is encoded by another genetic locus not affected in ADA-deficient SCID (Hirschhorn and Ratech, 1980; see Biochemistry of ADA, below). Late-onset patients may retain 2%–5% of normal activity, with the highest residual activity reported in subjects with adult-onset disease (Shovlin et al., 1993). In most patients, ADA protein, assessed with anti-ADA antibodies, has been undetectable, a finding suggesting that most *ADA* gene mutations result in no protein production or unstable proteins (Wiginton and Hutton, 1982; Arredondo-Vega et al., 2001; Otsu et al., 2002). However, it is possible that the antibodies used did not recognize some mutant proteins.

Our own unpublished experiments using quantitative immunoprecipitation with a polyclonal antibody and a series of mutants did detect protein in quantities proportional to the relative enzyme activity. One patient originally reported to have normal protein for the amount of enzyme activity seen was demonstrated to be a somatic mosaic, with some cells expressing normal ADA (Hirschhorn, 1994b; see Molecular Biology of ADA, below).

As mentioned above, partially ADA-deficient individuals lack ADA activity in erythrocytes but express 5%–80% normal activity in nonerythroid cells, such as cultured EBV-transformed lymphoid cells. These individuals were ascertained as a result of population screening undertaken in both normal adults and newborns (Hirschhorn, 1979b, 1990). They have been designated partial ADA deficients and have not presented with immunodeficiency. However, one of the same mutations that expresses approximately 5% of normal activity has recently been identified in patients with adult-onset immunodeficiency. This finding suggests that some of the mutations present in partially ADA deficients may not be benign when heteroallelic with a mutation that totally abolishes activity (see Genotype–Phenotype Correlations, below).

Enzymatic activity of PNP in RBC lysates of affected patients is universally absent. Immunoreactive protein, measured by Western blot analysis, may be present or absent. In one family, the mutant protein could not be demonstrated in the patient's cells but was present in both consanguineous parents; thus the mutated protein may be unstable (Osborne et al., 1977; Gudas et al., 1978).

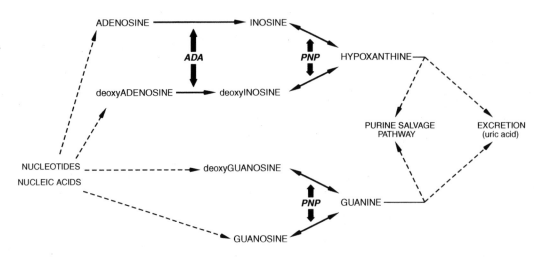

Figure 12.1. Schematic representation of adenosine deaminase (ADA) and purine nucleoside phospho-rylase (PNP) metabolic pathways.

Metabolic consequences of ADA and PNP deficiency

Adenosine deaminase is an enzyme of the purine salvage pathway that catalyzes the deamination of adenosine and 2-deoxyadenosine, as well as several naturally occurring methylated adenosine compounds (Hirschhorn and Ratech, 1980; Ratech et al., 1981, 1982). The deamination of adenosine and deoxyadenosine gives rise to inosine and to deoxyinosine, respectively (Fig. 12.1). These compounds can be further converted into hypoxanthine and then either enter a nonreversible pathway to uric acid in humans or, by the initial action of hypoxanthine phosphoribosyl transferase (HPRT), are salvaged back from hypoxanthine into other purines. The absence of ADA would be expected to result in diminution of the products of the reaction, inosine and 2-deoxyinosine. However, the presence of alternative "bypass" pathways apparently results in normal concentrations of these two products of the enzyme reaction in patients with ADA deficiency and, in contrast to PNP deficiency, in normal concentrations of uric acid, the final product of the pathway. Conversely, the absence of the enzyme would be expected to result in accumulation of the substrates adenosine and 2-deoxyadenosine. Not only are these substrates found in increased amounts in plasma and urine, but they also "spill over" into additional pathways that are normally only minimally used (Cohen et al., 1978; Coleman

et al., 1978; Kuttesch et al., 1978; Simmonds et al., 1978, 1982; Hirschhorn et al., 1981, 1982; Mills et al., 1982; Morgan et al., 1987; Fairbanks et al., 1994).

Deoxyadenosine is a component of DNA and primarily derives from the breakdown of DNA (Fig. 12.1 and 12.2). Therefore, deoxyadenosine would be expected to be in highest concentrations at sites of cell death, such as the thymus, where lymphocytes undergo apoptotic death during the course of differentiation and selection. Adenosine is a component of adenine nucleotides including ATP and RNA, and can be made both from the normal intracellular breakdown of ATP and from degradation of RNA following cell death. Both adenosine and deoxyadenosine are normally present in plasma with normal concentrations of approximately $1\,\mu M$ for adenosine and $0.5\,\mu M$ for deoxyadenosine.

In patients with ADA-deficient SCID, there are elevated concentrations of adenosine and deoxyadenosine in plasma ($1–6\,\mu M$ for adenosine and $1\,\mu M$ for deoxyadenosine). The actual concentrations in plasma are difficult to determine by ordinary procedures, as both compounds are almost instantaneously taken up by erythrocytes during drawing of a blood sample and are trapped intracellularly by phosphorylation. The most striking alteration in ADA deficiency is the accumulation of massive amounts of dATP in erythrocytes and lymphocytes (Hirschhorn et al., 1992). This results from uptake of the increased deoxyadenosine present in

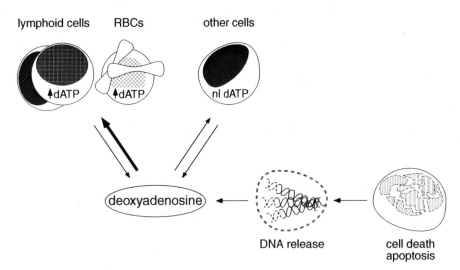

Figure 12.2. Adenosine deaminase deficiency: cellular and metabolic interactions. RBCs, red blood cells.

surrounding body fluids with subsequent intracellular phosphorylation and trapping. In cases with the most marked accumulation of dATP, ATP concentrations fall. The accumulation of dATP in a particular cell type or tissue is dependent on the rate of phosphorylation vs. the rate of dephosphorylation. There has been only one published study of dATP in additional tissues (in a patient dying with lymphoma and previously treated with partial exchange transfusions). This study of heart, brain, liver, and spleen reported only modest elevations in dATP (recalculated as 2–20 vs. the 500–2000 found in RBCs; Coleman et al., 1985). Surprisingly, among several nonlymphoid tissues examined, massive accumulation of phosphorylated deoxyadenosine was found only in the kidney (R. Hirschhorn, unpublished studies).

Patients with ADA deficiency additionally show a massive increase in excretion of deoxyadenosine in urine, where it is normally undetectable. By comparison, excretion of adenosine is only minimally elevated over that found in normal individuals. Several naturally occurring methylated adenosine compounds that are substrates for ADA are also excreted in urine in increased amounts in ADA-deficient individuals (Hirschhorn et al., 1982).

The increased concentrations of deoxyadenosine also inactivate SAH hydrolase, resulting in a secondary deficiency of that enzyme activity in erythrocytes (Hershfield et al., 1979; Hershfield and Mitchell, 2001). Normalization of SAH hydrolase activity appears to be the most sensitive indicator of normalization of metabolite concentrations (see Treatment and Prognosis, below). Although several other alterations in metabolites have been proposed, on the basis of in vitro investigations of proposed pathophysiologic mechanisms, none of these additional alterations has been demonstrated in vivo.

In general, adenosine metabolite concentrations correlate with severity of disease. In partially ADA-deficient individuals who are healthy, metabolite concentrations are on average greater than normal but markedly lower than those found in immunodeficient patients. Red blood cell dATP in partially deficient subjects ranges from 5 to 40 nmol/ml, compared to 25-fold increased in adult-onset patients and over 1000 fold-increased concentrations in infantile-onset patients (Table 12.2) (Hirschhorn et al., 1982, 1997). Deoxyadenosine excretion parallels concentrations of dATP, whereas adenosine concentration in urine is a poor discriminator between different types of individuals (R. Hirschhorn, unpublished results).

Different therapeutic maneuvers lower the concentrations of metabolites to differing degrees. Following bone marrow transplantation, metabolites in red cells, plasma, and urine are dramatically decreased. However, sensitive measurements indicate that metabolites are still elevated compared to normal, and in particular that plasma adenosine remains very high. Whether this is influenced by the bone marrow donor being a carrier or homozygous normal for the disorder is unknown. Metabolite concentrations following polyethylene glycol (PEG)-ADA therapy (see Treatment and Prognosis) are lower with respect to dATP in red cells than seen following bone marrow transplantation or vigorous partial-exchange transfusion (Hirschhorn et al., 1980a, 1981). It is not surprising that adenosine concentrations are less diminished since the affinity of ADA is greater for deoxyadenosine than for adenosine.

Purine nucleoside phosphorylase catalyzes the reversible phosphorylation of inosine, deoxyinosine, guanosine, and deoxyguanosine to their respective bases plus deoxyribose-1-phosphate (Fig. 12.1). The purine bases hypoxanthine and guanine may then be recycled by the action of HPRT to inosine monophosphate (IMP) and guanosine monophosphate (GMP), respectively, or excreted

as uric acid by the action of xanthine oxidase. The reverse reaction is not likely to occur in vivo because of the low levels of deoxyribose-1-phosphate and the rapid metabolism of the bases hypoxanthine and guanine by HPRT. PNP deficiency results in accumulation of its substrates with high serum levels of inosine and guanosine, and high urinary excretion of inosine, deoxyinosine, guanosine, and deoxyguanosine (Hershfield and Mitchell, 2001). These findings are accompanied by low serum and urinary levels of uric acid.

Biochemical and Pathophysiology Basis

Biochemistry of ADA

Adenosine deaminase (EC 3.5.4.4) is an enzyme of the purine salvage pathway that catalyzes the irreversible deamination of adenosine and, perhaps more significantly, deoxyadenosine, to inosine and deoxyinosine, respectively. The enzyme is an ubiquitous "housekeeping" enzyme that exists as a 40 kDa monomer predominantly in the cytoplasm (Daddona and Kelley, 1977; Schrader and Stacy, 1977). A small proportion of the enzyme is present on the surface of fibroblasts, T lymphocytes, and probably most cells, as a dimer complexed to two molecules of a combining protein, now identified as CD26 in T lymphocytes (Nishihara et al., 1973; Hirschhorn, 1975; Kameoka et al., 1993). It is hypothesized that ADA on the cell surface serves to regulate local concentrations of adenosine and thus engagement of the various cellular stimulatory and inhibitory adenosine receptors. ADA is also genetically polymorphic, with two common biochemical variants, or allozymes, segregating in the normal population (Spencer et al., 1968).

Although ADA is present in all cell types, enzyme activity differs considerably in different tissues. The highest amounts in humans are found in lymphoid tissues, particularly intrathymic immature T cells, as well as the brain and gastrointestinal tract, whereas the lowest activity is seen in erythrocytes (Hirschhorn et al., 1978). In lymphoid cells, enzyme activity declines with maturation of T cells but is higher in peripheral blood T cells than in B cells (Tung et al., 1976). In addition to the ADA encoded on chromosome 20 and deficient in ADA deficiency, there is an additional isozyme of ADA that accounts for 1–2% of total ADA activity but that deaminates adenosine only at higher than physiologic concentrations and is not inhibited by EHNA, an inhibitor of the major ADA isozyme (Daddona, 1981).

Murine ADA has been crystallized, and areas of evolutionary conservation from *E. coli* to humans have been identified (Chang et al., 1991; Wilson et al., 1991; Sharff et al., 1992; Wilson and Quiocho, 1993). The enzyme is composed of a motif of eight β-pleated sheets alternating with eight α helices. There are also five clearly defined additional α helices, three following the first β sheet, and the fourth and fifth following the last β sheet. The β sheets form a barrel shape surrounding the catalytic site which lies at the carboxyl end of the barrel. There is a zinc ion coordinately bound at the bottom of the β barrel, under the substrate-binding site. The unexpected presence of zinc within the catalytic pocket of ADA and other enzymes of the purine and pyrimidine salvage pathways could potentially illuminate the immunodeficiency associated with zinc deficiency. Several amino acids have been identified that are significant for binding of zinc and for catalysis. The precise mechanism of catalysis is under investigation by analysis of effect of mutations as measured by various parameters, including crystallography (Bhaumik et al., 1993; Ibrahim et al., 1995; Mohamedali et al., 1996; Sideraki et al., 1996).

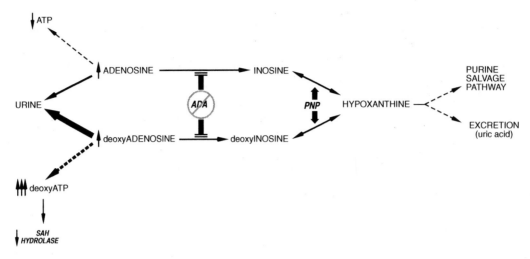

Figure 12.3. Metabolic consequences of enzyme deficiency found in adenosine deaminase-deficient patients.

Proposed Mechanisms for ADA Deficiency

Although much is known about the biochemistry of ADA, the mechanism(s) whereby deficiency of a ubiquitous enzyme results in predominantly lymphospecific pathology remains an area of investigation (reviewed in Hirschhorn, 1993; Benveniste and Cohen, 1995; Sekhsaria et al., 1996; Hershfield and Mitchell, 2001). On the basis of metabolic consequences of ADA deficiency (Fig. 12.3), several pathophysiologic mechanisms have been proposed and supported by in vivo or in vitro findings (Table 12.3). Deoxy ATP is known to be a feedback inhibitor of ribonucleotide reductase, an enzyme required for normal DNA synthesis. The observed marked elevation of dATP could explain the lack of lymphocyte proliferation required for further differentiation to mature cells. The lymphospecific toxicity has been explained by in vitro studies showing that in lymphocytes, and particularly immature T cells, the pathway for phosphorylation of deoxyadenosine is more active than the reverse pathway leading to dephosphorylation; this results in intracellular trapping of the phosphorylated compound. However, while this simplistic explanation is easily remembered and therefore attractive, more recent observations suggest that preferential trapping of dATP is more closely correlated with maturity of lymphoid cells than subtype, which is further supported by the greater sensitivity of chronic lymphocytic leukemia cells and hairy cell leukemia cells

(both usually derived from B cells) to ADA inhibitors or toxic adenosine analogues (Dillman, 2004).

An additional mechanism is suggested by the finding of marked diminution of SAH hydrolase activity. Deoxyadenosine irreversibly inactivates SAH hydrolase; markedly reduced activity of this enzyme is found in untreated ADA-deficient children. In vitro, this has been shown to result in accumulation of the substrate S-adenosylhomocysteine. Elevated concentrations of SAH result in feedback inhibition of the conversion of S-adenosylmethionine to S-adenosylhomocysteine and therefore prevent the transfer of methyl groups required for virtually all essential methylation reactions. The role of SAH hydrolase inactivation in the pathogenesis of the clinical findings in ADA deficiency remains to be determined. Interestingly, genetic deficiency of SAH hydrolase is not associated with any immune abnormalities, but with profound psychomotor delay, hypotonia, and defects of myelination (Baric et al., 2004).

Elevation of SAH has not been demonstrated in vivo in ADA-deficient patients, and inhibition of SAH hydrolase is still found in bone marrow–transplanted children who have normal immune function. However, administration of deoxycoformycin, a known inhibitor of ADA, to patients with leukemia was accompanied by elevations of SAH in vivo. The significance of this observation for patients with ADA deficiency is difficult to evaluate for several reasons. Deoxycoformycin also inhibits at least one other relevant enzyme, AMP deaminase, and the elevations of deoxyadenosine resulting from death of malignant cells in the presence of ADA inhibition (and of uric acid) far exceeded that observed in any SCID patients. No explanation for this mechanism leading to lymphospecific toxicity has been advanced.

Elevation of cyclic AMP, known to inhibit lymphocyte function, has also been demonstrated in lymphocytes in vitro but not in vivo. A proposed mechanism, inhibition of pyrimidine biosynthesis by elevation of ATP, can no longer be supported because, in fact, decreased rather than increased ATP is found in SCID patients with the most marked elevations of dATP (the original report of elevated ATP used an assay that measured dATP as well as ATP). Additional pathophysiological mechanisms have been proposed on the basis of in vitro observations (e.g., activation of ATP catabolism by deoxyadenosine and interference with terminal transferase by dATP), which, however, have not yet found confirmation in vivo. In summary, while the bulk of data support dATP as an important toxic metabolite, several in vitro observations

Table 12.3. Proposed Pathophysiologic Mechanisms

Elevated deoxy ATP	Inhibition of ribonucleotide reductase (required for DNA synthesis) and block of DNA replication
Elevated deoxyadenosine	Inhibition of DNA repair, leading to chromosome breakage. Induction of apoptosis
Elevated adenosine	Interaction with adenosine receptors. Induction of apoptosis
Inhibition of SAH hydrolase	Inhibition of methylation reactions (may play a role in neurologic changes and not in immunodeficiency, based on phenotype of SAH hydrolase–deficient humans)

SAH, S-adenosylhomocysteine.

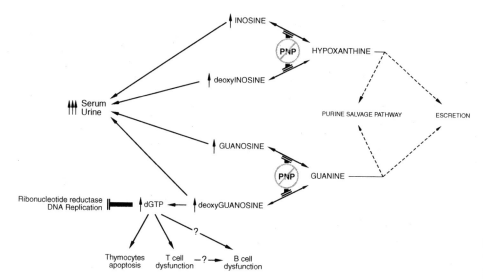

Figure 12.4. Metabolic and proposed cellular consequences of purine nucleoside phosphorylase (PNP) deficiency.

remain unexplained. It is likely that additional mechanisms are operative. However, all pathophysiologic mechanisms in ADA deficiency result from the presence of increased concentrations of substrates of ADA. These concentrations are particularly high in tissues, within which lymphoid cells normally undergo division and apoptosis, such as the thymus and infected or inflamed tissues. Deoxyadenosine has been reported to result in chromosome breakage and to induce apoptosis in immature thymic lymphocytes by a pathway found after DNA breakage, requiring expression of p53 and reversible by overexpression of Bcl-1. These studies correlate with the relatively high expression of p53 and low expression of Bcl-1 in immature intrathymic lymphocytes and suggest that the major block in lymphocyte differentiation resulting from ADA deficiency is intrathymic (Benveniste and Cohen, 1995). However granulocytemonoeyte–colony stimulating factor (G-CSF)–stimulated recovery of CD34[+] hematopoietic progenitors is lower in ADA-deficient patients than in normal individuals, a finding suggesting that there is also a block at an earlier stage (Sekhsaria et al., 1996).

Biochemistry of PNP

Human PNP is a trimer with a molecular weight of about 90 kDa (Osborne, 1980; Markert, 1991). The three-dimensional structure of human red cell PNP was resolved at 3.2 Å (Ealick et al., 1990) and confirmed a trimeric structure for the native enzyme. A motivation for determining the crystallographic structure of PNP was to provide a tool for computer-assisted design inhibitors of PNP (Ealick et al., 1991, 1993) for the selective abrogation of T cell function in vivo. Several groups have synthesized high-affinity inhibitors of PNP (Sircar et al., 1987; Ealick et al., 1993). By simulating the enzyme deficiency, PNP inhibitors may selectively depress T cell function to prevent allograft rejection or treat leukemia. Inhibition of PNP in rats correlated with increased levels of deoxyguanosine triphosphate (dGTP) selectively in proliferating thymocytes (Osborne and Barton, 1986). In dogs, inhibition of PNP prevented rejection of allogeneic platelets and appeared to induce tolerance (Osborne et al., 1986). The recent determination of high-resolution crystal structure (2.3 Å) provides a more reliable model for substrate binding and thus for designing PNP inhibitor molecules (de Azevedo et al., 2003).

PNP activity of RBC lysates can be estimated radiochemically or spectrophotometrically at 292 nm with coupled conversion of inosine to uric acid in the presence of xanthine oxidase (Osborne, 1980; Chu et al., 1989; Hershfield and Mitchell, 2001). Through this assay, the mean normal erythrocyte PNP activity has been determined to be 18.6 U/ml packed red cells. An estimation of the quantity of PNP protein can be obtained by Western blotting. Other readily available cell types for enzyme analysis include peripheral blood lymphocytes, EBV-induced B lymphoblastoid cell lines, and fibroblasts.

Proposed Mechanisms for PNP Deficiency

In inherited PNP deficiency, PNP substrates, which are normally low or undetectable, accumulate in the plasma and are excreted in the urine (Rich et al., 1980). DeoxyGTP has been found in patients' RBCs, in contrast to normal cells, where it is not measurable (Cohen et al., 1978).

Pathogenic mechanisms proposed in PNP deficiency (Fig. 12.4) have focused on the nucleoside substrates that accumulate, implicating either the nucleosides themselves or their metabolic products (Hershfield and Mitchell, 2001). Of the four PNP substrates that accumulate in PNP deficiency, deoxyguanosine and, to a lesser extent, guanosine, are toxic to cultured lymphoid cells (Chen et al., 1979; Henderson et al., 1980; Hershfield and Mitchell, 2001). Human lymphoblastoid cell lines with T cell characteristics are particularly sensitive to deoxyguanosine. At low micromolar concentrations of deoxyguanosine (e.g., 1 μM), ^{3}H-thymidine and ^{3}H-leucine incorporation into T-cell lines is markedly decreased, and at concentrations of 10 μM, no cell growth occurs and 50% of the cells are killed. Growth and incorporation of ^{3}H-thymidine and ^{3}H-leucine are decreased at higher deoxyguanosine concentrations in human B cell lines. Patients with PNP deficiency accumulate deoxyguanosine at levels that adversely affect dividing T lymphocytes. The extreme sensitivity of the T lymphoblasts and relative resistance of B lymphoblasts to the toxicity of deoxyguanosine may explain the selective loss of T cell function over time and the relatively mild effect on B cell function in patients with PNP deficiency (Ochs et al., 1979).

In support of this mechanism, virtually all cell types, including lymphocytes, exhibit facilitated nucleoside transport with a broad specificity (Plagemann et al., 1988). Inside the cell, deoxynucleosides are subject to enzymes with kinase activity to produce monophosphate metabolites. Once phosphorylated to deoxynucleoside monophosphate (dNMP), the nucleotide is effectively trapped in the cell, if the pathway to dNDP and dNTP formation is more active than the catabolic pathway mediated by nucleotidase to reform nucleosides. Because lymphocytes possess high deoxynucleoside kinase activity toward purine and pyrimidine deoxynucleosides (Barton and Osborne, 1986; Osborne, 1986), nucleotide formation is favored. Furthermore, deoxyguanosine kinase activity is higher in T cells than in B cells, consistent with the predominant T lymphocyte defect in PNP deficiency (Osborne, 1986; Osborne and Scott, 1983). This can result in accumulation of dGTP, which in turn will inhibit ribonucleotide reductase, the enzyme responsible for the production of a balanced supply of DNA precursors (Thelander and Reichard, 1979). There may be other mechanisms contributing to the lymphopenia in PNP deficiency, and the focus on ribonucleotide reductase inactivation may be overly simplistic (Hershfield and Mitchell, 2001).

Molecular Biology

Molecular Organization of the ADA Gene

The human *ADA* gene (MIM*608958) is localized on the long arm of chromosome 20 at 20q12–q13.1. Both the cDNA and the genomic DNA have been isolated and analyzed (Daddona et al., 1984; Wiginton et al., 1984, 1986; Valerio et al., 1984, 1985; Aronow et al., 1995). The cDNA for human ADA contains a coding region of 1089 nucleotides, including the initiation methionine codon ATG, and predicting a polypeptide of 363 amino acids with a calculated molecular weight of 40,638 Daltons. The *ADA* cDNA is contained in 12 exons within 32,040 nucleotides of genomic DNA, from the major cap site at position 95 from the ATG to the polyadenylation site. The first 230 bp upstream of the coding region are sufficient to promote expression of the *ADA* cDNA, as tested by DNA-mediated gene transfer of a minigene construct. The promoter is of the GC-rich type with binding sites for Sp1, now recognized in many housekeeping genes, and lacks obvious CAAT or TATA boxes. Additional regulatory sequences are present in the large (15 kb) first intron, including an enhancer responsible for high expression in T cells. Studies with transgenic mice indicate that sequences controlling differences in tissue expression are contained in the first intron, with enhancer elements and elements directing high expression in T lymphocytes as well as an element responsive to the transcription activator cMyb (Aronow et al., 1995). The seventh intron is very small and appears to be unspliced in a small, but detectable, portion of *ADA* mRNA in normals. The gene is very rich in repetitive sequences of the Alu type; 23 copies of Alu account for 1890 of the total genomic sequence. Seventeen Alu repeats are in the first two introns, with three additional Alu repeats in the 5′ upstream region. Alu repeats throughout the genome are known to be sites for gene deletions and duplications resulting from misalignment when homologous chromosomes pair during meiosis followed by unequal recombination. Alu repeats have been shown to be involved in causing deletions in the *ADA* gene (see below).

Mutation Analysis of ADA

The types and variety of mutations are not the same in all genetic diseases (see Chapter 2). The predominant mutations seen can vary at different genetic loci or with differing phenotypes at the same locus. Moreover, at different genetic loci there can be many different mutations or a few major mutations causing the majority of the disease cases. Finally, even when there are multiple different mutations, a particular population or ethnic group may demonstrate only a few of them.

Mutations in immunodeficient patients

In ADA deficiency there are multiple different mutations, but some are more common than others and have been found in unrelated individuals (Fig. 12.5). Several of the more common mutations share ancestral origins, whereas others represent independent recurrences of mutation at "hot spots" within the *ADA* gene. In the initial cases reported, there was a predominance of single base-pair changes resulting in amino acid substitutions, or missense mutations, at mutational hot spots. In late-onset patients, there appears to be an increased incidence of splice-site mutations. There is also an increasing number of recognized small deletions and insertions, as the methods of ADA patient diagnosis have turned to examination of genomic DNA sequence. Some ethnic concentrations of particular mutations appear to be emerging.

Over 50 deleterious mutations have been identified in ADA-deficient immunodeficient patients. An additional 11 "partial" mutations have been identified. Table 12.4 lists published mutations, and Table 12.5 indicates mutations found in multiple unrelated patients by the Hirschhorn laboratory. Additional mutations have been identified, but are not yet published from this laboratory, and not all reported mutations have been seen in this laboratory. Approximately two-thirds of the deleterious mutations have been reported by the Hershfield group (Duke University Medical Center). With respect to type of mutation, most of the clearly deleterious mutations (31) are missense mutations, followed by 10 splice-site mutations, 9 deletions or insertions, and 4 nonsense mutations. The missense mutations appear to be concentrated in exons 4, 5, and 7, regions known to encode amino acids involved in substrate binding or catalysis. Despite the multiplicity of mutations, 12 mutations account for almost two-thirds of

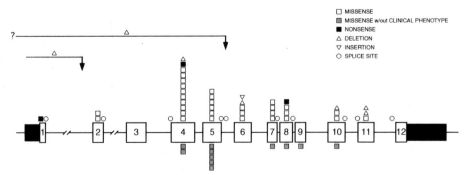

Figure 12.5. Mutations at the adenosine deaminase (ADA) locus.

Table 12.4. Mutations at the Adenosine Deaminase (ADA) Locus

Effect	Site	nt Change	ATG/Cap Site	Reference
A. Missense Mutations				
1. In immunodeficient patients				
His15Asp	Exon 2	CAT-GAT	43/138	Santisteban et al., 1995a
Gly20Arg	Exon 2	GGA-AGA	58/153	Yang et al., 1994
Gly74Cys	Exon 4	GGC-TGC	220/315	Arrendondo-Vega et al., 1998
Gly74Val	Exon 4	GGC-GTC	221/316	Bollinger et al., 1996
Gly74Asp	Exon 4	GGC-GAC	221/316	Ariga et al., 2001a
Ala83Asp	Exon 4	GCC-GAC	248/343	Santisteban et al., 1995a
Tyr97Cys	Exon 4	TAT-TGT	290/385	Jiang et al., 1997
Arg101Trp	Exon 4	CGG-TGG	301/396	Akeson et al., 1988
Arg101Gln	Exon 4	CGG-CAG	302/397	Bonthron et al., 1985
Arg101Leu	Exon 4	CGG-CTG	302/397	Santisteban et al., 1993
Pro104Leu	Exon 4	CCG-CTG	311/406	Atasoy et al., 1993
Leu107Pro	Exon 4	CTG-CCG	320/415	Hirschhorn et al., 1990
Pro126Gln	Exon 5	CCG-CTG	377/472	Ozsahin et al., 1997
Val129Met	Exon 5	GTG-ATG	385/480	Arrendondo-Vega et al., 1998
Gly140Glu	Exon 5	GGG-GAG	419/514	Arrendondo-Vega et al., 1998
Arg149Trp	Exon 5	CGG-TGG	445/540	Arrendondo-Vega et al., 1998
Arg156Cys	Exon 5	CGC-TGC	466/561	Hirschhorn, 1992a
Arg156His	Exon 5	CGC-CAC	467/562	Santisteban et al., 1993
Val177Met	Exon 6	GTG-ATG	529/624	Santisteban et al., 1993
Ala179Asp	Exon 6	GCC-GAC	536/631	Santisteban et al., 1995a
Gln199Pro	Exon 6	CAG-CCG	596/691	Arrendondo-Vega et al., 1998
Arg211Cys*	Exon 7	CGT-TGT	631/726	Hirschhorn et al., 1990
Arg211His	Exon 7	CGT-CAT	632/727	Akeson et al., 1988
Gly216Arg	Exon 7	GGG-AGG	646/741	Hirschhorn et al., 1991
Glu217Lys	Exon 7	GAG-AAG	649/744	Hirschhorn et al., 1992
Arg235Trp	Exon 8	CGG-TGG	703/798	R. Hirschhorn, unpublished report
Arg235Gln	Exon 8	CGG-CAG	704/799	Ariga et al., 2001b
Arg253Pro	Exon 8	CGG-CCG	758/853	Hirschhorn et al., 1993b
Ser291Leu	Exon 10	TCG-TTG	872/967	Hirschhorn, 1992a
Leu304Arg	Exon 10	CTG-CGG	912/1007	Valerio et al., 1986
Ala329Val	Exon 11	GCG-GTG	986/1081	Akeson et al., 1988
2. In clinically normal individuals with diminished RBC ADA ("partial ADA deficiency")				
Arg76Trp	Exon 4	CGG-TGG	226/321	Hirschhorn et al., 1990
Leu106Val	Exon 4	CTG-GTG	316/411	Jiang et al., 1997
Arg142Gln	Exon 5	CGA-CAG	425/520	Santisteban et al., 1995b
Arg149Gln	Exon 5	CGG-CAG	446/541	Hirschhorn et al., 1990
Leu152Met	Exon 5	CTG-ATG	454/549	Hirschhorn et al., 1997
Ala215Thr	Exon 7	GCC-ACC	643/738	Hirschhorn et al., 1990; Ozsahin et al., 1997
Thr233Ile	Exon 8	ACA-ATA	698/793	Hirschhorn et al., 1997
Gly239Ser	Exon 8	GGC-AGC	715/810	Ariga et al., 2001a
Pro274Leu	Exon 9	CCG-CTG	821/916	Hirschhorn et al., 1990
Pro297Gln	Exon 10	CCG-CAG	890/985	Hirschhorn et al., 1989
Met310Thr	Exon 10	ATG-ACG	930/1025	Ariga et al., 2001a
3. In normals (common SNPs)				
Asp8Asn	Exon 1	GAC-AAC	22/117	Hirschhorn et al., 1994a
Lys80Arg	Exon 4	AAA-AGA	239/334	Valerio et al., 1986
B. Nonsense Mutations				
Gln3Stop	Exon 1	CAG-TAG	7/102	Santisteban et al., 1995a
Gln119Stop	Exon 4	CAG-TAG	355/450	Ariga et al., 2001b
Arg142Stop	Exon 5	CGA-TGA	424/519	Santisteban et al., 1995a
Gln254Stop	Exon 8	CAG-TAG	760–855	Hirschhorn, 1993
C. Splice-Site Mutations				
Unstable mRNA	IVS 1	(+1) GT-CT		Hirschhorn et al., 1994b
Unstable mRNA (deletes exon 2; + use of cryptic site)	IVS 2	(+1) GT-AT		Arredondo-Vega et al., 1994 Onodera et al., 1998
Deletes exon 4	IVS 3	(+2) AG-GG		Akeson et al., 1987, 1988

(continued)

Table 12.4. (*continued*)

Effect	Site	nt Change	ATG/Cap Site	Reference
Unstable mRNA (deletes exon 5)	IVS 5	(+1) GT-AT		Santisteban et al., 1995a
Deletes exon 5	IVS 5	(+6) T-A		Santisteban et al., 1993
Unstable mRNA (deletes exon 7)	IVS 7	(+1) GT-AT		Kawamoto et al., 1993
Unstable mRNA (deletes exon 9)	IVS 8	3' 17 bp rearrangement insertion/deletion		Arredondo-Vega et al., 1994
Unstable mRNA	IVS 10	(+1) G-A (+ use of cryptic splice)		Santisteban et al., 1993
+32 bp and 100 aa	IVS 10	(−34) G-A		Santisteban et al., 1993
+13 bp and 43 aa	IVS 11	(−15) T-A		Arredondo-Vega et al., 2001

D. Deletions/Insertions

Effect	Site	nt Change	ATG/Cap Site	Reference
No mRNA		Promoter and exon 1 (Alu-Alu recombination)		Markert et al., 1988 Berkvens et al., 1990
Pro104fsX132	Exon 4	del A (314/409)		Ariga et al., 2001b
No mRNA		Promoter and exons 1–5		Hirschhorn et al., 1992
	Exon 5	del G (367/462)		Arrendondo-Vega et al., 1998
No mRNA	Exon 6	del TT (539–40/634–5) Stop (TGA) codon 185		Kawamoto et al., 1993
	Exon 6	ins C (577–8/672–3) Premature stop		Unpublished
Unstable mRNA	Exon 10	del gaaga (955–9/1050–4) Stop codon 320		Hirschhorn et al., 1993a Gossage et al., 1993
	Exon 11	del AG (1019–20/1114–5) Stop codon 348		Santisteban et al., 1993
	Exon 11	del Glu337 (1009–1011/1104–1106)		Arrendondo-Vega et al., 1998

*Mutation originally found in ADA-deficient child without immunodeficiency, heteroallelic with null missense mutation. Also found in ADA-deficient patient diagnosed in adulthood, heteroallelic with promoter-exon1 deletion. Probably the lowest activity of mutant enzymes is found in immunodeficient patients.

Unpublished data are from R. Hirschhorn, D. Yang, and C. Jiang.

mutant chromosomes in 47 patients studied in the Hirschhorn laboratory (Table 12.5). The majority of patients carried 1 of these 12 mutations on at least one chromosome. Additionally, the leucine-to-proline mutation at amino acid 107 (Leu107Pro) and neighboring proline to leucine at position 104 (Pro104Leu) have also been found in more than one patient, as has the Gln3stop mutation (two Somali patients). As more patients from different areas are studied, this distribution is likely to change. Over two-thirds of patients are compound heterozygotes with two different mutations, the remainder being homozygous for a single mutation. Homozygosity is typical of rare autosomal recessive diseases, for

Table 12.5. Mutations Found in Multiple Patients

Mutation	Number of Patients	Chromosomes
Ala329Val	9	12
del promoter-exon 1	7	9
Gly216Arg	6	7
Exon 10 5bp del	4	5
Arg156His	4	4
IVS5 +1 G-A	4	4
Ser291Leu	4	4
Arg211His	4	5
Arg142Stop	3	6
Gly20Arg	2	3
Gly74Val	3	3
Arg211Cys	2	2
Total	45/47	63/94

which consanguinity is an important risk factor. In the case of ADA deficiency, many patients with homozygous mutations are from populations with a history of reproductive isolation, including the American Amish community in Pennsylvania (Gly216Arg), Swiss and French Canadians (deletion of five nucleotides of exon10), inhabitants of Newfoundland (Gly20Arg), African Americans (Ala329Val), Canadian Mennonites (Arg142Stop), and Somalis (Gln3Stop).

The presence of the same mutation in unrelated individuals can result from descent from an unidentified common ancestor or from independent recurrence, usually at a site that is a hot spot for mutation. Descent from a common ancestor can be suspected if there is a common ethnic background or if both patients are also identical for other uncommon DNA polymorphic markers within the *ADA* gene, suggesting an ancestral haplotype (Chapter 2). Conversely, independent recurrence is indicated by differences in alleles at closely associated polymorphic DNA markers. Hot spots for independent recurrence of mutations include CpG dinucleotides (representing 30 of all human disease–related mutations), highly repetitive sequences (such as Alu sequences), and small repeat sequences that have been identified empirically. Over half of the missense mutations described to date in ADA-deficient patients are at CpG dinucleotides, a frequency much greater than that reported for many other diseases and setting the stage for independent recurrence. As an example, the Ala329Val mutation, the single-most commonly occurring *ADA* mutation, is at a CpG hot spot, in which the C residue of the GCG codon for alanine is changed to T. The mutation is found on two different haplotypes, one in African Americans and the second in Caucasians, consistent with independent recurrence in each of these groups at some time in the past.

One of the two reported large deletions, including the gene promoter region and exon 1, is relatively common and also appears to have arisen independently in different patients (Table 12.4) (Shovlin et al., 1994; Jiang et al., 1997). This deletion occurs through homologous recombination between two Alu repeats surrounding the promoter and first exon. Such a deletion has been reported in three patients, but with different sequences at the junctions of the deletion, indicating independent recurrence. Presence of this deletion can be easily missed unless tested for specifically such as single-strand conformation polymorphism (SSCP) or analysis of cDNA or of polymerase chain reaction (PCR)-amplified genomic DNA. In a study of 29 patients we found this mutation in 4 patients in whom we had been initially unable to identify a mutation on the second allele (R. Hirschhorn, unpublished data). By contrast with the independent recurrence of the promoter/exon 1 deletion, a 5 bp deletion in exon 10 has been identified in at least four unrelated patients but appears to have derived from a common ancestor in these apparently unrelated individuals. In all four patients, the deletion is found on an extremely rare chromosomal background defined by the presence of two rare nondeleterious missense mutations (normal variants) and, in the three patients studied more fully, a rare combination of restriction fragment length polymorphisms (RFLPs) (haplotype V) (Tzall et al., 1989). Nonetheless, the deletion occurs at a site empirically identified with increased frequency of small deletions and has homology with a site for topoisomerase; the deletion of five bases would fit with loss of a half turn of the helix due to breaks associated with topoisomerase. It is therefore possible for this mutation to recur independently.

Splice-site mutations have been reported particularly in individuals with later onset of disease. It can be expected that more nonsense mutations, small deletions, small insertions, and splice-site mutations (all of which can result in unstable mRNA) will be found as the predominant method of analysis changes from examination of cDNA to direct sequencing of genomic DNA.

Identification of the specific *ADA* mutation(s) present in a newly diagnosed patient may be aided by considering the frequency of different mutations in the relevant ancestral background.

Mutations in partially deficient individuals

In addition to mutations found in immunodeficient patients, 11 different missense mutations retaining differing amounts of easily detectable enzyme activity in nonerythroid cells have been identified in the course of screening erythrocytes from clinically normal individuals. These individuals were categorized as having partial ADA deficiency, based on absence of RBC ADA but presence of residual (5%–80% of normal) ADA in nonerythroid cell types, and identification either by screening of normal individuals or as an incidental finding in apparently healthy relatives of ADA deficients. Several of their *ADA* mutations have been found in multiple individuals, many of whom derive from the same geographic area in the Carribean or share African descent (Hirschhorn et al., 1990). One of these partial mutations, Arg211Cys, is listed with mutations in immunodeficient patients (Table 12.4). Originally identified through population screening of newborns, heteroallelic with a null-mutant allele, this mutation has now been identified in siblings with adult-onset immunodeficiency whose mutation on their opposite *ADA* allele is the del promoter-exon 1 (Table 12.4) (Daddona et al., 1983; Hirschhorn et al., 1990, 1997; Shovlin et al., 1993). It is possible that the original unaffected child identified through screening with the Arg211Cys mutation will develop immunodeficiency. The remaining two missense mutations were identified in healthy relatives of ADA-deficient patients (Gly239Ser and Met310Thr), as was a second instance of the Ala215Thr mutation. It is also possible that additional partial mutations that express very low, but easily detectable, ADA activity (Leu152Met), when heteroallelic with null mutations, will be found in patients with late-onset immunodeficiency. It is noteworthy that the majority of patients are of African descent (including a Kung tribesman), and a selective advantage for malaria is possible.

Effect of Different Mutations on Residual ADA Activity

As is most readily apparent from study of mutations found in partially ADA-deficient immunocompetent individuals, ADA mutations may not totally abolish enzyme activity (Table 12.6). This is also true for mutations found in immunodeficient individuals. In published and unpublished studies, we have compared the ability of over 20 different missense mutations to code for ADA proteins with residual activity in vitro. The mutations fall into four different groups:

1. Approximately half of the mutations found in immunodeficient patients do not express enzyme activity detectable by the methods used.
2. The remainder of the missense mutations found in immunodeficient patients express detectable residual ADA activity ranging from 0.5% to 2% of normal. (An exception is the mutation Arg211Cys, found in adult-onset immunodeficiency, which expresses somewhat more than 2% of normal activity.)
3. A borderline group of mutations encoding *ADA* expressing 3%–6% of normal activity; this group contains the above mutation Arg211Cys,

Table 12.6. Relative Ability of Mutant Enzymes to Express Residual ADA Activity

Enzyme Activity*			
Not Detectable	*0.5%–2%*	*2.5%–6%*	*10%–80%*
Gly20Arg	Arg156His	Arg211Cys	Arg149Gln
Pro104Leu	Arg253Pro	Leu152Met	Pro297Gln
Gly216Arg	Arg156Cys		Thr233Ile
Glu217Lys	Ala329Val		Arg76Trp
Arg235Trp	Gly74Val		Pro274Leu
Ser291Leu	Arg211His		Ala215Thr
Arg101Trp	Leu107Pro		
	Leu304Arg		

*Mutations listed in order of decreasing activity.

originally found in heterozygosity in a child ascertained by newborn screening, but more recently found heteroallelic with a large deletion in adult-onset immunodeficiency in siblings. Also in this category is the Leu152Met mutation present in homozygosity in a child ascertained by newborn screening who is currently healthy at 12 years of age, but had a prior sibling who died in infancy with an infectious disease (Hirschhorn et al., 1997).

4. Mutations expressing 10%–80% of normal, all found by screening of normal individuals. The effect of mutations on residual enzyme activity may be due to instability of the mutant enzyme, a direct effect on the binding of substrate, disruption of the zinc-interacting residues, or changing residues central to the catalytic mechanism. Although some of these effects can be hypothesized on the basis of crystal structure of the murine ADA molecule, definitive conclusions must await direct examination of mutant enzymes.

Analysis of activity of different mutant protein, has also been measured by expression in *E. coli* that are genetically devoid of endogenous ADA activity (Arredondo-Vega et al., 1998; Hershfield and Mitchell, 2001). On the basis of activity expressed in *E. coli*, various mutations were divided into four different groups that appear to correlate well with clinical and biochemical phenotype. Fourteen of the 29 mutations tested in *E. coli* had also been tested for expression in mammalian cells (Table 12.6, R. Hirschhorn and D. Yang, unpublished results). Mutations with the highest activity (class IV and class III) were seen in patients with partial deficiency. In general, the results of expression in mammalian cells correlated well with the results from the *E. coli* experiments.

Genotype–Phenotype Correlations

Correlations of phenotype with genotype are being examined for many inherited disorders with the increased definition of mutations at multiple different disease loci. However, other genetic and nongenetic factors can greatly modify the disease phenotype of patients with identical mutations. Phenotypic differences between siblings carrying the same mutation(s) could be due to modifying genes unlinked to the primary disease locus. Differences between unrelated individuals carrying the same mutation have been attributed to differences in chromosomal background within the gene. Environmental factors can also modify genetic disease phenotypes to a greater or lesser extent, depending on the particular disease. Lastly, a milder phenotype than predicted by the specific mutation can result from somatic mosaicism.

In an autosomal recessive disorder due to defects in a monomeric enzyme, such as ADA, presence of a null allele with a mutant allele expressing residual ADA activity is expected to result in a mild phenotype. Homozygosity for two such mutant alleles could theoretically result in an even milder phenotype. The expression of residual ADA could result from a missense mutation that doesn't totally abolish enzyme activity or of a mutation at a splice site that demonstrates "leakiness"—that is, allows some degree of normal splicing. Critical evaluation of phenotype vs. genotype would be best carried out by comparing patients with identical homozygous mutations to siblings carrying the same mutations. However, for a disorder as rare as ADA deficiency in which there exist multiple different mutations, definitive correlations may not be possible. Moreover, in ADA deficiency, environment, particularly exposure infections, could play a major modifying role. Additionally, as discussed more fully below, somatic mosaicism, due to *de novo* mutations during embryogenesis or to reversion of one of the inherited mutations to normal, can dramatically modify the phenotype.

Despite these caveats, correlations on a less stringent basis between specific mutations, metabolite concentrations, residual ADA activity, age of onset, and severity of disease appear to be present in ADA deficiency. Several mutations in homozygosity or quasi-homozygosity have been recognized in neonatal-onset patients that are consistent with the phenotype. These include a Gly20Arg, Glu217Lys, and Gly216Arg (heteroallelic with a large deletion including the promoter through exon 5), all of these missense mutations being at critical areas of the molecule. The deletion of five nucleotides in exon 10 and possibly the Arg142Stop mutations may also be associated with neonatal-onset SCID. As noted above, several splice-site mutations and the Arg211Cys mutation expressing some activity appear to be associated with later onset and milder perturbations of immune function and metabolites. While relative concordance between siblings (modified by early institution of supportive therapy) has been noted, marked discordance between one set of siblings has also been reported, suggesting the existence of modifying genes or other factors (Arredondo-Vega et al., 1994). The discordant siblings were heterozygous for two different splice mutations. One allele had in intron 2, at the invariant position IVS2(+1), a guanine changed to an adenosine nucleotide. The other allele bore a complex 17-bp rearrangement in intron 8 of the 3' splice site of IVS8; this mutation involved insertion of the purine-rich antisense strand of the poly-pyrimidine tract between the conserved CAG and the normal pyrimidine tract of the 3' splice-site junction (Arredondo-Vega et al., 1994). Presence of mRNA with normal splicing indicated that one or both mutations were somewhat leaky, and the difference in phenotype between the siblings was attributed to genetic variation in splicing efficiency. Although it would not be surprising to find that there are modifying genes, in this family the more severely affected sibling was retrospectively diagnosed, having a hepatoblastoma at the time of diagnosis of immunodeficiency. Interestingly, this tumor manifested trisomy of chromosome 20, characteristic of hepatoblastomas, and this is the chromosome on which the *ADA* gene resides. The presence of the tumor could well have contributed to the earlier development of immunological manifestations (Umetsu et al., 1994).

Somatic mosaicism: de novo and by reversion to normal of inherited mutations

Somatic mosaicism has clearly been identified as a modifier of phenotype, most commonly in autosomal dominant genetic disorders. In such cases, somatic mosaicism is caused by occurrence of a de novo mutation at some point during embryogenesis, resulting in a proportion of cells that carry a mutation and a proportion that are normal. Individuals with somatic mutation in general have a milder phenotype, but if the mutation is present in their germ cells, their offspring, to whom they transmit the mutation, carry the mutation in all cells and have a more severe phenotype. Somatic mosaicism is more difficult to identify for autosomal recessive disorders, but has been found in relatively common disorders such as cystic fibrosis and thalassemia. We have identified somatic mosaicism in two patients with ADA deficiency (Hirschhorn et al., 1994b, 1996); in one of them it occurred by reversion to normal of an inherited mutation. In both patients, mosaicism was uncovered during investigations directed at understanding why there had been improvement of the clinical phenotype, rather than deterioration, over time despite absence of any form of therapy. In the first patient, somatic mosaicism was demonstrated by isolation of B cell lines that expressed ADA and lacked one of the two mutations (IVS1(+1)c) carried by this child (but retained the Arg101Gln mutation), as well as by demonstration of absence of the splice-site mutation in a proportion of peripheral blood DNA. DNA was not available from the parents; we therefore could not prove or disprove that mosaicism had resulted from the usual mechanism of a de novo mutation during embryogenesis (Hirschhorn et al., 1994b).

In the second child, we determined that somatic mosaicism had occurred because of the unexpected reversion to normal of an inherited point mutation (Hirschhorn et al., 1996). A prior sibling had died of an immunodeficiency disorder that would now be categorized as SCID but was designated Nezeloff syndrome by his physicians at the time. Each parent carried a different point mutation at the *ADA* locus, each of which had been identified in other ADA-deficient patients with SCID (maternal = Arg156His; paternal = IVS5(+1)a). However, the child's concentrations of abnormal metabolites were relatively low, and residual ADA activity in peripheral blood cells was relatively high. Moreover, instead of deteriorating clinically without therapy, which had been refused for religious reasons, the child progressively improved. We identified multiple B cell lines that expressed ADA and determined that these carried only the paternal mutation. However, the maternal chromosome that originally bore the maternal mutation (Arg156His) was still present in these B cell lines, as evidenced by presence of a unique maternally derived RFLP linked to the mutation. Approximately 15 clones isolated from peripheral blood also contained the maternal marker but did not carry a mutation, confirming that reversion had occurred in vivo. The detectability of this reversion to normal probably required a selective advantage for survival of revertant cells. Whether there was an additional specific mechanism increasing the frequency of reversion at specific sites remains to be investigated.

Reversion to normal in additional cases of ADA deficiency has now been reported (Ariga et al., 2001b). In one case, probable reversion of the paternal Gln119stop mutation was demonstrated in a polyclonal population of herpesvirus saimiri-immortalized T cells that expressed half the normal level of ADA. Revertant cells were not recovered from the peripheral blood of the patient and therefore could represent an in vitro event. The observation of the revertant was made before the patient had started PEG-ADA treatment. Evidence supporting the occurrence of the reversion event in vivo included markedly lower dAXP levels in the patient's RBC at diagnosis than those expected in ADA-deficient patients carrying the same mutation. In addition, ADA activity was detectable at diagnosis at ~8 nmol/min/10^8 cells and decreased to ~3 nmol/min/10^8 cells after PEG-ADA, which could be explained by the reduction in numbers of the revertant, ADA-expressing cells that lost their selective advantage over the deficient cells after the initiation of enzyme replacement treatment. In the second case, reversion of an Arg235Gln maternal mutation was detected; however, because the sample studied was a monoclonal T cell line, the possibility could not be excluded that the reversion had occurred in vitro (Ariga et al., 2001b).

More recently, somatic mosaicism was demonstrated in a 16-year-old patient from a family in which ADA deficiency was to due to homozygosity for an intronic mutation in the last splice acceptor site of the ADA gene (IVS11(−15)a). Aberrant splicing due to the original mutation resulted in change of the last four *ADA* residues and added a stretch of 43 amino acids that rendered the protein unstable. The genotypic characteristics of the mosaic patient were investigated because he had greater residual immune function and less elevated erythrocyte deoxyadenosine nucleotides than his 4-year-old affected sister. Studies revealed that the patient's T cells and EBV B cell line had 75% of normal ADA activ-

ity and ADA protein of normal size by Western blot. In addition, DNA from peripheral blood mononuclear cells showed two mutant *ADA* alleles, both carrying the IVS11(−15)a splice site mutation, but one with an acquired deletion of the 11 adjacent nucleotides (del IVS11(−4 to −14)), which suppressed aberrant splicing and restored protein expression and function. Interestingly, enzyme replacement therapy with PEG-ADA in this case was also followed by a reduction of ADA activity in T cells, as well as a marked decrease of the peripheral blood lymphocytes carrying the "second-site" revertant allele (Arredondo-Vega et al., 2001).

Reversion to normal of inherited mutations has now been reported in several different disorders, including dermatologic and metabolic disorders and various immunologic disorders additional to ADA deficiency. These disorders include X-linked SCID, Wiskott Aldrich syndrome, Fanconi syndrome, Bloom syndrome, tyrosinemia, and epidermolysis bullosa (reviewed in Hirschhorn, 2003). Mosaicism with or without reversion should be suspected in patients with atypical or mild presentation of immunodeficiency. Reversion is probably a more frequent occurrence in other disorders, in addition to those reported, but is most easily ascertained in disorders such as those involving hematopoetic cells and skin, where phenotypic reversion can most easily be detected. The mechanisms that could be involved include intragenic recombination, mitotic gene conversion (both requiring heterozygosity), second-site compensating mutations, DNA slippage, and site-specific reversion of a mutated nucleotide to normal by undefined mechanisms (probably involving DNA breakage and repair). True reversions or involvement of second-site mutations may be a more common event than currently appreciated and could explain both published and anecdotal reports of T cell lines that, even though derived from immunodeficient patients, unexpectedly express ADA. In addition, somatic mosaicism has been described in other primary immunodeficiencies.

Molecular Organization of the PNP Gene

The disease gene for PNP, designated *NP* (MIM + 164050), is encoded by a single structural gene on human chromosome 14q13 (Ricciuti and Ruddle, 1973 George and Francke, 1976; Aitken and Ferguson-Smith, 1978). The human *NP* gene is about 7.5 kb in length and contains six exons (Williams et al., 1984). A cDNA of 1.7 kb has been cloned that contains a 289-codon open reading frame, encoding a 32 kDa protein (Goddard et al., 1983). The human *NP* promoter has been defined in 2 kb of the 5′ flanking region, containing a TATA box, an inverted CCAAT sequence, and two GC-rich regions within a 216 bp segment. Interestingly, although PNP is ubiquitously expressed in human tissues, the *NP* promoter does not conform to a normal GC-rich, constitutively expressed housekeeping promoter. The PNP protein is a homotrimer, therefore it is possible that dominant negative effects will be seen.

Mutational Analysis of PNP

Similar to ADA deficiency, mutation analysis of PNP has to examine both alleles. In some patients' cells, neither PNP protein nor PNP biochemical activity can be detected; in others, protein detectable by antibody assay but without enzymatic activity is found. In one family, the mutant protein could not be demonstrated in the patient's cells but was present in both consanguineous parents, a finding suggesting that mutated protein was unstable or may not have formed stable trimers (Osborne et al., 1977; Gudas et al., 1978). Results of mutation analysis, carried out so far

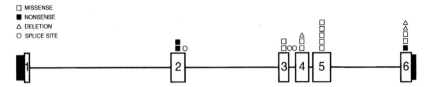

Figure 12.6. Mutations at the purine nucleoside phosphorylase (PNP) locus.

in 15 patients, are summarized in Figure 12.6 and Table 12.7. A homozygous mutation affecting codon 89 (Glu89Lys) was the first PNP mutation recognized (Williams et al., 1987). The affected patient from a second family was found to have a deletion of 170 bp in the *NP* mRNA due to a G-to-T transversion at the terminal nucleotide of exon 2 in the maternal allele, which caused skipping of exon 2 during mRNA processing. The paternal allele of this patient was found to carry a point mutation (Arg234Pro) in exon 6 (Andrews and Markert, 1992; Markert et al., 1997). The affected patient from a third family was found to be a compound heterozyte for an Asp-to-Gly substitution at codon 128 and an Arg-to-Pro substitution at codon 234; these mutations resulted in absence of immunoreactive protein with complete loss of functional activity (Aust et al., 1992; Buckley et al., 1997). Compound heterozygosity for a missense mutation (Tyr192Cys) and a 1 nucleotide deletion in exon 6 were later demonstrated in a patient with PNP deficiency and severe immunodeficiency (Pannicke et al., 1996). The mutations of four additional unrelated patients were also reported (Markert et al., 1997). These included two novel missense mutations (Ala174Pro

and Gly190Val) and a single amino acid deletion in exon 4 (del Ile129). One patient of this series had a point mutation in intron 3 (−18 g to a) resulting in an alternative splice site, frameshift, and premature stop codon, producing an unstable truncated protein; however, a small amount of normally spliced product could be detected, explaining the patient's late onset and mild course. Finally, two additional Arg234Pro mutations were also found, suggesting that codon 234 may be a mutational hot spot or, alternatively, that the affected individuals have a common ancestor (Markert et al., 1997). Nonsense mutations (Arg24Stop, Arg57Stop) have also been found in two unrelated patients in the homozygous state (Sasaki et al., 1998) and in heterozygosity with a splicing defect of the donor site of intron 3 (Dalal et al., 2001). Two additional reports on mutation analysis of PNP-deficient patients described the presence of novel homozygous missense mutations (Tyr166Cys and Gly156Ala). A recent report identified His257Asp and Arg234Stop mutations (Grunebaum et al., 2004). Of the 30 mutated alleles studied, 19 had missense mutations, 19 had nonsense mutations, 6 had splice-site mutations resulting in frameshift, and 2 had nucleotide deletions.

Table 12.7. Mutated Alleles of the Purine Nucleoside Phosphorylase (PNP) Gene

Effect	Site	nt Change	cDNA position	Reference
A. Missense Mutations				
Leu73Pro	Exon 3	CTG-CCG	218	Baguette et al., 2002
Glu89Lys	Exon 3	GAA-AAA	265	Williams et al., 1987
Ala117Thr	Exon 4	GCA-ACA	349	Tabarki et al., 2003
Asp128Gly	Exon 4	GAT-GGT	383	Markert et al., 1997
Gly156Ala	Exon 5	GGA-GCA	467	Moallem et al., 2002
Tyr166Cys	Exon 5	TAC-TGC	497	Tsuda et al., 2002
Ala174Pro	Exon 5	GCT-CCT	520	Markert et al., 1997
Gly190Val	Exon 5	GGC-GTC	569	Markert et al., 1997
Tyr192Cys	Exon 5	TAT-TGT	575	Pannicke et al., 1996
Arg234Pro	Exon 6	CGA-CCA	701	Aust et al., 1992
His257Asp	Exon 6	CAT-GAT	769	Grunebaum et al., 2004
B. Nonsense Mutations				
Arg24Stop	Exon 2	CGA-TGA	70	Sasaki et al., 1998
Arg58Stop	Exon 2	CGA-TGA	172	Dalal et al., 2001
Arg234Stop	Exon 6	CGA-TGA	700	Grunebaum et al., 2004
C. Splice-Site Mutations				
Deletes exon 3 and frameshift	Exon 2	G-T	181	Andrews and Markert, 1992
Deletes exon 3 and frameshift	IVS 3	(+1) G-A		Dalal et al., 2001
+16 bp and frameshift	IVS 3	(−18) G-A		Markert et al., 1997
D. Deletions/Insertions				
Ile129del	Exon 4	del ATC (385–387)		Markert et al., 1997
Gly156fs × 170	Exon 6	del A (468)		Baguette et al., 2002
Asn243fs × 261	Exon 6	del A (730)		Pannicke et al., 1996
E. Polymorphisms (SNPs) at the PNP locus				
Dup 10bp	−41	Ins CGGATCGGAG	5′ UT	Williams et al., 1984, 1987
Silent	Exon 2	CAT-CAC	60	Aust et al., 1992
Ser51Gly	Exon 2	AGT-GGT	151	Aust et al., 1992
Silent	Exon 2	CCT-CCC	171	Aust et al., 1992
Val217Ile	Exon 5	GTT-ATT	649	Moallem et al., 2002
	+903	Ins A	3′ UT	Williams et al., 1984, 1987

Because of the low numbers of PNP-deficient patients described to date, no clear genotype–phenotype correlations can be established for this disease. No PNP patients with somatic mosaicism have been described.

Strategies for Diagnosis

Given the emerging phenotype of late- and adult-onset immunodeficiency disease due to ADA deficiency, any individual with lymphopenia of unexplained etiology and frequent infections of any type, with or without autoimmunity, should be tested for ADA deficiency. In this setting an initial abnormal screening result obtained on erythrocytes should be followed by assay of ADA in nonerythroid cells.

Diagnosis of ADA deficiency in immunodeficient patients can be made by enzyme assay of several easily available cell types, including erythrocytes, lymphocytes, EBV-transformed B cells, and fibroblasts. If the patient has received a transfusion, erythrocytes are unreliable, and assay of a transformed B cell line or of fibroblasts should be used. If the diagnosis is suggested by abnormal assay of RBC, assay of lymphocytes and/or fibroblasts should also be performed to rule out the (unlikely) possibility of partial ADA deficiency, which would not be expected to give rise to immunodeficiency. Alternatively, analysis of DNA and identification of previously reported deleterious mutations can be performed. While there may not be sufficient lymphocytes for assay in the intial blood sample, there is usually sufficient DNA in the buffy coat that is removed prior to assay of RBCs. This DNA should be saved and can be used to sequence all exons and flanking regions. Determination of dATP and of deoxyadenosine in urine can also aid in diagnosis.

A variety of assays can measure the hydrolytic deamination of adenosine (Zielke and Sueltre, 1971). We have not found assays measuring release of ammonia to be reliable. For initial screening, we routinely use a linked spectrophotometric assay in which uric acid is the final end product (Edwards et al., 1971; Hirschhorn, 1979b). This assay is relatively sensitive, rapid, and easily performed. A second spectrophotometric method measuring the conversion of adenosine to inosine by loss of absorbance at the peak for adenosine is also simple and widely used, but it is much less sensitive because of the limitation in the concentration of substrate and in the amount of cell lysate that can be included in the assay. The most sensitive and specific assays are those that use radiolabeled adenosine as substrate in the presence and absence of the inhibitor EHNA and separate the products from the substrate by methods such as thin-layer chromatography (Hirschhorn, 1979b). The amount of enzyme activity inhibited by EHNA measures the activity resulting from the *ADA* locus affected in ADA-deficient immunodeficiency. The alternate isozyme of ADA is encoded by a distinct locus not affected in ADA-deficient immunodeficiency. Although this locus accounts for only 1%–2% of ADA activity in normal cells, its presence can confuse detailed characterization of residual ADA in diagnosis of ADA deficiency. We have also used a high-performance liquid chromatography (HPLC) assay using unlabeled adenosine and standard methods of separation (Hirschhorn et al., 1982), but this requires expensive machinery not commonly available. However, this assay could be easily automated with current available technology; it does not require radioactivity, and it is sensitive. Other methods amenable to automation have also been described (Carlucci et al., 2003).

Patients presenting with recurrent bacterial, viral, and fungal infections, neurologic deficits, lymphopenia due predominantly to the absence of T lymphocytes, abnormal T cell function, and defective antibody responses should be investigated for PNP deficiency. Absence of PNP enzymatic activity in RBC lysates, determined by radiochemical or spectrophotometric assays, will confirm the diagnosis. The linked spectrophotometric assay described above also measures PNP activity. Indeed, all patients must be tested for both deficiencies if the linked assay is used. The linked ADA assay depends on endogenous PNP, and therefore absence of PNP can resemble ADA deficiency. Immunoreactive protein, measured by Western blot analysis, may be present or absent. The diagnosis of PNP deficiency is strongly supported by low uric acid in serum (<2 mg/dl, and usually <1 mg/dl) and urine. High serum levels of inosine and guanosine and high urinary excretion of inosine, deoxyinosine, guanosine, and deoxyguanosine are characteristic for PNP deficiency (Cohen et al., 1978; Hershfield and Mitchell, 2001). An increase of dGTP has been reported in red cells of PNP-deficient patients (Cohen et al., 1978).

Prenatal Diagnosis and Carrier Detection

Prenatal diagnosis

Prenatal diagnosis of ADA deficiency has been made by enzyme assay on chorionic villous samples, amniotic cells, and fetal blood (Hirschhorn et al., 1975, 1992; Hirschhorn, 1979b, 1979c; Durandy et al., 1982; Simmonds et al., 1983; Linch et al., 1984; R. Hirschhorn, unpublished results). We have performed prenatal diagnosis in over 20 cases by enzyme assay of amniotic cells and correctly diagnosed the expected 25% to be affected. Predictions were confirmed either by postnatal ADA assay of erythrocytes and/or identification of mutations on both chromosomes in amniotic cells; infants predicted to be unaffected had ADA activity by assay of erythrocytes after birth. There was a clear separation between affected fetuses and fetuses at risk, but not affected. However, homozygous normals vs. carriers could not be definitively identified by enzyme assay in cases where we could identify carriers by heterozygosity for a mutation.

DNA-based diagnosis can definitively diagnose carriers, affected subjects, and normals in a setting where both ADA mutant alleles are known; this is feasible if the mutations have been studied in a previously affected child in the family or can be rapidly determined in the parents or samples preserved from a deceased affected child. Although RFLPs, when informative, could in theory also be used for diagnosis, we suggest that the AluVpA polymorphism described upstream of the first exon not be used for diagnosis, as we have identified a crossover in this region (Hirschhorn et al., 1994b). Direct detection of the specific pathologic mutations or enzyme assay is preferable, and identification of the mutations present can be performed given the availability of PCR and rapid sequence analysis.

Prenatal diagnosis can be valuable not only if parents wish to terminate an affected pregnancy but also for facilitating therapy of an affected infant after birth. A number of families have chosen to carry the pregnancy of an affected child to term (Jiang et al., 1997). HLA typing has then allowed rapid bone marrow transplantation (both histocompatible and T-depleted haploidentical) before onset of infections (Pollack et al., 1983). Prenatal diagnosis has also made possible harvest of cord blood for gene therapy (Kohn et al., 1995, 1998).

Similar to ADA deficiency, both amniotic cell culture and chorionic villus sampling have been used successfully to identify PNP deficient fetuses by assessing PNP activity (Carapella De Luca et al., 1986; Perignon et al., 1987; Kleijer et al., 1989).

Obviously, if the mutations of the *NP* gene are known in an affected family member, direct sequence analysis of fetal DNA will identify the PNP status of the fetus.

Carrier detection

Determination of heterozygotes can be attempted by assay of ADA in erythrocytes and demonstration of anomalous inheritance within the family of the normal ADA polymorphism (Chen et al., 1974; Scott et al., 1974; Hirschhorn et al., 1975; Hirschhorn, 1992). There is a large range of normal ADA activity; values follow a normal distribution only after log conversion. Most obligate carriers demonstrate, as expected, approximately half-normal ADA activity. However, approximately 10%–20% of carriers fall within the normal range, and 1% of normals have activity in the carrier range. Most troubling are those individuals at risk for being carriers who are at the borderline of normal. A definitive means for identification of carriers is demonstration of anomalous inheritance of the normal ADA polymorphism in a family at risk. However, the frequency of this normal polymorphism is low, therefore the number of families in which this approach is useful is also low.

We no longer attempt carrier identification as a definitive diagnostic measure, for several reasons. First, the problem of overlap does not allow the test to be definitive except in cases where both parents have markedly reduced activity (25% of absolute values; 50% of log conversion). Second, if heterozygote testing is being performed for relatives of a patient with known ADA deficiency, mutation detection now offers a definitive test. Third, in the case of a pregnancy at risk for SCID of unknown etiology, the prenatal diagnosis of SCID can be made by examination of lymphocytes in fetal blood, at which time ADA deficiency can be diagnosed with the erythrocytes obtained. Alternatively, and preferably, if amniocentesis has been performed for other reasons, ADA can be assayed in cultured amniocytes. Clearly a consensus is needed on the most efficient, sensitive, and specific strategies to be used for prenatal diagnosis of SCID that would avoid the danger of fetal blood sampling.

Carriers for PNP deficiency frequently have decreased PNP activity in red cell and white cell lysates. The distribution of PNP activity is much narrower than for ADA. If the mutations of the affected offspring are known, mutation analysis will definitively determine carrier status.

Treatment and Prognosis

Several management options are available for ADA deficiency. These are listed in Table 12.8 and include both prevention (e.g., prenatal diagnosis with selective pregnancy termination) and therapeutic approaches based on hematopoietic bone marrow/stem cell transplantation (HSCT), enzyme replacement, and gene therapy. For PNP deficiency, prevention and bone marrow transplantation are currently the only available alternatives.

Hematopoietic Bone Marrow/Stem Cell Transplantation

Allogeneic HSCT from a histocompatible sibling or other close relative in inbred communities is the therapy of choice for ADA deficiency (Parkman et al., 1975; Chen et al., 1978; Zegers and Stoop, 1983; Friedrich et al., 1985; Buckley et al., 1986, 1993, 1999; Fischer et al., 1986, 1990; Markert et al., 1987; Silber et al., 1987; Boulieu et al., 1988; Wijnaendts et al., 1989; Gaines

Table 12.8. Therapeutic Options for ADA Deficiency

1. Preventive
   a. Prenatal diagnosis with selective pregnancy termination
   b. Prenatal diagnosis to assist postnatal therapy: HLA typing, germ-free delivery
   c. Preimplantation diagnosis with selective implantation of nonmutant embryos
2. Hematopoietic stem cell transplantation
   a. Potential donors
      i. Histocompatible-related donor (usually sibling)*
      ii. Haploidentical-related donor (usually parent)
      iii. Matched unrelated donor
   b. Potential sources of hematopoietic stem cells
      i. Bone marrow
      ii. Mobilized peripheral blood
      iii. Cord blood
3. Enzyme replacement
   a. Partial-exchange transfusion (no longer used)
   b. PEG-conjugated calf intestinal ADA (ADAGEN)
4. Gene therapy
   a. Into cultured expanded T cells
   b. Into CD34+ stem cells
      i. Cord blood
      ii. Bone marrow

*Therapy of choice if available.

et al., 1991; Parkman, 1991; Fischer, 1992; Haddad et al., 1998; Bertrand et al., 1999; Amrolia et al., 2000; Rubocki et al., 2001; Antoine et al., 2003). This therapeutic maneuver has the greatest efficacy, does not necessarily require prior marrow ablation or permanent ongoing therapy, and has a relatively low morbidity and mortality. After successful HSCT, deoxyadenosine-based metabolites are dramatically lower than in untreated patients, but are still detectably higher than normal (Hirschhorn et al., 1981). The diminution of adenosine concentrations is not as dramatic, and this observation is to be expected because the ADA enzyme has a greater affinity (lower Km) for deoxyadenosine than for adenosine. Surprisingly, adenosine in plasma can remain very high without apparent adverse effects, although in ADA-deficient mice, elevated adenosine has significant effects (see Animal Models, below). Additionally, SAH hydrolase activity remains low, reflecting retention of increased amounts of metabolites (Hirschhorn et al., 1981). The incomplete metabolic correction may explain the persistence of nonimmunologic manifestations in transplanted patients, such as sensorineural deafness and cognitive and behavioral abnormalities (Tanaka et al., 1996; Rogers et al., 2001; Albuquerque and Gaspar, 2004), despite the fact that the bony abnormalities disappear rapidly. Genetic deficiency of SAH hydrolase is now known to result in mental deterioration, hypotonicity, and myopathy as well as multiple biochemical aberrations including hypermethionemia, but without signs of immunodeficiency (Baric et al., 2004). The ability of dietary manipulation to reverse the metabolic abnormalities and apparently the mental deterioration in SAH-deficient patients (Baric et al., 2004) raises the need to assess the correction of SAH pathway in ADA deficients after HSCT and offers a possible role for dietary manipulation in ADA- but also PNP-deficient patients at risk for cognitive defects. Finally, it is also not known if transplantation from an ADA-heterozygous carrier donor is less efficacious than from a donor who is homozygous normal. Metabolites have not been reported in patients transplanted following marrow ablation sufficient to result in replacement of all hematopoietic elements with donor-derived precursors.

Unfortunately, in an outbred population with small family size, as typically exists in the United States, fewer than 25% of patients have an HLA-matched related donor. Haploidentical transplantation from a related donor has higher morbidity and mortality in all forms of SCID than HLA-matched transplantation. It usually requires pre–treatment myeloablation, but it is performed in the absence of preparative chemotherapy in some centers (Buckley et al., 1999) and can result in permanent engraftment (see Chapter 47). The European Bone Marrow Transplantation (EMBT) working party has recently published the analysis of 30 years of cumulative experience with haploidentical transplantation for ADA deficiency, which showed a 3-year survival of only ~25% compared to 81% after HLA-identical HSCT (Antoine et al., 2003). Currently, therefore, it appears that ADA-deficient patients are poorer candidates for haploidentical transplantation than those with other forms of SCID, in which the average survival is >54% (Antoine et al., 2003). HSCT from matched unrelated donors has been successfully used in a few cases of ADA deficiency (Amrolia et al., 2000; Kane et al., 2001); however, the limited experience thus far does not allow us to draw definitive conclusions on safety and efficacy of this procedure, compared to use of related donors. Similar considerations also apply to use of cord blood from unrelated donors; despite initial encouraging results, more extensive investigation is still needed.

Bone marrow transplantation is the treatment of choice for PNP deficiency (see Chapter 47). There is, however, only limited clinical experience because of the rarity of the disease. Only about half of the transplanted PNP-deficient cases reported in the literature showed full engraftment and cure of their immunodeficiency (Markert, 1991; Broome et al., 1996; Carpenter et al., 1996; Hallett et al., 1999; Classen et al., 2001; Baguette et al., 2002). The procedure appears most successful if carried out at an early age and if the patient is conditioned prior to transplantation (Rich et al., 1980; Staal et al., 1980; Carpenter et al., 1996). Low-toxicity conditioning should probably be considered, as it can result in successful engraftment while avoiding the risk of further neurological deterioration (Classen et al., 2001). Unfortunately, however, even in successfully transplanted patients, the neurologic deficits have not improved (Markert, 1991; Carpenter et al., 1996; Hallett et al., 1999; Baguette et al., 2002). In view of these disappointing results,

whether PNP-deficient patients with severe neurological deficits should be considered candidates for HSCT is unclear. Attempts at treating PNP deficiency with fetal thymus transplants have also generated discouraging results (Markert, 1991).

Overall, the long-term prognosis of PNP deficiency remains poor. Thirty-one of 39 patients in published reports have died (Markert, 1991; Carpenter et al., 1996; Banzhoff et al., 1997; Hallett et al., 1999; Classen et al., 2001; Baguette et al., 2002; Tsuda et al., 2002). Seventeen deaths were due to infections, including four that were caused by varicella. Six were due to tumors (five lymphoma/lymphosarcoma) and three patients died of GVHD following bone marrow transplantation. Because of the abnormal antibody responses, clinical management of PNP-deficient patients should include regular treatment with intravenous immunoglobulin (IVIG). Prophylaxis against *Pneumocystis jiroveci* infection is also indicated.

Enzyme Replacement Therapy

Enzyme replacement therapy for ADA-deficient SCID does not require uptake of the enzyme into cells. Therapy is based first on the fact that metabolites are present in plasma and body fluids, where they can be degraded by administered enzyme present in the plasma. Second, additional toxic metabolites such as dATP are in equilibrium with the precursors in plasma (Polmar et al., 1976; Hirschhorn et al., 1980a; Hopp et al., 1985; Hershfield et al., 1987, 1993; Ochs et al., 1992; Weinberg et al., 1993; Hershfield, 1995a, 1995b, 2000).

Therefore, lowering of substrate concentrations in plasma results in lowering of intracellular concentrations of metabolites as well (Fig. 12.7). The first attempts at enzyme therapy used partial-exchange transfusion with normal, irradiated erythrocytes, because erythrocytes have transport sites for both adenosine and deoxyadenosine and contain ADA. Partial-exchange transfusion lowered metabolite concentrations dramatically, restored normal growth and development, and prolonged survival in at least six patients. However, this treatment did not alter immunologic responsiveness in most patients and, moreover, any improvement in immunologic parameters was often short-lived (Ochs et al., 1992). Additionally, transfusion carried the risk of transmission of infec-

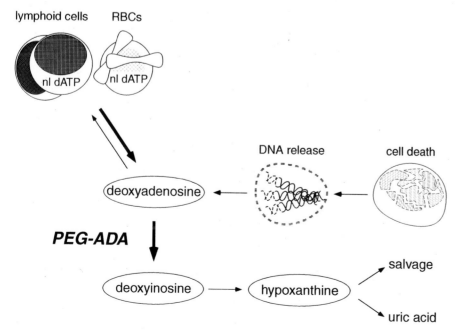

Figure 12.7. Adenosine deaminase deficiency: effects of enzyme replacement therapy. PEG-ADA, polyethylene glycol–adenosine deaminase; RBCs, red blood cells.

tious agents and resulted in iron overload. Three patients first treated with transfusion therapy survived until over 10 years of age and were then placed on PEG-ADA therapy. Two of these patients were siblings and were still alive at approximately 20 years of age.

The development of PEG-ADA enzyme replacement therapy (polyethylene-glycol-modified calf intestinal ADA; ADAGEN®) has replaced the original enzyme replacement treatments. The modification, involving addition of PEG to lysine residues, is designed to mask the enzyme from endogenous antibody-mediated destruction so that its half-life is markedly prolonged. While dosages recommended are from 15 to 30 U/kg of body weight weekly, regimens may be individualized, based on monitoring of plasma ADA activity. In practice, early-onset SCID patients are treated with twice-weekly intramuscular injections of 30–60 U/kg, based on ideal body weight, for the first several months of therapy. There may be a diminished half-life of the enzyme in very ill infants and/or poorer responses to usual doses. Monitoring of dATP, total deoxyadenosine nucleotides, and SAH hydrolase activity is recommended since increases in deoxynucleotides and decreases in SAH hydrolase activity have been associated with a reduction in lymphocyte counts and function (Chun et al., 1993). Periodic testing for development of anti-ADA antibodies is also advisable.

PEG-ADA therapy has completely replaced partial-exchange transfusion because it is safer; it can deliver greater amounts of enzyme and therefore more completely lower metabolites. In addition to restoration of normal growth and development and prolongation of life, it results in the development of protective, although not normal, T cell immunity in ~80% of treated patients. To date, more than 120 patients have been treated with PEG-ADA worldwide, with a survival rate of approximately 80%. Virtually all patients on PEG-ADA develop antibody against the bovine ADA protein. In ~10% of cases neutralizing antibodies impair the function of the injected enzyme and require an increase in the dosage or discontinuation of PEG-ADA in an attempt of achieving desensitazion (Chaffee et al., 1992; Chun et al., 1993; Hershfield, 2004). Other complications in patients on PEG-ADA treatment include autoimmune hemolytic anemia and EBV-positive lymphoproliferative syndrome, which require therapeutic attempts with HSCT. In one case, a patient responsive to transfusion treatment died of uncontrollable autoimmune hemolytic anemia following a viral infection (Ratech et al., 1985). A second patient died at 6 years of age of overwhelming varicella when exposure was not recognized in time to administer appropriate antiviral therapy. Of note, elective HSCT after PEG-ADA treatment has resulted in survival of ~50% of cases. This finding suggests the use of PEG-ADA to stabilize the metabolic status of patients after diagnosis so that transplantation can have the best chance of benefit.

Overall, clinical response of children on PEG-ADA has been good, as measured by normal growth and development, ability to attend school, absence of opportunistic infections, and normal recovery from varicella and other viral infections. Early mortality appears to be limited to early-onset cases with severe infectious complications. Immune reconstitution, as measured by lymphocyte counts and in vitro function, has been less complete, and approximately 20% of patients, predominantly with infantile-onset disease, show slower and lesser improvement. An increase in B cells usually precedes the increase in T cells and appearance of mitogen responses. Although mitogen responses improve from the initial 0%–10% of normal, they then fluctuate between 25% and 90% of normal. After the first year, most patients remain lymphopenic. Specific antibody responses have been detected in half of the patients, and half no longer receive regular IVIG replacement (Hershfield, 2004). Elegant studies of two patients with ADA-deficient SCID of early onset during their first year of enzyme therapy have provided evidence that the therapy results in apparent rescue of immature lymphocyte progenitors. It was shown that mature immunocompetent lymphocytes were recruited from progenitors, recapitulating ontogeny, rather than merely expanding a small pool of relatively mature cells (Weinberg et al., 1993). Thus PEG-ADA therapy, adjusted as needed to normalize SAH hydrolase activity, resulted in the sequential appearance of CD3^{dim} cells, followed by transient appearance of cells expressing both CD4 and CD8, and finally the mature phenotype of CD3^{bright} cells expressing either CD4 or CD8. These changes were observed between 3 and 5 months following the start of therapy. The appearance of mature T cells was then followed by IL-2-dependent mitogen responses and then rapidly by IL-2-independent responses and antigen-specific responses, also initially transiently IL-2 dependent. Other studies have demonstrated normalization of the antibody response, as indicated by appearance of reactivity to the bacteriophage $\Phi \times 174$ (Ochs et al., 1992).

Enzyme replacement therapy results in dramatic lowering of metabolites, most notably in returning SAH hydrolase activity to normal or almost normal. Activity of SAH hydrolase appears to be the most sensitive indicator of total body concentration of toxic metabolites. The major questions remaining about PEG-ADA therapy are whether immune function will remain improved over the years and whether the efficacy will be limited by the underlying phenotype or by prior history of infections that have presumably destroyed a significant portion of the pool of "rescueable" lymphocyte precursors. Follow-up studies in nine ADA-deficient patients treated with PEG-ADA for ~10 years have been recently published and showed that despite initial improvements, a gradual decline of lymphocyte counts and mitogenic proliferative responses occurred after a few years of treatment. ADA-deficient patients on PEG-ADA therefore should be followed closely to detect declining immune function with aging (Chan et al., 2005).

The major disadvantages of PEG-ADA therapy are its high cost, the necessity for weekly, lifelong therapy (requiring ongoing monitoring of metabolites for adjustment of dose), and the possibility of developing clinically significant anti-enzyme antibody. The cost and need for ongoing therapy are important although not insurmountable. A recombinant human form of the enzyme could solve or reduce the problems of anti-ADA antibody. The major question is that of long-term efficacy; until that is defined, further investigation of alternative or adjunctive therapies appears justified.

In contrast to ADA deficiency, enzyme replacement therapy for PNP by means of irradiated RBC transfusions (Zegers et al., 1978; Rich et al., 1980; Staal et al., 1980) has not been definitively proven beneficial for PNP deficiency. A purified form of the enzyme conjugated to polyethylene glycol (PEG-PNP) could potentially find a role in the clinical management of this disease (Hershfield et al., 1991). Alternative approaches with administration of deoxycytidine and tetrahydrouridine, oral uridine or guanine, or thymosin fraction 5 have been unsuccessful (Markert, 1991).

Gene Therapy

Adenosine deaminase–deficient SCID has been the pioneer disorder for development of human gene therapy (Blaese et al.,

1995; Bordignon et al., 1995; Kohn et al., 1995; Hoogerbrugge et al., 1996; Onodera et al., 1998; Aiuti et al., 2002a). This deficiency appeared to be an excellent candidate for gene therapy, based on the knowledge that the disease could be corrected by HSCT manipulation of bone marrow cells ex vivo prior to transplantation is routine and could be easily adapted to allow for introduction of the ADA cDNA into cells, and regulated expression did not appear to be required. Additionally, experiments in mice and humans suggested a selective survival advantage for cells carrying a functional ADA allele. Experiments in mice indicated that lymphoid cells containing the ADA gene have a marked advantage over ADA-deficient cells in an ADA-sufficient environment, a surrogate model for enzyme therapy (Ferrari et al., 1991). In humans, results of bone marrow transplantation were also consistent with the hypothesis that endogenous ADA is more effective than exogenous ADA. HSCT, while lowering metabolite concentrations, results in selective engraftment of donor T cells, rather than both rescue of host cells and engraftment of donor cells. Host B cells are often "rescued" without engraftment of donor B cells. These data superficially are also consistent with the finding of a lack of host T cell precursors to be rescued but a relative sufficiency of host B cells. This would imply that multipotential lymphoid stem cells are not engrafted or that T cell precursors have a stronger selective advantage than their B lineage counterparts.

These observations provided a rationale for attempts at gene therapy for ADA deficiency despite the availability of alternative modes of therapy (e.g., bone marrow transplantation, PEG-ADA). Gene therapy has important theoretical advantages, such as avoidance of the threat of GVHD and a potential reduction in therapeutic maneuvers required. To be successful, efficient and stable gene transfer into patients' cells is a prerequisite and, ideally, genetic correction of hematopoietic stem cells should be achieved. Achieving efficient transduction into stem cells and maintaining multipotentiality of this elusive cell type throughout the required manipulations are areas under active investigation (see Chapter 48).

Gene therapy for treatment of ADA deficiency by introduction into hematopoietic cells of a normal ADA cDNA contained in a retroviral vector has been pursued in the United States, the Netherlands, Italy, and Japan. As of 2004, approximately 25 patients had enrolled in these trials, although published data are available for only about half of the cases. All patients were treated with a retroviral vector containing the normal ADA cDNA and with ex vivo gene transfer. In all but one of the most recent trials reported to date, PEG-ADA was concurrently administered. The greatest amount of published information is available for the U.S. and Italian trials. The U.S. trials initially used T cells expanded in vitro as the recipient cells in two patients (Blaese et al., 1995; Mullen et al., 1996) and subsequently CD34+ cells isolated from the patients' cord blood in three newborns diagnosed prenatally (Kohn et al., 1995, 1998). Patients treated with T cell gene therapy showed improvement of immunologic parameters (Blaese et al., 1995), although the concomitant PEG-ADA treatment made it difficult to attribute these results to gene therapy alone. Nevertheless, this trial demonstrated that retroviral-mediated ADA gene transfer into T cells can achieve long-term (12+ years) presence and expression of the exogenous gene (Muul et al., 2003).

In the Italian trial, multiple injections were given over several months in two patients to simultaneously introduce peripheral blood cells containing the ADA cDNA, and T cell–depleted bone marrow cells containing the same construct marked with a different restriction site to obtain information about safety and possible efficacy. Both of these patients were 2 years of age before initiation

of PEG-ADA therapy, having been previously supported with irradiated red cell transfusions. They were considered to have failed PEG-ADA therapy, despite marked clinical and immunological improvement, because of failure to maintain lymphocyte counts and antigen-specific and nonspecific proliferative responses. One of these patients had delayed-onset disease (Notarangelo et al., 1992). The results indicated that short-term reconstitution was achieved from cells derived from peripheral blood, whereas reconstitution after 1 year was from bone marrow–derived cells. Reconstitution ranged from 0.8% to 30% of normal, depending on the assay used (Bordignon et al., 1995). In the face of continued enzyme replacement therapy, it is difficult to assess the contribution of gene-corrected cells to any improvement in immunologic function. However, on the basis of preliminary data indicating a selective advantage for gene-corrected cells, PEG-ADA was withdrawn in one of the treated patients. There was a consequent progressive increase in the proportion of gene-corrected T lymphocytes that ultimately replaced the ADA-negative cells and led to improvement of T cell functions (Aiuti et al., 2002b).

More recently, multilineage engraftment of gene-corrected cells, metabolic correction, and improvement of immune function were achieved in two ADA-deficient patients who were not treated with PEG-ADA and received genetically modified CD34+ cells after preparative nonmyeloablative chemotherapy (Aiuti et al., 2002a). These results suggest that gene therapy may soon become a real alternative treatment option for ADA deficiency. However, the occurrence of two cases of T cell leukemia in patients with X-linked SCID treated with gene therapy (Hacein-Bey-Abina et al., 2003) has provided an important word of caution on the possible secondary risks of retroviral gene addition.

Because PNP and ADA deficiency are caused by similar biochemical aberrations, it seems likely that gene therapy could also be beneficial for PNP-deficient patients. In preclinical studies using retroviral-mediated gene transfer, "in vitro" reconstitution of PNP activity in T lymphocytes derived from PNP-deficient subjects has been described (Nelson et al., 1995). These results suggest that T cells could potentially be used as vehicles for therapeutic *NP* gene expression. A clinical protocol testing this hypothesis was proposed in the mid-1990s, although technical difficulties have prevented it from entering the clinical stage. Because most PNP-deficient patients are profoundly lymphopenic and, in contrast to ADA deficients, this disease cannot be improved with enzyme replacement treatment, one expected problem in T lymphocyte–directed gene therapy for PNP deficiency is that patients will not have a sufficiently developed peripheral T cell repertoire before treatment to achieve meaningful immune reconstitution after gene correction. Moreover, the major neurologic abnormalities are not affected by either enzyme replacement in the form of exchange transfusions nor by HSCT.

Animal Models

ADA Knockout Mice

Although there are no known naturally occurring models of ADA deficiency, at least two groups have succeeded in generating ADA knockout mice (Blackburn et al., 1995; Migchielsen et al., 1995, 1996; Wakamiya et al., 1995). However, absence of ADA in mice leads to perinatal lethality. This finding is in contrast to the situation in humans; individuals homozygous for deletion of the promoter and exon 1 have been born alive and presented with a disease indistinguishable from that in other patients with ADA-deficient SCID. Pathologically, newborn knockout mice exhibit marked hepatocellular degeneration, atelectasis, and intestinal abnormalities. In contrast to humans with ADA-deficient SCID, in whom marked lymphopenia is evident by 18–20 weeks of gestation, there were only minor reductions in CD4+/CD8+ lymphoid cells in livers of ADA knockout mice.

The mice were rescued from perinatal lethality by two different approaches. Expression of a human ADA transgene containing human regulatory elements made them viable (Migchielsen et al., 1996), demonstrating that the lethality was not due to disruption of a gene within the ADA gene. More significantly, however, mice were rescued by expression of a transgene containing a promoter element restricting expression to the placenta and gastrointestinal tract organs with very high ADA activity in mice (Blackburn et al., 1995). Several of the metabolic abnormalities seen in humans were reproduced in these mice, including increased deoxyadenosine and dAMP in thymus and reduced SAH hydrolase in thymus, spleen, and liver. The mice showed moderate reductions in size of the thymus and spleen and in absolute numbers of lymphocytes in these organs. In summary, evidence for a mild immunodeficiency was found. It is possible that the postnatal expression of intestinal ADA provided partial immunologic rescue, suggesting that oral therapy might be ameliorative in human ADA deficiency. As an alternative explanation for the absence of profound immunodeficiency in the partially corrected mice, compensating pathways may exist in the mouse that alter the pathophysiology of ADA deficiency. It is well recognized that the final common pathway for purine metabolism, ending in uric acid, is quite different in mice from that in humans. Not infrequently, immunologic knockouts give phenotypes that differ between humans and mice.

More recently, a mouse deficient for ADA that does manifest combined immunodeficiency has been created by a two-stage genetic engineering strategy (Blackburn et al., 1998). These mice appear to reproduce not only the biochemical but also the immunologic abnormalities of the human disease. This model may therefore help clarify the role of enzyme deficiency in production of various human phenotypic features. ADA-deficient splenic B lymphocytes show defects in proliferation and activation with high propensity to undergo B cell receptor–mediated apoptosis. As a result, profound loss of germinal center architecture is noted, which may be responsible for impaired B cell development (Aldrich et al., 2003). In addition, the finding of renal pathology in these animals suggests that the renal abnormalities previously reported in humans with ADA deficiency are a manifestation of ADA deficiency (Ratech et al., 1985). Treatment of these mice with PEG-ADA showed that, while low doses could prevent the pulmonary insufficiency, the immunodeficiency could only be ameliorated by high doses, thus demonstrating a different impact of the therapy in different tissues (Blackburn et al., 2000). Further, these mice provided evidence that the respiratory failure was attributable to IL-13-mediated accumulation of activated alveolar macrophages and eosinophils and mast cell degranulation with airway hyperresponsiveness (Blackburn et al., 2000, 2003; Chunn et al., 2001). This finding offers insights into the mechanisms potentially responsible for asthmatic conditions and pulmonary insufficiency observed in some ADA-deficient humans.

PNP Knockout Mice

There are no known naturally occurring models for PNP deficiency. Attempts to develop PNP-deficient mice by mutagenizing drugs resulted in the identification of three missense mutations leading to severely reduced (1%–4.6%) but not absent PNP activity in erythrocytes (Mably et al., 1989; Snyder et al., 1997). Progressive thymic hypocellularity due to a reduction in CD4+/CD8+ double-positive cells was observed in these mice, which also showed a marked reduction in peripheral T lymphocyte numbers and function. Altough these mice were similar to humans with PNP deficiency, the delayed onset of the immune deficiency and the residual PNP activity were considered reasons to pursue total knockout models by gene targeting. PNP knockout animals were recently generated and show impaired thymic differentiation due to apoptotic signals originating in the mitochondria and decreased numbers of mature, dysfunctional T lymphocytes (Arpaia et al., 2000). As in humans with PNP deficiency, the B cell compartment in these mice is less affected with an increase in immature splenic pre-B cells. However, frequency of mature B lymphocytes is normal (Arpaia et al., 2000). These mice should prove useful for the testing of potential therapies such as PEG-PNP (Hershfield et al., 1991) and gene therapy.

Mouse models undoubtedly provide valuable insights into the pathogenesis of immunodeficiency due to defects of purine nucleotide metabolism. However, important differences may exist between mice and humans regarding both critical metabolic networks and alternative biochemical pathways. Conclusions on the significance of the findings observed in ADA and PNP knockout animals will have to be supported by confirmatory results obtained from studies in human patients.

Future Directions and Challenges

Even though ADA and PNP deficiency have been known to be the molecular basis of immunodeficiency and have been extensively investigated, major challenges remain from diagnostics to therapy to insights into the basic biology.

The discovery of the molecular basis of the various immunodeficiency disorders discussed in this volume makes it important to develop an overall strategy for diagnosing immune disorders. Currently, in a severely ill child, the first step is to determine the presence or absence of ADA deficiency, as enzyme replacement can provide a life-saving intervention. With development of other diagnostic and therapeutic options for additional disorders, this commonly used strategy may become outdated. With respect to diagnostics, ADA deficiency as an inherited disorder involves a family. The importance of experienced genetic counselors in helping family members deal with issues of identification as a carrier cannot be overemphasized. We are often contacted by family members to determine if they are carriers of the mutations(s) in their families. Currently, these investigations are "cottage industry" in approach. The development of "chip" technology for rapid scanning for mutations, now being applied on a research basis, could revolutionize diagnosis. However, given the rarity of the disease, automated mutation detection is unlikely to be developed by industry. Should there be an "orphan drug" equivalent for diagnostics to facilitate relatively noninvasive prenatal diagnosis not only for prevention but also for early institution of therapy when available? These concerns apply to virtually all primary immunodeficiency disorders.

With respect to basic biology, the role of ADA and adenosine is increasingly being investigated. Adenosine interacts with multiple receptors that have opposing actions in different cell types. ADA bound to CD26 at the cell surface plays a role in regulating local concentrations of adenosine. The potential role of adenosine in the clinical aspects of ADA deficiency has been ignored for some time. Because of the observation that children were immunocompetent after bone marrow transplantation, despite persistently elevated plasma adenosine concentrations, we have assumed there is no major role for adenosine in the pathophysiology of immunodeficiency. However, adenosine appears to be important in the pathogenesis of asthma, which may be more common in ADA-deficient patients than in the general population. Adenosine also has important roles in the cardiovascular and nervous systems. ADA shows localization to the nervous system, and recent experiments indicate a role for adenosine in regulating intracellular signaling pathways. An additional line of evidence of the importance of adenosine at the central nervous system (CNS) level comes from the clinical observation that methotrexate-induced coma is caused by elevated levels of adenosine and can be resolved by administration of an adenosine receptor antagonist (i.e., aminophylline). One of the most widespread clinical observations made by physicians treating ADA-deficient children for immunodeficiency has been that alertness improves when enzyme replacement therapy is instituted. Insufficient data are available, however, on long-term survivors of ADA-deficient SCID after HSCT to know whether these patients may have an intellectual or attention deficit.

With respect to therapy, the challenges are obvious. Roles for PEG-ADA and gene therapy exist for ADA-deficient patients lacking suitable donors for HSCT, but the risks of gene transfer into the hematopoietic stem cells for this disease must be defined.

Progress in clinical management of PNP deficiency is acutely needed to modify what is currently a poor prognosis. Even if successful HSCT can correct the immunodeficiency, the procedure most likely cannot reverse the CNS injury. An alternative therapy that needs to be explored is enzyme replacement with PEG-PNP, analogous to the use of PEG-ADA in ADA deficiency. In PNP knockout animals, PEG-PNP has been reported to raise the whole-blood PNP activity to 20% of wild-type levels and improve the metabolic abnormalities. PNP may also be a disease for hematopoietic stem cell gene therapy. With availability of PNP knockout mice, preclinical safety studies are now likely to begin.

References

Aitken DA, Ferguson-Smith MA. Regional assignment of nucleoside phosphorylase by exclusion to 14q13. Cytogenet Cell Genet 22:490–492, 1978.

Aiuti A, Slavin S, Aker M, Ficara F, Deola S, Mortellaro A, Morecki S, Andolfi G, Tabucchi A, Carlucci F, Marinello E, Cattaneo F, Vai S, Servida P, Miniero R, Roncarolo MG, Bordignon C. Correction of ADA-SCID by stem cell gene therapy combined with nonmyeloablative conditioning. Science 296:2410–2413, 2002a.

Aiuti A, Vai S, Mortellaro A, Casorati G, Ficara F, Andolfi G, Ferrari G, Tabucchi A, Carlucci F, Ochs HD, Notarangelo LD, Roncarolo MG, Bordignon C. Immune reconstitution in ADA-SCID after PBL gene therapy and discontinuation of enzyme replacement. Nat Med 8:423–425, 2002b.

Akeson AL, Wiginton DA, Dusing MR, States JC, Hutton JJ. Mutant human adenosine deaminase alleles and their expression by transfection into fibroblasts. J Biol Chem 263:16291–16296, 1988.

Akeson AL, Wiginton DA, States JC, Perme CM, Dusing MR, Hutton JJ. Mutations in the human adenosine deaminase gene that affect protein structure and RNA splicing. Proc Natl Acad Sci USA 84:5947–5951, 1987.

Albuquerque W, Gaspar HB. Bilateral sensorineural deafness in adenosine deaminase-deficient severe combined immunodeficiency. J Pediatr 144:278–280, 2004.

Aldrich MB, Chen W, Blackburn MR, Martinez-Valdez H, Datta SK, Kellems RE. Impaired germinal center maturation in adenosine deaminase deficiency. J Immunol 171:5562–5570, 2003.

Amrolia P, Gaspar HB, Hassan A, Webb D, Jones A, Sturt N, Mieli-Vergani G, Pagliuca A, Mufti G, Hadzic N, Davies G, Veys P. Nonmyeloablative stem cell transplantation for congenital immunodeficiencies. Blood 96:1239–1246, 2000.

Andrews LG, Markert ML. Exon skipping in purine nucleoside phosphorylase mRNA processing leading to severe immunodeficiency. J Biol Chem 267:7834–7838, 1992.

Antoine C, Muller S, Cant A, Cavazzana-Calvo M, Veys P, Vossen J, Fasth A, Heilmann C, Wulffraat N, Seger R, Blanche S, Friedrich W, Abinun M, Davies G, Bredius R, Schulz A, Landais P, Fischer A. Long-term survival and transplantation of haemopoietic stem cells for immunodeficiencies: report of the European experience 1968–99. Lancet 361:553–560, 2003.

Antony FC, Webster AD, Bain MD, Harland CC. Recalcitrant palmoplantar warts associated with adult-onset adenosine deaminase deficiency. Br J Dermatol 147:182–183, 2002.

Ariga T, Oda N, Sanstisteban I, Arredondo-Vega FX, Shioda M, Ueno H, Terada K, Kobayashi K, Hershfield MS, Sakiyama Y. Molecular basis for paradoxical carriers of adenosine deaminase (ADA) deficiency that show extremely low levels of ADA activity in peripheral blood cells without immunodeficiency. J Immunol 166:1698–1702, 2001a.

Ariga T, Oda N, Yamaguchi K, Kawamura N, Kikuta H, Taniuchi S, Kobayashi Y, Terada K, Ikeda H, Hershfield MS, Kobayashi K, Sakiyama Y. T-cell lines from 2 patients with adenosine deaminase (ADA) deficiency showed the restoration of ADA activity resulted from the reversion of an inherited mutation. Blood 97:2896–2899, 2001b.

Aronow BJ, Ebert CA, Valerius MT, Potter SS, Wiginton DA, Witte DP, Hutton JJ. Dissecting a locus control region: facilitation of enhancer function by extended enhancer-flanking sequences. Mol Cell Biol 15:1123–1135, 1995.

Arpaia E, Benveniste P, Di Cristofano A, Gu Y, Dalal I, Kelly S, Hershfield M, Pandolfi PP, Roifman CM, Cohen A. Mitochondrial basis for immune deficiency. Evidence from purine nucleoside phosphorylase-deficient mice. J Exp Med 191:2197–2208, 2000.

Arredondo-Vega FX, Santisteban I, Daniels S, Toutain S, Hershfield MS. Adenosine deaminase deficiency: genotype–phenotype correlations based on expressed activity of 29 mutant alleles. Am J Hum Genet 63:1049–1059, 1998.

Arredondo-Vega FX, Santisteban I, Kelly S, Schlossman CM, Umetsu DT, Hershfield MS. Correct splicing despite mutation of the invariant first nucleotide of a 5′ splice site: a possible basis for disparate clinical phenotypes in siblings with adenosine deaminase deficiency. Am J Hum Genet 54:820–830, 1994.

Arrendondo-Vega FX, Santisteban I, Notarangelo LD, El Dahr J, Buckley R, Roifman C, Conley ME, Hershfield MS. Seven novel mutations in the adenosine deaminase (ADA) gene in patients with severe and delayed onset combined immunodeficiency: G74C, V129M, G140E, R149W, Q199P, 462delG, and E337del. Mutations in brief no. 142. Online. Hum Mutat 11:482, 1998.

Arredondo-Vega FX, Santisteban I, Richard E, Bali P, Koleilat M, Loubser M, Al-Ghonaium A, Al-Helali M, Hershfield MS. Adenosine deaminase deficiency with mosaicism for a "second-site suppressor" of a splicing mutation: decline in revertant T lymphocytes during enzyme replacement therapy. Blood 99:1005–1013, 2001.

Atasoy U, Norby-Slycord CJ, Markert ML, Blaese RM, Culver KW, Chang L, Anderson WF, Mullen C, Nienhuis A, Carter C, Dunbar C, Leitman S, Berger M, et al. A missense mutation in exon 4 of the human adenosine deaminase gene causes severe combined immunodeficiency. Hum Mol Genet 2:1307–1308, 1993.

Aust MR, Andrews LG, Barrett MJ, Norby-Slycord CJ, Markert ML. Molecular analysis of mutations in a patient with purine nucleoside phosphorylase deficiency. Am J Hum Genet 51:763–772, 1992.

Baguette C, Vermylen C, Brichard B, Louis J, Dahan K, Vincent MF, Cornu G. Persistent developmental delay despite successful bone marrow transplantation for purine nucleoside phosphorylase deficiency. J Pediatr Hematol Oncol 24:69–71, 2002.

Banzhoff A, Schauer U, Riedel F, Gahr M, Rieger CH. Fatal varicella in a 5-year-old boy. Eur J Pediatr 156:333–334, 1997.

Baric I, Fumic K, Glenn B, Cuk M, Schulze A, Finkelstein JD, James SJ, Mejaski-Bosnjak V, Pazanin L, Pogribny IP, Rados M, Sarnavka V, Scukanec-Spoljar M, Allen RH, Stabler S, Uzelac L, Vugrek O, Wagner C, Zeisel S, Mudd SH. S-adenosylhomocysteine hydrolase deficiency in a human: a genetic disorder of methionine metabolism. Proc Natl Acad Sci USA 101:4234–4239, 2004.

Barton RW, Osborne WR. The effects of PNP inhibition on rat lymphoid cell populations. Adv Exp Med Biol 195(Part B):429–435, 1986.

Benveniste P, Cohen A. p53 expression is required for thymocyte apoptosis induced by adenosine deaminase deficiency. Proc Natl Acad Sci USA 92: 8373–8377, 1995.

Berkvens TM, van Ormondt H, Gerritsen EJ, Khan PM, van der Eb AJ. Identical 3250-bp deletion between two AluI repeats in the ADA genes of unrelated ADA-SCID patients. Genomics 7:486–490, 1990.

Bertrand Y, Landais P, Friedrich W, Gerritsen B, Morgan G, Fasth A, Cavazzana-Calvo M, Porta F, Cant A, Espanol T, Muller S, Veys P, Vossen J, Haddad E, Fischer A. Influence of severe combined immunodeficiency phenotype on the outcome of HLA non-identical, T-cell-depleted bone marrow transplantation: a retrospective European survey from the European Group for Bone Marrow Transplantation and the European Society for Immunodeficiency. J Pediatr 134:740–748, 1999.

Bhaumik D, Medin J, Gathy K, Coleman MS. Mutational analysis of active site residues of human adenosine deaminase. J Biol Chem 268:5464–5470, 1993.

Blackburn MR, Aldrich M, Volmer JB, Chen W, Zhong H, Kelly S, Hershfield MS, Datta SK, Kellems RE. The use of enzyme therapy to regulate the metabolic and phenotypic consequences of adenosine deaminase deficiency in mice. Differential impact on pulmonary and immunologic abnormalities. J Biol Chem 275:32114–32121, 2000.

Blackburn MR, Datta SK, Kellems RE. Adenosine deaminase-deficient mice generated using a two-stage genetic engineering strategy exhibit a combined immunodeficiency. J Biol Chem 273:5093–5100, 1998.

Blackburn MR, Lee CG, Young HW, Zhu Z, Chunn JL, Kang MJ, Banerjee SK, Elias JA. Adenosine Mediates IL-13-induced inflammation and remodeling in the lung and interacts in an IL-13-adenosine amplification pathway. J Clin Invest 112:332–344, 2003.

Blackburn MR, Wakamiya M, Caskey CT, Kellems RE. Tissue-specific rescue suggests that placental adenosine deaminase is important for fetal development in mice. J Biol Chem 270:23891–23894, 1995.

Blaese RM, Culver KW, Miller AD, Carter CS, Fleisher T, Clerici M, Shearer G, Chang L, Chiang Y, Tolstoshev P, Greenblatt JJ, Rosenberg SA, Klein H, Berger M, Mullen CA, Ramsey WJ, Muul L, Morgan RA, Anderson WF. T lymphocyte-directed gene therapy for ADA- SCID: initial trial results after 4 years. Science 270:475–480, 1995.

Bollinger ME, Arredondo-Vega FX, Santisteban I, Schwarz K, Hershfield MS, Lederman HM. Brief report: hepatic dysfunction as a complication of adenosine deaminase deficiency. N Engl J Med 334:1367–1371, 1996.

Bonthron DT, Markham AF, Ginsburg D, Orkin SH. Identification of a point mutation in the adenosine deaminase gene responsible for immunodeficiency. J Clin Invest 76:894–897, 1985.

Bordignon C, Notarangelo LD, Nobili N, Ferrari G, Casorati G, Panina P, Mazzolari E, Maggioni D, Rossi C, Servida P, Ugazio AG, Mavilio F. Gene therapy in peripheral blood lymphocytes and bone marrow for ADA-immunodeficient patients. Science 270:470–475, 1995.

Borkowsky W, Gershon AA, Shenkman L, Hirschhorn R. Adenosine deaminase deficiency without immunodeficiency: clinical and metabolic studies. Pediatr Res 14:885–889, 1980.

Boulieu R, Bory C, Souillet G. Purine metabolism in a bone-marrow transplanted adenosine deaminase deficient patient. Clin Chim Acta 178:349–352, 1988.

Broome CB, Graham ML, Saulsbury FT, Hershfield MS, Buckley RH. Correction of purine nucleoside phosphorylase deficiency by transplantation of allogeneic bone marrow from a sibling. J Pediatr 128:373–376, 1996.

Buckley RH. Advances in the understanding and treatment of human severe combined immunodeficiency. Immunol Res 22:237–251, 2000.

Buckley RH, Schiff RI, Schiff SE, Markert ML, Williams LW, Harville TO, Roberts JL, Puck JM. Human severe combined immunodeficiency: genetic, phenotypic, and functional diversity in one hundred eight infants. J Pediatr 130:378–387, 1997.

Buckley RH, Schiff SE, Sampson HA, Schiff RI, Markert ML, Knutsen AP, Hershfield MS, Huang AT, Mickey GH, Ward FE. Development of immunity in human severe primary T cell deficiency following haploidentical bone marrow stem cell transplantation. J Immunol 136:2398–2407, 1986.

Buckley RH, Schiff SE, Schiff RI, Markert L, Williams LW, Roberts JL, Myers LA, Ward FE. Hematopoietic stem-cell transplantation for the treatment of severe combined immunodeficiency. N Engl J Med 340:508–516, 1999.

Buckley RH, Schiff SE, Schiff RI, Roberts JL, Markert ML, Peters W, Williams LW, Ward FE. Haploidentical bone marrow stem cell transplantation in human severe combined immunodeficiency. Semin Hematol 30: 92–101; discussion 102–104, 1993.

Carapella De Luca E, Stegagno M, Dionisi Vici C, Paesano R, Fairbanks LD, Morris GS, Simmonds HA. Prenatal exclusion of purine nucleoside phosphorylase deficiency. Eur J Pediatr 145:51–53, 1986.

Carlucci F, Tabucchi A, Aiuti A, Rosi F, Floccari F, Pagani R, Marinello E. Capillary electrophoresis in diagnosis and monitoring of adenosine deaminase deficiency. Clin Chem 49:1830–1838, 2003.

Carpenter PA, Ziegler JB, Vowels MR. Late diagnosis and correction of purine nucleoside phosphorylase deficiency with allogeneic bone marrow transplantation. Bone Marrow Transplant 17:121–124, 1996.

Cederbaum SD, Kaitila I, Rimoin DL, Stiehm ER. The chondro-osseous dysplasia of adenosine deaminase deficiency with severe combined immunodeficiency. J Pediatr 89:737–742, 1976.

Chaffee S, Mary A, Stiehm ER, Girault D, Fischer A, Hershfield MS. IgG antibody response to polyethylene glycol-modified adenosine deaminase in patients with adenosine deaminase deficiency. J Clin Invest 89:1643–1651, 1992.

Chan B, Wara D, Bastian J, Hershfield MS, Bohnsack J, Azen CG, Parkman R, Weinberg K, Kohn DB. Long-term efficacy of enzyme replacement therapy for adenosine deaminase (ADA)-deficient severe combined immunodeficiency (SCID). Clin Immunol 117:133–143, 2005.

Chang ZY, Nygaard P, Chinault AC, Kellems RE. Deduced amino acid sequence of *Escherichia coli* adenosine deaminase reveals evolutionarily conserved amino acid residues: implications for catalytic function. Biochemistry 30:2273–2280, 1991.

Chen SH, Ochs HD, Scott CR, Giblett ER. Adenosine deaminase and nucleoside phosphorylase activity in patients with immunodeficiency syndromes. Clin Immunol Immunopathol 13:156–160, 1979.

Chen SH, Ochs HD, Scott CR, Giblett ER, Tingle AJ. Adenosine deaminase deficiency: disappearance of adenine deoxynucleotides from a patient's erythrocytes after successful marrow transplantation. J Clin Invest 62: 1386–1389, 1978.

Chen SH, Scott R, Giblett ER. Adenosine deaminase: demonstration of a "silent" gene associated with combined immunodeficiency disease. Am J Hum Genet 26:103–107, 1974.

Chu SY, Cashion P, Jiang M. Purine nucleoside phosphorylase in erythrocytes: determination of optimum reaction conditions. Clin Biochem 22:3–9, 1989.

Chun JD, Lee N, Kobayashi RH, Chaffee S, Hershfield MS, Stiehm ER. Suppression of an antibody to adenosine-deaminase (ADA) in an ADA-deficient patient receiving polyethylene glycol modified adenosine deaminase. Ann Allergy 70:462–466, 1993.

Chunn JL, Young HW, Banerjee SK, Colasurdo GN, Blackburn MR. Adenosine-dependent airway inflammation and hyperresponsiveness in partially adenosine deaminase-deficient mice. J Immunol 167:4676–4685, 2001.

Classen CF, Schulz AS, Sigl-Kraetzig M, Hoffmann GF, Simmonds HA, Fairbanks L, Debatin KM, Friedrich W. Successful HLA-identical bone marrow transplantation in a patient with PNP deficiency using busulfan and fludarabine for conditioning. Bone Marrow Transplant 28:93–96, 2001.

Cohen A, Gudas LJ, Ammann AJ, Staal G.E, Martin DW Jr. Deoxyguanosine triphosphate as a possible toxic metabolite in the immunodeficiency associated with purine nucleoside phosphorylase deficiency. J Clin Invest 61: 1405–1409, 1978.

Coleman MS, Danton MJ, Philips A. Adenosine deaminase and immune dysfunction. Biochemical correlates defined by molecular analysis throughout a disease course. Ann NY Acad Sci 451:54–65, 1985.

Coleman MS, Donofrio J, Hutton JJ, Hahn L, Daoud A, Lampkin B, Dyminski J. Identification and quantitation of adenine deoxynucleotides in erythrocytes of a patient with adenosine deaminase deficiency and severe combined immunodeficiency. J Biol Chem 253:1619–1626, 1978.

Daddona PE. Human adenosine deaminase. Properties and turnover in cultured T and B lymphoblasts. J Biol Chem 256:12496–12501, 1981.

Daddona PE, Kelley WN. Human adenosine deaminase. Purification and subunit structure. J Biol Chem 252:110–115, 1977.

Daddona PE, Mitchell BS, Meuwissen HJ, Davidson BL, Wilson JM, Koller CA. Adenosine deaminase deficiency with normal immune function. An acidic enzyme mutation. J Clin Invest 72:483–492, 1983.

Daddona PE, Shewach DS, Kelley WN, Argos P, Markham AF, Orkin SH. Human adenosine deaminase. cDNA and complete primary amino acid sequence. J Biol Chem 259:12101–12106, 1984.

Dalal I, Grunebaum E, Cohen A, Roifman CM. Two novel mutations in a purine nucleoside phosphorylase (PNP)-deficient patient. Clin Genet 59:430–437, 2001.

de Azevedo WFe Jr, Canduri F, dos Santos DM, Silva RG, de Oliveira JS, de Carvalho LP, Basso LA, Mendes MA, Palma MS, Santos DS. Crystal structure of human purine nucleoside phosphorylase at 2.3A resolution. Biochem Biophys Res Commun 308:545–552, 2003.

Dillman RO. Pentostatin (Nipent(R)) in the treatment of chronic lymphocyte leukemia and hairy cell leukemia. Expert Rev Anticancer Ther 4:27–36, 2004.

Dror Y, Grunebaum E, Hitzler J, Narendran A, Ye C, Tellier R, Edwards V, Freedman MH, Roifman CM. Purine nucleoside phosphorylase deficiency associated with a dysplastic marrow morphology. Pediatr Res 55: 472–477, 2004.

Durandy A, Oury C, Griscelli C, Dumez Y, Oury JF, Henrion R. Prenatal testing for inherited immune deficiencies by fetal blood sampling. Prenat Diagn 2:109–113, 1982.

Ealick SE, Babu YS, Bugg CE, Erion MD, Guida WC, Montgomery JA, Secrist JA, 3rd. Application of crystallographic and modeling methods in the design of purine nucleoside phosphorylase inhibitors. Proc Natl Acad Sci USA 88:11540–11544, 1991.

Ealick SE, Babu YS, Bugg CE, Erion MD, Guida WG, Montgomery JA, Secrist JA, 3rd. Application of X-ray crystallographic methods in the design of purine nucleoside phosphorylase inhibitors. Ann NY Acad Sci 685: 237–247, 1993.

Ealick SE, Rule SA, Carter DC, Greenhough TJ, Babu YS, Cook WJ, Habash J, Helliwell JR, Stoeckler JD, Parks RE, Jr, et al. Three-dimensional structure of human erythrocytic purine nucleoside phosphorylase at 3.2 A resolution. J Biol Chem 265:1812–1820, 1990.

Edwards YH, Hopkinson DA, Harris H. Adenosine deaminase isozymes in human tissues. Ann Hum Genet 35:207–219, 1971.

Fairbanks LD, Shovlin CL, Webster AD, Hughes JM, Simmonds HA. Adenosine deaminase deficiency with altered biochemical parameters in two sisters with late-onset immunodeficiency. J Inherit Metab Dis 17: 135–137, 1994.

Ferrari G, Rossini S, Giavazzi R, Maggioni D, Nobili N, Soldati M, Ungers G, Mavilio F, Gilboa E, Bordignon C. An in vivo model of somatic cell gene therapy for human severe combined immunodeficiency. Science 251: 1363–1366, 1991.

Fischer A. Primary immunodeficiencies: molecular aspects and treatment. Bone Marrow Transplant 9(Suppl 1):39–43, 1992.

Fischer A, Griscelli C, Friedrich W, Kubanek B, Levinsky R, Morgan G, Vossen J, Wagemaker G, Landais P. Bone-marrow transplantation for immunodeficiencies and osteopetrosis: European survey, 1968–1985. Lancet 2:1080–1084, 1986.

Fischer A, Landais P, Friedrich W, Morgan G, Gerritsen B, Fasth A, Porta F, Griscelli C, Goldman SF, Levinsky R, Vossen J. European experience of bone-marrow transplantation for severe combined immunodeficiency. Lancet 336:850–854, 1990.

Fleischman A, Hershfield MS, Toutain S, Lederman HM, Sullivan KE, Fasano MB, Greene J, Winkelstein JA. Adenosine deaminase deficiency and purine nucleoside phosphorylase deficiency in common variable immunodeficiency. Clin Diagn Lab Immunol 5:399–400, 1998.

Fox IH, Andres CM, Gelfand EW, Biggar D. Purine nucleoside phosphorylase deficiency: altered kinetic properties of a mutant enzyme. Science 197: 1084–1086, 1977.

Friedrich W, Goldmann SF, Ebell W, Blutters-Sawatzki R, Gaedicke G, Raghavachar A, Peter HH, Belohradsky B, Kreth W, Kubanek B, et al. Severe combined immunodeficiency: treatment by bone marrow transplantation in 15 infants using HLA-haploidentical donors. Eur J Pediatr 144:125–130, 1985.

Gaines AD, Schiff SE, Buckley RH. Donor type natural killer cells after haploidentical T cell-depleted bone marrow stem cell transplantation in a patient with adenosine deaminase-deficient severe combined immunodeficiency. Clin Immunol Immunopathol 60:299–304, 1991.

Geffner ME, Stiehm ER, Stephure D, Cowan MJ. Probable autoimmune thyroid disease and combined immunodeficiency disease. Am J Dis Child 140: 1194–1196, 1986.

George DL, Francke U. Gene dose effect: regional mapping of human nucleoside phosphorylase on chromosome 14. Science 194:851–852, 1976.

Giblett ER, Ammann AJ, Wara DW, Sandman R, Diamond LK. Nucleoside-phosphorylase deficiency in a child with severely defective T-cell immunity and normal B-cell immunity. Lancet 1:1010–1013, 1975.

Giblett ER, Anderson JE, Cohen F, Pollara B, Meuwissen HJ. Adenosine-deaminase deficiency in two patients with severely impaired cellular immunity. Lancet 2:1067–1069, 1972.

Goddard JM, Caput D, Williams SR, Martin DW Jr. Cloning of human purine-nucleoside phosphorylase cDNA sequences by complementation in *Escherichia coli*. Proc Natl Acad Sci USA 80:4281–4285, 1983.

Gossage DL, Norby-Slycord CJ, Hershfield MS, Markert ML. A homozygous 5 base-pair deletion in exon 10 of the adenosine deaminase (ADA) gene in a child with severe combined immunodeficiency and very low levels of ADA mRNA and protein. Hum Mol Genet 2:1493–1494, 1993.

Grunebaum E, Zhang J, Roifman CM. Novel mutations and hot-spots in patients with purine nucleoside phosphorylase deficiency. Nucleosides Nucleotides, Nucleic Acids 23:1411–1415, 2004.

Gudas LJ, Zannis VI, Clift SM, Ammann AJ, Staal GE, Martin DW Jr. Characterization of mutant subunits of human purine nucleoside phosphorylase. J Biol Chem 253:8916–8924, 1978.

Hacein-Bey-Abina S, Von Kalle C, Schmidt M, McCormack MP, Wulffraat N, Leboulch P, Lim A, Osborne CS, Pawliuk R, Morillon E, Sorensen R, Forster A, Fraser P, Cohen JI, de Saint Basile G, Alexander I, Wintergerst U, Frebourg T, Aurias A, Stoppa-Lyonnet D, Romana S, Radford-Weiss I, Gross F, Valensi F, Delabesse E, Macintyre E, Sigaux F, Soulier J, Leiva LE, Wissler M, Prinz C, Rabbitts TH, Le Deist F, Fischer A, Cavazzana-Calvo M. LMO2-associated clonal T cell proliferation in two patients after gene therapy for SCID-X1. Science 302:415–419, 2003.

Haddad E, Landais P, Friedrich W, Gerritsen B, Cavazzana-Calvo M, Morgan G, Bertrand Y, Fasth A, Porta F, Cant A, Espanol T, Muller S, Veys P, Vossen J, Fischer A. Long-term immune reconstitution and outcome after HLA-nonidentical T- cell-depleted bone marrow transplantation for severe combined immunodeficiency: a European retrospective study of 116 patients. Blood 91:3646–3653, 1998.

Hallett RJ, Gaspar B, Duley JA, et al. Allogeneic bone marrow transplantation corrects the immunodeficiency in PNP deficiency but does nor reverse the neurological abnormalities. Cell Mol Biol Lett 4:374, 1999.

Henderson JF, Scott FW, Lowe JK. Toxicity of naturally occurring purine deoxyribonucleosides. Pharmacol Ther 8:573–604, 1980.

Hershfield MS. PEG-ADA replacement therapy for adenosine deaminase deficiency: an update after 8.5 years. Clin Immunol Immunopathol 76: S228–232, 1995a.

Hershfield MS. PEG-ADA: an alternative to haploidentical bone marrow transplantation and an adjunct to gene therapy for adenosine deaminase deficiency. Hum Mutat 5:107–112, 1995b.

Hershfield MS. Adenosine deaminase deficiency: clinical expression, molecular basis, and therapy. Semin Hematol 35:291–298, 1998.

Hershfield MS. Immunodeficiency caused by adenosine deaminase deficiency. Immunol All Clin North Am 20:161–175, 2000.

Hershfield MS. Combined immune deficiencies due to purine enzyme defects. In: Stiehm ER, Ochs HD, Winkelstein JA, eds. Immunologic Disorders in Infants and Children. New York: editor Elsevier, pp. – , 2004.

Hershfield MS, Buckley RH, Greenberg ML, Melton AL, Schiff R, Hatem C, Kurtzberg J, Markert ML, Kobayashi RH, Kobayashi AL, Abuchowski A. Treatment of adenosine deaminase deficiency with polyethylene glycol-modified adenosine deaminase. N Engl J Med 316:589–596, 1987.

Hershfield MS, Chaffee S, Koro-Johnson L, Mary A, Smith AA, Short SA. Use of site-directed mutagenesis to enhance the epitope-shielding effect of covalent modification of proteins with polyethylene glycol. Proc Natl Acad Sci USA 88:7185–7189, 1991.

Hershfield MS, Chaffee S, Sorensen RU. Enzyme replacement therapy with polyethylene glycol-adenosine deaminase in adenosine deaminase deficiency: overview and case reports of three patients, including two now receiving gene therapy. Pediatr Res 33:S42–47; discussion S47–48, 1993.

Hershfield MS, Kredich NM, Ownby DR, Ownby H, Buckley R. In vivo inactivation of erythrocyte S-adenosylhomocysteine hydrolase by 2′-deoxyadenosine in adenosine deaminase-deficient patients. J Clin Invest 63:807–811, 1979.

Hershfield MS, Mitchell BS. Immunodeficiency diseases caused by adenosine deaminase deficiency and purine nucleoside phosphorylase deficiency. In: Scriver CR, Beaudet AL, Sly WS, Valle D, eds. The Metabolic and Molecular Bases of Inherited Disease. New York: McGraw-Hill, pp. 2585–2625, 2001.

Hirschhorn R. Conversion of human erythrocyte-adenosine deaminase activity to different tissue-specific isozymes. Evidence for a common catalytic unit. J Clin Invest 55:661–667, 1975.

Hirschhorn R. Clinical Delineation of Adenosine Deaminase Deficiency. Amsterdam: Excerpta Medica, Ciba Foundation Symposium, 1979a.

Hirschhorn R. Incidence and prenatal detection of adenosine deaminase deficiency and purine nucleoside phosphorylase deficiency. In: Pollara B, Pickering RJ, Meuwissen HG, Porter I, eds. Inborn Errors of Specific Immunity. New York: Academic Press pp. 5–15, 1979b.

Hirschhorn R. Prenatal diagnosis and heretozygote detection in adenosine deaminase deficiency. In: Guttler F, Seakins JWT, Harkness RA, eds. Inborn Errors of Immunity and Phagocytosis. Lancaster: MTP Press, pp. 121–128, 1979c.

Hirschhorn R. Adenosine deaminase deficiency. Immunodefic Rev 2:175–198, 1990.

Hirschhorn R. Identification of two new missense mutations (R156C and S291L) in two ADA- SCID patients unusual for response to therapy with partial exchange transfusions. Hum Mutat 1:166–168, 1992a.

Hirschhorn R. Prenatal diagnosis of adenosine deaminase deficiency and other selected immunodeficiencies. In: Milunski A, ed. Genetic Disorders and the Fetus: Diagnosis, Prevention, and Treatment. New York: Plenum Press, pp. 453–464, 1992b.

Hirschhorn R. Overview of biochemical abnormalities and molecular genetics of adenosine deaminase deficiency. Pediatr Res 33:S35–41, 1993.

Hirschhorn R. In vivo reversion to normal of inherited mutations in humans. J Med Genet 40:721–728, 2003.

Hirschhorn R, Beratis N, Rosen FS, Parkman R, Stern R, Polmar S. Adenosine-deaminase deficiency in a child diagnosed prenatally. Lancet 1:73–75, 1975.

Hirschhorn R, Borkowsky W, Jiang CK, Yang DR, Jenkins T. Two newly identified mutations (Thr233Ile and Leu152Met) in partially adenosine deaminase–deficient (ADA−) individuals that result in differing biochemical and metabolic phenotypes. Hum Genet 100:22–29, 1997.

Hirschhorn R, Chakravarti V, Puck J, Douglas SD. Homozygosity for a newly identified missense mutation in a patient with very severe combined immunodeficiency due to adenosine deaminase deficiency (ADA-SCID). Am J Hum Genet 49:878–885, 1991.

Hirschhorn R, Chen AS, Israni A, Yang DR, Huie ML. Two new mutations at the adenosine deaminase (ADA) locus (Q254X and del nt1050–54) unusual for not being missense mutations. Hum Mutat 2:320–323, 1993a.

Hirschhorn R, Ellenbogen A. Genetic heterogeneity in adenosine deaminase (ADA) deficiency: five different mutations in five new patients with partial ADA deficiency. Am J Hum Genet 38:13–25, 1986.

Hirschhorn R, Martiniuk F, Roegner-Maniscalco V, Ellenbogen A, Perignon JL, Jenkins T. Genetic heterogeneity in partial adenosine deaminase deficiency. J Clin Invest 71:1887–1892, 1983.

Hirschhorn R, Martiniuk F, Rosen FS. Adenosine deaminase activity in normal tissues and tissues from a child with severe combined immunodeficiency and adenosine deaminase deficiency. Clin Immunol Immunopathol 9:287–292, 1978.

Hirschhorn R, Nicknam MN, Eng F, Yang DR, Borkowsky W. Novel deletion and a new missense mutation (Glu 217 Lys) at the catalytic site in two adenosine deaminase alleles of a patient with neonatal onset adenosine deaminase–severe combined immunodeficiency. J Immunol 149:3107–3112, 1992.

Hirschhorn R, Paageorgiou PS, Kesarwala HH, Taft LT. Amelioration of neurologic abnormalities after "enzyme replacement" in adenosine deaminase deficiency. N Engl J Med 303:377–380, 1980a.

Hirschhorn R, Ratech H. Isozymes of adenosine deaminase. Isozymes Curr Top Biol Med Res 4:131–157, 1980.

Hirschhorn R, Ratech H, Rubinstein A, Papageorgiou P, Kesarwala H, Gelfand E, Roegner-Maniscalco V. Increased excretion of modified adenine nucleosides by children with adenosine deaminase deficiency. Pediatr Res 16:362–369, 1982.

Hirschhorn R, Roegner V, Jenkins T, Seaman C, Piomelli S, Borkowsky W. Erythrocyte adenosine deaminase deficiency without immunodeficiency. Evidence for an unstable mutant enzyme. J Clin Invest 64:1130–1139, 1979a.

Hirschhorn R, Roegner V, Rubinstein A, Papageorgiou P. Plasma deoxyadenosine, adenosine, and erythrocyte deoxyATP are elevated at birth in an adenosine deaminase-deficient child. J Clin Invest 65:768–771, 1980b.

Hirschhorn R, Roegner-Maniscalco V, Kuritsky L, Rosen FS. Bone marrow transplantation only partially restores purine metabolites to normal in adenosine deaminase–deficient patients. J Clin Invest 68:1387–1393, 1981.

Hirschhorn R, Tzall S, Ellenbogen A. Hot spot mutations in adenosine deaminase deficiency. Proc Natl Acad Sci USA 87:6171–6175, 1990.

Hirschhorn R, Tzall S, Ellenbogen A, Orkin SH. Identification of a point mutation resulting in a heat-labile adenosine deaminase (ADA) in two unrelated children with partial ADA deficiency. J Clin Invest 83:497–501, 1989.

Hirschhorn R, Vawter GF, Kirkpatrick JA Jr., Rosen FS. Adenosine deaminase deficiency: frequency and comparative pathology in autosomally recessive severe combined immunodeficiency. Clin Immunol Immunopathol 14:107–120, 1979b.

Hirschhorn R, Yang DR, Insel RA, Ballow M. Severe combined immunodeficiency of reduced severity due to homozygosity for an adenosine deaminase missense mutation (Arg253Pro). Cell Immunol 152:383–393, 1993b.

Hirschhorn R, Yang DR, Israni A. An Asp8Asn substitution results in the adenosine deaminase (ADA) genetic polymorphism (ADA 2 allozyme): occurrence on different chromosomal backgrounds and apparent intragenic crossover. Ann Hum Genet 58:1–9, 1994a.

Hirschhorn R, Yang DR, Israni A, Huie ML, Ownby DR. Somatic mosaicism for a newly identified splice-site mutation in a patient with adenosine deaminase–deficient immunodeficiency and spontaneous clinical recovery. Am J Hum Genet 55:59–68, 1994b.

Hirschhorn R, Yang DR, Puck JM, Huie ML, Jiang CK, Kurlandsky LE. Spontaneous in vivo reversion to normal of an inherited mutation in a patient with adenosine deaminase deficiency. Nat Genet 13:290–295, 1996.

Hoogerbrugge PM, van Beusechem VW, Fischer A, Debree M, Le Deist F, Perignon JL, Morgan G, Gaspar B, Fairbanks LD, Skeoch CH, Moseley A, Harvey M, Levinsky RJ, Valerio D. Bone marrow gene transfer in three patients with adenosine deaminase deficiency. Gene Ther 3:179–183, 1996.

Hopp RJ, Kobayashi RH, Antonson DL. Iron overload as a result of transfusion therapy in a patient with adenosine deaminase deficiency. Nebr Med J 70:95–97, 1985.

Ibrahim MM, Weber IT, Knudsen TB. Mutagenesis of human adenosine deaminase to active forms that partially resist inhibition by pentostatin. Biochem Biophys Res Commun 209:407–416, 1995.

Jiang C, Hong R, Horowitz SD, Kong X, Hirschhorn R. An adenosine deaminase (ADA) allele contains two newly identified deleterious mutations (Y97C and L106V) that interact to abolish enzyme activity. Hum Mol Genet 6:2271–2278, 1997.

Kameoka J, Tanaka T, Nojima Y, Schlossman SF, Morimoto C. Direct association of adenosine deaminase with a T cell activation antigen, CD26. Science 261:466–469, 1993.

Kane L, Gennery AR, Crooks BN, Flood TJ, Abinun M, Cant AJ. Neonatal bone marrow transplantation for severe combined immunodeficiency. Arch Dis Child Fetal Neonatal Ed 85:F110–113, 2001.

Kawamoto H, Ito K, Kashii S, Monden S, Fujita M, Norioka M, Sasai Y, Okuma M. A point mutation in the 5' splice region of intron 7 causes a deletion of exon 7 in adenosine deaminase mRNA. J Cell Biochem 51:322–325, 1993.

Kleijer WJ, Hussaarts-Odijk LM, Los FJ, Pijpers L, De Bree PK, Duran M. Prenatal diagnosis of purine nucleoside phosphorylase deficiency in the first and second trimesters of pregnancy. Prenat Diagn 9:401–407, 1989.

Kohn DB, Hershfield MS, Carbonaro D, Shigeoka A, Brooks J, Smogorzewska EM, Barsky LW, Chan R, Burotto F, Annett G, Nolta JA, Crooks G, Kapoor N, Elder M, Wara D, Bowen T, Madsen E, Snyder FF, Bastian J, Muul L, Blaese RM, Weinberg K, Parkman R. T lymphocytes with a normal ADA gene accumulate after transplantation of transduced autologous umbilical cord blood CD34+ cells in ADA-deficient SCID neonates. Nat Med 4:775–780, 1998.

Kohn DB, Weinberg KI, Nolta JA, Heiss LN, Lenarsky C, Crooks GM, Hanley ME, Annett G, Brooks JS, el-Khoureiy A, Lawrence K, Wells S, Moen RC, Bastian J, Williams-Herman DE, Elder M, Wara D, Bowen T, Hershfield MS, Mullen CA, Blaese RM, Parkman R. Engraftment of gene-modified umbilical cord blood cells in neonates with adenosine deaminase deficiency. Nat Med 1:1017–1023, 1995.

Kuttesch JF, Schmalstieg FC, Nelson JA. Analysis of adensine and other adenine compounds in patients with immunodeficiency diseases. J Liquid Chromatogr 1:97–109, 1978.

Levy Y, Hershfield MS, Fernandez-Mejia C, Polmar SH, Scudiery D, Berger M, Sorensen RU. Adenosine deaminase deficiency with late onset of recurrent infections: response to treatment with polyethylene glycol-modified adenosine deaminase. J Pediatr 113:312–317, 1988.

Linch DC, Levinsky RJ, Rodeck CH, Maclennan KA, Simmonds HA. Prenatal diagnosis of three cases of severe combined immunodeficiency: severe T cell deficiency during the first half of gestation in fetuses with adenosine deaminase deficiency. Clin Exp Immunol 56:223–232, 1984.

Mably ER, Fung E, Snyder FF. Genetic deficiency of purine nucleoside phosphorylase in the mouse. Characterization of partially and severely enzyme deficient mutants. Genome 32:1026–1032, 1989.

Markert ML. Purine nucleoside phosphorylase deficiency. Immunodefic Rev 3:45–81, 1991.

Markert ML. Molecular basis of adenosine deaminase deficiency. Immunodeficiency 5:141–157, 1994.

Markert ML, Finkel BD, McLaughlin TM, Watson TJ, Collard HR, McMahon CP, Andrews LG, Barrett MJ, Ward FE. Mutations in purine nucleoside phosphorylase deficiency. Hum Mutat 9:118–121, 1997.

Markert ML, Hershfield MS, Schiff RI, Buckley RH. Adenosine deaminase and purine nucleoside phosphorylase deficiencies: evaluation of therapeutic interventions in eight patients. J Clin Immunol 7:389–399, 1987.

Markert ML, Hutton JJ, Wiginton DA, States JC, Kaufman RE. Adenosine deaminase (ADA) deficiency due to deletion of the ADA gene promoter and first exon by homologous recombination between two Alu elements. J Clin Invest 81:1323–1327, 1988.

McGinniss MH, Wasniowska K, Zopf DA, Straus SE, Reichert CM. An erythrocyte Pr auto-antibody with sialoglycoprotein specificity in a patient with purine nucleoside phosphorylase deficiency. Transfusion 25:131–136, 1985.

Meuwissen HJ, Pollara B, Pickering RJ. Combined immunodeficiency disease associated with adenosine deaminase deficiency. Report on a workshop held in Albany, New York, October 1, 1973. J Pediatr 86:169–181, 1975.

Migchielsen AA, Breuer ML, Hershfield MS, Valerio D. Full genetic rescue of adenosine deaminase-deficient mice through introduction of the human gene. Hum Mol Genet 5:1523–1532, 1996.

Migchielsen AA, Breuer ML, van Roon MA, te Riele H, Zurcher C, Ossendorp F, Toutain S, Hershfield MS, Berns A, Valerio D. Adenosine-deaminase-deficient mice die perinatally and exhibit liver-cell degeneration, atelectasis and small intestinal cell death. Nat Genet 10:279–287, 1995.

Mills GC, Schmalstieg FC, Koolkin RJ, Goldblum RM. Urinary excretion of purines, purine nucleosides, and pseudouridine in immunodeficient children. Biochem Med 27:37–45, 1982.

Moallem HJ, Taningo G, Jiang CK, Hirschhorn R, Fikrig S. Purine nucleoside phosphorylase deficiency: a new case report and identification of two novel mutations (Gly156A1a and Val217Ile), only one of which (Gly156A1a) is deleterious. Clin Immunol 105:75–80, 2002.

Mohamedali KA, Kurz LC, Rudolph FB. Site-directed mutagenesis of active site glutamate-217 in mouse adenosine deaminase. Biochemistry 35:1672–1680, 1996.

Morgan G, Levinsky RJ, Hugh-Jones K, Fairbanks LD, Morris GS, Simmonds HA. Heterogeneity of biochemical, clinical and immunological parameters in severe combined immunodeficiency due to adenosine deaminase deficiency. Clin Exp Immunol 70:491–499, 1987.

Mullen CA, Snitzer K, Culver KW, Morgan RA, Anderson WF, Blaese RM. Molecular analysis of T lymphocyte–directed gene therapy for adenosine deaminase deficiency: long-term expression in vivo of genes introduced with a retroviral vector. Hum Gene Ther 7:1123–1129, 1996.

Muul LM, Tuschong LM, Soenen SL, Jagadeesh GJ, Ramsey WJ, Long Z, Carter CS, Garabedian EK, Alleyne M, Brown M, Bernstein W, Schurman SH, Fleisher TA, Leitman SF, Dunbar CE, Blaese RM, Candotti F. Persistence and expression of the adenosine deaminase gene for 12 years and immune reaction to gene transfer components: long-term results of the first clinical gene therapy trial. Blood 101:2563–2569, 2003.

Nelson DM, Butters KA, Markert ML, Reinsmoen NL, McIvor RS. Correction of proliferative responses in purine nucleoside phosphorylase (PNP)-deficient T lymphocytes by retroviral-mediated PNP gene transfer and expression. J Immunol 154:3006–3014, 1995.

Nishihara H, Ishikawa S, Shinkai K, Akedo H. Multiple forms of human adenosine deaminase. II. Isolation and properties of a conversion factor from human lung. Biochim Biophys Acta 302:429–442, 1973.

Nonoyama S, Hollenbaugh D, Aruffo A, Ledbetter JA, Ochs HD. B cell activation via CD40 is required for specific antibody production by antigen-stimulated human B cells. J Exp Med 178:1097–1102, 1993.

Notarangelo LD, Stoppoloni G, Toraldo R, Mazzolari E, Coletta A, Airo P, Bordignon C, Ugazio AG. Insulin-dependent diabetes mellitus and severe atopic dermatitis in a child with adenosine deaminase deficiency. Eur J Pediatr 151:811–814, 1992.

Ochs HD, Buckley RH, Kobayashi RH, Kobayashi AL, Sorensen RU, Douglas SD, Hamilton BL, Hershfield MS. Antibody responses to bacteriophage phi X174 in patients with adenosine deaminase deficiency. Blood 80:1163–1171, 1992.

Ochs UH, Chen SH, Ochs HD, Osborne WR, Scott CR. Purine nucleoside phosphorylase deficiency: a molecular model for selective loss of T cell function. J Immunol 122:2424–2429, 1979.

Onodera M, Ariga T, Kawamura N, Kobayashi I, Ohtsu M, Yamada M, Tame A, Furuta H, Okano M, Matsumoto S, Kotani H, McGarrity GJ, Blaese RM, Sakiyama Y. Successful peripheral T lymphocyte–directed gene transfer for a patient with severe combined immune deficiency due to adenosine deaminase deficiency. Blood 91:30–36, 1998.

Osborne WR. Human red cell purine nucleoside phosphorylase. Purification by biospecific affinity chromatography and physical properties. J Biol Chem 255:7089–7092, 1980.

Osborne WR. Nucleoside kinases in T and B lymphoblasts distinguished by autoradiography. Proc Natl Acad Sci USA 83:4030–4034, 1986.

Osborne WR, Barton RW. A rat model of purine nucleoside phosphorylase deficiency. Immunology 59:63–67, 1986.

Osborne WR, Chen SH, Giblett ER, Biggar WD, Ammann AA, Scott CR. Purine nucleoside phosphorylase deficiency. Evidence for molecular heterogeneity in two families with enzyme-deficient members. J Clin Invest 60:741–746, 1977.

Osborne WR, Deeg HJ, Slichter SJ. A canine model of induced purine nucleoside phosphorylase deficiency. Clin Exp Immunol 66:166–172, 1986.

Osborne WR, Scott CR. The metabolism of deoxyguanosine and guanosine in human B and T lymphoblasts. A role for deoxyguanosine kinase activ-

ity in the selective T-cell defect associated with purine nucleoside phosphorylase deficiency. Biochem J 214:711–718, 1983.

Otsu M, Hershfield MS, Tuschong LM, Muul LM, Onodera M, Ariga T, Sakiyama Y, Candotti F. Flow cytometry analysis of adenosine deaminase (ADA) expression: a simple and reliable tool for the assessment of ADA-deficient patients before and after gene therapy. Hum Gene Ther 13:425–432, 2002.

Ozsahin H, Arredondo-Vega FX, Santisteban I, Fuhrer H, Tuchschmid P, Jochum W, Aguzzi A, Lederman HM, Fleischman A, Winkelstein JA, Seger RA, Hershfield MS. Adenosine deaminase deficiency in adults. Blood 89:2849–2855, 1997.

Pannicke U, Tuchschmid P, Friedrich W, Bartram CR, Schwarz K. Two novel missense and frameshift mutations in exons 5 and 6 of the purine nucleoside phosphorylase (PNP) gene in a severe combined immunodeficiency (SCID) patient. Hum Genet 98:706–709, 1996.

Parkman R. The biology of bone marrow transplantation for severe combined immune deficiency. Adv Immunol 49:381–410, 1991.

Parkman R, Gelfand EW, Rosen FS, Sanderson A, Hirschhorn R. Severe combined immunodeficiency and adenosine deaminase deficiency. N Engl J Med 292:714–719, 1975.

Perignon JL, Durandy A, Peter MO, Freycon F, Dumez Y, Griscelli C. Early prenatal diagnosis of inherited severe immunodeficiencies linked to enzyme deficiencies. J Pediatr 111:595–598, 1987.

Plagemann PG, Wohlhueter RM, Woffendin C. Nucleoside and nucleobase transport in animal cells. Biochim Biophys Acta 947:405–443, 1988.

Pollack MS, Maurer DH, Mattes MJ, LeBlanc D, Horowitz SD, Hong R. HLA typing of amniotic fluid cells for the prenatal determination of therapeutic transplantation options for a fetus affected with adenosine deaminase deficiency. Transplantation 36:336–337, 1983.

Polmar SH, Stern RC, Schwartz AL, Wetzler EM, Chase PA, Hirschhorn R. Enzyme replacement therapy for adenosine deaminase deficiency and severe combined immunodeficiency. N Engl J Med 295:1337–1343, 1976.

Ratech H, Greco MA, Gallo G, Rimoin DL, Kamino H, Hirschhorn R. Pathologic findings in adenosine deaminase–deficient severe combined immunodeficiency. I. Kidney, adrenal, and chondro-osseous tissue alterations. Am J Pathol 120:157–169, 1985.

Ratech H, Hirschhorn R, Greco MA. Pathologic findings in adenosine deaminase deficient–severe combined immunodeficiency. II. Thymus, spleen, lymph node, and gastrointestinal tract lymphoid tissue alterations. Am J Pathol 135:1145–1156, 1989.

Ratech H, Kuritsky L, Thorbecke GJ, Hirschhorn R. Suppression of human lymphocyte DNA and protein synthesis in vitro by adenosine and eight modified adenine nucleosides in the presence or in the absence of adenosine deaminase inhibitors, 2′-deoxycoformycin (DCF) and erythro-9-(2-hydroxy-3-nonyl) adenine (EHNA). Cell Immunol 68:244–251, 1982.

Ratech H, Thorbecke GJ, Meredith G, Hirschhorn R. Comparison and possible homology of isozymes of adenosine deaminase in Aves and humans. Enzyme 26:74–84, 1981.

Ricciuti F, Ruddle FH. Assignment of nucleoside phosphorylase to D-14 and localization of X-linked loci in man by somatic cell genetics. Nat New Biol 241:180–182, 1973.

Rich KC, Majias E, Fox IH. Purine nucleoside phosphorylase deficiency: improved metabolic and immunologic function with erythrocyte transfusions. N Engl J Med 303:973–977, 1980.

Rogers MH, Lwin R, Fairbanks L, Gerritsen B, Gaspar HB. Cognitive and behavioral abnormalities in adenosine deaminase deficient severe combined immunodeficiency. J Pediatr 139:44–50, 2001.

Rubocki RJ, Parsa JR, Hershfield MS, Sanger WG, Pirruccello SJ, Santisteban I, Gordon BG, Strandjord SE, Warkentin PI, Coccia PF. Full hematopoietic engraftment after allogeneic bone marrow transplantation without cytoreduction in a child with severe combined immunodeficiency. Blood 97:809–811, 2001.

Santisteban I, Arredondo-Vega FX, Kelly S, Debre M, Fischer A, Perignon JL, Hilman B, elDahr J, Dreyfus DH, Gelfand EW, et al. Four new adenosine deaminase mutations, altering a zinc-binding histidine, two conserved alanines, and a 5' splice site. Hum Mutat 5:243–250, 1995a.

Santisteban I, Arredondo-Vega FX, Kelly S, Loubser M, Meydan N, Roifman C, Howell PL, Bowen T, Weinberg KI, Schroeder ML, et al. Three new adenosine deaminase mutations that define a splicing enhancer and cause severe and partial phenotypes: implications for evolution of a CpG hotspot and expression of a transduced ADA cDNA. Hum Mol Genet 4:2081–2087, 1995b.

Santisteban I, Arredondo-Vega FX, Kelly S, Mary A, Fischer A, Hummell DS, Lawton A, Sorensen RU, Stiehm ER, Uribe L, et al. Novel splicing, missense, and deletion mutations in seven adenosine deaminase–deficient patients with late/delayed onset of combined immunodeficiency disease.

Contribution of genotype to phenotype. J Clin Invest 92:2291–2302, 1993.

Sasaki Y, Iseki M, Yamaguchi S, Kurosawa Y, Yamamoto T, Moriwaki Y, Kenri T, Sasaki T, Yamashita R. Direct evidence of autosomal recessive inheritance of Arg24 to termination codon in purine nucleoside phosphorylase gene in a family with a severe combined immunodeficiency patient. Hum Genet 103:81–85, 1998.

Schrader WP, Stacy AR. Purification and subunit structure of adenosine deaminase from human kidney. J Biol Chem 252:6409–6415, 1977.

Schwartz AL, Polmar SH, Stern RC, Cowan DH. Abnormal platelet aggregation in severe combined immunodeficiency disease with adenosine deaminase deficiency. Br J Haematol 39:189–194, 1978.

Scott CR, Chen SH, Giblett ER. Detection of the carrier state in combined immunodeficiency disease associated with adenosine deaminase deficiency. J Clin Invest 53:1194–1196, 1974.

Sekhsaria S, Fleisher TA, Vowells S, Brown M, Miller J, Gordon I, Blaese RM, Dunbar CE, Leitman S, Malech HL. Granulocyte colony-stimulating factor recruitment of CD34+ progenitors to peripheral blood: impaired mobilization in chronic granulomatous disease and adenosine deaminase–deficient severe combined immunodeficiency patients. Blood 88: 1104–1112, 1996.

Sharff AJ, Wilson DK, Chang Z, Quiocho FA. Refined 2.5 A structure of murine adenosine deaminase at pH 6.0. J Mol Biol 226:917–921, 1992.

Shovlin CL, Hughes JM, Simmonds HA, Fairbanks L, Deacock S, Lechler R, Roberts I, Webster AD, Markert ML, Hirschhorn R, Yang DR, Israni A. Adult presentation of adenosine deaminase deficiency. Lancet 341:1471, 1993.

Shovlin CL, Simmonds HA, Fairbanks LD, Deacock SJ, Hughes JM, Lechler RI, Webster AD, Sun XM, Webb JC, Soutar AK. Adult onset immunodeficiency caused by inherited adenosine deaminase deficiency. J Immunol 153:2331–2339, 1994.

Sideraki V, Mohamedali KA, Wilson DK, Chang Z, Kellems RE, Quiocho FA, Rudolph FB. Probing the functional role of two conserved active site aspartates in mouse adenosine deaminase. Biochemistry 35:7862–7872, 1996.

Silber GM, Winkelstein JA, Moen RC, Horowitz SD, Trigg M, Hong R. Reconstitution of T- and B-cell function after T-lymphocyte-depleted haploidentical bone marrow transplantation in severe combined immunodeficiency due to adenosine deaminase deficiency. Clin Immunol Immunopathol 44:317–320, 1987.

Simmonds HA, Fairbanks LD, Webster DR, Rodeck CH, Linch DC, Levinsky RJ. Rapid prenatal diagnosis of adenosine deaminase deficiency and other purine disorders using foetal blood. Biosci Rep 3:31–38, 1983.

Simmonds HA, Levinsky RJ, Perrett D, Webster DR. Reciprocal relationship between erythrocyte ATP and deoxy-ATP levels in inherited ADA deficiency. Biochem Pharmacol 31:947–951, 1982.

Simmonds HA, Sahota A, Potter CF, Cameron JS. Purine metabolism and immunodeficiency: urinary purine excretion as a diagnostic screening test in adenosine deaminase and purine nucleoside phosphorylase deficiency. Clin Sci Mol Med 54:579–584, 1978.

Sircar JC, Kostlan CR, Pinter GW, Suto MJ, Bobovski TP, Capiris T, Schwender CF, Dong MK, Scott ME, Bennett MK, et al. 8-Amino-9-substituted guanines: potent purine nucleoside phosphorylase (PNP) inhibitors. Agents Actions 21:253–256, 1987.

Snyder FF, Jenuth JP, Mably ER, Mangat RK. Point mutations at the purine nucleoside phosphorylase locus impair thymocyte differentiation in the mouse. Proc Natl Acad Sci USA 94:2522–2527, 1997.

Spencer N, Hopkinson DA, Harris T. Adenosine deaminase polymorphysm in man. Ann Hum Genet 32:9–14, 1968.

Staal GE, Stoop JW, Zegers BJ, Siegenbeek van Heukelom LH, van der Vlist MJ, Wadman SK, Martin DW. Erythrocyte metabolism in purine nucleoside phosphorylase deficiency after enzyme replacement therapy by infusion of erythrocytes. J Clin Invest 65:103–108, 1980.

Suetsugu S, Miki H, Takenawa T. Identification of two human WAVE/SCAR homologues as general actin regulatory molecules which associate with the Arp2/3 complex. Biochem Biophys Res Commun 260:296–302, 1999.

Tabarki B, Yacoub M, Tlili K, Trabelsi A, Dogui M, Essoussi AS. Familial spastic paraplegia as the presenting manifestation in patients with purine nucleoside phosphorylase deficiency. J Child Neurol 18:140–141, 2003.

Tam DA Jr, Leshner RT. Stroke in purine nucleoside phosphorylase deficiency. Pediatr Neurol 12:146–148, 1995.

Tanaka C, Hara T, Suzaki I, Maegaki Y, Takeshita K. Sensorineural deafness in siblings with adenosine deaminase deficiency. Brain Dev 18:304–306, 1996.

Thelander L, Reichard P. Reduction of ribonucleotides. Annu Rev Biochem 48:133–158, 1979.

Tsuda M, Horinouchi K, Sakiyama T, Owada M. Novel missense mutation in the purine nucleoside phosphorylase gene in a Japanese patient with purine nucleoside phosphorylase deficiency. Pediatr Int 44:333–334, 2002.

Tung R, Silber R, Quagliata F, Conklyn M, Gottesman J, Hirschhorn R. Adenosine deaminase activity in chronic lymphocytic leukemia. Relationship to B-and T-cell subpopulations. J Clin Invest 57:756–761, 1976.

Tzall S, Ellenbogen A, Eng F, Hirschhorn R. Identification and characterization of nine RFLPs at the adenosine deaminase (ADA) locus. Am J Hum Genet 44:864–875, 1989.

Umetsu DT, Schlossman CM, Ochs HD, Hershfield MS. Heterogeneity of phenotype in two siblings with adenosine deaminase deficiency. J Allergy Clin Immunol 93:543–550, 1994.

Valerio D, Dekker BM, Duyvesteyn MG, van der Voorn L, Berkvens TM, van Ormondt H, van der Eb AJ. One adenosine deaminase allele in a patient with severe combined immunodeficiency contains a point mutation abolishing enzyme activity. EMBO J 5:113–119, 1986.

Valerio D, Duyvesteyn MG, Dekker BM, Weeda G, Berkvens TM, van der Voorn L, van Ormondt H, and van der Eb AJ. Adenosine deaminase: characterization and expression of a gene with a remarkable promoter. EMBO J 4:437–443, 1985.

Valerio D, McIvor RS, Williams SR, Duyvesteyn MG, van Ormondt H, van der Eb AJ, Martin DW Jr. Cloning of human adenosine deaminase cDNA and expression in mouse cells. Gene 31:147–153, 1984.

Wakamiya M, Blackburn MR, Jurecic R, McArthur MJ, Geske RS, Cartwright J, Jr, Mitani K, Vaishnav S, Belmont JW, Kellems RE, et al. Disruption of the adenosine deaminase gene causes hepatocellular impairment and perinatal lethality in mice. Proc Natl Acad Sci USA 92:3673–3677, 1995.

Weinberg K, Hershfield MS, Bastian J, Kohn D, Sender L, Parkman R, Lenarsky C. T lymphocyte ontogeny in adenosine deaminase–deficient severe combined immune deficiency after treatment with polyethylene glycol–modified adenosine deaminase. J Clin Invest 92:596–602, 1993.

Wiginton DA, Adrian GS, Hutton JJ. Sequence of human adenosine deaminase cDNA including the coding region and a small intron. Nucl Acids Res 12:2439–2446, 1984.

Wiginton DA, Hutton JJ. Immunoreactive protein in adenosine deaminase deficient human lymphoblast cell lines. J Biol Chem 257:3211–3217, 1982.

Wiginton DA, Kaplan DJ, States JC, Akeson AL, Perme CM, Bilyk IJ, Vaughn AJ, Lattier DL, Hutton JJ. Complete sequence and structure of the gene for human adenosine deaminase. Biochemistry 25:8234–8244, 1986.

Wijnaendts L, Le Deist F, Griscelli C, Fischer A. Development of immunologic functions after bone marrow transplantation in 33 patients with severe combined immunodeficiency. Blood 74:2212–2219, 1989.

Williams SR, Gekeler V, McIvor RS, Martin DW Jr. A human purine nucleoside phosphorylase deficiency caused by a single base change. J Biol Chem 262:2332–2338, 1987.

Williams SR, Martin DW Jr. Human purine nucleoside phosphorylase cDNA sequence and genomic clone characterization. Nucl Acids Res 12:5779–5787, 1984.

Wilson DK, Quiocho FA. A pre-transition-state mimic of an enzyme: X-ray structure of adenosine deaminase with bound 1-deazaadenosine and zinc-activated water. Biochemistry 32:1689–1694, 1993.

Wilson DK, Rudolph FB, Quiocho FA. Atomic structure of adenosine deaminase complexed with a transition-state analog: understanding catalysis and immunodeficiency mutations. Science 252:1278–1284, 1991.

Yamamoto T, Moriwaki Y, Matsui K, Takahashi S, Tsutsui H, Yoshimoto T, Okamura H, Nakanishi K, Kurosawa Y, Yamaguchi S, Sasaki Y, Higashino K. High IL-18 (interferon-gamma inducing factor) concentration in a purine nucleoside phosphorylase deficient patient. Arch Dis Child 81:179–180, 1999.

Yang DR, Huie ML, Hirschhorn R. Homozygosity for a missense mutation (G20R) associated with neonatal onset adenosine deaminase–deficient severe combined immunodeficiency (ADA-SCID). Clin Immunol Immunopathol 70:171–175, 1994.

Zegers BJ, Stoop JW. Therapy in adenosine deaminase and purine nucleoside phosphorylase deficient patients. Clin Biochem 16:43–47, 1983.

Zegers BJ, Stoop JW, Staal GE, Wadman SK. An approach to the restoration of T cell function in a purine nucleoside phosphorylase deficient patient. Ciba Found Symp 231–253, 1978.

Zielke CL, Sueltre CH. Purine, purine nucleoside, and purine nucleotide aminihydrolases. In: Boyer PD, ed. The Enzymes. New York: Academic Press, Vol. 4, pp. 47–78, 1971.

13

Severe Combined Immunodeficiency Due to Mutations in the CD45 Gene

TALAL A. CHATILA and MARKKU HEIKINHEIMO

The protein tyrosine phosphatase CD45, also known as protein-tyrosine phosphatase, receptor type, C (PTPRC), and leukocyte common antigen (LCA), is a high–molecular weight type I transmembrane protein that is exclusively expressed on all nucleated hematopoietic cells (Tonks et al., 1988; Thomas, 1989; Trowbridge and Thomas, 1994). It is an abundant protein estimated to comprise up to 10% of the cell surface areas of B and T lymphocytes. Despite its abundance and potentially high catalytic capacity, CD45 activity is directed at a limited number of physiologically relevant substrates that include Src and Janus kinases (Jak). CD45 plays a pivotal role in promoting signaling via lymphocyte antigen receptors by regulating the activity of receptor-associated Src-type tyrosine kinases (Ashwell and D'Oro, 1999; Thomas, 1999; Thomas and Brown, 1999; Alexander, 2000; Penninger et al., 2001; Hermiston et al., 2002). Its absence is associated with a profound block in signaling via antigen receptors (Pingel and Thomas, 1989; Koretzky et al., 1990; Desai et al., 1994). CD45 also serves to negatively regulate the function of integrin-mediated adhesion and cytokine receptor signaling by dephosphorylating integrin-associated Src kinases (Roach et al., 1997) and cytokine receptor–associated Jak kinases, respectively (Irie-Sasaki et al., 2001).

CD45 deficiency in humans (MIM 151460) results from rare deleterious point mutations and deletions that are inherited in an autosomal recessive manner. Two patients have been described to date, both of whom presented in infancy with severe combined immunodeficiency (SCID) associated with T cell depletion and failure of the residual T cells in the periphery to respond to mitogenic stimuli (Cale et al., 1997; Kung et al., 2000; Tchilian et al., 2001). The B cells, whose development was spared, failed to develop germinal centers or to sustain normal immunoglobulin production. The immunological abnormalities suffered by these patients mirrored those noted in genetically engineered animal models of CD45 deficiency (Kishihara et al., 1993; Byth et al., 1996; Mee et al., 1999), and reflect an obligate requirement for CD45 in antigen receptor signaling during T cell development and upon T and B cell activation in the periphery.

Regulatory Functions of CD45

The CD45 gene is located on chromosome 1q31–32 and contains 34 exons (Hall et al., 1988). The extracellular portion of CD45 is long (up to 51 nm) and heavily O-glycosylated. It can be divided into an amino-terminal region containing the O-linked glycosylation sites and cysteine rich region containing fibronectin type III sequence motifs. Cell type–specific alternative splicing of exons 4/A, 5/B, and 6/C, encoding sequences at the NH2-terminal region of the protein, results in the generation of up to eight CD45 isoforms. These isoforms vary in size of the extracellular region (ranging from 391 to 552 amino acids) and the extent of O-glycosylation (Rogers et al., 1992), and may differentially interact with other proteins either in *cis* or in *trans*. This interaction may in turn influence cell migration patterns and alter biochemical signaling events regulated by CD45.

In T cells, different CD45 isoforms are expressed in a developmental stage- and activation state-specific manner (reviewed in Trowbridge and Thomas, 1994). Immature thymocytes express low–molecular weight CD45 isoforms. Naive T cells express high–molecular weight, CD45RA-containing isoforms. Following activation, T cells switch to express a lower–molecular weight isoform lacking all three alternatively spliced exons (CD45RO). The CD45RO phenotype, frequently used to denote memory T cells, is reversible in that CD45RO T cells can reexpress the high–molecular weight isoforms. B cells express the largest CD45 isoform of 220 kD molecular weight (also known as B220) containing all three exonic sequences (CD45RABC).

The CD45 cytoplasmic region contains two prototypic phosphatase domains in tandem. The membrane-proximal domain is catalytically active whereas the membrane-distal domain is inactive (pseudophosphatase domain) but promotes recruitment of substrate proteins (Kashio et al., 1998). Reconstitution of the cytoplasmic domain of CD45 as part of chimeric molecules restores signaling via the T cell antigen receptor in CD45-deficient cell lines, indicating that the lack of CD45 phosphatase activity is the fundamental abnormality underlying the failure of antigen receptor signaling in CD45 deficiency (Desai et al., 1994).

The role of CD45 in lymphocyte antigen receptor signaling centers on regulating the activity of antigen receptor–associated Src family kinases: p56Lck and p59Fyn in T cells, and Lyn in B cells (Thomas and Brown, 1999). A major function of CD45 is to maintain these kinases in a quiescent state yet poised for activation upon engagement of antigen receptors. The activity of Src kinases is regulated by the phosphorylation status of two tyrosine residues: one at the carboxyl terminus, which serves a negative regulatory function, and the other within the kinase domain, which serves a positive regulatory function. In CD45-deficient cells, the C-terminal regulatory tyrosine residue is consistently found hyperphosphorylated, indicating that CD45 functions to maintain this site in a dephosphorylated form. Phosphorylation of the C-terminal regulatory tyrosine residue results in its intramolecular association with the SH2 domain of the same Src kinase, which locks the kinase in a closed conformation that renders it inactive. The deleterious impact of hyperphosphorylation Src kinase C-terminal inhibitory tyrosine in CD45 deficiency is highlighted by the observation that a constitutively active Lck mutant, in which the C-terminal tyrosine residue is changed into a phenylalanine, rescues the profound block in T cell development in CD45-deficient mice (Pingel et al., 1999; Seavitt et al., 1999; see below).

The positive regulatory tyrosine residue in the catalytic domain of Src kinases also serves as a substrate for CD45. This role is particularly important in regulating the function of Lck activity in thymocyte development and in down-regulating the activity of the Src kinases Hck and Lyn during integrin-mediated adhesion in macrophages.

Given that the net effect of CD45 is to maintain Src kinases in a dephosphorylated, yet primed state, how are the positive effects of CD45 on antigen receptor signaling mediated? One answer to this question was provided by the finding that CD45 is excluded from the immunological synapse, the supramolecular structure formed at the interface of T cells with antigen-presenting cells that includes the T cell receptor (TCR), CD4 and CD8 coreceptors, antigen-presenting major histocompatibility complex (MHC) molecules, and a variety of signaling molecules (Johnson et al., 2000). Lipid rafts containing the TCR, Lck, and the adapter protein LAT but excluding CD45 cluster at the immunological synapse, allowing effective src kinase activation.

A second mechanism by which CD45 activity is regulated involves receptor dimerization. On the basis of crystal structure of a related phosphatase, RPTPα, it was predicted that the juxtamembrane and proximal catalytic domain of CD45 form dimers in which the catalytic site of one catalytic domain is blocked by a wedge formed by the juxta-membrane region of its partner. Consistent with this model, mice carrying a mutation in which a highly conserved glutamic amino acid residue predicted to lie at the tip of the CD45 wedge domain is changed into arginine develop a lymphoproliferative disease and severe autoimmune nephritis. This phenotype is associated with hyperactive src kinases in lymphocytes (Majeti et al., 2000). While molecular interactions governing CD45 dimer formation and dissolution remain unclear, it has been hypothesized that different CD45 isoforms may vary in their capacity to form dimers (Hermiston et al., 2002). According to this hypothesis, the extensive O-linked glycosylation and sialylation found on the alternatively spliced exons 4–6 render the large CD45RA isoforms expressed on naive T cells more resistant to dimerization because of electrostatic repulsion. In contrast, the absence of this electrostatic barrier in the CD45RO isoform found on memory T cells promotes dimerization. This may explain the more effective signaling in memory T cells.

While CD45 promotes signaling via antigen receptors, it can dampen signaling by other receptor complexes. For example, CD45 negatively regulates integrin-mediated adhesion, an effect related to its ability to dephosphorylate Src kinases at integrin focal adhesion sites (Roach et al., 1997). Consistent with this function is the observation that CD45-deficient T cells and macrophages are abnormally adherent, a phenotype that is reversed by reconstitution of CD45 expression. As in the case of lymphocyte antigen receptor, a topological explanation underlies the regulatory function of CD45 in integrin-mediated adhesion (Thomas and Brown, 1999). Unlike the case of signaling via antigen receptors, where CD45 is excluded from the immunological synapse, CD45 colocalizes with integrin-centered focal adhesion sites. This serves to maintain Src kinases clustered at these sites under negative dephosphorylation pressure.

Another system in which CD45 exerts negative regulatory pressure is signaling via cytokine receptors, where CD45 acts to dephosphorylate receptor–associated Jak kinases (Irie-Sasaki et al., 2001; Penninger et al., 2001). Consistent with this finding, CD45-deficient mice exhibit increased cytokine-dependent myelopoiesis and erythropoiesis and are resistant to otherwise fatal cardiomyopathy associated with Coxsackie virus B3 infection. Given that other molecules such as SOCS (suppressor of cytokine signaling) and nonreceptor phosphotyrosine phosphatases SHP1 and SHP2 also contribute to negative regulation of Jak kinase activation, the precise role of CD45 in negative regulation of Jak kinase activation remains to be fully mapped.

Clinical and Pathological Manifestations

The clinical and pathological features are summarized in Table 13.1. Of the two reported cases of CD45 deficiency, one was a boy born to unrelated Finnish parents (Kung et al., 2000), and the other was a girl born to consanguineous Kurdish parents (Cale et al., 1997; Tchilian et al., 2001). Both children exhibited clinical features typical of SCID. The Finnish child suffered from recurrent infections starting at 6 weeks of age, including candidal skin and oral infections, recurrent otitis media, bronchitis, conjunctivitis, impetigo, gluteal abcess, and chronic rotavirus diarrhea. At around that time, he was noted to have severe anemia requiring transfusions in the face of marrow erythroplasia. He was also noted to have leukopenia and lymphopenia. Reticulocytes appeared in the blood at the age of 3 months and his hemoglobin levels normalized thereafter, but his lymphopenia persisted. He was vaccinated with Bacillus Calmette-Guerin (BCG) at birth. Generalized BCG infection was noted at age 4 months and isoniazide treatment was instituted. Despite supportive therapy, he suffered from severe malnutrition and failure to thrive. He had unrelenting chronic diarrhea associated with persistent Clostridium difficile and rotavirus infection. Respiratory syncytial virus antigen test was repeatedly positive in his

Table 13.1. Clinical Findings in CD45-Deficient Patients

Factor	Finnish Patient	Kurdish Patient
Age at presentation	6 weeks	2 months
Failure to thrive	Yes	Yes
Recurrent bacterial or viral infections	Yes	NR
Chronic rotaviral diarrhea	Yes	NR
Opportunistic infections	BCG, oral candidiasis	CMV
Bone marrow transplant	No	Yes
Terminal event	B cell lymphoma	Reactivated CMV infection

Data on the Finnish and Kurdish patients are from the reports of Kung et al. (2000), and Cale et al. (1997) and Tchilian et al. (2001), respectively. BCG, *Bacillus* Calmette-Guerin; CMV, cytomegalovirus; NR, not reported.

nasopharyngeal aspirate. He was evaluated for bone marrow transplantation at the age 1 year and 5 months. His weight at that time was only 5.5 kg, and the height was 66.5 cm (−3 SD). He died soon thereafter from an aggressive B cell lymphoma.

The Kurdish child presented at the age of 2 months with disseminated, postnatally acquired cytomegalovirus infection associated with fever, rash, pneumonitis, lymphadenopathy, hepatosplenomegaly, and pancytopenia. On the basis of her clinical phenotype and laboratory investigation, she was determined to have SCID and underwent bone marrow transplantation at the age of 8 months. Despite T cell engraftment, her cytomegalovirus infection was reactivated and she died 55 days after the bone marrow transplant.

Laboratory Findings

The laboratory findings of children with CD45 deficiency were in good concordance with the results obtained in the genetically engineered animal models of this disease (Table 13.2). Both children exhibited absolute lymphopenia resulting from depletion of the T cell population (8.9% in the Finnish infant, 15% in the Kurdish infant). The CD4 population was particularly affected (0.9% and 4%, respectively). The B cell population was normal in number. The natural killer (NK) cell population was decreased in the Finnish infant (3%) but undetermined in the Kurdish infant. CD45 expression as determined by flow cytometry was

Table 13.2. Lymphocyte Subpopulations in Human and Murine CD45 Deficiency

	Cell Count (% of Peripheral Lymphocytes)		
	CD45 knockout mice	Finnish Patient	Kurdish Patient
CD3	Depleted	Depleted (8.9%)	Depleted (14.9%)
CD3/4	Depleted	Depleted (0.9%)	Depleted (4%)
CD3/8	Depleted	Depleted (4.9%)	Decreased (20%)*
TCRαβ	Depleted	Depleted (2.2%)	NR
TCRγδ	Preserved	Normal (6.7%)	NR
NK	Preserved	Decreased (3%)	NR
B cells	Preserved	Normal (84.5%)	Normal (68.9%)

Murine data are derived from studies in mice deficient in exons 6, 9, and 12 (Byth et al., 1996; Kishihara et al., 1993; Mee et al., 1999). Data on the Finnish and Kurdish patients are from the reports of Kung et al. (2000), and Cale et al. (1997) and Tchilian et al. (2001), respectively. NR, not reported. *Percentage refers to total CD8+ cells in the periphery.

either totally absent (Finnish infant) or minimally present (Kurdish infant) (Fig. 13.1). Parents of both children exhibited normal levels of CD45 expression. Proliferative responses to mitogenic lectins were totally absent. Hypogammaglobulinemia was noted in both infants.

Molecular Basis

Both children suffered from autosomal recessive defects in the CD45 gene (Fig. 13.2). In the Finnish infant, the allele inherited from the mother carried a large deletion localized to the 3' region of the gene, while the other allele had a G-to-A transition at position +1 of the donor splice site of intron 13 (Kung et al., 2000). Sequencing of reverse transcribed and polymerase chain reaction (RT-PCR)-amplified CD45 transcripts derived from a patient with Epstein-Barr virus–transformed B lymphoblastic cell line demonstrated that the splice junction mutation interfered with splicing at the donor splice site of intron 13. Whereas aberrantly spliced CD45 transcripts resulting from the intron 13 donor splice junction mutation were detected by RT-PCR, no CD45 mRNA transcripts were detected by Northern blot analysis, indicating that truncated and/or aberrant CD45 mRNA are rapidly degraded. In the Kurdish infant with SCID, a 6 bp deletion was identified at nucleotide 1168 in exon 11 of the CD45 gene. This results in the deletion of two amino acids (glutamic acid 339 and tyrosine 340) in the first fibronectin type III module of the CD45 extracellular domain (Tchilian et al., 2001). Both parents were heterozygous for the deletion. Expression analysis studies in which a mutant CD45 cDNA carrying the 6 bp deletion was transfected into Chinese Hamster Ovary (CHO) and mouse EL-4 thymoma cells revealed that the mutant protein failed to express at the cell surface, although it was detected at reduced levels intracellularly. This finding indicated that the deleted amino acids may contribute to the proper folding, stability, and/or correct localization of the mutant protein.

Strategies for Diagnosis

Both cases of CD45 deficiency presented with a characteristic picture of SCID with profound but not total T cell depletion, absent proliferative responses to T cell mitogens, and normal B cell numbers. In both cases, definitive diagnosis of CD45 deficiency was made by flow cytometry, which revealed little or no expression of CD45 on the surface of peripheral blood mononuclear cells. Because CD45 staining is routinely included as part of flow cytometric screening of patients suspected of immunodeficiency, identification of patients with absent CD45 expression would be easy to make. However, two caveats should be noted. The first involves cases suffering from loss-of-function CD45 mutations associated with only partial loss of CD45 expression. These may be easily missed unless careful attention is paid to the mean fluorescence intensity of CD45 staining. The second involves even more challenging cases, those associated with loss-of-function mutations in CD45 cytoplasmic tail, including the active phosphatase domain. These cases may present with normal CD45 expression levels despite absent or near-absent phosphatase function. In this situation, the clinical picture may overlap with atypical forms of X-linked SCID (in boys) or Jak3 kinase deficiency. It will useful to place CD45 deficiency in the differential diagnosis of such cases. Such cryptic CD45 abnormalities can be excluded by evidence of normal signaling events triggered via TCR/CD3, including calcium mobilization and tyrosine phosphorylation.

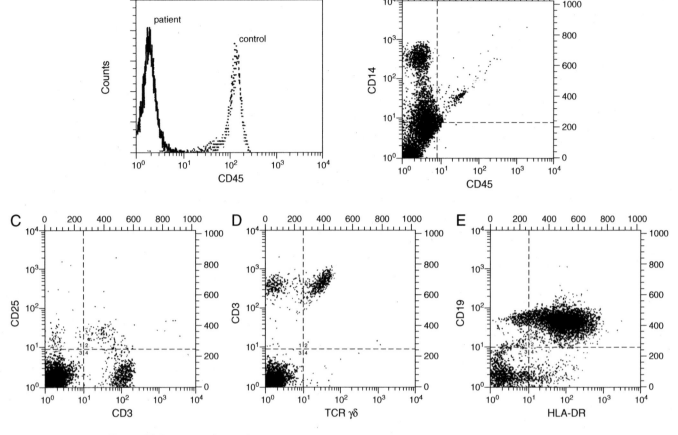

Figure 13.1. Flow cytometry analysis of peripheral lymphocytes of CD45-deficient Finnish infant. (A) Single-color analysis of CD45 expression in the index patient and a control subject. (B–E) Two-color analysis of patient lymphocytes: (B) CD14 and CD45, (C) CD25 and CD3, (D) CD3 and TCRγδ, (E) CD19 and HLA-DR.

Treatment and Prognosis

Definitive therapy for CD45 deficiency is similar to that for other SCID disease—namely, bone marrow transplantation. The fatal outcome in the two patients reported to date, including one who died with cytomegalovirus infection after bone marrow transplant, point to the lethal nature of this immunodeficiency and the urgent need for timely immune reconstitution. As in other cases of SCID, the ideal transplant would be with bone marrow from a human leukocyte antigen (HLA)-matched sibling, followed by bone marrow from matched unrelated donors or HLA-mismatched family members. Problems relating to T cell deficiency dominated the clinical presentation of the two patients, and it remains possible that partial immune reconstitution may be achieved upon infusion of donor marrow in the absence of a conditioning regimen. However, because CD45 is expressed on

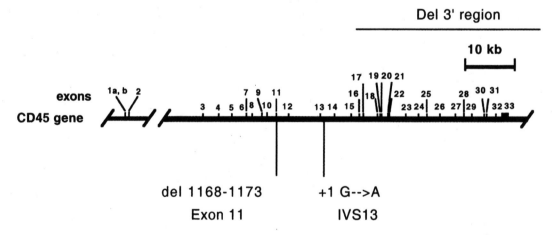

Figure 13.2. Genomic organization of CD45 gene organization. The mutations found in the respectively affected infant are indicated. The Finnish infant suffered from a large deletion in the 3' region of the gene, and a

G → A substitution in the splice donor junction of intervening sequence (IVS) 13. The Kurdish infant suffered from a homozygous 6 bp deletion in exon 11, corresponding to nucleotides 1168–1173 of CD45 cDNA.

nucleated cells of all hematopoietic lineages, it can be predicted that effective immune reconstitution will require a conditioning regimen to enable replacement of all recipient lineages with those of donor origin.

Animal Models

Studies on three different CD45 knockout mice, targeting exons 6, 9, and 12, respectively, have revealed a critical function for CD45 in thymocyte development (Byth et al., 1996; Kishihara et al., 1993; Mee et al., 1999). The most pronounced defect in the development in CD45-deficient thymocytes involves positive selection at the $CD4^+CD8^+$ stage. This results in the exit into the periphery of only 5%–10% of the expected number of mature T cells. Negative selection is also impaired, though less severely. Both defects reflect reduced, though not totally absent, T cell receptor signaling in CD45-deficient thymocytes, leading to a raised selection threshold. As noted above, a constitutive active p56Lck mutant rescues thymocyte development in CD45-deficient animals, consistent with impaired activation of Lck as the principal underlying mechanism involved in ineffective selection of CD45-deficient thymocytes (Pingel et al., 1999; Seavitt et al., 1999). In the periphery, T cell activation via the TCR is completely abrogated. Both T cell proliferation and cytokine secretion in response to TCR ligation are abolished.

B cell development is spared in CD45-deficient mice. However, the B cell receptor (BCR) signaling threshold is increased, leading to impaired proliferation of B cells in response to cross-linking of surface IgM (Benatar et al., 1996). Heightened signaling threshold also leads to defects in positive and negative selection of maturing B cells (Cyster et al., 1996). The transition for IgM^{hi} IgD^{lo} B cells to IgD^{hi} cells during the final maturation stage, which reflects positive selection by constitutive BCR signaling, is impaired. Negative selection at this stage is also impaired, also a reflection of attenuated BCR signaling. T cell–independent responses continue to proceed, but T cell–dependent responses are compromised.

Conclusions and Future Directions

CD45 deficiency is the first protein-tyrosine phosphatase deficiency identified in humans and may be the protype of a novel class of human immunodeficiencies due to defects in protein phosphatases. The SCID phenotype associated with CD45 deficiency reflects the critical role played by this phosphatase in promoting antigen receptor signaling and in regulating the function of other signaling complexes including cytokine receptors and integrins. CD45 deficiency expands the spectrum of immunodeficiency diseases associated with phosphotyrosine signaling pathways, including ZAP-70 and IL-7 receptor/common gamma chain/Jak3 kinase deficiency syndromes in T cells and Btk deficiency in B cells. It is plausible that CD45 deficiency represents the extreme end of a spectrum of CD45-related diseases associated with immunodeficiency, autoimmunity, and/or inflammation. Such disorders may result from selective defects in the expression of individual CD45 isoforms or abnormalities in CD45 function related to one or more receptor complexes. In mice, enhanced expression of particular CD45 isoforms in T cell subsets has been associated with a number of autoimmune diseases (Penninger et al., 2001). In humans, a C → G polymorphism at nucleotide 77 in exon 4/A of CD45 that results in defective alternative splicing of exon 4/A has been associated with multiple sclerosis, although this association was not reproduced by other studies (Jacobsen et al., 2000; Barcellos et al., 2001; Vorechovsky et al., 2001). Future studies will further clarify mechanisms by which CD45 deficiency leads to SCID and the role of CD45 in other immunological diseases.

Acknowledgments

We dedicate this publication to the memory of Dr. Matthew L. Thomas (1953–1999). We would like to thank our collaborators at Washington University School of Medicine, St. Louis, MO, USA; University of Helsinki, Finland; and University of Oulu, Finland. This work was supported by grants from the National Institutes of Health (HD35694) to T.A.C. and from Sigrid Juselius Foundation to M.H.

References

Alexander DR. The CD45 tyrosine phosphatase: a positive and negative regulator of immune cell function. Semin Immunol 12:349–359, 2000.

Ashwell JD, D'Oro U. CD45 and Src-family kinases: and now for something completely different. Immunol Today 20:412–416, 1999.

Barcellos LF, Caillier S, Dragone L, Elder M, Vittinghoff E, Bucher P, Lincoln RR, Pericak-Vance M, Haines JL, Weiss A, Hauser SL, Oksenberg JR. PTPRC (CD45) is not associated with the development of multiple sclerosis in U.S. patients. Nat Genet 29:23–24, 2001.

Benatar T, Carsetti R, Furlonger C, Kamalia N, Mak T, Paige CJ. Immunoglobulin-mediated signal transduction in B cells from CD45-deficient mice. J Exp Med 183:329–334, 1996.

Byth KF, Conroy LA, Howlett S, Smith AJ, May J, Alexander DR, Holmes N. CD45-null transgenic mice reveal a positive regulatory role for CD45 in early thymocyte development, in the selection of CD4+CD8+ thymocytes, and B cell maturation. J Exp Med 183:1707–1718, 1996.

Cale CM, Klein NJ, Novelli V, Veys P, Jones AM, Morgan G. Severe combined immunodeficiency with abnormalities in expression of the common leucocyte antigen, CD45. Arch Dis Child 76:163–164, 1997.

Cyster JG, Healy JI, Kishihara K, Mak TW, Thomas ML, Goodnow CC. Regulation of B-lymphocyte negative and positive selection by tyrosine phosphatase CD45. Nature 381:325–328, 1996.

Desai DM, Sap J, Silvennoinen O, Schlessinger J, Weiss A. The catalytic activity of the CD45 membrane-proximal phosphatase domain is required for TCR signaling and regulation. EMBO J 13:4002–4010, 1994.

Hall LR, Streuli M, Schlossman SF, Saito H. Complete exon–intron organization of the human leukocyte common antigen (CD45) gene. J Immunol 141:2781–2787, 1988.

Hermiston ML, Xu Z, Majeti R, Weiss A. Reciprocal regulation of lymphocyte activation by tyrosine kinases and phosphatases. J Clin Invest 109: 9–14, 2002.

Irie-Sasaki J, Sasaki T, Matsumoto W, Opavsky A, Cheng M, Welstead G, Griffiths E, Krawczyk C, Richardson CD, Aitken K, Iscove N, Koretzky G, Johnson P, Liu P, Rothstein DM, Penninger JM. CD45 is a JAK phosphatase and negatively regulates cytokine receptor signalling. Nature 409: 349–354, 2001.

Jacobsen M, Schweer D, Ziegler A, Gaber R, Schock S, Schwinzer R, Wonigeit K, Lindert RB, Kantarci O, Schaefer-Klein J, Schipper HI, Oertel WH, Heidenreich F, Weinshenker BG, Sommer N, Hemmer B. A point mutation in PTPRC is associated with the development of multiple sclerosis. Nat Genet 26:495–499, 2000.

Johnson KG, Bromley SK, Dustin ML, Thomas ML. A supramolecular basis for CD45 tyrosine phosphatase regulation in sustained T cell activation. Proc Natl Acad Sci USA 97:10138–10143, 2000.

Kashio N, Matsumoto W, Parker S, Rothstein DM. The second domain of the CD45 protein tyrosine phosphatase is critical for interleukin-2 secretion and substrate recruitment of TCR-zeta in vivo. J Biol Chem 273:33856–33863, 1998.

Kishihara K, Penninger J, Wallace VA, Kundig TM, Kawai K, Wakeham A, Timms E, Pfeffer K, Ohashi PS, Thomas ML, et al. Normal B lymphocyte development but impaired T cell maturation in CD45-exon6 protein tyrosine phosphatase–deficient mice. Cell 74:143–156, 1993.

Koretzky GA, Picus J, Thomas ML, Weiss A. Tyrosine phosphatase CD45 is essential for coupling T-cell antigen receptor to the phosphatidyl inositol pathway. Nature 346:66–68, 1990.

Kung C, Pingel JT, Heikinheimo M, Klemola T, Varkila K, Yoo LI, Vuopala K, Poyhonen M, Uhari M, Rogers M, Speck SH, Chatila T, Thomas ML. Mutations in the tyrosine phosphatase CD45 gene in a child with severe combined immunodeficiency disease. Nat Med 6:343–345, 2000.

Majeti R, Xu Z, Parslow TG, Olson JL, Daikh DI, Killeen N, Weiss A. An inactivating point mutation in the inhibitory wedge of CD45 causes lymphoproliferation and autoimmunity. Cell 103:1059–1070, 2000.

Mee PJ, Turner M, Basson MA, Costello PS, Zamoyska R, Tybulewicz VL. Greatly reduced efficiency of both positive and negative selection of thymocytes in CD45 tyrosine phosphatase-deficient mice. Eur J Immunol 29:2923–2933, 1999.

Penninger JM, Irie-Sasaki J, Sasaki T, Oliveira-dos-Santos AJ. CD45: new jobs for an old acquaintance. Nat Immunol 2:389–396, 2001.

Pingel JT, Thomas ML. Evidence that the leukocyte-common antigen is required for antigen-induced T lymphocyte proliferation. Cell 58:1055–1065, 1989.

Pingel S, Baker M, Turner M, Holmes N, Alexander DR. The CD45 tyrosine phosphatase regulates CD3-induced signal transduction and T cell development in recombinase-deficient mice: restoration of pre-TCR function by active p56(lck). Eur J Immunol 29:2376–2384, 1999.

Roach T, Slater S, Koval M, White L, Cahir McFarland ED, Okumura M, Thomas M, Brown E. CD45 regulates Src family member kinase activity associated with macrophage integrin-mediated adhesion. Curr Biol 7:408–417, 1997.

Rogers PR, Pilapil S, Hayakawa K, Romain PL, Parker DC. CD45 alternative exon expression in murine and human CD4+ T cell subsets. J Immunol 148:4054–4065, 1992.

Seavitt JR, White LS, Murphy KM, Loh DY, Perlmutter RM, Thomas ML. Expression of the p56(Lck) Y505F mutation in CD45-deficient mice rescues thymocyte development. Mol Cell Biol 19:4200–4208, 1999.

Tchilian EZ, Wallace DL, Wells RS, Flower DR, Morgan G, Beverley PC. A deletion in the gene encoding the CD45 antigen in a patient with SCID. J Immunol 166:1308–1313, 2001.

Thomas ML. The leukocyte common antigen family. Annu Rev Immunol 7:339–369, 1989.

Thomas ML. The regulation of antigen-receptor signaling by protein tyrosine phosphatases: a hole in the story. Curr Opin Immunol 11:270–276, 1999.

Thomas ML, Brown EJ. Positive and negative regulation of Src-family membrane kinases by CD45. Immunol Today 20:406–411, 1999.

Tonks NK, Charbonneau H, Diltz CD, Fischer EH, Walsh KA. Demonstration that the leukocyte common antigen CD45 is a protein tyrosine phosphatase. Biochemistry 27:8695–8701, 1988.

Trowbridge IS, Thomas ML. CD45: an emerging role as a protein tyrosine phosphatase required for lymphocyte activation and development. Annu Rev Immunol 12:85–116, 1994.

Vorechovsky I, Kralovicova J, Tchilian E, Masterman T, Zhang Z, Ferry B, Misbah S, Chapel H, Webster D, Hellgren D, Anvret M, Hillert J, Hammarstrom L, Beverley PC. Does 77C → G in PTPRC modify autoimmune disorders linked to the major histocompatibility locus? Nat Genet 29:22–23, 2001.

14

Severe Combined Immunodeficiency Due to Defects in T Cell Receptor–Associated Protein Tyrosine Kinases

MELISSA E. ELDER

ZAP-70 is a ζ chain–associated protein of 70,000 kDa, (MIM+ 176947). Deficiency of ZAP-70 leads to a rare autosomal recessive form of severe combined immunodeficiency (SCID) characterized by the selective absence of CD8[+] T cells and by abundant CD4[+] T cells in the peripheral blood that are unresponsive to T cell receptor (TCR)–mediated stimuli in vitro. Peripheral T lymphocytes from most affected patients demonstrate defective signaling following TCR engagement by antigen because of inherited mutations within the kinase domain of the cytoplasmic protein tyrosine kinase (PTK) ZAP-70. ZAP-70 deficiency provided the first evidence that PTKs, and ZAP-70 in particular, are required for normal human T cell development and function. More recently, deficiency of another critical PTK, Lck, has been associated with a SCID phenotype in isolated patients as well.

T Cell Signal Transduction

The processes involved in CD4 vs. CD8 selection during T cell ontogeny are not fully understood, but are known to require intact signal transduction through the TCR of the differentiating thymocyte (Pfeffer and Mak, 1994; Robey and Fowlkes, 1994). The signal transduction events mediated by the TCR on thymocytes are thought to be similar to those responsible for the activation of mature T cells. Propagation of antigen-binding signals from the TCR to the nucleus is dependent on the activation of the PTKs Lck and ZAP-70 (reviewed in Chan et al., 1994a; Weiss and Littman, 1994; Cantrell, 1996; Wange and Samelson, 1996; Kane et al., 2000). PTK activation is a rapid and critical event that results in phosphorylation of numerous downstream molecules, including phospholipase Cγl (PLCγl), linker for activation of T cells (LAT), Src homology 2 (SH2) domain–containing 76 kDa leukocyte protein (SLP-76), and the Vav guanine nucleotide exchange

factor (reviewed in Wange and Samelson, 1996; Qian and Weiss, 1997; Rudd, 1999; van Leeuwen and Samelson, 1999; van Oers, 1999; Kane et al., 2000). These tyrosine phosphorylation events are required for mobilization of intracellular free calcium ($[Ca^{2+}]_i$) and activation of the Ras/mitogen-activated protein kinase (MAPK) and phosphatidylinositol-3 (PI3) kinase pathways. These downstream reactions culminate in activation of T cells and initiation of T cell–specific responses, described in more detail in Chapter 6.

T Cell Receptor–Associated Protein Tyrosine Kinases

Stimulation of either the TCR or the B cell receptor (BCR) results in the activation of certain nonreceptor cytoplasmic PTKs whose functions are critical for lymphocyte responses to antigens (see Chapter 6). The importance of these PTKs to T cell development and function has been established by findings of immunodeficiency in both humans and PTK-deficient mice. Of the PTKs that have been described in T cells, the function of Lck is best understood. Lck is a 56 kDa Src family PTK that is expressed at high levels in peripheral T cells and in thymocytes at all stages of maturation (Perlmutter et al., 1988). Numerous in vivo and in vitro studies have confirmed the importance of Lck to normal T cell signal transduction. Recruitment of ZAP-70 to the TCR is dependent on the phosphorylation of consensus immunoreceptor tyrosine-based activation motifs (ITAMs) in the ε and ζ chains of CD3 by Lck (Gauen et al., 1994; Iwashima et al., 1994; Weiss and Littman, 1994; van Oers and Weiss, 1995; Weil et al., 1995). The ITAMs are found either singly or multiply in the CD3ε and ζ chains and mediate TCR interactions with PTKs involved in signal transduction and with ZAP-70 in particular (Irving et al., 1993; Gauen et al., 1994; Weiss and Littman,

1994; van Oers and Weiss, 1995). Lck is also primarily responsible for mediating ZAP-70 phosphorylation, thereby triggering critical downstream signaling events required for T cell activation (Watts et al., 1994; Chan et al., 1995).

Studies in genetically altered mice demonstrate that Lck is also required for differentiation events in the transition of double-negative (pre-TCR$^+$CD4$^-$CD8$^-$) thymocytes to double-positive (TCR$^+$CD4$^+$CD8$^+$) thymocytes (Molina et al., 1992; Levin et al., 1993). Disruption of Lck results in SCID in mice characterized by markedly decreased numbers of double-positive thymocytes and few single-positive (CD4$^+$ or CD8$^+$) thymocytes or peripheral T cells (Molina et al., 1992). This block in T cell development is related to a requirement for Lck in signaling through the pre-TCR CD3 complex (Mombaerts et al., 1994; Anderson and Perlmutter, 1995; Levelt et al., 1995). Lck is activated upon successful TCR β chain rearrangement; once activated, Lck functions to initiate TCR α chain rearrangement and prevent further TCR β chain rearrangement events.

Fyn, a 59 kDa Src family PTK expressed predominantly in neuronal cells and T lymphocytes, also participates in TCR signaling (Cooke et al., 1991). However, mice deficient in Fyn have relatively normal T cell development, although mature single-positive thymocytes exhibit some defects in signal transduction (Appleby et al., 1992; Stein et al., 1992). Even though Fyn does not appear to be essential for peripheral T cell function and its absence is not associated with a SCID phenotype in animals, mice lacking both Lck and Fyn have no thymocytes more mature than those at the double-negative stage. This finding suggests that Fyn can partially compensate for loss of Lck, and Fyn alone is sufficient to allow some T cell development (van Oers et al., 1996).

Another PTK involved in TCR signaling is Syk, a 72 kDa PTK with structural homology to ZAP-70. Syk is expressed predominantly in B cells, myeloid cells, and thymocytes, and is expressed only at very low levels in peripheral T cells (Chan et al., 1994c). Syk is critical to BCR signaling and may function in B cells in a role similar to that of ZAP-70 in T cells (Reth, 1995; DeFranco, 1997). Syk-deficient mice die shortly after birth from severe bleeding and demonstrate arrested B cell development at the pro-B cell stage (Cheng et al., 1995; Turner et al., 1995). Although ZAP-70 is not physiologically expressed in B lymphocytes, it can reconstitute BCR function in Syk-deficient mice (Kong et al., 1995). Similarly, there appears to be a role for Syk in TCR signaling. Syk has been shown to bind phosphorylated ζ and to be activated in response to TCR stimulation in thymocytes (Chan et al., 1994c; Gelfand et al., 1995; van Oers and Weiss, 1995), but absence of Syk does not affect T cell development in mice other than the maturation of Vγ3$^+$ thymocytes and γδ T cells in epithelial tissues (Mallick-Wood et al., 1996). Studies in mice have demonstrated that Syk expression is highest in thymocytes in which the pre-TCR is first expressed and is down-regulated when pre-TCR signals induce transition from the double-negative to the double-positive thymocyte stage (Chu et al., 1999). In contrast to ZAP-70-deficient mice, which are blocked at the double-positive stage of thymocyte development, mice made doubly deficient in ZAP-70 and Syk demonstrate complete arrest of thymic development at this pre-TCR checkpoint (Cheng et al., 1997), a finding suggesting that Syk does play a role in pre-TCR signaling and early αβ T cell differentiation.

ZAP-70 is a 70 kDa Syk family PTK expressed exclusively in T cells and in natural killer (NK) cells (Chan et al., 1992). ZAP-70 is expressed in all thymocyte subpopulations and is constitutively associated with phosphorylated CD3ζ in thymocytes and T cells in vivo (Chan et al., 1994c; van Oers et al., 1994, 1996). This association is in contrast to findings in vitro, in which ZAP-70 is not constituitively localized with the TCR, but rapidly binds phosphorylated ζ and CD3ε following TCR stimulation (Chan et al., 1991). Recruitment of ZAP-70 to the TCR is essential for its subsequent activation and for induction of downstream signaling events critical for induction of T cell–specific responses (Wange et al., 1995b; Weil et al., 1995; Weiss and Littman, 1994). As described above, Lck mediates the phosphorylation of both tyrosine residues within each ITAM of CD3ζ and CD3ε that occurs prior to ZAP-70 recruitment to the TCR (see Fig. 6.2 in Chapter 6) (Straus and Weiss, 1992; Gauen et al., 1994; Iwashima et al., 1994; van Oers and Weiss, 1995; Weil et al., 1995). High-affinity binding of ZAP-70 to ζ and CD3ε requires the cooperative binding of both ZAP-70 SH2 domains (Hatada et al., 1993; Wange et al., 1993; Gauen et al., 1994; Iwashima et al., 1994; Isakov et al., 1995). However, association of ZAP-70 with the phosphorylated ITAM-containing subunits of the TCR alone is insufficient to induce ZAP-70 kinase activity (van Oers et al., 1994; Madrenas et al., 1995). ZAP-70 itself must be phosphorylated at specific tyrosine residues to increase its catalytic function (Watts et al., 1994; Chan et al., 1995; Neumeister et al., 1995; Wange et al., 1995a, 1995b). Tyrosine phosphorylation of ZAP-70 is mediated by Src family PTKs and by autophosphorylation activity (Watts et al., 1994; Chan, et al., 1995; Neumeister et al., 1995; Wange et al., 1995a). Much of the increase in ZAP-70 catalytic function following TCR stimulation is associated with specific phosphorylation of tyrosine residue 493 by Lck (Watts et al., 1994; Chan et al., 1995). However, ZAP-70 enzymatic activity is also negatively regulated by phosphorylation of the adjacent tyrosine residue 492 (Chan et al., 1995; Wange et al., 1995a; Zhao and Weiss, 1996). Additional tyrosines within interdomain B bridging the SH2 and kinase domains of ZAP-70 are also phosphorylated and function as positive regulators of TCR signaling; these include tyrosine 315 (the putative binding site for the Vav guanine nucleotide exchange factor) and tyrosine 319, which may interact with PLCγ1 and Lck (Zhao and Weiss, 1999; Wu et al., 1997; Di Bartolo et al., 1999; Williams et al., 1999; Gong et al., 2001). In contrast, phosphorylation of tyrosine 292 within interdomain B of the ZAP-70 protein inhibits TCR signaling by serving as a binding site for the ubiquitin ligase Cbl, which targets ZAP-70 for ubiquitination and degradation (Lupher et al., 1996; Rao et al., 2000).

Following ZAP-70 phosphorylation and activation, multiple downstream signaling events occur that result in T cell activation. Phosphorylated ZAP-70 triggers recruitment of other molecules to the signaling complex, resulting in transduction of the TCR-mediated signal. Specific in vivo substrates for ZAP-70 include LAT and SLP-76 (Wardenburg et al., 1996; Raab et al., 1997; Williams et al., 1998, 1999; Zhang et al., 1998). Recruitment to the signaling complex is most likely mediated by the SH2 domains contained within each protein. Additional SH2 domain–containing signaling molecules recruited to the TCR via interactions with ZAP-70 or ZAP-70 substrates include PLCγ1, Cbl, Vav, Grb2, SOS, Gads, Itk, Ras-GTP, and the p85 subunit of PI3 kinase (Duplay et al., 1994; Katzav et al., 1994; Neumeister et al., 1995; Straus et al., 1996; Wardenburg et al., 1996; Wu et al., 1997; Finco et al., 1998; Yablonski et al., 1998; van Oers, 1999; Yablonski and Weiss, 2001). Formation of these protein complexes at the plasma membrane results in signal amplification and culminates in the transcription of genes involved in T cell activation, such as interleukin (IL)-2.

Table 14.1. Clinical Findings in Eight Patients with ZAP-70 Deficiency

Findings	Number of Affected Children
Infections	
Bacterial (otitis media, pneumonia)	4
P. jiroveci pneumonia	3
Cytomegalovirus retinitis or other infection	2
Parainfluenza pneumonitis	1
Chronic diarrhea or rotaviral enteritis	6
Severe or disseminated varicella	1
Oral or cutaneous candidiasis	3
Failure to Thrive	4
Physical Findings	
Presence of lymph tissue	5
Hepatosplenomegaly	1
Chronic eczematoid rash	2
Thymic shadow on chest X-ray	8

Clinical and Pathologic Manifestations of ZAP-70 Deficiency

Eight children from five families were originally described with SCID due to ZAP-70 deficiency (Arpaia et al., 1994; Chan et al., 1994b; Elder et al., 1994; Gelfand et al., 1995). These patients included six children from three genetically isolated Mennonite kindreds and two children from separate, unrelated (Hispanic and Caucasian) families, who were both products of consanguineous relationships. Similar to other forms of SCID, each affected child presented within the first 2 years of life with a history of recurrent infections and failure to thrive (Table 14.1) (Roifman et al., 1989; Monafo et al., 1992; Elder et al., 1995; Gelfand et al., 1995). Seven of these children are well following allogeneic bone marrow transplantation (BMT); one child of Mennonite background died 2 months after BMT (Monafo et al., 1992). Additional patients with ZAP-70 deficiency have since been described and have had similar clinical presentations (Matsuda et al., 1999; Noraz et al., 2000; Elder et al., 2001; Toyabe et al., 2001).

Most ZAP-70-deficient patients have detectable lymphoid tissue along with their normal or elevated peripheral blood lymphocyte counts. Thymic histology in ZAP-70 deficiency is remarkable for normal structural organization and normal percentages of double-positive and single-positive CD4+ thymocytes. In contrast, there are very few, if any, single-positive CD8+ cells (Gelfand et al., 1995; Roifman et al., 1989).

Laboratory Findings in ZAP-70 Deficiency

All patients have normal to elevated numbers of circulating lymphocytes (Table 14.2). Phenotypic analysis of their peripheral blood lymphocytes by flow cytometry reveals normal or increased percentages of CD3+ (38%–80%) and CD4+ T cells (37%–75%) because of the lack of CD8+ T cells (0%–3%) (Roifman et al., 1989; Monafo et al., 1992; Elder et al., 1995, 2001; Gelfand et al., 1995; Matsuda et al., 1999; Noraz et al., 2000). Expression of T cell surface proteins other than CD8 is normal. In those patients in whom human leukocyte antigen (HLA) typing and Southern blot analysis have been performed, the peripheral blood T cells were demonstrated to be polyclonal and not maternal in origin (Arpaia et al., 1994; Elder et al., 1995). Absent

proliferative responses to alloantigen and to a variety of mitogens in vitro, including phytohemagglutinin (PHA), pokeweed mitogen (PWM), concanavalin A, *Candida albicans*, and anti-CD3 monoclonal antibody (MAb), are noted on testing of patient lymphocytes, confirming the diagnosis of SCID. Lack of response to *Candida* skin testing and failure to reject an allogeneic skin graft were also demonstrated in one ZAP-70-deficient patient (Roifman et al., 1989). NK cell numbers and activity are relatively normal (Elder et al., 1994). All patients have normal numbers of B cells, but some differences in the level of B cell function have been noted between patients. One affected child from a Mennonite family was able to make specific antibodies to tetanus and had normal levels of serum immunoglobulins (Roifman et al., 1989), and another child had IgE reactive with food allergens, but did not demonstrate atopy or intestinal symptoms related to food ingestion (Toyabe et al., 2001). In contrast, most patients have low-serum IgG and lack specific antibody production, necessitating monthly intravenous immunoglobulin administration (Elder et al., 1995, 2001; Gelfand et al., 1995).

In the original eight patients with ZAP-70 deficiency, the markedly abnormal distribution of peripheral T cell subsets and the absence of T cell proliferation to any stimulus transduced by the TCR led to further studies that documented defects within the proximal TCR signaling pathway, later proven to be due to absence of ZAP-70 function. The patients' T lymphocytes exhibited diminished or absent $[Ca^{2+}]_i$ mobilization after stimulation with anti-CD3 MAb (Arpaia et al., 1994; Chan et al., 1994b; Gelfand et al., 1995; Elder et al., 2001). Furthermore, induction of most cytoplasmic tyrosine phosphoproteins was defective after co-cross-linking of the TCR on patient T cells with either anti-CD3 or a combination of anti-CD4 and anti-CD3 MAbs (Arpaia et al., 1994; Elder et al., 1995, 2001). In contrast to their absence of cell proliferation to TCR-mediated stimuli, ZAP-70-deficient lymphocytes proliferate normally to phorbol myristic acetate (PMA) plus ionomycin, agents that bypass proximal TCR signaling events by mimicking actions of the second messengers Ras and $[Ca^{2+}]_i$, respectively. In addition, IL-2 production is detected when lymphocytes are stimulated with PMA plus ionomycin, in contrast to the lack of detectable IL-2 production when T cells are incubated with anti-CD3 or PHA (Arpaia et al., 1994; Elder et al., 1995).

Molecular Basis of ZAP-70 Deficiency

In most affected patients, ZAP-70 protein is not detected by immunoblot (Arpaia et al., 1994; Chan et al., 1994b; Elder et al., 1994; Gelfand et al., 1995; Matsuda et al., 1999; Noraz et al., 2000; Toyabe et al., 2001). In contrast, normal levels of other PTKs are present in patient T cells. Additional studies in one patient demonstrated that Lck function was normal: it could be coprecipitated with CD4, was inducibly phosphorylated in response to cross-linking of surface CD3 and CD4, and exhibited normal autophosphorylation activity in vitro (Elder et al., 1995). Fyn kinase activity was shown to be intact in vitro in two Mennonite kindreds as well (Arpaia et al., 1994). One child with SCID, born to a consanguineous union, had undetectable ZAP-70 mRNA levels, but his underlying mutation(s) have not yet been identified (Gelfand et al., 1995). In contrast, the remaining patients have normal levels of full-length ZAP-70 mRNA compared to controls.

At least eight separate mutations in the gene encoding ZAP-70 (gene symbol *ZAP70* or *SRK*, Syk-related tyrosine kinase) have been identified in affected children (Arpaia et al., 1994; Chan

Table 14.2. Laboratory Findings in Patients with ZAP-70 Deficiency

Tests	Range of Patient Values	Normal Range
Lymphocyte Phenotype		
Absolute lymphocyte count	$4.0–20.0 \times 10^9/1$	$3.5–8.0 \times 10^9/1$
CD3+ cells	38%–80%	53%–85%
CD4+ cells	37%–75%	25%–68%
CD8+ cells	0%–10%	12%–40%
CD3+CD8+ cells	0%–3%	12%–37%
TCRα/β+ cells	53%–79%	50%–85%
TCRγ/δ+ cells	0.2%–?%	1%–12%
CD3+CD69+ cells	0%–3%	25%–55%
CD16+CD56+ cells	5%–13%	5%–29%
CD8+/CD56+ cells	1%–10%	8%–27%
CD19+ cells	13%–41%	6%–24%
Serum Immunoglobulin Levels		
IgG (pre-IVIG)	63–1870 mg/dl	340–1210 mg/dl
IgA	39–160 mg/dl	10–50 mg/dl
IgM	67–170 mg/dl	40–200 mg/dl
Isohemagglutinins	0–<1:1 titer	0–1:128 titer
Specific antibody production	1 pt (levels not reported)	
Lymphocyte Proliferative Function		
Mitogens (PHA, PWM)	0–1,077 cpm	35,000–230,000 cpm
Soluble antigen (tetanus, candida)	0–704 cpm	1300–89,000 cpm
Alloantigen (MLC)	124–4620 cpm	14,000–150,000 cpm
Anti-CD3	185–900 cpm	21,000–93,300 cpm
IL-2	1280–19,759 cpm	1390–5900 cpm
PMA	15,882–50,322 cpm	1645–110,000 cpm
PMA plus ionomycin	39,308–187,000 cpm	26,649–168,000 cpm
PMA plus IL-2	100,000–134,000 cpm	64,000–120,000 cpm
SAC (B cell mitogen)	5000–21,679 cpm	5000–17,000 cpm
IL-2 Production		
PHA, anti-CD3	none	
PMA plus ionomycin	normal	
NK cell cytotoxicity	20%–30%	20%–50%

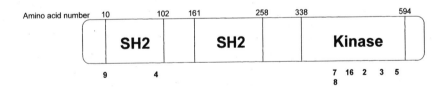

Mutant allele	DNA Mutation	Consequence to Protein
1	13 bp deletion (nts 1719-1731)	Deletion/frameshift/premature termination after 35 codons (K504_P508delfsX35)
2	C to A transition at nt 1763	Missense (S518R)
3	G to A transition at nt 1833	Splicing error (K541_K542insLEQ)
4	C to A transition at nt 448	Missense (P80Q)
5	A to T transition at nt 1923	Missense (M572L)
6	C to T at nt 1729	Missense (A507V)
7	C to T at nt 1602	Missense (R465C)
8	G to A at nt 1603	Missense (R465H)
9	? (no ZAP-70 mRNA)	

Figure 14-1. Schematic depiction of wild-type ZAP-70 protein and the identified mutant alleles. GenBank accession number is L05148 for the human AP-70 cDNA sequence.

et al., 1994b; Elder et al., 1994, 2001; Matsuda et al., 1999; Noraz et al., 2000; Toyabe et al., 2001). Interestingly, most mutations occur within the kinase domain of the ZAP-70 protein and significantly affect both protein stability and catalytic activity (Fig. 14.1).

ZAP-70 Mutation Analysis

Pedigree analyses have confirmed that ZAP-70 deficiency is an autosomal recessive genetic syndrome and that affected children have failed to inherit a normal allele of the *ZAP70* gene, located on human chromosome 2q12 (Chan et al., 1994b). The molecular defects reported to date are listed in Figure 14.1. All six children from the three genetically related Mennonite families inherited at least one mutant *ZAP70* allele with a splicing error due to a G-to-A transition within an intron, generating a new splice acceptor site upstream of the normal splice site. Specifically, three children from two families were homozygous for a 9 bp insertion (CTTGAGCAG) into the coding sequence after nucleotide 1832. This mutation results in the addition of three amino acid residues, leucine, glutamic acid, and glutamine (LEQ), within the ZAP-70 catalytic domain following residue 541 (K541insLEQ) (Arpaia et al., 1994). Three children from the remaining Mennonite family inherited this mutant allele along with a second mutant allele and were thus compound heterozygotes for two *ZAP70* mutations (Chan et al., 1994b). The second mutation in these Mennonite cases is a C-to-A transition at position 1763, which results in a serine-to-arginine substitution at amino acid 518 (S518R) within a highly conserved region of all Syk family PTK catalytic domains.

In a fourth affected and unrelated family, a single patient with ZAP-70 deficiency was homozygous for a 13 bp deletion at nucleotides 1719 to 1731 (Elder et al., 1994). This deletion results in a translational frameshift after residue 503 and introduces a premature stop 35 codons downstream, yielding a mutant protein truncated by 82 amino acids (K504_P508delfsX35). Interestingly, two siblings from an unrelated family were recently found to be homozygous for a C-to-T transition at position 1729 that results in an alanine-to-valine substitution at residue 507 (A507V), which is within the 13 bp deletion sequence (Noraz et al., 2000).

One Japanese patient with CD8 deficiency was a compound heterozygote for temperature sensitive mutations in *ZAP70*: a C-to-A transition at position 448 that results in a proline-to-glutamine substitution at residue 80 (P80Q), and an A-to-T transition at position 1923 that substitutes a leucine for methionine at amino acid 572 (M572L) within the ZAP-70 protein (Matsuda et al., 1999).

Most recently, two infants with SCID were demonstrated to have inherited a homozygous missense mutation within the highly conserved DLAARN motif in the ZAP-70 kinase domain (Elder et al., 2001; Toyabe et al., 2001). In one child, the mutation was a C-to-T transition at bp 1602, which results in an arginine-to-cysteine conversion at residue 465 (R465C). Unlike other described ZAP-70 mutations, this mutation only modestly affected protein stability, but it abrogated ZAP-70 catalytic function. Moreover, R465C is comparable to the mutation (R464C) that spontaneously arose in the inbred Strange (ST) mouse colony (Wiest et al., 1997). In contrast to ST mice, which lack any single-positive thymocytes and peripheral T cells, the R465C patient had typical findings of ZAP-70 deficiency and lacked only circulating CD8$^+$ T lymphocytes (Elder et al., 2001). This patient's case provides the first description of identical mutations in ZAP-70 having distinct T cell developmental consequences in

humans and mice. Subsequently, an unrelated patient was determined to be homozygous for a G-to-A transition at position 1603, resulting in an arginine-to-histidine (R465H) conversion at the same critical residue within the DLAARN motif (Toyabe et al., 2001). In contrast to the previous case and ST mice, this patient lacked ZAP-70 protein expression.

With the exception of the mutation R465C, all identified mutations significantly decrease the stability of the ZAP-70 protein in vitro and when transfected into cell lines in vitro (Chan et al., 1994b; Elder et al., 1994; Matsuda et al., 1999; Noraz et al., 2000). Furthermore, most mutations that change the sequence of the kinase domain of ZAP-70 affect its enzymatic activity. In vitro kinase assays have confirmed that mutant forms of ZAP-70 are catalytically inactive (Chan et al., 1994b; Elder et al., 1994, 2001; Noraz et al., 2000).

Functional Aspects of ZAP-70 Deficiency

The phenotype of ZAP-70 deficiency in humans presents a notable paradox: although a single signaling pathway had previously been assumed to be required for both thymic selection and peripheral T cell activation, the abundant CD4$^+$ T cells in this disorder, which presumably were selected positively in the thymus, are refractory to TCR-mediated activation in the periphery. Thymic tissue from three ZAP-70-deficient patients revealed mostly double-positive thymocytes and normal numbers of single-positive CD4$^+$ cells, but very few if any CD8$^+$ thymocytes (Roifman et al., 1989; Gelfand et al., 1995).

These results suggest that ZAP-70 is critical for CD8 selection and peripheral CD4$^+$ and CD8$^+$ T cell signaling, but is dispensable for CD4 selection in the thymus. One possible explanation for the presence of normal numbers of CD4$^+$ T cells is that the related PTK, Syk, which is expressed at higher levels in the thymus than in the periphery, may be able to rescue CD4 selection in the absence of ZAP-70 (Chan et al., 1994c; Gelfand et al., 1995). A role for Syk in thymocyte signaling is suggested by findings that double-positive thymocytes from one patient were able to mobilize [Ca^{2+}]$_i$ upon CD3 cross-linking (Gelfand et al., 1995). Comparable induction of tyrosine phosphoproteins was also seen in a human T-cell leukemia virus (HTLV)-1-transformed CD4$^+$ thymocyte line from the same patient. This thymocyte line demonstrated higher basal levels of Syk expression and increased Syk phosphorylation after TCR stimulation than in control HTLV-1-transformed thymocytes. Increased Syk activity in ZAP-70-deficient thymocytes may thus compensate at least in part for the lack of ZAP-70 function. The differential ability of Syk to replace ZAP-70 in CD4 vs. CD8 selection events may be related to the requirement for Lck in the recruitment of Syk family PTKs to the TCR and in their subsequent activation. Since more Lck is associated with the CD4 than with the CD8 coreceptor in double-positive thymocytes, CD4 cells may be preferentially selected if Syk is unable to fully substitute for loss of ZAP-70 function. Similarly, Syk activity, which is downregulated in mature T cells, is insufficient to compensate for ZAP-70 deficiency in peripheral CD4$^+$ T cell signal transduction. Peripheral T cells from two ZAP-70-deficient patients were shown to express high levels of Syk and be capable of partial TCR signaling after long-term culture (Noraz et al., 2000). However, findings have been variable in freshly isolated ZAP-70-deficient T cells and suggest that survival of these cells does not necessarily depend on ZAP-70-mediated TCR signaling or on up-regulation of Syk expression (Elder et al., 2001; Toyabe et al., 2001).

Alternatively, the level of Syk activity required for peripheral T cell survival may be less than that required for propagation of TCR signals. Further studies are needed to characterize the antigen specificity and TCR repertoire of CD4$^+$ T cells in ZAP-70 deficiency and to clarify the role of Syk in thymocyte selection and peripheral T cell activation.

Strategies for Diagnosis of ZAP-70 Deficiency

Patients with SCID characterized by variable hypogammaglobulinemia, relatively normal numbers of peripheral blood lymphocytes, normal or only modestly decreased T cells, but notable absence of CD8$^+$ T cells (<5%) should be screened for ZAP-70 deficiency. The diagnosis would be suggested by lack of T cell proliferation in vitro to TCR stimuli, such as PHA and anti-CD3 MAb, whereas proliferation to PMA plus ionomycin ought to be comparable to that of normal T cells. Further studies to confirm a proximal TCR signaling defect include defective [Ca^{2+}]$_i$ mobilization and poor tyrosine phosphoprotein induction after stimulation through the TCR. In most cases, blotting for ZAP-70 protein will demonstrate lack of ZAP-70 protein expression. If phosphotyrosine induction is abnormal but ZAP-70 protein is present, cDNA or genomic DNA sequencing would be required to characterize the mutation(s). To date, cDNA sequencing has been used primarily to determine ZAP-70 mutations; however, as the structure of the human *ZAP70* gene is now available, single-strand conformational polymorphism analysis and genomic DNA sequencing undoubtedly will be used more often because less blood will be required from the affected child.

Carrier Detection and Prenatal Diagnosis

If the ZAP-70 mutations are known in an affected proband, then both carrier detection in relatives and prenatal diagnosis of an at risk fetus can be performed. Individuals heterozygous for a mutant ZAP-70 allele are immunologically normal. Therefore, molecular techniques would be required to establish heterozygosity. However, since ZAP-70 deficiency is extremely rare and has primarily been demonstrated in consanguineous and genetically inbred families, carrier detection is useful for only a very few individuals in certain isolated population groups.

Treatment and Prognosis

Patients with ZAP-70 deficiency require hematopoietic stem cell transplantation for cure of SCID. Six of the original ZAP-70-deficient patients who were successfully transplanted received one of the following regimens: (1) a histocompatible bone marrow transplant (BMT) from a sibling after conditioning with busulfan and cytoxan (BuCy) and antithymocyte globulin (ATG) (one child; A.H. Filipovich, personal communication); (2) a T cell–depleted BMT from a parent either without prior conditioning (one child; E.W. Gelfand, personal communication) or after cytoxan/ATG conditioning (one child; Elder et al., 1995) or after BuCy/ATG conditioning (one child; A.H. Filipovich, personal communication); (3) an HLA-matched unrelated BMT after BuCy/ATG conditioning (one child; A.H. Filipovich, personal communication); or (4) a partial HLA-matched unrelated BMT after BuCy/ATG conditioning (one child; A.H. Filipovich, personal communication). Mobilized peripheral blood stem cells from a parent have also been used with variable success to reconstitute ZAP-70-deficient children (Elder et al., 2001; Skoda-Smith et al., 2001; Toyabe et al., 2001). In one case, a paternal mobi-

lized peripheral blood stem cell transplant followed by treatment with anti-CD20 MAb (Rituximab) successfully reconstituted a ZAP-70-deficient child who had developed an Epstein-Barr virus (EBV)-negative non-Hodgkin's B cell lymphoma following attempted T cell–depleted maternal haploidentical BMT (Skoda-Smith et al., 2001). Monthly intravenous gammaglobulin therapy is required in most cases for variable periods of time after hematopoietic stem cell transplantation.

Animal Model of ZAP-70 Deficiency

Genetically altered mice lacking the entire ZAP-70 locus exhibit markedly defective T cell activation and development (Negishi et al., 1995). In contrast to findings in ZAP-70-deficient patients, T cell ontogeny in ZAP-70 knockout mice is blocked at the double-positive stage of thymocyte differentiation. Thymocytes from mutant mice fail to mobilize [Ca^{2+}]$_i$ after TCR cross-linking by anti-CD3 MAb, and neither single-positive CD4$^+$ nor CD8$^+$ thymocytes develop, and peripheral T cells are absent. These findings as well as the demonstration that single-positive CD4$^+$ and CD8$^+$ T cell development could be rescued by expression of a functional human ZAP-70 cDNA in mutant thymocytes suggest that ZAP-70 is required for selection of both major thymocyte subsets in mice (Negishi et al., 1995). A comparable lymphocyte phenotype is seen in ST mice, which develop SCID due to a spontaneously arising mutation (R464C) within the highly conserved DLAARN motif of ZAP-70 that is essential for PTK enzymatic function (Wiest et al., 1997). Analysis of TCR signaling in ST thymocytes demonstrates that R464C abrogates ZAP-70 kinase activity, but the mutant protein is expressed and can be phosphorylated. These results confirm that ZAP-70 function is absolutely required for TCR activation and development of mature murine T lymphocytes.

The absence of CD4$^+$ T cells in ZAP-70-deficient mice contrasts with their presence in humans with ZAP-70 deficiency. Although the nature of the underlying mutations in human ZAP-70 deficiency conceivably might allow for some residual PTK activity in vivo, the disparate effects of identical ZAP-70 mutations suggest instead that human and murine thymocytes have different dependencies on ZAP-70 function during development. As stated above, both ZAP-70 knockout and ST mice exhibit markedly defective T cell activation, and in contrast to findings in ZAP-70-deficient patients (Gelfand et al., 1995), ST murine thymocytes do not mobilize [Ca^{2+}]$_i$ after TCR cross-linking (Negishi et al., 1995; Wiest et al., 1997). One explanation for this discrepancy is that the ability of Syk to contribute to pre-TCR and TCR signaling is substantially different between humans and mice; in particular, the level of Syk activity in double-positive thymocytes of ZAP-70-deficient mice may not be sufficient to rescue CD4 selection in the absence of ZAP-70. Although it remains to be established whether Syk expression is significantly higher in human than in mouse thymocytes, this explanation is supported by evidence that peripheral CD4$^+$ and CD8$^+$ T cell development in ZAP-70-deficient mice can be restored with human Syk transgene expression in the thymus (Gong et al., 1997). Moreover, in contrast to findings in murine double-positive thymocytes in which Syk expression is comparable to that seen in peripheral T cells, human double-positive thymocytes express significant levels of Syk and do not down-regulate this PTK to levels seen in peripheral T lymphocytes until after positive selection has commenced (Chu et al., 1999). As a consequence of its relative abundance in human double-positive thymocytes, Syk may partially compensate for loss of ZAP-70 during positive selection in ZAP-70-deficient patients. However, final conclusions regarding the distinct phenotypes of mice and humans deficient in ZAP-70 await more detailed analyses of the comparative expression and function of the Syk and ZAP-70 PTKs.

Lck Deficiency

In contrast to ZAP-70, in which SCID patients lack peripheral CD8+ T cells, human Lck deficiency has been associated with a selective CD4 lymphopenia (Goldman et al., 1998; Hubert et al., 2000; Sawabe et al., 2001). The underlying genetic defects resulting in observed decreased expression of functional Lck protein in a small number of sporadic cases are unknown. The clinical presentation of patients with selective CD4 lymphopenia and Lck deficiency is variable and may include SCID or common variable immunodeficiency (Goldman et al., 1998; Hubert et al., 2000; Sawabe et al., 2001).

Clinical and Laboratory Findings in Lck Deficiency

In addition to CD4 lymphopenia (range 4%–22%; 100–350 cells/mm³), affected individuals have decreased numbers of peripheral blood lymphocytes (780–1890 cells/mm³) and CD3+ T cells (507–1200 cells/mm³); CD8+ cell percentages and numbers are normal or increased (27%–65%, or 430–1058 cells/mm³). However, CD8+ T cells from the Lck-deficient SCID patient poorly expressed the costimulatory molecule, CD28 (Goldman et al., 1998). Although mildly to significantly less responsive than control lymphocytes, Lck-deficient T cells do proliferate to mitogens, anti-CD3 MAb, and IL-2, and have demonstrated normal alloantigen responses (Goldman et al., 1998; Hubert et al., 2000; Sawabe et al., 2001). B cell and NK cell numbers are appropriate for age, but some patients have had panhypogammaglobulinemia and required intravenous immunoglobulin therapy.

Clinically, the single Lck-deficient child with SCID had infections similar to those of other children with combined primary immunodeficiencies and eventually was successfully treated with a BMT from a matched, unrelated donor (Goldman et al., 1998). One elderly adult with CD4 lymphopenia and decreased Lck function presented initially with cryptococcal meningitis (Hubert et al., 2000).

Lck Mutation Analysis

The single child reported with Lck-deficient SCID was found to express an aberrantly spliced Lck mRNA lacking exon 7, which encodes the PTK ATP binding site and kinase domain (Straus and Weiss, 1992). Expression of a similar Lck mRNA lacking exon 7 is also found in the Jurkat cell line JCaM.1 (Straus and Weiss, 1992). As a result, the JCaM.1 cell line does not express Lck protein and exhibits profoundly defective proximal TCR signal transduction. A decreased but detectable amount of Lck protein was seen in the SCID patient's T cells by immunoblot; this signal was attributed to expression of the unstable mRNA lacking exon 7. Although less than in control lymphocytes, a significant amount of normal Lck mRNA was found in patient T cells as well. A relatively normal pattern of tyrosine phosphorylation was induced by TCR engagement despite defective expression of Lck; this is in obvious contrast to the JCaM.1 line (Straus and Weiss, 1992). Although TCR stimulation resulted in MAPK activation and $[Ca^{2+}]_i$ mobilization at levels comparable to that of control cells, significant up-regulation of CD69 expression was

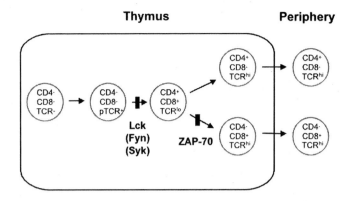

Figure 14-2. T cell ontogeny in humans. The developmental stages at which activities of certain protein tyrosine kinases (PTKs) have been identified as being critical for normal ontogeny are indicated.

not observed in the patient's CD8+ T cells. The underlying genetic defect resulting in defective Lck expression has not yet been identified in this or any patient with selective CD4 lymphopenia and abnormal Lck expression or function.

Conclusions and Future Directions

The defective TCR signaling observed in ZAP-70-deficient patients has established a critical role for a functional ZAP-70 PTK in normal TCR-mediated signal transduction. The failure of the TCR to mediate signals in thymocytes from mice deficient in ZAP-70 further supports the requisite role of ZAP-70 in TCR signal transduction. Despite findings that activation of Lck alone via co-cross-linking of CD4 or CD8 does not fully induce the PTK cascade and the other signaling reactions that occur as a result of TCR stimulation, a critical role for Lck in TCR signaling has been established on the basis of findings in mutant cell lines and Lck-deficient mice and one patient. These observations indicate that both Src and Syk family PTKs play unique and critical roles in TCR signal transduction.

In summary, TCR-associated PTKs are pivotally involved in distinct developmental events required for T cell maturation (Fig. 14.2). Lck and, to a lesser extent, Fyn are required for signaling in thymocytes; moreover, disruption of Lck severely affects peripheral T cell development and function in mice and humans. ZAP-70 deficiency has provided the first evidence that PTKs, and ZAP-70 in particular, are required for development of normal human T cell number and function. Further elucidation of the role of ZAP-70 in TCR signal transduction should be invaluable to the understanding of CD4 and CD8 selection in the thymus, as well as the pathogenesis of this form of SCID. Whether mutations in other molecules involved in TCR signaling produce abnormal T cell phenotypes in humans remains to be determined. Possible use of gene therapy as an alternative to BMT for cure of ZAP-70 deficiency remains to be explored.

Acknowledgments

The author wishes to thank A. Weiss for his invaluable support and A.H. Filipovich, E.W. Gelfand, and S. Skoda-Smith for their assistance in the clinical and laboratory descriptions of ZAP-70-deficient patients.

References

Anderson SJ, Perlmutter RM. A signaling pathway governing early thymocyte maturation. Immunol Today 16:99–105, 1995.

Appleby MW, Gross JA, Cook MP, Levine SD, Qian X, Perlmutter RM. Defective T cell receptor signaling in mice lacking the thymic isoform of p59^{fyn}. Cell 70:751–763, 1992.

Arpaia E, Shahar M, Dadi H, Cohen A, Roifman CM. Defective T cell receptor signaling and CD8$^+$ thymic selection in humans lacking ZAP-70 kinase. Cell 76:947–958, 1994.

Cantrell D. T cell antigen receptor signal transduction pathways. Annu Rev Immunol 14:259–274, 1996.

Chan AC, Dalton M, Johnson R, Kong G-H, Wang T, Thoma R, Kurosaki T. Activation of ZAP-70 kinase activity by phosphorylation of tyrosine 493 is required for lymphocyte antigen receptor function. EMBO J 14:2499–2598, 1995.

Chan AC, Desai DM, Weiss A. The role of protein tyrosine kinases and protein tyrosine phosphatases in T cell antigen receptor signal transduction. Annu Rev Immunol 12:555–592, 1994a.

Chan AC, Irving BA, Fraser JD, Weiss A. The ζ chain is associated with a tyrosine kinase and upon T-cell antigen receptor stimulation associates with ZAP-70, a 70-kDa tyrosine phosphoprotein. Proc Natl Acad Sci, USA 88:9166–9170, 1991.

Chan AC, Iwashima M, Turck CW, Weiss A. ZAP-70: A 70 kd protein tyrosine kinase that associates with the TCR ζ chain. Cell 71:649–662, 1992.

Chan AC, Kadlecek TA, Elder ME, Filipovich AH, Kuo W-L, Iwashima M, Parslow TG Weiss A. ZAP-70 deficiency in an autosomal recessive form of severe combined immunodeficiency. Science 264:1599–1601, 1994b.

Chan AC, van Oers NSC, Tran A, Turka L, Law C-L, Ryan JC, Clark EA, Weiss A. Differential expression of ZAP-70 and Syk protein tyrosine kinases, and the role of this family of protein tyrosine kinases in TCR signaling. J Immunol 152:4758–4766, 1994c.

Cheng, AM, Negishi I, Anderson SJ, Chan AC, Bolen J, Loh DY, Pawson T. Arrested development of double negative thymocytes in mice lacking both the Syk and ZAP-70 kinases. Proc Natl Acad Sci USA 94:9797–9801, 1997.

Cheng AM, Rowley B, Pao W, Hayday A, Bolen JB, Pawson T. Syk tyrosine kinase required for mouse viability and B-cell development. Nature 378:303–306, 1995.

Chu DH, van Oers NSC, Malissen M, Harris J, Elder M, Weiss A. Pre-T cell receptor signals are responsible for the down-regulation of Syk protein tyrosine kinase expression. J Immunol 163:2610–2620, 1999.

Cooke MP, Abraham KM, Forbush KA, Perlmutter RM. Regulation of T cell receptor signaling by a src family protein-tyrosine kinase (p59^{fyn}). Cell 65:281–291, 1991.

DeFranco AL. The complexity of signaling pathways activated by the BCR. Curr Opin Immunol 9:296–308, 1997.

Di Bartolo V, Mege D, Germain V, Pelosi M, Dufour E, Michel F, Magistrelli G, Isacchi A, Acuto O. Tyrosine 319, a newly identified phosphorylation site of ZAP-70, plays a critical role in T cell antigen receptor signaling. J Biol Chem 274:6285–6294, 1999.

Duplay P, Thome M, Herve F, Acuto O. p56^{lck} interacts via its src homology 2 domain with the ZAP-70 kinase. J Exp Med 179:1163–1172, 1994.

Elder M, Lin D, Clever J, Chan AC, Hope TJ, Weiss A, Parslow TG. Human severe combined immunodeficiency due to a defect in ZAP 70, a T cell tyrosine kinase. Science 264:1596–1599, 1994.

Elder ME, Hope TJ, Parslow TG, Umetsu DT, Wara DW, Cowan MJ. Severe combined immunodeficiency with absence of peripheral blood CD8$^+$ T cells due to ZAP-70 deficiency. Cell Immunol 165:110–117, 1995.

Elder ME, Skoda-Smith S, Kadlecek TA, Wang F, Wu J, Weiss A. Distinct T cell developmental consequences in humans and mice expressing identical mutations in the DLAARN motif of ZAP-70. J Immunol 166:656–661, 2001.

Finco TS, Kadlecek T, Zhang W, Samelson LE, Weiss A. LAT is required for TCR-mediated action of PLCγ1 and the Ras pathway. Immunity 9:617–626, 1998.

Gauen LK, Zhu Y, Letourneur F, Hu Q, Bolen JB, Matis LA, Klausner RD, Shaw AS. Interactions of p59^{fyn} and ZAP-70 with T-cell receptor activation motifs: defining the nature of a signalling motif. Mol Cell Biol 14:3729–3741, 1994.

Gelfand EW, Weinberg K, Mazer BD, Kadlecek TA, Weiss A. Absence of ZAP-70 prevents signaling through the antigen receptor on peripheral blood T cells but not on thymocytes. J Exp Med 182:1057–1066, 1995.

Goldman FD, Ballas ZK, Schutte BC, Kemp J, Hollenback C, Noraz N, Taylor N. Defective expression of p56^{lck} in an infant with severe combined immunodeficiency. J Clin Invest 102:421–429, 1998.

Gong Q, Jin X, Akk AM, Foger N, White M, Gong G, Wardenberg JB, Chan AC. Requirement for tyrosine residues 315 and 319 within ζ chain-associated protein 70 for T cell development. J Exp Med 194:507–518, 2001.

Gong Q, White L, Johnson R, White M, Negishi I, Thomas M, Chan AC. Restoration of thymocyte development and function in ZAP-70-deficient mice by the Syk protein tyrosine kinase. Immunity 7:369–377, 1997.

Hatada MH, Lu X, Laird ER, Green J, Morgenstern JP, Lou M, Marr CS, Phillips TB, Ram MK, Theriault K, Zoller MJ, Karas JL. Molecular basis for interaction of the protein tyrosine kinase ZAP-70 with the T-cell receptor. Nature 377:32–38, 1995.

Irving BA, Chan AC, Weiss A. Functional characterization of a signal transducing motif present in the T cell receptor ζ chain. J Exp Med 177:1093–1103, 1993.

Hubert P, Bergeron F, Ferreira V, Seligmann M, Oksenhendler E, Debre P, Autran B. Defective p56^{lck} activity in T cells from an adult patient with idiopathic CD4$^+$ lymphocytopenia. Int Immunol 12:449–457, 2000.

Isakov N, Wange RL, Burgess WH, Watts JD, Aebersold R, Samelson L. ZAP-70 binding specificity to T cell receptor tyrosine-based activation motifs: the tandem SH2 domains of ZAP-70 bind distinct tyrosine-based activation motifs with varying affinity. J Exp Med 181:375–380, 1995.

Iwashima M, Irving B, van Oers NSC, Chan AC, Weiss A. The sequential interaction of the T cell antigen receptor with two distinct cytoplasmic protein tyrosine kinases. Science 263:1136–1139, 1994.

Kane LP, Lin J, Weiss A. Signal transduction by the TCR for antigen. Curr Opin Immunol 12:242–249, 2000.

Katzav S, Sutherland M, Packham G, Yi T, Weiss A. The protein tyrosine kinase ZAP-70 can associate with the SH2 domain of proto-Vav. J Biol Chem 51:32579–32585, 1994.

Kong G-H, Bu J-Y, Kurosaki T, Shaw AS, Chan AC. Reconstitution of Syk function by the ZAP-70 protein tyrosine kinase. Immunity 2:485–492, 1995.

Levelt CN, Mombaerts P, Wang B, Kohler H, Tonegawa S, Eichmann K, Terhorst C. Regulation of thymocyte development through CD3: Functional dissociation between p56^{lck} and CD3 sigma in early thymic selection. Immunity 3:215–222, 1995.

Levin SD, Anderson SJ, Forbush KA, Perlmutter RM. A dominant-negative transgene defines a role for p56^{lck} in thymopoiesis. EMBO J 12:1671–1680, 1993.

Lupher ML, Reedquist KA, Miyake S, Langdon WY, Band H. A novel Phosphotyrosine-binding domain in the N-terminal transforming region of Cbl interacts directly and selectively with ZAP-70 in T cells. J Biol Chem 271:24063–24068, 1996.

Madrenas J, Wange RL, Wang JL, Isakov N, Samelson LE, Germain RN. ζ phosphorylation without ZAP-70 activation induced by T cell receptor antagonists or partial agonists. Science 267:515–518, 1995.

Mallick-Wood CA, Pao W, Cheng AM, Lewis JM, Kulkarni S, Bolen JB, Rowley B, Tigelaar RE, Pawson T, Hayday AC. Disruption of epithelial γδ T cell repertoires by mutation of the Syk tyrosine kinase. Proc Natl Acad Sci USA 93:9704–9709, 1996.

Matsuda S, Suzuki-Fujimoto T, Minowa A, Ueno H, Katamura K, Koyasu S. Temperature-sensitive ZAP70 mutants degrading through a proteasome-independent pathway. J Biol Chem 274:34515–34518, 1999.

Molina TJ, Kishihara K, Siderovski DP, van Ewijk W, Narendran A, Timms E, Wakeham A, Paige CJ, Hartmann K-U, Veillette A, Davidson D, Mak TW. Profound block in thymocyte development in mice lacking p56lck. Nature 357:161–164, 1992.

Mombaerts P, Anderson SJ, Perlmutter RM, Mak TW, Tonegawa S. An activated lck transgene promotes thymocyte development in RAG-1 mutant mice. Immunity 1:261–267, 1994.

Monafo WJ, Polmar SH, Neudorf S, Mather A, Filipovich AH. A hereditary immunodeficiency characterized by CD8$^+$ T lymphocyte deficiency and impaired lymphocyte activation. Clin Exp Immunol 90:390–393, 1992.

Negishi I, Motoyama N, Nakayama K-I, Nakayama K, Senju S, Hatakeyama S, Zhang Q, Chan AC, Loh DY. Essential role for ZAP-70 in both positive and negative selection of thymocytes. Nature 376:435–438, 1995.

Neumeister EN, Zhu Y, Richard S, Terhorst C, Chan A C, Shaw AS. Binding of ZAP-70 to phosphorylated T-cell receptor ζ and η enhances its autophosphorylation and generates specific binding sites for SH2 domain-containing proteins. Mol Cell Biol 15:3171–3178, 1995.

Noraz N, Schwarz K, Steinberg M, Dardalhon V, Rebouissou C, Hipskind R, Friedrich W, Yssel H, Bacon K, Taylor N. Alternative antigen receptor (TCR) signaling in T cells derived from ZAP-70-deficient patients expressing high levels of Syk. J Biol Chem 275:15832–15838, 2000.

Perlmutter RM, Marth JD, Lewis DB, Peet R, Ziegler SF, Wilson CB. Structure and expression of lck transcripts in human lymphoid cells. J Cell Biochem 38:117–126, 1988.

Pfeffer K, Mak TW. Lymphocyte ontogeny and activation in gene targeted mutant mice. Annu Rev Immunol 12:367–411, 1994.

Qian D, Weiss A. T cell antigen receptor signal transduction. Curr Opin Cell Biol 9:205–212, 1997.

Raab M, da Silva AJ, Findell PR, Rudd CE. Regulation of Vav-SLP-76 by ZAP-70 and its relevance to TCRzeta/CD3 induction of interleukin-2. Immunity 67:155–164, 1997.

Rao N, Lupher MLJ, Ota S, Reedquist KA, Druker BJ, Band H. The linker phosphorylation site Tyr 292 mediates the negative regulatory effect of Cbl on ZAP-70 in T cells. J Immunol 164:4616–4626, 2000.

Reth M. The B-cell antigen receptor complex and co-receptors. Immunol Today 16:310–313, 1995.

Robey E, Fowlkes BJ. Selective events in T cell development. Annu Rev Immunol 12:675–705, 1994.

Roifman CM, Hummel D, Martinez-Valdez H, Thorner P, Doherty PJ, Pan S, Cohen F, Cohen A. Depletion of CD8+ cells in human thymic medulla results in selective immune deficiency. J Exp Med 170:2177–2182, 1989.

Rudd CE. Adaptors and molecular scaffolds in immune cell signaling. Cell 96:5–8, 1999.

Sawabe T, Horiuchi T, Nakamura M, Tsukamoto H, Nakahara K, Harashima SI, Tsuchiya T, Nakano S. Defect of lck in a patient with common variable immunodeficiency. Int J Mol Med 7:609–614, 2001.

Skoda-Smith S, Douglas VK, Mehta P, Graham-Pole J, Wingard JR. Treatment of post-transplant lymphoproliferative disease with induction chemotherapy followed by haploidentical peripheral blood stem cell transplantation and Rituximab. Bone Marrow Transplant 27:329–332, 2001.

Stein PL, Lee H-M, Rich S, Soriano P. pp59fyn mutant mice display differential signaling in thymocytes and peripheral T cells. Cell 70:741–750, 1992.

Straus DB, Chan AC, Patai B, Weiss A. SH2 domain function is essential for the role of the Lck tyrosine kinase in T cell receptor signal transduction. J Biol Chem 271:9976–9981, 1996.

Straus DB, Weiss A. Genetic evidence for the involvement of the lck tyrosine kinase in signal transduction through the T cell antigen receptor. Cell 70:585–593, 1992.

Toyabe S-I, Watanabe A, Hirada W, Karasawa T, Uchiyama M. Specific immunoglobulin E responses in ZAP-70-deficient patients are mediated by Syk-dependent T-cell receptor signaling. Immunology 103:164–171, 2001.

Turner M, Mee PJ, Costello PS, Williams O, Price AA, Duddy LP, Furlong MT, Geahlen RL, Tybulewicz VL. Perinatal lethality and blocked B-cell development in mice lacking the tyrosine kinase Syk. Nature 378:298–302, 1995.

van Leeuwen JEM, Samelson LE. T cell antigen receptor-signal transduction. Curr Opin Immunol 11:242–248, 1999.

van Oers NSC. T cell receptor-mediated signs and signals governing T cell development. Semin Immunol 11:227–237, 1999.

van Oers NSC, Killeen N, Weiss A. ZAP-70 is constitutively associated with tyrosine-phosphorylated TCR ζ in murine thymocytes and lymph node T cells. Immunity 1:675–685, 1994.

van Oers NSC, Killeen N, Weiss A. Lck regulates the tyrosine phosphorylation of the T cell receptor subunits and ZAP-70 in murine thymocytes. J Exp Med 183:1053–1062, 1996.

van Oers NS, Weiss A. The Syk/ZAP-70 protein tyrosine kinase connection to antigen receptor signaling processes. Semin Immunol 7:227–236, 1995.

Wange RL, Guitian R, Isakov N, Watts JD, Aebersold R, Samelson LE. Activating and inhibitory mutations in adjacent tyrosines in the kinase domain of ZAP-70. J Biol Chem 270:18730–18733, 1995a.

Wange RL, Isakov N, Burke TR, Otaka A, Roller PP, Watts JD, Aebersold R, Samelson LE. F2(Pmp)2TAMζ3, a novel competitive inhibitor of the binding of ZAP-70 to the T cell antigen receptor, blocks early T cell signaling. J Biol Chem 270:944–948, 1995b.

Wange RL, Malek SN, Desiderio S, Samelson LE. The tandem SH2 domains of ZAP-70 bind to TCRζ and CD3ε from activated Jurkat T cells. J Biol Chem 268:19797–19801, 1993.

Wange RL, Samelson LE. Complex complexes: signaling at the TCR. Immunity 5:197–205, 1996.

Wardenburg JB, Fu C, Jackman JK, Flotow H, Wilkinson SE, Williams BL, Johnson R, Kong G, Chan AC, Findell PR. Phosphorylation of SLP-76 by the ZAP-70 protein-tyrosine kinase is required for T-cell receptor function. J Biol Chem 271:19641–19644, 1996.

Watts JD, Affolter M, Krebs DL, Wange RL, Samelson L, Aebersold R. Identification by electrospray ionization mass spectrometry of the sites of tyrosine phosphorylation induced in activated Jurkat T cells on the protein tyrosine kinase ZAP-70. J Biol Chem 269:29520–29529, 1994.

Weil R, Cloutier J-F, Fournel M, Viellette A. Regulation of Zap-70 by src family tyrosine protein kinases in an antigen-specific T-cell line. J Biol Chem 270:2791–2799, 1995.

Weiss A, Kadlecek T, Iwashima M, Chan A, van Oers N. Molecular and genetic insights into T-cell antigen receptor signaling. Ann NY Acad Sci 766:149–156, 1995.

Weiss A, Littman DR. Signal transduction by lymphocyte antigen receptors. Cell 76:263–274, 1994.

Wiest DL, Ashe JM, Howcraft TK, Lee T-M, Kemper DM, Negishi I, Singer DS, Singer A, Abe R. A spontaneously arising mutation in the DLAARN motif of murine ZAP-70 abrogates kinase activity and arrests thymocyte development. Immunity 6:663–667, 1997.

Williams BL, Irvin BJ, Sutor SL, Chini CC, Yacyshyn E, Bubeck Wardenburg J, Dalton M, Chan AC, Abraham RT. Phosphorylation of Tyr319 in ZAP-70 is required for T-cell antigen receptor–dependent phospholipase C-ras activation. EMBO J 18:1832–1844, 1999.

Williams BL, Schreiber KL, Zhang W, Wange RL, Samelson LE, Leibson PJ, Abraham RT. Genetic evidence for differential coupling of Syk family kinases to the T-cell receptor: reconstitution studies in a ZAP-70-deficient Jurkat T-cell line. Mol Cell Biol 18:1388–1399, 1998.

Wu J, Zhao Q, Kurosaki T, Weiss A. The Vav binding site (Y315) in ZAP-70 is critical for antigen receptor–mediated signal transduction. J Exp Med 185:1877–1882, 1997.

Yablonski D, Kuhne MR, Kadlecek T, Weiss A. Uncoupling of nonreceptor tyrosine kinases from PLCγl in an SLP-76-deficient T cell. Science 281:413–416, 1998.

Yablonski D, Weiss A. Mechanisms of signaling by the hematopoietic-specific adaptor proteins, SLP-76 and LAT and their B cell counterpart, BLNK/SLP-65. Adv Immunol 79:93–128, 2001.

Zhang W, Sloan-Lancaster J, Kitchen J, Trible RP, Samelson LE. LAT: the ZAP-70 tyrosine kinase substrate that links T cell receptor to cellular activation. Cell 92:83–92, 1998.

Zhao Q, Williams BL, Abraham RT, Weiss A. Interdomain B in ZAP-70 regulates but is not required for ZAP-70 signaling function in lymphocytes. Mol Cell Biol 19:948–956, 1999.

Zhao Q, Weiss A. Enhancement of lymphocyte responsiveness by a gain-of-function mutation of ZAP-70. Mol Cell Biol 16:6765–6774, 1996.

15

Human Interleukin-2 Receptor α Deficiency

CHAIM M. ROIFMAN

Regulation of the immune system requires communication among its cellular components. Such cell-to-cell interplay occurs in microenvironments in the lymphoid organs and sites of inflammation. A major mechanism of communication includes the secretion of a vast number of soluble mediators, of which the most extensively studied is interleukin-2 (IL-2). Originally identified as a T cell growth factor (Gillis and Smith, 1977a, 1977b) IL-2 was also later implicated in promoting growth of natural killer (NK) cells and B cells.

A better understanding of the effect of IL-2 was rendered by studying the structure of its receptor (IL-2R) and the signals generated by its perturbation. The IL-2R is multimeric, consisting of two obligate subunits, IL-2Rβ (CD122) and IL-2Rγ or γc (CD132), and a variably expressed IL-2Rα subunit (CD25) (Siegel et al., 1987; Wang and Smith, 1987; Waldmann, 1989; Kondo et al., 1994; Nakamura et al., 1994; Nelson et al., 1994). Similar to other cytokine receptor systems, IL-2R components are shared by other receptors including IL-4, -7, -9, and -15 (Leonard et al., 1994), accounting for some overlap in the function and characteristics of these lymphokines (see Chapters 9, 10).

Corresponding to which of the three IL-2R chains is expressed, different binding affinities for IL-2 can be recorded. The α chain alone binds IL-2 with low affinity (Kd ~ 10 nM), whereas IL-2Rβ binds with an even lower affinity (Kd ~ 100 nM) and the γ chain by itself has no measurable affinity. However, when coexpressed, the α and β chains form an intermediate affinity complex (Kd ~ 30 pM) (Arima et al., 1991; Anderson et al., 1995). Only the coexpression of all three chains forms the high-affinity IL-2R complex (Kd ~ 10 pM) (Takeshita et al., 1992). Signaling activity through the IL-2R occurs with only two of the possible combinations of components. The combination of β and γ chains expressed on macrophages, resting T cells and NK cells, responds to high concentrations of IL-2, whereas the

complete αβγ complex with the highest affinity can relay activation signals intracellularly at low concentrations of IL-2 (Smith, 1988). Indeed, because the phenotypes of IL-2$^{-/-}$ and IL-2Rα$^{-/-}$ mice are almost identical (Schorle, et al., 1991; Willerford et al., 1995), most of the biologic effects of IL-2 are likely mediated through the high-affinity complex. Thus, the α chain of the IL-2R appears critical for a full response to IL-2 in vivo.

Interleukin-2 Receptor α

Interleukin-2 receptor α was the first chain of the IL-2R complex to be cloned (Leonard et al., 1984; Cosman et al., 1984; Nikaido et al., 1984). It is a 55 kDa protein with an extracellular portion containing 219 amino acid residues, a transmembrane segment of 19 residues, and a short cytoplasmic portion containing only 13 residues. Unlike the other chains of this receptor, IL-2Rα has no similarity to the cytokine receptor superfamily, but it appears to have structural homology to the α chain of the IL-15 receptor (Giri et al., 1995). The genes encoding IL-2Rα and IL-15α are located in proximity to each other on chromosome 10 in humans and chromosome 2 in mice (Anderson et al., 1995), which suggests that they may have arisen by gene duplication.

Of the three chains of the IL-2R, IL-2Rα shows the most tightly regulated expression. During T cell development, IL-2Rα is already expressed on the earliest triple-negative (CD3$^-$CD4$^-$CD8$^-$) thymocytes (Godfrey and Zlotnick, 1993), but subsequently is dramatically down-regulated. Thymocytes do not express IL-2Rα for the remainder of their development into T cells.

In resting, mature T cells IL-2Rα is not expressed; it is induced by stimulation through the T cell receptor or by IL-1 and tumor necrosis factor-α (TNF-α) (Crabtree, 1989; Rothenberg, 1991). Similarly, mature B cells newly express IL-2Rα following stimulation through the B cell receptor (Jung et al., 1984; Tsudo et al., 1984; Waldmann et al., 1984). IL-2Rα is also up-regulated in response to IL-2.

The regulation of IL-2Rα gene expression appears to be dependent on several potent enhancers, including positive regulatory region I (PRRI) (Lin et al., 1990; Plaetinck et al., 1990), which binds NF-κB; the serum response factor; PRRII, which contains binding sites for Elf-1 and the chromatin-associated protein HMG-I; and PRRIII, which can bind Elf-1, HMG-1, and STAT5 (John et al., 1996; L'ecine et al., 1996).

Clinical and Immunological Phenotype of IL-2Rα Deficiency

To date, only two human subjects with IL-2Rα deficiency have been identified; both were from the same family (Sharfe et al., 1997; Roifman, 2000; C. Roifman, unpublished observations). The parents of both patients were first cousins. The index patient, a male, presented with persistent thrush, *Candida* esophagitis, and cytomegalovirus (CMV) pneumonitis at 6 months of age (Table 15.1). By 8 months, chronic diarrhea and failure to thrive were associated with adenovirus gastroenteritis and frequent hospitalizations for exacerbations of pulmonary disease. Lymphadenopathy and hepatosplenomegaly became increasingly apparent during the second year of life, and by the third year he developed frequent otitis media, gingivitis, and chronic mandibu-

Table 15.1. Clinical Immunological and Pathological Features of IL-2Rα Deficiency

Factor	Clinical Manifestations
Growth and Development	Failure to thrive (decreased height and weight for age)
Infections	
Viral	CMV pheumonitis, adenavirus entertitis
Fungal	*Candida* stomatitis and esophagitis
Bacterial	Otitis media
Lymphoid Tissue	
Lymph nodes	Generalized lymphadenopathy
Liver/spleen	Hepatosplenomegaly with normal liver function
Thymus	Normal size

Factor	Laboratory and Pathological Features
Markers	
CD3+ cells	Reduced (<1000 cells/ml)
CD3+, CD4+ cells	Reduced (300–450 cells/ml)
Mitogenic Responses	
Anti-CD3 and PHA	Markedly reduced (11% to 20% of normal)
Tissue Pathology	
Lymphocytic infiltrates	Heavy infiltrates in mandible, lungs, gastrointestinal tract, liver in absence of demonstrable infectious agents
Thymus	
Morphology	Loss of corticomedullary distinction, no Hassall's corpuscles
Immunohistochemistry	Lack of expression of CD1 and CD25 High bcl-2 expression Reduced apoptosis

lar inflammation. While serum IgM and IgG levels were normal, IgA level was low. The absolute number of peripheral CD3+ T cells was reduced, with a significant reduction in CD4+ T cells. In vitro assays of peripheral lymphocyte function demonstrated reduced proliferation after stimulation by anti-CD3 (11% of control), phytohemagglutinin (20% of control), and other mitogens. Addition of exogenous IL-2 did not significantly rescue these proliferative responses. An allogenic skin graft from a healthy donor (negative for Epstein-Barr virus, CMV, HIV, and hepatitis B) was not rejected. Biopsies of lung and upper gastrointestinal tissue revealed dense lymphocytic infiltrates in the absence of infectious agents. The presentation was thus that of a combined immunodeficiency with increased susceptibility to viral, bacterial, and fungal infections, and evidence of dysregulated lymphocytic inflammatory disease.

Absence of IL-2R α Chain (CD25) Expression

Epstein-Barr virus–transformed cells from these patients did not express detectable CD25 by flow cytometry, whereas EBV-transformed lines from normal individuals typically contain 20%–40% CD25-positive cells (Fig. 15.1A). Western blot analysis of lysates from peripheral blood lymphocytes confirmed the absence of CD25 protein (Fig. 15.1B). In contrast, expression of the common γ chain was normal and the IL-2Rβ chain was elevated, possibly reflecting compensation for the lack of the α chain, CD25.

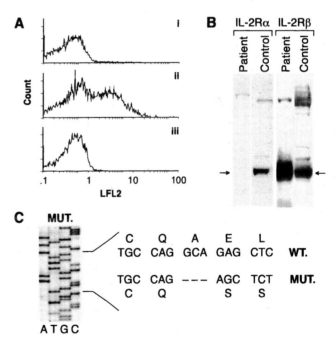

Figure 15.1. (A) Epstein-Barr virus–transformed patient B lymphocytes (trace i) and normal control B lymphocytes (trace ii) were stained with anti-CD25 and analyzed by flow cytometry, demonstrating the absence of CD25 expression on patient cells (1.1% positive) compared with a normal control (44% positive). Isotype-matched antibody control staining of patient cells (1.8% positive) is shown in trace iii. (B) Western blot analysis demonstrates the absence of IL-2Rα protein and elevated IL-2Rβ expression in patient peripheral blood lymphocytes compared with normal. (C) A 4 bp deletion in the patient's CD25 gene results in a frameshift in protein translation. The sequence around the deletion (cDNA 60–64) is shown (MUT.) and compared with the sequence and reading frame of normal CD25 (WT.).

Molecular Analysis

Two forms of CD25 cDNA were isolated from patient peripheral blood cells by reverse transcriptase-polymerase chain reaction, representing the full-length sequence (coding the active receptor) and a secondary splicing product lacking exon 4 (coding an inactive receptor) (Cosman et al., 1984; Leonard et al., 1984; Nikaido et al., 1984). Both forms of the patient's CD25 cDNA had a 4 bp deletion at cDNA 60–64, resulting in a translational frameshift (Fig. 15.1C). Predicted translation would proceed for only 20 amino acids before the deletion and resultant frameshift, with a further 25 irrelevant amino acids before termination. Thus even if this mRNA were stable, functional expression of CD25 would be effectively ablated. Consistent with autosomal recessive inheritance, the parents each demonstrated a normal and 4 bp–deleted allele.

Requirement of IL-2Rα for Normal Expression of CD1 in the Thymus

Atypically for profound cellular immunodeficiency, the thymus in IL-2Rα deficiency was of normal size, although displaying no Hassall's corpuscles and a lack of distinct cortical-medullary demarcation (Color Plate 15.I). Whereas immunohistochemical staining of thymus sections showed normal expression of CD3, CD2, CD4, CD8, and class I and class II major histocompatibility complex (MHC) proteins, staining for CD1 was completely negative (Color Plate 15.I).

In the normal thymus, CD1a is highly expressed on cortical thymocytes and dramatically down-regulated upon progression into the medullary antigen-presenting region. Because the CD1a gene itself was normal, a failure to provide appropriate signals for CD1 up-regulation in thymocytes may explain this phenomenon. It is possible that rather than serving simply as a nonclassical antigen-presenting molecule, CD1a may participate in mediating interactions between thymocytes and thymic epithelium, and absence of CD1a may be related to the loss of the distinct corticomedullary boundary.

Normally the induction of CD1 expression in cortical thymocytes precedes a dramatic decrease in the cellular level of the bcl-2 protein (Alvarez-Vallina et al., 1993; Fujii et al., 1994; Gratiot-Deans et al., 1994; Vanhecke et al., 1995). The presence of bcl-2 acts to protect cells against programmed cell death, without promoting proliferation (Cory, 1995). Early, immature triple-negative thymocytes and more mature double-positive (CD1+, CD3hi, CD4+, CD8+) medullary thymocytes express high levels of bcl-2 and are relatively resistant to apoptosis (Fujii et al., 1994; Gratiot-Deans et al., 1994; Cory, 1995). To permit immature thymocytes to undergo positive and negative selection, both of which result in the induction of programmed cell death 95% of the time, a reduction in bcl-2 levels is believed to be required. Whereas normal thymocytes demonstrated distinct areas of low (cortical) and high (medullary) bcl-2 expression, staining of patient thymus sections revealed that all CD25-deficient thymocytes expressed high levels of bcl-2 protein (Color Plate 15.I). The lack of regulation of bcl-2 expression in CD25 deficiency suggests that bcl-2 expression may be dependent on downstream events following either CD1 or CD25 signaling.

Sakaguchi et al. (1995) reported that CD25+ CD4+ T cells maintain self-tolerance in mice by suppressing autoreactive cells. Indeed, even in the absence of thymic irregularities, autoreactive responses emerged in the absence of CD25+ T cells. This finding suggests that the lymphocytic infiltrates observed in human CD25 deficiency could be autoimmune in nature. The persistence of high bcl-2 expression in cortical thymocytes supports this view; bcl-2 may permit some thymocytes bearing autoreactive T cell antigen receptors to escape deletion, as seen in some transgenic mice overexpressing bcl-2 (Siegel et al., 1992).

Normally, thymocytes expressing T cell receptors that bind avidly to an MHC molecule, which is presumably presenting self-derived antigens, are eliminated by apoptosis. Apoptosis in the CD25-deficient patient's thymus was low as demonstrated by decreased DNA degradation (Color Plate 15.1.) (Schmitz et al., 1991).

The heavy tissue infiltrates of lymphocytes found in a CD25-deficient patient suggest the involvement of autoreactive clones reminiscent of the oligoclonal expansion observed in multiple autoimmune disorders. Further, the higher than normal expression of bcl-2 in the thymus gland suggests that such autoreactive clones might escape selection because of reduced ability of these cells to undergo apoptosis. Thus IL-2Rα appears to be critical for the physiologic negative selection of thymocytes. In its absence, autoreactive clones that normally should be destined to die by apoptosis fail to do so, and instead expand and cause damage to peripheral tissues.

In conclusion, a combination of at least two events, one intrathymic and another peripheral, may have combined to create the phenotype observed in humans with CD25 deficiency.

IL-2Rα-Deficient Mice

Targeted disruption of IL-2Rα in the mouse showed that development of T and B cells appeared intact in these animals, including the distribution of thymocyte subpopulations in the thymus (Willerford et al., 1995). In addition, development of NK cells also appeared to be normal (Nelson and Willerford, 1998). However, as with IL-2 deficient mice, older IL-2Rα knockout mice developed polyclonal expansion of peripheral T cells that highly expressed CD44 but had a low expression of CD62L. Activated B cells present in young animals initially led to hypergammaglobulinemia, but in older animals a progressive loss of B cells was noted. The major phenotype of IL-2Rα knockout mice was autoimmune disease, including hemolytic anemia, severe colitis (reminiscent of human ulcerative colitis), and lymphadenopathy.

Treatment

The lymphadenopathy and tissue infiltrates of the CD25-deficient patient were partially ameliorated by the administration of corticosteroids. However, to effect a cure an allogeneic bone marrow transplant was performed, using an HLA-matched sibling as the donor. Engraftment was rapid and a complete resolution of symptoms ensued. On follow-up, the patient was free of symptoms without any treatment; over 95% of peripheral blood mononuclear cells were of donor origin, and growth and development were appropriate for age.

References

Alvarez-Vallina L, Gonzalez A, Gambon F, et al. Delimitation of the proliferative stages in the human thymus indicates that cell expansion occurs before the expression of CD3 (T cell receptor). J Immunol 150:8–16, 1993.

Anderson DM, Kumaki S, Ahdieh M, et al. Functional characterization of the human interleukin-15 receptor alpha chain and close linkage of IL15RA and IL2RA genes. J Biol Chem 270:29862–29869, 1995.

Arima N, Daitoku Y, Hidaka S, et al. Interleukin-2 production by primary adult T cell leukemia tumor cells is macrophage dependent. Am J Hematol 41:258–263, 1991.

Calabi F, Milstein C. A novel family of human major histocompatibility complex-related genes not mapping to chromosome 6. Nature 323:540–543, 1986.

Cory S. Regulation of lymphocyte survival by the bcl-2 gene family. Annu Rev Immunol 13:513–543, 1995.

Cosman D, Ceretti DP, Larsen A, et al. Cloning, sequence and expression of human interleukin-2 receptor. Nature 312:768–771, 1984.

Crabtree GR. Contingent genetic regulatory events in T lymphocyte activation. Science 243:355–361, 1989.

Fujii Y, Okumura M, Takeuchi Y, et al. Bcl-2 expression in the thymus and periphery. Cell Immunol 155:335–344, 1994.

Gillis S, Smith KA. In vitro generation of tumor-specific cytotoxic lymphocytes. Secondary allogeneic mixed tumor lymphocyte culture of normal murine spleen cells. J Exp Med 146:468–482, 1977a.

Gillis S, Smith KA. Long-term culture of tumour-specific cytotoxic T cells. Nature 268:164–166, 1977b.

Giri J, Kumaki S, Ahdieh M, et al. Identification and cloning of a novel IL-15 binding protein that is structurally related to the alpha chain of the IL-2 receptor. EMBO J 14:3654–3663, 1995.

Godfrey DI, Zlotnick A. Control points in early T-cell development. Immunol Today 14:547–552, 1993.

Gratiot-Deans J, Merino R, Nunez G, et al. Bcl-2 expression during T-cell development: early loss and late return occur at specific stages of commitment to differentiation and survival. Proc Natl Acad Sci USA 91:10685–10689, 1994.

John S, Robbins CM, Leonard WJ. An IL-2 response element in the human IL-2 receptor alpha chain promoter is a composite element that binds Stat5, Elf-1, HMG-I(Y) and a GATA family protein. EMBO J 15:5627–5635, 1996.

Jung LKL, Hara T, Fu SM. Detection and functional studies of p60–65 (Tac antigen) on activated human B cells. J Exp Med 160:1597–1602, 1984.

Kasinrerk W, Baumruker T, Majdic O, et al. CD1 molecule expression on human monocytes induced by granulocyte-macrophage colony-stimulating factor. J Immunol 150:579–584, 1993.

Kondo M, Ohashi Y, Tada K, et al. Expression of the mouse interleukin-2 receptor gamma chain in various cell populations of the thymus and spleen. Eur J Immunol 24:2026–2030, 1994.

L'ecine P, Algart'e M, Rameil P, et al. Elf-1 and Stat5 bind to a critical element in a new enhancer of the human interleukin-2 receptor alpha gene. Mol Cell Biol 16:6829–6840, 1996.

Leonard WJ, Depper JM, Crabtree GR, et al. Molecular cloning and expression of cDNAs for the human interleukin-2 receptor. Nature 311:626–631, 1984.

Leonard WJ, Noguchi M, Russell SM, et al. The molecular basis of X-linked severe combined immunodeficiency: the role of the interleukin-2 receptor gamma chain as a common gamma chain, gamma c. Immunol Rev 138:61–66, 1994.

Lin BB, Cross SL, Halden NF, et al. Delineation of an enhancerlike positive regulatory element in the interleukin-2 receptor alpha-chain gene. Mol Cell Biol 10:850–853, 1990.

Nakamura Y, Russell SM, Mess SA, et al. Heterodimerization of the IL-2 receptor beta- and gamma-chain cytoplasmic domains is required for signaling. Nature 369:330–333, 1994.

Nelson BH, Lord JD, Greenberg PD. Cytoplasmic domains of the interleukin-2 receptor beta and gamma chains mediate the signal for T-cell proliferation. Nature 369:333–336, 1994.

Nelson BH, Willerford DM. Biology of the interleukin-2 receptor. Adv Immunol 70:1–81, 1998.

Nikaido T, Shimizu A, Ishida N, et al. Molecular cloning of cDNA encoding human interleukin-2 receptor. Nature 311:631–35, 1984.

Plaetinck G, Combe MC, Corth'esy P, et al. Control of IL-2 receptor-alpha expression by IL-1, tumor necrosis factor, and IL-2. Complex regulation via elements in the 5′ flanking region. J Immunol 145:3340–3347, 1990.

Roifman CM. Human IL-2 receptor alpha chain deficiency. Pediatr Res 48:6–11, 2000.

Rothenberg EV. The development of functionally responsive T cells. Adv Immunol 51:85–214, 1991.

Sakaguchi S, Sakaguchi N, Asano M, et al. Immunologic self-tolerance maintained by activated T cells expressing IL-2 receptor alpha-chains (CD25). Breakdown of a single mechanism of self-tolerance causes various autoimmune diseases. J Immunol 155:1151–1164, 1995.

Schmitz GG, Walter T, Seibl R, et al. Non-radioactive labeling of oligonucleotides in vitro with the hapten digoxigenin by tailing with terminal transferase. Anal Biochem 192:222–223, 1991.

Schorle H, Holtschke T, Hunig T, et al. Development and function of T cells in mice rendered interleukin-2 deficient by gene targeting. Nature 352:621–624, 1991.

Sharfe N, Dadi HK, Shahar M, Roifman CM. Human immune disorder arising from mutation of the α chain of the interleukin-2 receptor. Proc Natl Acad Sci USA 94:3168–3171, 1997.

Siegel JP, Sharon M, Smith PL, Leonard WJ. The IL-2 receptor beta chain (p70): role in mediating signals for LAK, NK, and proliferative activities. Science 238:75–78, 1987.

Siegel RM, Katsumata M, Miyashita T, et al. Inhibition of thymocyte apoptosis and negative antigenic selection in bcl-2 transgenic mice. Proc Natl Acad Sci USA 89:7003–7007, 1992.

Smith KA. Interleukin-2: inception, impact, and implications. Science 240:1169–1176, 1988.

Takeshita T, Ohtani K, Asao H, et al. An associated molecule, p64, with IL-2 receptor beta chain-its possible involvement in the formation of the functional intermediate-affinity IL-2 receptor complex. J Immunol 148:2154–2158, 1992.

Tsudo M, Uchiyama T, Uchino H. Expression of Tac antigen on activated normal human B cells. J Exp Med 160:612–617, 1984.

Vanhecke D, Leclercq G, Plum J, et al. Characterization of distinct stages during the differentiation of human CD69+CD3+ thymocytes and identification of thymic emigrants. J Immunol 155:1862–1872, 1995.

Waldmann TA. The multi-subunit interleukin-2 receptor. Annu Rev Biochem 58:875–911, 1989.

Waldmann TA, Goldman CK, Robb RJ, et al. Expression of interleukin 2 receptors on activated human B cells. J Exp Med 160:1450–1466, 1984.

Wang HM, Smith KA. The interleukin 2 receptor. Functional consequences of its bimolecular structure. J Exp Med 166:1055–1069, 1987.

Willerford DM, Chen J, Ferry JA, et al. Interleukin-2 receptor alpha chain regulates the size and content of the peripheral lymphoid compartment. Immunity 3:521–530, 1995.

16

CD3 and CD8 Deficiencies

JOSÉ R. REGUEIRO and TERESA ESPANOL

Mature T cells detect the presence of antigens by way of a variable surface heterodimer (either $\alpha\beta$ or $\gamma\delta$) termed the *T cell receptor* (TCR) (Fig. 16.1). TCR molecules require association with a group of invariant proteins collectively called *CD3* and organized as dimers (Call et al., 2002). Since the first description of the T cell antigen receptor complex (TCR/CD3) in 1981, at least four different CD3 proteins have been reported: CD3γ, δ, ϵ and ζ. CD3 proteins participate in TCR/CD3 assembly and surface expression. They also aid in the delivery of intracellular signals that drive T cell maturation or apoptosis in the thymus (see Chapter 4), and T cell activation, proliferation, and effector function or anergy/apoptosis after antigen recognition (see Chapter 6; Malissen et al., 1999). During early T cell development, some CD3 chains may act alone or assist immature TCR ensembles, such as those containing pre-TCR chains. CD3 chains lack intrinsic enzymatic activity for signal transduction. Rather, they rely on phosphorylation–dependent recruitment and activation of a number of cytosolic and transmembrane protein tyrosine kinases (PTK) and adaptors such as ZAP-70, Fyn, Lck, TRIM, LAT, SLP-76, and SIT (Schraven et al., 1999). Most $\alpha\beta$ TCR-bearing T cells recognize processed peptides associated with major histocompatibility complex (MHC) molecules. This interaction is facilitated by the T cell coreceptor proteins CD4 and CD8, which show considerable affinity for the MHC but not peptide moiety. Coreceptor association thus increases the stability of TCR–MHC interactions extracellularly and recruits the crucial PTK Lck intracellularly through a conserved binding motif within its cytoplasmic tail, resulting in rapid T cell activation.

CD8 serves as a coreceptor for TCR recognition of MHC class I–associated peptides (Zamoyska, 1998), which leads to cytotoxic $\alpha\beta$ T lymphocyte (CTL) activation and lysis of the antigen-presenting cell. This mechanism enables CTLs to recognize and eliminate infected cells, tumor cells, and allogeneic graft cells. CD8 molecules are expressed on the cell surface either as an $\alpha\alpha$ homodimer (in natural killer [NK] cells, in intraepithelial $\alpha\beta$ T cells, and in $\gamma\delta$ T lymphocytes) or as an $\alpha\beta$ heterodimer (in $\alpha\beta$ T lymphocytes and thymocytes). Surface expression of CD8β is dependent on expression of CD8α, as CD8β polypeptides are otherwise retained in the endoplasmic reticulum and degraded. Both chains (α and β) are composed of a single extracellular immunoglobulin-like domain (also present in CD3γ, δ, and ϵ), a membrane-proximal hinge region, a transmembrane domain, and a cytoplasmic tail (Fig. 16.1). Expression of CD8 is characteristic of CTLs and is critical for their progression through the process of positive selection during differentiation in the thymus. However, other cell types can also express CD8 molecules.

Because of the central role of T cells in specific immune responses and the central role of the TCR/CD3 complex in T cell function, the description of a human familial CD3 deficiency in 1986 was in many ways surprising due to its phenotypic spectrum (Regueiro et al., 1986). Four years later, a second CD3 deficiency was reported (Thoenes et al., 1990). As it turned out, the former was due to a selective CD3γ deficiency (Arnaiz-Villena et al., 1992) and became the first primary TCR immunodeficiency for which the genetic basis had been elucidated, whereas the latter was caused by a partial CD3ϵ deficiency (Soudais et al., 1993). A further CD3γ deficiency case has been characterized biochemically and genetically (van Tol et al., 1997). Recently, complete CD3δ or CD3ϵ deficiencies have also been reported in patients with severe combined immunodeficiency (SCID) (Dadi et al., 2003; de Saint-Basile et al., 2004a). In addition, a human selective CD8 deficiency, caused by mutations in *CD8A*, has been reported (de la Calle-Martin et al., 2001). Taken together, CD3 and CD8 deficiencies provide insights into the redundant and unique roles of these transmembrane molecules for T cell antigen recognition and signal transduction.

In humans, CD3 deficiencies present as very rare autosomal recessive diseases characterized by a prominent TCR/CD3 expression defect that may be associated with a mild (CD3γ) or severe (CD3δ, ε) peripheral blood T but not B or NK lymphopenia. It is caused by mutations in the genes encoding for CD3γ (Chr 11q23 *CD3G*); CD3δ (Chr 11q23 *CD3D*); or CD3ε (Chr 11q23.3 *CD3E*). Also, a CD3ζ deficiency of French origin, with severe lung infections, low T cell counts, and low TCR/CD3 expression, has recently been characterized (de Saint-Basile et al., 2004b; A. Fischer, personal communication). A Dutch TCR/CD3 expression defect with SCID symptoms but no mutations in *CD3G, E* or *Z* has been reported but not fully characterized

(Brooimans et al., 2000). Human CD8 deficiency is also a very rare autosomal recessive disorder showing an absolute CD8 expression defect by mature peripheral blood T and NK lymphocytes. As a consequence, the αβ CTL lineage becomes CD4⁻CD8⁻ (double negative, DN). It is caused by a point mutation (Gene Bank number AY039664) in the gene encoding for CD8α (Chr 2p12 *CD8A*).

Mutation databases have been established at http://bioinf.uta.fi/CD3Gbase, CD3Dbase, CD3Ebase, and CD8Abase. OMIM (Online Mendelian Inheritance in Man) sites can be found at http://www3.ncbi.nlm.nih.gov/entrez/dispomim.cgi?id=186740 (for *CD3G*), 186790 (for *CD3D*), 186830 (for *CD3E*),

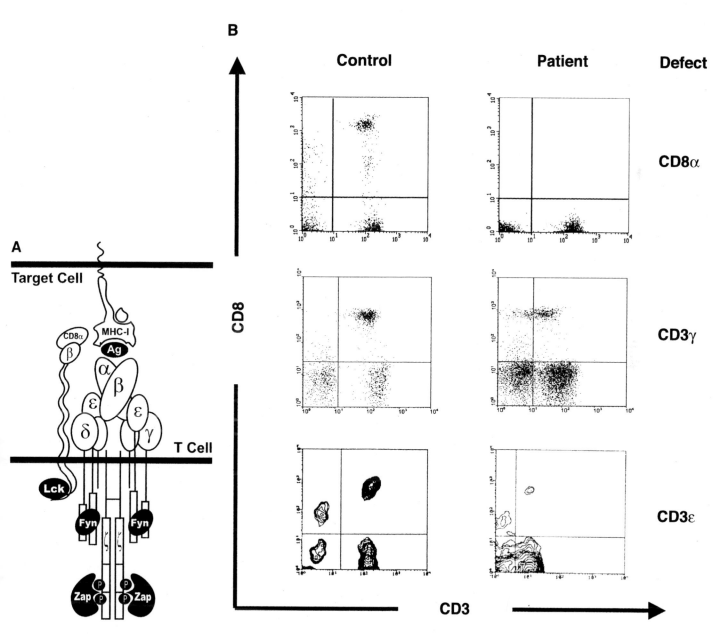

Figure 16.1. (A) Immunological synapse between a mature cytolytic αβT lymphocyte and an antigen-presenting target cell. Variable αβTCR heterodimers bind antigen (Ag) on major histocompatibility complex class I (MHC-I) molecules with aid from the CD8αβ coreceptor. CD3 dimers (γε, δε, and ζζ) and CD8 dimers then recruit intracellular enzymes (Fyn, Zap, Lck) to initiate signal transduction. (B) Representative lymphocyte phenotypes of human CD8α, CD3γ, and partial CD3ε deficiencies (the latter from cultured cell blasts, reproduced with permission from Soudais et al., 1993). The lack of mature T cells in complete human CD3δ or ε deficiency precluded obtaining a similar histogram. (C) Lymphocyte phenotype of a human TCR/CD3 expression defect (Dutch patient DS, molecular basis still unknown) and of her healthy father, who showed 50% expression levels compared to controls.

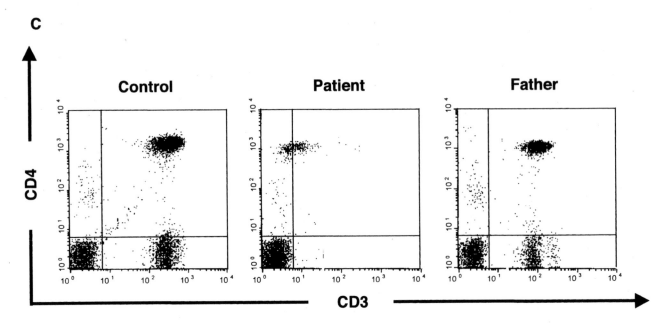

Figure 16.1. (*continued*)

and 186910 (*CD8A*), and genecard sites at www.genecards.org. For diagnostic support on these and other immunodeficiency, http://bioinf.uta.fi/IDdiagnostics/ should be consulted.

Clinical and Pathological Manifestations

CD3 Deficiency

The incidence of CD3 deficiencies is very low; 13 patients (8 males, 5 females) have been reported in 7 unrelated kindreds (Table 16.1). Age of onset, when symptoms are present, is early in life (before 3 years of age), essentially as recurrent bacterial or viral respiratory infections (all patients), as well as otitis (individuals DSF, PT in Table 16.1). Bacterial infections included *Hemophilus influenzae* in individuals VSF and PT (lung, ear), and *Salmonella enteritidis* (stool) and Yersinia enterocolitica (blood) in VSF. Viral infections included adenovirus (P2, PI-3), cytomegalovirus (CMV) (P3, PI-2, PII-1), parainfluenza (VSF), and Epstein-Barr virus (EBV) (PIII-1). Fungus was detected through oral or perineal candidiasis (PI-2, PIII-1) and presence of aspergillus (PII-2). Other symptoms included chronic diarrhea (VSF, P3, PII-1, PIII-1); failure to thrive (PII-1, VSF); autoimmune enteropathy (VSF); respiratory distress (P2, P3); asthmatic bronchitis (DSF, FK); diarrhea, allergic rhinitis, atopic eczema, vitiligo, lymphocytary—most likely viral in nature—meningitis, and dilated cardiomyopathy (DSF); urinary tract infections, nonatopic hyperreactive airway, and maxillary sinusitis (FK); and chronic sinusitis (PT). The patients had no history of chronic pyogenic infections or eczema. No dysmorphic features or bone abnormalities were reported. Patients followed normal vaccination schedules without complications. Five of 13 patients are presently alive. The rest shared SCID features and died early in life, most likely as a consequence of viral infections. A gut biopsy of patient VSF at 18 months of age showed a flat mucosa with crypt hypertrophy consistent with celiac disease. A gluten-free diet–resistant malabsorption syndrome with gut epithelial cell autoantibodies (autoimmune enteropathy) was finally diagnosed. The autopsy demonstrated bilateral bronchopneumonia and the presence of giant cells usually seen in Hecht's pneumonia, as well as mesenteric and mediastinic adenopathies. No thymus was evident on gross inspection, but microscopically the thymus rudiment (0.5×1.2 cm) and the lymph nodes, spleen, and bone marrow showed a marked lymphoid depletion, with no Hassal's corpuscles in the thymus, no plasma cells in the lymph nodes, and no lymphoid follicles in the spleen. Hassal's corpuscles were also absent in patients P1 and P3, despite a normal shadow on chest radiography. The Dutch patient with TCR/CD3 expression defect (DS), born to consanguineous parents, suffered two episodes of viral pneumonia at 7 months of age, and at 12 months showed SCID symptoms (failure to thrive, diarrhea, and *Pneumocystis carinii* pneumonia).

CD8 Deficiency

To date, CD8 deficiency has only been described in a consanguineous Spanish family (Fig. 16.2). The proband, a 25-year-old male (EP, II-4 in Table 16.1), presented with repeated respiratory infections and had two asymptomatic sisters (II-5 and II-7). The patient had suffered repeated bronchitis and otitis media from childhood. Chest X-ray and computed tomography revealed disseminated bronchiectases. Sputum culture was positive for *Haemophilus influenzae*. Functional respiratory tests showed severe mixed ventilatory disturbance. The patient's clinical status improved after intravenous antibiotic therapy. He has required further admissions because of respiratory reinfections. The parents and the remaining siblings have had no relevant medical history.

Laboratory Findings

CD3 Deficiency

Table 16.1 summarizes the main laboratory findings in CD3 deficiencies, mostly at the time of diagnosis (see also Zapata et al., 2000). Some of the abnormal features, however, may not be stable over time. For instance, many T cell proliferative responses in

Table 16.1. Characteristics of CD3 and CD8 Deficiencies

Deficiency in

Factor	CD3γ			CD3δ						CD3ε			CD3?	CD8α
Individual (family number)	DSF (1)	VSF (1)	FK (2)	P3 (3)	P1 (3)	P2 (3)	PII-1 (4)	PII-2 (4)	PIII-1 (5)	PT (6)	PI-2 (7)	PI-3 (7)	DS	EP (8)*
Nationality/consanguinity	Spanish/−	Spanish/−	Turkish/+	Canadian Mennonite/+	Canadian Mennonite/+	Canadian Mennonite/+	French/+	French/+	French/+	French/−	French/+	French/+	Dutch/+	Spanish/+
Gender	Male	Male	Male	Male	Female	Male	Female	Female	Male	Male	Male	Female	Female	Male
Age at diagnosis	4 years	1 year	4 years	2.5 months	0 month	2 months	3 months	0.1 month	2 months	2 years	1 month	0.1 month	1 year	25 years
Status/age in 2004 or when deceased (+)	Alive/23 years	+/32 months	Alive/14 years	+/3.5 months	Alive/4 years†	+/2 months	+/5 months	+/6 months†	+/6 months†	Alive/19 years	+/3 months	+/1 month†	Alive/8 years†	Alive/31 years
CD3 (Leu4, OKT3) expression	Low	Low	Undetectable	Undetectable	Undetectable	Undetectable	NT	Undetectable	Undetectable	Very low	NT	Undetectable	Very Low	Normal
On CD4+ PBL	Low (1/5)	NT	Low (1/3–1/4)	Undetectable	Undetectable	Undetectable	NT	Undetectable	Undetectable	Very low (1/10)	NT	Undetectable	Very Low (1/7)	Normal
On CD8+ PBL	Very low (1/10)	NT	Low (1/4–1/6)	Undetectable	Undetectable	Undetectable	NT	Undetectable	Undetectable	Very low (1/10)	NT	Undetectable	Very low (<1%)	Normal
TCR Expression														
αβ: BMA031, WT31	Very low (1/10)	NT	Low (1/4)	Undetectable	Undetectable	Undetectable	NT	NT	NT	Very low	NT	NT	Very low (<1%)	Normal
Vβ12	Low (1/4)	NT	NT	Undetectable	Undetectable	Undetectable	NT	NT	NT	NT	NT	NT	NT	Normal
γδ: TCRδ1	Low (1/4)	NT	Low (1/2)	Undetectable	Undetectable	Undetectable	NT	NT	NT	Very low	NT	NT	Very low (<1%)	Normal
PBL Counts	Normal/low	Normal	Normal	Low	Normal/low	Normal/low	Normal/high	Normal/high	Normal/high	Normal	Low	Low/normal	Normal/low	Normal
B cells	Normal	Normal	Normal	Normal	Normal	High	High/normal	High/normal	High/normal	Normal	NT	High/normal	High	Normal
NK cells	Normal	Normal	Normal	Normal	Normal	Normal	NT	High	NT	High	NT	Normal	Low	Normal
T cells	Normal/low	Normal/low	Low/normal	Absent	Absent	Absent	NT	Absent	Absent	Normal	NT	Absent	Very low	Normal
CD2+	Normal	Normal	Low	Very low	Very low	Very low	NT	NT	NT	Normal	NT	NT	NT	Normal
CD3-‡	Low	Low	Low	Absent	Absent	Absent	NT	Absent	Absent	Low	NT	Absent	Very low	Normal
CD4+	Normal/low	Normal	Low	Absent	Absent	Absent	NT	Absent	Absent	Low	NT	Absent	Low	Normal
CD8+	Low	Normal	Low	Absent	Absent	Absent	NT	Very low	Very low	Normal	NT	Very low	Very low	Absent
CD4-CD8- (DN)	Normal	Normal	Normal	NT	NT	NT	NT	NT	NT	Normal	NT	NT	NT	Very high
CD45RA+	Very low	NT	Very low	NT	NT	NT	NT	NT	NT	Normal	NT	NT	NT	Normal
CD45RO+	Normal	NT	Normal	NT	NT	NT	NT	NT	NT	Normal	NT	NT	NT	Normal
γδ‡	Low/normal	NT	Low/normal	Absent	Absent	Absent	NT	NT	NT	Low/normal	NT	NT	Very low	Normal
TCRVβ usage	NT	NT	Normal	NT	NT	NT	NT	NT	NT	Normal	NT	NT	NT	Normal

(continued)

Table 16.1. (continued)

Factor	CD3γ			CD3δ		CD3ε			CD3ζ	CD8α
	Deficiency in									
Lymphocyte Function										
B cells: IgG, A, E	Normal	Normal	Normal	Normal	Normal	Normal	Normal	Normal	Normal	Normal
IgM	Normal/low	Normal	Low	Normal	Normal	Normal/high	Normal/high	Normal/low	Normal/low	Normal
IgG2	Low/normal**	Low**	Normal	Normal	Normal	Low	Normal	Normal	Normal	Normal
Isohemagglutinins	Low (B)	Normal (B)	Normal (B)	NT	NT	Low	NT	NT	Low	Normal
Antibody responses to:										
Proteins	Normal	Normal	Normal	Normal	Low	Low	NT	NT	Low	Normal
Polysaccharides	Low	Low	Normal	Low	Low	Low	NT	NT	Low	Normal
NK cells (K562 lysis)	Normal	Normal	Normal	NT	NT	Normal	NT	NT	Normal	Normal
T cells										
PHA	Low	Low	Low	Absent	Absent	Low	Low	Absent	Low	Normal
Anti-CD3 (OKT3)	Low	Low	NT	NT	NT	Low	Low	Absent	Absent	Normal
Anti-CD2 + PMA	L/normal††	Normal	NT	NT	NT	Low	NT	NT	NT	NT
Tetanus toxoid	Low	Low	Low	NT	NT	Normal	NT	NT	Normal	Normal
Alloantigens	Low	Low	Low	NT	NT	Normal	NT	NT	Normal	Normal
Candidin	NT	NT	NT	NT	NT	Normal	NT	NT	Absent	Absent
PMA + ionomycin	Normal	NT	NT	NT	NT	Normal	NT	NT	Normal	Normal
Autoimmune features	Present‡‡	Present‡‡	Absent	NT	NT	Absent	NT	NT	Absent	Normal	Absent

DN, double negative; NT, not tested; PBL, peripheral blood lymphocyte; PHA, phytohemagglutinin; PMA, phorbol myristate acetate.

*Two healthy female sibs showed similar results.

†After bone marrow transplantation.

‡T cell counts by use of TCR/CD3 antibodies are not reliable in CD3 defects because of the expression defect of the whole complex. (αβ + γδ) T cells should be counted as CD2+ CD16−, and αβ T cells as CD4+ + CD8bright lymphocytes.

**The father was also IgG2 deficient.

††Recent (2003) in vitro evaluation of PBL response to bacterial (tuberculin, tetanus toxoid, diphtheria) and viral (cytomegalovirus, herpes simplex virus, rubella, varicella, mumps, measles, influenza A and B) antigens was normal.

‡‡Low-titer thyroglobulin and thyroid peroxidase autoantibodies have been present since June 1999 (DSF). Gut epithelial cell, smooth muscle, and mitochondrial autoantibodies, and autoimmune hemolytic anemia (VSF), and low-titer microsomal and thyroglobulin autoantibodies (FK) were present.

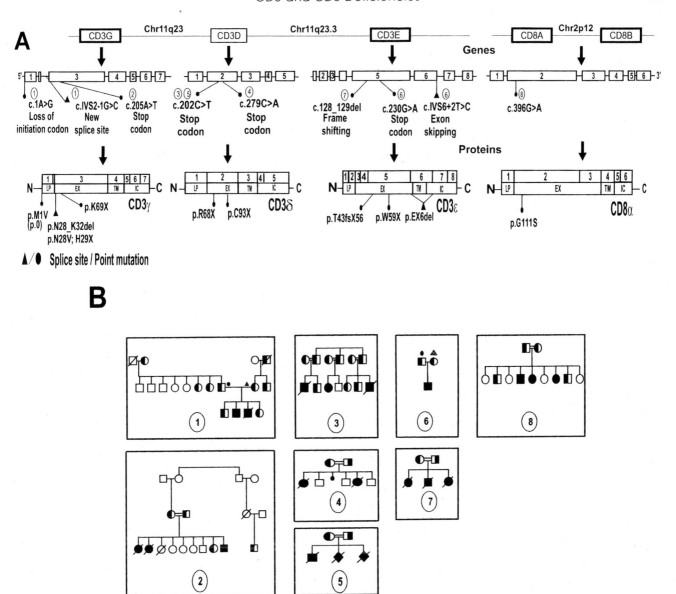

Figure 16.2. (A) The human *CD3GDE* and *CD8AB* gene complexes (from Genatlas http://www.dsi.univ-paris5.fr/genatlas) and their mutations. LP, EX, TM, and IC indicate the leader peptide, extracellular, transmembrane, and intracellular domains, respectively. Nomenclature follows published recommendations (http://archive.uwcm.ac.uk/uwcm/mg/docs//mut_nom.html). (B) Fate of each mutation along the family trees. For nonconsanguineous families, the paternal and maternal mutations are indicated. Three untested deceased individuals are shown as presumed heterozygote (maternal grandfather in family 1) or homozygotes (two females in family 2, based on clinical data). Female 6 in family 8 was not tested. In family 5, two homozygote fetuses from terminated pregnancies were also studied.

patient DSF became normal as he grew older. Also, immunoglobulin levels and lymphocyte counts may fluctuate from infections. The most consistent laboratory finding (when peripheral blood T cells are present) is a TCR/CD3 expression defect on otherwise phenotypically normal and polyclonal CD4+ and CD8+ (bright, to exclude NK cells) lymphocytes (Fig. 16.1B). However, monoclonal-specific, CD3 chain–specific, and/or T cell subset–specific differences may be observed. Lymphocyte counts are grossly normal or slightly diminished in venous blood, but lymphocyte subset–specific imbalances may be observed, sometimes dramatically. These include absence of T cells (both CD4+ and CD8+) in CD3δ or CD3ε deficiency (Dadi et al., 2003; de Saint-Basile et al., 2004a), or a very low number of CD45RA+ T cells in CD3γ deficiency (Zapata et al., 2000), which suggests a defective supply of naive T cells from the thymus

(Mackall et al., 1993) or poor peripheral survival due to weak homeostatic TCR–MHC interaction (Freitas and Rocha, 2000). Normal numbers of CD45R0+ T cells in CD3γ deficiency reflect a significant expansion of memory T cells, which are thought to be TCR-independent. TCR/CD3–induced T lymphocyte functions are very low, low, or normal, depending on the stimulus, whereas transmembrane stimuli (phorbol myristate acetate [PMA] + calcium ionophore) elicit normal responses. Skin tests with phytohemagglutinin (PHA), tetanus toxoid, PPD, or Candida are weak or absent. Some B cell functions may be low, manifested by serum IgG2 levels in two of three tested cases, isohemagglutinins in two of four, and in vivo responses to polysaccharides, but not to proteins. Immunoglobulin levels are generally normal, but may be low in SCID patients. Autoantibodies have been reported only in CD3γ deficiency. The Dutch TCR/CD3 expression defect

(Fig. 16.1C) showed some distinct laboratory features, such as a very severe T (particularly CD8$^+$) lymphopenia.

CD8 Deficiency

The main laboratory findings are shown in Table 16.1. Antibodies to tetanus, toxoplasma, mycoplasma pneumoniae, CMV, herpes zoster, herpes simplex, and rubella were present. Serologies to HIV and EBV, legionella pneumophila, aspergillus, and brucella were negative. Autoantibodies were negative. Lymphocyte phenotyping detected a total absence of surface CD8$^+$ (α or β) cells (Fig. 16.1B), presence of both CD3$^+$ ($\alpha\beta$ and $\gamma\delta$ T cells) and CD3$^-$ (NK cells), and a higher percentage of CD4$^-$ CD8$^-$ (DN) cells than that in normal donors. This increase was due to the rise in DN $\alpha\beta$ T cells (16%; reference range, 0.1%–2%), with a large Vβ repertoire and mostly CD3^{hi} CD5$^+$ CD2$^+$ CD45RA$^+$ CD57$^+$ CD11b$^+$ CD28$^-$. Upon stimulation, the DN T cells were positive for intracellular interferon-γ (IFN-γ), but not for interleukin-2 (IL-2) or IL-4. The percentage of DN $\gamma\delta$ T cells was normal (6%; reference range, 1%–8%). CD4$^+$ T cell, B cell, and NK cell percentage and absolute numbers were normal (Table 16.1). Intracellular CD8β was weakly positive.

Family Studies

Siblings with likely symptoms of CD3γ and CD8 deficiencies were found within two probands' families. Upon careful investigation, a healthy CD3γ-deficient sibling (individual DSF in Table 16.1) did show early clinical symptoms starting at 12 months of age, such as bacterial infections, asthmatic bronchitis, allergic rhinitis, diarrhea, vitiligo, atopic eczema, otitis, lymphocytary meningitis, and a mildly dilated cardiomyopathy that was probably secondary to unrecorded viral infections (Allende et al., 2000). Computerized axial tomography at the age of 6 revealed the presence of a thymus ($3 \times 1.2 \times 4.7$ cm). In contrast to this individual, three female siblings of the Turkish proband died before the age of 2 from chickenpox (at 18 months), measles (at 15 months), and (probably) leukemia (at 11 months), respectively. A definitive diagnosis of CD3γ deficiency was not made, but the first two siblings might be considered to have had CD3γ deficiencies (Sanal et al., 1996). Heterozygotes for CD3γ or ϵ deficiencies did not show TCR/CD3 expression defects, but the Dutch case did (Fig. 16.1C), suggesting a different molecular basis.

Two (females) of eight siblings of the CD8-deficient proband (EP) also lacked surface CD8$^+$ (α or β) expression and showed weak intracellular CD8β and high numbers of DN $\alpha\beta$ T cells (10% and 4%, respectively). Immunoglobulin levels were normal in all siblings studied. Antibody responses to varicella zoster, tetanus, herpes simplex, and natural antibodies were also present in a tested heterozygote (II-2) and in a homozygote (II-7). Mean fluorescence intensity of CD8α surface expression and soluble CD8 levels in serum (by ELISA) were decreased in the parents and in two heterozygous brothers (II-2 and II-8) but were normal in the remaining four siblings. These results indicate a good phenotype–genotype correlation (Fig. 16.2).

Molecular Basis

CD3 Deficiency

The lack of CD3γ, δ, or ϵ impairs both $\alpha\beta$ and $\gamma\delta$ TCR/CD3 assembly and surface expression. The expression defect is more severe in CD3ϵ (and probably CD3δ) than in CD3γ deficiency

(Fig. 16.1B). TCRα strictly associates with CD3$\delta\epsilon$ dimers, whereas TCRβ has been shown to interact with $\gamma\epsilon$ as well as $\delta\epsilon$ dimers (Call et al., 2002). This finding may explain the differential effect of the lack of CD3δ and ϵ, compared to γ, on surface TCR/CD3 expression. T cell development was blocked in complete CD3δ or ϵ deficiency and impaired in human CD3γ deficiency, but not in partial CD3ϵ deficiency. However, substantial numbers of mature T cells can be found in peripheral blood of CD3γ- or partially CD3ϵ-deficient patients, who in fact can show several normal immunological responses in vivo and relatively mild clinical symptoms. Therefore, repertoire shaping during intrathymic selection seems to adjust to available TCR/CD3 levels to populate peripheral lymphoid organs with fairly functional T cells in these cases.

CD8 Deficiency

Transfection studies were performed to establish a direct correlation between the mutation found in the CD8 immunoglobulin domain and the absence of any detectable CD8 antigen in homozygous family members. Wild-type and mutated CD8, as well as chimeric CD8 molecules (CD8 MUT/WT and WT/MUT), were subcloned into the *Xba*I/*Sac*I sites of pCDL-SRα296 vector (de la Calle-Martin et al., 2001). CD8 single-point mutants were generated by site-directed mutagenesis of the wild-type (wt CD8 > CD8^{ser111} or CD8^{arg111}) and mutated CD8 (mutant CD8 > CD8^{gly111}). The different constructs were transiently transfected in COS-7 cells and analyzed 48 hours later by immunofluorescence. The results demonstrated that the presence of serine or another amino acid at position 111 (CD8^{ser111} in the MUT/MUT and the MUT/WT construct) precludes CD8 expression, thereby suggesting that the presence of the evolutionary conserved glycine at this position may be important for appropriate folding of the protein. However, the lack of CD8 surface expression did not prevent development of a peripheral DN T cell lineage with functional features resembling CD8$^+$ T cells, such as IFN-γ synthesis. Similar results have been reported in mice (see Animal Models, below).

Functional Aspects

CD3 Deficiency

CD3δ and ϵ are essential for $\alpha\beta$ and $\gamma\delta$ T cell development in humans, therefore, no mature T cells have been available for the functional analysis of TCR/CD3 complexes lacking those chains. The study of mature T cells lacking CD3γ or partially lacking CD3ϵ has been complicated by two factors that hinder meaningful comparisons with normal individuals: (1) mild lymphopenia and/or differential T cell subset representation, and (2) defective surface expression of TCR/CD3 complexes. Nonetheless, it is clear that normal signaling is possible in vivo because antibody responses to T cell–dependent protein antigens were normal in these cases. Also, normal proliferative responses in vitro to certain antigens have been recorded (tetanus toxoid). Thus it seems that more subtle T lymphocyte functions will have to be studied in purified and/or cultured T cells.

Our studies in human CD3γ-deficient primary T cells, IL-2-dependent T cell lines, and herpesvirus saimiri-transformed T lymphocytes have indicated that CD3γ contributes to but is not absolutely required for the regulation of TCR trafficking in resting and antigen-stimulated mature T lymphocytes (Torres et al.,

2003). Despite its effects on TCR/CD3 expression (likely due to impaired recycling), CD3γ is not needed for several TCR/CD3-induced mature T cell responses, such as calcium flux, cytotoxicity, up- or down-regulation of several surface molecules, proliferation, and synthesis of certain cytokines (TNF-α). In contrast, PMA-induced TCR/CD3 down-regulation and TCR/CD3-induced synthesis of other cytokines (IL-2) as well as adhesion and polarization were severely impaired (Perez-Aciego et al., 1991; Arnaiz-Villena et al., 1992; Pacheco-Castro et al., 1998; Torres et al., 2002). The lack of CD3γ caused a stronger impairment of αβTCR/CD3 expression in CD8+ than that in CD4+ T cells in humans (Table 16.1) and in mice. We have shown that this is due to biochemical differences in the intracellular control of αβTCR/CD3 assembly, maturation, or transport between the two lineages, which result in conformational lineage-specific differences regulated by activation or differentiation in both normal and CD3γ-deficient primary T cells (Zapata et al., 1999, 2004).

CD8 Deficiency

Clinical manifestations, when present, are not severe, as shown in the murine homologue (see Animal Models, below). CD8 deficiency is thus compatible with life and less aggressive than HLA class I deficiencies. We believe that the absence of classical CD8+ CTL may be partially compensated for by the presence of a high percentage of αβ DN T cells in our patient, and by the cytolytic function of NK cells (Brown et al., 2001). The DN T cells were CD11b+ CD57+ CD45RA+ CD28− IFN-γ+ IL-2− IL-4−, a phenotype associated with effector CD8+ CTL (Hamann et al., 1999). The high antibody titers to many viral infections (CMV, herpes zoster, herpes simplex, rubella) in the patient seem to demonstrate that he has been in contact with these viruses and is immunocompetent enough to overcome these infections. Although analysis of recent infections in the proband showed only those of a bacterial nature, viral infections suffered at an early age might have been responsible for the alveolar lesions that later became overinfected and produced bronchiectases, as has also been reported in TAP-deficient adult patients (de la Salle et al., 1999). Further studies will be required to establish the functional features of CD8-deficient CTL.

Mutation Analysis

Mutation analysis was started by probing T cell RNA with CD3- or CD8-specific sequences. For CD3δ deficiency, microarray analysis of thymocyte RNA revealed low specific transcript levels. In all cases, cDNA was synthesized and used to amplify and sequence *CD3G*, *CD3D*, *CD3E*, or *CD8A*. This process revealed the presence of point mutations or small deletions in all cases (Fig. 16.2A), which could be traced with mutation-specific oligonucleotides, restriction enzymes, or direct sequencing. Small deletions were due to splice site mutations, which were identified on genomic DNA by sequencing relevant exon boundaries. Six of eight CD3 mutations caused early protein truncation at the extracellular domain, one caused loss of the initiation codon, and another caused skipping of the transmembrane domain. As a consequence, no mature CD3γ, δ, or ε proteins could be detected biochemically, and a TCR/CD3 expression defect ensued (ε ≥ δ > γ, Fig. 16.1B). The *CD8A* point mutation caused a missense substitution in the immunoglobulin domain at a very conserved position. Thus no intracellular or surface CD8α protein could be detected with several monoclon-

als, a finding suggesting that the mutant protein was degraded. CD8β surface expression is dependent on CD8α, thus CD8β was also undetectable extracellularly, although it could be detected intracellularly.

Strategies for Diagnosis

A definitive diagnosis of CD3 deficiency can be made in a male or female infant with a selective surface TCR/CD3 expression defect on mature peripheral blood T lymphocytes, or severe T lymphocytopenia, and mutations in *CD3G*, *D*, or *E* (or *Z*). CD8 deficiency is determined when either a male or female patient has an absolute surface CD8 expression defect on mature peripheral blood T and NK lymphocytes, high CD4−CD8− T cell numbers, and mutations in *CD8A*.

A probable diagnosis can be made in a male or female patient with selective T lymphocytopenia (T−B+NK+ SCID) or selective surface TCR/CD3 or CD8 expression defect on mature peripheral blood T lymphocytes.

Spectrum of Disease

Patients with CD3 or CD8 deficiency usually develop recurrent bacterial or viral respiratory infections as well as otitis. *Hemophilus influenzae* is frequently isolated. CD3-deficient SCID patients may develop fungal infections. The clinical course ranges from benign (CD3γ, partial CD3ε, CD8α) to severe (CD3δ, CD3ε, CD3γ), and asymptomatic siblings with CD3γ or CD8 deficiencies have been reported.

Differential Diagnosis

CD3 and CD8 deficiencies need to be differentiated from deficiencies in (1) ZAP-70; (2) TAP; (3) MHC class I; (4) IL7Rα; (5) purine nucleoside phosphorylase (PNP); and (6) adenosine deaminase (ADA). CD3γ and CD8 deficiencies may be misdiagnosed as patients may be fairly healthy. Testing for percentage of CD3 cells may not be enough to detect mild CD3 deficiencies (Fig. 16.1B). Analisis of the mean fluorescence intensity is mandatory, as is use of a range of TCR/CD3–specific monoclonals. The expression defect is more severe in CD3δ or CD3ε than in CD3γ deficiency. Lymphopenia, when present, affects only T cells (defined as CD2+CD16−), particularly CD45RA+, which are more thymus-dependent (Mackall et al., 1993). Biopsy specimens from lymphoid tissues should be thoroughly studied (Arnaiz-Villena et al., 1991; Dadi et al., 2003; de Saint-Basile et al., 2004a) and CD4+ and CD8+ T cells preserved (Perez-Aciego et al., 1991; Rodriguez-Gallego et al., 1996; Pacheco et al., 1998) and analyzed by immunoprecipitation (Alarcon et al., 1988; Perez-Aciego et al., 1991; Thoenes et al., 1992) and molecular biology techniques (Arnaiz-Villena et al., 1992; Soudais et al., 1993). In CD3ζ deficiency, reversion of some T cell clones to normal expression was observed in vivo as a consequence of additional mutations in T cell precursors (de Saint-Basile et al., 2004b).

Mode of Inheritance, Carrier detection, and Prenatal Diagnosis

CD3 and CD8 deficiencies are autosomal recessive disorders. Heterozygotes for CD3 deficiencies cannot be distinguished from normals by standard laboratory tests. Thus mutation analysis must be performed in each case, as explained above. In CD3 deficiencies, restriction fragment length polymorphism (RFLP) analysis with *Taq*I and a *CD3E* probe (50% heterozygosity) or polymorphic markers may help to define *CD3GDE* haplotype inheritance for carrier detection and/or prenatal diagnosis, since recombinations within the *CD3* gene complex are rare. In contrast, carriers for CD8 deficiency can be determined by cytometry or ELISA, because the levels of membrane-bound and soluble CD8 have correlated strictly with the genotype of the family members (see Laboratory Findings, above). Similarly, both healthy parents of the Dutch patient with TCR/CD3 expression defect whose molecular basis is still undetermined showed half-normal CD3 expression levels (Fig. 16.1C).

Treatment and Prognosis

The clinical manifestations and prognosis of CD3 and CD8 deficiencies are disparate even among siblings, ranging from early lethal SCID before 3 years of age (individuals VSF, P2, P3, II-1, II-2, III-1, I-2, I-3 in Table 16.1) to mild or no immunodeficiency and survival beyond 10 years of age (individuals PT, DSF, FK, EP in Table 16.1). Specific antibiotics were used in many cases, with clear clinical benefit. Lethality among CD3 deficiencies, however, may be high (8 of 13). Bone marrow transplantation was successfully performed in patient P1 with CD3δ deficiency and in the Dutch patient (DS) with TCR/CD3 expression defect before 15 months of age. Haploidentical bone marrow grafts have frequently failed (patients PII-2, PIII-1, PI-2). Mild CD3 deficiencies have been treated with prophylactic intravenous immunoglobulin treatment (400 mg/kg/month) with (Deist et al., 1991) or without (van Tol et al., 1997) antibiotics. Bronchial asthma in patient FK was treated with ketotifen and cromolyn sodium between 3.5 and 7 years of age (Sanal et al., 1996). He has been using salbutamol sulphate and sodium chromoglycate intermittently since he was 7 to treat his nonatopic hyperreactive airway, and eformoterol with occasionally inhaled steroids for the last 7 months. A patient who had CD3γ deficiency with SCID (VSF) was treated with antibiotics but died, probably from a viral infection. The healthy Spanish CD3γ deficiency patient (DSF) was treated with antibiotics only when symptoms developed and received treatment for his dilated cardiomyopathy. The observation that most antibody responses were normal in vivo prompted a comprehensive vaccination program, excluding attenuated viruses, for this individual. No secondary effects were recorded. Thus, this approach may be helpful on a preventive basis for other mild CD3 deficiencies. Gene therapy protocols are being developed in vitro (Sun et al., 1997). However, transfer of CD3γ into mature T cells may disrupt their intrathymic fine-tuning (Pacheco-Castro et al., 2003). Lymphoid progenitors may be better targets in this case, although the selective advantage of transduced over untransduced T cells remains to be established.

Animal Models

CD3 Deficiency

Single and multiple CD3 deficiencies have been created in mice through gene targeting of CD3 genes (reviewed by Malissen et al., 1999). Ablation of any CD3 protein essentially blocked T cell development, although at different intrathymic checkpoints and to a different extent. Indeed, all CD3 proteins, except CD3δ, are required for T cell selection at the pre-TCR (TCR-β) checkpoint, with the following level of importance: ε > γ > ζ. Interestingly, CD3δ is also dispensable for γδ T cell selection and for γδTCR surface expression in mice (but not in humans; Dadi et al., 2003).

However, all CD3 chains, including CD3δ, are required for T cell selection at the TCRαβ checkpoint and for αβTCR surface expression. The murine models of CD3 deficiency are similar to human CD3 deficiencies in some aspects (ε > γ in αβTCR expression, no peripheral T cells when CD3δ is lacking), but not in others (peripheral blood T lymphocyte numbers are clearly higher in humans lacking γ). However, comparisons between human and murine deficiencies must be made with be caution, particularly when analyzing peripheral lymphocyte subsets. For instance, ZAP70- or CIITA-deficient humans show normal or significant numbers of peripheral CD4+ T cells, respectively, and γc- or JAK3-deficient humans have normal numbers of B cells, whereas their murine counterparts do not. This discrepancy could be explained if we consider that deficient humans, but not mice, available for analysis may constitute a small surviving subset of those produced and thus may show different phenotypes from those of mice grown in special germ-free facilities. Alternatively, peripheral lymphoid expansion mechanisms may differ between species. Also, comparing human venous blood with murine spleens or lymph nodes may be unsuitable: the spleen and lymph nodes of a human CD3 deficiency (individual VSF in Table 16.1) with normal venous blood lymphocyte counts were severely depleted, as observed in all murine CD3 deficiencies (see Clinical and Pathological Manifestations, above). CD3 gene inactivation in mice, even when kept in pathogen-free facilities, may cause pathological manifestations (enteropathy in CD3ζ/η- or CD3δ-deficient mice) that resemble those observed in some humans (CD3γ or δ deficiency).

CD8 Deficiency

CD8 (α or β) knockout mice showed a severe reduction in MHC class I–restricted CTL development and function (Fung-Leung et al., 1991), but infections were mainly bacterial, with little incidence in survival. The CD8 glycoprotein plays an important role in the maturation and function of MHC class I–restricted T lymphocytes, but its presence does not appear to be essential for either CD8 lineage commitment or peripheral cytolytic function. It has been reported that TCR transgenic thymocytes from CD8α-deficient mice were able to restore positive selection of CD8 lineage cells (as shown by CD8β expression) in the absence of surface CD8, thereby compensating for the lack of CD8 expression by increasing the affinity of TCR for the positively selecting ligand (Goldrath and Hogquist, 1997). It is therefore possible that in humans the DN cells are in fact MHC class I–restricted, high-affinity T cells with cytolytic functions.

Concluding Remarks

Immature T lymphocytes cannot predict the isotype (αβ or γδ and surrogates thereof) or the specificity (MHC class I, MHC class II, CD1) of the particular TCR they will be endowed with. They may thus carry a range of adaptor CD3 chains capable of both supporting and signaling for different TCR ensembles in different phenotypic backgrounds. Indeed, the clear structural differences between the constant domains of αβ and γδ TCR involved in interactions with CD3 and other cell surface molecules strongly suggest that they may build different signaling complexes (Allison et al., 2001). Recently it has been shown that the γδ TCR does not contain CD3δ but rather a differentially glycosylated form of CD3γ upon T cell activation (Hayes et al., 2002). In addition, αβ T lymphocytes carry appropriate coreceptors (CD4 and CD8) to increase the likelihood of being rescued in the event that their

TCR has low affinity for MHC class II or class I, respectively. CD3 and CD8 chains are thus first expressed and used by T cells early during their intrathymic development. Accordingly, CD3 and CD8 deficiencies strongly influence early T cell differentiation events in both humans and mice. However, available data from some human deficiencies (CD3γ and partial CD3ε) indicate that significant or normal numbers of T lymphocytes can populate the peripheral blood compartment despite their low TCR/CD3 surface levels or lack of CD8 expression, respectively (probably after a strong post-thymic expansion of selected, but polyclonal, cells). T cell clones that fulfil the functional requirements for intrathymic survival may display aberrant phenotypes in the periphery (abnormal TCR/CD3 complexes, DN cells), but when tested they have been shown to be functional in vivo and in vitro. The adaptive value of the CD3 (particularly δ and ε) is nevertheless dramatically illustrated in SCID patients, whose survival is reduced without treatment. The healthy deficient siblings in CD3γ and CD8α deficiencies reflect the high redundancy of the immune system, or perhaps the existence of undefined modifying genes in these individuals (Foster et al., 1998). Further functional studies in peripheral blood T cells in these cases should clarify the specific extracellular and intracellular structural and signaling roles of the absent proteins at the last developmental checkpoint along T cell differentiation—namely, antigen recognition.

Note Added in Proof

Additional complete CD3δ- and CD3γ-deficient patients with SCID symptoms have been characterized recently (Takada et al., Eur J. Pediatr 164: 311–314, 2005, and Recio et al., unpublished). Also the G111S mutation in the *CD8A* gene has been shown recently to generate an ectopic glycosylation site, which may cause the lack of surface CD8 protein (Vogt et al. Nat Genet 37:692–700, 2005).

Acknowledgments

Antonio Arnaiz-Villena and Luis M. Allende (Hospital 12 de Octubre, Madrid), Oscar de la Calle-Martin (Hospital Sant Pau, Barcelona), and Manuel Hernandez (Hospital Vall d'Hebron, Barcelona) are joint coauthors of this work.

The following grants supported the work reviewed here: BFU2005-1738 (Dirección General de Investigación Científica), 8.3/21/01 and 570/04 (Comunidad Autónoma de Madrid), and BMC2002-3247 (Ministerio de Ciencia y Tecnología) to J.R.R. We thank Ozden Sanal (Hacettepe University Children's Hospital, Ankara, Turkey), Maarten J.M. van Tol (Leiden University Medical Center, The Netherlands), Alain Fischer (Hôpital Necker Enfants-Malades, Paris, France), Rik A. Brooimans (Wilhelmina Children's Hospital, University Medical Center Utrech, The Netherlands), and Jesús Ruiz-Contreras and Julián Clemente (Hospital 12 de Octubre, Madrid) for patient updates and for sharing unpublished data, and Ramón Rodríguez, Juan G. Cabanillas, and A. Pacheco-Castro (Universidad Complutense, Madrid) for help with the figures.

References

Alarcon B, Regueiro JR, Arnaiz-Villena A, Terhorst C. Familial defect in the surface expression of the T-cell receptor-CD3 complex. N Engl J Med 319:1203–1208, 1988.

Allende LM, Garcia-Perez MA, Moreno A, Ruiz-Contreras J, Arnaiz-Villena A. Fourteen years' follow-up of an autoimmune patient lacking the CD3γ subunit of the T-lymphocyte receptor. Blood 96:4007–4008, 2000.

Allison TJ, Winter CC, Fournie JJ, Bonneville M, Garboczi DN. Structure of a human γδ T-cell antigen receptor. Nature 411:820–824, 2001.

Arnaiz-Villena A, Perez-Aciego P, Ballestin C, Sotelo T, Perez-Seoane C, Martin-Villa JM, Regueiro JR. Biochemical basis of a novel T lymphocyte receptor immunodeficiency by immunohistochemistry: a possible CD3γ abnormality. Lab Invest 64:675–681, 1991.

Arnaiz-Villena A, Timon M, Corell A, Perez-Aciego P, Martin-Villa JM, Regueiro JR. Brief report: primary immunodeficiency caused by muta-

tions in the gene encoding the CD3-γ subunit of the T-lymphocyte receptor. N Engl J Med 327:529–533, 1992.

Brooimans RA, Rijkers GT, Wulffraat NM, Zegers BJM. Severe combined immunodeficiency in a patient with defective expression of CD3. Exp Clin Immunobiol 203:463, 2000.

Brown MG, Dokun AO, Heusel JW, Smith HR, Beckman DL, Blattenberger EA, Dubbelde CE, Stone LR, Scalzo AA, Yokoyama WM. Vital involvement of a natural killer cell activation receptor in resistance to viral infection. Science 292:934–937, 2001.

Call ME, Pyrdol J, Wiedmann M, Wucherpfennig KW. The organizing principle in the formation of the T cell receptor–CD3 complex. Cell 11: 967–979, 2002.

Dadi HK, Simon AJ, Roifman CM. Effect of CD3delta deficiency on maturation of alpha/beta and gamma/delta T-cell lineages in severe combined immunodeficiency. N Engl J Med 349:1821–1828, 2003.

de la Calle-Martin O, Hernandez M, Ordi J, Casamitjana N, Arostegui JI, Caragol I, Ferrando M, Labrador M, Rodriguez-Sanchez JL, Espanol T. Familial CD8 deficiency due to a mutation in the CD8α gene. J Clin Invest 108:117–123, 2001.

de la Salle H, Zimmer J, Fricker D, Angenieux C, Cazenave JP, Okubo M, Maeda H, Plebani A, Tongio MM, Dormoy A, Hanau D. HLA class I deficiencies due to mutations in subunit 1 of the peptide transporter TAP1. J Clin Invest 103:R9–R13, 1999.

de Saint-Basile G, Geissman F, Flori E, Uring-Lambert B, Soudais C, Jabado N, Fischer A, Le Deist F. Severe combined immunodeficiency caused by deficiency in either the δ or the ε subunit of CD3. J Clin Invest 114: 1512–1517, 2004a.

de Saint-Basile G, Geissman F, Rieux-Laucat F, Hivroz C, Soudais C, Jabado N, Fischer A, Le Deist F. Severe combined immunodeficiency caused by CD3 subunit δ, ε, and ζ deficiency. Abstract A2. Presented at the 11th meeting of the ESID, Versailles, France, 2004b.

Foster CB, Lehrnbecher T, Mol F, Steinberrg S, Venzon D, Walsh T, Noack D, Rae J, Winkelstein J, Curnutte JT, Chanock SJ. Polymorphism in host defense molecules influence the risk for immune-mediated complications in chronic granulomatous disease. J Clin Invest 102:2146–2155, 1998.

Freitas AA, Rocha B. Population biology of lymphocytes: the flight for survival. Annu Rev Immunol 18:83–111, 2000.

Fung-Leung WP, Schilham MW, Rahemtulla A, Kündig TM, Vollenweider M, Potter J, Van Ewijk W, Mak TW. CD8 is needed for development of cytotoxic T cells but not helper T cells. Cell 65:443–449, 1991.

Goldrath AW, Hogquist KA, Bevan MJ. CD8 lineage commitment in the absence of CD8. Immunity 6:633–642, 1997.

Hamann D, Roos MThL, Lier RAW. Faces and phases of human CD8+ T-cell development. Immunol Today 20:177–179, 1999.

Hayes SM, Laky K, El-Khoury D, Kappes DJ, Fowlkes BJ, Love PE. Activation-induced modification in the CD3 complex of the γδ T cell receptor. J Exp Med 196:1355–1361, 2002.

Le Deist F, Thoenes G, Corado J, Lisowska-Grospierre B, Fischer A. Immunodeficiency with low expression of the T cell receptor/CD3 complex. Effect on T lymphocyte activation. Eur J Immunol 21:1641–1647, 1991.

Mackall CL, Granger L, Sheard MA, Cepeda R, Gress RE. T-cell regeneration after bone marrow transplantation: differential CD45 isoform expression on thymic-derived versus thymic-independent progeny. Blood 82: 2585–2594, 1993.

Malissen B, Ardouin L, Lin SY, Malissen M. Function of the CD3 subunits of the pre-TCR and TCR complexes during T development. Adv Immunol 72:103–148, 1999.

Pacheco-Castro A, Martín JM, Millan R, Sanal O, Allende L, Regueiro JR. Toward gene therapy for human CD3 deficiencies. Hum Gene Therapy 14:1653–1661, 2003.

Pacheco-Castro A, Zapata DA, Torres PS, Regueiro JR. Signaling through a CD3γ-deficient TCR-CD3 complex in immortalized mature CD4+ and CD8+ T lymphocytes. J Immunol 161:3152–3160, 1998.

Perez-Aciego P, Alarcon B, Arnaiz-Villena A, Terhorst C, Timon M, Segurado OG, Regueiro JR. Expression and function of a variant T cell receptor complex lacking CD3-γ. J Exp Med 174:319–326, 1991.

Regueiro JR, Arnaiz-Villena A, Ortiz de Landazuri M, Martin-Villa JM, Vicario JL, Pascual-Ruiz V, Guerra-Garcia F, Alcami J, Lopez-Botet M, Manzanares J. Familial defect of CD3 (T3) expression by T cells associated with rare gut epithelial cell autoantibodies. Lancet i:1274–1275, 1986.

Rodriguez-Gallego C, Corell A, Timon M, Regueiro JR, Allende LM, Madrono A, Arnaiz-Villena A. Herpesvirus Saimiri transformation of T cells in a CD3γ immunodeficiency: phenotypical and functional characterization. J Immunol Methods 198:177–186, 1996.

Sanal O, Yel L, Ersoy F, Tezcan I, Berkel AI. Low expression of the T-cell receptor–CD3 complex: a case with a clinical presentation resembling humoral immunodeficiency. Turk J Pediatr 38:81–84, 1996.

Schraven B, Cardine AM, Hübener C, Bruyns E, Ding I. Integration of receptor-mediated signals in T cells by transmembrane adaptor proteins. Immunol Today 20:431–434, 1999.

Soudais C, Villartay JP, Deist FL, Fischer A, Lisowska-Grospierre B. Independent mutations of the human CD3-ε gene resulting in a T cell receptor/CD3 complex immunodeficiency. Nat Genet 3:77–81, 1993.

Sun J, Pacheco-Castro A, Borroto A, Alarcon B, Alvarez-Zapata D, Regueiro JR. Construction of retroviral vectors carrying human CD3γ cDNA and reconstitution of CD3γ expression and T cell receptor surface expression and function in a CD3-γ deficient mutant T cell line. Hum Gene Ther 8:1041–1048, 1997.

Thoenes G, Deist FL, Fisher A, Griscelli C, Lisowska-Grospierre B. Immunodeficiency associated with defective expression of the T-cell receptor–CD3 complex. N Engl J Med 322:1399, 1990.

Thoenes G, Soudais C, Deist FL, Griscelli C, Fischer A, Lisowska-Grospierre B. Structural analysis of low TCR–CD3 complex expression in T cells of an immunodeficient patient. J Biol Chem 267:487–493, 1992.

Torres PS, Alcover A, Zapata DA, Arnaud J, Pacheco A, Martín-Fernández JM, Villasevil EM, Sanal O, Regueiro JR. TCR dynamics in human mature T lymphocytes lacking CD3γ. J Immunol 170:5947–5955, 2003.

Torres PS, Zapata DA, Pacheco-Castro A, Rodríguez-Fernandez JL, Cabañas C, Regueiro JR. Contribution of CD3γ to TCR regulation and signaling in human mature T lymphocytes. Int Immunol 14:1357–1367, 2002.

van Tol MJD, Sanal O, Langlois van den Bergh R, van de Wal Y, Roos MTL, Berkel AI, Vossen JM, Koning F. CD3γ chain deficiency leads to a cellular immunodeficiency with mild clinical presentation. Immunologist (Suppl 1):41, 1997.

Zamoyska R. CD4 and CD8: modulators of T-cell receptor recognition of antigen and of immune responses? Curr Opin Immunol 10:82–87, 1998.

Zapata DA, Pacheco-Castro A, Torres PS, Millan R, Regueiro JR. CD3 immunodeficiencies. Immunol Aller Clin North Am 20:1–17, 2000.

Zapata DA, Pacheco-Castro A, Torres PS, Ramiro AR, San Jose E, Alarcon B, Alibaud L, Rubin B, Toribio ML, Regueiro JR. Conformational and biochemical differences in the TCR.CD3 complex of CD8+ versus CD4+ mature lymphocytes revealed in the absence of CD3γ. J Biol Chem 274: 35119–35128, 1999.

Zapata DA, Schamel WW, Torres PS, Alarcon B, Rossi NE, Navarro MN, Toribio ML, Regueiro JR. Biochemical differences in the αβ TCR–CD3 surface complex between CD8+ and CD4+ human mature T lymphocytes. J Biol Chem 279:24485–24492, 2004.

17

Molecular Basis of Major Histocompatibility Complex Class II Deficiency

WALTER REITH, BARBARA LISOWSKA-GROSPIERRE, and ALAIN FISCHER

Major histocompatibility complex class II (MHCII) molecules, also called human leukocyte antigens (HLA) in humans, are heterodimeric transmembrane glycoproteins consisting of α and β chains. The different human MHCII isotypes (HLA-DR, HLA-DQ, and HLA-DP) are encoded by distinct α chain and β chain genes that are clustered in the D region of the MHC on the short arm of chromosome 6. MHCII molecules play a pivotal role in the control of the immune system: they present exogenous peptide antigens to $CD4^+$ T lymphocytes, thereby leading to the antigen-specific T helper cell activation required for the initiation and propagation of adaptive immune responses. Given this essential function, it is not surprising that defects in the expression of MHCII molecules have profound immunopathological consequences.

Patients suffering from a rare primary immunodeficiency syndrome caused by the absence of MHCII expression were first identified in the late 1970s and early 1980s (Touraine et al., 1978; Schuurmann et al., 1979; Griscelli et al., 1980; Kuis et al., 1981; Touraine, 1981; Lisowska-Grospierre et al., 1983; Hadam et al., 1984, 1986). The lack of MHCII expression results in a severe defect in both cellular and humoral immune responses to foreign antigens and is consequently characterized by an extreme susceptibility to viral, bacterial, fungal, and protozoal infections, primarily of the respiratory and gastrointestinal tracts (reviewed in Griscelli et al., 1993; Klein et al., 1993; Elhasid and Etzioni, 1996). Severe malabsorption with failure to thrive ensues, often leading to death in early childhood.

The disease was formally named *major histocompatibility complex class II deficiency* (MHCII deficiency) (Rosen et al., 1992) and has been assigned the MIM (Mendelian Inheritance in Man) number 209920. It is also frequently referred to as the bare lymphocyte syndrome (BLS). However, the term *BLS* was first used to describe a defect in MHC class I (MHCI) expression in patients in which MHCII expression was not examined (Touraine et al., 1978), and it has been used synonymously for all defects involving expression of MHCI (BLS type I), MHCII (BLS type II), or both (BLS type III) (Touraine et al., 1992). Here we will discuss only the immunodeficiency syndrome associated with a constant and profound defect in MHCII expression, and we will thus use the term *MHCII deficiency*.

The disease is rare; fewer than 100 unrelated patients have been reported worldwide. The majority of patients are of North African origin (Algeria, Tunisia, Morocco) (Griscelli et al., 1993; Klein et al., 1993; Lisowska-Grospierre et al., 1994). The remaining patients are of diverse ethnic backgrounds that include Spain, Italy, Turkey, France, Holland, the United States, Israel, Saudia Arabia, and Pakistan (Kuis et al., 1981; Haas and Stiehm, 1987; Clement et al., 1988; Hume et al., 1989; Casper et al., 1990; Hadam et al., 1984, 1986; Lisowska-Grospierre et al., 1994; Peijnenburg et al., 1995). As expected for a rare disease, there is a high incidence of consanguinity in the affected families (Lisowska-Grospierre et al., 1994).

MHCII deficiency has an autosomal recessive mode of inheritance. A comparison between the pattern of inheritance of the disease and the MHC genotype in affected families has demonstrated that the genetic lesions responsible for the MHCII-deficient phenotype lie outside of the MHC (de Preval et al., 1985; Griscelli et al., 1993). This finding suggested that the disease is due to defects in *trans*-acting regulatory factors required for expression of MHCII genes. Elucidation of the molecular defects responsible for MHCII deficiency has confirmed this. The affected genes are now indeed known to encode regulatory factors controlling transcription of MHCII genes. Four regulatory genes—*MHC2TA* (MIM number 600005), *RFXANK* (MIM number 603200), *RFX5*

(MIM number 601863), and *RFXAP* (MIM number 601861)—have been isolated and shown to be mutated in MHCII deficiency patients (reviewed in Masternak et al., 2000a; Reith and Mach, 2001).

Clinical and Pathological Manifestations

Comprehensive accounts of the clinical and pathological manifestations associated with MHCII deficiency have been published previously (Griscelli et al., 1993; Klein et al., 1993; Elhasid and Etzioni, 1996). The major findings are summarized in Table 17.1. Clinical manifestations include primarily septicemia and recurrent infections of the gastrointestinal, pulmonary, upper respiratory, and urinary tracts. The patients are prone to bacterial, fungal, viral, and protozoal infections. Although the most frequently isolated bacteria were *Pseudomonas* and *Salmonella*, and the most frequent virus was cytomegalovirus (CMV), the type of infecting agent is by no means pathognomonic. Infections start within the first year of life; the mean age at first infection is 4.1 months. Subsequent evolution of the disease is characterized by an inexorable progression of the infectious complications until death ensues. Few children reach puberty; the majority die between the age of 6 months and 5 years. All of the pathological manifestations of MHCII deficiency are related to the infectious complications, and with the exception of the absence of MHCII expression there are no features that are specific for this particular immunodeficiency.

Bacterial infections in various locations are dominant. These include intestinal infections, pneumonitis, bronchitis, and septicemia. The most frequently isolated bacteria include *Pseudomonas, Salmonella, E. coli, Streptococcus,* and *Staphylococcus. Haemophilus* and *Proteus* species have also been isolated. In almost all patients, bacterial infections of the intestinal tract, together with *Candida albicans, Giardia lamblia,* and *Cryptosporidium* infection, are responsible for protracted diarrhea, malabsorption, and failure to thrive. Intestinal and hepatic involvement due to *Cryptosporidium* colonization appears to be more frequent in MHCII deficiency than it is in other immunodeficiencies. Protracted diarrhea is the most common gastrointestinal manifestation. Histological examinations of the intestinal mucosa typically reveal a variable degree of villous atrophy. There is also frequently an intraepithelial infiltration by lymphocytes, macrophages, and some plasma cells, and a severe colitis.

Hepatic involvement is frequent, but the manifestations are not uniform. Many patients exhibit either symptoms suggestive of viral hepatitis, or hepatic involvement resulting from cholangitis, parenteral nutrition, and the use of hepatotoxic drugs. The most frequent cause of hepatitis is infection with CMV. Pseudosclerosing cholangitis is a frequent complication of chronic *Cryptosporidium* infection, and bacterial cholangitis due to *Pseudomonas, Enterococcus,* and *Streptococcus* infections have been diagnosed in a number of patients.

Recurrent bronchopulmonary infections have been observed in all patients. Many had one or more episodes of pneumonia. The infectious agents identified include viruses (CMV, respiratory syncytial virus, enterovirus), bacteria (*Streptococcus, Haemophilus, Staphylococcus, Pseudomonas, Proteus*), *Pneumocystis carinii,* and *Candida albicans.*

Neurological manifestations due to viral infections have been diagnosed in a number of patients. These include poliomyelitis, meningoencephalitis, and chronic lymphocytic meningitis caused by enterovirus, herpes simplex virus, or poliovirus vaccination. Coxsackie virus, adenovirus, and poliovirus were frequently responsible for meningoencephalitis. Two patients developed poliomyelitis despite previous vaccination with inactivated virus. Another patient died of postvaccinal poliomyelitis with encephalitis after vaccination with live attenuated virus.

Hematologic manifestations are characterized by neutropenia and severe autoimmune cytopenia.

The clinical features vary considerably from one patient to another. This variability does not show any correlation with the genetic heterogeneity in the cause of the disease (see below). Interestingly, several patients having an atypical clinical course have been identified (Hauber et al., 1995, Wolf et al., 1995; Wiszniewski et al., 2001; B. Lisowska-Grospierre, unpublished data). Although these patients have classical MHCII deficiency, the clinical manifestations they suffer from are less severe or even absent, and their survival is considerably longer. Several patients over 20 years of age have been identified. The unusual capacity of these patients to cope with infections depends on genetic, immunological, and/or environmental differences that remain largely unknown.

Laboratory Findings—Immunological Features

The immunological manifestations characteristic of MHCII deficiency (reviewed in Griscelli et al., 1993; Klein et al., 1993) are summarized in Table 17.2. All of the immunological manifestations can be accounted for by the absence of antigen presentation via MHCII molecules. The most striking and constant consequence of the defect in MHCII expression is, as expected, the absence of cellular and humoral immune responses to foreign antigens. All patients are unable to mount T cell–mediated immune responses to specific antigens, as assessed by delayed-type hypersensitivity skin tests. This correlates with an absence of T cell responses in vitro in the presence of antigens with which the patients had been immunized or sensitized to by infections. Also consistent with the absence of MHCII expression is the finding that lymphocytes from patients have a decreased capacity to stimulate HLA-nonidentical lymphocytes in the mixed lymphocyte reaction.

Table 17.1. Clinical Manifestations

Manifestation	Patients	
	n	*%*
Repeated severe infections	63	(100)
Protracted diarrhea	54	(86)
Lower respiratory tract infections	54	(86)
Failure to thrive	46	(73)
Severe viral infections	40	(63)
Upper respiratory infections	35	(56)
Mucocutaneous candidiasis	19	(30)
Progressive liver disease	11	(17)
Cryptosporidiosis	11	(17)
Autoimmune cytopenia	4	(6)
Sclerosing cholangitis	6	(10)

Mean age at first infection is 4.1 months (range, 6 weeks to 12 months). Included are 43 patients from Hospital Necker-Enfants Malades, 1 patient from Hospital Robert Debré (Pickard et al., unpublished), 9 Tunisian patients (Bejaoui et al., 1998), and 10 patients reported by Saleem et al. (2000). Not included are four patients with an atypical clinical presentation in two unrelated families belonging to complementation group A (Quan et al., 1999; Wiszniewski et al., 2001).

Table 17.2. Summary of Immunological Findings*

Factor Measured	Findings	Patients[†]
HLA Class II Expression[‡]		
B cells	Absent (0%)	43/45
Monocytes	Residual (0–17%)**	6/37
PHA-activated T cells	Absent (0%)	32/37
	Residual (0–32%)**	5/37
HLA Class I Expression[‡]		
Mononuclear cells	Reduced	29/37
CD4+ Lymphopenia		*34/39*
Lymphocyte Proliferative Response to		
PHA	Normal	37/39
Antigen	Decreased	2/39
Serum Immunoglobulins		
IgG	Normal	6/30
	Decreased	24/30
IgM	Normal	9/40
	Decreased	28/40
	Increased	3/40
IgA	Normal	8/40
	Decreased	31/40
	Increased	3/40
Antibody Production Response to:		
Immunizations	Normal	1/20
	Decreased	2/20
	Negative	17/20
Microbial antigens	Decreased	5/27
	Negative	22/27

*Data are from 44 patients treated at Hospital Necker-Enfants Malades and 1 patient from Hospital Robert Debré, between 1977 and 2001 (Pickard et al., unpublished data).

[†]Results for all parameters are not available for all 45 patients. Only results for the number of patients tested are provided.

[‡]Tested by fluorescence-activated cell sorting (FACS) or microscopy.

**Numbers in parentheses indicate the percentage of "dull" stained cells.

Humoral immunity is severely impaired. Most patients are pan-hypogammaglobulinemic, almost agammaglobulinemic, or have a decrease in one or two immunoglobulin isotypes. Antibody responses to immunizations and infections by microbial agents are generally absent or strongly reduced. Interestingly, autoantibodies associated with autoimmune disorders have been found in several patients.

Patients have normal numbers of circulating T and B lymphocytes. In most patients, however, CD4+ T cell counts are reduced, whereas CD8+ T cell counts are proportionally increased. This reflects abnormal selection and maturation of CD4+ T cells resulting from a lack of MHCII expression in the thymus. Surprisingly, however, the remaining CD4+ T cell population appears to be phenotypically and functionally normal. The patient's CD4+ T cells exhibit only relatively minor differences with respect to the normal TCR repertoire (Rieux Laucat et al., 1993; Henwood et al., 1996) and behave normally in terms of alloreactivity and proliferative responses to mitogens (Griscelli et al., 1993; Klein et al., 1993).

The immunological features summarized above vary considerably from one patient to another. It is remarkable, however, that this variability does not show any correlation with the genetic heterogeneity in the cause of the disease (see below).

Molecular Basis

Abnormal Expression of MHCII Molecules

The hallmark of MHCII deficiency is the absence of MHCII molecules on the surface of all cells that normally express them, and the demonstration of this lack of expression remains the mainstay of diagnosis. In normal individuals, two modes of MHCII expression, constitutive and inducible, are observed (reviewed in Glimcher and Kara, 1992; Guardiola and Maffei, 1993; Mach et al., 1996). Constitutive expression is largely restricted to professional antigen-presenting cells (B lymphocytes, cells of the monocyte/macrophage lineage, and dendritic cells) and epithelial cells in the thymus. Inducible expression, by contrast, can be observed in virtually all cell types in response to a variety of stimuli, of which the most potent and well known is interferon-γ (IFN-γ). In MHCII-deficient patients, both the constitutive and inducible expression modes are abolished (reviewed in Griscelli et al., 1993; Klein et al., 1993). The absence of MHCII molecules concerns all professional antigen-presenting cells including B lymphocytes, cells of the macrophage/monocyte lineage such as Kupffer cells, and dendritic cells such as skin Langerhans cells. Activated T cells also remain MHCII negative. In addition, cells not derived from the bone marrow, such as thymic epithelial cells and endothelial and epithelial cells of the intestinal or bronchial mucosa, also lack MHCII molecules. Expression of MHCII cannot be restored in any cell type by IFN-γ.

The inability of patients' cells to express MHCII molecules constitutively or in response to IFN-γ has been demonstrated in vitro using peripheral blood lymphocytes (PBL), Epstein-Barr virus (EBV)-transformed B cell lines, interleukin-2 (IL-2)-dependent T cell lines, and primary or transformed fibroblasts derived from MHCII deficiency patients (de Preval et al., 1985, 1988; Lisowska-Grospierre et al., 1985; Griscelli et al., 1993; Klein et al., 1993). Studies on EBV-transformed B cell lines from patients indicated that expression of MHCII genes could not be detected at levels of the cell surface, intracellular protein, or mRNA (de Preval et al., 1985; Lisowska-Grospierre et al., 1985). In fibroblasts, the expression of MHCII genes cannot be induced by IFN-γ (de Preval et al., 1988). The lack of constitutive and inducible expression concerns all MHCII genes (encoding the DR, DP, and DQ α and β chains) (de Preval et al., 1985, 1988; Lisowska-Grospierre et al., 1985). In addition, there is a defect in expression of the invariant chain (*Ii*) gene (*CD74*) and the *HLA-DM* genes, which encode proteins required for antigen presentation by MHCII molecules (Cresswell, 1996; Alfonso and Karlsson, 2000); the *HLA-DMA* and *HLA-DMB* genes are silent and expression of the *Ii* gene is reduced (Nocera et al., 1993; Kern et al., 1995).

Although a complete absence of MHCII molecules is the general rule, certain patients appear to have a "leaky" phenotype (Griscelli et al., 1993; Klein et al., 1993). Low residual levels of MHCII expression have been observed in several patients on various cell types, including B cells, monocytes, activated T cells, Langerhans cells, intestinal endothelial cells, and thymic stromal and dendritic cells (Schuurman et al., 1985; Hadam et al., 1986; Klein et al., 1993). Very low levels of expression of certain MHCII genes have also been observed in EBV-transformed B cell lines and IFN-γ-treated fibroblasts derived from several patients (Griscelli et al., 1993; Klein et al., 1993; Peijnenburg et al., 1995).

In addition to the profound defect in MHCII expression, a reduction in cell surface expression of MHCI and β2 microglobulin is observed on fresh PBL, cultured fibroblasts, SV40-transformed fibroblasts, and EBV-transformed B cell lines from MHCII deficiency patients (Touraine et al., 1978; Schuurmann et al., 1979; Griscelli et al., 1980; Hadam et al., 1984, 1986; Sabatier et al., 1996). A reduction in MHCI expression is observed to a variable degree in over 75% of the patients (Table 17.2) (Klein et al., 1993).

MHCII Deficiency Is Due to Regulatory Defects in MHCII Gene Transcription

Direct measurements of the transcriptional activity of MHCII genes have demonstrated that the lack of expression in patients is due to a deficiency in transcription (Reith et al., 1988). This finding suggested that the disease is due to defects in regulatory factors controlling transcriptional activation of MHCII genes. Direct evidence for this interpretation was provided by four independent observations. First, family studies demonstrated that the genetic lesions responsible for the disease do not cosegregate with the MHC (de Preval et al., 1985; Griscelli et al., 1993). Second, reporter genes fused to the DNA sequences controlling transcription of MHCII genes (see below) remain silent upon transfection into cells from patients (Hasegawa et al., 1993; Riley and Boss, 1993). Third, nuclear extracts from patients' cells are unable to activate transcription from MHCII promoters in in vitro transcription experiments (Durand et al., 1994). Finally, expression of endogenous MHCII genes of patients' cells can be reactivated in somatic cell fusion experiments (see below).

Genetic Heterogeneity in MHCII Deficiency

It is now clear that defects in several distinct MHCII regulatory factors can give rise to MHCII deficiency. This genetic heterogeneity was first demonstrated by means of somatic cell fusion experiments performed with cell lines derived from different patients (Hume and Lee, 1989; Benichou and Strominger, 1991; Seidl et al., 1992; Lisowska-Grospierre et al., 1994). Several experimentally generated cell lines (Gladstone and Pious, 1978; Accolla, 1983; Calman and Peterlin, 1987) exhibiting an MHCII-negative phenotype indistinguishable from the patients' cell lines were also included in these studies. The results of these experiments indicate that the patients and experimentally derived cell lines can be assigned to four different complementation groups (Table 17.3, groups A to D), reflecting the existence of mutations in four distinct MHCII regulatory genes. Most patients (27 unrelated families) fall into complementation group B (reviewed in Masternak et al., 2000a). Group A contains patients from five different families (reviewed in Masternak et al., 2000a) as well as three experimentally derived mutants, most well-known one being RJ2.2.5 (Accolla, 1983). Group C contains patients from six families (reviewed in Masternak et al., 2000a). Group D was first defined by cell fusion experiments with the experimentally generated cell line 6.1.6 (Gladstone and Pious, 1978). Subsequent cell fusion experiments and isolation of the gene affected in 6.1.6 permitted the classification of patients from six unrelated families in this group (reviewed in Masternak et al., 2000a).

The spectrum of clinical manifestations and immunopatholologies associated with the disease encompasses all four complementation groups (Klein et al., 1993; Griscelli et al., 1993). No distinctive phenotype restricted to one of these complementation groups has been identified. Despite the genetic heterogeneity in the cause of MHCII deficiency, the syndrome is therefore clinically homogeneous.

Atypical Form of MHCII Deficiency

Twin brothers (Ken and Ker) exhibiting an atypical and less severe form of MHCII deficiency have been described (Hauber

Table 17.3. Phenotypical, Biochemical, and Molecular Defects of MHCII Deficiency Patients and Regulatory Mutants from Complementation Groups A to D

| | Wild Type | MHCII Deficiency Complementation Groups* | | | |
		A (II)	B (I)	C (IV)	D (III)
Prototypical patient		BLS-2	BLS-1, Ra	SJO	DA, ABI, ZM
Number of unrelated families[†]		5	27	6	6
Prototypical in vitro mutant		RJ2.2.5	None	G1B	6.1.6
Number of in vitro mutants[†]		3	None	1	1
MHCII expression	+	−	−	−	−
MHCII promoter activity[‡]	+	−	−	−	−
Binding of RFX[‡]	+	+	−	−	−
DNAseI hypersensitive sites[‡]	+	+	−	−	−
Promoter occupancy in vivo[‡]	+	+	−	−	−
Affected gene		*MHC2TA*	*RFXANK*	*RFX5*	*RFXAP*
MIM number		600005	603200	601863	601861
mRNA sequence entry		X74301	AF094760	X85786	Y12812
Chromosomal localization		16p13	19p12	1q21.1–21.3	13q14
Protein		CIITA	RFXANK**	RFX5	RFXAP
Size of protein (amino acids)		1130	269	616	272

*A–D, nomenclature for complementation groups used in Bénichou and Strominger (1991) and Lisowska-Grospierre et al. (1994); I–IV, alternative nomenclature used in Seidl et al. (1992).

[†]Numbers are based on somatic cell fusion experiments and/or mutation analysis of the affected genes.

[‡]Tested on at least one cell line in each complementation group.

**Also called RFX-B in Nagarajan et al. (1999).

et al., 1995; Wolf et al., 1995; Douhan et al., 1996). In contrast to the situation observed in the "classical" form of MHCII deficiency, defective expression in these patients does not concern all MHCII genes equally and does not affect all cell types to the same extent. In EBV-transformed B cells from these patients, the *HLA-DRB*, *HLA-DQB*, and *HLA-DPA* genes are silent whereas the *HLA-DRA*, *HLA-DQA*, and *HLA-DPB* genes are expressed. In mononuclear cells, by contrast, there is a significant level of *HLA-DRB*, *HLA-DQB*, and *HLA-DPA* gene expression. Moreover, impairment of the immune response is much less evident than in classical MHCII deficiency. In fact, investigations of MHCII-dependent immune functions in these patients indicate the presence of competent MHCII-positive antigen-presenting cells (Hauber et al., 1995; Wolf et al., 1995). Characterization of the genetic defect in these patients has demonstrated that they do not represent a fifth complementation group, as was initially believed. They belong in fact to complementation group C (Nekrep et al., 2002).

Biochemical Heterogeneity in MHCII Deficiency

MHCII expression is regulated primarily at the level of transcription by a short DNA segment situated immediately upstream of the transcription initiation site of each MHCII gene (reviewed in Benoist and Mathis, 1990; Mach et al., 1996). This promoter proximal region contains four *cis*-acting DNA elements—called the *S, X, X2,* and *Y* boxes—that are highly conserved in their sequence and in their organization with respect to orientation, order, and spacing relative to each other (Fig. 17.1A). This conservation is apparent not only in all MHCII genes from all species that have been examined but also in the invariant chain and *DM* genes. Finally, a similar region is also found in the promoters of the MHCI and β2 microglobulin (β2m) genes (van den Elsen et al., 1998).

In the hope of elucidating the molecular mechanisms controlling transcription of MHCII genes and identifying the regulatory genes that are mutated in MHCII deficiency, numerous studies were performed to identify and isolate DNA binding proteins that interact specifically with MHCII promoters (reviewed in Mach et al., 1996). These studies led to the identification of several key transcription factors, particularly the X box binding complex called *RFX* (regulatory factor X) (Reith et al., 1988).

RFX is a protein complex that was first identified in nuclear extracts from MHCII-positive B cell lines on the basis of its ability to bind in vitro to the X box of MHCII promoters (Reith et al., 1988). It has been purified to near homogeneity by affinity chromatography and shown to be a heteromeric protein consisting of three subunits of 75 kDa, 36 kDa, and 33 kDa (Durand et al., 1994; Masternak et al., 1998). The DNA-binding activity of this RFX complex has been analyzed extensively by in vitro studies using nuclear extracts prepared from MHCII deficiency cell lines and from the experimentally generated regulatory mutants (Reith et al., 1988; Stimac et al., 1991; Herrero-Sanchez et al., 1992; Hasegawa et al., 1993; Durand et al., 1994). Based on the presence or absence of RFX binding activity, two types of mutant cells were recognized (Table 17.3, Fig. 17.1); RFX binding activity is normal in cell lines classified in complementation group A but is deficient in cell lines assigned to complementation groups B, C, and D (reviewed in Mach et al., 1996). The lack of RFX binding activity in cells from complementation groups B–D

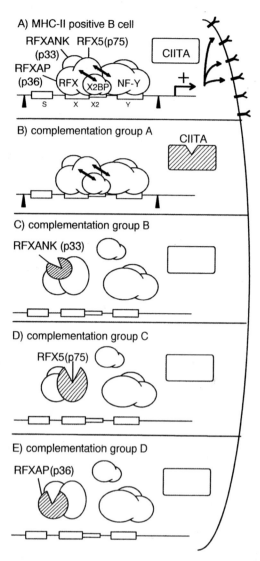

Figure 17.1. Molecular defects in MHCII deficiency. MHCII promoter occupancy and transcription status in normal B cells (A) and in B cells from complementation groups A to D (B–E). Open boxes represent the S, X, X2, and Y sequences. RFX, X2BP, and NF-Y bind to the X, X2, and Y boxes to form a nucleoprotein complex called the *MHCII enhanceosome*. Proteins binding to the S box remain poorly characterized. The MHCII enhanceosome forms a "landing pad" for CIITA. Cooperative protein–protein interactions between RFX, X2BP, and NF-Y are indicated by double-headed arrows. Arrowheads represent DNAseI hypersensitive sites. MHC2TA is mutated in complementation group A. Mutations in *MHC2TA* do not modify promoter occupation in vivo. In complementation groups B, C, and D, the 75 kDa (RFX5), 33 kDa (RFXANK), and 36 kDa (RFXAP) subunits of RFX are mutated. A deficiency in RFX leads to a bare promoter in vivo.

is specific since other known MHCII promoter binding proteins are detected normally in these cells (Reith et al., 1988; Stimac et al., 1991; Herrero-Sanchez et al., 1992; Hasegawa et al., 1993). The absence of RFX is functionally relevant because MHCII promoter activity can be restored to normal levels in in vitro transcription experiments when transcriptionally silent extracts from cells in groups B and C are supplemented with purified RFX (Durand et al., 1994).

Examination of DNAse I hypersensitive sites (Gonczy et al., 1989) and in vivo footprint experiments (Kara and Glimcher,

1991, 1993) have revealed that the lack of RFX binding activity observed in vitro correlates with a bare promoter in vivo (Table 17.3, Fig. 17.1), (reviewed in Mach et al., 1996). In RFX-positive cells (normal MHCII-positive B cells as well as B cells from complementation group A), MHCII promoters exhibit characteristic DNaseI hypersensitive sites and are occupied by DNA-binding proteins in vivo. In RFX-deficient B cells (complementation groups B–D), on the other hand, the DNaseI hypersensitive sites are missing and all of the MHCII promoter elements, including the X, X2, and Y boxes, are unoccupied.

The Gene Affected in Complementation Group A

A genetic approach based on cDNA expression cloning was developed to identify the genes affected in MHCII deficiency (Steimle et al., 1993). This approach is based on functional complementation of the genetic defects. Briefly, cell lines established from patients, or experimentally generated cell lines, were transfected with cDNA expression libraries and cells carrying cDNA clones capable of restoring MHCII expression were selected for. This approach was first successful in the case of RJ2.2.5 (Accolla, 1983), an experimentally generated cell line from complementation group A. Complementation of RJ2.2.5 led to isolation of the MHCII transactivator CIITA, a novel 1130–amino acid protein (Steimle et al., 1993).

Transfection with the CIITA cDNA restores expression of all MHCII isotypes (DR, DQ, DP) to wild-type levels in cell lines from complementation group A (Steimle et al., 1993). It also restores normal expression of the Ii (CD74), HLA-DMA, and HLA-DMB genes in these cells (Chang and Flavell, 1995; Kern et al., 1995).

The human MHC2TA gene is localized on chromosome 16 (16p13), and the corresponding mouse gene is situated in a syntenic region of mouse chromosome 16. This localization is in accordance with the findings that regulatory genes present on human and mouse chromosomes 16 are required for expression of MHCII genes (Accolla et al., 1986; Bono et al., 1991).

The Gene Affected in Complementation Group B

The gene affected in complementation group B, which contains the largest number of patients (Table 17.3), was isolated by a biochemical approach based on purification of the RFX complex. It was baptized RFXANK (Masternak et al., 1998) because it contains four ankyrin repeats. Ankyrin repeats constitute a well-known protein–protein interaction motif. The same gene was subsequently also called RFX-B (Nagarajan et al., 1999). RFXANK encodes the 33 kDa subunit of the RFX complex (Fig. 17.1). Transfection of the RFXANK cDNA restores RFX binding activity and thus reactivates expression of all MHCII isotypes (DR, DQ, DP) in cell lines from patients in complementation group B (Masternak et al., 1998; Nagarajan et al., 1999). The chromosomal localization of RFXANK is 19p12.

The Gene Affected in Complementation Group C

The same complementation approach used to isolate CIITA was successful in elucidating the molecular defect leading to a lack of RFX binding activity in patients from complementation group C. Complementation of a cell line derived from patient SJO

(Casper et al., 1990) led to the isolation of a cDNA encoding the 75 kDa subunit of RFX (Fig. 17.1) (Steimle et al., 1995). The gene was called RFX5 because it encoded the fifth member of a family of X box binding proteins sharing a highly characteristic DNA binding domain (DBD) (Steimle et al., 1995; Emery et al., 1996). This RFX DBD has been strongly conserved in evolution and has been identified in a variety of different proteins having diverse regulatory functions in organisms ranging from yeast to humans (Emery et al., 1996). The structure of the DBD of one member of the RFX family (RFX1) has been determined and shown to belong to the winged helix subfamily of the helix-turn-helix (HTH) proteins (Gajiwala et al., 2000). Surprisingly, the RFX1 DBD binds DNA in a fashion that is radically different from that observed for all other known HTH proteins (Gajiwala et al., 2000). The amino acids implicated in site-specific binding of the RFX1 DBD are strongly conserved in RFX5, implying that the latter interacts with its X box target site in a similar fashion (Gajiwala et al., 2000).

Transfection of the RFX5 cDNA restores RFX binding activity and thus reactivates expression of all MHCII isotypes (DR, DQ, DP) in cell lines from patients in complementation group C (Steimle et al., 1995). It also restores expression of the Ii (CD74), HLA-DMA, and HLA-DMB genes in these cells (Kern et al., 1995).

The human RFX5 gene is situated in a subcentromeric region of the long arm of chromosome 1 (Villard et al., 1997b). The corresponding mouse gene maps to a syntenic region of chromosome 3.

The Gene Affected in Complementation Group D

The experimentally generated cell line 6.1.6 (Gladstone and Pious, 1978) was initially the only representative of complementation group D (Hume and Lee, 1989; Benichou and Strominger, 1991; Seidl et al., 1992; Lisowska-Grospierre et al., 1994). The gene affected in 6.1.6 was isolated and shown to encode a novel protein corresponding to the 36 kDa subunit of the RFX complex (Fig. 17.1) (Durand et al., 1997). This protein was called RFX-associated protein (RFXAP) because it is a subunit of the RFX complex but does not contain the DBD characteristic of the RFX family of DNA binding proteins (Durand et al., 1997). Transfection of the RFXAP cDNA restores RFX binding activity and thus reactivates expression of all MHCII isotypes (DR, DQ, DP) in the 6.1.6 cell line.

Isolation of the RFXAP gene permitted the identification of MHCII deficiency patients belonging to complementation group D. Transfection of the RFXAP cDNA was found to complement cell lines derived from several patients (Durand et al., 1997; Villard et al., 1997a). The RFXAP gene is localized on the long arm of chromosome 13 (Villard et al., 1997a).

The Molecular Defect in Atypical Patients

Surprisingly, the gene affected in the atypical twins has recently been shown to be RFX5, thereby placing these patients in complementation group C (Nekrep et al., 2002). The defect is a point mutation changing a critical DNA contact residue within the DBD of RFX5. The unusual pattern of residual MHCII expression and atypical phenotype of these patients are probably a result of the mutation not compromising binding of RFX to all MHCII promoters to the same extent (Nekrep et al., 2002).

Function of the Affected MHCII Regulatory Factors

Structure and Mode of Action of CIITA

The primary sequence of CIITA exhibits four major features of interest (see Fig. 17.3A) (reviewed in Harton and Ting, 2000; Reith and Mach, 2001; Ting and Trowsdale, 2002). First, the N terminus of the protein contains a region rich in acidic amino acids. Second, downstream of this acidic region lie three segments rich in proline, serine, and threonine. Third, there is a centrally placed GTP binding domain that contains three characteristic sequences, a motif involved in nucleotide binding, a magnesium binding site, and a sequence believed to confer GTP binding specificity. Finally, there is a leucine-rich repeat (LRR)–based protein–protein interaction motif near the C terminus of the protein. All four features are required for the function of CIITA.

CIITA does not contain a recognizable DNA-binding domain and does not have affinity for DNA. Yet chromatin immunoprecipitation experiments have demonstrated that CIITA is physically associated in vivo with MHCII promoters and with the promoters of the *Ii, HLA-DM*, MHCI, and β2m genes (Hake et al., 2000; Masternak et al., 2000b, 2003; Beresford and Boss, 2001; Masternak and Reith, 2002). Recruitment of CIITA to MHCII promoters is mediated by multiple protein–protein interactions with DNA-bound factors (Fig. 17.2A). Factors bound to the S, X, X2, and Y boxes are all required for recruitment of CIITA (DeSandro et al., 2000; Hake et al., 2000; Masternak et al., 2000b; Zhu et al., 2000).

Once tethered to MHCII promoters, CIITA activates transcription via N-terminal transcription activation domains (Fig. 17.2A) (reviewed in Harton and Ting, 2000; Reith and Mach, 2001; Ting and Trowsdale, 2002). The acidic and proline/serine/threonine–rich regions in the N terminus of CIITA resemble the transcription activation domains found in transcription factors. Moreover, they can activate transcription when fused to heterologous DNA-binding proteins and can be replaced by activation domains from other transcription factors (Riley et al., 1995; Zhou and Glimcher, 1995). How these domains of CIITA function to activate transcription remains an open question. Three different but not mutually exclusive mechanisms have been proposed (Fig. 17.2A). First, CIITA can contact the general transcription factors TFIIB, hTAF$_{II}$32, and hTAF$_{II}$70, and may therefore activate transcription initiation by recruiting the general transcription machinery (Fontes et al., 1997; Mahanta et al., 1997; Masternak and Reith, 2002; Masternak et al., 2003). Second, CIITA may affect promoter clearance or transcription elongation by interacting with such factors as TFIIH or P-TEFb (Mahanta et al., 1997; Kanazawa et al., 2000). Finally, CIITA may facilitate chromatin remodeling at the promoter by recruiting coactivators having histone acetylase activity (Kretsovali et al., 1998; Fontes et al., 1999; Spilianakis et al., 2000; Beresford and Boss, 2001; Masternak and Reith, 2002; Masternak et al., 2003).

Analysis of the intracellular distribution of CIITA has shown that a substantial portion of the protein is localized in the nucleus. Several regions within CIITA have been implicated in nuclear targeting of the protein. First, three nuclear localization signals have been identified. One of these lies within the region deleted in patient BLS-2 (see Fig. 17.3A) (Cressman et al., 1999). Second, the GTP-binding domain appears to be required for nuclear import (Harton et al., 1999). Finally, a detailed mutational analysis of the LRR region has shown that it is important for directing CIITA to the nucleus (Hake et al., 2000).

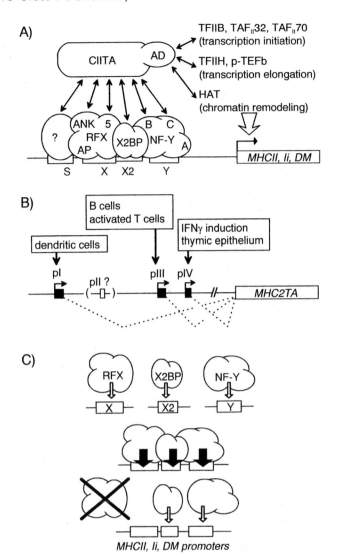

Figure 17.2. Function of CIITA and RFX. (A) CIITA is a non–DNA-binding coactivator that functions via protein–protein interactions (double-headed arrows). CIITA is tethered to the promoters by contacts with a poorly defined S box binding factor (?), the RFXANK and RFX5 subunits of RFX, X2BP (CREB), and the B and C subunits of NF-Y. CIITA is believed to activate transcription by recruiting other factors via its N-terminal activation domains (AD). Candidate factors include TFIIB, TAF$_{II}$32, TAF$_{II}$70, TFIIH, p-TEFb, and HAT (histone acetyl transferases). The roles of these factors in transcription initiation and elongation and in chromatin remodeling are indicated. (B) Cell type–specific and inducible expression of MHCII and related genes is controlled at the level of transcription of the *MHC2TA* gene. Transcription of *MHC2TA* is controlled by four independent promoters (pI, pII, pIII, and pIV) preceding four alternative first exons. These promoters exhibit different cell type specificity and responsiveness to IFN-γ. pII is not conserved in the mouse and its specificity is not known. (C) RFX participates in cooperative binding interactions required for promoter occupation in vivo. RFX, X2BP, and NF-Y have only low affinity (thin open arrows) for their respective target sites when bound on their own (top). This affinity is strongly enhanced (thick solid arrows) when the proteins bind cooperatively to the same DNA fragment (middle). In RFX-deficient cells, cooperative binding is lost and the promoters remain unoccupied in vivo (bottom).

CIITA shares a similar architecture and low sequence homology with a family of proteins containing a nucleotide-binding domain (NBD) coupled to a C-terminal LRR domain (reviewed in Harton and Ting, 2000; Harton et al., 2002). Although the

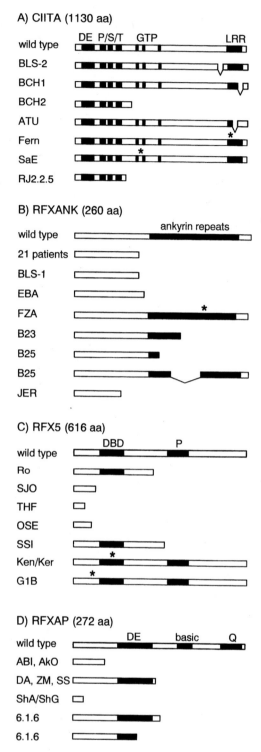

Figure 17.3. Mutations in MHCII deficiency. (A) Mutations in *MHC2TA* have been characterized in five unrelated patients and one experimentally generated cell line (RJ2.2.5). The ATP/GTP-binding domain, the leucine-rich repeat domain (LRR), the acidic region (DE), and the proline/serine/threonine–rich regions (P/S/T) are indicated. (B) Mutations in *RFXANK* have been characterized in 27 unrelated patients. The region containing ankyrin repeats is indicated. (C) Mutations in *RFX5* have been characterized in six unrelated patients and one experimentally generated cell line (G1B). The DNA-binding domain (DBD) and a proline-rich region (P) are indicated. (D) Mutations in *RFXAP* have been characterized in the experimentally generated 6.1.6 cell line and in six unrelated patients. Acidic (DE), basic, and glutamine (Q)-rich regions are indicated. In each case, the repercussion of the mutation on the

functions of many of these proteins are unknown, several have functions that are very different from that of CIITA. Conservation of the NBD-LRR domain organization in proteins having very different functions is intriguing. It is tempting to speculate that the similar structure of these proteins reflects an analogy in their mode of action.

Several studies have shown that CIITA can self-associate to form homomeric complexes. Although there is some controversy concerning the precise sequences that mediate self-association, the LRR and GTP binding domains have been implicated. (Kretsovali et al., 2001; Linhoff et al., 2001; Sisk et al., 2001). There is growing evidence that self-association is important for CIITA function, but there is as yet no consensus on its precise role.

Function and Expression of CIITA

MHCII genes, and the *Ii* (CD74), *HLA-DMA*, and *HLA-DMB* genes required for antigen presentation by MHCII molecules, are the major target genes of CIITA. In addition, CIITA contributes to, but is not essential for, expression of the MHCI and β2m genes (Gobin et al., 1997; Martin et al., 1997; van den Elsen et al., 1998). It is unlikely that CIITA plays an essential role in other systems, because all of the clinical manifestations exhibited by patients in which the *MHC2TA* gene is mutated can be attributed to the deficiency in MHC expression.

CIITA functions as a "master regulator" controlling cell type specificity, induction, and level of MHCII expression (reviewed in Harton and Ting, 2000; Reith and Mach 2001; Ting and Trowsdale, 2002). This is clearly demonstrated by the following findings.

1. The *MHC2TA* gene is expressed in a cell type–specific manner that correlates closely with MHCII expression.
2. Constitutive expression of MHCII genes in B cells is determined by constitutive expression of CIITA (Steimle et al., 1993).
3. CIITA expression is essential for the activation of MHCII gene transcription in response to IFN-γ, and induction of MHCII expression by IFN-γ is mediated by induction of CIITA expression (Chang et al., 1994; Chin et al., 1994; Steimle et al., 1994).
4. Differentiation of B cells into mature plasma cells is accompanied by the loss of MHCII expression, a process believed to be mediated by a dominant repression mechanism. This loss of MHCII expression has been shown to result from silencing of the *MHC2TA* gene (Silacci et al., 1994).
5. It has long been a puzzle that MHCII gene expression is induced in activated human T cells but not in activated mouse T cells. This discrepancy has been shown to be due to a species-specific difference in CIITA expression; CIITA is expressed in activated human T cells but not in activated mouse T cells (Chang et al., 1996b).
6. Repression of MHCII expression in trophoblast cells is caused by inhibition of CIITA expression (Morris et al., 1998, 2000).
7. The level of MHCII expression is modulated by the level of CIITA. Analysis of a large number of human and mouse cell lines and tissues has demonstrated that there is a tight quantitative correlation between the level of MHCII expression and that of CIITA expression. In addition, experimental modulation of CIITA expression using a tetracycline-inducible system has shown that the level of CIITA expression directly determines the level of MHCII expression (Otten et al., 1998).

protein is indicated schematically. Most mutations lead to internal deletions or C-terminal truncations. For JER (Lennon-Dumenil et al., 2001) only the truncated protein derived from the major splice variant is shown. Asterisks (Fern, SaE, G1B, FZA, Ken/Ker) indicate missense mutations. Mutations are described in detail in Masternak et al. (2000a).

8. Finally, an important emerging concept is that a variety of pathogens have developed the ability to inhibit CIITA expression—and thus MHCII expression—as a strategy to evade recognition by the immune system. Examples include CMV, varicella-zoster virus, *Mycobacterium bovis*, and *Chlamydia* (Miller et al., 1998; Le Roy et al., 1999; Wojciechowski et al., 1999; Zhong et al., 1999; Abenroth et al., 2000). This last point emphasizes the functional importance of CIITA as an essential immunomodulator.

Expression of the *MHC2TA* gene is directed by at least four independent promoters (I, II, III, and IV), which precede four alternative first exons (Fig. 17.2B). These promoters differ in their cell type specificity and response to IFN-γ (Muhlethaler-Mottet et al., 1997, 1998). It is thus the differential activity of the different CIITA promoters that ultimately determines the cell type specificity and inducibility of MHCII gene expression (reviewed in Harton and Ting, 2000; Reith and Mach, 2001; Ting and Trowsdale, 2002). Promoter I is used in dendritic cells (Muhlethaler-Mottet et al., 1997; Landmann et al., 2001). Promoter III primarily drives expression of CIITA in B cells and activated T cells, but also contributes to expression in dendritic cells. Promoter IV is essential for IFN-γ–induced expression in non–bone marrow–derived cells and for expression in epithelial cells of the thymic cortex (Waldburger et al., 2001, 2003).

Function and Mode of Action of RFX

In contrast to CIITA, the RFX complex is expressed ubiquitously in all cell types examined, even in MHCII-negative cells. However, like CIITA, the MHCII, *Ii* (*CD74*), *HLA-DMA*, and *HLA-DMB* genes are the major target genes of RFX. RFX is also implicated in expression of MHCI and β2m genes (Gobin et al., 1998; van den Elsen et al., 1998). It is unlikely that RFX plays a major essential role in other systems because the clinical manifestations in patients characterized by a defect in RFX (groups B, C and D) can all be attributed to the deficiency in MHC expression.

In vivo footprint experiments (Kara and Glimcher, 1991, 1993) and DNaseI hypersensitivity studies (Gonczy et al., 1989) have shown that the entire MHCII promoter, including the X, X2, and Y boxes, are unoccupied in RFX-deficient patients (Table 17.3, Fig. 17.1). This indicates that occupation of the promoter by DNA-binding factors such as the X2 box binding protein X2BP (Hasegawa and Boss, 1991), which has been shown to contain CREB (Moreno et al., 1999), and the Y box binding protein NF-Y (Mantovani, 1999) is dependent on binding of RFX to the adjacent X box. An explanation for these findings has been provided by in vitro binding studies demonstrating that RFX binds cooperatively with X2BP(CREB) and NF-Y to form a higher-order protein/DNA complex containing all three proteins (Fig. 17.2C) (Durand et al., 1994; Reith et al., 1994a, 1994b; Moreno et al., 1995; Louis-Plence et al., 1997). This nucleoprotein complex has recently been coined the *MHCII enhanceosome* (Masternak et al., 2000b). In the MHCII enhanceosome, the interactions of RFX, X2BP(CREB), and NF-Y with their respective target sites are strongly stabilized (Reith et al., 1994a, 1994b; Moreno et al., 1995; Louis-Plence et al., 1997). This stabilization is sufficiently strong to permit recruitment of RFX, X2BP(CREB), and NF-Y to all MHCII promoters, even to those that contain only very low–affinity binding sites for these proteins (Reith et al., 1994a; Louis-Plence et al., 1997). These cooperative binding interactions are essential for stable occupation of MHCII promoters in vivo (Wright et al., 1994). The bare promoter phenotype observed in groups B, C, and D is thus a direct consequence of the deficiency in RFX (Figs. 17.1 and 17.2C).

In addition to enhancing stability, the cooperative binding interactions between RFX, X2BP(CREB), and NF-Y are highly specific (W. Reith, unpublished data). For example, cooperative binding is not observed between RFX and proteins such as c-Jun and c-Fos, which are known to be able to bind to the X2 box in vitro, or between X2BP(CREB) and other X box binding proteins such as RFX1. This specificity ensures that RFX, X2BP(CREB), and NF-Y, rather than other related DNA binding proteins capable of recognizing the same DNA sequences, are recruited to MHCII promoters in vivo.

The fact that occupation of the MHCII promoter requires cooperative binding interactions between RFX, X2BP(CREB), NF-Y, and possibly other unidentified proteins, such as those recognizing the S box, explains the observation that the order, orientation, and spacing of the S, X, X2, and Y regulatory sequences are highly conserved in MHCII promoters and are critical for their activity (Vilen et al., 1991, 1992; Reith et al., 1994b).

Mutation Analysis

At the present time, six different mutations of the *MHC2TA* gene have been characterized in five unrelated BLS patients (Fig. 17.3A) (reviewed in Masternak et al., 2000a). One of these is a nonsense mutation leading to a severely truncated protein lacking the last two-thirds. Four of the mutations lie near the C terminus of the protein, in the vicinity of the protein–protein interaction domain consisting of LRRs. One of the latter is a missense mutation, while the other three are splice site mutations leading to the skipping of short in-frame exons. The most recent mutation to be identified is a missense mutation lying at amino acid 469 (Wiszniewski et al., 2001). The mutations affecting the two alleles of *MHC2TA* in the in vitro–generated RJ2.2.5 cell line have also been defined: one allele contains a large deletion within the CIITA gene (Fig. 17.3A), while the second allele is deleted entirely.

To date, eight different mutations of the *RFXANK* gene have been characterized in 27 unrelated patients (Fig. 17.3B) (reviewed in Masternak et al., 2000a). All mutations affect the integrity of the ankyrin repeat region. One is a missense mutation lying within the third repeat. The other six are nonsense mutations, deletions, or splice site mutations leading to proteins lacking all or part of the ankyrin repeat region. One of the mutations has been found in 21 unrelated patients, indicating the existence of a founder effect (Wiszniewski et al., 2000).

Mutations disrupting the *RFX5* gene have been identified in five classical patients in complementation group C (Fig. 17.3C) (reviewed in Masternak et al., 2000a). All are nonsense mutations or splice site mutations leading to the synthesis of severely truncated RFX5 proteins lacking the DBD and/or the C-terminal moiety of the protein. The atypical twins exhibiting an unusual mild form of MHCII deficiency have a point mutation in the DBD of RFX5 (Ken and Ker, Fig. 17.3C) (Nekrep et al., 2002). A mutation within RFX5 has also been identified in G1B, which is an in vitro–generated MHCII regulatory mutant. The RFX5 gene in G1B contains a missense mutation situated just upstream of the DNA binding domain (Brickey et al., 1999).

Only three different mutations disrupting the *RFXAP* gene have been identified in six unrelated families in complementation group D (Fig. 17.3D) (reviewed in Masternak et al., 2000a). Each allele of the *RFXAP* gene in the 6.1.6 cell line contains a frameshift mutation resulting from the insertion of a single G nucleotide (Fig. 17.3D) (Durand et al., 1997). All of these mutations lead to the synthesis of severely truncated RFXAP proteins.

Strategies for Diagnosis

Early diagnosis is critical because it increases the chances of successful bone marrow transplantation (BMT). Young children presenting with clinical and immunological features typical of MHCII deficiency should be referred by their physicians to specialized centers as soon as possible. The decisive criteria for the diagnosis of MHCII deficiency are the absence of MHCII expression and the inability to produce specific antibodies in response to immunization. These parameters should be tested in children having recurrent upper respiratory tract infections, diarrhea, and failure to thrive. Additional criteria warranting an investigation of MHCII expression include hypogammaglobulinemia and the absence of delayed-type hypersensitivity (DTH) skin tests.

Mode of Inheritance, Carrier Detection, and Prenatal Diagnosis

MHCII deficiency is inherited as an autosomal recessive disease. Carriers are healthy and exhibit no known phenotype. Considering the rarity of the disease, carrier detection is of no interest unless a consanguineous union is envisaged despite genetic counseling. In this case it could be performed either by using polymorphic markers flanking the affected gene or by a direct search for known mutations. Given the severity of MHCII deficiency, prenatal diagnosis in affected families is a valid ethical option. Previously, prenatal diagnosis has been carried out safely between the 20th and 22nd week of gestation by analyzing MHCII expression on fetal leukocytes obtained by means of an umbilical vein puncture guided by echography (Durandy et al., 1987). However, characterization of the mutations affecting the *MHC2TA, RFXANK, RFX5,* and *RFXAP* genes in families from complementation groups A, B, C, and D now offers a better option for prenatal diagnosis. The presence of these mutations could be assessed directly on trophoblastic cells obtained from a chorionic villi biopsy.

Treatment and Prognosis

Treatment of infections and other complications can at best reduce the frequency and severity of the clinical problems associated with MHCII deficiency. The optimal symptomatic care available consists of the prophylactic use of antibiotics, intravenous administration of immunoglobulins, and parenteral nutrition. However, these means do not prevent progressive organ dysfunction and death. In the absence of curative treatment—namely, BMT—prognosis is poor. As indicated in Table 17.4, the majority of patients who do not undergo BMT die at a young age from various infections, with or without autoimmune manifestations. Only a minority of patients characterized by a less severe clinical picture survives beyond the age of 14 years. Protracted diarrhea, malnutrition, the requirement for total parenteral nutrition, and the associated complications are the major causes of progressive clinical deterioration. There is no obvious difference in prognosis for patients belonging to the four different genetic complementation groups. The leaky phenotype characteristic of atypical patients is associated with a better outcome (Hauber et al., 1995; Wolf et al., 1995).

As for other combined immunodeficiency disorders, allogeneic BMT is currently the only available curative treatment for MHCII deficiency. The outcome of BMT in patients with MHCII

Table 17.4. Outcome with and without Bone Marrow Transplantation (BMT)

Without BMT (14 Patients)		After BMT (27 Patients)	
Outcome	n	Outcome	n
Chronic diarrhea	14	Well 1–11 years after BMT	11
Pneumonia	13	Persistnt immunodeficiency	1
Meningoencephalitis	5	Death <2 months after BMT	7
Hepatitis, cholangitis	6	Death <1 year after BMT	12
Sepsis	7	Death >1 year after BMT	3
Autoimmunity	4		
Death at age 6 months to 16 years	10		

Patients from Hospital Necker-Enfants Malades.

deficiency is summarized in Table 17.4. The success rate is relatively poor since less than half of the patients were cured by the procedure (Table 17.4; Klein et al., 1995). Results were much better in patients undergoing BMT before the age of 2 years, probably because the viral burden and organ dysfunction are less intense (Klein et al., 1995). When an HLA-identical sibling is available, the chances of success are fairly good. They are considerably lower when BMT is performed with matched unrelated donors or with partially HLA-compatible related donors. Although several patients have now been cured by BMT with such non–HLA-identical donors (Klein et al., 1995), the success rate remains lower than in other immunodeficiency syndromes. The two main obstacles are intractable persistent viral infections caused by a long-lasting T cell immunodeficiency, and graft failure or rejection resulting from the allogenic response in patients being normal.

Four conclusions can be drawn from our current experience with BMT in MHCII deficiency (Klein et al., 1995). First, despite the lack of MHCII expression, the risk of graft-versus-host disease is similar to that observed in patients with other forms of immunodeficiency. Second, CD4+ T cell counts remain low (albeit functional) in long-term survivors because of defective MHCII expression by the thymic epithelial cells of the host. Third, the lack of MHCII expression in nonhematopoietic cells does not appear to be detrimental for patients having undergone successful allogeneic BMT. Finally, given the invariably fatal course of typical MHCII deficiency and the poor outcome of BMT performed after the age of 2–4 years, it is highly recommended that BMT be performed in young children independent of whether an HLA-identical sibling is available.

Now that the four genes affected in MHCII deficiency have been identified, gene therapy has become a potential alternative to BMT. Introduction of the wild-type *MHC2TA, RFXANK, RFX5,* or *RFXAP* genes into the hematopoietic stem cells of patients in complementation groups A, B, C, and D, respectively, would represent a logical therapeutic strategy. It should be mentioned, however, that current gene therapy protocols remain hampered by the inefficiency of gene transfer into human hematopoietic stem cells. Moreover, in normal individuals MHCII expression is tightly controlled in a cell type–specific and inducible manner, and ectopic or nonphysiological levels of MHCII expression induced by the transgene should therefore be avoided in these patients. This should not represent a major problem in gene therapy with *RFX5, RFXANK,* and *RFXAP,* which are expressed ubiquitously at relatively constant levels in all cell types. Expression of CIITA is, on the other hand, tightly regulated. Correct expression of a *MHC2TA* transgene will be difficult to obtain unless the endogenous promoters of the *MHC2TA* gene are used. *Mhc2ta* and *Rfx5* knockout mice (see below) will be invaluable for evaluating the feasibility of gene therapy for MHCII deficiency.

Mouse Models for MHCII Deficiency

There are no spontaneous animal models for MHCII deficiency. However, three mouse models have been constructed by gene targeting. The first model to become available was the MHCII knockout mouse, which reproduced many of the immunopathological features of the human disease, including hypogammaglobulinemia, decreased CD4+ T cell counts, and a deficiency in cellular and humoral immune responses to foreign antigens (reviewed in Dardell et al., 1994; Grusby and Glimcher, 1995). A more faithful model reproducing the molecular defect exhibited by patients in complementation group A has been obtained by gene targeting of the mouse *Mhc2ta* gene (Chang et al., 1996a; Williams et al., 1998; Itoh-Lindstrom et al., 1999). The phenotype exhibited by the *Mhc2ta* knockout mouse is very similar to that of human MHCII deficiency patients. Both constitutive and IFN-γ-induced MHCII expression is strongly reduced. The mice are consequently impaired in CD4+ T cell–dependent immune responses and their immune system is severely compromised. The only major difference from the human disease concerns the mature CD4+ T cell population; the number of mature CD4+ T cells is drastically reduced in *Mhc2ta* knockout mice whereas only a minor reduction is observed in MHCII deficiency patients (see below). A third model reproducing the molecular defect exhibited by patients in complementation group C has been constructed by disruption of the mouse *Rfx5* gene (Clausen et al., 1998). The phenotype of *Rfx5* knockout mice is similar to that of *Mhc2ta* knockout mice. Constitutive and IFN-γ-inducible MHCII expression is strongly affected. There is also a severe reduction in the number of mature CD4+ T cells.

Unresolved Issues and Future Directions

Residual MHCII Expression

Both the CIITA and RFX5 knockout mice exhibit residual MHCII expression in certain tissues and cell types (reviewed in Reith and Mach, 2001), which implies that there must be RFX5- and/or CIITA-independent pathways for MHCII expression in specific cellular compartments. The precise pattern of residual expression differs between the two mice. RFX5−/− mice retain MHCII expression in the thymic medulla and significant, albeit weak, expression on a fraction of splenic and bone marrow–derived dendritic cells, and on B cells activated in vitro with lipopolysaccharide (LPS) and/or IL-4 (Clausen et al., 1998). In contrast, residual MHCII expression in CIITA−/− mice concerns primarily dendritic cells in the lymph nodes, B cells in germinal centers, and a subset of thymic epithelial cells (Chang et al., 1996a; Williams et al., 1998). This difference in residual expression pattern is surprising because the human disease is phenotypically homogeneous. Leaky expression has been observed in cells from certain BLS patients, but no characteristic residual expression pattern distinguishing RFX5-deficient patients from those with defects in CIITA have been described. This discrepancy could reflect species-specific differences in the respective roles of the two MHCII regulatory genes. However, because of the rarity and severity of the disease, only relatively few patients from defined complementation groups have been studied in detail

with respect to residual MHCII expression. Consequently, it is also possible that the phenotypic differences observed in the mouse system exist in the human disease as well but have escaped attention until now.

Modest Reduction in CD4+ T Lymphocytes

Normal development of mature CD4+ T lymphocytes requires the expression of MHCII molecules on cortical thymic epithelial cells (Viret and Janeway, 1999). The fact that the CD4+ T cell population is almost completely absent in MHCII, *Mhc2ta*, and *Rfx5* knockout mice is consistent with this finding (Dardell et al., 1994; Grusby and Glimcher, 1995; Chang et al., 1996a; Clausen et al., 1998). It is therefore quite surprising that the levels of CD4+ T lymphocytes are only mildly reduced in MHCII deficiency patients (Griscelli et al., 1993; Klein et al., 1993). This discrepancy between MHCII deficiency and the existing mouse models for the human disease remains unresolved. One possible explanation is that, in humans, mutations in *MHC2TA* or *RFX5* genes may permit a low residual level of MHCII expression on cortical epithelial cells of the thymus, and this residual expression is sufficient to drive positive selection of CD4+ T lymphocytes. In this context it may be relevant that residual MHCII expression in the thymus has indeed been described in certain patients (Schuurman et al., 1985; Griscelli et al., 1993). A subset of thymic epithelial cells retaining the ability to express MHCII molecules has also been observed in *Mhc2ta* knockout mice (Chang et al., 1996a) and in *Rfx5* knockout mice (Clausen et al., 1998). An alternative explanation could be that CD4+ T cell selection in humans can be driven by alternative mechanisms that differ from those most prominent in the mouse. Interestingly, an analysis of the CD4+ T cell repertoire in MHCII deficiency patients has revealed alterations suggesting that CD4+ T cells in these patients may have escaped the normal selection processes in the thymus (Henwood et al., 1996). It should be mentioned, however, that the same alterations were not observed in another study (Rieux Laucat et al., 1993).

Therapeutic Modulation of MHCII Expression

RFX5, RFXANK, RFXAP, and CIITA exhibit two features that are unusual for transcription factors. First, mutations in these factors almost completely abolish MHCII expression, indicating that they are essential and that no major bypass or alternative pathways can compensate for their absence. Second, they are highly specific for the *MHCII*, *Ii*, and *DM* genes. These characteristics suggest that inhibition of the synthesis or activity of CIITA, RFXANK, RFXAP, and RFX5 should result in a highly selective and efficient down-regulation of MHCII expression. This down-regulation would have profound effects on the control of the immune response. CIITA, RFXANK, RFXAP, and RFX5 may thus represent prime targets for novel immunomodulatory drugs having wide applications in situations such as organ transplantation and autoimmune diseases.

Acknowledgments

The literature cited here is only a small selection of all the contributions that have been made to the fields of MHCII gene regulation and the molecular basis of MHCII deficiency. We sincerely apologize to all colleagues whose work we have been unable to cite for reasons of lack of space. We thank all past and present members of our laboratories for helpful discussions and their contributions to the work reviewed here.

References

Abendroth A, Slobedman B, Lee E, Mellins E, Wallace M, Arvin AM. Modulation of major histocompatibility class II protein expression by varicella-zoster virus. J Virol 74:1900–1907, 2000.

Accolla RS. Human B cell variants immunoselected against a single Ia antigen subset have lost expression in several Ia antigen subsets. J Exp Med 157:1053–1058, 1983.

Accolla RS, Jotterand-Bellomo M, Scarpellino L, Maffei A, Carra G, Guardiola J. aIr-1, a newly found locus on mouse chromosome 16 encoding a trans-acting activator factor for MHC class II gene expression. J Exp Med 164:369–374, 1986.

Alfonso C, Karlsson L. Nonclassical MHC class II molecules. Annu Rev Immunol 18:113–142, 2000.

Bejaoui M, Barbouche MR, Mellouli F, Largueche B, Dellagi K. Primary immunologic deficiency by deficiency of HLA class II antigens: nine new Tunisian cases. Arch Pediatr 5:1089–1093, 1998.

Bénichou B, Strominger JL. Class II-antigen-negative patient and mutant B-cell lines represent at least three, and probably four, distinct genetic defects defined by complementation analysis. Proc Natl Acad Sci USA 88:4285–4288, 1991.

Benoist C, Mathis D. Regulation of major histocompatibility complex class-II genes: X, Y and other letters of the alphabet. Annu Rev Immunol 8:681–715, 1990.

Beresford GW, Boss JM. CIITA coordinates multiple histone acetylation modifications at the HLA-DRA promoter. Nat Immunol 2:652–657, 2001.

Bono MR, Alcaide-Loridan C, Couillin P, Letouze B, Grisard MC, Jouin H, Fellous M. Human chromosome 16 encodes a factor involved in induction of class II major histocompatibility antigens by interferon gamma. Proc Natl Acad Sci USA 88:6077–6081, 1991.

Brickey WJ, Wright KL, Zhu XS, Ting JP. Analysis of the defect in IFN-gamma induction of MHC class II genes in G1B cells: identification of a novel and functionally critical leucine-rich motif (62-LYLYLQL-68) in the regulatory factor × 5 transcription factor. J Immunol 163:6622–6630, 1999.

Calman AF, Peterlin BM. Mutant human B cell lines deficient in class II major histocompatibility complex transcription. J Immunol 139:2489–2495, 1987.

Casper JT, Ash RA, Kirchner P, Hunter JB, Havens PL, Chusid MJ. Successful treatment with an unrelated-donor bone marrow transplant in an HLA-deficient patient with severe combined immune deficiency ("bare lymphocyte syndrome"). J Pediatr 116:262–265, 1990.

Chang CH, Flavell RA. Class II transactivator regulates the expression of multiple genes involved in antigen presentation. J Exp Med 181:765–767, 1995.

Chang C-H, Fontes JD, Peterlin M, Flavell RA. Class II transactivator (CIITA) is sufficient for the inducible expression of major histocompatibility complex class II genes. J Exp Med 180:1367–1374, 1994.

Chang C-H, Guerder S, Hong S-C, van Ewijk W, Flavell RA. Mice lacking the MHC class II transactivator CIITA show tissue-specific impairment of MHC class II expression. Immunity 4:167–178, 1996a.

Chang C-H, Hong S-C, Hughes CCW, Janeway CAJ, Flavell RA. CIITA activates the expression of MHC class II genes in mouse T cells. Int Immunol 17:1515–1518, 1996b.

Chin K, Mao C, Skinner C, Riley JL, Wright KL, Moreno CS, Stark GR, Boss JM, Ting JP. Molecular analysis of G1B and G3A IFN-gamma mutants reveals that defects in CIITA or RFX result in defective class II MHC and Ii gene induction. Immunity 1:687–697, 1994.

Clausen BE, Waldburgen J-M, Schwenk F, Barras E, Mach B, Rajewsky K, Forster I, Reith W. Residual MHC class II expression on mature dentitic cells and activated B cells in RFX5-deficient mice. Immunity 8:143–155, 1998.

Clement LT, Plaeger Marshall S, Haas A, Saxon A, Martin AM. Bare lymphocyte syndrome. Consequences of absent class II major histocompatibility antigen expression for B lymphocyte differentiation and function. J Clin Invest 81:669–675, 1988.

Cressman DE, Chin KC, Taxman DJ, Ting JP. A defect in the nuclear translocation of CIITA causes a form of type II bare lymphocyte syndrome. Immunity 10:163–171, 1999.

Cresswell P. Invariant chain structure and MHC class II function. Cell 84:505–507, 1996.

Dardell S, Merkenschlager M, Bodmer H, Chan S, Cosgrove D, Benoist C, Mathis D. The immune system of mice lacking conventional MHC class II molecules. Adv Immunol 55:423–440, 1994.

de Preval C, Hadam MR, Mach B. Regulation of genes for HLA class II antigens in cell lines from patients with severe combined immunodeficiency. N Engl J Med 318:1295–1300, 1988.

de Preval C, Lisowska-Grospierre B, Loche M, Griscelli C, Mach B. A trans-acting class II regulatory gene unlinked to the MHC controls expression of HLA class II genes. Nature 318:291–293, 1985.

DeSandro AM, Nagarajan UM, Boss JM. Associations and interactions between bare lymphocyte syndrome factors. Mol Cell Biol 20:6587–6599, 2000.

Douhan J III, Hauber I, Eibl MM, Glimcher LH. Genetic evidence for a new type of major histocompatibility complex class II combined immunodeficiency characterized by a dyscoordinate regulation of HLA-D and chains. J Exp Med 183:1063–1069, 1996.

Durand B, Kobr M, Reith W, Mach B. Functional complementation of MHC class II regulatory mutants by the purified X box binding protein RFX. Mol Cell Biol 14:6839–6847, 1994.

Durand B, Sperisen P, Emery P, Barras E, Zufferey M, Mach B, Reith W. RFXAP, a novel subunit of the RFX DNA binding complex, is mutated in MHC class II deficiency. EMBO J 16:1045–1055, 1997.

Durandy A, Cerf-Bensussan N, Dumez Y, Griscelli C. Prenatal diagnosis of severe combined immunodeficiency with defective synthesis of HLA molecules. Prenat Diagn 7:27–34, 1987.

Elhasid R, Etzioni A. Major histocompatibility complex class II deficiency: a clinical review. Blood Rev 10:242–248, 1996.

Emery P, Durand B, Mach B, Reith W. RFX proteins, a novel family of DNA binding proteins conserved in the eukaryotic kingdom. Nucl Acids Res 24:803-807, 1996.

Fontes JD, Jiang B, Peterlin BM. The class II trans-activator CIITA interacts with the TBP-associated factor TAF II 32. Nucl Acids Res 25:2522–2528, 1997.

Fontes JD, Kanazawa S, Jean D, Peterlin BM. Interactions between the class II transactivator and CREB binding protein increase transcription of major histocompatibility complex class II genes. Mol Cell Biol 19:941–947, 1999.

Gajiwala KS, Chen H, Cornille F, Roques BP, Reith W, Mach B, Burley SK. Structure of the winged-helix protein hRFX1 reveals a new mode of DNA binding. Nature 403:916–921, 2000.

Gladstone P, Pious D. Stable variants affecting B cell alloantigens in human lymphoid cells. Nature 271:459–461, 1978.

Glimcher LH, Kara CJ. Sequences and factors: a guide to MHC class-II transcription. Annu Rev Immunol 10:13–49, 1992.

Gobin SJ, Peijnenburg A, Keijsers V, van den Elsen PJ. Site alpha is crucial for two routes of IFN gamma-induced MHC class I transactivation: the ISRE-mediated route and a novel pathway involving CIITA. Immunity 6:601–611, 1997.

Gobin SJ, Peijnenburg A, Van Eggermond M, van Zutphen M, van den Berg R, van den Elsen PJ. The RFX complex is crucial for the constitutive and CIITA-mediated transactivation of MHC class I and beta2-microglobulin genes. Immunity 9:531–541, 1998.

Gonczy P, Reith W, Barras E, Lisowska-Grospierre B, Griscelli C, Hadam MR, Mach B. Inherited immunodeficiency with a defect in a major histocompatibility complex class II promoter-binding protein differs in the chromatin structure of the HLA-DRA gene. Mol Cell Biol 9:296–302, 1989.

Griscelli C, Durandy A, Virelizier JL, Hors J, Lepage V, Colombani J. Impaired cell-to-cell interaction in partial combined immunodeficiency with variable expression of HLA antigens. In: Seligman M, Hitzig WH, eds. Primary Immunodeficiencies. Amsterdam: Elsevier/North Holland, pp. 499–503, 1980.

Griscelli C, Lisowska-Grospierre B, Mach B. Combined immunodeficiency with defective expression in MHC class II genes. In: Rosen FS, Seligman M, eds. Immunodeficiencies. Chur, Switzerland: Harwood Academic, pp. 141–154, 1993.

Grusby MJ, Glimcher LH. Immune responses in MHC class II-deficient mice. Annu Rev Immunol 13:417–435, 1995.

Guardiola J, Maffei A. Control of MHC class II gene expression in autoimmune, infectious, and neoplastic diseases. Crit Rev Immunol 13:247–268, 1993.

Haas A, Stiehm ER. Failure to thrive, thrush and hypogammaglobulinemia in a 6-month-old child. Ann Allergol 59:141–144, 1987.

Hadam MR, Dopfer R, Dammer G, Derau C, Niethammer D. Expression of MHC antigens in MHC-class-II-deficiency. In: Vossen J, Griscelli C, eds. Progress in Immunodeficiency Research and Therapy II. Amsterdam: Elsevier Science B.V., pp. 89–96, 1986.

Hadam MR, Dopfer R, Dammer G, Peter HH, Schlesier M, Muller C, Niethammer D. Defective expression of HLA-D-region determinants in children with congenital agammaglobulinemia and malabsorption: a new syndrome. In: Albert ED, Baur MP, Mayr WR, eds. Histocompatibility Testing 1984. Berlin: Springer-Verlag, pp. 645–650, 1984.

Hake, S, Masternak K, Kammerbauer C, Reith W, Steimle V. CIITA leucine-rich repeats control nuclear localization, in vivo recruitment to the major histocompatibility complex (MHC) class II enhanceosome and MHC class II gene transactivation. Mol Cell Biol 20:7716–7725, 2000.

Harton JA, Cressman DE, Chin KC, Der CJ, Ting JP. GTP binding by class II transactivator: role in nuclear import. Science 285:1402–1405, 1999.

Harton JA, Linhoff MW, Zhang J, Ting JP. Cutting edge: CATERPILLER: a large family of mammalian genes containing CARD, pyrin, nucleotide-binding, and leucine-rich repeat domains. J Immunol 169:4088–4093, 2002.

Harton JA, Ting JP. Class II transactivator: mastering the art of major histocompatibility complex expression. Mol Cell Biol 20:6185–6194, 2000.

Hasegawa SL, Boss JM. Two B cell factors bind the HLA-DRA X box region and recognize different subsets of HLA class II promoters. Nucl Acids Res 19:6269–6276, 1991.

Hasegawa SL, Riley JL, Sloan JH III, Boss JM. Protease treatment of nuclear extracts distinguishes between class II MHC X1 box DNA-binding proteins in wild-type and class II–deficient B cells. J Immunol 150:1781–1793, 1993.

Hauber I, Gulle H, Wolf HM, Maris M, Eggenbauer H, Eibl MM. Molecular characterization of major histocompatibility complex class II gene expression and demonstration of antigen-specific T cell response indicate a new phenotype in class II-deficient patients. J Exp Med 181:1411–1423, 1995.

Henwood J, van Eggermond MCJA, van Boxel-Dezaire AHH, Schipper R, den Hoedt M, Peijnenburg A, Sanal O, Ersoy F, Rijkers GT, Zegers BJM, Vossen JM, van Tol MJD, van den Elsen PJ. Human T cell repertoire generation in the absence of MHC class II expression results in a circulating CD4⁺CD8⁻ population with altered physicochemical properties of complementarity-determining region 3. J Immunol 156:895–906, 1996.

Herrero-Sanchez C, Reith W, Silacci P, Mach B. The DNA-binding defect observed in major histocompatibility complex class II regulatory mutants concerns only one member of a family of complexes binding to the X boxes of class II promoters. Mol Cell Biol 12:4076–4083, 1992.

Hume CR, Lee JS. Congenital Immunodeficiencies associated with absence of HLA class II antigens on lymphocytes result from distinct mutations in *trans*-acting factors. Hum Immunol 26:288–309, 1989.

Hume CR, Shookster LA, Collins N, O'Reilly R, Lee JS. Bare lymphocyte syndrome: altered HLA class II expression in B cell lines derived from two patients. Hum Immunol 25:1–11, 1989.

Itoh-Lindstrom Y, Piskurich JF, Felix NJ, Wang Y, Brickey WJ, Platt JL, Koller BH, Ting JP. Reduced IL-4-, lipopolysaccharide-, and IFN-gamma-induced MHC class II expression in mice lacking class II transactivator due to targeted deletion of the GTP-binding domain. J Immunol 163:2425–2431, 1999.

Kanazawa S, Okamoto T, Peterlin BM. Tat competes with CIITA for the binding to P-TEFb and blocks the expression of MHC class II genes in HIV infection. Immunity 12:61–70, 2000.

Kara CJ, Glimcher LH. In vivo footprinting of MHC class II genes: bare promoters in the bare lymphocyte syndrome. Science 252:709–712, 1991.

Kara CJ, Glimcher LH. Three in vivo promoter phenotypes in MHC class II deficient combined immunodeficiency. Immunogenetics 37:227–230, 1993.

Kern I, Steimle V, Siegrist C-A, Mach B. The two novel MHC class II transactivators RFX5 and CIITA both control expression of HLA-DM genes. Int Immunol 7:1295–1300, 1995.

Klein C, Cavazzana-Calvo M, Le Deist F, Jabado N, Benkerrou M, Blanche S, Lisowska-Grospierre B, Griscelli C. Bone marrow transplantation in major histocompatibility complex class II deficiency: a single-center study of 19 patients. Blood 85:580–587, 1995.

Klein C, Lisowska Grospierre B, LeDeist F, Fischer A, Griscelli C. Major histocompatibility complex class II deficiency: clinical manifestations, immunologic features, and outcome. J Pediatr 123:921–928, 1993.

Kretsovali A, Agalioti T, Spilianakis C, Tzortzakaki E, Merika M, Papamatheakis J. Involvement of CREB binding protein in expression of major histocompatibility complex class II genes via interaction with the class II transactivator. Mol Cell Biol 18:6777–6783, 1998.

Kretsovali A, Spilianakis C, Dimakopoulos A, Makatounakis T, Papamatheakis J. Self-association of class II transactivator correlates with its intracellular localization and transactivation. J Biol Chem 276:32191–32197, 2001.

Kuis W, Roord J, Zegers BJM, Schuurmann RKB, Heijnen CJ, Baldwin WM, Goulmy E, Claas F, van de Griend RJ, Rijkers GT, Van Rood JJ, Vossen JM, Ballieux RE, Stoop RJ. Clinical and immunological studies in a patient with the "bare lymphocyte" syndrome. In: Touraine JL, Gluckman E, Griscelli C, eds. Bone Marrow Transplantation in Europe. Amsterdam: Excerpta Medica, pp. 201–208, 1981.

Landmann S, Muhlethaler-Mottet A, Bernasconi L, Suter T, Waldburger JM, Masternak K, Arrighi JF, Hauser C, Fontana A, Reith W. Maturation of dendritic cells is accompanied by rapid transcriptional silencing of class II transactivator (CIITA) expression. J Exp Med 194:379–392, 2001.

Lennon-Dumenil AM, Barbouche MR, Vedrenne J, Prod'Homme T, Bejaoui M, Ghariani S, Charron D, Fellous M, Dellagi K, Alcaide-Loridan C. Uncoordinated HLA-D gene expression in a RFXANK-defective patient with MHC class II deficiency. J Immunol 166:5681–5687, 2001.

Le Roy E, Muhlethaler-Mottet A, Davrinche C, Mach B, Davignon JL. Escape of human cytomegalovirus from HLA-DR-restricted CD4(+) T-cell response is mediated by repression of gamma interferon-induced class II transactivator expression. J Virol 73:6582–6589, 1999.

Linhoff MW, Harton JA, Cressman DE, Martin BK, Ting JP. Two distinct domains within CIITA mediate self-association: involvement of the GTP-binding and leucine-rich repeat domains. Mol Cell Biol 21:3001–3011, 2001.

Lisowska-Grospierre B, Charron DJ, de Preval C, Durandy A, Griscelli C, Mach B. A defect in the regulation of major histocompatibility complex class II gene expression in human HLA-DR negative lymphocytes from patients with combined immunodeficiency syndrome. J Clin Invest 76:381–385, 1985.

Lisowska-Grospierre B, Durandy A, Virelizier JL, Fischer A, Griscelli C. Combined immunodeficiency with defective expression of HLA: modulation of an abnormal HLA synthesis and functional studies. Birth Defects 19:87–92, 1983.

Lisowska-Grospierre B, Fondaneche MC, Rols MP, Griscelli C, Fischer A. Two complementation groups account for most cases of inherited MHC class II deficiency. Hum Mol Genet 3:953–958, 1994.

Louis-Plence P, Moreno CS, Boss JM. Formation of a regulatory factor X/X2 box-binding protein/nuclear factor-Y multiprotein complex on the conserved regulatory regions of HLA class II genes. J Immunol 159:3899–3909, 1997.

Mach B, Steimle V, Martinez-Soria E, Reith W. Regulation of MHC class II genes: lessons from a disease. Annu Rev Immunol 14:301–331, 1996.

Mahanta SK, Scholl T, Yang FC, Strominger JL. Transactivation by CIITA, the type II bare lymphocyte syndrome–associated factor, requires participation of multiple regions of the TATA box binding protein. Proc Natl Acad Sci USA 94:6324–6329, 1997.

Mantovani R. The molecular biology of the CCAAT-binding factor NF-Y. Gene 239:15–27, 1999.

Martin BK, Chin KC, Olsen JC, Skinner CA, Dey A, Ozato K, Ting JP. Induction of MHC class I expression by the MHC class II transactivator CIITA. Immunity 6:591–600, 1997.

Masternak K, Barras E, Zufferey M, Conrad B, Corthals G, Aebersold R, Sanchez JC, Hochstrasser DF, Mach B, Reith W. A gene encoding a novel RFX-associated transactivator is mutated in the majority of MHC class II deficiency patients. Nat Genet 20:273–277, 1998.

Masternak K, Muhlethaler-Mottet A, Villard J, Peretti M, Reith W. Molecular genetics of the bare lymphocyte syndrome. Rev Immunogenet 2:267–282, 2000a.

Masternak K, Muhlethaler-Mottet A, Villard J, Zufferey M, Steimle V, Reith W. CIITA is a transcriptional coactivator that is recruited to MHC class II promoters by multiple synergistic interactions with an enhanceosome complex. Genes Dev 14:1156–1166, 2000b.

Masternak K, Peyraud N, Krawczyk M, Barras E, Reith W. Chromatin remodeling and extragenic transcription at the MHC class II locus control region. Nat Immunol 4:132–137, 2003.

Masternak K, Reith W. Promoter-specific functions of CIITA and the MHC class II enhanceosome in transcriptional activation. EMBO J 21:1379–1388, 2002.

Miller DM, Rahill BM, Boss JM, Lairmore MD, Durbin JE, Waldman JW, Sedmak DD. Human cytomegalovirus inhibits major histocompatibility complex class II expression by disruption of the Jak/Stat pathway. J Exp Med 187:675–683, 1998.

Moreno CS, Beresford GW, Louis-Plence P, Morris AC, Boss JM. CREB regulates MHC class II expression in a CIITA-dependent manner. Immunity 10:143–151, 1999.

Moreno CS, Emery P, West JE, Durand B, Reith W, Mach B, Boss JM. Purified X2 binding protein (X2BP) cooperatively binds the class II MHC X box region in the presence of purified RFX, the X box factor deficient in the bare lymphocyte syndrome. J Immunol 155:4313–4321, 1995.

Morris AC, Riley JL, Fleming WH, Boss JM. MHC class II gene silencing in trophoblast cells is caused by inhibition of CIITA expression. Am J Reprod Immunol 40:385–394, 1998.

Morris AC, Spangler WE, Boss JM. Methylation of class II trans-activator promoter IV: a novel mechanism of MHC class II gene control. J Immunol 164:4143–4149, 2000.

Muhlethaler-Mottet A, Di Berardino W, Otten LA, Mach B. Activation of the MHC class II transactivator CIITA by gamma interferon requires cooperative interaction between STAT1 and USF-1. Immunity 8:157–166, 1998.

Muhlethaler-Mottet A, Otten LA, Steimle V, Mach B. Expression of MHC class II molecules in different cellular and functional compartments is controlled by differential usage of multiple promoters of the transactivator CIITA. EMBO J 16:2851–2860, 1997.

Nagarajan UM, Louis-Plence P, DeSandro A, Nilsen R, Bushey A, Boss JM. RFX-B is the gene responsible for the most common cause of the bare lymphocyte syndrome, an MHC class II immunodeficiency. Immunity 10:153–162, 1999.

Nekrep N, Jabrane-Ferrat N, Wolf HM, Eibl MM, Geyer M, Peterlin BM. Mutation in a winged-helix DNA-binding motif causes atypical bare lymphocyte syndrome. Nat Immunol 3:1075–1081, 2002.

Nocera A, Barocci S, Depalma R, Gorski J. Analysis of transcripts of genes located within the HLA-D region in B-cells from an HLA-severe combined immunodeficiency individual. Hum Immunol 38:231–234, 1993.

Otten LA, Steimle V, Bontron S, Mach B. Quantitative control of MHC class II expression by the transactivator CIITA. Eur J Immunol 28:473–478, 1998.

Peijnenburg A, Godthelp B, van Boxel-Dezaire A, van den Elsen PJ. Definition of a novel complementation group in MHC class II deficiency. Immunogenetics 41:287–294, 1995.

Quan V, Towey M, Sacks S, Kelly AP. Absence of MHC class II gene expression in a patient with a single amino acid substitution in the class II transactivator protein CIITA. Immunogenetics 49:957–963, 1999.

Reith W, Kobr M, Emery P, Durand B, Siegrist CA, Mach B. Cooperative binding between factors RFX and X2bp to the X and X2 boxes of MHC class II promoters. J Biol Chem 269:20020–20025, 1994a.

Reith W, Mach B. The bare lymphocyte syndrome and the regulation of MHC expression. Annu Rev Immunol 19:331–373, 2001.

Reith W, Satola S, Herrero Sanchez C, Amaldi I, Lisowska-Grospierre B, Griscelli C, Hadam MR, Mach B. Congenital immunodeficiency with a regulatory defect in MHC class II gene expression lacks a specific HLA-DR promoter binding protein, RF-X. Cell 53:897–906, 1988.

Reith W, Siegrist CA, Durand B, Barras E, Mach B. Function of major histocompatibility complex class II promoters requires cooperative binding between factors RFX and NF-Y. Proc Natl Acad Sci USA 91:554–558, 1994b.

Rieux Laucat F, Le Deist F, Selz F, Fischer A, de Villartay JP. Normal T cell receptor V beta usage in a primary immunodeficiency associated with HLA class II deficiency. Eur J Immunol 23:928–934, 1993.

Riley JL, Boss JM. Class II MHC transcriptional mutants are defective in higher order complex formation J Immunol 151:6942–6953, 1993.

Riley JL, Westerheide SD, Price JA, Brown JA, Boss JM. Activation of class II MHC genes requires both the X box and the class II transactivator (CIITA). Immunity 2:533–543, 1995.

Rosen FS, Wedgwood RJ, Eibl M, Griscelli C, Seligmann M, Aiuti F, Kishimoto T, Matsumoto S, Khakhalin LN, Hanson LA, Hitzig WH, Thompson RA, Cooper MD, Good RA, Waldman TA. Primary immunodeficiency diseases: report of a WHO scientific group. Immunodefic Rev 3:195–236, 1992.

Sabatier C, Gimenez C, Calin-Laurens V, Rabourdin-Combe C, Touraine J-L. Type III bare lymphocye syndrome: lack of HLA class II gene expression and reduction in HLA class I gene expression. C R Acad Sci Paris 319:789–798, 1996.

Saleem MA, Arkwright PD, Davies EG, Cant AJ, Veys PA. Clinical course of patients with major histocompatibility complex class II deficiency. Arch Dis Child 83:356–359, 2000.

Schuurmann HJ, van de Wijngaert FP, Huber J, Schuurman RK, Zegers BJ, Roord JJ, Kater L. The thymus in "bare lymphocyte" syndrome: significance of expression of major histocompatibility complex antigens on thymic epithelial cells in intrathymic T-cell maturation. Hum Immunol 13:69–82, 1985.

Schuurman RKB, Van Rood JJ, Vossen JM, Schellekens PTA, Feltkamp-Vroom TM, Doyer E, Gmelig-Meyling F, Visser HKA. Failure of lymphocyte-membrane HLA A and B expression in two siblings with combined immunodeficiency. Clin Immunol Immunopathol 14:418–434, 1979.

Seidl C, Saraiya C, Osterweil Z, Fu YP, Lee JS. Genetic complexity of regulatory mutants defective for HLA class-II gene-expression J Immunol 148:1576–1584, 1992.

Silacci P, Mottet A, Steimle V, Reith W, Mach B. Developmental extinction of major histocompatibility complex class II gene expression in plasmo-

cytes is mediated by silencing of the transactivator gene CIITA. J Exp Med 180:1329–1336, 1994.

Sisk TJ, Roys S, Chang CH. Self-association of CIITA and its transactivation potential. Mol Cell Biol 21:4919–4928, 2001.

Spilianakis C, Papamatheakis J, Kretsovali A. Acetylation by PCAF enhances CIITA nuclear accumulation and transactivation of major histocompatibility complex class II genes. Mol Cell Biol 20:8489–8498, 2000.

Steimle V, Durand B, Barras E, Zufferey M, Hadam MR, Mach B, Reith W. A novel DNA binding regulatory factor is mutated in primary MHC class II deficiency (bare lymphocyte syndrome). Genes Dev 9:1021–1032, 1995.

Steimle V, Otten LA, Zufferey M, Mach B. Complementation cloning of an MHC class II transactivator mutated inhereditary MHC class II deficiency (or bare lymphocyte syndrome). Cell 75:135–146, 1993.

Steimle V, Siegrist C, Mottet A, Lisowska-Grospierre B, Mach B. Regulation of MHC class II expression by interferon-gamma mediated by the transactivator gene CIITA. Science 265:106–109, 1994.

Stimac E, Urieli-Shoval S, Kempin S, Pious D. Defective HLA DRA X box binding in the class II transactive transcription factor mutant 6.1.6 and in cell lines from class II immunodeficient patients. J Immunol 146: 4398–4405, 1991.

Ting JP, Trowsdale J. Genetic control of MHC class II expression. Cell 109 (Suppl):S21–33, 2002.

Touraine JL. The bare-lymphocyte syndrome report on the registry. Lancet 7:319–321, 1981.

Touraine JL, Betuel H, Souillet G. Combined immunodeficiency disease associated with absence of cell surface HLA A and B antigen. J Pediatr 93:47–51, 1978.

Touraine JL, Marseglia GL, Betuel H, Souillet G, Gebuhrer L. The bare lymphocyte syndrome. Bone Marrow Transpl 9(Suppl 1):54–56, 1992.

van den Elsen PJ, Peijnenburg A, van Eggermond MC, Gobin SJ. Shared regulatory elements in the promoters of MHC class I and class II genes. Immunol Today 19:308–312, 1998.

Vilen BJ, Cogswell JP, Ting JP. Stereospecific alignment of the X and Y elements is required for major histocompatibility complex class II DRA promoter function. Mol Cell Biol 11:2406–2415, 1991.

Vilen BJ, Penta JF, Ting JP. Structural constraints within a trimeric transcriptional regulatory region: constitutive and interferon-γ inducible expression of the HLA-DRA gene. J Biol Chem 267:23728–23734, 1992.

Villard J, Lisowska-Grospierre B, van den Elsen P, Fischer A, Reith W, Mach B. Mutation of RFXAP, a regulator of MHC class II genes, in primary MHC class II deficiency. N Engl J Med 337:748–753, 1997a.

Villard J, Reith W, Barras E, Gos A, Morris MA, van den Elsen PJ, Antonorakis A, Mach B. Chromosomal localization of the gene encoding RFX5, a novel transcription factor that is mutated in major histocompatibility complex class II deficiency. Hum Mutat 10:430–435, 1997b.

Viret C, Janeway CAJ. MHC and T cell development. Rev Immunogenet 1: 91–104, 1999.

Waldburger J-M, Rossi S, Hollander GA, Rodewald HR, Reith W, Acha-Orbea H. Promoter IV of the class II transactivator gene is essential for positive selection of CD4+ T cells. Blood 101:3550–3559, 2003.

Waldburger J-M, Suter T, Fontana A, Acha-Orbea H, Reith W. Selective abrogation of MHC class II expression on extra-hematopoietic cells in mice lacking promoter IV of the CIITA gene. J Exp Med 194:393–406, 2001.

Williams GS, Malin M, Vremec D, Chang CH, Boyd R, Benoist C, Mathis D. Mice lacking the transcription factor CIITA—a second look. Int Immunol 10:1957–1967, 1998.

Wiszniewski W, Fondaneche MC, Lambert N, Masternak K, Picard C, Notarangelo L, Schwartz K, Bal J, Reith W, Alcaide C, de Saint B, Fischer A, Lisowska-Grospierre B. Founder effect for a 26-bp deletion in the RFXANK gene in North African major histocompatibility complex class II–deficient patients belonging to complementation group B. Immunogenetics 51:261–267, 2000.

Wiszniewski W, Fondaneche MC, Le Deist F, Kanariou M, Selz F, Brousse, N, Steimle V, Barbieri G, Alcaide-Loridan C, Charron D, Fischer A, Lisowska-Grospierre B. Mutation of the class II transactivator leading to a mild immunodeficiency. J Immunol 167:1787–1794, 2001.

Wojciechowski W, DeSanctis J, Skamene E, Radzioch D. Attenuation of MHC class II expression in macrophages infected with *Mycobacterium bovis* bacillus Calmette-Guerin involves class II transactivator and depends on Nramp1 gene. J Immunol 163:2688–2696, 1999.

Wolf HM, Hauber I, Gulle H, Thon V, Eggenbauer H, Fischer MB, Fiala S, Eibl MM. Twin boys with major histocompatibiliy complex class II deficiency but inducible immune responses. N Engl J Med 332:86–90, 1995.

Wright KL, Vilen BJ, Itoh Lindstrom Y, Moore TL, Li G, Criscitiello M, Cogswell P, Clarke JB, Ting JP. CCAAT box binding protein NF-Y facilitates in vivo recruitment of upstream DNA binding transcription factors. EMBO J 13:4042–4053, 1994.

Zhong G, Fan T, Liu L. Chlamydia inhibits interferon gamma-inducible major histocompatibility complex class II expression by degradation of upstream stimulatory factor 1. J Exp Med 189:1931–1938, 1999.

Zhou H, Glimcher LH. Human MHC class II gene transcription directed by the carboxyl terminus of CIITA, one of the defective genes in type II MHC combined immune deficiency. Immunity 2:545–553, 1995.

Zhu XS, Linhoff MW, Li G, Chin KC, Maity SN, Ting JP. Transcriptional scaffold: CIITA interacts with NF-Y, RFX, and CREB to cause stereospecific regulation of the class II major histocompatibility complex promoter. Mol Cell Biol 20:6051–6061, 2000.

18

Peptide Transporter Defects in Human Leukocyte Antigen Class I Deficiency

HENRI DE LA SALLE, LIONEL DONATO, and DANIEL HANAU

Human leukocyte antigen (HLA) class I molecules present peptides derived from proteins that are synthesized in the cell to cytotoxic $\alpha\beta$ CD8[+] T lymphocytes. In this way, these molecules are involved in immune responses against intracellular pathogens and cancer cells. Although these molecules should a priori be essential to immune defense and thus to survival, a few cases have been described of children or adults who live with a defect in the expression of HLA class I molecules.

HLA class I deficiency, also called *type I bare lymphocyte syndrome* (BLS), is detected when HLA class I molecules on lymphocytes cannot be typed by serological methods because of their low expression at the plasma membrane. Complete HLA class I deficiency has never been reported, which suggests that low expression of class I molecules may be sufficient to ensure immune responses against pathogens; while total deficiency would be lethal. The first case of HLA class I deficiency was identified at a time when HLA class II typing techniques were unreliable. This case was later found to be an HLA class II deficiency associated with low expression of class I molecules (type III BLS) (Touraine et al., 1978; Sabatier et al., 1996), resulting from a defect in the RFXAP transcription factor (Durand et al., 1997). Two cases without immunodeficiency were subsequently described in a nonconsanguineous family (Payne et al., 1983). One was discovered when bone marrow transplantation was being considered to treat aplastic anemia, and the second was a younger brother who displayed the same defect of HLA class I expression and was healthy. Four other cases were identified in patients who had first-cousin parents and suffered from unexplained lung disease (Maeda et al., 1985; Sugiyama et al., 1986; de la Salle et al., 1994). Apart from one patient who experienced recurrent fever (Sugiyama et al., 1986), these patients did not seem to be abnormally susceptible to viral infections. Moreover,

when complete clinical data were available, they appeared to have been healthy during the first years of life. Thus, the pathology associated with type I BLS appears not to be a direct consequence of the deficiency—i.e., an expected susceptibility to viral infections or cancer—but rather a result of secondary effects. Because of this absence of a direct link between clinical manifestations and deficiency, the discovery of the first cases of type I BLS was fortuitous. Since the first genetic and clinical descriptions of two patients in 1994, other HLA class I–deficient individuals have been discovered among previous and new clinical cases.

Clinical and Pathological Manifestations

Only 20 well-documented cases of HLA class I molecule deficiency with normal expression of class II molecules have been identified; 13 of them result from a defect in the transporter of peptides associated with antigen processing (TAP) (Table 18.1). Contrary to types II and III BLS, which are characterized by the early onset of severe combined immunodeficiency, HLA class I deficiencies do not lead to any particular pathological manifestations during the first years of life. Pathology of the gut (diarrhea) is not observed, unlike in type II or III BLS. The clinical course of the known cases (reviewed in Gadola et al., 2000), summarized in Table 18.1, varies among individuals. A chronic inflammatory lung disease, developing generally in late childhood, is the most common, though not requisite, trait of TAP-deficient patients. It begins with infections with *Hemophilus influenza* during the first decade of life, is confined to the respiratory tract, and extends from the upper to lower airways. Other bacterial pathogens may also be found (*Streptoccocus pneumoniae, Klebsiella, Pseudomonas aeroginosa*). The high frequency of nasosinusal involvement and nasal polyposis, uncommon for noncystic

Table 18.1. Characteristics of HLA Class I Deficiencies (Type I Bare Lymphocyte Syndrome)

Cases	Symptoms	HLA Genotype	Defect	References*
M 9 years	Unexplained anemia	Heterozygous	Transcription	1
M 6 years	None	Heterozygous	Transcription	1
M 2 years	None	Heterozygous	Transcription	Unpublished
M 49 years	Chronic sinusitis, bilateral bronchiectasis	U	U	2
	Bacterial infections of the RT			
F 33 years	Nasal polyposis, panbronchiolitis	Homozygous	TAP1	3
	Bacterial infections of the RT			
	PFT: obstructive impairment			
	Localized cutaneous necrobiotic lipoidica			
M 24 years	Nasal polyps, pansinusitis	Homozygous	TAP1	4
	Bilateral bronchiectasis with emphysema			
	Granulomatous lesions, ectopia lentis			
F U	Chronic sinusitis, bronchitis and bronchiectasis	Homozygous	TAP1	5
F U	Chronic sinusitis, bronchitis and bronchiectasis, granulomatous lesions	Homozygous	TAP1	5
F U	Absence of lung disease, granulomatous lesions	Homozygous	TAP1	5, 6
F 20 years	Nasal polyposis, pansinusitis	Homozygous	TAP2	7
M 15 years	Bilateral bronchiectasis, chronic otitis media	Homozygous	TAP2	7
	Bacterial infections of the RT			
	PFT: obstructive impairment; F: emphysema			
M 36 years	Bacterial infections of the RT	Homozygous	TAP2	8
	Bilateral bronchiectasis			
F 36 years	Sinusitis and bronchitis, bronchiectasis	Homozygous	TAP2	5, 9
F U	Granulomatous lesions, vasculitis	Homozygous	TAP2	5
F U	Chronic sinusitis, bronchitis and bronchiectasis, granulomatous lesions	Homozygous	TAP2	5
M 46	Minor granulomatous lesions	Homozygous	TAP2	10
F 30	None	Homozygous	TAP2	10
M 15	Retinal toxoplasmosis	Homozygous	TAP1	12
M 14	Asymtomatic	Homozygous	TAP1	12
F 56	Primary chronic glomerulonephritis	Homozygous	Tapasin	11

F, female; M, male; PFT, pulmonary function tests; RT, respiratory tract; U, unknown. Years: age corresponding to clinical descriptions.

*1, Payne et al., 1983; Sullivan et al., 1985; 2, Sugiyama et al., 1986; 3, Maeda et al., 1985; Watanabe et al., 1987; Sugiyama et al., 1989; de la Salle et al., 1999[†]; Furukawa et al., 1999a[†], 1999b, 1999c, 2000; Azuma et al., 2001; 4, Plebani et al., 1996; de la Salle et al., 1999[†]; 5, Moins-Teisserenc et al., 1999[†]; 6, Willemsen et al., 1995[†]; 7, de la Salle et al., 1994[†]; Donato et al., 1995; Zimmer et al., 1998, 1999; 8, Matamoros et al., 2001[†]; 9, Teisserenc et al., 1997; 10, de la Salle et al., 2002[†]; 11, Yabe et al., 2002[†]; 12, unpublished observations.

[†]Reference in which mutation is described.

fibrosis in children, is noteworthy. The pathology inevitably evolves to a respiratory insufficiency resulting in bronchiectasis, emphysema, panbronchiolitis, or bronchial obstruction. In the early stages of the disease, computerized tomography (CT) scans of the chest may show bronchiolectasis, which later leads to bronchiectasis (Fig. 18.1). Hypoxemia can occur during infectious exacerbation. Skin lesions have been described in several patients and start with local inflammation, most often on the legs, developing into necrotizing granulomas. These lesions may be related to vasculitis (Watanabe et al., 1987; Plebani et al., 1996; Teisserenc et al., 1997). In a number of cases, lesions occurring in the upper respiratory tract led to mutilation of the midface (Moins-Teisserenc et al., 1999). One of these patients did not display inflammation of the airways. Recently, two adults without inflammatory lung disease were also described, one totally asymptomatic and the other with minor skin lesions on one leg (de la Salle et al., 2002). Definitive healing of the skin lesions has never been reported, except in this last case. Two other TAP1-deficient brothers were recently identified in our laboratory (de la Salle, unpublished results). In contrast to all previously described TAP-deficient individuals, these patients have unrelated parents, who nevertheless share a rare HLA haplotype. One of the patients is 14 years old and asymptomatic. The other patient is 15 and suffered a retinal toxoplasmosis, which, despite surgery, led to the loss of one eye.

The two HLA class I–deficient brothers described by Payne et al. were free of lung and upper-airway disease, although respiratory involvement could not be excluded because the patients were young, no ear-nose-throat or pulmonary investigations had been carried out, and long-term data were lacking. One of these children suffered from unexplained anemia but recovered under prolonged corticosteroid treatment. Another case has since been discovered in France (de la Salle, unpublished data). As shown in the next section, this type of deficiency is not caused by a TAP defect.

Finally, a moderate HLA class I deficiency resulting from a tapasin defect was recently characterized. Although the patient did not display any of the symptoms associated with TAP deficiency, he suffered from chronic primary glomerulonephritis (Yabe et al., 2002).

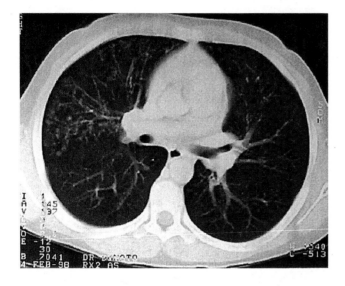

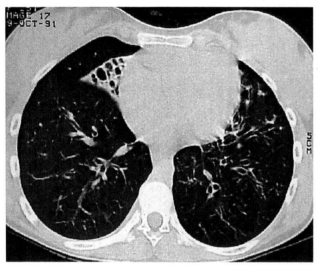

Figure 18.1. Chest CT scans. (Top) Bronchiolectasis in a 15-year-old TAP2-deficient patient. Patchy opacities spread out along the bronchovascular axes within the right middle lobe. (Bottom) Bilateral bronchiectasis in patient's eldest sister. Lesions extend to the right middle lobe, lingula, and left lower lobe and probably represent a later stage of the disease.

Molecular Basis of TAP Deficiency

Classical HLA class I molecules are composed of a polymorphic heavy chain, encoded by HLA-A, HLA-B, and HLA-C genes, associated with β2-microglobulin (β2m). The assembly of heavy chains with β2m (Creswell et al., 1999) occurs in the lumen of the endoplasmic reticulum under the control of chaperone molecules such as calnexin, calreticulin, and thiol oxidoreductase Erp57. After assembly the complexes are loaded with peptides derived from degradation of intracellular proteins. The peptides are transported from the cytosol into the lumen of the endoplasmic reticulum by TAP, a protein composed of two subunits, TAP1 and TAP2. These proteins belong to the ATP-binding cassette (ABC) family of transporters, which display common features in the cytoplasmic domain. The cytoplasmic part includes two sites (Walker sites A and B) involved in ATP binding and necessary for the transport of substrates (the structure of ABC

transporters is reviewed in Schneider and Hunke, 1998). However, in the case of TAP, the ATP binding site of TAP1 is dispensable (Kartunen et al., 2001). The N-terminal halves of the TAP subunits form their luminal and transmembrane domains. In general, peptide loading depends on interaction of the TAP1 subunit with a complex comprised of class I heavy chains, β2m and calreticulin, an interaction controlled by tapasin (TAP-associated glycoprotein).

Studies in tumor and mutant cell lines have shown that defective HLA class I expression may arise from the down-regulation of HLA class I genes or TAP genes, or from the absence of β2m, TAP, or tapasin. In TAP-deficient cell lines, most HLA class I molecules remain blocked between the endoplasmic reticulum and the *cis*-Golgi compartment and therefore stay endoglycosidase H sensitive and unsialylated. The HLA class I heavy chain/β2m complexes are peptide-free and unstable at 37°C, resulting in poor expression of HLA class I molecules on the cell surface. In the absence of TAP, the presentation of most peptides of intracellular origin is blocked, although TAP-independent presentation of some antigens can occur. The genes encoding the TAP subunits are located in the HLA class II genetic region on chromosome 6 and are polymorphic; up to six TAP1 and four TAP2 human alleles having been described to date (http://www.anthonynolan.com/HIG/nomenc.html). Calnexin is not essential for normal expression of HLA class I molecules (Scott and Dawson, 1996). In contrast, the processing of these molecules is altered in the tapasin-defective 721.220 cell line, in a manner similar to that in TAP-deficient cells, the effect of the mutation depending on the biophysical characteristics of the HLA variants. Thus, in transfected 721.220 cells, depending on the alleles, HLA class I molecules are more or less retained in the endoplasmic reticulum (Greenwood et al., 1994).

Genetic and biochemical studies of HLA class I deficiencies have revealed three kinds of defect. In two cases (Payne et al., 1983), molecular genetic analyses demonstrated that HLA class I genes were constitutively poorly expressed in lymphocytes (Sullivan et al., 1985). This deficiency was probably not linked to chromosome 6, as the two brothers had inherited different HLA haplotypes and the causative genetic defect has not yet been elucidated. In most instances of the second type of HLA class I deficiency, the patients were born to consanguineous parents. When HLA typing could be performed, patients were shown to be HLA homozygous, which suggests that the genetic defect was carried on chromosome 6 (Table 18.1). Biochemical studies of cell lines derived from these patients showed that their HLA class I heavy chains remained unsialylated (Maeda et al., 1985; de la Salle et al., 1994, 1999). Most of the heavy chains remained endoglycosidase H sensitive, whereas HLA class I molecules were unstable at 37°C (de la Salle et al., 1994, 1999, 2002; Teisserenc et al., 1997). All of these properties point to a defect in the peptide loading of HLA class I molecules. Additional complementation experiments demonstrated that the deficiencies resulted from a defect in either TAP1 or TAP2 (Table 18.1 and Fig. 18.2). Three mutations have been characterized in the TAP1 and four in the TAP2 gene; the MIM (Mendelian Inheritance in Man) numbers for these deficiencies are 170260 and 170261. All the mutations generate truncated subunits, and those in the transmembrane domains may be expected to have profound effects on the TAP complex. It has been shown that the amount of TAP2 protein is decreased in TAP1-deficient cell lines (Furukawa et al., 1999a, Moins-Teisserenc et al., 1999). In one patient, a mutation occurred in the ATP-binding domain of the TAP2 subunit (de la Salle et al., 2002). The third type of HLA class I deficiency identified arose

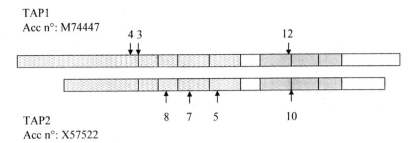

Figure 18.2. Structure of TAP1 and TAP2 genes and positions of known mutations. The Genbank accession numbers of the normal sequences are given. The exons are shown as boxes. Wavy boxes correspond to the luminal and transmembrane domains of the subunits and shaded boxes to the cytosolic ABC homology domains. The amino acid (aa) positions and sequences of the mutated codons are as follows: 3, aa 273, GAC to GA-; 4, aa 260, GGG to GG-; 5, aa 326, AGG to –GG; 7, aa 274, CGA to TGA; 8, aa 219, CGA to TGA; 10, aa 543, GTG to –TG; 12, aa 522, TAC to TAG. The numbering of the mutations corresponds to the reference numbers in Table 18.1.

from a tapasin defect. In this patient, HLA class I expression was reduced 10-fold. Additional biochemical and immunological investigations have not been reported.

Functional Aspects

Expression of HLA Class I Molecules

The expression of HLA class I molecules can be quantified by flow cytometry after staining of the cells with a pan-anti–HLA class I monoclonal antibody such as W6/32. On peripheral blood mononuclear cells (PBMCs) of the two individuals described by Payne et al., the expression of HLA class I molecules was reduced 10-fold, whereas this expression was normal on platelets (Sullivan et al., 1985). The latter observation would appear to contradict the fact that HLA typing could not be performed on platelets (Payne et al., 1983). Epstein-Barr virus–transformed B (EBV-B) cell lines derived from the patients progressively expressed higher levels of HLA class I molecules after a few weeks of culture. In an analogous case, we observed that the PBMCs of a 2-year-old child displayed low HLA class I expression while the EBV-B cell line gradually expressed higher levels of these molecules, although still 10 times less than normal EBV-B cells. Additional experiments demonstrated that HLA class I genes were induced in activated T cells, their expression being up-regulated by tumor necrosis factor-α (TNF-α) and interferon-α (IFN-α) or IFN-γ (de la Salle, unpublished observations). Thus, in this type of deficiency, HLA class I genes can be induced by inflammatory cytokines. As a result, HLA class I–mediated immune responses can be increased when necessary and, for this reason, the defect may be qualified as conditional. Although HLA class I expression in other tissues of these individuals has not been documented, it is remarkable that the expression of HLA class II molecules is normal.

On the surface of cells from TAP-deficient patients, the expression of HLA class I molecules is reduced 100-fold (de la Salle et al., 1994, 1999; Teisserenc et al., 1997) and the same level of reduction is found on lymphocytes, monocytes, neutrophils, and skin fibroblasts. This expression was slightly increased on lymphocytes and fibroblasts through treatment with IFN-α or IFN-γ, whereas TNF-α induced weak up-regulation on fibroblasts only. These observations probably reflect merely the capacity of these cytokines to up-regulate HLA class I genes. A similar effect was reported when the PBMCs of another patient were incubated with phytohemagglutinin (PHA) and IFN-γ

(Plebani et al., 1996). Two adults with a TAP2 deficiency were recently described who surprisingly expressed five times more HLA class I molecules than those in other TAP-deficient patients (de la Salle et al., 2002). This discrepancy results from a moderate TAP-independent cell surface expression of probably empty HLA-B7 molecules, which is 20% that on normal HLA-B7 cells. Interestingly, one of these individuals had mild symptoms, whereas the other was asymptomatic.

HLA class I molecules were found to be absent from the skin of TAP-deficient patients (Hanau et al., 1994). Immunohistochemical studies of skin biopsies from two other patients showed that these molecules were not expressed in normal skin but were present in skin lesions. In one case, HLA class I expression was lower than that in skin from normal individuals (Watanabe et al., 1987), whereas in the other case the location of these molecules within cells or at the cell surface was uncertain (Plebani et al., 1996).

Soluble HLA Class I Molecules

Soluble HLA class I molecules circulate in plasma (normal values, 160 ng to 3 μg/ml) and are observed in HLA class I–deficient patients, although at relatively low levels. TAP-deficient patients and the child described above who had a low but inducible HLA class I expression on lymphocytes displayed 0.15 and 0.31 μg/ml of soluble HLA class I molecules, respectively (de la Salle, unpublished data).

Expression of Nonclassical HLA Class I Molecules

Nonclassical HLA class I molecules are composed of a nonpolymorphic heavy chain associated with β2m, and unlike the ubiquitous classical HLA class I molecules, the nonclassical molecules are expressed only on specialized cells. In particular, CD1 molecules are expressed on dendritic cells, including epidermal Langerhans cells. In two TAP-deficient patients, immunocytochemical staining of skin biopsies showed HLA class I molecules to be undetectable but CD1a antigens to be normally expressed on Langerhans cells. Flow cytometry further demonstrated that CD1 antigens were present at normal levels on dendritic cells derived in vitro from monocytes (Hanau et al., 1994). In another case, CD1a molecules were likewise normally expressed on epidermal Langerhans cells in biopsies taken from nonlesional skin, but were not detectable in biopsies taken from ulcers (Plebani et al., 1996). This absence of CD1a from lesion biopsies might only result from the local inflammation and not be linked to the genetic defect.

Another important HLA class I–like molecule is HLA-E, which presents, in a TAP-dependent manner, peptides derived from signal peptides of classical HLA class I molecules. This protein interacts with the NKG-2A/CD94 inhibitory receptor expressed on natural killer (NK) cells and a subset of T cells and thereby acts as a sensor in the biosynthetic pathway of HLA class I molecules. HLA-E/NKG-2A/CD94 interactions suppress the cytolytic responses of NK and T cells and their cytokine release. Surprisingly, through immunofluorescence techniques, HLA-E was found to be expressed on the PHA-induced T cell blasts but not on the EBV-B cells of a TAP-deficient patient (Furukawa et al., 1999a). Because of the confidential distribution of the anti-HLA-E monoclonal antibody used in the study, these results could not be challenged except in one case where HLA-E molecules were shown to be nearly undetectable on the surface of PBMCs and EBV-B cells (Matamoros et al., 2001).

T Lymphocyte Subpopulations

Experiments in transgenic mice have shown that the positive selection of $\alpha\beta$ CD8$^+$ T cells is dependent on interaction of their T cell receptor with HLA class I molecules expressed on thymic epithelial cells. Consequently, MHC class I–deficient mice have very low numbers of CD8$^+$ T cells. Most analyses of T cell subpopulations in type I BLS patients have been limited to determination of the ratio of CD8$^+$ to CD4$^+$ T cells. This ratio frequently appears to lie within normal values (Maeda et al., 1985; Sugiyama et al., 1986; Plebani et al., 1996; Teisserenc et al., 1997; Moins-Teisserenc et al., 1999), although the absolute number of T cells decreased progressively in one case (Plebani et al., 1996). No data are available on T cell subsets in the patients described by Payne et al. In the apparently similar case identified in our laboratory, the numbers of CD4$^+$ and CD8$^+$ $\alpha\beta$ T lymphocytes were normal (unpublished observations).

T cell subpopulations have been analyzed in PBMCs from some TAP-deficient patients (de la Salle et al., 1994, 2002; Moins-Teisserenc et al., 1999). In two cases (Table 18.2) the ratio of CD8$^+$ to CD4$^+$ T cells in patient 1 appeared to be somewhat diminished compared to that in normal individuals. Approximately one-third of T cells were $\gamma\delta$ T cells, one-third of which were CD8$^+$. A high proportion of CD8$^+$ T cells expressed $\gamma\delta$ receptors and the absolute number of CD8$^+$ $\alpha\beta$ T cells was low, although it was significantly higher than that in MHC class I–deficient transgenic mice. In contrast, the proportion of CD8$^+$ $\alpha\beta$ T cells in PBMCs of this patient's younger brother (patient 2), who was considered at the time to be healthy, was very low whereas the number of $\gamma\delta$ T cells was normal. Soon after identification of the deficiency, patient 2 also developed lung pathology. During progression of the disease, an expansion of $\alpha\beta$ CD8$^+$ and $\gamma\delta$ T cells was observed, a finding suggesting that these two subsets can be recruited in immune responses. An expansion of $\gamma\delta$ T cells has been observed in several but not all cases (Moins-Teisserenc et al., 1999; de la Salle et al., 2002; Matamoros et al., 2001). Because a large proportion of CD8$^+$ cells may correspond to HLA-unrestricted $\gamma\delta$ T cells in type I BLS patients, relevant assessment and interpretation of CD8$^+$ T cell frequencies and CD8$^+$-to-CD4$^+$ ratios are possible only by analyzing exclusively $\alpha\beta$ T cells. On this basis, the numbers of CD8$^+$ $\alpha\beta$ T cells appear to be generally decreased, although they sometimes remain within the lower limits. Finally, the repertoire of CD8$^+$ $\alpha\beta$

Table 18.2. Evolution of T Cell Subpopulations in TAP-Deficient Patients

Lymphocyte Subpopulations	Patient 1		Patient 2	
CD8$^+$	22.5	16	5	16.5
CD4$^+$	42.5	43	60.5	53
CD4$^+$CD8$^+$	7.5	10	0.3	1
$\alpha\beta$	45	59	60	69
$\alpha\beta$ CD8$^+$	11	15	2.4	11
$\alpha\beta$ CD8$^-$CD4$^-$	<1	<1	<1	<1
$\gamma\delta$	27	16	5	11
$\gamma\delta$ CD8$^+$	11	6	1.2	5
NK	11	8.5	5	8

Results are given as percentages of total lymphocyte population and were obtained on two different blood samples taken at a 2-year interval. Patient 2 was considered to be healthy when the first sample was taken but suffered from chronic lung inflammation at the time of the second one.

T cells is oligoclonal and quite similar to that of CD4$^+$ cells (de la Salle, unpublished observations). This finding suggests that the deficiency has only a weak incidence in the CD8$^+$ T cell repertoire.

Lymphocyte Natural Killer Subpopulations

The number of NK cells seems to stay within normal ranges in HLA class I–deficient patients, varying from lower to higher values, depending on the individual (de la Salle et al., 1994, 2001; Moins-Teisserenc et al., 1999; Furukawa et al., 1999a; Matamoros et al., 2001). A study of the phenotype of NK cells in two TAP2-deficient patients showed that these cells express the type III receptor for IgG (CD16) and the CD56 adhesion molecule. In addition, 40% to 50% of NK cells were found to express high levels of CD56, compared to less than 10% in normal subjects. In TAP$^+$ individuals, these cells must be activated with IL-2 to become cytotoxic.

The cytolytic activity of NK cells is controlled by a balance of activating and inhibitory receptors (Moretta et al., 2000), and the latter receptors block the cytolytic process when they interact with HLA class I molecules on the target cells. Resting TAP-deficient NK cells display a normally diverse repertoire of inhibitory receptors (Zimmer et al., 1998; Furukawa et al., 1999c). Levels of expression of these receptors are similar to those on normal cells, except for the NKG-2A/CD94 and ILT2 receptors, which were found to be overexpressed on NK cells but not on T cells in three cases (Zimmer et al., 1998 and unpublished observations; Matamoros et al., 2001). This overexpression of NKG-2A/CD94 was not found in another study (Furukawa et al., 1999b), whereas in the two patients from the first study, it seemed to decrease with age or improvement of clinical status (unpublished data). The inhibitory receptors negatively regulate the cytolytic activity of TAP$^-$ NK cells and are therefore functional.

In a more recent study (Markel et al., 2004), the repertoire of inhibitory receptors on NK clones derived from three patients from the same family was compared to that on NK clones from an unaffected sister. The number of clones expressing higher levels of inhibiting receptors was increased on TAP$^-$ clones. Interestingly, whereas TAP$^+$ NK cells rarely express the carcinogen embryonic antigen-related cell adhesion molecule 1 (CEA-CAM1), an inhibitory receptor, most of the TAP$^-$ clones express this molecule.

This work demonstrates that the repertoire of inhibitory receptors on the activated NK cells of these patients is unique.

The repertoire of most activating receptors is also normal on peripheral TAP$^-$ NK cells (Vitale et al., 2002). Thus, these cells express receptors involved in the killing of tumor cells (NKp30, 40, and 46) or virally infected cells (NKG2-D). On polyclonal NK cell lines derived from TAP-deficient patients, the repertoire of activating receptors nevertheless displays some abnormality, since the expression of NKp80 is low on many cells. Moreover, the same abnormality is observed at a clonal level. Triggering of these receptors induces normal cytolytic responses, except for 2B4 and NKp80, which were found to be functional on only a limited number of NK clones. Hence, the deficiency appears to have an observable incidence on a restricted spectrum of NK receptors and only in some cells.

Humoral Immune Response

The effects of HLA class I deficiency on the levels of immunoglobulin (Ig) classes and subclasses have not yet been fully investigated. Hypergammaglobulinemia with low levels of IgG2 and an absence of IgG4 was observed in one case (Plebani et al., 1996) and IgG2 deficiency was found in another (Matamoros et al., 2001).

Titration of antibodies in the sera of two TAP2-deficient patients showed them to have been infected by most common viruses: measles, mumps, herpes, cytomegalovirus, influenza, varicella, and EBV (Donato et al., 1995). Since these viral infections did not lead to an exaggerated pathology or require special care, the TAP-independent immune responses of these individuals must be to some extent efficient. This contrasts with the pathologies of herpes, cytomegalovirus, and EBV observed in patients lacking NK cells (Biron at al., 1989) or with diminished NK cell activity (Caligiuri et al., 1987). The fact that TAP-deficient patients can have high titers of antibodies against measles, mumps, herpes, cytomegalovirus, or varicella suggests that antibodies are important in their immune defense against these viruses. High levels of antiviral antibodies have not been reported in all patients. Moreover, normal titers of antibodies against EBV, respiratory syncytial virus, and influenza were found (Donato et al., 1985; unpublished data), which would suggest that cell-mediated immune responses are effective against these three viruses. In contrast, vaccinations failed to induce antibody responses to polysaccharides (Matamoros et al., 2001). Antibodies against herpes and EBV were detected in serum from one case of "conditional" HLA class I deficiency (de la Salle, unpublished observations).

Cell-Mediated Immune Responses

The cytotoxicity of TAP-deficient NK and T cells has been investigated in several patients. Although resting NK cells did not appear to kill the HLA class I–negative K562 cells classically used in NK cytotoxicity assays, they were able to mediate a weak antibody-dependent cytotoxicity. After activation in vitro with IL-2 or IL-12, these NK cells killed K562 cells, but not other HLA class I–negative cells such as Daudi or 721.221 cells (Furukawa et al., 1999c). When TAP-deficient NK cells were stimulated with EBV-B cells and IL-2, they proliferated and developed cytotoxicity against several target cells in the same manner as NK cells from normal donors, although with lower efficiency. More importantly, these activated cells were cytotoxic to autologous EBV-B cells and skin fibroblasts. Cytokines, which increase HLA

class I expression and consequently protect normal fibroblasts from lysis by activated autologous NK cells, did not protect the TAP-deficient cells (Zimmer et al., 1999). This reactivity toward autologous EBV-B cells and fibroblasts is mediated by an NK cell subset expressing high levels of NKp46 (Vitale et al., 2002). Thus, it would appear that in vivo the NK cells of these patients can be activated by cytokines released during antiviral responses, while the activated NKp46 bright NK cells are aggressive to surrounding uninfected cells.

In contrast, activated TAP-deficient NK cells do not kill autologous T cell blasts, whereas less than 10% of TAP$^+$ NK cell clones are unable to kill TAP$^-$ T cell blasts. This tolerance of autologous T cells in TAP-deficient patients could be mediated by an inhibitory receptor expressed by all TAP$^-$ NK cells, but by no more than a few TAP$^+$ NK cells (Vitale et al., 2002). This hypothesis was confirmed by the demonstration that CEA-CAM1 is expressed by most of the activated TAP$^-$ NK cells and inhibits the lysis of autologous PHA T cell blasts by homotypic interaction (Markel et al., 2004).

Autoreactive γδ T cells have also been described in TAP-deficient patients. Interestingly, biopsies of skin lesions revealed the presence of foci of activated NK cells and γδ T cells in the dermis, suggesting a role of these cells in the development of skin lesions (Moins-Teisserenc et al., 1999).

TAP-independent anti-EBV αβ T cell responses have been demonstrated in two cases of TAP deficiency. In one study, a cytotoxic CD8$^+$ αβ T cell clone was characterized that recognized a peptide of latent membrane protein 2 (LMP2) presented by HLA-B molecules (de la Salle et al., 1997). The LMP2 antigen was also found to be presented by HLA-A2 on TAP-deficient cell lines (Lee et al., 1996). More recently, an anti-EBV T cell clone recognizing the EBV transcription factor BMFR1 presented by HLA-B7 was isolated from another TAP-deficient patient (de la Salle et al., 2002). Therefore, CD8$^+$ αβ T cells can contribute to immune responses against viruses in TAP-deficient patients through recognition of TAP-independent antigens presented by classical HLA class I molecules.

A Model for the Pathology

At first glance, the absence of susceptibility to viruses and predominance of pulmonary bacterial infections in TAP-deficient patients may appear surprising. Our analysis nevertheless demonstrates that cytotoxic CD8$^+$ αβ T cells recognizing TAP-independent viral antigens can be stimulated in vivo and suggests that activated NK cells could also play a role in immune defense. These cell-mediated cytotoxic responses are less efficient than in normal individuals because (1) TAP-independent antigens are more rare and (2) the activated NK cells are less cytotoxic than those from normal subjects. Although a higher production of antibodies may partly compensate for these weaker cell-mediated responses, the overall immune response is unlikely to be sufficient. Consequently, TAP deficiency should lead to a delayed clearance of viral infections, as observed in β2m-deficient animals (Raulet, 1994).

Several viruses, including respiratory syncytial virus, are known to induce synthesis of IL-8, a chemoattractant for neutrophils and for a subpopulation of T lymphocytes. Because the lungs are probably more subject to viral infections than other tissues, these organs would be attacked (1) by the viruses inefficiently cleared and (2) by proteolytic enzymes released from neutrophils present in large numbers due to the sustained production of IL-8. Activated NK cells, and probably also cytotoxic CD8$^+$ αβ or γδ

T cells expressing NK inhibitory receptors, could further kill uninfected HLA class I–deficient autologous cells because of the absence of counterregulation by the inhibitory receptors. This would lead to destruction of ciliary cells and fibrosis of the lungs, with the result that bacteria and/or bacterial endotoxins would be inefficiently eliminated, thereby increasing the chemotaxis of neutrophils and maintaining a state of chronic inflammation in the lungs. It has been shown that cystic fibrosis patients display inflammation of the lungs that involves an associated increased neutrophil count within the first weeks of life, several years before the appearance of lung insufficiency (Kahn et al., 1995). Similarly, the progressive degradation of lung tissues of TAP-deficient patients is probably mediated by neutrophils and may begin long before any observable pathology.

One poorly understood aspect of the pathology is the development of skin lesions at an any age and only in some patients. No pathogens could be detected in these lesions (Gadola et al., 2000). The activated NK and γδ T cells present in inflamed tissues, which kill autologous cells in TAP-deficient patients, may be involved in this process. Histological studies support this hypothesis (Moins-Teisserenc et al., 1999).

Strategies for Diagnosis

HLA class I deficiency is generally diagnosed by serological HLA typing, but it can also be easily identified by flow cytometric analysis of PBMCs labeled with the anti–class I monomorphic monoclonal antibody W6/32. This test should also be carried out on PBMCs from other members of the family (parents and co-laterals). The type of defect, particularly whether it involves transcription or assembly of HLA class I molecules, may be investigated in a few experiments. In consanguinous families HLA typing can reveal linkage of the deficiency to chromosome 6. Stimulation of T lymphocytes with allogeneic PBMCs, PHA, and IL-2 will show whether HLA class I expression can be induced, indicating whether the defect is transcriptional. If the expression of HLA class I molecules remains low on activated T cells, intracellular class I molecules can be analyzed by metabolic labeling of proteins with ^{35}S-methionine, immunoprecipitation of cell lysates with W6/32, optional treatment of the immunoprecipitates with neuraminidase, and separation of the proteins by isoelectric focusing. This test will give information on the sialylation of HLA class I heavy chains and their association with β2m. Absence of sialylation would strongly suggest a defect of peptide loading. In this case, infection of a cell line derived from the patient with a recombinant vaccinia virus expressing either TAP1, TAP2, or both subunits (constructed by Russ et al., 1995), followed by flow cytometry of cells stained with W6/32, will determine whether the deficiency results from a TAP defect.

Treatment and Prognosis

Bronchiectasis and bacterial colonization of the respiratory tract lead to chronic respiratory failure and a strong reduction in life expectancy. As in cystic fibrosis and other inherited dysfunctions of the respiratory mucosae, the evolution of bronchiectasis is closely linked to the bacterial charge. Since no specific therapy can yet be proposed for HLA class I–deficient patients, the only way to limit the inflammatory process and hence the neutrophil-mediated lung damage is to strongly treat and, if possible, prevent the episodes of bronchial infection. When the diagnosis is made in infancy—for instance, in the case of early

detection in the family of a known patient—nurseries and other infant communities should be avoided to reduce the risk of early viral contamination. Immunizations against measles, pertussis, and influenza must be carefully controlled and exposure to tobacco smoke in the home environment should be prohibited. Bacteriological examination of the sputum is mandatory as soon as bacterial colonization becomes effective to provide guidelines for antimicrobial therapy. *Haemophilus influenzae* and *Streptococcus pneumoniae* strains, which are commonly found in repeated sputum tests from such patients, can be treated with oral antibiotics (β-lactamines, macrolides, penicillinase inhibitors), while intravenous treatment can be useful in the event of a major bacterial inoculum (bronchorrhea). Some other types of gram-negative bacilli such as enterobacteria and nonmucoid *Pseudomonas aeruginosa* strains may also be found in sputum and require intravenous administration of third-generation β-lactamines and aminosides. Low doses of erythromycin have been reported to improve and stabilize chronic inflammation of the respiratory tract in a patient treated for 19 years (Furukawa et al., 2000; Azuma et al., 2001). This antibiotic is also an inhibitor of neutrophil functions and used in the treatment of diffuse pan-bronchiolitis in Far-East countries, which supports the hypothesis that lung disease of TAP-deficient patients is mediated by neutrophils.

A long-term policy for antimicrobial therapy is difficult to define, as the bronchial colonization does not immediately endanger the survival of these HLA class I–deficient individuals. However, continuous or alternate use of oral antibiotics becomes necessary when bronchiectasis develops. Regular intravenous administration of high-dose antibiotics increases patients' level of comfort and probably slows their progressive functional impairment. One of the cases followed in Strasbourg was diagnosed when the patient was 12. At this time the bacterial charge was of major concern, requiring continuous oral antibiotics and some intravenous treatment during infectious exacerbations. This policy did not induce any bacterial resistance and enabled stabilization of the bronchiectasis. The bronchorrhea gradually disappeared and antibiotics were withdrawn at the age of 20 with no further functional impairment, as is the usual pattern in bronchiectasis caused by noncystic fibrosis.

Pulmonary function tests, which should be performed at regular intervals, will initially show bronchial obstruction unresponsive to inhaled bronchodilators. Inhaled corticosteroids have been tried at this stage, but without clear clinical benefit. Overdistention of the chest and chronic respiratory failure occur secondarily and lead to end-stage disease.

Computed tomography (CT) scans and 99m-Technetium pulmonary scintigraphies are useful tools for assessment of bronchiectasis. If localized lesions are suspected, preoperative bronchography and surgical lobectomy should be considered, although to our knowledge no HLA class I–deficient patient has to date undergone thoracic surgery. Since the mucosal injuries of type I BLS also involve the upper airways, nasal endoscopy and a sinusal CT scan can be proposed in the case of suspected sinusitis with nasosinusal polyps. The treatment of such lesions is either surgical (polypectomy, ethmoidectomy) or medical (local washing, high-dose topical corticosteroids), or requires both types of intervention. Surgical treatment of chronic sinusitis was reported to accelerate the nasal disease in one case (Gadola et al., 2000), but not in another (Azuma et al., 2001). Chronic otitis media must be carefully checked on regular audiograms and tympanograms. Surgical operations should only be performed under high doses of intravenous antibiotics. Use of tympanostomy tubes necessitate prolonged antibiotic therapy to avoid middle ear suppuration.

The skin ulcers are difficult to cure. Trials with IFN-α or IFN-γ made the lesions worse, and skin grafting was followed by the reappearance of lesions at the same sites (Willemsen et al., 1995). Only basic antiseptic care can be recommended (Gadola et al., 2000).

Animal Models

MHC class I–deficient transgenic mice have been generated by disrupting the genes encoding β2m (Koller et al., 1990; Zijlstra et al., 1990), the TAP1 subunit (Van Kaer et al., 1992), or tapasin (Grandea et al., 2000). Findings obtained with the first two models are discussed in detail in three reviews (Raulet, 1994; Ljunggren et al., 1996; Hoglund et al., 1997). These two deficient strains express low levels of MHC class I molecules on the plasma membranes and have very low absolute numbers of CD8$^+$ αβ T cells. In β2m-deficient mice, CD8$^+$ αβ T cells can reject allogeneic tumor cells and syngeneic tumor cells expressing minor antigens (Apasov and Sitkovski, 1994). The mice can fight viral infections but with lower efficiency than that of normal animals. Thus, attenuated influenza viruses are cleared more slowly and virulent strains inflict a higher rate of mortality. β2m-deficient mice, by contrast, cannot eliminate Theiler's virus although they survive early infection. The mechanisms of resistance to these and other viruses, such as Sendai virus, rotavirus, reovirus, and herpes simplex virus, appear to involve CD4$^+$ T cells and antibody production. More recent studies have analyzed the immune responses of TAP-deficient mice. In these animals, HSV gB-specific cytotoxic T cells were induced by immunization with a recombinant vaccinia virus or naked DNA, but not following HSV infection (Paliard et al., 2001). TAP-deficient animals were more susceptible to infection by the intracellular pathogen *Mycobacterium tuberculosis* (Behar et al., 1999). In contrast, they were not particularly susceptible to tumor formation (Johnsen et al., 2001). NK cells from β2m-deficient mice displayed reduced cytotoxicity but could be activated in vivo by viral infection (Su et al., 1994; Tay et al., 1995). TAP-deficient mice have been widely studied to characterize the development of CD8$^+$ αβ T cells (reviewed in Ljunggren et al., 1996). Their NK cells, like those of β2m-deficient mice, display reduced activity (Ljunggren et al., 1994).

Future Directions

Most of the identified HLA class I deficiencies result from a defect in one of the two TAP subunits. Although the associated lung and skin pathologies are highly characteristic, some individuals remain asymptomatic for decades, hence the true frequency of the disease is unknown. Therefore, HLA class I deficiency should be more systematically investigated in cases of unexplained chronic inflammation of the respiratory tract that lead to development of nasal polyps, granulomatous lesions of the midface or legs, bronchiectasis, or chronic bacterial infection of the lungs, notably with *Haemophilus influenzae*. On the other hand, the fact that TAP-deficient adults can be healthy indicates that TAP deficiency could come to the fore in atypical situations. In the absence of clinical data on "conditional" HLA class I deficiencies, the discovery of such defects is at present incidental. It will be necessary to collect data on the health status of these individuals and elucidate the genetic defect(s) responsible for their deficiency.

The process of lung degradation in HLA class I deficiency is likewise not yet fully understood. Efficient methods of treating the lung disease need to be developed, for example, through testing of drugs modulating neutrophil activity. The etiology of the skin lesions requires investigation, as does effective care of these lesions. Interestingly, the lesions of one patient transiently regressed when she was pregnant (Furukawa et al., 2000), as is often observed for other clinical manifestations of autoimmune diseases. This regression suggests that favorable regulatory responses controlling NK and T cell activity are induced during pregnancy and remain to be discovered. Finally, the influence of HLA class I deficiency on the production of antibacterial antibodies requires clarification.

At a more fundamental level, as suggested by our own studies of anti-EBV T cell responses in TAP-deficient patients, analysis of antiviral responses mediated by CD8$^+$ αβ T cells in these individuals might lead to the identification of a large number of viral proteins presented in a TAP-independent manner. Such observations could provide insight into the molecular bases and physiological relevance of these TAP-independent presentation pathways.

References

Apasov SG, Sitkovsky MV. Development and antigen specificity of CD8 cytotoxic T lymphocytes in beta 2-microglobulin-negative, MHC class I-deficient mice in response to immunization with tumor cells. J Immunol 152:2087–2097, 1994.

Azuma A, Keicho N, Furukawa H, Yabe T, Kudoh S. Prolonged survival of a bare lymphocyte syndrome type I patient with diffuse panbronchiolitis treated with erythromycin. Sarcoidosis Vasc Diffuse Lung Dis 18:312–313, 2001.

Behar SM, Dascher CC, Grusby MJ, Wang CR, Brenner MB. Susceptibility of mice deficient in CD1D or TAP1 to infection with *Mycobacterium tuberculosis*. J Exp Med 189:1973–1980, 1999.

Biron CA, Byron KS, Sullivan JL. Severe herpes virus infections in an adolescent without natural killer cells. N Engl J Med 320:1731–1735, 1989.

Caligiuri M, Murray C, Buchwald D, Levine H, Cheney P, Peterson D, Komaroff AL, Ritz J. Phenotypic and functional deficiency of natural killer cells in patients with chronic fatigue syndrome. J Immunol 139:3306–3313, 1987.

Cresswell P, Bangia N, Dick T, Diedrich G. The nature of the MHC class I peptide loading complex. Immunol Rev 172:21–28, 1999.

de la Salle H, Hanau D, Fricker D, Urlacher A, Kelly A, Salamero J, Powis SH, Donato L, Bausinger H, Laforet M, Jeras M, Spehner D, Bieber T, Falkenrodt A, Cazenave JP, Trowsdale J, Tongio MM. Homozygous human TAP peptide transporter mutation in HLA class I deficiency. Science 265:237–241, 1994.

de la Salle H, Houssaint E, Peyrat M-A, Arnold D, Salamero J, Pinczon D, Stevanovic S, Bausinger H, Fricker D, Gomard E, Biddison W, Lehner P, UytdeHaag F, Sasportes M, Donato L, Rammensee H-G, Cazenave J-P, Hanau D, Tongio M-M, Bonneville M. Human peptide transporter deficiency. Importance of HLA-B in the presentation of TAP-independent EBV antigens. J Immunol 158:4555–4563, 1997.

de la Salle H, Saulquin X, Mansour I, Klaymé S, Fricker D, Zimmer J, Cazenave J-P, Hanau D, Bonneville M, Houssaint E, Lefranc G, Naman R. Asymptomatic deficiency in the peptide transporter associated to antigen processing (TAP). Clin Exp Immunol 128: 525–531, 2002.

de la Salle H, Zimmer J, Fricker D, Angenieux C, Cazenave J-P, Okubo M, Maeda H, Plebani A, Tongio M-M, Dormoy A, Hanau D. HLA class I deficiencies due to mutations in the subunit 1 of the peptide transporter TAP1. J Clin Invest 103:R9–R13, 1999.

Donato L, de la Salle H, Hanau D, Tongio MM, Oswald M, Vandevenne A, Geisert J. Association of HLA class I antigen deficiency related to TAP2 gene mutation with familial bronchiectasis. J Pediatr 127:895–900, 1995.

Durand B, Sperisen P, Emery P, Barras E, Zufferey M, Mach B, Reith W. RFXAP, a novel subunit of the RFX DNA binding complex is mutated in MHC class II deficiency. EMBO J 16:1045–1055, 1997.

Furukawa H, Murata S, Yabe T, Shimbara N, Keicho N, Kashiwase K, Watanabe K, Ishikawa Y, Akaza T, Tadokoro K, Tohma S, Inoue T, Tokunaga K, Yamamoto K, Tanaka K, Juji T. Splice acceptor site mutation of the transporter associated with antigen processing-1 gene in human bare lymphocyte syndrome. J Clin Invest 103:755–758, 1999a.

Furukawa H, Yabe T, Akaza T, Tadokoro K, Tohma S, Inoue T, Tokunaga K, Yamamoto K, Geraghty DE, Juji T. Cell surface expression of HLA-E molecules on PBMC from a TAP1-deficient patient. Tissue Antigens 53: 292–295, 1999b.

Furukawa H, Yabe T, Inoue T, Yamamoto K, Juji T. HLA class I deficiency: NK cell and skin lesions. Mod Asp Immunobiol 1:166–168, 2000.

Furukawa H, Yabe T, Watanabe K, Miyamoto R, Miki A, Akaza T, Tadokoro K, Tohma S, Inoue T, Yamamoto K, Juji T. Tolerance of NK and LAK activity for HLA class I-deficient targets in a TAP1-deficient patient (bare lymphocyte syndrome type I). Hum Immunol 60:32–40, 1999c.

Gadola SD, Moins-Teisserenc HT, Trowsdale J, Gross WL, Cerundolo V. TAP deficiency syndrome. Clin Exp Immunol 121:173–178, 2000.

Grandea AG, Golovina TN, Hamilton SE, Sriram V, Spies T, Brutkiewicz RR, Harty JT, Eisenlohr LC, Van Kaer L. Impaired assembly yet normal trafficking of MHC class I molecules in Tapasin mutant mice. Immunity 13:213–222, 2000.

Greenwood R, Shimizu Y, Sekhon GS, DeMars R. Novel allele specific, post-translational reduction in HLA class I surface expression in a mutant human B cell line. J Immunol 153:5525–5536, 1994.

Hanau D, Fricker D, Bieber T, Esposito-Farese M-E, Bausinger H, Cazenave J-P, Donato L, Tongio M-M, de la Salle H. CD1 expression is not affected by human peptide transporter deficiency. Hum Immunol 41:61–68, 1994.

Hoglund P, Sundback J, Olsson-Alheim MY, Johansson M, Salcedo M, Ohlen C, Ljunggren H-G, Sentman CL, Karre K. Host MHC class I gene control of NK-cell specificity in the mouse. Immunol Rev 155:11–28, 1997.

Johnsen AK, France J, Nagy N, Askew D, Abdul-Karim FW, Gerson SL, Sy MS, Harding CV. Systemic deficits in transporter for antigen presentation (TAP)-1 or proteasome subunit LMP2 have little or no effect on tumor incidence. Int J Cancer 91:366–372, 2001.

Karttunen JT, Lehner PJ, Gupta SS, Hewitt EW, Cresswell P. Distinct functions and cooperative interaction of the subunits of the transporter associated with antigen processing (TAP). Proc Natl Acad Sci USA. 98: 7431–7436, 2001.

Khan TZ, Wagener JS, Bost T, Martinez J, Accurso FJ, Riches DWH. Early pulmonary inflammation in infants with cystic fibrosis. Am J Respir Crit Care Med 151:1075–1082, 1995.

Koller BH, Marrack P, Kappler JW, Smithies O. Normal development of mice deficient in beta 2 microglobulin, MHC class I proteins, and CD8 T cells. Science 248:1227–1230, 1990.

Lee S, Thomas W, Blake N, Rickinson A. Transporter (TAP)-independent processing of a multiple membrane-spanning protein, the Epstein-Barr virus latent membrane protein 2. Eur J Immunol 26:1875–1883, 1996.

Ljunggren H-G, Glas R, Sandberg JK, Karre K. Reactivity and specificity of CD8 T cells in mice with defects in the MHC class I antigen-presenting pathway. Immunol Rev 151:123–148, 1996.

Ljunggren HG, Van Kaer L, Ploegh HL, Tonegawa S. Altered natural killer cell repertoire in Tap-1 mutant mice. Proc Natl Acad Sci USA 91: 6520–6524, 1994.

Maeda H, Hirata R, Chen RF, Suzaki H, Kudoh S, Tohyama H. Defective expression of HLA class I antigens: a case of the bare lymphocyte without immunodeficiency. Immunogenetics 21:549–558, 1985.

Markel G, Mussaffi H, Ling KL, Salio M, Gadola S, Steuer G, Blau H, Achdout H, de Miguel M, Gonen-Gross T, Hanna J, Arnon TI, Qimron U, Volovitz I, Eisenbach L, Blumberg RS, Porgador A, Cerundolo V, Mandelboim O. The mechanisms controlling NK cell autoreactivity in TAP2-deficient patients. Blood 103:1770–1778, 2004.

Matamoros N, Milà J, Llano M, Bals A, Vicario JL, Pons J, Crespí C, Martinez N, Iglesias-Alzueta J, López-Botet M. Molecular studies and NK cell function of a new case of TAP2 homozygous human deficiency. Clin Exp Immunol 125:274–282, 2001.

Moins-Teisserenc HT, Gadola SD, Cella M, Dunbar PR, Exley A, Blake N, Baykal C, Lambert J, Bigliardi P, Willemsen M, Jones M, Buechner S, Colonna M, Gross WL, Cerundolo V, Baycal C. Association of a syndrome resembling Wegener's granulomatosis with low surface expression of HLA class-I molecules. Lancet 354:1598–1603, 1999.

Moretta A, Biassoni R, Bottino C, Moretta L. Surface receptors delivering opposite signals regulate the function of human NK cells. Semin Immunol 12:129–138, 2000.

Paliard X, Doe B, Selby MJ, Hartog K, Lee AY, Burke RL, Walker CM. Induction of herpes simplex virus gB-specific cytotoxic T lymphocytes in

TAP1-deficient mice by genetic immunization but not HSV infection. Virology 282:56–64, 2001.

Payne R, Brodsky FM, Peterlin BM, Young LM. "Bare lymphocytes" without immunodeficiency. Hum Immunol 6:219–227, 1983.

Plebani A, Monafo V, Cattaneo R, Carella G, Brugnoni D, Facchetti F, Battocchio S, Meini A, Notarangelo LD, Duse M, Ugazio AG. Defective expression of HLA class I and CD1a molecules in a boy with Marfan-like phenotype and deep skin ulcers. J Am Acad Dermatol 35:814–818, 1996.

Raulet DH. MHC class I deficient mice. Adv Immunol 55:381–421, 1994.

Russ G, Esquivel F, Yewdell JW, Cresswell P, Spies T, Bennink JR. Assembly, intracellular localization, and nucleotide binding properties of the human peptide transporters TAP1 and TAP2 expressed by recombinant vaccinia viruses. J Biol Chem 270:21312–21318, 1995.

Sabatier C, Gimenez C, Calin-Laurens V, Rabourdin-Combe C, Touraine JL. Type III bare lymphocyte syndrome: lack of HLA class II gene expression and reduction in HLA class I gene expression. C R Acad Sci Paris Life Sci 319:789–798, 1996.

Schneider E, Hunke S. ATP-binding-cassette (ABC) transport systems: functional and structural aspects of the ATP-hydrolyzing subunits/domains. FEMS Microbiol Rev 22:1–20, 1998.

Scott JE, Dawson JR. MHC class I expression and transport in a calnexin deficient cell line. J Immunol 155:143–148, 1996.

Su HC, Orange JS, Fast LD, Chan AT, Simpson JS, Terhorst C, Biron CA. IL-2-dependent NK cell responses discovered in virus-infected beta 2-microglobulin–deficient mice. J Immunol 153:5674–5681, 1994.

Sugiyama Y, Kudoh S, Kitamura S. A case of the bare lymphocyte syndrome with clinical manifestations of diffuse panbronchiolitis. Nippon Kyobu Shikkan Gakkai Zasshi 27:980–983, 1989.

Sugiyama Y, Maeda H, Okumura K, Takaku F. Progressive sinobronchiectasis associated with the "bare lymphocyte syndrome" in an adult. Chest 89: 398–401, 1986.

Sullivan KE, Stobo JD, Peterlin BM. Molecular analysis of the bare lymphocyte syndrome. J Clin Invest 76:75–79, 1985.

Tay HC, Welsh RM, Brutkiewicz RR. NK cell response to viral infections in beta 2-microglobulin-deficient mice. J Immunol 154:780–789, 1995.

Teisserenc H, Schmitt W, Blake N, Dunbar R, Gadola S, Gross WL, Exley A, Cerundolo V. A case of primary immunodeficiency due to a defect of the major histocompatibility gene complex class I processing and presentation pathway. Immunol Lett 57:183–187, 1997.

Touraine JL, Betuel H, Souillet G, Jeune M. Combined immunodeficiency disease associated with absence of cell surface HLA-A and-B antigens. J Pediatr 93:47–51, 1978.

Van Kaer L, Ashton-Rickardt PG, Ploegh HL, Tonegawa S. TAP1 mutant mice are deficient in antigen presentation, surface class I molecules, and CD4-CD8 T cells. Cell 71:1205–1214, 1992.

Vitale M, Zimmer J, Castriconi R, Hanau D, Donato L, Bottino C, Moretta L, de la Salle H, Moretta A. Analysis of natural killer cells in TAP2-deficient patients: expression of functional triggering receptors and evidence for the existence of inhibitory receptor(s) that prevent lysis of normal autologous cells. Blood 99:1723–1729, 2002.

Watanabe S, Iwata M, Maeda H, Ishibashi Y. Immunohistochemical studies of major histocompatibility antigens in a case of the bare lymphocyte syndrome without immunodeficiency. J Am Acad Dermatol 17:895–902, 1987.

Willemsen M, De Coninck A, Goossens A, DeCree J, Roseeuw D. Unusual clinical manifestation of a disfiguring necrobiotic granulomatous disease. J Am Acad Dermatol 33:887–890, 1995.

Yabe T, Kawamura S, Sato M, Kashiwase K, Tanaka H, Ishikawa Y, Asao Y, Oyama J, Tsuruta K, Tokunaga K, Tadokoro K, Juji T. A subject with a novel type I bare lymphocyte syndrome has tapasin deficiency due to deletion of 4 exons by Alu-mediated recombination. Blood 100:1496–1498, 2002.

Zijlstra M, Bix M, Simister NE, Loring JM, Raulet RH, Jaenisch R. Beta 2-microglobulin mice lack CD4-8 cytolytic T cells. Nature 344:742–746, 1990.

Zimmer J, Donato L, Hanau D, Cazenave J-P, Tongio M-M, Moretta A, de la Salle H. Activity and phenotype of natural killer cells in peptide transporter (TAP)-deficient patients (type I bare lymphocyte syndrome). J Exp Med 187:117–122, 1998.

Zimmer J, Donato L, Hanau D, Cazenave JP, Moretta A, Tongio MM, de la Salle H. Inefficient protection of human TAP-deficient fibroblasts from autologous NK cell-mediated lysis by cytokines inducing HLA class I expression. Eur J Immunol 29:1286–1291, 1999.

19

CD40, CD40 Ligand, and the Hyper-IgM Syndrome

RAIF S. GEHA, ALESSANDRO PLEBANI, and LUIGI D. NOTARANGELO

Immunodeficiency with hyper-IgM (HIGM) is a rare congenital disorder, characterized by recurrent infections and very low levels of serum IgG, IgA, and IgE, with normal or elevated IgM (Notarangelo et al., 1992). Both primary and acquired forms of the disease have been reported. Among primary HIGM, X-linked (Krantman et al., 1980; Benkerrou et al., 1990), autosomal recessive (Pascual-Salcedo et al., 1983; Benkerrou et al., 1990; Revy et al., 2000; Ferrari et al., 2001, Imai et al., 2003b), and possibly autosomal dominant (Beall et al., 1980; Brahmi et al., 1983) variants are known, accounting for genetic heterogeneity. Acquired HIGM may be secondary to congenital rubella (Schimke et al., 1969; Espanol et al., 1986; Benkerrou et al., 1990), neoplasia (Raziuddin et al., 1989), or use of antiepileptic drugs (Mitsuya et al., 1979). The disease, originally named *dysgammaglobulinemia*, was first described in 1961 in a 15-year-old boy with recurrent pneumonia, meningitis, and lymphadenopathy (Burtin, 1961), and in two male brothers with a history of recurrent bacterial infections (Rosen et al., 1961).

The primary immunological defect in HIGM had long remained elusive. On the basis of immunoglobulin profile and demonstration that peripheral B lymphocytes from patients with HIGM uniquely express IgM and/or IgD at the cell surface (Schwaber et al., 1981; Levitt et al., 1983), it was originally hypothesized that B lymphocytes from HIGM patients have an intrinsic inability to undergo immunoglobulin isotype switch (Geha et al., 1979; Levitt et al., 1983). However, the observation that patients with the X-linked form of the disease (XHIGM) are uniquely prone to opportunistic infections (Hong et al., 1962) suggested a T cell defect despite laboratory evidence for a humoral immune deficiency. The hypothesis of a primary T cell defect in XHIGM was elegantly supported by studies of Mayer et al. (1986), who demonstrated that B cells from XHIGM patients can be driven to secrete immunoglobulins of various isotypes in the presence of pokeweed mitogen when cocultured with "helper T lymphoblasts" from a patient with a Sezary-like syndrome.

Experiments aimed at characterizing the helper T cell signals involved in B cell differentiation led to the discovery that monoclonal antibodies to CD40 (a surface protein constitutively expressed on B cells) are able to induce isotype switch in the presence of appropriate costimulatory cytokines (Rousset et al., 1991; Zhang et al., 1991). The gene encoding the natural ligand for CD40 (CD40L, also designated CD154) was cloned first in the mouse (Armitage et al., 1992) and then in humans (Graf et al., 1992; Hollenbaugh et al., 1992; Lederman et al., 1992; Gauchat et al., 1993a). CD40L was shown to be a surface molecule transiently expressed on activated T cells, mainly belonging to the CD4+ subset (Lane et al., 1992). The *CD40L* gene (also designated tumor necrosis factor superfamily member 5, or *TNFSF5*) was mapped to the X chromosome region q26 (Graf et al., 1992), where the XHIGM locus had been assigned (Padayachee et al., 1992, 1993), and was thus investigated as a candidate gene for XHIGM. Indeed, within a few weeks, five groups independently demonstrated that mutations of the *CD40L/TNFSF5* gene account for XHIGM (MIM #308220) (Allen et al., 1993a; Aruffo et al., 1993; DiSanto et al., 1993; Fuleihan et al., 1993b; Korthauer et al., 1993).

More recently, another group of HIGM patients have been identified whose clinical and immunological features are similar to those of XHIGM, but with an autosomal recessive inheritance (Ferrari et al., 2001). In these patients, mutations of the *CD40* gene (CD40 deficiency; MIM #606843) have been identified, as discussed below. These findings reinforce the importance of the fundamental role that CD40L–CD40 interaction and downstream signaling events play in regulating T cell–dependent B cell responses.

251

An X-linked HIGM phenotype may also be associated with ectodermal dysplasia (MIM #300291); this disease (described in more detail in Chapter 36) is due to mutations of the IKK-γ (NEMO) gene, involved in nuclear factor (NF)-κB activation (Zonana et al., 2000; Döffinger et al., 2001; Jain et al., 2001).

While defects of CD40L, CD40, and NEMO also affect immune cells other than B lymphocytes (e.g., T lymphocytes and dendritic cells), some forms of HIGM syndrome reflect intrinsic B cell defects that impair the processes of class switch recombination (CSR) and somatic hypermutation (SHM). In particular, Revy et al. (2000) have shown that an autosomal recessive variant of HIGM (activation-induced cytidine deaminase [AID] deficiency; MIM #605258) is due to mutations of the activation-induced cytidine deaminase (AICD) gene that is selectively expressed in germinal-center B cells and participates in immunoglobulin isotype switching and somatic hypermutation. In contrast to patients with mutations of CD40L, those with mutations of AID have enlarged lymph nodes and tonsils, with prominent germinal centers, and suffer mainly from recurrent bacterial but not opportunistic infections. Similar features are also observed in patients with the uracil-N-glycosylase (UNG) deficiency (MIM #608106), an enzyme also involved in CSR and SHM (Imai et al., 2003b). Finally, at least one other variant of autosomal recessive HIGM with defective CSR has been recognized (selective CSR deficiency), but its gene defects remain obscure (Imai et al., 2003a).

In this chapter, we will focus on CD40L and CD40 defects. Deficiencies of AID, UNG, and NEMO will be discussed in Chapters 20 and 36, respectively.

Biology of CD40 and CD40 Ligand

CD40

CD40, a 50 κDa glycoprotein, is a member of the tumor necrosis factor receptor (TNFR) family of surface molecules. The gene, TNFRSF5 (*109535), encodes a type I transmembrane protein of 277 amino acids (a.a.) (Stamenkovic et al., 1989). CD40 is expressed on all B cells, but also on other cells that include follicular dendritic cells, thymic epithelial cells, some endothelial and epithelial cells, and neurons. CD40 plays an important role in B cell survival, growth, and differentiation. CD40 ligation on the surface of B cells in the presence of interleukin-4 (IL-4) initiates proliferation and growth and induces homotypic cell adhesion and up-regulation of the expression of CD23, CD54, CD80, CD86, and lymphotoxin-α on B cells. CD40 ligation also up-regulates Fas expression on B cells, making them susceptible to killing by Fas ligand$^+$ (FasL$^+$)-activated T cells (Banchereau et al., 1994; van Kooten and Banchereau, 2000). However, CD40 also delivers an antiapoptotic signal to B cells by inducing antiapoptotic genes that include Bcl-xL and A20 (Ishida et al., 1995; Sarma et al., 1995). Recently it has been shown that C4 binding protein (C4BP), a regulator component of the classical complement pathway, binds directly to CD40 on human B cells at a site that differs from that used by CD40L. Engagement of CD40 by C4BP triggers signaling pathways similar to those triggered by CD40L, as demonstrated by the fact that this interaction induces proliferation, up-regulation of CD54 and CD86 expression, and IL-4–dependent IgE isotype switching in normal B cells (Brodeur et al., 2003). These findings unequivocally suggest that C4BP is an activating ligand for CD40 and establish a novel interface between complement and B cell activation.

CD40 and isotype switching

Heavy-chain class switching results from deletional recombination between characteristic repetitive sequences (switch regions) located 5′ of the Cμ gene and of each C$_H$ gene, except Cδ. IL-4 and IL-13, the switch factors for IgE, induce the transcription of a 1.8 kb ε germ-line mRNA that initiates 5′ of the Sε region. This transcript is sterile, as it is not translated into a functional protein. Induction of a mature 2.0 kb εmRNA and of IgE protein synthesis requires a second signal, provided by T cells, via CD40L–CD40 interactions (Oettgen, 2000). CD40$^{-/-}$ mice fail to undergo T cell–dependent isotype switching and fail to develop germinal centers following immunization with T cell–dependent antigens (Castigli et al., 1994; Kawabe et al., 1994). Similar results were obtained in mice with disrupted CD40L genes (Xu et al., 1994; Borrow et al., 1996). Crosslinking of CD40 induces the expression of activation-induced deaminase (AID), which plays a critical role in isotype switching. B cells from AID$^{-/-}$ mice and from patients with AID deficiency are unable to undergo isotype switching (Muramatsu et al., 2000; Revy et al., 2000). Several molecules that play a role in DNA repair have been found to be important or essential for isotype switching; these include Ku70, Ku80, DNA-PK, Msh2, and others (Stavnezer, 2000).

Structure of CD40 receptor complex

The intracellular sequences of murine and human CD40 are shown below:

Mu: 216KRVVKKPRDNEMLPPAARRQDPQEMEDYPGH------NTA
    APVQETLHGCQPVTQEDGKESRLSVQERQVTDSLALRPLV

Hu: 216KKVAKKPTNKAPHP--------KQEPQE INFPDDLPGS---NTA
    APVQETLHGCQPVTQEDGKESRISVQERQ

The intracellular domain of human CD40, which starts at a.a. 216 from the initiating methionine, has a binding site for Jak3 in its proline-rich Box 1 membrane proximal region (a.a. 222–229), a binding site for tumor necrosis factor receptor–associated factor 6 (TRAF6) that spans the sequence KQEPQE (a.a. 230–236) (Ishida et al., 1996), and a consensus core binding sequence, PxQxT (a.a. 250–254), that binds TRAF2 and TRAF3 directly (Cheng et al., 1995; Pullen et al., 1998; Lee et al., 1999; Sutherland et al., 1999). Amino acid residues surrounding this core sequence are also involved in TRAF2,3 binding. The sites of TRAF2 and TRAF3 binding overlap but are not identical. Indeed, mutation of Pro250 to Ala destroys TRAF2 binding but does not affect TRAF3 binding. The reverse is true for mutations of L255, Q263, and E264. These mutations destroy TRAF3 binding but do not affect TRAF2 binding. Furthermore, the C-terminal 18 a.a., which contain the sequence PxxQxD, contribute to TRAF2 but not to TRAF3 binding (Ye et al., 1999). There is a debate as to whether TRAF6 binds directly to CD40. It has been suggested that an adaptor protein, possibly related to MyoD88, that links the IL-1 receptor recruited protein IRAK to TRAF6 facilitates TRAF6 binding to CD40. TRAF1 is probably recruited to CD40 by TRAF2, whereas TRAF5 is recruited by TRAF3 (Leo et al., 1999).

The intracellular domain of murine CD40 also starts at a.a. 216 from the initiating methionine. Like human CD40, it has a proline-rich membrane proximal region (a.a. 222–230). More importantly, it has a highly conserved putative TRAF 6 binding sequence, RQDPQE (a.a. 234–239), and a 32–a.a stretch (a.a. 247–278) that is 100% homologous to a.a. 246–277 of human CD40 (shaded sequence above). This stretch contains the PxQxT core motif (a.a. 251–255) and all the residues that have been shown to differentially influence TRAF2 and TRAF3 binding.

Murine CD40 has an additional C-terminal 11–a.a. sequence (a.a. 279–289) that is not present in human CD40. Murine CD40, like its human counterpart, binds TRAF2, TRAF3, and TRAF6.

Signal transduction following CD40 engagement

CD40 ligation causes an increase in protein tyrosine phosphorylation (Ren et al., 1994; Faris et al., 1994), enhanced association of CD40 with TRAF proteins (Pullen et al., 1999), activation of NF-κB, AP-1, STAT3, and STAT5 transcription factors (Berberich et al. 1994; Hanissian et al., 1997; Iciek et al., 1997; Revy et al., 1999), and activation of the mitogen-activated protein (MAP) kinases Erk, JNK, and p38 (Li et al., 1996). Jak3 activation is thought to mediate STAT activation by CD40 (Karras et al., 1997). CD40 ligation also causes the recruitment of CD40 into lipid rafts (Hostager et al., 2000; Vidalain et al., 2000). There is evidence that CD40, like TNFR1, may already be trimerized by its extracellular pre-ligand association domain (PLAD) (Chan et al., 2000; Kaykas et al., 2001). CD40 ligation by membrane-bound trimeric CD40L causes a higher degree of oligomerization and, most importantly, a conformational change that results in its translocation with associated TRAF proteins to lipid rafts.

A truncated derivative of TRAF2 lacking an amino-terminal RING finger domain is a dominant-negative inhibitor of NF-κB activation mediated by CD40 (Rothe et al., 1995). An 11–a.a. motif in the intracellular domain of CD40 that spans the core PxQxT TRAF2,3 binding sequence was found to be sufficient for the activation of Jun, p38, and NF-κB. TRAF6 has been reported to synergize with TRAF2 in NF-κB activation (Lee et al., 1999; Tsukamoto et al., 1999). However, in another study TRAF6 was found not to be important for NF-κB activation in B cells (Jalukar et al., 2000). Furthermore, a CD40 mutant that binds TRAF2 but not TRAF3 (or TRAF5) was shown to activate NF-κB. This finding, together with the inability of TRAF1 to activate NF-κB, suggests that TRAF2 is the most important element in CD40-mediated activation of NF-κB. However, the mechanism of NF-κB activation by TRAF2 is still unclear. Oligomerization of the TRAF2 effector domain results in specific binding to MEKK1, a protein kinase capable of activating JNK, p38, and the IKK complex (Baud et al., 1999). TRAF2 has also been found to bind to the kinase NIK, which can also phosphorylate and activate the IKK complex. TRAF2 also binds to RIP, a protein that is central to NF-κB activation by TNFR1 and to the protection of cells from TNF-mediated death. RIP was recently found to bind to MEKK3, which then phosphorylates and activates IKK (Wang et al., 2001). It has been shown that TRAF6 functions as an E3 ubiquitin ligase to catalyze, together with Ubc13/Uev1A, the synthesis of polyubiquitin chains linked through lysine-63 (K63) of ubiquitin and the activation of a TAK1–TAB1/2 complex, which phosphorylates and activates IKK (Deng et al., 2000; Yang et al., 2000; Shuto et al., 2001). Blockade of this polyubiquitin chain synthesis prevents TRAF6-mediated activation of IKK. However, TRAF6 does not appear to activate NF-κB in B cells (Jalukar et al., 2000).

Data from knockout mice and from patients with IKKγ/NEMO mutations (Zonana et al., 2000; Döffinger et al., 2001; Jain et al., 2001) strongly suggest that NF-κB plays an important role in CD40-mediated isotype switching. The point mutation in NIK in *aly* mice and null mutations in IKKα are associated with low-serum IgG and absent-serum IgA. B cells from p50, RelA, c-Rel, p52, and IKKα knockout mice, but not from RelB knockout mice, have defects in class switching and in germinal center formation (Sha, 1998). TRAF2⁻/⁻ mice die perinatally but TRAF2⁻/⁻ TNFR1⁻/⁻ and TRAF2⁻/⁻ TNF⁻/⁻ double-mutant mice are viable

(Yeh et al., 1997). Isotype switching to IgG is impaired in TRAF2⁻/⁻ TNFR1⁻/⁻ mice. This finding further supports the idea that a pathway consisting of TRAF2-mediated activation of NF-κB in CD40-activated B cells is critical for isotype switching. Importantly, both type 1 (p50-dependent) and type 2 (p52-dependent) NF-κB signaling pathways are triggered following CD40 activation and contribute to the gene expression and biological program unique to CD40 in B cell activation (Zarnegar et al., 2004).

TRAF6 and TRAF2 have been reported to be involved in JNK and p38 activation by CD40 (Reinhard et al., 1997; Song et al. 1997; Leo et al., 1999). Both synergize in the activation of JNK, but TRAF6 appears to be the most important factor for activation of p38 (Leo et al., 1999). TRAF3 has been reported to activate the JNK and p38 pathways (Grammer et al., 1998). There is also evidence for a TRAF-independent pathway of CD40-mediated JNK activation. A deletion mutant of TRAF6 lacking the NH2-terminal domain acted as a dominant-negative mutant to suppress ERK activation by full-length CD40 and by a deletion mutant of CD40, only containing the binding site for TRAF6 in its cytoplasmic tail (Kashiwada et al., 1998). This result suggests that TRAF6 may be the most important element in CD40-mediated activation of ERK. A model for CD40 signaling is presented in Figure 19.1.

Finally, the redox factor APE/Ref-1 has been reported to act as a key signaling intermediate in response to CD40-mediated B cell activation. Upon CD40 cross-linking, APE/Ref-1 translocates from the cytoplasm to the nucleus, where it modulates the DNA-binding activity of the Pax5 and EBF transcription factors. APE/Ref-1 appears to be required for CD40-mediated Pax5 activation, as the repression of APE/Ref-1 protein production is able to block CD40-induced Pax5 binding activity (Merluzzi et al., 2003).

CD40 Ligand

The murine CD40L has been identified and the gene cloned as an EL4 thymoma cell surface molecule that binds to soluble CD40 (Armitage et al., 1992). Subsequently, the human *CD40L* gene (*TNFSF5*, 300386) was cloned from activated T cells (Graf et al., 1992; Hollenbaugh et al., 1992; Spriggs et al., 1992). Independently, Lederman and coworkers identified a subclone of Jurkat T cells that is able to provide contact-dependent helper function to B cells (Lederman et al., 1992); this molecule has since been cloned and confirmed to be CD40L (CD154, also referred to as *gp39*). The human cDNA has an open reading frame of 783 base pairs (bp) that codes for a type II membrane protein 261 a.a. long. The extracellular domain is 215 a.a. long, the transmembrane domain is 24 a.a. in length, and the intracellular domain is 22 a.a. long. The extracellular domain immediately proximal to the transmembrane region has a putative proteolytic cleavage site (His-Arg-Arg-Leu), which suggests that the extracellular domain may be "shed." Molecular modeling of CD40L based on the crystal structure of TNF indicates that a.a. residues 189–209 are critical for the binding of CD40L to CD40 (Peitsch and Jongeneel, 1993).

Detailed organization of the murine (Tsitsikov et al., 1994) and human (Villa et al., 1994; Shimadzu et al., 1995) *CD40L* genes has been reported. The gene consists of five exons. Exon 1 encodes for the 5′ untranslated region and the first 52 a.a., including 22 a.a. of the intracytoplasmic tail, 24 a.a. of the transmembrane domain, and 6 a.a. of extracellular domain. Exons 2, 3, and 4 encode a.a. 53–96, a.a. 97–114, and a.a. 115–135 a.a.,

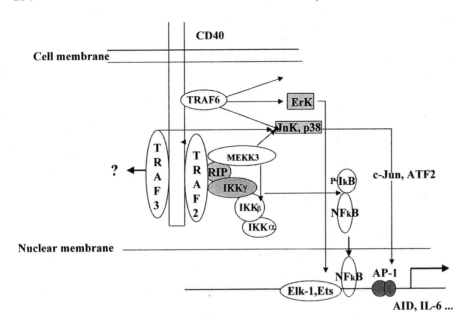

Figure 19.1. Hypothetical model of CD40 signaling. CD40 ligation causes enhanced association of CD40 with tumor necrosis factor receptor–associated factor (TRAF) proteins. Oligomerization of TRAF2 effector domain results in specific binding to MEKK3, a kinase capable of activating JNK, p38, and the IKK complex. TRAF2 also binds to RIP, a protein central to NF-kB activation. Subsequently, RIP binds to MEKK3, which then activates the IKK complex. JNK and p38 are also activated by CD40-activated TRAF6. TRAF6 is known to be the most important element in CD40-mediated activation of ERK. JNK and p38 transduce their activation signal to the nucleus through c-Jun and ATF2, whereas ERK binds to Elk-Ets binding sites. As a result of CD40-mediated signaling, a number of critical genes involved in terminal B cell differentiation and inflammation (such as AID and IL-6) are transcribed.

respectively. Exon 5 encodes the rest of the protein (a.a. 136–260) and the 3′ untranslated region. There is no homology in the position of the exons between CD40L and any of the known genes from the TNF family, but in all these genes the sequence encoding the receptor binding domain is located in the last exon. Sequences up to 1.5 kb upstream from the murine gene lack the TATAA or CCAAT boxes but have an Sp1 sequence, six nuclear factor of activated T cells (NFAT)-like sequences, and one OAP-like site. The 3′ untranslated region of the murine gene has two adjacent microsatellite repeats (a 50-bp-long CT and a 90-bp-long CA repeat) as well as two ATTTA elements that are putatively responsible for the stability of mRNA.

Several studies have illustrated the importance of CD40 and its ligand, CD40L, in humoral immunity. Recombinant CD40L mimics the action of CD40 monoclonal antibody (MAb) and is able to stimulate B cell proliferation in the presence of phorbol myristate acetate (PMA) and to induce immunoglobulin synthesis (Spriggs et al., 1992; Lane et al., 1993). Immunoglobulin secretion by B cells is highly modulated by cytokines. In the presence of recombinant CD40L, IL-2 and IL-10 induce specifically the secretion of IgM, IgG1, and IgA (Durandy et al., 1993) whereas IL-4 is necessary for the secretion of IgG4 and IgE. Antibody to CD40L can block T cell–dependent B cell activation (Noelle et al., 1992a, 1992b). Likewise, soluble CD40, a product of the fusion of cDNA segments encoding the extracellular domain of CD40 to genomic DNA segments encoding human IgG1, inhibits IgE synthesis (Fanslow et al., 1992). Immunization of mice with KLH (a thymus-dependent antigen) or DNP-Ficoll (a thymus-independent antigen) induces the expression of CD40L by T helper (TH) cells, and this induction coincides with the development of cytokine-producing cells. Through the use of immunocytochemical techniques, it was elegantly demonstrated that CD40L cells and cytokine-producing cells are juxtaposed in the lymphoid organs (Van den Eertwegh et al., 1993). Short-term treatment with anti-CD40L antibody suppressed the immune response against these antigens, but adoptive transfer of cells from anti-CD40L–treated mice could fully reconstitute TH function in irradiated recipient mice, showing that immune suppression does not involve clonal anergy or deletion (Foy et al., 1993). Thus it appears that CD40L expression is essential for both thymus-dependent and thymus-independent antigens.

However, in mice with targeted disruption of the CD40 or CD40L gene, only the antibody response against the T-dependent antigen is impaired. This finding suggests that stimulation via CD40/CD40L may not be critical for antibody responses to T-independent antigens, at least in the murine model.

Soluble CD40L also acts as T cell growth factor, being a costimulatory molecule for both α/β and γ/δ T cells (Armitage et al., 1993; Fanslow et al., 1994; Ramsdell et al., 1994). In the presence of submitogenic concentrations of Con A, phytohemagglutinin (PHA), CD3 MAb, or MAbs to the T cell receptor (TCR), addition of soluble CD40L increased the expression of CD25 and CD69. CD40L is also essential for the activation of macrophage effector function by T cells. CD40L$^{-/-}$ mice are less effective in stimulating allogenic macrophages to produce inflammatory cytokines and reactive nitrogen intermediates (Stout et al., 1996).

Regulation of CD40 ligand expression

CD40L is a highly inducible gene and is mainly expressed by CD4$^+$ T cells, although polymerase chain reaction (PCR) products have been identified using mRNA derived from CD8$^+$ cells, monocytes, and natural killer (NK) cells (Cocks et al., 1993). In addition, mast cells, basophils (Gauchat et al., 1993b), and eosinophils (Gauchat et al., 1995) have been shown to express functional CD40L on their surface. The T cell expression of CD40L is well regulated; resting T lymphocytes do not express CD40L. In α/β T cells, CD40L mRNA becomes detectable as early as 1 hour after stimulation with PMA and ionomycin, peaks at 3 hours, and disappears by 24 hours. Surface CD40L is detected as early as 3 hours after stimulation with PMA and ionomycin, peaks at 6 hours after stimulation, starts to decline by 8 hours, and is barely detectable by 16 hours. However, murine TH cells activated by anti-CD3 displayed sustained expression of CD40L, showing 50% of the maximal staining even 24 hours poststimulation, but fell rapidly by 48 hours (Castle et al., 1993; Roy et al., 1993). Simultaneous engagement of the T cell costimulatory molecule CD28 by MAb enhances CD40L expression (Klaus et al, 1994; Ding et al 1995). Highly purified peripheral blood γ/δ T cells also express CD40L after stimulation (Horner et al., 1995). The kinetics of mRNA synthesis and surface expression closely resembles that of α/β T cells, but the levels are much lower. Although the physiological significance of this observation needs to be assessed, it suggests a mechanism by which γ/δ T cells might be able to provide helper function in isotype switching.

Mature thymocytes express functional CD40L on their surface, and CD40 is also functionally expressed on thymic epithelial cells and dendritic cells, a finding suggesting that the CD40/CD40L system may play a role in T cell development. Indeed, negative selection of endogenously expressed antigens and superantigens were blocked by the administration of antibodies to CD40 ligand, illustrating a role for CD40 ligand in thymic selection (Foy et al., 1995).

CD40L expression is developmentally regulated. Immature CD4+ CD8+ human thymocytes obtained from infants (3 months to 2 years of age) failed to express CD40L upon activation. In contrast, CD4+ thymocytes, but not CD8+ thymocytes, expressed CD40L and could induce B cells to undergo isotype switching to IgE in the presence of IL-4 (Fuleihan et al., 1995). Newborn T cells were found to be deficient in CD40L expression and in their ability to induce isotype switching in B cells (Brugnoni et al., 1994; Fuleihan et al., 1994a; Durandy et al., 1995; Nonoyama et al., 1995). The ability of T cells to express CD40L improved by 1 month of age and reached a plateau by late adolescence (Brugnoni et al., 1996). In keeping with this finding, infants below 6 months of age tend to express low amounts of CD40L compared to that in older subjects (Gilmour et al., 2003).

Cyclosporin A (CsA) inhibits the surface and mRNA expression of CD40L in human (Fuleihan et al., 1994b) and murine (Roy et al., 1993) T cells. CsA is a naturally occurring immunosupressant that binds to its cellular receptor(s), cyclophilin, forming a complex that inhibits the activity of the phosphoprotein phosphatase calcineurin. Calcineurin dephosphorylates the cytoplasmic subunit of the transcription factor, NFAT, which translocates into the nucleus to form the functional NFAT complex and regulates the expression of the gene encoding IL-2 (Jain et al., 1993). The transcription of CD40L mRNA and the surface expression of the protein is inhibited by pretreatment of T cells with CsA in a dose-dependent manner. The ability of CsA analogues to inhibit CD40L expression correlated with the affinity of the cyclophilin drug complex to calcineurin and not with the affinity of the drug to cyclophilin. These results suggest that transcription factors activated by calcineurin, such as NFAT, regulate the transcription of the CD40L gene. This regulatory mechanism was borne out experimentally as described below.

The corticosteroid hydrocortisone up-regulates CD40L mRNA expression in peripheral blood mononuclear cells (PBMCs) and surface expression of CD40L in PBMCs as well as in purified populations of T and B cells. Furthermore, hydrocortisone induces IgE synthesis in IL-4-stimulated normal human B cells but fails to induce IgE synthesis in B cells from CD40L-deficient patients. Disruption of CD40L–CD40 interaction by soluble CD40–Ig fusion protein or anti-CD40L MAb blocked the capacity of hydrocortisone to induce IgE synthesis in normal B cells. Up-regulation of CD40L mRNA and induction of IgE synthesis by hydrocortisone were inhibited by the steroid hormone receptor antagonist RU-486 (Jabara et al., 2001). These results indicate that ligand-mediated activation of the glucocorticoid receptor (GR) up-regulates CD40L expression in human lymphocytes. It is possible that hydrocortisone acts by inducing GR binding to glucocorticoid-responsive elements present in the CD40L promoter.

Table 19.1. NFAT-Like Sequences in Murine and Human *CD4OL* Gene Promoter/Enhancer Region

Orientation Relative to ORF	Sequence	Position From Transcription Start Site
Murine		
NM-1 (+)	-AAGCACATTTTCCAGGAA-	−57 to −74
NM-2 (−)	-GCAGTATTTTCCTATTG-	−266 to −283
NLM-1 (+)	-TTTGTCACTTTCCTTGAA-	−327 to −310
NM-3 (+)	-AAAGTCTTTTTCCTTAGC-	−935 to −918
NM-4 (−)	-AAATGAGTTTTCCAAATG-	−999 to −1016
NLM-2 (+)	-AAGCAATTTTACCAGTTT-	−1152 to −1169
Human		
1 (+)	-AAGCACATTTTCCAGGAA-	−57 to −74
2 (−)	-GCAGTATTTTCCTATCAC-	−254 to −269
3 (+)	-TTTGTCACTTTCCTTGAA-	−296 to −314

NM, NFAT motifs; NLM, NFAT-like motifs; ORF, open reading frame; +, orientation same as that of ORF; −, opposite orientation.

The organization of the murine and human *CD40L* genes shows remarkable conservation even in the 5′ upstream regulatory sequences. The transcription originates from a G residue 68 bp upstream from the A of the initiation codon in both species (Tsitsikov et al., 1994; Schubert et al., 1995). Within 1.2 kb from the transcription start site, the mouse gene has four motifs that contain the invariant TTTTCC sequence found in the two NFAT binding motifs (NM) and two NFAT-like motifs (NLM) of the murine IL-2 gene (Table 19.1). The NM-1, NM-2, and the NLM-1 motifs are conserved in the human gene; however, the NM-3, NM-4, and NLM-2 motifs are not. It may be noted that the position and orientation of the NFAT binding motifs in the human gene are identical to those of the equivalent NFAT motifs in the murine gene. A detailed study of the most proximal NM sites in the murine system showed that this sequence formed two complexes on electrophoretic mobility shift analyses (EMSA) and that mutation of the TTTTCC sequence but not of the flanking sequences abolished the capacity to inhibit complex formation (Tsytsykova et al., 1996). Both complexes were sensitive to CsA and contained NFATc and NFATp as revealed by supershift analyses. Short (18 bp) oligonucleotides containing the NFAT sites were not supershifted by antisera to Fos and Jun proteins; however, long oligonucleotides (30 bp) bound to AP-1 proteins (Fos and Jun). Trimers of the proximal NFAT (long oligonucleotides) homologous sites were transcriptionally active. These results suggest that NFATp and/or related proteins play an important role in expression of the CD40L gene. Similar results have been obtained with human CD4 cells (Schubert et al., 1995).

Clinical and Pathological Manifestations of CD40 Ligand Deficiency

Most patients with CD40L deficiency (XHIGM) present in infancy with recurrent upper and lower respiratory tract infections and have a unique predisposition to *Pneumocystis carinii* pneumonia (PCP) (Levitt et al., 1983; Benkerrou et al., 1990; Notarangelo et al., 1992; Banatvala et al., 1994; Conley et al., 1994; Kraakman et al., 1995). In some cases, PCP may even mark the clinical onset of the disease (Marshall et al., 1964; Ochs and Wedgwood, 1989; Levy et al., 1997; Winkelstein et al., 2003). The frequency of PCP in XHIGM varies from 31.7% to

48.1% in the European and U.S. series of patients (Winkelstein et al., 2003; L. Notarangelo et al., unpublished observation). Lung infections may also be due to cytomegalovirus, cryptococcus, and mycobacteria, including bacillus Calmette-Guerin (Levy et al., 1997). In some cases, disseminated cryptococcosis, histoplasmosis, or mycobacterial infection may ensue (Kyong et al., 1978; Tu et al., 1991; Banatvala et al., 1994; Hostoffer et al., 1994; Iseki et al., 1994; Tabone et al., 1994; Levy et al., 1997).

Diarrhea, a frequent finding, occurs in over 50% of XHIGM patients (Notarangelo et al., 1992; Levy et al., 1997; Winkelstein et al., 2003) and may become chronic, requiring total parenteral nutrition to avoid severe growth failure. Chronic watery diarrhea is often associated with *Cryptosporidium* infection (Stiehm et al., 1986) that may also contribute to sclerosing cholangitis—a severe and often fatal complication (DiPalma et al., 1986; Banatvala et al., 1994; Hayward et al., 1997; Levy et al., 1997; Winkelstein et al., 2003). The incidence of liver and biliary tract disease increases with age (Hayward et al., 1997).

Oral ulcers and proctitis are common manifestations (Hong et al., 1962; Kyong et al., 1978; Rieger et al., 1980; Benkerrou et al., 1990; Notarangelo et al., 1992; Banatvala et al., 1994; Macchi et al., 1995) and are usually associated with neutropenia, either chronic (Aruffo et al., 1993; Levy et al., 1997) or cyclic (Notarangelo et al., 1992; Wang et al., 1994; Shimadzu et al., 1995).

Patients with mutations of CD40L are at increased risk for neoplasms, most often lymphomas (Filipovich et al., 1994) but also liver/biliary tract and gastrointestinal tumors, which are rarely observed in other primary immunodeficiencies (Facchetti et al., 1995; Hayward et al., 1997). Autoimmune manifestations may occur in X-linked forms of HIGM but more so in autosomal forms. These may lead to arthritis, thrombocytopenia, hemolytic anemia, hypoparathyroidism, or immune complex–mediated nephritis (Pascual-Salcedo et al., 1983; Benkerrou et al., 1990; Hollenbaugh et al., 1994). Anemia is present in about 25% of XHIGM patients (Notarangelo et al., 1992) and may be secondary to chronic infections or to parvovirus B19-induced red blood cell aplasia. The latter may even be the only manifestation of disease in patients with a mild phenotype (Seyama et al., 1998a).

Severe neurological involvement has also been reported (Banatvala et al., 1994; Levy et al., 1997, Ziegner et al., 2002). Meningoencephalitis due to enterovirus infection may occur, despite regular administration of intravenous immunoglobulins (IVIG) (Cunningham et al., 1999; Halliday et al., 2003).

Lymph nodes of XHIGM patients lack germinal centers (Rosen et al., 1961; Hong et al., 1962; Stiehm and Fudenberg, 1966; Facchetti et al., 1995) (Color Plate 19. I). This is the consequence of ineffective CD40–CD40L interaction in the extrafollicular areas, resulting in poor recruitment of germinal-center precursors. In addition, severe depletion and phenotypic abnormalities of follicular dendritic cells have been reported in XHIGM that may contribute to poor antigen trapping and result in inefficient rescue of the few germinal-center B cells from apoptosis (Facchetti et al., 1995). Bone marrow examination in patients with concurrent neutropenia often reveals a block of myeloid differentiation at the myelocyte/promyelocyte stage (Hong et al., 1962; Kyong et al., 1978; Benkerrou et al., 1990; Notarangelo et al., 1992). By contrast, serum levels of granulocyte colony-stimulating factor (G-CSF) in neutropenic XHIGM patients are normal or elevated (Wang et al., 1994).

A European registry of CD40L-deficient patients has been organized that includes clinical, immunological, and molecular data. The registry is fully accessible through at http://bioinf

.uta.fi/CD40Lbase/index2.html. A similar registry has been set up in the United States by USIDnet.

Laboratory Findings

Immunoglobulin levels

Like all forms of HIGM, XHIGM is characterized by markedly reduced serum IgG, IgA, and IgE with normal to elevated IgM levels and a normal number of circulating B cells (Geha et al., 1979; Levy et al., 1987; Notarangelo et al., 1992; Winkelstein et al., 2003). Variability of IgM serum levels has been reported among affected members of the same family, indicating that increased IgM may reflect chronic antigenic stimulation rather than the direct effect of a molecular defect (Kroczek et al., 1994).

In a series of 56 XHIGM patients, the majority (53%) had normal IgM serum levels at the time of diagnosis (Levy et al., 1997). It appears that IgM serum levels increase with age, particularly if initiation of IVIG substitution therapy is delayed (Levy et al., 1997). In a recent study, however, as many as one-quarter of patients with confirmed CD40L deficiency had low concentrations of serum IgM, indicating that even low-serum IgM should not preclude testing for CD40L deficiency (Gilmour et al., 2003). Although serum levels of IgG, IgA, and IgE are normally very low, exceptional cases with elevated IgA, IgE, or even IgG have been reported in patients with severe defects in the CD40L gene (Levy et al., 1997; L. Notarangelo, unpublished observation), indicating that environmental and/or additional molecular mechanisms other than CD40L are involved in isotype switch.

Levels of specific antibodies of the IgM isotype (e.g., isohemagglutinins, Forssman antibodies) are normal (Rosen et al., 1961; Kyong et al., 1978; Benkerrou et al., 1990). Immunization with T-dependent antigens (e.g., bacteriophage ϕx174) leads to reduced primary and secondary IgM antibody responses, whereas there is little or no production of IgG-specific antibodies following recall immunization (Stiehm and Fudenberg, 1966; Benkerrou et al., 1990; Nonoyama et al., 1993). In addition, analysis of V_H gene segments in patients with CD40L mutations has revealed a lower frequency of somatic mutations in IgM-expressing B cells than that in controls (Chu et al., 1995; Razanajaona et al., 1996). This finding is in keeping with the observed lower affinity of antibodies produced by XHIM patients in response to vaccination.

Defects of immunoglobulin isotype switching and of somatic mutations are a direct consequence of the underlying genetic defect. Because of the inability to express functional CD40L trimers, activated T cells are unable to provide a key helper signal for terminal B cell differentiation. The functional integrity of XHIGM B cells, by contrast, initially suggested by the historical experiments performed by Mayer et al. (1986), is best illustrated by intact CSR and the production of IgG, IgA, or IgE upon in vitro coculture of PBMCs with anti-CD40 MAb (or soluble CD40L) and appropriate cytokines, such as IL-4 and IL-10 (Allen et al., 1993a; Aruffo et al., 1993; Durandy et al., 1993; Fuleihan et al., 1993a; Korthauer et al., 1993; Callard et al., 1994; Saiki et al., 1995).

B and T lymphocytes

The demonstration of normal numbers of circulating B cells allows differentiation from X-linked agammaglobulinemia. As a rule, circulating B cells from XHIGM patients express IgM

Table 19.2. Synopsis of Laboratory Findings in X-Linked Form of Hyper-IgM (CD40L Deficiency)

Assay	Typical Phenotype	Percent of XHIGM Patients Showing Phenotype*
Immunological Features		
Serum IgG	<2 SD below normal range	100
Serum IgA (mg/dl)	Undetectable	93
Serum IgM (mg/dl)	Normal	53 (at diagnosis)[†]
	Elevated	47 (at diagnosis)[†]
Antibody response to T-dependent antigens ($\phi \times 174$)	Lack of specific IgG production	100[‡]
B cell count	Normal	90
CD4[+] cell count	Normal	94
CD8[+] cell count	Normal	98
Proliferative response to PHA	Normal (>50,000 cpm)	93
Proliferative response to T-dependent antigens	Often reduced (<5000 cpm)	37
CD40L expression**		
As assessed with CD40-Ig	Absent	Nearly 100[††]
As assessed with MAb	Usually absent	95
As assessed with polclonal antiserum	Detectable in some cases	23
Hematological Features		
Neutropenia	Generally present (mostly chronic)	68
Anemia	Often present	32

*Unless differently specified, data are from Levy et al. (1997).

[†]Elevated levels of IgM are detected in 70% of patients during follow-up.

[‡]From Nonoyama et al. (1993).

**From a series of 22 patients analyzed at the Department of Pediatrics, University of Brescia, Italy.

[††]Activated CD4[+] T cells from patients with missense mutations in intracytoplasmic or transmembrane domains of CD40L may occasionally react with CD40-Ig (Seyama et al., 1998b).

and/or IgD, but not other isotypes (Levitt et al., 1983; Benkerrou et al., 1990). Since CD40L–CD40 interaction is essential for memory B cell generation, the number of circulating IgD⁻CD27⁺ switched memory B cells is strongly diminished in patients with CD40L mutations (Agematsu et al., 1998).

In spite of the T cell nature of the defect in XHIGM, the number and distribution of T cell subsets are normal, although the proportion of CD45R0⁺ primed T cells is reduced (Jain et al., 1999). In vitro proliferative responses to mitogens are also normal in these patients (Benkerrou et al., 1990; Ameratunga et al., 1997; Levy et al., 1997). In contrast, in vitro proliferative response to antigens is often reduced (Ameratunga et al., 1997; Levy et al., 1997). A defect in TH1 responses has been reported, with reduced secretion of interferon-γ (IFN-γ) and failure to induce antigen-presenting cells to synthesize IL-12 (Jain et al., 1999; Subauste et al., 1999). Finally, T cells from patients with CD40L mutations are unable to provide help for the antibody response to polysaccharide antigens. This deficit further contributes to the susceptibility to infections observed in patients with XHIGM (Jeurissen et al., 2004). A summary of laboratory features typically observed in XHIGM is shown in Table 19.2.

Molecular Basis of CD40 Ligand Deficiency

By means of linkage analysis, the XHIGM locus was originally assigned to Xq24–27 (Mensink et al., 1987) and subsequently mapped to Xq26.3–27 (Padayachee et al., 1992, 1993). Cloning of the human *CD40L/TNFSF5* gene and coincidental mapping to the same region of the X chromosome (Graf et al., 1992) were

soon followed by the recognition that mutations of *CD40L* account for XHIGM (Allen et al., 1993a; Aruffo et al., 1993; DiSanto et al., 1993; Fuleihan et al., 1993b; Korthauer et al., 1993). More accurate mapping (Pilia et al., 1994) and elucidation of the organization of the *CD40L/TNFSF5* gene (Villa et al., 1994; Shimadzu et al., 1995) have since been provided. The human *CD40L/TNFSF5* gene encompasses about 13 kb of genomic DNA and is organized in five exons and four introns. Definition of the exon–intron boundaries has enabled a search for mutations at the genomic level (Villa et al., 1994; Lin et al., 1996).

CD40L mutations

Since 1993, a long list of distinct mutations of the *CD40L/TN-FSF5* gene have been identified in multiple unrelated XHIGM families. Figure 19.2 illustrates the mutations identified in 128 patients included in the European CD40Lbase Registry. Although mutations may affect the entire gene, they are unequally distributed and the majority are located in exon 5, which contains most of the TNF-homology domain (Hollenbaugh et al., 1992).

Missense mutations are the most common cause of the disease. In addition, one single amino acid change (Arg81Trp) that does not lead to diminished CD40 binding or to clinical or immunological abnormalities has been described and should therefore be considered a rare polymorphism (Bajorath et al., 1996). In some cases, for example, the Trp140stop mutation, premature termination is compatible with expression of a truncated molecule at the cell surface, as shown by staining with polyclonal anti-CD40L antibody (Korthauer et al., 1993, Seyama et al., 1998b). Small insertions or deletions are also common; these

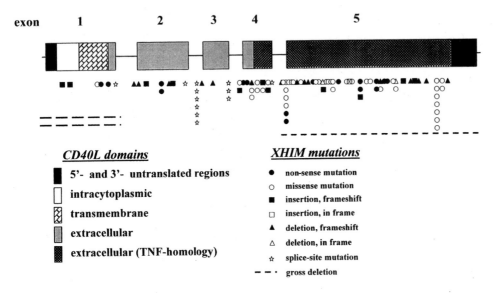

exon   1   2   3   4   5

CD40L domains

- ■ 5'- and 3'- untranslated regions
- ▢ intracytoplasmic
- ▨ transmembrane
- ▦ extracellular
- ■ extracellular (TNF-homology)

XHIM mutations

- ● non-sense mutation
- ○ missense mutation
- ■ insertion, frameshift
- ▢ insertion, in frame
- ▲ deletion, frameshift
- △ deletion, in frame
- ☆ splice-site mutation
- – – · gross deletion

Figure 19.2. Description of CD40L mutations identified in 128 patients enrolled in the European CD40Lbase Registry. The various mutations reported in families with X-linked form of hyper-IgM syndrome are shown with different symbols, as indicated in the figure, and aligned along the CD40L cDNA schema.

may be due to polymerase slippage, occurring at sites of nucleotide duplications or tandem repeats in the CD40L sequence (Macchi et al., 1995). A few patients with two different mutations have been described (Aruffo et al., 1993; Grammer et al., 1995; Lin et al., 1996).

The finding that several apparently unrelated families share mutations at the same codon has led to the hypothesis that hotspot mutations in the *CD40L/TNFSF5* gene exist. In particular, several families have been reported with mutations affecting codon 140 (Korthauer et al., 1993; Iseki et al., 1994; Macchi et al., 1995; Saiki et al., 1995; Bajorath et al., 1996; Notarangelo et al., 1996; Seyama et al., 1998b; Lee et al., 2005) or with the Leu155Pro mutation (Allen et al., 1993a; Lin et al., 1996; Notarangelo et al., 1996) or the Thr254Met substitution (Bajorath et al., 1996; Notarangelo et al., 1996, Lee et al., 2005). Recurrence of mutations at these codons is not due to the presence of CpG dinucleotides.

Investigation of the effect of amino acid substitutions on CD40L expression and function, studied through several approaches, has contributed to definition of the role that single residues play in determining folding, assembling, and CD40-binding properties of CD40L. For some naturally occurring mutations, transfectants that express surface membrane or soluble forms of mutant CD40L molecules have been generated. The mutagenized recombinants fail to bind CD40-Ig or to induce B cell proliferation and immunoglobulin secretion in the presence of IL-4 (Allen et al., 1993a; Aruffo et al., 1993).

Functional aspects of CD40L deficiency

Human CD40L belongs to the TNF family (Hollenbaugh et al., 1992). Interestingly, when one considers the missense mutations that affect the TNF-like domain of CD40L, a remarkable proportion (9 out of 24, or 37.5%) affect residues that are identical between CD40L and TNF, whereas the sequence identity between these molecules in the region is only 24.7%. Despite the rather limited sequence identity of the CD40L TNF-like domain with TNF (27.3%), the homology is sufficient to allow computer modeling based on the crystal structures available for TNF and for the TNF/TNFR complex (Jones et al., 1989; Eck and Sprang, 1991; Banner et al., 1993). Thus, models have been generated for

murine (Peitsch and Jongeneel, 1993) and human (Bajorath et al., 1995a, 1995b; Notarangelo et al., 1996) CD40L, and an X-ray structure of the extracellular portion of human CD40L has been produced (Karpusas et al., 1995). Analogous to TNF, CD40L forms a trimer and exhibits a remarkably similar overall fold, with the extracellular portion assuming the shape of a truncated pyramid (Karpusas et al., 1995). A disulfide bond between Cys178 and Cys218 stabilizes the top of the molecule. The CD40 binding site consists of a shallow groove formed between two monomers. Buried and solvent-accessible residues of the CD40L molecule have been identified (Bajorath et al., 1995a, 1995b; Karpusas et al., 1995). Interestingly, of several residues predicted to be directly involved in CD40 binding, only one (Gly144) has been found mutated in an XHIGM patient (Macchi et al., 1995). In addition, only a few residues (Lys143, Tyr145, Tyr146, Arg203, and Gln220) appear to be really critical for CD40 binding, as shown by in vitro mutagenesis studies (Bajorath et al., 1995a, 1995b). The crystal structure of the extracellular portion of CD40L has indeed shown that both hydrophobic and hydrophilic residues form the surface of the CD40 binding site (Karpusas et al., 1995). In addition, a number of buried residues appear to be important for proper monomer folding and trimer formation. The location of mutations that occur in XHIGM patients has been compared to that in the CD40L model. Ser128 and Glu129 (which have both been reported to be mutated) lie close to Lys143 in the three-dimensional structure. Since Lys143 is involved in CD40 binding, it is likely that mutations at codons 128 and 129 disturb ligand–receptor interaction (Karpusas et al., 1995; Bajorath et al., 1996). Similarly, Val126 and Leu155 (also mutated in XHIGM) participate in the formation of a hydrophobic core that is very close to residues 143–145, which are involved in CD40 binding; it is predicted that these mutations also affect the CD40 binding property of CD40L. Finally, three additional mutations (Thr147Asn, Thr211Asp, Gly250Ala) involve residues that are either buried (Thr147) or exposed (Thr211, Gly250) and are located at the interface between monomers; they participate in the formation of three equivalent CD40 binding sites, one per interface between monomers. Mutation at these residues should also affect CD40 binding (Bajorath et al., 1996).

However, the majority of missense mutations reported in XHIGM do not involve the CD40 binding site. The amino acids affected may participate in the generation of the hydrophobic core, so mutations at these residues compromise core packing and folding of the monomer (this is the case for Trp140Arg, Trp140Cys, Trp140Gly, Leu232Ser, Ala235Pro, Val237Glu, Thr254Met, and Leu258Ser) (Bajorath et al., 1996). Alternatively, they may involve buried residues at the interface between monomers; mutations at these sites are likely to disturb trimer formation, as predicted for Ala123Glu, Tyr170Cys, Tyr172His, and Gly227Val (Karpusas et al., 1995; Bajorath et al., 1996). Finally, the single amino acid substitution Met36Arg in the transmembrane domain of CD40L introduces a polar residue in a very hydrophobic sequence, thus inhibiting membrane expression of the protein (Korthauer et al., 1993).

Strategy for Diagnosis

The diagnosis of XHIGM is usually accomplished by demonstrating in vitro the inability of activated patient CD4$^+$ T cells to express functional CD40L (CD154) molecules, as assessed by binding soluble CD40-Ig chimeric constructs. Monoclonal antibodies to CD40L are often used to stain activated CD4$^+$ T cells in flow cytometry assays. However, false-negative results may be obtained because occasionally monoclonal antibodies recognize mutant forms of CD40L expressed at the cell surface. This phenomenon is even more common when polyclonal antisera to CD40L are used in the staining procedure, as they may recognize even truncated forms of the protein (Seyama et al., 1998b). Therefore, polyclonal antisera to CD40L should not be used for diagnosis. Although rare, even the chimeric CD40-Ig molecule may bind to mutant CD40L, particularly in patients with missense mutations in the transmembrane or cytoplasmic domains, which are permissive for membrane protein expression (Seyama et al., 1998a, 1998b; Lee et al., 2005). Ultimately, mutation analysis at the CD40L/TNFSF5 locus may be required for a definitive diagnosis.

A number of critical factors should be considered when performing diagnostic assays for XHIGM. First, appropriate controls for T cell activation (e.g., expression of CD69) should be included. This is particularly important to distinguish XHIGM from common variable immunodeficiency (CVID); a subgroup of CVID patients have defective CD40L expression in the context of a broader T cell activation defect (Farrington et al., 1994). Second, because CD40L is preferentially expressed by activated CD4$^+$ cells (Lane et al., 1992), the proportion of CD4$^+$ T cells in the patient should be analyzed. This is particularly important when a more simple whole-blood assay is used to evaluate CD40L expression (Gilmour et al., 2003). It has been recognized that activated T cells from patients with major histocompatibility complex (MHC) class II deficiency fail to express CD40L because of the markedly reduced proportion of CD4$^+$ T lymphocytes (Callard et al., 1994). Third, the age of the proband has to be considered. There is ample evidence showing that expression of CD40L by activated neonatal T cells is physiologically reduced (Brugnoni et al., 1994; Fuleihan et al., 1994a; Durandy et al., 1995; Nonoyama et al., 1995), making flow cytometry unsuitable for diagnosis of XHIGM in neonates. Defects of CD40L could not be demonstrated in autosomal forms of HIGM (Callard et al., 1994; Oliva et al., 1995), therefore, analysis of CD40L expression is particularly important for the correct diagnosis of sporadic HIGM in males, as it

allows distinction between XHIGM and autosomal forms of HIGM.

As mentioned above, definitive confirmation of CD40L deficiency can be achieved through molecular studies. Investigation of mutations at the DNA level has become possible following elucidation of the genomic structure of the CD40L/TNFSF5 gene (Villa et al., 1994; Shimadzu et al., 1995). This information has in turn allowed diagnosis even when viable lymphocytes for studying CD40L expression are not available.

Carrier Detection and Prenatal Diagnosis

In contrast to carriers of other X-linked immunodeficiencies (e.g., X-linked agammaglobulinemia [XLA]; X-linked severe combined immunodeficiency [X-SCID]; Wiskott-Aldrich Syndrome [WAS]), carrier females of XHIGM exhibit a random pattern of X inactivation. This was originally established in mature, IgG- and IgA-positive B lymphocytes (Hendricks et al., 1990), indicating the integrity of the B cell machinery for isotype switching. Following the demonstration that XHIGM is caused by mutations of the CD40L/TNFSF5 gene, it was shown that two populations of circulating T lymphocytes (one expressing the wild-type CD40L allele and the other expressing the mutated one) are present in XHIGM carriers (Hollenbaugh et al., 1994). In carriers with skewed lyonization, no clinical or immunological abnormalities are found, indicating that limited CD40L expression is sufficient to induce isotype switching and normal generation of memory B cells (Callard et al., 1994; Hollenbaugh et al., 1994). However, extreme lyonization with selective expression of the mutant form of CD40L may result in an overt clinical phenotype (de Saint Basile et al., 1999).

Carrier detection is best achieved with molecular assays targeted at the CD40L/TNFSF5 locus. In families with clear X-linked inheritance linkage analysis can be performed, taking advantage of two sets of hypervariable microsatellites at the 3′ untranslated region of the CD40L/TNFSF5 gene (Allen et al., 1993b; DiSanto et al., 1993, 1994; Gauchat et al., 1993a; Ramesh et al., 1994; Shimadzu et al., 1995). Whenever the mutation is known, DNA sequencing, with a search for heterozygosity for the specific mutation, is the most simple and direct way to attempt carrier detection (Villa et al., 1994; Shimadzu et al., 1995; Lin et al., 1996). Occasionally, heterozygosity for the mutation (e.g., carrier detection) can also be performed at the cDNA level, as for splice-site mutations that cause exon skipping (DiSanto et al., 1993; Hollenbaugh et al., 1994).

In families with clear X-linked inheritance, prenatal diagnosis can be safely attempted at 10 weeks gestation on chorionic villi DNA by means of segregation analysis with hypervariable microsatellites at the 3′ untranslated region of the CD40L gene (DiSanto et al., 1994). Characterization of organization of the CD40L/TNFSF5 gene allows prenatal diagnosis even in families with sporadic presentation, provided that the mutation is known (Villa et al., 1994).

Despite the reduced ability of activated T cells from neonates to express CD40L (Brugnoni et al., 1994; Fuleihan et al., 1994a; Durandy et al., 1995; Nonoyama et al., 1995), surface membrane CD40L was detected on activated T cells from 19 to 28-week-old fetuses (Durandy et al., 1995). However, because of the obviously complex developmental control of CD40L expression, staining for CD40L on fetal cord blood T lymphocytes should not be used as the sole technique for prenatal diagnosis of XHIGM.

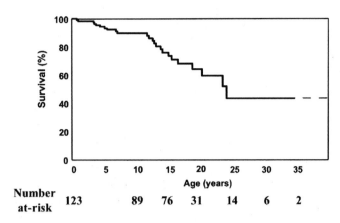

Figure 19.3. Cumulative survival curve of 128 patients with the X-linked form of hyper-IgM enrolled in the European Registry. The number of patients at various ages is shown at the bottom of the panel.

Treatment and Prognosis

The long-term prognosis of XHIGM appears to be worse than that in other forms of congenital hypogammaglobulinemia, for example, XLA. The cumulative survival curve for 128 XHIGM patients enrolled in the European Registry is shown in Figure 19.3, with 30 of 128 patients having died. The mortality is somewhat lower in the U.S. series (8 deceased out of 79 subjects), possibly reflecting a lower incidence of sclerosing cholangitis and irreversible liver damage (Winkelstein et al., 2003). The main causes of death include infections early in life and, later on, severe liver disease and malignant tumors (Hayward et al., 1997; Levy et al., 1997).

The complex array of clinical manifestations and the increased risk of opportunistic infections and chronic neutropenia require multiple therapeutic approaches. Regular infusion of IVIG (400–600 mg/kg every 21 to 28 days) is the most important form of treatment. It significantly reduces the severity and frequency of infections (Levy et al., 1997) and may occasionally correct neutropenia (Banatvala et al., 1994; Levy et al., 1997). In view of the higher risk for severe clinical manifestations, patients suffering from XHIGM often require more aggressive treatment. Continuous prophylaxis with cotrimoxazole has been advocated to prevent PCP (Notarangelo et al., 1992; Banatvala et al., 1994) and has in fact proven effective (Levy et al., 1997). Long-term treatment with amphotericin B and flucytosine are necessary for cryptococcosis (Iseki et al., 1994; Tabone et al., 1994). Patients with severe neutropenia may benefit from treatment with recombinant G-CSF; in some cases, this approach has caused a change from chronic to cyclic neutropenia (Wang et al., 1994; Shimadzu et al., 1995). Total parenteral nutrition may be necessary in patients with protracted diarrhea and malabsorption, particularly if these are due to *Cryptosporidium* (Benkerrou et al., 1990). *Cryptosporidium* infection should be prevented by using filtered or sterile water and treated with azythromycin or nitazoxanide. Early detection of *Cryptosporidium* infection is best achieved by PCR-based amplification of stool DNA and microscopy of bile fluid (McLauchlin et al., 2003).

Despite these efforts, the mortality rate remains high (Levy et al., 1997), as illustrated in Figure 19.3. Therefore, more radical forms of treatment have been proposed. Successful hematopoietic stem cells transplantation (HSCT) from a human leukocyte antigen (HLA)-identical sibling or matched unrelated donor (Thomas et al., 1995; Levy et al., 1997; Bordigoni et al., 1998;

Scholl et al., 1998; Kato et al., 1999; Kawai et al., 1999; Gennery et al., 2000; Duplantier et al., 2001) or partially matched cord blood (Ziegner et al., 2001) have been reported. However, in a recent series of 38 XHIGM patients treated by HSCT, a high mortality rate (31.6%) was observed (Gennery et al., 2004). In all cases, death was from infections. Importantly, preexisting lung disease was associated with a poor outcome. Nonmyeloablative HSCT has been successfully used in an XHIGM patient with severe liver disease (Jacobsohn et al., 2004). It should be noted that lack of a strict genotype–phenotype correlation in XHIGM prevents selection for bone marrow transplantation of those patients at high risk for mortality.

While attempts to treat severe liver disease (sclerosing cholangitis, cirrhosis) with liver transplantation usually fail because of relapse of the disease in the transplanted organ (Hayward et al., 1997; Levy et al., 1997), more promising results have been achieved in severely ill patients with a combined bone marrow and cadaveric orthotopic liver transplantation (Hadzic et al., 2000).

The recognition that expression of the *CD40L/TNFSF5* gene is under tight regulatory control makes gene therapy a less viable option, particularly since deregulated expression of CD40L in transgenic mice has been shown to result in tumor development (Brown et al., 1998; Sacco et al., 2000). Use of lentiviral vectors might enable insertion of autologous regulatory gene elements (Barry et al., 2000), thus making gene therapy–based treatment with acceptable risks possible in the future. However, the finding that mutant forms of CD40L interact with wild-type molecules and prevent expression of functional trimers (Seyama et al., 1999; Su et al., 2001) raises further doubts that gene therapy could become an effective form of treatment for XHIGM. These problems may be circumvented by *trans*-splicing (a process by which two different pre-mRNAs are joined by the cellular splicing apparatus), which allows complementation of the gene defect while preserving the natural regulation and cell specificity of CD40L expression. Indeed, this strategy has been successfully used to correct a murine model of CD40L deficiency (Tahara et al., 2004).

Clinical and Pathological Manifestations of CD40 Deficiency

Defective expression of CD40 by B lymphocytes (CD40 deficiency, HIGM3) has been detected in four children from three unrelated families with autosomal recessive HIGM (Ferrari et al., 2001; Kutukculer et al., 2003). Clinical and immunological data at presentation (Table 19.3) were very similar to those observed in XHIGM, but autosomal recessive inheritance was indicated by parental consanguinity and by the fact that three of the four patients are female. Patient 1, an 8-year-old Italian girl, suffered from PCP at 4 months of age and had another episode of pneumonia at age 2, when she was found to be panhypogammaglobulinemic and was started on IVIG treatment. Patients 2 and 3 are first cousins from a multiply related Arabian family. Patient 2 is a 5-year-old male who suffered from recurrent pneumonia, hypogammaglobulinemia with elevated IgM, and neutropenia. Patient 3 is a 7-year-old female who also experienced recurrent lower respiratory tract infections. She was diagnosed with HIGM at 8 months of age, and substitution treatment with IVIG was started. At 3 years of age, she was admitted to a pediatric intensive care unit for severe interstitial pneumonia. Patient 4, a 12-month-old Turkish girl born to consanguineous parents, was hospitalized for respiratory distress. She developed necrotizing pneumonia caused by *Pseudomonas aeruginosa* and

Table 19.3. Clinical and Immunological Features of Four Patients with CD40 Deficiency

	Patient 1	Patient 2*	Patient 3*	Patient 4
Clinical Features				
Current age (years)/gender	8/F	5/M	7/F	Deceased/F
Age at onset (months)	4	6	8	12
Recurrent URTI/LRTI	+	+	+	+
Interstitial pneumonia	+(PCP)	−	+	+
Immunological Investigations				
Serum IgG (mg/dl)	180	<100	<100	<146
Serum IgA	<6.6	<6.6	<6.6	<5.6
Serum IgM	81	400	200	80
CD3 (%)	73	75	76	56
CD4 (%)	55	35	34	24
CD8 (%)	13	24	19	34
CD19(%)	16	19	20	35
CD40 (%)	0	0	0	0
In vitro response to PHA (cpm)	124,200	122,000	138,000	115,000

*Patient 2 and Patient 3 are first cousins.

PCP, *Pneumocystis carinii* pneumonia; PHA, phytohemagglutinin; URTI/LRTI, Upper and lower respiratory tract infections.

chronic watery diarrhea due to *Cryptosporidium parvum*, which was also isolated from tracheal aspirates, indicating disseminated infection. She received a matched-sibling stem cell transplantation but died of cardiorespiratory arrest at day 16 post-transplant. All four children had very low levels of IgG and IgA, and two had increased serum IgM levels. Lymphocyte numbers and subset distributions were normal, as were in vitro proliferative responses to mitogens. In contrast to observations consistently seen in XHIGM, B cells from these patients could not be induced to secrete IgG and IgA upon in vitro activation with anti-CD40 MAb and IL-10, a result indicating a B cell intrinsic defect.

Functional Aspects of CD40 Deficiency

Immunophenotypic analysis showed that circulating B cells and monocytes lacked surface membrane CD40. The protein was also undetectable intracellularly in patient 1 (as shown by Western blot analysis of lymphoblastoid B cell lines), whereas an aberrant pattern of migration of the CD40 protein was detected in patient 2. Mutation analysis showed that patient 1 was homozygous for a silent mutation (A-to-T substitution at nucleotide 408, corresponding to the fifth nucleotide of exon 5). However, this mutation involves and disrupts an exonic splicing enhancer, thus preventing incorporation of exon 5 in the mRNA. Consequently, cDNA from this patient lacked 94 nucleotides (matching exon 5), resulting in frameshift and premature termination. Patients 2 and 3 were both homozygous for a C-to-T change at nucleotide 247, resulting in a nonconserved Cys83-to-Arg amino acid substitution. The mutation in patient 4 occurred at position −2 of the acceptor site of intron 3; the resulting use of a cryptic splice site caused a 6 bp deletion in exon 4.

Further investigation of the functional consequences of CD40 deficiency showed that both memory B cell generation and somatic mutation were affected. Dendritic cells, cultured with TNF-α or with lipopolysaccharide (LPS) combined with IFN-γ, displayed a consistent defect in their ability to induce proliferation of allogeneic T cells and secretion of IFN-γ. The defective costimulatory activity of dendritic cells derived from patients with CD40 deficiency was associated with lower cell surface levels of MHC class II antigen and with a decreased release of IL-12. These findings support the notion that CD40 deficiency is not an exclusive defect of humoral immunity but should be considered a combined defect of B and T cell compartments (Fontana et al., 2003).

Strategy for Diagnosis

The diagnosis of CD40 deficiency is usually made by demonstrating the inability of peripheral blood B cells to constitutively express CD40 molecules, assessed by staining with MAbs to CD40 in patients with clinical features and an immunoglobulin profile suggestive of HIGM. Cytofluorimetric analysis could be considered a reliable technique, as all patients reported with mutations of the *CD40* gene lacked expression of CD40 at the cell surface. However, the possibility of false-negative results, due to recognition of mutant CD40 molecules by the monoclonal antibody, exists. Furthermore, because CD40 is expressed as a trimer, is it theoretically possible that heterozygous mutations that allow expression of CD40 but affect its function may result in an HIGM phenotype through a dominant-negative effect. Ultimately, diagnosis of CD40 deficiency requires mutation analysis.

Treatment and Prognosis

Management of patients with CD40 deficiency is similar to that outlined for patients with CD40L deficiency. Treatment includes regular infusions of IVIG, PCP phrophylaxis, water purification measures to prevent *Cryptosporidium* infection, and monitoring of liver status by ultrasound scanning and biochemical analysis. Compared to CD40L deficiency, the benefits of HSCT in CD40 deficiency are less obvious and remain to be proven, as this strategy would not correct defective CD40 expression on nonhematopoietic cells. Successful immune reconstitution has been recently achieved in a fifth patient with CD40 deficiency by means of hematopoietic stem cell transplantation from a matched sibling (E. Mazzolari, L. Notarangelo, and N. Kutukculer unpublished observation).

Animals Models of CD40 and CD40L Deficiency

Gene Disruption

Mice with disruption of the CD40L gene

CD40L$^{-/-}$ mice exhibit normal percentages of B and T cell subpopulations but display selective deficiencies in humoral immunity. Basal serum immunoglobulin isotype levels are significantly lower than in normal mice, and IgE is undetectable. Furthermore, CD40L-deficient mice fail to mount secondary antigen-specific responses to immunization with T-dependent antigens. By contrast, they produce antigen-specific antibody of all isotypes except IgE in response to thymus-independent antigens. These results underscore the requirement of CD40L for T cell–dependent antibody responses (Renshaw et al., 1994; Xu et al., 1994). Moreover, Ig class switching to isotypes other than IgE can occur in vivo in the absence of CD40L, a phenomenon supporting the notion that alternative B cell signaling pathways regulate responses to thymus-independent antigens.

CD4$^+$ T cells from CD40L$^{-/-}$ mice were fourfold less effective than normal T cells in activating the nitric oxide response in allogeneic macrophages. CD40L$^{-/-}$ T cells fixed with paraformaldehyde after a 6-hour activation period, a time point at which CD40L dominates the macrophage-activating capability of T cells, failed to activate the production of inflammatory cytokines (TNF-α) or the generation of reactive nitrogen intermediates. After 24 hours of activation, however, both CD40L$^{-/-}$ and normal T cells could induce similar but weak responses from activated macrophages (Stout et al., 1996). These studies demonstrate that CD40L$^{-/-}$ mice have a deficient T cell–dependent macrophage-mediated immune response. However, CD40L-deficient mice are able to generate normal primary cytotoxic T cell responses (in spite of a defective humoral response) to a viral infection (Whitmire et al., 1996).

CD40L$^{-/-}$ mice are susceptible to *Pneumocystis carinii* infection (as are CD40$^{-/-}$ mice). Treatment of wild-type mice with soluble CD40L-fusion protein evokes a pulmonary inflammatory response that is not observed in identically treated CD40$^{-/-}$ mice (Wiley et al., 1997). This finding supports evidence that ligation of CD40 results in inflammatory responses and that soluble CD40L is a potent inflammagen that may be important for protection against *P. carinii* infection.

Finally, when injected with *Cryptococcus neoformans*, CD40L$^{-/-}$ mice show increased fungal growth in the brain, associated with reduced production of IL-12, IFN-γ, and nitrites (Pietrella et al., 2004).

Mice with disruption of the CD40 gene

CD40$^{-/-}$ mice have normal numbers of T and B cells, indicating that CD40 is not essential for B cell development. Their B cells fail to proliferate and undergo isotype switching in response to soluble CD40 ligand (sCD40L) and IL-4 but respond normally to LPS in the presence of IL-4. CD40$^{-/-}$ mice completely fail to mount an antigen-specific antibody response or to develop germinal centers following immunization with T cell–dependent antigens, but they respond normally to the T cell–independent antigens. The most noticeable alteration in the serum immunoglobulin levels of young CD40$^{-/-}$ animals is absence of IgE and severe decrease of IgG1 and IgG2a (Castigli et al., 1994; Kawabe et al., 1994). These results indicate an essential role of CD40–CD40L interactions in the antibody response to T cell–dependent antigens and in isotype switching.

B cells deficient in CD40 expression are unable to elicit the proliferation of allogeneic T cells in vitro. More importantly, mice immunized with CD40$^{-/-}$ B cells become tolerant to allogeneic MHC antigens as measured by a mixed lymphocyte reaction and cytotoxic T cell assay. The failure of CD40$^{-/-}$ B cells to serve as antigen-presenting cells in vitro is corrected by the addition of anti-CD28 MAb. Moreover, LPS stimulation, which up-regulates B7 expression, reverses the inability of CD40$^{-/-}$ B cells to stimulate an alloresponse in vitro and abrogates the capacity of these B cells to induce tolerance in vivo (Hollander et al., 1996). These results suggest that CD40 engagement by CD40 ligand expressed on antigen-activated T cells is critical for the up-regulation of B7 molecules on antigen-presenting B cells that subsequently deliver the costimulatory signals necessary for T cell proliferation and differentiation.

In addition to susceptibility to *Pneumocystis carinii* infection, CD40-deficient mice are also prone to *Mycobacterium avium* infection (Florido et al., 2004). Furthermore, when inoculated with the defective murine leukemia retrovirus LP-BM5def, CD40$^{-/-}$ mice become infected and show virus expression similar to that in wild-type mice. However, unlike the wild-type mice, CD40-deficient mice do not develop symptoms of immunodeficiency, lymphoproliferation, and the typical histological changes in the lymphoid tissue (Yu et al., 1999). These results show that the CD40–CD40L interaction in vivo is essential for anergy induction and the subsequent development of immunodeficiency and pathologic expansion of lymphocytes.

Recently it has been shown that CD40$^{-/-}$ adult mice develop neuronal cell dysfunction and gross central nervous system abnormalities with age. These findings suggest that CD40 signaling plays an important role in normal neuronal cell maintenance and confers resistance to aging-induced stress (Tan et al., 2002).

Conclusion

Detailed clinical, molecular, and immunological analysis of patients with XHIGM has been instrumental in unraveling the complex effects that CD40L (CD154) exerts in vivo upon interaction with CD40. For many years considered a prototypic humoral immunodeficiency, XHIGM is now viewed as a combined defect of cognate immunity. Similarly, CD40–CD40L interaction, originally thought to play a major role in terminal B cell differentiation only, is now widely recognized as a key signal in a variety of biological systems, particularly TH1-related inflammatory responses. Not surprisingly, anti-CD40L MAbs are coming into clinical practice as a potent anti-inflammatory drug (Durie et al., 1993) and as a powerful tool to prevent graft rejection and graft-vs.-host disease (Durie et al., 1994). Furthermore, recent observations indicate that CD40L is indeed a real cytokine, as it may also be released in an active, secretory form. It is expected that this profound change in perspective may lead to further therapeutic approaches based on disruption of CD40–CD40L interaction. Soluble CD40L is presently being explored at the National Institutes of Health (NIH) as a possible form of treatment for XHIGM. However, it remains to be seen if continuous administration of CD40L is safe and effective.

Since the first edition of this text, much has been written on the molecular pathophysiology of autosomal recessive HIGM syndromes. The genetic heterogeneity has been well documented. In patients with mutations of the *AICD* or the *UNG* gene, the disease is intrinsic to B cells, and the overall clinical manifestations are compatible with defective CSR and SHM (see Chapter 20). In contrast, patients with a mutation of CD40 are clinically and immunologically indistinguishable from patients with CD40L deficiency. This observation confirms the critical role that CD40L–CD40 interaction plays in protecting patients from not only bacteria but also opportunistic pathogens.

Acknowledgments

This work was partially supported by the Ministero dell'Istruzione Universita'e Ricerca (MIUR-COFIN 2004 to L.D.N. MIUR-CONIN 2004) and Fondo per gli Investimenti della Ricerca di Base-Ministero dell'Istruzione Universita'e Ricerca funding (project code RBNE0189JJ_004) to L.D.N.; the European Union Integrating and Strengthening the European Research Area Programme, proposal 006411 (EURO-Policy-PID) funding to L.D.N., European Union Grant QLG1-CT-2001-01536 to A.P., and by the Associazione per le Immunodeficienze Primitive.

References

Agematsu K, Nagumo H, Shinozaki K, Hokibara S, Yasui K, Terada K, Kawamura N, Yoba T, Nonoyama S, Ochs HD, Komiyama A. Absence of IgD–CD27+ memory B cell population in X-linked hyper-IgM syndrome. J Clin Invest 102:853–860, 1998.

Allen RC, Armitage RJ, Conley ME, Rosenblatt H, Jenkins NA, Copeland NG, Bedell MA, Edelhoff S, Disteche CM, Simoneaux DK, Fanslow WC, Belmont J, Spriggs MK. CD40 ligand gene defects responsible for X-linked hyper-IgM syndrome. Science 259:990–993, 1993a.

Allen RC, Spriggs M, Belmont JW. Dinucleotide repeat polymorphism in the human CD40 ligand gene. Hum Mol Genet 2:828, 1993b.

Ameratunga R, Lederman HM, Sullivan KE, Seyama K, French JK, Prestidge R, Marbrook J, Fanslow WC, Ochs HD, Winkelstein JA. Defective antigen induced lymphocyte proliferation in the X-linked hyperimmunoglobulin M syndrome. J Pediatr 131:147–150, 1997.

Armitage RJ, Fanslow WC, Strockbine L, Sato TA, Clifford KN, Macduff BM, Anderson DM, Gimpel SD, Davis-Smith T, Maliszewski CR, Clark EA, Smith CA, Grabstein KH, Cosman D, Spriggs MK. Molecular and biological characterization of a murine ligand for CD40. Nature 357:80–82, 1992.

Armitage RJ, Tough TW, Macduff BM, Fanslow WC, Spriggs MK, Ramsdell F, Alderson MR. CD40 ligand is a T cell growth factor. Eur J Immunol 23:2326–2331, 1993.

Aruffo A, Farrington M, Hollenbaugh D, Li X, Milatovich A, Nonoyama S, Bajorath J, Grosmaire LS, Stenkamp R, Neubauer M, Roberts RL, Noelle RJ, Ledbetter JA, Francke U, Ochs HD. The CD40 ligand, gp39, is defective in activated T cells from patients with X-linked hyper-IgM syndrome. Cell 72:291–300, 1993.

Bajorath J, Chalupny NJ, Marken JS, Siadak AW, Skonier J, Gordon M, Hollenhaugh D, Noelle RJ, Ochs HD, Aruffo A. Identification of residues on CD40 and its ligand which are critical for the receptor–ligand interaction. Biochemistry 34:1833–1844, 1995a.

Bajorath J, Marken JS, Chalupny NJ, Spoon TL, Siadak AW, Gordon M, Noelle RJ, Hollenbaugh D, Aruffo A. Analysis of gp39/CD40 interactions using molecular models and site-directed mutagenesis. Biochemistry 34:9884–9892, 1995b.

Bajorath J, Seyama K, Nonoyama S, Ochs HD, Aruffo A. Classification of mutations in the human CD40 ligand, gp39, that are associated with X-linked hyper IgM syndrome. Protein Sci 5:531–534, 1996.

Banatvala N, Davies J, Kanariou M, Strobel S, Levinsky R, Morgan G. Hypogammaglobulinaemia associated with normal or increased IgM (the hyper-IgM syndrome): a case series review. Arch Dis Child 71:150–152, 1994.

Banchereau J, Bazan F, Blanchard D, Briere F, Galizzi JP, van Kooten C, Liu YJ, Rousset F, Saeland S. The CD40 antigen and its ligand. Annu Rev Immunol 12:881–922, 1994.

Banner DW, D'Arcy A, Janes W, Gentz R, Schoenfeld H-J, Broger C, Loetscher H, Lesslauer W. Crystal structure of the soluble human 55kD

TNF receptor–human TNF complex: implications for TNF receptor activation. Cell 73:431–445, 1993.

Barry SC, Seppen J, Ramesh N, Foster JL, Seyama K, Ochs HD, Garcia JV, Osborne WRA. Lentiviral and murine retroviral transduction of T cells for expression of human CD40 ligand. Hum Gene Ther 11:323–332, 2000.

Baud V, Liu ZG, Bennett B, Suzuki N, Xia Y, Karin M. Signaling by proinflammatory cytokines: oligomerization of TRAF2 and TRAF6 is sufficient for JNK and IKK activation and target gene induction via an amino-terminal effector domain. Genes Dev 13:1297–1308, 1999.

Beall GN, Ashman RF, Miller ME, Easwaran C, Raghunathan R, Louie J, Yoshikawa T. Hypogammaglobulinemia in mother and son. J Allergy Clin Immunol 65:471–481, 1980.

Benkerrou M, Gougeon ML, Griscelli C, Fischer A. Hypogammaglobulinemie G et A avec hypergammaglobulinemie M. A propos de 12 observations. Arch Fr Pediatr 47:345–349, 1990.

Berberich I, Shu GL, Clark EA. Cross-linking CD40 on B cells rapidly activates nuclear factor-κB. J Immunol 153:4357–4366, 1994.

Bordigoni P, Auburtin B, Carret AS, Schuhmacher A, Humbert JC, Le Deist F, Sommelet D. Bone marrow transplantation as treatment for X-linked immunodeficiency with hyper-IgM. Bone Marrow Transplant 22:1111–1114, 1998.

Borrow P, Tishon A, Lee S, Xu J, Grewal IS, Oldstone MB, Flavell RA. CD40L-deficient mice show deficits in antiviral immunity and have an impaired memory CD8+ CTL response. J Exp Med 183:2129–2142, 1996.

Brahmi Z, Lazarus KH, Hodes ME, Baehner RL. Immunologic studies of three family members with the immunodeficiency with hyper-IgM syndrome. J Clin Immunol 3:127–134, 1983.

Brodeur SR, Angelini F, Bacharier LB, Blom AM, Mizoguchi E, Fujiwara H, Plebani A, Notarangelo LD, Dahlback B, Tsitsikov E, Geha RS. C4b-binding protein (C4BP) activates B cells through the CD40 receptor. Immunity 18:837–848, 2003.

Brown MP, Topham DJ, Sangster MY, Zhao J, Flynn KJ, Surman SL, Woodland DL, Doherty PC, Farr AG, Pattengale PK, Brenner MK. Thymic lymphoproliferative disease after successful correction of CD40 ligand deficiency by gene transfer in mice. Nat Med 4:1253–1260, 1998.

Brugnoni D, Airò P, Graf D, Marconi M, Lebowitz M, Plebani A, Giliani S, Malacarne F, Cattaneo R, Ugazio A, Albertini A, Kroczek RA, Notarangelo LD. Ineffective expression of CD40 ligand on cord blood T cells may contribute to poor immunoglobulin production in the newborn. Eur J Immunol 24:1919–1924, 1994.

Brugnoni D, Airo P, Graf D, Marconi M, Molinari C, Braga D, Malacarne F, Soresina A, Ugazio AG, Cattaneo R, Kroczek RA, Notarangelo LD. Ontogeny of CD40L expression by activated peripheral blood lymphocytes in humans. Immunol Lett 49:27–30, 1996.

Burtin P. Un exemple d'agammaglobulinemie atypique (un cas de grande hypogammaglobulinemie avec augmentation de la 2-macroglobuline). Rev Fr Etud Clin Biol 6:286–289, 1961.

Callard RE, Smith SH, Herbert J, Morgan G, Padayachee M, Lederman S, Chess L, Krockzek RA, Fanslow WC, Armitage RJ. CD40 ligand (CD40L) expression and B cell function in agammaglobulinemia with normal or elevated levels of IgM (HIM). Comparison of X-linked, autosomal recessive, and non-X-linked forms of disease and obligate carriers. J Immunol 153:3295–3306, 1994.

Castigli E, Alt F, Davidson L, Bottaro A, Mizoguchi E, Bhan AK, Geha RS. CD40 deficient mice generated by RAG-2 deficient blastocyst complementation. Proc Natl Acad Sci USA 91:12135–12139, 1994.

Castle BE, Kishimoto K, Stearns C, Brown ML, Kehry MR. Regulation of expression of the ligand for CD40 on T helper cells. J Immunol 151:1777–1788, 1993.

Chan FK, Chun HJ, Zheng L, Siegel RM, Bui KL, Lenardo MJ. A domain in TNF receptors that mediates ligand-independent receptor assembly and signaling. Science 288:2351–2354, 2000.

Cheng G, Cleary AM, Ye Z, Hong DI, Lederman S, Baltimore D. Involvement of CRAF1, a relative of TRAF, in CD40 signaling. Science 267:1494–1498, 1995.

Chu YW, Marin E, Fuleihan R, Ramesh N, Rosen FS, Geha RS, Insel RA. Somatic mutations of human immunoglobulin V genes in the X-linked hyper IgM syndrome. J Clin Invest 95:1389–1393, 1995.

Cocks BG, de Waal Malefyt R, Galizzi J-P, de Vries JE, Aversa G. IL-13 induces proliferation and differentiation of human B cells activated by the CD40 ligand. Int Immunol 6:657–663, 1993.

Conley ME, Larche M, Bonagura VR, Lawton AR, Buckley RH, Fu SM, Coustan-Smith E, Herrod HG, Campana D. Hyper IgM syndrome associated with defective CD40-mediated B cell activation. J Clin Invest 94: 1404–1409, 1994.

Cunningham CK, Bonville CA, Ochs HD, Seyama K, John PA, Rotbart HA, Weiner LB. Enteroviral meningoencephalitis as a complication of X-linked hyper IgM syndrome. J Pediatr 134:584–588, 1999.

Deng L, Wang C, Spencer E, Yang L, Braun A, You J, Slaughter C, Pickart C, Chen ZJ. Activation of the IkappaB kinase complex by TRAF6 requires a dimeric ubiquitin-conjugating enzyme complex and a unique polyubiquitin chain. Cell 103:351–361, 2000.

De Saint Basile G, Tabone MD, Durandy A, Phan F, Fischer A, Le Deist F. CD40 ligand expression deficiency in a female carrier of the X-linked hyper-IgM syndrome as a result of X chromosome lyonization. Eur J Immunol 29:367–373, 1999.

Ding L, Green JM, Thompson CB, Shevach EM. B7/CD28-dependent and independent induction of CD40 ligand expression. J Immunol 155: 5124–5132, 1995.

DiPalma JA, Strobel CT, Farrow JG. Primary sclerosing cholangitis associated with hyperimmunoglobulin M immunodeficiency (dysgammaglobulinemia). Gastroenterology 91:464–468, 1986.

DiSanto JP, Bonnefoy JY, Gauchat JF, Fischer A, de Saint Basile G. Brief report: CD40 ligand mutations in X-linked immunodeficiency with hyper-IgM. Nature 361:541–543, 1993.

DiSanto JP, Markiewicz S, Gauchat JF, Bonnefoy JY, Fischer A, de Saint Basile G. Brief report: prenatal diagnosis of X-linked hyper IgM syndrome. N Engl J Med 330:969–973, 1994.

Döffinger R, Smahi A, Bessia C, Geissmann F, Feinberg J, Durandy A, Bodemer C, Kenwrick S, Dupuis-Girod S, Blanche S, Wood P, Rabia SH, Headon DJ, Overbeek PA, Le Deist F, Holland SM, Belani K, Kumararatne DS, Fischer A, Shapiro R, Conley ME, Reimund E, Kalhoff H, Abinun M, Munnich A, Israël A, Coutois G, Casanova J-L. X-linked anhidrotic ectodermal dysplasia with immunodeficiency is caused by impaired NF-κB signaling. Nat Genet 27:277–285, 2001.

Duplantier JE, Seyama K, Day NK, Hitchcock R, Nelson RP Jr, Ochs HD, Haraguchi S, Klemperer MR, Good RA. Immunologic reconstitution following bone marrow transplantation for X-linked hyper IgM syndrome. Clin Immunol 98:313–318, 2001.

Durandy A, de Saint Basile G, Lisowska-Grospierre B, Gauchat JF, Forvielle M, Kroczek RA, Bonnefoy J-Y, Fischer A. Undetectable CD40 ligand expression on T cells and low B cell responses to CD40 binding agonists in human newborn. J Immunol 154:1560–1568, 1995.

Durandy A, Schiff C, Bonnefoy JY, Forveille M, Rousset F, Mazzei G, Milili M, Fischer A. Induction by anti-CD40 antibody or soluble CD40 ligand and cytokines of IgG, IgA, and IgE production by B cells from patients with X-linked hyper IgM syndrome. Eur J Immunol 23:2294–2299, 1993.

Durie FH, Aruffo A, Ledbetter J, Crassi KM, Green WR, Fast LD, Noelle RJ. Antibody to the ligand of CD40, gp39, blocks the occurrence of the acute and chronic forms of graft-vs-host disease. J Clin Invest 94:1333–1338, 1994.

Durie FH, Fava RA, Foy TM, Aruffo A, Ledbetter JA, Noelle RJ. Prevention of collagen-induced arthritis with an antibody to gp39, the ligand for CD40. Science 261:1328–1330, 1993.

Eck MJ, Sprang SR. The structure of tumor necrosis factor at 2.6Å resolution: implications for receptor binding. J Biol Chem 264:17595–17606, 1991.

Espanol T, Canals C, Bofill A, Moreno A, Sentis M. Immunological abnormalities in late-onset rubella syndrome and correction with gammaglobulin treatment. In: Vossen J, Griscelli C, eds. Progress in Immunodeficiency Research and Therapy II. Amsterdam: Elsevier, pp. 405–410, 1986.

Facchetti F, Appiani C, Salvi L, Levy J, Notarangelo LD. Immunohistologic analysis of ineffective CD40–CD40 ligand interaction in lymphoid tissues from patients with X-linked immunodeficiency with hyper-IgM. J Immunol 154:6624–6633, 1995.

Fanslow WC, Anderson DM, Grabstein KH, Clark EA, Cosman D, Armitage RJ. Soluble forms of CD40 inhibit biologic responses of human B cells. J Immunol 149:655–660, 1992.

Fanslow WC, Clifford KN, Seaman M, Alderson MR, Spriggs MK, Armitage RJ, Ramsdell F. Recombinant CD40 ligand exerts potent biologic effects on T cells. J Immunol 152:4262–4269, 1994.

Faris M, Gaskin F, Parsons JT, Fu SM. CD40 signaling pathway: anti-CD40 monoclonal antibody induces rapid dephosphorylation and phosphorylation of tyrosine-phosphorylated proteins including protein tyrosine kinase Lyn, Fyn, and Syk and the appearance of a 28-kD tyrosine phosphorylated protein. J Exp Med 179:1923–1931, 1994.

Farrington M, Grosmaire LS, Nonoyama S, Fischer SH, Hollenbaugh D, Ledbetter JA, Noelle RJ, Aruffo A, Ochs HD. CD40 ligand is defective in a subset of patients with common variable immunodeficiency. Proc Natl Acad Sci USA 91:1099–1103, 1994.

Ferrari S, Giliani S, Insalaco A, Al-Ghonaium A, Soresina AR, Loubser M, Avanzini MA, Marconi M, Badolato R, Ugazio AG, Levy Y, Catalan N, Durandy A, Tbakhi A, Notarangelo LD, Plebani A. Mutations of CD40 gene cause an autosomal recessive form of immunodeficiency with hyper IgM. Proc Natl Acad Sci USA 98:12614–12619, 2001.

Filipovich AH, Mathur A, Kamat D, Kersey JH, Shapiro RS. Lymphoproliferative disorders and other tumors complicating immunodeficiencies. Immunodeficiency 5:91–112, 1994.

Florido M, Goncalves AS, Gomes MS, Appelberg R. CD40 is required for the optimal induction of protective immunity to Mycobacterium avium. Immunology 111:323–327, 2004.

Fontana S, Moratto D, Mangal S, De Francesco M, Vermi W, Ferrari S, Facchetti F, Kutukculer N, Fiorini C, Duse M, Das PK, Notarangelo LD, Olebani A, Badolato R. Functional defects of dendritic cells in patients with CD40 deficiency. Blood 102:4099–4106, 2003.

Foy TM, Page DM, Waldschmidt TJ, Schoneveld A, Laman JD, Masters SR, Tygrett L, Ledbetter JA, Aruffo A, Claassen E, Xu JC, Flavell RA, Oehen S, Hedrick SM, Noelle RJ. An essential role for gp39, the ligand for CD40, in thymic selection. J Exp Med 182:1377–1388, 1995.

Foy TM, Shepherd DM, Durie FH, Aruffo A, Ledbetter JA, Noelle RJ. In vivo CD40–gp39 interactions are essential for thymus-dependent humoral immunity. II. Prolonged suppression of the humoral immune response by an antibody to the ligand for CD40, gp39. J Exp Med 178: 1567–1575, 1993.

Fuleihan R, Ahern D, Geha RS. Decreased expression of the ligand for CD40 in newborn lymphocytes. Eur J Immunol 24:1925–1928, 1994a.

Fuleihan R, Ahern D, Geha RS. CD40 ligand expression is developmentally regulated in human thymocytes. Clin Immunol Immunopathol 76:52–58, 1995.

Fuleihan R, Ramesh N, Geha R. Role of CD40–CD40 ligand interaction in immunoglobulin isotype switching. Curr Opin Immunol 5:963–967, 1993a.

Fuleihan R, Ramesh N, Horner A, Ahern D, Belshaw PJ, Alberg DG, Stanemkovic I, Harmon W, Geha RS. Cyclosporin A inhibits CD40L expression in T lymphocytes. J Clin Invest 93:1315–1320, 1994b.

Fuleihan R, Ramesh N, Loh R, Jabara H, Rosen FS, Chatila T, Fu SM, Stamenkovic I, Geha RS. Defective expression of the CD40 ligand in X chromosome–linked immunoglobulin deficiency with normal or elevated IgM. Proc Natl Acad Sci USA 90:2170–2173, 1993b.

Gauchat J-F, Aubry J-P, Mazzei G, Life P, Jomotte T, Elson G, Bonnefoy J-Y. Human CD40-ligand: molecular cloning, cellular distribution, and regulation of expression by factors controlling IgE production. FEBS Lett 315:259–266, 1993a.

Gauchat J-F, Henchoz S, Fattah D, Mazzei G, Aubry J-P, Jomotte T, Dash L, Page K, Solari R, Aldebert D, Capron M, Dahinden C, Bonnefoy J-Y. CD40 ligand is functionally expressed on human eosinophils. Eur J Immunol 25:863–865, 1995.

Gauchat J-F, Henchoz S, Mazzei G, Aubry J-P, Brunner T, Blasey H, Life P, Talabot D, Flores-Romo L, Thompson J, Kishi K, Butterfield J, Dahinden C, Bonnefoy J-Y. Induction of human IgE synthesis in B cells by mast cells and basophils. Nature 365:340–343, 1993b.

Geha RS, Hyslop N, Alami S, Farah F, Schneeberger EE, Rosen FS. Hyper immunoglobulin M immunodeficiency (dysgammaglobulinemia): presence of immunoglobulin M–secreting plasmacytoid cells in peripheral blood and failure of immunoglobulin M–immunoglobulin G switch in B-cell differentiation. J Clin Invest 64:385–391, 1979.

Gennery AR, Clark JE, Flood TJ, Abinun M, Cant A. T-cell-depleted bone marrow transplantation from allogeneic sibling for X-linked hyperimmunoglobulin M syndrome. J Pediatr 137:290, 2000.

Gennery AR, Khawaja K, Veys P, Bredius RG, Notarangelo LD, Mazzolari E, Fischer A, Landais P, Cavazzana-Calvo M, Friedrich W, Fasth A, Wulffrraat NM, Matthes-Martin S, Bensoussan D, Bordigoni P, Lange A, Pagliuca A, Andolina M, Cant AJ, Davies EG. Treatment of CD40 ligand deficiency by hematopoietic stem cell transplantation: a survey of the European experience, 1993–2002. Blood 103:1152–1157, 2004.

Gilmour KC, Walshe D, Heath S, Monaghan G, Loughlin S, Lester T, Norbury G, Cale CM. Immunological and genetic analysis of 65 patients with a clinical suspicion of X-linked hyper-IgM. J Clin Pathol 56: 256–262, 2003.

Graf D, Korthauer U, Mages HW, Senger G, Kroczek RA. Cloning of TRAP, a ligand for CD40 on human T cells. Eur J Immunol 22:3191–3194, 1992.

Grammer AC, Bergman MC, Miura Y, Fujita K, Davis LS, Lipsky PE. The CD40 ligand expressed by human B cells costimulates B cell responses. J Immunol 154:4996–5010, 1995.

Grammer AC, Swantek JL, McFarland RD, Miura Y, Geppert T, Lipsky PE. TNF receptor–associated factor-3 signaling mediates activation of p38 and Jun N-terminal kinase, cytokine secretion, and Ig production following ligation of CD40 on human B cells. J Immunol 161:1183–1193, 1998.

Hadzic N, Pagliuca A, Rela M, Portmann B, Jones A, Veys P, Heaton ND, Mufti GJ, Mieli-Vergani G. Correction of hyper-IgM syndrome after liver and bone marrow transplantation. N Engl J Med 342:320–324, 2000.

Halliday E, Winkelstein J, Webster ADB. Enteroviral infections in primary immunodeficiency (PID): A survey of morbidity and mortality. J Infect 46:1–8, 2003.

Hanissian S, Geha RS. Jak3 is associated with CD40 and is critical for CD40 induction of gene expression in B cells. Immunity 6:379–388, 1997.

Hayward AR, Levy J, Facchetti F, Notarangelo L, Ochs HD, Etzioni A, Bonnefoy JY, Cosyns M, Weinberg A. Cholangiopathy and tumors of the pancreas, liver, and biliary tree in boys with X-linked immunodeficiency with hyper-IgM. J Immunol 158:977–983, 1997.

Hendriks RW, Kraakman MEM, Craig IW, Espanol T, Schuurman RKB. Evidence that in X-linked immunodeficiency with hyperimmunoglobulinemia M the intrinsic immunoglobulin heavy chain class switch mechanism is intact. Eur J Immunol 20:2603–2608, 1990.

Hollander GA, Castigli E, Kulbacki R, Su M, Burakoff SJ, Gutierrez-Ramos JC, Geha RS. Induction of alloantigen-specific tolerance by B cells from CD40-deficient mice. Proc Natl Acad Sci USA 93:4994–4998, 1996.

Hollenbaugh D, Grosmaire LS, Kullas CD, Chalupny NJ, Braesch-Andersen S, Noelle RJ, Stamenkovic I, Ledbetter JA, Aruffo A. The human T cell antigen gp39, a member of the TNF gene family, is a ligand for the CD 40 receptor: expression of a soluble form of gp39 with B cell co-stimulatory activity. EMBO J 11:4313–4321, 1992.

Hollenbaugh D, Wu LH, Ochs HD, Nonoyama S, Grosmaire LS, Ledbetter JA, Noelle RJ, Hill H, Aruffo A. The random inactivation of the X-chromosome carrying the defective gene responsible for X-linked hyper IgM syndrome (X-HIM) in female carriers of HIGM1. J Clin Invest 94:616–622, 1994.

Hong R, Schubert WK, Perrin EV, West CD. Antibody deficiency syndrome associated with beta-2 macroglobulinemia. J Pediatr 61:831–842, 1962.

Horner AA, Jabara H, Ramesh N, Geha RS. T lymphocytes express CD40 ligand and induce isotype switching in B lymphocytes. J Exp Med 181:1239–1244, 1995.

Hostager BS, Catlett IM, Bishop GA. Recruitment of CD40 and tumor necrosis factor receptor–associated factors 2 and 3 to membrane microdomains during CD40 signaling. J Biol Chem 275:15392–15398, 2000.

Hostoffer RW, Berger M, Clark HT, Schreiber JR. Disseminated histoplasma capsulatum in a patient with hyper IgM immunodeficiency. Pediatrics 94:234–236, 1994.

Iciek LA, Delphin SA, Stavnezer J CD40 cross-linking induces Ig epsilon germline transcripts in B cells via activation of NF-kappaB: synergy with IL-4 induction. J Immunol 158:4769–4779, 1997.

Imai K, Catalan N, Plebani A, Marodi L, Sanal O, Kumaki S, Nagendran V, Wood P, Glastre C, Sarrod-Reynauld F, Hermine O, Forveille M, Revy P, Fischer A, Durandy A. Hyper-IgM type 4 with a B lymphocyte–intrinsic selective deficiency in Ig class-switch recombination. J Clin Invest 112:136–142, 2003a.

Imai K, Sluppaug G, Lee WI, Revy P, Nonoyama S, Catalan N, Yel L, Forveille M, Kavli B, Krokan HE, Ochs HD, Fischer A, Durandy A. Human uracil DNA-glycosylase deficiency associated with profoundly impaired immunoglobulin class switch recombination. Nat Immunol 4:1023–1028, 2003b.

Iseki M, Anzo M, Yamashita N, Matsuo N. Hyper-IgM immunodeficiency with disseminated cryptococcosis. Acta Pediatr 83:780–782, 1994.

Ishida T, Kobayashi N, Tojo T, Ishida S, Yamamoto T, Inoue J. CD40 signaling-mediated induction of Bcl-XL, Cdk4, and Cdk6. Implication of their cooperation in selective B cell growth. J Immunol 155:5527–5535, 1995.

Ishida T, Mizushima S, Azuma S, Kobayashi N, Tojo T, Suzuki K, Aizawa S, Watanabe T, Mosialos G, Kieff E, et al. Identification of TRAF6, a novel tumor necrosis factor receptor–associated factor protein that mediates signaling from an amino-terminal domain of the CD40 cytoplasmic region. J Biol Chem 271:28745–28748, 1996.

Jabara HH, Brodeur SR, Geha RS. Glucocorticoids upregulate CD40 ligand expression and induce CD40L-dependent immunoglobulin isotype switching. J Clin Invest 107:371–378, 2001.

Jacobsohn DA, Emerick KM, Scholl P, Melin-Aldana H, O'Gorman M, Duerst R, Kletzel M. Nonmyeloablative hematopoietic stem cell transplant for X-linked hyper-immunoglobulin M syndrome with cholangiopathy. Pediatrics 113:122–127, 2004.

Jain A, Atkinson TP, Lipsky PE, Slater JE, Nelson DL, Strober W. Defects of T-cell effector function and post-thymic maturation in X-linked hyper-IgM syndrome. J Clin Invest 103:1151–1158, 1999.

Jain A, Ma AC, Liu S, Brown M, Cohen J, Strober W. Specific missense mutations in *NEMO* result in hyper-IgM syndrome with hypohydrotic ectodermal dysplasia. Nat Immunol 2:223–228, 2001.

Jain J, McCaffrey PG, Miner Z, Kerppola TK, Lambert JN, Verdine GL, Curran T, Rao A. The T-cell transcription factor NFATp is a substrate for calcineurin and interacts with Fos and Jun. Nature 365:352–355, 1993.

Jalukar SV, Hostager BS, Bishop GA. Characterization of the roles of TNF receptor–associated factor 6 in CD40-mediated B lymphocyte effector functions. J Immunol 164:623–630, 2000.

Jeurissen A, Wuyts G, Kasran A, Ramdien-Murli S, Blanckaert N, Boon L, Ceuppens JL, Bossuyet X. The human antibody response to pneumococcal capsular polysaccharide is dependent on the CD40–CD40 ligand interaction. Eur J Immunol 34:850–858, 2004.

Jones EY, Stuart DI, Walker NPC. Structure of tumor necrosis factor. Nature 338:225–228, 1989.

Karpusas M, Hsu YM, Wang JH, Thompson J, Lederman S, Chess L, Thomas D. 2A crystal structure of an extracellular fragment of human CD40 ligand. Structure 3:1031–1039, 1995.

Karras JG, Wang Z, Huo L, Frank DA, Rothstein TL. Induction of STAT protein signaling through the CD40 receptor in B lymphocytes: distinct STAT activation following surface Ig and CD40 receptor engagement. J Immunol 159:4350–4355, 1997.

Kashiwada M, Shirakata Y, Inoue JI, Nakano H, Okazaki K, Okumura K, Yamamoto T, Nagaoka H, Takemori T. Tumor necrosis factor receptor–associated factor 6 (TRAF6) stimulates extracellular signal–regulated kinase (ERK) activity in CD40 signaling along a ras-independent pathway. J Exp Med 187:237–244, 1998.

Kato T, Tsuge I, Inaba J, Kato K, Matsuyama T, Kojima S. Successful bone marrow transplantation in a child with X-linked hyper-IgM syndrome. Bone Marrow Transplant 23:1081–1083, 1999.

Kawabe T, Naka T, Yoshida K, Tanaka T, Fujiwara H, Suematsu S, Yoshida N, Kishimoto T, Kikutani H. The immune responses in CD40-deficient mice: impaired immunoglobulin class switching and germinal center formation. Immunity 1:167–178, 1994.

Kawai S, Sasahara Y, Minegishi M, Tsuchiya S, Fujie H, Ohashi Y, Kumaki S, Konno T. Immunological reconstitution by allogeneic bone marrow transplantation in a child with the X-linked hyper-IgM syndrome. Eur J Pediatr 158:394–397, 1999.

Kaykas A, Worringer K, Sugden B. CD40 and LMP-1 both signal from lipid rafts but LMP-1 assembles a distinct, more efficient signaling complex. EMBO J 20:2641–2654, 2001.

Klaus SJ, Pinchuk LM, Ochs HD, Law CL, Fanslow WC, Armitage RJ, Clark EA. Costimulation through CD28 enhances T-cell dependent B cell activation via CD40–CD40L interaction. J Immunol 152:5643–5652, 1994.

Korthauer U, Graf D, Mages HW, Briere F, Padayachee M, Malcolm S, Ugazio AG, Notarangelo LD, Levinsky RJ, Kroczek RA. Defective expression of T-cell CD40 ligand causes X-linked immunodeficiency with hyper-IgM. Nature 361:539–541, 1993.

Kraakman MEM, de Weers M, Espanol T, Shuurman RKB, Hendriks RW. Identification of a CD40L gene mutation and genetic counseling in a family with immunodeficiency with hyperglobulinemia M. Clin Genet 48:46–48, 1995.

Krantman HJ, Stiehm ER, Stevens RH, Saxon A, Seeger RC. Abnormal B cell differentiation and varible increased T cell suppression in immunodeficiency with hyper-IgM. Clin Exp Immunol 40:147–156, 1980.

Kroczek RA, Graf D, Brugnoni D, Giliani S, Korthauer U, Ugazio A, Senger G, Mages HW, Villa A, Notarangelo LD. Defective expression of CD40 ligand on T cells causes X-linked immunodeficiency with hyper-IgM (HIGM1). Immunol Rev 138:39–59, 1994.

Kutukculer N, Moratto D, Aydinok Y, Lougaris V, Aksoylar S, Plebani A, Genel F, Notarangelo LD. Disseminated *Cryptosporidium* infection in an infant with hyper-IgM syndrome caused by CD40 deficiency. J Pediatr 142:194–196, 2003.

Kyong CU, Virella G, Fudenberg HH, Darby CP. X-linked immunodeficiency with increased IgM: clinical, ethnic, and immunologic heterogeneity. Pediatr Res 12:1024–1026, 1978.

Lane P, Brocker T, Hubele S, Padovan E, Lanzavecchia A, McConnell F. Soluble CD40 ligand can replace the normal T cell–derived CD40 ligand signal to B cells in T-dependent activation. J Exp Med 177:1209–1213, 1993.

Lane P, Traunecker A, Hueble S, Inui S, Lanzavecchia A, Gray D. Activated human T cells express a ligand for the human B cell–associated antigen CD40 which participates in T-dependent activation of B lymphocytes. Eur J Immunol 22:2573–2578, 1992.

Lederman S, Yellin MJ, Krichevsky A, Belko J, Lee JJ, Chess L. Identification of a novel surface protein on activated CD4 T cells that induces contact-dependent B cell differentiation (Help). J Exp Med 175:1091–1101, 1992.

Lee HH, Dempsey PW, Parks TP, Zhu X, Baltimore D, Cheng G. Specificities of CD40 signaling: involvement of TRAF2 in CD40-induced NF-kappaB activation and intercellular adhesion molecule-1 up-regulation. Proc Natl Acad Sci USA 96:1421–1426, 1999.

Lee WI, Torgerson TR, Schumacher MJ, Yel L, Zhu Q, Ochs HD. Molecular analysis of a large cohort of patients with the hyper IgM syndrome (HIGM). Blood 105:1881–1890, 2005.

Leo E, Welsh K, Matsuzawa S, Zapata JM, Kitada S, Mitchell RS, Ely KR, Reed JC. Differential requirements for tumor necrosis factor receptor–associated factor family proteins in CD40-mediated induction of NF-kappaB and Jun N-terminal kinase activation. J Biol Chem 274:22414–22422, 1999.

Levitt D, Haber P, Rich K, Cooper MD. Hyper IgM immunodeficiency. A primary dysfunction of B lymphocyte isotype switching. J Clin Invest 72:1650–1657, 1983.

Levy J, Espanol-Boren T, Thomas C, Fischer A, Tovo P, Bordigoni P, Reznick I, Fasth A, Baer M, Gomez L, Sanders EAM, Tabone M-D, Plantaz D, Etzioni A, Monafo V, Hammarstrom L, Abrahamsen T, Jones A, Finn A, Klemola T, De Vries E, Sanal O, Peitsch MC, Notarangelo LD. The clinical spectrum of X-linked hyper IgM syndrome. J Pediatr 131:47–54, 1997.

Li YY, Baccam M, Waters SB, Pessin JE, Bishop GA, Koretzky GA. CD40 ligation results in protein kinase C–independent activation of ERK and JNK in resting murine splenic B cells. J Immunol 157:1440–1447, 1996.

Lin Q, Rohrer J, Allen RC, Larche M, Greene JM, Shigeoka AO, Gatti RA, Derauf DC, Belmont JW, Conley ME. A single-strand conformation polymorphism study of CD40 ligand. J Clin Invest 97:196–201, 1996.

Macchi P, Villa A, Strina D, Sacco MG, Morali F, Brugnoni D, Giliani S, Mantuano E, Fasth A, Andersson B, Zegers BJM, Cavagni G, Reznick I, Levy J, Zan-Bar I, Porat Y, Airo P, Plebani A, Vezzoni P, Notarangelo LD. Characterization of nine novel mutations in the CD40 ligand gene in patients with X-linked hyper IgM syndrome of various ancestry. Am J Hum Genet 56:898–906, 1995.

Marshall WC, Waston JJ, Bodian M. Pneumocystis carinii pneumonia and congenital hypogammaglobulinemia. Arch Dis Child 39:18–25, 1964.

Mayer L, Kwan SP, Thompson C, Ko HS, Chiorazzi N, Waldmann T, Rosen F. Evidence for a defect in "switch" T cells in patients with immunodeficiency and hyperimmunoglobulinemia M. N Engl J Med 314:409–413, 1986.

McLauchlin J, Amar CF, Pedraza-Diaz S, Mieli-Vergani G, Hadzic N, Davies EG. Polymerase chain reaction–based diagnosis of infection with Cryptosporidium in children with primary immunodeficiencies. Pediatr Infect Dis J 22:329–334, 2003.

Mensink EJBM, Thompson A, Sandkuijl LA, Kraakman ME, Schot JD, Espanol T, Schuurman RK. X-linked immunodeficiency with hyper IgM appears to be linked to DXS42 RFLP locus. Hum Genet 76:96–99, 1987.

Merluzzi S, Moretti S, Altamura S, Zwollo P, Sigvardsson M, Vitale G, Pucillo C. CD40 stimulation induces Pax5/BSAP and EBF activation through a APE/Ref-1 dependent redox mechanism. J Biol Chem 279:1777–1786, 2003.

Mitsuya H, Tomino S, Hisamitsu S, Kishimoto S. Evidence for the failure of IgA specific T helper activity in patients with immunodeficiency with hyper IgM. J Clin Lab Immunol 2:337–342, 1979.

Muramatsu M, Kinoshita K, Fagarasan S, Yamada S, Shinkai Y, Honjo T. Class switch recombination and hypermutation require activation-induced cytidine deaminase (AID), a potential RNA editing enzyme. Cell 102:553–563, 2000.

Noelle RJ, Ledbetter JA, Aruffo A. CD40 and its ligand, an essential ligand–receptor pair for thymus-dependent B-cell activation. Immunol Today 13:431–433, 1992a.

Noelle RJ, Shepherd DM, Fell HP. Cognate interaction between T helper cells and B cells: VII. Role of contact and lymphokines in the expression of germ-line and mature 1 transcripts. J Immunol 149:1164–1169, 1992b.

Nonoyama S, Hollenbaugh D, Aruffo A, Ledbetter JA, Ochs HD. B cell activation via CD40 is required for specific antibody production by antigen-stimulated human B cells. J Exp Med 178:1097–1102, 1993.

Nonoyama S, Penix LA, Edwards CP, Lewis DB, Ito S, Aruffo A, Wilson CB, Ochs HD. Diminished expression of CD40 ligand by activated neonatal T cells. J Clin Invest 95:66–75, 1995.

Notarangelo LD, Duse M, Ugazio AG. Immunodeficiency with hyper-IgM (HIM). Immunodefic Rev 3:101–122, 1992.

Notarangelo LD, Peitsch MC, Abrahamsen TG, Bachelot C, Bordigoni P, Cant AJ, Chapel H, Clementi M, Deacock S, de Saint Basile G, Duse M, Espanol T, Etzioni A, Fasth A, Fischer A, Giliani S, Gomes L, Hammarstrom L, Jones A, Kanariou M, Kinnon C, Kelmola T, Kroczek RA,

Levy J, Matamoros N, Monafo V, Paolucci P, Reznick I, Sanal O, Smith CIE, Thompson RA, Tovo P, Villa A, Vihinen M, Vossen J, Zegers BJM, Ochs HD, Conley ME, Iseki M, Ramesh N, Shimadzu M, Saiki O. CD40Lbase: a database of CD40L gene mutations causing X-linked hyper-IgM syndrome. Immunol Today 17:511–516, 1996.

Ochs HD, Wedgwood RJ. Disorders of the B cell system. In: Stiehm ER, ed. Immunologic Disorders in Infants and Children, 3rd ed. Philadelphia: WB Saunders, pp. 226–256, 1989.

Oettgen HC. Regulation of the IgE isotype switch: new insights on cytokine signals and the functions of epsilon germline transcripts. Curr Opin Immunol 12:618–623, 2000.

Oliva A, Quinti I, Scala E, Fanales-Belasio E, Rainaldi L, Pierdominici M, Giovannetti A, Paganelli R, Aiuti F, Pandolfi F. Immunodeficiency with hyper immunoglobulinemia M in two female patients is not associated with abnormalities of CD40 or CD40 ligand expression. J Allergy Clin Immunol 96:403–410, 1995.

Padayachee M, Feighery C, Finn A, McKeown C, Levinsky RJ, Kinnon C, Malcolm S. Mapping of the X-linked form of hyper IgM syndrome (HIGM1) to Xq26 by close linkage to HPRT. Genomics 14:551–553, 1992.

Padayachee M, Levinsky RJ, Kinnon C, Finn A, Mckeown C, Feighery C, Notarangelo LD, Hendriks RW, Read AP, Malcolm S. Mapping of the X-linked form of hyper IgM syndrome (HIGM1). J Med Genet 30:202–205, 1993.

Pascual-Salcedo D, de la Concha EG, Garcia-Rodriguez MC, Zabay JM, Sainz T, Fontan G. Cellular basis of hyper IgM immunodeficiency. J Clin Lab 10:29–34, 1983.

Peitsch MC, Jongeneel CV. A 3-D model for the CD40 ligand predicts that it is a compact trimer similar to the tumor necrosis factors. Int Immunol 5:233–238, 1993.

Pietrella D, Lupo P, Perito S, Mosci P, Bistoni F, Vecchiarelli A. Disruption of CD40/CD40L interaction influences the course of Cryptococcus neoformans infection. FEMS Immunol Med Microbiol 40:63–70, 2004.

Pilia G, Porta G, Padayachee M, Malcolm S, Zucchi I, Villa A, Macchi P, Vezzoni P, Schlessinger D. Human CD40L maps between DXS144E and DXS300 in Xq26. Genomics 22:249–251, 1994.

Pullen SS, Labadia ME, Ingraham RH, McWhirter SM, Everdeen DS, Alber T, Crute JJ, Kehry MR. High-affinity interactions of tumor necrosis factor receptor–associated factors (TRAFs) and CD40 require TRAF trimerization and CD40 multimerization. Biochemistry 38:10168–10177, 1999.

Pullen SS, Miller HG, Everdeen DS, Dang TT, Crute JJ, Kehry MR. CD40–tumor necrosis factor receptor–associated factor (TRAF) interactions: regulation of CD40 signaling through multiple TRAF binding sites and TRAF hetero-oligomerization. Biochemistry 37:11836–11845, 1998.

Ramesh N, Fuleihan R, Geha R. Molecular pathology of X-linked immunoglobulin deficiency with normal or elevated IgM (HIGMX-1). Immunol Rev 138:87–104, 1994.

Ramsdell F, Seaman M, Clifford KN, Fanslow WC. CD40 ligand acts as a costimulatory signal for neonatal thymic γδ cells. J Immunol 152:2190–2197, 1994.

Razanajaona D, van Kooten C, Lebecque S, Bridon J-M, Ho S, Smith S, Callard R, Banchereau J, Brière F. Somatic mutations in human Ig variable genes correlate with a partially functional CD40-ligand in the X-linked hyper-IgM syndrome. J Immunol 157:1492–1498, 1996.

Raziuddin S, Assaf HM, Teklu B. T cell malignancy in Richter's syndrome presenting as hyper IgM. Induction and characterization of a novel CD3, CD4, CD8, T cell subset from phytohemaglutinin-stimulated patient's CD3, CD4, CD8 leukemic T cells. Eur J Immunol 19:469–474, 1989.

Reinhard C, Shamoon B, Shyamala V, Williams LT. Tumor necrosis factor alpha–induced activation of c-jun N-terminal kinase is mediated by TRAF2. EMBO J 16:1080–1092, 1997.

Ren CL, Morio T, Fu SM, Geha RS. Signal transduction via CD40 involves activation of lyn kinase and phosphatidylinositol-3-kinase, and phosphorylation of phospholipase C gamma 2. J Exp Med 179:673–680, 1994.

Renshaw BR, Fanslow WC 3rd, Armitage RJ, Campbell KA, Liggitt D, Wright B, Davison BL, Maliszewski CR. Humoral immune responses in CD40 ligand–deficient mice. J Exp Med 180:1889–1900, 1994.

Revy P, Hivroz C, Andreu G, Graber P, Martinache C, Fischer A, Durandy A. Activation of the Janus kinase 3–STAT5a pathway after CD40 triggering of human monocytes but not resting B cells. J Immunol 163:787–793, 1999.

Revy P, Muto T, Levy Y, Geissmann F, Plebani A, Sanal O, Catalan N, Forveille M, Dufourcq-Lagelouse R, Gennery A, Tezcan I, Ersoy F, Kayserili H, Ugazio A, Brousse N, Muramatsu M, Notarangelo LD, Kinoshita K, Honjo T, Fischer A, Durandy A. Activation-induced cytidine deaminase (AID) deficiency causes the autosomal recessive form of the hyper-IgM syndrome (HIGM2). Cell 102:565–575, 2000.

Rieger CH, Nelson LA, Peri BA, Lustig JV, Newcomb RW. Transient hypogammaglobulinemia of infancy. J Pediatr 91:601–603, 1980.

Rosen FS, Kevy SV, Merler E, Janeway CA, Gitlin D. Recurrent bacterial infections and dysgammaglobulinemia: deficiency of 7S gammaglobulins in the presence of elevated 19S gamma-globulins. Report of two cases. Pediatrics 28:182–195, 1961.

Rothe M, Sarma V, Dixit VM, Goeddel DV. TRAF2-mediated activation of NF-kappa B by TNF receptor 2 and CD40. Science 269:1424–1427, 1995.

Rousset F, Garcia E, Banchereau J. Cytokine-induced proliferation and immunoglobulin production of human lymphocytes triggered through their CD40 antigen. J Exp Med 235:705–710, 1991.

Roy M, Waldschmidt T, Aruffo A, Ledbetter JA, Noelle RJ. The regulation of the expression of gp39, the CD40 ligand, on normal and cloned CD4 T cells. J Immunol 151:2497–2510, 1993.

Sacco MG, Ungari M, Catò EM, Villa A, Strina D, Notarangelo LD, Jonkers J, Zecca L, Facchetti F, Vezzoni P. Lymphoid abnormalities in CD40 ligand transgenic mice suggest the need for tight regulation in gene therapy approaches to hyper-immunoglobulin M (IgM) syndrome. Cancer Gene Ther 7:1299–1306, 2000.

Saiki O, Tanaka T, Wada Y, Uda H, Inoue A, Katada Y, Izeki M, Iwata M, Nunoi H, Matsuda I, Kinoshita N, Kishimoto T. Signaling through CD40 rescues IgE but not IgG or IgA secretion in X-linked immunodeficiency with hyper-IgM. J Clin Invest 95:510–514, 1995.

Sarma V, Lin Z, Clark L, Rust BM, Tewari M, Noelle RJ, Dixit VM. Activation of the B-cell surface receptor CD40 induces A20, a novel zinc finger protein that inhibits apoptosis. J Biol Chem 270:12343–12346, 1995.

Schimke RN, Bolano C, Kirkpatrick CH. Immunologic deficiency in the congenital rubella syndrome. Am J Dis Child 118:626–633, 1969.

Scholl PR, O'Gorman MR, Pachman LM, Haut P, Kletzel M. Correction of neutropenia and hypogammaglobulinemia in X-linked hyper-IgM syndrome by allogeneic bone marrow transplantation. Bone Marrow Transplant 22:1215–1218, 1998.

Schubert LA, King G, Cron RQ, Lewis DB, Aruffo A, Hollenbaugh D. The human gp39 promoter. Two distinct nuclear factors of activated T cell protein-binding elements contribute to transcriptional activation. J Biol Chem 270:29624–29627, 1995.

Schwaber JF, Lazarus H, Rosen FS. IgM-restricted production of immunoglobulin by lymphoid cell lines from patients with immunodeficiency with hyper IgM (dysgammaglobulinemia). Clin Immunol Immunopathol 19:91–97, 1981.

Seyama K, Kobayashi R, Hasle H, Apter A, Rutledge J, Rosen D, Ochs HD. Parvovirus B19-induced anemia as presenting manifestation of X-linked hyper-IgM syndrome. J Infect Dis 178:318–324, 1998a.

Seyama K, Nonoyama S, Gangsaas I, Hollenbaugh D, Pabst HF, Aruffo A, Ochs HD. Mutations of the CD40 ligand gene and its effects on CD40 ligand expression in patients with X-linked hyper-IgM syndrome. Blood 92:2421–2434, 1998b.

Seyama K, Osborne WRA, Ochs HD. CD40 ligand mutants responsible for X-linked hyper-IgM syndrome associate with wild-type CD40 ligand. J Biol Chem 274:11310–11320, 1999.

Sha WC. Regulation of immune responses by NF-kappa B/Rel transcription factor. J Exp Med 187:143–146, 1998.

Shimadzu M, Nunoi H, Terasaki H, Ninomiya R, Iwata M, Kanegasaka S, Matsuda I. Structural organization of the gene for CD40 ligand: molecular analysis for diagnosis of X-linked hyper-IgM syndrome. Biochim Biophy Acta 1260:67–72, 1995.

Shuto T, Xu H, Wang B, Han J, Kai H, Gu XX, Murphy TF, Lim DJ, Li JD. Activation of NF-kappa B by nontypeable Hemophilus influenzae is mediated by toll-like receptor 2-TAK1-dependent NIK-IKK alpha/beta-I kappa B alpha and MKK3/6-p38 MAP kinase signaling pathways in epithelial cells. Proc Natl Acad Sci USA 98:8774–8779, 2001.

Song H, Regnier C, Kirschning C, Goeddel D, Rothe M. Tumor necrosis factor (TNF)–mediated kinase cascades: bifurcation of nuclear factor-κB and c-jun N-terminal kinase (JNK/SAPK) pathways at TNF receptor–associated factor 2. Proc Natl Acad Sci USA 94:9792–9796, 1997.

Spriggs MK, Armitage RJ, Strockbine L, Clifford KN, Macduff BM, Sato TA, Maliszewski CR, Fanslow WC. Recombinant human CD40 ligand stimulates B cell proliferation and immunoglobulin E secretion. J Exp Med 176:1543–1550, 1992.

Stamenkovic I, Clark EA, Seed B. A B-lymphocyte activation molecule related to the nerve growth factor receptor and induced by cytokines in carcinomas. EMBO J 8:1403–1410, 1989.

Stavnezer J. Molecular processes that regulate class switching. Curr Top Microbiol Immunol 245:127–168, 2000.

Stiehm ER, Chin TW, Haas A, Peerless AG. Infectious complications of the primary immunodeficiencies. Clin Immunol Immunopathol 40:69–86, 1986.

Stiehm ER, Fudenberg HH. Clinical and immunologic features of dysgammaglobulinemia type I: report of a case diagnosed in the first year of life. Am J Med 40:805–815, 1966.

Stout RD, Suttles J, Xu J, Grewal IS, Flavell RA. Impaired T cell–mediated macrophage activation in CD40 ligand-deficient mice. J Immunol 156:8–11, 1996.

Su L, Garber EA, Hsu Y-M. CD154 variant lacking tumor necrosis factor homologous domain inhibits cell surface expression of wild-type protein. J Biol Chem 276:1673–1676, 2001.

Subauste CS, Wessendarp M, Sorensen RU, Leiva LE. CD40–CD40 ligand interaction is central to cell-mediated immunity against Toxoplasma gondii: patients with hyper-IgM syndrome have a defective type 1 immune response that can be restored by soluble CD40 ligand trimer. J Immunol 162:6690–6700, 1999.

Sutherland CL, Krebs DL, Gold MR. An 11–amino acid sequence in the cytoplasmic domain of CD40 is sufficient for activation of c-Jun N-terminal kinase, activation of MAPKAP kinase-2, phosphorylation of I kappa B alpha, and protection of WEHI-231 cells from anti–IgM-induced growth arrest. J Immunol 162:4720–4730, 1999.

Tabone M-D, Leveger G, Landman J, Aznar C, Boccon-Gibod L, Lasfargues G. Disseminated lymphonodular cryptococcosis in a child with X-linked hyper-IgM immunodeficiency. Pediatr Infect Dis J 13:77–79, 1994.

Tahara M, Pergolizzi RG, Kobayashi H, Krause A, Luettich K, Lesser M, Crystal RG. Trans-splicing repair of CD40 ligand deficiency results in naturally regulated correction of a mouse model of hyper-IgM X-linked immunodeficiency. Nat Med 10:835–841, 2004.

Tan J, Town T, Mori T, Obregon D, Wu Y, DelleDonne A, Rojiani A, Crawfird F, Flavell RA, Mullan M. CD40 is expressed and functional on neuronal cells. EMBO J 21:643–652, 2002.

Thomas C, de Saint Basile G, LeDeist F, Theophile D, Benkerrou M, Haddard E, Blanche S, Fischer A. Brief report; correction of X-linked hyper-IgM syndrome by allogeneic bone marrow transplantation. N Engl J Med 333:426–429, 1995.

Tsitsikov EN, Ramesh N, Geha RS. Structure of the murine CD40 ligand gene. Mol Immunol 31:895–900, 1994.

Tsukamoto N, Kobayashi N, Azuma S, Yamamoto T, Inoue J. Two differently regulated nuclear factor kappaB activation pathways triggered by the cytoplasmic tail of CD40. Proc Natl Acad Sci USA 96:1234–1239, 1999.

Tsytsykova AV, Tsitsikov EN, Geha RS. The CD40L promoter contains nuclear factors of activated T cell–binding motifs which require AP-1 binding for activation of transcription. J Biol Chem 271:3763–3770, 1996.

Tu RK, Peters ME, Gourley GR, Hong R. Esophageal histoplasmosis in a child with immunodeficiency with hyper-IgM. AJR Am J Roentgenol 157:381–382, 1991.

Van den Eertwegh AJM, Noelle RJ, Roy M, Shepard DM, Aruffo A, Ledbetter JA, Boersma WJA, Claassen E. In vivo CD40–gp39 interactions are essential for thymus-dependent humoral immunity. I. In vivo expression of CD40 ligand, cytokines, and antibody production delineates sites of cognate T-B interactions. J Exp Med 178:1555–1565, 1993.

van Kooten C, Banchereau J. CD40–CD40 ligand. J Leukoc Biol 67:2–17, 2000.

Vidalain PO, Azocar O, Servet-Delprat C, Rabourdin-Combe C, Gerlier D, Manie S. CD40 signaling in human dendritic cells is initiated within membrane rafts. EMBO J 19:3304–3313, 2000.

Villa A, Notarangelo LD, DiSanto JP, Macchi PP, Strina D, Frattini A, Lucchini F, Patrosso CM, Giliani S, Mantuano E, Agosti S, Nocera G, Kroczek RA, Fischer A, Ugazio AG, de Saint Basile G, Vezzoni P. Organization of the human CD40L gene: implications for molecular defects in X chromosome–linked hyper-IgM syndrome and prenatal diagnosis. Proc Natl Acad Sci USA 91:2110–2114, 1994.

Wang C, Deng L, Hong M, Akkaraju GR, Inoue J, Chen ZJ. TAK1 is a ubiquitin-dependent kinase of MKK and IKK. Nature 412:346–351, 2001.

Wang WC, Cordoba J, Infante AJ, Conley ME. Successful treatment of neutropenia in hyper immunoglobulinemia M syndrome with granulocyte colony-stimulating factor. Am J Pediatr Hematol Oncol 16:160–163, 1994.

Whitmire JK, Slifka MK, Grewal IS, Flavell RA, Ahmed R. CD40 ligand–deficient mice generate a normal primary cytotoxic T-lymphocyte response but a defective humoral response to a viral infection. J Virol 70:8375–8381, 1996.

Wiley JA, Geha R, Harmsen AG. Exogenous CD40 ligand induces a pulmonary inflammation response. J Immunol 158:2932–2938, 1997.

Winkelstein JA, Marino MC, Ochs H, Fuleihan R, Scholl PR, Geha R, Stiehm ER, Conley ME. The X-linked hyper-IgM syndrome: clinical and immunological features of 79 patients. Medicine 82:373–384, 2003.

Xu J, Foy TM, Laman JD, Elliott EA, Dunn JJ, Waldschmidt TJ, Elsemore J, Noelle RJ, Flavell RA. Mice deficient for the CD40 ligand. Immunity 1:423–431, 1994.

Yang J, Boerm M, McCarty M, Bucana C, Fidler IJ, Zhuang Y, Su B. Mekk3 is essential for early embryonic cardiovascular development. Nat Genet 24:309–313, 2000.

Ye H, Park YC, Kreishman M, Kieff E, Wu H. The structural basis for the recognition of diverse receptor sequences by TRAF2. Mol Cell 4:321–330, 1999.

Yeh WC, Shahinian A, Speiser D, Kraunus J, Billia F, Wakeham A, de la Pompa JL, Ferrick D, Hum B, Iscove N, et al. Early lethality, functional NF-kappaB activation, and increased sensitivity to TNF-induced cell death in TRAF2-deficient mice. Immunity 7:715–725, 1997.

Yu P, Morawetz RA, Chattopadhyay S, Makino M, Kishimoto T, Kikutani H. CD40-deficient mice infected with the defective murine leukemia virus LP-BM5def do not develop murine AIDS but produce IgE and IgG1 in vivo. Eur J Immunol 29:615–625, 1999.

Zarnegar B, He JQ, Oganesyan G, Hoffman A, Baltimore D, Cheng G. Unique CD40-mediated biological program in B cell activation requires both type 1 and type 2 NF-kappaB activation pathways. Proc Natl Acad Sci USA 101:8108–8113, 2004.

Zhang K, Clark EA, Saxon A. CD40 stimulation provides an IFN-γ-independent and IL-4-dependent differentiation signal directly to human B cells for IgE production. J Immunol 146:1836–1842, 1991.

Ziegner UH, Kobayashi RH, Cunningham-Rundles C, Español T, Fasth A, Huttenlocher A, Krogstad P, Marthinsen L, Notarangelo LD, Pasic S. Rieger CH, Rudge P, Sankar R. Shigeoka AO, Stiehm ER, Sullivan KE, Webster AD, Ochs HD. Progressive neurodegeneration in patients with primary immunodeficiency disease on IVIG treatment. Clin Immunol 102:19–24, 2002.

Ziegner UH, Ochs HD, Schanen C, Feig SA, Seyama K, Futatani T, Gross T, Wakim M, Roberts RL, Rawlings DJ, Dovat S, Fraser JK, Stiehm ER. Unrelated umbilical cord stem cell transplantation for X-linked immunodeficiencies. J Pediatr 138:570–573, 2001.

Zonana J, Elder ME, Schneider LC, Orlow SJ, Moss C, Golabi M, Shapira SK, Farndon PA, Wara DW, Emmal SA, et al. A novel X-linked disorder of immune deficiency and hypohidrotic ectodermal dysplasia is allelic to incontinentia pigmenti and due to mutations in IKK-gamma (NEMO). Am J Hum Genet 67:1555–1562, 2000.

20

Autosomal Hyper-IgM Syndromes Caused by an Intrinsic B Cell Defect

ANNE DURANDY, PATRICK REVY, and ALAIN FISCHER

The study of inherited hyper-IgM syndromes (HIGM) has greatly contributed to our understanding of the normal processes of antibody maturation, because these syndromes have in common a defect in immunoglobulin (Ig) class switch recombination (CSR), as demonstrated by normal or elevated serum IgM levels. This is in contrast to absent or strongly decreased levels of the other immunoglobulin (Ig) isotypes. Antibody maturation leads to the production of antibodies of different isotypes and formation of B cell receptors (BCR) with high affinity for antigen. This event usually takes place in the secondary lymphoid organs (spleen, lymph nodes, tonsils) in an antigen- and T lymphocyte–dependent manner. When mature (but still naive) IgM+IgD+ B cells, after emigrating from the bone marrow (or fetal liver), encounter an antigen that is specifically recognized by their BCR, they proliferate vigorously and give birth to a unique lymphoid formation, the germinal center. In this location, B cells undergo the two major events of maturation: CSR and somatic hypermutation (SHM).

Class Switch Recombination and Somatic Hypermutation

Class switch recombination is a process of DNA recombination between two different switch (S) regions located upstream of the constant (C) regions, while the intervening DNA is deleted by forming excision circles (Iwasato et al., 1990; Matsuoka et al., 1990; von Schwedler et al., 1990; Kinoshita and Honjo, 2000; Manis et al., 2002). Replacement of the Cμ region by a Cx region from another class of Ig results in the production of antibodies of different isotypes (IgG, IgA, and IgE) with the same variable (V) region and thus the same antigen specificity and affinity. The different Ig isotypes vary in activities (half-life, binding to Fc receptors, ability to activate the complement system) and tissue localization (IgA is secreted by mucosal membranes). Thus CSR is necessary for an optimal humoral response against pathogens.

Through SHM, missense mutations and, less frequently, deletions or insertions are introduced into the V regions of immunoglobulins. This process is triggered by activation of the BCR and signaling via CD40 (Storb et al., 1998; Jacobs et al., 2001). These mutations occur at a high frequency in the V regions and their proximal flanks (1×10^{-3} bases/generation). SHM is required as a basis for the selection and proliferation of B cells expressing a BCR with a high affinity for antigen in close interaction with follicular dendritic cells (Rajewsky, 1996; Frazer et al., 1997). The CSR and SHM processes occur simultaneously in germinal centers, but neither is a prerequisite for the other because IgM may be mutated whereas IgG or IgA can remain unmutated (Kaartinen et al., 1983; Jacob and Kelsoe, 1992).

Three successive steps are required for the process of CSR and SHM:

1. Transcription of the targeted DNA (S and V regions). In S regions, this step leads to the formation of RNA–DNA hybrids, known as stable R-loops, on the template DNA strand, leaving the single nontemplate strand accessible for cleavage (Bransteitter et al., 2003; Chaudhuri et al., 2003; Dickerson et al., 2003; Ramiro et al., 2003; Yu et al., 2003).
2. DNA cleavage. During CSR, single-stranded DNA breaks result in double-stranded DNA breaks (DSB) by a mechanism currently unknown. It has been suggested that the template DNA strand may also be attacked in transcription bubbles (Bransteitter et al., 2003), resulting in scattered DSB, eventually processed by exonucleases and error-prone polymerases into blunt DSB. This error-prone DNA processing is suggested by the high frequency of mutations found in Sμ-Sx junctions (Chen et al., 2001). In V regions, single-stranded DNA breaks are either directly repaired or processed into scattered DSB. Alternatively, recent data suggest that blunt DSB could occur spontaneously in V regions and secondarily lead to scattered DSB (Catalan et al., 2003; Zan et al., 2003).

3. DNA repair. The mechanisms involved in DNA repair differ for CSR and SHM. During CSR, histone H2AX is phosphorylated, and the repair protein 53BP1 and the complex MRE11/RAD50/NBS1 are recruited at DSB in repair foci. Thereafter, the DNA repair machinery joins Sμ and Sx sequences by means of the widespread, constitutively expressed nonhomologous end-joining (NHEJ) enzymes, including the KU proteins that act on DNA blunt DSB (Rolink et al., 1996; Casellas et al., 1998; Manis et al., 1998). In contrast, SHM DNA repair does not require the NHEJ complex (Bemark et al., 2000), but probably the error-prone polymerases η and ζ (Zan et al., 2001) and the mismatch repair (MMR) enzymes (Cascalho et al., 1998; Wiesendanger et al., 1998; Kenter, 1999; Schrader et al., 1999; Evans and Alani, 2000).

CSR and SHM are initiated by T and B cell interaction, involving CD40 ligand (CD40L or CD154), a molecule transiently expressed on activated CD4+ T cells, and CD40, constitutively expressed on B lymphocytes. The CD40L–CD40 interaction is required for B cell proliferation, germinal center formation, CSR, and SHM, as demonstrated by the phenotype of patients with loss of function of either the *CD40L* (Aruffo et al., 1993; DiSanto et al., 1993) (see Chapter 19) or *CD40* gene (Ferrari et al., 2001). The role of the CD40 activation pathway in antibody maturation has been underscored by the recent demonstration of a profound immune deficiency, including the HIGM phenotype, as the result of defective nuclear factor-κB (NF-κB) signaling following CD40 activation. This is illustrated by the fact that hypomorphic mutations in the zinc finger domain of the nuclear factor-κB essential modulator gene (also called *NEMO* or *IKKγ*) (Zonana et al., 2000; Döffinger et al., 2001; Jain et al., 2001) or mutation producing a gain of function of the NF-κB inhibitor IκBα (Courtois et al., 2003) result, respectively, in a syndrome of X-linked or autosomal dominant anhydrotic ectodermal dysplasia (AED) associated with a T cell immunodeficiency and the HIGM condition.

HIGM syndromes with an autosomal recessive mode of inheritance have been described over the years by a number of investigators (Callard et al., 1994; Conley et al., 1994; Durandy et al., 1997). This condition is characterized by a specific B cell defect, resulting in increased susceptibility to bacterial infections (but not to opportunistic infections) that can be easily controlled by regular intravenous Ig (IVIG) substitution. Lymphadenopathy is frequent (50%–75%) and autoimmunity is reported in 25% of patients. SHM is found to be either normal or defective, according to the molecular defect. B cells are intrinsically defective; although they normally proliferate, they are unable to undergo CSR after activation by CD40L and cytokines. The precise delineation of the defects leading to abnormal CSR allowed the definition of molecularly defined autosomal recessive HIGM conditions.

Activation-Induced Cytidine Deaminase (AID) Deficiency

The activation-induced cytidine deaminase (*AICDA*) gene (*605257) was first identified in mice (Muramatsu et al., 1999) and cloned by substractive hybridization between murine lymphoma CH12F-2 B cells with and without induction of CSR in vitro. The AICDA RNA transcripts are detected only in B cells undergoing CSR or SHM either in vivo (in germinal center B cells) or in vitro (Muramatsu et al., 1999; Revy et al., 2000; Diaz and Casali, 2002; Faili et al., 2002; Papavasiliou and Schatz, 2002). The activation-induced cytidine deaminase (AID) protein is structurally similar (34% amino acid sequence identity) to the apoB mRNA-editing enzyme APOBEC-1. RNA editing is widely used to create new functional RNAs from a single gene. APOBEC-1 edits ApoB mRNA by deamination of a cytosine into a uracil

residue at a specific site, resulting in a stop codon. ApoB100 and ApoB48, the translation products of the unedited and edited apoB mRNAs, respectively, have entirely different functions and expression profiles (Navaratnam et al., 1993; Teng et al., 1993; Mehta et al., 2000). APOBEC-1 requires an auxiliary factor (ACF) for the site-specific editing of apoB mRNA. This auxiliary factor is widely expressed, including in tissues that do not express APOBEC-1 (Navaratnam et al., 1993; Teng et al., 1993; Yamanaka et al., 1994).

The open reading frame of the *AICDA* cDNA encodes a 198-residue protein with a molecular mass of approximately 24 kDa. This protein contains an active site for cytidine deamination, whose the sequence is conserved throughout the large cytidine deaminase family, and has been shown to display cytidine deaminase activity in vitro (Muramatsu et al., 1999). The C-terminal domain also contains a leucine-rich region that may be important for protein–protein interaction. This region is thought to bind accessory factors required for AID activity and may be important in AID tetramerization (Dickerson et al., 2003). Recently, a nuclear localization signal (NLS) and a nuclear export signal (NES) have been described in the N and C termini of the molecule (Ito et al., 2004), although the function of this NLS is still debated (Brar et al., 2004; McBride et al., 2004). An APOBEC-1-like domain is also described but its exact function remains unknown (Fig. 20.1).

AID-deficient patients and AID−/− mice display a defect in both CSR and SHM, which demonstrates the crucial role of AID in both these processes required for B cell terminal differentiation. The mechanism of action of AID, however, remains open to debate. Because the sequence of AID is similar to that of the RNA-editing enzyme APOBEC-1, originally it was proposed that AID edits an mRNA encoding a substrate common to CSR and SHM, probably an endonuclease (Chen et al., 2001; Kinoshita and Honjo, 2001; Honjo et al., 2002). The recently described requirement for de novo protein synthesis downstream of AID expression in CSR, compatible with the synthesis of a recombinase, is consistent with the RNA-editing model (Doi et al., 2003).

However, recent data strongly indicate that AID exerts a DNA-editing activity. Following the transfection of *E. coli*, AID deaminates deoxycytidine (dC) residues within DNA into deoxyuridine (dU) (Petersen-Mahrt et al., 2002). Subsequently, several groups have demonstrated in cell-free assays a direct role for AID on single-stranded DNA but not on double-stranded DNA, RNA–DNA hybrids, or RNA (Bransteitter et al., 2003; Chaudhuri et al., 2003; Dickerson et al., 2003; Ramiro et al., 2003). The transcription of S regions increases AID activity (Ramiro et al., 2003; Shinkura et al., 2003), probably by generating the secondary structures required for this activity (Yu et al., 2003). R loops are generated by the formation of RNA–DNA hybrids on the template DNA strand, rendering the single nontemplate strand a target for AID to generate the first lesion required for DNA cleavage. Although these observations provide strong evidence that AID has DNA-editing activity, they were obtained in nonphysiological conditions (overexpression in *E. coli*, using in vitro assays) in which the well-known RNA-editing protein APOBEC-1 exerts a similar effect (Harris et al., 2002; Petersen-Mahrt and Neuberger, 2003).

Clinical and Pathological Manifestations of AID Deficiency

Four reports describing AID deficiency (MIM #605258) have been published in the literature (Minegishi et al., 2000; Revy et al., 2000; Quartier et al., 2004; Lee et al., 2005). Although the onset of symptoms occurs during early childhood (mean age, 5 years), the diagnosis is frequently established at a later age.

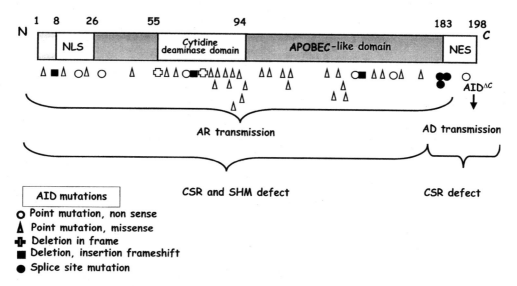

Figure 20.1. Schematic representation of activation-induced cytidine deaminase (AID) and localization of mutations in AID deficiency. Mutations are scattered throughout the entire gene. Each symbol represents a unique mutation. Mutations in the C-terminal domain do not affect somatic hypermutation (SHM). A mutation of the C-terminal region (AID$^{\Delta C}$) results in truncation of the last nine amino acids of the nuclear export signal (NES) and is responsible for an autosomal dominant (AD) form of HIGM. AR, autosomal recessive; CSR, class switch recombination; NLS, nuclear localization signal.

According to clinical data from 51 AID-deficient patients, all presented with recurrent bacterial infections; more than half (58%) had respiratory tract infections, with 14% of the patients reporting bronchiectasis. Gastrointestinal infections were observed in 27%, sometimes related to persistent *Giardia* infections. Such infections may result in failure to thrive. Infections of the central nervous system (e.g., meningitis) have been reported in 25% of AID-deficient patients, often associated with inadequate Ig substitution. One case each of herpes virus encephalitis and poliomyelitis have been described. Two adult patients died prematurely, one of pulmonary hemorrhage at 47 years of age, the other of septicemia at age 63.

A striking lymphoid hyperplasia is present in the majority (75%) of patients, affecting predominantly the cervical lymph nodes and tonsils. In one case, mesenteric lymph node hyperplasia resulted in intestinal obstruction. Hepatosplenomegaly has been reported in 10% of the patient cohort. Other manifestations include arthritis (12%) and autoimmune manifestations (hemolytic anemia, thrombopenia, and autoimmune hepatitis) (21%); autoantibodies of the IgM isotypes are detectable in some cases. Systematic lupus erythematous, diabetes mellitus, and Crohn's disease have been reported in one patient each (Table 20.1).

Laboratory Findings in AID Deficiency

All patients had normal or elevated IgM at the time of diagnosis and markedly diminished or, most often, undetectable serum levels of IgG and IgA. In some patients, 7S IgM can be demonstrated. In agreement with the aberrant serum immunoglobulin levels, antigen-specific (vaccine or infectious agents) antibodies of the IgG isotype were not detectable. When analyzed, IgM isohemagglutinins and antipolysaccharide IgM antibodies were present. IgM serum levels often diminish after Ig substitution, a finding suggesting that increased IgM reflects chronic antigenic stimulation rather than a direct effect of the AID deficiency.

Numbers of peripheral blood T cells (CD3$^+$) and T cell subsets (CD4$^+$ and CD8$^+$) as well as in vitro T cell proliferation to mitogens and antigens are normal. Peripheral blood B cells (CD19$^+$) are normal in number and express wild-type CD40 in normal concentrations. All CD19$^+$ B cells coexpress sIgM and sIgD, in contrast to age-matched controls, who have a population of CD19$^+$ B cells that express sIgG or sIgA and not sIgM/sIgD.

Soluble CD40-L (sCD40L)-induced B cell proliferation in vitro is normal. However, in vitro activation of B lymphocytes by sCD40L and interleukin-4 (IL-4), which induces IgE production in controls and CD40L-deficient patients (Durandy et al., 1993), is ineffective in AID-deficient patients. Under the same culture conditions, S-region transcription is normally induced, whereas DNA DSB are not detected in Sμ regions, providing evidence that the CSR defect is located downstream from transcription and upstream from DNA cleavage (Catalan et al., 2003). A normal fraction (20%–50%) of B cells express the CD27 marker, which indicates mutated memory B cells, even if limited to the IgM$^+$/IgD$^+$ B cell compartment (Klein et al., 1998). However, the frequency of SHM on CD19$^+$CD27$^+$ B cells is dramatically reduced. Thus, AID deficiency leads to not only lack of CSR but also defective SHM (Revy et al., 2000) (Table 20.2).

Most of the patients exhibit enlarged secondary lymphoid organs, which may require surgical resection (tonsils) or biopsy (cervical lymph nodes); histological evaluation shows marked follicular hyperplasia. Germinal centers are giant, being 2 to more than 10 times larger than those from control reactive lymph nodes (Plate 20.I). The mantle zone and interfollicular areas appear thin. The giant germinal centers contain a normal follicular dendritic cell network and B cells that are PNA$^+$, CD38$^+$, CD23$^+$, CD83$^+$, CD95$^+$, CD40$^+$, IgM$^+$, Bcl2$^-$, and Ki67$^+$. Strikingly, many germinal-center B cells coexpress sIgD, in contrast to normal reactive germinal centers, in which IgD$^+$ B cells are rarely found. The high proliferation index of germinal center B cells is associated with a dense network of macrophages filled with apoptotic bodies giving a starry-sky appearance. The characteristic markers and size of the germinal-center B cells identify them as proliferating (Ki67$^+$) germinal-center founder cells (CD38$^+$, sIgM$^+$, sIgD$^+$), prone to undergo SHM and selection (Lebecque et al., 1997). Occasional CD27$^+$ B cells as well as IgM- and IgD-expressing

Table 20.1. Clinical Manifestations in Hyper-IgM Syndrome Due to an Intrinsic B Cell Defect

Clinical Manifestations	AID Deficiency (%)	UNG Deficiency (%)	Specific Defect of CSR located	
			Upstream (%)	Downstream (%)
			From DNA Cleavage	
Patients (n)	55	3	16	15
Mean age at diagnosis in years (range)	5 (0.3–53)	6 (3–9)	7 (1–15)	9 (0.3–23)
Recurrent infections				
Upper respiratory tract	93	100	100	100
Lower respiratory tract	58	100	87	93
Digestive tract	17	66	31	20
Urinary tract	6	33	0	13
Central nervous system	14	0	0	0
Lymphoid hyperplasia	75	66	50	40
Autoimmunity	21	0	0	27
Lymphoma	0	0	0	13

AID, activation-induced cytidine deaminase; CSR, class switch recombination; UNG, uracil-*N*-glycosylase.

Table 20.2. Laboratory Findings in Hyper-IgM Syndrome Due to an Intrinsic B Cell Defect

Assay	Phenotype	AID Deficiency (%)	UNG Deficiency (%)	Specific CSR Defect	
				Upstream (%)	Downstream (%)
				From DNA Cleavage	
Patients		55	3	16	15
Ig Levels					
IgM	Normal	5	0	25	20
IgM	Elevated	95	100	75	80
IgG	<2 SD below normal	15	66	25	30
IgG	Undetectable	85	33	75	70
IgA	<2 SD below normal	17	66	30	30
IgA	Undetectable	83	33	70	70
Antibody Production					
Allohemagglutinins	Present	100	ND	100	100
Polysaccharid IgM antibody	Present	100	ND	100	100
IgG antibody production	Undetectable	100	100	100	100
B Cell Count and Function					
B cell count	Normal	100	100	100	100
CD27+ B cell count	Normal	100	100	95	0
	Decreased	0	0	5	100
sCD40L-induced proliferation	Normal	100	100	100	100
sCD40L- induced CSR	Undetectable	100	100	100	100
SHM	Normal	10	100 (biased)	100	100*
	Decreased	90	0	0	0

CSR, class switch recombination; ND, not done; SHM, somatic hypermutation.

*Measured on a decreased CD27+ B cell population.

plasma cells are found in germinal centers and T cell areas; however, neither IgG- nor IgA-expressing plasma cells are observed.

Molecular Basis of AID Deficiency

Because the analysis of informative pedigrees suggested an autosomal recessive inheritance, genetic mapping was attempted by studying the segregation of polymorphic microsatellite markers in several consanguineous families. Random screening of the genome indicated that disease segregation was compatible in all studied families with the telomeric region of the short arm of chromosome 12 at p13 with a multipoint LOD score of 10.45

(Revy et al., 2000). Recombination analysis defined the critical genetic interval as a 4.5 cM region, in which a gene coding for AID had recently been localized (Muto et al., 2000). The human *AICDA* gene encompasses about 10 kb of genomic DNA and is organized in five exons and four introns. Definition of the exon–intron boundaries allowed a search for mutations at the genomic level. Deleterious mutations were found in all regions of the gene, including the cytidine deaminase domain (Minegishi et al., 2000; Revy et al., 2000; Quartier et al., 2004; Lee et al., 2005).

Forty different mutations have been found in 45 families, most often as homozygous defects (29 families), less frequently as

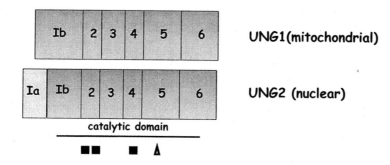

Figure 20.2. Schematic representation of uracil-*N*-glycosylase (UNG) and localization of mutations in UNG deficiency. Mutations affect the catalytic domain of both UNG1 (mitochondrial isoform) and UNG2 (nuclear isoform).

compound heterozygous mutations (16 families). They include missense mutations (28 families), nonsense mutations, and small deletions (6 families) (Fig. 20.1). In addition, deletions of the entire coding region (3 families) or splice-site mutations (3 families) leading to either a longer RNA transcript or to frameshift and premature stop codon were reported. The same mutations were found in a number of unrelated families of the same ethnic origin (e.g., French Canadians, Turkish); analysis of flanking polymorphic markers in these families indicated a common ancestral origin of the mutation (Minegishi et al., 2000; Revy et al., 2000).

Several mutations, located in the C-terminal part of the *AICDA* gene, were recently shown to result in defective CSR, whereas SHM is not affected (Ta et al., 2003). This observation suggests that, in addition to its cytidine deaminase activity, AID acts on CSR by binding a CSR-specific cofactor. Because mutations are normally found in Sμ regions, a defect in targeting AID to the S regions is unlikely and a defect in DNA repair can be suspected (Barreto et al., 2003). Another unexpected finding recently reported (Kasahara et al., 2003; Imai et al., 2005) is that a heterozygous nonsense mutation, also located in the C-terminal domain, results in the loss of the nine last amino acids of NES (AID$^{\Delta C}$) and a variable HIGM condition transmitted as an autosomal dominant disease (Fig. 20.1). Haploinsufficiency is higly unlikely because subjects heterozygous for AID deficiency always exhibit normal Ig levels. Two nonexclusive explanations for this dominant effect have been proposed: (1) the mutated allele, which is devoid of a normal nuclear export signal, accumulates in the nucleus, overriding the wild-type allele (Ito et al., 2004), or (2) in order to induce CSR, AID has to form homodimeric or multimeric complexes while the mutated allele cannot multimerize (Ta et al., 2003).

Uracil-*N* Glycosylase (UNG) Deficiency

Uracil-*N* Glycosylase

Uracil-*N*-glycosylase belongs to the family of uracil-DNA-glycosylases capable of deglycosylating uracil residues that are misintegrated into DNA. Each of the two different UNG promoters creates a different isoform: UNG1 (305 amino acids), which is mitochondrial and ubiquitously expressed, and UNG2 (314 amino acids), which is nuclear and expressed in proliferating cells, including B cells undergoing CSR. The catalytic domain binds the replication protein RPA and the proliferating cell nu-

clear antigen (PCNA) in a multimolecular complex involved in DNA base excision repair (Fig. 20.2). According to a model proposed by Petersen-Mahrt and Neuberger (2002), AID deaminates cytosine into uracil residues on single-stranded DNA. Following the deglycosylation and removal of uracil residues by UNG, an abasic site is created that can be attacked by an apyrimidinic endonuclease (APE), leading to single-stranded DNA breaks. The processing and repair of the DNA nicks complete both CSR and SHM. In the absence of UNG, this pathway is impaired, resulting in defective CSR and abnormal SHM. The presence of SHM with a skewed pattern of G/C residues may arise from the replication of U/G lesions in the absence of U removal. MMR enzymes may also recognize and repair these lesions, introducing mutations on neighboring nucleotides that result in transitions and transversions of A/T residues (Petersen-Mahrt et al., 2002; Rada et al., 2002). Alternatively it has been proposed that rather than UNG's enzymatic activity on DNA, the UNG protein is required for CSR by its involvement in the recruitment of DNA repair molecules or its role in folding the CSR-induced DSB (Honjo et al., 2004). However, this hypothesis does not explain the defect in DSB formation within Sμ regions observed in UNG-deficient B cells (Imai et al., 2003b).

Clinical and Pathological Manifestations of UNG Deficiency

To date, only three UNG-deficient patients (MIM #608106, gene *191525) have been reported (Imai et al., 2003b); two were diagnosed during childhood, the other as an adult. All three patients have had a history of frequent bacterial infections of the respiratory tract that are easily controlled by regular IVIG infusions. Lymphadenopathy was observed in two of three patients, one with impressive enlargement of mediastinal lymph nodes. The adult patient has developed Sjögren syndrome in recent years. The absence of metabolic abnormality suggests that UNG deficiency is compensated in mitochondria by other uracil-DNA glycosylases (Table 20.1).

Laboratory Findings in UNG Deficiency

At the time of diagnosis, all three patients presented with HIGM, defined by markedly diminished serum levels of IgG and IgA and an increased serum level of IgM. No antibodies of the IgG isotype were detected to vaccines nor to infectious agents.

Peripheral blood T cell and T cell subset numbers as well as in vitro T cell proliferation to mitogens and antigens were normal. Peripheral blood B cells (CD19[+]) were normal in number, expressed CD40, which was of wild type, and coexpressed sIgM and sIgD with a normal fraction expressing CD27.

When cultured in the presence of sCD40-L, B cells proliferate normally but fail to undergo CSR and secrete IgG, IgA, or IgE in the presence of appropriate cytokines. As in AID deficiency, the CSR defect occurs downstream from S-region transcription and upstream from DSB in Sμ regions.

Somatic hypermutations were found in normal frequency in CD19[+]CD27[+] B cells but exhibited a biased pattern. Almost all mutations are transitions at G/C residues (G>A, C>T), although transitions and transversions are equally present on A/T nucleotides (Table 20.2).

The association of an HIGM phenotype with UNG deficiency, together with the description of a mild CSR defect and a similarly biased SHM in UNG-deficient mice, provides a strong argument for DNA-editing activity of AID (Di Noia and Neuberger, 2002; Rada et al., 2002).

Molecular Basis of UNG Deficiency

Four different mutations affecting the catalytic domain of UNG1 and UNG2 have been found. Two patients have small deletions leading to a premature stop codon (homozygous mutation in one patient born in a consanguineous family and two heterozygous mutations in the other). The third patient carries a homozygous missense mutation (Fig. 20.3). UNG expression and function were defective in Epstein-Barr virus (EBV) B cell lines, providing evidence for the lack of any compensatory UNG-DNA glycosylase activity, at least in B cells.

Hyper-Igm Syndromes with Unknown Molecular Defect(s)

Not all cases of HIGM due to an intrinsic B cell defect are related to AID or UNG deficiency. Although most of these cases are sporadic, the mode of inheritance observed in a few multiplex or consanguineous families is compatible with an autosomal recessive pattern. The clinical phenotype is similar to that of AID deficiency, including increased susceptibility to bacterial infections of the respiratory and gastrointestinal tracts. Lymphoid hyperplasia is milder and less frequent (50%), consisting of moderate follicular hyperplasia without the giant germinal centers typical of AID deficiency (Table 20.1).

The CSR defect appears to be milder, as residual serum levels of IgG can be detected in some patients. While isohemagglutinins and IgM antipolysaccharide antibodies are present in normal amounts, IgG antibodies against immunization antigens or infectious agents cannot be detected. Upon activation with sCD40L and cytokines, B cells proliferate but do not undergo CSR (Table 20.2).

The definition of the precise location of the CSR defect has led to the delineation of two distinct groups.

Class Switch Recombination Defect Located Upstream from S Region DNA Cleavage

We are following a subgroup of 16 patients with an HIGM phenotype characterized by good prognosis, lack of autoimmune manifestations, and no increased risk of lymphoma or other malignancies. No CSR-induced DSB occur in Sμ regions of patients' B cells, although both AID and UNG transcripts are normally expressed. The defect, located downstream from S-region transcription and upstream from the S-region DNA cleavage, is restricted to CSR, as SHM is normal in both frequency and pattern in the CD27[+] B cell subset, which is represented in normal numbers.

This type of HIGM could thus be caused by a direct or indirect impairment of AID targeting on S regions. Although targeting factors of AID are presently unknown, they most likely exist because AID deaminates cytosines only in the S and V regions in B cells. AID shares sequence similarity with the RNA-editing enzyme APOBEC-1, which is only expressed in the gut and requires a cofactor, ACF (APOBEC-1-cofactor), which targets APOBEC-1 on a unique C residue in ApoB mRNA. In addition, specific switch factors have been described in CSR-activated B cells. Although their role remains elusive, it has been proposed that these cofactors act as docking proteins for the recruitment of the recombinase complexes to DNA-specific regions (Shanmugam et al., 2000; Ma et al., 2002).

Class Switch Recombination Defect Located Downstream from S Region DNA Cleavage

This condition has been found in 15 patients thus far (Imai et al., 2003a). The prognosis of this HIGM subgroup is complicated by the occurrence of autoimmune manifestations that were found in 4 of 15 patients and were sometimes life threatening (severe autoimmune hemolytic anemia). Double-strand breaks are normally detected in Sμ regions in CSR-activated B cells, suggesting a defect downstream from DNA cleavage. The subsequent step, DNA repair, is impaired because excision circles and functional transcripts of switched isotypes cannot be detected. The normal presence of DSB and of mutations in Sμ regions rules out a defect in AID-targeting to S regions. SHM is present in normal frequency and pattern in the purified CD27[+] B cell population. However, the CD27[+] B cell count is decreased compared to that of controls (<10% of the B cell population).

Two hypotheses can account for this unique phenotype: (1) a defect in survival signals delivered to switched B cells—this does not fit with the observed defective in vitro CSR—and (2) a DNA repair defect, because CSR-induced DSB occur normally. CSR and SHM are known to use different pathways for DNA repair. NHEJ enzymes and the MRE11/hRad50/NBS1 protein complex have been shown to be involved in CSR DNA repair (Rolink et al., 1996; Casellas et al., 1998). Nevertheless, a defect in one of these proteins is unlikely given the phenotype of patients carrying mutations in *MRE11* or *NBS1* genes (ataxia-like disease or Nijmegen breakage syndrome, respectively; see Chapters 29 and 30). A defective CSR with normal SHM has been reported in H2AX and 53BP1 knockout mice (Petersen et al., 2001; Manis et al., 2004; Ward et al., 2004) but a defect in one of these genes has been ruled out in our patients by sequence analysis. Thus, other DNA repair factor(s) have to be considered, including the undefined cofactor that binds to the C-terminal part of AID. Two of our 15 patients have developed Hodgkin lymphoma. Although the number is small, this observation is compatible with a DNA repair defect, which could facilitate illegitimate recombination leading to oncogene activation.

Strategy for Diagnosis of Hyper-IgM Syndrome Due to an Intrinsic B Cell Defect

Like all patients with the diagnosis of HIGM, this group of patients with an intrinsic B cell defect is defined by markedly diminished serum levels of IgG and IgA and a normal or increased level of IgM. Assessment of CD27+ B cell count and analysis of the frequency and pattern of SHM allow identification of these different autosomal recessive HIGM conditions (Table 20.2). A precise diagnosis is required for optimal prognosis assessment.

Other HIGM syndromes not caused by a B cell–specific abnormality are associated with T cell defects, which strongly worsens the prognosis. Defects of CD40L and CD40 are excluded by assessing membrane expression of these two molecules and/or direct gene sequencing (see Chapter 19). A defect in the NF-κB activation pathway (due to mutations in *NEMO*, also designated IKK-γ, or in IκBα) is often responsible for an HIGM phenotype characterized by a T cell defect and frequently associated with hypohidrotic ectodermal dysplasia (see Chapter 36).

Other causes of HIGM that should be excluded are the following:

1. Ataxia telangiectasia (AT), in which elevated IgM can develop before the onset of neurological manifestations (Meyts et al., 2003). It has been proposed that the HIGM condition in AT is caused by a T cell activation abnormality (Gatti et al., 1991) or, more likely, by a B cell defect, since AT-mutated (*ATM*), the gene responsible for this syndrome, plays a role in CSR (but not SHM) DNA repair (Pan-Hammarstrom et al., 2003; see Chapter 29).
2. Congenital rubella, in which a defect of T cell activation leads to defective CD40L expression on CD4+ T cells (Kawamura et al., 2000).
3. Patients with major histocompatibility complex (MHC) class II deficiency have diminished expression of CD40L by activated CD4+ T cells and can present with elevated serum IgM (Nonoyama et al., 1998; see Chapter 17).
4. An HIGM phenotype has been observed as part of a syndrome associated with microcephaly, mental retardation, and combined immunodeficiency. B cells from these patients are unable to proliferate in response to CD40 signaling and BCR activation. In spite of progressive B cell lymphopenia, serum IgM levels remain elevated. Circulating CD4+ lymphocytes are limited to expression of the memory marker CD45RO and the T cell proliferative response to mitogens is defective. These features suggest a DNA repair defect not restricted to the B cell compartment (A. Durandy, unpublished observation).

Prenatal Diagnosis

Prenatal diagnosis can be performed by sequence analysis of the *AID* or *UNG* gene with genomic DNA obtained from the fetus. Prenatal diagnosis could raise ethical problems since the prognosis is generally good and nearly all patients reach adulthood with only a few recurrent bacterial infections, provided that prophylactic treatment with IVIG is started early and given on a regular basis. However, other life-threatening complications (autoimmunity, lymphoma) can occur.

Prognosis and Treatment

As soon as the diagnosis of HIGM is established, treatment with regular IVIG infusions (400–600 mg/kg every 21–28 days) must be initiated with the aim of maintaining a trough IgG level of 700–800 mg/dl. This protocol results in a significant reduction in the severity and frequency of infections and often reduces or even normalizes serum IgM levels. However, the lymphoid hyperplasia does not seem to be reduced by IVIG therapy.

With adequate prophylactic treatment, patients with HIGM due to intrinsic B cell deficiency are protected from infections and can reach adulthood without developing bronchiectasis. Surprisingly, they do not appear to be unusually susceptible to enteroviral infections, a serious complication observed in patients with X-linked agammaglobulinemia (Quartier et al., 2000; see also Chapter 21). This observation suggests a protective role of IgM (even without SHM) as a first barrier against some pathogens.

Autoimmunity has been reported in AID deficiency and in the HIGM condition characterized by a CSR defect located downstream from the S-region cleavage. Both conditions are characterized by an SHM defect (in the latter condition the B cell memory subset is decreased). In contrast, autoimmunity has not been reported in the HIGM condition characterized by a CSR defect located upstream from the S-region cleavage, in which both SHM and memory B cell numbers are normal. Autoimmunity could thus be related to defective SHM. It may be that autoimmunity, initiated by germ-line Ig sequences, is caused by the lack of negative selection in germinal centers.

A more serious complication, the occurrence of tumors, has to be considered for the prognostic assessment. The subgroup of HIGM characterized by a CSR defect located downstream from the S-region cleavage may be directly related to a DNA repair defect and patients could become susceptible to an increased risk of malignancy. UNG is part of the DNA base excision repair and is thus involved in the repair of spontaneously occurring base lesions as part of a major antimutagenic defense strategy. Interestingly, UNG-deficient mice develop B cell lymphomas when aging (Nilsen et al., 2003), so UNG deficiency may predispose to maliganancies in adulthood (Table 20.3).

Animal Models of AID and UNG Deficiencies

No naturally occurring mutants defective in AID or UNG have been described in animals. However, AID- and UNG-deficient mice, as well as AID-transgenic mice, have been generated by gene-targeting techniques.

Table 20.3. Main Clinical and Laboratory Findings in Hyper-IgM Syndrome Due to an Intrinsic B Cell Defect

Molecular Defect	Transmission	S DNA Cleavage	B CD27+	SHM Frequency	Autoimmunity	Lymphoma
AID	AR	–	+	–	+	–
AID-C ter	AR	Not done	+	+	–	–
AID$^{\Delta c}$	AD	+	+	+*	–	–
UNG	AR	–	+	+ (bias)	–	?
Other HIGM	AR	–	+	+	–	–
Other HIGM	AR	+	Diminished	+†	+	+

AD, autosomal dominant; AR, autosomal recessive; SHM, somatic hypermutation.

*In six of seven patients.

†Normal in frequency in the diminished B CD27+ population.

AID-Deficient Mice

The phenotype of AID$^{-/-}$ mice resembles completely that observed in patients and is associated with the three main features of AID deficiency:

1. Defective CSR in vivo and in vitro. The CSR defect has been shown to occur downstream from S-region transcription and upstream from the occurrence of repair foci at DSB on the Ig locus (Petersen et al., 2001).
2. Defective somatic hypermutation.
3. Giant germinal-center formation in spleen and lymph nodes with accumulation of IgM$^+$/IgD$^+$/PNA$^+$ proliferating B cells (Muramatsu et al., 2000).

AID-Transgenic Mice

AID-transgenic mice express mutations in the T cell receptor, a finding indicating that aberrantly and overexpressed AID can exert its activity outside the B cell compartment. All of these mice develop tumors affecting the lymphoid compartment (T lymphoma) and nonlymphoid tissues (e.g., epithelium of respiratory bronchioles). Interestingly, these transgenic mice do not develop B cell lymphomas, an observation suggesting that AID activity and/or nuclear localization can be regulated effectively only in B cells (Okazaki et al., 2003).

UNG-Deficient Mice

UNG-deficient mice have been generated to study the effects of base excision repair defects on the incidence of tumors (Nilsen et al., 2000). No striking biologic effects could be shown, most likely because of compensatory mechanisms provided by other uracil-N glycosylases. A more recent study of CSR and SHM provided evidence for a mild in vivo and a profound in vitro CSR defect. The remaining CSR observed in vivo is likely related to MMR enzymes, which are known to be involved in CSR in mice (Rada et al., 2002). This study also showed a normal frequency of SHM that exhibit a skewed pattern. Since all mutations at G/C residues are transitions, likely occurring on U/G nucleotides after replication, mutations observed on A/T residues could be the consequence of the recognition and repair of U/G lesions by MMR. Both observations, confirmed by similar data in humans (although the CSR defect is much more pronounced in UNG-deficient patients), are a strong argument for a DNA-editing activity of AID.

Without exception, UNG-deficient mice develop B lymphomas when aging, an observation that could reflect the lack of compensatory uracil-DNA glycosylases in B cells (Nilsen et al., 2003). Another adverse consequence has been reported in UNG-deficient mice: compared with wild-type mice, postischemic brain injury is much more severe, a complication likely related to the mitochondrial DNA repair defect (Endres et al., 2004).

Conclusions

The ongoing investigation of inherited HIGM syndromes is shedding new light on the process of antibody maturation in human B cells. This is especially true for the evaluation of HIGM due to an intrinsic B cell defect, which has illustrated the complex mechanisms involved in both events of B cell maturation—CSR and SHM. On the basis of clinical phenotypes, the following mode of action of AID and UNG is proposed: AID, at center stage of CSR and SHM, deaminates cytosine nucleotides to uracil in S and V

regions of Ig genes. The integrated uridine nucleosides are deglycosylated and removed from DNA by UNG, resulting in an abasic site that becomes a target for an endonuclease. This DNA cleavage step appears to be sufficient for SHM, at least on G/C residues, but not for CSR, which require DSB. Beyond its cytidine deaminase activity, AID requires specific cofactors. A CSR-specific cofactor, which could be involved in DSB DNA repair, is expected to bind to the C-terminal part of multimeric AID. It is likely that the molecular definition of the HIGM entity caused by a CSR defect located downstream from S-region cleavage will lead to the identification of this cofactor. Taken together, these observations indicate that AID acts in a multimolecular complex composed of individual partners that have yet to be defined. The precise diagnosis of these HIGM conditions, in addition to contributing to a better understanding of the antibody maturation processes, provides science-based guidelines for better prognosis assessment and treatment management.

Acknowledgments

This work was supported by INSERM, l'Association de la Recherche contre le Cancer (ARC), la Ligue Contre le Cancer; CEE contract EURO-Policy-PID no. SP23-CT-2005-006411; the Institut des Maladies Rares (GIS); and Assistance-Publique-Hopitaux de Paris (AP-HP). Patrick Revy is a scientist from CNRS.

References

Aruffo A, Farrington M, Hollenbaugh D, Li X, Milatovich A, Nonoyama S, Bajorath J, Grosmaire LS, Stenkamp R, Neubauer M, et al. The CD40 ligand, gp39, is defective in activated T cells from patients with X-linked hyper-IgM syndrome. Cell 72:291–300, 1993.

Barreto V, Reina-San-Martin B, Ramiro AR, McBride KM, Nussenzweig MC. C-terminal deletion of AID uncouples class switch recombination from somatic hypermutation and gene conversion. Mol Cell 12:501–508, 2003.

Bemark M, Sale JE, Kim HJ, Berek C, Cosgrove RA, Neuberger MS. Somatic hypermutation in the absence of DNA-dependent protein kinase catalytic subunit (DNA-PK(cs)) or recombination-activating gene (RAG)1 activity. J Exp Med 192:1509–1514, 2000.

Bransteitter R, Pham P, Scharff MD, Goodman MF. Activation-induced cytidine deaminase deaminates deoxycytidine on single-stranded DNA but requires the action of RNase. Proc Natl Acad Sci USA 100:4102–4107, 2003.

Brar S, Watson M, Diaz M. Activation-induced cytosine deaminase, AID, is actively exported out of the nucleus but retained by the induction of DNA breaks. J Biol Chem 279:26395–26401, 2004.

Callard RE, Smith SH, Herbert J, Morgan G, Padayachee M, Lederman S, Chess L, Kroczek RA, Fanslow WC, Armitage RJ. CD40 ligand (CD40L) expression and B cell function in agammaglobulinemia with normal or elevated levels of IgM (HIM). Comparison of X-linked, autosomal recessive, and non-X-linked forms of the disease, and obligate carriers. J Immunol 153:3295–3306, 1994.

Cascalho M, Wong J, Steinberg C, Wabl M. Mismatch repair co-opted by hypermutation. Science 279(5354):1207–1210, 1998.

Casellas R, Nussenzweig A, Wuerffel R, Pelanda R, Reichlin A, Suh H, Qin XF, Besmer E, Kenter A, Rajewsky K, Nussenzweig MC. Ku80 is required for immunoglobulin isotype switching. EMBO J 17:2404–2411, 1998.

Catalan N, Selz F, Imai K, Revy P, Fischer A, Durandy A. The block in immunoglobulin class switch recombination caused by activation-induced cytidine deaminase deficiency occurs prior to the generation of DNA double strand breaks in switch mu region. J Immunol 171:2504–2509, 2003.

Chaudhuri J, Tian M, Khuong C, Chua K, Pinaud E, Alt FW. Transcription-targeted DNA deamination by the AID antibody diversification enzyme. Nature 422(6933):726–730, 2003.

Chen X, Kinoshita K, Honjo T. Variable deletion and duplication at recombination junction ends: implication for staggered double-strand cleavage in class-switch recombination. Proc Natl Acad Sci USA 98:13860–13865, 2001.

Conley ME, Larche M, Bonagura VR, Lawton AR 3rd, Buckley RH, Fu SM, Coustan-Smith E, Herrod HG, Campana D. Hyper IgM syndrome associated with defective CD40-mediated B cell activation [see comments]. J Clin Invest 94:1404–1409, 1994.

Courtois G, Smahi A, Reichenbach J, Doffinger R, Cancrini C, Bonnet M, Puel A, Chable-Bessia C, Yamaoka S, Feinberg J, Dupuis-Girod S, Bodemer C, Livadiotti S, Novelli F, Rossi P, Fischer A, Israel A, Munnich A, Le Deist F, Casanova JL. A hypermorphic IκBα mutation is associated with autosomal dominant anhidrotic ectodermal dysplasia and T cell immunodeficiency. J Clin Invest 112:1108–1115, 2003.

Diaz M, Casali P. Somatic immunoglobulin hypermutation. Curr Opin Immunol 14:235–240, 2002.

Dickerson SK, Market E, Besmer E, Papavasiliou FN. AID mediates hypermutation by deaminating single stranded DNA. J Exp Med 197:1291–1296, 2003.

Di Noia J, Neuberger MS. Altering the pathway of immunoglobulin hypermutation by inhibiting uracil-DNA glycosylase. Nature 419(6902):43–48, 2002.

DiSanto JP, Bonnefoy JY, Gauchat JF, Fischer A, de Saint Basile G. CD40 ligand mutations in X-linked immunodeficiency with hyper-IgM. Nature 361(6412):541–543, 1993.

Döffinger R, Smahi A, Bessia C, Geissmann F, Feinberg J, Durandy A, Bodemer C, Kenwrick S, Dupuis S, Blanche S, Wood P, Headon DJ, Overbeek PA, Holland SM, Kumararatne DS, Fischer A, Shapiro R, Conley ME, Reimund E, Kalhoff H, Abinum M, Munnich A, Israel A, Courtois G, Casanova JL. X-linked ectodermal dysplasia anhydrotic and immunodeficiency is caused by hypo-functional NEMO mutations. Nat Genet 27:277–285, 2001.

Doi T, Kinoshita K, Ikegawa M, Muramatsu M, Honjo T. De novo protein synthesis is required for the activation-induced cytidine deaminase function in class-switch recombination. Proc Natl Acad Sci USA 100:2634–2638, 2003.

Durandy A, Hivroz C, Mazerolles F, Schiff C, Bernard F, Jouanguy E, Revy P, DiSanto JP, Gauchat JF, Bonnefoy JY, Casanova JL, Fischer A. Abnormal CD40-mediated activation pathway in B lymphocytes from patients with hyper-IgM syndrome and normal CD40 ligand expression. J Immunol 158:2576–2584, 1997.

Durandy A, Schiff C, Bonnefoy JY, Forveille M, Rousset F, Mazzei G, Milili M, Fischer A. Induction by anti-CD40 antibody or soluble CD40 ligand and cytokines of IgG, IgA and IgE production by B cells from patients with X-linked hyper IgM syndrome. Eur J Immunol 23:2294–2299, 1993.

Endres M, Biniszkiewicz D, Sobol RW, Harms C, Ahmadi M, Lipski A, Katchanov J, Mergenthaler P, Dirnagl U, Wilson SH, Meisel A, Jaenisch R. Increased postischemic brain injury in mice deficient in uracil-DNA glycosylase. J Clin Invest 113:1711–1721, 2004.

Evans E, Alani E. Roles for mismatch repair factors in regulating genetic recombination. Mol Cell Biol 20:7839–7844, 2000.

Faili A, Aoufouchi S, Flatter E, Gueranger Q, Reynaud CA, Weill JC. Induction of somatic hypermutation in immunoglobulin genes is dependent on DNA polymerase iota. Nature 419(6910):944–947, 2002.

Ferrari S, Giliani S, Insalaco A, Al-Ghonaium A, Soresina AR, Loubser M, Avanzini MA, Marconi M, Badolato R, Ugazio AG, Levy Y, Catalan N, Durandy A, Tbakhi A, Notarangelo LD, Plebani A. Mutations of CD40 gene cause an autosomal recessive form of immunodeficiency with hyper IgM. Proc Natl Acad Sci USA 98:12614–12619, 2001.

Frazer JK, LeGros J, de Bouteiller O, Liu YJ, Banchereau J, Pascual V, Capra JD. Identification and cloning of genes expressed by human tonsillar B lymphocyte subsets. Ann NY Acad Sci 815:316–318, 1997.

Gatti RA, Boder E, Vinters HV, Sparkes RS, Norman A, Lange K. Ataxia-telangiectasia: an interdisciplinary approach to pathogenesis. Medicine (Baltimore) 70:99–117, 1991.

Harris RS, Petersen-Mahrt SK, Neuberger MS. RNA editing enzyme APOBEC1 and some of its homologs can act as DNA mutators. Mol Cell 10:1247–1253, 2002.

Honjo T, Kinoshita K, Muramatsu M. Molecular mechanism of class switch recombination: linkage with somatic hypermutation. Annu Rev Immunol 20:165–196, 2002.

Honjo T, Muramatsu M, Fagarasan S. AID: how does it aid antibody diversity? Immunity 20:659–668, 2004.

Imai K, Catalan N, Plebani A, Marodi L, Sanal O, Kumaki S, Nagendran V, Wood P, Glastre C, Sarrot-Reynauld F, Forveille M, Revy P, Fischer A, Durandy A. Hyper-IgM syndrome type 4 with a B-lymphocyte intrinsic selective deficiency in immunoglobulin class switch recombination. J Clin Invest 112:136–142, 2003.

Imai K, Slupphaug G, Lee WI, Revy P, Nonoyama S, Catalan N, Yel L, Forveille M, Kavli B, Krokan HE, Ochs HD, Fischer A, Durandy A. Human uracil-DNA glycosylase deficiency associated with profoundly impaired immunoglobulin class-switch recombination. Nat Immunol 7:7, 2003.

Imai K, Zhu Y, Revy P, Morio T, Mizutani S, Fischer A, Nonoyama S, Durandy A. Analysis of class switch recombination and somatic hypermutation in patients affected with autosomal dominant hyper-IgM syndrome type 2. Clin Immunol 115:277–285, 2005.

Ito S, Nagaoka H, Shinkura R, Begum N, Muramatsu M, Nakata M, Honjo T. Activation-induced cytidine deaminase shuttles between nucleus and cytoplasm like apolipoprotein B mRNA editing catalytic polypeptide 1. Proc Natl Acad Sci USA 101:1975–1980, 2004.

Iwasato T, Shimizu A, Honjo T, Yamagishi H. Circular DNA is excised by immunoglobulin class switch recombination. Cell 62:143–149, 1990.

Jacob J, Kelsoe G. In situ studies of the primary immune response to (4-hydroxy-3-nitrophenyl)acetyl. II. A common clonal origin for periarteriolar lymphoid sheath-associated foci and germinal centers. J Exp Med 176:679–687, 1992.

Jacobs H, Rajewsky K, Fukita Y, Bross L. Indirect and direct evidence for DNA double-strand breaks in hypermutating immunoglobulin genes. Philos Trans R Soc Lond B Biol Sci 356(1405):119–125, 2001.

Jain A, Ma CA, Liu S, Brown M, Cohen J, Strober W. Specific missense mutations in NEMO result in hyper-IgM syndrome with hypohydrotic ectodermal dysplasia. Nat Immunol 2:223–228, 2001.

Kaartinen M, Griffiths GM, Markham AF, Milstein C. mRNA sequences define an unusually restricted IgG response to 2-phenyloxazolone and its early diversification. Nature 304(5924):320–324, 1983.

Kasahara Y, Kaneko H, Fukao T, Terada T, Asano T, Kasahara K, Kondo N. Hyper-IgM syndrome with putative dominant negative mutation in activation-induced cytidine deaminase. J Allergy Clin Immunol 112:755–760, 2003.

Kawamura N, Okamura A, Furuta H, Katow S, Yamada M, Kobayashi I, Okano M, Kobayashi K, Sakiyama Y. Improved dysgammaglobulinaemia in congenital rubella syndrome after immunoglobulin therapy: correlation with CD154 expression. Eur J Pediatr 159:764–766, 2000.

Kenter AL. The liaison of isotype class switch and mismatch repair: an illegitimate affair. J Exp Med 190:307–310, 1999.

Kinoshita K, Honjo T. Unique and unprecedented recombination mechanisms in class switching. Curr Opin Immunol 12:195–198, 2000.

Kinoshita K, Honjo T. Linking class-switch recombination with somatic hypermutation. Nat Rev Mol Cell Biol 2:493–503, 2001.

Klein U, Rajewsky K, Kuppers R. Human immunoglobulin (Ig)M+IgD+ peripheral blood B cells expressing the CD27 cell surface antigen carry somatically mutated variable region genes: CD27 as a general marker for somatically mutated (memory) B cells. J Exp Med 188:1679–1689, 1998.

Lebecque S, de Bouteiller O, Arpin C, Banchereau J, Liu YJ. Germinal center founder cells display propensity for apoptosis before onset of somatic mutation. J Exp Med 185:563–571, 1997.

Lee WI, Torgerson TR, Schumacher MJ, Yel L, Zhu Q, Ochs HD. Molecular analysis of a large cohort of patients with the hyper IgM syndrome (HIGH). Blood 105:1881–1890, 2005.

Ma L, Wortis HH, Kenter AL. Two new isotype-specific switching activities detected for Ig class switching. J Immunol 168:2835–2846, 2002.

Manis JP, Dudley D, Kaylor L, Alt FW. IgH class switch recombination to IgG1 in DNA-PKcs-deficient B cells. Immunity 16:607–617, 2002.

Manis JP, Gu Y, Lansford R, Sonoda E, Ferrini R, Davidson L, Rajewsky K, Alt FW. Ku70 is required for late B cell development and immunoglobulin heavy chain class switching. J Exp Med 187:2081–2089, 1998.

Manis JP, Morales JC, Xia Z, Kutok JL, Alt FW, Carpenter PB. 53BP1 links DNA damage–response pathways to immunoglobulin heavy chain class-switch recombination. Nat Immunol 5:481–487, 2004.

Matsuoka M, Yoshida K, Maeda T, Usuda S, Sakano H. Switch circular DNA formed in cytokine-treated mouse splenocytes: evidence for intramolecular DNA deletion in immunoglobulin class switching. Cell 62:135–142, 1990.

McBride KM, Barreto V, Ramiro AR, Stavropoulos P, Nussenzweig MC. Somatic hypermutation is limited by CRM1-dependent nuclear export of activation-induced deaminase. J Exp Med 199:1235–1244, 2004.

Mehta A, Kinter MT, Sherman NE, Driscoll DM. Molecular cloning of APOBEC-1 complementation factor, a novel RNA-binding protein involved in the editing of apolipoprotein B mRNA. Mol Cell Biol 20:1846–1854, 2000.

Meyts I, Weemases C, DeWolf-Peeters C, Proesmans M, Renard M, Yuttebroeck A, DeBoeck K. Unusual and severe disease discourse in a child with ataxia-telangiectasia. Pediatr Allergy Immunol 14:330–333, 2003.

Minegishi Y, Lavoie A, Cunningham-Rundles C, Bedard PM, Hebert J, Cote L, Dan K, Sedlak D, Buckley RH, Fischer A, Durandy A, Conley ME. Mutations in activation-induced cytidine deaminase in patients with hyper IgM syndrome. Clin Immunol 97:203–210, 2000.

Muramatsu M, Kinoshita K, Fagarasan S, Yamada S, Shinkai Y, Honjo T. Class switch recombination and hypermutation require activation-induced cytidine deaminase (AID), a potential RNA editing enzyme. Cell 102:553–563, 2000.

Muramatsu M, Sankaranand VS, Anant S, Sugai M, Kinoshita K, Davidson NO, Honjo T. Specific expression of activation-induced cytidine deaminase

(AID), a novel member of the RNA-editing deaminase family in germinal center B cells. J Biol Chem 274:18470–18476, 1999.

Muto T, Muramatsu M, Taniwaki M, Kinoshita K, Honjo T. Isolation, tissue distribution, and chromosomal localization of the human activation-induced cytidine deaminase (AID) gene. Genomics 68:85–88, 2000.

Navaratnam N, Morrison JR, Bhattacharya S, Patel D, Funahashi T, Giannoni F, Teng BB, Davidson NO, Scott J. The p27 catalytic subunit of the apolipoprotein B mRNA editing enzyme is a cytidine deaminase. J Biol Chem 268:20709–20712, 1993.

Nilsen H, Rosewell I, Robins P, Skjelbred CF, Andersen S, Slupphaug G, Daly G, Krokan HE, Lindahl T, Barnes DE. Uracil–DNA glycosylase (UNG)–deficient mice reveal a primary role of the enzyme during DNA replication. Mol Cell 5:1059–1065, 2000.

Nilsen H, Stamp G, Andersen S, Hrivnak G, Krokan HE, Lindahl T, Barnes DE. Gene-targeted mice lacking the UNG uracil–DNA glycosylase develop B-cell lymphomas. Oncogene 22:5381–5381, 2003.

Nonoyama S, Etzioni A, Toru H, et al. Diminished expression of CD40 ligand may contribute to the defective humoral immunity in patients with MHC class II deficiency. Eur J Immunol 28:589–598, 1998.

Okazaki IM, Hiai H, Kakazu N, Yamada S, Muramatsu M, Kinoshita K, Honjo T. Constitutive expression of AID leads to tumorigenesis. J Exp Med 197:1173–1181, 2003.

Pan-Hammarstrom Q, Dai S, Zhao Y, van Dijk-Hard IF, Gatti RA, Borresen-Dale AL, Hammarstrom L. ATM is not required in somatic hypermutation of VH, but is involved in the introduction of mutations in the switch mu region. J Immunol 170:3707–3716, 2003.

Papavasiliou FN, Schatz DG. Somatic hypermutation of immunoglobulin genes: merging mechanisms for genetic diversity. Cell 109(Suppl):S35–44, 2002.

Petersen S, Casellas R, Reina-San-Martin B, Chen HT, Difilippantonio MJ, Wilson PC, Hanitsch L, Celeste A, Muramatsu M, Pilch DR, Redon C, Ried T, Bonner WM, Honjo T, Nussenzweig MC, Nussenzweig A. AID is required to initiate Nbs1/gamma-H2AX focus formation and mutations at sites of class switching. Nature 414(6864):660–665, 2001.

Petersen-Mahrt SK, Harris RS, Neuberger MS. AID mutates E. coli suggesting a DNA deamination mechanism for antibody diversification. Nature 418(6893):99–104, 2002.

Petersen-Mahrt SK, Neuberger MS. In vitro deamination of cytosine to uracil in single-stranded DNA by APOBEC1. J Biol Chem 14:14, 2003.

Quartier P, Bustamante J, Sanal O, Plebani A, Debre M, Deville A, Litzman J, Levy J, Fermand JP, Lane P, Horneff G, Aksu G, Yalcin I, Davies G, Tezcan I, Ersoy F, Catalan N, Imai K, Fischer A, Durandy A. Clinical, immunologic and genetic analysis of 29 patients with autosomal recessive hyper-IgM syndrome due to activation-induced cytidine deaminase deficiency. Clin Immunol 110:22–29, 2004.

Quartier P, Foray S, Casanova JL, Hau-Rainsard I, Blanche S, Fischer A. Enteroviral meningoencephalitis in X-linked agammaglobulinemia: intensive immunoglobulin therapy and sequential viral detection in cerebrospinal fluid by polymerase chain reaction. Pediatr Infect Dis J 19:1106–1108, 2000.

Rada C, Williams GT, Nilsen H, Barnes DE, Lindahl T, Neuberger MS. Immunoglobulin isotype switching is inhibited and somatic hypermutation perturbed in UNG-deficient mice. Curr Biol 12:1748–1755, 2002.

Rajewsky K. Clonal selection and learning in the antibody system. Nature 381(6585):751–758, 1996.

Ramiro AR, Stavropoulos P, Jankovic M, Nussenzweig MC. Transcription enhances AID-mediated cytidine deamination by exposing single-stranded DNA on the nontemplate strand. Nat Immunol 4:452–456, 2003.

Revy P, Muto T, Levy Y, Geissmann F, Plebani A, Sanal O, Catalan N, Forveille M, Dufourcq-Labelouse R, Gennery A, Tezcan I, Ersoy F, Kayserili H, Ugazio AG, Brousse N, Muramatsu M, Notarangelo LD, Kinoshita K, Honjo T, Fischer A, Durandy A. Activation-induced cytidine deaminase (AID) deficiency causes the autosomal recessive form of the hyper-IgM syndrome (HIGM2). Cell 102:565–575, 2000.

Rolink A, Melchers F, Andersson J. The SCID but not the RAG-2 gene product is required for S mu-S epsilon heavy chain class switching. Immunity 5:319–330, 1996.

Schrader CE, Edelmann W, Kucherlapati R, Stavnezer J. Reduced isotype switching in splenic B cells from mice deficient in mismatch repair enzymes. J Exp Med 190:323–330, 1999.

Shanmugam A, Shi MJ, Yauch L, Stavnezer J, Kenter AL. Evidence for class-specific factors in immunoglobulin isotype switching. J Exp Med 191:1365–1380, 2000.

Shinkura R, Tian M, Smith M, Chua K, Fujiwara Y, Alt FW. The influence of transcriptional orientation on endogenous switch region function. Nat Immunol 4:435–441, 2003.

Storb U, Klotz EL, Hackett J Jr, Kage K, Bozek G, Martin TE. A hypermutable insert in an immunoglobulin transgene contains hotspots of somatic mutation and sequences predicting highly stable structures in the RNA transcript. J Exp Med 188:689–698, 1998.

Ta VT, Nagaoka H, Catalan N, Durandy A, Fischer A, Imai K, Nonoyama S, Tashiro J, Ikegawa M, Ito S, Kinoshita K, Muramatsu M, Honjo T. AID mutant analyses indicate requirement for class-switch-specific cofactors. Nat Immunol 4:843–848, 2003.

Teng B, Burant CF, Davidson NO. Molecular cloning of an apolipoprotein B messenger RNA editing protein. Science 260(5115):1816–1819, 1993.

von Schwedler U, Jack HM, Wabl M. Circular DNA is a product of the immunoglobulin class switch rearrangement. Nature 345(6274):452–456, 1990.

Ward IM, Reina-San-Martin B, Olaru A, Minn K, Tamada K, Lau JS, Cascalho M, Chen L, Nussenzweig A, Livak F, Nussenzweig MC, Chen J. 53BP1 is required for class switch recombination. J Cell Biol 165:459–464, 2004.

Wiesendanger M, Scharff MD, Edelmann W. Somatic hypermutation, transcription, and DNA mismatch repair. Cell 94:415–418, 1998.

Yamanaka S, Poksay KS, Balestra ME, Zeng GQ, Innerarity TL. Cloning and mutagenesis of the rabbit ApoB mRNA editing protein. A zinc motif is essential for catalytic activity, and noncatalytic auxiliary factor(s) of the editing complex are widely distributed. J Biol Chem 269:21725–21734, 1994.

Yu K, Chedin F, Hsieh CL, Wilson TE, Lieber MR. R-loops at immunoglobulin class switch regions in the chromosomes of stimulated B cells. Nat Immunol 4:442–451, 2003.

Zan H, Komori A, Li Z, Cerutti A, Schaffer A, Flajnik MF, Diaz M, Casali P. The translesion DNA polymerase zeta plays a major role in Ig and bcl-6 somatic hypermutation. Immunity 14:643–653, 2001.

Zan H, Wu X, Komori A, Holloman WK, Casali P. AID-dependent generation of Resected double-strand DNA breaks and recruitment of Rad52/Rad51 in somatic hypermutation. Immunity 18:727–738, 2003.

Zonana J, Elder ME, Schneider LC, Orlow SJ, Moss C, Golabi M, Shapira SK, Farndon PA, Wara DW, Emmal SA, Ferguson BM. A novel X-linked disorder of immune deficiency and hypohidrotic ectodermal dysplasia is allelic to incontinentia pigmenti and due to mutations in IKK-gamma (NEMO). Am J Hum Genet 67:6, 2000.

21

X-Linked Agammaglobulinemia: A Disease of Btk Tyrosine Kinase

C. I. EDVARD SMITH, ANNE B. SATTERTHWAITE, and OWEN N. WITTE

X-linked agammaglobulinemia (XLA) is caused by a B lymphocyte differentiation arrest and was originally described in 1952 by the American physician Dr. (Colonel) Ogden C. Bruton. XLA is frequently recognized as the prototype primary immunodeficiency (PID) (Rosen et al., 1984) and was the first human immune disorder in which an underlying defect was clearly identified. The locus designation is *BTK* and the Mendelian Inheritance in Man (MIM) number is 300300. XLA is characterized by an increased susceptibility to extracellular bacterial infections (Lederman and Winkelstein, 1985; Sideras and Smith, 1995; Ochs and Smith, 1996). Enteroviral infections also frequently run a severe course, often resist therapy, and have therefore become increasingly important (Lederman and Winkelstein, 1985; McKinney et al., 1987; Ochs and Smith, 1996; Plebani et al., 2002). Through different approaches, the gene affected in XLA was isolated simultaneously by two groups and found to encode a novel cytoplasmic tyrosine kinase designated *Bruton's agammaglobulinemia tyrosine kinase*, or Btk (Tsukada et al., 1993; Vetrie et al., 1993).

Bruton's initial report described an 8-year-old boy highly susceptible to bacterial infections, in particular *Streptococcus pneumoniae*, from the age of 4 1/2 years. As reviewed in greater detail (Sideras and Smith, 1995; Smith and Notarangelo, 1997), the analysis of serum through electrophoresis, which had only recently been applied in a clinical setting, revealed the absence of detectable immunoglobulins (Ig). This finding prompted Bruton to coin the term *agammaglobulinemia*, a name that has been kept in spite of the observation that minute and sometimes even considerable amounts of Ig are detectable in XLA patients. Bruton not only realized that there was a connection between the absence of Ig and the susceptibility to infections, he also initiated substitution treatment with subcutaneous γ-globulin and demonstrated its efficacy.

It has been noticed that the patient initially described by Bruton had some characteristics that are not typical for classical XLA (reviewed in Sideras and Smith, 1995). However, certain patients with XLA, as confirmed by mutation analysis, have demonstrated a mild disease phenotype similar to or even milder than that of Bruton's case (Vihinen et al., 1995a, 1996b, 2001; Bykowsky et al., 1996; Jones et al., 1996; Hashimoto et al., 1999; Stewart et al., 2001; Wood et al., 2001; Plebani et al., 2002). In a collaborative study, Bruton and coworkers reported on additional patients in whom the diagnosis of XLA seems indisputable (Bruton et al., 1952); but, more importantly, the original report inspired a great number of investigators to look for patients with antibody deficiency. As a result, within a few years, many patients were identified worldwide with not only XLA but also many other forms of Ig abnormality (reviewed in Good et al., 1962). The recognition of different forms of antibody deficiency disease was a gradual process, and it was not until the early 1970s that a classification as we know it today was generally accepted (Cooper et al., 1973).

In the 1950s the relationship between lymphocytes and plasma cells was still debated, and studies on XLA were crucial to this analysis (Good and Zak, 1956). More than a decade later, Naor et al. (1969) first described absence of antigen-binding cells in patients with XLA. This observation was followed by a number of investigations using technologies based on fluorochrome-labeled anti-Ig preparations that conclusively demonstrated a B lineage differentiation defect (reviewed in Sideras and Smith, 1995; Smith and Notarangelo, 1997). Over the years, hematopoietic cells other than B lymphocytes have been characterized in XLA. Although occasional reports have described non–B lineage cells to be affected, only granulocytopenia has been a frequent finding, and this is secondary to infections (Janeway, 1954; Koslowski and Evans, 1991; Sideras and Smith, 1995; Farrar et al., 1996). Thus, in spite

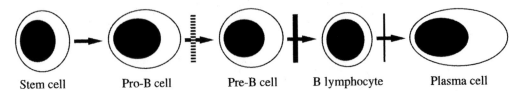

Stem cell   Pro-B cell   Pre-B cell   B lymphocyte   Plasma cell

Figure 21.1. Schematic representation of B lymphocyte development and the differentiation block/growth arrest in XLA. The broken line represents a partial block and the filled line an almost total block in B lineage differentiation in XLA (modified from Mattsson et al., 1996). The thin broken line demonstrates the second block affecting B cell differentiation as detected in mice with a targeted deletion of the *Btk* gene (Hendriks et al., 1996).

of the demonstration that Btk is expressed outside the B cell lineage (Tsukada et al., 1993; de Weers et al., 1993; Smith et al., 1994a, Müller et al., 1999), there is no evidence demonstrating that a functional defect in non–B cells contributes to the XLA phenotype.

XLA is characterized by an increased susceptibility to infections, with onset most often during the first year of life, when transferred maternal Ig has been catabolized. Analysis of serum demonstrates a pronounced decrease in Ig levels of all isotypes; IgA is usually undetectable. There is a virtual absence of humoral response to recall antigens. B lymphocyte and plasma cell numbers are markedly decreased, whereas T lymphocyte subsets show a relative increase. The defect is caused by a differentiation arrest confined to the B cell lineage (Fig. 21.1), distinguishing XLA from several other Ig deficiencies. B lineage cells in all organs are affected, resulting in a reduced size of lymph nodes and tonsils.

The defective gene encodes a cytoplasmic tyrosine kinase designated *Btk*. Mutation analysis will confirm the diagnosis and may be used to identify healthy carriers. Treatment consists of antibiotics to combat ongoing infections and γ-globulin substitution as prophylaxis.

Clinical and Pathological Manifestations

Incidence

The incidence of XLA has been investigated in several ethnic populations (Sideras and Smith, 1995). Most of these studies were performed during the 1980s prior to the cloning of many of the genes defective in primary Ig deficiencies, including the *BTK* gene, thus preventing definitive diagnosis (reviewed in Sideras and Smith, 1995). Furthermore, these investigations were usually not specifically aimed at studying XLA but were general surveys of PID, often carried out for the first time on a national basis. Thus, several parameters may have influenced the actual patient numbers identified. An incidence for XLA of about 5 in 10⁶ individuals was frequently reported. Ethnic differences were considered, since in the Japanese survey by Hayakawa et al. (1981) only 56 XLA cases were reported. Low numbers were found also in Malaysia (Noh et al., 1995) and in black populations in the United States and South Africa. However, lethal X-linked traits are believed to occur by de novo mutations in approximately one-third of the cases (Haldane, 1935; Chase and Murphy, 1973), a finding arguing against incidence variations in mutation frequency among different ethnic populations. In support of this notion, the number of Japanese patients with verified mutations in the *BTK* gene has increased considerably (Kanegane et al., 2001). However, even if racial differences in incidence do not exist, delayed diagnosis in non-Caucasians has been reported (Conley and Howard, 2002).

Onset of Symptoms and Age at Diagnosis

Onset of symptoms, mainly manifested as respiratory and/or gastrointestinal tract infections, is normally within the first year of life, after the disappearance of maternal IgG transported across the placenta. In a survey of 96 North American patients with XLA, Lederman and Winkelstein (1985) noted that 25% had symptoms by the age of 4 months, 50% by 8 months, 75% by 12 months, and 90% by 18 months. In a British study comprising 44 patients with XLA, symptoms did not present in 40% of affected boys during their first year of life and 20% remained asymptomatic until the age of 3–5 years, whereas in common variable immunodeficiency (CVID), a biphasic distribution was found with symptoms beginning at 1–5 and 16–20 years, respectively (Hermaszewski and Webster, 1993). In an Italian study of 73 patients with mutation-verified XLA the mean age of onset of symptoms was 2 years (Plebani et al., 2002). In reports from recent years there seems to be a tendency toward later onset of symptoms. This phenomenon may be caused by a generous contemporary usage of more efficient antibiotics. As expected, there was no difference in age when symptoms appeared between familial and sporadic cases of XLA (Lederman and Winkelstein, 1985; Hansel et al., 1987), although diagnosis may be delayed among sporadic cases.

Lederman and Winkelstein (1985) reported a mean age at diagnosis of 2½ years in familial and 3½ in sporadic cases. Hansel et al. (1987) found 2½ years to be the average age of diagnosis among 69 patients not subdivided according to familial or nonfamilial cases, whereas Plebani et al. (2002) found 3.5 years to be the mean age. Hansel et al. (1987) and Plebani et al. (2002) reported that earlier diagnosis was made in more recent years, perhaps reflecting the rarity of an initial diagnosis being made later than during childhood. This development is likely to continue, especially in familial cases, because of the availability of mutation analysis. However, some patients with mutation-verified diagnosis do not present with symptoms until much later in life (Vihinen et al., 1995, 1996b, 2001; Hashimoto et al., 1999, Wood et al., 2001), whereas others have symptoms but are not diagnosed until later for other reasons (Stewart et al., 2001; Morwood et al., 2004). It is noteworthy that onset may also vary among individuals within the same family carrying the same mutation (Wedgewood and Ochs, 1980), demonstrating that other factors may influence this process.

The presenting symptoms in XLA vary among patients. Pneumonia, otitis media, and diarrhea are frequent clinical presentations. Sinusitis, conjunctivitis, and pyoderma are also prevalent (Table 21.1). Hematogenic dissemination of the infection may result in septicemia, meningitis, septic arthritis, or osteomyelitis. Thus, a highly increased frequency of infections is seen in all organ systems, with the possible exception of the urinary tract, in which infections seem to be limited to *Mycoplasma* or, more

Table 21.1. Infections in Patients with X-Linked Agammaglobulinemia

	Patients in Each Study (%)			
Presenting Infection	Lederman and Winkelstein (1985) (n = 96)	Hansel et al. (1987) (n = 69)	Hermaszewski and Webster (1993) (n = 44)	Plebani et al. (2002) (n = 73)
Ear, nose, and throat	75	22	52	50
Pneumonia	56	67	32	39
Gastrointestinal infection	35	16	11	13
Bacterial skin infection	28	DC*	14	27
Meningitis	10	17	5	4
Septicemia	10	dc	7	6
Osteomyelitis	3	dc	5	—

*DC, different classification used, preventing direct comparison.

Modified from Sideras and Smith (1995).

rarely, *Chlamydia* species. Arthritis, affecting large joints, was found in about 20% of patients, central nervous system (CNS) infections in 4%–16%, and septicemia in 6%–10% of patients before or at the time of diagnosis (Lederman and Winkelstein, 1985; Hansel et al., 1987; Hermaszewski and Webster, 1993; Plebani et al., 2002), although the presenting symptoms are rarely limited to a single manifestation. Conley and Howard (2002) found a high frequency of *Pseudomonas* infections in children diagnosed before the age of 12 months, one of whom died prior to diagnosis. Hansel et al. (1987) reported that hypogammaglobulinemia was initially misdiagnosed as juvenile chronic arthritis in two children and delays in diagnosis were noticed in several others presenting with arthritis.

In sum, the onset and type of symptoms may vary extensively. Most patients will show an increased frequency of infections during their first year of life, whereas a few may be asymptomatic until adolescence.

Pathology of Lymphoid Organs

The B lineage defect is manifested as a virtual absence of B lymphocytes and plasma cells in all organs. In the affected newborn, lymphoid hypoplasia may not be apparent, since in healthy infants the antigen-induced expansion of B lymphocytes in secondary lymphoid organs has not yet taken place. Adenoids and tonsils are frequently rudimentary and lymph nodes are reduced in size. Secondary lymphoid organs, such as lymph nodes and appendix, lack germinal centers and follicles (Good, 1954; Sideras and Smith, 1995). In the lamina propria of the gut, plasma cells are typically absent in patients with XLA, this is not the case in most other primary immunodeficiencies (Ochs et al., 1972; Ament et al., 1973; Buckley and Rowlands, 1973). A low number of plasma cells in the gut is also a typical finding in CVID. However, biopsies of lymphoid organs for diagnostic reasons are now rarely indicated, with the exception of sampling for isolation of an infectious agent.

Analysis of bone marrow has revealed a maturation block between terminal deoxynucleotidyl transferase (TdT) Cμ-negative early pre-B cells and Cμ-positive pre-B cells (Campana et al., 1990; Nomura et al., 2000). The severity of the block is variable, thus normal pre-B cells can develop in some patients. The proliferative activity of these pre-B cells is impaired, however (Pearl et al., 1978; Campana et al., 1990; Noordzij et al., 2002a). Furthermore, although the differentiation block is manifested in the early stages of B lymphocyte development, it is likely that the

defect in XLA also affects the later stages of B cell development (Conley, 1985). Experiments in mice indicate that this is indeed the case (Hendriks et al., 1996).

Spectrum of Infections

Bacterial respiratory tract and gastrointestinal infections are the predominant manifestations of XLA, as they are of other antibody deficiencies. What distinguishes XLA from most other humoral defects is the increased frequency of chronic enteroviral infections. Pyogenic bacteria, such as *Hemophilus influenzae*, *Streptococcus pneumoniae*, and *Staphylococcus aureus*, for which antibodies act as opsonins, typically cause infections. In normal individuals, antibody binding to microorganisms contributes to the inflammatory reaction, which causes the clinical symptoms. Because XLA patients lack antibodies, clinical symptoms are often mild and do not reflect the severity of the infections. As in other immunodeficiencies, infections typically are recurrent or chronic in nature. Another hallmark of XLA is the observation that infections are often found in more than one location and may be atypical, such as *Mycoplasma*-associated arthritis.

Lederman and Winkelstein (1985) reported that 71% of investigated XLA patients presented with chronic infections. Chronic pulmonary disease was found in almost half of the patients, complicated in some by hypoxemia and corpulmonale. Hearing loss secondary to chronic otitis media and meningoencephalitis as well as delayed speech acquisition also occurred frequently. However, patients diagnosed early in life and receiving adequate treatment rarely developed sensory-neurologic complications caused by bacterial infections. It should also be noted that certain XLA patients have a mutation extending from the *BTK* gene into the adjacent *TIMM8A* (formerly *DDP*) gene causing sensory-neurologic manifestations (see Chromosomal Region Containing the *BTK* gene, below).

Chronic progressive encephalitis caused by enteroviral infection is an often fatal complication of XLA patients, who are uniquely susceptible to enteroviruses causing meningoencephalitis. This disease is described in more detail in below. Bacterial infections, found in all patients displaying antibody deficiency, are discussed briefly in the following section and in more detail in Chapters 43 and 46.

Other viral infections, such as measles, and infections with intracellular microorganisms, such as *Mycobacteria* or the protozoan *Toxoplasma gondii*, run a normal course that is not different from that in immunologically normal individuals. For these infectious agents cellular immunity is believed to constitute the main defense. Patients with XLA seem not to be infected by Epstein-Barr virus (EBV), a finding pointing to the crucial role of B lymphocytes for this virus (Faulkner et al., 1999). Infections with *Pneumocystis carinii*, a major pathogen in patients with impaired cellular immunity, may occur in XLA, although rarely (Alibrahim et al., 1998; Dittrich et al., 2003). Increased susceptibility to other fungal infections has not been reported (see also Miscellaneous Infections, below).

Bacterial infections

Bacterial infections are the major complications in XLA and other antibody deficiencies (Lederman and Winkelstein, 1985; Stiehm et al., 1986; Spicket et al., 1991; Hermaszewski and Webster, 1993; Ochs and Smith, 1996). The typical sites of infections are presented in Table 21.1. In a survey of patients with XLA, Lederman and Winkelstein (1985) reported that respiratory tract and/or gastrointestinal tract infections caused the presenting symptoms in 91% of patients. Similar findings were obtained by Hermaszewski and Webster (1993).

The most frequently observed organisms include *H. influenzae*, a chronic sputum isolate in 82% of cases; *S. aureus*, in 27%; and *S. pneumoniae*, in 21% (Lederman and Winkelstein, 1985). In chronic conjuctivitis, *H. influenzae* was found in more than half of the investigated patients. In septic arthritis, *H. influenzae* and *S. pneumoniae* were most frequently reported prior to diagnosis, whereas a viral etiology was predominantly observed after the diagnosis of XLA had been established; *Mycoplasma* species were isolated in some cases. A similar pattern was noted in bacterial meningitis, with *H. influenzae* and *S. pneumoniae* being the predominant organisms prior to diagnosis, followed by a higher frequency of viral agents in diagnosed patients. In septicemia *Pseudomonas* was the most frequently isolated microorganism, with *H. influenzae*, *S. pneumoniae*, and *S. aureus* being isolated less consistently.

Infections with the nonsporulating gram-negative rod *Campylobacter jejuni* have been reported to cause gastrointestinal disease, erysipelas-like skin lesions, pericarditis, and recurrent fever in patients with XLA (Kerstens et al., 1992; Rafi and Matz, 2002). The diarrhea may be of long duration, but in some cases patients are asymptomatic (Melamed et al., 1983; van der Meer et al., 1986; Chusid et al., 1987; Hermaszewski and Webster, 1993; Schuster et al., 1996). Excretion of *C. jejuni* in the stool, which in untreated non–immune-deficient subjects normally persists for 2–3 weeks, may be prolonged. As for many other bacterial species, human serum is bactericidal for *Campylobacter* isolates and antibodies seem to constitute an important line of defense (Blaser et al., 1985; Cover and Blaser, 1989). Infection with fastidious organisms such as *H. cinaedi* (previously known as *C. cinaedi*) has been reported in XLA (reviewed in Simons et al., 2004). The presentation was hyperpigmented macules, without increased local warmth, fever, or any other signs of illness.

Systemic *Ureaplasma urealyticum* infections or infections with other *Mycoplasma* species are also frequent and may primarily cause symptoms in the respiratory tract, joints, and urogenital tract (Stuckey et al., 1978; Webster et al., 1978; Lederman and Winkelstein, 1985; Roifman et al., 1986; Gelfand, 1993; Hermaszewski and Webster, 1993). These organisms are often difficult to identify, and the course of disease may be prolonged, with an insidious onset. Symptoms may be severe, with accompanying weight loss. Significantly milder symptoms are associated with *Mycoplasma* infections of the respiratory tract compared to normal individuals, and there are minimal or no changes on chest X-ray despite prolonged periods of cough (Foy et al., 1973). Combined infections of *Mycoplasma* and other bacterial species may also contribute to disease severity. Urogenital tract infections can cause urethral strictures and result in epididymitis and prostatitis (Hermaszewski and Webster, 1993; Ochs and Smith, 1996).

Enterovirus infections

Most viral infections run a normal course in XLA (Janeway et al., 1953; Lederman and Winkelstein, 1985; Ochs and Smith, 1996). However, enteroviral infections frequently cause chronic meningoencephalitis often associated with a dermatomyositis/fasciitis-like syndrome in patients with agammaglobulinemia. Thus, although viral infections are the hallmark of abnormalities in cellular immunity, enteroviral infections are found in patients with severe agammaglobulinemia, particularly in XLA. The most comprehensive review in the field describes 42 patients with antibody deficiency, 18 of whom have classic XLA and 14 with clinical features typical for XLA but devoid of a family history (McKinney et al., 1987). Enteroviral disease presenting with a similar clinical picture to that in XLA was also seen in some patients with CVID and in patients with thymoma and hypogammaglobulinemia. However, the frequency of patients affected was considerably lower than in XLA. Hermaszewski and Webster (1993) reported a 10-fold increased risk in patients with XLA compared to those with CVID. Also, in CD40 ligand defects enteroviral meningoencephalitis has been reported (Cunningham et al., 1999). In agammaglobulinemia caused by mutations in the μ heavy–chain gene, resulting in undetectable B cells, chronic enteroviral infection seems to occur as frequently as in XLA, although the number of identified patients is still limited (Lopes Granados et al., 2002). Recently, enteroviral meningoencephalitis was reported after treatment with monoclonal antibodies directed against the B lymphocyte cell surface antigen CD20 (Quartier et al., 2003).

The reason for this high susceptibility is unknown, but it may be the result of the virtual complete absence of antibodies in XLA, compared to several other Ig deficiencies. As for most viral infections, immunoglobulins have a protective effect against enteroviruses, as demonstrated over 60 years ago (Kramer, 1943; Hammon et al., 1952). Alternatively, the lack of B lymphocytes may impair the removal of viral particles, impede antigen presentation, or affect other parameters in the immune defense. Enteroviral infection is frequently manifested as chronic encephalomyelitis (McKinney et al., 1987) and insidious onset of neurologic symptoms and altered cognitive function are typical. Almost any symptom in an agammaglobulinemic patient may be caused by an enteroviral infection of the CNS.

Types of enteroviruses causing disease in XLA. Echovirus is the predominant pathogen among the enteroviruses causing meningoencephalitis in agammaglobulinemic patients. Coxsackieviruses A and B have also been reported to cause disease (McKinney et al., 1987; Lederman and Winkelstein, 1985). Patients with agammaglobulinemia are also highly susceptible to poliovirus infection, as reviewed by Wyatt (1973), who calculated that vaccine-associated poliomyelitis was increased by a factor of 10^4 in this patient category. Lederman and Winkelstein (1985) observed one case of poliovirus vaccination–associated death in their survey. Hermaszewski and Webster (1993) reported one patient with paralytic poliomyelitis and one who suffered foot drop following oral polio virus vaccination, and McKinney et al. (1987) described two patients with paralytic poliomyelitis prior to their echoviral infections. Sarpong et al. (2002) reported one patient who survived infection with wild poliomyelitis in childhood many years before the diagnosis of XLA was made. Vaccine-associated poliomyelitis may also occur in nonvaccinated individuals, since the oral live vaccine may spread in the population (Hidalgo et al., 2003). McKinney et al. (1987) reported a close correlation between the prevalence of echoviral serotypes in agammaglobulinemic patients and that observed in the general population. During the period 1970–1983, the most common echoviral serotypes in both populations were 11, 9, and 30 (Strikas et al., 1986).

Clinical features and investigation of enteroviral infection in agammaglobulinemia. In XLA patients demonstrating neurological symptoms, enteroviral infection should always be suspected. Agammaglobulinemic patients developing meningoencephalitic enteroviral disease often present with slowly progressing neurologic symptoms, including ataxia, loss of cognitive skills, and paresthesias. Some patients show an acute onset with fever, headache, and seizures. Nearly all patients display pleocytosis in their cerebrospinal fluid (CSF), with a predominance of lymphocytes. Leukocyte numbers are usually $<10^3$ cells/mm^3, and protein concentration is typically between 0.5 and 5 g/l (McKinney et al., 1987). Imaging with magnetic resonance imaging (MRI) or computed tomography (CT) scanning was found to be normal initially in patients with early encephalopathy, thus having a limited diagnostic value. Cultures for enterovirus are frequently negative. However, the use of reverse-transcription polymerase chain reaction (PCR) has improved the identification of enterovirus in the CNS (Rotbart, 1990; Zoll et al., 1992; Rotbart et al., 1994), including patients with XLA (Webster et al., 1993; Rudge et al., 1996). Bacterial infections of the CNS have to be differentiated from the less common, fulminant, acute-onset encephalomyelitis caused by enteroviruses. Since bacterial infections in XLA generally respond well to prompt treatment with antibiotics, it is important to exclude a bacterial origin.

Enteroviral infection may also present as a dermatomyositis-like syndrome associated with dissemination of enterovirus (McKinney et al., 1987; Thyss et al., 1990). This form of the disease is characterized by peripheral edema, erythematous rash, and evidence of inflammation in skin and muscle biopsy specimens. The infection in the CNS seems to occur prior to dissemination of the virus. Edema or myositis with fasciitis may be found as the only manifestation of viral dissemination. Enteroviral hepatitis resulting in hepatomegaly and an increase in liver enzymes such as alanine aminotransferase are frequently seen in affected patients, usually associated with erythematous rashes and fever.

Most patients with long-standing enteroviral disease have similar symptomatology. More than half will show weakness, hearing loss, headache, lethargy/coma, seizures, ataxia, or paresthesias. Personality changes appear to be common, including depression and emotional lability, and the interval between onset of viral infection in the CNS and the appearance of overt symptoms may be considerable (McKinney et al., 1987).

Pathology of enteroviral disease in X-linked agammaglobulinemia. Histological examination of enteroviral meningoencephalitis demonstrates meningeal inflammation with perivascular mononuclear cell infiltrates and edematous thickening of the leptomeninges (McKinney et al., 1987; Rudge et al., 1996). Cerebral edema is extensive and diffuse encephalitis with glial reaction including microglial nodules and focal neuronal degeneration is evident. Astrogliosis in association with perivascular lymphocytic cuffs and elongated microglial cells have also been observed. In

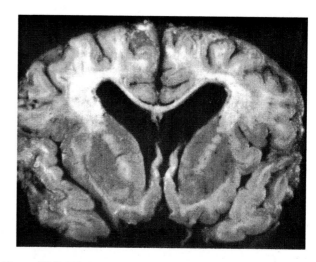

Figure 21.2. Whole brain section of a patient with XLA having an enteroviral infection presumably contracted at 8 years of age. Autopsy performed at 17 years of age, after several years of progressing dementia, shows severe thinning of the cerebral cortex, reduced subcortical and deep white matter, and marked dilatation of the lateral ventricles (reproduced from Rudge et al., 1996).

particular the cerebellum but also the brain stem and the spinal cord show loss of neurons. Eventually, most patients display profound cerebral atrophy with enlargement of the ventricles, which can be detected with CT. At autopsy the histologic appearance is sometimes consistent with that seen in an end-stage, severe encephalitic process of long duration (Fig. 21.2). Some patients do not show features of encephalitis but instead have evidence of long-standing leptomeningitis.

Hepatic involvement is manifested as centrilobular congestion and periportal lymphocytic infiltrates. Lymphocytic infiltrates may be found in multiple organs, including heart, lung, and kidney, whereas enteroviral infections in normal individuals do not become chronic. Furthermore, XLA patients may not only become chronically infected but also excrete enterovirus for extended periods of time (McKinney et al., 1987). As reported in a recent workshop (Halsey, 2002), 17 persons with B cell immune deficiency disorders, primarily XLA or CVID, who excreted polio vaccine viruses for 6 months or more, sometimes for many years, have been identified over the past 40 years. Most of these patients became paralyzed from the viruses, often after several years of poliovirus excretion. To this end, a recent Italian study found long-term excretors to be rare (Fiore et al., 2004). No effective therapy has been identified; some affected individuals have spontaneously stopped excreting polioviruses after several years.

Treatment and prevention of enteroviral disease. Initial attempts using high-dose treatment or intraventricular delivery of immunoglobulins were considered successful (Mease et al., 1981; Erlendsson et al., 1985; reviewed in McKinney et al., 1987; Misbah et al., 1992). However, treatment failures have been reported (Johnsson et al., 1985) and long-term follow-up has demonstrated that the enteroviral infection is not always eradicated, although in selected patients all symptoms disappeared when receiving adequate Ig treatment (Mease et al., 1985; Crennan et al., 1986; Rudge et al., 1996). Quartier et al. (1999, 2000) treated three patients with enteroviral meningoencephalitis. Residual IgG levels were increased to 31–63 g/l—i.e., considerably higher levels than those in healthy controls. In two patients clinical symptoms and CSF abnormalities resolved. The third patient died despite intraventricular infusion of Ig through an Omaya reservoir.

It has been suggested that high-dose intravenous immunoglobulin (IVIG) substitution therapy slows the development of cerebral disease. However, the number of patients is limited, rendering statistical evaluation impossible (Erlendsson et al., 1985; Mease et al., 1985). It has been considered important to try and identify the virus causing the infection to select Ig preparations with high specific antibody titers (H.D. Ochs, J.M. Puck, personal communication). Some practitioners prefer intrathecal delivery, whereas others use the IV route. Liese et al. (1992) reported that neither low- nor high-dose IVIG therapy improved the clinical course and that intraventricular administration of IVIG was ineffective. Misbah et al. (1992) have suggested that the significant clinical improvement seen in their patient following high-dose IVIG may have been due to an anti-inflammatory effect. Oral treatment with ribavirin had no effect. These authors also recommend the use of serial CSF albumin-level determinations to monitor the blood–brain barrier permeability.

As of 2003, and 2005, respectively two patients treated with a combination of Ig therapy and pleconaril (Quartier et al., 2000) have shown no signs of recurrence of the enteroviral infection with a follow-up of >4 and >6 years (P. Quartier, personal communication). Pleconaril treatment was found to cause clinical improvement in 78% of patients with potentially life-threatening enterovirus infection, including 12 of 16 with chronic enterovirus meningoencephalitis (Rotbart and Webster, 2001). Recently, a mutation in polio virus was found to accompany reduced susceptibility to pleconaril in a patient with CVID, known to be a long-term excretor of the virus (MacLennan et al., 2004).

There is clinical evidence that substitution therapy resulting in high serum levels of IgG protects against enteroviral meningoencephalitis, because the frequency of patients developing this infection has decreased over the years (Liese et al., 1992; Misbah et al., 1992; A.D.B. Webster, personal communication). Liese et al. (1992) did not find symptoms of chronic encephalitis in any of eight patients in whom high-dose IVIG was started before the age of 5 years. Rudge et al. (1996) have suggested that Ig treatment resulting in serum IgG levels maintained above 8 g/l may provide protection. However, although this is the general trend, fatal enteroviral infections may still occur during high-dose Ig substitution therapy (Misbah et al., 1992; Quartier et al., 1999). It could be anticipated that rare forms of enteroviruses would be more prone to cause infections because γ-globulin preparations would lack neutralizing antibodies.

Miscellaneous Infections

Gastrointestinal infection caused by the flagellate *Giardia lamblia* has been found in many patients with XLA, although it appears to be more common in CVID (Ochs et al., 1972; Hermaszewski and Webster, 1993; Lavilla et al., 1993). The infection may cause abdominal pains, diarrhea, and malabsorption. *P. carinii* infection has been identified in most forms of PID but is more common in patients with a defect in cellular immunity (Masur et al., 1989; Walzer, 1991). Infections may preferentially occur in XLA patients who are debilitated or otherwise compromised (Lederman and Winkelstein, 1985). A recent outbreak of *P. carinii* pneumonia in a colony of mice specifically lacking B lymphocytes caused death in more than 50 of the animals (Marcotte et al., 1996). Although species differences may exist, this finding further indicates that humoral immunity to this protozoan is of importance (see also Spectrum of Infections, above).

Arthritis

Arthritis is frequently observed in XLA. It may be the presenting symptom and has been mistaken for chronic juvenile arthritis (Hansel et al., 1987). The arthritis is normally nonseptic, monoarthritic, and affects the large joints, causing hydroarthritis with relatively little pain (McLaughlin et al., 1972; Ochs and Smith, 1996). The arthritis frequently responds to γ-globulin treatment (Webster et al., 1976; Plebani et al., 2002) and there is usually no apparent joint destruction. Residual IgG levels of >8 g/l were associated with improvement of clinical symptoms, whereas in patients with 5–8 g/l recurrences were seen (Quartier et al., 1999). The erythrocyte sedimentation rate is normal, as are serological tests for rheumatoid factor and antinuclear antibodies. (Because these patients essentially lack immunoglobulins, autoantibody analysis is of no value.) The cause of the arthritis is frequently unknown, since an infectious origin has not been verified. Lederman and Winkelstein (1985) reported arthritis, including polyarthritis, in 20% of XLA patients. Less than half of the episodes were due to acute pyogenic infections. Conley and Howard (2002) reported pneumococcal arthritis in two patients diagnosed after >40 months of age. Enteroviruses or *Mycoplasma* species have also been identified in affected joints from some patients (Ackerson et al., 1987; Hermaszewski and Webster, 1993). Recently, an atypical case of rheumatoid arthritis with infiltrating CD8 cells was reported (Verbruggen et al., 2005).

Autoimmunity

In contrast CVID (Cunningham-Rundles et al., 1987; Hermaszewski et al., 1991), XLA does not seem to predispose to autoimmune disorders (Sideras and Smith, 1995). Type 1 diabetes has only been reported in a single patient with XLA, but this finding suggests that humoral immunity is not required for development of this form of autoimmunity (Martin et al., 2001). Whether humoral immunity may still contribute to the disease process in humans is not known, but in the animal diabetes model, nonobese diabetic (NOD) mice, this is the case. As mentioned in the Arthritis section above, a case of rheumatoid arthritis in XLA has also been reported (Verbruggen et al., 2005).

Allergic Reactions

Few allergic reactions have been reported in XLA patients. After repeated treatment with intravenous infusions of ceftriaxone for an *H. influenzae* infection, a child developed diffuse, maculopapular rash with minimal pruritus, hyperthermia, flushing, and lethargy (Collins and Assa'ad, 2002). A skin biopsy showed the presence of infiltrating CD4+, CD45RO+ memory T cells in the absence of detectable IgE.

Tumors

Predisposition to tumors is the hallmark of several PIDs, such as the Wiskott-Aldrich syndrome and ataxia-telangiectasia (Filipovich et al., 1994; Smith and Notarangelo, 1997). In XLA this relationship is less obvious (Sideras and Smith, 1995; Ochs and Smith, 1996), although 4.2% of a total of 500 patients with neoplasia in a primary immunodeficiency disease registry were reported to have XLA (Filipovich and Shapiro, 1991). Lymphoreticular malignancies may be slightly increased (Kersey et al., 1973; Lederman and Winkelstein, 1985; Filipovich et al., 1994). The incidence of rectosigmoid cancer has been suggested to show a 30-fold increment, and mortality was 59-fold greater in a survey of 52 Dutch patients (van der Meer et al., 1993). Rectosigmoid cancer was also observed in a Swedish (Sideras and Smith, 1995) and a North American patient (H.D. Ochs, personal communication). Glutathione-S-transferase activity, possibly reflecting detoxification capacity, in gastrointestinal mucosa was found to significantly correlate with tumor incidence in humans, and decreased levels were also identified in patients with XLA (Grubben et al., 2000). However, the causal relationship to XLA, if any, remains elusive, and human adenocarcinoma cell lines were found not to express Btk (Smith et al., 1994a). Two patients with pituitary adenoma have been identified (Hermaszewski and Webster, 1993; Ochs and Smith, 1996). In case reports, von Recklinghausen disease was noticed at the age of 33 (Hirata et al., 2002) whereas extranodal cytotoxic T cell lymphoma was observed in another patient (Kanavaros et al., 2001). These findings indicate that there is a minor increase in malignacies in patients with XLA.

Lavilla et al. (1993) and Paller (1995) have suggested that complete gastrointestinal studies and examination for lymphomas should be performed regularly in all patients with XLA. In view of the minor increase in tumor frequency seen in XLA, most investigators seem to favor a more modest approach (H.D. Ochs; A.D.B. Webster; J.W.M. van der Meer, personal communication). However, owing to the high frequency of atrophic gastritis, pernicious anemia, and gastric adenocarcinoma in CVID (Kinlen et al., 1985; Cunninghan-Rundles et al., 1987), it seems reasonable to implement careful monitoring with regular endoscopic screening of XLA patients in whom atrophic gastritis was diagnosed. The risk of cancer of the stomach in nonimmunoimpaired patients with pernicious anemia who suffer from chronic gastritis and achlorhydria was estimated to be increased by a factor of 3 (Elsborg and Mosbech, 1979).

As discussed in the section Animal Models below, a mutation resulting in the substitution of arginine at position 41 with glutamine, designated BTK*, has a transforming capacity (Li et al., 1995). This effect is manifested in transduced fibroblast 3T3 cells and also in the form of IL-5-independent growth of a pro-B cell line. Initial studies of patients with various forms of B lymphoid tumors did not indicate any abnormal expression of Btk (Katz et al., 1994; Vorechovsky et al., 1994b). Furthermore, an increased frequency of chromosomal abberations in the Xq22 region (in which the BTK gene is located) has to date not been reported in B lineage tumors. However, in a recent report, defective expression of Btk in acute lymphoblastic leukemia was reported, although the biological significance, if any, of this phenomenon is unknown (Goodman et al., 2003).

Causes of Death

Among 170 patients observed by Lederman and Winkelstein (1985), Hermaszewski and Webster (1993) and Ochs and Smith (1996), 29 deaths were recorded (Table 21.2). The major cause of death was viral infections, which occurred in about half the patients. Enteroviral infections predominated, with echoviruses being the major agent causing disseminated disease, including meningoencephalitis. The disease progression is characterized by slow deterioration with increasing loss of cerebral function. Chronic pulmonary disease, amyloidosis, septicemia with osteomyelitis, and inflammatory bowel disease were other causes of death. Approximately one-third of the deaths reported by Lederman and Winkelstein (1985) were caused by cardiorespiratory failure, secondary to chronic pulmonary disease and corpul-

Table 21.2. Cause of Death in X-Linked Agammaglobulinemia*

Cause of Death	Patients (n)	Age at Death (Years)
Pulmonary infections (acute, chronic)	9	Mean 20 (10–27)
Enterovirus infections		
ECHO	10	12 (6–23)
Coxsackie	1	28
Polio (attenuated vaccine)	1	4
Advenovirus infections	1	14
Hepatitis	3	12 (10–24)
Staphylococcus (percarditis/sepsis)	2	23 (20–26)
Amyloidosis	1	Unknown
Inflammatory bowel disease	1	Unknown

*Premature death occured in 30 of 170 XLA patients studied longitudinally in the United States and Canada (n = 96) (Lederman and Winkelstein, 1985), Great Britain (n = 44) (Hermaszewski and Webster, 1993), and Seattle, WA (n = 30) (H.D. Ochs unpublished data).

Reproduced from Ochs and Smith (1996).

monale. Hermaszewski and Webster (1993) reported a single patient who died from respiratory disease. This patient did not suffer from corpulmonale. Iatrogenic disease in the form of hepatitis C contracted during globulin substitution treatment was fatal in one patient. However, patients with XLA normally seem to develop a less fulminant hepatitis than that in CVID patients (Hermaszewski and Webster, 1993; Bjøro et al., 1994; J. Björkander, personal communication). As discussed elsewhere in this chapter, malignancies constitute a rare cause of death in XLA.

Laboratory Findings

The laboratory findings characteristic for XLA reflect the B lineage defect and are manifested as severely decreased numbers of B lymphocytes and absence of serum immunoglobulins (Table 21.3). Rarely, XLA patients may have near-normal or normal Ig levels and numbers of B lymphocytes. In these patients analysis of the spectrum of antibodies and investigation of antigen-specific antibody responses are recommended (Table 21.3).

Table 21.3. Characteristic Laboratory Findings in Patients with X-Linked Agammaglobulinemia

Serum Ig levels*	IgM	IgG	IgA
g/l	<0.1	<2	Often undetectable
Isohemagglutinins[†]	Undetectable		
Antibody responses to foreign antigens[†]	Undetectable or markedly reduced		
Peripheral blood[‡]	CD19	CD20	Surface Ig+
B lymphocyte markers	<2%	<2%	<2%

*Normal values vary somewhat among different laboratories, but are typically as follows: IgM: 0.5–2 g/l; IgG, 7–16 g/l; IgA: 0.5–3 g/l in adults. Normal values for IgA may vary extensively until adolescence. The IgG level is typically >4 g/l at all ages. In the newborn it is similar to what is seen in adults, as a consequence of placental transfer; it will thereafter decrease until about 6 months of age.

[†]Analysis is not obligatory for diagnosis. However, analysis is recommended in patients having essentially normal Ig levels. For definitive diagnosis of XLA, mutation analysis has to be carried out.

[‡]Normal values vary somewhat among different laboratories, but are typically 5%–20%, corresponding to $0.08–0.4 \times 10^9$ cells/l. As surface Ig determination may be influenced by Fc receptor binding, the inclusion of CD marker analysis is recommended.

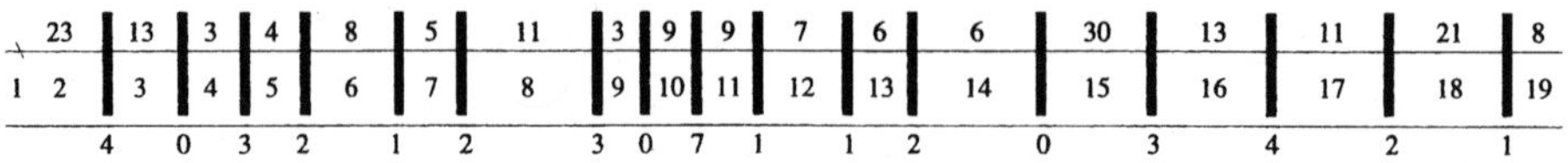

23	13	3	4	8	5	11	3	9	9	7	6	6	30	13	11	21	8
1	2	3	4	5	6	7	8	9	10	11	12	13	14	15	16	17	18	19
4	0	3	2	1	2	3	0	7	1	1	2	0	3	4	2	1		

Figure 21.3. Schematic representation of the Btk protein. Boxes represent functional regions or domain structures. The protein is composed of the following domains: PH (pleckstrin homology), TH (Tec homology), SH3 (Src homology 3), SH2 (Src homology 2) and kinase (SH1). The numbers denote amino acids numbered from the N-terminus. For simplicity the linker regions between functional domains are not denoted.

Molecular Basis of X-Linked Agammaglobulinemia

The Gene Defective in X-Linked Agammaglobulinemia Encodes a Tyrosine Kinase

The molecular basis of XLA was identified using two different modes of gene cloning: positional cloning by applying cDNA selection on yeast artificial chromosomes from the implicated region, and investigation of novel protein tyrosine kinases (PTKs) expressed in B lymphocytes (Tsukada et al., 1993; Vetrie et al., 1993). These studies demonstrated that a gene, *BTK*, encoding a novel cytoplasmic PTK was defective in XLA. PTKs are enzymes that catalyze the phosphorylation of tyrosine residues in proteins with ATP or other nucleotides as phosphor donors and belong to the enzyme classification (EC) group EC 2.7.1.112. PTKs are subdivided into receptor PTKs, which are membrane-spanning proteins such as the receptor for platelet-derived growth factor (PDGF), and cytoplasmic, or nonreceptor PTKs, exemplified by the cellular homologue of Rous sarcoma virus, c-Src (Manning et al., 2002). The current estimate of human PTKs is 58 receptor PTKs and 32 nonreceptor PTKs.

When the *BTK* gene was isolated, it was also the first time a cytoplasmic PTK was implicated in a hereditary human disease. Subsequently, mutations in the genes encoding both the Jak3 and Zap-70 cytoplasmic kinases have been shown to cause PID (see Chapters 10 and 14, respectively).

Btk is composed of 659 amino acids with a total molecular weight of 77 kDa; the corresponding mRNA is normally found as a single species of 2.7 kb (Tsukada et al., 1993; Vetrie et al., 1993; Smith et al., 1994b). Btk carries three domains, which are also found in Src. These are from the C terminus, the kinase domain of about 280 amino acids, also referred to as *Src homology 1* (SH1); a region of about 100 residues, which binds to phosphorylated tyrosine residues, designated *SH2*; and a domain of about 65 amino acids known to interact with proline-rich stretches, referred to as *SH3*, as depicted in Figure 21.3 (Pawson, 1995).

In addition, Btk contains two regions in the N terminus, designated *Pleckstrin homology* (PH), with 140 amino acids, and *Tec homology* (TH), containing approximately 80 residues (Fig. 21.3). The PH domain is found in more than 100 proteins and is believed to have a membrane-targeting function (Salim et al., 1996; Rameh et al., 1997). The TH region is composed of an extension of the PH domain, designated the *Btk motif* (27 residues), and a proline-rich stretch (Vihinen et al., 1994b; Smith et al., 1994b). The Btk motif in the TH region has been shown to bind a Zn^{2+} ion (Vihinen et al., 1997b). This region was named after Tec, which was the first member to be identified in the family of PTKs to which Btk belongs (Mano et al., 1990). The other family members are Itk (also called Tsk and Emt) and Bmx (also called Etk). The kinase Txk (also Rlk) lacks the PH domain but is related to the Tec family of kinases. For comprehensive reviews of the Tec family see Smith et al. (2001) and Takesono et al. (2002).

Chromosomal region containing the *BTK* gene

The human *BTK* gene is located on the long arm of the X chromosome in a region designated Xq22.1 (Fig. 21.4). It is transcribed in a telomere ($\rightarrow$) centromere direction (Vorechovsky et al., 1994a) and the human gene encompasses 37.5 kb (Hagemann et al., 1994; Ohta et al., 1994; Rohrer et al., 1994; Sideras et al., 1994) as depicted in Figure 21.4. Use of cDNA selection technology enabled identification of several RNA species expressed from this region in B cells and in B cell progenitors (Vorechovsky et al., 1994a). A deletion extending into the closest flanking gene, the centromerically located gene initially referred to as *DXS1274E*, was found in a family with XLA and sensorineural deafness (Vorechovsky et al., 1994a). Mutations in this gene, later renamed *DDP* (deafness dystonia protein) and then officially called *TIMM8A*, because it encodes a conserved mitochondrial protein, were found to cause Mohr-Tranebjaerg syndrome (Jin et al., 1996). Subsequently, patients with various deletions extending from the *BTK* gene into the *DDP* gene have been reported (Richter et al., 2001). A map of this chromosomal region is depicted in Figure 21.4.

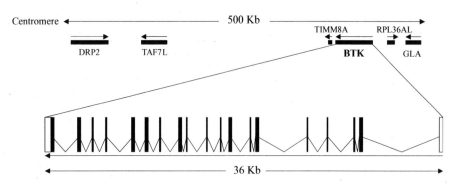

Figure 21.4. Physical map of the Xq22.1 region showing the *BTK* gene and adjacent genes (top) and how they are transcribed. Deletions encompassing the 3′ end of the *BTK* gene and extending into the *TIMM8A* gene cause XLA and Mohr-Tranebjaerg syndrome. Below is the organization of the *BTK* gene, showing the 19 exons. Filled squares represent translated exonic regions.

Genomic organization of the *BTK* gene

Btk was the first member of the Tec family for which the genomic organization was established. The related *TXK* gene, which encodes a kinase lacking a PH domain, has shown an organizational pattern similar to that of *BTK* (Ohta et al., 1996). The human *BTK* gene comprises 19 exons, including a 5′ untranslated region (exon 1) and a 3 exon containing both the C-terminal coding and a 3′ untranslated part (Hagemann et al., 1994; Ohta et al., 1994; Rohrer et al., 1994; Sideras et al., 1994), as depicted in Figure 21.4. The sizes of the exons vary from 55 to 560 bp, and the introns range from 164 bp to 9 kb. In the mouse, a similar genomic organization was observed (Sideras et al., 1994), the difference being mainly an increased size of introns 4 and 12. The number of exons was identical in humans and mice, as were the exon–intron boundaries. Furthermore, the human, mouse, and rat Btk proteins are highly conserved, being 98%–99% identical at the amino acid level (Sideras et al., 1994; Lindvall et al., 2005).

The promoter region of the *BTK* gene was initially inferred from sequence motifs in the DNA stretch 5 of the start site (Sideras et al., 1994). Through functional analysis of this region, binding sites for members of two families of transcription factors have been identified—namely, Sp1 and Spi-1/PU.1, respectively (Himmelmann et al., 1996; Müller et al., 1996, 1999). Tissue specificity seems to be provided by the Spi-1/PU.1 factors, which are selectively expressed among hematopoietic cells. Btk is expressed in all hematopoietic cells with the exception of T cells and plasma cells. This indicates that the *BTK* gene is turned on early during differentiation, and Btk expression has been observed in cells carrying the early progenitor marker CD34 (Smith et al., 1994a).

The first mutations identified resulted from amino acid substitutions in the kinase domain (Vetrie et al., 1993). However, mutations have been found scattered all over the gene, afflicting all the domains of the protein.

Functional Aspects of Btk Signaling

Multiple receptors connect to Btk in B and non-B hematopoietic cell types.

Immunoglobulin-Based Receptors

The ordered rearrangement of immunoglobulin heavy-chain segments and expression of associated signaling molecules like Igβ (CD79b) is a critical step in the production and selection of diverse immature B lineage cells. The transition from pro-B to pre-B phenotype cells can be induced by cross-linking of the CD79b molecule, even in cells from *Rag2* knockout mice that lack productive Ig rearrangements. However, in *Btk/Rag2* double-knockout mice this induced transition does not occur, a result supporting a role for Btk in one of the earliest steps in B lineage development (Kouro et al., 2001).

Proper assembly and signaling from the pre-B cell receptor is needed to progress through B cell development for selection of the heavy chain repertoire and to signal for light-chain rearrangements (Conley et al., 2000). Btk and other signaling molecules including Lyn, Syk, BLNK (also known as Slp-65), phosphatidylinositol 3-kinase (PI3K), Vav, and PLCγ2 can all be associated in a lipid raft signaling complex with the pre-B cell receptor (Guo et al., 2000) necessary for effective Ca^{2+} signaling.

The most intensively studied receptor on the surface of B lineage cells is the Ig receptor complex, or B cell receptor (BCR), which contains both heavy and light chains and the associated signaling molecules, Igα and Igβ. Peripheral resting B cells with a IgM^{low}/IgD^{high} phenotype are reduced in numbers in X-linked immunodeficiency (Xid) mice and nearly absent in most patients with XLA. Activation by cross-linking with anti-immunoglobulin is defective in Xid B cells, with failure to sustain a strong flux of Ca^{2+} and progress through the cell cycle. Early steps downstream of BCR activation include tyrosine phosphorylation of the immunreceptor tyrosine-based activation motif (ITAM) sequences on Igα and β by Src family kinases (predominantly Lyn). This eventually results in the assembly of a membrane-associated signaling complex that includes Lyn, Syk, PI3K, PLCγ2, BLNK, and Btk (reviewed in Fruman et al., 2000) (Fig. 21.5). The joint activity of these proteins in a common complex or pathway is strongly supported by the striking finding that knockouts causing absence of Btk, PLCγ, BLNK, and the p85 form of PI3K all show the common phenotype of the Xid mouse (reviewed in Fruman et al., 2000; Leitges et al., 1996; Fruman et al., 1999; Hashimoto et al., 1999; Jumaa et al., 1999; Minegishi et al., 1999; Pappu et al., 1999; Suzuki et al., 1999; Wang et al., 2000; Xu et al., 2000).

BCR cross-linking and Lyn activation also activates PI3K, resulting in the production of inositol lipids that bind to PH domain–containing proteins such as Btk and stabilize their membrane association (Fukuda et al., 1996; Salim et al., 1996; Li et al., 1997a, 1997b; Rameh et al., 1997; Bolland et al., 1998; Scharenberg et al., 1998; Nore et al., 2000). This lipid–enzyme interaction may also directly influence the kinase activity of Btk (Saito et al., 2001). Pathways that deplete these PI3K-generated lipids, like activation of the SHIP phosphatase via inhibitory receptors, antagonize the assembly and stability of the BCR-directed signalosome complex (Bolland et al., 1998; Scharenberg et al., 1998). A recent addition to the PI3K pathway is the phosphatidylinositol-4-phosphate 5-kinases (PIP5Ks) (Saito et al., 2003). This signaling assembly is thought to segregate to a specialized lipid domain or raft critical for efficient and sustained signaling.

Lyn and other Src family kinases can transphosphorylate Btk on tyrosine 551, located within the kinase activation loop, resulting in a dramatic increase in enzyme activity (Rawlings et al., 1996). This process is followed by autophosphorylation at tyrosine 223 within the SH3 domain (Park et al., 1996), resulting in stronger downstream signaling by altering binding interactions of the SH3 domain (Morrogh et al., 1999) and relieving negative control of Btk. Several Btk SH3-binding partners have been identified. Some, such as Sab, interact with the SH3 domain and serve to inhibit the kinase activity (Yamadori et al., 1999). An attractive model to consider for further analysis is an inactive pool of Btk existing in the cytoplasm with a bound regulator released upon kinase activation and autophosphorylation within the SH3 domain. This two-step activation mechanism is highly conserved among the Tec family of kinases in mammals (Heyeck et al., 1997) and similar interactions are seen for Src and Tec family kinases in *Drosophila* (Guarnieri et al., 1998; Roulier et al., 1998). Antibodies specific for the phosphotyrosine-modified sequences around residues 551 and 223 of Btk have been useful in defining the pathway of activation and inactivation of Btk and demonstrating that the active fraction of Btk moves into the receptor signaling complex (Wahl et al., 1997; Nisitani et al., 1999).

Postreceptor Control of Btk Activity

A variety of mechanisms to control Btk activity within the cytoplasm and signalosome structure have been described. Like other tyrosine kinases, Btk can be directly activated inside of cells by

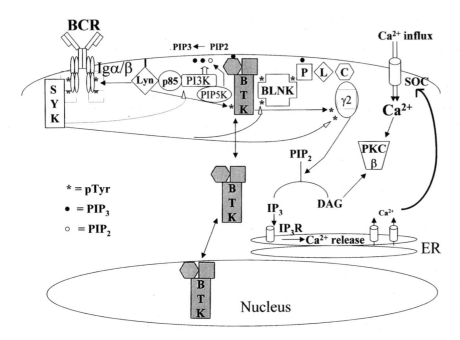

Figure 21.5. Schematic representation of signaling pathways in which Btk has been implicated. Since Btk may be found in different subcellular locations, this is also depicted.

the addition of strong oxidizing agents such as hydrogen peroxide (Qin et al., 2000). This seems to effect the function of Btk in coordinating the transphosphorylation of PLCγ to regulate Ca²⁺ flux and other signals (Qin and Chock, 2001).

Serine phosphorylation of Btk by PKCβ can down-regulate its tyrosine kinase activity (Yao et al., 1994; Kang et al., 2001). However, the phenotype of a *Pkcb* knockout is almost identical to that of the Xid mouse at the whole-animal level (Leitges et al., 1996). These findings may relate to the need to maintain an optimal dose and timing of activation for Btk within the B cell. Alternatively, PKCβ may be part of a feedback loop to limit the extent of Btk signaling. PKCβ is activated downstream of PLCγ2, which itself is regulated by Btk (Humphries et al., 2004). Thus, PKCβ may be required to transmit Btk signals in addition to down-regulating them.

Selected Cytokine and Other Classes of Receptors Require Btk for Signaling in B Lineage Cells

The interleukin-5 (IL-5) receptor mediates important growth and developmental choices for the B and eosinophil cell lineages in the mouse. Although this class of receptors acts predominantly through the activation of specific members of the Jak family of kinases to transphosphorylate Stat proteins to activate gene expression, the IL-5 α subunit can also activate Src family kinases and Btk (Sato et al., 1994; Pazdrak et al., 1995). Certain Jak family kinases have been reported to directly phosphorylate Btk (Takahashi-Tezuka et al., 1997). Studies with the Xid mouse strain have shown that full-signal responses through this receptor in B cells require the function of Btk (Hitoshi et al., 1993; Koike et al., 1995). Similarly, function of the IL-10 receptor on B cell survival and activation is Btk-dependent (Go et al., 1990).

Other receptors of quite different types, including CD38 (Kikuchi et al., 1995; Santos-Argumedo et al., 1995; Yamashita et al., 1995), RP105 (Miyake et al., 1994), CD72 (Venkataraman et al., 1998), and CD40 (Hasbold and Klaus, 1994), have been

linked to Btk by showing defective signaling in Xid B cells under some experimental conditions. Failure to efficiently transmit signals from some or all of these receptors likely contributes to the Xid phenotype, although the relative requirement for each signaling pathway has not been defined.

Activation of Btk by Receptors in Non-B Cells

Btk is broadly expressed among hematopoietic cell types with the exception of T cells (Smith et al., 1994a). Important receptors, such as the Fcε receptor of mast cells, which mediates degranulation responses via IgE and allergen complex–induced binding, have been clearly linked to Btk activation by genetic and biochemical criteria (Kawakami et al., 1994; Hata et al., 1998a; Setoguchi et al., 1998). Although Xid mice and XLA patients demonstrate competent mast cell responses through this receptor, Btk appears to play an important quantitative role in the efficiency of the response (Hata et al., 1998b). Sustained Ca²⁺ flux influenced by Btk and other members of the Tec family of kinases appears crucial for these events (Kawakami et al., 2000).

A very different type of receptor activation is exemplified by the collagen-mediated activation of platelet aggregation via non integrin glycoprotein receptors. Although Xid mice and XLA patients show no gross defect in blood clotting, Btk is clearly activated by this mechanism and likely plays an additive role with other Tec family kinases in mediating effective platelet activation (Quek et al., 1998).

Cross-Talk Between the G Protein–Coupled Receptor Family and Btk

The largest family of receptors in the human or mouse genomes is the multimembrane spanning G protein–coupled receptors that mediate an enormous range of cellular responses (Gether, 2000). Activation of one of these receptors results in signaling though a specific subset of the Gα and Gβ/γ components of the heterotrimeric G protein complex. The range of downstream signals is broad, with activation of downstream second messengers and transcriptional responses. Several reports have connected activation of G protein subunits to activation of Btk by a direct protein interaction mechanism (Tsukada et al., 1994; Langhans-Rajasekaran et al., 1995; Bence et al., 1997; Jiang et al., 1998b). Most studies have used either cotransfection analysis or in vitro activation assays to monitor changes in the phosphorylation status of Btk or its specific activity as a tyrosine kinase. Associations between the activity of $G\alpha12$ (Jiang et al., 1998b) and $G\alpha q$ (Bence et al., 1997; Ma and Huang, 1998) subtypes and $G\beta/\gamma$ subunits (Tsukada et al., 1994; Langhans-Rajasekaran et al., 1995) with Btk have been noted. There is some genetic evidence from transfection studies that shows the quantitative importance of such cross-talk between G protein–coupled receptors and Btk signaling (Satterthwaite et al., 2000). This is an important area for future study. Furthermore, activation of G protein–coupled receptors stimulate PI3K activation, which recruits Btk to the cell membrane (Nore et al., 2000), linking it to small GTPases.

Downstream Signaling Events Mediated by Btk

The broad range of receptors that require Btk for effective signal transduction and the Xid-like phenotype generated by loss-of-function mutations affecting PLCγ2, BLNK, PI3K, and PKCβ presage the complexity of assigning a precise and limited set of downsteam signals to Btk. Since evidence exists to support Btk's participation in a "signalosome"-type complex for receptors like the BCR, one must first define those signals regulated by the complex. The clearest signal is the regulated increase in intracytoplasmic calcium following BCR receptor engagement. A strikingly common cellular phenotype for loss-of-function mutants of Btk and the other molecules mentioned above is the loss of sustained calcium flux by oscillatory calcium pumps using capacitive-type mechanisms (Rigley et al., 1989; Takata et al., 1995; Takata and Kurosaki, 1996; Kurosaki and Kurosaki, 1997; Fluckiger et al., 1998; Ishiai et al., 1999; Jumaa et al., 1999; Pappu et al., 1999; Wen et al., 2004).

The tyrosine phosphorylation of PLCγ by several enzymes including Btk and Syk is known to activate calcium flux through the production of inositol 1, 4, 5-triphosphate (IP3) and diacylglycerol (DAG) (Humphries et al., 2004) through release of Ca^{2+} from intracellular stores, primarily in the endoplasmic reticulum. In a yet-to-be-defined mechanism, this released Ca^{2+} and other signals control capacitive (or store operated) channels that regulate the sustained influx of Ca^{2+} from the extracellular fluid (reviewed in Scharenberg and Kinet, 1998). Candidates for these capacitive pumps have been defined (Harteneck et al., 2000). The sustained flux of Ca^{2+} would be expected to influence a broad range of cellular events including specific transcription factor activation, and cytoskeletal rearrangement needed for entry into S phase.

A variety of cytoplasmic molecules have been linked to Btk by physical or genetic means, including Wiskott-Aldrich syndrome protein (WASP) (Guinamard et al., 1998), Cbl (Cory et al., 1995), Akt (Craxton et al., 1999; Kitaura et al., 2000), phospholipase D (Hitomi et al., 2001), Ras (Deng et al., 1998), JNK (Kawakami et al., 1997, 1998; Deng et al., 1998; Hata et al., 1998b; Jiang et al., 1998a), Bcl-2 (Woodland et al., 1996), and Bcl-x (Anderson et al., 1996; Solvason et al., 1998). This collection implicates a broad variety of signal transduction processes as working with Btk. These include the mitogen-activated protein kinase (MAPK) cascades, antiapoptotic pathways, and regulators of the cytoskeletion. The precise and quantitative role of Btk in these processes,

compared to that of other factors, is hard to assess at this point in time.

Role of Btk in the Nucleus

Through its actions in the cytoplasm, some signals from Btk should influence processes within the nucleus. Evidence for Btk directly modifying transcription factors such as STAT5 (Mahajan et al., 2001) and TFII-I (Yang and Desiderio, 1997; Novina et al., 1999; Egloff and Desiderio, 2001) by tyrosine phosphorylation is one mode of control. The nuclear factor (NF)-κB transcription factor pathway has also been connected to Btk. BCR-induced activation of IKK and subsequent degradation of I-κB and activation of the NF-κB pathway is impaired in B cells lacking Btk, BLNK, or PLCγ2 (Bajpai et al., 2000; Petro et al., 2000; Petro and Khan, 2001; Tan et al., 2001). At least one transcription factor called Bright is reported to bind directly with Btk (Webb et al., 2000) and relocalize as a complex within the nucleus. Such mechanisms could dramatically increase the range of actions for Btk within the nucleus (Mohamed et al., 2000).

Mutation Analysis

Techniques for Mutation Analysis

Several techniques for mutation analysis exist, such as single-strand conformation polymorphism (SSCP), denaturing gradient gel electrophoresis (DGGE), and chemical cleavage of mismatch (CCM). Mutation detection has greatly improved over the years, and this development is likely to continue. Most of the techniques are highly reliable and identify the majority but rarely all of the mutations in affected genes. Thus, in selected patients alternative techniques may have to be employed. Knowledge of the genomic organization of the *BTK* gene now allows the use of DNA as a template (Conley et al., 1994; Hagemann et al., 1994; Ohta et al., 1994; Vorechovsky et al., 1995a, 1995b), whereas in the initial mutation reports reverse-transcribed RNA was applied. The use of DNA is advantageous, as it is more resistant to degradation than RNA, facilitating transport conditions. Furthermore, it allows the identification of splice-site mutations and other mutations, which are not encoded in the mRNA sequence.

Mutation analysis is often carried out on an international basis, and active laboratories can be found in the mutation database reports (Vihinen et al., 1995, 1998; Lindvall et al., 2005). It is advisable to contact the laboratory performing mutation determination prior to sampling as certain requirements may have to be fulfilled. Samples, frequently peripheral blood, may be sent as either a fresh, unprocessed specimen or as purified DNA. In some instances RNA and protein analysis may also be indicated.

In certain patients with an XLA phenotype a mutation will not be found. This may be due to an inability of the technique used to identify the mutation, but, as is the case in rare females, locus heterogeneity (other genes affected) is also expected to cause an XLA phenotype in certain males. Moreover, the selective absence of Btk RNA or protein should be regarded as XLA until proven otherwise.

Spectrum of Mutations in the *BTK* Gene

Although all DNA is subject to mutagenic alteration, gene-related patterns exist. Preferentially in diseases with an autosomal recessive inheritance pattern founder effects may be seen, resulting in the overrepresentation of one or a few mutations. However, for sex-linked traits, representing about 10% of genetic disease in newborns (Baird et al., 1988), this is not the case, and in XLA patients mutations are spread out over the entire *BTK* gene. This pattern is reflected by the fact that the frequency of new mutations reported to the BTKbase (see below) has been only marginally reduced over time.

The first mutations identified resulted from amino acid substitutions in the kinase domain (Vetrie et al., 1993). However, mutations are scattered all over the gene, afflicting every domain of the protein. In 1994 an international study group for XLA was formed with the aim of collecting all mutations into a common database. This database is designated *BTKbase* and is continuously updated and available through the Internet (http://bioinf.uta.fi/BTKbase/). Investigators carrying out mutation analyses are encouraged to contact the study group and report new information. Instructions are available at the BTKbase Web site or through one of the authors (C.I.E.S.). For further information on immunodeficiency disease mutation databases, including instructions for data submission, see Chapter 45.

The first report contained 122 unique mutations (78%) from 157 families in Europe and the United States (Vihinen et al., 1995). The 1996 updates also include patients from Japan and Australia and list 175 unique mutations (74%) in 236 families (Vihinen et al., 1996a, 1996b). The last edition lists 554 unique molecular events (67%) in 823 unrelated families (Lindvall et al., 2005). Thus, the frequency of unique mutations among new cases is only slowly decreasing.

Various forms of genetic abnormalities have been found in the *BTK* gene, representing all major types of alterations (Vihinen et al., 1996a, 1996b, 1997a). These include missense (amino acid substitution) and nonsense (stop codon formation) mutations, deletions, and insertions. The majority of deletions and insertions are out of frame, resulting in stop codon formation, but in-frame variants have also been identified. Most of the mutations are located in exonic regions (affecting coding sequence), whereas about 16% affect splice sites (Table 21.4). Large deletions have also been found encompassing several exons and introns, some of which also extend into neighboring genes (Vetrie et al., 1993; Vorechovsky et al., 1994a; Richter et al., 2001). A single mutation confined to the promoter region has been found (Holinski-Feder et al., 1998), but these are normally very rare, typically corresponding to a few percent or less (Gianelli et al.,

1996). Gianelli et al. found 17 of 1380 patient entries (1.2%) to be caused by molecularily unique events in the promoter of the hemophilia B gene (*F9*), another X-linked disease.

Most mutations affect single base pairs and a predilection for certain sites exists. Thus, CpG sites are highly prone to mutagenic events. The 5-methylcytosine bases frequently spontaneously deaminate to thymine, causing transitions (Duncan and Miller, 1980). These sites are also the major mutational hot spots for the sex-linked primary immunodeficiencies, including XLA (Smith and Vihinen, 1996; Lindvall et al., 2005).

Figure 21.6 depicts the location of different mutations in relation to the amino acid sequence of the Btk protein. As can be seen, missense mutations are not uniformly distributed but are preferentially found in the kinase domain, and especially in the C-terminal portion of the kinase domain. A number of missense mutations also exist in the PH and SH2 domains, whereas the TH-SH3 region is much less affected. Conversely, mutations altering the reading frame, resulting in stop codon formation and frequent loss of protein expression due to unstable conformation, are, as expected, evenly distributed. Structural information has allowed the use of molecular modeling to interpret the consequences of mutations that are in-frame for all domains of Btk with the exception of the TH region, for which there is as yet no template (Lindvall et al., 2005).

Genotype–phenotype analyses have been performed without initially establishing firm correlations (Vihinen et al., 1996a; Holinski-Feder et al., 1998). A modest number of mutations with mild phenotypes have been observed, most of which are caused by substitutions. However, in some patients frameshift mutations perturbing the expression of Btk protein were found to be compatible with mild disease. Especially splice site mutations yielding low levels of normal mRNA are expected to result in a mild phenotype, but this has so far not been documented (Noordzij et al., 2002b). Occasionally, the identical genetic change may cause both mild and severe disease. This phenomenon is of no surprise, as a phenotypic variation among family members, presumably carrying an identical genetic abnormality, was known in XLA many years prior to the disease gene cloning (Buckley and Sidbury, 1968; Goldblum et al., 1974; Wedgwood and Ochs, 1980) and has also been verified by mutation analysis (Bykowsky et al., 1996; Kornfeld et al., 1997). This variation also demonstrates that confounding parameters exist, possibly of both genetic and environmental origin. Nevertheless, recent

Table 21.4. Number of Unique Mutations per Number of Families Affected

Mutation type	Upstream	Downstream	PH	TH	SH3	SH2	TK	Other	Total
Missense	0/0	0/0	35/67	7/7	0/0	28/58	110/194	0/0	180/326
Nonsense	0/0	0/0	13/25	5/8	11/29	10/17	28/56	0/0	67/135
In-frame insertion	0/0	0/0	0/0	0/0	0/0	0/0	2/2	0/0	2/2
In-frame deletion	0/0	0/0	6/6	2/2	0/0	3/4	8/11	0/0	19/23
Frameshift insertion	0/0	0/0	7/14	9/14	3/3	3/3	16/19	0/0	38/53
Frameshift deletion	0/0	0/0	29/33	17/18	15/16	14/14	42/47	0/0	117/128
Splice-site in-frame	0/0	0/0	3/5	0/0	4/6	1/1	3/4	0/0	11/16
Splice-site frameshift	0/0	0/0	7/7	0/0	1/1	3/3	9/10	0/0	20/21
Splice-site undefined	4/5	0/0	19/22	4/7	5/6	13/14	28/37	0/0	73/91
Gross deletion	0/0	0/0	0/0	0/0	0/0	0/0	0/0	14/14	14/14
Insertion	0/0	0/0	0/0	0/0	0/0	0/0	2/2	1/2	3/4
Other	4/4	0/0	2/2	2/2	0/0	1/1	0/0	1/1	10/10
Total	8/9	0/0	121/181	46/58	39/61	76/115	248/382	16/17	554/823

PH, pleckstrin homology; SH, Src homology; TH, Tec homology; TK, tyrosine kinase.

Data from BTKbase V7.50. Reproduced with permission from Lindvall et al. (2005).

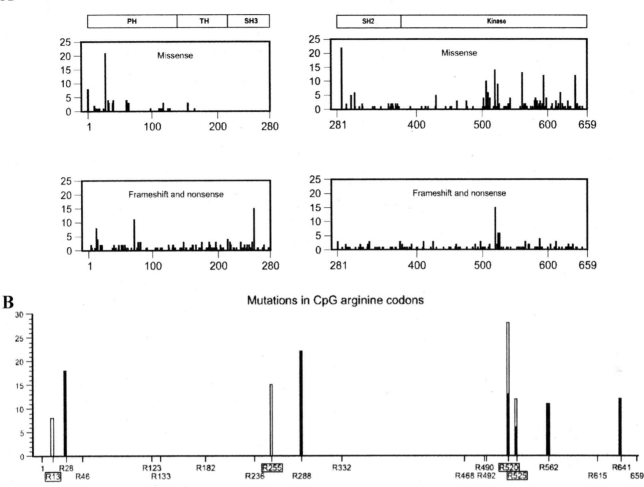

Figure 21.6. Distribution of different mutations in the *BTK* gene. (A) Distribution of different codon mutations. The number of unrelated families with missense vs. frameshift + nonsense mutations in the different domains of Btk is shown. (B) Distribution of CpG-arginine codons in Btk and the location and number of mutations at these sites. Boxed codons represent CGA sequences, which are prone to generate nonsense mutations. The Y axis denotes the number of unrelated families having mutations and the X axis, the codon number. Open bars represent nonsense and filled bars missense mutations. Reproduced with permission from Lindvall et al. (2005).

analysis conclusively demonstrates that many residues will not cause XLA when affected by missense mutations (Lindvall et al., 2005). Moreover, among the highly mutation-prone CpG sites, only some are sensitive to replacements, whereas stop codon formation without any known exception causes XLA (Lindvall et al., 2004).

Mutations Affecting *BTK* and *TIMM8A* Genes

Certain XLA patients have a mutation extending from the *BTK* gene into the adjacent *TIMM8A* gene causing sensory-neurologic manifestations (see Chromosomal Region Containing the *BTK* Gene, above).

Agammaglobulinemia with Growth Hormone Deficiency

Agammaglobulinemia with growth hormone deficiency (MIM number 307200) was originally reported in four males in an American family (Fleisher et al., 1980). In contrast to most pa-

tients with XLA, the affected individuals demonstrated the presence of some tonsillar tissue. Moreover, when mutation analysis was performed in the prototype family, sequencing of the complete cDNA did not reveal any mutation, and normal-sized Btk protein is expressed at a level comparable to that of healthy controls (Stewart et al., 1995). Recent findings implicate that the *ELF4* gene (E74-like factor 4; ets domain transcription factor; formerly MEF) located in Xq26 may be involved, although these findings should still be treated as nonconclusive (Stewart et al., 2005). At least five additional patients with agammaglobulinemia and growth hormone deficiency have been reported by different investigators (reviewed in Sideras and Smith, 1995), and in those patients undergoing mutation analysis alterations were confined to the *BTK* gene (Conley et al., 1994; Vihinen et al., 1994c). Furthermore, identical mutations have also been found in patients lacking evidence of growth hormone deficiency (Vihinen et al., 1996a, 1997a). The cause of the growth hormone deficiency in these patients remains elusive, and the criteria for establishing this form of hormone deficiency may vary.

Females With an XLA Phenotype and Autosomal Recessive Inheritance

With a single reported exception, females carrying a mutation of the *BTK* gene on one of their X chromosomes are healthy and show no evidence of XLA. A strong selection of B lymphocytes expressing the nonaffected *BTK* gene has been reported in both mice (Nahm et al., 1983) and humans (Conley et al., 1986; Fearon et al., 1987). Thus, it is unlikely that females displaying even a highly skewed X-chromosome inactivation pattern would be affected, since the selective growth and differentiation advantage of B lineage cells using the X chromosome with a normal *BTK* gene would preclude disease. In the single reported female with XLA, the mutation is heterozygous and inherited from her father (Takada et al., 2004). Because of the unexpected phenotype and the finding of an exclusive inactivation of the maternal X chromosome in both hematopoietic and mucosal cells, basic mechanisms for lyonization were analyzed. Defects in the *XIST* gene regulating X-inactivation were not detected.

An array of other genetic abnormalities could, theoretically, result in female XLA, such as X-chromosome translocations, Turner's syndrome (females with a single X and no Y chromosome), and uniparental disomy (two copies of the same, affected X chromosome) (Conley and Sweinberg, 1992).

Over the past few years several autosomally recessive disorders causing B cell deficiency have been identified. Previously it was demonstrated in mice that mutations precluding the expression of surface IgM would result in the absence of B cells (Kitamura et al., 1991). Eight different mutations in the human IgH chain locus (*IGHM*) preventing expression of membrane protein were found to result in the virtual absence of B cells in 12 human families (Lopez Granados et al., 2002). Furthermore, mutations in the human 5/14.1 gene (*IGLL1*) encoding the pre-B cell receptor surrogate light chain, as well as in the Igα gene (*CD79A*) and the linker protein *BLNK* gene result in B cell deficiency and agammaglobulinemia (see Chapter 22).

Strategies for Diagnosis

An X-linked inheritance (only males having the disease) with more than one generation affected and laboratory findings demonstrating severely decreased B lymphocyte and Ig levels make the diagnosis of XLA highly probable. However, about one-third of XLA cases are sporadic and caused by de novo mutations. Diagnosis is confirmed by mutation analysis. In mild forms of XLA, B lymphocyte and Ig levels may be only partially decreased, thus resembling X-linked hyper-IgM syndrome and CVID. Another differential diagnosis may be X-linked lymphoproliferative syndrome.

The physical examination normally reveals markedly hypoplastic or absent tonsils, adenoids, and lymph nodes. In healthy newborns and infants peripheral lymphoid organs are hypoplastic, frequently preventing the inclusion of this diagnostic criterion. Untreated patients are generally infected once the maternally transferred Ig has been catabolized; the symptoms depend on the site and severity of the infection. Patients often get used to carrying infections, including having symptoms such as frequent coughing and rhinorrhea, and tiredness is a frequent complaint. A common finding is that adult patients perceive restrictions in several areas of their daily life (Gardulf et al., 1993).

In patients receiving adequate treatment, most of the time there will not be any firm evidence of overt infections; however, the lymphoid hypoplasia will persist. Growth and development are generally age appropriate. However, infections may still occur even during optimal treatment, and many patients will continue to experience some restrictions in areas of their daily life.

Mode of Inheritance, Carrier Detection, and Prenatal Diagnosis

X-linked agammaglobulinemia is a typical X-linked disease affecting males inheriting the defective gene, whereas females are healthy carriers. A defective gene in females can be detected at the level of X-chromosome usage. In females only one X chromosome is functional in each cell (Lyon, 1966; Migeon, 1994). Early during embryogenesis one of the two X chromosomes is inactivated in a random fashion in all mammals, providing a mechanism for gene dosage compensation. Thus, in an individual cell, or clone, the same X chromosome will be active, whereas in a cell lineage the X-chromosome usage is typically random. However, in females carrying a defective *BTK* gene, virtually all mature B cells use the normal X chromosome; in other lineages, such as the T lymphocyte, the inactivation is random (Conley et al., 1986). This demonstrates that Btk is essential for B lymphocyte differentiation or survival.

The technique of determining X chromosome inactivation was used for carrier detection prior to the cloning of the *BTK* gene. For prenatal diagnosis, measurement of fetal B lymphocytes was used prior to the cloning of the *BTK* gene (Journet et al., 1992). DNA markers linked to the disease locus were also employed (reviewed in Sideras and Smith, 1995) and may still be applied in families in whom a mutation in *BTK* has not been identified. Methods to identify inactivated vs. noninactivated X chromosomes via PCR-based techniques may be used for genetic counseling by assessing carrier status for mothers of isolated affected males (Allen et al., 1994). In families with known mutations in the *BTK* gene, unambiguous identification of carrier females and affected fetal males can be made. A protein-based flow-cytometric technique enabling the analysis of the majority of carriers, irrespective of knowledge of the exact mutation, has been developed (Futatani et al., 1998). Flow cytometry and Western blotting with Btk-specific antisera will identify the majority of patients, since frameshifts, stop codons, and a large fraction of missense mutations will not yield a stable protein.

Treatment and Prognosis

γ-Globulin Replacement Therapy

Therapeutic effect of γ-Globulin replacement

Substitution therapy with high-dose γ-globulin is essential in XLA as in other Ig deficiencies (Roifman et al., 1985) and is described in detail in Chapter 46. Normal serum IgG levels may be obtained using high-dose intravenous or subcutaneous treatment; intramuscular administration is insufficient. In a study comprising 29 patients with XLA, a beneficial effect of high-dose vs. low-dose IVIG therapy on the incidence of pneumonias and the number of days spent in the hospital was documented (Liese et al., 1992). Improvements in therapeutic outcome were particularly evident when replacement therapy was initiated before the age of 5 years. In a retrospective study of 31 XLA patients, Quartier et al. (1999) reported a significant decrease from 0.4 bacterial infections annually prior to IVIG to 0.06 during treatment. These authors also found that a residual serum IgG level of >8 g/l was significantly more protective than 5–8 g/l.

In a retrospective analysis of the incidence of pulmonary disease in hypogammaglobulinemia, it was found that XLA patients had on average only 0.1 pneumonias per treatment year compared to 0.18 in patients with CVID (Sweinberg et al., 1991). Seven of 10 patients with XLA had normal chest X-ray films 8–15 years after diagnosis, and none had bronchiectasies. Pulmonary disease was more common and more severe in CVID. In contrast, Curtin et al. (1991) reported that eight patients with XLA developed bronchiectasis at a significantly earlier age than those who had CVID. Since the mean age of patients reported by Sweinberg et al. (1991) was lower, these differences may either represent pathological changes developing over time or, more likely, reflect the improved therapy and improved diagnostic tools currently available. In a prospective study, Kainulainen et al. (1999) reported that IgG preinfusion levels of 5 g/l did not protect against silent progression of bronchiectasies in 5 of 14 patients with primary hypogammaglobulinemia receiving IVIG.

In a series of patients treated with high-dose subcutaneous γ-globulin, the majority of whom had CVID, only 0.2 patient days/year were spent in the hospital for respiratory tract infections (Gardulf et al., 1991). Furthermore, a significantly increased health-related function and improved self-rated health were reported (Gardulf et al., 1993, 1995). Subcutaneous delivery may also be in the form of express infusions, further decreasing the time (Hansen et al., 2002).

Because patients with normal IgG levels during replacement therapy may be resistant to acquiring fatal enteroviral disease (Liese et al., 1992; Misbah et al., 1992), it is important that XLA patients at all times receive appropriate doses of IgG. Once enteroviral meningoencephalitis has been contracted it is frequently therapy-resistant.

Viral Hepatitis Transferred with Contaminated Immunoglobulin Batches

Hepatitis C infection has so far only occurred after treatment with IVIG and not following substitution with intramuscular preparations, the products also used for subcutaneous administration. Hepatitis C has been observed after the infusion of experimental IVIG preparations (Lever et al., 1984; Ochs et al., 1985; Yap et al., 1994) and commercial IVIG batches (Björkander et al., 1988; Bjøro et al., 1994; Healey et al., 1996).

Patients with PID seem to be unduly susceptible to this infection, possibly because they cannot mount a sufficient immune response against the virus. However, XLA patients with hepatitis C may develop a less fulminant hepatitis than that in CVID patients (Hermaszewski and Webster, 1993; Bjøro et al., 1994; J. Björkander, personal communication). In one series reported by Bjøro et al. (1994), all five infected CVID patients developed severe cirrhosis, including one with fatal outcome, whereas only one of six XLA patients developed cirrhosis and end-stage liver disease. This patient was coinfected with hepatitis B and D viruses. However, in a study by Razvi et al. (2001), the outcome of a hepatitis C infection did not differ between CVID and XLA patients, whereas Quinti et al. (2002) reported a better prognosis in XLA than that in CVID.

Antibiotics

Treatment of infections is essential in all forms of PIDs. The use of antibiotics to combat bacterial infections represents one of the cornerstones in the management of XLA, and prolonged administration is often necessary. However, as in CVID, it is frequently

not possible to eradicate an infectious agent completely. Thus, DNA fingerprinting and the use of antilipopolysaccharide monoclonal antibodies have revealed that the same strain of *H. influenzae* may colonize a patient for many years despite long-term therapy with adequate doses of different antibiotics (Samuelson et al., 1995). For a more detailed description of treatment with antibiotics, see Chapter 46.

Bone Marrow Transplantation and Gene Therapy

Bone marrow transplantation is an option for XLA, as for other PIDs. However, transplantation is not a risk-free procedure, as graft-vs.-host reactions and severe infections may ensue. The stem cell grafting procedure may or may not be ablative. Thus, conditioning increases the chance for engraftment, whereas under nonablative conditions insufficient chimerism may develop. Howard et al. (2003) recently reported three patients receiving cord blood or bone marrow grafts from human leukocyte antigen (HLA)-matched siblings without receiving any preparative regimen or antirejection drugs, and another three who received treatment with cyclosporin A and mycophenolate mophetil. However, none of the patients showed an increase in serum IgM or peripheral B cell counts.

Gene therapy was suggested as a future treatment in both the original reports on cloning of the *BTK* gene (Tsukada et al., 1993; Vetrie et al., 1993). In theory, the defect underlying XLA makes this disease particularly suitable for gene therapy, since the differentiation defect would enable gene-corrected cells to selectively survive. This characteristic is seen also in adenosine deaminase (ADA) deficiency and SCID caused by mutations in the common γ-chain (*XSCID1*), mainly affecting T lineage development. For both these disorders, successful gene therapy has been conducted (see Chapter 48).

Because permanent correction of hematopoietic stem cells would be desirable and current retroviral delivery systems may cause tumor formation (Hacein-Bey-Abina et al., 2003; Dave et al., 2004), gene therapy for XLA may be more distant than previously thought. Thus, in contrast to ADA, the Btk protein could be hazardous if produced in excess amounts or expressed incorrectly in terms of lineage restriction or temporal control. Several other kinases have been implicated in tumor formation when mutated or overexpressed (Heisterkamp et al., 1990; Abraham et al., 1991). This phenomenon may necessitate the use of endogenous-control elements to ensure correct expression or, alternatively, techniques involving disease gene repair rather than the transfer of an intact copy of the defective gene. Nevertheless, retroviral vectors have been developed for the potential treatment of XLA (Islam et al., 1999; Yu et al., 2004).

Since only a single X chromosome is active in each cell, the potential dominant-negative effect of an abnormal Btk protein would not be seen in carriers. However, it could be inferred from other signaling pathways that mutated cytoplasmic tyrosine kinases may exert dominant-negative effects. Furthermore, the dominant-negative effect could be stronger than in the absence of a gene product, as examplified by the Src family member Lck (Levin et al., 1993). The underlying mechanism may be that the abnormal protein could also affect other signaling pathways. This means that the transfer of a normal copy of the *BTK* gene to hematopoietic stem or progenitor cells might only have a therapeutic effect in the approximately 85% of XLA patients lacking Btk protein. In patients with a dominant-negative mutation, repair of the defective gene and gene transfer combined with degradation of an abnormal transcript are potential treatment modalities. In several dominant-negative systems, a gene product needs to be overexpressed, as compared to the nonmutated, wild-type protein suggesting that the level of expression of the transferred gene is crucial.

Furthermore, the expression of Btk in early hematopoietic progenitors makes the Btk promoter (Himmelmann et al., 1996; Müller et al., 1996, 1999) of potential interest in gene therapy for diseases other than XLA. Tissue-specific expression of other therapeutic genes might be provided by the use of this endogenous promoter.

Prognosis

Prior to antibiotic therapy and γ-globulin substitution therapy, the prognosis was poor. Analysis of patients born before 1950 in a large Dutch pedigree revealed that there was a 90% probability of children with XLA dying between 2 months and 8 years of age (Mensink et al., 1984). With the advent of antibiotics and γ-globulin replacement therapy in the 1950s, the prognosis improved considerably (Lederman and Winkelstein, 1985), and this development seems to have continued (Hermaszewski and Webster, 1993; Ochs and Smith, 1996). This trend is also likely to continue because future therapies such as gene replacement have curative potential.

Animal Models of Btk Loss of Function

Overview

The syntenic arrangement of mouse and human X chromosome regions suggests that murine Xid and human XLA are both caused by deficiencies of Btk expression or function. The Xid mutation is defined as a point mutation in the PH domain that leaves kinase activity intact (Rawlings et al., 1993; Thomas et al., 1993). Xid is a relatively mild immune deficiency with loss of some B cell subpopulations and humoral responses (Scher, 1982; Wicker and Scher, 1986). Allele-specific variation in disease severity seemed a plausible explanation until the phenotype of mice with null mutations of Btk were created and shown to have a mild Xid-like phenotype (Kerner et al., 1995; Khan et al., 1995; Hendriks et al., 1996), rather than the severe loss of B cells seen in XLA. This set of observations and other studies described below strongly support the concept that the penetrance of the B cell–immune deficit due to loss of Btk function is strongly influenced by genetic context.

Xid Affects Multiple Stages of B Cell Development and Function

The Xid mutation was first defined in the early 1970s by abnormal responses to polysaccharide antigens in the highly inbred CBA/N strain of mice, a defect that segregated in a sex-linked manner (Amsbaugh et al., 1972). This strain of mice and congenic derivatives of the Xid mutation on other backgrounds show normal fecundity and have minimal if any elevation of cancer risk. They also do not have to be housed in specialized animal facilities.

Detailed analysis of the immune defects in Xid show cell-autonomous defects only for the B cell lineage. These include the loss of specific cell subpopulations such as CD5+ or B1 cells that normally accumulate in the peritoneum. The remaining B cells that emigrate from the marrow to peripheral sites show an immature phenotype exemplified by a high IgM-to-IgD ratio, low major histocompatibility complex (MHC) class II antigen expression, and inability to secrete IgM or class switch for certain isotypes such as IgG3. In Xid mice, responses to type II T cell–independent antigens, exemplified by the trinitrophenyl-derivatived Ficoll, are absent, and B cells cannot form multicellular colonies in response to certain mitogens (Scher, 1982; Wicker and Scher, 1986).

Responses to T cell–dependent antigens are normal. If T cell help is removed through neonatal thymectomy or because of simultaneous presence of the nu/nu gene, B cell development in the bone marrow is blunted, and the immune deficit is severe (Wortis et al., 1982; Karagogeos et al., 1986). The presence of the Xid allele can relieve the systemic lupus-like autoimmune disease complex seen in mouse strains such as NZB/NZW (Taurog et al., 1979), reduce the susceptibility to S. aureus–induced arthritis (Zhao et al., 1995) and M. pulmonis pneumonia (Sandstedt et al., 1997), and modify the antibody production seen in the lymphoproliferative disorder caused by defects in the Motheaten tyrosine phosphatase (Scribner et al., 1987). All of these effects can be rationalized by the altered production of pathogenic antibodies associated with the Xid allele.

More subtle and complex genetic interactions are seen when the severity of the Xid allele is evaluated in the context of specific backcrosses or different congenic strains that do not harbor any obvious immune or developmental defect. The Xid allele on a C3H background is more severe than that of the original CBA/N strain (Bona et al., 1980; Mond et al., 1983a). Similar effects of strain background were noted in analysis of germ-line knockouts of the Btk gene, discussed below (Khan et al., 1995). The number and function of predicted modifier loci are not known.

Genetically Engineered Btk Knockout Strains Display a Phenotype Similar to Those of Xid Strains

Three groups have published analyses of lymphocyte development and function in the absence of Btk expression (Kerner et al., 1995; Khan et al., 1995; Hendriks et al., 1996). Null mutations of Btk created in embryonic stem cells by homologous recombination were passaged to the lymphocyte lineage by transfer into the blastocysts of immune-defective Rag2 knockout mice and the germ line of otherwise immune-competent mice. Detailed analyses of the B cell developmental pathways and functional responses to a variety of cell surface cross-linking antibodies, mitogens, and chemical mediators showed a phenotype that is remarkably similar to that seen in Xid strains. Some minor variation in the subpopulations of early B cell precursors in the marrow and variation in immune responses according to strain background were described, but the overall picture strongly suggests that the point mutation in the PH domain found in Xid is as severe an allele as no expression of Btk at all. Recently it was demonstrated that there was no survival difference between cells carrying an active Xid allele and an active knockout allele in heterozygous females (Lindvall et al., 2005). This clearly demonstrates that there is no residual activity in Btk with an Xid alteration, nor is there any dominant negative effect on other signalling molecules. Moreover, expression profiling has been used to study the effect of the Xid mutation and of the Btk loss-of-function allele (Lindvall et al., 2004).

Development of wild-type levels of Btk by transgenesis experiments can reconstitute normal B cell function and development (Drabek et al., 1997). Transgenes that express less than endogenous levels of Btk show partial rescue and support a dose-limiting role for Btk in Ig receptor signaling (Satterthwaite et al., 1997).

Some insight into the pathways Btk likely uses in connecting surface stimulation to the cellular responses comes from analyses of selected knockout strains of mice. A large number of genes involved in Ig gene structural rearrangement, components of the Ig receptor complex, and some downstream signal transduction components have been shown to be essential for normal B cell development. Many of these block B cell differentiation at an early stage in the marrow, and few B cells are available for detailed functional analyses. However, apart from the defect in the transition from small pre-B cells to immature B cells in the bone marrow, through replacement of the *Btk* gene by insertion of *lacZ*, Hendriks et al. (1996) demonstrated a second differentiation arrest during maturation from IgD^{low}IgM^{high} cells to IgD^{high}-IgM^{low} stages in the periphery.

Several studies have combined the Xid mutation with loss of function in a second gene to create more severe B cell phenotypes and help define pathways that are likely rate limiting for Btk function. A striking result is the severe block in B cell development at the pre-B cell stage observed when a loss of Btk function is combined with a loss of Tec function (Ellmeier et al., 2000). This can be most simply interpreted as Btk and Tec serving essential but redundant roles in the pathways connected to the pre-B cell Ig receptor. The phenotype of this mouse closely resembles the general changes seen in human XLA.

Other mutations can be combined with a loss of function of Btk to produce a severe XLA-like phenotype in the mouse. The transcription factor OBF1 regulates B cell–specific genes and germinal-center responses. When combined with the Xid mutation, the *OBF1* mutation results in agammaglobulinemia secondary to a block at the bone marrow stage of development (Schubart et al., 2000). Although both genes express cell-autonomous effects within the B cell lineage, the precise biochemical connection between their signal transduction pathways and the final phenotype of the whole mouse are not yet defined.

Even more difficult to understand is the dramatic effect of mutation at the nude locus when combined with Xid (Karagogeos et al., 1986). The nude gene encodes a transcription factor of the winged helix class that has an impact on T cell development and thymic function, but has no discernable phenotype within the B cell lineage as a single knockout. When combined with Xid, however, there is a severe block in B cell development at the pro-B to pre-B transition. The cellular and molecular circuitry of this strong genetic effect is not understood. These and other studies described below point out the importance of having whole-animal models to combine with biochemical and cellular tests of Btk function. They also suggest potential mechanisms for the difference in severity of Xid and XLA.

A most striking example of convergence toward a common function comes from genetic and phenotypic analysis of the collection of single gene knockouts that result in a Xid-like phenotype. Mutation affecting PLCγ2, the p85 form of PI3K, PKCβ, or the adaptor protein BLNK all show a very similar Xid-like phenotype with selective loss of B cells and antigen responses, defective activation from the Ig receptor, and loss of Ca^{2+} flux in residual peripheral B cells (reviewed in Fruman et al., 2000; Leitges et al., 1996; Fruman et al., 1999; Hashimoto et al., 2000; Jumaa et al., 1999; Minegishi et al., 1999; Pappu et al., 1999; Suzuki et al., 1999; Wen et al., 2004). Much additional evidence, described below, suggests that these proteins all work in a complex or signalosome that mediates signals from cell membrane receptors including but not limited to the BCR (Fig. 21.5).

Normal B cell Responses Require an Optimal Dose of Btk

Correction of the Xid phenotype can be accomplished by transgenic expression of a cDNA of the wild-type *Btk* gene controlled by an MHC class II region promoter (Drabek et al., 1997). Another transgenic strain used an Ig promoter and enhancer to express a Btk cDNA at about 25% of the normal level of Btk protein in peripheral B cells (Satterthwaite et al., 1997). These mice showed full correction of the numerical deficit in mature, IgM^{low}IgD^{high} peripheral B2 cells, but only partial recovery of signal response to BCR stimulation as measured with in vitro stimulation assays or in vivo immunizations (Satterthwaite et al., 1997; Pinschewer et al., 1999). Increasing the dose of Btk by creating mice homozygous for the transgene crossed over Xid or wild-type background demonstrated that Btk-dependent responses were optimal at the wild-type level of enzyme, with lower responses seen either below or above the wild-type level of expression.

This concept of an optimal dose of Btk is supported by the phenotype of a transgenic strain of mice expressing a mutant (E41K) form of the enzyme (Dingjan et al., 1998; Maas et al., 1999). This mutation was first isolated by random mutagenesis and selection for an allele of Btk that could transform fibroblast cells to grow suspended in agar. The mutation increases the ability of the enzyme to associate with membranes and the fraction of enzyme chronically modified by phosphotyrosine, indicating that it is an activated allele (Li et al., 1995). Surprisingly, the transgenic E41K strain did not overproduce B cells or have hyperactivated B cells, but rather produced a more severe block in B cell development at the pre-B cell stage similar to that in the human XLA phenotype. However, this phenotype was only seen in transgenic animals carrying several copies of the mutated gene fragment. This finding suggests that too much Btk activity can create negative signals as potently as loss-of-function mutations. Consistent with this model, we have observed that specific XLA patient mutations produce Btk enzymes with intact tyrosine kinase function and increased levels of activity for calcium flux after BCR stimulation in a reconstructed cell system (M. Wahl et al., unpublished observations). Strategies for defining genetic modifiers should help quantify genes and pathways that are most important for Btk function.

Unexpectedly, loss-of-function mutations in the *Btk* gene result in susceptibility to B lymphoma development. This is seen in mice homozygous for inactivating double mutations in *Blnk/Slp-65* and *Btk* genes (Kerssebom et al., 2003). Recently, the tumor-promoting effect was found to be independent of Btk kinase activity (Middendorp et al., 2005).

The availability of mouse strains with hemi- or homozygous loss-of-function mutations for numerous lymphocyte-specific or more generally expressed proteins allows the formal testing of pairwise combinations for genetic interaction and the modification of the Btk-defined Xid phenotype. Complete loss-of-function mutations of Btk or a transgenic strain expressing low levels of Btk have been used as genetic partners in such crosses. Strong evidence of such quantitatively important interactions have been defined for Btk and the transcription factor OBF-1 (Schubart et al., 2000), the Lyn tyrosine kinase (Satterthwaite et al., 1998, 2000; Takeshita et al., 1998), the nude winged-helix transcription factor (Karagogeos et al., 1986), the Motheaten SHP-1 phosphatase (Scribner et al., 1987), the Tec tyrosine kinase (Ellmeier et al., 2000), the CD19 coreceptor (Satterthwaite et al., 2000) and CD40 (Oka et al., 1996; Khan et al., 1997). Such genetic tests of function indicate that both components are important but require biochemical analyses to unravel the potential mechanistic connections or parallel signals that may be involved.

Some help in expediting our understanding of the mechanisms of Btk action are likely to come from studies in *Drosophila*. Both the Src family and Tec family of kinases are found in flies and have already been connected genetically in pathways that influence structures like the ring canal of the fly oocyte, the structure of the male sexual organ, and longevity (Guarnieri et al., 1998; Roulier et al., 1998, Baba et al., 1999). It was recently demonstrated that the human *Btk* gene can partially substitute for the *Drosophila* Btk29A gene defect (Hamada et al., 2005). Our desire to understand the signal transduction pathways of B lymphocytes regulated by Btk, which may influence normal B cell function, autoimmune states, immune deficiencies in addition to XLA, and malignant lymphomas, should hopefully be moved forward by analysis of alternative genetic systems.

Acknowledgments

This work was supported by the Swedish Science Council and the Euro-Policy-PID grant. Owen N. Witte is an investigator at the Howard Hughes Medical Institute. Anne B. Satterthwaite is the Southwestern Medical Foundation Scholar in biomedical research. We are indebted to Leonardo Vargas and Jessica Lindvall for skillful assistance.

References

Abraham KM, Levin SD, Marth JD, Forbush KA, Perlmutter RM. Thymic tumorigenesis induced by overexpression of p56lck. Proc Natl Acad Sci USA 88:3977–3981, 1991.

Ackerson BK, Raghunathan R, Keller MA, Bui RHD, Phinney PR, Imagawa DT. Echovirus 11 arthritis in a patient with X-linked agammaglobulinemia. Pediatr Infect Dis J 6:485–488, 1987.

Alibrahim A, Lepore M, Lierl M, Filipovich A, Assaad A. *Pneumocystis carinii* pneumonia in an infant with X-linked agammaglobulinemia. J Allergy Clin Immunol 101:552–553, 1998.

Allen RC, Nachtman RG, Rosenblatt MM, Belmont JW. Application of carrier testing to genetic counseling for X-linked agammaglobulinemia. Am J Hum Genet 54:25–35, 1994.

Amsbaugh DF, Hansen CT, Prescott B, Stashak PW, Barthold DR, Baker PJ. Genetic control of the antibody response to type 3 pneumococcal polysaccharide in mice. I. Evidence that an X-linked gene plays a decisive role in determining responsiveness. J Exp Med 136:931–949, 1972.

Ament ME, Ochs HD, Davis SD. Structure and function of the gastrointestinal tract in primary immunodeficiency syndromes. A study of 39 patients. Medicine 52:227–248, 1973.

Anderson JS, Teutsch M, Dong Z, Wortis HH. An essential role for Bruton's tyrosine kinase in the regulation of Bruton's B-cell apoptosis. Proc Natl Acad Sci USA 93:10966–10971, 1996.

Baba K, Takeshita A, Majima K, Ueda R, Kondo S, Juni N, Yamamoto D. The *Drosophila* Bruton's tyrosine kinase (Btk) homolog is required for adult survival and male genital formation. Mol Cell Biol 19:4405–4413, 1999.

Baird PA, Anderson TW, Newcombe HB, Lowry RB. Genetic disorders in children and young adults: a population study. Am J Hum Genet 42:677–693, 1988.

Bajpai UD, Zhang K, Teutsch M, Sen R, Wortis HH. Bruton's tyrosine kinase links the B cell receptor to nuclear factor κB activation. J Exp Med 191:1735–1744, 2000.

Bence K, Ma W, Kozasa T, Huang X-Y. Direct stimulation of Bruton's tyrosine kinase by G_q-protein α-subunit. Nature 389:296–299, 1997.

Björkander J, Cunningham-Rundles C, Lundin P, Olsson R, Soderstrom R, Hanson L-A. Intravenous immunoglobulin prophylaxis causing liver damage in 16 of 77 patients with hypogammaglobulinemia or IgG subclass deficiency. Am J Med 84:107–111, 1988.

Bjøro K, Frland SS, Yun Z, Samdal HH, Haaland T. Hepatitis C infection in patients with primary hypogammaglobulinemia after treatment with contaminated immune globulin. N Engl J Med 331:1607–1611, 1994.

Blaser MJ, Smith PF, Kohler PF. Susceptibility of *Campylobacter* isolates to the bactericidal activity of human serum. J Infect Dis 151:227–235, 1985.

Bolland S, Pearse RN, Kurosaki T, Ravetch JV. SHIP modulates immune receptor responses by regulating membrane association of Btk. Immunity 8:509–516, 1998.

Bona C, Mond JJ, Paul WE. Synergistic genetic defect in B-lymphocyte function. J Exp Med 151:224–234, 1980.

Bruton OC. Agammaglobulinemia. Pediatrics 9:722–727, 1952.

Bruton OC, Apt L, Gitlin D, Janeway CA. Absence of serum gamma globulins. Am J Dis Child 84:632–636, 1952.

Buckley RH, Rowlands DT Jr. Agammaglobulinemia, neutropenia, fever, and abdominal pain. J Allergy Clin Immunol 51:308–318, 1973.

Buckley RH, Sidbury JB Jr. Hereditary alterations in the immune response: coexistence of "agammaglobulinemia", acquired hypogammaglobulinemia and selective immunoglobulin deficiency in a sibship. Pediatr Res 2:72–84, 1968.

Bykowsky MJ, Haire RN, Ohta Y, Tang H, Sung SS, Veksler ES, Greene JM, Fu SM, Litman GW, Sullivan KE. Discordant phenotype in siblings with X-linked agammaglobulinemia. Am J Hum Genet 58:477–483, 1996.

Campana D, Farrant J, Inamdar N, Webster ADB, Janossy G. Phenotypic features and proliferative activity of B cell progenitors in X-linked agammaglobulinemia. J Immunol 145:1675–1680, 1990.

Chase GA, Murphy EA. Risk of recurrence and carrier frequency for X-linked lethal recessives. Hum Hered 23:19–26, 1973.

Chusid MJ, Colemann CM, Dunne WM. Chronic asymptomatic *Campylobacter* bacteremia in a boy with X-linked hypogammaglobulinemia. Pediatr Infect Dis 6:943–944, 1987.

Collins MH, Assa'ad AH. Drug reaction to ceftriaxone in a child with X-linked agammaglobulinemia. J Allergy Clin Immunol 109:888–889, 2002.

Conley ME. B cells in patients with X-linked agammaglobulinemia. J Immunol 134:3070–3074, 1985.

Conley ME, Brown P, Pickard AR, Buckley RH, Miller DS, Raskind WH, Singer JW, Fialkow PJ. Expression of the gene defect in X-linked agammaglobulinemia. N Engl J Med 315:564–567, 1986.

Conley ME, Fitch-Hilgenberg ME, Cleveland JL, Parolini O, Rohrer J. Screening of genomic DNA to identify mutations in the gene for Bruton's tyrosine kinase. Hum Mol Genet 3:1751–1756, 1994.

Conley ME, Howard V. Clinical findings leading to the diagnosis of X-linked agammaglobulinemia. J Pediatr 141:566–571, 2002.

Conley ME, Rohrer J, Rapalus L, Boylin EC, Minegishi Y. Defects in early B-cell development: comparing the consequences of abnormalities in pre-BCR signaling in the human and the mouse. Immunol Rev 178:75–90, 2000.

Conley ME, Sweinberg SK. Females with a disorder phenotypically identical to X-linked agammaglobulinemia. J Clin Immunol 12:139–143, 1992.

Cooper MD, Faulk PW, Fudenberg HH, Hitzig W, Good RA, Kunkel H, Rosen FS, Seligmann M, Soothill J, Wedgwood RJ. Classification of primary immunodeficiencies. N Engl J Med 288:966–967, 1973.

Cory GOC, Lovering RC, Hinshelwood S, MacCarthy-Morrogh L, Levinsky RJ, Kinnon C. The protein product of the c-cbl protooncogene is phosphorylated after B cell receptor stimulation and binds the SH3 domain of Bruton's tyrosine kinase. J Exp Med 182:611–615, 1995.

Cover TL, Blaser MJ. The pathobiology of *Campylobacter* infection in humans. Annu Rev Med 40:269–285, 1989.

Craxton A, Jiang A, Kurosaki T, Clark EA. Syk and Bruton's tyrosine kinase are required for B cell antigen receptor–mediated activation of the kinase Akt. J Biol Chem 274:30644–30650, 1999.

Crennan JM, van Scoy RE, McKenna CH, Smith TF. Echovirus polymyositis in patients with hypogammaglobulinemia. Failure of high-dose intravenous gammaglobulin therapy and review of the literature. Am J Med 81:35–42, 1986.

Cunningham CK, Bonville CA, Ochs HD, Seyama K, John PA, Rotbart HA, Weiner LB. Enteroviral meningoencephalitis as a complication of X-linked hyper IgM syndrome. J Pediatr 134:584–588, 1999.

Cunningham-Rundles C, Siegal FP, Cunningham-Rundles S, Lieberman P. Incidence of cancer in 98 patients with common varied immunodeficiency. J Clin Immunol 7:294–299, 1987.

Curtin JJ, Webster ADB, Farrant J, Katz D. Bronchiectasis in hypogammaglobulinaemia—a computed tomography assessment. Clin Radiol 44:82–84, 1991.

Dave UP, Jenkins NA, Copeland NG. Gene therapy insertional mutagenesis insights. Science 303:333, 2004.

Deng J, Kawakami Y, Hartman SE, Satoh T, Kawakami T. Involvement of Ras in Bruton's tyrosine kinase–mediated JNK activation. J Biol Chem 273:16787–16791, 1998.

de Weers M, Verschuren MC, Kraakman ME, Mensink RG, Schuurman RK, van Dongen JJ, Hendriks RW. The Bruton's tyrosine kinase gene is expressed throughout B cell differentiation, from early precursor B cell stages preceding immunoglobulin gene rearrangement up to mature B cell stages. Eur J Immunol 23:3109–3114, 1993.

Dingjan GM, Maas A, Nawijn MC, Smit L, Voerman JS, Grosveld F, Hendriks RW. Severe B cell deficiency and disrupted splenic architecture in transgenic mice expressing the E41K mutated form of Bruton's tyrosine kinase. EMBO J 17:5309–5320, 1998.

Dittrich AM, Schulze I, Magdorf K, Wahn V, Wahn U. X-linked agammaglobulinaemia and *Pneumocystis carinii* pneumonia—an unusual coincidence? Eur J Pediatr 162:432–433, 2003.

Drabek D, Raguz S, DeWit TPM, Dingjan GM, Savelkoul HFJ, Grosveld F, Rudolf WH. Correction of the X-linked imunodeficiency phenotype by transgenic expression of human Bruton tyrosine kinase under the control of the class II major histocompatibility complex Ea locus control region. Proc Natl Acad Sci USA 94:610–615, 1997.

Duncan BK, Miller JH. Mutagenic deamination of cytosine residues in DNA. Nature 287:560–561, 1980.

Egloff AM, Desiderio S. Identification of phosphorylation sites for Bruton's tyrosine kinase within the transcriptional regulator BAP/TFII-I. J Biol Chem 276:27806–27815, 2001.

Ellmeier W, Jung S, Sunshine MJ, Hatam F, Xu Y, Baltimore D, Mano H, Littman DR. Severe B cell deficiency in mice lacking the Tec kinase family members Tec and Btk. J Exp Med 192:1611–1624, 2000.

Elsborg L, Mosbech J. Pernicious anaemia as a risk factor in gastric cancer. Acta Med Scand 206:315–318, 1979.

Erlendsson K, Swartz T, Dwyer JM. Successful reversal of echovirus encephalitis in X-linked hypogammaglobulinemia by intraventricular administration of immunoglobulin. N Engl J Med 312:351–353, 1985.

Farrar JE, Rohrer J, Conley ME. Neutropenia in X-linked agammaglobulinemia. Clin Immunol Immunopathol 81:271–276, 1996.

Faulkner GC, Burrows SR, Khanna R, Moss DJ, Bird AG, Crawford DH. X-Linked agammaglobulinemia patients are not infected with Epstein-Barr virus:implications for the biology of the virus. J Virol 73:1555–1564, 1999.

Fearon ER, Winkelstein JA, Civin CI, Pardoll D, Vogelstein, B. Carrier detection in X-linked agammaglobulinemia by analysis of X-chromosome inactivation. N Engl J Med 316:427–431, 1987.

Ferguson KM, Lemmon MA, Schlessinger J, Sigler PB. Structure of the high affinity complex of inositol triphosphate with a phospholipase C pleckstrin homology domain. Cell 83:1037–1046, 1995.

Filipovich AH, Mathur A, Kamat D, Kersey JH, Shapiro RS. Lymphoproliferative disorders and other tumors complicating immunodeficiencies. Immunodeficiency 5:91–112, 1994.

Filipovich AH, Shapiro RS. Tumors in patients with common variable immunodeficiency. J Immunol Immunopharmacol 11:43–46, 1991.

Fiore L, Plebani A, Buttinelli G, Fiore S, Donati V, Marturano J, Soresina A, Martire B, Azzari C, Nigro G, Cardinale F, Trizzino A, Pignata C, Alvisi P, Anastasio E, Bossi G, Ugazio AG. Search for poliovirus long-term excretors among patients affected by agammaglobulinemia. Clin Immunol 111:98–102, 2004.

Fleisher TA, White R, Broder S, Nissley SP, Blaese RM, Mulvihill JJ, Olive G, Waldmann TA. X-linked agammaglobulinemia and isolated growth hormone deficiency. N Engl J Med 302:1429–1434, 1980.

Fluckiger AC, Li Z, Kato RM, Wahl MI, Ochs HD, Longnecker R, Kinet JP, Witte ON, Scharenberg AM, Rawlings DJ. Btk/Tec kinases regulate sustained increases in intracellular Ca^{2+} following B-cell receptor activation. EMBO J 17:1973–1985, 1998.

Foy HJ, Ochs H, Davis SD, Kenny GE, Luce RR. *Mycoplasma pneumoniae* infections in patients with immunodeficiency syndromes: report of four cases. J Infect Dis 127:388–393, 1973.

Fruman D, Satterthwaite AB, Witte ON. Xid-like phenotypes: a B cell signalosome takes shape. Immunity 13:1–3, 2000.

Fruman DA, Snapper SB, Yballe CM, Davidson L, Yu JY, Alt FW, Cantley LC. Impaired B cell development and proliferation in absence of phosphoinositide 3-kinase p85α. Science 283:393–397, 1999.

Fukuda M, Kojima T, Kabayama H, Mikoshiba K. Mutation of the pleckstrin homology domain of Bruton's tyrosine kinase in immunodeficiency-impaired inositol 1,3,4,5-tetrakisphosphate binding capacity. J Biol Chem 271:30303–30306, 1996.

Futatani T, Miyawaki T, Tsukada S, Hashimoto S, Kunikata T, Arai S, Kurimoto M, Niida Y, Matsuoka H, Sakiyama Y, Iwata T, Tsuchiya S, Tatsuzawa O, Yoshizaki K, Kishimoto T. Deficient expression of Bruton's tyrosine kinase in monocytes from X-linked agammaglobulinemia as evaluated by a flow cytometric analysis and its clinical application to carrier detection. Blood 91:595–602, 1998.

Gardulf A, Andersen V, Bjorkander J, Ericson D, Frland SS, Gustafson R, Hammarstrom L, Jacobsen MB, Jonsson E, Moller G, Nystrom T, Seberg B, Smith CIE. Subcutaneous immunoglobulin replacement in patients with primary antibody deficiencies: safety and costs. Lancet 345:365–369, 1995.

Gardulf A, Bjorvell H, Gustafson R, Hammarstrom L, Smith CIE. The life situation in patients with primary antibody deficiency—untreated or treated with subcutaneous gammaglobulin infusions. Clin Exp Immunol 92:200–204, 1993.

Gardulf A, Hammarstrom L, Smith CIE. Home treatment of hypogammaglobulinemia with subcutaneous gammaglobulin by rapid infusions. Lancet 338:162–166, 1991.

Gelfand EW. Unique susceptibility of patients with antibody deficiency to *Mycoplasma* infection. Clin Infect Dis 17 (Suppl):250–253, 1993.

Gether U. Uncovering molecular mechanisms involved in activation of G protein-coupled receptors. Endocrine Rev 21:90–113, 2000.

Giannelli F, Green PM, Sommer SS, Poon M-C, Ludwig M, Schwaab R, Reitsma PH, Goossens M, Yoshioka A, Brownlee GG. Hemophilia B (sixth edition): a database of point mutations and short additions and deletions. Nucl Acids Res 24:103–118, 1996.

Go NF, Castle BE, Barret R, Kastelein R, Dang W, Mosmann TR, Moore KW, Howard M. Interleukin 10, a novel B cell stimulatory factor: unresponsiveness of X chromosome–linked immunodeficiency B cells. J Exp Med 172:1625–1631, 1990.

Goldblum RM, Lord RA, Cooper MD, Gathings WE, Goldman AS. X-linked B lymphocyte deficiency. I. Panhypoglobulinemia and dysglobulinemia in siblings. J Pediatr 85:188–191, 1974.

Good RA. Clinical investigations in patients with agammaglobulinemia. J Lab Clin Med 44:803, 1954.

Good RA, Kelly WD, Rotstein J, Varco RL. Immunological deficiency diseases. Agammaglobulinemia, hypogammaglobulinemia, Hodgkin's disease and sarcoidosis. Prog Allergy 6:187–319, 1962.

Good RA, Zak SJ. Disturbances in gamma globulin synthesis as "experiments of nature". Pediatrics 18:109–149, 1956.

Goodman PA, Wood CM, Vassilev AO, Mao C, Uckun FM. Defective expression of Bruton's tyrosine kinase in acute lymphoblastic leukemia. Leuk Lymphoma 44:1011–1018, 2003.

Grubben MJ, van den Braak CC, Peters WH, van der Meer JW, Nagengast FM. Low levels of colonic glutathione S-transferase in patients with X-linked agammaglobulinaemia. Eur J Clin Invest 30:642–645, 2000.

Guarnieri DJ, Dodson GS, Simon MA. SRC64 regulates the localization of a Tec-family kinase required for *Drosophila* ring canal growth. Mol Cell 1:831–840, 1998.

Guinamard R, Aspenstrom P, Fougereau M, Chavrier P, Guillemot JC. Tyrosine phosphorylation of the Wiskott-Aldrich syndrome protein by Lyn and Btk is regulated by CDC42. FEBS Lett 434:431–436, 1998.

Guo B, Kato RM, Garcia-Lloret M, Wahl MI, Rawlings DJ. Engagement of the human pre-B cell receptor generates a lipid raft–dependent calcium signaling complex. Immunity 13:243–253, 2000.

Hacein-Bey-Abina S, Von Kalle C, Schmidt M, McCormack MP, Wulffraat N, Leboulch P, Lim A, Osborne CS, Pawliuk R, Morillon E, Sorensen R, Forster A, Fraser P, Cohen JI, de Saint Basile G, Alexander I, Wintergerst U, Frebourg T, Aurias A, Stoppa-Lyonnet D, Romana S, Radford-Weiss I, Gross F, Valensi F, Delabesse E, Macintyre E, Sigaux F, Soulier J, Leiva LE, Wissler M, Prinz C, Rabbitts TH, Le Deist F, Fischer A, Cavazzana-Calvo M. LMO2-associated clonal T cell proliferation in two patients after gene therapy for SCID-X1. Science 302:415–419, 2003; erratum in Science 302:568, 2003.

Hagemann TL, Chen Y, Rosen FS, Kwan S-P. The genomic structure of the *BTK* gene and its use in direct DNA sequence analysis for mutations in patients with X-linked agammaglobulinemia. Hum Mol Genet 3:1743–1749, 1994.

Haldane JBS. The rate of spontaneous mutation of a human gene. J Genet 31:317–326, 1935.

Halsey N. Workshop on persistent poliovirus excretion in persons with primary immune deficiency diseases, San Francisco, June 28, 2002.

Hammon W McD, Coriell LL, Stokes J Jr. Evaluation of Red Cross gammaglobulin as a prophylactic agent for poliomyelitis. I. Plan of controlled field tests and results of 1951 pilot study in Utah. JAMA 150:739–749, 1952.

Hamada N, Backesjo C-M, Smith CIE, Yamamoto D. Functional replacement of *Drosophila* Btk29A with human Btk in male genital development and survival. FEBS Lett 2005 (in press).

Hansel TT, Haeney MR, Thompson RA. Primary hypogammaglobulinemia and arthritis. BMJ 295:174–175, 1987.

Hansen S, Gustafson R, Smith CI, Gardulf A. Express subcutaneous IgG infusions: decreased time of delivery with maintained safety. Clin Immunol 104:237–241, 2002.

Harteneck C, Plant TD, Schultz G. From worm to man: three subfamilies of TRP channels. Trends Neurosci 23:159–166, 2000.

Hasbold J, Klaus GG. B cells from CBA/N mice do not proliferate following ligation of CD40. Eur J Immunol 24:152–157, 1994.

Hashimoto S, Miyawaki T, Futatani T, Kanegane H, Usui K, Nukiwa T, Namiuchi S, Matsushita M, Yamadori T, Suemura M, Kishimoto T,

Tsukada S. Atypical X-linked agammaglobulinemia diagnosed in three adults. Intern Med 38:722–725, 1999.

Hashimoto A, Takeda K, Inaba M, Sekimata M, Kaisho T, Ikehara S, Homma Y, Akira S, Kurosaki T. Cutting Edge: Essential role of phospholipase C-2 in B cell development and function. J Immunol 165:1738–1742, 2000.

Hata D, Kawakami Y, Inagaki N, Lantz CS, Kitamura T, Khan WN, Maeda-Yamamoto M, Miura T, Han W, Hartman SE, et al. Involvement of Bruton's tyrosine kinase in FcεRI-dependent mast cell degranulation and cytokine production. J Exp Med 187:1235–1247, 1998a.

Hata D, Kitaura J, Hartman SE, Kawakami Y, Yokota T, Kawakami T. Bruton's tyrosine kinase–mediated interleukin-2 gene activation in mast cells. J Biol Chem 273:10979–10987, 1998b.

Hayakawa H, Iwata T, Yata J, Kobayashi N. Primary immunodeficiency syndrome in Japan. I. Overview of the nationwide survey on primary immunodeficiency syndrome. J Clin Immunol 1:31–39, 1981.

Healey CJ, Sabharwal NK, Daub J, Davidson F, Yap P-L, Fleming KA, Chapman RWG, Simmonds P, Chapel H. Outbreak of hepatitis C following the use of anti-hepatitis C virus–screened intravenous immunoglobulin therapy. Gastroenterology 110:1120–1126, 1996.

Heisterkamp N, Jenster G, ten Hoeve J, Zovich D, Pattengale PK, Groffen J. Acute leukaemia in bcr/abl transgenic mice. Nature 344:251–253, 1990.

Hendriks RW, de Bruijn MFTR, Maas A, Dingjan GM, Karis A, Grosveld F. Inactivation of Btk by insertion of lacZ reveals defects in B cell development past the pre-B cell stage. EMBO J 15:4862–4872, 1996.

Hermaszewski RA, Ratnavel RC, Denman DJ, Denman AM, Webster ADB. Immunodeficiency and lymphoproliferative disorders. Baillieres Clin Rheumatol 5:277–300, 1991.

Hermaszewski RA, Webster ADB. Primary hypogammaglobulinaemia: a survey of clinical manifestations and complications. Q J Med 86:31–42, 1993.

Heyeck SD, Wilcox HM, Bunnell SC, Berg LJ. Lck phosphorylates the activation loop tyrosine of the Itk kinase domain and activates Itk kinase activity. J Biol Chem 272:25401–25408, 1997.

Hidalgo S, Erro MC, Cisterna D, Freire MC. Paralytic poliomyelitis caused by a vaccine-derived polio virus in an antibody-deficient Argentinian child. Pediatr Infect Dis J 22:570–571, 2003.

Himmelmann A, Thevenin C, Harrison K, Kehrl JH. Analysis of the Bruton's tyrosine kinase gene promoter reveals critical PU.1 and Sp1 sites. Blood 87:1036–1044, 1996.

Hirata D, Nara H, Inaba T, Muroi R, Kanegane H, Miyawaki T, Okazaki H, Minota S. Recklinghausen disease in a patient with X-linked agammaglobulinemia. Intern Med 41:1039–1043, 2002.

Hitomi T, Yanagi S, Inatome R, Ding J, Takano T, Yamamura H. Requirement of Syk-phospholipase C-γ2 pathway for phorbol ester–induced phospholipase D activation in DT40 cells. Genes Cells 6:475–485, 2001.

Hitoshi Y, Sonoda E, Kikuchi Y, Yonehara S, Nakauchi H, Takatsu K. IL-5 receptor positive B cells, but not eosinophils, are functionally and numerically influenced in mice carrying the X-linked immune defect. Int Immunol 5:1183–1192, 1993.

Holinski-Feder E, Weiss M, Brandau O, Jedele KB, Nore B, Backesjo CM, Vihinen M, Gotz G, Hubbard SR, Belohradsky BH, Smith CIE, Meindl A. Mutation screening of the BTK gene in 56 families with X-linked agammaglobulinemia (XLA): 47 unique mutations without correlation to clinical course. Pediatrics 101:276–284, 1998.

Howard V, Myers LA, Williams DA, Wheeler G, Turner EV, Cunningham JM, Conley ME. Stem cell transplants for patients with X-linked agammaglobulinemia. Clin Immunol 107:98–102, 2003.

Humphries LA, Dangelmaier C, Sommer K, Kipp K, Kato RM, Griffith N, Bakman I, Turk CW, Daniel JL, Rawlings DJ. Tec kinases mediate sustained calcium influx via site-specific tyrosine phosphorylation of the phospholipase Cgamma Src homology 2-Src homology 3 linker. J Biol Chem 279:37651–37661, 2004.

Ishiai M, Kurosaki M, Pappu R, Okawa K, Ronko I, Fu C, Shibata M, Iwamatsu A, Chan AC, Kurosaki T. BLNK required for coupling Syk to PLCγ2 and Rac1-JNK in B cells. Immunity 10:117–125, 1999.

Islam TC, Branden LJ, Kohn DB, Islam KB, Smith CI. BTK-mediated apoptosis, a possible mechanism for failure to generate high-titer retroviral producer clones. J Gene Med 2:204–209, 1999.

Janeway CA. Cases from the medical grand rounds. Massachusetts General Hospital. Am Pract Digest Treat 5:487–492, 1954.

Janeway CA, Apt L, Gitlin D. Agammaglobulinemia. Trans Assoc Am Physicians 66:200–202, 1953.

Jiang A, Craxton A, Kurosaki T, Clark EA. Different protein tyrosine kinases are required for B cell antigen receptor–mediated activation of extracellular signal-regulated kinase, c-Jun NH2-terminal kinase 1, and p38 mitogen-activated protein kinase. J Exp Med 188:1297–1306, 1998a.

Jiang Y, Ma W, Wan Y, Kozasa T, Hattori S, Huang X-Y. The G protein G alpha 12 stimulates Bruton's tyrosine kinase and a ras GAP through a conserved PH/BM domain. Nature 395:808–813, 1998b.

Jin H, May M, Tranebjaerg L, Kendall E, Fontan G, Jackson J, Subramony SH, Arena F, Lubs H, Smith S, Stevenson R, Schwartz C, Vetrie D. A novel X-linked gene, DDP, shows mutations in families with deafness (DFN-1), dystonia, mental deficiency and blindness. Nat Gen 14:177–180, 1996.

Johnson PR, Edwards KM, Wright PF. Failure of intraventricular γ-globulin to eradicate echovirus encephalitis in a patient with X-linked agammaglobulinemia. N Engl J Med 313:1546–1547, 1985.

Jones A, Bradley L, Alterman L, Tarlow M, Thompson R, Kinnon C, Morgan G. X-linked agammaglobulinaemia with a 'leaky' phenotype. Arch Dis Child 74:548–549, 1996.

Journet O, Durandy A, Doussau M, Le Deist F, Couvreur J, Griscelli C, Fischer A, de Saint Basile G. Carrier detection and prenatal diagnosis of X-linked agammaglobulinemia. Am J Med Genet 43:885–887, 1992.

Jumaa H, Wollscheid B, Mitterer M, Wienands J, Reth M, Nielsen PJ. Abnormal development and function of B lymphocytes in mice deficient for the signaling adaptor protein SLP-65. Immunity 11:547–554, 1999.

Kainulainen L, Varpula M, Liippo K, Svedstrom E, Nikoskelainen J, Ruuskanen O. Pulmonary abnormalities in patients with primary hypogammaglobulinemia. J Allergy Clin Immunol 104:1031–1036, 1999.

Kanavaros P, Rontogianni D, Hrissovergi D, Efthimiadoy A, Argyrakos T, Mastoris K, Stefanaki K. Extranodal cytotoxic T-cell lymphoma in a patient with X-linked agammaglobulinaemia. Leuk Lymphoma 42:235–238, 2001.

Kanegane H, Futatani T, Wang Y, Nomura K, Shinozaki K, Matsukura H, Kubota T, Tsukada S, Miyawaki T. Clinical and mutational characteristics of X-linked agammaglobulinemia and its carrier identified by flow cytometric assessment combined with genetic analysis. J Allergy Clin Immunol 108:1012–1020, 2001.

Kang SW, Wahl MI, Chu J, Kitaura J, Kawakami Y, Kato RM, Tabuchi R, Tarakhovsky A, Kawakami T, Turck CW, Witte ON, Rawlings DJ. PKCβ modulates antigen receptor signaling via regulation of Btk membrane localization. EMBO J 20:5692–5702, 2001.

Karagogeos D, Rosenberg N, Wortis HH. Early arrest of B cell development in nude, X-linked immune-deficient mice. Eur J Immunol 16:1125–1130, 1986.

Katz FE, Lovering RC, Bradley LAD, Rigley KP, Brown D, Cotter F, Chessells JM, Levinsky RJ, Kinnon C. Expression of the X-linked agammaglobulinemia gene, Btk in B-cell acute lymphoblastic leukemia. Leukemia 8:574–577, 1994.

Kawakami Y, Hartman SE, Holland PM, Cooper JA, Kawakami T. Multiple signaling pathways for the activation of JNK in mast cells: involvement of Bruton's tyrosine kinase, protein kinase C, and JNK kinases, SEK1 and MKK7. J Immunol 161:1795–1802, 1998.

Kawakami Y, Kitaura J, Satterthwaite AB, Kato RM, Asai K, Hartman SE, Maeda-Yamamoto M, Lowell CA, Rawlings DJ, Witte ON, Kawakami T. Redundant and opposing functions of two tyrosine kinases, Btk and Lyn, in mast cell activation. J Immunol 165:1210–1210, 2000.

Kawakami Y, Miura T, Bissonnette R, Hata D, Khan WN, Kitamura T, Maeda-Yamamoto M, Hartman SE, Yao L, Alt FW, Kawakami T. Bruton's tyrosine kinase regulates apoptosis and JNK/SAPK kinase activity. Proc Natl Acad Sci USA 94:3938–3942, 1997.

Kawakami Y, Yao L, Miura T, Tsukada S, Witte ON, Kawakami T. Tyrosine phosphorylation and activation of Bruton tyrosine kinase (Btk) upon FcεRI cross-linking. Mol Cell Biol 14:5108–5113, 1994.

Kerner JD, Appleby MW, Mohr RN, Chien S, Rawlings DJ, Maliszewski CR, Witte ON, Perlmutter RM. Impaired expansion of mouse B cell progenitors lacking Btk. Immunity 3:301–312, 1995.

Kersey JH, Spector BD, Good RA. Primary immunodeficiency diseases and cancer: the Immunodeficiency-Cancer Registry. Int J Cancer 12:333–347, 1973.

Kersseboom R, Middendorp S, Dingjan GM, Dahlenborg K, Reth M, Jumaa H, Hendriks RW. Bruton's tyrosine kinase cooperates with the B cell linker protein SLP-65 as a tumor suppressor in pre-B cells. J Exp Med 198:91–98, 2003.

Kerstens PJSM, Endtz HP, Meis JFGM, Oyen WJG, Koopman RJI, van den Broek PJ, van der Meer JWM. Erysipelas-like skin lesions associated with Campylobacter jejuni septicemia in patients with hypogammaglobulinemia. Eur J Clin Microbiol Infect Dis 11:842–847, 1992.

Khan WN, Alt FW, Gerstein RM, Malynn BA, Larsson I, Rathbun G, Davidson L, Muller S, Kantor AB, Herzenberg LA, Rosen FS, Sideras P. Defective B-cell development and function in Btk-deficient mice. Immunity 3:283–299, 1995.

Khan WN, Nilsson A, Mizoguchi E, Castigli E, Forsell J, Bhan AK, Geha R, Sideras P, Alt FW. Impaired B cell maturation in mice lacking Bruton's tyrosine kinase (Btk) and CD40. Int Immunol 9:395–405, 1997.

Kikuchi Y, Yasue T, Miyake K, Kimoto M, Takatsu K. CD38 ligation induces tyrosine phosphorylation of Bruton tyrosine kinase and enhanced expression of interleukin 5-receptor alpha chain: synergistic effects with interleukin 5. Proc Natl Acad Sci USA 92:11814–11818, 1995.

Kinlen LJ, Webster ADB, Bird AG, Haile R, Peto J, Soothill JF, Thompson RA. Prospective study of cancer in patients with hypogammaglobulinaemia. Lancet 1:263–266, 1985.

Kitamura D, Roes J, Kuhn R, Rajewsky K. A B-cell-deficient mouse by targetted disruption of the membrane exon of the immunoglobulin chain gene. Nature 350:423–426, 1991.

Kitaura J, Asai K, Maeda-Yamamoto M, Kawakami Y, Kikkawa U, Kawakami T. Akt-dependent cytokine production in mast cells. J Exp Med 192:729–740, 2000.

Koike M, Kikuchi Y, Tominage A, Takaki S, Akagi K, Miyazaki JI, Yamamura KI, Takatsu K. Defect of IL-5-receptor–mediated signaling in B cells of X-linked immunodeficient (Xid) mice. Int Immunol 7:21–30, 1995.

Kornfeld SJ, Zeffren B, Christodoulou CS, Day NK, Cawkwell G, Good RA. Extreme variation in X-linked agammaglobulinemia phenotype in a three-generation family. J Allergy Clin Immunol 100:702–706, 1997.

Kouro T, Nagata K, Takaki S, Nisitani S, Hirano M, Wahl MI, Witte ON, Karasuyama H, Takatsu K. Bruton's tyrosine kinase is required for signaling the CD79b-mediated pro-B to pre-B cell transition. Int Immunol 13:485–493, 2001.

Kozlowski C, Evans DIK. Neutropenia associated with X-linked agammaglobulinaemia. J Clin Pathol 44:388–390, 1991.

Kramer SD. Protection in white mice with human post-convalescent serum against infection with poliomyelitis virus (Armstrong strain). II. J Immunol 47:67–76, 1943.

Kurosaki T, Kurosaki M. Transphosphorylation of Bruton's tyrosine kinase on tyrosine 551 is critical for B cell antigen receptor function. J Biol Chem 272:15595–15598, 1997.

Langhans-Rajasekaran SA, Wan Y, Huang Xin-Y. Activation of Tsk and Btk tyrosine kinases by G protein subunits. Proc Natl Acad Sci USA 92:8601–8605, 1995.

Lavilla P, Gil A, Rodriguez MCG, Dupla ML, Pintado V, Fontan G. X-linked agammaglobulinemia and gastric adenocarcinoma. Cancer 72:1528–1531, 1993.

Lederman HM, Winkelstein JA. X-linked agammaglobulinemia: an analysis of 96 patients. Medicine (Baltimore) 64:145–156, 1985.

Leitges M, Schmedt C, Guinamard R, Davoust J, Schaal S, Stabel S, Tarakhovsky A. Immunodeficiency in protein kinase C–deficient mice. Science 273:788–791, 1996.

Lever AML, Webster ADB, Brown D, Thomas HC. Non-A, non-B hepatitis occurring in agammaglobulinaemic patients after intravenous immunoglobulin. Lancet 2:1062–1064, 1984.

Levin SD, Anderson SJ, Forbush KA, Perlmutter RM. A dominant-negative transgene defines a role for p56lck in thymopoiesis. EMBO J 12:1671–1680, 1993.

Li T, Rawlings DJ, Park H, Kato RM, Witte ON, Satterthwaite AB. Constitutive membrane association potentiates activation of Bruton's tyrosine kinase. Oncogene 15:1375–1383, 1997a.

Li T, Tsukada S, Satterthwaite A, Havlik MH, Park H, Takatsu K, Witte ON. Activation of Bruton's tyrosine kinase (Btk) by a point mutation in its pleckstrin homology (PH) domain. Immunity 2:451–460, 1995.

Li Z, Wahl MI, Euginoa A, Stephens LR, Hawkins PT, Witte ON. Phosphatidylinositol 3-kinase activates Bruton's tyrosine kinase in concert with Src family kinases. Proc Natl Acad Sci USA 94:13820–13825, 1997b.

Liese JG, Wintergerst U, Tympner KD, Belohradsky BH. High- vs low-dose immunoglobulin therapy in the long-term treatment of X-linked agammaglobulinemia. Am J Dis Child 146:335–339, 1992.

Lindvall JM, Blomberg KE, Berglof A, Yang Q, Smith CI, Islam TC. Gene expression profile of B cells from Xid mice and Btk knockout mice. Eur J Immunol 34:1981–1991, 2004.

Lindvall J, Blomberg KEM, Valiaho J, Vargas L, Heinonen JE, Berglof A, Mohamed AJ, Nore BF, Vihinen M, Smith CIE. Bruton's tyrosine kinase: cell biology, sequence conservation, mutation spectrum, siRNA modifications and expression profiling. Immunol Rev 203:200–215, 2005.

Lopez Granados E, Porpiglia AS, Hogan MB, Matamoros N, Krasovec S, Pignata C, Smith CI, Hammarstrom L, Björkander J, Belohradsky BH, Casariego GF, Garcia Rodriguez MC, Conley ME. Clinical and molecular analysis of patients with defects in μ heavy chain gene. J Clin Invest 110:1029–1035, 2002.

Lyon MF. X-chromosome inactivation in mammals. Adv Teratol 1:25–54, 1966.

Ma YC, Huang XY. Identification of the binding site for gqalpha on its effector Bruton's tyrosine kinase. Proc Natl Acad Sci USA 95:12197–12201, 1998.

Maas A, Dingjan GM, Grosveld F, Hendriks RW. Early arrest in B cell development in transgenic mice that express the E41K Bruton's tyrosine kinase mutant under the control of the CD19 promoter region. J Immunol 162:6526–6533, 1999.

MacLennan C, Dunn G, Huissoon AP, Kumararatne DS, Martin J, O'Leary P, Thompson RA, Osman H, Wood P, Minor P, Wood DJ, Pillay D. Failure to clear persistent vaccine-derived neurovirulent poliovirus infection in an immunodeficient man. Lancet 363:1509–1513, 2004.

Mahajan S, Vassilev A, Sun N, Ozer Z, Mao C, Uckun FM. Transcription factor STAT5A is a substrate of Bruton's tyrosine kinase in B cells. J Biol Chem 276:31216–31228, 2001.

Manning G, Whyte DB, Martinez R, Hunter T, Sudarsanam S. The protein kinase complement of the human genome. Science 6:298:1912–1934, 2002.

Mano H, Ishikawa F, Nishida J, Hara H, Takaku F. A novel protein-tyrosine kinase, Tec, is preferentially expressed in the liver. Oncogene 5:1781–1786, 1990.

Marcotte H, Levesque D, Delanay K, Bourgeault A, de la Durantaye R, Brochu S, Lavoie MC. *Pneumocystis carinii* infection in transgenic B cell–deficient mice. J Infect Dis 173:1034–1037, 1996.

Martin S, Wolf-Eichbaum D, Duinkerken G, Scherbaum WA, Kolb H, Noordzij JG, Roep BO. Development of type 1 diabetes despite severe hereditary B-lymphocyte deficiency. N Engl J Med 345:1036–1040, 2001.

Masur H, Lane HC, Kovacs JA, Allegra JC, Edman JC. Pneumocystis pneumonia: from bench to clinic. Ann Intern Med 111:813–826, 1989.

Mattsson PT, Vihinen M, Smith CIE. X-linked agammaglobulinemia (XLA): a genetic tyrosine kinase (Btk) disease. Bioessays 18:825–834, 1996.

McKinney RE Jr, Katz SL, Wilfert CM. Chronic enteroviral meningoencephalitis in agammaglobulinemic patients. Rev Infect Dis 9:334–356, 1987.

McLaughlin JF, Schaller J, Wedgwood RJ. Arthritis and immunodeficiency. J Pediatr 81:801–803, 1972.

Mease PJ, Ochs HD, Corey L, Dragavon J, Wedgwood RJ. Echovirus encephalitis/myositis in X-linked agammaglobulinemia. N Engl J Med 313:758, 1985.

Mease PJ, Ochs HD, Wedgwood RJ. Successful treatment of echovirus meningoencephalitis and myositis-fasciitis with intravenous immune globulin therapy in a patient with X-linked agammaglobulinemia. N Engl J Med 304:1278–1281, 1981.

Melamed I, Bujanover Y, Igra YS, Schwartz D, Zakuth V, Spirer Z. *Campylobacter* enteritis in normal and immunodeficient children. Am J Dis Child 137:752–753, 1983.

Mensink EJBM, Schot JDL, Tippett P, Ott J, Schuurman RKB. X-linked agammaglobulinemia and the red blood cell determinants Xg and 12E7 are not closely linked. Hum Genet 68:303–309, 1984.

Middendorp S, Zijlstra AJ, Kersseboom R, Dingjan GM, Jumaa H, Hendriks RW. Tumor suppressor function of Bruton tyrosine kinase is independent of its catalytic activity. Blood 105:259–265, 2005.

Migeon BR. X chromosome inactivation: molecular mechanisms and genetic consequences. Trends Genet 10:230–235, 1994.

Minegishi Y, Rohrer J, Coustan-Smith E, Lederman HM, Pappu R, Campana D, Chan AC, Conley ME. An essential role for BLNK in human B cell development. Science 286:1954–1957, 1999.

Misbah SA, Spickett GP, Ryba PJC, Hockaday JM, Kroll JS, Sherwood C, Kurtz JB, Moxon ER, Chapel HM. Chronic enteroviral meningoencephalitis in agammaglobulinemia: case report and review of the literature. J Clin Immunol 12:266–270, 1992.

Miyake K, Yamashita Y, Hitoshi Y, Takatsu K, Kimoto M. Murine B cell proliferation and protection from apoptosis with an antibody against a 105-kD molecule: unresponsiveness of X-linked immunodeficient B cells. J Exp Med 180:1217–1224, 1994.

Mohamed AJ, Vargas L, Nore BF, Backesjo CM, Christensson B, Smith CI. Nucleocytoplasmic shuttling of Bruton's tyrosine kinase. J Biol Chem 275:40614–40619, 2000.

Mond JJ, Norton G, Paul WE, Scher I, Finkelman FD, House S, Schaeffer M, Mongini PKA, Hansen C, Bona C. Establishment of an inbred line of mice that express a synergistic immune defect precluding in vitro responses to type 1 and type 2 antigens, B cell mitogens, and a number of T cell–derived helper factors. J Exp Med 158:1401–1414, 1983a.

Mond JJ, Schaefer M, Smith J, Finkelman FD. Lyb-5 B cells of CBA/N mice can be induced to synthesize DNA by culture with insolubilized but not soluble anti-Ig. J Immunol 131:2107–2109, 1983b.

Morrogh LM, Hinshelwood S, Costello P, Cory GO, Kinnon C. The SH3 domain of Bruton's tyrosine kinase displays altered ligand binding properties when auto-phosphorylated in vitro. Eur J Immunol 29:2269–2279, 1999.

Morwood K, Bourne H, Gold M, Gillis D, Benson EM. Phenotypic variability:clinical presentation between the 6th year and the 60th year in a family with X-linked agammaglobulinemia. J Allergy Clin Immunol 113:783–785, 2004.

Müller S, Maas A, Islam TC, Sideras P, Suske G, Philipsen S, Xanthopoulos KG, Hendriks RW, Smith CI. Synergistic activation of the human Btk promoter by transcription factors Sp1/3 and PU.1. Biochem Biophys Res Commun 259:364–369, 1999.

Müller S, Sideras P, Smith CIE, Xanthopoulos KG. Cell-specific expression of human Bruton's agammaglobulinemia tyrosine kinase (Btk) gene is regulated by Sp1-and Spi-1/PU.1-family members. Oncogene 13:1955–1964, 1996.

Nahm MH, Paslay JW, Davie JM. Unbalanced X chromosome mosaicism in B cells of mice with X-linked immunodeficiency. J Exp Med 158:920–931, 1983.

Naor D, Bentwich Z, Cividalli G. Inability of peripheral lymphoid cells of agammaglobulinaemic patients to bind radioiodinated albumins. Aust J Exp Biol Med Sci 47:759–761, 1969.

Nisitani S, Kato RM, Rawlings DJ, Witte ON, Wahl MI. In situ detection of activated Bruton's tyrosine kinase in the immunoglobulin signaling complex by phosphopeptide-specific monoclonal antibodies. Proc Natl Acad Sci USA 96:2221–2226, 1999.

Noh LM, Ismaik Z, Zainudin B, Low SM, Azizi B, Noah RM, Nasaruddin BA. Clinical patterns of X-linked agammaglobulinemia in Malaysian children. Acta Paediatr Jpn 37:331–335, 1995.

Nomura K, Kanegane H, Karasuyama H, Tsukada S, Agematsu K, Murakami G, Sakazume S, Sako M, Tanaka R, Kuniya Y, Komeno T, Ishihara S, Hayashi K, Kishimoto T, Miyawaki T. Genetic defect in human X-linked agammaglobulinemia impedes a maturational evolution of pro-B cells into a later stage of pre-B cells in the B-cell differentiation pathway. Blood 96:610–617, 2000.

Noordzij JG, de Bruin-Versteeg S, Comans-Bitter WM, Hartwig NG, Hendriks RW, de Groot R, van Dongen JJ. Composition of precursor B-cell compartment in bone marrow from patients with X-linked agammaglobulinemia compared with healthy children. Pediatr Res 51:159–168, 2002a.

Noordzij JG, de Bruin-Versteeg S, Hartwig NG, Weemaes CM, Gerritsen EJ, Bernatowska E, van Lierde S, de Groot R, van Dongen JJ. XLA patients with BTK splice-site mutations produce low levels of wild-type BTK transcripts. J Clin Immunol 22:306–318, 2002b.

Nore BF, Vargas L, Mohamed AJ, Branden LJ, Backesjo CM, Islam TC, Mattsson PT, Hultenby K, Christensson B, Smith CI. Redistribution of Bruton's tyrosine kinase by activation of phosphatidylinositol 3-kinase and Rho-family GTPases. Eur J Immunol 30:145–154, 2000.

Novina CD, Kumar S, Bajpai U, Cheriyath V, Zhang K, Pillai S, Wortis HH, Roy AL. Regulation of nuclear localization and transcriptional activity of TFII-I by Bruton's tyrosine kinase. Mol Cell Biol 19:5014–5024, 1999.

Ochs HD, Ament ME, Davis SD. Giardiasis with malabsorption in X-linked agammaglobulinemia. N Engl J Med 287:341–342, 1972.

Ochs HD, Fisher SH, Virant FS, Lee ML. Non-A, non-B hepatitis after intravenous immunoglobin. Lancet i:322–323, 1985.

Ochs HD, Smith CIE. X-linked agammaglobulinemia. A clinical and molecular analysis. Medicine 75:287–299, 1996.

Ohta Y, Haire RN, Amemiya CT, Litman RT, Trager T, Riess O, Litman GW. Human Txk: genomic organization, structure and contiguous linkage with the Tec gene. Oncogene 12:937–942, 1996.

Ohta Y, Haire RN, Litman RT, Fu SM, Nelson RP, Kratz J, Kornfeld SJ, de la Morena M, Good RA, Litman GW. Genomic organisation and structure of Bruton agammaglobulinemia tyrosine kinase: localisation of mutations associated with varied clinical presentations and course in X-linked agammaglobulinemia. Proc Natl Acad Sci USA 91:9062–9066, 1994.

Oka Y, Rolink AG, Andersson J, Kamanaka M, Uchida J, Yasui T, Kishimoto T, Kikutani H, Melchers F. Profound reduction of mature B cell numbers, reactivities and serum Ig levels in mice which simultaneously carry the XID and CD40 deficiency genes. Int Immunol 8:1675–1685, 1996.

Paller AS. Immunodeficiency syndromes. X-linked agammaglobulinemia, common variable immunodeficiency, Chediak-Higashi syndrome, Wiskott-Aldrich syndrome, and X-linked lymphoproliferative disorder. Dermatol Clin 13:65–71, 1995.

Pappu R, Cheng AM, Li B, Gong Q, Chiu C, Griffin N, White M, Sleckman BP, Chan AC. Requirement for B cell linker protein (BLNK) in B cell development. Science 286:286, 1999.

Park H, Wahl MI, Afar DE, Turck CW, Rawlings DJ, Tam C, Scharenberg AM, Kinet J-P, Witte ON. Regulation of Btk function by a major autophosphorylation site within the SH3 domain. Immunity 4:515–525, 1996.

Pawson T. Protein modules and signalling networks. Nature 373:573–580, 1995.

Pazdrak K, Stafford S, Alam R. The activation of the Jak-STAT 1 signaling pathway by IL-5 in eosinophils. J Immunol 155:397–402, 1995.

Pearl ER, Vogler LB, Okos AJ, Crist WM, Lawton AR III, Cooper MD. B lymphocyte precursors in human bone marrow: an analysis of normal individuals and patients with antibody-deficiency states. J Immunol 120:1169–1175, 1978.

Petro JB, Khan WN. Phospholipase C-gamma 2 couples Bruton's tyrosine kinase to the NF-κB signaling pathway in B lymphocytes. J Biol Chem 276:1715–1719, 2001.

Petro JB, Rahman SM, Ballard DW, Khan WN. Bruton's tyrosine kinase is required for activation of IκB kinase and nuclear factor κB in response to B cell receptor engagement. J Exp Med 191:1745–1754, 2000.

Pinschewer DD, Ochsenbein AF, Satterthwaite AB, Witte ON, Hengartner H, Zinkernagel RM. A Btk transgene restores the antiviral TI-2 antibody responses of Xid mice in a dose-dependent fashion. Eur J Immunol 29:2981–2987, 1999.

Plebani A, Soresina A, Rondelli R, Amato GM, Azzari C, Cardinale F, Cazzola G, Consolini R, De Mattia D, Dell'Erba G, Duse M, Fiorini M, Martino S, Martire B, Masi M, Monafo V, Moschese V, Notarangelo LD, Orlandi P, Panei P, Pession A, Pietrogrande MC, Pignata C, Quinti I, Ragno V, Rossi P, Sciotto A, Stabile A. Clinical, immunological, and molecular analysis in a large cohort of patients with X-linked agammaglobulinemia: an Italian multicenter study. Clin Immunol 104:221–230, 2002.

Quartier P, Debre M, De Blic J, de Sauverzac R, Sayegh N, Jabado N, Haddad E, Blanche S, Casanova JL, Smith CI, Le Deist F, de Saint Basile G, Fischer A. Early and prolonged intravenous immunoglobulin replacement therapy in childhood agammaglobulinemia: a retrospective survey of 31 patients. J Pediatr 13:589–596, 1999.

Quartier P, Foray S, Casanova JL, Hau-Rainsard I, Blanche S, Fischer A. Enteroviral meningoencephalitis in X-linked agammaglobulinemia: intensive immunoglobulin therapy and sequential viral detection in cerebrospinal fluid by polymerase chain reaction. Pediatr Infect Dis J 19:1106–1108, 2000.

Quartier P, Tournilhac O, Archimbaud C, Lazaro L, Chaleteix C, Millet P, Peigue-Lafeuille H, Blanche S, Fischer A, Casanova JL, Travade P, Tardieu M. Enteroviral meningoencephalitis after anti-CD20 (rituximab) treatment. Clin Infect Dis 3:e47–49, 2003.

Quek LS, Bolen J, Watson SP. A role for Bruton's tyrosine kinase (Btk) in platelet activation by collagen. Curr Biol 8:1137–1140, 1998.

Qin S, Chock PB. Bruton's tyrosine kinase is essential for hydrogen peroxide–induced calcium signaling. Biochemistry 40:8085–8091, 2001.

Quinti I, Pierdominici M, Marziali M, Giovannetti A, Donnanno S, Chapel H, Bjorkander J, Aiuti F. European surveillance of immunoglobulin safety—results of initial survey of 1243 patients with primary immunodeficiencies in 16 countries. Clin Immunol 104:231–236, 2002.

Rafi A, Matz J. An unusual case of Campylobacter jejuni pericarditis in a patient with X-linked agammaglobulinemia. Ann Allergy Asthma Immunol 89:362–367, 2002.

Rameh LE, Arvidsson AK, Carraway KL 3rd, Couvillon AD, Rathbun G, Crompton A, VanRenterghem B, Czech MP, Ravichandran KS, Burakoff SJ, Wang DS, Chen CS, Cantley LC. A comparative analysis of the phosphoinositide binding specificity of pleckstrin homology domains. J Biol Chem 272:22059–22066, 1997.

Rawlings DJ, Saffran DC, Tsukada S, Largaespada DA, Grimaldi JC, Cohen L, Mohr RN, Bazan JF, Howard M, Copeland NG, Jenkins NA, Witte ON. Mutation of the unique region of Bruton's tyrosine kinase in immunodeficient XID mice. Science 261:358–361, 1993.

Rawlings DJ, Scharenberg AM, Park H, Wahl MI, Lin S, Kato RM, Fluckiger AC, Witte ON, Kinet JP. Activation of BTK by a phosphorylation mechanism initiated by Src family kinases. Science 271:822–825, 1996.

Razvi S, Schneider L, Jonas MM, Cunningham-Rundles C. Outcome of intravenous immunoglobulin–transmitted hepatitis C virus infection in primary immunodeficiency. Clin Immunol 101:284–288, 2001.

Richter D, Conley ME, Rohrer J, Myers LA, Zahradka K, Kelecic J, Sertic J, Stavljenic-Rukavina A. A contiguous deletion syndrome of X-linked agammaglobulinemia and sensorineural deafness. Pediatr Allergy Immunol 12:107–111, 2001.

Rigley KP, Harnett MM, Phillips RJ, Klaus GGB. Analysis of signaling via surface immunoglobulin receptors on B cells from CBA/N mice. Eur J Immunol 19:2081–2086, 1989.

Rohrer J, Parolino O, Belmont JW, Conley ME. The genomic structure of human BTK, the defective gene in X-linked agammaglobulinemia. Immunogenetics 40:319–324, 1994.

Roifman CM, Lederman HM, Lavi S, Levison H, Gelfand EW. Benefit of intravenous IgG replacement in hypogammaglobulinemic patients with chronic sinopulmonary disease. Am J Med 79:171–174, 1985.

Roifman CM, Rao CP, Lederman HM. Increased susceptibility to *Mycoplasma* infection in patients with hypogammaglobulinemia. Am J Med 80:590–594, 1986.

Rosen FS, Cooper MD, Wedgwood RJP. The primary immunodeficiencies (first of two papers). N Engl J Med 311:235–242, 1984.

Rotbart HA. Diagnosis of enteroviral meningitis with the polymerase chain reaction. J Pediatr 117:85–89, 1990.

Rotbart HA, Sawyer MH, Fast S, Lewinsky C, Murphy N, Keyser EF, Spadoro J, Kao SY, Loeffelholz M. Diagnosis of enteroviral meningitis by PCR with a colorimetric microwell detection assay. J Clin Microbiol 32:2590–2592, 1994.

Rotbart HA, Webster ADB. Treatment of potentially life-threatening enterovirus infections with pleconaril. Clin Infect Dis 32:228–235, 2001.

Roth PE, DeFranco AL. Receptor tails unlock developmental checkpoints for B lymphocytes. Science 272:1752–1754, 1996.

Roulier EM, Panzer S, Beckendorf SK. The Tec29 tyrosine kinase is required during *Drosophila* embryogenesis and interacts with Src64 in ring canal development. Mol Cell 1:819–829, 1998.

Rudge P, Webster ADB, Revesz T, Warner T, Espanol T, Cunningham-Rundles C, Hyman N. Encephalomyelitis in primary hypogammaglobulinaemia. Brain 119:1–15, 1996.

Saito K, Scharenberg AM, Kinot JP. Interaction between the Btk PH domain and phosphatidylinositol-3,4,5-trisphosphate directly regulates Btk. J Biol Chem 276:16201–16206, 2001.

Saito K, Tolias KF, Saci A, Koon HB, Humphries LA, Scharenberg A, Rawlings DJ, Kinet JP, Carpenter CL. BTK regulates PtdIns-4,5-P2 synthesis: importance for calcium signaling and PI3K activity. Immunity 19:669–678, 2003.

Salim K, Bottomley MJ, Querfurth E, Zvelebil MJ, Gout I, Scaife R, Margolis RL, Gigg R, Smith CIE, Driscoll PC, Waterfield MD, Panayotou G. Distinct specificity in the recognition of phosphoinositides by the pleckstrin homology domains of dynamin and Bruton's tyrosine kinase. EMBO J 15:6241–6250, 1996.

Samuelson A, Borrelli S, Gustafson R, Hammarstrom L, Smith CIE, Jonasson J, Lindberg AA. Characterization of *Haemophilus influenzae* isolates from the respiratory tract of patients with primary antibody deficiencies: evidence for persistent colonizations. Scand J Infect Dis 27:303–313, 1995.

Sandstedt K, Berglof A, Feinstein R, Bolske G, Evengard B, Smith CIE. Differential susceptibility to *Mycoplasma pulmonis* intranasal infection in X-linked immunodeficient (Xid), severe combined immunodeficient (SCID), and immunocompetent mice. Clin Exp Immunol 108:490–496, 1997.

Santos-Argumedo L, Lund FE, Heath AW, Solvason N, Wu WW, Grimaldi JC, Parkhouse RME, Howard M. CD38 unresponsiveness of Xid B cell implicates Bruton's tyrosine kinase (Btk) as a regulator of CD38-induced signal transduction. Int Immunol 7:163–170, 1995.

Sarpong S, Skolnick HS, Ochs HD, Futatani T, Winkelstein JA. Survival of wild polio by a patient with XLA. Ann Allergy Asthma Immunol 88:59–60, 2002.

Sato S, Katagiri T, Takaki S, Kikuchi Y, Hitoshi Y, Yonehara S, Tsukada S, Kitamura D, Watanabe T, Witte O, Takatsu K. IL-5 receptor–mediated tyrosine phosphorylation of SH2/SH3-containing proteins and activation of Btk and JAK2 kinases. J Exp Med 180:2101–2111, 1994.

Satterthwaite A, Cheroutre H, Khan WN, Sideras P, Witte ON. Btk dosage determines sensitivity to B cell antigen receptor cross-linking. Proc Natl Acad Sci USA 94:13152–13157, 1997.

Satterthwaite AB, Lowell CA, Khan WN, Sideras P, Alt FW, Witte ON. Independent and opposing roles for Btk and Lyn in B and myeloid signaling pathways. J Exp Med 188:833–844, 1998.

Satterthwaite AB, Willis F, Kanchanastit P, Fruman D, Cantley LC, Helgason CD, Humphries RK, Lowell CA, Simon M, Leitges M, et al. A sensitized genetic system for the analysis of murine B lymphocyte signal transduction pathways dependent on Bruton's tyrosine kinase. Proc Natl Acad Sci USA 97:6687–6692, 2000.

Scharenberg AM, El-Hillal O, Fruman DA, Beitz LO, Li Z, Lin S, Gout I, Cantley LC, Rawlings DJ, Kinet JP. Phosphatidylinositol-3,4,5-trisphosphate (PtdIns-3,4,5-P3)/Tec kinase-dependent calcium signaling pathway: a target for SHIP-mediated inhibitory signals. EMBO J 17:1961–1972, 1998.

Scharenberg AM Kinet JP. PtdIns-3,4,5-P3: a regulatory nexus between tyrosine kinases and sustained calcium signals. Cell 94:5–8, 1998.

Scher I. The CBA/N mouse strain: an experimental model illustrating the influence of the X-chromosome on immunity. Adv Immunol 33:1–71, 1982.

Schubart DB, Rolink A, Schubart K, Matthias P. Cutting edge: lack of peripheral B cells and severe agammaglobulinemia in mice simultaneously lacking Bruton's tyrosine kinase and the B cell–specific transcriptional coactivator OBF-1. J Immunol 164:18–22, 2000.

Schuster V, Seidenspinner S, Kreth HW. Detection of a novel mutation in the Src homology domain 2 (SH2) of Bruton's tyrosine kinase and direct female carrier evaluation in a family with X-linked agammaglobulinemia. Am J Med Genet 63:318–322, 1996.

Scribner CL, Hansen CT, Klinman DM, Steinberg AD. The interaction of the XID and ME genes. J Immunol 138:3611–3617, 1987.

Setoguchi R, Kinashi T, Sagara H, Hirosawa K, Takatsu K. Defective degranulation and calcium mobilization of bone-marrow derived mast cells from Xid and Btk-deficient mice. Immunol Lett 64:109–118, 1998.

Sideras P, Muller S, Shiels H, Jin H, Khan WN, Nilsson L, Parkinson E, Thomas JD, Branden L, Larsson I, Paul WE, Rosen FS, Alt FW, Vetrie D, Smith CIE, Xanthopoulos KG. Genomic organisation of mouse and human Bruton's agammaglobulinemia tyrosine kinase (Btk) loci. J Immunol 153:5607–5618, 1994.

Sideras P, Smith CIE. Molecular and cellular aspects of X-linked agammaglobulinemia. Adv Immunol 59:135–223, 1995.

Simons E, Spacek LA, Lederman HM, Winkelstein JA. *Helicobacter cinaedi* bacteremia presenting as macules in an afebrile patient with X-linked agammaglobulinemia. Infection 32:367–368, 2004.

Smith CIE, Baskin B, Humire-Greiff P, Zhou J-N, Olsson PG, Maniar HS, Kjellen P, Lambris JD, Christensson B, Hammarstrom L, Bentley D, Vetrie D, Islam KB, Vorechovsky I, Sideras P. Expression of Bruton's agammaglobulinemia tyrosine kinase gene, BTK, is selectively down-regulated in T lymphocytes and plasma cells. J Immunol 152:557–565, 1994a.

Smith CIE, Islam TC, Mattsson PT, Mohamed AJ, Nore BF, Vihinen M. The Tec family of cytoplasmic tyrosine kinases: mammalian Btk, Bmx, Itk, Tec, Txk and homologs in other species. Bioessays 23:436–446, 2001.

Smith CIE, Islam KB, Vorechovsky I, Olerup O, Wallin E, Rabbani H, Baskin B, Hammarstrom L. X-linked agammaglobulinemia and other immunoglobulin deficiencies. Immunol Rev 138:159–183, 1994b.

Smith CIE, Notarangelo LD. Molecular basis for X-linked immunodeficiencies. Adv Genet 35:57–115, 1997.

Smith CIE, Vihinen M. Immunodeficiency mutation databases—a new research tool. Immunol Today 17:495–496, 1996.

Solvason N, Wu WW, Kabra N, Lund-Johansen F, Roncarolo MG, Behrens TW, Grillot DAM, Nunez G, Lees E, Howard M. Transgene expression of bcl-xL permits anti-immunoglobulin (Ig)-induced proliferation in Xid B cells. J Exp Med 187:1081–1091, 1998.

Spickett GP, Misbah SA, Chapel HM. Primary antibody deficiency in adults. Lancet 337:281–284, 1991.

Stewart DM, Notarangelo LD, Kurman CC, Staudt LM, Nelson DL. Molecular genetic analysis of X-linked hypogammaglobulinemia and isolated growth hormone deficiency. J Immunol 155:2770–2774, 1995.

Stewart DM, Tian L, Nelson DL. A case of X-linked agammaglobulinemia diagnosed in adulthood. Clin Immunol 99:94–99, 2001.

Stewart DM, Tian L, Notarangelo LD, Nelson DL. Update on X-linked hypogammaglobulinemia with isolated growth hormone deficiency. Curr Opin Allergy Clin Immunol. 5:510–512, 2005.

Stiehm ER, Chin TW, Haas A, Peerless AG. Infectious complications of the primary immunodeficiencies. Clin Immunol Immunopathol 40:69–86, 1986.

Strikas RA, Anderson LJ, Parker RA. Temporal and geographic patterns of isolates of nonpolio enterovirus in the United States, 1970–1983. J Infect Dis 153:346–351, 1986.

Stuckey M, Quinn PA, Gelfand EW. Identification of ureaplasma urealyticum (T-strain mycoplasma) in patients with polyarthritis. Lancet 2:17–20, 1978.

Suzuki H, Terauchi Y, Fujiwara M, Aizawa S, Yazaki Y, Kadowaki T, Koyasu S. Xid-like immunodeficiency in mice with disruption of the p85α subunit of phosphoinositide 3-kinase. Science 283:390–392, 1999.

Sweinberg SK, Wodell RA, Grodofsky MP, Greene JM, Conley ME. Retrospective analysis of the incidence of pulmonary disease in hypogammaglobulinemia. J Allergy Clin Immunol 88:96–104, 1991.

Takata M, Homma Y, Kurosaki T. Requirement of phospholipase C-gamma2 activation in surface IgM-induced B cell apoptosis. J Exp Med 182:907–914, 1995.

Takada H, Kanegane H, Nomura A, Yamamoto K, Ihara K, Takahashi Y, Tsukada S, Miyawaki T, Hara T. Female agammaglobulinemia due to Bruton's tyrosine kinase deficiency caused by extremely skewed X chromosome inactivation. Blood 103:185–187, 2004.

Takahashi-Tezuka M, Hibi M, Fujitani Y, Fukada T, Yamaguchi T, Hirano T. Tec tyrosine kinase links the cytokine receptors to PI-3 kinase probably through JAK. Oncogene 14:2273–2282, 1997.

Takata M, Kurosaki T. A role for Bruton's tyrosine kinase in B cell antigen receptor–mediated activation of phospholipase C-2. J Exp Med 184:31–40, 1996.

Takeshita H, Taniuchi I, Kato J, Watanabe T. Abrogation of autoimmune disease in Lyn-deficient mice by the mutation of the *Btk* gene. Int Immunol 10:435–444, 1998.

Takesono A, Finkelstein LD, Schwartzberg PL. Beyond calcium: new signaling pathways for Tec family kinases. J Cell Sci 115:3039–3048, 2002.

Tan JE, Wong SC, Gan SK, Xu S, Lam KP. The adaptor protein BLNK is required for B cell antigen receptor-induced activation of nuclear factor-kappa B and cell cycle entry and survival of B lymphocytes. J Biol Chem 276:20055–20063, 2001.

Taurog JD, Moutsopoulos HM, Rosenberg YJ, Chused TM, Steinberg AD. CBA/N X-linked B-cell defect prevents NZB B-cell hyperactivity in F1 mice. J Exp Med 150:31–43, 1979.

Thomas JD, Sideras P, Smith CIE, Vorechovsky I, Chapman V, Paul WE. A missense mutation in the X-linked agammaglobulinemia gene colocalizes with the mouse X-linked immunodeficiency gene. Science 261:355–358, 1993.

Thyss A, El Baze P, Lefebvre J-C, Schnedier M, Ortonne J-P. Dermatomyositis-like syndrome in X-linked hypogammaglobulinemia. Case report and review of the literature. Acta Derm Venereol (Stockh) 70:309–313, 1990.

Tsukada S, Saffran DC, Rawlings DJ, Parolini O, Allen RC, Klisak I, Sparkes RS, Kubagawa H, Mohandas T, Quan S, Belmont JW, Cooper MD, Conley ME, Witte ON. Deficient expression of a B cell cytoplasmic tyrosine kinase in human X-linked agammaglobulinemia. Cell 72:279–290, 1993.

Tsukada S, Simon M, Witte O, Katz A. Binding of the subunits of heterotrimeric G-proteins to the PH domain of Bruton's tyrosine kinase. Proc Natl Acad Sci USA 91:11256–11260, 1994.

van der Meer JWM, Mouton RP, Daha MR, Schuurman RKB. *Campylobacter jejuni* bacteraemia as a cause of recurrent fever in a patient with hypogammaglobulinemia. J Infect 12:235–239, 1986.

van der Meer JWM, Weening RS, Schellekens PTA, van Muster IP, Nagengast FM. Colorectal cancer in patients with X-linked agammaglobulinemia. Lancet 341:1439–1440, 1993.

Venkataraman C, Muthusamy N, Muthukkumar S, Bondada S. Activation of lyn, Blk, and Btk but not syk in CD72-stimulated B lymphocytes. J Immunol 160:3322–3329, 1998.

Verbruggen G, De Backer S, Deforce D, Demetter P, Cuvelier C, Veys E, Elewaut D. X-linked agammaglobulinemia and rheumatoid arthritis. Ann Rheum Dis 64:1075–1078, 2005.

Vetrie D, Vorechovsky I, Sideras P, Holland J, Davies A, Flinter F, Hammarstrom L, Kinnon C, Levinsky R, Bobrow M, Smith CIE, Bentley DR. The gene involved in X-linked agammaglobulinemia is a member of the Src family of protein-tyrosine kinases. Nature 361:226–233, 1993.

Vihinen M, Brandau O, Branden LJ, Kwan S-P, Lappalainen I, Lester T, Noordzij JG, Ochs HD, Ollila J, Pienaar SM, Riikonen P, Saha BK, Smith CIE. BTKbase, mutation database for X-linked agammaglobulinemia (XLA). Nucl Acids Res 26:242–247, 1998.

Vihinen M, Cooper MD, de Saint Basile G, Fischer A, Good RA, Hendriks RW, Kinnon C, Kwan S-P, Litman GW, Notarangelo LD, Ochs HD, Rosen FS, Vetrie D, Webster ADB, Zegers BJM, Smith CIE. BTKbase: a database of XLA-causing mutations. Immunol Today 16:460–465, 1995.

Vihinen M, Nilsson L, Smith CIE. Structural basis of SH2 mutations in X-linked agammaglobulinemia. Biochem Biophys Res Commun 205:1270–1277, 1994a.

Vihinen M, Nilsson L, Smith CIE. Tec homology (TH) adjacent to PH domain. FEBS Lett 350:263–265, 1994b.

Vihinen M, Nore B, Mattsson PT, Backesjo C-M, Nars M, Koutaniemi S, Watanabe C, Lester T, Jones A, Ochs HD, Smith CIE. Missense mutations affecting a conserved cysteine pair in the TH domain of Btk. FEBS Lett 413:205–210, 1997b.

Vihinen M, Vetrie D, Maniar HS, Ochs HD, Zhu Q, Vorechovsky I, Webster ADB, Notarangelo LD, Nilsson L, Sowadski JM, Smith CIE. Structural basis for chromosome X-linked agammaglobulinemia. A tyrosine kinase disease. Proc Natl Acad Sci USA 91:12803–12807, 1994c.

Vorechovsky I, Luo L, de Saint Basile G, Hammarström L, Webster ADB, Smith CIE. Improved oligonucleotide primer set for molecular diagnosis of X-linked agammaglobulinemia. Predominance of amino acid substitutions in the catalytic domain of Bruton's tyrosine kinase. Hum Mol Genet 4:2403–2405, 1995a.

Vorechovsky I, Vetrie D, Holland J, Bentley DR, Thomas K, Zhou J-N, Notarangelo LD, Plebani A, Fontan G, Ochs HD, Hammarstrom L, Sideras

P, Smith CIE. Isolation of cosmid and cDNA clones in the region surrounding the BTK gene at Xq21.3–q22. Genomics 21:517–524, 1994a.

Vorechovsky I, Vetrie D, Merup M, Zhou J-N, Hammarstrom L, Bentley DR, Smith CIE. A novel protein-typrosine kinase gene BTK mutated in patients with X-linked agammaglobulinemia: no evidence for DNA rearrangements in B-cell neoplasias. In: Borden EC, Goldman JM, Grignani F, eds. Molecular Diagnosis and Monitoring of Leukemia and Lymphoma, Vol. 2, Ares-Serono Symposia, Challenges of Modern Medicine. Rome: Ares Serono Symposia Publications, pp. 205–209, 1994b.

Vorechovsky I, Vihinen M, de Saint Basile G, Honsova S, Hammarstrom L, Muller S, Nilsson L, Fischer A, Smith CIE. DNA-based mutation analysis of Bruton's tyrosine kinase gene in patients with X-linked agammaglobulinemia. Hum Mol Genet 4:51–58, 1995b.

Wahl MI, Fluckiger AC, Kato RM, Park H, Witte ON, Rawlings DJ. Phosphorylation of two regulatory tyrosine residues in the activation of Bruton's tyrosine kinase via alternative receptors. Proc Natl Acad Sci USA 94:11526–11533, 1997.

Walzer PD. Immunopathogenesis of *Pneumocystis carinii* infection. J Lab Clin Med 118:206–216, 1991.

Wang D, Feng J, Wen R, Marine J-C, Sangster MY, Parganas E, Hoffmeyer A, Jackson CW, Cleveland JL, Murray PJ, Ihle JN. Phospholipase Cgamma2 is essential in the functions of B cell and several Fc receptors. Immunity 13:25–35, 2000.

Webb CF, Yamashita Y, Ayers N, Evetts S, Paulin Y, Conley ME, Smith EA. The transcription factor Bright associates with Bruton's tyrosine kinase, the defective protein in immunodeficiency disease. J Immunol 165:6956–6965, 2000.

Webster AD, Loewi G, Dourmashkin RD, Golding DN, Ward DJ, Asherson GL. Polyarthritis in adults with hypogammaglobulinemia and its rapid response to immunoglobulin treatment. BMJ 1(6021):13–14, 1976.

Webster ADB, Rotbart HA, Warner T, Rudge P, Hyman N. Diagnosis of enterovirus brain disease in hypogammaglobulinemic patients by polymerase chain reaction. Clin Infect Dis 17:657–661, 1993.

Webster ADB, Taylor-Robinson D, Furr PM, Asherson GL. Mycoplasmal (ureaplasmal) septic arthritis in hypogammaglobulinemia. BMJ 1(6111):478–480, 1978.

Wedgwood RJ, Ochs HD. Variability in the expression of X-linked agammaglobulinemia: the co-existence of classic X-LA (Bruton type) and "common variable immunodeficiency" in the same families. In: Seligmann M, Hitzig WH, eds. Primary Immunodeficiencies. Amsterdam: Elsevier, North-Holland Biomedical Press, pp. 69–78, 1980.

Wen R, Chen Y, Schuman J, Fu G, Yang S, Zhang W, Newman DK, Wang D. An important role of phospholipase Cγ1 in pre-B-cell development and allelic exclusion. EMBO J 23:4007–4017, 2004.

Wicker LS, Scher I. X-linked immune deficiency (Xid) of CBA/N mice. Curr Top Microbiol Immunol 124:87–101, 1986.

Wood PMD, Mayne A, Joyce H, Smith CIE, Granoff DM, Kumararatne DS. A mutation in Bruton's tyrosine kinase as a cause of selective anti-polysaccharide antibody deficiency. J Pediatr 139:148–151, 2001.

Woodland RT, Schmidt MR, Korsmeyer SJ, Gravel KA. Regulation of B cell survival in Xid mice by the proto-oncogene bcl-2. J Immunol 156:2143–2154, 1996.

Wortis HH, Burkly L, Hughes D, Roschelle S, Waneck G. Lack of mature B cells in nude mice with X-linked immune deficiency. J Exp Med 155:903–917, 1982.

Wyatt HV. Poliomyelitis in hypogammaglobulinemics. J Infect Dis 128:802–806, 1973.

Xu S, Tan JE, Wong EP, Manickam A, Ponniah S, Lam KP. B cell development and activation defects resulting in Xid-like immunodeficiency in BLNK/SLP-65-deficient mice. Int Immunol 12:397–404, 2000.

Yamadori T, Baba Y, Matsushita M, Hashimoto S, Kurosaki M, Kurosaki T, Kishimoto T, Tsukada S. Bruton's tyrosine kinase activity is negatively regulated by Sab, the Btk-SH3 domain–binding protein. Proc Natl Acad Sci USA 96:6341–6346, 1999.

Yamashita Y, Miyake K, Kikuchi Y, Takatsu K, Noda T, Kosugi A, Kimoto M. A monoclonal antibody against murine CD38 delivers a signal into B cells for prolongation of survival and protection against apoptosis in vitro: unresponsiveness of XID B cells to MAb. Immunology 85:248–255, 1995.

Yang W, Desiderio S. BAP-135, a target for Bruton's tyrosine kinase in response to B cell receptor engagement. Proc Natl Acad Sci USA 94:604–609, 1997.

Yang W, Malek SN, Desiderio S. An SH3-binding site conserved in Bruton's tyrosine kinase and related tyrosine kinases mediates specific protein interactions in vitro and in vivo. J Biol Chem 270:20832–20840, 1995.

Yang W-C, Collette Y, Nunes JA, Olive D. Tec kinase: a family with multiple roles in immunity. Immunity 12:373–382, 2000.

Yao L, Kawakami Y, Kawakami T. The pleckstrin homology domain of Bruton tyrosine kinase interacts with protein kinase C. Proc Natl Acad Sci USA 91:9175–9179, 1994.

Yap PL, McOmish F, Webster ADB, Hammarstrom L, Smith CIE, Bjorkander J, Ochs HD, Fischer SH, Quinti I, Simmonds P. Hepatitis C virus transmission by intravenous immunoglobulin. J Hepatol 21:455–460, 1994.

Yu PW, Tabuchi RS, Kato RM, Astrakhan A, Humblet-Baron S, Kipp K, Chae K, Ellmeier W, Witte ON, Rawlings DJ. Sustained correction of B-cell development and function in a murine model of X-linked agammaglobulinemia (XLA) using retroviral-mediated gene transfer. Blood 104: 1281–1290, 2004.

Zhao YX, Abdelnour A, Holmdahl R, Tarkowski A. Mice with the Xid B cell defect are less susceptible to developing *Staphylococcus aureus*–induced arthritis. J Immunol 155:2067–2076, 1995.

Zoll GJ, Melchers WJ, Kopecka H, Jambroes G, van der Poel HJ, Galama JM. General primer-mediated polymerase chain reaction for detection of enteroviruses: application for diagnostic routine and persistent infections. J Clin Microbiol 30:160–165, 1992.

22

Autosomal Recessive Agammaglobulinemia

MARY ELLEN CONLEY

Normal development of the B cell lineage is dependent on appropriate expression and extinction of a panoply of genes, some of which are B cell–specific and some of which are more broadly expressed (Billips et al., 1995; Rajewsky, 1996; Yankee and Clark, 2000; Rolink et al., 2001). These genes encode B cell–specific transcription factors, proteins required for the rearrangement of the immunoglobulin gene segments, signal transduction molecules, receptors for growth factors and adhesion molecules, and many others. The immunoglobulin genes and proteins encoded by these genes obviously play a central role.

The classic disorder of B cell development, X-linked agammaglobulinemia (XLA), was first described in the 1950s (Bruton, 1952; Janeway et al., 1953; Good, 1954a, 1954b). It is characterized by the early onset of bacterial infections, profound hypogammaglobulinemia, and markedly reduced numbers of B cells (Ochs and Winkelstein, 1996; Conley et al., 2000a). The defective gene in this disorder encodes a cytoplasmic tyrosine kinase, Btk, that is involved in signal transduction (Tsukada et al., 1993; Vetrie et al., 1993). It is not yet clear, however, how defects in this protein result in impaired B cell proliferation, differentiation, or survival.

The incidence of other genetic disorders that result in a failure of B cell development is difficult to determine. Only about half of the males with the clinical features of XLA have a positive family history of the disease (Lederman and Winkelstein, 1985; Conley et al., 1998). The remaining patients may be the first members of their families to show manifestations of a new mutation in Btk or they may be patients with disorders that are clinically similar to XLA but caused by defects in different genes or by combinations of genetic and environmental factors. The frequency of XLA-like disorders in females provides some clues to the overall incidence; however, because physicians may be less likely to consider antibody deficiency in a girl, the numbers calculated in this manner may represent an underestimate.

Defects in Btk are rarely responsible for immunodeficiency in females with an XLA phenotype. Studies using X chromosome inactivation analysis of B cells, T cells, neutrophils, and platelets of women who are heterozygous for mutations in Btk indicate that even a small number of B cell precursors that have the nonmutant X as the active X can provide normal B cell immunity because of the strong selective advantage conferred on these cells by a normal Btk (Conley et al., 1986; Fearon et al., 1987; Conley and Puck, 1988). However, it should be noted that an exception has been reported by Takada et al. (2004), who described a girl with XLA who had a mutation in Btk on one X chromosome and an inability to use the other X chromosome as the active X chromosome.

When techniques were developed to identify B cells in the early 1970s, it became clear that some of the patients with hypogammaglobulinemia and absent B cells were girls. In 1973 Aiuti et al. described three patients with infantile onset of hypogammaglobulinemia and absent B cells; one was a girl. Hoffman et al. reported two sisters with a disorder phenotypically identical to XLA in 1977; these authors postulated that their patients might have an autosomal recessive form of the disease. In a study on chronic enteroviral encephalitis that included 36 patients with agammaglobulinemia and absent B cells, McKinney et al. (1987) noted that 18 of the patients had a family history of disease consistent with XLA, and 18 had sporadic disease. Three of the latter 18 patients were females. In 1992 we reported two unrelated girls who were included in our patient population of 17 individuals with a disorder that was indistinguishable from XLA. Extensive evaluation of one of these girls indicated that it was highly unlikely that she had a defect in a gene at Xq22, the site of the XLA gene (Conley and Sweinberg, 1992). Both maternal and paternal alleles could be detected in this region and both X chromosomes could be used as the active X chromosome. Because XLA is a relatively uncommon disorder, the probability of a new mutation in the Btk gene in both parental gametes was extremely small. Two more recent studies have examined early events in B cell differentiation in girls with an XLA phenotype (De La Morena et al., 1995; Meffre et al., 1996). On the basis of these observations, we have estimated that approximately 10% of patients with congenital hypogammaglobulinemia and markedly reduced numbers of B cells are females (Conley and Sweinberg, 1992; Conley et al., 1994). It can be assumed that there is a similar number of males with an XLA phenotype who do not have mutations in Btk.

Approaches to Identification of Mutant Genes in Patients with Defects in B Cell Development

It cannot be concluded that all of the patients with an XLA phenotype who do not have mutations in Btk have an autosomal recessive disorder causing their disease. There may be environmental factors or combinations of susceptibility genes that result in immunodeficiency. We have evaluated several young adult males with the diagnosis of common variable immunodeficiency who have had markedly reduced numbers of B cells and no mutations in Btk or other genes associated with B cell development. Hypogammaglobulinemia and absent B cells may be the presenting findings in patients with myelodysplasia and monosomy 7 (Srivannaboon et al., 2001), trisomy 8, or dyskeratosis congenita. However, in families with more than one affected sibling or when there is parental consanguinity, the disease is very likely to be caused by an autosomal recessive disorder.

Several approaches could be used to identify candidate genes that might be responsible for autosomal recessive defects in B cell development. Murine models of immunodeficiency have been created by "knocking out" the function of a gene by homologous recombination (Loffert et al., 1994). In several of these models, the affected mice demonstrate hypogammaglobulinemia and a complete absence of B cells or a phenotype similar to that seen in Btk-deficient mice (Kitamura et al., 1991, 1992; Chen et al., 1993; Bain et al., 1994; Urbanek et al., 1994; Zhuang et al., 1994; Cheng et al., 1995; Lin and Grosschedl, 1995; Gong and Nussenzweig, 1996; Leitges et al., 1996; Nagasawa et al., 1996; Schilham et al., 1996; Torres et al., 1996; Jumaa et al., 1999; Pappu et al., 1999; Suzuki et al., 1999; Wang et al., 2000; Mundt et al., 2001; Tokimasa et al., 2001; Clayton et al., 2002; Jou et al., 2002; Yamazaki et al., 2002). Most of the genes that are targeted in these studies encode transcription factors important for B cell development, components of the B cell antigen receptor complex, or signal transduction molecules. There are several caveats to this approach. First, defects in the same gene may cause a different phenotype in mice and humans (Conley et al., 2000b). Abnormalities in the gene for Btk, which result in a severe B cell defect in humans and a much milder defect in mice, are an excellent example of this phenomenon. Second, spontaneously occurring mutations seen in patients may include amino acid substitutions in addition to the null phenotypes usually created in knockout mice. These more subtle mutations may have a wider range of consequences. Finally, it should be noted that while defects in several of the transcription factors, E2A, PAX5, EBF, and Sox4, result in abnormalities restricted to the B cell lineage in the immune system, they also caused runting, brain defects, or heart abnormalities (Bain et al., 1994; Urbanek et al., 1994; Zhuang et al., 1994; Lin and Grosschedl, 1995; Schilham et al., 1996), making it less likely that these genes are involved in

patients who have defects of B cell development but no additional morphologic defects.

Another approach to the identification of defective genes is based on the possibility that two different inherited disorders that result in the same clinical phenotype may involve genes that encode functionally related proteins (Conley and Sweinberg, 1992). For example, males with X-linked severe combined immunodeficiency (SCID) have absent T cells and natural killer (NK) cells but a normal or elevated number of B cells (Conley et al., 1990). Approximately 10% of the patients with SCID who have this laboratory profile are females, who were suspected to have an autosomal recessive form of the disease (Conley et al., 1990). After *IL2RG*, encoding the common γ chain, was identified as the abnormal gene in X-linked SCID, defects in the next protein involved in the common γ-chain signaling cascade, JAK3, were sought and found (Macchi et al., 1995; Russell et al., 1995). Although it is not clear that all of the crucial downstream targets of Btk have been identified, Btk is phosphorylated and activated by cross-linking of several cell surface receptors including IL-5R (Sato et al., 1994), IL-6R (Matsuda et al., 1995), the high-affinity receptor for IgE (Kawakami et al., 1994), the collagen receptor glycoprotein VI in platelets (Quek et al., 1998; Oda et al., 2000), and, perhaps most importantly, surface IgM on B cells (Aoki et al., 1994; de Weers et al., 1994; Saouaf et al., 1994).

To identify autosomal recessive disorders of B cell development, we have used an approach that combines evaluation of candidate genes with linkage analysis. Because it is likely that the most important role for Btk in B cell development relates to signaling through the B cell or pre-B cell receptor, we have focused on genes encoding proteins in this pathway. This includes the components of the B cell and pre-B cells receptor: the immunoglobulin heavy chain, the surrogate light chain, and the signal transduction molecules Igα and Igβ, as well as downstream signal transduction molecules such as Syk, PI3K, PLCγ2, and the adaptor protein BLNK. All of these genes have been mapped to specific sites within the human genome. This allows the selection of highly polymorphic markers linked to each gene. In a consanguineous family, the parents of a patient will share an allele (by common descent) at the correct locus and the affected patients will be homozygous for those polymorphic markers. In any family with more than one affected child, the affected siblings should have inherited the same polymorphic alleles near the gene of interest whereas the unaffected siblings should differ.

Detection of Mutations in μ Heavy-Chain Gene

In our initial efforts to identify autosomal recessive causes of severe hypogammaglobulinemia and absent B cells, we studied two consanguineous families that included affected girls as well as boys (Fig. 22.1). Linkage studies using highly polymorphic markers near the immunoglobulin heavy-chain locus at chromosome 14q32.3 (Benger et al., 1991) showed that the affected children in each family were identical to each other and were homozygous for the polymorphic markers at this locus. Using a probe for the μ constant region gene to analyze DNA by Southern blotting techniques, we identified a complete deletion of the μ chain in the affected children in family 1, a Turkish family (Yel et al., 1996). Probes both proximal and distal to this portion of the heavy-chain locus demonstrated a 75 kb deletion that included most of the D region genes, the J region genes, the immunoglobulin enhancer region, and all of the coding regions of the μ constant region gene but not the δ constant region gene (Fig. 22.2).

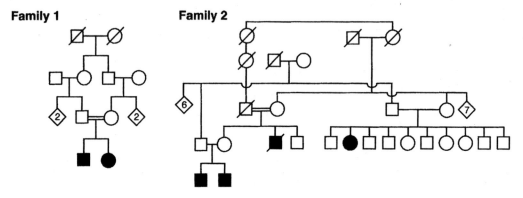

Figure 22.1. Pedigrees for two families in which the affected individuals, shown as filled symbols, had early-onset hypogammaglobulinemia and absent B cells. Circles denote female family members and squares indicate male family members; symbols with a slash represent deceased family members. Figure adapted from Yel et al. (1996). Copyright 1996, Massachusetts Medical Society. All rights reserved.

Southern blot analysis of DNA from members of the second family, a family from Appalachia, did not demonstrate gross deletions or rearrangements of the immunoglobulin locus. However, because of the high probability of a mutation in this region indicated by the linkage studies, we screened genomic DNA from an affected child from this family by single-strand conformational polymorphism (SSCP; see Chapter 44) for alterations in the four constant region exons and two membrane exons of the μ heavy-chain gene. The use of a screening evaluation allowed us to examine DNA from not only members of family 2 but also other patients who were thought to have sporadic XLA but in whom we had not found mutations in Btk. Analysis of exon 4 of the μ constant-region gene, the exon that encodes the C-terminal immunoglobulin domain, demonstrated altered migrations of bands from the affected girl in family 2 and from a boy with presumed sporadic XLA (Yel et al., 1996) (Fig. 22.2). DNA from both samples showed the absence of bands seen in controls, indicating that the alterations were either homozygous or hemizygous (only one allele present).

Exon 4 from the affected girl in family 2 was sequenced and a single base pair substitution, a G-to-A transition at position 1831 (according to the numbering system of Friedlander et al. (1990), was identified. This substitution occurs at the −1 position for the alternative splice site used to link the two membrane exons to the μ constant region transcript so that the cell surface form of μ chain can be produced, rather than the secreted form. This alteration causes the substitution of serine for glycine at codon 557 in the secreted form of μ chain and the substitution of lysine for aspartic acid at the same codon in the membrane form of μ chain. More importantly, the mutated splice site is expected to result in inefficient or absent production of the transcript for the membrane form of μ heavy chain.

The sequence of exon 4 of the μ heavy-chain gene in the boy with no family history of immunodeficiency demonstrated a T-to-G substitution at nucleotide 1768 in codon 536. This alteration causes a replacement of the wild-type cysteine with glycine. The cysteine at this position is the 3′ cysteine involved in the intradomain disulfide bridge that is conserved in all immunoglobulin domains of all isotypes (Beale and Feinstein, 1976). The loss of this cysteine would be expected to make the immunoglobulin protein unstable. Because this patient's parents were from different ethnic backgrounds, it was thought to be unlikely that he was homozygous for this mutation. Therefore we sought evidence for a deletion on the other chromosome. When genomic DNA from the patient was analyzed by Southern blot, using a probe from the μ constant region gene, there was a 50% decrease in the intensity

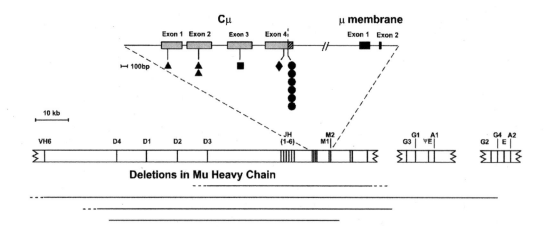

Figure 22.2. Mutations in μ heavy-chain gene in patients with agammaglobulinemia. The approximate lengths of the five large deletions are shown below the drawing of the immunoglobulin heavy-chain locus. The sites of the frameshift mutations in exons 1 and 2 (triangle), the premature stop codon in exon 3 (square), the amino acid substitution (diamond), and the alternative splice defects (circle) in exon 4 are shown in the magnified region of this locus at the top of the figure. The alternative splice site at the end of exon 4, which is marked by a dashed line, allows the constant region domains to be spliced to the membrane exons.

of the μ-specific band. Probes from the V_H, D_H, J_H, and constant regions indicated that this deletion included part of the V_H region, all of the D_H and J_H regions, and all of the constant-region genes except for the IgA2 heavy-chain gene.

Since the original report of these mutations, 11 additional families with defects in μ heavy chain have been reported (Lopez et al., 2002; Milili et al., 2002; Schiff et al., 2000) (Fig. 22.2). In five of the families, the affected patients were homozygous for the same single base pair substitution at the alternative splice site seen in family 2. Analysis of polymorphic markers within the immunoglobulin locus indicated that this mutation, a G-to-A substitution, occurred at least three separate times. This alteration is found at a vulnerable site, a CpG dinucleotide (Cooper and Youssoufian, 1988). Two unrelated Spanish families had a 2–base pair deletion, an AA deletion, at codon 168 within exon 2 of the constant region of μ heavy chain. Immunoglobulin haplotype analysis in these families indicated that they shared an ancestor (Lopez et al., 2002). A premature stop codon at codon 258 in exon 3 was seen in a child from Argentina. A frameshift mutation, a C insertion at codon 23 in exon 1 of μ heavy chain, was reported by Schiff et al. (2000). Five different large deletions within the μ heavy-chain locus have been described (Lopez et al., 2002; Milili et al., 2002). All of these deletions remove the D and J regions as well as the μ constant-region gene.

There are several factors that make the μ heavy-chain locus susceptible to mutation. During normal B cell development, the 1000 kb immunoglobulin heavy-chain locus undergoes chromosomal breakage and rearrangement associated with both VDJ joining and isotype switching. The nature of the DNA structures that permits these rearrangements, including a high frequency of repeated or highly homologous sequences, may make this region susceptible to unequal crossover in meiosis resulting in deletions. Deletions within the V region (Cook et al., 1994) and within the region encoding the constant-region genes (Olsson et al., 1993; Chen et al., 1995) are well recognized.

Normal functioning of the μ heavy-chain protein requires the ability to interact with many proteins, including the surrogate light chains, the classic light chains, and the immunoglobulin-associated chains, Igα and Igβ. The μ heavy chain expressed on the cell surface must transmit signals to the cell interior and it must interact with other cell surface proteins, including the CD19/CD21 complex. These interactions place structural constraints throughout the μ heavy-chain molecule and suggest that mutations at many sites may destroy the ability of the μ heavy chain to function in B cell differentiation.

Detection of Mutations in the $\lambda_{5/14.1}$ Gene

Because mutations in μ heavy chain and Btk did not account for all of the patients with agammaglobulinemia and absent B cells, we tested the hypothesis that defects in other components of the B cell or pre-B cell receptor complex might result in an XLA phenotype. The genes for the surrogate light chain, V_{preB} and $\lambda_{5/14.1}$, were particularly attractive gene candidates because they are B cell–specific (Sakaguchi and Melchers, 1986; Kudo and Melchers, 1987; Melchers et al., 1993), they are functionally required at exactly the same point in B cell differentiation as the rearranged μ heavy chain, and, as a practical point, they are small genes and therefore relatively easy to analyze (Kudo and Melchers, 1987).

The proteins encoded by the V_{preB} and $\lambda_{5/14.1}$ genes assemble to produce a complex very similar to the λ light chain. The amino-terminal portion of V_{preB} has high homology to the variable region of an immunoglobulin molecule, and the carboxy-terminal portion of $\lambda_{5/14.1}$ has homology to the J region and constant region of λ light chain (Sakaguchi and Melchers, 1986; Kudo and Melchers, 1987). These two proteins are noncovalently linked to each other (Kerr et al., 1989; Minegishi et al., 1999b) and covalently linked to the μ heavy chain via a cysteine residue in the carboxy-terminal portion of $\lambda_{5/14.1}$ (Pillai and Baltimore, 1987; Kerr et al., 1989). Together, V_{preB} and $\lambda_{5/14.1}$ form a surrogate light chain that escorts the rearranged μ heavy chain to the cell surface prior to the rearrangement of the conventional light-chain genes. This allows the B cell precursor to test the integrity of the rearranged μ heavy chain before investing in extensive proliferation or additional gene rearrangements.

To screen for mutations in the V_{preB} and $\lambda_{5/14.1}$ genes, both of which are located within the λ light-chain locus at chromosome 22q11.2 (Erikson et al., 1981; Bossy et al., 1991; Bauer et al., 1993), polymerase chain reaction (PCR) primers were designed to flank the two exons of V_{preB} and the three exons of $\lambda_{5/14.1}$. Because there are two λ_5 pseudogenes that have over 95% homology with exons 2 and 3 of $\lambda_{5/14.1}$, care was taken to develop primers for exon 2 that would amplify only the functional gene, and the PCR product for exon 3 was digested with BstUI, an enzyme that would be expected to cleave the functional sequence but not the sequence from the pseudogenes (Minegishi et al., 1998). The PCR products were separated on a nondenaturing gel and analyzed by SSCP. DNA from one patient, a 5-year-old boy with the clinical signs and symptoms of sporadic XLA, demonstrated both normal and abnormal bands for exon 1 and exon 3 of $\lambda_{5/14.1}$ (Minegishi et al., 1998). Family studies and sequence analysis showed that the abnormality in exon 1, which was derived from the maternal allele, was due to a C-to-T transition in codon 22, resulting in the substitution of a premature stop codon for the wild-type glutamine. The alterations in exon 3, from the paternal allele, were caused by 3 base pair substitutions in codons 131, 140, and 142. The first two substitutions would not be expected to alter the coding sequence; however, the C-to-T transition at nucleotide 425 would be predicted to replace the invariant proline at codon 142 with a leucine. Protein-folding studies demonstrated that this alteration resulted in an inability of the $\lambda_{5/14.1}$ protein to fold properly (Minegishi et al., 1998).

Of interest, the three base pair substitutions in the paternal allele of $\lambda_{5/14.1}$ are the same as those found at the corresponding site in exon 3 of the $\lambda_{5/14.1}$ pseudogene 16.1, a finding suggesting that this mutation was the result of a gene conversion event (Minegishi et al., 1998). To determine whether the alterations represented a normal polymorphic variant, we used SSCP to analyze genomic DNA from normal controls. Although an allele identical to that seen in the patient was not seen in controls, the $\lambda_{5/14.1}$ locus was found to be highly polymorphic. Thirteen variant alleles of $\lambda_{5/14.1}$, the majority of which could be attributed to gene conversion events, were found in 134 unrelated individuals (Conley et al., 1999). Nine of these variants resulted in amino acid substitutions. Although gene conversion is an unusual mechanism of mutation, some species use gene conversion to generate diversity in the variable region of immunoglobulin loci (Reynaud et al., 1987; Thompson, 1992). Immunoglobulin and immunoglobulin-like genes may be unusually susceptible to gene conversion events.

Detection of Mutations in the Igα Gene

The signal transduction molecules Igα and Igβ (also called CD79a and CD79b or mb-1 and B29) are essential components of the pre-B cell and B cell receptor complex (Hombach et al., 1990). Both molecules are B cell–specific proteins with structural similarities to the CD3γ, δ, and ε chains in T cells. Both have a single extracellular immunoglobulin domain, a transmembrane domain, and an intracytoplasmic domain containing an immunoreceptor tyrosine-based activation motif (ITAM) characterized by the sequence YXXL(X)$_7$YXXL, in which Y represents tyrosine, L represents leucine, and X denotes any amino acid. Igα and Igβ form a covalently linked heterodimer that masks the hydrophilic transmembrane domain of μ heavy chain and escorts it to the cell surface. When the B cell receptor is cross-linked, a protein in the src family phosphorylates the tyrosines in the ITAM motif, converting this sequence into a docking site for the downstream tyrosine kinase, Syk.

SSCP analysis of genomic DNA has been used to screen patients for mutations in Igα, a 5 exon gene at chromosome 19q13.2 (Ha et al., 1994), and Igβ, a 6 exon gene at chromosome 17q23 (Wood et al., 1993). Three patients with defects in Igα have been identified. The first, a Turkish girl, was found to have a homozygous A-to-G substitution at the invariant −2 position of the splice acceptor site for exon 3 (Minegishi et al., 1999a). Reverse transcription PCR analysis of cDNA derived from this patient's bone marrow showed that the majority of Igα transcripts deleted exon 3. Because exon 3 contains 119 base pairs, this change results in a frameshift mutation. A small number of transcripts used a cryptic splice acceptor site within exon 3, resulting in a 13–base pair deletion. Exon 3 of Igα encodes for the transmembrane domain; therefore, these frameshift mutations can be considered functional null mutations. A different splice defect, a G-to-A substitution at the +1 position of the splice donor site for exon 2, was identified in another Turkish child (Wang et al., 2002). The third mutation, a premature stop codon due to a G-to-T substitution in codon 48 in exon 2 in Igα, was identified in a Mexican child (M.E. Conley, unpublished results).

To determine if a null defect in Igα results in a block in B cell differentiation before V-to-DJ recombination, we used primers that could amplify members of the largest human V$_H$ families, VH1, VH3, and VH4, to analyze cDNA from the bone marrow of the first Igα-deficient patient and the patient with an amino acid substitution in the CH4 domain of μ heavy chain. The PCR products were separated on a sequencing gel to allow discrimination of transcripts with CDR3 regions of varying length. Both patients had markedly decreased transcripts for rearranged μ heavy chains compared to controls; however, the amount and the diversity of the transcripts were approximately equal in the two patients (Minegishi et al., 1999a). These findings suggest that both defects block B cell differentiation at the same stage of maturation.

Detection of Mutations in the BLNK Gene

Cross-linking of the B cell receptor complex initiates a cascade of tyrosine phosphorylation events. One of the first proteins to be phosphorylated is a 456–amino acid adaptor protein referred to as BLNK (Fu and Chan, 1997; Fu et al., 1998; Goitsuka et al., 1998; Wienands et al., 1998) (also called SLP-65 and BASH), which has significant homology to SLP-76, a protein expressed in T cells, myeloid cells, and platelets (Jackman et al., 1995; Clements et al., 1998a). Once BLNK is phosphorylated by Syk, it acts as a scaffold to assemble the downstream targets of B cell receptor–mediated activation including Grb2, Vav, Nck, and PLCγ2.

Several observations suggested that mutations in BLNK might result in a selective defect in B cell development. First, expression of BLNK is limited to B cells and myeloid cells (Fu et al., 1998). Second, absence of BLNK in a chicken B cell line, DT40, like absence of Btk, results in defective calcium mobilization (Ishiai et al., 1999; Kurosaki, 1999). Third, mice that are

null for the T cell homolog of BLNK, SLP-76, fail to develop T cells (Clements et al., 1998b; (Pivniouk et al., 1998).

To determine whether mutations in BLNK might cause immunodeficiency, the gene was mapped to chromosome 10q23.22 using fluorescence in situ hybridization (FISH) and the genomic organization was determined (Minegishi et al., 1999c). PCR primers flanking each of the 17 exons were used to screen genomic DNA from patients with B cell defects of unknown etiology. One patient, a 20-year-old male from Appalachia who was previously thought to have XLA, was found to have a homozygous alteration in the first exon and associated flanking regions of BLNK. Sequencing of this region demonstrated two noncontiguous base pair substitutions. The first alteration, a C-to-A substitution at the third base pair in codon 10, does not change the proline encoded at this position and would not be expected to have functional consequences. The second alteration, an A-to-T substitution, was seen at the conserved +3 position of the splice donor site of intron 1, 20 base pairs downstream from the alteration in codon 10 (Minegishi et al., 1999c). Neither of the two base pair alterations seen in the patient were found in 100 normal controls. Analysis of cDNA from the bone marrow of this patient demonstrated a complete absence of BLNK transcripts.

B Cell Differentiation in Patients with Proven Autosomal Recessive Agammaglobulinemia

Although patients with XLA have markedly reduced numbers of B cells, a small number of B cells with an immature phenotype are usually present in the peripheral circulation (patients have 0.01%–0.50% CD19$^+$ lymphocytes compared to 5%–20% in controls) in patients less than 15 years of age (Conley, 1985; Nomura et al., 2000). Older patients with XLA are less likely to have detectable B cells. Analysis of six patients with mutations in μ heavy chain, or Igα, all of whom were less than 15 years old at the time of the study, showed that these patients had less than 0.01% B cells in the blood (Yel et al., 1996; Minegishi et al., 1999a). This suggests a complete block in B cell development early in the B cell lineage in these patients. The patient with mutations in the λ$_{5/14.1}$ gene has consistently had a small number of B cells (0.06%) in the peripheral circulation (Minegishi et al., 1998). The profound decrease in B cell numbers and antibody deficiency in the λ$_{5/14.1}$-deficient patient contrasts with findings in mice that fail to express λ$_5$. These mice have approximately 20% of the normal numbers of B cells by 4 months of age and they are able to make antibody to both T-dependent and T-independent antigens (Kitamura et al., 1992). The 20-year-old patient with BLNK deficiency was studied in parallel with an age-matched patient with XLA. There were fewer than 0.01% B cells in the peripheral circulation in either patient.

To compare the point in B cell differentiation at which the block occurs in patients with mutations in the genes for Btk, μ heavy chain, λ$_{5/14.1}$, Igα, or BLNK, we analyzed bone marrow samples from patients with each defect (Fig. 22.3) (Yel et al., 1996; Minegishi et al., 1998, 1999a, 1999c). In normal bone marrow, the earliest B cell precursors are identified by coexpression of surface CD34 and CD19 and cytoplasmic expression of terminal deoxynucleotidyl transferase (TdT) and RAG (Campana et al., 1990; Billips et al., 1995). At this stage in differentiation, the immunoglobulin genes are undergoing the first step in gene rearrangement, DJ joining. These pro-B cells give rise to a population of pre-B cells that are positive for CD19 but they have lost expression of CD34, TdT, and RAG. They have completed immunoglobulin heavy-chain gene rearrangement by joining a

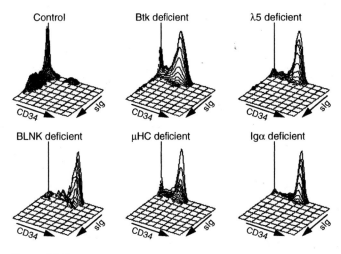

Figure 22.3. Bone marrow cells from a control and from patients with immunodeficiency were stained with antibodies to CD19, CD34, and human light chains. Cells stained for CD19 were analyzed for expression of CD34 and surface immunoglobulin. An equal number of CD19+ cells were evaluated in each sample. Figure is from Conley et al. (2000b). Copyright 2000, Munksgaard.

V gene to the DJ segment and they express cytoplasmic μ. In the normal individual, the ratio of pro-B cells to pre-B cells declines with age; however, there are usually 2 to 5 times more pre-B cells than pro-B cells (Campana et al., 1990; Nunez et al., 1996).

All of the patients had normal numbers of the earliest B cell precursors, pro-B cells that express both CD34 and CD19. However, cells at the next stage of differentiation, cells that express CD19 but are negative for CD34, were markedly decreased in number in the patients with mutations in Btk, $\lambda_{5/14.1}$, and BLNK, and were completely missing in patients with mutations in the μ heavy-chain gene or Igα (Yel et al., 1996; Minegishi et al., 1998, 1999a, 1999c) (Fig. 22.3). The patients with mutations in Btk (seven patients) or BLNK had an unusual population of B lineage cells that expressed cytoplasmic μ heavy chain but still expressed CD34 and TdT, which suggests incomplete but not absent signaling through the pre-B cell receptor complex. It is not surprising that mutations in μ heavy chain, $\lambda_{5/14.1}$, and Igα all resulted in a block in B cell development at the same point in differentiation as all three proteins are required to form the normal pre-B cell receptor complex. The results also demonstrate that the earliest point in B cell differentiation at which defects in Btk and BLNK impair B cell development coincides with expression of the pre-B cell receptor complex, suggesting that these two proteins are required for normal signaling through this complex.

Clinical Characteristics in Patients with Autosomal Recessive Agammaglobulinemia

It is the impression of many physicians who provide care for patients with hypogammaglobulinemia that girls with an XLA phenotype have a more severe disease than males. The 21 affected patients from 14 families with known mutations in the μ heavy-chain gene represent a small sample size. However, if we exclude the youngest affected child in family 2, who was evaluated in the first month of life because of the family history of immunodeficiency, the patients with mutations in this gene were recognized to have an immune deficiency at an earlier age than patients with mutations in Btk (mean of 11 months vs. 32 months) (Lederman and Winkelstein, 1985; Farrar et al., 1996; Meffre et al., 1996; Yel

et al., 1996; Lopez et al., 2002) and the majority experienced a life-threatening infection. Seven of the patients developed chronic enteroviral encephalitis, a complication seen in less than 10% of patients with XLA (Lederman and Winkelstein, 1985). Three of the patients died of chronic enteroviral encephalitis at 3 to 9 years of age. One of the remaining patients continues to have significant infections despite intravenous γ-globulin therapy. However, there is clear variability in the clinical course; two of the patients have survived more than 40 years.

The patient with mutations in $\lambda_{5/14.1}$ had recurrent otitis as an infant and was recognized to have immunodeficiency at 3 years of age, when he developed hemophilus influenza meningitis despite previous immunization with the conjugated vaccine. The Igα-deficient patients have had a clinical course similar to that of patients with defects in μ heavy chain. Two were recognized as having immunodeficiency at about 1 year of age and one died at 8 years of age of probable chronic enteroviral infection (Minegishi et al., 1999a; Milili et al., 2002). The patient with BLNK deficiency had the onset of recurrent otitis at 8 months of age and was diagnosed as having XLA at 16 months of age, after his second episode of pneumonia. He has done moderately well after γ-globulin, therapy was started; however, he has had chronic otitis and sinusitis, hepatitis C acquired from intravenous γ-globulin, and an episode of protein-losing enteropathy in adolescence. It is noteworthy that this patient had an older brother who died of pseudomonas sepsis and neutropenia at 16 months of age, probably due to BLNK deficiency.

If patients with complete blocks in B cell differentiation, like the patients with mutations in μ heavy-chain gene or Igα, have a more severe clinical disease than patients with mutations in Btk, then the small amount of immunoglobulin found in patients with XLA may play a protective role, perhaps through complement activation or FcR binding.

The treatment for patients with autosomal recessive agammaglobulinemia is currently the same as that for other patients with hypogammaglobulinemia, including patients with XLA. Immunoglobulin replacement and aggressive use of antibiotics provide excellent but not perfect protection from infection. Consideration of gene therapy to treat mutations in μ heavy-chain gene presents unusual problems because of the size and complexity of the immunoglobulin heavy-chain locus. In patients with single base pair substitutions, correction by homologous recombination (Rice et al., 2001) or by ribozyme-mediated repair of a defective transcript (Lan et al., 1998) might be successful.

Defects in B Cell Development Associated with Morphologic Abnormalities

Several reports have described patients with markedly reduced numbers of peripheral blood B cells and morphologic defects (Adderson et al., 2000; Revy et al., 2000; Hoffman et al., 2001; Verloes et al., 2001). All of these patients have had microcephaly and some are described as having dysmorphic facial features and abnormalities of the hands (Hoffman et al., 2001; Verloes et al., 2001). Progressive pancytopenia has been reported in others (Adderson et al., 2000; Revy et al., 2000). It is not clear whether these patients represent a single gene defect or several different disorders. In at least one case, the parents were consanguineous, increasing the probability that the child had a single gene defect. Most of these patients have been analyzed for defects in the gene for PAX5, a transcription factor that is essential for normal central nervous system and B cell development (Urbanek et al., 1994); however, no abnormalities have been found.

Conclusions

Although a larger sample size could permit a more accurate estimate, we calculate that mutations in μ heavy-chain gene, $\lambda_{5/14.1}$, Igα, or BLNK account for approximately half of all patients with defects in early B cell development who do not have abnormalities in the gene for Btk. It is not clear at this point whether the remaining half represent one or a small number of genetic defects or whether they are a heterogeneous group in which almost every patient may be unique.

Over the next few years it is likely that additional gene defects responsible for abnormal B cell development will be elucidated. Identification of these genes is of obvious importance to the families of affected patients. However, it also provides new perspectives on normal B cell development and the functional relationship between the various genes required for normal B cell development. For example, a comparison of B cell development in patients with mutations in μ heavy-chain gene with that seen in patients with XLA supports the hypothesis that Btk, the defective protein in XLA, plays a major role in signal transduction through the pre-B cell receptor complex. Comparison of human disorders in B cell development with murine models of immunodeficiency also highlights the aspects of B cell signaling that are invariant and those that may be influenced by other genetic or environmental factors.

References

Adderson EE, Viskochil DH, Carey JC, Shigeoka AO, Christenson JC, Bohnsack JF, Hill HR. Growth failure, intracranial calcifications, acquired pancytopenia, and unusual humoral immunodeficiency: a genetic syndrome? Am J Med Genet 95:17–20, 2000.

Aiuti F, Fontana L, Gatti RA. Membrane-bound immunoglobulin (Ig) and in vitro production of Ig by lymphoid cells from patients with primary immunodeficiencies. Scand J Immunol 2:9–16, 1973.

Aoki Y, Isselbacher KJ, Pillai S. Bruton tyrosine kinase is tyrosine phosphorylated and activated in pre-B lymphocytes and receptor-ligated B cells. Proc Natl Acad Sci USA 91:10606–10609, 1994.

Bain G, Maandag ECR, Izon DJ, Amsen D, Kruisbeek AM, Weintraub BC, Krop I, Schlissel MS, Feeney AJ, van Roon M, van der Valk M, te Riele HPJ, Berns A, Murre C. E 2A proteins are required for proper B cell development and initiation of immunoglobulin gene rearrangements. Cell 79:885–892, 1994.

Bauer TR Jr, McDermid HE, Budarf ML, Van Keuren ML, Blomberg BB. Physical location of the human immunoglobulin lambda-like genes, 14.1, 16.1, and 16.2. Immunogenetics 38:387–399, 1993.

Beale D, Feinstein A. Structure and function of the constant regions of immunoglobulins. Q Rev Biophys 9:135–180, 1976.

Benger JC, Teshima I, Walter MA, Brubacher MG, Daouk GH, Cox DW. Localization and genetic linkage of the human immunoglobulin heavy chain genes and the creatine kinase brain (CKB) gene: identification of a hot spot for recombination. Genomics 9:614–622, 1991.

Billips LG, Lassoued K, Nunez C, Wang J, Kubagawa H, Gartland GL, Burrows PD, Cooper MD. Human B-cell development. Ann NY Acad Sci 764:1–8, 1995.

Bossy D, Milili M, Zucman J, Thomas G, Fougereau M, Schiff C. Organization and expression of the lambda-like genes that contribute to the mu-surrogate light chain complex in human pre-B cells. Int Immunol 3:1081–1090, 1991.

Bruton OC. Agammaglobulinemia. Pediatrics 9:722–728, 1952.

Campana D, Farrant J, Inamdar N, Webster ADB, Janossy G. Phenotypic features and proliferative activity of B cell progenitors in X-linked agammaglobulinemia. J Immunol 145:1675–1680, 1990.

Chen J, Trounstine M, Alt FW, Young F, Kurahara C, Loring JF, Huszar D. Immunoglobulin gene rearrangement in B cell deficient mice generated by targeted deletion of the JH locus. Int Immunol 5:647–656, 1993.

Chen ZQ, Hofker MH, Cox DW. Defining the breakpoint of a multigene deletion in the immunoglobulin heavy chain gene cluster. Immunogenetics 41:69–73, 1995.

Cheng AM, Rowley B, Pao W, Hayday A, Bolen JB, Pawson T. Syk tyrosine kinase required for mouse viability and B-cell development. Nature 378:303–306, 1995.

Clayton E, Bardi G, Bell SE, Chantry D, Downes CP, Gray A, Humphries LA, Rawlings D, Reynolds H, Vigorito E, Turner M. A crucial role for the p110δ subunit of phosphatidylinositol 3-kinase in B cell development and activation. J Exp Med 196:753–763, 2002.

Clements JL, Ross-Barta SE, Tygrett LT, Waldschmidt TJ, Koretzky GA. SLP-76 expression is restricted to hemopoietic cells of monocyte, granulocyte, and T lymphocyte lineage and is regulated during T cell maturation and activation. J Immunol 161:3880–3889, 1998a.

Clements JL, Yang B, Ross-Barta SE, Eliason SL, Hrstka RF, Williamson RA, Koretzky GA. Requirement for the leukocyte-specific adapter protein SLP-76 for normal T cell development. Science 281:416–419, 1998b.

Conley ME. B cells in patients with X-linked agammaglobulinemia. J Immunol 134:3070–3074, 1985.

Conley ME, Brown P, Pickard AR, Buckley RH, Miller DS, Raskind WH, Singer JW, Fialkow PJ. Expression of the gene defect in X-linked agammaglobulinemia. N Engl J Med 315:564–567, 1986.

Conley ME, Buckley RH, Hong R, Guerra-Hanson C, Roifman CM, Brochstein JA, Pahwa S, Puck JM. X-linked severe combined immunodeficiency: diagnosis in males with sporadic severe combined immunodeficiency and clarification of clinical findings. J Clin Invest 85:1548–1554, 1990.

Conley ME, Mathias D, Treadaway J, Minegishi Y, Rohrer J. Mutations in Btk in patients with presumed X-linked agammaglobulinemia. Am J Hum Genet 62:1034–1043, 1998.

Conley ME, Parolini O, Rohrer J, Campana D. X-linked agammaglobulinemia: new approaches to old questions based on the identification of the defective gene. Immunol Rev 138:5–21, 1994.

Conley ME, Puck JM. Carrier detection in typical and atypical X-linked agammaglobulinemia. J Pediatr 112:688–694, 1988.

Conley ME, Rapalus L, Boylin EC, Rohrer J, Minegishi Y. Gene conversion events contribute to the polymorphic variation of the surrogate light chain gene lambda 5/14.1. Clin Immunol 93:162–167, 1999.

Conley ME, Rohrer J, Minegishi Y. X-linked agammaglobulinemia. Clin Rev Allergy Immunol 19:183–204, 2000a.

Conley ME, Rohrer J, Rapalus L, Boylin EC, Minegishi Y. Defects in early B-cell development: comparing the consequences of abnormalities in pre-BCR signaling in the human and the mouse. Immunol Rev 178:75–90, 2000b.

Conley ME, Sweinberg SK. Females with a disorder phenotypically identical to X-linked agammaglobulinemia. J Clin Immunol 12:139–143, 1992.

Cook GP, Tomlinson IM, Walter G, Riethman H, Carter NP, Buluwela L, Winter G, Rabbitts TH. A map of the human immunoglobulin VH locus completed by analysis of the telomeric region of chromosome 14q. Nat Genet 7:162–168, 1994.

Cooper DN, Youssoufian H. The CpG dinucleotide and human genetic disease. Hum Genet 78:151–155, 1988.

De La Morena M, Haire RN, Ohta Y, Nelson RP, Litman RT, Day NK, Good RA, Litman GW. Predominance of sterile immunoglobulin transcripts in a female phenotypically resembling Bruton's agammaglobulinemia. Eur J Immunol 25:809–815, 1995.

de Weers M, Brouns GS, Hinshelwood S, Kinnon C, Schuurman RKB, Hendriks RW, Borst J. B-cell antigen receptor stimulation activates the human Bruton's tyrosine kinase, which is deficient in X-linked agammaglobulinemia. J Biol Chem 269:23857–23860, 1994.

Erikson J, Martinis J, Croce CM. Assignment of the genes for human lambda immunoglobulin chains to chromosome 22. Nature 294:173–175, 1981.

Farrar JE, Rohrer J, Conley ME. Neutropenia in X-linked agammaglobulinemia. Clin Immunol Immunopathol 81:271–276, 1996.

Fearon ER, Winkelstein JA, Civin CI, Pardoll DM, Vogelstein B. Carrier detection in X-linked agammaglobulinemia by analysis of X-chromosome inactivation. N Engl J Med 316:427–431, 1987.

Friedlander RM, Nussenzweig MC, Leder P. Complete nucleotide sequence of the membrane form of the human IgM heavy chain. Nucl Acids Res 18:4278, 1990.

Fu C, Chan AC. Identification of two tyrosine phosphoproteins, pp70 and pp68, which interact with phospholipase Cγ, Grb2, and Vav after B cell antigen receptor activation. J Biol Chem 272:27362–27368, 1997.

Fu C, Turck CW, Kurosaki T, Chan AC. BLNK: a central linker protein in B cell activation. Immunity 9:93–103, 1998.

Goitsuka R, Fujimura Y, Mamada H, Umeda A, Morimura T, Uetsuka K, Doi K, Tsuji S, Kitamura D. BASH, a novel signaling molecule preferentially expressed in B cells of the bursa of Fabricius. J Immunol 161:5804–5808, 1998.

Gong S, Nussenzweig MC. Regulation of an early developmental checkpoint in the B cell pathway by Ig beta. Science 272:411–414, 1996.

Good RA. Agammaglobulinemia: a provocative experiment of nature. Bull Univ Minnesota Hosp 26:1–19, 1954a.

Good RA. Clinical Investigations in patients with agammaglobulinemia. J Lab Clin Med 44:803, 1954b.

Ha H, Barnoski BL, Sun L, Emanuel BS, Burrows PD. Structure, chromosomal localization, and methylation pattern of the human mb-1 gene. J Immunol 152:5749–5757, 1994.

Hoffman HM, Bastian JF, Bird LM. Humoral immunodeficiency with facial dysmorphology and limb anomalies: a new syndrome. Clin Dysmorphol 10:1–8, 2001.

Hoffman H, Winchester R, Schulkind M, Frias JL, Ayoub EM, Good RA. Hypoimmunoglobulinemia with normal T cell function in female siblings. Clin Immunol Immunopathol 7:364–371, 1977.

Hombach J, Tsubata T, Leclercq L, Stappert H, Reth M. Molecular components of the B-cell antigen receptor complex of the IgM class. Nature 343:760–762, 1990.

Ishiai M, Kurosaki M, Pappu R, Okawa K, Ronko I, Fu C, Shibata M, Iwamatsu A, Chan AC, Kurosaki T. BLNK required for coupling Syk to PLC gamma 2 and Rac1-JNK in B cells. Immunity 10:117–125, 1999.

Jackman JK, Motto DG, Sun Q, Tanemoto M, Turck CW, Peltz GA, Koretzky GA, Findell PR. Molecular cloning of SLP-76, a 76-kDa tyrosine phosphoprotein associated with Grb2 in T cells. J Biol Chem 270: 7029–7032, 1995.

Janeway CA, Apt L, Gitlin D. Agammaglobulinemia. Trans Assoc Am Physician 66:200–202, 1953.

Jou ST, Carpino N, Takahashi Y, Piekorz R, Chao JR, Carpino N, Wang D, Ihle JN. Essential, nonredundant role for the phosphoinositide 3-kinase p110delta in signaling by the B-cell receptor complex. Mol Cell Biol 22:8580–8591, 2002.

Jumaa H, Wollscheid B, Mitterer M, Wienands J, Reth M, Nielsen PJ. Abnormal development and function of B lymphocytes in mice deficient for the signaling adaptor protein SLP-65. Immunity 11:547–554, 1999.

Kawakami Y, Yao L, Miura T, Tsukada S, Witte ON, Kawakami T. Tyrosine phosphorylation and activation of Bruton tyrosine kinase upon FcεRI cross-linking. Mol Cell Biol 14:5108–5113, 1994.

Kerr WG, Cooper MD, Feng L, Burrows PD, Hendershot LM. Mu heavy chains can associate with a pseudo-light chain complex (psi L) in human pre-B cell lines. Int Immunol 1:355–361, 1989.

Kitamura D, Kudo A, Schaal S, Muller W, Melchers F, Rajewsky K. A critical role of lambda 5 protein in B cell development. Cell 69:823–831, 1992.

Kitamura D, Roes J, Kuhn R, Rajewsky K. A B cell–deficient mouse by targeted disruption of the membrane exon of the immunoglobulin mu chain gene. Nature 350:423–426, 1991.

Kudo A, Melchers F. A second gene, VpreB in the lambda 5 locus of the mouse, which appears to be selectively expressed in pre-B lymphocytes. EMBO J 6:2267–2272, 1987.

Kurosaki T. Genetic analysis of B cell antigen receptor signaling. Annu Rev Immunol 17:555–592, 1999.

Lan N, Howrey RP, Lee SW, Smith CA, Sullenger BA. Ribozyme-mediated repair of sickle beta-globin mRNAs in erythrocyte precursors. Science 280:1593–1596, 1998.

Lederman HM, Winkelstein JA. X-linked agammaglobulinemia: an analysis of 96 patients. Medicine 64:145–156, 1985.

Leitges M, Schmedt C, Guinamard R, Davoust J, Schaal S, Stabel S, Tarakhovsky A. Immunodeficiency in protein kinase cβ-deficient mice. Science 273:788–791, 1996.

Lin H, Grosschedl R. Failure of B-cell differentiation in mice lacking the transcription factor EBF. Nature 376:263–267, 1995.

Loffert D, Schaal S, Ehlich A, Hardy RR, Zou YR, Muller W, Rajewsky K. Early B-cell development in the mouse: insights from mutations introduced by gene targeting. Immunol Rev 137:135–153, 1994.

Lopez GE, Porpiglia AS, Hogan MB, Matamoros N, Krasovec S, Pignata C, Smith CI, Hammarstrom L, Bjorkander J, Belohradsky BH, Casariego GF, Garcia Rodriguez MC, Conley ME. Clinical and molecular analysis of patients with defects in micro heavy chain gene. J Clin Invest 110: 1029–1035, 2002.

Macchi P, Villa A, Gillani S, Sacco MG, Frattini A, Porta F, Ugazio AG, Johnston JA, Candotti F, O'Shea JJ, Vezzoni P, Notarangelo LD. Mutations of Jak-3 gene in patients with autosomal severe combined immune deficiency (SCID). Nature 377:65–68, 1995.

Matsuda T, Takahashi-Tezuka M, Fukada T, Okuyama Y, Fujitani Y, Tsukada S, Mano H, Hirai H, Witte ON, Hirano T. Association and activation of Btk and Tec tyrosine kinases by gp130, a signal transducer of the interleukin-6 family of cytokines. Blood 85:627–633, 1995.

McKinney RE Jr, Katz SL, Wilfert CM. Chronic enteroviral meningoencephalitis in agammaglobulinemic patients. Rev Infect Dis 9:334–356, 1987.

Meffre E, LeDeist F, de Saint-Basile G, Deville A, Fougereau M, Fischer A, Schiff C. A human non-XLA immunodeficiency disease characterized by blockage of B cell development at an early proB cell stage. J Clin Invest 98:1519–1526, 1996.

Melchers F, Karasuyama H, Haasner D, Bauer S, Kudo A, Sakaguchi N, Jameson B, Rolink A. The surrogate light chain in B-cell development. Immunol Today 14:60–68, 1993.

Milili M, Antunes H, Blanco-Betancourt C, Nogueiras A, Santos E, Vasconcelos J, Castro e Melo, Schiff C. A new case of autosomal recessive agammaglobulinaemia with impaired pre-B cell differentiation due to a large deletion of the IGH locus. Eur J Pediatr 161:479–484, 2002.

Minegishi Y, Coustan-Smith E, Rapalus L, Ersoy F, Campana D, Conley ME. Mutations in Igα (CD79a) result in a complete block in B cell development. J Clin Invest 104:1115–1121, 1999a.

Minegishi Y, Coustan-Smith E, Wang Y-H, Cooper MD, Campana D, Conley ME. Mutations in the human λ5/14.1 gene result in B cell deficiency and agammaglobulinemia. J Exp Med 187:71–77, 1998.

Minegishi Y, Hendershot LM, Conley ME. Novel mechanisms control the folding and assembly of lambda5/14.1 and VpreB to produce an intact surrogate light chain. Proc Natl Acad Sci USA 96:3041–3046, 1999b.

Minegishi Y, Rohrer J, Coustan-Smith E, Lederman HM, Pappu R, Campana D, Chan AC, Conley ME. An essential role for BLNK in human B cell development. Science 286:1954–1957, 1999c.

Mundt C, Licence S, Shimizu T, Melchers F, Martensson IL. Loss of precursor B cell expansion but not allelic exclusion in VpreB1/VpreB2 double-deficient mice. J Exp Med 193:435–445, 2001.

Nagasawa T, Hirota S, Tachibana K, Takakura N, Nishikawa S, Kitamura Y, Yoshida N, Kikutani H, Kishimoto T. Defects of B-cell lymphopoiesis and bone-marrow myelopoiesis in mice lacking the CXC chemokine PBSF/SDF-1. Nature 382:635–638, 1996.

Nomura K, Kanegane H, Karasuyama H, Tsukada S, Agematsu K, Murakami G, Sakazume S, Sako M, Tanaka R, Kuniya Y, Komeno T, Ishihara S, Hayashi K, Kishimoto T, Miyawaki T. Genetic defect in human X-linked agammaglobulinemia impedes a maturational evolution of pro-B cells into a later stage of pre-B cells in the B-cell differentiation pathway. Blood 96:610–617, 2000.

Nunez C, Nishimoto N, Gartland GL, Billips LG, Burrows PD, Kubagawa H, Cooper MD. B cells are generated throughout life in humans. J Immunol 156:866–872, 1996.

Ochs HD, Winkelstein. Disorders of the B-cell system. In: Stiehm ER, ed. Immunologic Disorders in Infants and Children, 4th ed. Philadelphia: WB Saunders, pp 296–338, 1996.

Oda A, Ikeda Y, Ochs HD, Druker BJ, Ozaki K, Handa M, Ariga T, Sakiyama Y, Witte ON, Wahl MI. Rapid tyrosine phosphorylation and activation of Bruton's tyrosine/Tec kinases in platelets induced by collagen binding or CD32 cross-linking. Blood 95:1663–1670, 2000.

Olsson PG, Rabbani H, Hammarstrom L, Smith CI. Novel human immunoglobulin heavy chain constant region gene deletion haplotypes characterized by pulsed-field electrophoresis. Clin Exp Immunol 94:84–90, 1993.

Pappu R, Cheng AM, Li B, Gong Q, Chiu C, Griffin N, White M, Sleckman BP, Chan AC. Requirement for B cell linker protein (BLNK) in B cell development. Science 286:1949–1954, 1999.

Pillai S, Baltimore D. Formation of disulphide-linked mu 2 omega 2 tetramers in pre-B cells by the 18K omega-immunoglobulin light chain. Nature 329:172–174, 1987.

Pivniouk V, Tsitsikov E, Swinton P, Rathbun G, Alt FW, Geha RS. Impaired viability and profound block in thymocyte development in mice lacking the adaptor protein SLP-76. Cell 94:229–238, 1998.

Quek LS, Bolen J, Watson SP. A role for Bruton's tyrosine kinase (Btk) in platelet activation by collagen. Curr Biol 8:1137–1140, 1998.

Rajewsky K. Clonal selection and learning in the antibody system. Nature 381:751–758, 1996.

Revy P, Busslinger M, Tashiro K, Arenzana F, Pillet P, Fischer A, Durandy A. A syndrome involving intrauterine growth retardation, microcephaly, cerebellar hypoplasia, B lymphocyte deficiency, and progressive pancytopenia. Pediatrics 105:E39, 2000.

Reynaud CA, Anquez V, Grimal H, Weill JC. A hyperconversion mechanism generates the chicken light chain preimmune repertoire. Cell 48:379–388, 1987.

Rice MC, Czymmek K, Kmiec EB. The potential of nucleic acid repair in functional genomics. Nat Biotechnol 19:321–326, 2001.

Rolink AG, Schaniel C, Andersson J, Melchers F. Selection events operating at various stages in B cell development. Curr Opin Immunol 13:202–207, 2001.

Russell SM, Tayebi N, Nakajima H, Riedy MC, Roberts JL, Aman MJ, Migone TS, Noguchi M, Markert ML, Buckley RH, O'Shea JJ, Leonard WJ. Mutation of Jak3 in a patient with SCID: essential role of Jak3 in lymphoid development. Science 270:797–800, 1995.

Sakaguchi N, Melchers F. Lambda 5, a new light-chain-related locus selectively expressed in pre-B lymphocytes. Nature 324:579–582, 1986.

Saouaf SJ, Mahajan S, Rowley RB, Kut SA, Fargnoli J, Burkhardt AL, Tsukada S, Witte ON, Bolen JB. Temporal differences in the activation of three classes of non-transmembrane protein tyrosine kinases following B-cell antigen receptor surface engagement. Proc Natl Acad Sci USA 91: 9524–9528, 1994.

Sato S, Katagiri T, Takaki S, Kikuchi Y, Hitoshi Y, Yonehara S, Tsukada S, Kitamura D, Watanabe T, Witte O, Takatsu K. IL-5 receptor–mediated tyrosine phosphorylation of SH2/SH3-containing proteins and activation of Bruton's tyrosine and Janus 2 kinases. J Exp Med 180:2101–2111, 1994.

Schiff C, Lemmers B, Deville A, Fougereau M, Meffre E. Autosomal primary immunodeficiencies affecting human bone marrow B-cell differentiation. Immunol Rev 178:91–98, 2000.

Schilham MW, Oosterwegel MA, Moerer P, Ya J, de Boer PA, van de Wetering M, Verbeek S, Lamers WH, Kruisbeek AM, Cumano A, Clevers H. Defects in cardiac outflow tract formation and pro-B-lymphocyte expansion in mice lacking Sox-4. Nature 380:711–714, 1996.

Srivannaboon K, Conley ME, Coustan-Smith E, Wang WC. Hypogammaglobulinemia and reduced numbers of B cells in children with myelodysplastic syndrome. Pediatr Hematol Oncol 23:122–125, 2001.

Suzuki H, Terauchi Y, Fujiwara M, Aizawa S, Yazaki Y, Kadowaki T, Koyasu S. Xid-like immunodeficiency in mice with disruption of the p85α subunit of phosphoinositide 3-kinase. Science 283:390–392, 1999.

Takada H, Kanegane H, Nomura A, Yamamoto K, Ihara K, Takahashi Y, Tsukada S, Miyawaki T, Hara T. Female agammaglobulinemia due to the Bruton tyrosine kinase deficiency caused by extremely skewed X-chromosome inactivation. Blood 103:185–187, 2004.

Thompson CB. Creation of immunoglobulin diversity by intrachromosomal gene conversion. Trends Genet 8:416–422, 1992.

Tokimasa S, Ohta H, Sawada A, Matsuda Y, Kim JY, Nishiguchi S, Hara J, Takihara Y. Lack of the Polycomb-group gene rae28 causes maturation arrest at the early B-cell developmental stage. Exp Hematol 29:93–103, 2001.

Torres RM, Flaswinkel H, Reth M, Rajewsky K. Aberrant B cell development and immune response in mice with a compromised BCR complex. Science 272:1804–1808, 1996.

Tsukada S, Saffran DC, Rawlings DJ, Parolini O, Allen RC, Klisak I, Sparkes RS, Kubagawa H, Mohandas T, Quan S, Belmont JW, Cooper MD, Conley ME, Witte ON. Deficient expression of a B cell cytoplasmic tyrosine kinase in human X-linked agammaglobulinemia. Cell 72:279–290, 1993.

Urbanek P, Wang ZQ, Fetka I, Wagner EF, Busslinger M. Complete block of early B cell differentiation and altered patterning of the posterior midbrain in mice lacking Pax5/BSAP. Cell 79:901–912, 1994.

Verloes A, Dresse MF, Keutgen H, Asplund C, Smith CI. Microphthalmia, facial anomalies, microcephaly, thumb and hallux hypoplasia, and agammaglobulinemia. Am J Med Genet 101:209–212, 2001.

Vetrie D, Vorechovsky I, Sideras P, Holland J, Davies A, Flinter F, Hammarstrom L, Kinnon C, Levinsky R, Bobrow M, Smith CIE, Bentley DR. The gene involved in X-linked agammaglobulinemia is a member of the src family of protein-tyrosine kinases. Nature 361:226–233, 1993.

Wang D, Feng J, Wen R, Marine JC, Sangster MY, Parganas E, Hoffmeyer A, Jackson CW, Cleveland JL, Murray PJ, Ihle JN. Phospholipase Cγ2 is essential in the functions of B cell and several Fc receptors. Immunity 13: 25–35, 2000.

Wang Y, Kanegane H, Sanal O, Tezcan I, Ersoy F, Futatani T, Miyawaki T. Novel Igα (CD79a) gene mutation in a Turkish patient with B cell–deficient agammaglobulinemia. Am J Med Genet 108:333–336, 2002.

Wienands J, Schweikert J, Wollscheid B, Jumaa H, Nielsen PJ, Reth M. SLP-65: a new signaling component in B lymphocytes which requires expression of the antigen receptor for phosphorylation. J Exp Med 188:791–795, 1998.

Wood WJ, Thompson AA, Korenberg J, Chen XN, May W, Wall R, Denny CT, Wood WJ Jr. Isolation and chromosomal mapping of the human immunoglobulin-associated B29 gene (IGB). Genomics 16:187–192, 1993.

Yamazaki T, Takeda K, Gotoh K, Takeshima H, Akira S, Kurosaki T. Essential immunoregulatory role for BCAP in B cell development and function. J Exp Med 195:535–545, 2002.

Yankee TM, Clark EA. Signaling through the B cell antigen receptor in developing B cells. Rev Immunogenet 2:185–203, 2000.

Yel L, Minegishi Y, Coustan-Smith E, Buckley RH, Trubel H, Pachman LM, Kitchingman GR, Campana D, Rohrer J, Conley ME. Mutations in the mu heavy chain gene in patients with agammaglobulinemia. N Engl J Med 335:1486–1493, 1996.

Zhuang Y, Soriano P, Weintraub H. The helix-loop-helix gene E2A is required for B cell formation. Cell 79:875–884, 1994.

23

Genetic Approach to Common Variable Immunodeficiency and IgA Deficiency

LENNART HAMMARSTRÖM and C. I. EDVARD SMITH

Common variable immunodeficiency (CVID), Mendelian Inheritance in Man (MIM) number 240500, affects approximately 1 in 10,000–100,000 individuals. The patients display a marked reduction in serum levels of both immunoglobulin G (IgG) and IgA. In half of the patients, IgM is also reduced. The onset of disease shows two peaks, around 1–5 and 16–20 years of age (Hermaszewski and Webster, 1993) and is equally distributed between the two sexes. The disorder may appear in previously immunologically normal individuals, although the induction phase has been documented only in a few cases (Smith et al., 1985). Usually the patients present with clinical symptoms due to the hypogammaglobulinemia, as they suffer from frequent respiratory and gastrointestinal tract infections (see Table 23.2). In addition to the B cell defect, variable degrees of T cell dysfunction have frequently been noted in CVID patients. Low or normal proportions of CD19-positive cells are also often observed, a finding that distinguishes "classical" CVID patients from those with a concomitant thymoma.

With 0.05 g/l of serum IgAD as the upper limit for diagnosis, selective IgA deficiency (IgAD), MIM number 137100, is the most common form of immunodeficiency in the Western world and affects approximately 1 in 600 individuals. Great variability in the prevalence can, however, be found in different ethnic groups, and a markedly lower frequency has been reported in mongoloid populations (Table 23.1), suggesting a genetic influence. In about two-thirds of cases, the deficiency does not lead to an increased occurrence of infections, whereas the remaining patients suffer from bacterial infections in both the upper and lower respiratory tract (Table 23.2). The defect is manifested already at the stem cell level, and transfer of bone marrow from an IgA-deficient donor to a normal recipient results in IgA deficiency in the recipient (Hammarstrom et al., 1985c) whereas transfer of bone marrow from a normal individual to an

IgA-deficient patient will correct the defect (Kurobane et al., 1991).

The genes for $\alpha 1$ and $\alpha 2$ can readily be demonstrated in the genome of both CVID (Smith and Hammarstrom, 1984) and IgAD patients (Hammarstrom et al., 1985a), and the silent genes can be re-expressed in the children of IgA-deficient parents (Hammarstrom et al., 1987). These findings strongly suggest that the defect is due to dysregulation of the expression of the Ig genes. In a few selected cases, the defect is restricted to one of the two subclasses, and these cases are most often although not invariably due to deletions of the corresponding α chain gene (Migone et al., 1984; Lefranc et al., 1991). Some of these mutations have been identified by screening of healthy blood donors (Lefranc et al., 1982, 1991; Rabbani et al., 1996), whereas a few have been found in patients prone to infections. Thus, selective IgG1 and IgG2 deficiency caused by homozygous gene deletions have both been reported in patients with an increased susceptibility to infections (Smith et al., 1989; Tashita et al., 1998).

By definition, IgAD is expected to be selective and confined to the IgA class. In many cases, however, a simultaneous change in the IgG subclass pattern is seen with a lack of specific anti-polysaccharide antibodies of the IgG2 subclass (Hammarstrom et al., 1985d) or a total lack of serum IgG2 (Oxelius et al., 1981), IgG4, and IgE (Hammarstrom et al., 1986), reflecting a relative or absolute block in switching to genes downstream of the $\gamma 1$. Progression from IgAD to CVID has been observed in a number of cases, suggesting that the two diseases are related and may represent faults of the same underlying defect.

During the past few years, mutations in a number of genes associated with B cell differentiation, including *ICOS, TACI, BAFF-R,* and *CD19*, have been found in patients with CVID and IgAD. However, the molecular basis still remains unknown in the vast majority of patients.

313

Table 23.1. Frequency of IgA Deficiency in Different Ethnic Populations*

Reference	Population	No.	IgA Cutoff	Frequency
Hobbs, 1968	England	11,000	<0.05	1/480
Frommel et al., 1973	France	15,200	<0.05	1/2172
Pai et al., 1974	Canada	15,500	<0.05	1/1300
Koistinen, 1975	Finland	64,588	<0.01	1/396
Vyas et al., 1975	USA	73,569	<0.1	1/650
Holt et al., 1977	England	29,745	<0.04	1/522
Hammarstrom and Smith[†]	Sweden	34,440	<0.05	1/574
Ulfarsson et al., 1982	Iceland	15,663	<0.1	1/633
Yadav and Iyngkaran, 1979	Malaysia	2025	<0.05	0/2025
Kanoh et al., 1986	Japan	222,597	<0.05	1/18,500
Ozawa et al., 1986	Japan	93,020	<0.03	1/23,255
Ezeoke, 1988	Nigeria	3772	<0.01	1/629[‡]
Carneiro-Sampaio et al., 1989	Brazil	11,576	<0.05	1/965
Feng, 1992	China	33,171	<0.05	1/4100

*Only data from major studies on Caucasians have been included.
[†]Unpublished data.
[‡]Only children were studied.

Table 23.2. Clinical Variables in Immunoglobulin-Deficient Patients

Symptom	CVID	IgAD	Common Pathogens
Sinusitis	+++	++	Hemophilus influenzae
	+++	+	Streptococcus pneumonie
	++		Moraxella catharralis
Pneumonia	+++	(+)	Hemophilus influenzae
	+++		Streptococcus pneumonie
Bronchiectasies	++		
Gastrointestinal	+	(+)	Giardia lamblia
infections	+		Campylobacter jejuni
belong together			
Splenomegaly	+		
Lymphadenopathy	++		
Conjunctivitis	+		
Meningitis	+		ECHO virus
Viral infections	+		Hepatitis C, varicella-zoster virus
Cancer risk	+		
Autoimmunity	+	+	
Hemolytic anemia	(+)		
Thrombocytopenia	(+)		
Urogenital infection	(+)		Ureaplasma urealyticum

(+), infrequent; +, occasional; ++, frequent; +++, very frequent.

Historical Overview

In 1952 the first report of Ig deficiency appeared (Bruton, 1952). This report inspired a large number of investigators to analyze Ig levels in patients prone to infections (reviewed in Good et al., 1962; Sideras and Smith, 1995; Smith and Notarangelo, 1997). At the time, knowledge on lymphocyte subsets was lacking, and patients with autosomal recessive severe combined immunodeficiency were sometimes referred to as having agammaglobulinemia (Keidan et al., 1953). Females with CVID had already been reported the year after Bruton's original description (Olhagen, 1953). Both adult-onset (Olhagen, 1953; Grant and Wallace, 1954; Jacobsen, 1954; Lang et al., 1954; Prasad and Koza, 1954; Saslaw and Wall 1954) and congenital agammaglobulinemia in females (Pearce and Perinpanayagam, 1957) were described. Adult onset in male patients with a CVID phenotype was also reported (Olhagen, 1953), as reviewed in Citron (1957), who described additional patients suffering from agammaglobulinemia with concomitant splenomegaly.

The first study on selective Ig deficiency reported the absence of IgG in the hyper-IgM syndrome (Israel-Asselain et al., 1960; Rosen et al., 1961). In 1964, IgA deficiency was observed in two healthy laboratory workers, clearly demonstrating that IgA may be dispensable in certain individuals (Rockey et al., 1964). However, on the basis of a review of 30 cases, it was later determined that this defect frequently results in a propensity for infections (Ammann and Hong, 1971).

The classification of Ig deficiencies was often complicated by the lack of suitable techniques. In the mid-1960s Rosen and Janeway subdivided the antibody deficiency syndromes into six forms. Among these were congenital forms, including sex-linked and sporadic/autosomal recessive inheritance; acquired agammaglobulinemia; and a third subgroup, congenital and acquired dysgammaglobulinemia, which included IgAD and the hyper-IgM syndrome (Rosen and Janeway, 1966). The present classification of Ig deficiency dates back to 1973 (Cooper et al., 1973).

Mode of Inheritence

Familial inheritance of the deficiency is observed in approximately 20% of cases, and CVID and IgAD may both be present in the same family. In rare instances, patients with IgAD may progress to CVID, a phenomenon suggesting that the disorders reflect facets of the same underlying disease (Schaffer et al., 1989). These data therefore strongly argue that the two disorders represent an allelic condition with a variable expression of a common defect, and there is substantial evidence supporting a common genetic susceptibility. The finding of Ig deficiency in only one of two monozygotic twins (Huntley and Stephenson, 1968, Lewkonia et al., 1976, Ulfarsson et al., 1982) suggests an environmental, possibly infectious, agent as a triggering factor.

Clinical and Pathological Manifestations

Infections

Patients with IgAD and CVID suffer from a variety of respiratory and gastrointestinal tract infections (Table 23.2). The severity of infections reflects the degree of immune dysfunction and is thus more pronounced in patients with hypogammaglobulinemia. Enlarged lymph nodes and spleen are noted in up to half of patients with CVID, but not in patients with X-linked agammaglobulinemia (XLA) (Curtin et al., 1995), and may reflect persistence of low-grade infections. The lymph nodes may show a striking reactive follicular hyperplasia, and non-caseating granulomas in the liver (Color Plate 23.I) and skin (Color Plate 23.II) occur. The gastrointestinal tract may also be involved in this process with a characteristic nodular lymphoid hyperplasia. The spectrum of infections in IgAD and CVID patients is, however, usually rather limited. Some of these are highlighted below.

Hemophilus influenzae is a common pathogen in the human respiratory tract. The majority of isolates are non-encapsulated and fall into the category of serologically nontypable strains, which often cause acute otitis media, acute sinusitis, conjunctivitis, pneumonia, and bronchitis in immunocompetent patients. These bacteria also constitute the major pathogen in CVID patients who suffer from frequent upper respiratory tract infections. Patients may remain colonized for years with the same strain in spite of "adequate" γ-globulin therapy and antibiotics (Samuelson et al., 1995) and may develop multiple bouts of symptoms. It is still unclear why the bacteria are poorly cleared by antimicrobial therapy but intracellular growth may occur in crypt cells in the adenoid and tonsils.

Moraxella catharralis and *Streptococcus pneumoniae* are the second and third most common pathogens in patients with CVID; both organisms give rise to upper respiratory tract infections. In earlier published series of patients, serious pulmonary manifestations such as bronchiectasis, pulmonary fibrosis, and respiratory failure were not uncommon (Dukes et al., 1978; Hausser et al., 1983; Bjorkander et al., 1984). However, increasing awareness of immunodeficiency disorders, early diagnosis, and prompt institution of antibiotic therapy and γ-globulin substitution have resulted in far lower frequency of severe respiratory tract complications (Sweinberg et al., 1991; Hermaszewski and Webster, 1993).

Mycoplasmas have been increasingly recognized as pathogens in humans. *Mycoplasma pneumoniae* is a common cause of pneumonia in both normal and immunodeficient individuals. Two additional species, *Mycoplasma hominis* and *Ureaplasma urealyticum*, have also been implicated in a variety of infections, particularly in the urogenital tract. Each of these species has also been isolated from synovial fluid of patients with acute arthritis (Color Plate 23.III), and a role for these organisms in chronic arthritis has therefore been suggested.

Hypogammaglobulinemic patients appear to be highly susceptible to systemic mycoplasma infections, but the diagnosis may be delayed because of the insidious onset of symptoms. As antibodies are of major importance to combat these infections, CVID patients may suffer a protracted clinical course, and severe sequelae have been reported (Webster et al., 1978; Taylor-Robinson et al., 1985; Vogler et al., 1985; Roifman et al., 1986; Kraus et al., 1988; Jorup-Ronstrom et al., 1989; Mohiuddin et al., 1991) with extensive joint destruction (Fig. 23.I).

The use of contaminated γ-globulin preparations has been responsible for several outbreaks of hepatitis C infections in CVID patients. The long-term prognosis for these patients is poor, with about one-third developing cirrhosis within 10 years and ultimately dying of liver failure. In the latest outbreak, identical sequences for the envelope protein genes could be identified in the incriminated batch of γ-globulin and in the sera from infected patients (Widell et al., 1997).

Transient recovery of the ability to produce immunoglobulins at the time of hepatitis C infection has been reported in a few patients (Hammarstrom and Smith, 1986; Osur et al., 1987) and has also been demonstrated in patients infected with HIV (Morell et al., 1986; Webster et al., 1986; Wright et al., 1987). These findings strongly suggest an immunoregulatory dysfunction as a cause of CVID.

Lack of immunoglobulins might affect the acquisition and persistence of hepatitis C infections, and an increased prevalence of hepatitis C in IgAD patients has previously been suggested (Benbassat et al., 1973; Ilan et al., 1993). However, because IgAD may develop during the course of the hepatitis infection (Hishitani et al., 1980), the association of hepatitis C and IgAD probably reflects an effect rather than a cause.

Inflammatory Bowel Disease

An infectious etiology of inflammatory bowel diseases (IBD) has previously been strongly suspected but no microorganism has been etiologically linked to these disorders. Mice in which the genes for interleukin (IL)-2 or IL-10 or the T cell receptor (Mombaerts et al., 1993) genes have been inactivated (knockout mice) exhibit an inflammatory reaction in the gastrointestinal tract, which both histologically and "clinically" resembles human IBD. An infectious origin of the intestinal symptoms in these mice is likely, since the animals do not suffer from IBD if kept under germ-free conditions (Kuhn et al., 1993; Sadlack et al., 1993). These observations support the involvement of a microbial agent in the pathogenetic process.

A few IgAD and CVID patients have previously been described who suffer from Crohn's disease (Eggert et al., 1969; Douglas et al., 1971; Soltoft et al., 1972; Hodgson and Jewell, 1977; Saxon et al., 1977; Elson et al., 1984; Abramowsky and Sorensen, 1988; Teahon et al., 1994) or ulcerative colitis (Hollinger, 1967; Kaplinsky et al., 1973; Matuchansky et al., 1977; Curzio et al., 1985), but an association has not been ascertained because of the lack of a sufficiently large patient population.

Cancer Incidence

A high frequency of cancer, especially malignant lymphomas, has been described among patients with primary immunodeficiencies, but there are few investigations following patients over time and comparing cancer incidence with a background population for

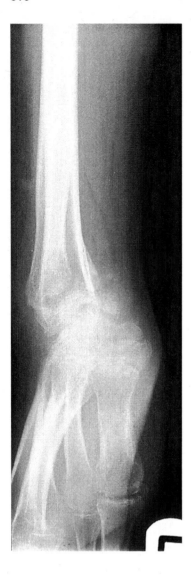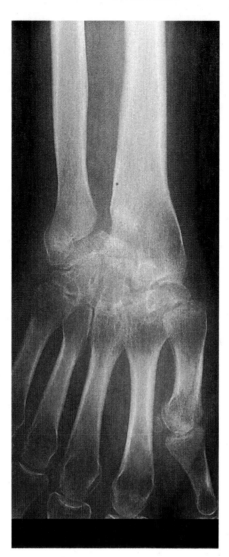

Figure 23.1. Destruction of carpal bones and subluxation of the wrist joint in a 42-year-old patient with common variable immunodeficiency and *M. hominis* infection.

estimation of a relative risk. A British prospective study from 1985 (Kinlen et al.) reported a 23-fold increased risk for malignant lymphoma and 50-fold increase for gastric cancer among 377 patients with hypogammaglobulinemia, primarily CVID. Patients were followed for an average of 10 years. In another study, 98 patients with CVID were followed for up to 13 years, and the risk for lymphomas was estimated to be more than 100-fold increased (Cunningham-Rundles et al., 1987). This is comparable to the relative risk for non-Hodgkin's lymphoma found among 301 patients with combined immunodeficiencies such as the Wiskott-Aldrich syndrome (Perry et al., 1980). However, in a recent study on a large number of IgA-deficient individuals, followed for 20 years, no increased risk for malignancy could be observed (Mellemkjaer et al., 2002), although a slightly increased incidence in malignant lymphoma and stomach cancer was noted in CVID patients followed for a similar time. The etiology of lymphoproliferative malignancy in primary immunodeficiency may involve infection with Epstein-Barr virus (EBV), defects in immunoregulations, and/or genetic instability, and previous experiments in γ-globulin-treated SCID mice repopulated with human peripheral blood lymphocytes from EBV-positive donors show a strong inhibitory effect of this therapy on tumor formation (Abedi et al., 1993). The excess of gastric cancer in immunodeficient patients may be related to a reduced immune response against *Helicobacter pylori*. However, we did not ob-

serve an increased prevalence in IgAD patients or healthy IgAD blood donors, nor was there any evidence for a higher titer of IgG antibodies against the microorganism in carriers. These findings argue against a pivotal role for IgA in the protection against infection (Bogstedt et al., 1996). Long-term studies are, however, not available to answer the question of whether the risk for ulcer development or gastric cancer is greater in IgAD-seropositive individuals than in a control population.

Autoimmunity

The list of autoimmune disorders associated with IgAD and CVID has grown to include systemic lupus erythematosus, rheumatoid arthritis, Sjögren syndrome, dermatomyositis, thyroiditis, celiac disease, insulin-dependent diabetes mellitus, pernicious anemia, Addison disease, idiopathic thrombocytopenic purpura (ITP), and autoimmune hemolytic anemia. This is in stark contrast to XLA, in which autoimmunity is rare (see Chapter 21). In an early survey of IgAD patients, 37% were in fact found to have autoimmune disease or autoimmune phenomena (Amman and Hong, 1971). Similar data on the prevalence of autoantibodies in IgAD patients have been obtained through use of a panel of antinuclear antibody-related antigens (Goshen et al., 1989) and may suggest a predisposition to autoimmune symptoms in antibody-deficient individuals. Whether this is related to genetic factors (see below) or caused by increased exposure to putatively cross-reactive antigens through an increased permeability of the respiratory and gastrointestinal mucosa remains unknown.

Anti-IgA Antibodies

Antibodies against IgA are a common finding in patients with IgAD or CVID and up to 60% show demonstrable titers. The etiology of this immune response is unknown; it could be due to an autoimmune reaction against autologous IgA (Mochizuki et al., 1993) or occur through immunization via exposure to blood products containing IgA (Cunningham-Rundles et al., 1986; Frankel et al., 1986) or induced by IgA epitope-mimicking food products. Approximately 20–40% of the patients with IgAD have developed anti-IgA antibodies at the time of diagnosis without being exposed to IgA-containing blood products. Antibodies against IgA are usually of the IgG class, mainly IgG1 and IgG4 (Hammarstrom et al., 1983), but IgM anti-IgA antibodies may also be present (Bjorkander et al., 1987). In exceptional cases, the antibodies have been suggested to be of the IgE class (Burks et al., 1986; Ferreira et al., 1988), which may give rise to serious anaphylactic phenomena upon injection of IgA-containing blood products. Several severe reactions have indeed been reported after infusion of IgA-containing preparations (Vyas et al., 1968; Schmidt et al., 1969), and different methods have been tried to reduce or eliminate the concentration of anti-IgA antibodies in selected patients. Development of antibodies of differing specificities is genetically determined, and the induction of anti-IgA antibodies has also been suggested to be associated both with major histocompatibility complex (MHC) alleles (Strothman et al., 1989; Olerup et al., 1990) and Gm allotypes (Hammarstrom et al., 1985b).

Maternal transmission of IgAD, mediated by placentally transferred anti-IgA antibodies, could theoretically contribute to induction of the deficiency in selected cases of IgAD (Petty et al., 1985; de Laat et al., 1991). Human anti-IgA antibodies are transferred to the fetus and have been shown to inhibit IgA production in human cells in vitro (Warrington et al., 1982; Hammarstrom et al., 1983).

Laboratory Findings

The pathognomonic hallmark of IgAD is a low level of serum IgA with normal levels of IgM and IgG (Table 23.3). However, raised levels of IgG, mainly IgG1 and IgG3, may be seen in up to a third of the patients. In most instances IgAD is defined as <0.05 g/l of serum IgA in adults. Almost invariably, there is a concomitant lack of secretory IgA, although a dichotomy has been documented in exceptional cases, and in small children, a saliva sample may suffice for determination of IgA status, thus avoiding blood sampling.

In CVID, IgA is usually absent and IgG levels are decreased, whereas IgM is low or absent in only half of the cases (Table 23.3). There is currently no recognized diagnostic level of IgG in CVID, although our working definition would suggest <3 g/l in adults.

Surface IgA-expressing B cells are usually low in patients with IgAD, and most cells express an immature phenotype with most IgA-positive cells simultaneously expressing IgD (Conley and Cooper, 1981). In contrast, the proportion of surface Ig-positive cells remains unaffected in most CVID patients. However the B cells do not mature properly, and plasma cell numbers are low in the bone marrow. A large number of additional cell surface CD markers have been analyzed in IgAD and CVID, but their diagnostic value is limited, although fluorescence-activated cell sorter (FACS) profiles have been suggested for subclassification of CVID patients (Warnatz et al., 2002). Similar restrictions

Table 23.3. Characteristic Laboratory Findings in IgA Deficiency and Common Variable Immunodeficiency

Parameter	CVID	IgAD
Serum IgM levels	Low/normal	Normal
Serum IgG levels	Low	Normal/high
Serum IgA levels	Low	Low
Secretory IgA	Low	Low
Surface IgM+ cells	Normal	Normal
Surface IgG+ cells	Normal	Normal
Surface IgA+ cells	Normal	Low/normal
Autoantibodies (anti-IgA)	20%–30%	40%–60%
Lymphocyte CD markers	(Normal)	Normal
Mitogen responsiveness	Low/normal	Normal
Plasma cells (bone marrow)	Low	Normal

apply to in vitro testing with a panel of mitogens such as phytohemagglutinin (PHA), although it may aid in determining the extent of the T cell defect seen in a proportion of CVID patients.

The age at which the disease manifests itself may vary. In IgAD, most cases are probably manifest at birth, although formal studies on this point are lacking. Induction of "idiopathic" IgAD has actually been described in a few children.

CVID may develop in children, although most patients present with symptoms as adults. A biphasic distribution, with incidence peaks at 1–5 and 16–20 years of age, has been suggested (Hermaszewski and Webster, 1993).

Antibodies against IgA are also typical markers of IgAD and CVID. These autoantibodies are not seen in individuals with normal levels of IgA.

Genetic Component of IgA Deficiency and Common Variable Immunodeficiency

Heritability of IgA Deficiency and Common Variable Immunodeficiency

Most cases of IgAD and CVID described to date have been sporadic, but familial cases have been observed, and a susceptibility trait can occasionally be traced back for many generations (Wollheim et al., 1964). Thus far, more than 100 families with multiple cases of IgAD have been reported in the literature (for references see Vorechovsky et al., 1995; Kralovicova et al., 2003). The mode of inheritance of the deficiency has been suggested to be either recessive or dominant. In 20% of the published cases, both IgAD and CVID occurred in the same family, usually presenting with CVID in the parental generation and IgAD in the children.

On the basis of extensive segregation analysis in hundreds of families, it was recently shown that a single gene is likely responsible for the regulation of serum levels of IgA (Borecki et al., 1994). Since no skewed sex ratio has been found in IgAD patients, it is possible that a single, autosomally inherited gene with a limited penetrance is responsible for the development of the defect. This hypothesis has prompted a search for the implicated gene.

Chromosome 6

The human leukocyte antigens (HLA) are implicated in the genetic susceptibility to a large number of diseases. Some of the diseases associated with HLA class II are related to specific amino acids or epitopes on the domain of the DR or DQ molecules.

As early as the late 1970s, an association between IgAD and certain HLA types was suggested. However, because these investigations were carried out on groups of patients with a variety of diseases, the findings may have been secondary and due to an association with the primary diseases. In the early 1980s, it was shown for the first time that there was an association between isolated IgA deficiency and the MHC region (Oen et al., 1982), in particular the HLA class II region (Hammarstrom and Smith, 1983). A genetic predisposition similar to that found in IgA deficiency has also been observed in patients with CVID (Schaffer et al., 1989; Olerup et al., 1992), although the gene(s) implicated varies.

A report by Wilton et al. (1985) provided the first suggestion that genes within the MHC class III region are associated with IgA deficiency, as they found that deletions, duplications, or defects at the C4A or 21-hydroxylase (CYP21) loci were present on the majority of independent MHC haplotypes in the studied IgAD subjects. It was later reported that IgAD and CVID share polymorphisms of MHC class III complement genes (Schaffer et al., 1989). In a subsequent study by Volanakis and coworkers (1992), 12 IgAD and 19 CVID individuals from 21 families and their relatives were investigated. They found that a small number of MHC haplotypes were shared between most of the immunodeficient individuals and that at least one of two of these haplotypes was present in 77% of these individuals. These authors later confirmed their findings in a report on a family with two IgAD and three CVID members (Ashman et al., 1992). Similar results have been reported by Howe and coworkers (1991), who found a striking increase of *C4A* gene deletions in CVID patients, which were associated with specific HLA or tumor necrosis factor-α (TNF-α) gene polymorphisms.

We have previously investigated 110 Swedish IgAD subjects by C4 and factor B typing (Bucin et al., 1991). Of these individuals, 18% were C4A deficient compared to 5.8% of the controls ($p < 0.01$). No significant deviations in the distribution of factor B variants were observed. Results from C4 typing in CVID patients showed a similar change to that in the IgAD patients compared to controls (Truedsson et al., 1995). Because of the strong linkage disequilibrium within the MHC, most haplotypes with C4A gene deletion are examples of an extended haplotype (Schneider et al., 1986).

The strong linkage disequilibrium of the MHC region makes the location of the locus associated with IgAD and CVID difficult to determine, and this question is still not answered. On the basis of data on MHC class III variants in these immunodeficiencies, a possible location in the class III region between the C4B and the C2 genes has been suggested (Volanakis et al., 1992).

Our own work suggests instead that the class II region, and in particular the DQ locus, is involved in mediating both susceptibility and resistance to development of IgAD (Olerup et al., 1990, 1991; Kralovicova et al., 2003) and CVID (Olerup et al., 1992; Kralovicova et al., 2003). A comparison of the sequences of the polymorphic amino-terminal domain of the DQ chain showed that the three susceptibility haplotypes all had a neutral alanine or valine at position 57, whereas the protective allele carried the negatively charged aspartic acid at this position. Recently, independent reports have suggested that two distinct loci, one in the class II region and one in the class III region, located on different MHC haplotypes, confer susceptibility to development of IgAD and CVID (de la Concha et al., 2002; Gual et al., 2004; Schroeder et al., 2004).

Chromosome 18

IgAD in patients with aberrations of chromosome 18 was first recognized in the mid-1960s. Deletions of the short arm, long arm, or ring chromosome 18 all result in Ig deficiency in approximately

half of the reported cases (for references see Hammarstrom and Smith, 1999). Because the exact breakpoint has not been delineated in most of these patients, it is possible that the extent of the deletion determines whether a deficient state will ensue or not. However, the results achieved to date suggest that the size of the lost fragment does not correlate directly to the immunoglobulin phenotype. Since one of the chromosomes is structurally normal, the deficiency must result from a hemizygous deletion or malfunction of the gene in question, and similar gene dose effects have been noted in other diseases. Li et al. (1995) have previously suggested an involvement of NFATc, a transcription factor in activated T cells that is involved in the expression of cytokines and surface molecules required for an immune response, in 18q patients lacking IgA. Because the defective gene in the immunodeficient wst/wst mouse resides in the corresponding syntenic region, a relationship could be possible. However, the mouse model does not clinically resemble IgAD or CVID (Kaiserlian et al., 1985), arguing in favor of the involvement of a different gene in the human disease. Furthermore, extensive analysis of a large number of families with IgAD/CVID shows no association with chromosome 18 markers in "idiopathic" IgAD (Vorechovsky et al., 1999).

An analysis of serum levels in our own patients with chromosome 18p deletions showed that one of them also lacked IgG2 and IgG4, giving rise to a CVID phenotype (Truedsson et al., 1995). This finding suggests a relation between the two different forms of defect in Ig production also in this category of patients.

Functional Aspects

Defective Immunoglobulin Class Switch in IgA Deficiency and Common Variable Immunodeficiency

Switching is preceded by transcription of the I and switch regions upstream of the Ig heavy-chain constant-region gene, giving rise to germ-line transcripts. These transcripts are also referred to as *sterile transcripts* as they do not contain V region sequences. The I region is thought to play an important although not crucial role in the induction of switch, as mice with a targeted deletion of this genetic element still produce normal levels of IgA (Harriman et al., 1996). Germ-line I transcripts are easily detected in unstimulated peripheral blood mononuclear cells from normal donors whereas they are absent in cells from IgAD individuals (Islam et al., 1994). However, they can be readily induced by the addition of transforming growth factor-β (TGF-β), demonstrating that the locus is accessible for transcription provided that additional signals are supplied. These transcripts, which are generated early after activation of the cells, also include α. However, all subsequent stages of IgA production, including the switch at the genomic level, appear to be impaired (Islam et al., 1994). Although TGF-β has been suggested as a switch factor for IgA, we could not find any difference in the steady-state production of this cytokine in cells from IgAD individuals. Still, a dysregulation of TGF-β was suggested to be involved in the pathogenesis of IgAD because serum levels of the cytokine were markedly lower in patients than in controls (Müller et al., 1995).

IL-5 is a pleiotropic molecule with effects on both granulocytes and lymphocytes. In the mouse, this cytokine has been demonstrated to be of major importance for IgA production (Harriman et al., 1988; Stavnezer et al., 1988). Expression of IL-5 in the mouse appears to be regulated by genes within the MHC complex (Dieli et al., 1993), and in vivo administration of the cytokine to low-responder mice results in an enhanced IgA response (Dieli et al., 1995). Human B cells also produce IgA when stimulated with IL-5 (Yokota et al., 1987), and in view of the association between genes within the HLA complex and IgAD and CVID, an involvement in the etiology may be envisaged. However, we have failed to demonstrate any decrease in the frequency of IL-5-producing cells or in the level of mRNA in individual cells from IgA-deficient individuals (Smith et al., 1990), thus diminished production of IL-5 may not be part of the pathophysiological process.

A cultivation system that allows the expression of immunoglobulins of both cells from IgA-deficient (Briere et al., 1994) and CVID (Zielen et al., 1993) patients has been previously described. In this system anti-CD40 antibodies are used in conjunction with IL-10. Although the physiology of this in vitro system—i.e., the induction of switching at the molecular level—still remains to be proven, it clearly demonstrates that secretion of IgG1, IgG3, IgG4 (Fujieda et al., 1995), and IgA (Zielen et al., 1993; Briere et al., 1994), with a biased expression of IgA1 (Friman et al., 1996), can indeed be achieved if the appropriate stimuli are added. Again, however, the basis of the inability to switch in vivo remains elusive as the gp39 (CD40 ligand) is expressed on T cells from CVID patients (Farrington et al., 1994), although at a slightly lower level in a subgroup of patients. This expression may be the cause of their long-recognized ability to support IgA synthesis in normal B cells (Smith and Hammarstrom, 1987). Thus, although the timing and concentration of cytokines may play a crucial role in the switching process, there is no strong evidence to implicate any cytokine or cytokine receptor in the disease process.

Drug-Induced Immunoglobulin Deficiencies

IgA deficiency is infrequently seen in patients treated with a variety of antirheumatic and antiepileptic drugs (Table 23.4) (for references see Truedsson et al., 1995; Zhou et al., 2006) In approximately half of the reported patients the deficiency is reversible after cessation of treatment, although full recovery requires months or even years. The deficient state can be induced by multiple drugs in a given patient (Farr et al., 1991), thus selected individuals may be predisposed to develop drug-induced Ig deficiency. Recent findings clearly suggest that selected drugs

Table 23.4. Pattern of Drug-Induced Immunoglobulin Deficiencies

Drug	CVID	IgG2-IgAD	IgAD
Sulfasalazine	X	X	X
Gold			X
Chloroquine			X
Penicillamine			X
Captopril			X
Fenclofenac			X
Hydantonin	X	X	X
Carbamazepine	X		X
Valproate			X
Thyroxine*			X
Levamisol*	X		
Ibuprofen*			X
Salicylic acid*			X
Cyclosporin A*			X

*Requires independent confirmation.

such as hydantoin act late in B cell differentiation through a mechanism distinct from the idiopathic form of IgAD (Zhou et al., 2006).

CVID and IgG2-IgA deficiency have also been shown to be induced by some of the above drugs (for references see Truedsson et al., 1995), and the recent identification of unifying links between drug-induced CVID and IgAD suggests that the iatrogenic form may be similar to the idiopathic form of Ig deficiency and that the etiological process involves common steps.

The mechanism underlying the drug-induced form of IgAD and CVID has not been determined. There is as yet no common molecular denominator in the drugs used, and identification of novel drugs, or category of drugs, would therefore be of marked benefit for our understanding of the phenomenon. Some of them contain a highly reactive sulfhydryl group. It is therefore possible that the immunological dysregulation induced by these agents, including the formation of immune complexes and induction of autoimmune disorders such as systemic lupus and pemphigus (for references see Smith and Hammarstrom, 1985), plays a role in development of the deficiency in genetically susceptible patients.

Strategies for Diagnosis

Selective IgAD hardly presents any diagnostic problems in adults. But because serum IgA levels may remain low for a protracted time period in children (Plebani et al., 1986), a diagnosis of IgAD cannot be made before the teens, using <0.05 g/l as a cutoff. A simultaneous absence of IgG2 and IgG4, even in early childhood, is a strong indicator of persistent IgAD.

CVID probably represents a mixture of diseases with different etiologies. Recently, a deletion in the *ICOS* gene, encoding the inducible costimulator expressed on T cells and required for late B cell differention, class switching, and memory B cell generation, was shown to result in a disorder resembling adult-onset CVID (Grimbacher et al., 2003). However, only a minority of CVID patients is affected by mutations of *ICOS*, and all patients described to date show the same genetic alteration.

Genes on chromosome 5 have also been suggested to be involved in the pathophysiological process in selected CVID patients (Braig et al., 2003), as have mutations in the *LRRC8* gene on chromosome 9 (Sawada et al., 2003).

Surface Ig-positive cells remain unaffected in the blood of most patients with CVID. However, in patients with XLA, these cells are low or absent, which may aid in the differential diagnosis in young boys. The cloning of the *BTK* gene (see Chapter 21) enables the differential diagnosis in a vast majority of XLA patients by mutation screening. The spectrum of infections also differs slightly, and patients with CVID are prone to nonbacterial infections, as a proportion of patients show a concomitant T cell defect.

A distinction between CVID and hyper-IgM syndrome can be made on the basis of gender, as most patients show an X-linked inheritance pattern, and through levels of immunoglobulins where IgM levels are elevated in typical cases. Again, the spectrum of infections appears slightly different, and since most genes involved have been cloned (see Chapter 19), a correct diagnosis is possible by mutation screening.

X-linked lymphoproliferative disease (XLP) is a primary immunodeficiency caused by a defect in the *SH2D1A* gene. The disease is characterized by severe, often fatal infectious mononucleosis, lymphomas, and Ig deficiencies. Although typical cases (see Chapter 32) are easily distinguishable from CVID patients, problems in the differential diagnosis may occur (Morra et al., 2001; Soresina et al., 2002), and sequencing of the *SH2D1A* gene may therefore be warranted.

The warts, hypogammaglobulinemia, immunodeficiency, myelokathexis (WHIM) syndrome represents yet another potential differential diagnosis to CVID. The genetic defect of the WHIM syndrome was recently identified as truncating mutations in the cytoplasmic portion of the G protein–coupled, chemokine receptor *CXCR4* gene, which is located on chromosome 2q21 (Hernandez et al., 2003). CXCR4 is the receptor for CXCL12, also known as stromal-derived factor 1 (SDF-1). Coined by Wetzler et al. (1990), this autosomal dominant disease is characterized by recurrent bacterial infections and extensive human papillomavirus infections, whereas infection with cytomegalovirus or *Toxoplasma gondii* runs a normal course (Diaz, 2005). The phenotype is not identical among affected individuals, because warts are not seen in all patients and the hypogammaglobulinemia may be variable. Nonimmunological phenotypes may also exist, since at least one patient and deficient mice have cardiac abnormalities. In terms of the immunological phenotype, both mice (Ma et al., 1998; Zou et al., 1998) lacking the protein and humans with truncating mutations show B cell lymphopenia. There is a special lack of memory B cells and a restricted T cell repertoire (Gulino et al., 2004) in the mouse, and myeloid progenitors fail to migrate to the bone marrow. In affected humans, myeloid cells fail to exit the bone marrow (myelokathexis) in the absence of inflammation, resulting in neutropenia. Treatment consists of granulocyte colony–stimulating factor (G-CSF) (not used by all centers) and intravenous immunoglobulin (IVIG). Lymphoid tumors have been reported, which suggests the importance of intact CXCL12–CXCR4 signaling for proper regulation of lymphocyte proliferation (Chae et al., 2001; Imashuku et al., 2002). Certain patients have abnormalities in the CXCL12–CXCR4 pathway that are not caused by *CXCR4* mutations, thus the genetic basis may be diverse (Balabanian et al., 2005).

TACI and BAFF-R are TNF-like receptors, responding to a number of ligands (BAFF, BCMA, and APRIL) involved in maturation and differention of B cells. In view of the impaired Ig class switching recently described in APRIL- (Castigli et al., 2004) and BAFF-deficient mice (Schiemann et al., 2001), it seems likely that similar defects involving this family of receptors and ligands will also be involved in the pathogenesis of selected cases of CVID in humans. Indeed, truncating and mismatch mutations have been described in both TACI (Salzer et al., 2004b; Castigli et al., 2005, Salzer et al., 2005) and BAFF-R (Salzer et al., 2004a) and shown to be associated with a CVID phenotype. The former may account for up to 10% of all patients, whereas the latter seems much more rare.

The CD19 molecule is expressed by B lymphocytes and follicular dendritic cells of the hematopoetic system and it is the earliest of the B lineage–restricted antigens. It is present on the cell surface associated with CD21, CD81, CD225, and the B cell receptor (BCR) complex, and acts to lower the threshold for antigen-mediated signaling. In mice, the CD19 molecule is involved in development of B1 and marginal-zone B cells and, when lacking, antibody responses and B cell memory are strongly affected. The first mutations in CD19 in patients with CVID were recently described in two separate families (van Zelm et al., 2006). It is likely, however, that this is a rare cause of CVID.

In patients with hypogammaglobulinemia due to thymoma, B cells are lacking altogether in both peripheral blood and the bone marrow, and a scan of the thymus may indicate presence of a tumor. Age at onset may also be of some help in the differential

diagnosis of hypogammaglobulinemia. Adult onset of infections clearly suggests CVID rather than XLA, and thymomatous patients are usually although not invariably older than the average CVID patient.

Treatment Options

The foundation of therapy for CVID and IgAD patients is antibiotics and Ig replacement. Gammaglobulin infusions have been used for decades in patients with CVID, but only recently have infectious-prone patients with IgAD received γ-globulin therapy (Gustafson et al., 1997). The doses employed have gradually risen, and today a weekly dose of 100–150 mg/kg body weigth is recommended (Rosen et al., 1995).

Prior to the introduction of γ-globulin replacement therapy in XLA patients, γ-globulin had been given intramuscularly primarily as prophylaxis against various viral diseases. Bruton (1952) however, started his patients on prophylactic treatment using subcutaneous injections of γ-globulin, a treatment regimen that was later altered to intramuscular administration. The intramuscular injections remained the mode of therapy for immunodeficiency patients for almost two decades. However, because of the limited amount that could be given, IVIG preparations were developed.

Treatment with slow, subcutaneous infusions of γ-globulin was reintroduced by Berger et al. (1980), and a number of reports on the treatment of hypogammaglobulinemic patients followed (for references, see Gardulf et al., 1991). However, because of the slow rate of infusion, this form of treatment did not meet with widespread appreciation.

Home treatment of hypogammaglobulinemia in patients with primary immunodeficiency disorders with γ-globulin for intravenous use (IVIG) was introduced in 1986 (Ochs et al., 1986) and represented a significant step forward in the prophylactic use of γ-globulin. This initial report was soon followed by additional reports (Ashida and Saxon, 1986; Chapel et al., 1988; Ryan et al., 1988) showing the effectiveness of the method. This form of treatment is limited, however, to patients with no prior history of adverse reactions to γ-globulin treatment, requires the training and continuous presence of a partner during infusions, and is dependent on easy access to suitable blood vessels.

Rapid subcutaneous infusion of γ-globulin preparations intended for intramuscular administration was first described by Gardulf et al. (1991) and can be used in patients with a previous history of adverse reactions even in a home setting, requires no presence of a trained partner, results in a very low incidence of adverse reactions (Gardulf et al., 1995), and is markedly cheaper than home treatment with IVIG. This treatment therefore represents a preferred form of prophylaxis in patients with CVID (Gardulf and Hammarstrom, 1996).

In spite of replacement therapy with intravenous or subcutaneously administered γ-globulin, some patients still suffer from respiratory and gastrointestinal tract infections. Topical application of γ-globulin preparations might therefore be of benefit, as it provides a high local concentration of specific antibodies at the site of infection. In five patients with CVID who were chronic nasopharyngeal carriers of non-encapsulated *Hemophilus influenzae*, nose drops containing human immunoglobulins were provided as treatment. The preparation of IgA and IgG was given as nose drops and the results showed that two of the five patients cleared their infection and remained culture negative for a prolonged period of time (Lindberg et al., 1993). Coughing was also alleviated in all patients, thus nasally administered Ig may be of potential use in treating immunodeficient patients.

Oral administration of polyclonal human Ig has also been shown to be therapeutically effective against intestinal infections in immunodeficient patients (Melamed et al., 1991; Hammarstrom et al., 1993; Tjellstrom et al., 1993). Although this form of therapy remains experimental, it may constitute a valuable therapeutic option in selected cases.

During the past few years, we have witnessed a remarkable increase in our knowledge of the molecular basis of a variety of immunodeficiency disorders in humans. As a result of these efforts, novel findings on point mutations, deletions, and splicing abnormalities have been described in a number of diseases, including XLA, hyper-IgM syndrome, Wiskott-Aldrich syndrome, and ataxia-telangiectasia (AT). It is clear from the published studies not only that different mutations may give rise to varying phenotypical appearances, but the very same mutation can be associated with quite diverse clinical pictures, depending on the presence of modifying "background" genes.

Diseases such as IgAD, IgAD combined with IgG2 and IgG4 deficiency, and CVID all seem to share a common genetic background and may therefore be related diseases, expressing different facets of the same underlying defect. This finding is important not only for a conceptual understanding of these disorders and the development of a correct nomenclature but also for mapping of disease genes. Induction of IgAD and CVID probably requires the presence of a predisposing gene and a triggering factor, the nature of which is still unknown. In most of the multicase families, affected family members are found in more than one generation, a pattern compatible with an autosomal dominant inheritance with a limited penetrance. It is not clear whether a predisposing gene would have to be present in a heterozygous or a homozygous state. If disease symptoms occur from a heterozygous state, the immunoglobulin deficiency–associated protein could be part of a multimer complex—perhaps a receptor involved in cell proliferation, differentiation, and class switching, where an improper balance in concentrations of the subcomponents may perturb its function. It is thus likely that the key to understanding the true basis of IgAD and CVID is the identification of the gene(s) involved in their pathogenesis. A genome-wide search for susceptibility genes in a large cohort of multiplex families is required to solve the questions of etiology and pathogenesis of these forms of immunological defects.

Animal Models

Although there are a number of reports on IgA-deficient dogs (Felsburg et al., 1985; Moroff et al., 1986; Glickman et al., 1988) and chickens (Luster et al., 1976), the molecular basis of these deficiencies has not been elucidated.

There is as yet no rodent model available that resembles the human disease, although knockout mice with a deleted J chain (Hendrickson et al., 1995), Iα region (Harriman et al., 1996), or Cα region (Harriman et al., 1999) have been described. In J chain–deficient mice, only secretion of IgA is impaired, and serum levels of IgA are up to 30-fold higher than in normal wild-type mice. Interestingly, there seems to be a J chain–independent IgA transport in the intestinal, mammary, and respiratory epithelial cells of these mice (Hendrickson et al., 1996), adding to the complexity of the secretory IgA machinery. Contrary to what might have been expected from mice with deleted I regions or I region promoters for γ1, γ2b, and ε, mice with an I region deletion produced normal levels of IgA. This observation suggests that the I region as such is redundant and can be replaced by other gene sequences (Lorenz et al., 1995). Thus splicing of germ-line

transcripts rather than transcription per se may control DNA rearrangement leading to class switch.

Mice with a targeted inactivation of the α heavy-chain constant-region gene and part of the Sα region have also been produced (Harriman et al., 1999). These mice are profoundly deficient in both systemic and secretory IgA and show a perturbed pattern of expression of immunoglobulins, manifested as an increased level of IgM and IgG (primarily IgG2b) and decreased levels of IgG3 and IgE in both serum and secretions. These mice are, however, largely normal in development of their lymphoid tissues and proliferative responses. Cytokine profiles in response to antigenic challenge (influenza virus) are altered with a down-regulation of Th1-mediated immune responses (Zhang et al., 2002).

Acknowledgments

This work was supported by the Swedish Research Council and EU grant QLG1-CT-2001-01536. We are indebted to Dr. David Webster at the Royal Free and University College Medical School, London, for kindly providing the figures presented in this chapter.

References

Abedi MR, Christensson B, Al-Masud S, Hammarstrom L, Smith CIE. γ-Globulin modulates the growth of EBV derived B cell tumors in SCID mice reconstituted with human lymphocytes. Int J Cancer 55:824–829, 1993.

Abramowsky CR, Sorensen RU. Regional enteritis-like enteropathy in a patient with agammaglobulinemia: histologic and immunocytologic studies. Hum Pathol 19:483–486, 1988.

Ammann AJ, Hong R. Selective IgA deficiency: presentation of 30 cases and a review of the literature. Medicine 50:223–236, 1971.

Ashida ER, Saxon A. Home intravenous immunoglobulin therapy by self-administration. J Clin Immunol 6:306–309, 1986.

Ashman RF, Schaffer FM, Kemp JD, Yokoyama WM, Zhu Z-B, Cooper MD, Volanakis JE. Genetic and immunologic analysis of a family containing five patients with common-variable immune deficiency or selective IgA deficiency. J Clin Immunol 12:406–414, 1992.

Balabanian K, Lagane B, Pablos JL, Laurent L, Planchenault T, Verola O, Lebbe C, Kerob D, Dupuy A, Hermine O, Nicolas JF, Latger-Cannard V, Bensoussan D, Bordigoni P, Baleux F, Le Deist F, Virelizier JL, Arenzana-Seisdedos F, Bachelerie F. WHIM syndromes with different genetic anomalies are accounted for by impaired CXCR4 desensitization to CXCL12. Blood 105:2449–2457, 2005.

Benbassat J, Keren L, Zlotnic A. Hepatitis in selective IgA deficiency. BMJ 4:762–763, 1973.

Berger M, Cupps TR, Fauci AS. Immunoglobulin replacement therapy by slow subcutaneous infusion. Ann Intern Med 93:55–56, 1980.

Bjorkander J, Bake B, Hanson L-A. Primary hypogammaglobulinemia: impaired lung function and body growth with delayed diagnosis and inadequate treatment. Eur J Resp Dis 65:529–536, 1984.

Bjorkander J, Hammarstrom L, Smith CIE, Buckley RH, Cunningham-Rundles C, Hanson L-A. Immunoglobulin prophylaxis in patients with antibody deficiency syndromes and anti-IgA antibodies. J Clin Immunol 7:8–15, 1987.

Bogstedt A, Nava S, Wadstrom T, Hammarstrom L. *Helicobacter pylori* infections in IgA deficiency: lack of role for the secretory immune system. Clin Exp Immunol 105:202–204, 1996.

Borecki IB, McGue M, Gerrard JW, Lebowitz MD, Rao DC. Familial resemblance for immunoglobulin levels. Hum Genet 94:179–185, 1994.

Braig DU, Schaffer AA, Glocker E, Salzer U, Warnatz K, Peter HH, Grimbacher B. Linkage of autosomal dominant common variable immunodeficiency to chromosome 5p and evidence for locus heterogeneity. Hum Genet 112:369–378, 2003.

Briere F, Bridon J-C, Chevet D, Souillet G, Bienvenu F, Guret C, Martinez-Valdez H, Banchereau J. Interleukin-10 induces B lymphocytes from IgA-deficient patients to secrete IgA. J Clin Invest 94:97–104, 1994.

Bruton OC. Agammaglobulinemia. Pediatrics 9:722–727, 1952.

Bucin D, Truedsson L, Hammarstrom L, Smith CIE, Sjoholm AG. C4 polymorphism and major histocompatibility complex haplotypes in IgA deficiency: association with C4A null haplotypes. Exp Clin Immunogenet 8:223–241, 1991.

Burks AW, Sampson HA, Buckley RH. Anaphylactic reactions after γ-globulin administration in patients with hypogammaglobulinemia. Detection of IgE antibodies to IgA. N Engl J Med 314:560–564, 1986.

Carneiro-Sampaio MM, Carbonare SB, Rozentraub RB, de Araujo MN, Riberiro MA, Porto MH. Frequency of selective IgA deficiency among Brazilian blood donors and healthy pregnant women. Allergol Immunopathol 17:213–216, 1989.

Castigli E, Scott S, Dedeoglu F, Bryce P, Jabara H, Bhan AK, Mizoguchi E, Geha RS. Impaired IgA class switching in APRIL-deficient mice. Proc Natl Acad Sci USA 101:3903–3908, 2004.

Castigli E, Wilson SA, Garibyan L, Rachid R, Bonilla F, Schneider L, Geha RS. TACI is mutant in common variable immunodeficiency and IgA deficiency. Nature Genet 37:829–834, 2005.

Chae KM, Ertle JO, Tharp MD. B-cell lymphoma in a patient with WHIM syndrome. J Am Acad Dermatol 44:124–128, 2001.

Chapel H, Brennan P, Delson E. Immunoglobulin replacement therapy by self-infusion at home. Clin Exp Immunol 73:160–162, 1988.

Citron KM. Agammaglobulinemia with splenomegaly. BMJ 1:1148–1151, 1957.

Conley ME, Cooper MD. Immature B cells in IgA-deficient patients. N Engl J Med 305:495–497, 1981.

Cooper MD, Faulk PW, Fudenberg HH, Hitzig W, Good RA, Kunkel H, Rosen FS, Seligmann M, Soothill J, Wedgwood RJ. Classification of primary immunodeficiencies. N Engl J Med 288:966–967, 1973.

Cunningham-Rundles C, Siegal FP, Cunningham-Rundles S, Lieberman P. Incidence of cancer in 98 patients with common varied immunodeficiency. J Clin Immunol 7:294–299, 1987.

Cunningham-Rundles C, Wong S, Bjorkander J, Hanson L-A. Use of an IgA-depleted intravenous immunoglobulin in a patient with an anti-IgA antibody. Clin Immunol Immunopathol 38:141–149, 1986.

Curtin JJ, Murray JG, Apthorp LA, Franz AM, Webster ADB. Mediastinal lymph node enlargement and splenomegaly in primary hypogammaglobulinemia. Clin Radiol 50:489–491, 1995.

Curzio M, Bernasconi G, Gullotta R, Ceriani A, Sala G. Association of ulcerative colitis, sclerosing cholangitis and cholangiocarcinoma in a patient with IgA deficiency. Endoscopy 17:123–125, 1985.

de Laat PC, Weemaes CM, Bakkeren JA, van den Brandt FC, van Lith TG, de Graaf R, van Munster PJ, Stoelinga GB. Familial selective IgA deficiency with circulating anti-IgA antibodies: a distinct group of patients. Clin Immunol Immunopathol 58:92–101, 1991.

De la Concha EG, Fernandez-Arquero M, Gual L, Vigil P, Martinez A, Urcelay E, Ferreira A, Garcia-Rodriguez MC, Fontan G. MHC susceptibility genes to IgA deficiency are located in different regions on different HLA haplotypes. J Immunol 169:4637–4643, 2002.

Diaz GA. CXCR4 mutations in WHIM syndrome: a misguided immune system? Immunol Rev 203:235–243, 2005.

Dieli F, Asherson GL, Sireci G, Lio D, Bonanno CT, Salerno A. IL-5 enhances in vitro and in vivo antigen-specific IgA production in MHC genetically determined low IL-5 responder mice. Cell Immunol 163:309–313, 1995.

Dieli F, Sireci G, Lio D, Bonanno CT, Salerno A. Major histocompatibility complex regulation of interleukin-5 production in the mouse. Eur J Immunol 23:2897–2902, 1993.

Douglas SD, Goldberg LS, Fudenberg HH. Familial selective deficiency of IgA. J Pediatr 78:873–875, 1971.

Dukes RJ, Rosenow EC, Heremans PE. Pulmonary manifestations of hypogammaglobulinemia. Thorax 33:603–607, 1978.

Eggert RC, Wilson ID, Good RA. Agammaglobulinemia and regional enteritis. Ann Intern Med 71:581–585, 1969.

Elson CO, James SP, Graeff AS, Berendson RA, Strober W. Hypogammaglobulinemia due to abnormal suppressor T-cell activity in Crohn's disease. Gastroenterology 86:569–576, 1984.

Ezeoke AC. Selective IgA deficiency in eastern Nigeria. Afr J Med Sci 17:17–21, 1988.

Farr M, Kitas GD, Tuhn EJ, Bacon PA. Immunodeficiencies associated with sulphasalazine therapy in inflammatory arthritis. Br J Rheumatol 30:413–417, 1991.

Farrington M, Grosmaire LS, Nonoyama S, Fisher SH, Hollenbaugh D, Ledbetter JA, Noelle RJ, Aruffo A, Ochs HD. CD40 ligand expression is defective in a subset of patients with common variable immunodeficiency. Proc Natl Acad Sci USA 91:1099–1103, 1994.

Felsburg PJ, Glickman LT, Jezyk PF. Selective IgA deficiency in the dog. Clin Immunol Immunopathol 36:297–305, 1985.

Feng L. Epidemiological study of selective IgA deficiency among 6 nationalities in China. Chin Med J 72:88–90, 1992.

Ferreira A, Rodriguez MCG, Lopez-Trascasa M, Salcedo DP, Fontan G. Anti-IgA antibodies in selective IgA deficiency and in primary immunod-

eficient patients treated with γ-globulin. Clin Immunol Immunopathol 47:199–207, 1988.

Frankel SJ, Polmar SH, Grumet FC, Wedner HJ. Anti-IgA antibody associated reactions to intravenous gammaglobulin in a patient who tolerated intramuscular gammaglobulin. Ann Allergy 56:436–439, 1986.

Friman V, Hanson L-A, Bridon J-M, Tarkowski A, Banchereau J, Briere F. IL-10 driven immunoglobulin production by B lymphocytes from IgA-deficient individuals correlates to infection proneness. Clin Exp Immunol 104:432–438, 1996.

Frommel D, Moullec J, Lambin P, Fine JM. Selective serum IgA deficiency. Frequency among 15,200 French blood donors. Vox Sang 25:513–518, 1973.

Fujieda S, Zhang K, Saxon A. IL-4 plus CD40 monoclonal antibody induces human B cells subclass-specific isotype switch: switching to γ1, γ3 and γ4, but not γ2. J Immunol 155:2318–2328, 1995.

Gardulf A, Andersen V, Bjorkander J, Ericson D, Frøland S, Gustafson R, Hammarstrom L, Jacobsen MR, Jonsson E, Moller G, Nystrom T, Seberg B, Smith CIE. Subcutaneous immunoglobulin replacement in patients with primary antibody deficiencies: safety and cost. Lancet 345:365–369, 1995.

Gardulf A, Hammarstrom L. Subcutaneous administration of immunoglobulins. What are the advantages? Clin Immunother 6:108–116, 1996.

Gardulf A, Hammarstrom L, Smith CIE. Home treatment of hypogammaglobulinemia with subcutaneous gammaglobulin by rapid infusion. Lancet 338:162–166, 1991.

Glickman LT, Shofer FS, Payton AJ, Laster LL, Felsburg PJ. Survey of serum IgA, IgG, and IgM concentrations in a large beagle population in which IgA deficiency had been identified. Am J Vet Res 49:1240–1245, 1988.

Good RA, Kelly WD, Rotstein J, Vargo RL. Immunological deficiency diseases. Agammaglobulinemia, hypogammaglobulinemia, Hodgkin's disease and sarcoidosis. Prog Allergy 6:184–319, 1962.

Goshen E, Livne A, Krupp M, Hammarstrom L, Dighiero G, Slor H, Schoenfeld Y. Antinuclear and related autoantibodies in sera of healthy subjects with IgA deficiency. J Autoimmun 2:51–60, 1989.

Grant GH, Wallace WD. Agammaglobulinemia. Lancet ii:671–673, 1954.

Grimbacher B, Hutloff A, Schlesier M, Glocker E, Warnatz K, Drager R, Eibel H, Fischer B, Schaffer AA, Mages HW, Kroczek RA, Peter HH. Homozygous loss of ICOS is associated with adult-onset common variable immunodeficiency. Nat Immunol 4:261–268, 2003.

Gual L, Martinez A, Fernandez-Arquero M, Garcia-Rodriguez MC, Ferreria A, Fontan G, de la Concha EG, Urcelay E. Major histocompatibility complex haplotypes in Spanish immunoglobulin A deficiency patients: a comparative fine-mapping microsattelite study. Tissue Antigens 64: 671–677, 2004.

Gulino AV, Moratto D, Sozzani S, Cavadini P, Otero K, Tassone L, Imberti L, Pirovano S, Notarangelo LD, Soresina R, Mazzolari E, Nelson DL, Notarangelo LD, Badolato R. Altered leukocyte response to CXCL12 in patients with warts hypogammaglobulinemia, infections, myelokathexis (WHIM) syndrome. Blood 104:444–452, 2004.

Gustafson R, Gardulf A, Granert C, Hansen S, Hammarstrom L. Prophylactic therapy for selective IgA deficiency. Lancet 350:865, 1997.

Hammarstrom L, Carlsson B, Smith CIE, Wallin J, Wieslander L. Detection of IgA heavy chain constant region genes in IgA deficient donors: evidence against gene deletions. Clin Exp Immunol 60:661–664, 1985a.

Hammarstrom L, de Lange G, Smith CIE. IgA2 allotypes in IgA deficiency. Re-expression of the silent IgA2m2 allotype in the children of IgA deficient patients. J Immunogenet 14:197–201, 1987.

Hammarstrom L, Grubb R, Jakobsen BK, Oxelius V, Persson U, Smith CIE. Concomitant deficiency of IgG4 and IgE in IgA-deficient donors with high titres of anti-IgA. Monogr Allergy 20:234–235, 1986.

Hammarstrom L, Grubb R, Smith CIE. Gm allotypes in IgA deficiency. J Immunogenet 12:125–130, 1985b.

Hammarstrom L, Lonnqvist B, Ringden O, Smith CIE, Wiebe T. Transfer of IgA deficiency to a bone marrow grafted patient with aplastic anaemia. Lancet 1:778–781, 1985c.

Hammarstrom L, Persson MAA, Smith CIE. Anti-IgA in selective IgA deficiency: in vitro effects and Ig subclass pattern of human anti-IgA. Scand J Immunol 18:509–513, 1983.

Hammarstrom L, Persson MAA, Smith CIE. Immunoglobulin subclass distribution of human anti-carbohydrate antibodies: aberrant pattern in IgA-deficient donors. Immunology 54:821–826, 1985d.

Hammarstrom L, Smith CIE. HLA-A, B, C and DR antigens in immunoglobulin A deficiency. Tissue Antigens 21:75–79, 1983.

Hammarstrom L, Smith CIE. IgM production in hypogammaglobulinemic patients during non-A, non-B hepatitis. Lancet 1:743, 1986.

Hammarstrom V, Smith CIE, Hammarstrom L. Oral immunoglobulin treatment in Campylobacter jejuni enteritis. Lancet 341:1036, 1993.

Hammarstrom L, Smith CIE. Genetic approach to common variable immunodeficiency and IgA deficiency. In: Ochs H, Smith CIE, Puck J, eds. Primary Immunodeficiency Diseases, A Molecular and Genetic Approach. New York: Oxford University Press, pp. 250–262, 1999.

Harriman GR, Bogue M, Rogers P, Finegold M, Pacheo S, Bradley A, Zhang Y, Mbawuike IN. Targeted deletion of the IgA constant region in mice leads to IgA deficiency with alterations in expression of other Ig isotypes. J Immunol 162:2521–2529, 1999.

Harriman GR, Bradley A, Das S, Rogers-Fani P, Davis AC. IgA class switch in I exon-deficient mice. Role of germline transcription in class switch recombination. J Clin Invest 97:477–485, 1996.

Harriman GR, Kunimoto DY, Elliott JF, Paetkau V, Strober W. The role of IL-5 in IgA B cell differentiation. J Immunol 140:3033–3039, 1988.

Hausser C, Virelizier JL, Buriot D, Griscelli C. Common variable hypogammaglobulinemia in children. Am J Child 137:833–837, 1983.

Hendrickson BA, Conner DA, Ladd DJ, Kendall D, Casanova JE, Corthesy B, Max EE, Neutra MR, Seidman CE, Seidman JG. Altered hepatic transport of immunoglobulin A mice lacking the J chain. J Exp Med 182:1905–1912, 1995.

Hendrickson BA, Rindisbacher L, Corthesy B, Kendall D, Waltz DA, Neutra MR, Seidman JG. Lack of association of secretory component with IgA in J chain–deficient mice. J Immunol 157:750–754, 1996.

Hermaszewski RA, Webster ADB. Primary hypogammaglobulinemia: a survey of clinical manifestations and complications. Q J Med 86:31–42, 1993.

Hernandez PA, Gorlin RJ, Lukens JN, Taniuchi S, Bohinjec J, Francois F, Klotman ME, Diaz GA. Mutations in the chemokine receptor gene *CXCR4* are associated with WHIM syndrome, a combined immunodeficiency disease. Nat Genet 34:70–74, 2003.

Hishitani Y, Nakamura Y, Inui M, Kakehi K, Mozai T, Kanoh T. Development of IgA deficiency in the course of chronic active hepatitis. Jpn J Gastroenterol 77:789–793, 1980.

Hobbs JR. Immune imbalance in dysgammaglobulinemia type IV. Lancet i:110–114, 1968.

Hodgson HJ, Jewell DP. Selective IgA deficiency and Crohn's disease: report of two cases. Gut 18:644–646, 1977.

Hollinger HZ. Hypogammaglobulinemia, thymoma and ulcerative colitis. CMAJ 96:1584–1586, 1967.

Holt PD, Tandy NP, Anstee DJ. Screening of blood donors for IgA deficiency: a study of the donor population of southwest England. J Clin Pathol 30:1007–1010, 1977.

Howe HS, So AKL, Farrant J, Webster ADB. Common variable immunodeficiency is associated with polymorphic markers in the human major histocompatibility complex. Clin Exp Immunol 84:387–390, 1991.

Huntley CC, Stephenson RL. IgA deficiency: family studies. N C Med J 29:325–331, 1968.

Ilan Y, Shouval D, Ashur Y, Manns M, Naparstek. Y. IgA deficiency associated with chronic hepatitis C virus infection. A cause or an effect? Arch Intern Med 153:1588–1592, 1993.

Imashuku S, Miyagawa A, Chiyonobu T, Ishida H, Yoshihara T, Teramura T, Kuriyama K, Imamura T, Hibi S, Morimoto A, Todo S. Epstein-Barr virus–associated T-lymphoproliferative disease with hemophagocytic syndrome, followed by fatal intestinal B lymphoma in a young adult female with WHIM syndrome. Warts, hypogammaglobulinemia, infections, and myelokathexis. Ann Hematol 81:470–473, 2002.

Islam KB, Baskin B, Nilsson L, Hammarstrom L, Sideras P, Smith CIE. Molecular analysis of IgA deficiency: evidence for impaired switching to IgA. J Immunol 152:1442–1452, 1994.

Israel-Asselain R, Burtin P, Chebat J. Un trouble biologique noveau: lagammaglobulinemie (un cas). Bull Soc Med Hop Paris 76:519–523, 1960.

Jacobsen HEL. Agammaglobulinemia. Nord Med 52:1278, 1954.

Jorup-Ronstrom C, Ahl T, Hammarstrom L, Smith CIE, Rylander M, Hallander H. Septic osteomyelitis and polyarthritis with ureaplasma in hypogammaglobulinemia. Infection 17:301–303, 1989.

Kaiserlian D, Delacroix D, Bach JF. The wasted mouse mutant. I. An animal model of secretory IgA deficiency with normal serum IgA. J Immunol 135:1126–1131, 1985.

Kanoh T, Mizumoto T, Yasuda N, Koya M, Ohno Y, Uchino H, Yoshimura K, Ohkubo Y, Yamaguchi H. Selective IgA deficiency in Japanese blood donors. Frequency and statistical analysis. Vox Sang 50:81–86, 1986.

Kaplinsky N, Pras M, Frankl O. Case reports. Severe enterocolitis complicating crysotherapy. Ann Rheum Dis 32:574–577, 1973.

Keidan SE, McCarthy K, Haworth JC. Fatal generalized vaccinia with failure of antibody production and absence of serum gamma globulin. Arch Dis Child 28:110–116, 1953.

Kinlen LJ, Webster ADB, Bird AG, Haile R, Peto J, Soothill JF, Thompson RA. Prospective study of cancer in patients with hypogammaglobulinemia. Lancet i:263–266, 1985.

Koistinen J. Selective IgA deficiency in blood donors. Vox Sang 29:192–202, 1975.

Kralovicova J, Hammarstrom L, Plebani A, Webster ADB, Vorechovsky I. Fine-scale mapping at *IGAD1* and genome-wide genetic linkage analysis implicate HLA-DQ/DR as a major susceptibility locus in selective IgA deficiency and common variable immunodeficiency. J Immunol 170:2765–2775, 2003.

Kraus VB, Baraniuk JN, Hill GB, Allen NB. *Ureaplasma urealyticum* septic arthritis in hypogammaglobulinemia. J Rheumatol 15:369–371, 1988.

Kuhn R, Lohler J, Rennick D, Rajewsky K, Muller W. Interleukin-10-deficient mice develop chronic enterocolitis. Cell 75:263–274, 1993.

Kurobane I, Riches PG, Sheldon J, Jones S, Hobbs JR. Incidental correction of severe IgA deficiency by displacement bone marrow transplantation. Bone Marrow Transplant 7:494–495, 1991.

Lang N, Schettler G, Wildhack R. Uber einen Fall von Agammaglobulinamie und das Verhalten parenteral zugefuhrten radioaktiv markierten Gammaglobulins im Serum. Klin Wochenschr 32:856–863, 1954.

Lefranc MP, Hammarstrom L, Smith CIE, Lefranc G. Gene deletions in the human immunoglobulin heavy chain constant region locus: molecular and immunological analysis. Immunodeficiency 2:265–281, 1991.

Lefranc MP, Lefranc G, Rabbitts TH. Inherited deletion of immunoglobulin heavy chain constant region genes in normal human individuals. Nature 300:760–762, 1982.

Lewkonia RM, Gairdner D, Doe WF. IgA deficiency in one of identical twins. BMJ 1:311–313, 1976.

Li X, Ho SN, Luna J, Giacalone J, Thomas DJ, Timmerman LA, Crabtree GR, Francke U. Cloning and chromosomal localization of the human and murine genes for the T-cell transcription factors NFATc and NFATp. Cytogenet Cell Genet 63:185–191, 1995.

Lindberg K, Samuelson A, Rynnel-Dagoo B, Smith CIE, Hammarstrom L. Nasal administration of IgA to individuals with hypogammaglobulinemia. Scand J Infect Dis 25:395–397, 1993.

Lorenz M, Jung S, Radbruch A. Switch transcripts in immunoglobulin class switching. Science 267:1825–1828, 1995.

Luster MI, Leslie GA, Cole RK. Selective IgA deficiency in chickens with spontaneous autoimmune thyroiditis. Nature 263:331, 1976.

Ma Q, Jones D, Borghesani PR, Segal RA, Nagasawa T, Kishimoto T, Bronson RT, Springer TA. Impaired B-lymphopoiesis, myelopoiesis, and derailed cerebellar neuron migration in CXCR4- and SDF-1-deficient mice. Proc Natl Acad Sci USA 95:9448–9453, 1998.

Matuchansky C, Messing B, Tursz T, Galian A, Bernier JJ, Seligmann M, Preud'homme JL. Ulcerative colitis in a patient with anti-B lymphocytotoxin and hypogammaglobulinemia. Gastroenterology 73:578–582, 1977.

Melamed I, Griffiths AM, Roifman CM. Benefit of oral immune globulin therapy in patients with immunodeficiency and chronic diarrhea. J Pediatr 119:486–489, 1991.

Mellemkjaer L, Hammarstrom L, Andersen V, Yuen J, Heilmann C, Barington T, Bjorkander J, Olsen JH. Cancer risk among patients with IgA deficiency or common variable immunodeficiency and their relatives: a combined Danish and Swedish study. Clin Exp Immunol 130:495–500, 2002.

Migone N, Oliviero S, de Lange G, de Lacroix DL, Boschis D, Altruda F, Silengo L, De Marchi M, Carbonara AO. Multiple gene deletions within the human immunoglobulin heavy-chain cluster. Proc Natl Acad Sci USA 81:5811–5815, 1984.

Mochizuki S, Smith CIE, Hallgren R, Hammarstrom L. Systemic immunization against IgA in immunoglobulin deficiency. Clin Exp Immunol 94:334–336, 1993.

Mohiuddin AA, Corren J, Harbeck RJ, Teague JL, Volz M, Gelfand EW. *Ureaplasma urealyticum* chronic osteomyelitis in a patient with hypogammaglobulinemia. J Allergy Clin Immunol 87:104–107, 1991.

Mombaerts P, Mizoguchi E, Grusby MJ, Glimcher LH, Bhan AK, Tonegawa S. Spontaneous development of inflammatory bowel disease in T cell receptor mutant mice. Cell 75:275–282, 1993.

Morell A, Barandun S, Locher G. HTLV-III seroconversion in a homosexual patient with common variable immunodeficiency. N Engl J Med 315:456–457, 1986.

Moroff SD, Hurvitz AI, Peterson ME, Saunders L, Noone KE. IgA deficiency in Sharpei dogs. Vet Immunol Immunopathol 13:181–188, 1986.

Morra M, Silander O, Calpe S, Choi M, Oettgen H, Myers L, Etzioni A, Buckley R, Terhorst C. Alterations of the X-linked lymphoproliferative disease gene *SH2D1A* in common variable immunodeficiency syndrome. Blood 98:1321–1325, 2001.

Müller F, Aukrust P, Nilssen DE, Frøland SS. Reduced serum level of transforming growth factor-beta in patients with IgA deficiency. Clin Immunol Immunopathol 76:203–208, 1995.

Ochs HD, Fischer SH, Lee ML, Delson ES, Kingdon HS, Wedgwood RJ. Intravenous immunoglobulin home treatment for patients with primary immunodeficiency diseases. Lancet i:610–611, 1986.

Oen K, Petty RE, Schroeder ML. Immunoglobulin A deficiency: genetic studies. Tissue Antigens 19:174–182, 1982.

Olerup O, Smith CIE, Bjorkander J, Hammarstrom L. Shared HLA class II associated genetic susceptibility and resistance, related to the HLA-DQB1 gene, in IgA deficiency and common variable immunodeficiency. Proc Natl Acad Sci USA 89:10653–10657, 1992.

Olerup O, Smith CIE, Hammarstrom L. Different amino acids at position 57 of the HLA-DQ chain associated with susceptibility and resistance to IgA deficiency. Nature 347:289–290, 1990.

Olerup O, Smith CIE, Hammarstrom L. Is selective IgA deficiency associated with central HLA genes or alleles of the DR-DQ region? Immunol Today 12:134, 1991.

Olhagen B. Recidiverande luftvägsinfektioner och agammaglobulinemi-ett nytt syndrom. Nord Med 50:1688–1689, 1953.

Osur SL, Lillie MA, Chen PB, Ambrus JL, Wilson ME. Evaluation of serum IgG levels and normalization of T4/T8 ratio after hepatitis in a patient with common variable immunodeficiency. J Allergy Clin Immunol 79:969–975, 1987.

Oxelius V-A, Laurell AB, Lindqvist B, Henryka G, Axelsson U, Bjorkander J, Hanson L-A. IgG subclasses in selective IgA deficiency. Importance of IgG2-IgA deficiency. N Engl J Med 304:1476–1477, 1981.

Ozawa N, Shimizu M, Imai M, Miyawaka Y, Mayumi M. Selective absence of immunoglobulin A1 or A2 among blood donors and hospital patients. Transfusion 26:73–76, 1986.

Pai MK, Davidson M, Bedritis I, Zipursky A. Selective IgA deficiency in Rh-negative women. Vox Sang 27:87–91, 1974.

Pearce KM, Peripanyagam MS. Congenital idiopathic hypogammaglobulinemia. Arch Dis Child 32:422–430, 1957.

Perry GS III, Spector B, Schuman LM, Mandel JS, Anderson VE, McHugh RB, Hanson MR, Fahlstrom SM, Krivit W, Kersey JH. The Wiskott-Aldrich syndrome in USA and in Canada (1892–1979). J Pediatr 97:72–78, 1980.

Petty RE, Sherry DD, Johansson J. Anti-IgA in pregnancy. N Engl J Med 313:1620–1625, 1985.

Plebani A, Monafo V, Ugazio AG, Burgio GR. Clinical heterogeneity and reversibility of selective immunoglobulin A in 80 children. Lancet i:829–831, 1986.

Prasad AS, Koza DW. Agammaglobulinemia. Ann Intern Med 41:629–639, 1954.

Rabbani H, Pan Q, Kondo N, Smith CIE, Hammarstrom L. Duplications and deletions of the human IGHC locus: evolutionary implications. Immunogenetics 45:136–141, 1996.

Rockey JH, Hanson L, Heremans JF, Kunkel HG. Beta-2A aglobulinemia in two healthy men. J Lab Clin Med 63:205–212, 1964.

Roifman CM, Rao CP, Lederman HM, Lavi S, Quinn P, Gelfand EW. Increased susceptibility to *Mycoplasma* infection in patients with hypogammaglobulinemia. Am J Med 80:590–594, 1986.

Rosen FS, Cooper MD, Wedgwood RJ. The primary immunodeficiencies. N Engl J Med 333:431–440, 1995.

Rosen FS, Janeway CA. The gamma globulins. III. The antibody deficiency syndromes. N Engl J Med 275:709–715, 1966.

Rosen FS, Kevy S, Merler E, Janeway CA, Gitlin D. Recurrent bacterial infections and dysgammaglobulinemia: deficient 7S gammaglobulin in the presence of elevated 19S gammaglobulins: report of two cases. Pediatrics 28:182–195, 1961.

Ryan A, Thompson BJ, Webster ADB. Home intravenous immunoglobulin therapy for patients with primary hypogammaglobulinemia. Lancet 2:793, 1988.

Sadlack B, Merz H, Schorle H, Schimpl A, Feller AC, Horak I. Ulcerative colitis–like disease in mice with a disrupted interleukin-2-gene. Cell 75:283–292, 1993.

Salzer U, Gutenberger L, Bossaller L, Schlesier M, Grimbacher B, Eibel H, Peter HH. Finally found: Human BAFF-R deficiency causes CVID. Abstract B72. Presented at the XIth meeting for the European Society for Immunodeficiencies, Versailles, 2004a.

Salzer U, Schlesier M, Ferry B, Woellner C, Rockstroh J, Chapel H, Grimbacher B. Mutations in *TACI* are associated with an immunodeficient phenotype in humans. Abstract B73. Presented at the XIth meeting for the European Society for Immunodeficiencies, Versailles, 2004b.

Salzer U, Chapel HM, Webster ADB, Pan-Hammarström Q, Schmitt-Graeff A, Schlesier M, Peter HH, Rockstroh JK, Schneider P, Schäffer AA, Hammarström L, Grimbacher B. Mutations in *TNFRSF13B* encoding TACI are associated with common variable immunodeficiency in humans. Nat Genet 37:820–828, 2005.

Samuelson A, Borrelli S, Gustafson R, Hammarstrom L, Smith CIE, Jonasson J, Lindberg AA. Characterization of *Haemophilus influenzae* isolates from the respiratory tract of patients with primary antibody deficiencies: evidence for persistent colonization. Scand J Infect Dis 27:303–313, 1995.

Saslaw S, Wall RL. Adult agammaglobulinemia. Proc Centr Soc Clin Res 27:104–109, 1954.

Sawada A, Takihara Y, Kim JY, Matsuda-Hashii Y, Tokimasa S, Fujisaki H, Kubota K, Endo H, Onodera T, Ohta H, Ozono K, Hara J. A congenital mutation of the novel gene *LRRC8* causes agammaglobulinemia in humans. J Clin Invest 112:1707–1713, 2003.

Saxon A, Stevens RH, Ashman RF, Parker NH. Dual immune defects in nongranulomatous ulcerative jejunoileitis with hypogammaglobulinemia. Clin Immunol Immunopathol 8:272–279, 1977.

Schaffer FM, Palermos J, Zhu ZB, Barger BO, Cooper MD, Volonakis JE. Individuals with IgA deficiency and common variable immunodeficiency share polymorphisms of major histocompatibility complex class III genes. Proc Natl Acad Sci USA 86:8015–8019, 1989.

Schiemann B, Gommerman JL, Vora K, Cachero TG, Shulga-Morskaya S, Dobles M, Frew E, Scott ML. An essential role for BAFF in the normal development of B cells through a BCMA-independent pathway. Science 293:2111–2114, 2001.

Schmidt AP, Taswell HF, Gleich GJ. Anaphylactic transfusion reactions associated with anti-IgA antibody. N Engl J Med 280:188–193, 1969.

Schneider PM, Carroll MC, Alper CA, Rittner C, Whitehead AS, Yunis EJ, Colten HR. Polymorphism of the human complement C4 and steroid 21-hydroxylase genes. J Clin Invest 78:650–657, 1986.

Schroeder HW Jr, Schroeder HW 3rd, Sheikh SM. The complex genetics of common variable immunodeficiency. J Invest Med 52:90–103, 2004.

Sideras P, Smith CIE. Molecular and cellular aspects of X-linked agammaglobulinemia. Adv Immunol 59:135–223, 1995.

Smith CIE, Hammarstrom L. Detection of α1 and α2 heavy chain constant region genes in common variable hypogammaglobulinemia patients with undetectable IgA. Scand J Immunol 20:361–363, 1984.

Smith CIE, Hammarstrom L. Immunologic abnormalities induced by D-penicillamine. In: Dukor P, Kallos P, Schlumberger HD, West GB, eds. Pseudoallergic Reactions. Involvement of Drugs and Chemicals 4. Basel: S Karger, pp. 138–180, 1985.

Smith CIE, Hammarstrom L. Cellular basis of immunodeficiency. Ann Clin Res 19:220–229, 1987.

Smith CIE, Hammarstrom L, Henter J-I, de Lange G. Molecular and serological analysis of IgG1 deficiency caused by new forms of the constant region of the IgH chain gene deletion. J Immunol 142:4514–4519, 1989.

Smith CIE, Hammarstrom L, Lindahl M, Lockner D. Kinetics of spontaneously occurring common variable hypogammaglobulinemia. An analysis of two individuals with previously normal immunoglobulin levels. Clin Immunol Immunopathol 37:22–29, 1985.

Smith CIE, Moller G, Severinson E, Hammarstrom L. Frequencies of IL-5 mRNA producing cells in normal individuals and in immunoglobulin-deficient patients as measured by in situ hybridization. Clin Exp Immunol 81:417–422, 1990.

Smith CIE, Notarangelo LD. Molecular basis for X-linked immunodeficiencies. Adv Genet 35:57–116, 1997.

Soltoft J, Petersen L, Kruse P. Immunoglobulin deficiency and regional enteritis. Scand J Gastroenterol 7:233–236, 1972.

Soresina A, Lougaris V, Giliani S, Cardinale F, Armenio L, Cattalini M, Notarangelo LD, Plebani A. Mutations of the X-linked lymphoproliferative disease gene *SH2D1A* mimicking common variable immunodeficiency. Eur J Pediatr 161:656–659, 2002.

Stavnezer J, Radcliffe G, Lin Y-C, Nietupski J, Berggren L, Sitia R, Severinson E. Immunoglobulin heavy-chain switching may be directed by prior induction of transcripts from constant-region genes. Proc Natl Acad Sci USA 85:7704–7708, 1988.

Strothman RA, Sedestrom LM, Ball MJ, Chen SN. HLA association of anti-IgA antibody production. Tissue Antigens 34:141–144, 1989.

Sweinberg SK, Wodell RA, Grodofsky MP, Greene JM, Conley ME. Retrospective analysis of the incidence of pulmonary disease in hypogammaglobulinemia. J Allergy Clin Immunol 88:96–104, 1991.

Tashita H, Fukao T, Kaneko H, Teramoto T, Inoue R, Kasahara K, Kondo N. Molecular basis of selective IgG2 deficiency: the mutated membrane-bound form of γ2 heavy chain caused complete IgG2 deficiency in two Japanese siblings. J Clin Invest 101:677–681, 1998.

Taylor-Robinson D, Furr PM, Webster ADB. *Ureaplasma urealyticum* causing persistent urethritis in a patient with hypogammaglobulinemia. Genitourin Med 61:404–408, 1985.

Teahon K, Webster AD, Price AB, Weston J, Bjarnason I. Studies on the enteropathy associated with primary hypogammaglobulinemia. Gut 35:1244–1249, 1994.

Tjellstrom B, Stenhammar L, Eriksson S, Magnusson K-E. Oral immunoglobulin A supplement in treatment of *Clostridium difficile* enteritis. Lancet 341:701–702, 1993.

Truedsson L, Baskin B, Pan Q, Rabbani H, Vorechovsky I, Smith CIE, Hammarstrom L. Genetics of IgA deficiency. APMIS 103:833–842, 1995.

Ulfarsson J, Gudmundsson S, Birgisdottir B, Kjeld JM, Jensson O. Selective serum IgA deficiency in Icelanders. Frequency, family studies and Ig levels. Acta Med Scand 211:481–487, 1982.

van Zelm MC, Reisli I, van der Burg M, Castano D, van Noesel CJM, van Tol MJD, Woellner C, Grimbacher B, Patino PJ, van Dongen JJM, Franco JL. Novel antibody deficiency in patients with CD19 gene defects. N Engl J Med 2006 in press.

Vogler LB, Waites KB, Wright PF, Perrin JM, Cassell GH. *Ureaplasma urealyticum* polyarthritis in agmmaglobulinemia. Pediatr Inf Dis J 4:687–691, 1985.

Volanakis JE, Zhu Z-B, Schaffer FM, Macon KJ, Palermos J, Barger BO, Go R, Campbell RD, Schroeder HW Jr, Cooper MD. Major histocompatibility complex class III genes and susceptibility to immunoglobulin A deficiency and common variable immunodeficiency. J Clin Invest 89:1914–1922, 1992.

Vorechovsky I, Blennow E, Nordenskjold M, Webster ADB, Hammarstrom L. A putative susceptibility locus on chromosome 18 is not a major contributor to human selective IgA deficiency: evidence from meiotic mapping of 83 multiple-case families. J Immunol 163:2236–2242, 1999.

Vorechovsky I, Zetterquist H, Paganelli R, Koskinen S, Webster ADB, Bjorkander J, Smith CIE, Hammarstrom L. Family and linkage study of selective IgA deficiency and common variable immunodeficiency. Clin Immunol Immunopathol 77:214–218, 1995.

Vyas GN, Perkins HA, Fudenberg HH. Anaphylactoid transfusion reactions associated with anti-IgA. Lancet ii:312–315, 1968.

Vyas GN, Perkins HA, Yang Y-M, Basantani GK. Healthy blood donors with selective absence of immunoglobulin A: prevention of anaphylactic transfusion reactions caused by antibodies to IgA. J Lab Clin Med 85:838–842, 1975.

Warnatz K, Denz A, Drager R, Braun M, Groth C, Wolff-Vorbeck G, Eibel H, Schlesier M, Peter HH. Severe deficiency of switched memory B cells (CD27(+)IgM(−)IgD(−)) in subgroups of patients with common variable immunodeficiency: a new approach to classify a heterogeneous disease. Blood 99:1544–1551, 2002.

Warrington RJ, Rutherford WJ, Sauder PJ, Bees WCH. Homologous antibody to immunoglobulin (Ig)-A suppresses in vitro mitogen-induced IgA synthesis. Clin Immunol Immunopathol 23:698–703, 1982.

Webster ADB, Dalgleish AG, Malkowsky M, Beattie R, Patterson S, Asherson GL, North M, Weiss RA. Isolation of retroviruses from two patients with "common variable" hypogamma-globulinaemia. Lancet i:581–583, 1986.

Webster ADB, Taylor-Robinson D, Furr P, Asherson G. *Mycoplasma* (ureaplasma) septic arthritis in hypogammaglobulinemia. BMJ 1:478–479, 1978.

Wetzler M, Talpaz M, Kleinerman ES, King A, Huh YO, Gutterman JU, Kurzrock R. A new familial immunodeficiency disorder characterized by severe neutropenia, a defective marrow release mechanism, and hypogammaglobulinemia. Am J Med 89:663–672, 1990.

Widell A, Zhang Y-Y, Andersson-Gare B, Hammarstrom L. At least three hepatitis C virus strains implicated in Swedish and Danish patients with intravenous immunoglobulin-associated hepatitis. Transfusion 37:313–320, 1997.

Wilton AN, Cobain TJ, Dawkins RL. Family studies of IgA deficiency. Immunogenetics 21:333–342, 1985.

Wollheim FA, Belfrage S, Coster C, Lindholm H. Primary "acquired" hypogamma-globulinemia. Clinical and genetic aspects of nine cases. Acta Med Scand 176:1–16, 1964.

Wright JJ, Birx DL, Wagner DK, Waldmann TA, Blaese RM, Fleisher TA. Normalization of antibody responsiveness in a patient with common variable hypogammaglobulinemia and HIV infection. N Engl J Med 317:1516–1520, 1987.

Yadav M, Iyngkaran N. Low incidence of selective IgA deficiency in normal Malaysians. Med J Malaysia 34:145–148, 1979.

Yokota T, Coffman R L, Hagiwara H, Rennick D, Takebe Y, Yokota K, Gemmell L, Shrader B, Yang G, Meyerson P, Luh J, Hoy P, Pene J, Briere F, Banchereau J, de Vries J, Lee F, Arai N, Arai K. Isolation and characterization of lympoike cDNA clones encoding mouse and human IgA enhancing factor and eosinophil colony stimulating factor activities: relationship to interleukin 5. Proc Natl Acad Sci USA 84:7378–7382, 1987.

Zhang Y, Pacheco S, Acuna CL, Switzer KC, Wang Y, Gilmore X, Harriman GR, Mbawuike IN. Immunoglobulin A–deficient mice exhibit altered T helper 1–type immune responses but retain mucosal immunity to influenza virus. Immunology 105:286–294, 2002.

Zhou W, Pan-Hammarstrom Q, Freidin M, Aarli JA, Webster ADB, Olerup O, Hammarström L. Drug-induced immunoglobulin deficiency. Chem Immunol in press, 2006.

Zielen S, Bauscher P, Hofmann D, Meur SC. Interleukin 10 and immune restoration in common variable immunodeficiency. Lancet 342:750–751, 1993.

Zou YR, Kottmann AH, Kuroda M, Taniuchi I, Littman DR. Function of the chemokine receptor CXCR4 in haematopoiesis and in cerebellar development. Nature 393:595–599, 1998.

24

Autoimmune Lymphoproliferative Syndrome

JENNIFER M. PUCK, FREDERIC RIEUX-LAUCAT, FRANÇOISE LE DEIST, and STEPHEN E. STRAUS

Immunodeficiency disorders have traditionally been thought of as conditions resulting from the inability to mount effective host responses to infectious agents. However, immune dysregulation and autoimmune phenomena are seen in many inherited and acquired immunodeficiency disorders. Particular alleles of the major histocompatibility (MHC) locus have long been associated with increased susceptibility to a variety of diseases with an autoimmune basis, for example, insulin-dependent diabetes mellitus and celiac disease (Bodmer, 1996; Hammer et al., 1997; Thorsby, 1997). The detailed mechanisms that allow tolerance to be broken so that immune reactions can be directed against one's own tissues are becoming better understood. The composition of the lymphocyte antigen recognition repertoire and the potential for cross-reactivity between self-antigens in one's tissues and foreign antigens from the environment is defined in part by an individual's MHC haplotypes. With improved understanding of the processes directing selection, expansion, and control of an appropriate lymphocyte repertoire, several non–MHC-linked heritable immune disorders are now recognized in which disruption of regulatory functions is a predominant feature. For example, autoimmune polyendocrinopathy with candidiasis and ectodermal dystrophy, or APECED (see Chapter 25), is due to defects in an inducer of presentation of self-antigens in the thymus to provide for central tolerization (Anderson et al., 2002; Liston et al., 2003). Autoimmunity is also a hallmark of interleukin (IL)-2 receptor α-chain deficiency (Chapter 15), common variable immunodeficiency (Chapter 23), Wiskott-Aldrich syndrome (Chapter 31), and X-linked immunodysregulation–polyendocrinopathy–enteropathy (IPEX, Chapter 26). The present chapter concentrates on a discrete class of inherited autoimmune disorders due to impaired apoptosis of activated peripheral lymphocytes.

After leaving the thymus, mature T cells normally undergo a life cycle of activation and effector responses followed by apoptosis, or programmed cell death. Apoptosis maintains immune homeostasis and minimizes potential reactions against self-antigens by limiting lymphocyte accumulation after appropriate expansion in response to antigenic challenge. It is not surprising that a process as important as apoptosis is tightly regulated by interactions among multiple components. Two major mechanisms for the death of lymphocytes after their stimulation are recognized (Lenardo et al., 1999). Passive apoptosis mediated by mitochondrial mechanisms follows withdrawal of IL-2 after clearance of antigen, whereas active apoptosis requires the engagement of specific cell surface molecules, principally the Fas receptor, a member of the tumor necrosis factor receptor (TNFR) gene superfamily also known as CD95 or APO-1.

After lymphocytes have been stimulated and are proliferating, a second encounter with antigen induces expression of both the transmembrane receptor Fas and its ligand, Fas ligand (FasL). Extracellular engagement of a trimer of FasL chains with homotrimeric Fas triggers a cascade of intracellular molecular events leading to alterations in the cell membrane, DNA fragmentation, and ultimately the death of the cell. Two animal models that reveal the in vivo importance of this pathway in maintaining lymphocyte homeostasis are mice with lpr and gld mutations, genetic defects in Fas and FasL expression, respectively (Nagata and Goldstein, 1995). These mice develop lymphoproliferation, autoantibody formation, and autoimmune nephritis. The relevance of the Fas apoptotic pathway to human disease was postulated in 1992 with a description of two children with massive, nonmalignant lymphoid hyperplasia and autoimmune disease (Sneller et al., 1992). Subsequently, Rieux-Laucat et al. (1995) from INSERM, in Paris, and Fisher et al. (1995) from the U.S. National Institutes of Health (NIH) documented that this disorder, now called *autoimmune lymphoproliferative syndrome* (ALPS), is associated with inherited mutations in the gene encoding Fas, *FAS* or *TNFRSF6* (for tumor necrosis factor receptor superfamily member 6, MIM #601859, *134637). The condition has also been called *lymphoproliferative syndrome with autoimmunity* and *Canale-Smith syndrome*, named for the authors of an early clinical description of the condition (Canale and Smith, 1967). Further reports by these and other teams of investigators have enlarged the number of known patients with ALPS to well over 200 and documented that the syndrome can be associated with defects in apoptosis pathway members other than the transmembrane Fas receptor. While the series of patients followed at the NIH is currently the largest (Sneller et al., 1997, 2003; Jackson et al., 1999; Bleesing et al., 2001), patients have been reported worldwide (Drappa et al., 1996; Bettinardi et al., 1997; Le Diest et al., 2003; Rieux-Laucat et al., 2003), providing an increasingly comprehensive picture of the clinical, genetic, and immunologic features of ALPS and its consequences for a patient bearing this defect in lymphocyte apoptosis over a period of decades.

Even among the cohorts of ALPS patients bearing Fas mutations, the story is a complex one. The majority of patients with ALPS have heterozygous *TNFRSF6* mutations, but compound heterozygous or homozygous mutations have been found in a few severely affected patients with early-onset disease in infancy. Most of the mutant Fas alleles from patients with ALPS have a dominant negative effect on apoptosis by normal alleles coexpressed in the same cell. The relatives of ALPS patients who share the same Fas defects may have mild or undetectable lymphoproliferation and autoimmunity, or may be severely affected. These considerations suggest that factors in addition to heterozygous defects of Fas are required for the full clinical expression of ALPS. In addition, individuals with inherited Fas defects are at increased risk of lymphoma and possibly other malignancies. Thus, as the first human immune disorder to be associated with defective lymphocyte apoptosis, ALPS illuminates the critical role of cell death in health and disease.

Diagnostic Criteria and Classification by Genotype

Autoimmune lymphoproliferative syndrome is defined as an impairment of lymphocyte apoptosis that includes chronic, nonmalignant lymphadenopathy and/or splenomegaly, plus expansion of a normally rare subset of lymphocytes in the peripheral blood and tissues—T cells that express α/β T cell receptors (TCRα/β+) but express neither CD4 nor CD8 coreceptors (CD4− CD8−), cells that are referred to as *double-negative T* (DNT) cells. The

Table 24.1. Defining Features of Autoimmune Lymphoproliferative Syndrome

I Required

Chronic (>6 months duration) accumulation of nonmalignant lymphocytes
    Splenomegaly
    Noninfectious lymphadenopathy
Elevated numbers of CD4− CD8− T cells expressing α/β T cell receptors (DNT cells)
    >1% of T cells in peripheral blood
        Demonstrated in histological specimens such as spleen or lymph nodes
Defective lymphocyte apoptosis by in vitro assay

II Nearly Universal

Autoimmunity, including one or more of the following:
    Autoimmune hemolytic anemia
    Autoimmune thrombocytopenia
    Autoimmune neutropenia
    Other autoimmune manifestations
    Autoantibodies, especially positive direct Coombs test

III Supporting

Positive family history of
    Lymphoproliferation, with or without documented autoimmunity
    Lymphoma
Deleterious mutation of *TNFRSF6* or other gene encoding apoptosis mediator proteins

DNT, double-negative T (cells).

strict case definition of ALPS (Table 24.1) requires lymphocyte accumulation, DNT expansion, and defective lymphocyte apoptosis as assayed in vitro. Autoimmune phenomena occur at some time in many individuals manifesting these required elements. Subjects in whom all ALPS criteria cannot be met because of the nonavailability of suitable specimens for analysis can be considered to have a presumptive diagnosis of ALPS. Both the definitive and presumptive diagnoses are further supported by a family history consistent with an autosomal dominant disorder, by occurrence of lymphoma in the patient or his or her relatives, and by molecular diagnostic studies discussed below.

A classification system for genotypes of ALPS has been established by the NIH group (Puck and Straus, 2004), with variations suggested by others (Rieux-Laucat et al., 2003; Holzelova et al., 2004). As shown in Table 24.2, *ALPS Ia* includes the originally reported patients, in whom germ-line *TNFRSF6* mutations produce deleterious consequences for the expression or function of the Fas protein. This type accounts for two-thirds to three-quarters of all

Table 24.2. Genotypic Classification of Autoimmune Lymphoproliferative Syndrome in Unrelated Probands

ALPS Type	Defective Gene	Protein	Percent of ALPS Cases*
Ia	*TNFRSF6*	Fas, major apoptosis receptor in lymphocytes	79
Ia (somatic mutant)	*TNFRSF6*	Same as type Ia	Unknown
Ib	*TNFSF6*	Fas ligand	<1
II	*CASP10, CASP8*	Caspase-10 or caspase-8, intracellular protease in apoptosis cascade	3
III[†]	Unknown	Unknown	17

*NIH cohort (Zhu et al., 2006, and unpublished data).

[†]May include individuals with ALPS Ia, somatic mutant.

ALPS cases in various series. The majority of ALPS Ia patients have dominant, heterozygous *TNFRSF6* mutations, but two patients with compound heterozygous mutations and a patient with homozygous null mutation of Fas have been reported (Rieux-Laucat et al., 1995; Jackson et al., 1999; van der Burg et al., 2000). A few patients reported more recently have had somatic changes in Fas without germ-line mutations (Holzelova et al., 2004), and these are designated *ALPS Ia, somatic*.

Patients who meet the defining criteria for ALPS but lack Fas defects may have deleterious mutations in genes encoding other components of apoptosis pathways. A defect in FasL in an adult patient with atypical lupus defined *ALPS Ib* (Wu et al., 1996). Patients with ALPS and defects in caspase-10 are known as having *ALPS II* (Wang et al., 1999; Zhu et al., 2006). Two siblings with defects in caspase-8 and a phenotype including mild ALPS features plus immunodeficiency can also be considered to have ALPS II (Chun et al., 2002). Patients who meet all the clinical and laboratory criteria for ALPS but in whom mutations in apoptosis pathway genes have not been identified are termed *ALPS III*. Additional patients have been described who have some features of ALPS, but no demonstrable defects of in vitro apoptosis; these are not included in the strictly defined syndrome (Dianzani et al., 1997; unpublished data).

Epidemiology

Autoimmune lymphoproliferative syndrome occurs in both sexes and in persons of diverse racial backgrounds. Because it is a rare condition that has been defined only within the past few years, no figures estimating incidence have yet been generated. However, patients with idiopathic lymphoproliferation and autoimmune phenomena, sometimes inherited as autosomal dominant

traits, have appeared in multiple literature reports and clinical series from the 1960s onward (Randall et al., 1965; Canale and Smith, 1967; Holimon and Madge, 1971; Rao et al., 1974; Cheng et al., 1980). Some of these individuals are likely to have been suffering from ALPS, and in at least three cases ALPS has been proven in follow-up by detection of mutations in *TNFRSF6* (Drappa et al., 1996). Patients with medical findings consistent with ALPS have been under the care of physicians in many specialties: hematologists, called upon to manage the thrombocytopenia and hemolytic anemia; oncologists, who have biopsied the enlarged lymph nodes and sometimes felt compelled to treat patients with persistent adenopathy as if they had lymphoma; and rheumatologists, who have evaluated and managed some of their autoimmune phenomena.

In patients with defined mutations of *TNFRSF6* it has been possible to recognize multiple relatives bearing identical mutations, but with highly variable clinical penetrance. However, similar mutations have not been detected in large numbers of healthy individuals screened at random. In some ALPS families most or all individuals with Fas mutations meet strict criteria for ALPS, as listed in Table 24.1, whereas in other genetically affected persons few or no clinical, immunological, or hematological manifestations can be found.

Clinical Manifestations

Clinical features of ALPS Ia due to mutations in *TNFRSF6* are listed in Table 24.3. The frequencies of each feature are given for probands, defined as unrelated individuals who were the first in their kindred to be referred to the NIH, and their relatives who carry the same *TNFRSF6* mutations as the probands (Sneller et al., 2003, unpublished data). Other series are similar in overall

Table 24.3. Clinical Findings in Probands with ALPS Ia and Their *TNFRSF6* mutation–Positive Relatives (NIH Cohort)

Clinical Finding	Probands* (n = 79)	Relatives† (n = 164)
Age of diagnosis	Birth to 15 years (mean, 2 years)	NA
Gender	36 males, 43 females	
Lymphoproliferation	100%	44%
Lymphadenopathy	92%	30%
Splenomegaly	88%	23%
Splenectomy	51%	17%
Hepatomegaly	72%	NA
Autoantibodies in significant titer	69%	24%
Overt autoimmune disease	70%	24%
Hemolytic anemia, Coombs positive	51%	12%
Idiopathic thrombocytopenic purpura	47%	12%
Neutropenia	23%	2%
Heptatitis, biliary cirrhosis	2–3%	1%–2%
Optic neuritis, uveitis, epscleritis	2–3%	0%
Thyroiditis, hypothyroidism	1–2%	2%
Glomerulonephritis	1–2%	0%
Polyneuroradiculitis (Guillain-Barré)	1%	1%–2%
Encephalomyelitis	1%–2%	0%
Skin rashes, including urticaria, vasculitis	common	NA
Malignancy		
Lymphoma	9%	4%

NA, not available.

*Proband, the first member of each family referred to the NIH.

†While some relatives with *TNFRSF6* mutations meet the criteria for the full definition of ALPS, others do not, because of reduced penetrance and variable expressivity.

range and frequency of clinical features (Le Deist et al., 1996; Vaishnaw et al., 1999b). The presentation of probands with splenomegaly and adenopathy is most often in infancy or early childhood, with a mean age of 2 years; only rarely do patients present with adenopathy as late as 15 years. At least three children were clinically affected at birth (Le Deist et al., 1996, 2003; Bettinardi et al., 1997).

Lymphoproliferation

Lymphoproliferation is the most dramatic and consistent physical feature of ALPS (Table 24.3). In addition, patients almost always develop splenomegaly of moderate to massive proportions before age 5. Although the dimensions of the spleen may fluctuate over time in a given patient, palpable splenomegaly almost always persists. The spleen may extend only 2 to 4 cm below the left costal margin or past the umbilicus and into the pelvis with commensurate degrees of abdominal distention. Splenectomy, originally performed in most patients to manage blood cytopenias, is now discouraged unless severe hypersplenism is refractory to other measures. Splenectomy has been necessitated in ALPS patients by traumatic rupture of their enlarged spleens.

Mild to moderate hepatomegaly is observed in most patients at some point in time. However, clinical signs of liver dysfunction are uncommon in the absence of hepatitis C virus infection, which has complicated the course of some patients who have received blood transfusions for management of severe hemolytic anemia.

Lymphadenopathy is a consistent feature of ALPS. Virtually all patients have experienced protracted periods of palpable, nontender lymph node enlargement, but the dimensions of the nodes can fluctuate, tending to become relatively less impressive through adolescence and adulthood. On the other hand, lymphadenopathy may be massive, distorting anatomical landmarks, as seen in the 5-year-old child depicted in Color Plate 24.I, in whom the lymphoid mass varied but did not abate through 10 years of serial clinical observations. The anterior, posterior cervical, and axillary chains in this patient were the primary sites of enlarged lymph nodes, but as seen in the rear view, there was also enlargement of posterior nodes. Some patients have had enlargement of preauricular and submental nodes as well as nodes in the axillary, epitrochlear, and inguinal chains. Mediastinal and retroperitoneal adenopathy can be detected on imaging studies (Avila et al., 1999; Rao et al., 2006). Canale and Smith (1967) observed that intercurrent infections were associated with reductions in lymph node size, and patients followed at the NIH have had similar paradoxical decreases in lymph nodes in a few, but not most, instances of documented infections.

Autoimmunity

Autoimmunity in ALPS is largely directed against blood cells. Direct Coombs-positive autoimmune hemolytic anemia (AIHA) is the most common autoimmune complication (Table 24.3), immune-mediated thrombocytopenia (ITP) second, while autoimmune neutropenia has been proven less frequently, possibly because of a lack of sensitive standardized tests for antineutrophil antibodies. Episodes of hemolysis may be severe; many patients have experienced at least one occasion on which hemoglobin levels fell below 7 mg/dl. Similarly, platelet counts below 10,000/μl have been seen one or more times in almost half of the patients followed at the NIH (Sneller et al., 1997, unpublished results).

Glomerulonephritis with renal compromise has been severe enough to require dialysis, and Guillain-Barré polyneuroradiculi-

tis has occurred without any recognized predisposing infectious illness (Sneller et al., 1997; Rieux-Laucat et al., 2003). In addition, many patients suffer from recurring rashes, including urticaria and nonspecific cutaneous vasculitis. Other infrequently reported findings of unclear, but presumably immune-mediated pathogenesis in ALPS patients have immune-mediated included arthralgia, arthritis, hepatitis, biliary cirrhosis, iridocyclitis or uveitis, mucosal ulcers, panniculitis, pulmonary infiltrates, seizures, and vasculitis (Rieux-Laucat et al., 2003; Sneller et al., 2003).

Autoimmunity is a hallmark in ALPS. However, it can be difficult to document for three reasons. First, not all patients are tested for many recognized types of autoantibodies. Second, some patients manifest overt autoimmune phenomena only after many years of lymph node and spleen enlargement. For example, one patient seen at the NIH first developed ITP at age 31, while another first manifested AIHA at age 54. Finally, in the absence of demonstrable antiplatelet, antineutrophil, or anti–red cell antibodies, one cannot diagnose with certainty an immune basis for blood cytopenias in a setting of ongoing hypersplenism. Additional patients such as those in reports of Le Deist et al. (1996) and Bettinardi et al. (1997), who were recognized because of their more severely affected siblings, are so far without overt autoimmune disease but do have circulating autoantibodies.

Malignancy

In some patients who later proved to have ALPS a lymphoreticular malignancy had been diagnosed and even treated with multidrug chemotherapy, but this diagnosis was later reversed upon review of the histology in lymph node biopsies. However, in one of the earliest reports of ALPS, Hodgkin disease (HD) and non-Hodgkin lymphoma (NHL) were confirmed in two young adult brothers with ALPS, one of whom died (Fisher et al., 1995). An unrelated ALPS patient treated for confirmed NHL has had an affected cousin who developed HD at age 7, and another unrelated woman and her son with ALPS both had HD (Infante et al., 1998; NIH, unpublished data). A multicenter study determined that in patients with ALPS Ia, the risk of NHL was 14-fold and that of HD was 51-fold above that of the general population (Straus et al., 2001). Lymphomas are almost exclusively B cell derived and include various subtypes of HD, Burkitt lymphoma, follicular B lymphoma, and T cell–rich B cell lymphoma. The overall rate of lymphoma among ALPS Ia patients followed at the NIH is 9% (Table 24.3) (Sneller et al., 2003). Lymphoma has been diagnosed in patients up to 51 years of age; as young patients are followed for increasing durations of time, the overall rate of lymphoma may increase.

Two older ALPS patients reported by Drappa et al. (1996) had malignancy. One, who died of hepatocellular carcinoma at age 43, had risk factors including hepatitis C and a history of prior cytotoxic chemotherapy for his adenopathy. The other had multiple thyroid and breast adenomas and two basal cell carcinomas, all between the ages of 15 and 41. Other solid-organ malignancies have occurred in some of the older relatives of ALPS patients, but neither their frequency nor any other features recognized to date clearly distinguish them from malignancies in the general population.

Overlap Between Autoimmune Lymphoproliferative Syndrome and Other Syndromes

With increased awareness in the medical community, patients previously diagnosed with other conditions have been recognized to have ALPS. Evans syndrome is a hematologic disorder of unknown etiology consisting of multiple autoimmune blood cytopenias, most commonly hemolytic anemia and thrombocytopenia. Enlargement of lymph nodes, spleen, and liver occurs in over half of the cases. First described by Evans et al. (1951), this syndrome is clinically similar to ALPS. A recent examination of 12 patients with Evans syndrome confirmed ALPS in half of them (Teachey et al., 2005). The authors of this study suggested enumeration of αβ DNT cells in all cases of Evans syndrome as an initial screening test for ALPS.

Children with sinus histiocytosis with massive lymphadenopathy (SHML), also known as Rosai-Dorfman disease, share some clinical features with ALPS, including prominent adenopathy, hypergammaglobulinemia, and autoimmune phenomena in 10%–15% of cases (Rosai and Dorfman, 1969, 1972; Grabczynska et al., 2001). Histological examination of tissues from 44 patients with confirmed ALPS Ia revealed in 18 cases the characteristic SHML histiocytic proliferation with emperipolesis (enlarged histiocytes that have engulfed other blood cells) and prominent expression of the S-100 antigen that typifies Rosai-Dorfman syndrome (Maric et al., 2005). A preliminary report has also noted *TNFRSF6* mutations in DNA isolated from tissues of SHML patients (George et al., 2004).

Although the original mouse with Fas deficiency was developed as a model for human systemic lupus erythematosus (SLE), *TNRFSF6* mutations have not been found commonly in patients with SLE. Nonetheless, at least one patient each with ALPS Ia, Ib, and II confirmed by mutation analysis has fulfilled the diagnostic criteria for SLE (Wu et al., 1996; Vaishnaw et al., 1999b; Gill et al., 2003; Zhu et al., 2006).

Finally, the recognition of increased risk of lymphoma in ALPS Ia suggests that with other forms of ALPS, inherited mutations in the receptor-mediated apoptosis pathway may underlie a proportion of sporadic occurrences of this malignancy, and possibly a considerable proportion of familial lymphomas. Somatic mutations in Fas are already well known to occur in some 10% of cases of B cell lymphomas and leukemias. The recent demonstration of somatic mutations in ALPS (Holzelova et al., 2004) indicates that clinical features of autoimmunity and lymphoproliferation can long predate the actual emergence of clonal lymphoproliferation.

Pathological Features

Histopathological analysis of lymph nodes of patients affected with ALPS shows characteristic pathologic changes (Sneller et al., 1992; Lim et al., 1998), as seen in Color Plate 24.II. There is architectural preservation, but with a florid reactive follicular hyperplasia and marked paracortical expansion with immunoblasts and plasma cells. The features resemble those of viral lymphadenitis except for the conspicuous absence of histiocytes normally seen to contain apoptotic debris. The paracortical expansion in ALPS is in some cases extensive enough to consider a differential diagnosis of immunoblastic lymphoma, with many cells expressing the Ki-67 antigen indicative of active proliferation (Gerdes et al., 1984).

Analysis of splenic tissue from patients demonstrates lymphoid hyperplasia of the white pulp with histological features similar to those of the lymph nodes. B cells expand the lymphoid follicles while DNT cells accumulate in the paracortical areas. Bone marrow aspirates are generally unremarkable, although trilineage hematopoiesis is seen in patients with autoimmune cytopenias.

Although many of the T cells in both spleen and lymph nodes are CD4+ or CD8+, the remarkable and most characteristic feature of the lymphoid histology in ALPS is the large proportion of TCR α/β CD4⁻ CD8⁻ cells in the paracortical areas. Given the underlying defects in apoptosis in ALPS, it was surprising when histological analyses showed many splenic lymphocytes undergoing apoptosis (Le Deist et al., 1996). It is presumed that alternative pathways of lymphocyte apoptosis may be up-regulated in an attempt to compensate for a defect in the Fas-mediated apoptosis pathway. As discussed above, histiocytic infiltrates and emperipolesis of lymphocytes and plasma cells, as seen in SHML, are found in biopsied lymph nodes of about 40% of ALPS cases. The enlarged histiocytes, located in paracortical areas and sinusoids, are strongly positive for the S-100 antigen (Maric et al., 2005).

In ALPS II associated with defects in caspase-10, impairment of dendritic cell apoptosis was noted and associated in one patient with expansion of dentritic cells in a lymph node biopsy (Wang et al., 1999).

Laboratory Findings

Immunologic Findings

Lymphocyte phenotyping provided the first clues as to the unique nature of ALPS. There is an increase of peripheral blood CD3+ T cells that exceeds the sum of CD4+ plus CD8+ cells, indicating expansion of a normally minor DNT cell subset. Such cells can be found in the blood of some patients with malignancy, HIV infection, acute viral infections, and certain other inflammatory states. However, in these disorders, the expanded cell subpopulation bears TCR γ/δ T cell receptors. In contrast, the subpopulation that is increased in virtually all patients with ALPS on virtually every occasion includes α/β CD4⁻ CD8⁻ T cells. This population is less than 1% of CD3+ T cells in normal controls and Fas-normal relatives of ALPS patients, whereas ALPS patients typically have 5% to 20% DNT cells, with a range from 1% to 68% (Bleesing et al., 2001). These cells are also generally CD45RA+, CD45RO⁻, CD57+, and many of them express DR, or HLA class II, antigens (Sneller et al., 1997). Unlike CD4⁻ CD8⁻ thymocytes, the DNT cells of ALPS, when isolated and studied in vitro, are poorly responsive to mitogens and antigens and fail to produce cytokines such as IL-2 upon activation (Sneller et al., 1992). Rather than immature cells, they appear to be a population of aged T cells that have escaped elimination by apoptosis. Thus they are a marker for the ALPS disease state, but are probably not themselves a primary cause of autoimmunity.

Patients with ALPS also show other abnormalities in their immunological profiles (Bleesing et al., 2001, 2002) (Table 24.4). In addition to CD4+ and CD8+ T cells displaying DR and CD57, ALPS patients average a five-fold or greater expansion of B cell numbers relative to normal subjects. Natural killer (NK) cell numbers are normal. ALPS patients have a characteristic TH2 T helper cell–oriented cytokine profile, with reduced in vitro release of the TH1 cytokines IL-12, IL-2, and interferon-γ (IFN-γ) and increased TH2 cytokines IL-4, IL-5, and IL-10. Levels of IL-10 in serum are profoundly elevated in some patients with ALPS, especially those with Fas mutations, whereas they are usually undetectable in normal subjects and patients without ALPS, even those who have a variety of autoimmune disorders characterized by autoantibodies, such as SLE (Fuss et al., 1997). The TH2 cytokine profile is thought to promote the development of autoimmune features of ALPS.

Table 24.4. Laboratory Findings in Autoimmune Lymphoproliferative Syndrome

Immunology

Lymphocytes
  Relative, if not absolute lymphocytosis involving both B and T cells
  Excess of CD4− CD8− T cells, specifically >1% α/β TCR CD4− CD8− cells
  Increased proportions of HLA DR+ and CD57+ T cells
  Decreased CD4+ CD25+ regulatory cells
  Decreased CD27 expression on B cells (with increased soluble CD27 in serum)
Decreased delayed-type hypersensitivity to skin test antigens
Granulocytes
  Neutropenia
  Eosinophilia
Immunoglobulins
  Elevated levels of IgG, IgA, and/or IgM
  Monoclonal IgG1 spike in one severely affected patient with homozygous Fas deficiency
  Poor and/or unsustained specific antibody responses to polysaccharide antigens
Autoantibodies to the following:
  Erythrocytes (direct Coombs)
  Platelets
  Neutrophils
  Phospholipids
  Smooth muscle
  Rheumatoid factor
  Antinuclear antigens
Cytokines
  Elevated serum IL-10

Hematology

Anemia
  Hypersplenism
  Autoimmune hemolysis
  Iron deficiency
Elevated vitamin B_{12} levels

Chemistry

Elevated aminotransferases (in cases of hepatitis)
Proteinuria (in cases of glomerulonephritis)

Despite a dramatic and at times alarming degree of lymphoid organ enlargement, immunity in ALPS is surprisingly intact unless disease complications are being treated with immunosuppressive medications. Except for frequent pneumococcal sepsis following splenectomy and a distinctive immunodeficient profile in the two siblings reported with caspase-8 defects, ALPS patients have rarely experienced unusual or severe opportunistic infections. Nonetheless, abnormalities in both humoral and cellular immunity can be demonstrated. Of eight NIH patients tested, four failed to respond to a panel of three delayed-type hypersensitivity skin test antigens. Although antibody responses to T-dependent antigens appear to be intact, patients with ALPS respond poorly to polysaccharide antigens, such as those in the pneumococcal polysaccharide vaccines. Moreover, several patients have failed to sustain initially protective antibody levels to pneumococcal polysaccharides, a concern in asplenic individuals who are susceptible to bacterial sepsis. Antibodies to the T-dependent antigen tetanus toxoid have also been noted to be poorly sustained. Immunoglobulin levels are usually elevated, with IgG concentrations as high as 8 g/dl. IgA or other isotypes may be elevated. The immunoglobulin is almost invariably polyclonal, but Rieux-Laucat et al. (1995) reported one child with a monoclonal IgG-1 spike.

Autoantibody production is very common in ALPS, with most antibodies directed against red cells or platelets. Antineutrophil antibodies and low titers of anti–smooth muscle, antiphospholipid, antinuclear antibodies, and rheumatoid factor can also be seen.

Hematology

Most ALPS patients are anemic on the basis of one or more of three mechanisms: hypersplenism, Coombs-positive hemolysis, and iron deficiency. Prior to splenectomy it is not uncommon for hemoglobin levels to average 7–8 mg/dl. Hemoglobin concentrations below 3 mg/dl can be seen in acute hemolytic crises. Red cell indices are mostly normocytic, but microcytosis is common, and red cell survival is short.

Platelet counts can be normal, but in the presence of hypersplenism are typically low, and they are elevated post-splenectomy. Thrombocytopenic crises with bruising and epistaxis are frequent immune-mediated events.

Nearly all patients with ALPS sustain an absolute lymphocytosis ranging from 8000 to 90,000 cells/µl or even higher, but averaging about 14,000 cells/µl after splenectomy. Granulocytosis can occur, although an absolute neutropenia is common prior to splenectomy. Post-splenectomy immune-mediated neutropenia is well documented (Kwon et al., 2003). Most patients also exhibit a relative, if not absolute, eosinophilia ranging from 3% to 32% and averaging about 7%.

For unknown reasons, vitamin B_{12} levels are modestly to markedly elevated in subjects with ALPS.

Chemistry

The blood chemistry profile in ALPS is largely normal, but occasional patients have persistently elevated aminotransferases in the 100–300 IU/ml range. One individual in the NIH series had hypercholesterolemia associated with lymphocytic infiltration into the hepatic sinusoids and portal triads; liver transplantation was eventually required (S.E. Straus, unpublished). While this patient did not have any evidence of viral hepatitis, a patient with ALPS and hepatitis C has been reported to develop hepatocellular carcinoma (Drappa et al., 1996).

Molecular Basis

The similarity between humans with ALPS and mice with *lpr* and *gld* mutations was postulated in 1992 in a report from the NIH of two children with massive, nonmalignant lymphoid hyperplasia, autoimmune disease, and markedly elevated numbers of DNT cells (Sneller et al., 1992). The *lpr* mouse had been studied for many years as a model for immune complex diseases, particularly lupus, and was known to have lymphoid hyperplasia and expanded DNT cells as well as nephritis due to renal deposition of autoantibodies (Theofilopoulos et al., 1981; Cohen and Eisenberg, 1991). Shortly after the NIH patients were reported in 1992, the genetic cause of the murine *lpr* phenotype was discovered to be a homozygous autosomal recessive mutation causing extremely reduced levels of the protein designated Fas (for *FS*-7 cell line–*a*ssociated *s*urface antigen) (Yonehara et al., 1989; Watanabe-Fukunaga et al., 1992). The same protein was independently identified and named APO-1 (Trauth et al., 1989; Dhein et al., 1992; Oehm et al., 1992), and a third name, CD95, was subsequently assigned.

In both the Japanese group led by S. Yonehara and S. Nagata and the German group led by P.H. Krammer, monoclonal antibodies were developed that induced apoptosis upon binding to the surface of cells. In addition to their effect of cross-linking a cell surface apoptosis receptor, these antibodies were used to purify the Fas/APO-1/CD95 protein, which in turn was partially sequenced, leading to isolation of the human cDNA for the apoptosis gene *TNFRSF6* (previously called *APT1*). Furthermore, the same antibodies were used to demonstrate the absence of Fas on lymphocytes of the *lpr* mouse, indicating that defective lymphocyte apoptosis was the basis of the autoimmune phenotype of this mouse. In related studies, the defect in *gld* mice proved to be in FasL, which cross-links Fas under physiological conditions to induce apoptosis (Fig. 24.1) (Takahashi et al., 1994). Both Rieux-Laucat et al. (1995) and Fisher et al. (1995) described defects in the human *TNFRSF6* gene in patients with autoimmunity, lymphoproliferation, and excess CD4⁻ CD8⁻ T cells, including one of the original NIH patients described by Sneller et al. (1992).

Fas and FasL are members of two superfamilies of receptors and ligands that are important in immune regulation (reviewed in Nagata and Goldstein, 1995; Lenardo et al., 1999). Fas is a member of the tumor necrosis factor receptor superfamily, which includes TNFRSF1A (p55) (see Chapter 27) and TNFRSF1B (p75); CD40, important in B cell activation (see Chapter 19); CD30, found on Reed-Sternberg cells in Hodgkin lymphoma; and several other receptors. These type 1 membrane-spanning proteins share up to 25% amino acid identity and contain variable numbers of conserved extracellular cysteine-rich domains (CRDs). Fas and TNFRSF1A share an intracellular region of homology as well, a 70–amino acid "death domain," around which is assembled a death-inducing signal complex (DISC) that propagates intracellular signals for apoptosis.

Protein structural studies indicate that FasL, which occurs in membrane-bound and secreted forms, self-associates into homotrimers with a conical configuration to become functionally active (Fig. 24.1). The FasL trimer engages a trimeric complex of Fas chains displayed on the surface of lymphocytes. Fas chains self-assemble at the cell surface by means of their pre-ligand association domains in the first CRD of the Fas molecules (Siegel et al., 2000). Upon ligand engagement, the extracellular projections of the Fas trimeric complex extend and embrace the FasL trimer. Disulfide bonds between the cysteine residues of the CRDs stabilize the conformation of the extracellular portion of Fas.

Extracellular binding of a FasL trimer to a Fas trimer results in the formation at the intracellular side of the cell membrane a DISC that consists of the trimeric Fas death domains, the Fas-associated death domain protein FADD (also called *MORT1*), TRADD, RIP, and associated partners that possess proteolytic ICE-like domains (named for their homology to interleukin-1β converting enzyme) (Enari et al., 1995; Hsu et al., 1995, 1996; Los et al., 1995). These ICE-like proteases, now collectively referred to as *caspases*, cleave proteins at specific amino acid recognition sites. Procaspase-8 (originally called FLICE and MACH by different independent groups of discoverers) and procaspase-10 can be cleaved by the proteolytic domain of FADD. After cleavage, caspase-8 and caspase-10 themselves become active proteases that cleave further protease precursors in a cascade, eventually leading to activation of effectors caspase-3 and caspase-9, which in turn bring about the cellular

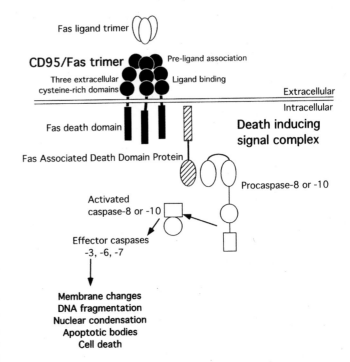

Figure 24.1. Lymphocyte apoptosis pathways (Nagata, 1997). After Fas is linked by trimeric Fas ligand, its intracellular death domain transduces signals to cytoplasmic death domain–containing protein FADD. Caspase protease domains of FADD cleave downstream proteases caspase −8 and −10, which in turn signal the activation of proteolytic enzymes and DNAses.

events that constitute the apoptosis program. Characteristic lethal cellular events collectively known as *apoptosis* include early membrane permeabilization and exposure of proteins not normally detectable at the cell surface; DNA cleavage between nucleosome units into fragments of incremental sizes, visible on electrophoresis gels as "ladders"; condensation and segmentation of nuclei; and shedding of "apoptotic bodies," nuclear particles encased in membrane that are rapidly phagocytosed by macrophages (Nagata and Goldstein, 1995; Lenardo, 1996). Apoptosis, in contrast to necrosis, the other major physiologic mechanism for removal of cells in the body, does not incite local inflammation.

Figure 24.2 shows the organization of the *TNFRSF6* gene encoding Fas; the gene has nine exons within a genomic span of about 25 kb on human chromosome 10q23 (Behrmann et al., 1994). The open reading frame, beginning in exon 2, encodes a signal peptide of 16 amino acids. After directing transmembrane expression this peptide is cleaved off of the mature protein. Exons 2 through 5 encode the three extracellular CRDs of Fas; the sequences encoding the transmembrane domain lie within exon 6. The intracellular domain of *TNFRSF6* includes in exon 9 a death domain with homology to the intracellular portion of *TNFRSF1A*. A number of single nucleotide polymorphisms (SNPs) that do not alter amino acid sequence have been defined within the *TNFRSF6* gene (Neimela et al., 2005). Particularly common SNPs in exon 3 and exon 7 (Fiucci and Ruberti, 1994) make possible allotype assignment for family genetic studies. The Fas protein is expressed in heart and liver as well as in lymphocytes. Particularly high amounts are found in T cells activated by T cell receptor (TCR) engagement and IL-2.

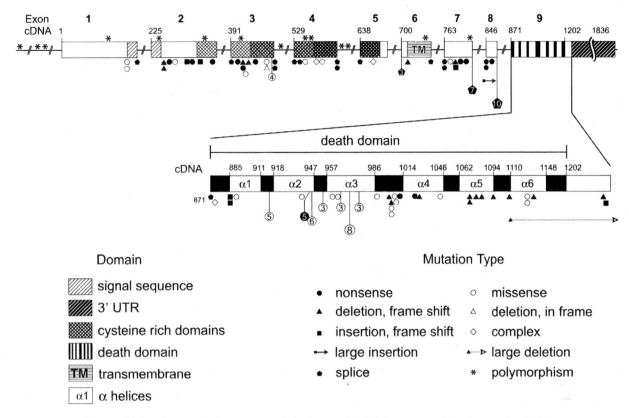

Figure 24.2. Diagram of the structure of the human *TNFRSF6* gene encoding the protein CD95/ Fas/APO-1, showing mutations in patients with ALPS. Asterisks above gene, single nucleotide polymorphisms; symbols below, disease-causing mutations. Symbols containing numbers indicate multiple independent mutations at the same site. Genbank accession number M67454.

Mutation Analysis and Genotype–Phenotype Correlations in ALPS Ia

To date, well over 200 patients with ALPS have been identified (Kasahara et al., 1998; Jackson et al., 1999; Vaishnaw et al., 1999a, 1999b; Le Deist et al., 2003; Puck, 2005). Among these, *TNFRSF6* gene mutations causing ALPS Ia have been found in over 136 families, and several families have more than one affected member (Drappa et al., 1996; Le Deist et al., 1996; Bettinardi et al., 1997; Sneller et al., 1997; Infante et al., 1998; Puck, 2005). There are 107 unique mutations and a minority of recurrent mutations, as indicated in Figure 24.2, which depicts the sites and types of mutations in *TNFRSF6* in patients with ALPS Ia. These mutations, other than the polymorphisms mentioned above and other SNPs that do not alter the predicted amino acid sequence of the Fas protein, have not been detected upon screening over 200 alleles of chromosome 10 from unrelated healthy individuals.

All of the mutations causing ALPS Ia to date are changes of a single nucleotide or a few nucleotides in *TNFRSF6*, except for one 331 bp insertion 5′ of exon 8 that disrupts splicing and one 290 bp terminal deletion in exon 9 (Fig. 24.2). The latter deletion was found in homozygosity in a very severely affected daughter of consanguinous parents (Rieux-Laucat et al., 1995; Le Deist et al., 1996). The infant had massive lymphoproliferation at birth, evidenced by hydrops fetalis with massive hepatosplenomegaly. The spleen had to be removed at the age of 2 months, at which time it weighed 1.8 kg. Other findings were pulmonary infiltrates, intra-abdominal lymph node enlargement as shown by

computed tomographic scanning, and lymphocytosis up to 150,000/µl. Although a *TNFRSF6* mRNA signal of reduced length was detected by Northern analysis in this patient, consistent with deletion of the 3′ end of the gene, Fas protein was not detectable by cell surface staining with anti-Fas antibody, a finding suggesting a defect either in protein synthesis or in stability or transport to the cell membrane. The heterozygous parents of this patient were healthy, and their lymphocytes had normal Fas-mediated apoptosis according to the in vitro testing method employed (Le Deist et al., 1996). Thus, this human null mutation was most reminiscent of the *lpr* mouse mutation in that it resulted in nonexpression of Fas and a recessive, severe disease phenotype.

The three brothers with striking lymphoproliferation characteristic of ALPS reported by Bettinardi et al. (1997) were compound heterozygotes for two missense mutations, one in the extracellular CRD2 domain and the other at the proximal end of the intracellular death domain. One brother had autoimmune thrombocytopenia and hemolytic anemia, while the others had no overt autoimmune disease but did have autoantibodies. Interestingly, their parents, each a heterozygous carrier with one wild-type Fas allele, were reported to be healthy and without elevated DNT cells or defective apoptosis. The mechanism by which the two mutations in these brothers might combine to produce ALPS with recessive phenotype is not clear.

By far the most common form of type Ia ALPS is that associated with heterozygous Fas mutations; ALPS is inherited in an autosomal dominant fashion along with Fas defects in most kindreds, although de novo mutations in probands have been documented. Patients with this form of ALPS have one mutant and one normal, functional Fas allele. As shown in Figure 24.2, the most common region of the *TNFRSF6* gene to be mutated in ALPS Ia is the intracellular death domain in exon 9, expanded in the figure to show the large number of mutations clustered within it. The heterozygous death domain mutations occur in and around the six α-helical regions of the peptide structure (Huang et al., 1996). These mutations are predicted to result in either early termination of protein synthesis (frameshifting insertions and deletions; amino acids changed to stop codons) or single amino acid substitutions (missense mutations) as shown in Figure 24.2. They occur in portions of the death domain that are highly conserved in other death domain proteins and in other species such as the mouse. For example, a point mutation in murine Fas in the *lpr^{cg}* mouse strain has been identified and found to predispose to lymphoproliferation and autoimmune disease similar to that in mice with the *lpr* and *gld* mutations (Watanabe-Fukunaga et al., 1992; Kimura and Matsuzawa, 1994). This missense point mutation in the *lpr^{cg}* mouse introduces a nonconserved asparagine residue corresponding to human Fas amino acid 238, between the second and third α helices. Immediately adjacent to the position of this mouse mutation, three human missense mutations—G237V, G237S, and G237D—have been identified in patients with ALPS. The heterozygous death domain substitution mutations are compatible with expression of mRNA and protein, which suggests that mutant protein molecules may inhibit apoptosis by normal Fas expressed concurrently. Ultrastructural studies have indicated disruption of the death domain architecture by some mutations, whereas others appear to affect contact points between Fas and FADD (Huang et al., 1996).

Many other mutations in the extracellular domains of *TNFRSF6* as well as in the more proximal intracellular regions result in clinical and immunological presentations similar to those of ALPS patients with death domain mutations, but often of milder clinical severity. As an example, one patient with a splice mutation immediately following exon 3 was shown to make in-frame abnormal mRNA and protein that skipped exon 3 (Fisher et al., 1995; this individual is pictured in Color Plate 24.I). Two other patients had mutations within exon 3, a nonsense mutation, and a single base deletion with a frameshift. Curiously, unlike the splice mutation described above, analysis of cDNA clones showed that these mutant alleles were not associated with exon 3 skipping (Jackson et al., 1999; J.M. Puck, unpublished results). If translated, they would produce truncated proteins corresponding only to the first CRD. Splice mutations of exons encoding intracellular domains have also been found, in some cases producing a shortened mRNA and protein terminating immediately after the transmembrane region, but without intracellular charged amino acids to anchor it (Fisher et al., 1995). The possibility that some mutations encode shortened Fas proteins that are secreted from the cell needs to be explored. These mutations may cause disease through the mechanism of haploinsufficiency. Expression and function of mutant alleles must be addressed experimentally to determine whether and by what mechanism they are deleterious.

Satisfactory correlations between the Fas genotype and the clinical presentation or phenotype of each individual are complicated by several factors. First, as indicated above, ALPS may be recessive, but it is more often a dominant disorder associated with heterozygous mutations; the mode of inheritance is at least in part dependent on the type of mutation itself, with homozygous or compound heterozygous mutations expected to produce

more severe, recessive disease. Second, penetrance and expressivity of phenotypes associated with heterozygous Fas mutations are also variable, in that mutation-bearing relatives of ALPS probands may have all of the defining criteria for ALPS or may instead have milder or even completely undetectable clinical and immunological abnormalities (Infante et al., 1998; Jackson et al., 1999; Vaishnaw et al., 1999a).

Functional Aspects: In Vitro Assay of Apoptosis

Defective apoptosis is the hallmark of peripheral blood lymphocytes of patients with ALPS. Activated, cultured T cells from ALPS patients exhibit reduced rates of apoptotic death when stimulated through the TCR CD3 or through the Fas pathway (Fig. 24.3A). To assay apoptosis, peripheral blood mononuclear cells in vitro are initially exposed to a strong activating stimulus such as phytohemagglutinin (PHA). Then the activated T cells from these cultures are maintained and expanded in IL-2, and after 1 to 3 weeks the cells are subjected to cross-linking with an

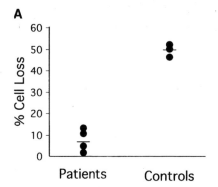

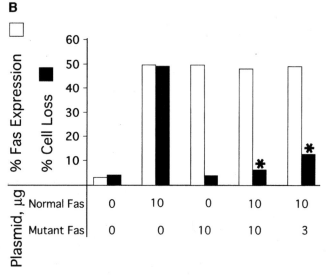

Figure 24.3. Fas-mediated apoptosis. (A) Fas-mediated killing of activated, interleukin-2–dependent T cells derived from ALPS patients vs. normal controls. The percent cell loss reflects the difference between cells exposed to an anti-CD3 monoclonal antibody and cells not exposed to the antibody (Fisher et al., 1995). (B) Expression (open bars) and apoptosis (black bars) in cells transfected in vitro with mixtures of plasmids expressing *TNFRSF6* cDNA constructs, followed by exposure to anti-Fas antibody to induce cell loss. Transfection with normal Fas leads to killing of all cells expressing Fas, whereas essentially no cell loss occurs with mutant Fas. Mixtures of normal and mutant Fas show the dominant negative inhibition of apoptosis by mutated Fas (*) despite the presence of normal Fas.

anti-CD3 antibody, Fas ligand, or an anti-Fas monoclonal antibody, such as CH11 or Apo-1 (Fisher et al., 1995). Apoptosis can be quantitated by a variety of means, perhaps most directly by measuring loss of viable cells in culture wells exposed to antibody vs. no antibody for 24 hours. As shown in Figure 24.3A, after anti-CD3 cross-linking, activated cultures of lymphocytes from four ALPS patients exhibited rates of cell loss averaging only 7% compared to an average of 50% for cultures from three healthy control subjects. Other methods of demonstrating apoptosis include staining free DNA ends that result from DNA fragmentation and demonstrating characteristic membrane changes. Assay conditions and normal ranges for all apoptosis tests must be established and monitored in each laboratory.

By definition, lymphocytes from all ALPS patients with deleterious Fas mutations have defective Fas-specific apoptosis. ALPS patient B cell lines transformed with Epstein Barr virus likewise show defective apoptosis after anti-Fas exposure, indicating that both B and T lymphocytes express the defect in Fas-mediated programmed cell death (Sneller et al., 1997). In addition, mutation-bearing family members, even those with no clinical abnormalities and no elevations of CD4⁻ CD8⁻ T cells, demonstrate defective apoptosis in vitro. Thus the impairment in cellular apoptosis associated with Fas mutation is inherited as a dominant trait.

The NIH group (Fisher et al., 1995) studied the mechanism by which a heterozygous mutant Fas allele can exert a dominant inhibition of apoptosis by using an in vitro transfection system (Fig. 24.3B). *TNRFSF6* cDNA in an expression plasmid introduced into a Fas-negative mouse thymoma cell line by electroporation achieved measurable cell surface expression of mutant or normal Fas in about 50% of the target cells (Fig. 24.3B, open bars). When the human-specific CH11 anti-Fas monoclonal antibody was added (black bars), 50% of cells treated with 10 μg of normal Fas plasmid were killed; thus virtually all of the Fas-expressing cells died. When thymoma cells were transfected with *TNFRSF6* cDNA bearing the death domain mutation T225P found in an ALPS patient, protein was expressed at the cells surface, but there was no apoptotic cell loss after treatment with CH11. As shown on the right of the figure, when mixtures of normal and mutant *TNFRSF6* cDNA were transfected together, the mutant allele inhibited transmission of a death signal by the normal, wild-type allele (Fig. 24.3B, asterisks). With equal amounts of wild-type and mutated Fas cDNA, apoptosis was almost completely interrupted; this dominant inhibitory effect was still seen with a 3:1 wild type–to–mutant ratio.

The dominant interfering effect on apoptosis of Fas proteins with a death domain mutation is consistent with the model of Fas as a functional trimer (Fisher et al., 1995). Three Fas molecules form a trimeric complex to interact with a FasL trimer at the cell surface, and the intracellular death domains of the Fas molecules must interact properly with downstream mediators in the DISC to accomplish cell killing. If there is equal expression of normal and mutant Fas mRNA, normal and defective protein chains are expected to be synthesized and expressed equally at the cell surface. Assembly of these Fas monomer chains into trimers at random will yield only one out of every eight trimer complexes with three normal Fas subunits. Following this model, the presence of one, two, or three defective Fas molecules in a complex is predicted to render that complex nonfunctional. Thus, heterozygous interfering mutations are expected to have a profound inhibitory effect on apoptosis, as is actually observed.

Some Fas proteins with mutations outside of the death domain may also have a dominant inhibitory effect (Fisher et al., 1995;

Jackson et al., 1999). Similarly, truncated Fas protein terminating before or within the death domain may impair apoptosis in a dominant negative fashion (Jackson et al., 1999; Rieux-Laucat et al., 1999; Vaishnaw et al., 1999a). On the other hand, certain mutations, and indeed some splice variants of normal Fas, produce a protein that lacks the transmembrane region and thus may be secreted rather than membrane bound (Cheng et al., 1994; Papoff et al., 1996; Ruberti et al., 1996). In vitro studies by some investigators indicate that peptides containing the first 49 amino acids of Fas are sufficient to inhibit apoptosis in cultured cells (Papoff et al., 1996). However, the pathophysiologic role of secreted Fas in ALPS or in other autoimmune disorders, whether produced by mutant alleles or splice variants, remains unclear. Furthermore, some *TNFRSF6* mutations, such as termination codons at the far 5′ end of the gene are null, resulting in loss of function rather than dominant interference (Jackson et al., 1999; Vaishnaw et al., 1999a). These mutations appear to cause ALPS by producing haploinsufficiency, implying that the amount of Fas at the cell surface is a critical parameter for induction of apoptosis in physiologic conditions.

Autoimmune Lymphoproliferative Syndrome Due to Somatic Mutations of Fas

Holzelova et al. (2004) studied a group of six children presenting by 2 years of age with typical clinical features of ALPS, including lymphadenopathy, splenomegaly, elevated DNT cells, hypergammaglobulinemia, and, in four of six cases, autoimmune disease. Interestingly, none of the patients had affected relatives; moreover, they lacked demonstrable defects in lymphocyte Fas-mediated apoptosis and did not have germ-line mutations of *TNRFSF6*. The DNT cells of these patients were isolated by flow-cytometric sorting, and DNA prepared from this cell subset was subjected to *TNFRSF6* sequence analysis. In all six DNT samples, deleterious Fas mutations either identical to or having the same effects as previously known dominant interfering mutations were found. T cells from these patients that had been activated in vitro and cultured in IL-2 did not harbor the mutations, nor did the patients' buccal mucosal cells, indicating that the Fas defects had arisen by somatic mutation and were subject to positive selective pressure because of their resistance to physiologic apoptosis signals in vivo. ALPS due to Fas defects arising by somatic mutation in T cell precursors, common lymphoid progenitors, or hematopoietic progenitors is designated *ALPS Ia (somatic mutant)* (Table 24.2). It is not yet clear what proportion of patients currently diagnosed as ALPS III may actually have somatic defects in Fas.

ALPS-Like Illnesses Without Fas Defects

Both children and adults who have autoimmune lymphoproliferation but no mutations in *TNFRSF6* have been observed. Some of these individuals have modestly expanded numbers of DNT cells. Among this group are patients with impaired in vitro apoptosis via the Fas pathway, those with normal apoptosis after anti-Fas antibody exposure but impairment of apoptosis by TCR restimulation, and patients with no demonstrable apoptosis defects (Dianzani et al., 1997; Sneller et al., 1997; S.E. Straus and J.M. Puck, unpublished observations; J.P. Villartay, unpublished observations). Additional patients with clinical findings similar to those of ALPS patients have failed to show elevations of DNT cells, although not all have been studied over long time periods with consistent staining protocols. A variety of patients with autoimmune blood cytopenias have splenomegaly with or without adenopathy; they are not considered to have ALPS unless the required features in Table 24.1 are fully met.

Of probands (the first subject enrolled in each kindred) in the NIH cohort who met the criteria for ALPS in Table 24.1, 79% had specific Fas defects (ALPS Ia), as shown in Table 24.2. The remaining patients, however, had normal *TNFRSF6* gene sequences, and were thus investigated for mutations in other components of lymphocyte apoptosis pathways, many of which are depicted in Figure 24.1. A single patient had a mutation in FasL, similar to the patient reported by Wu et al. (1996), and was designated as having ALPS Ib (Bi et al., 2001). No humans to date have been found with mutations in FADD, consistent with the finding that mice with targeted disruptions of this gene are nonviable. However, patients with either caspase-10 or caspase-8 defects have been recognized, and are designated as ALPS II (Table 24.2).

Two heterozygous, dominant-interfering caspase-10 mutations have been found to cause ALPS II in three families (Wang et al., 1999; Zhu et al., 2006). The missense mutations are L285F, located in the proximal portion of the p17 protease domain, and I406L, very near the active site made up of conserved amino acids QACQG at 399–403. An additional mutation V410I was initially noted in homozygosity in a subject with recurrent fevers, noninfectious lymphocytic meningitis, optic neuritis, and no Fas defect (Wang et al., 1999). However, the patient's disease may have been caused in part by a subsequently identified TNF receptor–associated periodic fever mutation (see Chapter 27). Furthermore, the V410I variant of caspase-10 is now known to be a polymorphism in healthy populations, with an allele frequency of 6.8% in Danish, 3.4% in U.S. Caucasian, and 0.5% in African American unrelated individuals (Gronbaek et al., 2000; Zhu et al., 2006). Zhu et al. also confirmed that individuals with caspase-10 V410I, including homozygotes, are healthy, and even found statistical evidence that caspase-10 V410I may have a protective effect against severe disease in subjects with Fas mutations that can cause ALPS Ia. Zhu et al. further reported another caspase-10 population variant, Y446C, present in 1.6% of Caucasian alleles, for which no functional role has yet been demonstrated.

A single family has been found in which a son and daughter of a consanguineous marriage were homozygous for the caspase-8 mutation R248W, a nonconserved amino acid substitution in the proximal p18 protease subunit. Both children had features of ALPS, including adenopathy, mildly increased DNTs, autoantibodies, and impaired lymphocyte apoptosis, whereas heterozygous relatives were unaffected. Moreover, unlike other ALPS cases, these children also manifested T and B cell immunodeficiency with growth retardation, recurrent sinopulmonary and herpes simplex virus infections, eczema, and poor responses to immunizations. The caspase-8 mutation not only abrogated the cleavage activity of experimental protease substrates and failed to mediate apoptosis when transfected into epithelial cell lines, it also rendered the patients' lymphocytes refractory to stimulation in vitro (Chun et al., 2002). Further studies confirmed a requirement for full-length caspase-8 in the NF-κB activation phase of normal T, B, and NK cell responses (Su et al., 2005). Thus caspase-8 has dual functions, in both apoptotic and cell activation pathways.

Patients with ALPS type III are those who meet the criteria for ALPS but have no defined molecular defect. Whereas some have defective Fas-mediated apoptosis, others have been studied whose lymphocytes demonstrate reduced TCR-mediated killing, while Fas-mediated apoptosis is intact by in vitro assay (Sneller et al., 1997). Although some of these individuals may belong to

the ALPS Ia somatic mutant group of patients, lymphocyte apoptosis pathways other than the Fas pathway but still activated by TCR restimulation could be the site of a genetic defect in some of these individuals. It is possible that the majority of such patients described by Dianzani et al. (1997), who had ALPS with Fas pathway apoptosis defects but normal Fas gene sequences, also carry as-yet unidentified mutations in other apoptosis pathway genes.

Strategies for Diagnosis

Unexplained splenomegaly and lymphadenopathy of early onset, particularly when accompanied by overt autoimmune disease and/or a positive family history, are the clinical features that lead to a suspicion of ALPS. More than 1% of α/β CD4− CD8− T cells are a defining characteristic of ALPS, but may not be counted correctly if only CD4, CD8, and CD3 are quantified because several more common conditions are associated with increased γ/δ T cells lacking CD4 and CD8. Hypergammaglobulinemia and elevated numbers of B cells and autoantibodies are further important clues and are more widely assayed. Since Fas membrane expression is absent only in rare patients with null mutations in both alleles, its assessment is of little help in diagnosis. Histological examination of enlarged lymph node biopsies yields a fairly characteristic appearance in ALPS, especially in cases associated with Fas mutations, and special stains revealing DNT cells can be diagnostic even in subjects who are not available to provide fresh blood samples (Lim et al., 1998). In vitro evaluation of lymphocyte apoptosis as triggered by agonistic Fas-specific or anti-CD3–specific antibodies can help establish the diagnosis.

Abnormal Fas-mediated apoptosis should lead first to investigation for causative mutations in the *TNFRSF6* gene transcript and sequence. Single-strand confirmation polymorphism (SSCP) analysis or dideoxy fingerprinting can be used to screen the nine *TNFRSF6* exons (Hyashi, 1992; Sarkar et al., 1992; Fisher et al., 1995). DNA sequencing can be performed on segments of the gene that exhibit abnormal migration in screening assays, characteristic of altered primary sequence. Alternatively, exon 9, the most frequently mutated portion of the gene, can be sequenced first, with subsequent attention to the remaining eight exons if no deleterious mutation is found. Special attention should be given to establishing the significance of missense mutations. SNPs in *TNFRSF6* have been delineated that are not associated with ALPS (Niemela et al., 2006). For previously unreported changes a panel of 100 chromosomes from 50 unrelated, healthy individuals helps to suggest that a missense mutation is not merely a polymorphism without functional consequences. However, functional assays of apoptosis must be combined with sequence abnormalities to prove the deleterious nature of any Fas mutation.

In a patient with clinical and immunologic features of ALPS, a constitutional *TNFRSF6* mutation associated with defective Fas and impaired lymphocyte apoptosis would confirm the diagnosis of ALPS Ia. Patients with Fas defects only in a sublineage of their hematopoietic cells, designated ALPS Ia (somatic mutant), can be diagnosed on the basis of deleterious *TNFRSF6* mutations in isolated DNT cells (Holtzelova et al., 2004). If the sequence of both *TNFRSF6* alleles is normal, deleterious mutations in the genes encoding caspase-10 and caspase-8 (ALPS II) can be sought, as well as FasL (ALPS Ib) if apoptosis in response to anti-Fas stimulation is intact. Remaining patients without defined defects receive a diagnosis of ALPS III.

It is not yet clear to what extent defects in Fas or other lymphocyte apoptosis mediators, particularly caspase-8, contribute to

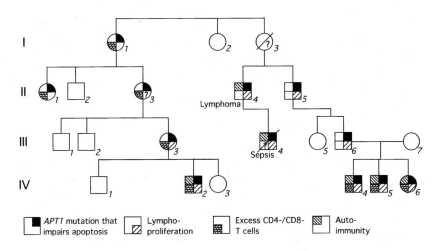

Figure 24.4. Dominant inheritance of *TNFRSF6* mutation and features of ALPS in a large kindred (adapted from Infante et al., 1998). Squares, males; circles females; slash, deceased; ?, could not be ascertained.

common variable immunodeficiency (CVID) (see Chapter 23) or autosomal hyper-IgM syndrome (see Chapter 20), both syndromes representing collections of defects with diverse genetic etiologies. Up to one-third of CVID and autosomal hyper-IgM patients may experience chronic lymphadenopathy and/or splenomegaly, and autoimmune features are commonly present in both conditions. However, it is not common for CVID to be diagnosed as early in life as ALPS, and CVID frequently becomes more severe in the teen years to adulthood, when the findings of ALPS, if anything, tend to regress. Nonetheless, potential overlap between several features of ALPS and other primary immunodeficiency syndromes is an area for further investigation.

The differential diagnosis of ALPS vs. malignancy and the apparent increased risk of lymphomas in ALPS remain major concerns for patients presenting with enlarged lymphoid organs or those who exhibit significant new lymph node enlargement. A biopsy of consistently large or rapidly growing nodes should reveal the characteristic histological features of ALPS (Color Plate 24.II), whereas in lymphoma a homogenous monoclonal cell population disrupts the normal architecture. Study of clonality of immunoglobulin or TCR gene rearrangements and cytogenetic investigation for chromosomal translocations must be done to identify true lymphomas in patients with a history of prolonged adenopathy.

Findings in Relatives of ALPS Probands

Studies of family members of ALPS Ia probands have been undertaken to find additional individuals who might carry the same mutations as ALPS probands (Fisher et al., 1995; Rieux-Laucat et al., 1995, 1999; Drappa et al., 1996; Bettinardi et al., 1997; Sneller et al., 1997; Infante et al., 1998; Jackson et al., 1999; Vaishnaw et al., 1999a). In some instances newly occurring *TNFRSF6* germ-line mutations have been found in probands whose healthy parents had normal *TNFRSF6* gene sequences (Sneller et al., 1997). In the rest of the families, regardless of whether the mode of inheritance was recessive or dominant, relatives with a mutated Fas allele have been identified. Some of these relatives proved completely free of symptoms and signs of ALPS, whereas others met the diagnostic criteria for ALPS (Table 24.1). Still other mutation-bearing relatives had some but not all of the features of ALPS, such as episodes of significant adenopathy or an enlarged spleen without autoimmune disease. For example, in the family of one ALPS patient followed by the NIH group, four relatives in addition to the patient were found to

share the same mutation on one *TNFRSF6* allele. All had defective in vitro lymphocyte apoptosis. However, none of the relatives experienced any clinical manifestations of ALPS and none had autoantibodies or any other laboratory abnormalities except for one individual with mildly increased (1.7%) DNT cells.

In contrast, a large kindred was studied in which 12 individuals in four generations were followed for over 30 years with a variety of findings including splenomegaly, adenopathy, and Coombs-positive anemia; affected subjects were recently proven to have a heterozygous mutation changing an aspartic acid to valine at position 244 (D244V) in the death domain of Fas (Fig. 24.4) (Infante et al., 1998). The diagnosis of ALPS was first confirmed in individual IV-5, who at age 2 was in general good health but had adenopathy and splenomegaly, Coombs-positive anemia, 2.1% DNT cells, and a plasma IgG of 2355 mg/dl. All of the surviving mutation-bearing members of this kindred (black upper right quadrants of pedigree symbols in Fig. 24.4) had impaired lymphocyte apoptosis. Furthermore, as shown in Figure 24.4 each of these individuals had features of ALPS in at least one category— lymphoproliferation, evidenced by splenomegaly and or adenopathy (lower right quadrant), ≥1% DNT cells (lower left quadrant), and autoimmunity, with either overt manifestations such as hemolytic anemia or ITP or significant titers of autoantibodies (upper left quadrant). By late adolescence or adulthood, lymphoproliferation and autoimmune manifestations tended to abate, and the only premature death in the family has been due to post-splenectomy sepsis at age 9 in individual III-4. However, the occurrence of NHL in individual II-4 at age 50 and his development of ITP at age 23 and hemolytic anemia at age 54 demonstrate the lifelong risk of malignancy and the unpredictable course in this and many other families with Fas defects. Since this kindred was reported, Hodgkin lymphoma was diagnosed in individual IV-4 at age 7 years.

Only limited family studies have been conducted in ALPS II, which, seems to have variable penetrance and severity similar to ALPS Ia (Zhu et al., 2006). Prenatal diagnosis has not been published by either mutational analysis of *TNFRSF6* or assessment of lymphocyte surface markers in fetal blood. The prenatal hydramnios of the severely affected recessive case reported by Le Deist et al. (1996) indicates that, at least in this patient, lymphoproliferation was ongoing before birth.

Prognosis and Treatment

Growing experience with ALPS indicates that patients can achieve a normal life span. Patient histories suggest that adenopathy may diminish with age; but while the most severe autoimmune disease appears to occur in early childhood, as indicated above, episodes can recur or, in fact, arise unpredictably at any age. In older individuals now recognized to have a longstanding history of ALPS, splenectomy was common, but recognition of the risks of infection in asplenic subjects has made this a procedure of last resort in current practice. Nonetheless, splenectomy has been required in about half of all of our patients with ALPS to manage their severe hypersplenism, severe hemolysis, or refractory thrombocytopenia without resorting to chronic use of steroids at doses that impair growth and development. Splenectomy has also been performed following splenic rupture and in some cases when lymphoma was suspected. Fatal post-splenectomy sepsis has been documented in multiple patients despite prior administration of polysaccharide vaccines and prescription of prophylactic antibiotics.

On the basis of studies suggesting efficacy in *lpr* mice with an ALPS-like phenotype (Mountz et al., 1987), one patient received sequential therapeutic trials of prednisone, IFN-α, IL-2, and cyclosporine-A for treatment of her disease (Sneller et al., 1997). Therapy with high-dose prednisone resulted in a transient decrease of lymphadenopathy, but the lymph nodes returned to their original size following reduction of the dose. None of the other treatments resulted in a change in the degree of lymphadenopathy or clinical status. In view of the substantial toxicity and lack of efficacy of the various agents used to treat this patient and the fact that the lymphoproliferative disease was not threatening any vital organ function, no attempt has been made to specifically treat lymphoproliferation in other patients seen by the NIH group.

However, many patients with ALPS, even after splenectomy, suffer severe episodes of AIHA, thrombocytopenia, and neutropenia requiring immunosuppressive therapy. Most episodes of ITP and some hemolytic crises respond to short courses of high-dose steroids, such as 1 mg/kg of prednisone daily. In these patients, like the one described above, lymph node size transiently decreases to some degree during treatment. In several patients, multiple courses of high-dose steroid pulses, or prolonged daily steroid plus intravenous immunoglobulin therapy may be required for control of autoimmune disease. At various times in patients with refractory autoimmunity, vincristine, azathioprine, methotrexate, and cyclophosphamide have been used.

Of 87 splenectomized patients followed at the NIH 5 have died. Two children had fatal sepsis due to *Streptococcus pneumoniae*, while three other patients developed opportunistic infections associated with multidrug immunosuppressive therapy for aggressive, infiltrative polyclonal lymphoproliferation (Rao et al., 2005). Efforts to avoid the complications of chronic steroids and immunosuppressive regimens in children with ALPS have led to investigation of alternative agents. The antimalarial drug combination of pyrimethamine and sulphadoxine (Fansidar) was suggested to be effective in a preliminary study of seven ALPS patients, two with ALPS Ia and five with ALPS III (van der Werff Ten Bosch et al., 2002). However, experience with Fansidar among NIH patients has not been as encouraging as suggested by this report. More recently, mycophenolate mofetil (MMF) was evaluated in NIH patients as a potential steroid-sparing immunosuppressive agent. MMF is a prodrug of mycophenolic acid, which inhibits a key enzyme in the purine synthetic pathway, an especially active pathway in T and B lymphocytes. MMF, previously shown to be effective in immune-mediated cytopenias (Howard et al., 2002; Hou et al., 2003), was used to treat cytopenias in 13 ALPS patients who were steroid-dependent (Rao et al., 2005). Twelve of 13 responded, making

possible a reduction or termination of steroid treatment and, in some cases, avoidance of splenectomy.

Most ALPS patients can be successfully weaned from treatment after an acute episode of an autoimmune cytopenia, and the rate of occurrence of episodes and their severity may dimminish as patients enter adolescence. Adults with ALPS may cease to experience autoimmune complications, but conversely, new onset of ITP has occurred in adulthood (Drappa et al., 1996; Infante et al., 1998).

In a patient with complete Fas deficiency, ALPS manifestations were so severe that several courses of antithymocyte globulin and then chemotherapy were given to reduce the lymphocyte burden (Le Deist et al., 1996). This treatment proved to be only transiently beneficial, so T cell–depleted, parental haploidentical bone marrow transplantation (BMT) was undertaken. A first attempt of marrow transplantation led to early rejection. However, a second transplant with T cell–depleted marrow from the second HLA haploidentical parent was successful. There was no recurrence of lymphoproliferation or of autoimmunity, although DNT cells continued to be detected in the child's blood for over 2 years. This child was well 3 years after the second BMT attempt (Benkerrou et al., 1997). Clearly, the role of BMT is not well defined in ALPS, and this treatment should be considered only for the rare patient in whom life-threatening complications prove refractory to more conservative measures.

Animal Models

The MRL *lpr* mouse pointed the way to the discovery of Fas defects in humans. This spontaneous mouse mutant strain has increased autoimmunity compared to the MRL parent strain; it was discovered to have high numbers of CD4$^-$ CD8$^-$ lymphocytes and defective apoptosis and was subsequently demonstrated to be Fas deficient (Watanabe-Fukunaga et al., 1992; Nagata and Goldstein, 1995). Originally described as having a lupus phenotype, the MRL *lpr* mouse actually lacks some of the more typical features of human lupus such as anti-DNA antibodies and frequent arthritis. However, these mice regularly develop antinuclear antibodies, hypergammaglobulinemia, adenopathy, and nephritis. Additional spontaneous mutant mouse strains with a similar phenotype are *gld*, found to have recessive defect of Fas ligand, and *lpr*^{cg}, a strain with a death domain point mutation causing a change in a conserved amino acid of Fas. Transgenic mice expressing dominant negative mutations in Fas corresponding to the mutations found in humans with ALPS had apoptosis defects and developed hepatosplenomegaly and lymphocytic liver infiltration (Choi et al., 1999).

Like the human, the phenotype in mice with *lpr* mutation is highly strain-dependent. For example, C57BL6 mice with the *lpr* mutation have much less severe disease than that of MRL *lpr* mice. Furthermore, the MRL strain is autoimmune-prone, even without defective apoptosis conferred by the *lpr* Fas defect, in part because it expresses a hypoactive variant of IL-2 (Choi et al., 2002). Both class I and class II MHC determinants are important in development of autoimmunity in Fas-deficient mice (Creech et al., 1996; Christianson et al., 1996).

The range of autoimmune findings in *lpr*, *gld*, and *lpr*^{cg} mice is not identical to that seen in humans with ALPS; for example, nephritis is uncommon in patients. While FasL defects are not a frequent cause of ALPS, an adult male with atypical lupus and adenopathy was reported to have a dominant heterozygous FasL mutation (Wu et al., 1996); one additional ALPS patient in the NIH series has a FasL defect (Bi et al., 2001).

Although the mouse is an excellent model system in which to evaluate relationships between Fas apoptosis and other modulators of immune responses, differences between species need to be recognized. For example, the mouse lacks caspase-10, which in humans is located adjacent to caspase-8 and probably arose by gene duplication. Thus the relative roles of these caspases in the Fas apoptosis pathway cannot readily be dissected in mice. Mice with targeted disruptions of caspase-8 have cardiac and hematopoietic defects and do not survive (Varfolomeev et al., 1998), whereas humans lacking caspase-8 activity have features of both ALPS and combined immunodeficiency.

Future Directions and Challenges

Molecular Events Controlling Apoptosis

The importance of programmed cell death in diverse physiologic processes involving dividing cells is widely recognized. We now understand that apoptosis is critical for maintenance of immune cell homeostasis, both by terminating an appropriate immune response and by preventing runaway responses by mature lymphocytes with cross-reactivity to self-antigens. However, all of the molecular events that deliver an apoptotic signal, the process of cell death itself, and the regulation of every step of the process are not yet fully understood (Chinnaiyan and Dixit, 1997; Nagata, 1997). Added insights into these processes have been garnered with extensive studies driven by the availability of cells with Fas defects and of increasingly sophisticated in vitro technologies. For example, the redistribution of Fas into lipid rafts at the cell surface has been highlighted as an important mechanism for making lymphocytes more sensitive to apoptosis (Muppidi and Siegel, 2004). The transmembrane molecules TNFR1 and Fas interact with their ligands as trimers and share intracellular death domain regions. Both the TNFR1 pathway and the Fas pathway are expressed in mature lymphocytes (Zheng et al., 1995). The TNFR1 pathway involves some genes with restricted specificity, such as TNFR1 itself, TRADD, and TRAF-2, but some of the other death domain interacting genes, and perhaps certain caspases and final nuclear effectors of apoptosis, may be shared with the Fas pathway. An additional apoptosis pathway through a distinct receptor DR3 (death receptor 3) has been identified in lymphocytes and additional receptors DR4 and DR5 have been isolated (Chinnaiyan et al., 1996). Other intracellular signal transducers are also involved. The pivotal molecule NF-κB can be activated and appears to have an antiapoptotic effect by up-regulating cellular survival factors, but its relationship with caspase-8 in cell activation is also essential. It is not entirely clear how mitochondrial apoptosis pathways interact with pathways of apoptosis involving TNFR family members, and defects in these pathways may underlie some cases of ALPS III as well as other clinical syndromes involving inflammation, lymphoproliferation, and immune dysregulation.

Modifiers of the ALPS Phenotype

Even among ALPS patients with a well-defined Fas defect, the clinical phenotype can be highly variable, as appreciated early in the course of work in the field. This variation suggests that additional genetic and or environmental factors must be required to interact with Fas defects to produce overt lymphoproliferation and autoimmunity. These putative ALPS-modifying factors might include other members of the Fas apoptosis pathway or related pathways, many of which are still being identified. An existing model for severe disease produced by complementation between two apoptosis pathway mutations is the mouse doubly heterozygous for *gld* and *lpr^cg* defects of FasL and Fas, respectively. Identification of critical intracellular signaling mediators in the caspase protease cascade provides additional candidate genes for modifiers of the ALPS phenotype. Moreover, a large number of gene products regulating lymphocyte signaling networks have been implicated in lymphoproliferation and autoimmunity in mice; many of these could be exacerbated by further impairment of apoptosis and therefore may also be candidates for second mutations in ALPS.

The MHC locus is a major modifier of risk for many autoimmune conditions, and HLA B44 appears to be protective against severe disease in individuals with ALPS Ia (Vacek et al., 2006). The caspase-10 variant V410I is also protective (Zhu et al., 2006). In contrast to many autoimmune diseases, ALPS appears to affect males somewhat more severely than females. Identification and an understanding of the mechanisms whereby these and other factors modify risk promise to clarify the genetic etiologies of further autoimmune syndromes, and perhaps provide new therapeutic approaches for autoimmune disorders.

Acknowledgments

We thank members of ALPS research teams at the NIH: Michael Lenardo, Koneti Rao, Janet Dale, Faith Dugan, Joie Davis, Roxanne Fischer, Thomas Fleisher, Amy Hsu, and Elaine Jaffe; and at INSERM and Hôpital Necker: Alain Fischer, J.P. de Villartay, J.F. Emiel, and N. Brousse. We also thank the families and their referring physicians who have participated in our studies.

References

Anderson MS, Venanzi ES, Klein L, Chen Z, Berzins SP, et al. Projection of an immunological self shadow within the thymus by the aire protein. Science 298:1395–1401, 2002.

Avila AN, Dwyer AJ, Dale JK, Lopatin UA, Sneller MD, Jaffe ES, Puck JM, Straus SE. Autoimmune lymphoproliferative syndrome: a syndrome associated with inherited genetic defects that impair lymphocytic apoptosis—CT and US features. Radiology 212:257–263, 1999.

Behrmann I, Walczak H, Krammer PH. Structure of the human APO-1 gene. Eur J Immunol 24:3057–3062, 1994.

Benkerrou M, Le Deist F, de Villartay JP, Caillat-Zucman S, Rieux-Laucat F, Jabado N, Cavazzana-Calvo M, Fischer A. Correction of Fas (CD95) deficiency by haploidentical bone marrow transplantation. Eur J Immunol 27:2043–2047, 1997.

Bettinardi A, Brugnoni D, Quiròs-Roldan E, Malagoli A, La Grutta S, Correra A, Notarangelo LD. Missense mutations in the Fas gene resulting in autoimmune lymphoproliferative syndrome: a molecular and immunological analysis. Blood 89:902–909, 1997.

Bi LL, Zheng L, Dale JK, Atkinson TP, Puck JM, Lenardo MJ, Straus SE. Autoimmune lymphoproliferative syndrome (ALPS) due to Fas-ligand mutations. Am J Hum Genet (Suppl2):A626, 2001.

Bleesing JJ, Brown MR, Novicio C, Guarraia D, Dale JK, Straus SE, Fleisher TA. A composite picture of TcR a/b (+) CD4(−)CD8(−) T cells (a/b-DNTCs) in humans with autoimmune lymphoproliferative syndrome. Clin Immunol 104:21–30, 2002.

Bleesing JJH, Brown MR, Straus SE, Dale JK, Siegel RM, Johnson M, Lenardo MJ, Puck JM, Fleisher TA. Immunophenotypic profiles in families with lymphoproliferative syndrome. Blood 98:2466–2473, 2001.

Bodmer J. World distribution of HLA alleles and implications for disease. Ciba Found Symp 197:233–253; discussion 253–281, 1996.

Canale VC, Smith CH. Chronic lymphadenopathy simulating malignant lymphoma. J Pediatr 70:891–899, 1967.

Cheng DS, Williams HJ, Kitahara M. Hereditary hepatosplenomegaly. West J Med 132:70–74, 1980.

Cheng J, Zhou T, Liu C, Shapiro JP, Brauer MJ, Kiefer MC, Barr PJ, Mountz JD. Protection from Fas-mediated apoptosis by a soluble form of the Fas molecule. Science 263:1759–1762, 1994.

Chinnaiyan AM, Dixit VM. Portrait of an executioner: the molecular mechanism of FAS/APO-1-induced apoptosis. Semin Immunol 9:69–76, 1997.

Chinnaiyan AM, O'Rourke K, Yu, G-L, Lyons RH, Garg M, Duan DR, Xing L, Gentz R, Ni J, Dixit VM. Signal transduction by DR#, a death domain–containing receptor related to TNFR-1 and CD95. Science 274: 990–992, 1996.

Choi Y, Ramnath VR, Eaton AS, Chen A, Simon-Stoos KL, Kleiner DE, Erikson J, Puck JM. Expression in transgenic mice of dominant interfering fas mutations: a model for human autoimmune lymphoproliferative syndrome. Clin Immunol 93:34–45, 1999.

Choi Y, Simon-Stoos K, Puck JM. Hypo-active variant of IL-2 and associated decreased T cell activation contribute to impaired apoptosis in autoimmune prone MRL mice. Eur J Immunol 32:677–685, 2002.

Christianson GL, Blankenburg RL, Duffy TM, Panka D, Roths JB, Marshak-Rothstein A, Roopenian DC. β2-microglobulin dependence of the lupus-like autoimmune syndrome of MRL-*lpr* mice. J Immunol 156:4932–4939, 1996.

Chun HJ, Zheng L, Ahmad M, Wang J, Speirs CK, et al. Pleiotropic defects in lymphocyte activation caused by caspase-8 mutations laead to human immunodeficiency. Nature 419:395–399, 2002.

Cohen PL, Eisenberg RA. *Lpr* and *gld*: single gene models of systemic autoimmunity and lymphoproliferative disease. Annu Rev Immunol 9: 243–269, 1991.

Creech EA, Nakul-Aquaronne D, Reap EA, Cheek RL, Wolthusen PA, Cohen PL, Eisenberg RA. MHC genes modify systemic autoimmune disease. J Immunol 156:812–817, 1996.

Dianzani U, Bragardo M, DiFranco D, Alliaudi C, Scagni P, Buonfiglio D, Redoglia V, Bonissoni S, Correra A, Dianzani I, Ramenghi U. Deficiency of the Fas apoptosis pathway without Fas gene mutations in pediatric patients with autoimmunity/lymphoproliferation. Blood 89:2871–2879, 1997.

Dhein J, Daniel PT, Trauth BC, Oehm A, Moller P, Krammer PH. Induction of apoptosis by monoclonal antibody anti-APO-1 class switch variants is dependent on cross-linking of APO-1 cell surface antigens. J Immunol 149:3166–3173, 1992.

Drappa J, Vaishnaw AK, Sullivan KE, Chu J-L, Elkon KB. Fas gene mutations in the Canale-Smith syndrome, an inherited lymphoproliferative disorder associated with autoimmunity. N Engl J Med 335:1643–1649, 1996.

Enari M, Hug H, Nagata S. Involvement of an ICE-like protease in Fas-mediated apoptosis. Nature 375:78–81, 1995.

Evans RS, Takahashi K, Duane RT, Payne R, Liu C. Primary thrombocytopenic purpura and acquired hemolytic anemia; evidence for a common etiology. AMA Arch Intern Med 87:48–65, 1951.

Fisher GH, Rosenberg FJ, Straus SE, Dale JK, Middleton LA, Lin AY, Strober W, Lenardo MJ, Puck JM. Dominant interfering Fas gene mutations impair apoptosis in a human autoimmune lymphoproliferative syndrome. Cell 81:935–946, 1995.

Fiucci G, Ruberti G. Detection of polymorphisms within the FAS cDNA gene sequence by GC-clamp denaturing gradient gel electrophoresis. Immunogenetics 39:437–439, 1994.

Fuss IJ, Strober W, Dale JK, Fritz S, Pearlstein G, Puck JM, Lenardo M, Straus S. Characteristic T helper 2 T cell cytokine abnormalities in autoimmune lymphoproliferative syndrome, a syndrome marked by defective apoptosis and humoral autoimmunity. J Immunol 158:1912–1918, 1997.

George T, Ma L, Nagy P, et al. *TNFRSF6* (Fas antigen) mutations in patients with sinus histiocytosis with massive lymphadenopathy. Blood 104 (Suppl):2389a, 2004.

Gerdes J, Lemke H, Baisch H, Wacker HH, Schwab U, Stein H. Cell cycle analysis of a cell proliferation-associated human nuclear antigen defined by the monoclonal antibody Ki-67. J Immunol 133:1710–1715, 1984.

Gill JM, Quisel AM, Rocca PV, Walters DT. Diagnosis of systemic lupus erythematosus. Am Fam Physician 68:2179–2186, 2003.

Grabczynska SA, Toh CT, Francis N, et al. Rosai-Dorfman disease complicated by autoimmune haemolytic anaemia: case report and review of a multisystem disease with cutaneous infiltrates. Br J Dermatol 145:323–326, 2001.

Gronbæk K, Dalby T, Zeuthen J, Ralfiaer E, Guldberg P. The V410I (G1228A) variant of the caspase-10 gene is a common polymorphism of the Danish population. Blood 95:2184–2185, 2000.

Hammer J, Sturniolo T, Sinigaglia F. HLA class II peptide binding specificity and autoimmunity. Adv Immunol 66:67–100. 1997.

Holimon JL, Madge GE. A familial disorder characterized by hepatosplenomegaly presenting as "preleukemia." Va Med Mon 98:644–648, 1971.

Holzelova E, Vonarbourg C, Stolzenberg MC, Arkwright PD, Selz F, Prieur AM, Blanche S, Bartunkova J, Vilmer E, Fischer A, Le Deist F, Rieux-Laucat F. Autoimmune lymphoproliferative syndrome with somatic Fas mutations. N Engl J Med 351:1409–1418, 2004.

Hou M, Peng J, Shi Y, Zhang C, Qin P, Zhao C, Ji X, Wang X, Zhang M. Mycophenolate mofitil (MMF) for the treatment of steroid-resistant idiopathic thrombocytopenic purpura. Eur J Haematol 70:353–357, 2003.

Howard J, Hoffbrand AV, Prentice HG, Mehta A. Mycophenolate mofetil for the treatment of refractory auto-immune haemolytic anaemia and autoimmune thrombocytopenia purpura. Br J Haematol 117:712–715, 2002.

Hsu H, Shu H-B, Pan M-G, Goeddel DV. TRADD–TRAF2 and TRADD–FADD interactions define two distinct TNF receptor 1 signal transduction pathways. Cell 84:299–308, 1996.

Hsu H, Xiong J, Goeddel D. The TNF receptor 1–associated protein TRADD signals cell death and NF-κB activation. Cell 81:495–504, 1995.

Huang B, Eberstadt M, Olejniczak ET, Meadows RP, Fesik S. NMR structure and mutagenesis of the Fas (APO-1/CD95) death domain. Nature 384:638–641, 1996.

Hyashi K. PCR-SSCP: a method for detection of mutations. PCR Genet Anal Tech Appl 9:73–79, 1992.

Infante AJ, Britton HA, DiNapoliT, Middelton LA, Lenardo MJ, Jackson CE, Wang J, Fleisher T, Straus SE, Puck JM. The clinical spectrum in a large kindred with autoimmune lymphoproliferative syndrome (ALPS), due to a Fas mutation that impairs lymphocyte apoptosis. J Pediatr 133:129–622, 1998.

Jackson CE, Fischer RE, Hsu AP, Anderson SM, Choi Y, et al. Autoimmune lymphoproliferative syndrome with defective Fas: genotype influences penetrance. Am J Hum Genet 64:1002–1014, 1999.

Kasahara Y, Wada T, Niida Y, Yachie A, Seki H, Ishida Y, et al. Novel Fas (CD95/APO-1) mutations in infants with a lymphoproliferative disorder. Int Immunol 10:195–202, 1998.

Kimura M, Matsuzawa A. Autoimmunity in mice bearing *lpr^cg*: a novel mutant gene. Int Rev Immunol 11:193–210, 1994.

Kwon S-W, Procter J, Dale JK, Straus SE, Stroncek DF. Neutrophil and platelet antibodies in autoimmune lymphoproliferative syndrome. Vox Sang 85:307–312, 2003.

Le Deist F, Emile J-F, Rieux-Laucat F, Benkerrou M, Roberts I, Brousse N, Fischer A. Clinical, immunological, and pathological consequences of Fas-deficient conditions. Lancet 348:719–723, 1996.

Le Deist F, Rieux-Laucat F, Fischer A. Autoimmune lymphoproliferative syndromes: genetic defects of apoptosis pathways. Cell Death Differ 10: 124–133, 2003.

Lenardo M. Fas and the art of lymphocyte maintenance. J Exp Med 183:721, 1996.

Lenardo M, Chan FKM, Hornung F, McFarland H, Siegel R, Wang J, Zheng L. Mature T lymphocyte apoptosis—immune regulation in a dynamic and unpredictable antigenic environment. Annu Rev Immunol 17:221–253, 1999.

Lim MS, Straus SE, Dale JK, Fleisher TA, Stetler-Stevenson M, et al. Pathological findings in human autoimmune lymphoproliferative syndrome. Am J Pathol 153:1541–1550, 1998.

Liston A, Lesage S, Wilson J, Peltonen L, Goodnow CC. Aire regulates negative selection of organ-specific T cells. Nat Immunol 4:350–354, 2003.

Los M, Van de Craen M, Penning LC, Schenk H, Westendorp M, Baeuerle PA, Droge W, Krammer PH, Fiers W, Schulze OK. Requirement of an ICE/CED-3 protease for Fas/APO-1-mediated apoptosis. Nature 375: 81–83, 1995.

Maric I, Pittaluga S, Dale JK, Delsol G, Niemela J, et al. Histologic features of sinus histiocytosis with massive lymphadenopathy in patients with autoimmune lymphoproliferative syndrome (ALPS). Am J Surg Pathol 29: 903–911, 2005.

Mountz JD, Smith HR, Wilder RL, Reeves JP, Steinberg AD. CS-A therapy in MRL-lpr/lpr mice: amelioration of immunopathology despite autoantibody production. J Immunol 138:157–163, 1987.

Muppidi JR, Siegel RM. Ligand-independent redistribution of Fas (CD95) into lipid rafts mediates clonotypic T cell death. Nat Immunol 5:182–189, 2004.

Nagata S. Apoptosis by death factor. Cell 88:355–365, 1997.

Nagata S, Goldstein P. The Fas death factor. Science 267:1449–1456, 1995.

Niemela JE, Hsu AP, Fleisher TA, Puck JM. Single nucleotide polymorphisms in *TNFRSF6*. Mol Cell Probes 20:21–26, 2006.

Oehm A, Behrmann I, Falk W, Pawlita M, Maier G, Klas C, Li-Weber M, Richards S, Dhein J, Trauth BC, et al. Purification and molecular cloning of the APO-1 cell surface antigen, a member of the tumor necrosis factor/nerve growth factor receptor superfamily. Sequence identity with the Fas antigen. J Biol Chem 267:10709–10715, 1992.

Papoff G, Cascino I, Eramo A, Starace G, Lynch DH, Ruberti G. An N-terminal domain shared by Fas/Apo-1 (CD95) soluble variants prevents cell death in vitro. J Immunol 156:4622–4630, 1996.

Puck JM. ALPSbase: Database of mutations causing human ALPS. http://research.nhgri.nih.gov/alps/, 2005.

Puck JM, Straus SE. Somatic mutations—not just for cancer anymore. N Engl J Med 351:1388–1390, 2004.

Randall DL, Reiquam CW, Githens JH, Robinson A. Familial myeloproliferative disease. Am J Dis Child 110:479–500, 1965.

Rao LM, Shahidi NT, Opitz JM. Hereditary splenomegaly with hypersplenism. Clin Genet 5:379–386, 1974.

Rao VK, Dugan F, Dale JK, Davis J, Tretler J, Hurley JK, Fleisher T, Puck J, Straus SE. Use of mycophenolate mofetil for chronic, refractory immune ctopenias in children with autoimmune lymphoproliferative syndrome. Br J Haematol 129:534–538, 2005.

Rao VK, Carrasquillo JA, Dale JK, Bacharach SL, Whatley M, Dugan F, Tretler J, Fleisher T, Puck JM, Wilson W, Jaffe ES, Avila N, Chen CC, Straus SE. Fluorodeoxyglucose positron emission tomography (FDG-PET) for monitoring lymphadenopathy in the autoimmune lymphoproliferative syndrome (ALPS). Am J Hematol 81:81–85, 2006.

Rieux-Laucat F, Blachere S, Danielan S, De Villartay JP, Oleastro M, Solary E, Bader-Meunier B, Arkwright P, Pondare C, Bernaudin F, Chapel H, Nielsen S, Berrah M, Fischer A, Le Deist F. Lymphoproliferative syndrome with autoimmunity: a possible genetic basis for dominant expression of the clinical manifestations. Blood 94:2575–2582, 1999.

Rieux-Laucat F, Le Deist F, Fischer A. Autoimmune lymphoproliferative syndromes: genetic defects of apoptosis pathways. Cell Death Differ 10:124–133, 2003.

Rieux-Laucat F, Le Deist F, Hivroz C, Roberts IAG, Debatin KM, Fischer A, de Villartay JP. Mutations in Fas associated with human lymphoproliferative syndrome and autoimmunity. Science 268:1347–1349, 1995.

Rosai J, Dorfman RF. Sinus histiocytosis with massive lymphadenopathy. A newly recognized benign clinicopathological entity. Arch Pathol 87:63–70, 1969.

Rosai J, Dorfman RF. Sinus histiocytosis with massive lymphadenopathy: a pseudolymphomatous benign disorder. Analysis of 34 cases. Cancer 30:1174–1188, 1972.

Ruberti G, Cascino I, Papoff G, Eramo A. Fas splicing variants and their effect on apoptosis. Adv Exp Med Biol 406:125–134, 1996.

Sarkar G, Yoon H, Sommer SS. Dideoxy fingerprinting (DDF): a rapid and efficient screen for the presence of mutations. Genomics 13:441, 1992.

Siegel RM, Frederiksen JK, Zacharias DA, Chan FK, Johnson M, Lynch D, Tsien RY, Lenardo MJ. Fas preassociation required for apoptosis signaling and dominant inhibition by pathogenic mutations. Science 288:2354–2357, 2000.

Sneller MC, Dale JK, Straus SE. Autoimmune lymphoproliferative syndrome. Curr Opin Rheumatol 15:417–421, 2003.

Sneller MC, Straus SE, Jaffe ES, Jaffe JS, Fleisher TA, Stetler SM, Strober W. A novel lymphoproliferative/autoimmune syndrome resembling murine lpr/gld disease. J Clin Invest 90:334–341, 1992.

Sneller MC, Wang J, Dale JK, Strober W, Middelton LA, Choi Y, Fleischer TA, Lim MS, Jaffe ES, Puck JM, Lenardo MJ, Straus SE. Clinical, immunologic and genetic features of an autoimmune lymphoproliferative syndrome associated with abnormal lymphocyte apoptosis. Blood 89:1341–1348, 1997.

Straus SE, Jaffe ES, Puck JM, Dale JK, Elkon KB, et al. The development of lymphomas in families with autoimmune lymphoproliferative syndrome with germline Fas mutations and defective lymphocyte apoptosis. Blood. 98:194–200, 2001.

Su H, Bidere N, Zheng L, Cubre A, Sakai K, Dale J, Salmena L, Hakem R, Straus S, Lenardo M. Requirement for caspase-8 in NF-κB activation by antigen receptor. Science 307:1465–1468, 2005.

Takahashi T, Tanaka M, Brannan CI, Jenkins NA, Copeland NG, Suda T, Nagata S. Generalized lymphoproliferative disease in mice, caused by a point mutation in the Fas ligand. Cell 76:969–976, 1994.

Teachey DT, Manno CS, Axsom KM, Andrews T, Choi JK, Greenbaum BH, McMann JM, Sullivan KE, Travis SF, Grupp SA. Unmasking Evans syndrome: T-cell phenotype and apoptotic response reveal autoimmune lymphoproliferative syndrome (ALPS). Blood 105:2443–2448, 2005.

Theofilopoulos AN, Balderas RS, Shawler DL, Lee S, Dixon FJ. Influence of thymic genotype on the systemic lupus erythematosus-like disease and T cell proliferation of MRL/Mp-lpr/lpr mice. J Exp Med 153:1405–1414, 1981.

Thorsby E. Invited anniversary review: HLA associated diseases. Hum Immunol 53:1–11, 1997.

Trauth BC, Klas C, Peters AMJ, Matzuku S, Möller P, Falk W, Debatin K-M, Krammer PH. Monoclonal antibody–mediated tumor regression by induction of apoptosis. Science 245:301–305, 1989.

Vacek MM, Schäffer AA, Davis J, Fischer RE, Dale JK, Straus SE, Puck JM. HLA B44 is associated with decreased severity of autoimmune lymphoproliferative syndrome in patients with CD95 mutations (ALPS Ia). Clin Immunol 118:59–65, 2006.

Vaishnaw AK, Orlinick JR, Chu J-L, Krammer PH, Chao MV, Elkon KB. The molecular basis for apoptotic defects in patients with CD95 (Fas/APO-1) mutations. J Clin Invest 103:355–363, 1999a.

Vaishnaw AK, Toubi E, Ohsako S, Drappa J, Buys S, Estrada J, Sitarz A, Zemel L, Chu J-L, Elkon KB. The spectrum of apoptotic defects and clinical manifestations, including systemic lupus erythematosus, in humans with CD95 (Fas/APO-1) mutations. Arthritis Rheum 42:1833–1842, 1999b.

van der Burg M, de Groot R, Comans-Bitter WM, den Hollander JC, Hooijkaas H, Neijens HJ, Berger RM, Oranje AP, Langerak AW, van Dongen JJ. Autoimmune lymphoproliferative syndrome (ALPS) in a child from consanguineous parents: a dominant or recessive disease? Pediatr Res 47:336–343, 2000.

van der Werff Ten Bosch J, Schotte P, Ferster A, Azzi N, Boehler T, Laurey G, Arola M, Demanet C, Beyaert R, Thielemans K, Otten J. Reversion of autoimmune lymphoproliferative syndrome with an antimalarial drug: preliminary results of a clinical cohort study and molecular observations. Br J Haematol 117:176–188, 2002.

Varfolomeev EE, Schuchmann M, Luria V, Chiannilkulchai N, Beckmann JS, Mett IL, Rebrikov D, Brodianski VM, Kemper OC, Kollet O, Lapidot T, Soffer D, Sobe T, Avraham KB, Goncharov T, Holtmann H, Lonai P, Wallach D. Targeted disruption of the mouse caspase 8 gene ablates cell death induction by the TNF receptors, Fas/Apo1, and DR3 and is lethal prenatally. Immunity 9:167–176, 1998.

Wang J, Zheng L, Lobito A, Chan FK-M, Dale J, Sneller M, Yao X, Puck JM, Straus SE, Lenardo MJ. Inherited human caspase 10 mutations underlie defective lymphocyte and dentritic cell apoptosis in autoimmune lymphoproliferative syndrome type II. Cell 98:47–58, 1999.

Watanabe-Fukunaga R, Brannan CI, Copeland NG, Jenkins NA, Nagata S. Lymphoproliferation disorder in mice explained by defects in Fas antigen that mediates apoptosis. Nature 356:314–318, 1992.

Wu J, Wilson J, He J, Xiang L, Schur PH, Mountz JD. Fas ligand mutation in a patient with systemic lupus erythematosus and lymphoproliferative disease. J Clin Invest 98:1107–1113, 1996.

Yonehara S, Ishii A, Yonehara M. A cell-killing monoclonal antibody (anti-Fas) to a cell surface antigen co-downregulated with the receptor of tumor necrosis factor. J Exp Med 169:1747–1756, 1989.

Zheng L, Fisher G, Miller RE, Peschon J, Lynch DH, Lenardo MJ. Induction of apoptosis in mature T cells by tumour necrosis factor. Nature 377:348–351, 1995.

Zhu S, Hsu AP, Vacek MM, Zheng L, Schäffer AA, Dale JK, Davis J, Fischer RE, Straus SE, Boruchov D, Saulsbury FT, Lenardo MJ, Puck JM. Genetic alterations in caspase-10 may be causative or protective in autoimmune lymphoproliferative syndrome. Hum Genet 119:284–294, 2006.

25

Autoimmune Polyendocrinopathy, Candidiasis, Ectodermal Dystrophy

LEENA PELTONEN-PALOTIE, MARIA HALONEN, and JAAKKO PERHEENTUPA

Autoimmune polyendocrinopathy–candidiasis–ectodermal dystrophy (APECED; OMIM 240300), an autosomal recessive disease, provides a unique model for molecular studies of autoimmunity because of the monogenic inheritance of this disorder, characterized by multiple features of abnormal immunological tolerance. APECED was first mentioned in the literature by Thorpe and Handley in 1929, and since then it has been given several names, such as APS1 or Whitaker's syndrome (Leonard, 1946; Whitaker et al., 1956; Neufeld et al., 1981; Ahonen, 1985). Patients with APECED have been identified in numerous populations and among multiple ethnicities. The disease occurs more frequently in isolated populations, the lifetime prevalence being rather high among the Finns, Iranian Jews, and Sardinians (1/25,000, 1/9000, and 1/14,500, respectively) (Zlotogora and Shapiro, 1992; Rosatelli et al., 1998).

The APECED locus was mapped in the Finnish families to 21q22.3 (Aaltonen et al., 1994). The locus homogeneity was confirmed in a multinational group of patients, although the mutations in patients with distinct origins are expected to be different because of different haplotypes of disease alleles (Björses et al., 1996). A novel gene, *AIRE* (for *AutoImmune REgulator*), which causes APECED, was positionally cloned in 1997 (Finnish-German APECED Consortium, 1997; Nagamine et al., 1997). *AIRE* contains 11.9 kb of genomic DNA and 14 exons with boundaries that follow the GT-AG rule (Mount, 1982). The last exon of the gene seems to overlap with the promoter region of the *PFKL* gene, transcribed from the same strand of DNA as *AIRE* (Levanon et al., 1995). Close to 50 mutations have been identified in APECED patients. The distribution of these mutations has guided analyses of the functional domains of the 545–amino acid–long Aire protein. This protein is targeted to both the nucleus and cytoplasm and its role as a transcription activator has been demonstrated in vitro. Analysis of the first knockout mouse models suggests a role for Aire in the development of both central and peripheral tolerance (Anderson et al., 2002; Ramsey et al., 2002b). Several excellent reviews on APECED and AIRE have been published (Anderson, 2002; Björses et al., 1998; Peterson et al., 1998a, 1998b; Aaltonen and Björses, 1999; Meriluoto et al., 2001).

Clinical and Pathological Manifestations

The clinical picture of APECED is highly variable (Ahonen et al., 1990; Betterle et al., 1998; Perheentupa and Miettinen, 1999; Myhre et al., 2001; Perheentupa, 2002) (Table 25.1) and the frequencies of the phenotype components vary from one population to another. Symptoms include components of three biological pathways: (1) autoaggressive destruction of tissues, predominantly endocrine glands; (2) consequences of a partial defect of cell-mediated immunity, most commonly superficial candidiasis; and (3) ectodermal dystrophies. Factors contributing to the complexity of the disease are not yet understood, but variation in symptoms among siblings suggests that factors other than the *AIRE* mutations play an important role. Unlike other APECED patients, Iranian Jewish patients (Zlotogora and Schapiro, 1992) have no keratopathy and have a lower prevalence of candidiasis and hypoadrenocorticism. Italian patients differ from Finnish patients in having less frequent keratoconjunctivitis (12% vs. 21%) and diabetes (2% vs. 18%) (Betterle et al., 1998).

A so-called Whitaker's triad of symptoms—hypoparathyroidism, adrenocortical failure (Addison's disease), and chronic mucocutaneous candidal infections—is pathognomonic for APECED (Ahonen et al., 1990). Other endocrinopathies include gonadal atrophy, type 1 diabetes, gastric parietal cell atrophy, and hypothyroidism (Ahonen et al., 1990; Betterle et al., 1993). The mucocutaneous candidiasis can affect the oral, ungual, esophagial,

Table 25.1. Frequency of Clinical Features of APECED

Disease Component	Prevalence (%)
Endocrine Components	
Hypoparathyroidism	79
Addison disease	72
Ovarian failure	60*
Hypothyroidism	4
Type 1 diabetes	12
Pernicious anemia	13
Nonendocrine Components	
Mucocutaneous candidiasis	100
Enamel hypoplasia	77
Vitiligo	13
Alopecia	72
Nail dystrophy	52
Malabsorption	18
Autoimmune hepatitis	12
Keratopathy	35
Rare Disease Components	*No. of cases*
Central diabetes insipidus	6
Growth hormone deficiency	8
Adrenocorticotropin deficiency	3
Gonadotropin deficiency	2
Hyperthyroidism	3
Autoimmune hemolytic anemia	3
IgA deficiency	>18
Asplenia	18
Cholelithiasis	7
Periodic fever with rash	11
Sjögren syndrome	20
Oral squamous cell carcinoma	8

*Calculated for postpubertal females.

and vaginal mucosa and nails. Autoimmune hepatitis, enamel hypoplasia, nail dystrophies, keratoconjunctivitis, vitiligo, and alopecia are other typical manifestations of APECED (Wagman et al., 1987; Lukinmaa et al., 1996; Perniola et al., 1998) (Table 25.1 and Color Plates 25.I to 25.VI). Candidiasis, hypoparathyroidism, and hypoadrenocorticism were found in 50% of Finnish patients at the age of 20 years, 55% at age 30, and 40% at age 40. It should be emphasized that the diagnostic criterion of having at least two elements of this triad would leave many cases missed. In some cases the rare components dominate with none of the triad present.

Candidiasis

Oral candidiasis usually appears first in the mildest cases as angular cheilosis (Color Plate 25.V). Presentations include acute inflammation of all oral mucosa, hyperplastic chronic candidiasis with thick, white tongue coating, and atrophic disease characterized by scant coatings and scarred thin mucosa with leukoplakia-like areas (Myllärniemi and Perheentupa, 1978). This chronic condition is carcinogenic. Candidal esophagitis is also common; it causes substernal pain and odynophagia and may lead to stricture with dysphagia. Perianal candidal eczema is common, and intestinal mucosal candidiasis may cause abdominal pain, meteorism, and diarrhea. The infection may spread to the skin of the hands and face and the nails. Candidal vulvovaginitis is also common after puberty. Humoral immunity against *Candida*

develops normally. Generalized candidiasis has only been reported in patients on immunosuppressive medication (Betterle et al., 1998). Serious lung disease may be more common (Brun, 1982). Extensive bilateral pneumonia was reported in one patient (Arvanitakis and Knouss, 1973). In a 30-year-old patient of ours who died of septicemia after hip joint replacement, the autopsy revealed *Candida* abscesses in the pericardium and small intestine, along with necrotizing inflammation of the large intestine and mesenterium.

Endocrinopathies and Associated Clinical Features

In some patients, hypoparathyroidism can be latent for years before a distinct manifestation occurs. In the Finnish series of 90 APECED patients, it remained the only endocrinopathy in 27% of patients at age 20 and in 18% at age 30. Adrenocortical insufficiency remained the only endocrinopathy in 15% of our patients at age 20 and in 14% at age 30. Hypogonadism manifested as primary gonadal failure in our patients. Half of the affected females had primary amenorrhea, many with partial pubertal development. All females with hypogonadism also had hypoadrenocorticism, and 92% of females over 15 years of age who had hypoadrenocorticism also had hypogonadism. Of 7 males who had hypogonadism, 5 had hypoadrenocorticism, whereas only 5 of 27 males with hypoadrenocorticism had hypogonadism.

Diabetes mellitus (DM) affected 12% of our APECED patients—4.5- to 9-fold more patients than in other large series (Neufeld et al., 1981; Betterle et al., 1998). This rate reflects the prevalence of type I DM in the general population. Hypothyroidism is relatively uncommon, but was the first endocrinopathy in one of our patients. Hyperthyroidism is rare. Hashimoto's thyroiditis may occur at the same frequency as that of hypothyroidism (Brun, 1982). Pernicious anemia (autoimmune gastritis) is the most common gastrointestinal problem, with a peak incidence at 10 to 20 years of age.

Periodic or chronic diarrhea, usually with steatorrhea, and severe obstipation (often alternating with diarrhea) are equally prevalent. In most cases the diarrhea is secondary to hypoparathyroidism and depends on the presence of hypocalcemia (Peracchi et al., 1998). However, most patients having equally severe hypocalcemia never develop diarrhea. Also, some patients develop hypoparathyroidism years after the onset of diarrhea, and some not at all. The diarrhea may become severely incapacitating through a vicious cycle with hypocalcemia: diarrhea impairs the ability to absorb calcium and the calciferol drugs, making the hypocalcemia difficult to control by oral medication. Apparently, hypocalcemia prevents secretion of cholecystokinin by the duodenal mucosa in response to a meal, leading to failure of the physiologic stimulus for normal gall bladder contraction and pancreatic enzyme secretion (Miettinen and Perheentupa, 1971; Heubi et al., 1983; Högenauer et al., 2001). In three cases secretory failure of the exocrine pancreas appeared to be the predominant mechanism, thus enzyme replacement was necessary (Scirè et al., 1991; Ward et al., 1999, 2001; J. Perheentupa, unpublished observations). The autoimmune destruction of enterochromaffin cells (EC) of duodenal mucosa, which produce cholecystokinin and serotonin, has been demonstrated (Ekwall et al., 1998; Ward et al., 1999). This condition has been treated with success using immunosuppressive medication (Padeh et al., 1997; Ward et al., 1999, 2001).

Autoimmune hepatitis may be the first manifestation of APECED. In most cases chronic and without symptoms, it may lead to cirrhosis or be fulminant and lethal. Three of our 15 patients died within 2 months of the diagnosis, despite intensive immunosuppressive therapy.

Keratoconjunctivitis is relatively common, seemingly independent of hypoparathyroidism, and typically develops before the age of 17. In some Finnish cases this was the first symptom or part of the initial manifestation, or it occurred after candidiasis. Initial symptoms are intense photophobia, blepharospasm, and lacrimation.

Skin Symptoms and Ectodermal Dystrophies

The most frequent manifestation of ectodermal dystrophy is enamel hypoplasia of permanent teeth (Color Plate 25.1) (Myllärniemi and Perheentupa, 1978; Lukinmaa et al., 1996). Alopecia was the first manifestation or among the initial symptoms in 4% of Finnish patients. Appearing as patchy loss of hair, in 21 of 28 of our patients it became universal, being transient in some cases. Vitiligo is highly variable. In a few patients initial spots fade, but in most patients they grow larger (Color Plate 25.VI). Urticaria-like erythema with fever recurred frequently over 2 months to 11 years in 8 of our 89 patients. In three cases, biopsy revealed lymphoplasmacytic vasculitis. Serum IgG levels were supranormal, and circulating immune complexes were detected in one patient. Hepatitis was 3.5-fold and iridocyclitis 30-fold more prevalent in these patients than in the others.

Pathological Manifestations

The autoimmune tissue destruction in APECED appears similar to that observed in the same tissues in non-APECED autoimmunity. Initial features include tissue infiltration by lymphocytes, plasma cells, and macrophages. The tissue structure is then gradually destroyed, resulting in atrophy or hyalinization. In some cases parenchymal cells are replaced by fat cells or fibrotic tissue. The atrophy may be focal (Williams and Wood, 1959) and its timing may differ among the three layers of the adrenal cortex (Craig et al., 1955). The parathyroid and adrenal glands often become undetectable and the adrenal medulla, initially unaffected, may dramatically atrophy (Gass, 1962). Early in the course of hepatitis, lymphocytic infiltration is confined to portal tracts and immediate periportal areas. With periportal lymphoplasmacytic infiltration necrosis of periportal hepatocytes may appear. At later stages, heavy infiltration of lymphocytes, macrophages, and polymorphonuclear leukocytes results in the widening of portal tracts and in a fibrotic process dominated by collagen fibers and lobular necroinflammation. Cirrhosis is followed by canalicular and intracellular cholestasis, ballooning degeneration of hepatocytes, and lobular disarray (Craig et al., 1955; Goldstein et al., 1996).

The keratitic corneas show irregular, initially slightly raised, confluent and grayish opacities, with mild bulbar injection of the conjunctiva, and subsequent superficial corneal neovascularization (Gass, 1962). In advanced cases, the corneal epithelium becomes severly atrophic with areas of incipient epidermalization. Bowman's membrane is destroyed and the anterior corneal stroma can be replaced by vascularized scar tissue and areas of chronic lymphoplasmacytic infiltration (Tarkkanen and Merenmies, 2001).

There are also reports of nontypical pathological tissue changes in APECED. In a patient with microscopic hematuria and significant proteinuria, a biopsy revealed focal segmental proliferative glomerulonephritis with crescentic glomeruli, and

Table 25.2. Autoantigens Characterized in Patients with APECED

Disease Component Endocrine	Autoantigen
Addison's disease	P450c21
	P450c17
	P450scc
Gonadal failure	P450scc
Hypoparathyroidism	Calcium sensing receptor
Hypothyroidism	TPO
	TG
IDDM	ICA
	GAD65, GAD67
	IA-2
Nonendocrine	
Alopecia	TH
Autoimmune hepatitis	P4501A2
	P4502A6
	AADC
Autoimmune gastritis	H+K+-ATPase
	intrinsic factor
Malabsorption	TPH
Vitiligo	Transcription factors SOX9 and SOX10

Abbreviations: AADC, aromatic L-amino acid decarboxylase; GAD, glutamic acid decarboxylase; H+K+ATPase, proton pump of the gastric mucosa; IA-2, tyrosine phosphatase; ICA, islet cell antigen; scc, side chain–cleaving enzyme; TG, thyroglobulin; TH, tyrosine hydroxylase; TPH, tryptophan hydroxylase; TPO, thyroid peroxidase.

irregular granular deposits of IgG and C3 on the basement membrane (Berberoglu et al., 2000). One patient with emotional lability associated with retrograde amnesia had patchy demyelination lesions in deep white matter, characteristic of progressive multifocal leukoencephalopathy (Parker et al., 1990). At the autopsy of a 6-year old patient with no apparent neurological clinical abnormalities, isolated focal perivascular collections of lymphocytes and large mononuclear cells were observed in the hippocampal gyrus and medulla. The olivary nucleus showed degeneration, neurophagia, loss of nerve cells, and accumulation of glial elements (Craig et al., 1955). Not surprisingly, this would imply a general autoimmune reaction manifesting in multiple tissues and showing wide individual variation.

Laboratory Findings

The autoimmune manifestations of APECED include not only infiltration of lymphocytes in affected organs but also the presence of various circulating, antigen-specific autoantibodies (Table 25.2) (Ahonen, 1993; Song et al., 1996; Perniola et al., 2000). The autoantibodies facilitate the clinical diagnosis and to some degree predict the course of the disease. The sensitivity of an APECED diagnosis obtained by detection of autoantibodies (P450c21, P450scc and AADC) is 89%. One group of autoantibodies is targeted against hydroxylases P450c17 (Krohn et al. 1992), P450c21 (Winqvist et al., 1992; Uibo et al., 1994b) and P450scc (Uibo et al., 1994a; Winqvist et al., 1995), which catalyse those chemical reactions required for the production of steroid hormones such as aldosterone, progesterone, and cortisol (Chen et al., 1996). The presence of P450c21 precedes the development of both adrenal and ovarian failure (Ahonen et al., 1987). Another group of enzymatic autoantigens is pteridine-dependent hydroxylases, and tryptophan, tyrosine, and phenylalanine hydroxylases (TPH, TH, and PAH respectively).

All enzymes of this group are involved in the catalysis of serotonin and dopamine, as is the aromatic L-amino acid decarboxylase (AADC), also a target autoantigen in APECED patients (Husebye et al., 1997; Ekwall et al., 1998, 2000; Hedstrand et al., 2000). The gastrointestinal dysfunction in APECED patients has been shown to be associated with the presence of TPH autoantibodies. The role of TH autoantibodies is linked to the development of alopecia areata. Various other autoantibodies have also been found. These are targeted against GAD65 and GAD67 (Bjork et al., 1994; Velloso et al., 1994), tyrosine phosphatase IA-2 (Gylling et al., 2000), CYP1A2 (Clemente et al., 1997; Gebre-Medhin et al., 1997), CYP2A6 (Clemente et al., 1998), thyroid peroxidase (Betterle et al., 1998), thyroglobulin (Betterle et al., 1998), the proton pump of the gastric mucosa H+K+ATPase (Karlsson et al., 1988), intrinsic factor (Mirakian and Bottazzo, 1994), and the calcium-sensing receptor (Li et al., 1996). Recently, two transcription factors, SOX9 and SOX10, were found to be targets for autoantibodies in APECED patients (Hedstrand et al., 2001). The autoantibodies against P4501A2 and P4502A6 associate weakly with active hepatitis and those against SOX9 and 10 with vitiligo in patients with APECED.

Molecular Basis of APECED

To date, 48 different mutations have been characterized in the *AIRE* gene of patients with APECED (Table 25.3). The mutations vary from single nucleotide substitutions, small insertions and deletions, splice-site donor or acceptor mutations, to gross deletions. Most APECED mutations lead to a premature termination codon and are predicted to delete the carboxy terminus of the AIRE protein. Another significant group is missense mutations, found in all functional domains of AIRE; the homogeneous staining region (HSR) domain (discussed below) shows a distinct clustering of disease mutations.

Functional Aspects of the AIRE Protein

Domains of the AIRE Polypeptide

The *AIRE* gene encodes a 545–amino acid protein, AIRE, with a molecular weight of 57.5 kDa and a calculated pI of 7.53. The AIRE protein consists of multiple functional domains suggested to be involved in nuclear import, transcriptional activity, DNA binding, and homomultimerization (reviewed in Kumar et al., 2002) (Fig. 25.1). The first 100 amino acids form the HSR, which is predicted to form a four-helix bundle structure (Pitkänen et al., 2000). The HSR defines a protein family including Sp100, Sp140 (the speckled proteins 100 and 140 kDa, respectively), and a putative human protein, AA431918 (Sternsdorf et al., 1999). Interestingly, the homomultimerization capacity of AIRE (Pitkänen et al., 2000) resides on the HSR domain (Sternsdorf et al., 1999). In the nucleus, AIRE is associated with dots that resemble promyelotic leukemia (PML) bodies (Zhong et al., 2000), whereas in the cytoplasm, it is attached to intermediate filaments that colocalize with vimentin and α-tubulin representing microtubules, and to aggregates of varying size (Björses et al., 1999; Heino et al., 1999a; Rinderle et al., 1999). The HSR domain of AIRE has been suggested to be responsible for the attachment of AIRE with cytoplasmic filaments (Pitkänen et al., 2001; Ramsey et al., 2002a), whereas the HSR of Sp100 is responsible for the targeting of Sp100 to the PML bodies (Sternsdorf et al., 1999).

The amino acids 189–290 of AIRE represent a SAND domain (amino acids 189–290), recently characterized as a novel DNA-binding structure (Gibson et al., 1998; Bottomley et al., 2001). The SAND domain is present in a family of proteins including members such as Sp100, AIRE, NucP41/75, and deformed epidermal autoregulatory factor-1 (DEAF-1) of *Drosophila melanogaster* (Gibson et al., 1998). The structure of the SAND domain of Sp100b contains a fold with five-stranded, twisted antiparallel β sheets that pack against four α helices (Bottomley et al., 2001). SAND is suggested to represent a DNA-binding domain particularly characteristic for chromatin-dependent transcriptional regulation, as it is often found in proteins carrying putative modules for association with chromatin—for example, plant homeodomain type (PHD) zinc fingers. Interestingly, the AIRE protein seems to bind to zinc finger consensus DNA sequence EGR as a homomultimer, and to oligo-TGG with high affinity when part of a large complex (Kumar et al., 2001). Nevertheless, the specific DNA-binding capacity of the SAND domain of AIRE has not yet been shown. In addition to DNA binding, the SAND domain of AIRE may be necessary for the nuclear localization (Ramsey et al., 2002a).

Two regions of AIRE (amino acids 296–343 and 434–475) contain PHD zinc fingers, predominantly found in proteins that regulate transcription at the chromatin level (Aasland et al., 1995). The PHD fingers are found in proteins that function in the regulation of transcription at the chromatin level (Aasland et al., 1995) and at present, one or more PHD fingers have been described in >400 proteins (Capili et al., 2001). The characteristic motif for PHD fingers consists of seven cysteines and a histidine arranged in a C4HC3 consensus (Aasland et al., 1995; Pascual et al., 2000). The presence of two PHD zinc finger domains in the carboxy-terminal half of AIRE suggests a role for AIRE in the regulation of gene expression. Indeed, AIRE has been characterized as a powerful transactivator of transcription (Björses et al., 2000, Pitkänen et al., 2000) and the PHD zinc fingers have been mapped as the transactivation domains of AIRE (Pitkänen et al., 2001; Halonen et al., 2002). The three-dimensional structure of the PHD zinc fingers supports their suggested role as mediators of protein–protein interactions (Capili et al., 2001). However, this function of PHD domains of the AIRE protein has not yet been demonstrated.

In addition to the HSR, SAND, and PHD domains, the AIRE protein harbors a leucine zipper motif within the first PHD domain (amino acids 319–341), a putative nuclear localization signal (NLS) (amino acids 113–133), and four LXXLL motifs (amino acids 7–11, 63–67, 414–418, 518–524). The leucine zipper motif characterizes a major class of eukaryotic transcriptional regulators. The leucine zipper motif of AIRE has been proposed to be involved in the homomultimerization of AIRE (Kumar et al., 2001), but this remains to be shown. The NLS of AIRE has been shown to be functional (Pitkänen et al., 2001), but so far, the nuclear import mechanisms have not been characterized. Our recent unpublished data suggest that the NLS of AIRE functions via the importin α-mediated mechanism. The LXXLL domains are found in a family of nuclear proteins. In addition, they have been shown to be necessary and sufficient for the binding of proteins to ligated nuclear receptors (Heery et al., 1997). As a result of this protein–protein interaction, the proteins containing LXXLL motifs mediate the transcriptional activity of nuclear receptors. No experimental data on the function of the LXXLL motifs of the AIRE protein have been presented thus far.

Several predicted domains of AIRE, together with its localization in nuclear dots, imply its role in the regulation of transcription, and it has been shown that AIRE acts as powerful transcriptional transactivators in vitro (Björses et al., 2000;

Table 25.3. Mutations Reported in AIRE Gene of Patients with APECED

No.	cDNA Change AIRE ORF	Effect on Coding Sequence	Affected Region of AIRE	Reference
1	30–52dup23bp	R15fsX19	HSR	Cihakova et al., 2001
2	43C > T	R15C	HSR	Sato et al., 2002
3	44G > T	R15L	HSR	Pearce et al., 1998
4	47C > T	T16M	HSR	Cihakova et al., 2001
5	62C > T	A21V	HSR	
6	83T > C	L28P	HSR	Pearce et al., 1998; Heino et al., 1999b
7	86T > C	L29P	HSR	Kogawa et al., 2002a
8	IVS1_IVS4	del exons 2–4	Intron 1	Cihakova et al., 2001
9	232T > A	W78R	HSR	Cihakova et al., 2001
10	238G > T	V80L	HSR	
11	247A > G	K83E	HSR	Nagamine et al., 1997
12	254A > G	Y85C	HSR	
13	269A > G	Y90C	HSR	Pearce et al., 1998
14	191–226del36bp	del64–75 and D76Y	HSR	Heino et al., 1999b
15	208^209insCAGG	D70fsX216	HSR	Heino et al., 1999b
16	278T > G	L93R	HSR	Ward et al., 1999
17	415C > T	R139X	HSR	Rosatelli et al., 1998; Cihakova et al., 2001
18	IVS3+2T	GT>GC	Intron 3	Wang et al., 1998
19	508^509ins 13bp	A170fsX219	Before SAND	
20	517C > T	Q173X	Before SAND	Heino et al., 1999b
21	607C > T	R203X	SAND	Scott et al., 1998
22	682T > G	G228W	SAND	Cetani et al., 2001
23	755C > T	P252L	SAND	Meloni et al., 2002
24	769C > T	R257X	SAND	Finnish-German Consortium, 1997; Nagamine et al., 1997; Scott et al., 1998; Wang et al., 1998; Heino et al., 1999b; Ward et al., 1999
25	901G > A	V301M	PHD1	Soderbergh et al., 2004
26	932G > A	C311Y	PHD1	
27	931delT	C311fsX376	PHD1	
28	967–979del13bp	C322fsX372	LZ	Finnish-German Consortium, 1997; Pearce et al., 1998; Rosatelli et al., 1998; Scott et al., 1998; Heino et al., 1999b; Ward et al., 1999; Cihakova et al., 2001
29	969^970InsCCTG	L323fsX372	LZ	Scott et al., 1998
30	977C < A	P326Q	LZ	Saugier-Veber et al., 2001
31	1072C > T	Q358X	PRR	Meloni et al., 2002
32	1103^1104insC	P370fsX370	PRR	Ishii et al., 2000
33	1163^1164insA	M388fsX422	PRR	Finnish-German Consortium, 1997
34	1189delC	L397fsX478	PRR	
35	1193delC	P398fsX478	PRR	Finnish-German Consortium, 1997
36	1244^1245insC	L417fsX422	LXXLL	
37	1242^1243insA	H416fsX422	LXXLL	Myhre et al., 1998
38	1249delC	L417fsX478	LXXLL	Pearce et al., 1998
39	1264delC	P422fsX478	PRR	Heino et al., 1999b
40	IVS9-1G > C	AG>AC	Skip exon 10	Heino et al., 2001
41	IVS9-1G > A	AG>AA	Skip exon 10	Heino et al., 1999b
42	1295InsAC	C434fsX479	PHD2	Wang et al., 1998
43	1296delGinsAC	R433fsX502	PHD2	Heino et al., 1999b
44	1344delCinsTT	C449fsX502	PHD2	Heino et al., 2001
45	IVS11+1G > A	GT>AT, X476	PHD2	Heino et al., 2001
46	1513delG	A502fsX519	C terminus	Ishii et al., 2000
47	1616C > T	P539L	C terminus	Meloni et al., 2002
48	1638A > T	X546C+ 59 aa	Stop codon	Scott et al., 1998

LZ, leucine zipper; ORF, open reading frame.

Pitkänen et al., 2001). Further, it seems that the carboxy-terminal part of AIRE, containing the PHD finger and leucine zipper domains, is important for the transactivation capacity. Homomultimerization may be required for specific molecular interactions; in the case of AIRE it may be required for DNA binding. A phosphorylated form of the AIRE protein has been found in mono-, di-, and tetrameric forms in vivo and in vitro and the amino-terminal HSR domain has been shown to be required for the homomultimerization of AIRE in vitro (Pitkänen et al., 2000; Kumar et al., 2001). So far, the only specific protein–protein interaction characterized for AIRE is that with CREB binding protein (CBP). However, the specific AIRE domain(s) responsible for this interaction has not been mapped (Pitkänen et al., 2000).

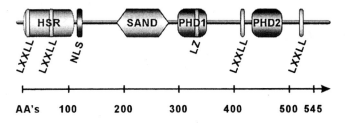

Figure 25.1. Domains of the AIRE protein. HSR, homogeneous staining region; LZ, leucine zipper; NLS, nuclear localization signal.

Subcellular Localization of the AIRE Protein

Charateristically, the in vitro–expressed AIRE polypeptides show two types of distribution in cells: (1) nuclear dot-like staining excluding the nucleoli, and (2) cytoplasmic filamentous or microtubular staining (Finnish-German APECED Consortium, 1997). Immunostaining of cells in tissue sections reveals mostly nuclear staining, although some cell types, including the interstitial cells of the testis and neurons in the trigeminal ganglions, exhibit specific smooth cytoplasmic staining. Both human and mouse cells show similar dual nuclear and cytoplasmic subcellular distribution.

Tissue Expression of AIRE

Human AIRE protein expression was initially found in the thymus and lymph node (Björses et al., 1999; Heino et al., 1999a), as well as in the spleen and peripheral blood cells (Björses et al., 1999). The mRNA expression pattern was similar, and appendix and fetal liver were found to express AIRE (Nagamine et al., 1997; Heino et al., 1999a).

By use of sensitive reverse transcription polymerase chain reaction (RT-PCR) techniques, low level of transcripts can be identified in most human and mouse tissues (Table 25.4). In the thymus, AIRE/Aire protein expression seems to be restricted to the medulla. Studies on expression of the mouse *Aire* gene indicate a wider tissue expression pattern than that detected in human tissue studies (Heino et al., 2001; Kogawa et al., 2002b). Most probably the mouse findings better reflect the real distribution of Aire expression because of multiple complications associated with accessing and handling human tissue samples. At the cellular level, Aire protein expression has been observed in thymic corpuscles, reticular epithelial cells, and a small subpopulation of medullary thymocytes. Consistent results show that in the mouse Aire is mainly expressed in the thymic epithelial cells (TEC) (Zuklys et al., 2000; Heino et al., 2001) and particularly in a subpopulation of corticomedullary and medullary 29$^+$ epithelial cells in the adult tissue (Zuklys et al., 2000).

Consequences of APECED Mutations

Several of the studied mutations change the distribution of the AIRE protein between the nucleus and cytoplasm. In particular, mutations of the predicted surface area of the HSR domain block the cytoplasmic localization of AIRE. Instead, the mutant proteins accumulate in the nucleus. This finding suggests that the mutations either enhance nuclear import or inhibit nuclear export (Björses et al., 2000). Since the NLS of the AIRE protein seems to be sufficient for nuclear import (Pitkänen et al., 2001), inhibition of nuclear export by these mutations seems more likely. AIRE seems to be exported from the nucleus by specific nuclear

export signal (NES)-dependent export, and the export signal is suggested to lie within the amino terminus of AIRE (Pitkänen et al., 2001). Mutations of the SAND domain appear to disturb the distribution of AIRE between the nucleus and cytoplasm and, when expressed in vitro, reveal excessive staining in the perinuclear region (Björses et al., 2000; Ramsey et al., 2002a). This finding suggests a role for the SAND domain in nuclear transport mechanisms. The most common APECED mutation, R257X, is a nonsense mutation that severely disturbs subcellular localization of the mutant protein, inhibits the transactivation function, and complex formation of AIRE, but exerts almost no effect on the homomultimerization capacity of the mutant protein.

AIRE Genotype–APECED Phenotype Associations

In a series of over 100 patients from Finland, Sweden, Norway, and Italy, an association between the absence of R257X mutation in *AIRE* and decreased frequency of mucocutaneous candidiasis was established (Halonen et al., 2002). Compared to the consequences of many other mutations, the R257X mutation results in a total loss of function, whereas the less dramatic truncations of the AIRE protein and many missense mutations, especially the predicted surface mutations of the HSR domain and the mutations in the leucine zipper domain, seem to have less severe effects on the function of the AIRE protein. Since a large proportion of patients from nonfounder populations represent compound heterozygotes, the genotype–phenotype associations may be difficult to assess. In addition, the effects of the mutations in vivo may be complicated to predict because of the multimer structure of AIRE.

The wide variation in phenotype of patients with APECED suggests that factors other than the diversity of mutations in the *AIRE* gene affect the phenotype. The linkage and association between the human leukocyte antigen (HLA) genes and the APECED phenotype were studied earlier, but no significant associations have been established (Maclaren and Riley, 1986; Ahonen et al., 1988; Aaltonen et al., 1993; Huang et al., 1996; Betterle et al., 1998). Many of the disease components of APECED are associated with specific HLA alleles when these appear as isolated diseases or as a part of polyglandular syndrome type II, and HLA class II alleles seem to modify the APECED phenotype. Associations with specific HLA haplotypes have been found for alopecia, Addison disease, and type 1 diabetes. These same associations have been established for non-APECED patients, indicating a significant dependence of these disease components on the HLA type (Maclaren and Riley, 1986; Weetman et al., 1991; Colombe et al., 1999; Yu et al., 1999) (Table 25.5). Alopecia is associated strongly with the DRB1*04 allele, which is also associated with severe forms of idiopathic alopecia. Increased risk for Addison disease is associated with the DRB1*03 allele, which together with the DRB1*04 allele has repeatedly been found associated with Addison disease in non-APECED patients. The haplotype DRB1*1501-DQB1*0602 is associated with protection from type 1 diabetes. Interestingly, this is the major protective haplotype for type 1 diabetes in non-APECED patients as well.

Only weak associations have been observed between HLA type and autoantibodies in APECED patients. Thus in APECED, the HLA alleles may not have a strong influence on autoantibody formation. This finding contrasts with those made in APECED trait components, isolated autoimmune diseases in which HLA alleles are often associated with the presence of autoantibodies.

Table 25.4. Expression of Aire Protein in Different Tissues as Detected by Immunohistochemistry

Organ System	Tissue	Cellular Level
Immune System		
Thymus	Medulla	Reticular epithelial
	Medulla	Thymic corpuscle cells
	Medulla	Medullary thymocytes
Spleen	Red pulp	Tissue macrophages
	Red pulp	Lymphocytes
	Red pulp	Reticular cells
Lymph nodes	Medulla	Lyphocytes
	Medulla	Reticular cells
Bone marrow		Megakaryocytes, lymphoblasts, myeloblasts
Peripheral blood		Lymphocytes, polymorphonuclear leukocytes Monocytes
Urinary Tract		
Kidney	Proximal and distal convoluted	Epithelial cells
	Glomeruli	Podocytes
	Kidney pelvis	Transitional epithelium
Bladder	Myometrium	Smooth muscle
Genital Organs		
Testes	Seminiferous tubules	Pachytene spermatocytes, round spermatids Peritubular cells, Sertoli cells—few
	Interstitial cells	
Epididymis		Epithelial cells
Seminal vesicle		Epithelial cells
Prostate		Epithelial cells
Ovary	Follicles	Granulosa cells, oocytes
Uterus	Mucosa	Epithelial cells
	Secretory glands	Epithelial cells
	Myometrium	Smooth muscle
Alimentary Tract		
Salivary glands	Acini	Secretory cells
	Secretory ducts	Epithelial cells
Stomach	Mucosa	Mucosal epithelial
		Parietal cells of gastric gland
Small Intestine and	Mucosa	Epithelial cells
Liver		Hepatocytes and Kuppfer cells
Pancreas		Exo- and endocrine cells
		Islets of Langerhans (most of the cells)
Respiratory Tract		
Lung	Bronchi	Epithelial cells
	Alveolar sacks	Epithelial and alveolar cells, macrophages
Trachea	Cartilage	Undifferentiated perichondrial cells
		Differentiating chondroblasts
Endocrine Organs		
Adrenal gland	Zona glomerulosa	
	Medulla	Chromaffin cells
	Zona fasciculata and reticulata	
Thyroid gland	Follicles	Epithelial and parafollicular cells
Pituitary gland	Anterior and intermediate lobe	
Nervous System		
Brain	Cerebral cortex	
	Hippocampus	Neurons
	Amygdala	Glial cells
	Hypothalamus	
	Cerebellar cortex	
	Spinal cord	
	Dorsal root ganglia	
Eye		
	Retina	Ganglial cells, Bipolar nerons

Data from Meriluoto et al., 2001.

Table 25.5. HLA Associations Between Disease Components and HLA Class II Alleles in Index Patients with APECED

Disease Component	HLA DRB1* Allele	p-value	HLA DQB1* Allele	p-value
Addison disease[†]	03	0.021		
Alopecia[†]	04	<0.001	0302	0.001
Type 1 diabetes[†]	15	0.036	0602	0.035
Candidiasis	01	0.019	0501	0.016
Keratopathy	04	0.032		
Keratopathy	11	0.037		
Vitiligo			0301	0.032

[†]Data from non-APECED patients supports the association (Halonen et al., 2002).

Mouse Models of APECED

Recently, two different *Aire*-deficient mouse models have been developed (Ramsey et al., 2002a; Anderson et al., 2002). In both models, the mice were kept in sterile conditions, they developed normally, and were clinically healthy. However, autoimmune features of APECED in *Aire*[−/−] mice were evident, including multiorgan lymphocytic infiltration, circulating autoantibodies, and infertility.

The first *Aire*-deficient mouse model was constructed through the targeted disruption of exon 6 of the mouse *Aire* gene (Ramsey et al., 2002b). Exon 6 was chosen, as the major Finnish mutation R257X leads to a premature stop codon in exon 6 of the human *AIRE* gene. Reproduction in the *Aire*-deficient mice was abnormal, and 85% of the males and females were found to be infertile. This is in concordance with findings in APECED patients, who develop ovarian failure in 39% of the cases at the age of 15 years; the incidence is estimated to increase up to 72% by the age of 36 years (Perheentupa, 2002). Histologic analyses in 2- to 3-month-old *Aire*-deficient mice revealed atrophy of the thymus, lymphocyte infiltrations in liver and in a single atrophied ovary, and atrophy of adrenal glands. The liver findings are consistent with the incidence of autoimmune hepatitis in 12% of patients with APECED. The variation in lymphocyte infiltrates and atrophy of the organs varied among mice, a result concordant with the highly variable phenotype of APECED patients.

The presence of autoantibodies was observed in liver, spermatogonia/spermatids, exocrine pancreas, adrenal cortex, and, in a single case, the β cells of the islets of Langerhans. These findings are consistent with the presence of various circulating autoantibodies in patients with APECED. The distribution of B and T lymphocytes in both thymus and periphery were normal. A normal number of apoptotic thymocytes and proliferating T and B cells in the *Aire*[−/−] mice was seen, whereas hyperproliferation of *Aire*-deficient T cells was detected after immunization.

Further, an alteration in spectra of the complementary determining region 3 (CD3) of the T cell receptor (TCR) vβ chain in *Aire*-deficient T cells after immunization was observed in splenic but not in thymic T cells; a clear alteration was found in 3 of the 24 Vβ families (MuBV18, MuBV19, and MuBV20). The overrepresentation of certain TCRs may cause imbalance in T cell homeostasis and trigger autoimmunity. The findings in this model suggest that the autoimmunity in *Aire*-deficient mice may at least partially be caused by defects in the peripheral regulation mechanisms of tolerance.

A second knockout mouse model for APECED was produced through conditional targeted disruption of exon 2, including parts of the surrounding intronic sequences (Anderson et al., 2002). Thus, the defect differs from that induced by Ramsey and colleagues in that (1) the deletion of exon 2 affects a different functional part of the Aire protein, the HSR domain, than that affected by the deletion of exon 6, and (2) recombination was induced by lox/cre-mediated recombination. However, the first difference may not have relevance, as the truncated Aire mRNA may not be translated to a protein or this protein may be unstable.

Also observed in this *Aire*-deficient mouse were lymphocyte infiltrations in particular structures of several organs, including the perivascular region of the salivary gland, ovarian follicles, and retina of the eye. Serum autoantibodies against particular structures of multiple organs were also observed, such as oocytes of the ovary, parietal cells in the stomach, and the outer layer of the retina of the eye. These findings suggest that the organs of the *Aire*-deficient mice are selectively attacked by autoimmune inflammation, and the defect in tolerance is broad, yet specific. The findings in the ovary are consistent with those in patients with APECED, but no defects in the retina or in the salivary glands have been reported in patients with APECED. Compared to the findings in the first mouse model, different organs or parts of organs were the targets of autoimmune attack; thus the phenotype of the two models may differ to some degree. Concerning the immune cells, the number of mTECs was twice as high as in controls and the number of activated memory T cells was doubled in the *Aire*-deficient mice. Four types of radiation bone marrow chimeras were produced: those that expressed Aire (1) only in radioresistant cells (i.e., nonhematopoietic), (2) only in radiosensitive cells (i.e., hematopoietic cells), (3) in neither cell type, or (4) in both cell types. Only type 2 and 3 chimeras exhibited autoimmune features, which suggests that Aire functions in nonhematopoietic cells (Anderson et al., 2002).

Thymus graft experiments were performed to explore whether Aire functions in the thymus or in the periphery. After 6 weeks, signs of autoimmunity similar to those in *Aire*-deficient mice were seen in those recipient mice transplanted by *Aire*-deficient thymus, whereas no signs of autoimmunity were present in the control mice (Anderson et al., 2000). These findings suggest that Aire would function in the radioresistant stromal cells of the thymus.

Anderson et al. (2000) also isolated *Aire*-deficient naive lymphocytes from the spleen and lymph nodes of *Aire*-deficient and control mice and transferred them into alymphoid recipients. After 12 weeks, autoimmunity similar to that in *Aire*-deficient mice was detected in the recipient mice of *Aire*-deficient lymphocytes. This result suggests that *Aire*-deficient lymphocytes educated in *Aire*-deficient thymus are sufficient to provoke autoimmunity. The authors concluded that Aire expression in peripheral parenchymal tissue is not the factor controlling autoimmune attack.

On the basis of the expression pattern of Aire in the epithelial cells of thymus, together with its probable role as a transcriptional regulator, an intriguing hypothesis was tested: Aire may control autoimmunity by regulating the expression of ectopic antigens in thymic medullary epithelial cells. Analysis of the transcriptional profiles of thymic epithelial cells from *Aire*-deficient mice revealed down-regulation of numerous genes, implying that Aire is a transcriptional activator of 100–300 genes represented on the array. Specifically, some previously established ectopically expressed genes (Derbinski et al., 2001) were found to be silenced or repressed. The 30 most strongly down-regulated genes were analyzed further, and all of these except for one were found to be genes encoding for tissue-restricted antigens expressed ectopically. Interestingly, the analysis of all the down-regulated genes showed that a significant number of the genes encoding for tissue-restricted antigens were from the target tissues of autoimmune attack in *Aire*-deficient mice.

Both mouse models for APECED seem to provide good murine models for organ-specific autoimmunity, although none of the most common phenotype components of APECED—i.e., mucocutaneous candidiasis, adrenocortical failure, and hypoparathyroidism—were manifested in these mice, and the mice did not have any symptoms of disease, except for infertility. However, future studies will show whether the APECED mice develop a more severe phenotype after being exposed to different pathogens and to specific environmental stimuli.

Diagnosis

Diagnostic DNA analysis of mutations in the *AIRE* gene should be considered in patients under 30 years of age with two of the typical disease components (or even one if additional features exist). All patients and their families should be provided with information on APECED and the possible development of new components. Certain autoantibodies help in predicting the development of new disease components (Perheentupa, 2002). Candidiasis of the mouth is diagnosed by findings of typical white coatings and abundant growth of *Candida albicans* on culture. Usually the determination of plasma parathyroid hormone is not necessary, and a diagnosis of hypoparathyroidism can be made by the presence of simultaneous hypocalcemia and hyperphosphatemia, if renal insufficiency is excluded. Addison disease is usually indicated by high serum titers of P450c21 antibodies. The inability of the zona fasciculata of the adrenal cortex to produce cortisol can be tested at an early stage with a short adrenocorticotropic hormone test, and later on the inability is indicated by low plasma cortisol levels. The inability of the zona glomerulosa to produce renin is indicated at early stages by supranormal plasma renin activity and at later stages by salt craving, hyponatremia, and hyperkalemia (Perheentupa, 2002). If the patient's serum contains antiadrenocortical or CYP450c21 antibodies, progress to adrenal insufficiency is almost certain. In females, circulating antibodies to CYP450scc or CYP450c17 predict ovarian atrophy. Gonadotropin deficiency and primary gonadal failure can be confirmed with the gonatropin-releasing hormone test. To predict DM, GAD autoantibodies are of value, although a patient with high levels may never develop the disease. Patients with these antibodies should be followed by monitoring blood glycohemoglobin levels. These will probably be supranormal before the onset of clinical diabetes.

Mutation diagnosis is available from several specialized laboratories internationally. The relatively large number of mutations creates the challenge for DNA-based diagnostics. APECED cannot be excluded even when *AIRE* mutation remains unidentified. This is probably a passing phase, until the sequencing methods and their full coverage of the gene become more efficient.

Treatment and Prognosis

Patients usually require continuous hormone replacement therapy, calcium and vitamin D supplements, and systemic antibiotics for candidal infections. Immunosuppressive therapy is used for treatment of autoimmune hepatitis. With careful treatment, patients can usually cope with the disease and their life expectancy is only slightly decreased. However, oral squamous cell carcinoma or a sudden onset of the disease by hypocalcemic or Addisonian crisis or acute hepatitis can sometimes be of a fulminant nature (Ahonen et al., 1990).

Management of patients for several diseases, particularly hypoparathyroidism, hypoadrenocorticism, diabetes, and chronic diarrhea, is more demanding than the sum of efforts for the isolated diseases. They and their therapies interfere with each other. Because of the basic immunodeficiency, live virus vaccines must be avoided. To identify persons with partial destruction of the parathyroids and risk of hypocalcemia during periods of hypocalcemic stress such as fasting, exceptionally low calcium intake, or high Pi intake or diuretics, the reserve capacity of the parathyroid glands can be evaluated with an EDTA infusion test.

Regular follow-up must include determination of serum alanine aminotransferase (ALT) activity to monitor liver function. Even slightly supranormal levels call for frequent follow-up, and very high levels justify needle biopsy. If a patient with chronic or recurrent diarrhea of steatorrhea has hypoparathyroidism, calcemia should be brought to a normal range to find out whether the disorder is simply secondary to hypacalcemia. If not, gastroenterological expertise is needed for duodenoscopy, chlocystokinin test of exocrine pancreatic function, bile concentration, and mucosal biopsy. Since asplenic patients need appropriate immunization and antibiotic coverage, patients with signs of splenic insufficiency on blood smear need an abdominal ultrasound for assessment of the spleen and detection of gallstones.

A systematic survival study has been carried out in 89 Finnish patients; 20 died of nonaccidental causes at 6–60 (median, 35.5) years of age. Three patients died of oral cancer at age 34–45 years and three died of fulminant hepatitis at 10–15 years of age. Six patients living alone were unexpectedly found dead at home, having died of unknown causes at ages 26–63 years. They all had hypoadrenocorticism and hypoparathyroidism, three had diabetes, and two were alcoholics. Six patients died of various APECED-related causes at 6–60 years of age. Three of them died before APECED was recognized, two had diabetes and hypoparathyroidism at age 6–60 years, and one had hypoparathyroidism at age 13. In retrospect, Addisonian crisis was possible. At autopsy, the 13-year-old had lymphocytic myocarditis. A 60-year-old man with hypoadrenocorticism, hypoparathyroidism, and Parkinson disease died after several months with high fever and unconsciousness. A 32-year-old woman with hypoadrenocorticism, diabetes, and hypoparathyroidism died of a pulmonary embolism after a 4.5-hour vacation flight. A 29-year-old woman with hypoadrenocorticism, hypoparathyroidism, renal insufficiency, and fulminant rheumatoid arthritis died of septicemia after replacement of necrotic hip joints. A 44-year-old man with hypoparathyroidism, hypoadrenocorticism, and tapetoretinal degeneration died of alcoholism.

Of the living Finnish patients, 44 are older than 20 (20–54, median 35) years of age. Of them, 38 have an approximately normal working capacity; two others work at a capacity limited by poor vision. One man retired after a career as a businessman at the age of 50 because he felt incapacitated. Two patients retired because of blindness, at ages 32 and 36 years. Of our 22 patients older than 20, 3 are partially incapacitated from APECED-related problems. Of our nine nonhypogonadal male patients older than 25 living in a steady heterosexual relationship, six had fathered children. Of the 10 nonhypogonadal female patients over 20 years of age, 5 had lived in a similar relationship. Four had given birth to a child—two in the natural way, and two through embryo transfer.

Conclusions And Future Challenges

APECED is one of the rare autoimmune diseases with monogenic inheritance. It provides a unique model for studies of more common autoimmune diseases. Furthermore, the sequence alterations in the *AIRE* gene may contribute to the pathogenesis of other, more common autoimmune diseases such as type 1 diabetes and Addison disease. In the future, the genetic association between the mutations and polymorphisms in the *AIRE* gene and the incidence of common autoimmune diseases should be analyzed.

Defective function of the *AIRE* gene may cause defects in the effector cells of the immune system and alter immune reactivity in general. Another level of disease phenotype modification is the presentation and recognition of self-antigens, which is affected by certain HLA alleles that either favor or disfavor the presentation of certain disease-associated self-antigens. Interestingly, new data indicate that AIRE may also function by regulating the expression of ectopic antigens in thymic medullar cells and, thus, by regulating efficient antigen presentation during negative selection in the thymus (Anderson et al., 2005; Kuroda et al., 2005).

The tissue expression pattern of Aire suggests that it functions in the regulation of central tolerance, but it may also function in the secondary lymphoid organs as well as in nonlymphoid peripheral tissues. AIRE acts as a powerful transactivator in vitro and the regions that regulate the transactivation function of AIRE have been initially identified in SAND and PHD finger domains. AIRE has been found to be present in a soluble form in large complexes of molecular weight over 670 kDa. One possibility is that AIRE functions as a co-activator in a large transcriptional complex. In general, transcriptional regulation may occur at the DNA, histone, nucleosome, or chromatin level. Identification of other protein–protein interactions is important; so far only one protein that interacts with AIRE, CBP, has been identified.

The *Aire*-deficient mouse models provide us with the possibility of introducing the deficiency of *Aire* to different genetic backgrounds and thus explore the genetic modifying factors of the APECED phenotype. In addition, these mice can be exposed to different environmental stimuli to identify the phenotype-modifying environmental factors. An understanding of the factors that modify the phenotype will provide clues to the pathogenesis of APECED and better tools to predict the disease course of an individual.

The recent findings concerning function of the AIRE protein in vitro and in vivo strongly support the idea that it provides a good model for general studies of immunological tolerance and its breakdown. The autoimmune reactions in patients with APECED are mostly targeted against endocrine glands, which have highly specialized functions and express a number of proteins that are unique for these organs. The mechanism of ectopic expression of rare tissue antigens may have evolved to protect the highly specialized organs with specific antigens from autoimmunity. A more detailed understanding of these features will increase our capacity to treat patients and control their tissue-specific symptoms.

References

Aaltonen J, Björses P. Cloning of the APECED gene provides new insight into human autoimmunity. Ann Med 31:111–116, 1999.

Aaltonen J, Björses P, Sandkuijl L, Perheentupa J, Peltonen L. An autosomal locus causing autoimmune disease: autoimmune polyglandular disease type I assigned to chromosome 21. Nat Genet 8:83–87, 1994.

Aaltonen J, Komulainen J, Vikman A, Palotie A, Wadelius C, Perheentupa J, Peltonen L. Autoimmune polyglandular disease type I. Exclusion map using amplifiable multiallelic markers in a microtiter well format. Eur J Hum Genet 1:164–171, 1993.

Aasland R, Gibson TJ, Stewart AF. The PHD finger: implications for chromatin-mediated transcriptional regulation. Trends Biochem Sci 20: 56–59, 1995.

Ahonen P. Autoimmune polyendocrinopathy–candidosis–ectodermal dystrophy (APECED): autosomal recessive inheritance. Clin Genet 27:535–542, 1985.

Ahonen P. Autoimmune polyendocrinopathy–candidiasis–ectodermal dystrophy (APECED). In: Childrens' Hospital. University of Helsinki, Helsinki, 1993.

Ahonen P, Koskimies S, Lokki ML, Tiilikainen A, Perheentupa J. The expression of autoimmune polyglandular disease type I appears associated with several HLA-A antigens but not with HLA-DR. J Clin Endocrinol Metab 66:1152–1157, 1988.

Ahonen P, Miettinen A, Perheentupa J. Adrenal and steroidal cell antibodies in patients with autoimmune polyglandular disease type I and risk of adrenocortical and ovarian failure. J Clin Endocrinol Metab 64:494–500, 1987.

Ahonen P, Myllarniemi S, Sipila I, Perheentupa J. Clinical variation of autoimmune polyendocrinopathy–candidiasis–ectodermal dystrophy (APECED) in a series of 68 patients. N Engl J Med 322:1829–1836, 1990.

Anderson MS. Autoimmune endocrine disease. Curr Opin Immunol 14: 760–764, 2002.

Anderson MS, Venanzi ES, Klein L, Chen Z, Berzins SP, Turley SJ, Von Boehmer H, Bronson R, Dierich A, Benoist C, Mathis D. Projection of an immunological self shadow within the thymus by the Aire protein. Science 298:1395–1401, 2002.

Anderson MS, Venanzi ES, Chen Z, Berzins SP, Benoist C, Mathis D. The cellular mechanism of Aire control of T cell tolerance. Immunity 23:227–239, 2005.

Arvanitakis C, Knouss RF. Selective hypopituitarism. Impaired cell-mediated immunity and chronic mucocutaneous candidiasis. JAMA 225:1492–1495, 1973.

Berberoglu M, Ocal G, Cetinkaya E, Ikinciogullari A, Babacan E, Kansu A, Adiyaman P, Akcurin S, Memioglu N. Polyglandular autoimmune syndrome accompanied by Munchausen syndrome. Pediatr Int 42:386–388, 2000.

Betterle C, Greggio NA, Volpato M. Autoimmune polyglandular syndrome type 1. J Clin Endocrinol Metab 83:1049–1055, 1998.

Betterle C, Rossi A, Dalla Pria S, Artifoni A, Pedini B, Gavasso S, Caretto A. Premature ovarian failure: autoimmunity and natural history. Clin Endocrinol (Oxf) 39:35–43, 1993.

Bjork E, Velloso LA, Kampe O, Karlsson FA. GAD autoantibodies in IDDM, stiff-man syndrome, and autoimmune polyendocrine syndrome type 1 recognize different epitopes. Diabetes 43:161–165, 1994.

Björses P, Aaltonen J, Horelli-Kuitunen N, Yaspo ML, Peltonen L. Gene defect behind APECED: a new clue to autoimmunity. Hum Mol Genet 7: 1547–1553, 1998.

Björses P, Aaltonen J, Vikman A, Perheentupa J, Ben-Zion G, Chiumello G, Dahl N, Heideman P, Hoorweg-Nijman JJ, Mathivon L, Mullis PE, Pohl M, Ritzen M, Romeo G, Shapiro MS, Smith CS, Solyom J, Zlotogora J, Peltonen L. Genetic homogeneity of autoimmune polyglandular disease type I. Am J Hum Genet 59:879–886, 1996.

Björses P, Halonen M, Palvimo JJ, Kolmer M, Aaltonen J, Ellonen P, Perheentupa J, Ulmanen I, Peltonen L. Mutations in the *AIRE* gene: effects on subcellular location and transactivation function of the autoimmune polyendocrinopathy–candidiasis–ectodermal dystrophy protein. Am J Hum Genet 66:378–392, 2000.

Björses P, Pelto-Huikko M, Kaukonen J, Aaltonen J, Peltonen L, Ulmanen I. Localization of the APECED protein in distinct nuclear structures. Hum Mol Genet 8:259–266, 1999.

Bottomley MJ, Collard MW, Huggenvik JI, Liu Z, Gibson TJ, Sattler M. The SAND domain structure defines a novel DNA-binding fold in transcriptional regulation. Nat Struct Biol 8:626–633, 2001.

Brun JM. Juvenile autoimmune polyendocrinopathy. Horm Res 16:308–316, 1982.

Capili AD, Schultz DC, Rauscher IF, Borden KL. Solution structure of the PHD domain from the KAP-1 corepressor: structural determinants for PHD, RING and LIM zinc-binding domains. EMBO J 20:165–177, 2001.

Cetani F, Barbesino G, Borsari S, Pardi E, Cianferotti L, Pinchera A, Marcocci C. A novel mutation of the autoimmune regulator gene in an Italian kindred with autoimmune polyedndocrinopathy-candidiasis-ectodermal dystrophy, acting in a dominant fashion and strongly cosegregating with hypothyroid autoimmune thyroiditis. J Clin Endocrinol Metab 86: 4747–4752, 2001.

Chen S, Sawicka J, Betterle C, Powell M, Prentice L, Volpato M, Rees Smith B, Furmaniak J. Autoantibodies to steroidogenic enzymes in autoimmune polyglandular syndrome, Addison's disease, and premature ovarian failure. J Clin Endocrinol Metab 81:1871–1876, 1996.

Cihakova D, Trebusak K, Heino M, Fadeyev V, Tiulpakov A, Battelino T, Tar A, Halasz Z, Blumel P, Tawfik S, Krohn K, Lebl J, Peterson P. Novel AIRE mutations and P450 cytochrome autoantibodies in Central and Eastern European patients with APECED. Hum Mutat 18:225–232, 2001.

Clemente MG, Meloni A, Obermayer-Straub P, Frau F, Manns MP, De Virgiliis S. Two cytochromes P450 are major hepatocellular autoantigens in autoimmune polyglandular syndrome type 1. Gastroenterology 114:324–328, 1998.

Clemente MG, Obermayer-Straub P, Meloni A, Strassburg CP, Arangino V, Tukey RH, De Virgiliis S, Manns MP. Cytochrome P450 1A2 is a hepatic autoantigen in autoimmune polyglandular syndrome type 1. J Clin Endocrinol Metab 82:1353–1361, 1997.

Colombe BW, Lou CD, Price VH. The genetic basis of alopecia areata: HLA associations with patchy alopecia areata versus alopecia totalis and alopecia universalis. J Investig Dermatol Symp Proc 4:216–219, 1999.

Craig JM, Schiff LM, Boone JE. Chronic moniliasis associated with Addison's disease. AMA J Dis Child 89:669–684, 1955.

Derbinski J, Schulte A, Kyewski B, Klein L. Promiscuous gene expression in medullary thymic epithelial cells mirrors the peripheral self. Nat Immunol 2:1032–1039, 2001.

Ekwall O, Hedstrand H, Grimelius L, Haavik J, Perheentupa J, Gustafsson J, Husebye E, Kampe O, Rorsman F. Identification of tryptophan hydroxylase as an intestinal autoantigen. Lancet 352:279–283, 1998.

Ekwall O, Hedstrand H, Haavik J, Perheentupa J, Betterle C, Gustafsson J, Husebye E, Rorsman F, Kampe O. Pteridin-dependent hydroxylases as autoantigens in autoimmune polyendocrine syndrome type I. J Clin Endocrinol Metab 85:2944–2950, 2000.

Finnish-German APECED Consortium. An autoimmune disease, APECED, caused by mutations in a novel gene featuring two PHD-type zinc-finger domains. The Finnish-German APECED Consortium. Autoimmune polyendocrinopathy–candidiasis–ectodermal dystrophy. Nat Genet 17:399–403, 1997.

Gass JDM. The syndrome of keratoconjunctivitis superficial moniliasis, idiopathic hypoparathyroidism and Addison's disease. Am J Ophthalmol 54:146–197, 1962.

Gebre-Medhin G, Husebye ES, Gustafsson J, Winqvist O, Goksoyr A, Rorsman F, Kampe O. Cytochrome P450IA2 and aromatic L-amino acid decarboxylase are hepatic autoantigens in autoimmune polyendocrine syndrome type I. FEBS Lett 412:439–445, 1997.

Gibson TJ, Ramu C, Gemund C, Aasland R. The APECED polyglandular autoimmune syndrome protein, AIRE-1, contains the SAND domain and is probably a transcription factor. Trends Biochem Sci 23:242–244, 1998.

Goldstein NS, Rosenthal P, Sinatra F, Dehner LP. Liver disease in polyglandular autoimmune disease type one: clinicopathological study of three patients and review of the literature. Pediatr Pathol Lab Med 16:625–636, 1996.

Gylling M, Tuomi T, Bjorses P, Kontiainen S, Partanen J, Christie MR, Knip M, Perheentupa J, Miettinen A. ss-cell autoantibodies, human leukocyte antigen II alleles, and type 1 diabetes in autoimmune polyendocrinopathy–candidiasis–ectodermal dystrophy. J Clin Endocrinol Metab 85:4434–4440, 2000.

Halonen M, Eskelin P, Myhre AG, Perheentupa J, Husebye ES, Kämpe O, Rorsman F, Peltonen L, Ulmanen I, Partanen J. AIRE mutations and human leukocyte antigen genotypes as determinants of the autoimmune polyendocrinopathy–candidiasis–ectodermal dystrophy phenotype. J Clin Endocrinol Metab 87:2568–2574, 2002.

Hedstrand H, Ekwall O, Haavik J, Landgren E, Betterle C, Perheentupa J, Gustafsson J, Husebye E, Rorsman F, Kampe O. Identification of tyrosine hydroxylase as an autoantigen in autoimmune polyendocrine syndrome type I. Biochem Biophys Res Commun 267:456–461, 2000.

Hedstrand H, Ekwall O, Olsson MJ, Landgren E, Kemp EH, Weetman AP, Perheentupa J, Husebye E, Gustafsson J, Betterle C, Kampe O, Rorsman F. The transcription factors SOX9 and SOX10 are vitiligo autoantigens in autoimmune polyendocrine syndrome type I. J Biol Chem 22:22, 2001.

Heery DM, Kalkhoven E, Hoare S, Parker MG. A signature motif in transcriptional co-activators mediates binding to nuclear receptors. Nature 387:733–736, 1997.

Heino M, Peterson P, Kudoh J, Shimizu N, Antonarakis SE, Scott HS, Krohn K. APECED mutations in the autoimmune regulator (AIRE) gene. Hum Mutat 18:205–211, 2001.

Heino M, Peterson P, Kudoh J, Nagamine K, Lagerstedt A, Ovod V, Ranki A, Rantala I, Nieminen M, Tuukkanen J, Scott HS, Antonarakis SE, Shimizu N, Krohn K. Autoimmune regulator is expressed in the cells regulating immune tolerance in thymus medulla. Biochem Biophys Res Commun 257:821–825, 1999.

Heino M, Scott HS, Chen Q, Peterson P, Mäenpää U, Papasavvas MP, Mittaz L, Barras C, Rossier C, Chrousos GP, Stratakis CA, Nagamine K, Kudoh J, Shimizu N, Maclaren N, Antonarakis SE, Krohn K. Mutation analyses of North American APS-1 patients. Hum Mutat 13:69–74, 1999.

Heubi JE, Partin JC, Schubert WK. Hypocalcemia and steatorrhea—clues to etiology. Digest Dis Sci 28:124–128, 1983.

Högenauer C, Meyer RL, Netto GJ, Bell D, Little KH, Ferries L, Ana CA, Porter JL, Fordtran JS. Malabsorption due to cholecystokinin deficiency in a patient with autoimmune polyglandular syndrome type I. N Engl J Med 344:270–274, 2001.

Huang W, Connor E, Rosa TD, Muir A, Schatz D, Silverstein J, Crockett S, She JX, Maclaren NK. Although DR3-DQB1*0201 may be associated with multiple component diseases of the autoimmune polyglandular syndromes, the human leukocyte antigen DR4-DQB1*0302 haplotype is implicated only in β-cell autoimmunity. J Clin Endocrinol Metab 81:2559–2563, 1996.

Husebye ES, Gebre-Medhin G, Tuomi T, Perheentupa J, Landin-Olsson M, Gustafsson J, Rorsman F, Kampe O. Autoantibodies against aromatic L-amino acid decarboxylase in autoimmune polyendocrine syndrome type I. J Clin Endocrinol Metab 82:147–150, 1997.

Ishii T, Suzuki Y, Ando N, Matsuo N, Ogata T. Novel mutations of the autoimmune regulator gene in two siblings with autoimmune polyendocrinopathy–candidiasis–ectodermal dystrophy. J Clin Endocrinol Metab 85:2922–2926, 2000.

Karlsson FA, Burman P, Loof L, Mardh S. Major parietal cell antigen in autoimmune gastritis with pernicious anemia is the acid-producing H+, K+-adenosine triphosphatase of the stomach. J Clin Invest 81:475–479, 1988.

Kogawa K, Kudoh J, Nagafuchi S, Ohga S, Katsuta H, Ishibashi H, Harada M, Hara T, Shimizu N. Distinct clinical phenotype and immunoreactivity in Japanese siblings with autoimmune polyglandular syndrome type 1 (APS-1) associated with compound heterozygous novel AIRE gene mutations. Clin Immunol 103:277–283, 2002a.

Kogawa K, Nagafuchi S, Katsuta H, Kudoh J, Tamiya S, Sakai Y, Shimizu N, Harada M. Expression of AIRE gene in peripheral monocyte/dendritic cell lineage. Immunol Lett 80:195–198, 2002.

Krohn K, Uibo R, Aavik E, Peterson P, Savilahti K. Identification by molecular cloning of an autoantigen associated with Addison's disease as steroid 17α-hydroxylase. Lancet 339:770–773, 1992.

Kumar PG, Laloraya M, She JX. Population genetics and functions of the autoimmune regulator (AIRE). Endocrinol Metab Clin North Am 31:321–338, vi, 2002.

Kumar PG, Laloraya M, Wang C-Y, Ruan Q-G, Davoodi-Semiromi A, Kao K-J, She J-X. The autoimmune regulator (AIRE) is a DNA binding protein. Biol Chem 276:41357–41364, 2001.

Kuroda N, Mitani T, Takeda N, Ishimaru N, Arakaki R, Hayashi Y, Bando Y, Izumi K, Takahashi T, Nomura T, Sakaguchi S, Ueno T, Takahama Y, Uchida D, Sun S, Kajiura F, Mouri Y, Han H, Matsushima A, Yamada G, Matsumoto M. Development of autoimmunity against transcriptionally unrepressed target antigen in the thymus of Aire-deficient mice. J Immunol 174:1862–1870, 2005.

Leonard F. Chronic idiopathic hypoparathyroidism with superimposed Addison's disease in a child. J Clin Endocrinol 6:493–506, 1946.

Levanon D, Brandeis M, Bernstein Y, Groner Y. Common promoter features in human and mouse liver type phosphofructokinase gene. Biochem Mol Biol Int 35:929–936, 1995.

Li Y, Song YH, Rais N, Connor E, Schatz D, Muir A, Maclaren N. Autoantibodies to the extracellular domain of the calcium sensing receptor in patients with acquired hypoparathyroidism. J Clin Invest 97:910–914, 1996.

Lukinmaa PL, Waltimo J, Pirinen S. Microanatomy of the dental enamel in autoimmune polyendocrinopathy–candidiasis–ectodermal dystrophy (APECED): report of three cases. J Craniofac Genet Dev Biol 16:174–181, 1996.

Maclaren N, Riley W. Inherited susceptibility to autoimmune Addison's disease is linked to human leukocyte antigens-DR3 and/or DR4, except when associated with type 1 autoimmune polyglandular syndrome. J Clin Endocrinol Metab 62:455–459, 1986.

Meloni A, Perniola R, Faa V, Corvaglia E, Cao A, Rosatelli MC. Delineation of the molecular defects in the AIRE gene in autoimmune polyendocrinopathy–candidiasis–ectodermal dystrophy patients from southern Italy. J Clin Endocrinol Metab 87:841–846, 2002.

Meriluoto T, Halonen M, Pelto-Huikko M, Kangas H, Korhonen J, Kolmer M, Ulmanen I, Eskelin P. The autoimmune regulator: a key toward understanding the molecular pathogenesis of autoimmune polyendocrinopathy–candidiasis–ectodermal dystrophy. Keio J Med 50:225–239, 2001.

Miettinen TA, Perheentupa J. Bile salt deficiency in fat malabsorption of hypoparathyroidism. Scand J Clin Lab Invest 27:116A, 1971.

Mount SM. A catalogue of splice junction sequences. Nucl Acids Res 10: 459–472, 1982.

Myhre AG, Bjorses P, Dalen A, Husebye ES. Three sisters with Addison's disease. J Clin Endocrinol Metab 83:4204–4206, 1998.

Myhre AG, Halonen M, Eskelin P, Ekwall O, Hedstrand H, Rorsman F, Kampe O, Husebye ES. Autoimmune polyendocrine syndrome type 1 (APS I) in Norway. Clin Endocrinol (Oxf) 54:211–217, 2001.

Myllärniemi S, Perheentupa J. Oral findings in the autoimmune polyendocrinopathy-candidiasis syndrome (APECED) and other forms of hypoparathyroidism. Oral Surg 45:721–729, 1978.

Nagamine K, Peterson P, Scott HS, Kudoh J, Minoshima S, Heino M, Krohn KJ, Lalioti MD, Mullis PE, Antonarakis SE, Kawasaki K, Asakawa S, Ito F, Shimizu N. Positional cloning of the APECED gene. Nat Genet 17:393–398, 1997.

Neufeld M, Maclaren NK, Blizzard RM. Two types of autoimmune Addison's disease associated with different polyglandular autoimmune (PGA) syndromes. Medicine (Baltimore) 60:355–362, 1981.

Padeh S, Theodor R, Jonas A, Passwell JH. Severe malabsorption in autoimmune polyendocrinopathy-candidosis-ectodermal dystrophy syndrome successfully treated with immunosuppression. Arch Dis Child 76:532–534, 1997.

Parker RI, O'Shea P, Forman EN, Acquired splenic atrophy in a sibship with the autoimmune polyendocrinopathy-candidiasis syndrome. J Pediatr 117: 591–593, 1990.

Pascual J, Martinez-Yamout M, Dyson HJ, Wright PE. Structure of the PHD zinc finger from human Williams-Beuren syndrome transcription factor. J Mol Biol 304:723–729, 2000.

Pearce SH, Cheetham T, Imrie H, Vaidya B, Barnes ND, Bilous RW, Carr D, Meeran K, Shaw NJ, Smith CS, Toft AD, Williams G, Kendall-Taylor P. A common and recurrent 13-bp deletion in the autoimmune regulator gene in British kindreds with autoimmune polyendocrinopathy type 1. Am J Hum Genet 63:1675–1684, 1998.

Peracchi M, Bardella MT, Conte D. Late-onset idiopathic hypoparathyroidism as a cause of diarrhoea. Eur J Gastroenterol Hepatol 10:163–165, 1998.

Perheentupa J. APS-I/APECED: the clinical disease and therapy. Endocrinol Metab Clin North Am 31:295–320, vi, 2002.

Perheentupa J, Miettinen A. Type 1 autoimmune polyglandular disease. Ann Med Intern (Paris) 150:313–325, 1999.

Perniola R, Falorni A, Clemente MG, Forini F, Accogli E, Lobreglio G. Organ-specific and non–organ-specific autoantibodies in children and young adults with autoimmune polyendocrinopathy-candidiasis-ectodermal dystrophy (APECED). Eur J Endocrinol 143:497–503, 2000.

Perniola R, Tamborrino G, Marsigliante S, De Rinaldis C. Assessment of enamel hypoplasia in autoimmune polyendocrinopathy-candidiasis-ectodermal dystrophy (APECED). J Oral Pathol Med 27:278–282, 1998.

Peterson P, Heino M, Krohn K. APECED-oireyhtymän immunologinen ja geneettinen tausta. Duodecim 114:1458–1464, 1998a.

Peterson P, Nagamine K, Scott H, Heino M, Kudoh J, Shimizu N, Antonarakis SE, Krohn KJ. APECED: a monogenic autoimmune disease providing new clues to self-tolerance. Immunol Today 19:384–386, 1998b.

Pitkänen J, Doucas V, Sternsdorf T, Nakajima T, Aratani S, Jensen K, Will H, Vähämurto P, Ollila J, Vihinen M, Scott HS, Antonarakis SE, Kudoh J, Shimizu N, Krohn K, Peterson P. The autoimmune regulator protein has transcriptional transactivating properties and interacts with the common coactivator CREB-binding protein. J Biol Chem 275:16802–16809, 2000.

Pitkänen J, Vahamurto P, Krohn K, Peterson P. Subcellular localization of the autoimmune regulator protein. Characterization of nuclear targeting and transcriptional activation domain. J Biol Chem 276:19597–19602, 2001.

Ramsey C, Bukrinsky A, Peltonen L. Systematic mutagenesis of the functional domains of AIRE reveals their role in intracellular targeting. Hum Mol Genet 11:3299–3308, 2002a.

Ramsey C, Winqvist O, Puhakka L, Halonen M, Moro A, Kampe O, Eskelin P, Pelto-Huikko M, Peltonen L. Aire-deficient mice develop multiple features of APECED phenotype and show altered immune response. Hum Mol Genet 11:397–409, 2002b.

Rinderle C, Christensen HM, Schweiger S, Lehrach H, Yaspo ML. AIRE encodes a nuclear protein co-localizing with cytoskeletal filaments: altered subcellular distribution of mutants lacking the PHD zinc fingers. Hum Mol Genet 8:277–290, 1999.

Rosatelli MC, Meloni A, Devoto M, Cao A, Scott HS, Peterson P, Heino M, Krohn KJ, Nagamine K, Kudoh J, Shimizu N, Antonarakis SE. A common mutation in Sardinian autoimmune polyendocrinopathy-candidiasis-ectodermal dystrophy patients. Hum Genet 103:428–434, 1998.

Sato K, Kankajima K, Imamura H, Deguchi T, Horinouchi S, Yamazaki K, Yamada E, Kanaji Y, Takano K. A novel missense mutation of AIRE gene in a patient with autoimmune polyendocrinopathy, candidiasis and ectodermal dystrophy (APECED), accompanied with progressive muscular atrophy: case report and review of the literature in Japan. Endocrine J 49: 625–633, 2002.

Saugier-Veber P, Drouot N, Wolf LM, Kuhn JM, Frebourg T, Lefebvre H. Identification of a novel mutation in the autoimmune regulator (AIRE-1) gene in a French family with autoimmune polyendocrinopathy-candidiasis-ectodermal dystrophy. Eur J Endocrinol 144:347–351, 2001.

Scirè G, Magliocca FM, Cianfarani S, Scalamandrè A, Petrozza V, Bonamico M. Autoimmune polyendocrine candidiasis syndrome with associated chronic diarrhea caused by intestinal infection and pancreas insufficiency. J Pediatrr Castroenterol 13:224–227, 1991.

Scott HS, Heino M, Peterson P, Mittaz L, Lalioti MD, Betterle C, Cohen A, Seri M, Lerone M, Romeo G, Collin P, Salo M, Metcalfe R, Weetman A, Papasavvas MP, Rossier C, Nagamine K, Kudoh J, Shimizu N, Krohn KJ, Antonarakis SE. Common mutations in autoimmune polyendocrinopathy-candidiasis-ectodermal dystrophy patients of different origins. Mol Endocrinol 12:1112–1119, 1998.

Söderbergh A, Myhre A, Ekwall O, Gebre-Medhin G, Hedstrand H, Landgren E, Miettinen A, Eskelin P, Halonen M, Tuomi T, Gustafsson J, Husebye E, Perheentupa J, Gylling M, Manns M, Rorsman F, Kämpe O, Nilsson T. Prevalence and clinical associations of ten defined autoantibodies in autoimmune polyendocrine syndrome type I. J Clin Endocrinol Metab 89:557–562, 2004.

Song YH, Li Y, Maclaren NK. The nature of autoantigens targeted in autoimmune endocrine diseases. Immunol Today 17:232–238, 1996.

Sternsdorf T, Jensen K, Reich B, Will H. The nuclear dot protein sp100, characterization of domains necessary for dimerization, subcellular localization, and modification by small ubiquitin-like modifiers. J Biol Chem 274: 12555–12666, 1999.

Tarkkanen A, Merenmies L. Corneal pathology and outcome of keratoplasty in autoimmune-candidiasis-ectodermal dystrophy. Acta Ophthalmol Scand 79:204–207, 2001.

Thorpe E, Handley H. Chronic tetany and chronic mucelial stomatitis in a child aged four and one-half years. Am J Dis Child 28:328–338, 1929.

Uibo R, Aavik E, Peterson P, Perheentupa J, Aranko S, Pelkonen R, Krohn KJ. Autoantibodies to cytochrome P450 enzymes P450scc, P450c17, and P450c21 in autoimmune polyglandular disease types I and II and in isolated Addison's disease. J Clin Endocrinol Metab 78:323–328, 1994a.

Uibo R, Perheentupa J, Ovod V, Krohn KJ. Characterization of adrenal autoantigens recognized by sera from patients with autoimmune polyglandular syndrome (APS) type I. J Autoimmun 7:399–411, 1994b.

Velloso LA, Winqvist O, Gustafsson J, Kampe O, Karlsson FA. Autoantibodies against a novel 51 kDa islet antigen and glutamate decarboxylase isoforms in autoimmune polyendocrine sxyndrome type I. Diabetologia 37: 61–69, 1994.

Wagman RD, Kazdan JJ, Kooh SW, Fraser D. Keratitis associated with the multiple endocrine deficiency, autoimmune disease, and candidiasis syndrome. Am J Ophthalmol 103:569–575, 1987.

Wang CY, Davoodi-Semiromi A, Huang W, Connor E, Shi JD, She JX. Characterization of mutations in patients with autoimmune polyglandular syndrome type 1 (APS1). Hum Genet 103:681–685, 1998.

Ward L, Ekwall O, Martin S, Oligny L, Kämpe O, Deal C. Severe gastrointestinal dysfunction in an adloscent girl with autoimmune-polyendocrinopathy-candidiasis-ectodermal dystrophy (APECED): additional evidence for enterochromaffin cell destruction as a cause of malabsorption. Pediatric Res 49:123A, 2001.

Ward L, Paquette J, Seidman E, Huot C, Alvarez F, Crock P, Delvin E, Kampe O, Deal C. Severe autoimmune polyendocrinopathy-candidiasis-ectodermal dystrophy in an adolescent girl with a novel AIRE mutation: response to immunosuppressive therapy. J Clin Endocrinol Metab 84: 844–852, 1999.

Weetman AP, Zhang L, Tandon N, Edwards OM. HLA associations with autoimmune Addison's disease. Tissue Antigens 38:31–3, 1991.

Whitaker J, Landing B, Esselborn V, Williams R. The syndrome of familial juvenile hypoadrenocorticism, hypoparathyroidism and superficial moniliasis. J Clin Endocrinol Metab 16:1374–1387, 1956.

Williams E, Wood C. The syndrome of hypoparathyroidism and steatorrhoea. Arch Dis Child 34:302–306, 1959.

Winqvist O, Gebre-Medhin G, Gustafsson J, Ritzen EM, Lundkvist O, Karlsson FA, Kampe O. Identification of the main gonadal autoantigens in patients with adrenal insufficiency and associated ovarian failure. J Clin Endocrinol Metab 80:1717–1723, 1995.

Winqvist O, Karlsson FA, Kampe O. 21-Hydroxylase, a major autoantigen in idiopathic Addison's disease. Lancet 339:1559–1562, 1992.

Yu L, Brewer KW, Gates S, Wu A, Wang T, Babu SR, Gottlieb PA, Freed BM, Noble J, Erlich HA, Rewers MJ, Eisenbarth GS. DRB1*04 and DQ alleles: expression of 21-hydroxylase autoantibodies and risk of progression to Addison's disease. J Clin Endocrinol Metab 84:328–335, 1999.

Zhong S, Salomoni P, Pandolfi PP. The transcriptional role of PML and the nuclear body. Nat Cell Biol 2:E85–90, 2000.

Zlotogora J, Shapiro MS. Polyglandular autoimmune syndrome type I among Iranian Jews. J Med Genet 29:824–826, 1992.

Zuklys S, Balciunaite G, Agarwal A, Fasler-Kan E, Palmer E, Hollander GA. Normal thymic architecture and negative selection are associated with *Aire* expression, the gene defective in the autoimmune–polyendocrinopathy–candidiasis–ectodermal dystrophy (APECED). J Immunol 165:1976–1983, 2000.

26

Immune Dysregulation, Polyendocrinopathy, Enteropathy, and X-Linked Inheritance

TROY R. TORGERSON, ELEONORA GAMBINERI, STEVEN F. ZIEGLER, and HANS D. OCHS

In 1982, Powell and colleagues reported on a large family with multiple affected males in a five-generation pedigree (Fig. 26.1). Affected males presented early in life with multiple endocrinopathies, severe chronic enteropathy, dermatitis, autoimmune hemolytic anemia, and antibody-induced neutropenia and thrombocytopenia. Most of the affected boys died before the age of 3 years of malabsorption, failure to thrive, infections, or other complications. Characteristic findings at autopsy of these and subsequently identified patients included lymphocytic infiltrates affecting the lungs and endocrine organs such as pancreas and thyroid, and increased lymphoid elements in lymph nodes and spleen (Powell et al., 1982; Wildin et al., 2002). Symptomatic therapy with immunosuppressive drugs provided some beneficial effects (Seidman et al., 1990).

More than 20 years before the initial description of this syndrome of immune dysregulation, polyendocrinopathy, enteropathy, with X-linked inheritance (IPEX), a spontaneously occurring mutant mouse strain called *scurfy* was identified at the Oakridge National Laboratory (Russell et al., 1959). Affected male mice have many phenotypic similarities to IPEX, including X-linked inheritance, polyendocrinopathy, enteropathy resulting in failure to thrive, and dermatitis. Death occurs invariably during the first 3–4 weeks of life.

The gene responsible for IPEX was mapped to Xp11.23–Xq13.3 by linkage analysis (Bennett et al., 2000; Ferguson et al., 2000). Using positional cloning, the gene responsible for the scurfy syndrome was identified and found to be a transcription factor, Foxp3, belonging to the forkhead/winged helix family (Brunkow et al., 2001). The human orthologue, *FOXP3*, was subsequently recognized as the causative gene for IPEX (Chatila et al., 2000; Bennett et al., 2001b; Wildin et al., 2001). Following this discovery, additional families with mutations of *FOXP3* were identified and the phenotype was characterized (Kobayashi

et al., 2001; Wildin et al., 2002; Gambineri et al., 2003; Owen et al., 2003).

Finally, using the scurfy mouse model, three independent groups have demonstrated that Foxp3 plays an essential role in generating CD4[+] CD25[+] regulatory T cells (Fontenot et al., 2003; Hori et al., 2003; Khattri et al., 2003), providing convincing evidence that the lack of regulatory T cells is the direct cause of the early onset of multiple autoimmune disorders in scurfy mice and patients with the IPEX phenotype.

Clinical and Pathologic Manifestations

Incidence, Onset of Symptoms, and Age at Diagnosis

Because of underreporting, the true incidence of IPEX is unknown. Following the discovery of the genetic defect in IPEX, more than 50 unrelated families with *FOXP3* mutations have been identified (Gambineri et al., submitted). A positive family history leads to an early diagnosis, based on the triad of severe diarrhea and failure to thrive due to villous atrophy, an eczema-like skin disease, and early-onset diabetes. As one would expect, there are milder, less characteristic phenotypes not readily recognized as IPEX. The oldest boy in our series was 11 years of age when the diagnosis of IPEX was considered and confirmed by mutation analysis.

Gastrointestinal Symptoms and Failure to Thrive

Early-onset diarrhea associated with villous atrophy and lymphocytic infiltrates in the small bowel mucosa are the most prominent clinical findings in patients with the IPEX phenotype (Meyer et al., 1970; Ellis et al., 1982; Hattevig et al., 1982;

355

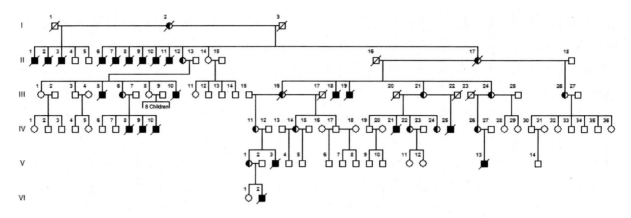

Figure 26.1. Updated pedigree of the IPEX kindred originally described by Powell et al. (1982), demonstrating X-linked inheritance and high mortality (half-filled circle, carrier female; filled square with slash, affected deceased male).

Powell et al., 1982; Savage et al., 1982; Walker-Smith et al., 1982; Seidman et al., 1990; Jonas et al., 1991, Satake et al., 1993; Zeller et al., 1994; Roberts and Searle, 1995; Finel et al., 1996; Di Rocco and Marta, 1996; Peake et al., 1996; Kobayashi et al., 1998; Chatila et al., 2000; Cilio et al., 2000; Ferguson et al., 2000; Baud et al., 2001; Bennett et al., 2001b; Levy-Lahad and Wildin, 2001; Wildin et al., 2002; Gambineri et al., 2003, submitted). Every patient in our series of 50 families with IPEX or IPEX-like phenotype presented with gastrointestinal symptoms of watery or mucoid-bloody diarrhea that does not respond to dietary manipulation. In many instances, total parenteral nutrition (TPN) is required to prevent severe failure to thrive. Severe villous atrophy and mucosal erosion with lymphocytic infiltrates of the submucosa or lamina propria are frequently observed in small-bowel biopsies, often leading to the diagnosis of Crohn disease or, if present in the colon, ulcerative colitis. In rare cases, gastrointestinal symptoms may occur at a later age, possibly resulting from a less severe mutation of *FOXP3* or, in some cases, non-FOXP3-related mechanisms. Treatment with immunosuppressive drugs may improve gastrointestinal symptoms in some patients.

Autoimmune Endocrinopathy

Early-onset (sometimes neonatal) insulin-dependent type 1 diabetes is a frequent initial finding (Meyer et al., 1970; Dodge and Lawrence, 1977; Hattevig et al., 1982; Powell et al., 1982; Jonas et al., 1991; Satake et al., 1993; Zeller et al., 1994; Roberts and Searle, 1995; Finel et al., 1996; Di Rocco and Marta, 1996; Peake et al., 1996; Bennett et al., 2000; Cilio et al., 2000; Ferguson et al., 2000; Levy-Lahad and Wildin, 2001; Wildin et al., 2002; Nieves et al., 2004; Gambineri et al., submitted). On appropriate evaluation, patients lack detectable insulin in the serum and often have anti–islet cell antibodies. At autopsy, chronic interstitial inflammation with lymphocytic infiltrates and absence of islet cells is a characteristic finding. Thyroid disease, initially presenting as either hypo- or hyperthyroidism, is a common complication (Powell et al., 1982; Satake et al., 1993; Wildin et al., 2001, 2002; Nieves et al., 2004) and may be associated with elevated thyrotropin levels or anti-thyroid microsomal antibodies (Savage et al., 1982; Kobayashi et al., 1998; Wildin et al., 2002).

In our own clinical survey of IPEX patients, type 1 diabetes was present in 78% and thyroid disease in 39% of patients with a

FOXP3 mutation. Interestingly, only 1 of 50 IPEX patients had adrenal insufficiency.

Autoimmune Hematologic Disorders

Coombs-positive hemolytic anemia, autoimmune thrombocytopenia, or neutropenia with early or late onset is a frequent complication (Powell et al., 1982; Satake et al., 1993; Roberts and Searle, 1995; Di Rocco and Marta, 1996; Baud et al., 2001; Levy-Lahad and Wildin, 2001; Wildin et al., 2002; Gambineri et al., 2003, submitted; Nieves et al., 2004). Specific autoantibodies (anti–red blood cell, antiplatelet, or antineutrophil antibodies) are frequently present in the circulation.

Dermatologic Abnormalities

Some of the most common clinical findings are lesions of the skin (Powell et al., 1982; Ellis et al., 1982; Zeller et al., 1994; Roberts and Searle, 1995; Di Rocco and Marta, 1996; Peake et al., 1996; Ferguson et al., 2000; Baud et al., 2001; Chatila et al., 2001; Levy-Lahad and Wildin, 2001; Nieves et al., 2004; Gambineri et al., submitted). Newborns may present with erythematous lesions involving the entire body; older patients may develop eczema (Color Plate 26.I) or localized psoriasiform dermatitis (Color Plate 26.IIA). Histologically, the psoriasiform lesions show irregular hyperplasia of the epidermis with overlying parakeratosis and lymphocytic infiltrates (Color Plate 26.IIB). Two patients have developed *alopecia universalis*, accompanied by longitudinal ridging of the nails (Nieves et al., 2004). Treatment with steroid ointment may improve the skin lesions.

Infections

It is unclear whether IPEX patients have a significantly increased susceptibility to infections as a function of their genetic defect as was suspected by Powell et al. (1982), or whether this susceptibility is secondary to other clinical features, such as decreased barrier function of the skin and gut, or to immunosuppressive therapy. In a large group of patients with the IPEX phenotype, half had serious infection including sepsis, meningitis, pneumonia, and osteomyelitis, many of these infections occurring prior to the initiation of immunosuppressive therapy (Gambineri et al., submitted). Sepsis due to line infections is a common complication. It is likely that autoimmune neutropenia, if present, contributes to the susceptibility to infections. The most common pathogens identified were *Enterococcus* and *Staphylococcus* species, cytomegalovirus, and *Candida* (Jonas et al., 1991; Roberts and Searle, 1995; Peake et al., 1996; Kobayashi et al., 1998; Ferguson et al., 2000; Levy-Lahad and Wildin, 2001; Gambineri et al., 2003).

Other Clinical Manifestations

Severe, acute reactions to routine immunizations have been reported (Powell et al., 1982). Such reactions suggest that FOXP3 and regulatory T cells are necessary to keep immune responses to foreign antigens under control and prevent the potential of "horror autotoxicus" or autoimmunity predicted by Paul Ehrlich (1910) more than 100 years ago.

Renal disease, described as glomerulonephropathy or interstitial nephritis, has been reported early on (Powell et al., 1982; Ellis et al., 1982; Zeller et al., 1994; Kobayashi et al., 1998). In our own IPEX series, more than 50% of the patients with *FOXP3* mutation had renal abnormalities (Gambineri et al., submitted). In some instances, renal disease may be directly caused or worsened by treatment with cyclosporin A, FK506, or sirolimus; however, renal disease has been described in patients not receiving any immunosuppressive drugs.

Hepatosplenomegaly and lymphadenopathy due to extensive lymphocytic infiltrates have been reported in patients at autopsy (Roberts and Searle, 1995; Peake et al., 1996; Levy-Lahad and Wildin, 2001; Wildin et al., 2002). Unexpectedly, almost half of the IPEX patients in our own series had neurologic problems including seizures and mental retardation (Gambineri et al., submitted).

Histopathology

Histologic evaluation of the intestinal tract is characterized by a striking loss of villi in the small bowel, associated with mucosal erosions and lymphocytic infiltrates in the lamina propria and submucosa. The large bowel may also be involved, demonstrating lymphocytic infiltrates. The pancreas of infants with insulin-dependent diabetes shows lymphocytic infiltrates and loss of Langerhans cells; the thyroid, if affected, is invaded by lymphocytes (Levy-Lehad and Wildin, 2001; Wildin et al., 2002).

Microscopic evaluations of skin biopsies are consistent with eczema. Some lesions resemble psoriasiform dermatitis showing hyperplasia of the epidermis with overlying confluent parakeratosis (Color Plate 26.IIB). The epidermis may contain large numbers of infiltrating lymphocytes that consist predominantly of CD4$^+$ and CD8$^+$ T cells (Nieves et al., 2004).

The liver is frequently enlarged with fatty changes, cholestasis, and lymphocytic infiltrates that suggest "autoimmune hepatitis." Some of these changes may be due to long-term hyperalimentation. The enlarged spleen and lymph nodes represent hyperplasia caused by infiltrating lymphocytes (Levy-Lehad and Wildin, 2001; Wildin et al., 2002). A hypotrophic thymus, often observed at autopsy, may be the result of chronic illness or prolonged immunosuppressive therapy. Sections of the lung often reveal lymphocytic infiltrates and hemorrhagic changes. Renal abnormalities include interstitial nephritis, focal tubular atrophy, membranous glomerulopathy, and lymphocytic infiltrates.

Laboratory Findings

The immunologic evaluation of IPEX patients is unremarkable except for elevated serum levels of IgE and IgA and marked eosinophilia. IgG and IgM levels, absolute lymphocyte counts, and subset numbers are within normal range, and in vitro lymphocyte proliferations are normal. In our series, 90% of IPEX patients had elevated IgE and 67% had elevated IgA (Gambineri et al., submitted).

Following immunization with protein and polysaccharide antigens, most patients, with a few exceptions, respond with normal antibody titers (for review, see Wildin et al., 2002). These evaluations are difficult since most patients are on systemic immunosuppressive therapy at the time of testing.

The presence of autoantibodies is a hallmark of this syndrome. Most patients with insulin-dependent diabetes have autoantibodies against pancreatic islet cells (Jonas et al., 1991; Roberts and Searle, 1995; Finel et al., 1996; Peake et al., 1996; Ferguson et al., 2000; Baud et al., 2001; Wildin et al., 2002). Anti-insulin and anti-glutamic acid decarboxylase (GAD) antibodies have also been reported (Cilio et al., 2000, Baud et al., 2001). In addition, antimicrosomal/antithyroglobulin antibodies and antibodies against smooth muscles have been demonstrated (Powell et al., 1982; Savage et al., 1982; Seidman et al., 1990; Satake et al., 1993; Di Rocco and Marta, 1996; Finel et al., 1996; Ferguson et al., 2000; Baud et al., 2001). Antibodies against human intestinal tissue and a circulating antibody specific for a 75 kDa gut- and kidney-specific antigen (AIE-75) have been observed (Walker-Smith et al., 1982; Satake et al., 1993; Kobayashi et al., 1998, 1999).

Peripheral blood lymphocytes expressing the CD4 and CD25 markers are present in IPEX patients with mutations of *FOXP3*. However, based on flow cytometric analysis, patients with mutations of *FOXP3* (even if the missense mutation allows expression of the mutated protein) completely lack CD4$^+$ CD25$^+$ cells expressing FOXP3 (Gavin et al., in press).

Molecular Basis of IPEX

Following the identification of a 2 bp insertion in the *Foxp3* gene of mice with the scurfy phenotype (Brunkow et al., 2001), several laboratories reported that symptomatic males of families with X-linked IPEX had mutations of the human *FOXP3* gene (Chatila et al., 2000; Bennett et al., 2001b; Wildin et al., 2001). The human *FOXP3* gene is located at the short arm of the X chromosome (Xp11.23) and consists of 11 translated exons that encode a protein of 431 amino acids (429 amino acids for the murine Foxp3). The two proteins, human and murine, have 86% sequence identity. The gene is expressed predominantly in lymphoid tissues (thymus, spleen, and lymph nodes), particularly in CD4$^+$ CD25$^{+(bright)}$ T cells (Roncador et al., 2005). In mice, Foxp3 is expressed at low levels in CD4$^+$ CD25$^-$ cells but not or at very low levels in CD8$^+$ cells (Brunkow et al., 2001; Hori et al., 2003; Fontenot et al., 2005). Human CD8$^+$ cells can express FOXP3, although typically at lower levels (Cosmi et al., 2003; Walker et al., 2003; Xystrakis et al., 2004; Roncador et al., 2005).

The Forkhead (FKH) BOX protein FOXP3 is a member of the P subfamily of Fox transcription factors, which, as a group, are characterized by the presence of a highly conserved winged helix/forkhead DNA binding domain. Proteins bearing a forkhead DNA-binding motif comprise a large family of related molecules that play diverse roles in enhancing or suppressing transcription. Studies in model organisms such as *Caenorhabditis elegans*, *Drosophila melanogaster*, and *Mus musculus* have demonstrated a pivotal role for Fox family transcription factors in embryonic patterning, development, and metabolism (Gajiwala and Burley,

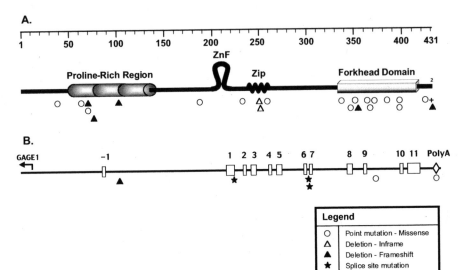

Figure 26.2. FOXP3 structure. (A) Schematic representation of FOXP3 protein, highlighting the proline-rich region at the N terminus, followed by a C2H2 zinc finger domain (ZnF), a leucine zipper (Zip), and the DNA-binding forkhead domain at the C terminus. (B) Genomic organization of the *FOXP3* gene. There are 11 coding exons, a Poly A region located 878–883 bp downstream of the FOXP3 stop codon, and the adjacent (upstream) gene (*GAGE1*). The location and type of *FOXP3* mutations identified to date are indicated by specific symbols. Nucleotide 1 is the first nucleotide of exon 1.

2000; Carlsson and Mahlapuu, 2002). A subset of these transcription factor family members was shown to play a role in the development and maintenance of normal immune responses and thymic development (Foxn1), in lineage commitment (Foxp3, e.g., CD4+ CD25+ regulatory T cells), and in the function of lymphocytes (Foxj1 and Foxo3).

The FOXP3 protein has a number of characteristic structural features including a proline-rich domain at the N terminus, a C2H2 zinc finger and a leucine zipper (both conserved structural motifs involved in protein-protein interaction) in the central portion, and a forkhead DNA-binding domain at the C terminus (Fig. 26.2). There is a putative nuclear localization signal at the C-terminal portion of the forkhead domain.

Function of FOXP3

The most essential functions of a transcription factor are nuclear import and binding to DNA. Transcription factors often interact with partners to form either homo- or heterodimers. Using N-terminal green fluorescent protein (GFP)-tagged c-DNA constructs, it is possible to transfect HEK293 cells and analyze the transfectants for the ability of the encoded FOXP3 protein fragments to enter the nucleus and bind to DNA. The intact forkhead domain is required for this process. If the forkhead domain is

deleted or mutated—for example, by point mutation that results in an amino acid substitution that leads to the IPEX phenotype—nuclear import and DNA binding are abolished (Fig. 26.3) (Lopes et al., submitted). To be functionally active, FOXP3 has to be in the homodimer formation, which depends on the intact leucine zipper sequence; naturally occurring mutations in this region interfere with this homodimerization. A novel functional domain within the amino-terminal region of FOXP3 seems to be required for FOXP3-mediated repression of nuclear factor of activated T cells (NFAT)-controlled gene transcription (Lopes et al., submitted).

FOXP3 Acts as a Transcriptional Repressor of Cytokine Promoters

Foxp3 was shown to localize to the nucleus in a forkhead domain–dependent manner. Overexpression of full-length Foxp3 was capable of suppressing transcription from a promoter construct consisting of multimers of either a consensus forkhead DNA-binding site or of a DNA-binding site for NFAT. Jurkat T cells overexpressing human FOXP3 produced less interleukin-2 (IL-2) in response to cross-linking of CD3 than did wild-type cells (Schubert et al., 2001). A recent study suggests that Foxp3, but not Foxp1 or Foxp2, physically associates and functionally interacts with NF-κB and NFAT protein, and as a result inhibits

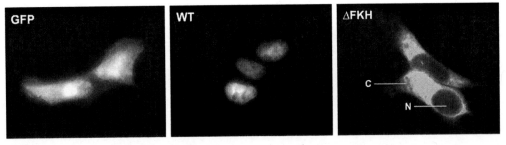

Figure 26.3. Nuclear import of FOXP3. The Forkhead (FKH) domain of FOXP3 is required for nuclear import. Constructs encoding N-terminal green fluorescent protein (GFP), GFP-FOXP3 (WT), or GFP-FOXP3 lacking the forkhead (ΔFKH) domain were transiently transfected into HEK 293 cells and evaluated by standard fluorescence microscopy for

the ability to translocate to the nucleus. GFP by itself is below the size-exclusion limit for the nuclear pore complex and therefore is present throughout the cell. WT FOXP3 is located entirely in the nucleus; if the forkhead domain is deleted (ΔFKH-FOXP3) the protein is excluded from the nucleus (N). C, cytoplasm.

IL-2, IL-4, and interferon-γ (IFN-γ) production by CD4[+] effector cells (Bettelli et al., 2005). Scurfy mice T cells have a substantial increase in NFAT and NF-κB transcriptional activity compared with T cells derived from wild-type mice. This overexpression of NFAT and NF-κB is reduced to normal levels by complementation of Foxp3 in scurfy-derived T cells (Bettelli et al., 2005). Thus Foxp3 functions as a specific transcription corepressor for the two pivotal transcription factors, NFAT and NF-κB, which play a key role in the expression of multiple cytokine genes.

FOXP3 as a Rheostat of the Immune Response

The generation of transgenic mice expressing multiple copies of the *Foxp3* gene results in a dramatic suppression of immune responses. Transgenic mice have markedly decreased numbers of CD4[+] T cells in the peripheral blood, and decreased cellularity in lymph nodes and the spleen. In contrast to the scurfy T cells, those derived from Foxp3 transgenic mice were hyporesponsive to stimulation both in vivo and in vitro. The suppressive effect was shown to be entirely dependent on peripheral T cells, as overexpression of wild-type Foxp3 in the thymus did not affect peripheral blood T cell numbers or functions (Khattri et al., 2001). In this model, Foxp3 functions as a rheostat of the immune system, with activation responses being inversely proportional to the amount of Foxp3 protein expressed by CD4[+] T cells. Combined with the findings reported by Bettelli et al. (2005, vide supra), this hypothesis postulates that Foxp3 has an important function in peripheral CD4[+] T cells, in addition to its role in generating regulatory T cells in the thymus. If Foxp3 directly interacts with NFAT and NF-κB, it is possible that this physical association recruits Foxp3 to the promoters of cytokine genes. Being a potent transcriptional repressor, the recruitment of Foxp3 to these promoters would turn off any transcriptional activity. Such a mechanism would explain the fact that scurfy T cells are hyperresponsive to T cell receptor (TCR) stimulators with anti-CD3 (Clark et al., 1999). The observation that myelin proteolipid protein-specific autoreactive T cells transduced with Foxp3 are no longer able to mediate experimental autoimmune encephalomyelitis supports the notion that Foxp3 suppresses the effector function of autoreactive T cells (Bettelli et al., 2005). A similar suppression of experimental allergic encephalomyelitis by Foxp3 positive regulatory T cells was reported by Yu et al. (2005).

FOXP3 and CD4[+] CD25[+] Regulatory T Cells

A small subset of CD4[+] T cells expressing the low-affinity IL-2 receptor α-chain (CD25) have been associated with antigen-specific suppression of T cell responses (Sakaguchi et al., 2001). CD4[+] CD25[+] regulatory T cells (Tregs) are anergic, but upon activation suppress the proliferation and IL-2 production of naive and memory CD4[+] T cells through a contact-dependent, cytokine-independent mechanism (Itoh et al., 1999; Shevach, 2002).

Regulatory T cells have been recognized as leading factors in the control of chronic human diseases. They play a major role in transplantation tolerance (reviewed by Wood and Sakaguchi, 2003) and seem to be low in numbers (and expression of FOXP3) in patients with chronic graft-versus-host disease (following bone marrow transplantation) (Zorn et al., 2005). Similarly, a lack of regulatory T cells has been associated with autoimmune diseases in both human and mice (Wei et al., 2004; Loser et al., 2005; Marinaki et al., 2005; Yu et al., 2005), and, as expected, treatment strategies to increase Treg function have improved transplantation tolerance and autoimmune symptoms (Bettelli et al., 2005; Loser et al., 2005). Protocols to expand human CD4[+] CD25[+] regulatory

T cells while maintaining their suppressive activity to inhibit effector T cell proliferation have been established. CD4[+] CD25[+] T cells, isolated from human peripheral blood, can be expanded up to 200-fold in vitro in the presence of anti-CD3 and anti-CD28 coated Dynabeads and high concentrations of exogenous IL-2 (Earle et al., 2005). These cells maintain markers of Tregs, including expression of CD25 and FOXP3, and maintain suppressor activity in regard to proliferation and cytokine secretion by effector T cells. Increased numbers and activities of Tregs have been associated with tumor progression (Karube et al., 2004; Viguier et al., 2004; Berger et al., 2005; Ormandy et al., 2005; Unitt et al., 2005), and therapies are being explored to reduce Treg activity (Wei et al., 2004; Beyer et al., 2005; Sharma et al., 2005).

Although the precise molecular events that lead to the production and regulation of these regulatory T cells are unknown, recently it was shown that Foxp3 plays a crucial role in the generation of Tregs in mice (Fontenot et al., 2003; Hori et al., 2003; Khattri et al., 2003). Foxp3 is preferentially expressed in the CD4[+] CD25[+] pool of cells, and mice that lack Foxp3 (scurfy or Foxp3 knockout mice) lack functional Tregs. Expression of FOXP3 in human or murine CD4[+] CD25[-] T cells, achieved by a transgene, is sufficient to convert these cells to a Treg-like phenotype regardless of CD25 expression (Hori et al., 2003; Khattri et al., 2003; Yagi et al., 2004). Murine CD4[+] CD25[-] cells, if activated in vitro by cross-linking CD3, do not express Foxp3 and do not acquire suppressor activity, despite strong expression of CD25 on the cell surface (Fontenot et al., 2003; Khattri et al., 2003). In contrast to the finding in mice, at least one group has reported that human CD4[+] CD25[-] cells can be activated in vitro to express FOXP3 and to suppress T cell proliferation (Walker et al., 2003); this finding could not be confirmed by a second group of investigators (Yagi et al., 2004), and the issue needs to be clarified.

Thus, Foxp3 is both required and sufficient to generate a population of Tregs, at least in mice. It is unknown at this time how this population of CD4[+] CD25[+] regulatory T cells exerts its -potent suppressive effect on the immune response and how regulatory T cells themselves are generated and modulated. Using a sophisticated staining technique, it was recently shown that IPEX patients with known FOXP3 mutations, including missense mutations that allow expression of mutated FOXP3 protein with a single amino acid substitution, lack CD4[+] CD25[+] T cells expressing FOXP3 (Color Plate 26-III and Fig. 26.4) (Gavin et al., 2006).

On the basis of available experimental data, *Tregs* can be defined as a subset of CD4[+] CD25[+] T cells that express Foxp3, are anergic, and suppress the proliferation and IL-2 production of naive and memory CD4[+] T cells through a contact-dependent, cytokine-independent mechanism (Itoh et al., 1994; Shevach, 2002). Tregs function in a dominant, *trans*-acting way to actively suppress immune activation. Tregs, therefore, play a critical role in establishing and maintaining self-tolerance and immune homeostasis (Fontenot and Rudensky, 2005).

In contrast to this "dominant tolerance" created by dedicated regulatory T cells, "recessive tolerance" refers to the passive mechanism of "negative selection" that leads to deletion or functional inactivation of autoreactive T and B cell clones in the thymus, bone marrow, and peripheral lymphoid organs, respectively, without affecting other self-reactive lymphocyte clones (see Chapters 24 and 25).

Although the Treg story is still in flux, several key facts are generally accepted. CD4[+] CD25[+] regulatory T cells have been demonstrated in the thymus of both mice and humans (Papiernik et al., 1998; Itoh et al., 1999; Stephens and Mason, 2000; Roncador et al., 2005). These CD4+ CD25+ thymocytes are capable of suppression in adoptive transfer models and in in vitro suppression assays (Itoh et al., 1999). Furthermore, the generation of Tregs in the thymus requires TCR signaling during thymocyte development (Hsieh and Rudensky, 2005). In this model of regulatory T cell lineage commitment, high-avidity TCR–self-peptide–MHC interactions take place in the thymus, augmented by CD28 signaling and perhaps additional, unidentified signals to induce Foxp3 expression. The human FOXP3 promoter was recently shown to be T cell specific and to exhibit a TATA and CAAT box approximately 6000 bp upstream of the translation start site. The basal promoter contains 3 NFAT and 3 AP-1 sites, which positively regulate the trans activation of the FOXP3 promoter in response to TCR engagement. This event is suppressed by cyclosporine A (Mantel et al., 2006). Such regulatory mechanisms ensures that Tregs represent a dedicated T cell lineage capable of controlling T cell self-reactivity and autoimmune disorders. The role of Foxp3, therefore, is that of being the single-most important Treg lineage specification factor (Fontenot and Rudensky, 2005). The lymphoproliferative autoimmune syndrome of scurfy and IPEX resulting from Foxp3 and FOXP3 deficiency, respectively, identifies Treg cells as guarantors of immunologic tolerance to self, and FOXP3 as the mediator of the genetic mechanism of dominant tolerance.

Mutation Analysis

In an effort to define the clinical and immunologic phenotype and to explore a possible genotype–phenotype correlation, we evaluated more than 70 patients from 50 families living in North or South America, Europe, or Asia with a clinical phenotype compatible with IPEX for mutations of FOXP3 (Gambineri et al., submitted). To date, we have identified over 25 novel mutations (Fig. 26.2), in addition to 6 mutations reported previously by others (Chatila et al., 2000; Wildin et al., 2001, 2002; Owen et al., 2003). These naturally occurring mutations have been invaluable for understanding the relative importance of the structural domains of FOXP3. The missense mutations identified thus far cluster in three specific functional domains: the proline-rich domain, the leucine zipper, and the forkhead domain (Fig. 26.2). No missense mutations have been discovered in the zinc finger domain, which suggests that it may not play a critical role in FOXP3 function. Other mutations identified include missense mutations, deletions, and splice site mutations. In one family with multiple

affected members, we found a large deletion upstream of exon 1 resulting in failure to initiate splicing. The family initially described by Powell in 1982 has a point mutation affecting the first canonical polyadenylation region (AAUAAA → AAUGAA) which resides 878–883 bp downstream of the FOXP3 stop codon (Bennett et al., 2001a). This mutation seems to result in a milder phenotype, sometimes with onset of symptoms at school age. Nevertheless, all affected members of that family eventually succumbed to this disease (Fig. 26.1). Not all patients who present with the IPEX phenotype have detectable mutations of FOXP3. Of 50 unrelated families with symptoms compatible with IPEX referred to our laboratory for sequencing of FOXP3, only 60% had identifiable mutations of FOXP3 (Gambineri et al., submitted). Through use of real-time polymerase chain reaction (PCR), half of these "IPEX-like" patients were shown to have low levels of mRNA, whereas the others had normal concentrations of FOXP3 mRNA, findings suggesting that at least some IPEX-like patients may have mutations involving regulatory sequences of the FOXP3 gene such as promoter or enhancer regions. Alternatively, there may be other genes or gene products that are directly or indirectly involved in the activation of FOXP3 itself.

Strategies for Diagnosis

Because of the wide spectrum of clinical findings, the diagnosis of IPEX should be considered in any young male patient presenting with intractable diarrhea, villous atrophy, and failure to thrive. The presence of an erythematous/eczematoid rash or a psoriasiform dermatitis supports the diagnosis (Color Plates 26.I and 26.II). Early onset of insulin-dependent diabetes and/or hypothyroidism in a patient with gastrointestinal symptoms and eczema is almost pathognomonic for IPEX. Autoimmune hemolytic anemia, neutropenia, or thrombocytopenia are not always present. The diagnosis of IPEX is confirmed by demonstrating the absence of CD4+ CD25+ FOXP3+ regulatory T cells (Fig. 26.4 and Color Plate 26. III) (Gavin et al., 2006) or by mutation analysis of FOXP3.

Differential Diagnosis

Other single-gene defects have been identified as cause of a clinical phenotype involving immune dysregulation in either humans or mice (Table 26.1). FAS/APO-1 (CD95) is a transmembrane receptor belonging to the tumor necrosis factor (TNF) receptor superfamily. Engagement of FAS/APO-1 by its ligand, FASL,

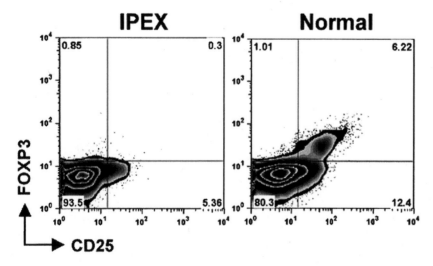

Figure 26.4. Identification of regulatory T cells in peripheral blood. A proportion of CD4+ CD25+(bright) T cells express FOXP3. The cells were stained for CD4 and CD25, permeabilized, and stained with anti-FOXP3 monoclonal antibody and submitted to flow cytometry.

Table 26.1 Single-Gene Defects Causing a Phenotype of Immune Dysregulation

Gene (Chapter)	FOXP3 (26)	FAS/FASL (24)	AIRE (25)	RAG1/RAG2; Artemis (9)	WASP (31)	CTLA-4	TGF-β1/TβRII
Human disease	IPEX	ALPS	APECED	Omenn syndrome	WAS	Not known	Not known
Mouse	Scurfy	MRLlpr/glp	Aire knockout	Not known	Wasp knockout	Ctla-4 knockout	Tgf-β1/TβRII conditional knockout
Onset of Symptoms							
Human	Early infancy	1–2 years	4–5 years	Infancy	Infancy	–	–
Mouse	First week of life	Early	Late (6–30 weeks)	–	(Asymptomatic)	2 weeks	2–3 weeks
Lethality							
Human	Infancy	Adulthood	Adulthood	Infancy	Infancy	–	–
Mouse	3 weeks	Late	Late	–	Late	3–4 weeks	3–4 weeks/8–10 weeks
Clinical Feature							
Endocrinopathy	+++ Diabetes, thyroiditis	(+)	++++ Adrenal failure, hypoparathyroidism	–	–	++	++
Enteritis	++++	(+)	(+)	++++	+++ (Bloody diarrhea)	++	++
Skin lesions	++++ Erythema, eczema, psoriasiform dermatitis, alopecia	–	+++ Ectodermal dystrophy, mucocutaneous candidiasis, vitiligo, alopecia	++++ Erythroderma	++++ Chronic eczema	–	–
Hemolytic anemia	++	++	+	–	+++	–	–
Thrombocytopenia		Episodic				–	–
Lymphadenopathy	++	++++	++	+++	++	++++	++++
Hepatosplenomegaly	++	++++	+ (Autoimmune hepatitis)	+++	++	++++	++++
Gonadal failure	–	–	++	–	–	–	–
Renal disease	++	(+)	–	–	++	–	–
Lab Abnormalities							
Elevated IgG, IgA, IgM	– (high IgA)	++	(+)	Low IgG, IgA, IgM, low number of B cells and elevated number of T cells, decreased lymphocyte proliferation	High IgA		–
Elevated IgE	+++	+	–	+++	+	–	–
Eosinophilia	++	+	–	+++	+	–	–
Autoantibodies	Anti-β cells Anti-blood cells Anti-enterocytes	Anti-blood cells	Anti-parathyroid, anti-adrenal cortex	–	Anti-blood cells IgA nephropathy	–	Nuclear antigens, activated T cells
Lymphocytic infiltrates	Activated T cells in lymph nodes, spleen, liver, pancreas, skin	Double-negative immature T cells; lymph nodes, spleen, liver	Adrenal gland, gonads	Skin	Skin	Activated T cells; heart and lungs	Activated T cells and neutrophils; heart and lungs

ALPS, autoimmune lymphoproliferative syndrome; APECED, autoimmune polyendocrinopathy, candidiasis, ectodermal dysplasia; IPEX, immune dysregulation, polyendocrinopathy, enteropathy, X-linked; WAS, Wiskott-Aldrich syndrome.

induces programmed cell death in a variety of cell lines including lymphocytes (Nagata, 1997). Programmed cell death is an important mechanism of regulating the immune response by deleting autoreactive lymphocyte clones from the peripheral lymphocyte pool ("recessive tolerance"). Mice with inactivating mutations in either Fas or FasL show dramatic lymphocytic proliferation and infiltration of multiple organs. Unlike scurfy mice, whose infiltrating lymphocytes have an activated phenotype, the majority of lymphocytes in the infiltrates of Fas/FasL mutant mice are immature, nonactivated double-negative T cells (Watanabe-Fukunaga et al., 1992; Takahashi et al., 1994). Fas/FasL mutants develop autoantibodies, including IgM rheumatoid factor and antichromatin antibodies (Weintraub et al., 1998). These mutant mice survive for prolonged periods of time, in contrast to mice with mutations of *Foxp3*. In humans, mutations in FAS or FASL cause a rare autosomal-dominant syndrome known as autoimmune lymphoproliferative syndrome (ALPS) or Canale-Smith syndrome, which presents in the first 1–2 years of life and is characterized by massive lymphadenopathy and splenomegaly caused by nonmalignant lymphocytic infiltrates and a variety of autoimmune phenomena (Fisher et al., 1995; Rieux-Laucat et al., 1995; Drappa et al., 1996) (see Chapter 24). The most frequent autoimmune disorders associated with ALPS are episodic hemolytic anemia, thrombocytopenia, or neutropenia. Patients with ALPS survive well into adulthood and, as they age, they continue to have autoimmune manifestations. Although the lymphoproliferative component of the syndrome often resolves with age, ALPS patients have a high incidence of B cell lymphoma.

Autoimmune regulator (AIRE) is a DNA-binding protein encoded by a single gene on chromosome 21 (Bjorses et al., 1998). The *Aire* gene is expressed in lymph nodes, spleen, testis, and thymus, particularly in the dendritic cell population of the murine thymus (Heino et al., 2000). Mutations in this gene cause the rare autosomal recessive human syndrome of autoimmune polyendocrinopathy, candidiasis, ectodermal dysplasia (APECED) (see Chapter 25). The three most common characteristics of this disease are mucocutaneous candidiasis, hypoparathyroidism, and adrenocortical insufficiency. Patients may develop a variety of other symptoms, including type 1 diabetes, Hashimoto's thyroiditis, vitiligo, and hemolytic anemia. The onset of APECED is less fulminant than that of IPEX, typically starting with candidiasis by age 5, hypoparathyroidism by age 10, and Addison disease by age 15 (Vogel et al., 2002). *Aire*-deficient mice, generated by targeted gene disruption, develop many of the typical APECED features (Anderson et al., 2002; Ramsey et al., 2002). Affected mice are born and develop normally but have lymphocytic infiltrates in liver and atrophy of adrenals and gonadal tissue. *Aire*-deficient mice often develop autoantibodies to liver, exocrine pancreas, testis, and adrenal glands. Recently it was demonstrated in mice that Aire expression by thymic dendritic cells is required for the expression of self-antigens by these antigen presenting cells (Anderson et al., 2002). Following presentation of self-antigens to autoreactive T cell clones, they are eliminated by negative selection (reviewed by Su and Anderson, 2004). Thus, Aire provides a mechanism for deletion of functional autoreactive T cells in the thymus, contributing substantially to "recessive tolerance."

Omenn syndrome is a clinically defined disorder characterized by early onset, a generalized erythematous rash, combined immune deficiency, elevated serum IgE, and eosinophilia (see Chapter 9). Most patients with Omenn syndrome have normal numbers of (oligoclonal) T cells and low numbers or absent circulating B cells. Because of severe gastrointestinal symptoms and failure to thrive, TPN is often required and line infection is a frequent complication. Hypomorphic mutations of *Rag1* and *Rag2* are frequently associated with Omenn syndrome, but mutations of Artemis or IL-7R have been reported.

Patients with the Wiskott-Aldrich syndrome (WAS), caused by mutations of WASP, frequently present during early infancy with bloody diarrhea, bacterial and viral infections, eczema, and bleeding due to congenital thrombocytopenia. Patients with WAS may develop autoimmune hemolytic anemia or thrombocytopenia, and neutropenia. As in IPEX, the inheritance is X-linked (see Chapter 31).

Carrier Detection and Prenatal Diagnosis

If the mutation in a given family is known, a suspected carrier female can be identified by mutation analysis. Similarly, prenatal diagnosis of a male fetus at risk can be determined by DNA analysis with chorionic villous biopsy or cultured amniocytes as DNA source. It is unclear if fetal blood contains regulatory T cells that express CD4, CD25, and FOXP3.

Treatment and Prognosis

Early, aggressive therapy is of utmost importance in treating IPEX patients. Often TPN is necessary to ensure adequate nutrition. This type of treatment requires placement of a central catheter, which may cause problems with line infection and septicemia. Red blood cell and platelet transfusions may be necessary. It is unclear if early immunosuppressive therapy can prevent the onset of type 1 diabetes. Long-term immunosuppression has proven effective in some patients, but usually only partially and for a limited period of time. Cyclosporin A or tacrolimus (FK506), often in combination with steroids, has been used with some success (Seidmann et al., 1990; Satake et al., 1993; Kobayashi et al., 1995; Di Rocco and Marta, 1996; Finel et al., 1996; Ferguson et al., 2000; Baud et al., 2001; Levy-Lahad and Wildin, 2001; Wildin et al., 2002). Sirolimus (rapamycin) is better tolerated and seems to be less nephrotoxic (Bindl et al., 2005). The combinations of a long list of immunosuppressive medications, including methotrexate, corticosteroids, infliximab and rituximab, have been tried but not with convincing success. Chronic immunosuppressive therapy may facilitate opportunistic infections.

Hematopoietic stem cell transplantation is currently the only effective cure for IPEX, and some patients have achieved complete remission of symptoms following bone marrow transplantation (Baud et al., 2001; Mazzolari et al., 2005), despite the fact that at least in one case only 20%–30% of the T cells were of donor origin (Baud et al., 2001). However, the long-term outcome of stem cell transplantation is often unfavorable (Baud et al., 2001; Wilden et al., 2002), although the number of reported transplants is small. The degree of symptomatic remission following stem cell transplantation depends on the transplant being initiated prior to irreversible damage that may have occurred to target organs such as the pancreas and thyroid. Interestingly, the patients reported by Baud et al. (2001) had complete symptomatic remission, including reversion of type 1 diabetes, during the conditioning regimen that consisted of anti–T lymphocyte globulin, busulfan, and cyclophosphamide. This result raises the possibility that cytotoxic or biologic agents that target T cells may be an effective treatment in patients who have failed other therapies. In general, the prognosis of IPEX is poor. Untreated, most patients die at an early age. Patients with unusual mutations, such as those affecting mRNA splicing or polyadenylation, may benefit from the generation of a small amount of normal mRNA, and present with a relatively mild clinical phenotype. However, even these patients do poorly in the long run, with most dying before 10 years of age, and a few surviving to the third decade of life (Powell et al., 1982; Bennett et al., 2001b) (Fig. 26.1). Treatment with potent immunosuppressive agents that target T cells in particular can make a difference, but because of toxicity and increased susceptibility to infection, these agents do not guarantee long-term amelioration of symptoms. Although bone marrow transplantation does provide hope for a cure, the risks are substantial. Stem cell transplantation has to be performed early in the course of the disease, before the pancreatic islet cells and other target organs have been irreversibly damaged. At this time, it is unclear how regulatory T cells are generated and maintained following stem cell transplantation.

Animal Models

The *Scurfy* (*sf*) Mutation, a Mouse Model for IPEX

The original *sf* mutation, a fatal X-linked condition, has occurred spontaneously in a partially in-bred strain of mice at the Oakridge National Laboratory (Russell et al., 1959). Shortly after birth, affected male mice present with a scaly skin rash and severe runting secondary to chronic diarrhea and malabsorption. They have scaling of the ears (Color Plate 26.IV), eyelids, feet, and tail, which is short, and are born with thickened ears. Characteristically, the mice exhibit lymph adenopathy, splenomegaly, massive lymphocytic infiltrates in the skin, liver, and lungs, and develop hemolytic anemia associated with a positive Coomb test (Godfrey et al., 1991b) suggesting that the *sf* mutation causes a "generalized autoimmune-like syndrome."

Immunologic Findings

After a systematic study of these mice, Godfrey and colleagues suggested that "the scurfy disease may be the result of immune dysfunction rather than being a classic immune deficiency" (Godfrey et al., 1991b). The thymus of young *sf* mice, although small in size, is densely populated with lymphocytes and has a distinct cortex and medulla. As the disease progresses, the thymic cortex is rapidly depleted of lymphocytes, and in mice older than 25 days, the thymus is a "shrunken stromal remnant lacking any corticomedullary distinction" (Godfrey et al., 1991b). Lymph nodes, spleen, and liver, however, are markedly enlarged from extramedullary hematopoiesis and cellular infiltrates. This lymphoproliferative disease is mediated by CD4$^+$ CD8$^-$ T lymphocytes (Godfrey et al., 1994). Serum IgG and IgM are markedly elevated; IgA, which is absent in young normal mice, is demonstrable in male pubs with the *sf* mutation (Godfrey et al., 1991a). Flow-cytometric analysis of cell suspensions from spleen or lymph nodes of *sf* mice reveal a characteristic increase in Mac-1$^+$ monocytic cells and a decrease in B220$^+$ cells; the latter population shows an increased expression of B7.1 and B7.2 costimulatory molecules, suggesting a state of activation (Clark et al., 1999). The activity of *sf* T cells appears up-regulated in vivo, as suggested by the spontaneous expression of CD69, CD25, CD80 (B7.1), and CD86 (B7.2). Although *sf* T cells are hyperresponsive to TCR ligation, they still require costimulation through CD28, albeit at decreased intensity (Clark et al., 1999).

Following successful activation, they produce large amounts of granulocyte-macrophage colony-stimulating factor (>1000-fold higher than wild-type CD4$^+$) as well as a number of other cytokines, including IL-2, IL-5, IL-6, IL-7, IL10, IFN-γ, and TNF-α (Blair et al., 1994; Kanangat et al., 1996; Clark et al., 1999). Interestingly, this hyperresponsiveness is resistant to suppression by inhibitors of tyrosine kinases, such as genistein and herbimycin A, and cyclosporin A (Clark et al., 1999). These observations suggest that the *sf* mutation interferes with a physiologic down-regulation of T cell activation and may have implications for the immunosuppressive therapy of IPEX patients.

Transfer Experiments in *sf* Mice

The effect of transplantation of lymphoid organs and cell suspensions from *sf* (or wild-type) mice into athymic nude or severe combined immunodeficiency disease (SCID) mice (Godfrey et al., 1994) can be summarized as follows. First, transplanted sf thymus transfers the sf phenotype to nude and SCID mice. Second, euthymic (immunologic competent) recipients of congenic sf thymus grafts remain clinically normal, as do all SCID and nude recipients of normal thymic transplants. Third, single-cell suspensions of thymus, lymph node, or spleen from *sf* mice transferred into histocompatible nude or SCID mice by intraperitoneal injection result in an *sf* phenotype in all recipients. Additional transfer experiments have demonstrated that the primary cause of the *sf* phenotype is the CD4$^+$ CD8$^-$ T cell population; CD4$^+$ but not CD8$^+$ lymph node T cells from *sf* mice transfer the disease to syngenic host nude mice (Blair et al., 1994). Finally, if normal CD4$^+$ T cells are added to the CD4$^+$ *sf* T cells, the host nude mice do not develop the *sf* phenotype. These in vivo experiments suggest that *sf* is the result of dysregulated CD4$^+$ T cells, which express activation markers, excrete large quantities of cytokines, and are capable of inducing autoimmune disorders. Thus, *sf* is most consistent with an autoimmune lymphoproliferative disease due to an inability to down-regulate antigen-driven T cell activation.

Mutation of Foxp3 as the Cause of sf

The *sf* locus was originally mapped to a 1.7 Cm interval between *DXWas70* and *Otc* in the proximal region of the mouse X chromosome (Lyon et al., 1990, Kanangat et al., 1996). Through combining high-resolution genetic and physical mapping with large-scale sequence analysis, the gene responsible for the *sf* mutation was identified and designated as Foxp3 (Brunkow et al., 2001). The protein encoded by *Foxp3* is a new member of the forkhead winged-helix family of transcriptional regulators and is highly conserved in different mammalian species. The spontaneous mutation of *Foxp3* in *sf* mice is a 2 bp insertion in exon 8, resulting in a frameshift that leads to a truncated protein product lacking the carboxy-terminal forkhead domain (Brunkow et al., 2001).

Foxp3 Transgenic Mice

To examine the in vivo consequences of Foxp3 overexpression, several different Foxp3-transgenic mouse lines were established, each with differing levels of transgene expression (Brunkow et al., 2001; Khattri et al., 2001). Each of these lines, when bred into an otherwise wild-type background, resulted in a reduction of lymph node size and cellularity. The extent of this reduction correlated with transgene copy number and expression, with higher Foxp3 levels resulting in a greater reduction in lymph node and splenic cellularity. Both CD4[+] and CD8[+] lymphocytes were reduced in number; thymic cellularity was unaffected. A transgenic line with 16 copies of the transgene had an expression level of Foxp3 that was approximately threefold higher than that in normal controls. This transgenic line had a 50% reduction in the number of peripheral blood CD4[+] T cells and a 75% reduction in CD8[+] T cells. Histologically, peripheral lymphoid organs lacked follicular structure and were without margins between follicular and interfollicular regions. To explore the effect of increased Foxp3 expression, mice from this transgenic line were studied for T cell function. Purified CD4[+] T cells displayed reduced proliferative responses when activated in vitro and lacked IL-2 production. Thus, Foxp3 is capable of regulating the ability of CD4[+] T cells to respond to TCR-mediated signals. As a direct consequence, T helper function is severely impaired in *Foxp3* transgenic mice that fail to respond to T-dependent antigen (Kasprowicz et al., 2003).

Finally, the *sf* mouse model was instrumental in the discovery of regulatory T cells (Fontenot et al., 2003; Hori et al., 2003; Khattri et al., 2003) (see FOXP3 and CD4[+] CD25[+] Regulatory T cells, above) and thus played a major role in understanding the molecular basis of IPEX. Using Foxp3 negative gene-targeted mice and a GFP-Foxp3 fusion–protein–reporter knock-in allele, it could be shown that expression of Foxp3 was highly restricted to αβ CD4[+] T cells and, irrespectively of CD25 expression, correlated with suppressor activity (Fontenot et al., 2005).

Ctla-4- and Tgf-β1-Deficient Mice

Two mouse models, both without a human counterpart, show many similarities to the scurfy mouse. Ctla-4-deficient mice develop a lymphoproliferative syndrome similar to that of scurfy mice; however, the lymphocytic infiltrates tend to be more widespread, with accumulation of activated T cells in heart, lungs, lymph nodes, thymus, spleen, liver, bone marrow, and pancreas. Mice are well until 2 weeks of age, then become ill and die by 3 to 4 weeks of age, probably of myocardinal infarction due to massive lymphocytic infiltrates in the heart muscle (Waterhouse et al., 1995; Tivol et al., 1995). CTLA-4 is a cell surface molecule that is expressed in activated T cells. When engaged by its ligand B7.1 or B7.2, CTLA-4 has an inhibitory effect on T cell activation responses including proliferation, cytokine secretion, and cell surface protein expression (Chambers and Allison, 1999). Although there is no human syndrome caused by mutations of CTLA-4, it has been suggested that specific polymorphisms may increase the risk of developing Graves disease or autoimmune diabetes (Cosentino et al., 2002; Yung et al., 2002). Transforming growth factor β1 (TGF-β1) belongs to a family of related growth factors that play diverse roles in cellular processes including wound healing, hematopoiesis, and immune regulation. Tgfβ1-deficient mice develop normally until 2 weeks of age, when they begin to waste, and die by 3 to 4 weeks of age. Deficient mice also develop lymphocytic infiltrates into major organs, particularly heart, lungs, and salivary glands, and die of cardiopulmonary symptoms secondary to massive lymphocytic infiltrates (Shull et al., 1992; Christ et al., 1994; Kulkarni et al., 1995). Tgfβ1 knockout mice develop high autoantibody titers to several nuclear antigens, including single and double-stranded DNA (Yaswen et al., 1996). Mice conditionally lacking the transforming growth factor beta type II receptor (TβRII), one of the two cell surface receptors for the TGF-β family of growth factors, have a phenotype of lym-

phocytic infiltration and autoimmunity but with a less fulminant course (Leveen et al., 2002). No human syndromes with mutations of Ctla-4, Tgfβ1, and TβRII have been described.

Conclusion and Future Directions

FOXP3 is the key mediator of regulatory T cell development in the thymus. Naturally occurring mutations of *FOXP3* interfere with this process, resulting in the generation of autoaggressive T lymphocyte clones that are directly responsible for IPEX in humans and scurfy in mice; both are lethal diseases. Bone marrow transplantation is the only cure for patients with IPEX. It is anticipated that exploitation of the scurfy mouse model and further evaluation of patients with IPEX will lead to a better understanding of the function of FOXP3 as a transcription factor and will facilitate the identification of genes that are regulated by FOXP3. Finally, we need an answer to the question of what regulates the regulator. Investigations along these lines will provide important insight into the mechanisms of immunosuppression, autoimmunity, and tolerance, and may lead to novel strategies to treat not only patients with IPEX but also those suffering from autoimmune diseases, graft versus host disease, or cancer.

References

Anderson MS, Venanzi ES, Klein L, Chen Z, Berzins SP, Turley SJ, von Boehmer H, Bronson R, Dierich A, Benoist C, Mathis D. Projection of an immunological self shadow within the thymus by the aire protein. Science 298:1395–1401, 2002.

Baud O, Goulet O, Canioni D, Le Deist F, Radford I, Rieu D, Dupuis-Girod S, Cerf-Bensussan N, Cavazzana-Calvo M, Brousse N, Fischer A, Casanova JL. Treatment of the immune dysregulation, polyendocrinopathy, enteropathy, X-linked syndrome (IPEX) by allogeneic bone marrow transplantation. N Engl J Med 344:1758–1762, 2001.

Bennett CL, Brunkow ME, Ramsdell F, O'Briant KC, Zhu Q, Fuleihan RL, Shigeoka AO, Ochs HD, Chance PF. A rare polyadenylation signal mutation of the *FOXP3* gene (AAUAAA → AAUGAA) leads to the IPEX syndrome. Immunogenetics 53:435–439, 2001a.

Bennett CL, Christie J, Ramsdell F, Brunkow ME, Ferguson PJ, Whitesell L, Kelly TE, Saulsbury FT, Chance PF, Ochs HD. The immune dysregulation, polyendocrinopathy, enteropathy, X-linked syndrome (IPEX) is caused by mutations of *FOXP3*. Nat Genet 27:20–21, 2001b.

Bennett CL, Yoshioka R, Kiyosawa H, Barker DF, Fain PR, Shigeoka AO, Chance PF. X-Linked syndrome of polyendocrinopathy, immune dysfunction, and diarrhea maps to Xp11.23–Xq13.3. Am J Hum Genet 66: 461–468, 2000.

Berger CL, Tigelaar R, Cohen J, Mariwalla K, Trinh J, Wang N, Edelson RL. Cutaneous T cell lymphonia: malignant proliferation of T regulatory cells. Blood 105:1640–1647, 2005.

Bettelli E, Dastrange M, Oukka M. Foxp3 interacts with nuclear factor of activated T cells and NF-κB to repress cytokine gene expression and effector functions of T helper cells. Proc Natl Acad Sci USA 102:5138–5143, 2005.

Beyer M, Kochanek M, Darabi K, Popov A, Jensen M, Endl E, Knolle PA, Thomas RK, von Bergwelt-Baildon M, Debey S, Hallek M, Schultze JL. Reduced frequencies and suppressive function of CD4[+] CD25 high regulatory T cells in patients with chronic lymphocytic leukemia after therapy with fludarabine. Blood 106:2018–2025, 2005.

Bindl L, Torgerson TR, Perroni L, Youssef N, Ochs HD, Goulet O, Ruemmele FM. Successful use of the new immune-suppressor sirolimus in IPEX (immune dysregulation polyendocrinopathy, enteropathy, X-linked syndrome). J Pediatr 147:256–259, 2005.

Bjorses P, Aaltonen J, Horelli-Kuitunen N, Yaspo ML, Peltonen L. Gene defect behind APECED: a new clue to autoimmunity. Hum Mol Genet 7: 1547–1553, 1998.

Blair PJ, Bultman SJ, Haas JC, Rouse BT, Wilkinson JE, Godfrey VL. CD4[+]CD8[-] T cells are the effector cells in disease pathogenesis in the scurfy (sf) mouse. J Immunol 153:3764–3774, 1994.

Brunkow ME, Jeffery EW, Hjerrild KA, Paeper B, Clark LB, Yasayko SA, Wilkinson JE, Galas D, Ziegler SF, Ramsdell F. Disruption of a new forkhead/winged-helix protein, scurfin, results in the fatal lymphoproliferative disorder of the scurfy mouse. Nat Genet 27:68–73, 2001.

Carlsson P, Mahlapuu M. Forkhead transcription factors: key players in development and metabolism. Dev Biol 250:1–23, 2002.

Chambers CA, Allison JP. Costimulatory regulation of T cell function. Curr Opin Cell Biol 11:203–210, 1999.

Chatila TA, Blaeser F, Ho N, Lederman HM, Voulgaropoulos C, Helms C, Bowcock AM. JM2, encoding a fork head-related protein, is mutated in X-linked autoimmunity-allergic disregulation syndrome. J Clin Invest 106:75–81, 2000.

Christ M, McCartney-Francis NL, Kulkarni AB, Ward JM, Mizel DE, Mackall CL, Gress RE, Hines KL, Tian H, Karlsson S, et al. Immune dysregulation in TGF-β1-deficient mice. J Immunol 153:1936–1946, 1994.

Cilio CM, Bosco S, Moretti C, Farilla L, Savignoni F, Colarizi P, Multari G, Di Mario U, Bucci G, Dotta F. Congenital autoimmune diabetes mellitus. N Engl J Med 342:1529–1531, 2000.

Clark LB, Appleby MW, Brunkow ME, Wilkinson JE, Ziegler SF, Ramsdell F. Cellular and molecular characterization of the scurfy mouse mutant. J Immunol 162:2546–2554, 1999.

Cosentino A, Gambelunghe G, Tortoioli C, Falorni A. CTLA-4 gene polymorphism contributes to the genetic risk for latent autoimmune diabetes in adults. Ann NY Acad Sci 958:337–340, 2002.

Cosmi L, Liotta F, Lazzeri E, Francalanci M, Angeli R, Mazzinghi B, Santarlasci V, Manetti R, Vanini V, Romagnani P, Maggi E, Romagnani S, Annunziato F. Human CD8+CD25+ thymocytes share phenotypic and functional features with CD4+CD25+ regulatory thymocytes. Blood 102: 4107–4114, 2003.

Di Rocco M, Marta R. X linked immune dysregulation, neonatal insulin dependent diabetes, and intractable diarrhoea. Arch Dis Child Fetal Neonatal Ed 75:144, 1996.

Dodge JA, Laurence KM. Congenital absence of islets of Langerhans. Arch Dis Child 52:411–413, 1977.

Drappa J, Vaishnaw AK, Sullivan KE, Chu JL, Elkon KB. Fas gene mutations in the Canale-Smith syndrome, an inherited lymphoproliferative disorder associated with autoimmunity. N Engl J Med 335:1643–1649, 1996.

Earle KE, Tang Q, Zhou X, Liu W, Zhu S, Bonyhadi ML, Bluestone JA. In vitro expanded human CD4+CD25+ regulatory T cells suppress effector T cell proliferation. Clin Immunol 115:3–9, 2005.

Ehrlich P. Collected Studies on Immunity. New York: J. Wiley and Sons, 1910.

Ellis D, Fisher SE, Smith WI Jr, Jaffe R. Familial occurrence of renal and intestinal disease associated with tissue autoantibodies. Am J Dis Child 136:323–326, 1982.

Ferguson PJ, Blanton SH, Saulsbury FT, McDuffie MJ, Lemahieu V, Gastier JM, Francke U, Borowitz SM, Sutphen JL, Kelly TE. Manifestations and linkage analysis in X-linked autoimmunity-immunodeficiency syndrome. Am J Med Genet 90:390–397, 2000.

Finel E, Giroux JD, Metz C, Robert JJ, Robert O, Sadoun E, Alix D, de Parscau L. Diabete neonatal vrai associe a une maladie auto-immune. Arch Pediatr 3:782–784, 1996.

Fisher GH, Rosenberg FJ, Straus SE, Dale JK, Middleton LA, Lin AY, Strober W, Lenardo MJ, Puck JM. Dominant interfering Fas gene mutations impair apoptosis in a human autoimmune lymphoproliferative syndrome. Cell 81:935–946, 1995.

Fontenot JD, Gavin MA, Rudensky AY. Foxp3 programs the development and function of CD4+CD25+ regulatory T cells. Nat Immunol 4:330–336, 2003.

Fontenot JD, Rasmussen JP, Williams LM, Dooley JL, Farr AG, Rudensky AY. Regulatory T cell lineage specification by the forkhead transcription factor foxp3. Immunity 22:329–341, 2005.

Fontenot JD, Rudensky AY. A well adapted regulatory contrivance: regulatory T cell development and the forkhead family transcription factor Foxp3. Nat Immunol 6:331–337, 2005.

Gajiwala KS, Burley SK. Winged helix proteins. Curr Opin Struct Biol 10: 110–116, 2000.

Gambineri E, Torgerson TR, Ochs HD. Immune dysregulation, polyendocrinopathy, enteropathy, and X-linked inheritance, a syndrome of systemic autoimmunity caused by mutations of FOXP3, a critical regulator of T-cell homeostasis. Curr Opin Rheumatol 15:430–435, 2003.

Gambineri E, Vijay S, Añover S, Fischer A, Gavin MA, Lederman HM, Notarangelo LD, Ruemmele FM, Sullivan K, Ochs HD, Torgerson TR. Clinincal and molecular analysis of a large cohort of patients with the IPEX phenotype. Submitted, 2006.

Gavin MA, Torgerson TR, Houston E, deRoos P, Ho WY, Ocheltree EL, Greenberg PD, Ochs HD, Rudensky AY. Single cell analysis of FOXP3 expression suggests FOXP3-dependent commitment of an in vivo generated regulatory T cell lineage in humans. Running title: FOXP3-dependent human regulatory T cell development. PNAS 2006, in press.

Godfrey VL, Rouse BT, Wilkinson JE. Transplantation of T cell–mediated, lymphoreticular disease from the scurfy (sf) mouse. Am J Pathol 145: 281–286, 1994.

Godfrey VL, Wilkinson JE, Rinchik EM, Russell LB. Fatal lymphoreticular disease in the scurfy (sf) mouse requires T cells that mature in a sf thymic environment: potential model for thymic education. Proc Natl Acad Sci USA 88:5528–5532, 1991a.

Godfrey VL, Wilkinson JE, Russell LB. X-linked lymphoreticular disease in the scurfy (sf) mutant mouse. Am J Pathol 138:1379–1387, 1991b.

Hattevig G, Kjellman B, Fallstrom SP. Congenital permanent diabetes mellitus and celiac disease. J Pediatr 101:955–957, 1982.

Heino M, Peterson P, Sillanpaa N, Guerin S, Wu L, Anderson G, Scott HS, Antonarakis SE, Kudoh J, Shimizu N, Jenkinson EJ, Naquet P, Krohn KJ. RNA and protein expression of the murine autoimmune regulator gene (Aire) in normal, RelB-deficient and in NOD mouse. Eur J Immunol 30:1884–1893, 2000.

Hori S, Nomura T, Sakaguchi S. Control of regulatory T cell development by the transcription factor Foxp3. Science 299:1057–1061, 2003.

Hsieh CS, Rudensky AY. The role of TCR specificity in naturally arising CD25+ CD4+ regulatory T cell biology. Curr Top Microbiol Immunol 293: 25–42, 2005.

Itoh M, Takahashi T, Sakaguchi N, Kuniyasu Y, Shimizu J, Otsuka F, Sakaguchi S. Thymus and autoimmunity: production of CD25+CD4+ naturally anergic and suppressive T cells as a key function of the thymus in maintaining immunologic self-tolerance. J Immunol 162:5317–5326, 1999.

Jonas MM, Bell MD, Eidson MS, Koutouby R, Hensley GT. Congenital diabetes mellitus and fatal secretory diarrhea in two infants. J Pediatr Gastroenterol Nutr 13:415–425, 1991.

Kanangat S, Blair P, Reddy R, Daheshia M, Godfrey V, Rouse BT, Wilkinson E. Disease in the scurfy (sf) mouse is associated with overexpression of cytokine genes. Eur J Immunol 26:161–165, 1996. Erratum in: Eur J Immunol 33:2064, 2003.

Karube K, Ohshima K, Tsuchiya T, Yamaguchi T, Kawano R, Suzumiya J, Utsunomiya A, Harada M, Kikuchi M. Expression of FoxP3, a key molecule in CD4CD25 regulatory T cells, in adult T-cell leukaemia/lymphoma cells. Br J Haematol 126:81–84, 2004.

Kasprowicz DJ, Smallwood PS, Tyznik AJ, Ziegler SF. Scurfin (FoxP3) controls T-dependent immune responses in vivo through regulation of CD4+ T cell effector function. J Immunol 171:1216–1223, 2003.

Khattri R, Cox T, Yasayko SA, Ramsdell F. An essential role for Scurfin in CD4+CD25+ T regulatory cells. Nat Immunol 4:337–342, 2003.

Khattri R, Kasprowicz D, Cox T, Mortrud M, Appleby MW, Brunkow ME, Ziegler SF, Ramsdell F. The amount of scurfin protein determines peripheral T cell number and responsiveness. J Immunol 167:6312–6320, 2001.

Kobayashi I, Imamura K, Kubota M, Ishikawa S, Yamada M, Tonoki H, Okano M, Storch WB, Moriuchi T, Sakiyama Y, Kobayashi K. Identification of an autoimmune enteropathy-related 75-kilodalton antigen. Gastroenterology 117:823–830, 1999.

Kobayashi I, Imamura K, Yamada M, Okano M, Yara A, Ikema S, Ishikawa N. A 75-kD autoantigen recognized by sera from patients with X-linked autoimmune enteropathy associated with nephropathy. Clin Exp Immunol 111:527–531, 1998.

Kobayashi I, Nakanishi M, Okano M, Sakiyama Y, Matsumoto S. Combination therapy with tacrolimus and betamethasone for a patient with X-linked auto-immune enteropathy. Eur J Pediatr 154:594–595, 1995.

Kobayashi I, Shiari R, Yamada M, Kawamura N, Okano M, Yara A, Iguchi A, Ishikawa N, Ariga T, Sakiyama Y, Ochs HD, Kobayashi K. Novel mutations of FOXP3 in two Japanese patients with immune dysregulation, polyendocrinopathy, enteropathy, X linked syndrome (IPEX). J Med Genet 38:874–876, 2001.

Kulkarni AB, Ward JM, Yaswen L, Mackall CL, Bauer SR, Huh CG, Gress RE, Karlsson S. Transforming growth factor-beta 1 null mice. An animal model for inflammatory disorders. Am J Pathol 146:264–275, 1995.

Leveen P, Larsson J, Ehinger M, Cilio CM, Sundler M, Sjostrand LJ, Holmdahl R, Karlsson S. Induced disruption of the transforming growth factor beta type II receptor gene in mice causes a lethal inflammatory disorder that is transplantable. Blood 100:560–568, 2002.

Levy-Lahad E, Wildin RS. Neonatal diabetes mellitus, enteropathy, thrombocytopenia, and endocrinopathy: further evidence for an X-linked lethal syndrome. J Pediatr 138:577–580, 2001.

Lopes JE, Torgerson TR, Schubert LA, Anover SD, Ochs HD, Ziegler SF. Analysis of FOXP3 reveals multiple domains required for its function as a transcriptional repressor. Submitted, 2006.

Loser K, Hansen W, Apelt J, Balkow S, Buer J, Beissert S. In vitro–generated regulatory T cells induced by Foxp3-retrovirus infection control murine contact allergy and systemic autoimmunity. Gene Ther 12:1294–1304, 2005.

Lyon MF, Peters J, Glenister PH, Ball S, Wright E. The scurfy mouse mutant has previously unrecognized hematological abnormalities and resembles Wiskott-Aldrich syndrome. Proc Natl Acad Sci USA 87:2433–2437, 1990.

Mantel PY, Quaked N, Ruckert B, Karagiannidis C, Welz R, Blaser K, Schmidt-Weber CB. Molecular mechanisms underlying FOXP3 induction in human T cells. J Immunol 176:3593–3602, 2006.

Marinaki S, Neumann I, Kalsch AI, Grimminger P, Breedijk A, Birck R, Schmitt W, Waldherr R, Yard BA, Van Der Woude FJ. Abnormalities of CD4 T cell subpopulations in ANCA-associated vasculitis. Clin Exp Immunol 140:181–191, 2005.

Mazzolari E, Forino C, Fontana M, D'Ippolito C, Lanfranchi A, Gambineri E, Ochs H, Badolato R, Notarangelo LD. A new case of IPEX receiving bone marrow transplantation. Bone Marrow Transplant 35:1033–1034, 2005.

Meyer B, Nezelof C, Lemoine, Charlas J, Caille B, Vialatte J. Apropos de deux cas de diabete neonatal. Ann Pediatr (Paris) 17:569–573, 1970.

Nagata S. Apoptosis by death factor. Cell 88:355–365, 1997.

Nieves DS, Phipps RP, Pollock SJ, Ochs HD, Zhu Q, Scott GA, Ryan CK, Kobayashi I, Rossi TM, Goldsmith LA. Dermatologic and immunologic findings in the immune dysregulation, polyendocrinopathy, enteropathy, X-linked syndrome. Arch of Dermatol 140:466–472, 2004.

Ormandy LA, Hillemann T, Wedemeyer H, Manns MP, Greten TF, Korangy F. Increased populations of regulatory T cells in peripheral blood of patients with hepatocellular carcinoma. Cancer Res 65:2457–2464, 2005.

Owen CJ, Jennings CE, Imrie H, Lachaux A, Bridges NA, Cheetham TD, Pearce SH. Mutational analysis of the *FOXP3* gene and evidence for genetic heterogeneity in the immunodysregulation, polyendocrinopathy, enteropathy syndrome. J Clin Endocrinol Metab 88:6034–6039, 2003.

Papiernik M, de Moraes ML, Pontoux C, Vasseur F, Penit C. Regulatory CD4 T cells: expression of IL-2R alpha chain, resistance to clonal deletion and IL-2 dependency. Int Immunol 10:371–378, 1998.

Peake JE, McCrossin RB, Byrne G, Shepherd R. X-linked immune dysregulation, neonatal insulin dependent diabetes, and intractable diarrhoea. Arch Dis Child Fetal Neonatal Ed 74:195–199, 1996.

Powell BR, Buist NR, Stenzel P. An X-linked syndrome of diarrhea, polyendocrinopathy, and fatal infection in infancy. J Pediatr 100:731–737, 1982.

Ramsey C, Winqvist O, Puhakka L, Halonen M, Moro A, Kampe O, Eskelin P, Pelto-Huikko M, Peltonen L. *Aire*-deficient mice develop multiple features of APECED phenotype and show altered immune response. Hum Mol Genet 11:397–409, 2002.

Rieux-Laucat F, Le Deist F, Hivroz C, Roberts IA, Debatin KM, Fischer A, de Villartay JP. Mutations in Fas associated with human lymphoproliferative syndrome and autoimmunity. Science 268:1347–1349, 1995.

Roberts J, Searle J. Neonatal diabetes mellitus associated with severe diarrhea, hyperimmunoglobulin E syndrome, and absence of islets of Langerhans. Pediatr Pathol Lab Med 15:477–483, 1995.

Roncador G, Brown PJ, Maestre L, Hue S, Martinez-Torrecuadrada JL, Ling KL, Pratap S, Toms C, Fox BC, Cerundolo V, Powrie F, Banham AH. Analysis of FOXP3 protein expression in human CD4+CD25+ regulatory T cells at the single-cell level. Eur J Immunol 35:1681–1691, 2005.

Russell WL, Russell LB, Gower JS. Exceptional inheritance of a sex-linked gene in the mouse explained on the basis that the X/O sex-chromosome constitution is female. Proc Natl Acad Sci USA 45:554–560, 1959.

Sakaguchi S, Takahashi T, Yamazaki S, Kuniyasu Y, Itoh M, Sakaguchi N, Shimizu J. Immunologic self tolerance maintained by T-cell-mediated control of self-reactive T cells: implications for autoimmunity and tumor immunity. Microbes Infect 3:911–918, 2001.

Satake N, Nakanishi M, Okano M, Tomizawa K, Ishizaka A, Kojima K, Onodera M, Ariga T, Satake A, Sakiyama Y, et al. A Japanese family of X-linked auto-immune enteropathy with haemolytic anaemia and polyendocrinopathy. Eur J Pediatr 152:313–315, 1993.

Savage MO, Mirakian R, Harries JT, Bottazzo GF. Could protracted diarrhoea of infancy have an autoimmune pathogenesis? Lancet 1:966–967, 1982.

Schubert LA, Jeffery E, Zhang Y, Ramsdell F, Ziegler SF. Scurfin (FOXP3) acts as a repressor of transcription and regulates T cell activation. J Biol Chem 276:37672–37679, 2001.

Seidman EG, Lacaille F, Russo P, Galeano N, Murphy G, Roy CC. Successful treatment of autoimmune enteropathy with cyclosporine. J Pediatr 117:929–932, 1990.

Sharma S, Yang SC, Zhu L, Reckamp K, Gardner B, Baratelli F, Huang M, Batra RK, Dubinett SM. Tumor cyclooxygenase-2/prostaglandin E2–dependent promotion of FOXP3 expression and CD4+ CD25+ T regulatory cell activities in lung cancer. Cancer Res 65:5211–5220, 2005.

Shevach EM. Certified professionals: CD4(+)CD25(+) suppressor T cells. J Exp Med 193:F41–46, 2002.

Shull MM, Ormsby I, Kier AB, Pawlowski S, Diebold RJ, Yin M, Allen R, Sidman G, Proetzel G, Calvin D, et al. Targeted disruption of the mouse transforming growth factor-β1 gene results in multifocal inflammatory disease. Nature 359:693–699, 1992.

Stephens LA, Mason D. CD25 is a marker for CD4+ thymocytes that prevent autoimmune diabetes in rats, but peripheral T cells with this function are found in both CD25+ and CD25– subpopulations. J Immunol 165:3105–3110, 2000.

Su MA, Anderson MS. Aire: an update. Curr Opin Immunol 16:746–752, 2004.

Takahashi T, Tanaka M, Brannan CI, Jenkins NA, Copeland NG, Suda T, Nagata S. Generalized lymphoproliferative disease in mice, caused by a point mutation in the Fas ligand. Cell 76:969–976, 1994.

Tivol EA, Borriello F, Schweitzer AN, Lynch WP, Bluestone JA, Sharpe AH. Loss of CTLA-4 leads to massive lymphoproliferation and fatal multiorgan tissue destruction, revealing a critical negative regulatory role of CTLA-4. Immunity 3:541–547, 1995.

Unitt E, Rushbrook SM, Marshall A, Davies S, Gibbs P, Morris LS, Coleman N, Alexander GJ. Compromised lymphocytes infiltrate hepatocellular carcinoma: the role of T-regulatory cells. Hepatology 41:722–730, 2005.

Viguier M, Lemaitre F, Verola O, Cho MS, Gorochov G, Dubertret L, Bachelez H, Kourilsky P, Ferradini L. Foxp3 expressing CD4+CD25(high) regulatory T cells are overrepresented in human metastatic melanoma lymph nodes and inhibit the function of infiltrating T cells. J Immunol 173:1444–1453, 2004.

Vogel A, Strassburg CP, Obermayer-Straub P, Brabant G, Manns MP. The genetic background of autoimmune polyendocrinopathy-candidiasis-ectodermal dystrophy and its autoimmune disease components. J Mol Med 80:201–211, 2002.

Walker MR, Kasprowicz DJ, Gersuk VH, Benard A, Van Landeghen M, Buckner JH, Ziegler SF. Induction of FoxP3 and acquisition of T regulatory activity by stimulated human CD4+CD25– T cells. J Clin Invest 112:1437–1443, 2003.

Walker-Smith JA, Unsworth DJ, Hutchins P, Phillips AD, Holborow EJ. Autoantibodies against gut epithelium in child with small-intestinal enteropathy. Lancet 1:566–567, 1982.

Watanabe-Fukunaga R, Brannan CI, Copeland NG, Jenkins NA, Nagata S. Lymphoproliferation disorder in mice explained by defects in Fas antigen that mediates apoptosis. Nature 356:314–317, 1992.

Waterhouse P, Penninger JM, Timms E, Wakeham A, Shahinian A, Lee KP, Thompson CB, Griesser H, Mak TW. Lymphoproliferative disorders with early lethality in mice deficient in Ctla-4. Science 270:985–988, 1995.

Wei WZ, Morris GP, Kong YC. Anti-tumor immunity and autoimmunity: a balancing act of regulatory T cells. Cancer Immunol Immunother 53:73–78, 2004.

Weintraub JP, Godfrey V, Wolthusen PA, Cheek RL, Eisenberg RA, Cohen PL. Immunological and pathological consequences of mutations in both Fas and Fas ligand. Cell Immunol 186:8–17, 1998.

Wildin RS, Ramsdell F, Peake J, Faravelli F, Casanova JL, Buist N, Levy-Lahad E, Mazzella M, Goulet O, Perroni L, Bricarelli FD, Byrne G, McEuen M, Proll S, Appleby M, Brunkow ME. X-linked neonatal diabetes mellitus, enteropathy and endocrinopathy syndrome is the human equivalent of mouse scurfy. Nat Genet 27:18–20, 2001.

Wildin RS, Smyk-Pearson S, Filipovich AH. Clinical and molecular features of the immunodysregulation, polyendocrinopathy, enteropathy, X linked (IPEX) syndrome. J Med Genet 39:537–545, 2002.

Wood KJ, Sakaguchi S. Regulatory T cells in transplantation tolerance. Nat Rev Immunol 3:199–210, 2003.

Xystrakis E, Dejean AS, Bernard I, Druet P, Liblau R, Gonzalez-Dunia D, Saoudi A. Identification of a novel natural regulatory CD8 T-cell subset and analysis of its mechanism of regulation. Blood 104:3294–3301, 2004.

Yagi H, Nomura T, Nakamura K, Yamazaki S, Kitawaki T, Hori S, Maeda M, Onodera M, Uchiyama T, Fujii S, Sakaguchi S. Crucial role of FOXP3 in the development and function of human CD25+CD4+ regulatory T cells. Int Immunol 16:1643–1656, 2004.

Yaswen L, Kulkarni AB, Fredrickson T, Mittleman B, Schiffman R, Payne S, Longenecker G, Mozes E, Karlsson S. Autoimmune manifestations in the transforming growth factor-β1 knockout mouse. Blood 87:1439–1445, 1996.

Yu P, Gregg RK, Bell JJ, Ellis JS, Divekar R, Lee HH, Jain R, Waldner H, Hardaway JC, Collins M, Kuchroo VK, Zaghouani H. Specific T regulatory cells display broad suppressive functions against experimental allergic encephalomyelitis upon activation with cognate antigen. J Immunol 174:6772–6780, 2005.

Yung E, Cheng PS, Fok TF, Wong GW. CTLA-4 gene A-G polymorphism and childhood Graves' disease. Clin Endocrinol (Oxf) 56:649–653, 2002.

Zeller J, Voyer M, Bougneres PF. Hyperglycemies et diabetes neonatals. Arch Pediatr 1:561–567, 1994.

Zorn E, Kim HT, Lee SJ, Floyd BH, Litsa D, Arumugarajah S, Bellucci R, Alyea EP, Antin JH, Soiffer RJ, Ritz J. Reduced frequency of FOXP3+ CD4+CD25+ regulatory T cells in patients with chronic graft-versus-host disease. Blood. 106:2903–2911, 2005.

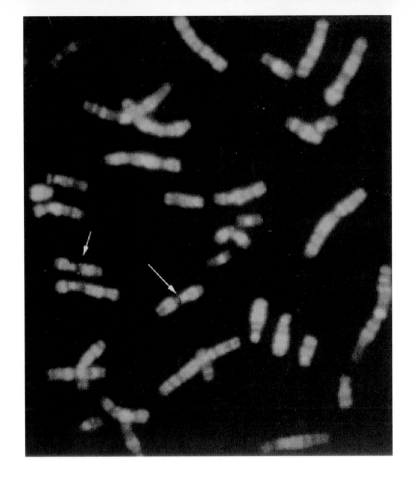

Color Plate 2.1 Fluorescence in situ hybridization with a probe consisting of DNA from a yeast clone containing a large human artificial chromosome (YAC) labeled with the fluorescent dye rhodamine. The chromosomes are counterstained with 4′,6-diamino-2-phenylindole (DAPI), and the images are recorded with a computer-assisted camera. Because the human YAC was selected to contain the gene for *FADD*, a Fas-interacting apoptosis signaling molecule in lymphocytes, this study shows that the *FADD* gene is located on the proximal long arm of chromosome 11 at location 11q13.3 (Kim et al., 1995).

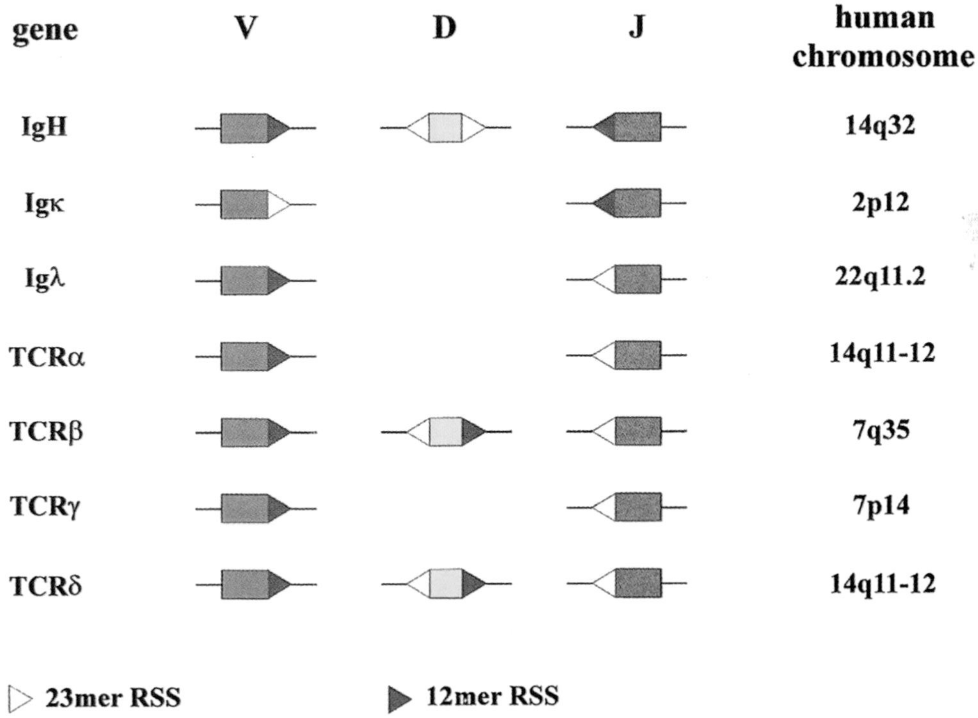

gene	V	D	J	human chromosome
IgH	▭	◁▷	◀	14q32
Igκ	▭▷		◀	2p12
Igλ	▭		◁	22q11.2
TCRα	▭		◁	14q11-12
TCRβ	▭	◁▷	◁	7q35
TCRγ	▭		◁	7p14
TCRδ	▭	◁▷	◁	14q11-12

▷ **23mer RSS**   ▶ **12mer RSS**

A

Color Plate 11.1 (A) Schematic structure and chromosomal localization of the human immunoglobulin (Ig) and T cell antigen receptor (TCR) segments. Each rectangle represents V, D, or J modules. D elements are only present in the IgH, TCRβ, and TCRδ loci. The exons of the constant region of the Ig or TCR are encoded 3′ of the J segments.

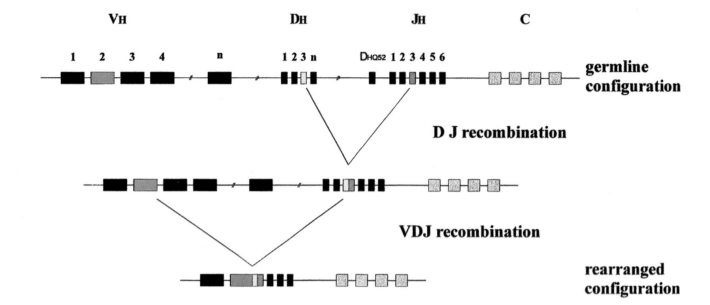

V_H   **D_H**   **J_H**   **C**

B

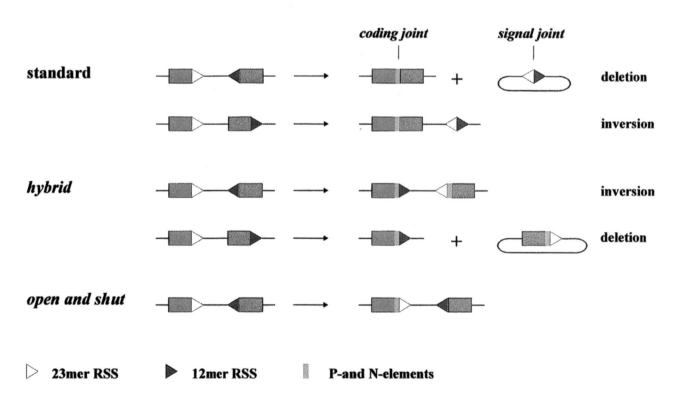

Color Plate 11.1 (continued) (B) Diagram of the rearrangement process on the human Ig heavy chain (IgH) locus. D-to-J joining is followed by V-to-DJ recombination. (C) Possible reaction pathways and resultant products in a single V(D)J recombination event.

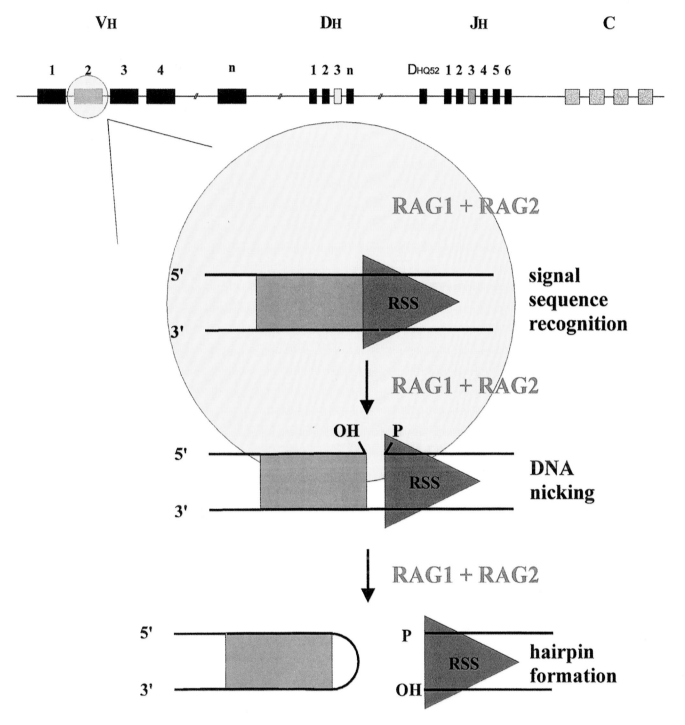

Color Plate 11.II Schematic drawing of RAG1 and RAG2 function: initiation of the V(D)J recombination through their endonuclease activity is followed by *trans*-esterification and hairpin formation.

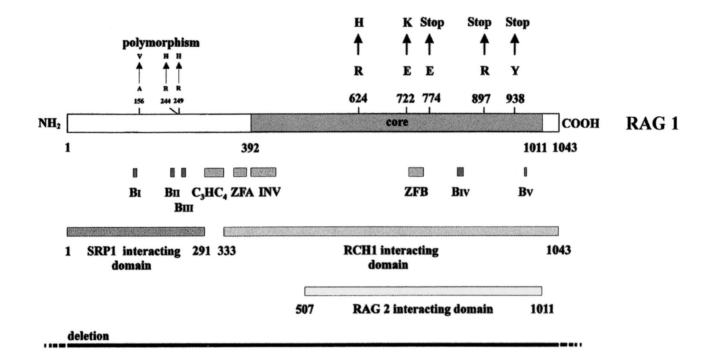

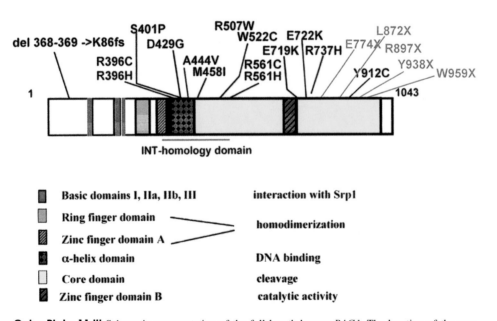

Color Plate 11.III Schematic representation of the full-length human *RAG1*. The location of the core domain is depicted. Some mutations associated with Omenn syndrome are represented in black, while T⁻B⁻ SCID mutations are shown in pink. The SRP1 interacting domain encompasses the N-terminal region (1–291) of *RAG1*. The amino acids necessary for RCH1 interaction (333–1043) are situated in the C terminus. The RAG2 interaction domain stretches from amino acids 507 to 1011.

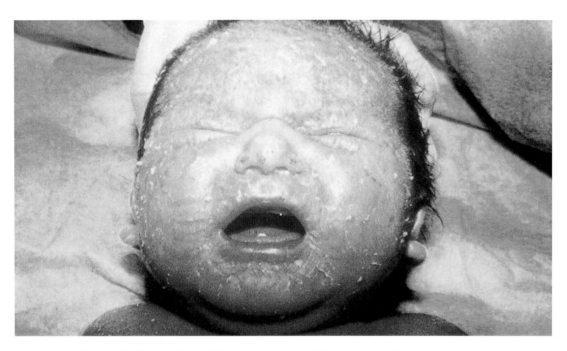

Color Plate 11.IV Infant with Omenn syndrome and characteristic erythromatous, scaly rash involving the entire body.

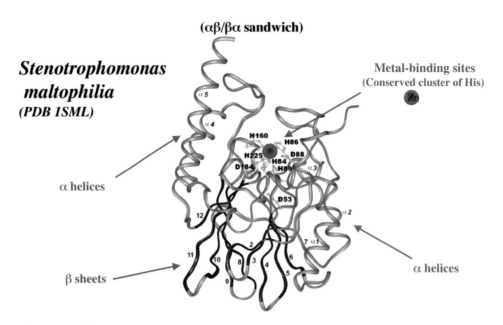

Color Plate 11.V Three-dimensional representation of the *Stenotrophomonas maltophilia* metallo-β-lactamase. Conserved residues of the active site are represented as ball-and-stick.

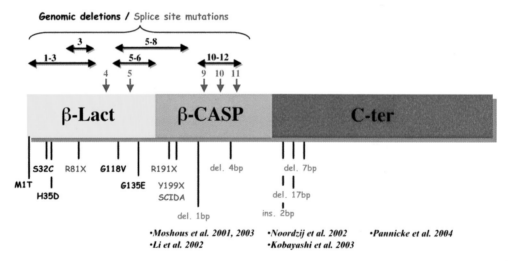

Color Plate 11.VI Genomic organization of the human Artemis gene with mutations identified in RS-SCID patients. Horizontal arrows indicate genomic deletions of exons, and vertical arrows indicate splice site mutations leading to exon skipping. Data from Li et al. (2002), Moshons et al. (2001, 2003), Noordzij et al. (2002), and Kobayashi et al. (2003).

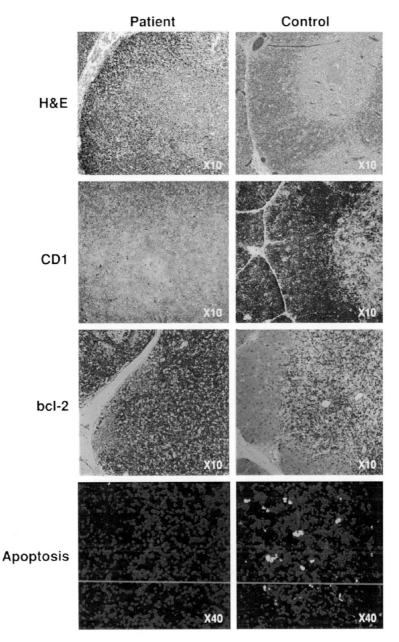

Color Plate 15.1 An immunohistological comparison of thymus sections from a patient lacking CD25 (IL2-Rα) (left) vs. a normal age-matched control (right). Hematoxylin and eosin (H&E) staining (top row) revealed fibrous septae separating lobules of lymphoid tissue in normal thymus, but loss of the normally distinct demarcation between the two areas in the patient, although cortex and medulla are present. Immunhistochemical analysis showed lack of expression of CD1 in the patient (second row), whereas control samples stained strongly for this marker. Expression of bcl-2 (third row) in the normal thymus is restricted to the medulla, with few positive cells present within the cortex, whereas the patient's sample displays a uniformly high level of bcl-2 expression. Consequently, apoptosis in the patient's thymus was reduced dramatically, illustrated by fluorescent labeling (yellow) of DNA ends (bottom row).

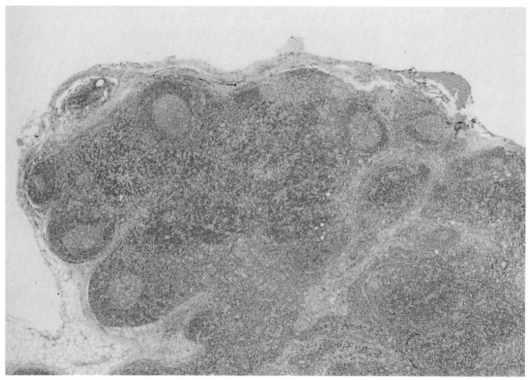

A

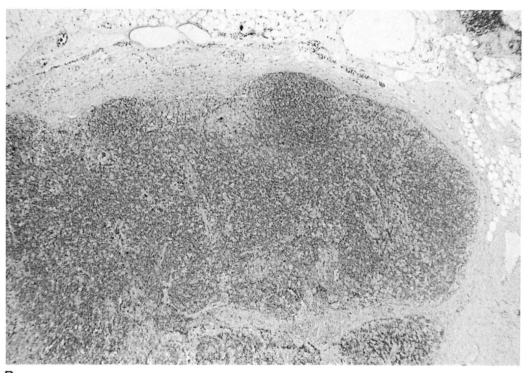

B

Color Plate 19.1 Pathology of lymph nodes in X-linked form of hyper-IgM (XHIM). (A) Morphology of a normal lymph node is shown, with presence of secondary follicles within germinal centers. (B) A lymph node from an XHIM patient shows primary follicles with no evidence of germinal centers. Sections were stained with hematoxylin-eosin. (Courtesy of Prof. F. Facchetti, Department of Pathology, University of Brescia, Italy.)

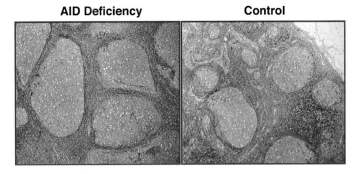

Color Plate 20.1 Giant germinal centers in the lymph node of an AID-deficient patient, compared with normal reactive lymph node germinal centers (×36 original magnification).

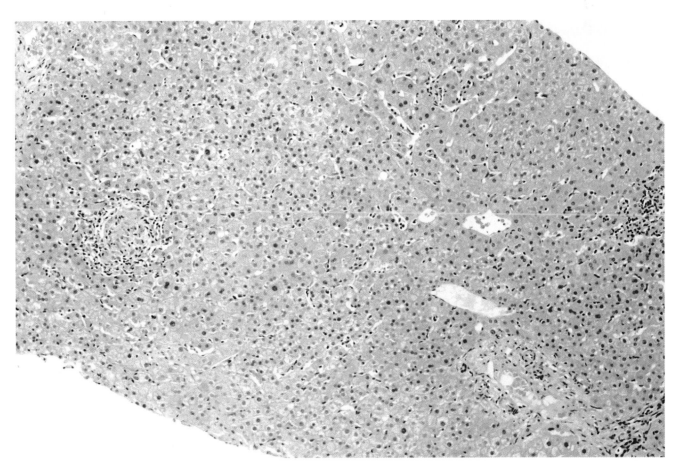

Color Plate 23.1 Granulomas in the liver of 47-year-old patient with common variable immunodeficiency.

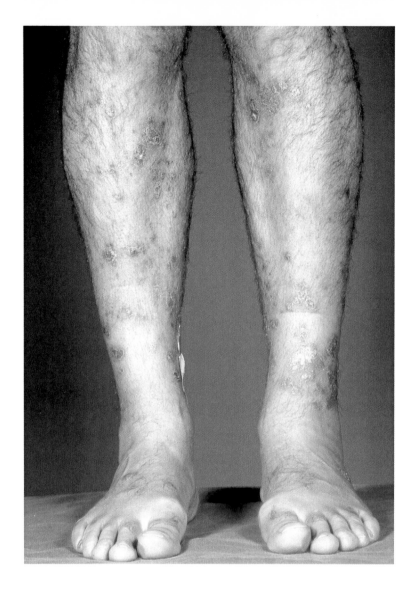

Color Plate 23.II Cutaneous granulomas on the legs of a 47-year-old man with common variable immunodeficiency.

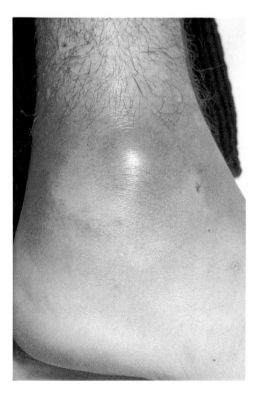

Color Plate 23.III Ureaplasma ankle joint arthritis in a 39-year-old patient with common variable immunodeficiency.

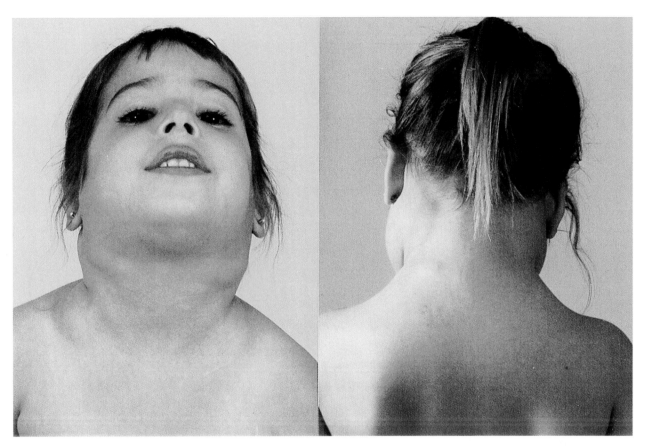

Color Plate 24.i Patient with autoimmune lymphoproliferative syndrome (ALPS) due to a heterozygous mutation of Fas. Note massive enlargement of anterior and posterior cervical lymph nodes, as well as nodes in right axillary, submandibular, and preauricular regions.

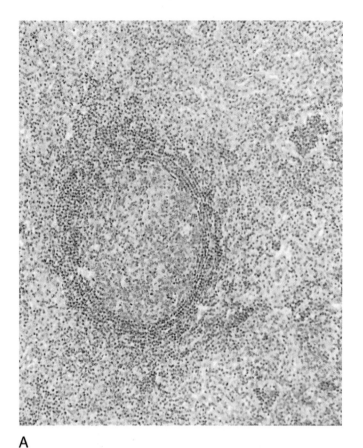

A

B

Plate 24.II Lymph node histology in autoimmune lymphoproliferative syndrome (ALPS). (A) Hematoxolyn and eosin staining demonstrating lymphocytic infiltration in a lymph node from a patient with heterozygous Fas deficiency and ALPS. There is preservation of follicular architecture, but marked reactive hyperplasia and paracortical expansion of lymphocytes, immunoblasts, and plasma cells; there are no histiocytes containing cellular debris as would be typically seen in viral adenitis. Immunostaining of parallel frozen sections showed the lymphocytes to be predominantly CD3⁺CD4⁻CD8⁻. (B) High-power magnification (100×) of lymph node frozen section from another patient (courtesy of Professor N. Brousse, Hôpital Necker, Paris). Immunostaining performed with an anti-CD3 monoclonal antibody coupled to alkaline phosphatase (blue) and both anti-CD4 and anti-CD8 antibodies coupled to peroxidase (brown) reveals a large proportion of T cells (CD3⁺) that are CD4⁻ and CD8⁻.

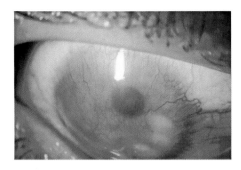

Color Plate 25.I Corneal cloudiness caused by failed treatment of keratopathy in a patient with autoimmune polyendocrinopathy, candidiasis, and ectodermal dysplasia (APECED).

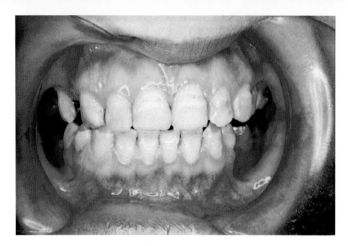

Color Plate 25.II Transverse ridges of enamel hypoplasia in permanent teeth in APECED.

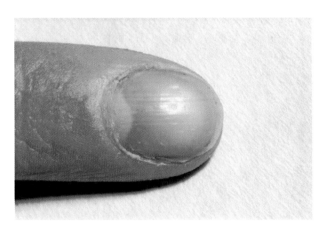

Color Plate 25.III Pitted nail dystrophy in APECED.

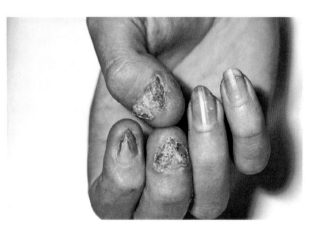

Color Plate 25.IV Nail candidiasis in APECED.

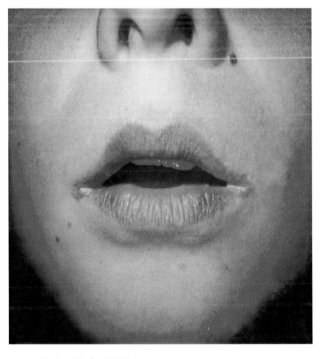

Color Plate 25.V Angular cheilosis, the most common sign of oral candidiasis in APECED.

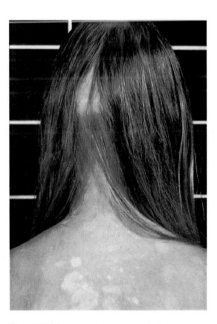

Color Plate 25.VI Patchy alopecia and vitiligo in APECED.

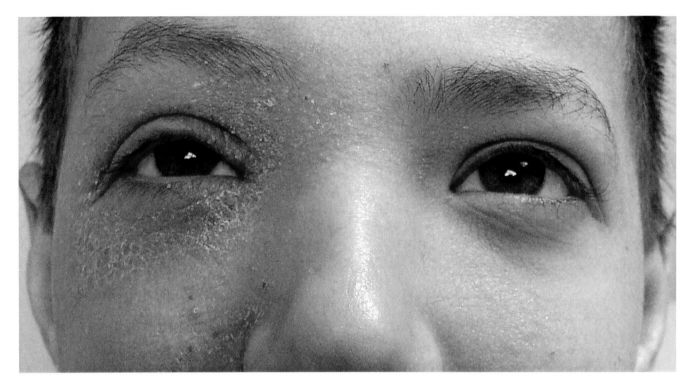

Color Plate 26.I Chronic eczema in a 14-year-old boy with IPEX and a splice site mutation in *FOXP3*.

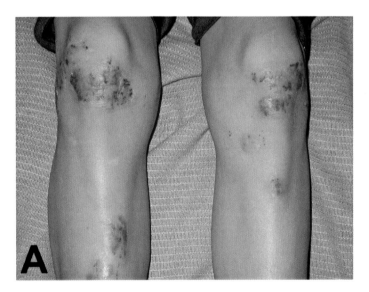

A

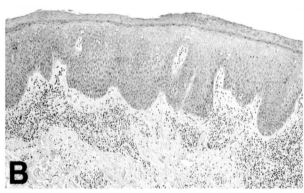

B

Color Plate 26.II (A) Psoriasiform dermatitis in a patient with IPEX due to an amino acid substitution in FOXP3 (Ala384Thr). Chronic scaly, erythematous plaques are present on the patient's legs. (B) A skin biopsy of a new skin lesion of the same patient shows irregular psoriasiform hyperplasia of the epidermis with overlying parakeratosis. Cell infiltrates consist mainly of T lymphocytes (CD8 > CD4) (hemotoxylin-eosin, ×10). (From Nieves et al., *Arch Dermatol* 140:466–472, 2004, with permission.)

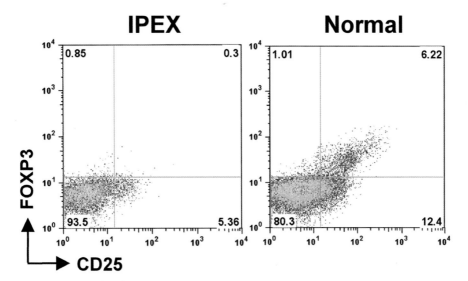

Color Plate 26.III Regulatory T cells (T regs) in human peripheral blood. Mononuclear cells were stained for CD4$^+$ and CD25$^+$, permeabilized incubated with anti-FOXP3 monoclonal antibody and submitted to flow cytometry. A small portion of CD4$^+$ and CD25$^{+ \text{(bright)}}$ normal T cells express FOXP3 (in this study 6.22%). This subset of CD4$^+$, CD25$^+$, FOXP3$^+$ cells are absent in the peripheral blood of a patient with IPEX.

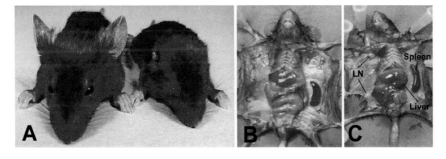

Color Plate 26-IV (A) Wild type (left) and scurfy (right) littermates, age 21 days. Note the small size of the scurfy mouse, the small and thickened ears, and the scaling of the feet. Compared to the wild type mouse (B), the scurfy mouse (C) has hepatosplenomegaly and enlarged lymph nodes (LN). Scurfy mice are deficient in FOXP3.

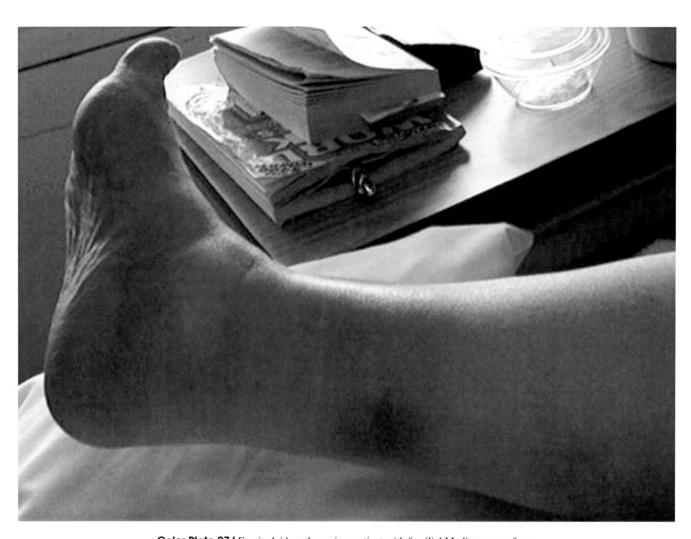

Color Plate 27.1 Erysipeloid erythema in a patient with familial Mediterranean fever.

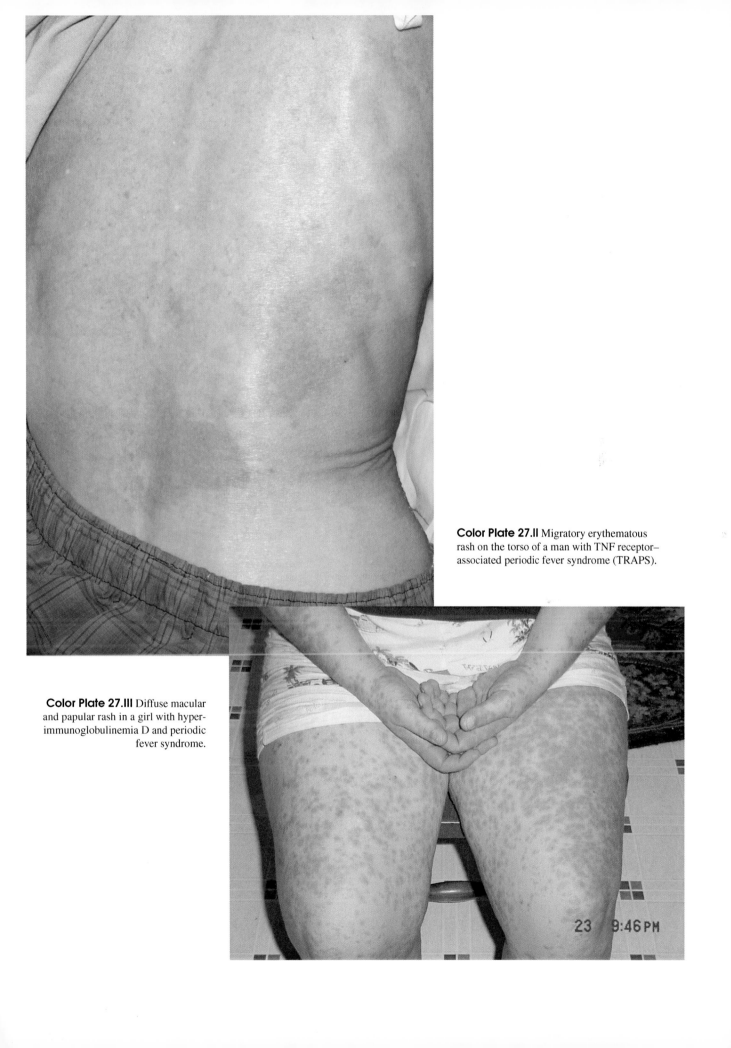

Color Plate 27.II Migratory erythematous rash on the torso of a man with TNF receptor–associated periodic fever syndrome (TRAPS).

Color Plate 27.III Diffuse macular and papular rash in a girl with hyper-immunoglobulinemia D and periodic fever syndrome.

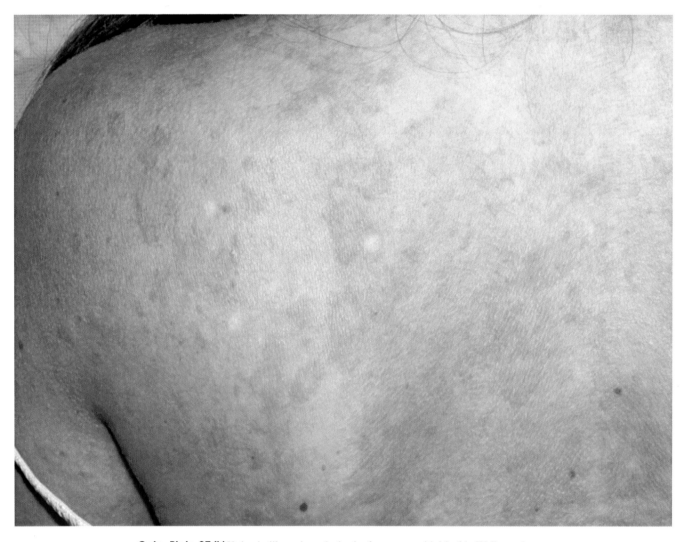

Color Plate 27.IV Urticaria-like rash on the back of a woman with Muckle-Wells syndrome.

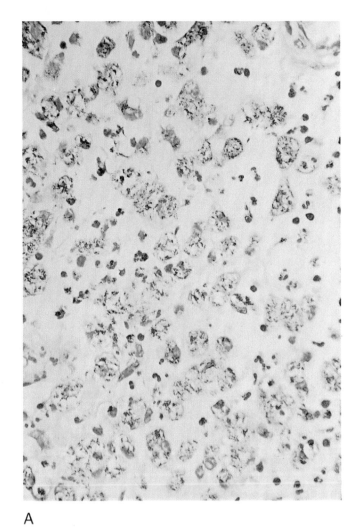

A

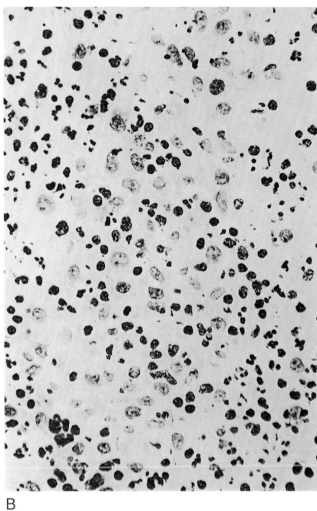

B

Color Plate 28.1 Ill-circumscribed and -differentiated mycobacterial granulomas in children with IFNγR1 deficiency. (A) Liver BCG granuloma in the 8-month-old Tunisian child with IFNγR1 deficiency. Macrophages are loaded with acid-fast bacilli (Ziehl ×400). (B) Liver *M. smegmatis* granuloma in the 4-year-old Italian child with IFNγR1 deficiency. No visible acid-fast bacilli (Ziehl ×400).

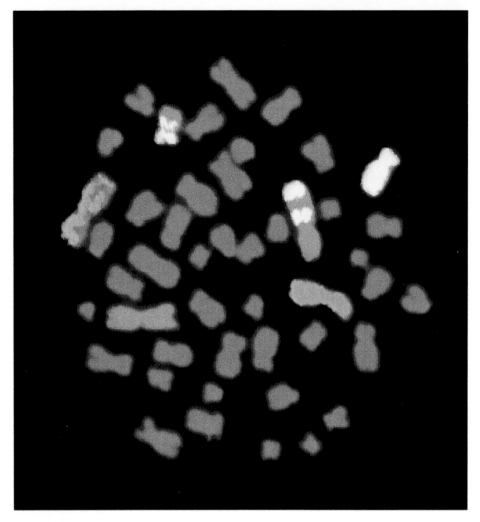

Color Plate 30.I Nijmegen breakage syndrome metaphase after three-color whole-chromosome painting. The cell was prepared 48 hours after exposure to 0.5 Gy. Red, whole-chromosome paint (WCP) 1; green, WCP 2; white, WCP 4. Note that insertion of chromatin from chromosome 4 (white) into chromosome 2 (red) could be made visible, which would escape detection by conventional Giemsa staining.

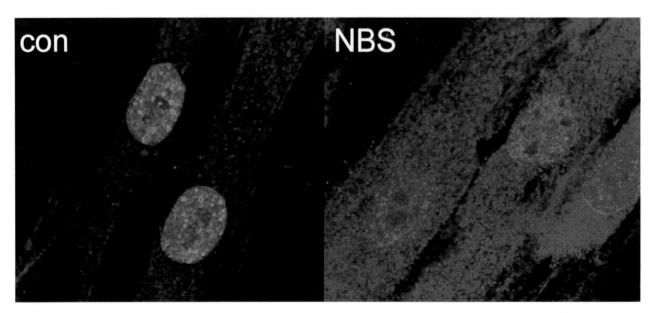

Color Plate 30.II Ionizing radiation-induced foci in primary fibroblasts detected by anti-MRE11. Control and Nijmegen breakage syndrome (NBS) cells were irradiated and subsequently fixed and stained for MRE11 (green). Cells were counterstained with the DNA stain TOTO3 (blue). Irradiated control (con) cells show discrete, bright green nuclear foci whereas NBS cells show diffuse cytoplasmic staining for MRE11.

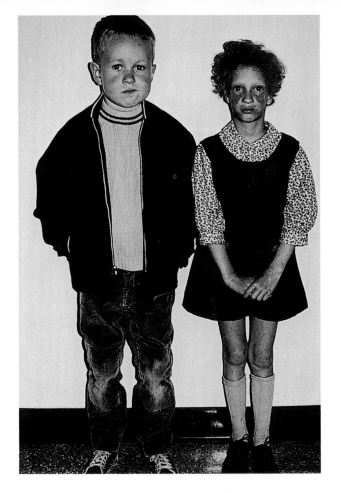

Color Plate 30.III A 7 1/2–year-old girl with Bloom syndrome, identified as 40(DoRoe) in the Bloom Syndrome Registry, standing beside a normal 6-year-old boy. 40(DoRoe) exhibits the characteristic short stature; a slightly disproportionately small head but otherwise normal body proportions; a paucity of subcutaneous adipose tissue; and a sun-sensitive, erythematous skin lesion affecting only the lips, the butterfly area of the face, and, minimally, the dorsa of the hands.

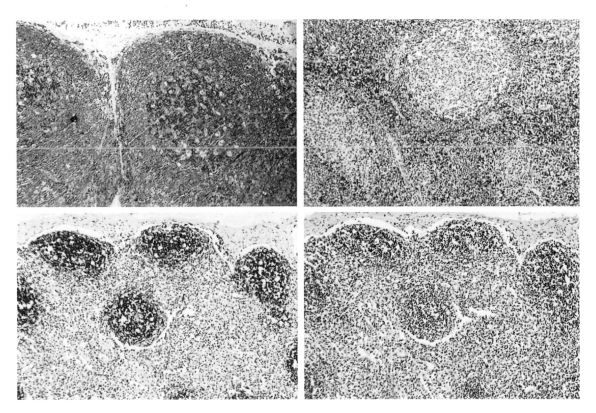

Color Plate 31.I Normal lymph node (top) and lymph node from a patient with the Wiskott-Aldrich syndrome (bottom). The left panels have been stained for B cells (in red). It can be seen that B cells are present in the poorly formed follicles of the WAS lymph node. The right panels have been stained for T cells (in red). The abundant numbers of T cells in the interfollicular area of the normal lymph node are sparse in the WAS lymph node (Perez-Atayde and Rosen, 1995).

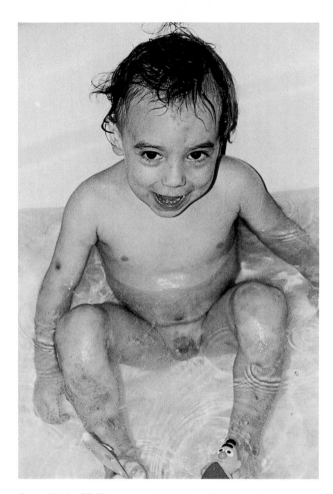

Color Plate 31.II Two-year-old Wiskott-Aldrich syndrome patient with a clinical score of 3. Note bruises and eczema of hands and legs.

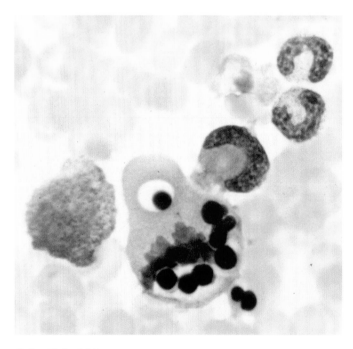

Color Plate 32.I Bone marrow aspirate from a 6-year-old boy with X-linked lymphoproliferative disease (XLP) who suffered from virus-associated hemophagocytic syndrome (VAHS). The figure shows an activated marrow histiocyte with erythrophagocytosis.

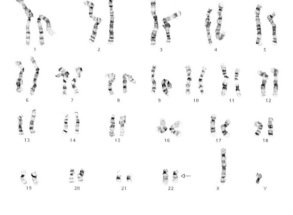

Color Plate 33.I Heterozygous deletion of chromosome 22q11 in DiGeorge syndrome. G-banded karyotype with visible shortening of 22q (arrow).

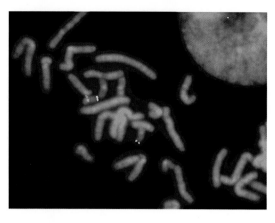

Color Plate 33.II Heterozygous deletion of chromosome 22q11in DiGeorge syndrome. Fluorescence in situ hybridization (FISH) of DiGeorge metaphase chromosomes with control probe (green signals) identifying both homologs of chromosome 22; TUPLE1 probe (red signal) was deleted from one homolog.

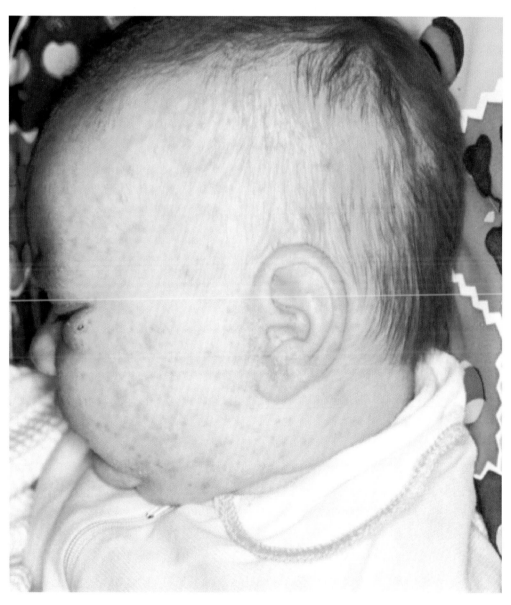

Color Plate 34.I Newborn rash of hyper-IgE syndrome (Job syndrome).

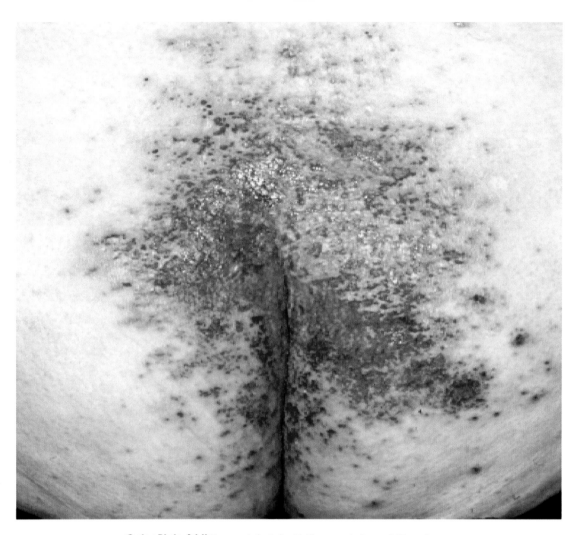

Color Plate 34.II Eczema infected with *S. aureus* in hyper-IgE syndrome.

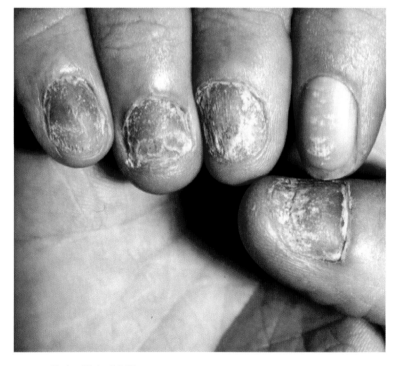

Color Plate 34.III Candida onychomycosis in hyper-IgE syndrome.

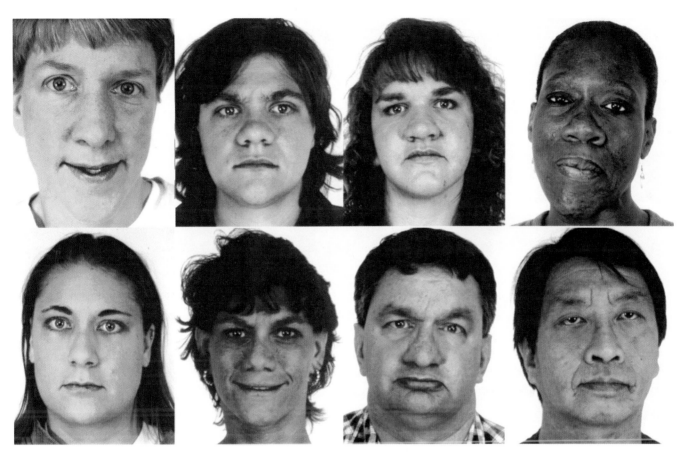

Color Plate 34.IV Characteristic facies of hyper-IgE syndrome. Note the mild facial asymmetry, prominent jaw, and wide nasal alae. (By permission, *New England Journal of Medicine*.)

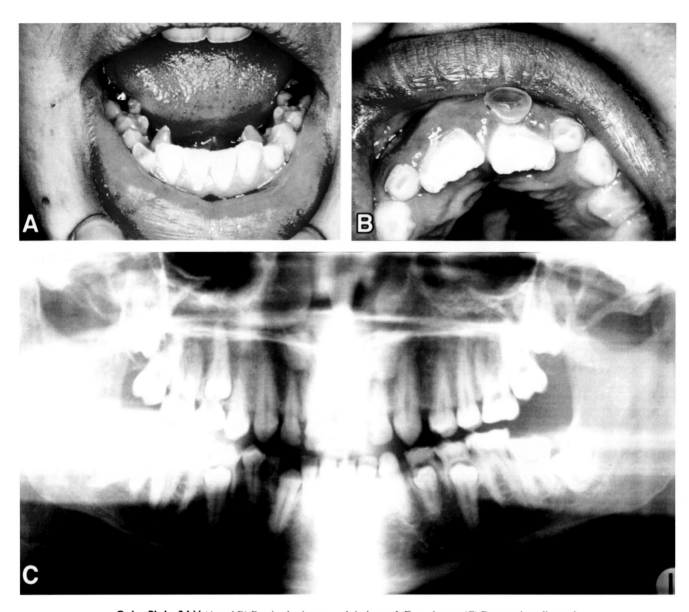

Color Plate 34.V (A and B) Retained primary teeth in hyper-IgE syndrome. (C) Panoramic radiograph of the teeth showing numerous retained primary teeth with secondary teeth unable to erupt.

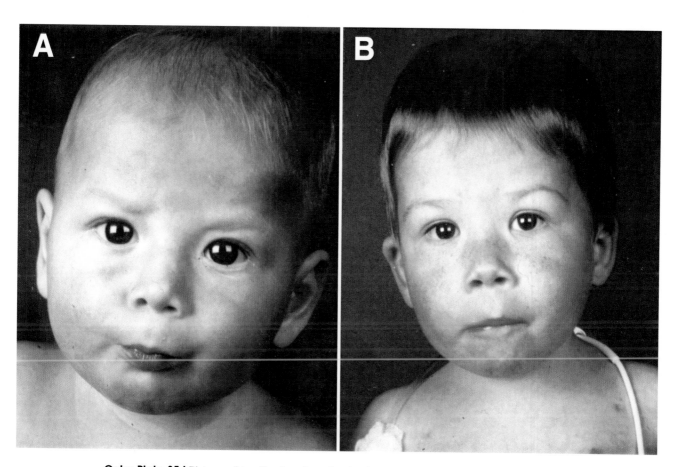

Color Plate 35.1 Pictures of two Dutch patients (brothers) with immunodeficiency with centromere instability and facial anomalies (ICF) syndrome. (A) Patient 2 (at age 1 year); (B) Patient 1 (at age 4–5 years) (Wijmenga et al., 1998).

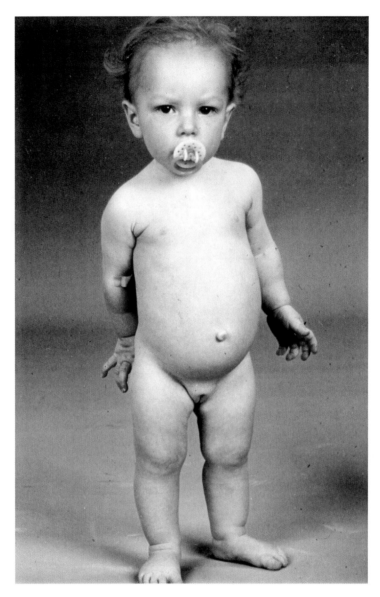

Color Plate 36.1 A 3-year-old girl with cartilage hair hypoplasia (CHH). Note the short-limbed, short stature (height, 74 cm, or −6 SD), sparse and thin hair, and bulging abdomen. She had exceptionally severe, hemorrhagic varicella at 2 years of age.

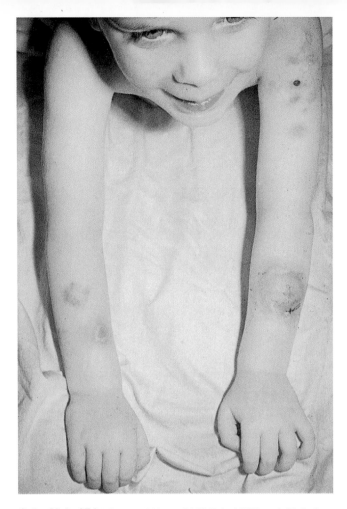

Color Plate 37.1 A 3-year-old boy with X-linked CGD and skin lesions caused by *Serratia marcescens*.

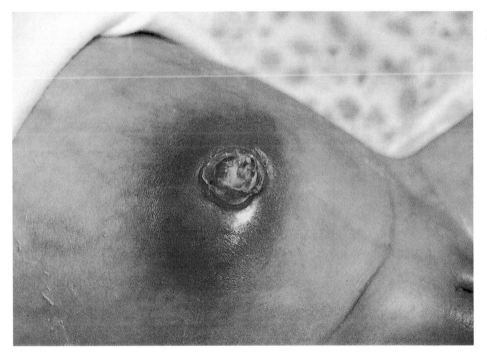

Color Plate 38.1 Omphalitis in a child with the severe phenotype of leukocyte adhesion deficiency (LAD I).

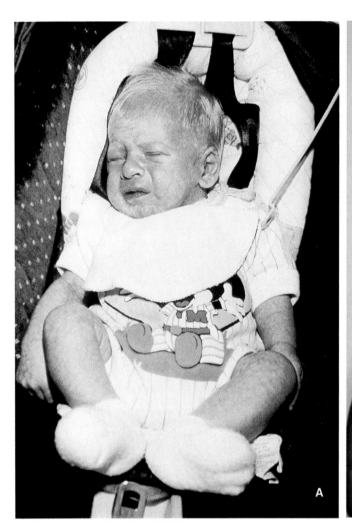

Color Plate 40.1 Two patients with Chediak-Higashi syndrome (CHS). (A) Caucasian patient; note severe hypopigmentation typical of oculocutaneous albinism and unusual silvery hair color characteristic of CHS.

(B) Japanese patient; note mild hypopigmentation, principally evident on the trunk.

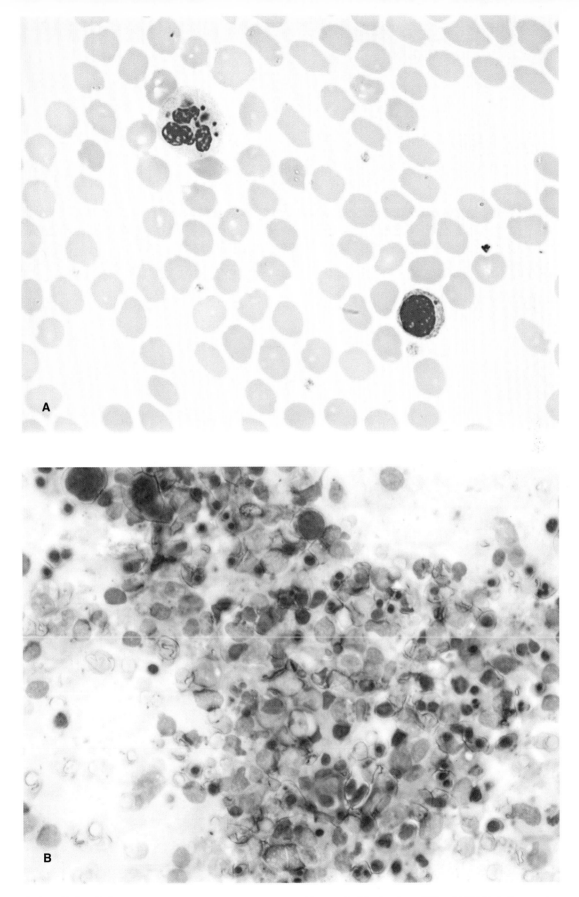

Color Plate 40.II Micrographic findings in Chediak-Higashi syndrome (CHS). (A) Peripheral blood smear from a patient with CHS. Note giant cytoplasmic inclusions in neutrophil, lymphocyte, and platelets. (B) Bone marrow biopsy of original patient of Higashi (1954) during accelerated phase. Note dense lymphohistiocytic infilitrate with erythrophagocytosis. (Original pathologic slide from 1950, courtesy of Ototaka Higashi, M.D.)

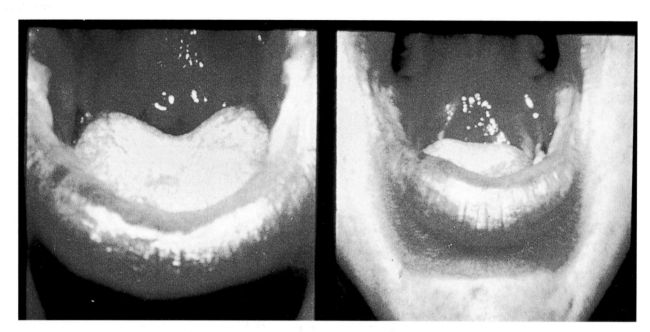

Color Plate 42.1 Hereditary angioedema in a patient with C1-inhibitor deficiency. C1-inhibitor deficiency results in the loss of regulation of macromolecular C1 function and normal kinin generation. Minor triggers activate the complement system and result in angioedema. The left panel demonstrates oropharyngeal involvement in a patient with C1-inhibitor deficiency. The right panel demonstrates return of normal anatomy after the episode. (Courtesy of Albert Sheffer, M.D.)

27

Periodic Fever Syndromes

DANIEL L. KASTNER, SUSANNAH BRYDGES, and KEITH M. HULL

The periodic fever syndromes are a heterogeneous group of inherited disorders characterized by recurrent episodes of fever and localized inflammation, most commonly affecting the serosal membranes, joints, and skin (Table 27.1). A significant minority of patients develop systemic deposition of amyloid A protein (AA amyloidosis) as a longer-term consequence of their inflammatory episodes. While at first glance these disorders appear to be similar to the more commonly recognized autoimmune disorders (e.g., systemic lupus erythematosus), they differ in several important respects, including the lack of high-titer autoantibodies or antigen-specific T cells, and the predominance of monocytes and neutrophils rather than lymphocytes as effector cells. Hence, the term *autoinflammatory disorders* has been proposed to describe the periodic fevers and related conditions (McDermott et al., 1999; Galon et al., 2000; Hull et al., 2003).

Advances in the past several years have significantly increased our understanding of these disorders, with four genes underlying six clinically distinct periodic fever syndromes having been identified. In 1997 a novel gene causing perhaps the most common of these illnesses, the recessively inherited familial Mediterranean fever (FMF; Mendelian Inheritance in Man [MIM] 249100), was identified by positional cloning (French FMF Consortium, 1997; International FMF Consortium, 1997). Within 2 years, mutations in the 55 kDa tumor necrosis factor (TNF) receptor were found in a group of patients with dominantly inherited periodic fever (the TNF receptor–associated periodic syndrome [TRAPS]; MIM 142680) (McDermott et al., 1999), and mutations in the mevalonate kinase gene (*MVK*) were identified in the recessively inherited hyperimmunoglobulinemia-D with periodic fever syndrome (HIDS; MIM 260920) (Drenth et al., 1999; Houten et al., 1999). A fourth periodic fever gene, which shares a functional domain with the FMF gene, was discovered by positional cloning in 2001 (Hoffman et al., 2001a). Mutations in this gene

were first shown to cause two dominantly inherited conditions, Muckle-Wells syndrome (MWS; MIM 191100) and familial cold autoinflammatory syndrome (FCAS; MIM 120100). The following year mutations in the same gene were discovered in patients with yet another recurrent fever disorder, neonatal-onset multisystem inflammatory disease (NOMID, also called chronic infantile neurologic cutaneous articular [CINCA] syndrome; MIM 607115) (Aksentijevich et al., 2002; Feldmann et al., 2002).

Although the precise mechanism by which mutations in each of these genes causes recurrent fever and inflammation is still under investigation, the available molecular genetic data suggest that the recurrent fever syndromes represent deficiencies in the regulation of innate immunity. There is an emerging body of data indicating that both pyrin, the FMF protein, and cryopyrin, the protein mutated in FCAS, MWS, and NOMID/CINCA, are regulators of interleukin (IL)-1β production, nuclear factor (NF)-κB activation, and leukocyte apoptosis, all critical components of innate immunity. Similarly, the mutations in the extracellular domain of the p55 TNF receptor lead to increased TNF signaling, due in part to a failure in TNF receptor ectodomain cleavage. And although mutations in mevalonate kinase, a key enzyme in cholesterol biosynthesis, were quite unexpected in HIDS, new data suggest a nexus between the mevalonate pathway and IL-1β regulation. The periodic fever syndromes thus represent yet another example of how Mendelian disorders can inform our understanding of normal immune function.

Familial Mediterranean Fever

Although molecular genetic data suggest that founder mutations causing FMF (MIM 249100) arose many centuries ago (International FMF Consortium, 1997), the first recognizable report of

Table 27.1. Characteristics of Periodic Fever Syndromes

	FMF	TRAPS	HIDS	FCAS	MWS	NOMID
Inheritance	Recessive	Dominant	Recessive	Dominant	Dominant	Dominant, de novo
Ethnicity	Turkish, Armenian, Arab, Jewish, Italian, Greek, other	Any ethnicity	Dutch, French, other European	Mostly European	Mostly European	Any ethnicity
Duration of attacks	12–72 hours	>7 days	3–7 days	12–24 hours	2–3 days	Continuous
Cutaneous	Erysipeloid erythematous rash on lower leg, ankle, foot	Migratory rash, often associated with underlying myalgia	Maculopapular rash on trunk and limbs, urticaria	Urticaria-like rash induced by cold temperatures	Urticaria-like rash	Urticaria-like rash
Abdominal	Sterile peritonitis, constipation	Peritonitis, diarrhea or constipation	Severe pain, vomiting, diarrhea, rarely peritonitis	Nausea	Abdominal pain	Not common
Pleural	Common	Common	Rare	Not seen	Rare	Rare
Arthropathy	Monoarthritis, occasionally protracted arthritis in knee or hip	Arthritis in large joints, arthralgia	Arthralgia, symmetric polyarthritis	Polyarthralgia	Polyarthralgia, oligoarthritis	Epiphyseal overgrowth, contractures, intermittent or chronic arthritis
Ocular	Rare	Conjunctivitis, periorbital edema	Uncommon	Conjunctivitis	Conjunctivitis, episcleritis	Uveitis, conjunctivitis, progressive vision loss
Neurologic	Rare	Rare	Headache	Headache	Sensorineural deafness	Sensorineural deafness, chronic aseptic meningitis, mental retardation, headache
Lymph/spleen	Splenomegaly more common than lymphadenopathy	Splenomegaly more common than adenopathy	Cervical adenopathy	Not seen	Rare	Hepatosplenomegaly, adenopathy
Vasculitis	Henoch-Schönlein purpura, polyarteritis nodosa	Henoch-Schönlein purpura, lymphocytic vasculitis	Cutaneous vasculitis common, rarely Henoch-Schönlein purpura	Not seen	Not seen	Occasional
Amyloidosis	Risk depends on *MEFV* and *SAA* genotypes, other factors	Occurs in ~10%	Case reports	Rare	Occurs in ~25%	May develop in a portion of patients reaching adulthood
Treatment	Colchicine	Etanercept, NSAIDs, steroids	Etanercept investigational, NSAIDs, steroids	Anakinra investigational, NSAIDs	Anakinra investigational, NSAIDs, prednisone	Anakinra investigational

FCAS, familial cold autoinflammatory syndrome; FMF, familial Mediterranean fever; HIDS, hyperimmunoglobulinemia-D with periodic fever syndrome; MWS, Muckle-Wells syndrome; NOMID, neonatal-onset multisystem inflammatory disease; NSAIDs, nonsteroidal anti-inflammatory drugs; TRAPS, TNF receptor-associated periodic syndrome.

a case of FMF was published in 1908 (Janeway and Mosenthal, 1908), and the first series of 10 cases of "benign paroxysmal peritonitis" was published in 1945 (Siegal, 1945). Subsequent descriptions of large numbers of North African and Iraqi Jewish cases in the newly formed state of Israel led to the proposal of the now widely accepted *familial Mediterranean fever* nomenclature (Heller et al., 1958; Sohar et al., 1967), although it should be noted that other names, such as *recurrent polyserositis, recurrent hereditary polyserositis,* and *periodic disease,* are sometimes used.

During the 1960s and 1970s, studies of FMF focused on the clinical phenotype, mode of inheritance, ethnic distribution, and treatment. Several large series, particularly from Israel (Sohar et al., 1967), described in detail the serosal, synovial, and cutaneous manifestations of FMF, and elucidated the connection between FMF and systemic AA amyloidosis. Although high carrier frequencies gave rise to pseudodominance, careful segregation analysis indicated that FMF is recessively inherited, with incomplete penetrance (Sohar et al., 1962, 1967). The preponderance of cases reported were of non-Ashkenazi Jewish, Armenian, Arab, and Turkish origin. Later epidemiologic and family-based studies among non-Ashkenazi Jews and Armenians demonstrated extremely high frequencies of FMF (Rogers et al., 1989; Yuval et al., 1995), suggesting a possible heterozygote advantage, and identified ethnic differences in the susceptibility to amyloidosis (Meyerhoff, 1980; Pras et al., 1982). Finally, the early 1970s saw the serendipitous discovery of colchicine as an effective prophylaxis for the inflammatory attacks of FMF (Goldfinger, 1972; Dinarello et al., 1974; Goldstein and Schwabe, 1974; Zemer et al., 1974). Ten years later colchicine was also established as effective in preventing the amyloidosis of FMF (Zemer et al., 1986).

Further advances in the understanding of FMF awaited the development of positional cloning techniques and the infrastructure of the Human Genome Project. In 1992 the FMF locus, *MEFV*, was mapped to chromosome 16p13 (Pras et al., 1992), and 5 years later two groups independently identified disease-associated missense mutations in a novel positional candidate gene (French FMF Consortium, 1997; International FMF Consortium, 1997), the protein product of which was termed *pyrin* or *marenostrin* by the respective consortia (and for simplicity will be denoted as *pyrin* in these pages). Availability of genetic testing has broadened the clinical and ethnic/geographic spectrum of FMF, while studies of pyrin have shed new light on the regulation of cytokine production, NF-κB activation, and apoptosis, and have defined a functional domain present in over 20 human proteins involved in the regulation of inflammation.

Clinical and Pathological Manifestations

This disorder is characterized by relatively discrete, usually 1- to 3-day episodes of fever with serositis, synovitis, or skin rash. In some patients attacks begin in infancy or very early childhood, and 80%–90% of patients experience their first episode by age 20. Young children sometimes present with fever alone. The frequency of FMF attacks is highly variable, both among patients and for any given patient, with the interval between attacks ranging from days to years. Moreover, the type of attack (abdominal, pleural, arthritic) may also vary over time. Some patients relate attacks to physical or emotional stress, although in many cases there is no obvious provocative event. There is a slight predominance of males in most series, possibly the result of underreporting in women for social reasons or underrecognition because of confounding gynecologic diagnoses. In some women attacks may occur at a specific point in the menstrual cycle (Ben-Chetrit and Ben-Chetrit, 2001) and sometimes remit during pregnancy (Sohar et al., 1967; Schwabe and Peters, 1974).

Attacks of fever and abdominal pain occur at some time in nearly all FMF patients, and range from a dull, aching pain to full-blown peritonitis. Constipation is usual during the attacks, sometimes with a diarrheal stool at the very end of the episode. Plain films may demonstrate air-fluid levels, and computed tomography (CT) may show thickened mesenteric folds, lymphadenopathy, splenomegaly, or mild ascites (Zissin et al., 2003). On laparoscopy there may be a neutrophil-rich exudate. Repeated episodes may lead to peritoneal adhesions.

Pleurisy may occur alone with fever or concurrently with abdominal pain. Pleuritic episodes are usually unilateral, with sharp, stabbing chest pain and, in some cases, diaphragmatic pain referred to the ipsilateral shoulder. Radiographic findings may include atelectasis (Brauman and Gilboa, 1987) due to splinting and, in a minority of cases, pleural effusion. Thoracentesis, when performed, yields a neutrophil-laden exudate. Pleural thickening sometimes develops after multiple attacks (Livneh et al., 1999).

Other forms of serosal inflammation may also be seen in FMF. Nonuremic pericarditis is much less common than peritoneal or pleural involvement (Kees et al., 1997; Tutar et al., 2003; Turkish FMF Study Group, 2005). Although small subclinical effusions are more frequent than symptomatic pericarditis, there have been rare reports of tamponade (Zimand et al., 1994). Unilateral acute scrotum occurs in about 5% of prepubertal boys with FMF (Livneh et al., 1994a; Majeed et al., 2000b), resulting from inflammation of the tunica vaginalis, an embryologic remnant of the peritoneal membrane.

Joint involvement in FMF is particularly common among North African Jews (Pras et al., 1998; Brik et al., 2001), and has been related to the M694V homozygous genotype (Brik et al., 1999; Cazeneuve et al., 1999; Gershoni-Baruch et al., 2002), which is very frequent in this population. Acute monoarticular arthritis is most characteristic in FMF (Heller et al., 1966), often affecting the knee, ankle, or hip. Such attacks tend to last somewhat longer than serosal episodes (often about 1 week), sometimes with large effusions, extreme pain, and inability to bear weight. Synovial fluid often appears septic, with as many as 100,000 polymorphonuclear leuckocytes/mm^3, but cultures are sterile. Soft tissue swelling may be apparent on X-rays taken during attacks, but erosive changes do not develop. A number of other less common oligo- or polyarticular patterns of arthritis may occur, especially in children (Majeed and Rawashdeh, 1997; Ince et al., 2002). Arthralgia is also very common in FMF.

In the precolchicine era, about 5% of patients with acute monoarticular arthritis went on to develop protracted arthritis, usually affecting the hip (Sneh et al., 1977). In such cases, symptoms could last for several months, sometimes leading to secondary osteoarthritic radiographic changes and/or osteonecrosis, and requiring total hip replacement surgery. Chronic sacroiliitis may also occur in FMF, regardless of the HLA-B27 status or colchicine therapy (Brodey and Wolff, 1975; Lehman et al., 1978; Langevitz et al., 1997).

The most characteristic cutaneous lesion of FMF is erysipeloid erythema (Color Plate 27.I), a sharply demarcated, erythematous, warm, tender, swollen area 10–15 cm in diameter occurring unilaterally or bilaterally, usually on the dorsum of the foot, ankle, or lower leg (Azizi and Fisher, 1976; Barzilai et al., 2000). On skin biopsy, there is a mixed perivascular infiltrate of polymorphonuclear leukocytes, histiocytes, and lymphocytes. As is the case for arthritis, the frequency of erysipeloid erythema may be increased among M694V homozygotes (Koné Paut et al., 2000).

Children with FMF frequently develop myalgia of the legs related to vigorous exertion (Majeed et al., 2000a). Much less commonly, FMF patients may experience attacks of febrile myalgia, with excruciating muscle pain unrelated to exertion, that can last from a few days to several weeks (Langevitz et al., 1994; Sidi et al., 2000). During these episodes the creatine kinase is normal, the erythrocyte sedimentation rate (ESR) is prolonged, and the electromyogram shows nonspecific myopathic changes. Histologic data suggest that febrile myalgia is a form of vasculitis. Other forms of vasculitis, including Henoch-Schönlein purpura and polyarteritis nodosum, are also seen at increased frequency in FMF (Gedalia et al., 1992; Rawashdeh and Majeed, 1996; Özdogan et al., 1997; Tinaztepe et al., 1997; Ozen, 1999; Tekin et al., 1999; Ozen et al., 2001; Turkish FMF Study Group, 2005).

Systemic amyloidosis develops in a subset of FMF patients, as a result of deposition of a fragment of serum amyloid A (SAA) in the kidneys, adrenals, intestine, spleen, lung, and testes (Sohar et al., 1967). SAA is an acute-phase reactant produced by the liver and found at high levels in the serum during FMF attacks. Patients with amyloid deposition in the kidneys progress from albuminuria to the nephrotic syndrome to renal failure, usually over the course of 3 to 5 years. Amyloid deposits in the gastrointestinal tract may cause malabsorption (Mor et al., 2003), and deposits in the testis may cause azoospermia and infertility (Ben-Chetrit et al., 1998). Cardiac involvement, neuropathy, and arthropathy are very uncommon with the amyloidosis of FMF. The diagnosis is usually established by renal or rectal biopsy.

The amyloidosis of FMF usually occurs after the onset of inflammatory attacks (phenotype I), but rarely can occur as the first manifestation of FMF (phenotype II) (Sohar et al., 1967; Turkish FMF Study Group, 2005), perhaps from subclinical elevations in the SAA. The overall risk of amyloidosis in FMF is the product of a complex interaction of factors. Prior to the cloning of *MEFV*, epidemiologic data indicated that among Jewish subpopulations, the risk was highest for North African Jews, intermediate for Iraqi Jews, and very low for Ashkenazi Jews (Pras et al., 1982). This gradient has subsequently been found to parallel the frequency of the M694V/M694V genotype, which in most studies is associated with an increased risk of amyloidosis (Brik et al., 1999; Cazeneuve et al., 1999; Mansour et al., 2001; Gershoni-Baruch et al., 2002, 2003; Majeed et al., 2002), although not in a large recent series from Turkey (Turkish FMF Study Group, 2005). Other risk factors for amyloidosis include male gender, the SAA1 α/α genotype, a positive family history for amyloidosis, and colchicine noncompliance (Cazeneuve et al., 2000; Akar et al., 2003; Gershoni-Baruch et al., 2003; Turkish FMF Study Group, 2005). There are also geographic and secular effects on amyloid susceptibility, perhaps reflecting improvements in general medical care that may modify the SAA load from intercurrent illness.

Laboratory Findings

During acute attacks of FMF, there is a leukocytosis, often with a left shift, an accelerated ESR, and increases in several serum acute-phase proteins, including SAA, C-reactive protein (CRP), fibrinogen, haptoglobin, and the C3 and C4 complement components. Urinalysis may demonstrate albuminuria and microscopic hematuria during attacks.

During the intercritical period, the white count and acute-phase reactants may normalize, but in some patients there is biochemical evidence of persistent subclinical inflammation, including abnormalities of the ESR, SAA, CRP, and fibrinogen (Tunca et al., 1999; Korkmaz et al., 2002; Duzova et al., 2003). Patients may also have a mild anemia of chronic disease and modest elevations in the serum immunoglobulins between attacks (Eliakim et al., 1981). A minority of patients have an increased serum IgD, although usually not to the level seen in HIDS (Medlej-Hashim et al., 2001).

A number of laboratory abnormalities are associated with the amyloidosis of FMF. The earliest finding is isolated albuminuria, without hematuria, with a normal or only slightly depressed serum albumin and normal renal function. As proteinuria increases, the serum albumin begins to fall, and renal function deteriorates over approximately 3 to 5 years to the point of renal failure. During this period laboratory findings of uremia evolve, including hyperphosphatemia, acidosis, hyperkalemia, and anemia.

Molecular Basis of Familial Mediterranean Fever: The Disease Gene, *MEFV*

The gene mutated in FMF, *MEFV*, is comprised of 10 exons, oriented $5' \to 3'$ centromere to telomere over an approximately 15 kb genomic interval on chromosome 16p13.3 (International FMF Consortium, 1997). *MEFV* encodes an ~3.7 kb transcript with a 781–amino acid open reading frame that is expressed in granulocytes, cytokine-activated monocytes, and synovial and peritoneal fibroblasts (Centola et al., 2000; Matzner et al., 2000; Papin et al., 2003; Diaz et al., 2004). Initial computational analysis of the conceptual protein identified a cassette comprising a B-box zinc finger (residues 375–407), an α-helical coiled-coil domain (residues 408–594), and a B30.2 domain (residues 598–774), all of which have been implicated in protein–protein interactions. Although not apparent at the time the gene was cloned, exon 1 encodes a 92–amino acid motif now called the *PYRIN domain* that facilitates homotypic interactions among proteins involved in the regulation of inflammation and apoptosis (Bertin and DiStefano, 2000; Inohara and Nuñez, 2000; Martinon et al., 2001; Pawlowski et al., 2001; Richards et al., 2001; Staub et al., 2001; Girardin et al., 2003).

Four single nucleotide substitutions in FMF patients were initially identified in exon 10, resulting in conservative missense mutations clustered in a 47–amino acid interval in the C-terminal B30.2 domain (French FMF Consortium, 1997; International FMF Consortium, 1997). One leads to the substitution of isoleucine for methionine at residue 680 (M680I), two others lead to the substitution of valine or isoleucine for methionine at residue 694 (M694V, M694I), and the fourth causes the substitution of alanine for valine at residue 726 (V726A). For each of the M680I, M694V, and V726A mutations, microsatellite and single nucleotide polymorphism haplotype analysis disclosed ancestral relationships among carrier chromosomes in populations that have been separated for centuries.

At the time of this writing, a total of 35 disease-associated *MEFV* mutations have been published (Fig. 27.1), and a substantial number of others have been directly communicated to a database available on the World Wide Web at http://fmf.igh.cnrs.fr/infevers/. Of the 35 published mutations, 30 are missense single amino acid substitutions, 2 are in-frame deletions, and 1 is an

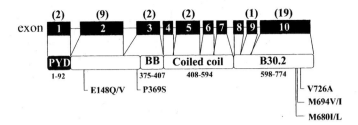

Figure 27.1. Schematic of *MEFV* gene and the encoded protein, pyrin (marenostrin). The number of published mutations for each exon is indicated in parentheses above the schematic. Protein domains are indicated: PYD, PYRIN domain; BB, B-box zinc finger. The amino acid residue range for each domain is indicated below the schematic. Mutational hot spots and mutations noted in the text are also shown.

in-frame insertion. Only 2 of the 35 mutations, a frameshift in exon 2 and a nonsense mutation in exon 10, would truncate the pyrin protein. Nineteen of the mutations (54%) are in exon 10, encoding the B30.2 domain, and there are two "hot spots" (M680 and M694) in exon 10 with more than one known mutation. The second major cluster of mutations is in exon 2, where there are nine mutations (26% of the total), and there is a mutational hot spot at E148.

Function of Pyrin, the *MEFV* Gene Product

Recent work on the function of pyrin, the *MEFV* gene product, has focused on interactions mediated by the N-terminal 92–amino acid domain encoded by exon 1. This motif, which has variously been denoted the *PYRIN domain* (Bertin and DiStefano, 2000), *PYD* (Martinon et al., 2001), *PAAD* (Pawlowski et al., 2001), or *DAPIN* (Staub et al., 2001), has now been recognized in a total of over 20 human proteins involved in the regulation of inflammation and apoptosis (Harton et al., 2002; Tschopp et al., 2003). Computational modeling and subsequent NMR spectroscopy have demonstrated that the PYRIN domain is the fourth member of the death domain–fold superfamily (Fairbrother et al., 2001; Richards et al., 2001; Eliezer, 2003; Hiller et al., 2003; Liepinsh et al., 2003; Liu et al., 2003), which also includes death domains, death effector domains, and caspase-recruitment domains (CARDs). All four assume a six α-helix three-dimensional structure that facilitates homotypic interactions through electrostatic charge interactions. Thus, the PYRIN domain of pyrin is a docking motif that facilitates cognate interactions with other PYRIN domain proteins.

The PYRIN domain of pyrin interacts specifically with the homologous domain of a protein called *ASC* (apoptosis-associated specklike protein with a CARD), a bipartite adaptor consisting solely of an N-terminal PYRIN domain and a C-terminal CARD in tandem (Masumoto et al., 1999, 2003; Richards et al., 2001; Chae et al., 2003; Dowds et al., 2003). Through its CARD, ASC binds caspase-1 (also known as *IL-1β converting enzyme* [ICE]) and other adaptor proteins, leading to the cleavage of caspase-1 into enzymatically active p20 and p10 subunits (Martinon et al., 2002; Srinivasula et al., 2002; Wang et al., 2002; Chae et al., 2003; Stehlik et al., 2003; Agostini et al., 2004; Martinon and Tschopp, 2004). Activated caspase-1, in turn, cleaves IL-1β from its 31 kDa precursor form to its 17 kDa biologically active fragment, which is a potent mediator of fever and inflammation. Data from mice expressing a hypomorphic pyrin mutant indicate that wild-type pyrin plays an important role in regulating the ASC-ICE-IL-1β cascade (Chae et al., 2003).

Although less completely understood, the interaction of pyrin with ASC also appears to regulate leukocyte apoptosis. Peritoneal macrophages from the pyrin-deficient mice exhibit a defect in apoptosis through a caspase-8-dependent, IL-1β-independent pathway, suggesting a role for wild-type pyrin in limiting the duration of the innate immune response through cell death (Chae et al., 2003). Nevertheless, underscoring the complexity of the process, in certain transfection systems wild-type pyrin exerts an antiapoptotic effect (Richards et al., 2001; Dowds et al., 2003; Masumoto et al., 2003).

Finally, again mediated through its interactions with ASC, pyrin modulates NF-κB activation, another important component of the innate immune response. ASC has been shown to bind to components of the IκB kinase complex, which regulates NF-κB through the phosphorylation of IκB (Stehlik et al., 2002). Depending on the cellular context, cotransfection of wild-type pyrin with ASC may potentiate or suppress NF-κB activation (Stehlik et al., 2002; Dowds et al., 2003; Masumoto et al., 2003).

While the interaction of the N-terminal domain of pyrin with ASC sheds new light on the regulation of inflammation, it does not yet explain the molecular mechanism by which missense mutations in pyrin, many of which are at the C-terminal end of the protein, lead to autoinflammatory disease. Possibly, these mutations indirectly influence the effect of pyrin on IL-1β processing, apoptosis, and/or NF-κB activation, perhaps conferring a selective advantage by pushing the balance, under some circumstances, toward heightened innate immunity.

Mutation Analysis

Prior to the identification of *MEFV*, FMF was thought to be primarily a disease of non-Ashkenazi Jews, Armenians, Arabs, and Turks. Availability of genetic testing has allowed unequivocal identification of numerous cases among several additional populations with Mediterranean roots, including Ashkenazi Jews (Samuels et al., 1998; Aksentijevich et al., 1999; Stoffman et al., 2000; Gershoni-Baruch et al., 2001; Kogan et al., 2001), Italians (Samuels et al., 1998; Aksentijevich et al., 1999; La Regina et al., 2003), Greeks (Konstantopoulos et al., 2003), Spaniards (Touitou, 2001), and Cypriots (Deltas et al., 2002), and of occasional cases in a broad range of other ethnicities (Dodé et al., 2000b; Touitou, 2001). In some of these newly recognized patients, the clinical phenotype is milder than that usually seen in the classically affected ethnic groups, perhaps owing to documented differences in the population distribution of specific *MEFV* mutations.

Direct screening for mutations has confirmed previous estimates of extraordinarily high carrier frequencies in several ethnic groups. Carrier frequencies of at least 20% have now been established among North African, Iraqi, and Ashkenazi Jews, Arabs, Turks, and Armenians (Stoffman et al., 2000; Gershoni-Baruch et al., 2001; Kogan et al., 2001; Yilmaz et al., 2001). Assuming complete penetrance, these data would predict a disease frequency of at least 1% among these populations. Since these figures overestimate the disease frequencies, where they are known, by at least a factor of 2 (Yuval et al., 1995; Ozen et al., 1998), it is likely that there are substantial numbers of individuals with two *MEFV* mutations but minimal symptoms. Recent family studies support this assertion (Tunca et al., 2002), but contrast with the almost absolute association of *MEFV* genotype with disease in the families analyzed in positional cloning studies. This discrepancy is most likely explained by the fact that the earlier families were chosen for disease severity and for sibships with multiple affected individuals, both factors that would favor the cosegregation of modifier alleles tending to increase the penetrance of *MEFV* mutations.

As noted above, over half of the known mutations in *MEFV* are located in exon 10, which encodes the C-terminal B30.2 domain of pyrin. When the frequencies of the various mutations among patients are taken into account, the bias toward exon 10 becomes much stronger (Touitou, 2001). Among certain populations, such as Ashkenazi Jews, E148Q (exon 2) and P369S (exon 3) are also observed at a relatively high frequency (Aksentijevich et al., 1999). For this reason, many commercial and academic laboratories screen for FMF by sequencing exon 10 and performing mutation-specific tests, such as restriction endonuclease assays, for E148Q and P369S. The diagnostic yield of this approach is comparable to that obtained with a more systematic mutational screen of the entire coding region by denaturing gradient gel electrophoresis (Cazeneuve et al., 2003).

FMF patients homozygous for the E148Q mutation alone are much less common than would be predicted on the basis of the observed frequency of this mutation (Ben-Chetrit et al., 2000; Ozen et al., 2002; Tchernitchko et al., 2003). Nevertheless, E148Q is frequently the only identifiable mutation in *trans* with an exon 10 mutation in patients with moderate to severe disease, indicating that this variant is more than a benign polymorphism (Samuels et al., 1998; Aksentijevich et al., 1999; Akar et al., 2001; Ben-Chetrit and Backenroth, 2001). At the other end of the genotype–phenotype spectrum is M694V. Studies of Jewish, Arab, and Armenian patients indicate that M694V homozygotes are at increased risk of amyloidosis (Brik et al., 1999; Cazeneuve et al., 1999; Mansour et al., 2001; Gershoni-Baruch et al., 2002, 2003; Majeed et al., 2002), although this appears not to be the case among Turks (Turkish FMF Study Group, 2005). As noted previously, M694V homozygotes may also be at increased risk for arthritis and erysipeloid erythema, as well as for an early age of onset and frequent attacks (Dewalle et al., 1998; Brik et al., 1999; Cazeneuve et al., 1999; Koné Paut et al., 2000; Gershoni-Baruch et al., 2002). Although the data are less extensive, the M694I mutation may also confer increased risk of amyloidosis (Ben-Chetrit and Backenroth, 2001; Mansour et al., 2001).

At least two additional factors complicate the interpretation of mutational studies in FMF. First, the E148Q mutation can be seen in *cis* with several exon 10 mutations, most commonly V726A. The V726A-E148Q complex allele is relatively common in the Ashkenazi Jewish population, and haplotype analysis suggests that it arose by recombination between FMF chromosomes carrying the respective individual mutations (Aksentijevich et al., 1999). There is also evidence that V726A-E148Q is a high-risk allele for amyloidosis (Gershoni-Baruch et al., 2002). From a practical standpoint, family studies would be required to determine phase in patients heterozygous for these two mutations and with no other demonstrable sequence changes.

A second problem is that up to 30% of patients with typical clinical findings of FMF, including a therapeutic response to colchicine, have only one demonstrable *MEFV* mutation (Aksentijevich et al., 1999; Cazeneuve et al., 1999; Akar et al., 2000; Medlej-Hashim et al., 2000; Mansour et al., 2001; Padeh et al., 2003), even when the entire coding region is screened (Cazeneuve et al., 2003). Noncoding mutations offer one possible explanation, but would not explain the divergence from Hardy-Weinberg equilibrium that has recently been described in Armenians from the Karabakh (Cazeneuve et al., 2003). Alternatively, it is possible that, at least on certain genetic backgrounds, a single

MEFV mutation is sufficient to manifest symptoms. Consistent with this view, it is now well established that FMF carriers often exhibit biochemical evidence of intermittent inflammation, and there are at least two rare *MEFV* mutations (ΔM694 and the M694I-E148Q complex allele) that transmit clinically typical FMF in a dominant fashion (Booth et al., 2000). Finally, on the basis of the findings of Turkish FMF families unlinked to chromosome 16 (Akarsu et al., 1997) and FMF patients from Palma de Mallorca having no demonstrable *MEFV* mutations (Domingo et al., 2000), some investigators have posited the existence of additional FMF genes besides *MEFV*, accounting for the "mutation deficit" in symptomatic heterozygotes.

Strategies for Diagnosis

In many instances, the possibility of FMF is first considered in a child with recurrent, unexplained episodes of fever, with or without localized inflammatory manifestations. In Western countries, patients often experience multiple episodes over a period of several months before the diagnosis is entertained, and it is not unusual for such patients to have already undergone extensive evaluations for infection, malignancy, and, in some cases, inflammatory bowel disease. In considering the diagnosis of FMF, it is important to recall that there are occasional FMF patients without known Mediterranean heritage, and because of the recessive mode of inheritance of FMF and the small family size and increased mobility of Western society, about half of the patients in most series have a negative family history.

A number of sets of clinical criteria were proposed prior to the identification of *MEFV*; the most widely quoted one was developed at a large center in Tel-Hashomer, Israel (Livneh et al., 1997b). The various sets of criteria agree that the cardinal features of FMF are short (12 hours to 3 days), recurrent (3 or more) episodes of fever (rectal temperature >38°C) with painful manifestations in the abdomen, chest, joints, or skin in the absence of any other demonstrable causative factors. The Tel-Hashomer criteria enumerate milder attacks, exertional leg pain, and a favorable response to colchicine as minor criteria, and a positive family history, age of onset <20 years, appropriate ethnicity, parental consanguinity, an acute-phase response during attacks, episodic proteinuria/hematuria, and an unproductive laparotomy as supportive criteria. The diagnosis is then established with appropriate combinations of major, minor, and supportive criteria.

Although the Tel-Hashomer criteria perform extremely well in high-risk populations, they probably do not work as well in Western nations, where the Bayesian pretest probabilities are much lower, the disease is milder (due to a different spectrum of mutations), physicians have had much less clinical experience with FMF, and the frequency of other hereditary periodic fevers may be higher than the frequency of FMF. These criteria nevertheless provide important guidance for physicians in the United States and Europe. Clinical features that may help differentiate FMF from the other hereditary periodic fevers include ethnicity, duration of attacks, type of skin rash, and responsiveness to colchicine (Table 27.1).

Genetic testing has assumed a major adjunctive role in the diagnosis of FMF, and, as previously noted, has extended both the clinical and the ethnic spectrum of FMF. Nevertheless, the previously issues of sensitivity (the "mutation deficit") and penetrance underscore the need to consider clinical information in the interpretation of *MEFV* genetic test results.

To date there are no protein-based tests or assays for pyrin expression or function that would aid in the diagnosis of FMF, although this goal now seems within reach. Twenty years ago a metaraminol infusion to provoke an attack was proposed as a diagnostic test (Barakat et al., 1984), but it is not generally used because of safety concerns (Cattan et al., 1984; Buades et al., 1989).

Mode of Inheritance, Carrier Detection, and Prenatal Diagnosis

Standard teaching is that FMF is inherited as an autosomal recessive disorder with reduced penetrance in females (M:F ratios are generally around 1.5 to 1). Hence, in a family with two unaffected parents whose first child is diagnosed with FMF, the recurrence risk to each subsequent male child would be 25%. For families in which one parent is affected and the other is not, if one child is affected the recurrence risk is 50%. In cases where an affected individual marries an unaffected individual of unknown carrier status from a high-risk ethnic group, the risk of having an affected child is one-half the carrier frequency for that ethnic group. Since the measured carrier frequencies for Jewish, Arab, Armenian, and Turkish populations are often >20%, in many cases this translates into a risk of 10% or more.

Because molecular diagnosis has broadened the FMF phenotype and ethnic distribution, the foregoing analysis may be oversimplified. We now know that some mutations, such as M694V, have greater penetrance than others, such as E148Q; that a few *MEFV* mutations truly show a dominant mode of inheritance; that there is a biochemical inflammatory phenotype associated with the FMF carrier state; and that a substantial number of patients (often with relatively mild symptoms) have only one demonstrable mutation. Such information complicates genetic counseling.

Given the rare occurrence of FMF phenotype II, in which patients present with amyloidosis as the first manifestation of the disease, the question may be raised whether asymptomatic relatives of FMF patients should be screened for *MEFV* mutations, perhaps with the intention of initiating prophylactic colchicine in those individuals who test positive for two mutations. In Western nations in which phenotype II is exceedingly rare, where the M694V frequency is low and amyloidosis is uncommon even in patients with FMF, screening of asymptomatic family members is generally not performed, since the discovery of "genetic FMF" may adversely affect the insurability of individuals who may never develop symptoms. There is still no consensus on presymptomatic screening in families with a strong history of amyloidosis, and some physicians would advocate careful follow-up rather than colchicine prophylaxis in asymptomatic family members with two mutations.

Prenatal diagnosis of FMF is feasible but requires careful genetic counseling to appropriately explain decreased penetrance and interpretation of heterozygous genotypes. In addition, given the relative effectiveness of colchicine therapy, prenatal diagnosis raises significant moral and ethical issues regarding the possible termination of pregnancy for what many regard to be a treatable disease.

Treatment and Prognosis

Daily oral colchicine therapy has been established as effective in preventing both the acute attacks of FMF and systemic amyloidosis. About three-fourths of adult FMF patients taking 1.2 to 1.8 mg of colchicine per day experience a near-complete remis-

sion of their attacks, and over 90% demonstrate a marked improvement. Colchicine may cause diarrhea or gastrointestinal upset, but this side effect can be minimized by starting at a low dose and gradually titrating upward, and by dividing the daily dose. In some patients the gastrointestinal effects of colchicine are aggravated by lactose intolerance (Fradkin et al., 1995), in which case a lactose-free diet may be helpful. Colchicine is safe in children but must be carefully titrated to efficacy and toxicity (Zemer et al., 1991; Özkaya and Yalçinkaya, 2003).

Oral colchicine may also prevent amyloid progression in FMF patients who already have proteinuria due to amyloidosis (Livneh et al., 1994b; Simsek et al., 2000; Öner et al., 2003). The prognosis is best if the serum creatinine is <1.5 mg/dl, and is adversely affected by tubulointerstitial disease at diagnosis and by noncompliance. Doses of 1.5 mg/day or more are most effective in these patients, as well as in patients who have already undergone renal transplantation (Livneh et al., 1992). The combination of colchicine and cyclosporine should be avoided when possible in transplant patients, since cyclosporine inhibits the MDR1 transport system required for hepatic and renal colchicine excretion (Speeg et al., 1992; Gruberg et al., 1999; Simkin and Gardner, 2000; Minetti and Minetti, 2003).

Agents that inhibit or compete for the hepatic cytochrome P450 system component CYP 3A4, such as cimetidine, erythromycin, lovastatin, and grapefruit juice, may also increase colchicine blood levels (Ben-Chetrit and Levy, 1998a). Colchicine toxicity other than diarrhea is rare in patients taking standard doses, but can occur in the presence of inhibitors of clearance in elderly patients with renal insufficiency (Kuncl et al., 1987; Altiparmak et al., 2002) or if colchicine is given intravenously to abort an attack in patients already receiving oral colchicine (Wallace and Singer, 1988; Putterman et al., 1991; Bonnel et al., 2002). Most experts advise continuing colchicine in female FMF patients during conception and pregnancy and performing an amniocentesis to screen for the slightly increased risk of trisomy 21 (Ben-Chetrit and Levy, 2003). Although small concentrations are present in the breast milk of women taking colchicine, breast-feeding is considered safe (Ben-Chetrit et al., 1996).

Colchicine may prevent the attacks of FMF through multiple mechanisms. Colchicine is concentrated in granulocytes, the major effector in FMF attacks, perhaps because these cells express only low levels of the *MDR1*-encoded P-glycoprotein pump (Ben-Chetrit and Levy, 1998b; c). Through its interaction with microtubules or other less well-defined mechanisms, colchicine inhibits L-selectin expression on neutrophils (Cronstein et al., 1995) and inhibits neutrophil chemotaxis (Dinarello et al., 1976; Bar-Eli et al., 1981). It is also of interest but of unknown significance that pyrin itself is expressed predominantly in neutrophils and associates with microtubules (Mansfield et al., 2001).

When FMF presents with polyarteritis nodosum, Henoch-Schönlein purpura, or febrile myalgia, additional therapy with high-dose corticosteroids, and sometimes cyclophosphamide, may be necessary (Langevitz et al., 1994; Tinaztepe et al., 1997; Majeed et al., 2000a; Ozen et al., 2001). For the subset of patients with FMF whose more typical attacks do not respond well to colchicine, several adjunctive approaches are under investigation, including subcutaneous interferon-α (Tunca et al., 1997; Calguneri et al., 2004a, 2004b; Tunca et al., 2004), weekly low-dose intravenous colchicine (Lidar et al., 2003), and biologic therapies targeted at TNF or IL-1β. Allogeneic bone marrow transplantation has recently been proposed as a treatment for refractory FMF (Milledge et al., 2002), but many experts regard the risk-benefit ratio as unacceptable (Touitou et al., 2003).

In a large majority of patients with FMF, the prognosis on standard colchicine therapy is excellent, allowing for a full range of activities and a normal life span. Amyloidosis is the major life-limiting manifestation of FMF, but fortunately the incidence is much reduced with colchicine prophylaxis. Renal transplantation has proven to be effective in patients who take adequate doses of colchicine in the post-transplant period. Patients who respond poorly to colchicine are often very impaired functionally and are a major therapeutic priority.

Animal Models

Chae and colleagues (2003) recently reported the development of a mouse line expressing a truncated, hypomorphic form of pyrin. Consistent with the previous discussion of the role of pyrin in IL-1β maturation, peritoneal macrophages from these mice exhibited increased caspase-1 activation, increased IL-1β processing and secretion and a defect in apoptosis that was independent of IL-1β but associated with impaired caspase-8 cleavage. Overall, the mice exhibited an inflammatory phenotype. Low doses of bacterial lipopolysaccharide (LPS) induced an accentuated body temperature response in homozygous mutant mice, and higher doses induced increased lethality in the homozygous mutants, relative to wild type. Moreover, the induction of inflammatory periotoneal exudates by thioglycollate was increased in homozygous mutants relative to heterozygotes or wild-type mice.

Thus murine pyrin plays an important role in the regulation of the innate immune response; mutants with diminished function may confer heightened inflammatory responses that could be beneficial in the heterozygous state. Additional studies with pyrin-null mice and knock-ins of FMF-associated mutants may further delineate these pathways.

TNF Receptor–Associated Periodic Fever Syndrome

The term *familial Hibernian fever* (FHF; MIM142680) was first proposed to describe a large family of Irish/Scottish ancestry afflicted with recurrent episodes of fever, abdominal pain, myalgia, and erythematous rash that responded to corticosteroid but not colchicine treatment (Williamson et al., 1982). Fifteen years later, a follow-up report confirmed a dominant mode of inheritance in this family, extended the clinical phenotype to include conjunctivitis and periorbital edema, and documented systemic AA amyloidosis in 1 of 16 living affected family members (McDermott et al., 1997). Several other reports described families with similar, although not completely identical, dominantly inherited inflammatory symptoms from several different ethnic backgrounds (Bergman and Warmenius, 1968; Gertz et al., 1987; Hawle et al., 1989; Karenko et al., 1992; Zweers and Erkelens, 1993; Gadallah et al., 1995; Mache et al., 1996; Zaks and Kastner, 1997), making it difficult to be certain whether these syndromes arose from distinct mutations at a common locus or occurred as a result of mutations in different genes.

In 1998, two independent groups mapped the susceptibility loci for FHF and an Australian (Scottish) variant denoted *familial periodic fever syndrome* to chromosome 12p13 (McDermott et al., 1998; Mulley et al., 1998), suggesting that the same locus was responsible for both syndromes. Plausible functional candidates in the linkage interval included *CD27, LAG-3, CD4, C1R, C1S,* and *TNFRSF1A. TNFRSF1A* encodes the 55 kDa receptor for TNF (also known as TNFR1, TNFRSF1A, p55, p60, and CD120a). Given the central role of TNF signaling in inflammation and the observation of reduced levels of the soluble p55 receptor in the serum of several patients with FHF, a collaborative effort was undertaken to sequence *TNFRSF1A* among affected and nonaffected members from seven families of various ethnicities with autosomal dominant recurrent fever syndromes.

Sequence analyisis demonstrated six distinct *TNFRSF1A* missense mutations, five of which resulted in substitutions at highly conserved cysteine residues (McDermott et al., 1999). The discovery of mutations in *TNFRSF1A* consolidated these clinical variants into a single nosologic entity denoted the TNF receptor–associated periodic syndrome (TRAPS), a name chosen to reflect the involvement of the p55 TNF receptor in the pathogenesis of the disease while avoiding the suggestion of a specific ethnic bias. Over 30 *TNFRSF1A* mutations have now been reported in patients with recurrent fever (McDermott et al., 1999; Dodé et al., 2000a, 2002a; Aganna et al., 2001, 2002b, 2003; Aksentijevich et al., 2001; Jadoul et al., 2001; Simon et al., 2001b, 2001c; Nevala et al., 2002; Kriegel et al., 2003; Weyhreter et al., 2003; Horiuchi et al., 2004), subsuming a wide range of ethnic groups, including African Americans, East Asians, and populations in which FMF and HIDS are common.

Clinical and Pathological Manifestations

In the largest single group of TRAPS patients reported to date (Hull et al., 2002b), the median age of onset was 3 years, ranging from 2 weeks to 53 years of age. Males and females are equally affected. In contrast with FMF, the duration of TRAPS attacks is quite variable (Dodé et al., 2002a), ranging from short episodes of 1 to 2 days to month-long flares, and in rare cases, patients experience nearly continuous, fluctuating symptoms (McDermott et al., 1997). At the onset of an attack, inflammatory symptoms, such as muscle cramping, abdominal pain, or pleuritic chest pain, may be relatively subtle, gradually increasing over the course of 1 to 3 days. Pain often persists at its maximum intensity for several days before gradual resolution. Some patients associate the onset of attacks with physical or emotional stress, menses, or local trauma, but in many cases there does not appear to be a definite stimulus that provokes an attack. In women, pregnancy is sometimes associated with remission (McDermott et al., 1997; Kriegel et al., 2003), with possible exacerbation during the postpartum period (Rösen-Wolff et al., 2001).

Nearly all patients develop fever in association with at least some of their attacks. Temperature >38°C (maximally 41°C) usually lasts for more than 3 days, often heralding the onset of other inflammatory symptoms. Young children invariably experience fever with their attacks, but fever may be absent during some attacks in adults.

Serosal involvement is a prominent feature of TRAPS (Hull et al., 2002b). Attacks consisting solely of fever and abdominal pain occur in over 90% of patients with TRAPS, and can be the result of inflammation of the peritoneum or of the abdominal musculature or both. Serosal inflammation often produces the physical findings of an acute abdomen, and approximately half of the patients in one series had undergone at least one laparoscopy or exploratory laparotomy. Findings frequently include mononuclear infiltrates in the bowel wall or peritoneal adhesions, which eventually can cause bowel necrosis. Pleuritic attacks, with or without radiographic evidence of effusion, occur in about 50% of TRAPS patients. Less common serosal manifestations include pericarditis and episodes of scrotal pain.

Localized myalgia is extremely common during TRAPS attacks. The myalgia of TRAPS manifests as cramp-like discomfort, fluctuating in severity but disabling at its worst. Affected areas are warm, tender to palpation, and often associated with an erythematous patch. When found on an extremity, the myalgia and rash of TRAPS characteristically migrate centrifugally (as opposed to spreading) from proximal to distal limb over several days. As the region of inflammation passes over a joint (e.g., knee or elbow), there is often evidence of synovitis and effusion, with transient contracture. Although most commonly affecting the limbs and torso, myalgia and rash can also occur on the face and neck. During the episodes of myalgia, serum creatine kinase and aldolase concentrations remain normal. Magnetic resonance imaging demonstrates focal areas of edema in the affected muscular compartments and intramuscular septa (Hull et al., 2002d). Biopsies in TRAPS patients with active myalgia have demonstrated monocytic fasciitis or lymphocytic vasculitis but not myositis (Hull et al., 2002d; Drewe et al., 2003a).

TRAPS attacks frequently lead to arthralgia or arthritis, either as a part of the migratory myalgia picture or independently. Polyarticular arthralgia is by far the most common rheumatic manifestation of TRAPS. The arthritis of TRAPS tends to be nonerosive and either monoarticular or pauciarticular and asymmetric, most commonly affecting the hips, knees, and ankles.

The most distinctive of the cutaneous manifestations of TRAPS is the centrifugally migratory erythematous rash (Color Plate 27.II) (Toro et al., 2000). Such lesions are warm, tender, and blanch on palpation and are sometimes as much as 30 cm in diameter. Histologically, there is a superficial and deep perivascular and interstitial mononuclear cell infiltrate, sometimes with a low-grade lymphocytic vasculitis (Toro et al., 2000). Other less unique rashes are also commonly observed in TRAPS. They include urticaria-like plaques and serpiginous erythematous patches and plaques (Toro et al., 2000). These variants often involve several different areas of the body simultaneously and are neither migratory nor associated with concurrent myalgia. Relapsing episodes of panniculitis have also been reported (Lamprecht et al., 2004).

Eye involvement is much more common in TRAPS than in FMF, occurring in over 75% of patients (Hull et al., 2002b). The most frequent ocular findings are conjunctivitis and periorbital edema. Uveitis is relatively rare, but should be considered in patients experiencing blurred vision or eye pain.

As in FMF, systemic amyloidosis is the most serious complication of TRAPS and is due to the deposition of an insoluble fragment of SAA (Jadoul et al., 2001; Simon et al., 2001b; Dodé et al., 2002b), as in other forms of secondary amyloidosis. As the clinical spectrum of mutation-positive TRAPS expands, the frequency of amyloidosis among reported cases has diminished and is currently about 10%. Nephrotic syndrome and renal failure are the most common consequences; there is also one case of hepatic transplantation due to TRAPS amyloidosis reported in the literature (Hull et al., 2002b).

Laboratory Findings

The attacks of TRAPS are nearly always associated with a vigorous acute-phase response (Hull et al., 2002b), including an accelerated ESR and increased CRP, haptoglobin, fibrinogen, C3 and C4 complement, and ferritin. Although not widely available, the SAA level represents the most sensitive and rapid measure of the acute-phase response and may be an important determinant to monitor in patients with systemic amyloidosis (Gillmore et al.,

2001). During attacks patients may have prominent leukocytosis and neutrophilia, sometimes with white counts >20,000/mm^3, and children often have thrombocytosis.

Patients with TRAPS frequently manifest biochemical evidence of ongoing inflammation even between their acute episodes, although the magnitude of laboratory abnormalities may be diminished. The anemia of chronic disease is common among patients with frequent attacks, and a moderate polyclonal gammopathy is often seen. Modest elevations in the serum IgD have been reported (Simon et al., 2001c; Dodé et al., 2002a). Low-titer anticardiolipin antibodies and antinuclear antibodies are seen in a minority of patients.

As in FMF, albuminuria, usually without significant hematuria, is the most common manifestation of systemic amyloidosis in TRAPS. Initially, renal function is normal, although TRAPS amyloidosis may progress to renal failure within 1 to 2 years. Hepatic involvement usually causes an elevated alkaline phosphatase with normal transaminases. The diagnosis of amyloidosis should be confirmed with appropriate tissue specimens.

Molecular Basis of TRAPS: The Disease Gene, *TNFRSF1A*

TNFRSF1A is a 10-exon gene with a 455-codon open reading frame (Loetscher et al., 1990; Fuchs et al., 1992). The encoded protein has a 29–amino acid leader, a 182–amino acid extracellular domain, a 21–amino acid transmembrane domain, and a 223-residue intracellular domain. At the time of this writing, 39 mutations in *TNFRSF1A* have been reported in patients with recurrent episodes of fever and inflammation, and an updated database of mutations is available on the World Wide Web at http://fmf.igh.cnrs.fr/infevers/. All of the known mutations affect the extracellular cysteine-rich domains of the p55 TNF receptor (Fig. 27.2). Nineteen cause missense substitutions at cysteine residues, 18 cause missense substitutions at noncysteine residues, 1 causes an in-frame single amino acid deletion, and one is a splice mutation that causes a 4–amino acid insertion. There are also several mutational hot spots, including five at cysteine residues (C30, C33, C52, C70, and C88, numbered relative to the leucine immediately following the cleavage of the signal peptide) and four noncysteine residues (Y20, H22, T50, and R92). To date, no patients have been identified with mutations in either the transmembrane or intracellular domains of the TNFRSF1A protein, null mutations, or mutations in the p75 TNF receptor (TNFRSF1B), which is encoded on chromosome 1p36. Several reports have described families or individuals with TRAPS-like clinical findings but no demonstrable mutations in *TNFRSF1A*, raising the possibility of locus heterogeneity (Aksentijevich et al., 2001; Dodé et al., 2002a; Aganna et al., 2003).

Function of the p55 TNF Receptor, the *TNFRSF1A* Gene Product

TNF is a proinflammatory cytokine with pleiotropic biologic effects (Vassalli, 1992). At a cellular level, TNF stimulation can lead either to NF-κB activation or apoptosis, depending on a number of contextual factors that have still not been completely defined. Administration of TNF to experimental animals can cause leukocyte activation, cytokine secretion, increased expression of adhesion molecules on leukocytes and endothelial cell surfaces, host resistance to intracellular pathogens, angiogenesis, pyrexia, anemia, and cachexia.

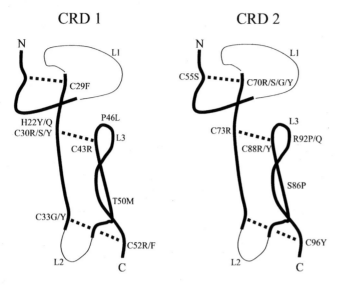

Figure 27.2. Structures of the first two cysteine-rich domains (CRDs) of the 55 kDa TNF receptor, TNFRSF1A. Loops (L1–L3) are indicated. Thick lines represent well-conserved regions, dotted lines depict disulfide bonds. Eighteen cysteine mutations causing the TNF receptor–associated periodic syndrome (TRAPS) are shown. A 19th cysteine mutation is in CRD 3 (C98Y). Several other noncysteine mutations are also shown. At the time of this writing a total of 39 TRAPS mutations have been published or presented in abstracts. All are in the extracellular domains of TNFRSF1A. To date, none are frameshift or nonsense mutations.

As noted above, there are two cellular receptors for TNF, a 55 kDa protein encoded on chromosome 12p13 (TNFRSF1A) and a 75 kDa receptor encoded on chromosome 1p36 (TNFRSF1B) (Smith et al., 1990). Both are members of a family of cell-surface receptors with repeating cysteine-rich extracellular domains (CRDs) (Bazzoni and Beutler, 1996). Both receptors have four extracellular CRDs comprising about 40 residues, with three intrachain disulfide bonds stabilizing the structure of each CRD. The intracellular segment of the p55 receptor also includes a death domain of around 70 residues that is involved in signal transduction (Hsu et al., 1995). The p55 receptor is expressed widely, whereas the p75 receptor is expressed predominantly on leukocytes and endothelial cells.

TNF forms homotrimers that in turn aggregate homotrimers of either p55 or p75 receptors on the cell surface (Engelmann et al., 1990). All of the cysteine mutations in the p55 receptor are predicted to have a major effect on its three-dimensional structure, since they would prevent the formation of highly conserved disulfide bonds important to maintaining proper folding of the molecule. In addition, noncysteine mutations, such as those at T50, may prevent the formation of hydrogen bonds (Aksentijevich et al., 2001). Because TNF signaling requires homotrimerization of receptors, the dominant inheritance of TRAPS may be explained by the fact that structural modifications of even one of the three molecules in the complex may disrupt necessary interactions. If equimolar amounts of wild-type and mutant receptor were present on the cell surface, only one of eight homotrimers would be expected to be composed solely of normal chains.

Nevertheless, it was somewhat surprising that mutations in the p55 TNF receptor caused autoinflammatory disease rather than a more conventional immunodeficiency phenotype. In the initial report describing TRAPS (McDermott et al., 1999), leukocytes from three patients with the C52F mutation were studied for in-

creased TNF binding or constitutive activation through the mutant receptors (possibly by the formation of interchain disulfide bonds). The data supported neither possibility.

Instead, evidence was presented that mutant p55 receptors are refractory to activation-induced cleavage of the ectodomain, a homeostatic process that normally limits repeated signaling at the cell surface and creates a pool of potentially antagonistic soluble receptors. Four lines of evidence were adduced: (1) patients with four different *TNFRSF1A* mutations had diminished levels of soluble p55 in the serum, relative to healthy controls or patients with other inflammatory disorders; (2) membrane p55 was increased on peripheral blood leukocytes from C52F patients; (3) activation-induced clearance of cell surface p55 was reduced in leukocytes from C52F patients; and (4) activation-induced soluble p55 in leukocyte culture supernatants was less for C52F patients than for normal controls. The mechanism by which disease-associated mutations impair cleavage most likely represents an indirect structural effect, since all but 1 of the 39 known mutations are remote from the Asn_{172}–Val_{173} site where metalloprotease-induced cleavage actually occurs (Gullberg et al., 1992).

Current evidence suggests that impaired ectodomain cleavage is unlikely to be the whole explanation for the TRAPS phenotype. Impaired receptor shedding has been observed by flow cytometry in leukocytes from patients with nine mutations (H22Y, C30S, C33G, P46L, T50M, T50K, C52F, F112I, and I170N) (McDermott et al., 1999; Aksentijevich et al., 2001; Nevala et al., 2002; Aganna et al., 2003), but not in patients with six other disease-associated variants (T37I, ΔD42, C52R, the splice mutation, N65I, and R92Q) (Aksentijevich et al., 2001; Aganna et al., 2003). The issue is further complicated by the observation that receptor shedding defects are in some cases cell type–dependent (Huggins et al., 2004). Although inappropriately low levels of soluble p55 are seen in a substantial subset of patients, this is also not a universal finding in mutation-proven TRAPS (Aganna et al., 2003). Other possible mechanisms of disease include effects on ligand-independent receptor self-association (Chan et al., 2000), effects on ligand-binding (Todd et al., 2004), abnormal intracellular trafficking of mutant receptors (Todd et al., 2004), and the relative balance of signaling through p55 and p75 receptors.

Mutation Analysis

Most specialty laboratories use automated DNA sequencing, with or without a screening step such as denaturing high-performance liquid chromatography, for mutation detection. Thirty-seven of the 39 mutations are in exons 2 to 4 of the 10 exon gene, and 37 of the 39 are in the first two CRDs. Mutational screening therefore usually focuses on these high-probability regions of the gene. The conventional system for numbering mutations in TRAPS found in this chapter and most published reports denotes the leucine that immediately follows the cleavage of the signal peptide as residue 1. Inclusion of the signal peptide would increase these numbers by 29.

In general, the penetrance of noncysteine mutations appears lower than that of cysteine substitutions (Aksentijevich et al., 2001). Moreover, cysteine mutations have been associated with a higher risk of amyloidosis.

Two specific noncysteine *TNFRSF1A* mutations are sufficiently common to be considered polymorphisms in some populations (Aksentijevich et al., 2001). R92Q, which is present in almost half of the independent TRAPS chromosomes identified in a large cohort followed at the U.S. National Institutes of Health, is also present in approximately 1% of Caucasian control chromosomes. Since the population frequency of TRAPS is far less than 1%, the penetrance of this variant must be low. However, data are accumulating that the TRAPS phenotype is but one end of a spectrum of inflammatory conditions associated with R92Q. Recent reports demonstrate an increased frequency of this *TNFRS1A* variant in an early arthritis clinic (Aksentijevich et al., 2001), in association with atherosclerosis (Poirier et al., 2004), and in patients with systemic amyloidosis complicating juvenile idiopathic arthritis (Aganna et al., 2004). Similarly, the P46L variant is found in approximately 2% of African-American control chromosomes (Aksentijevich et al., 2001) and at an even higher frequency among some sub-Saharran African populations (Tchernitchko et al., 2005).

Strategies for Diagnosis

Clinical suspicion is the cornerstone of the diagnosis of TRAPS. Among the clinical features of TRAPS that help distinguish it from the other periodic fever syndromes are the duration of attacks (episodes lasting more than 1 week suggest TRAPS, although shorter attacks can be seen), the migratory myalgia and overlying erythematous rash, presence of periorbital edema during attacks, a dominant pattern of inheritance, and the differential response to corticosteroids over colchicine. Also in the differential diagnosis are systemic-onset juvenile chronic arthritis (SOJCA) and adult-onset Still's disease. Distinguishing features include fever pattern (temperatures usually return to normal or below normal each day in SOJCA and adult Still's, rather than remaining elevated around the clock in TRAPS), clinical course of the arthritis (progressive, erosive polyarticular arthritis are common in SOJCA and adult Still's), and cutaneous manifestations (evanescent salmon-colored macular or maculopapular rash in SOJCA and adult Still's).

Once clinical suspicion has been established, the diagnosis of TRAPS is confirmed or refuted by *TNFRSF1A* sequence analysis. More complete sequencing may be entertained if the clinical suspicion is high but the yield is relatively low. There are numerous sporadic and some familial cases that clinically resemble TRAPS but do not have *TNFRSF1A* mutations, and it is probably best to reserve a term such as *idiopathic autoinflammatory disease* for such cases.

Serum levels of soluble p55 receptor, while of theoretical interest, have not proven to be an adequate substitute for genetic testing. Soluble p55 levels can be low, normal, or high among patients who are suspected of having TRAPS but are found to be mutation negative (Aganna et al., 2003). Moreover, although most mutation-positive TRAPS patients do have low levels of soluble p55, inflammatory attacks or renal insufficiency can spuriously normalize soluble p55 measurements.

Mode of Inheritance, Carrier Detection, and Prenatal Diagnosis

Although TRAPS is inherited in an autosomal dominant fashion, penetrance is not 100%, even for substitutions at cysteine residues. Further complicating the issue are reports of several cases of de novo *TNFRSF1A* mutations (Aganna et al., 2002b, 2003). Careful history-taking can sometimes identify unsuspected cases among the allegedly unaffected relatives of TRAPS patients, and genetic testing is of benefit in establishing the correct diagnosis in these individuals. Genetic testing may also be warranted for asymp-

tomatic relatives in families with a strong history of TRAPS-associated amyloidosis. However, in cases where the risk of amyloidosis is low, the possible benefits of identifying other mutation-positive asymptomatic relatives should be weighed against the potential impact of such information on insurability, especially for children. Similarly, the use of molecular techniques for prenatal diagnosis should be approached with great caution, since there are still insufficient data to make reliable estimates of penetrance, and since the field of targeted cytokine-inhibitory therapies is rapidly evolving.

Treatment and Prognosis

In contrast to FMF, colchicine prevents neither the acute attacks nor the amyloidosis of TRAPS (Dodé et al., 2002b; Hull et al., 2002b). The efficacy of nonsteroidal anti-inflammatory drugs is limited to mild attacks. Short courses of oral or parenteral corticosteroids may be effective in more severe episodes, but escalating doses are often required, with the attendant toxicities. There is a growing body of evidence that twice- or thrice-weekly administration of etanercept, the p75 TNFR:Fc fusion protein, is effective in reducing, although usually not eliminating, the clinical and laboratory manifestations of TRAPS (Kastner et al., 1999; Galon et al., 2000; Nigrovic and Sundel, 2001; Simon et al., 2001c; Hull et al., 2002a, 2002b; Drewe et al., 2003b; Weyhreter et al., 2003; Lamprecht et al., 2004). Etanercept also appears to have a role in preventing amyloid deposition, although monitoring of SAA levels may be necessary to titrate the dosage (Drewe et al., 2000, 2004; Hull et al., 2002c).

The prognosis of TRAPS is largely related to development of systemic amyloidosis, which is more frequent among patients with cysteine substitutions or a positive family history of amyloidosis (Aksentijevich et al., 2001; Kallinich et al., 2004). Infrequently, TRAPS patients develop life-threatening abdominal complications, such as bowel obstruction or necrosis.

Animal Models

Kollias and colleagues recently reported knock-in mice that express a nonsheddable p55 TNF receptor with a mutation at the cleavage site (Xanthoulea et al., 2004). These mice exhibited a dominantly inherited autoinflammatory phenotype that supports the hypothesis that TNF receptor shedding is an important negative homeostatic mechanism. Mutant mice developed chronic active hepatitis, were more susceptible to the toxic effects of bacterial LPS and TNF than wild-type animals, and exhibited increased susceptibility to experimental autoimmune encephalomyelitis and TNF-induced arthritis. Moreover, macrophages from these mice exhibited increased innate immune responses to Toll-like receptor stimulation. Nevertheless, differences between the phenotype of these mice and the clinical picture in TRAPS suggest that additional mechanisms are probably operative in the human disease. Development of mouse lines that are knock-ins for specific TRAPS-associated mutations may shed light on this issue.

Hyperimmunoglobulinemia D with Periodic Fever Syndrome

Among the currently recognized hereditary periodic fever syndromes, HIDS (MIM 260920) was the most recently described, with the initial study proposing a unique disorder in six Dutch patients in 1984 (van der Meer et al., 1984). Although these patients had a clinical picture similar to that of FMF, there were distinguishing features, including prominent lymphadenopathy, and less severe abdominal symptoms than usually seen with FMF. Moreover, all six Dutch patients were found to have polyclonal elevations in their serum IgD levels, and all five of the Dutch patients who underwent bone marrow aspiration and biopsy had markedly increased numbers of δ+ plasma cells in the marrow. In contrast, only one of eight patients with FMF had an increased serum IgD, and the one FMF patient who underwent a bone marrow examination had normal numbers of δ+ plasma cells. The HIDS nomenclature was proposed to describe this apparently new periodic fever syndrome.

Three of the initial patients had a positive family history, but it was only after additional patients and families were identified that a clear autosomal recessive mode of inheritance was apparent (Drenth et al., 1994c; Livneh et al., 1997a). Ten years after the first description of HIDS, a report of 50 cases with this disorder, most of them from the Netherlands and France, established HIDS as a clinical entity distinct from FMF (Drenth et al., 1994b). Two other studies demonstrated that the susceptibility locus for HIDS is not linked to the FMF locus on the short arm of chromosome 16 or to the immunoglobulin heavy-chain region on the long arm of chromosome 14 (Drenth et al., 1994c; Livneh et al., 1997a).

In 1999, 15 years after its initial description, two groups from the Netherlands independently discovered HIDS-associated mutations in *MVK*, the gene encoding mevalonate kinase, an enzyme involved in cholesterol and nonsterol isoprene biosynthesis (Fig. 27.3) (Drenth et al., 1999; Houten et al., 1999). Although not well understood, this surprising conclusion was strengthened by the complementary functional and positional cloning approaches employed by the competing groups, and *MVK* mutations still account for most patients with clinical HIDS (Simon et al., 2001a). Nevertheless, as is the case for both FMF and TRAPS, elucidation of the underlying gene has led to recognition of additional complexity. Thus, it is now clear that some patients with periodic fever have raised serum IgD levels without *MVK* mutations (Simon et al., 2001a), whereas others with *MVK* mutations have normal IgD levels (Houten et al., 1999; Frenkel et al., 2000; Saulsbury, 2003; Takada et al., 2003). Moreover, as we gain further insight into the role of the mevalonate pathway in regulating inflammation, the study of HIDS promises dividends that will extend far beyond these fascinating but relatively uncommon patients.

Clinical and Pathological Manifestations

HIDS was first recognized in the Netherlands, and even 20 years later the majority of reported cases are of Dutch or neighboring northern European ancestry (Drenth and van der Meer, 2001; Simon et al., 2003). Typically febrile attacks begin within the first year of life, often precipitated by childhood immunizations, and there is no gender bias (Drenth et al., 1994b). The duration of attacks, 3 to 7 days, is somewhat longer than the duration of FMF attacks, but shorter than the episodes sometimes seen in TRAPS. In addition to immunizations, minor infections, trauma, surgery, and menses may trigger attacks. On average, attacks occur about once or twice a month but usually without true periodicity in childhood and adolescence; attacks may become less frequent or severe in adults.

The attacks of HIDS often begin with chills and headache. In children, diffuse tender lymphadenopathy, particularly in the cervical chains, is common and is much more frequent than in FMF or TRAPS. As in the latter two disorders, abdominal pain is often

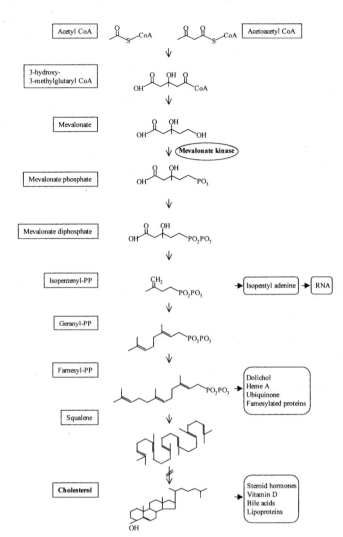

Figure 27.3. The mevalonate pathway. The hyperimmunoglobulinemia D with periodic fever syndrome (HIDS) is caused by recessively inherited mutations in the mevalonate kinase enzyme. HIDS-associated mevalonate kinase mutations typically leave 1%–3% residual enzymatic activity. More severe mutations in this enzyme cause mevalonic aciduria, a condition characterized by severe developmental delay as well as episodic inflammatory attacks.

present during attacks, although the incidence of peritoneal signs in HIDS is much lower than in FMF or TRAPS (Drenth et al., 1994b; Livneh et al., 1997a). Moreover, whereas the abdominal attacks of FMF and TRAPS are frequently associated with constipation, because of decreased peristalsis, the abdominal attacks of HIDS are often accompanied by diarrhea and vomiting. Nevertheless, some patients with HIDS do develop adhesions, probably from recurrent peritoneal inflammation. Scrotal pain, presumably due to inflammation of the tunica vaginalis, has been reported in HIDS (Saulsbury, 2003), but pleurisy and pericarditis have not been observed.

HIDS can present with a number of different mucocutaneous findings, including diffuse, painful, erythematous macules, a diffuse, erythematous macular and papular rash (Color Plate 27.III), erythematous papules and nodules, urticaria, and a morbilliform rash (Drenth et al., 1994a, 1994b). Unlike FMF, there is no predilection for the feet, ankles, or lower legs, and, unlike TRAPS, the rash of HIDS is not migratory. Histologically, cutaneous vasculitis, perivascular inflammatory cells, and deposits of IgD, IgM, or C3 may be present. Other forms of cutaneous vasculitis reported in HIDS include Henoch-Schönlein purpura (Haraldsson et al., 1992) and erythema elevatum diutinum (Miyagawa et al., 1993). Aphthous ulcers of the mouth and vagina may also be seen in HIDS, which, in combination with fever and cervical lymphadenopathy, may be confused with the syndrome of periodic fever, aphthous stomatitis, pharyngitis, and adenopathy (PFAPA), a common nongenetic cause of recurrent fever in children (Marshall et al., 1987, 1989; Thomas et al., 1999).

HIDS can also affect the joints (Haraldsson et al., 1992; Drenth and Prieur, 1993; Loeliger et al., 1993; Drenth et al., 1994b), most frequently with polyarthralgia. HIDS may also present with intermittent episodes of polyarticular arthritis of the large joints, usually but not always with fever, and sometimes coinciding with abdominal attacks. Arthritic attacks are more common in children and are usually nondestructive; synovial fluid is rich in granulocytes.

Systemic amyloidosis is uncommon in HIDS but has been reported (Obici et al., 2004; D'Osualdo et al., 2005). There is currently no explanation for the relative infrequency of amyloidosis in HIDS.

Laboratory Findings

Prior to the identification of the underlying gene, HIDS was defined by the polyclonal elevation of the serum IgD (>100 IU/ml or >14.1 mg/dl) on two occasions at least 1 month apart (Drenth et al., 1994b). While the vast majority of *MVK* mutation–positive patients with recurrent fevers meet this criterion, a small percentage of these patients do not. Serum IgD levels do not correlate with the severity of HIDS, either when following an individual patient or when comparing patients, and do not predictably fluctuate with attacks (Hiemstra et al., 1989; Drenth et al., 1994b). Over 80% of HIDS patients also have persistent polyclonal increases in serum IgA levels (Hiemstra et al., 1989; Haraldsson et al., 1992; Klasen et al., 2001).

As in FMF and TRAPS, during their inflammatory attacks HIDS patients present with leukocytosis and a left shift, an accelerated ESR, elevated acute-phase reactants (including CRP and SAA), and sometimes transient hematuria (Drenth et al., 1994b; Frenkel et al., 2000; Drenth and van der Meer, 2001). Serum levels of several proinflammatory cytokines may be increased during attacks, as is the urinary excretion of neopterin and leukotriene E_4 (Drenth et al., 1995; Frenkel et al., 2001b). Urinary levels of mevalonic acid are also markedly increased during attacks (Drenth et al., 1999; Houten et al., 1999; Frenkel et al., 2001a; Kelley and Takada, 2002).

Molecular Basis of HIDS: The Disease Gene, *MVK*

HIDS is caused by recessively inherited mutations in *MVK*, encoded on the long arm of human chromosome 12 (Drenth et al., 1999; Houten et al., 1999). HIDS-associated mutations lead to a marked reduction in mevalonate kinase enzymatic activity (vide infra), but fibroblasts from patients nevertheless typically demonstrate 1% to 3% of the activity seen in fibroblasts from healthy controls. *MVK* mutations leading to the complete loss of enzymatic activity cause mevalonic aciduria, an extremely rare condition that manifests not only the periodic fevers, lymphadenopathy,

abdominal pain, rash, and arthralgia seen in HIDS, but also hypotonia, mental retardation, cataracts, and failure to thrive (Hoffmann et al., 1986, 1993; Kelley, 2000).

MVK spans a genomic region of 22 kb, and is comprised of 11 exons, the first of which encodes most of the 5' untranslated region in the cDNA (Cuisset et al., 2001; Houten et al., 2001). The gene encodes a 396–amino acid protein (Schafer et al., 1992). At the time of this writing over 30 HIDS-associated mutations have been published, and an updated database of mutations (some of which have not yet been published) is available on the World Wide Web at fmf.igh.cnrs.fr/infevers/. HIDS-associated *MVK* mutations are distributed throughout the coding sequence, whereas mutations causing mevalonic aciduria are concentrated around sequences encoding the active sites of the mevalonate kinase enzyme (Cuisset et al., 2001; Houten et al., 2001).

Function of Mevalonate Kinase, the *MVK* Gene Product

Mevalonate kinase catalyzes the conversion of mevalonic acid to 5-phosphomevalonic acid in the synthesis of the sterols, which include cholesterol, vitamin D, bile acids, and steroid hormones (Goldstein and Brown, 1990; Brown and Goldstein, 1997; Valle, 1999). This pathway also leads to the production of nonsterol isoprenoids, which are involved in a host of cellular functions. It is unlikely that the autoinflammatory phenotype of HIDS is due to a deficiency in cholesterol, because patients with HIDS usually have cholesterol levels in the low to normal range, and the autoinflammatory phenotype is not seen in patients with other more profound disorders of the mevalonate pathway, such as Smith-Lemli-Opitz syndrome, in which cholesterol deficiency is more significant (Kelley, 2000).

There are two current hypotheses on the pathogenesis of HIDS. The first proposes that the inflammatory phenotype is due to the buildup of mevalonic acid, the substrate for the mevalonate kinase enzyme (Simon et al., 2004). The second hypothesis holds that the disorder is due to deficiencies in isoprenoids normally synthesized through the mevalonate pathway (Frenkel et al., 2002). Although there are in vitro data demonstrating accentuated IL-1β secretion in HIDS leukocytes that can be reversed by the addition of farnesol and geranyl-geraniol (isoprenoid compounds), the issue remains controversial. Some investigators have proposed that small GTP-binding proteins may provide the link between isoprenoids and inflammation (Takada et al., 2003), but this possibility awaits direct confirmation.

Both the isoprenoid deficiency and mevalonate accumulation hypotheses predict a worsening of symptoms with decreased mevalonate kinase enzymatic activity. In vitro studies of cell lines harboring wild-type or HIDS-mutant *MVK* indicate that the mutant enzyme functions best at 30°C, with a diminution at 37°C and further decreases at 39°C (Houten et al., 2002). This provocative finding may account for the association of HIDS attacks with immunizations and infections, and may also account for the increased urinary mevalonic acid levels seen during HIDS attacks.

Mutation Analysis

A very high percentage of HIDS patients harboring *MVK* mutations have at least one copy of the substitution of isoleucine for valine at residue 377 (V377I) (Cuisset et al., 2001; Houten et al., 2001; D'Osualdo et al., 2005). Population-based surveys of newborns in The Netherlands indicate a carrier frequency of 0.6% for the V377I mutation among the Dutch (Houten et al., 2003), with haplotype data supporting a founder effect (Houten et al., 2003). Analysis of *MVK* genotypes among HIDS patients indicate an underrepresentation of V377I homozygotes, relative to the expected Hardy-Weinberg distribution, suggesting a milder phenotype or reduced penetrance for V377I homozygotes (Houten et al., 2003).

Because many patients with HIDS are heterozygous for V377I, commercial and academic laboratories often perform an initial screen for the V377I mutation by restriction endonuclease analysis, sometimes also adding an assay for the second-most common mutation, the substitution of threonine for isoleucine at residue 268 (I268T). More extensive screening, usually by DNA sequencing, is reserved for patients who are heterozygous for either mutation (but not for compound heterozygotes, in whom the molecular diagnosis of HIDS would be already established).

Strategies for Diagnosis

There are currently three possible strategies for diagnosing HIDS: clinical, molecular, and biochemical. Consistent with practice before the identification of the underlying gene, the clinical diagnosis of HIDS is established by documenting elevations in serum IgD levels (>100 IU/ml, or >14.1 mg/dl) on two occasions at least a month apart, with a compatible clinical history. The molecular diagnosis is established by documenting two mutations in *MVK*, while the biochemical diagnosis is established by documenting elevations in urinary mevalonic acid during attacks, or decreased enzymatic activity in cells cultured from the patient. In many cases, all three strategies agree, in which case the patient is sometimes said to have "classic-type HIDS" (Simon et al., 2001a).

Although there is strong concordance between molecular and biochemical diagnosis, clinical and molecular diagnoses sometimes diverge. About one-quarter of patients satisfying clinical criteria for HIDS have no demonstrable *MVK* mutations (Simon et al., 2001a). These patients tend to have milder disease and lower IgD levels than patients with classic-type HIDS and are said to have "variant-type HIDS." There is also a small number of patients who meet genetic and biochemical criteria for HIDS, with a compatible clinical picture, except for persistently normal IgD levels (Houten et al., 1999; Frenkel et al., 2000; Saulsbury, 2003; Takada et al., 2003). This discrepancy is more frequent in young children, who may eventually exhibit increased serum IgD levels (Drenth and van der Meer, 2001). The term *Dutch-type periodic fever* has been proposed for periodic fever patients meeting genetic or biochemical criteria, regardless of their IgD levels (Frenkel et al., 2000).

Further complicating the picture is the finding that a small percentage of patients with FMF and TRAPS may have modest elevations in their serum IgD, although not to the very high levels seen in some HIDS patients (Livneh et al., 1997a; Medlej-Hashim et al., 2001; Simon et al., 2001c; Dodé et al., 2002a). The differential diagnosis of an elevated serum IgD level also includes IgD multiple myeloma, Hodgkin disease, cigarette smoking, diabetes mellitus, pregnancy, hyperimmunoglobulinemia E syndrome, ataxia telangiectasia, acquired immunodeficiency syndrome, and recurrent infections such as tuberculosis and aspergillosis (Hiemstra et al., 1989; Boom et al., 1990; Drenth et al., 1994b).

Given these complexities, it is reasonable to take a combined approach for patients in whom there is a suitable index of suspicion for HIDS/mevalonate kinase deficiency, combining serum IgD measurement with genetic and/or biochemical analysis. In light of the divergence between IgD and molecular findings and the apparent lack of correlation between IgD and disease severity, some investigators have suggested a change in nomenclature, but this appears unlikely in the face of firmly established convention.

Mode of Inheritance, Carrier Detection, and Prenatal Diagnosis

As noted above, HIDS is inherited as an autosomal recessive trait. There are currently no data on the penetrance of individual HIDS genotypes, although population–genetic studies suggest that V377I homozygotes may not always manifest HIDS symptoms. In light of the likelihood of reduced penetrance, the generally favorable prognosis for HIDS, and the possibility of genetic discrimination, genetic testing is usually reserved for symptomatic individuals. Prenatal diagnosis of HIDS is possible but raises a number of ethical issues if undertaken with the possibility of terminating a pregnancy for what is usually a nonfatal disorder with a number of new treatment options.

Treatment and Prognosis

Until recently, no cases of systemic amyloidosis had been associated with HIDS (Obici et al., 2004; D'Osualdo et al., 2004), and this still remains a very rare complication. Hence, the overwhelming majority of patients with HIDS have a normal life expectancy (Drenth et al., 1994b). Moreover, as noted above, symptoms usually ameliorate in adulthood.

Most patients with HIDS do not respond to colchicine, although a few patients do show some improvement with daily treatment. Corticosteroids, cyclosporine, and intravenous immunoglobulin are not generally effective in HIDS, although intra-articular steroids and nonsteroidal antiinflammatory drugs may be of benefit for HIDS arthritis.

Ongoing therapeutic trials in HIDS focus on the mevalonate pathway and on cytokine inhibition. The statin class of drugs inhibits HMG CoA reductase, the enzyme immediately preceding mevalonate kinase in the mevalonate pathway. Although one member of this pharmacologic family, lovastatin, caused exacerbations in the more severe mevalonic aciduria, simvastatin appears safe in HIDS, and preliminary data suggest a possible benefit (Simon et al., 2004). A small trial of thalidomide, which, among other effects, inhibits TNF-α production, resulted in a nonsignificant decrease in acute-phase reactants and no effect on the attack rate (Drenth et al., 2001). In contrast, the more potent TNF inhibitor etanercept produced substantial improvement in two patients with HIDS (Takada et al., 2003). IL-1 inhibition may represent yet another possible therapeutic strategy.

Animal Models

There are currently no animal models reported for HIDS.

The Cryopyrinopathies

The cryopyrinopathies—familial cold autoinflammatory syndrome (FCAS, MIM 120100), Muckle-Wells syndrome (MWS, MIM 191100), and neonatal-onset multisystem inflammatory disease (NOMID, MIM 607115, also called chronic infantile neurologic cutaneous and articular [CINCA] syndrome)—are a group of autosomal dominant autoinflammatory conditions consisting of episodic or fluctuating inflammation with associated cutaneous and synovial symptoms. Although some symptoms may resemble those of FMF or TRAPS, the cryopyrinopathies are distinct clinical phenotypes. A large family with what is now called FCAS was described first (Kile and Rusk, 1940), and Muckle and Wells reported on a family with their eponymous syndrome in 1962. NOMID/CINCA was first recognized as a clinical entity in the early 1980s (Prieur and Griscelli, 1981; Hassink and Goldsmith, 1983), although it was not initially apparent that this condition is a genetic disorder because of decreased reproductive fitness in patients carrying the diagnosis.

Between 1999 and 2000, genetic markers associated with FCAS, MWS, and a clinical overlap syndrome sharing features of both conditions were independently mapped to the distal region of the long arm of chromosome 1 (Cuisset et al., 1999; Hoffman et al., 2000; McDermott et al., 2000), a finding suggesting that all three disorders are linked to the same gene. In 2001, several missense mutations associated with FCAS and MWS were identified in an exon of a newly discovered gene denoted *CIAS1* (cold-induced auto-inflammatory syndrome-1) (Hoffman et al., 2001a). This gene, which is also called *PYPAF1* (Manji et al., 2002), *NALP3* (Aganna et al., 2002a), and *CATERPILLER1.1* (O'Connor et al., 2003), is expressed mainly in hematopoietic tissue. Similarities between clinical features of NOMID/CINCA and MWS led to the discovery in 2002 of de novo missense mutations in *CIAS1* in a significant percentage of patients with NOMID/CINCA as well (Aksentijevich et al., 2002; Feldmann et al., 2002). None of the mutations associated with FCAS, MWS, or NOMID/CINCA were found in healthy controls.

Currently, over 35 mutations linked to disease have been found in *CIAS1* (Hoffman et al., 2001a; Aganna et al., 2002a; Aksentijevich et al., 2002; Dodé et al., 2002c; Feldmann et al., 2002; Granel et al., 2003; Hoffman et al., 2003; Rösen-Wolff et al., 2003; Arostegui et al., 2004; Frenkel et al., 2004; Neven et al., 2004; Stojanov et al., 2004). As is the case for the other periodic fever syndromes, an updated list of mutations is available at http://fmf.igh.cnrs.fr/infevers/. Several mutations are shared by more than one condition and many patients evince symptoms that fall between the established diagnostic boundaries (Lieberman et al., 1998; McDermott et al., 2000; Aganna et al., 2002a; Granel et al., 2003; Hawkins et al., 2004b). Variability in phenotype among patients with the same mutation suggests that other genetic or environmental factors influence disease severity.

Clinical and Pathological Manifestations

Familial cold autoinflammatory syndrome

FCAS, also called familial polymorphous cold eruption and cold hypersensitivity, is considered the mildest of the cryopyrinopathies. Symptoms include episodes of fever, urticaria-like rash, arthralgia, and, less commonly, drowsiness, headache, nausea, and extreme thirst (Hoffman et al., 2001b; Johnstone et al., 2003; Wanderer and Hoffman, 2004). Febrile attacks are brought on by generalized exposure to cold temperatures. In one study, less than an hour on average of cold exposure was needed to precipitate symptoms (Hoffman et al., 2001b). Approximately 2.5 hours later, these patients experienced symptoms that lasted about 12 hours. Longer exposure to cold correlated with worse symptoms. In some individuals, attacks occur nearly daily, often worse in the evening and resolving by morning. Most patients have their first attack by 6 months of age.

The rash associated with FCAS can present as petechiae, erythematous patches, or confluent plaques, usually beginning on the face or extremities and spreading (Johnstone et al., 2003).

Although the rash appears hive-like, skin biopsies reveal infiltrates of neutrophils and lymphocytes (Hoffman et al., 2001b), rather than mast cells, indicating that the rash is not true urticaria. In areas of rash, there is also endothelial cell swelling and vacuolization, with capillary lumenal narrowing.

Polyarthralgia involving the hands, knees, ankles, and occasionally the feet, wrists, and elbows usually accompanies flares. Some patients may develop a nonerosive arthropathy with deformities of the metacarpalphalangeal and proximal interphalangeal joints (Commerford and Meyers, 1977). Some patients also complain of ocular symptoms, including watering and blurred vision.

Muckle-Wells syndrome

The first published description of MWS was a 1962 report on a Derbyshire kindred (Muckle and Wells, 1962). Affected individuals suffered from "aguey bouts" of inflammation consisting of fever, malaise, an urticaria-like rash, and stabbing pains in the large joints. In addition, affected members of the family developed bilateral sensorineural hearing loss and renal amyloidosis. Attacks were not usually linked to cold and tended to be more severe than those associated with FCAS.

Most patients with MWS have their first attack by adolescence. MWS-associated episodes last about 24–48 hours (Muckle and Wells, 1962; Muckle, 1979; Cuisset et al., 1999) and in addition to the symptoms noted above may also include abdominal pain, conjunctivitis, and episcleritis (Watts et al., 1994; Cuisset et al., 1999). Skin manifestations similar to those associated with FCAS usually accompany episodes (Color Plate 27.IV). Although arthralgia is much more common than arthritis, oligoarticular synovitis and sterile pyogenic arthritis occur occasionally (Schwarz et al., 1989; Watts et al., 1994). Approximately three-fourths of patients in one series developed sensorineural hearing loss, usually beginning in childhood with high-frequency hearing loss (Schwarz et al., 1989). About one-third of adult patients in the same series developed systemic AA amyloidosis (Muckle, 1979) affecting primarily the kidneys. Other target organs include the thyroid, adrenals, spleen, and testes (Schwarz et al., 1989). Hearing loss appears not to be due to amyloid deposition in the inner ear or auditory nerve, and current hypotheses focus on either possible inflammation of the inner ear or expression of *CIAS1* in the cochlea.

Neonatal-onset multisystem inflammatory disease/chronic infantile neurologic cutaneous articular syndrome

NOMID/CINCA is the most severe of the cryopyrinopathies. In addition to the fevers, arthralgias, hearing loss, and amyloidosis seen in MWS, patients with NOMID/CINCA may have a distinct, deforming arthropathy (Prieur and Griscelli, 1981; Hassink and Goldsmith, 1983; Hashkes and Lovell, 1997; Prieur, 2001) as well as chronic aseptic meningitis, intellectual impairment, and loss of vision. Approximately 20% of patients die before age 20 (Prieur et al., 1987; Hashkes and Lovell, 1997).

The rash associated with NOMID/CINCA is similar to that associated with FCAS and MWS and is nearly always present to some degree (Prieur, 2001). Articular symptoms are variable (Prieur et al., 1987; Hashkes and Lovell, 1997; Prieur, 2001), with some patients exhibiting mild swelling and pain, but no radiographic changes, whereas others have severe deformities involving symmetric overgrowth of the epiphyses and growth cartilage of the long bones, especially prominent in the knees, ankles, elbows, and hands. The latter changes may occur within the first year of life and contractures may severely restrict movement (Prieur et al., 1987; Hashkes and Lovell, 1997; Prieur, 2001). Joint radiographs from severe cases may show enlarged, irregular ossification of the epiphyses of the long bones, especially the tibias, often with a "bread crumb" appearance. There may be irregularity in the epiphyseal plates of the femur, radius, and tibia, as well as early growth plate closure and shortening of the long bones (Kaufman and Lovell, 1986; Hashkes and Lovell, 1997). Skull radiographs show frontal bosselation, delayed closure of the anterior fontanelle, and increased cranial volume. Synovial biopsy usually shows only modest inflammation.

The neurosensory manifestions of NOMID/CINCA are potentially of great concern. Many patients develop chronic aseptic meningitis, with increased cerebrospinal fluid (CSF) pressure, an elevation in CSF protein concentration, and a pleiocytosis consisting mostly of polymorphonuclear leukocytes (Torbiak et al., 1989). Brain imaging studies may reveal mild ventricular dilatation, cerebral atrophy, and prominent sulci (Prieur, 2001). Although some patients perform well at school, other children with NOMID/CINCA have developmental delays and learning deficits and still others exhibit mental retardation (Torbiak et al., 1989; Dollfus et al., 2000). As in MWS, sensorineural hearing loss is frequent. Ocular involvement may range from conjunctivitis to anterior or posterior uveitis, sometimes leading to blindness (Dollfus et al., 2000). Funduscopic examination frequently reveals optic disc edema, papilledema, or optic atrophy.

Other findings include hepatosplenomegaly and lymphadenopathy, as well as vasculitis, thrombosis, and the aforementioned amyloidosis (Prieur et al., 1987; Torbiak et al., 1989; Hashkes and Lovell, 1997; Prieur, 2001). Profound growth delay and reduced reproductive potential are also common.

Laboratory Findings in the Cryopyrinopathies

Laboratory features of the cryopyrinopathies include an accelerated ESR, polymorphonuclear leukocytosis, thrombocytosis, and anemia of chronic disease. Elevated acute-phase reactants, such as CRP and SAA, are also observed. High-titer autoantibodies are not observed, although some patients do have modest titers of anticardiolipin antibodies.

Molecular Basis of the Cryopyrinopathies: the CIAS1 Gene

CIAS1 is located on chromosome 1q44 and consists of nine exons, encoding a 3105 bp potential open reading frame (Hoffman et al., 2001a). Via alternative splicing, exons 1–3, 5, and 7–9 are included in the coding sequence for cryopyrin, producing a 920–amino acid, 106 kDa protein. Expression analyses detect the cryopyrin message in leukocytes and chondrocytes, with little expression in other tissues (Hoffman et al., 2001a; Feldmann et al., 2002).

The CIAS1 protein product was named cryopyrin to emphasize the existence of an N-terminal PYRIN domain, like that in the pyrin protein, as well as the association with cold-induced symptoms in FCAS (Hoffman et al., 2001a). Besides the PYRIN domain (amino acids [a.a.] 13–83), cryopyrin contains a central NACHT domain (a.a. 217–533) (Koonin and Aravind, 2000), named for its presence in neuronal apoptosis inhibitor protein (NAIP), the major histocompatibility complex class II transactivator (CIITA), the incompatibility locus protein from *Podospora anserina* (HET-E), and mammalian telomerase-associated proteins (TP1). At the C terminus of cryopyrin are seven leucine-rich repeats (LRRs) (a.a. 697–920). This arrangement of PYRIN–NACHT–LRRs is found in at least 14 proteins in the human genome (Harton et al., 2002; Tschopp et al., 2003), many of which are expressed in leukocytes and hematopoietic tissue.

Function of Cryopyrin, the CIAS1 Gene Product

The PYRIN domain of cryopyrin has been shown to interact specifically with ASC (Gumucio et al., 2002; Manji et al., 2002; Dowds et al., 2003), as noted with pyrin, a finding suggesting that cryopyrin too is involved in the caspase-1/IL-1β pathway. This macromolecular complex of cryopyrin (NALP3), ASC, and caspase-1, with a fourth protein called *Cardinal*, has been denoted the inflammasome (Agostini et al., 2004; Martinon and Tschopp, 2004). Transfection studies indicate that cryopyrin potentiates inflammation through its interaction with ASC. Cryopyrin regulates IL-1β secretion (Wang et al., 2002; Stehlik et al., 2003), NF-κB activation (Gumucio et al., 2002; Manji et al., 2002; Stehlik et al., 2002; Dowds et al., 2003; O'Connor et al., 2003), and apoptosis (Dowds et al., 2003).

The NACHT domain contains seven conserved motifs, including an ATPase-specific P loop and a Mg^{2+} binding site, and is involved in protein oligomerization (Koonin and Aravind, 2000). Disease-associated mutations are found almost exclusively in the NACHT domain, suggesting an important role for this motif in the function of cryopyrin.

LRRs are common components of the extracellular domains of Toll-like receptors (TLRs), as well as several cytoplasmic proteins. The LRRs of TLRs appear to recognize pathogen-associated molecular patterns (PAMPs), common molecules in bacterial cell walls, such as peptidoglycan and lipopolysaccharide (Inohara et al., 2002; Chamaillard et al., 2003; Girardin et al., 2003). Upon contact with a PAMP, TLRs transduce signals into the cell to up-regulate proinflammatory mediators such as costimulatory molecules, cytokines, and inducible nitric oxide synthase (iNOS). LRRs on cytoplasmic proteins such as cryopyrin may serve a similar purpose in detecting intracellular bacteria or bacterial products. Muramyl-dipeptide (MDP), a common PAMP, may activate formation of the cryopyrin (NALP3) inflammasome (Martinon et al., 2004). Thus, in this setting cryopyrin appears to be a proinflammatory molecule, up-regulating caspase-1 and IL-1β upon sensing bacterial MDP.

Under normal conditions, cryopyrin is kept from activating caspase-1 unnecessarily, possibly in two different ways. First, pyrin may compete with cryopyrin for binding to ASC (Dowds et al., 2003), preventing formation of the cryopyrin (NALP3) inflammasome. Second, studies of LRR deletion mutants of both cryopyrin and NALP1 (Martinon et al., 2002; Agostini et al., 2004), a related protein, suggest that the LRRs have an autoinhibitory function, maintaining the protein in an inactive state. Upon sensing intracellular bacteria, the LRRs may release the rest of the protein from inhibition, allowing formation of the cryopyrin (NALP3) inflammasome (Fig. 27.4).

Mutation Analysis

Nearly all of the known mutations occur in six small clusters in exon 3, encoding the NACHT domain (Hoffman et al., 2001a, 2003; Aganna et al., 2002a; Aksentijevich et al., 2002; Dodé et al., 2002c; Feldmann et al., 2002; Granel et al., 2003; Rösen-Wolff et al., 2003; Arostegui et al., 2004; Frenkel et al., 2004; Neven et al., 2004; Stojanov et al., 2004). Although the crystal

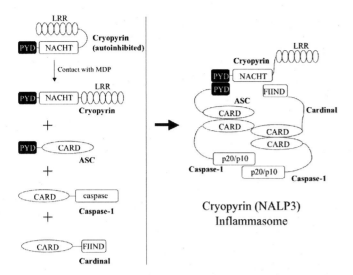

Figure 27.4. Formation of the cryopyrin (NALP3) inflammasome. Depicted on the left are the domain structures of the four proteins that comprise this macromolecular complex. At baseline, interaction of the leucine-rich repeats (LRR) with the NACHT domain of cryopyrin prevents assembly of the complex. Muramyl-dipeptide, a bacterial cell-wall product, may bind the LRR of cryopyrin, allowing assembly of the inflammasome. Mutations in the NACHT domain associated with familial cold autoinflammatory syndrome (FCAS), Muckle-Wells syndrome (MWS), and neonatal-onset multisystem inflammatory disease (NOMID) may alter the LRR–NACHT interaction in such a way that the threshold of activation is diminished. Assembly of the inflammasome leads to interaction of the catalytic domains (p20/p10) of caspase-1 molecules, leading to autocatalysis, release of p20 and p10, and subsequent IL-1β activation. PYD, PYRIN domain.

structure of cryopyrin has not been solved, computational modeling suggests that many of the disease-causing mutations are located along the nucleotide binding cleft or near a region that senses when a nucleotide is bound (Neven et al., 2004).

Mutations in cryopyrin appear to increase its proinflammatory properties, perhaps by increasing the binding affinity of cryopyrin for ASC or rendering the protein more labile, so that minor stimuli (such as cold temperatures) release the LRR-mediated autoinhibition. Such mutations may be considered gain-of-function genetic changes, consistent with the dominant inheritance patterns observed in the cryopyrinopathies.

Multiple substitutions at residues 260, 264, 303, 436, 439, and 523 exist. Only limited genotype–phenotype correlations can be made, as disease severity does not segregate among clusters of mutations. Although D303G/N, Q306L, and F309S are associated with NOMID/CINCA, L305P is associated with FCAS.

Strategies for Diagnosis

Similar to FMF, the diagnosis of these disorders is often a combination of clinical observations and genetic testing. For FCAS, a clinical diagnosis may be established by the presence of at least four of the following: fever and rash induced by generalized cold exposure, short (<24 hour) episodes, autosomal dominant inheritance, age of onset <6 months, conjunctivitis during attacks, and absence of deafness, periorbital edema, lymphadenopathy, and serositis (Johnstone et al., 2003). Longer episodes, hearing loss, lack of association with cold temperatures, and amyloidosis are more suggestive of MWS (Muckle, 1979), whereas aseptic meningitis, uveitis, and the characteristic arthropathy support the di-

agnosis of NOMID/CINCA (Hashkes and Lovell, 1997; Prieur, 2001; Neven et al., 2004). Genetic testing can provide an unequivocal diagnosis, if positive. However, the sensitivity is not 100%, and in fact only about half of patients meeting clinical criteria for NOMID/CINCA have demonstrable mutations in *CIAS1* (Aksentijevich et al., 2002; Neven et al., 2004). Possibly, *CIAS1* mutation-negative patients have defects in related genes. A positive genotyping result also may not distinguish among the three conditions, as several mutations are shared by more than one disease entity (Hoffman et al., 2001a; Aganna et al., 2002a; Aksentijevich et al., 2002; Dodé et al., 2002c; Feldmann et al., 2002; Granel et al., 2003; Rösen-Wolff et al., 2003; Neven et al., 2004).

Mode of Inheritance, Carrier Detection, Prenatal Diagnosis

CIAS1 mutations are inherited in an autosomal dominant fashion, a pattern recognized early in families with FCAS and MWS (Kile and Rusk, 1940; Muckle and Wells, 1962; Johnstone et al., 2003). The inheritance pattern for NOMID/CINCA is less clear, as patients have reduced reproductive potential. Most cases are sporadic, resulting from de novo mutations in children of healthy individuals, although a small number of familial cases have been documented (Feldmann et al., 2002).

Thus far, most mutations in *CIAS1* show a high degree of penetrance, such that carriers nearly always show some clinical manifestations. Disease severity may vary extensively, even among individuals harboring the same mutations, indicating that other factors influence phenotype. Findings in some patients blur the boundaries between diagnoses, with some features of FCAS, such as cold sensitivity, and other findings consistent with MWS, such as amyloid nephropathy (Hoffman et al., 2001a; Aganna et al., 2002a; Dodé et al., 2002c; Neven et al., 2004). Other patients may represent an overlap between MWS and NOMID/CINCA at the more severe end of the phenotypic continuum (Lieberman et al., 1998; Aksentijevich et al., 2002; Dodé et al., 2002c; Feldmann et al., 2002; Granel et al., 2003; Rösen-Wolff et al., 2003; Neven et al., 2004).

Recurrence risks to siblings depend on whether the mutation in the proband is de novo. If it is, then it is highly unlikely that another such event will occur, and hence the recurrence risk is low. However, if the affected child has inherited the mutation from either parent, then there is a 50% chance that any further child from that parent will also carry the mutation. Again, it should be noted that family members with the same mutations may not exhibit all the same signs and symptoms with equal severity.

Treatment and Prognosis

Patients with the cryopyrinopathies generally do not respond well to colchicine (Hoffman et al., 2001b). Corticosteroids are helpful in some cases, but carry a high risk of side effects and often have minimal effect on the arthropathy or central nervous system manifestations of NOMID/CINCA (Hashkes and Lovell, 1997; Prieur, 2001). Nonsteroidal anti-inflammatory drugs offer some relief for arthralgias and constitutional symptoms but do little to control overall inflammation. Recently, promising results have been obtained with the IL-1β receptor antagonist, anakinra (Dailey et al., 2004; Hawkins et al., 2004a, 2004b; Hoffman et al., 2004). Patients with FCAS and MWS reported essentially complete remission of all disease symptoms (Hoffman et al., 2004). NOMID/CINCA-induced uveitis, rash, and fever resolved and patients' cerebrospinal pressure dropped significantly at anakinra doses of 1–2 mg/kg per day (Dailey et al., 2004). It will be important to follow children with NOMID/CINCA on anakinra to observe long-term academic performance and physical growth, as well as to determine whether very early treatment can avert joint deformities.

Untreated, FCAS appears not to be associated with long-term sequelae, save for one report of renal amyloidosis occurring late in life (Hoffman et al., 2001b). Prognosis in MWS patients is highly dependent on the development of amyloidosis, which occurs in approximately one-third of individuals. Many patients with MWS develop significant bilateral sensorineural deafness. Patients with NOMID/CINCA often have a reduced life expectancy; currently, about 20% die before the age of 20 of infection or amyloidosis (Prieur et al., 1987; Hashkes and Lovell, 1997). Morbidities include intellectual impairment, vision loss, sensorineural hearing loss, and physical disability due to contractures.

Early and continued treatment with anakinra may reduce the risk of developing amyloidosis in both MWS and NOMID/CINCA patients, possibly averting or delaying renal failure and the attendant complications. The role of IL-1 inhibition in reversing preexisting deficits will probably depend on the circumstances. Since amyloidosis is thought to involve an equilibrium between deposition and resorption, it is possible that aggressive treatment soon after the discovery of proteinuria could prevent the progression to renal failure, but later intervention may not be as successful. A similar logic may apply to the hearing loss associated with MWS and NOMID/CINCA.

Animal Models

As yet, no animal models for the cryopyrinopathies have been reported. However, four groups recently reported the production of cryopyrin knockout mice (Kanneganti et al., 2006; Mariathasan et al., 2006; Martinon et al., 2006; Sutterwala et al. 2006). These animals confirm the importance of cryopyrin for caspase-1 and IL-1β activation in response to a number of stimuli, including LPS, bacterial RNA, *Staphylococcus aureus*, *Listeria monocytogenes*, and monosodium urate crystals.

References

Aganna E, Aksentijevich I, Hitman GA, et al. Tumor necrosis factor receptor–associated periodic syndrome (TRAPS) in a Dutch family: evidence for a *TNFRSF1A* mutation with reduced penetrance. Eur J Hum Genet 9:63–66, 2001.

Aganna E, Hammond L, Hawkins PN, et al. Heterogeneity among patients with tumor necrosis factor receptor–associated periodic syndrome phenotypes. Arthritis Rheum 48:2632–2644, 2003.

Aganna E, Hawkins PN, Ozen S, et al. Allelic variants in genes associated with hereditary periodic fever syndromes as susceptibility factors for reactive systemic AA amyloidosis. Genes Immun 5:289–293, 2004.

Aganna E, Martinon F, Hawkins PN, et al. Association of mutations in the *NALP3/CIAS1/PYPAF1* gene with a broad phenotype including recurrent fever, cold sensitivity, sensorineural deafness, and AA amyloidosis. Arthritis Rheum 46:2445–2452, 2002a.

Aganna E, Zeharia A, Hitman GA, et al. An Israeli Arab patient with a de novo *TNFRSF1A* mutation causing tumor necrosis factor receptor–associated periodic syndrome. Arthritis Rheum 46:245–249, 2002b.

Agostini L, Martinon F, Burns K, et al. NALP3 forms an IL-1β-processing inflammasome with increased activity in Muckle-Wells autoinflammatory disorder. Immunity 20:319–325, 2004.

Akar N, Akar E, Yalçinkaya F. E148Q of the *MEFV* gene causes amyloidosis in familial Mediterranean fever patients. Pediatrics 108:215, 2001.

Akar N, Hasipek M, Akar E, et al. Serum amyloid A1 and tumor necrosis factor-alpha alleles in Turkish familial Mediterranean fever patients with and without amyloidosis. Amyloid 10:12–16, 2003.

Akar N, Misiroglu M, Yalçinkaya F, et al. MEFV mutations in Turkish patients suffering from familial Mediterranean fever. Hum Mutat 15:118–119, 2000.

Akarsu AN, Saatçi Ü, Ozen S, et al. Genetic linkage study of familial Mediterranean fever (FMF) to 16p13.3 and evidence for genetic heterogeneity in the Turkish population. J Med Genet 34:573–578, 1997.

Aksentijevich I, Galon J, Soares M, et al. The tumor-necrosis-factor receptor–associated periodic syndrome: new mutations in *TNFRSF1A*, ancestral origins, genotype–phenotype studies, and evidence for further genetic heterogeneity of periodic fevers. Am J Hum Genet 69:301–314, 2001.

Aksentijevich I, Nowak M, Mallah M, et al. De novo CIAS1 mutations, cytokine activation, and evidence for genetic heterogeneity in patients with neonatal-onset multisystem inflammatory disease (NOMID): a new member of the expanding family of pyrin-associated autoinflammatory diseases. Arthritis Rheum 46:3340–3348, 2002.

Aksentijevich I, Torosyan Y, Samuels J, et al. Mutation and haplotype studies of familial Mediterranean fever reveal new ancestral relationships and evidence for a high carrier frequency with reduced penetrance in the Ashkenazi Jewish population. Am J Hum Genet 64:949–962, 1999.

Altiparmak MR, Pamuk ON, Pamuk GE, et al. Colchicine neuromyopathy: a report of six cases. Clin Exp Rheumatol 20:S13–16, 2002.

Arostegui JI, Aldea A, Modesto C, et al. Clinical and genetic heterogeneity among Spanish patients with recurrent autoinflammatory syndromes associated with the CIAS1/PYPAF1/NALP3 gene. Arthritis Rheum 50:4045–4050, 2004.

Azizi E, Fisher BK. Cutaneous manifestations of familial Mediterranean fever. Arch Dermatol 112:364–366, 1976.

Barakat MH, El-Khawad AO, Gumaa KA, et al. Metaraminol provocative test: a specific diagnostic test for familial Mediterranean fever. Lancet 1:656–657, 1984.

Bar-Eli M, Ehrenfeld M, Levy M, et al. Leukocyte chemotaxis in recurrent polyserositis (familial Mediterranean fever). Am J Med Sci 281:15–18, 1981.

Barzilai A, Langevitz P, Goldberg I, et al. Erysipelas-like erythema of familial Mediterranean fever: clinicopathologic correlation. J Am Acad Dermatol 42:791–795, 2000.

Bazzoni F, Beutler B. The tumor necrosis factor ligand and receptor families. N Engl J Med 334:1717–1725, 1996.

Ben-Chetrit E, Backenroth R. Amyloidosis induced, end stage renal disease in patients with familial Mediterranean fever is highly associated with point mutations in the *MEFV* gene. Ann Rheum Dis 60:146–149, 2001.

Ben-Chetrit E, Backenroth R, Haimov-Kochman R, et al. Azoospermia in familial Mediterranean fever patients: the role of colchicine and amyloidosis. Ann Rheum Dis 57:259–260, 1998.

Ben-Chetrit E, Ben-Chetrit A. Familial Mediterranean fever and menstruation. BJOG 108:403–407, 2001.

Ben-Chetrit E, Lerer I, Malamud E, et al. The *E148Q* mutation in the MEFV gene: is it a disease-causing mutation or a sequence variant? Hum Mutat 15:385–386, 2000.

Ben-Chetrit E, Levy M. Colchicine: 1998 update. Semin Arthritis Rheum 28:48–59, 1998a.

Ben-Chetrit E, Levy M. Familial Mediterranean fever. Lancet 351:659–664, 1998b.

Ben-Chetrit E, Levy M. Does the lack of the P-glycoprotein efflux pump in neutrophils explain the efficacy of colchicine in familial Mediterranean fever and other inflammatory diseases? Med Hypotheses 51:377–380, 1998c.

Ben-Chetrit E, Levy M. Reproductive system in familial Mediterranean fever: an overview. Ann Rheum Dis 62:916–919, 2003.

Ben-Chetrit E, Scherrmann JM, Levy M. Colchicine in breast milk of patients with familial Mediterranean fever. Arthritis Rheum 39:1213–1217, 1996.

Bergman F, Warmenius S. Familial perireticular amyloidosis in a Swedish family. Am J Med 45:601–606, 1968.

Bertin J, DiStefano PS. The PYRIN domain: a novel motif found in apoptosis and inflammation proteins. Cell Death Differ 7:1273–1274, 2000.

Bonnel RA, Villalba ML, Karwoski CB, et al. Deaths associated with inappropriate intravenous colchicine administration. J Emerg Med 22:385–387, 2002.

Boom BW, Daha MR, Vermeer BJ, et al. IgD immune complex vasculitis in a patient with hyperimmunoglobulinemia D and periodic fever. Arch Dermatol 126:1621–1624, 1990.

Booth DR, Gillmore JD, Lachmann HJ, et al. The genetic basis of autosomal dominant familial Mediterranean fever. Q J Med 93:217–221, 2000.

Brauman A, Gilboa Y. Recurrent pulmonary atelectasis as a manifestation of familial Mediterranean fever. Arch Intern Med 147:378–379, 1987.

Brik R, Shinawi M, Kasinetz L, et al. The musculoskeletal manifestations of familial Mediterranean fever in children genetically diagnosed with the disease. Arthritis Rheum 44:1416–1419, 2001.

Brik R, Shinawi M, Kepten I, et al. Familial Mediterranean fever: clinical and genetic characterization in a mixed pediatric population of Jewish and Arab patients. Pediatrics 103:e70, 1999.

Brodey PA, Wolff SM. Radiographic changes in the sacroiliac joints in familial Mediterranean fever. Radiology 114:331–333, 1975.

Brown MS, Goldstein JL. The SREBP pathway: regulation of cholesterol metabolism by proteolysis of a membrane-bound transcription factor. Cell 89:331–340, 1997.

Buades J, Bassa A, Altes J, et al. The metaraminol test and adverse cardiac effects. Ann Intern Med 111:259–260, 1989.

Calguneri M, Apras S, Ozbalkan Z, et al. The efficacy of interferon-alpha in a patient with resistant familial Mediterranean fever complicated by polyarteritis nodosa. Intern Med 43:612–614, 2004a.

Calguneri M, Apras S, Ozbalkan Z, et al. The efficacy of continuous interferon alpha administration as an adjunctive agent to colchicine-resistant familial Mediterranean fever patients. Clin Exp Rheumatol 22:S41–44, 2004b.

Cattan D, Dervichian M, Courillon A, et al. Metaraminol provocation test for familial Mediterranean fever. Lancet 1:1130–1131, 1984.

Cazeneuve C, Ajrapetyan H, Papin S, et al. Identification of *MEFV*-independent modifying genetic factors for familial Mediterranean fever. Am J Hum Genet 67:1136–1143, 2000.

Cazeneuve C, Hovannesyan Z, Genevieve D, et al. Familial Mediterranean fever among patients from Karabakh and the diagnostic value of *MEFV* gene analysis in all classically affected populations. Arthritis Rheum 48:2324–2331, 2003.

Cazeneuve C, Sarkisian T, Pêcheux C, et al. *MEFV*-gene analysis in Armenian patients with familial Mediterranean fever: diagnostic value and unfavorable renal prognosis of the M694V homozygous genotype–genetic and therapeutic implications. Am J Hum Genet 65:88–97, 1999.

Centola M, Wood G, Frucht DM, et al. The gene for familial Mediterranean fever, *MEFV*, is expressed in early leukocyte development and is regulated in response to inflammatory mediators. Blood 95:3223–3231, 2000.

Chae JJ, Komarow HD, Cheng J, et al. Targeted disruption of pyrin, the FMF protein, causes heightened sensitivity to endotoxin and a defect in macrophage apoptosis. Mol Cell 11:591–604, 2003.

Chamaillard M, Girardin SE, Viala J, et al. Nods, Nalps and Naip: intracellular regulators of bacterial-induced inflammation. Cell Microbiol 5:581–592, 2003.

Chan FK, Chun HJ, Zheng L, et al. A domain in TNF receptors that mediates ligand-independent receptor assembly and signaling. Science 288:2351–2354, 2000.

Commerford PJ, Meyers OL. Arthropathy associated with familial cold urticaria. S Afr Med J 51:105–108, 1977.

Cronstein BN, Molad Y, Reibman J, et al. Colchicine alters the quantitative and qualitative display of selectins on endothelial cells and neutrophils. J Clin Invest 96:994–1002, 1995.

Cuisset L, Drenth JP, Berthelot JM, et al. Genetic linkage of the Muckle-Wells syndrome to chromosome 1q44. Am J Hum Genet 65:1054–1059, 1999.

Cuisset L, Drenth JP, Simon A, et al. Molecular analysis of *MVK* mutations and enzymatic activity in hyper-IgD and periodic fever syndrome. Eur J Hum Genet 9:260–266, 2001.

Dailey NJ, Aksentijevich I, Chae JJ, et al. Interleukin-1 receptor antagonist anakinra in the treatment of neonatal onset multisystem inflammatory disease. Arthritis Rheum 50:S440, 2004.

Deltas CC, Mean R, Rossou E, et al. Familial Mediterranean fever (FMF) mutations occur frequently in the Greek-Cypriot population of Cyprus. Genet Test 6:15–21, 2002.

Dewalle M, Domingo C, Rozenbaum M, et al. Phenotype–genotype correlation in Jewish patients suffering from familial Mediterranean fever (FMF). Eur J Hum Genet 6:95–97, 1998.

Diaz A, Hu C, Kastner DL, et al. Lipopolysaccharide-induced expression of multiple alternatively spliced MEFV transcripts in human synovial fibroblasts: a prominent splice isoform lacks the C-terminal domain that is highly mutated in familial Mediterranean fever. Arthritis Rheum 50:3679–3689, 2004.

Dinarello CA, Chusid MJ, Fauci AS, et al. Effect of prophylactic colchicine therapy on leukocyte function in patients with familial Mediterranean fever. Arthritis Rheum 19:618–622, 1976.

Dinarello CA, Wolff SM, Goldfinger SE, et al. Colchicine therapy for familial mediterranean fever. A double-blind trial. N Engl J Med 291:934–937, 1974.

Dodé C, André M, Bienvenu T, et al. The enlarging clinical, genetic, and population spectrum of tumor necrosis factor receptor–associated periodic syndrome. Arthritis Rheum 46:2181–2188, 2002a.

Dodé C, Hazenberg BP, Pêcheux C, et al. Mutational spectrum in the *MEFV* and *TNFRSF1A* genes in patients suffering from AA amyloidosis and

recurrent inflammatory attacks. Nephrol Dial Transplant 17:1212–1217, 2002b.

Dodé C, Le Du N, Cuisset L, et al. New mutations of *CIAS1* that are responsible for Muckle-Wells syndrome and familial cold urticaria: a novel mutation underlies both syndromes. Am J Hum Genet 70:1498–1506, 2002c.

Dodé C, Papo T, Fieschi C, et al. A novel missense mutation (C30S) in the gene encoding tumor necrosis factor receptor 1 linked to autosomal-dominant recurrent fever with localized myositis in a French family. Arthritis Rheum 43:1535–1542, 2000a.

Dodé C, Pêcheux C, Cazeneuve C, et al. Mutations in the *MEFV* gene in a large series of patients with a clinical diagnosis of familial Mediterranean fever. Am J Med Genet 92:241–246, 2000b.

Dollfus H, Hafner R, Hofmann HM, et al. Chronic infantile neurological cutaneous and articular/neonatal onset multisystem inflammatory disease syndrome: ocular manifestations in a recently recognized chronic inflammatory disease of childhood. Arch Ophthalmol 118:1386–1392, 2000.

Domingo C, Touitou I, Bayou A, et al. Familial Mediterranean fever in the 'Chuetas' of Mallorca: a question of Jewish origin or genetic heterogeneity. Eur J Hum Genet 8:242–246, 2000.

D'Osualdo A, Picco P, Caroli F, et al. *MVK* mutations and associated clinical features in Italian patients affected with autoinflammatory disorders and recurrent fever. Eur J Hum Genet 13:314–320, 2005.

Dowds TA, Masumoto J, Chen FF, et al. Regulation of cryopyrin/Pypaf1 signaling by pyrin, the familial Mediterranean fever gene product. Biochem Biophys Res Commun 302:575–580, 2003.

Drenth JP, Boom BW, Toonstra J, et al. Cutaneous manifestations and histologic findings in the hyperimmunoglobulinemia D syndrome. International Hyper IgD Study Group. Arch Dermatol 130:59–65, 1994a.

Drenth JP, Cuisset L, Grateau G, et al. Mutations in the gene encoding mevalonate kinase cause hyper-IgD and periodic fever syndrome. International Hyper-IgD Study Group. Nat Genet 22:178–181, 1999.

Drenth JP, Haagsma CJ, van der Meer JW. Hyperimmunoglobulinemia D and periodic fever syndrome. The clinical spectrum in a series of 50 patients. International Hyper-IgD Study Group. Medicine (Baltimore) 73:133–144, 1994b.

Drenth JP, Mariman EC, Van der Velde-Visser SD, et al. Location of the gene causing hyperimmunoglobulinemia D and periodic fever syndrome differs from that for familial Mediterranean fever. International Hyper-IgD Study Group. Hum Genet 94:616–620, 1994c.

Drenth JP, Powell RJ, Brown NS, et al. Interferon-gamma and urine neopterin in attacks of the hyperimmunoglobulinaemia D and periodic fever syndrome. Eur J Clin Invest 25:683–686, 1995.

Drenth JP, Prieur AM. Occurrence of arthritis in hyperimmunoglobulinaemia D. Ann Rheum Dis 52:765–766, 1993.

Drenth JP, van der Meer JW. Hereditary periodic fever. N Engl J Med 345:1748–1757, 2001.

Drenth JP, Vonk AG, Simon A, et al. Limited efficacy of thalidomide in the treatment of febrile attacks of the hyper-IgD and periodic fever syndrome: a randomized, double-blind, placebo-controlled trial. J Pharmacol Exp Ther 298:1221–1226, 2001.

Drewe E, Huggins ML, Morgan AG, et al. Treatment of renal amyloidosis with etanercept in tumour necrosis factor receptor–associated periodic syndrome. Rheumatology (Oxford) 43:1405–1408, 2004.

Drewe E, Lanyon PC, Powell RJ. Emerging clinical spectrum of tumor necrosis factor receptor–associated periodic syndrome: comment on the articles by Hull et al. and Dodé et al. Arthritis Rheum 48:1768–1769; author reply 1769–1770, 2003a.

Drewe E, McDermott EM, Powell RJ. Treatment of the nephrotic syndrome with etanercept in patients with the tumor necrosis factor receptor–associated periodic syndrome. N Engl J Med 343:1044–1045, 2000.

Drewe E, McDermott EM, Powell PT, et al. Prospective study of anti-tumour necrosis factor receptor superfamily 1B fusion protein, and case study of anti-tumour necrosis factor receptor superfamily 1A fusion protein, in tumour necrosis factor receptor–associated periodic syndrome (TRAPS): clinical and laboratory findings in a series of seven patients. Rheumatology (Oxford) 42:235–239, 2003b.

Duzova A, Bakkaloglu A, Besbas N, et al. Role of A-SAA in monitoring subclinical inflammation and in colchicine dosage in familial Mediterranean fever. Clin Exp Rheumatol 21:509–514, 2003.

Eliakim M, Levy M, Ehrenfeld M. Laboratory examinations. In: Recurrent Polyserositis (familial Mediterranean Fever, Periodic Disease). Amsterdam: Elsevier, North Holland, pp. 87–95, 1981.

Eliezer D. Folding pyrin into the family. Structure (Camb) 11:1190–1191, 2003.

Engelmann H, Holtmann H, Brakebusch C, et al. Antibodies to a soluble form of a tumor necrosis factor (TNF) receptor have TNF-like activity. J Biol Chem 265:14497–14504, 1990.

Fairbrother WJ, Gordon NC, Humke EW, et al. The PYRIN domain: a member of the death domain-fold superfamily. Protein Sci 10:1911–1918, 2001.

Feldmann J, Prieur AM, Quartier P, et al. Chronic infantile neurological cutaneous and articular syndrome is caused by mutations in *CIAS1*, a gene highly expressed in polymorphonuclear cells and chondrocytes. Am J Hum Genet 71:198–203, 2002.

Fradkin A, Yahav J, Zemer D, et al. Colchicine-induced lactose malabsorption in patients with familial Mediterranean fever. Isr J Med Sci 31:616–620, 1995.

French FMF Consortium. A candidate gene for familial Mediterranean fever. Nat Genet 17:25–31, 1997.

Frenkel J, Houten SM, Waterham HR, et al. Mevalonate kinase deficiency and Dutch type periodic fever. Clin Exp Rheumatol 18:525–532, 2000.

Frenkel J, Houten SM, Waterham HR, et al. Clinical and molecular variability in childhood periodic fever with hyperimmunoglobulinaemia D. Rheumatology (Oxford) 40:579–584, 2001a.

Frenkel J, Rijkers GT, Mandey SH, et al. Lack of isoprenoid products raises ex vivo interleukin-1beta secretion in hyperimmunoglobulinemia D and periodic fever syndrome. Arthritis Rheum 46:2794–2803, 2002.

Frenkel J, van Kempen MJ, Kuis W, et al. Variant chronic infantile neurologic, cutaneous, articular syndrome due to a mutation within the leucine-rich repeat domain of CIAS1. Arthritis Rheum 50:2719–2720, 2004.

Frenkel J, Willemsen MA, Weemaes CM, et al. Increased urinary leukotriene E(4) during febrile attacks in the hyperimmunoglobulinaemia D and periodic fever syndrome. Arch Dis Child 85:158–159, 2001b.

Fuchs P, Strehl S, Dworzak M, et al. Structure of the human TNF receptor 1 (p60) gene (TNFR1) and localization to chromosome 12p13 [corrected]. Genomics 13:219–224, 1992.

Gadallah MF, Vasquez F, Abreo F, et al. A 38-year-old man with nephrotic syndrome, episodic fever and abdominal pain. J LA State Med Soc 147:493–499, 1995.

Galon J, Aksentijevich I, McDermott MF, et al. *TNFRSF1A* mutations and autoinflammatory syndromes. Curr Opin Immunol 12:479–486, 2000.

Gedalia A, Adar A, Gorodischer R. Familial Mediterranean fever in children. J Rheumatol Suppl 35:1–9, 1992.

Gershoni-Baruch R, Brik R, Shinawi M, et al. The differential contribution of *MEFV* mutant alleles to the clinical profile of familial Mediterranean fever. Eur J Hum Genet 10:145–149, 2002.

Gershoni-Baruch R, Brik R, Zacks N, et al. The contribution of genotypes at the *MEFV* and *SAA1* loci to amyloidosis and disease severity in patients with familial Mediterranean fever. Arthritis Rheum 48:1149–1155, 2003.

Gershoni-Baruch R, Shinawi M, Leah K, et al. Familial Mediterranean fever: prevalence, penetrance and genetic drift. Eur J Hum Genet 9:634–637, 2001.

Gertz MA, Petitt RM, Perrault J, et al. Autosomal dominant familial Mediterranean fever-like syndrome with amyloidosis. Mayo Clin Proc 62:1095–1100, 1987.

Gillmore JD, Lovat LB, Persey MR, et al. Amyloid load and clinical outcome in AA amyloidosis in relation to circulating concentration of serum amyloid A protein. Lancet 358:24–29, 2001.

Girardin SE, Boneca IG, Viala J, et al. Nod2 is a general sensor of peptidoglycan through muramyl dipeptide (MDP) detection. J Biol Chem 278:8869–8872, 2003.

Goldfinger SE. Colchicine for familial Mediterranean fever. N Engl J Med 287:1302, 1972.

Goldstein JL, Brown MS. Regulation of the mevalonate pathway. Nature 343:425–430, 1990.

Goldstein RC, Schwabe AD. Prophylactic colchicine therapy in familial Mediterranean fever. A controlled, double-blind study. Ann Intern Med 81:792–794, 1974.

Granel B, Philip N, Serratrice J, et al. *CIAS1* mutation in a patient with overlap between Muckle-Wells and chronic infantile neurological cutaneous and articular syndromes. Dermatology 206:257–259, 2003.

Gruberg L, Har-Zahav Y, Agranat O, et al. Acute myopathy induced by colchicine in a cyclosporine treated heart transplant recipient: possible role of the multidrug resistance transporter. Transplant Proc 31:2157–2158, 1999.

Gullberg U, Lantz M, Lindvall L, et al. Involvement of an Asn/Val cleavage site in the production of a soluble form of a human tumor necrosis factor (TNF) receptor. Site-directed mutagenesis of a putative cleavage site in the p55 TNF receptor chain. Eur J Cell Biol 58:307–312, 1992.

Gumucio DL, Diaz A, Schaner P, et al. Fire and ICE: the role of pyrin domain–containing proteins in inflammation and apoptosis. Clin Exp Rheumatol 20:S45–53, 2002.

Haraldsson A, Weemaes CM, De Boer AW, et al. Immunological studies in the hyper-immunoglobulin D syndrome. J Clin Immunol 12:424–428, 1992.

Harton JA, Linhoff MW, Zhang J, et al. Cutting edge: CATERPILLER: a large family of mammalian genes containing CARD, pyrin, nucleotide-binding, and leucine-rich repeat domains. J Immunol 169:4088–4093, 2002.

Hashkes PJ, Lovell DJ. Recognition of infantile-onset multisystem inflammatory disease as a unique entity. J Pediatr 130:513–515, 1997.

Hassink SG, Goldsmith DP. Neonatal onset multisystem inflammatory disease. Arthritis Rheum 26:668–673, 1983.

Hawkins PN, Bybee A, Aganna E, et al. Response to anakinra in a de novo case of neonatal-onset multisystem inflammatory disease. Arthritis Rheum 50:2708–2709, 2004a.

Hawkins PN, Lachmann HJ, Aganna E, et al. Spectrum of clinical features in Muckle-Wells syndrome and response to anakinra. Arthritis Rheum 50:607–612, 2004b.

Hawle H, Winckelmann G, Kortsik CS. Familial Mediterranean fever in a German family [in German]. Dtsch Med Wochenschr 114:665–668, 1989.

Heller H, Gafni J, Michaeli D, et al. The arthritis of familial Mediterranean fever (FMF). Arthritis Rheum 9:1–17, 1966.

Heller H, Sohar E, Sherf L. Familial Mediterranean fever. AMA Arch Intern Med 102:50–71, 1958.

Hiemstra I, Vossen JM, van der Meer JW, et al. Clinical and immunological studies in patients with an increased serum IgD level. J Clin Immunol 9:393–400, 1989.

Hiller S, Kohl A, Fiorito F, et al. NMR structure of the apoptosis- and inflammation-related NALP1 pyrin domain. Structure (Camb) 11:1199–1205, 2003.

Hoffman HM, Gregory SG, Mueller JL, et al. Fine structure mapping of *CIAS1*: identification of an ancestral haplotype and a common FCAS mutation, L353P. Hum Genet 112:209–216, 2003.

Hoffman HM, Mueller JL, Broide DH, et al. Mutation of a new gene encoding a putative pyrin-like protein causes familial cold autoinflammatory syndrome and Muckle-Wells syndrome. Nat Genet 29:301–305, 2001a.

Hoffman HM, Rosengren S, Boyle DL, et al. Prevention of cold-associated acute inflammation in familial cold autoinflammatory syndrome by interleukin-1 receptor antagonist. Lancet 364:1779–1785, 2004.

Hoffman HM, Wanderer AA, Broide DH. Familial cold autoinflammatory syndrome: phenotype and genotype of an autosomal dominant periodic fever. J Allergy Clin Immunol 108:615–620, 2001b.

Hoffman HM, Wright FA, Broide DH, et al. Identification of a locus on chromosome 1q44 for familial cold urticaria. Am J Hum Genet 66:1693–1698, 2000.

Hoffmann G, Gibson KM, Brandt IK, et al. Mevalonic aciduria—an inborn error of cholesterol and nonsterol isoprene biosynthesis. N Engl J Med 314:1610–1614, 1986.

Hoffmann GF, Charpentier C, Mayatepek E, et al. Clinical and biochemical phenotype in 11 patients with mevalonic aciduria. Pediatrics 91:915–921, 1993.

Horiuchi T, Tsukamoto H, Mitoma H, et al. Novel mutations in *TNFRSF1A* in patients with typical tumor necrosis factor receptor–associated periodic syndrome and with systemic lupus erythematosus in Japanese. Int J Mol Med 14:813–818, 2004.

Houten SM, Frenkel J, Rijkers GT, et al. Temperature dependence of mutant mevalonate kinase activity as a pathogenic factor in hyper-IgD and periodic fever syndrome. Hum Mol Genet 11:3115–3124, 2002.

Houten SM, Koster J, Romeijn GJ, et al. Organization of the mevalonate kinase (MVK) gene and identification of novel mutations causing mevalonic aciduria and hyperimmunoglobulinaemia D and periodic fever syndrome. Eur J Hum Genet 9:253–259, 2001.

Houten SM, Kuis W, Duran M, et al. Mutations in *MVK*, encoding mevalonate kinase, cause hyperimmunoglobulinaemia D and periodic fever syndrome. Nat Genet 22:175–177, 1999.

Houten SM, van Woerden CS, Wijburg FA, et al. Carrier frequency of the V377I (1129G > A) MVK mutation, associated with hyper-IgD and periodic fever syndrome, in the Netherlands. Eur J Hum Genet 11:196–200, 2003.

Hsu H, Xiong J, Goeddel DV. The TNF receptor 1–associated protein TRADD signals cell death and NF-κB activation. Cell 81:495–504, 1995.

Huggins ML, Radford PM, McIntosh RS, et al. Shedding of mutant tumor necrosis factor receptor superfamily 1A associated with tumor necrosis factor receptor–associated periodic syndrome: differences between cell types. Arthritis Rheum 50:2651–2659, 2004.

Hull KM, Aksentijevich I, Singh HK. Efficacy of etanercept for the treatment of patients with TNF receptor–associated periodic syndrome (TRAPS). Arthritis Rheum 46:S378(Abstract), 2002a.

Hull KM, Drewe E, Aksentijevich I, et al. The TNF receptor–associated periodic syndrome (TRAPS): emerging concepts of an autoinflammatory disorder. Medicine (Baltimore) 81:349–368, 2002b.

Hull KM, Kastner DL, Balow JE. Hereditary periodic fever. N Engl J Med 346:1415–1416; author reply 1415–1416, 2002c.

Hull KM, Shoham N, Chae JJ, et al. The expanding spectrum of systemic autoinflammatory disorders and their rheumatic manifestations. Curr Opin Rheumatol 15:61–69, 2003.

Hull KM, Wong K, Wood GM, et al. Monocytic fasciitis: a newly recognized clinical feature of tumor necrosis factor receptor dysfunction. Arthritis Rheum 46:2189–2194, 2002d.

Ince E, Çakar N, Tekin M, et al. Arthritis in children with familial Mediterranean fever. Rheumatol Int 21:213–217, 2002.

Inohara N, Nuñez G. Genes with homology to mammalian apoptosis regulators identified in zebrafish. Cell Death Differ 7:509–510, 2000.

Inohara N, Ogura Y, Nuñez G. Nods: a family of cytosolic proteins that regulate the host response to pathogens. Curr Opin Microbiol 5:76–80, 2002.

International FMF Consortium. Ancient missense mutations in a new member of the *RoRet* gene family are likely to cause familial Mediterranean fever. Cell 90:797–807, 1997.

Jadoul M, Dodé C, Cosyns JP, et al. Autosomal-dominant periodic fever with AA amyloidosis: novel mutation in tumor necrosis factor receptor 1 gene rapid communication. Kidney Int 59:1677–1682, 2001.

Janeway TC, Mosenthal HO. An unusual paroxysmal syndrome, probably allied to recurrent vomiting, with a study of the nitrogen metablolism. Trans Assoc Am Physicians 23:504–518, 1908.

Johnstone RF, Dolen WK, Hoffman HM. A large kindred with familial cold autoinflammatory syndrome. Ann Allergy Asthma Immunol 90:233–237, 2003.

Kallinich T, Briese S, Roesler J, et al. Two familial cases with tumor necrosis factor receptor–associated periodic syndrome caused by a non-cysteine mutation (T50M) in the *TNFRSF1A* gene associated with severe multiorganic amyloidosis. J Rheumatol 31:2519–2522, 2004.

Kanneganti TD, Özören N, Body-Malapel M, et al. Bacterial RNA and small antiviral compounds activate caspase-1 through cryopyrin/NALP3. Nature 440:233–236, 2006.

Karenko L, Pettersson T, Roberts P. Autosomal dominant 'Mediterranean fever' in a Finnish family. J Intern Med 232:365–369, 1992.

Kastner DL, Aksentijevich I, Galon J. TNF receptor associated periodic syndrome (TRAPS): novel TNFR1 mutations and early experience with etanercept therapy. Arthritis Rheum 42:S117(Abstract), 1999.

Kaufman RA, Lovell DJ. Infantile-onset multisystem inflammatory disease: radiologic findings. Radiology 160:741–746, 1986.

Kees S, Langevitz P, Zemer D, et al. Attacks of pericarditis as a manifestation of familial Mediterranean fever (FMF). Q J Med 90:643–647, 1997.

Kelley RI. Inborn errors of cholesterol biosynthesis. Adv Pediatr 47:1–53, 2000.

Kelley RI, Takada I. Hereditary periodic fever. N Engl J Med 346: 1415–1416; author reply 1415–1416, 2002.

Kile RM, Rusk HA. A case of cold urticaria with an unusual family history. JAMA 114:1067–1068, 1940.

Klasen IS, Goertz JH, van de Wiel GA, et al. Hyper-immunoglobulin A in the hyperimmunoglobulinemia D syndrome. Clin Diagn Lab Immunol 8: 58–61, 2001.

Kogan A, Shinar Y, Lidar M, et al. Common MEFV mutations among Jewish ethnic groups in Israel: high frequency of carrier and phenotype III states and absence of a perceptible biological advantage for the carrier state. Am J Med Genet 102:272–276, 2001.

Koné Paut I, Dubuc M, Sportouch J, et al. Phenotype–genotype correlation in 91 patients with familial Mediterranean fever reveals a high frequency of cutaneomucous features. Rheumatology (Oxford) 39:1275–1279, 2000.

Konstantopoulos K, Kanta A, Deltas C, et al. Familial Mediterranean fever associated pyrin mutations in Greece. Ann Rheum Dis 62:479–481, 2003.

Koonin EV, Aravind L. The NACHT family—a new group of predicted NTPases implicated in apoptosis and MHC transcription activation. Trends Biochem Sci 25:223–224, 2000.

Korkmaz C, Özdogan H, Kasapçopur O, et al. Acute phase response in familial Mediterranean fever. Ann Rheum Dis 61:79–81, 2002.

Kriegel MA, Huffmeier U, Scherb E, et al. Tumor necrosis factor receptor–associated periodic syndrome characterized by a mutation affecting the cleavage site of the receptor: implications for pathogenesis. Arthritis Rheum 48:2386–2388, 2003.

Kuncl RW, Duncan G, Watson D, et al. Colchicine myopathy and neuropathy. N Engl J Med 316:1562–1568, 1987.

Lamprecht P, Moosig F, Adam-Klages S, et al. Small vessel vasculitis and relapsing panniculitis in tumour necrosis factor receptor associated periodic syndrome (TRAPS). Ann Rheum Dis 63:1518–1520, 2004.

Langevitz P, Zemer D, Livneh A, et al. Protracted febrile myalgia in patients with familial Mediterranean fever. J Rheumatol 21:1708–1709, 1994.

Langevitz P, Livneh A, Zemer D, et al. Seronegative spondyloarthropathy in familial Mediterranean fever. Semin Arthritis Rheum 27:67–72, 1997.

La Regina M, Nucera G, Diaco M, et al. Familial Mediterranean fever is no longer a rare disease in Italy. Eur J Hum Genet 11:50–56, 2003.

Lehman TJ, Hanson V, Kornreich H, et al. HLA-B27-negative sacroiliitis: a manifestation of familial Mediterranean fever in childhood. Pediatrics 61:423–426, 1978.

Lidar M, Kedem R, Langevitz P, et al. Intravenous colchicine for treatment of patients with familial Mediterranean fever unresponsive to oral colchicine. J Rheumatol 30:2620–2623, 2003.

Lieberman A, Grossman ME, Silvers DN. Muckle-Wells syndrome: case report and review of cutaneous pathology. J Am Acad Dermatol 39: 290–291, 1998.

Liepinsh E, Barbals R, Dahl E, et al. The death-domain fold of the ASC PYRIN domain, presenting a basis for PYRIN/PYRIN recognition. J Mol Biol 332:1155–1163, 2003.

Liu T, Rojas A, Ye Y, et al. Homology modeling provides insights into the binding mode of the PAAD/DAPIN/pyrin domain, a fourth member of the CARD/DD/DED domain family. Protein Sci 12:1872–1881, 2003.

Livneh A, Drenth JP, Klasen IS, et al. Familial Mediterranean fever and hyperimmunoglobulinemia D syndrome: two diseases with distinct clinical, serologic, and genetic features. J Rheumatol 24:1558–1563, 1997a.

Livneh A, Langevitz P, Pras M. Pulmonary associations in familial Mediterranean fever. Curr Opin Pulm Med 5:326–331, 1999.

Livneh A, Langevitz P, Zemer D, et al. Criteria for the diagnosis of familial Mediterranean fever. Arthritis Rheum 40:1879–1885, 1997b.

Livneh A, Madgar I, Langevitz P, et al. Recurrent episodes of acute scrotum with ischemic testicular necrosis in a patient with familial Mediterranean fever. J Urol 151:431–432, 1994a.

Livneh A, Zemer D, Langevitz P, et al. Colchicine treatment of AA amyloidosis of familial Mediterranean fever. An analysis of factors affecting outcome. Arthritis Rheum 37:1804–1811, 1994b.

Livneh A, Zemer D, Siegal B, et al. Colchicine prevents kidney transplant amyloidosis in familial Mediterranean fever. Nephron 60:418–422, 1992.

Loeliger AE, Kruize AA, Bijilsma JW, et al. Arthritis in hyperimmunoglobulinaemia D. Ann Rheum Dis 52:81, 1993.

Loetscher H, Pan YC, Lahm HW, et al. Molecular cloning and expression of the human 55 kD tumor necrosis factor receptor. Cell 61:351–359, 1990.

Mache CJ, Goriup U, Fischel-Ghodsian N, et al. Autosomal dominant familial Mediterranean fever-like syndrome. Eur J Pediatr 155:787–790, 1996.

Majeed HA, Al-Qudah AK, Qubain H, et al. The clinical patterns of myalgia in children with familial Mediterranean fever. Semin Arthritis Rheum 30: 138–143, 2000a.

Majeed HA, El-Shanti H, Al-Khateeb MS, et al. Genotype/phenotype correlations in Arab patients with familial Mediterranean fever. Semin Arthritis Rheum 31:371–376, 2002.

Majeed HA, Ghandour K, Shahin HM. The acute scrotum in Arab children with familial Mediterranean fever. Pediatr Surg Int 16:72–74, 2000b.

Majeed HA, Rawashdeh M. The clinical patterns of arthritis in children with familial Mediterranean fever. Q J Med 90:37–43, 1997.

Manji GA, Wang L, Geddes BJ, et al. PYPAF1, a PYRIN-containing Apaf1-like protein that assembles with ASC and regulates activation of NF-κB. J Biol Chem 277:11570–11575, 2002.

Mansfield E, Chae JJ, Komarow HD, et al. The familial Mediterranean fever protein, pyrin, associates with microtubules and colocalizes with actin filaments. Blood 98:851–859, 2001.

Mansour I, Delague V, Cazeneuve C, et al. Familial Mediterranean fever in Lebanon: mutation spectrum, evidence for cases in Maronites, Greek orthodoxes, Greek catholics, Syriacs and Chiites and for an association between amyloidosis and M694V and M694I mutations. Eur J Hum Genet 9:51–55, 2001.

Mariathasan S, Weiss DS, Newton K, et al. Cryopyrin activates the inflammasome in response to toxins and ATP. Nature 440:228–232, 2006.

Marshall GS, Edwards KM, Butler J, et al. Syndrome of periodic fever, pharyngitis, and aphthous stomatitis. J Pediatr 110:43–46, 1987.

Marshall GS, Edwards KM, Lawton AR. PFAPA syndrome. Pediatr Infect Dis J 8:658–659, 1989.

Martinon F, Agostini L, Meylan E, et al. Identification of bacterial muramyl dipeptide as activator of the NALP3/cryopyrin inflammasome. Curr Biol 14:1929–1934, 2004.

Martinon F, Burns K, Tschopp J. The inflammasome: a molecular platform triggering activation of inflammatory caspases and processing of proIL-β. Mol Cell 10:417–426, 2002.

Martinon F, Hofmann K, Tschopp J. The pyrin domain: a possible member of the death domain–fold family implicated in apoptosis and inflammation. Curr Biol 11:R118–120, 2001.

Martinon F, Pétrilli V, Mayor A, Tardivel A, et al. Gout-associated uric acid crystals activate the NALP3 inflammasome. Nature 440:237–241, 2006.

Martinon F, Tschopp J. Inflammatory caspases: linking an intracellular innate immune system to autoinflammatory diseases. Cell 117:561–574, 2004.

Masumoto J, Dowds TA, Schaner P, et al. ASC is an activating adaptor for NF-κB and caspase-8-dependent apoptosis. Biochem Biophys Res Commun 303:69–73, 2003.

Masumoto J, Taniguchi S, Ayukawa K, et al. ASC, a novel 22-kDa protein, aggregates during apoptosis of human promyelocytic leukemia HL-60 cells. J Biol Chem 274:33835–33838, 1999.

Matzner Y, Abedat S, Shapiro E, et al. Expression of the familial Mediterranean fever gene and activity of the C5a inhibitor in human primary fibroblast cultures. Blood 96:727–731, 2000.

McDermott EM, Smillie DM, Powell RJ. Clinical spectrum of familial Hibernian fever: a 14-year follow-up study of the index case and extended family. Mayo Clin Proc 72:806–817, 1997.

McDermott MF, Aganna E, Hitman GA, et al. An autosomal dominant periodic fever associated with AA amyloidosis in a north Indian family maps to distal chromosome 1q. Arthritis Rheum 43:2034–2040, 2000.

McDermott MF, Aksentijevich I, Galon J, et al. Germline mutations in the extracellular domains of the 55 kDa TNF receptor, TNFR1, define a family of dominantly inherited autoinflammatory syndromes. Cell 97:133–144, 1999.

McDermott MF, Ogunkolade BW, McDermott EM, et al. Linkage of familial Hibernian fever to chromosome 12p13. Am J Hum Genet 62:1446–1451, 1998.

Medlej-Hashim M, Petit I, Adib S, et al. Familial Mediterranean fever: association of elevated IgD plasma levels with specific MEFV mutations. Eur J Hum Genet 9:849–854, 2001.

Medlej-Hashim M, Rawashdeh M, Chouery E, et al. Genetic screening of fourteen mutations in Jordanian familial Mediterranean fever patients. Hum Mutat 15:384, 2000.

Meyerhoff J. Familial Mediterranean fever: report of a large family, review of the literature, and discussion of the frequency of amyloidosis. Medicine (Baltimore) 59:66–77, 1980.

Milledge J, Shaw PJ, Mansour A, et al. Allogeneic bone marrow transplantation: cure for familial Mediterranean fever. Blood 100:774–777, 2002.

Minetti EE, Minetti L. Multiple organ failure in a kidney transplant patient receiving both colchicine and cyclosporine. J Nephrol 16:421–425, 2003.

Miyagawa S, Kitamura W, Morita K, et al. Association of hyperimmunoglobulinaemia D syndrome with erythema elevatum diutinum. Br J Dermatol 128:572–574, 1993.

Mor A, Gal R, Livneh A. Abdominal and digestive system associations of familial Mediterranean fever. Am J Gastroenterol 98:2594–2604, 2003.

Muckle TJ. The 'Muckle-Wells' syndrome. Br J Dermatol 100:87–92, 1979.

Muckle TJ, Wells M. Urticaria, deafness, and amyloidosis: a new heredofamilial syndrome. Q J Med 31:235–248, 1962.

Mulley J, Saar K, Hewitt G, et al. Gene localization for an autosomal dominant familial periodic fever to 12p13. Am J Hum Genet 62:884–889, 1998.

Nevala H, Karenko L, Stjernberg S, et al. A novel mutation in the third extracellular domain of the tumor necrosis factor receptor 1 in a Finnish family with autosomal-dominant recurrent fever. Arthritis Rheum 46: 1061–1066, 2002.

Neven B, Callebaut I, Prieur A M, et al. Molecular basis of the spectral expression of CIAS1 mutations associated with phagocytic cell–mediated autoinflammatory disorders CINCA/NOMID, MWS, and FCU. Blood 103: 2809–2815, 2004.

Nigrovic PA, Sundel RP. Treatment of TRAPS with etanercept: use in pediatrics. Clin Exp Rheumatol 19:484–485, 2001.

Obici L, Manno C, Muda AO, et al. First report of systemic reactive (AA) amyloidosis in a patient with the hyperimmunoglobulinemia D with periodic fever syndrome. Arthritis Rheum 50:2966–2969, 2004.

O'Connor W Jr, Harton JA, Zhu X, et al. CIAS1/cryopyrin/PYPAF1/NALP3/ CATERPILLER 1.1 is an inducible inflammatory mediator with NF-κB suppressive properties. J Immunol 171:6329–6333, 2003.

Öner A, Erdogan O, Demircin G, et al. Efficacy of colchicine therapy in amyloid nephropathy of familial Mediterranean fever. Pediatr Nephrol 18: 521–526, 2003.

Özdogan H, Arisoy N, Kasapcapur O, et al. Vasculitis in familial Mediterranean fever. J Rheumatol 24:323–327, 1997.

Ozen S. New interest in an old disease: familial Mediterranean fever. Clin Exp Rheumatol 17:745–749, 1999.

Ozen S, Ben-Chetrit E, Bakkaloglu A, et al. Polyarteritis nodosa in patients with familial Mediterranean fever (FMF): a concomitant disease or a feature of FMF? Semin Arthritis Rheum 30:281–287, 2001.

Ozen S, Besbas N, Bakkaloglu A, et al. Pyrin Q148 mutation and familial Mediterranean fever. Q J Med 95:332–333, 2002.

Ozen S, Karaaslan Y, Özdemir O, et al. Prevalence of juvenile chronic arthritis and familial Mediterranean fever in Turkey: a field study. J Rheumatol 25:2445–2449, 1998.

Özkaya N, Yalçinkaya F. Colchicine treatment in children with familial Mediterranean fever. Clin Rheumatol 22:314–317, 2003.

Padeh S, Shinar Y, Pras E, et al. Clinical and diagnostic value of genetic testing in 216 Israeli children with Familial Mediterranean fever. J Rheumatol 30:185–190, 2003.

Papin C, Cazeneuve C, Duquesnoy P, et al. The tumor necrosis factor α–dependent activation of the human mediterranean fever (MEFV) promoter is mediated by a synergistic interaction between C/EBP β and NF κB p65. J Biol Chem 278:48839–48847, 2003.

Pawlowski K, Pio F, Chu Z, et al. PAAD—a new protein domain associated with apoptosis, cancer and autoimmune diseases. Trends Biochem Sci 26:85–87, 2001.

Poirier O, Nicaud V, Gariepy J, et al. Polymorphism R92Q of the tumour necrosis factor receptor 1 gene is associated with myocardial infarction and carotid intima-media thickness—the ECTIM, AXA, EVA and GENIC Studies. Eur J Hum Genet 12:213–219, 2004.

Pras E, Aksentijevich I, Gruberg L, et al. Mapping of a gene causing familial Mediterranean fever to the short arm of chromosome 16. N Engl J Med 326:1509–1513, 1992.

Pras M, Bronspigel N, Zemer D, et al. Variable incidence of amyloidosis in familial Mediterranean fever among different ethnic groups. Johns Hopkins Med J 150:22–26, 1982.

Pras E, Livneh A, Balow JE Jr, et al. Clinical differences between North African and Iraqi Jews with familial Mediterranean fever. Am J Med Genet 75:216–219, 1998.

Prieur AM. A recently recognised chronic inflammatory disease of early onset characterised by the triad of rash, central nervous system involvement and arthropathy. Clin Exp Rheumatol 19:103–106, 2001.

Prieur AM, Griscelli C. Arthropathy with rash, chronic meningitis, eye lesions, and mental retardation. J Pediatr 99:79–83, 1981.

Prieur AM, Griscelli C, Lampert F, et al. A chronic, infantile, neurological, cutaneous and articular (CINCA) syndrome. A specific entity analysed in 30 patients. Scand J Rheumatol Suppl 66:57–68, 1987.

Putterman C, Ben-Chetrit E, Caraco Y, et al. Colchicine intoxication: clinical pharmacology, risk factors, features, and management. Semin Arthritis Rheum 21:143–155, 1991.

Rawashdeh MO, Majeed HA. Familial Mediterranean fever in Arab children: the high prevalence and gene frequency. Eur J Pediatr 155:540–544, 1996.

Richards N, Schaner P, Diaz A, et al. Interaction between pyrin and the apoptotic speck protein (ASC) modulates ASC-induced apoptosis. J Biol Chem 276:39320–39329, 2001.

Rogers DB, Shohat M, Petersen GM, et al. Familial Mediterranean fever in Armenians: autosomal recessive inheritance with high gene frequency. Am J Med Genet 34:168–172, 1989.

Rösen-Wolff A, Kreth HW, Hofmann S, et al. Periodic fever (TRAPS) caused by mutations in the TNFα receptor 1 (TNFRSF1A) gene of three German patients. Eur J Haematol 67:105–109, 2001.

Rösen-Wolff A, Quietzsch J, Schroder H, et al. Two German CINCA (NOMID) patients with different clinical severity and response to anti-inflammatory treatment. Eur J Haematol 71:215–219, 2003.

Samuels J, Aksentijevich I, Torosyan Y, et al. Familial Mediterranean fever at the millennium. Clinical spectrum, ancient mutations, and a survey of 100 American referrals to the National Institutes of Health. Medicine (Baltimore) 77:268–297, 1998.

Saulsbury FT. Hyperimmunoglobulinemia D and periodic fever syndrome (HIDS) in a child with normal serum IgD, but increased serum IgA concentration. J Pediatr 143:127–129, 2003.

Schafer BL, Bishop RW, Kratunis VJ, et al. Molecular cloning of human mevalonate kinase and identification of a missense mutation in the genetic disease mevalonic aciduria. J Biol Chem 267:13229–13238, 1992.

Schwabe AD, Peters RS. Familial Mediterranean fever in Armenians. Analysis of 100 cases. Medicine (Baltimore) 53:453–462, 1974.

Schwarz RE, Dralle H, Linke RP, et al. Amyloid goiter and arthritides after kidney transplantation in a patient with systemic amyloidosis and Muckle-Wells syndrome. Am J Clin Pathol 92:821–825, 1989.

Sidi G, Shinar Y, Livneh A, et al. Protracted febrile myalgia of familial Mediterranean fever. Mutation analysis and clinical correlations. Scand J Rheumatol 29:174–176, 2000.

Siegal S. Benign peroxysmal peritonitis. Ann Intern Med 23:1–21, 1945.

Simkin PA, Gardner GC. Colchicine use in cyclosporine treated transplant recipients: how little is too much? J Rheumatol 27:1334–1337, 2000.

Simon A, Cuisset L, Vincent MF, et al. Molecular analysis of the mevalonate kinase gene in a cohort of patients with the hyper-igd and periodic fever syndrome: its application as a diagnostic tool. Ann Intern Med 135:338–343, 2001a.

Simon A, Dodé C, van der Meer JW, et al. Familial periodic fever and amyloidosis due to a new mutation in the *TNFRSF1A* gene. Am J Med 110:313–316, 2001b.

Simon A, Drewe E, van der Meer JW, et al. Simvastatin treatment for inflammatory attacks of the hyperimmunoglobulinemia D and periodic fever syndrome. Clin Pharmacol Ther 75:476–483, 2004.

Simon A, Mariman EC, van der Meer JW, et al. A founder effect in the hyperimmunoglobulinemia D and periodic fever syndrome. Am J Med 114:148–152, 2003.

Simon A, van Deuren M, Tighe PJ, et al. Genetic analysis as a valuable key to diagnosis and treatment of periodic fever. Arch Intern Med 161:2491–2493, 2001c.

Simsek B, Islek I, Simsek T, et al. Regression of nephrotic syndrome due to amyloidosis secondary to familial mediterranean fever following colchicine treatment. Nephrol Dial Transplant 15:281–282, 2000.

Smith CA, Davis T, Anderson D, et al. A receptor for tumor necrosis factor defines an unusual family of cellular and viral proteins. Science 248:1019–1023, 1990.

Sneh E, Pras M, Michaeli D, et al. Protracted arthritis in familial Mediterranean fever. Rheumatol Rehabil 16:102–106, 1977.

Sohar E, Gafni J, Pras M, et al. Familial Mediterranean fever. A survey of 470 cases and review of the literature. Am J Med 43:227–253, 1967.

Sohar E, Pras M, Heller J, et al. Genetics of familial Mediterranean fever. Arch Intern Med 110:109–118, 1962.

Speeg KV, Maldonado AL, Liaci J, et al. Effect of cyclosporine on colchicine secretion by the kidney multidrug transporter studied in vivo. J Pharmacol Exp Ther 261:50–55, 1992.

Srinivasula SM, Poyet JL, Razmara M, et al. The PYRIN-CARD protein ASC is an activating adaptor for caspase-1. J Biol Chem 277:21119–21122, 2002.

Staub E, Dahl E, Rosenthal A. The DAPIN family: a novel domain links apoptotic and interferon response proteins. Trends Biochem Sci 26:83–85, 2001.

Stehlik C, Fiorentino L, Dorfleutner A, et al. The PAAD/PYRIN-family protein ASC is a dual regulator of a conserved step in nuclear factor κB activation pathways. J Exp Med 196:1605–1615, 2002.

Stehlik C, Lee SH, Dorfleutner A, et al. Apoptosis-associated speck-like protein containing a caspase recruitment domain is a regulator of procaspase-1 activation. J Immunol 171:6154–6163, 2003.

Stoffman N, Magal N, Shohat T, et al. Higher than expected carrier rates for familial Mediterranean fever in various Jewish ethnic groups. Eur J Hum Genet 8:307–310, 2000.

Stojanov S, Weiss M, Lohse P, et al. A novel *CIAS1* mutation and plasma/cerebrospinal fluid cytokine profile in a German patient with neonatal-onset multisystem inflammatory disease responsive to methotrexate therapy. Pediatrics 114:e124–127, 2004.

Sutterwala FS, Ogura Y, Szczepanik M, et al. Critical role for NALP3/CIAS1/cryopyrin in innate and adaptive immunity through its regulation of caspase-1. Immunity 24:317–327, 2006.

Takada K, Aksentijevich I, Mahadevan V, et al. Favorable preliminary experience with etanercept in two patients with the hyperimmunoglobulinemia D and periodic fever syndrome. Arthritis Rheum 48:2645–2651, 2003.

Tchernitchko D, Chiminqgi M, Galacteros F, et al. Unexpected high frequency of P46L TNFRSF1A allele in sub-Saharan West African populations. Eur J Hum Genet 13:513–515, 2005.

Tchernitchko D, Legendre M, Cazeneuve C, et al. The E148Q MEFV allele is not implicated in the development of familial Mediterranean fever. Hum Mutat 22:339–340, 2003.

Tekin M, Yalçinkaya F, Tumer N, et al. Familial Mediterranean fever—renal involvement by diseases other than amyloid. Nephrol Dial Transplant 14:475–479, 1999.

Thomas KT, Feder HM Jr, Lawton AR, et al. Periodic fever syndrome in children. J Pediatr 135:15–21, 1999.

Tinaztepe K, Gucer S, Bakkaloglu A, et al. Familial Mediterranean fever and polyarteritis nodosa: experience of five paediatric cases. A causal relationship or coincidence? Eur J Pediatr 156:505–506, 1997.

Todd I, Radford PM, Draper-Morgan KA, et al. Mutant forms of tumour necrosis factor receptor I that occur in TNF-receptor–associated periodic syndrome retain signalling functions but show abnormal behaviour. Immunology 113:65–79, 2004.

Torbiak RP, Dent PB, Cockshott WP. NOMID—a neonatal syndrome of multisystem inflammation. Skeletal Radiol 18:359–364, 1989.

Toro JR, Aksentijevich I, Hull K, et al. Tumor necrosis factor receptor-associated periodic syndrome: a novel syndrome with cutaneous manifestations. Arch Dermatol 136:1487–1494, 2000.

Touitou I. The spectrum of familial Mediterranean fever (FMF) mutations. Eur J Hum Genet 9:473–483, 2001.

Touitou I, Ben-Chetrit E, Gershoni-Baruch R, et al. Allogenic bone marrow transplantation: not a treatment yet for familial Mediterranean fever. Blood 102:409, 2003.

Tschopp J, Martinon F, Burns K. NALPs: a novel protein family involved in inflammation. Nat Rev Mol Cell Biol 4:95–104, 2003.

Tunca M, Akar S, Hawkins PN, et al. The significance of paired *MEFV* mutations in individuals without symptoms of familial Mediterranean fever. Eur J Hum Genet 10:786–789, 2002.

Tunca M, Akar S, Soyturk M, et al. The effect of interferon alpha administration on acute attacks of familial Mediterranean fever: a double-blind, placebo-controlled trial. Clin Exp Rheumatol 22:S37–40, 2004.

Tunca M, Kirkali G, Soyturk M, et al. Acute phase response and evolution of familial Mediterranean fever. Lancet 353:1415, 1999.

Tunca M, Tankurt E, Akbaylar Akpinar H, et al. The efficacy of interferon alpha on colchicine-resistant familial Mediterranean fever attacks: a pilot study. Br J Rheumatol 36:1005–1008, 1997.

Turkish FMF Study Group. Familial Mediterranean fever (FMF) in Turkey: results of a nationwide multicenter study. Medicine (Baltimore) 84:1–11, 2005.

Tutar E, Yalçinkaya F, Özkaya N, et al. Incidence of pericardial effusion during attacks of familial Mediterranean fever. Heart 89:1257–1258, 2003.

Valle D. You give me fever. Nat Genet 22:121–122, 1999.

van der Meer JW, Vossen JM, Radl J, et al. Hyperimmunoglobulinaemia D and periodic fever: a new syndrome. Lancet 1:1087–1090, 1984.

Vassalli P. The pathophysiology of tumor necrosis factors. Annu Rev Immunol 10:411–452, 1992.

Wallace SL, Singer JZ. Review: systemic toxicity associated with the intravenous administration of colchicine—guidelines for use. J Rheumatol 15:495–499, 1988.

Wanderer AA, Hoffman HM. The spectrum of acquired and familial cold-induced urticaria/urticaria-like syndromes. Immunol Allergy Clin North Am 24:259–286, vii, 2004.

Wang L, Manji GA, Grenier JM, et al. PYPAF7, a novel PYRIN-containing Apaf1-like protein that regulates activation of NF-κB and caspase-1-dependent cytokine processing. J Biol Chem 277:29874–29880, 2002.

Watts RA, Nicholls A, Scott DG. The arthropathy of the Muckle-Wells syndrome. Br J Rheumatol 33:1184–1187, 1994.

Weyhreter H, Schwartz M, Kristensen TD, et al. A new mutation causing autosomal dominant periodic fever syndrome in a Danish family. J Pediatr 142:191–193, 2003.

Williamson LM, Hull D, Mehta R, et al. Familial Hibernian fever. Q J Med 51:469–480, 1982.

Xanthoulea S, Pasparakis M, Kousteni S, et al. Tumor necrosis factor (TNF) receptor shedding controls thresholds of innate immune activation that balance opposing TNF functions in infectious and inflammatory diseases. J Exp Med 200:367–376, 2004.

Yilmaz E, Ozen S, Balci B, et al. Mutation frequency of familial Mediterranean fever and evidence for a high carrier rate in the Turkish population. Eur J Hum Genet 9:553–555, 2001.

Yuval Y, Hemo-Zisser M, Zemer D, et al. Dominant inheritance in two families with familial Mediterranean fever (FMF). Am J Med Genet 57:455–457, 1995.

Zaks N, Kastner DL. Clinical syndromes resembling familial Mediterranean fever. In: Sohar E, Gafni J, Pras M, eds. Familial Mediterranean Fever: First International Conference. London and Tel Aviv: Freund, pp. 211–215, 1997.

Zemer D, Livneh A, Danon YL, et al. Long-term colchicine treatment in children with familial Mediterranean fever. Arthritis Rheum 34:973–977, 1991.

Zemer D, Pras M, Sohar E, et al. Colchicine in the prevention and treatment of the amyloidosis of familial Mediterranean fever. N Engl J Med 314:1001–1005, 1986.

Zemer D, Revach M, Pras M, et al. A controlled trial of colchicine in preventing attacks of familial mediterranean fever. N Engl J Med 291:932–934, 1974.

Zimand S, Tauber T, Hegesch T, et al. Familial Mediterranean fever presenting with massive cardiac tamponade. Clin Exp Rheumatol 12:67–69, 1994.

Zissin R, Rathaus V, Gayer G, et al. CT findings in patients with familial Mediterranean fever during an acute abdominal attack. Br J Radiol 76:22–25, 2003.

Zweers EJ, Erkelens DW. A Dutch family with familial Mediterranean fever [in Dutch]. Ned Tijdschr Geneeskd 137:1570–1573, 1993.

28

Inherited Disorders of the Interleukin-12/23–Interferon Gamma Axis

MELANIE J. NEWPORT, STEVEN M. HOLLAND, MICHAEL LEVIN,
and JEAN-LAURENT CASANOVA

Over the past 50 years there have been a number of reported cases of severe disseminated infection with weakly virulent mycobacteria in individuals without recognized predisposing immunodeficiency. Mycobacterial species included various environmental mycobacteria (EM) and several *Mycobacterium bovis* bacillus Calmette-Guérin (BCG) vaccine substrains. High rates of affected siblings and parental consanguinity suggested the existence of a novel primary immunodeficiency syndrome, subsequently named *Mendelian susceptibility to mycobacterial disease* (MSMD, MIM 209950). Molecular investigation of these families has identified mutations in five genes in the interleukin (IL)-12/23–dependent interferon-gamma (IFN-γ) axis, highlighting the importance of this pathway in human immunity to mycobacteria. There remain a number of patients for whom a genetic etiology has yet to be identified; mutations in other genes await discovery.

Sporadic cases of disseminated EM infection in the absence of recognized immunodeficiency are well described (e.g., Buhler and Pollack, 1953; van der Hoeven et al., 1958). Familial-disseminated EM infection was first reported in 1964—three members of the same Danish family had fatal disseminated *M. avium* complex (MAC) (Engbaek, 1964). Uchiyama et al. (1981) identified two siblings with *M. avium* infection. More recently, Holland and colleagues reported three male members of one family with disseminated EM infection (Holland et al., 1994; Frucht and Holland, 1996; Frucht et al., 1999).

Idiopathic disseminated BCG infection following vaccination was first reported in 1951 (Mimouni, 1951). A sporadic case born to consanguinous parents was described in 1973 (Ulgenalp et al., 1973), and families with more than one affected member were first reported at around the same time (Sicevic, 1972; Fedak, 1974). That patients with inherited susceptibility to mycobacterial infections may also be at increased risk of *Salmonella* infection was first highlighted in a report by Heyne (1976), who described a

brother and sister from Germany who both developed generalized infection after neonatal BCG vaccination. The boy later developed *Salmonella* enteritis and osteomyelitis. In Prague, a 3-year-old boy who had been vaccinated with BCG at the age of 3 days developed disseminated *Salmonella* and BCG infection resulting in his death 3 years later (Doleckova et al., 1977). A first cousin of this child also had disseminated BCG infection (Dvoracek et al., 1959).

The first family in which the molecular basis of increased susceptibility to EM was elucidated was described in 1995 (Levin et al., 1995). Four children from the same village in Malta all developed disseminated EM infection. Two were brothers related to a third child as fourth cousins, while the fourth child was not knowingly related to the others. The parents of the brothers were second cousins and both related to both parents of the fourth cousin. Each child was infected with a different mycobacterial species (*M. chelonae, M. fortuitum*, and two different strains of MAC), a phenomenon suggesting that an innate defect in host immunity was responsible. However, extensive immunological investigation failed to identify any known defect predisposing to such infections. Patients had defective up-regulation of monocyte function in response to endotoxin and IFN-γ (Levin et al., 1995) and defective antigen presentation (D'Souza et al., 1996). The high degree of consanguinity within the Maltese family suggested that the children were homozygous for a rare recessive mutation inherited from a common ancestor. Through a whole-genome search for homozygosity in three of the affected children, the gene was mapped to the region of chromosome 6q containing the gene encoding the IFN-γ receptor ligand binding chain (IFN-γR1) of the IFN-γ receptor complex (Newport et al., 1996). A mutation in the coding region of this gene (*IFNGR1*), which resulted in complete absence of IFN-γR1 expression at the cell surface, was subsequently identified as the cause of the defect (Newport et al., 1996).

Table 28.1. Genes Involved in Defective Macrophage Activation

Gene	Gene Product	Chromosomal Location	MIM No.
IFNGR1	Interferon-γ receptor ligand binding chain	6q23–q24	107470
IFNGR2	Interferon-γ receptor signal transducing chain	21q22.1–22.2	145659
IL12RB1	Interleukin-12 receptor β-1 subunit	19p13.1	601604
IL12B	Interleukin-12p40 subunit	5q31.1–33.1	161561
STAT1	Signal transducer and activator of transcription 1	2q32.2–32.3	600555

Meanwhile, authors of a survey conducted in parallel to the work described above found that of 108 cases of disseminated infection following BCG vaccination reported since 1951, 50% were idiopathic (Casanova et al., 1995). A retrospective study of all cases of disseminated BCG infection following vaccination in France between 1974 and 1994 revealed that of 32 children identified, 16 had no recognized predisposing immunodeficiency (Casanova et al., 1996). Among a total of 60 children worldwide with idiopathic disseminated BCG infection for whom information was available, four pairs of siblings and one pair of first cousins were identified, and parental consanguinity was noted in 24 families. Clinical and histopathological features in a Tunisian child with disseminated BCG infection, born to consanguineous parents, were remarkably similar to those of the Maltese children with EM infections. A series of candidate genes involved in antimycobacterial immunity in the mouse model of BCG infection were tested by homozygosity mapping. The segregation of markers within *IFNGR1* suggested linkage, and a frameshift mutation resulting in the absence of IFN-γR1 was identified (Jouanguy et al., 1996).

Although mutations in *IFNGR1* were subsequently identified in other cases of MSMD, there were a number of patients in whom mutations within *IFNGR1* were not detected. Investigation of other candidate genes within the IFN-γ pathway led to the identification of mutations in four other genes (Table 28.1), all of which are involved in the IL-12-dependent, IFN-γ-mediated immunity (reviewed in Dorman and Holland, 2000; Lammas et al., 2000; Remus et al., 2001; Casanova and Abel, 2002, 2004).

Clinical and Pathological Manifestations

The central feature of MSMD is infection with weakly pathogenic mycobacteria. In keeping with the genetic heterogeneity there is a clinical spectrum of MSMD. At one end of the spectrum, mutations in *IFNGR1* or *IFNGR2*, which result in a lack of functional protein at the cell surface (complete receptor deficiency), have a very poor prognosis, with the development of disseminated infection in early childhood and progressively fatal disease (Jouanguy et al., 1996; Newport et al., 1996; Dorman and Holland, 1998; Dorman et al., 2004). At the other end, through screening of family members, individuals have been identified who carry mutations involving *IFNGR1*, *STAT1*, *IL12B*, and *IL12RB1* but have not developed infection with either mycobacteria or salmonella (Jouanguy et al., 1999b; Altare et al., 2001; Dupuis et al., 2001; Picard et al., 2002; Caragol et al., 2003). Other *IFNGR1* and *IFNGR2* mutations resulting in the expression of an abnormal protein causing partial receptor deficiency are associated with milder phenotypes and response to IFN-γ treatment (Jouanguy et al., 1997, 1999b; Doffinger et al., 2000; Dorman et al., 2004). Similarly, mutations in the genes encoding the IL-12p40 subunit (*IL12B*) or the IL-12 receptor β1 subunit (*IL12RB1*) resulting in complete deficiency of either protein result in a less severe phenotype and good

response to antimicrobial and IFN-γ treatment. The signal transducer and activator of transcription 1 (*STAT1*) mutation is phenotypically similar to partial IFN-γR deficiency (Dupuis et al., 2000).

A striking feature of MSMD is the specific susceptibility to poorly pathogenic mycobacterial species. Various mycobacteria species have been isolated, including slow-growing species such as *M. kansasii*, *M. avium*, and *M. szulgai*, and rapid-growing species such as *M. smegmatis*, *M. abscessus*, *M. chelonei*, *M. fortuitum*, and *M. peregrinum*. *M. smegmatis* (Pierre-Audigier et al., 1997) and *M. peregrinum* (Koscielniak et al., 2003) had not previously been documented as causes of disseminated EM disease. The more virulent *M. tuberculosis* has been implicated in or isolated from individuals with IFN-γR1, IL-12p40, and IL-12Rβ1 deficiency (Jouanguy et al., 1997; Altare et al., 2001; Picard et al., 2002). The mycobacterial species identified correlate with the genetic defect; for example, rapid-growing mycobacterial species are mostly observed in children with complete IFN-γR1 or IFN-γR2 deficiency (Table 28.2). Salmonella infections ranging from protracted gastroenteritis to septicemia and disseminated infection occurred in about a quarter of reported cases, more commonly in association with IL-12p40 and IL-12Rβ1 deficiency (MacLennan et al., 2004). Other pathogens isolated from MSMD cases include *Listeria monocytogenes* (Roesler et al., 1999), *Histoplasma capsulatum* (Jouanguy et al., 1999b), and *Norcardia asteroides* (Picard et al., 2002). Fungal and bacterial pathogens such as candida and staphylococci have not caused infection, despite the presence of indwelling intravenous catheters in many patients. Increased susceptibility to viral infections, particularly with herpes viruses, has been noted in some patients in whom MSMD has been shown to be due to IFN-γR1 deficiency (Dorman et al., 1999; Cunningham et al., 2000; Uzel et al., 2000; Novelli and Casanova, 2004). Recently, a 11-year-child with complete IFN-γR1 deficiency who had developed mycobacterial disease at the age of 5 months was diagnosed with Kaposi sarcoma (Camcioglu et al., 2004). Histologic appearance of the lesions was characteristic for Kaposi sarcoma; human herpesvirus-8 (HHV-8)–associated antigen was detected in situ by immunohistochemistry, and HHV-8 DNA was amplified by polymerase chain reaction (PCR) from the lesions. However, this situation is not universal, and most other patients have had classical childhood viral infections without problems. Mutation of *STAT1* has not resulted in increased susceptibility to viral infection despite the role of *STAT1* in both IFN-γ- and IFN-α-mediated immunity (see section Molecular Basis of Disease, below).

Patients with MSMD due to complete IFN-γR1 deficiency may present in childhood with a characteristic syndrome of chronic fever, weight loss, lymphadenopathy, hepatosplenomegaly, and evidence of disseminated infection that may involve bone, skin, soft tissues, lung, and meninges. The clinical presentation appears to vary according to the genetic defect involved. For example, dominant partial IFN-γR1 deficiency is almost always associated with osteomyelitis (Jouanguy et al., 1999b; Villela et al., 2001;

Table 28.2. Clinical Features of Inherited Disorders of Interleukin-12–Interferon-γ Axis: Pathogens Isolated and Organs Involved

Disorder	Infection	RES	Bone	CNS	GIS	RS	Skin	References
cIFN-γR1	MAC	+	+	+		+		Newport et al., 1996;
	M. fortuitum	+	+					Jouanguy et al., 1996, 2000;
	M. chelonae	+	+					Pierre-Audigier et al., 1997;
	BCG	+	+	+			+	Altare et al., 1998b;
	M. smegmatis	+		+				Holland et al., 1998;
	M. kansasii	+	+			+	+	Vesterhus et al., 1998;
	M. szulgai	+	+					Roesler et al., 1999;
	Salmonella	+			+			Cunningham et al., 2000;
	L. monocytogenes	+		+				Allende et al., 2001;
								Rosenzweig et al., 2002;
								Koscielnak et al., 2003
cIFN-γR2	*M. fortuitum*	+				+		Dorman and Holland, 1998
	MAC	+				+		
AR pIFN-γR1	BCG	+					+	Jouanguy et al., 1997
	Salmonella	+						
AR pIFN-γR2	BCG	+					+	Doffinger et al., 2000
	M. abcessus	+					+	
AD pIFN-γR1	*M. tuberculosis*	+				+		Jouanguy et al., 1999b;
	MAC		+			+	+	Villela et al., 2001
	BCG	+	+			+	+	
	M. kansasii	+						
	Salmonella		+					
	H. capsulatum	+						
cIL-12p40	BCG	+					+	Altare et al., 1998c; Picard et al., 2002
	M. tuberculosis	+						
	Salmonella spp.	+			+			
	Norcardia asteroides					+		
cIL-12Rβ1	BCG	+						Altare et al., 1998a, 2001;
	MAC	+				+		de Jong et al., 1998;
	M. fortuitum-chelonae	+			+	+		Asku et al., 2001; Sakai et al., 2001
	M. tuberculosis	+			+			
	Salmonella	+			+			
STAT1	BCG	+						Dupuis et al., 2001
	MAC	+						
	Lethal viral infection +/−							Dupuis et al., 2003

Abbreviations:

AD pIFN-γR1, autosomal dominant partial interferon-gamma receptor 1 deficiency; AR pIFN-γR1, autosomal recessive partial interferon-gamma receptor 1 deficiency; AR pIFN-γR2, autosomal recessive partial interferon-gamma receptor 2 deficiency; BCG, bacille Calmette-Guerin; cIFN-γR1, complete interferon-gamma receptor 1 deficiency; cIFN-γR2, complete interferon-gamma receptor 2 deficiency; cIL-12p40, complete interleukin-12 p40 deficiency; cIL-12β1, complete interleukin-12 receptor β1 deficiency; CNS, central nervous system; GIS, gastrointestinal system; MAC, *Mycobacterium avium* complex; RES, reticuloendothelial system; RS, respiratory system; STAT1, partial signal transducer and activator of transcription 1 deficiency.

Sasaki et al., 2002; Dorman et al., 2004), whereas lymphadenopathy is a very common feature of IL-12p40 or IL-12Rβ1 deficiency (Altare et al., 1998a, 1998c, 2001; de Jong et al., 1998; Aksu et al., 2001; Sakai et al., 2001; Picard et al., 2002). The clinical features of each genetic defect remain to be carefully described as more patients with MSMD are identified. The age of onset varies according to the gene involved, the type of mutation, and whether the affected individual received BCG vaccination at birth or acquired EM infection via natural routes (Dorman et al., 2004). A correlation between clinical phenotype and histopathological findings has been observed (Emile et al., 1997). Two distinct histological types have been documented that appear to be associated with distinct clinical phenotypes (Color Plate 28.I). Approximately half the patients with disseminated BCG infections had tuberculoid (type I) granulomata with well-defined epithelioid and giant cells surrounded by lymphocytes and fibrosis containing only occasional acid-fast bacilli. The remaining patients had lepromatous-like (type II) lesions with poorly formed granulomata containing large numbers of acid-fast bacilli. Patients with type I granulomata had a good prognosis but virtually all the children with poor granuloma formation (type II) died. EM granulomata tend to be poorly formed irrespective of the clinical outcome and underlying genetic defect.

Laboratory Findings

Chronic infection leads to normochromic, normocytic anemia and raised inflammatory markers. Immune function in patients with MSMD has been extensively investigated in an attempt to identify a known immunodeficiency and is in general remarkably normal. CD4[+] T helper cells are often normal but may be low secondary to chronic infection. Levels of serum immunoglobulin isotypes, including IgG subclasses, are normal or elevated, and antigen-specific antibody titers are normal. T cell proliferation in vitro in response to various mitogens and recall antigens are also normal. Polymorphonuclear cells are normal in terms of morphology, CD18 expression, chemotaxis, and respiratory burst. Delayed-type hypersensitivity (DTH) testing in vivo and

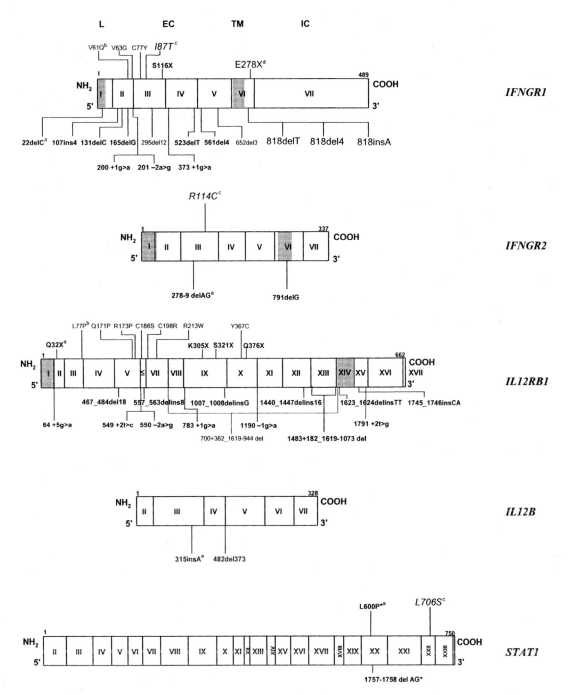

Figure 28.1. Mutations identified to date in the five MSMD genes. The gene-coding regions are indicated with vertical bars separating the exons, designated by roman numerals. [a]Nonsense, splice-site mutations and frameshift insertions and deletions (recessive) causing complete deficiency with no detectable protein expression at the cell surface (small font in bold); [b]missense mutations and in-frame deletions (recessive) causing complete deficiency with detectable surface protein expression (small font); [c,d]mutations that are recessive (large font, italic)[c] or dominant (large font),[d] causing partial deficiency; *indicates two patients with homozygous STAT1 mutation who were susceptible to not only mycobacterial but also severe or eventual lethal viral infections.

blastogenesis in vitro to purified protein derivative (PPD) are normal in patients with complete IFN-γR1 and IL-12Rβ1 deficiency, results indicating that IL-12 and IFN-γ are not required for DTH or blastogenesis to mycobacterial antigens.

Molecular Basis of the Disease

Mutations in five genes of the IL-12/IFN-γ axis causing increased susceptibility to mycobacteria have been identified to

date (summarized in Fig. 28.1). This pathway is central to the immune response to intracellular pathogens such as mycobacteria. The functions of these genes are described in more detail in Functional Aspects of the Proteins, below.

IFNGR1

Mutations in this gene were the first to be identified as the cause of MSMD (Jouanguy et al., 1996; Newport et al., 1996). Subsequent investigation of patients with increased susceptibility to poorly pathogenic mycobacteria has led to the identification of at least 15 null-recessive mutations in this gene (Fig. 28.1) (Pierre-Audigier et al., 1997; Altare et al., 1998b; Holland et al., 1998; Vesterhus et al., 1998; Roesler et al., 1999; Cunningham et al., 2000; Jouanguy et al., 2000; Allende et al., 2001; Rosenzweig et al., 2002; Koscielniak et al., 2003; Dorman et al., 2004). The identification of families in which mycobacterial infections occurred in more than one generation suggested dominant mutations might also exist (Jouanguy et al., 1999b). Investigation of 18 individuals from 12 kindreds led to the identification of a small deletion hot spot within *IFNGR1*. A 4 base pair (bp) deletion at nucleotide position 818 (818del4) was identified in 11 of the unrelated kindreds and the 12th family had a single nucleotide deletion (T) in this position (818delT). The 818del4 mutation leads to a premature stop codon at position 827–829 within the intracellular domain of the receptor. The receptor is expressed on the cell surface but the mutant receptor lacks the three motifs required for intracellular signaling (the JAK1 and STAT1 binding sites, and the tyrosine phosphorylation site). It also lacks a recycling motif, so the truncated receptor accumulates on the cell surface and interferes with signaling by the normal receptor encoded by the normal copy of *IFNGR1*. Thus, the mutant allele has a dominant effect (in comparison to the recessive form of IFN-γR1 deficiency, in which parents are healthy carriers of the mutations). Subsequently, other *IFNGR1* mutations resulting in a dominantly inherited phenotype were identified (Dorman et al., 1999; Villela et al., 2001; Sasaki et al., 2002). A second small deletion hot spot was recently identified in *IFNGR1*, in this case with a recessive phenotype (Rosenzweig et al., 2002).

In summary, a range of mutations including frameshift, insertion, deletion, nonsense, missense, and splice mutations have been identified in *IFNGR1* (Fig. 28.1). All recessive mutations identified to date occur in the part of the gene encoding the extracellular domain of the receptor chain, the majority of which result in complete lack of receptor expression. Two of the recessive mutations allow expression of a poorly functioning protein, leading to partial deficiency (Jouanguy et al., 1997). Partial receptor deficiency may also result from dominant mutations leading to a receptor being deprived of its intracytoplasmic segment.

IFNGR2

Complete deficiency of IFN-γR2 was found in a child with disseminated *M. fortuitum* and MAC infections in whom cell surface expression of IFN-γR1 and *IFNGR1* sequence was normal (Dorman and Holland, 1998). Sequence analysis of *IFNGR2* led to the identification of a 2 bp deletion (277–278delAG), which in turn led to a premature stop codon (Fig. 28.1). The truncated protein lacked both the transmembrane and intracellular (signaling) domains and was not expressed at the cell surface. Both parents, though unrelated, carried this mutation, for which the child was homozygous. A case of partial IFN-γR2 deficiency has also been described (Doffinger et al., 2000). A child born to related Portuguese parents developed disseminated infection following BCG vaccination. At the age of 16 she developed *M. abscessus* infection. A point mutation was identified in the *IFNGR2* sequence: the patient was homozygous for the mutation whereas both parents were heterozygous. This mutation results in an amino acid substitution at position 114 (arginine → cysteine) within the extracellular domain (Fig. 28.1). The mutant IFN-γR2 is expressed normally on the cell surface, but presumably the affinity between IFN-γR1 and IFN-γR2 is impaired.

IL12B

Complete IL-12B (IL-12p40) subunit deficiency leading to MSMD and *Salmonella* infections has also been described. The first case was born to consanguineous Pakistani parents and was immunized with BCG at birth (Altare et al., 1998c). Sequencing of *IL12B* revealed a large deletion involving two coding exons resulting in a frameshift deletion of 374 nucleotides between positions 482 and 854 (Fig. 28.1). The parents and a healthy sibling were carriers of this mutation; the affected child was homozygous. Eleven additional patients from five other families have been identified to date (Picard et al., 2002; Fieschi and Casanova, 2003). One child had only salmonellosis. All other patients had mycobacterial disease, BCG-osis in 10 children and *M. chelonei* in 1 child. Four children with BCG-osis also had salmonellosis, one had tuberculosis, and one has nocardiosis. Five children died but all survivors are well and no longer on treatment. Interestingly, one kindred from India had the same large deletion previously reported in the Pakistani kindred. A founder effect was documented and dated to approximately 29 generations ago (95% confidence interval [CI] 9–115) and 700 years ago (95% CI 216–2760) by means of a novel mutation dating method (Genin et al., 2004). The other four kindreds originated from the Arabic peninsula and were all found to carry the same *IL12B* frameshift insertion (315insA) (Picard et al., 2002). A founder effect was again documented and dated to 47 generations ago (95% CI 22–110) and 1100 years ago (95% CI 528–2640). The fact that all patients with IL-12B deficiency identified to date have *IL12B* mutations resulting from a founder effect, one in the Indian subcontinent and another in the Arabic peninsula, is consistent with the rarity of IL-12p40 deficiency among patients with MSMD. It is the first example of a founder effect among Mendelian mycobacterial susceptibility genes. IL-12p40 has recently been shown to be to be a component of IL-23. Thus IL-12p40 deficiency probably results in IL-23 deficiency; however, owing to the lack of human IL-23-specific antibodies, this cannot be ascertained as yet.

IL12RB1

Mutations in *IL12RB1* (which encodes the β1 subunit of the IL-12 receptor) have been identified in 41 patients from 29 different families (Altare et al., 1998a, 2001; de Jong et al., 1998; Verhagen et al., 2000; Asku et al., 2001; Sakai et al., 2001; Fieschi et al., 2003; Staretz-Haham et al., 2003). Most patients had BCG or nontuberculous mycobacteria (NTM) disease, often with salmonellosis, but several were found to suffer from salmonellosis only and some from tuberculosis only (Fieschi et al., 2003; Fieschi and Casanova, 2003). A significant fraction of patients were asymptomatic. A total of 21 unique mutations have been identified, including nonsense, splice, and frameshift mutations, which lead to premature termination of translation in the extracellular domain (Fig. 28.1). This abrogates cell surface expression resulting in complete IL-12Rβ1 deficiency. Two missense mutations, also resulting in a lack of receptor expression at the cell surface, were validated by gene transfer studies (Altare et al., 2001; Sakai et al., 2001). Recently, a complete IL-12/IL-23 receptor β1 deficiency with cell surface–expressed nonfunctional receptors was reported (Fieschi et al., 2004). IL-12 and IL-23 did not bind normally to the patient's cells; STAT4 was not phosphorylated and IFN-γ production was not induced in the patient's cells (upon stimulation with IL-12 or IL-23). Only recessive, loss-of-function mutations have been identified in *IL12RB1* to date. The recent observation that IL-12Rβ1 also serves as a subunit in the IL-23 receptor suggests that *IL12RB1* mutations prevent IL-23 activation, but this has not been experimentally tested as yet.

STAT1

The identification of two unrelated families presenting with MSMD in the absence of mutation in any of the genes discussed above led to the discovery of the fifth MSMD gene. A 33-year-old French woman with a history of disseminated BCG infection following childhood vaccination and a 10-year-old North American girl with disseminated *M. avium* infection were found to carry a de novo mutation (the parents of both patients had two wild-type copies of *STAT1*) in the coding region of *STAT1* (Dupuis et al., 2001). Both were heterozygous for a single T > C nucleotide change at position 2116, which results in L706S in the COOH-terminal region (Fig. 28.1). The abnormal protein exerts a dominant negative effect on the normal protein in terms of STAT-1 dimer (also known as gamma activating factor [GAF]) activation but not in terms of STAT-1/STAT-2/p48 trimer (also known as interferon-stimulated gamma factor 3 [ISGF3]) activation. The *STAT1* mutation is loss of function for the two cellular phenotypes (it impairs phosphorylation of tyrosine 701) but dominant for one (GAF activation) and recessive for another (ISGF3 activation) in heterozygous cells stimulated with either type of IFN. To our knowledge it is the first reported mutation in a human gene to be dominant and recessive for two cellular phenotypes. Vulnerability to mycobacteria and resistance to viruses thus imply that GAF mediates antimycobacterial IFN-γ activity, whereas the antiviral effects of IFNs are either STAT-1-independent or ISGF3-dependent. This novel disorder proves that IL-12-induced, IFN-γ-mediated immunity against mycobacteria is both STAT-1- and GAF-dependent.

The interpretation of the effect of the heterozygous *STAT1* mutation L706S on its function has recently been confirmed by the observation of two unrelated infants found to be homozygous for two unique mutations of *STAT1* in exon 20 (Fig. 28.1) (Dupuis et al., 2003). Neither IFN-α/β nor IFN-γ was able to activate STAT1-containing transcription factors in patient cells. Like individuals with IFN-γR deficiency, both infants suffered from mycobacterial disease. Unlike patients with IFN-γR deficiency, both died of viral disease. Furthermore, viral multiplication in vitro was not inhibited by adding recombinant IFN-α/β to cell lines from the two individuals. Thus, complete impairment of STAT1-dependent responses to human IFN-α/β results in increased susceptibility to both mycobacteria and viral disease.

Functional Aspects of the Proteins

The receptor for IFN-γ consists of two subunits: IFN-γR1, the ligand-binding chain (previously known as the α chain), and IFN-γR2, the signal-transducing chain (previously known as the β chain or accessory factor-1) (Bach et al., 1997). As the ligand-binding chains interact with IFN-γ homodimers, they dimerize and become associated with two signal transduction chains. This leads to the activation of specific members of two protein families—the Janus kinases (JAK) and the signal transducers and activators of transcription (STAT). JAK1 and JAK2 phosphorylate key tyrosine residues on the ligand-binding chains. This leads to the recruitment and activation of STAT1, which translocates to the nucleus as a phosphorylated homodimer (GAF) to activate a wide range of IFN-γ-responsive genes. After signaling, the receptor complex is internalized and dissociates. The IFN-γR1 chain is then recycled to the cell surface. IFN-γR1 is expressed constitutively at

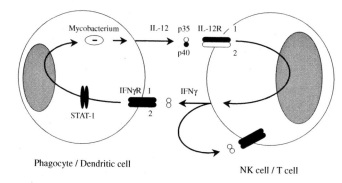

Figure 28.2. Cytokine interactions between the macrophage or dendritic cell and T or NK cell in the context of mycobacterial infection, illustrating the interaction between IL-12 and IFN-γ. Upon infection, primary host response cells such as macrophages release a range of cytokines including IL-12, which stimulate T and NK cells to secrete IFN-γ, activate macrophages to kill intracellular pathogens, and enhance the differentiation of IFN-γ-producing T helper cells.

moderate levels on the surface of all nucleated cells. IFN-γR2 is also constitutively expressed at low levels but expression is regulated by external stimuli, including IFN-γ itself (Bach et al., 1995).

Interleukin-12 is a heterodimeric cytokine comprised of two subunits, p40 and p35, which together form the biologically active p70 molecule. The IL-12p40 subunit is shared by IL-23 (Fieschi and Casanova, 2003). IL-12 and IL-23 are produced by activated antigen-presenting cells such as dendritic cells and macrophages in response to a number of microorganisms and microbial products, including lipopolysaccharide, lipoarabinomannan, and bacterial superantigens (Trinchieri, 1998). It can also be secreted upon stimulation by T cells in a CD154-CD40-dependent and IFN-γ-dependent manner. The stimulation of whole blood by live BCG was shown to trigger the IL-12/IFN-γ axis by an IRAK-4 and NEMO-dependent, noncognate interaction among monocytes and natural killer (NK) cells and T lymphocytes (Feinberg et al., 2004). It promotes cell-mediated immunity to intracellular pathogens by inducing the production of IFN-γ by both T and NK cells. The IL-12 receptor complex, expressed on activated T and NK cells, consists of two subunits known as the β1 and β2 subunits. Binding of IL-12 to the heterodimeric IL-12 receptor complex induces the phosphorylation of tyrosine kinase 2 (Tyk2) and JAK2 and subsequent activation of STAT4, which dimerises and translocates to the nucleus to activate IL-12-inducible genes. The IL-12Rβ1 subunit is also part of the IL-23 receptor. Figure 28.2 shows the cytokine interactions between the macrophage and T or NK cell in the context of mycobacterial infection, illustrating the interaction between IL-12 and IFN-γ.

Mutation Analysis

Mutations in *IFNGR1*, *IFNGR2*, *STAT1*, *IL12B*, and *IL12RB1* can be detected by single-strand conformation polymorphism (SSCP) and/or direct sequencing (Fig. 28.1). Primers to amplify and sequence all exons and flanking intron regions have been published and are available upon request.

Strategies for Diagnosis

Clinical Diagnosis

Inherited defects of the IL-12–IFN-γ axis may be considered in the differential diagnosis of all patients presenting with severe infection (including disseminated and recurrent diseases) with intracellular microorganisms, particularly when the organism is considered to be nonpathogenic in the "immunocompetent" individual. However, these defects should be sought aggressively in patients with severe nontuberculous mycobacterial or salmonella infections. Furthermore, a high index of suspicion is warranted in patients presenting with chronic fever, wasting, hepatosplenomegaly lymphadenopathy, and anemia in whom a pathogen is not isolated, as cultures may be persistently negative (Levin et al., 1995; Pierre-Audigier et al., 1997). Diagnosis may also be confounded by the lack of usually diagnostic granulomata, in which microbes may or may not be visible. An initial diagnosis of histiocytosis X has occasionally been made, hence MSMD should be considered in chemotherapy-resistant children with a tentative diagnosis of histiocytosis without formal histological criteria (Edgar et al., 2001). In many individuals, MSMD becomes apparent following BCG vaccination, thus vaccination history is essential. Because of the high incidence of parental consanguinity and affected relatives, family history is important. Specific attention must be directed at possible parental relatedness. Defects in the IL-12–IFN-γ axis should not only be sought in patients with disseminated or recurrent BCG/EM disease but also considered in patients with acute local BCG/EM, severe tuberculosis, severe histoplasmosis, listeriosis, and severe viral infections. Despite the progress outlined in this chapter, our understanding of the molecular basis of MSMD is still in its relative infancy; it is likely that there are many aspects of the disease that are yet to be unraveled. It is therefore prudent to consider the disorder in those diagnostic conundrums in which infectious, malignant, or inflammatory diagnoses are entertained.

Laboratory Diagnosis

In vitro testing is based on (1) circulating IFN-γ levels, (2) protein expression (FACS, ELISA), (3) functional studies, and (4) DNA analysis.

Measurement of circulating IFN-γ in either plasma or serum is a simple means of differentiating patients with complete IFN-γR deficiency from those with other MSMD mutations (Fieschi et al., 2001). These children have high levels of plasma IFN-γ, whereas IFN-γ is low or undetectable in plasma taken from healthy controls or from MSMD patients with IL-12p40 or IL-12Rβ1 receptor deficiency or partial IFNγR1 or 2 deficiency. These high levels are thought to be due to sustained production of IFN-γ in the most severe form of MSMD and/or the requirement for an intact IFN-γR for ligation and removal of IFN-γ from the circulation. This observation provides a simple diagnostic assay for individuals having severe BCG/EM disease. It should be kept in mind, however, that elevated plasma or local (e.g., pleural tuberculosis) IFN-γ levels may also be seen in normal hosts with tuberculosis.

The IFN-γR is expressed ubiquitously on all nucleated cells, whereas the IL-12 receptor is found only on NK and T cells. Analysis of Epstein-Barr virus (EBV)-induced B lymphoblasts, SV-40 fibroblasts, or peripheral blood mononuclear cells (PBMC) for IFN-γR cell surface expression by fluorescence-activated cell sorting (FACS) is a simple means to assess the presence or absence of these receptors, as demonstrated for the first reported cases of complete IFN-γR1 deficiency (Jouanguy et al., 1996; Newport et al., 1996). Mutations causing the dominant form of IFN-γR1 deficiency abrogate the receptor recycling motif leading to high levels of cell surface IFN-γR1 expression (up to 10-fold), which is easily detectable by FACS staining (Jouanguy et al., 1999b; Villela et al., 2001; Sasaki et al., 2002). Normal expression

of IFNγ-R1, as detected by FACS, even using blocking antibodies, does not exclude partial or even complete IFNγ-R1 deficiency from mutations that result in the surface expression of an abnormal protein (Jouanguy et al., 1997, 2000). Antibodies that recognize low levels of IFN-γR2 present on resting cells are not yet adapted to routine laboratory use. Antibodies that recognize IL-12Rβ1 work well on phytohemagglutinin (PHA) blasts and allow a diagnosis of IL-12Rβ1 deficiency. To date, all *IL12RB1* mutations identified cause a loss of expression of the encoded chain. Staining of *Herpesvirus saimiri*–transformed T cell lines also works well; this is not the case for other cell lines such as EBV-transformed B lymphoblasts and SV40-transformed fibroblasts. Secreted IL-12p40 and p70 can be detected by ELISA in the supernatant of PBMC stimulated by BCG or in the supernatant of EBV-transformed B lymphoblasts stimulated with phorbol 12,13-dibutyrate (PDBu). To date, all *IL12B* mutations identified have been associated with a lack of detectable IL-12p40 and IL-12p70. However, prolonged stimulation of IL-12Rβ1 deficient T cell lines appears to rescue some degree of IL-12 responsiveness (Verhagen et al., 2000).

Expression of IFN-γR or IL-12R does not imply function, and therefore other in vitro assays are required to identify which component(s) of the IL-12/IFN-γ pathway are defective. Upon binding to its receptor, IFN-γ induces pleiotropic effects, including the up-regulation of major histocompatibility complex (MHC) class II expression and TNF-α production by monocytes. These effects are mediated by the binding of phosphorylated STAT1 to gamma-activating-sequences (GAS) in gamma-responsive genes. Thus IFN-γR deficiency may be diagnosed functionally by studying in vitro responses to IFN-γ. A simple whole-blood assay was used to demonstrate defective responses to IFN-γ in the Maltese kindred (Levin et al., 1995), and this technique was modified to study PBMC responses in a patient with partial IFN-γR1 deficiency (Jouanguy et al., 1997). MHC class II expression is easily studied by flow cytometry (Altare et al., 1998b), whereas phosphorylation and nuclear translocation of STAT1 in response to IFN-γ can be assessed using electrophoretic mobility shift assays (Bach et al., 1997; Dupuis et al., 2001) or, more simply, by flow cytometry with a STAT1-specific monoclonal antibody (Fleischer et al., 1999). Cellular responses to IFN-γ should be tested at low and high concentrations of IFN-γ to differentiate between partial and complete receptor deficiency. In vitro studies in patients with IL-12p40 deficiency show defective IFN-γ production by PBMC or whole blood following stimulation with BCG. This defect was restored by the addition of recombinant IL-12 to the culture medium. IL-12Rβ1-deficient patients also have diminished mitogen-induced IFN-γ production, but IL-12 p70 production in response to lipopolysaccharide (LPS), tuberculin, or mycobacteria is normal. A flow-cytometric assay that detects phosphorylated STAT4 has also been developed (Uzel et al., 2001). Notably, children with complete IFN-γR deficiency have low in vitro production of IFN-γ because of impaired production of IL-12 (Holland et al., 1998).

With the exception of the dominant *IFNGR1* hot-spot mutations and the two *IL12B* mutations (founder effects), every MSMD family has a unique mutation. It is therefore not cost-effective to set up mutation screening assays looking for known mutations. A combination of in vitro phenotyping (expression and functional studies) and direct gene sequencing is recommended. Once the causative mutation has been established in a family, other family members can be screened directly for the mutation. Accurate molecular diagnosis by biochemical, functional, and genetic studies is of the utmost importance for predicting clinical outcome and guiding the treatment of patients.

Genetic Counseling and Prenatal Diagnosis

Defects in the IL-12–IFN-γ pathway may be inherited either as dominant or recessive disorders, depending on the mutation. All mutations reported in *IFNGR2*, *IL12RB1*, and *IL12B* are recessive: many patients are homozygous for recessive mutations, reflecting the high frequency of parental consanguinuity within this group of patients. *IFNGR1* mutations were initially identified as homozygous recessively inherited, but dominant mutations have subsequently been identified as well. Compound heterozygotes have also been identified. The *STAT1* mutation identified in three individuals to date is dominant. Finally, X-linked recessive inheritance has been suggested in one kindred, although the molecular basis of increased susceptibility to EM in this family has yet to be established (Holland et al., 1994; Frucht and Holland, 1996; Frucht et al., 1999).

Given the heterogeneity of this syndrome, coupled with its rarity, carrier detection or screening is not currently feasible. In one family with recessive IFN-γR1 deficiency, heterozygous carriers had an intermediate cellular phenotype in vitro (Levin et al., 1995; Newport et al., 1996), although this may have been dependent on the assay used. To date, there is no clinical phenotype associated with heterozygosity for any of the recessive alleles. Once the molecular basis is known within a family, it is simplest to screen other members by directly sequencing their DNA. Counseling within families where the mutation is known is straightforward in terms of the risk of inheriting a "susceptible" genotype (25% risk of an affected child if recessive, 50% risk of an affected child if dominant inheritance). However, any discussion must also take into account the following: (1) the clinical phenotype depends on the gene affected and whether the mutation leads to complete or partial protein deficiency; (2) development of disease is dependent on pathogen exposure; and (3) there are individuals who have inherited a susceptible genotype without developing disease, presumably thanks to the impact of modifyer genes that result in residual antimycobacterial immune function. To date, there are no known individuals with complete IFN-γR1, IFN-γR2, or STAT1 deficiency who have not been clinically affected. Complete IFN-γR1 or IFN-γR2 deficiency is the most severe phenotype and is frequently lethal despite the use of antibiotics. BCG vaccination must be withheld from potentially affected children until IFN-γR status is clarified. Bone marrow transplantation (BMT) has proved very difficult and less successful than would be anticipated (see below), perhaps because transplantation has typically been attempted after disseminated mycobacterial disease occurred.

Once a molecular diagnosis has been established, prenatal diagnosis can be offered to affected families with severe disease—i.e., complete IFN-γR deficiency. The role of prenatal diagnosis for other mutations is less obvious as the phenotype is less severe, disease is preventable, and many individuals carrying mutations are disease-free.

Treatment and Prognosis

The treatment of defects in the IL-12–IFN-γ axis should be tailored to the individual patient according to their mutation, the clinical pattern of disease, and the pathogens involved (Holland, 2000b). Established infection should be treated with appropriate antimicrobial drugs as determined by the genus and species. Thus microbiological isolation and characterization of the causative pathogen at an early stage are desirable. The role for in vitro susceptibilities in directing treatment of EM is still unproven and poorly defined. EM are notoriously resistant to a number of antimicrobials. Cytokine therapy has helped clear mycobacterial infection in patients with full or partial function of the IFN-γ receptor (Holland et al., 1994; Holland, 2000a). Patients with IL-12B (IL-12p40) or IL-12Rβ1 deficiency or partial IFN-γR deficiency respond well to IFN-γ treatment. However, intestinal, mesenteric, and splenic infections can be resistant to antibiotics and IFN-γ. Splenectomy was helpful in two children with splenic sequestration (IFN-γ induced in one child); on occasion abdominal lymph node resection may be indicated (Kaufman et al., 1998; J.-L. Casanova, unpublished report). Overall, patients with partial IFN-γR/STAT1 deficiency or complete IL-12Rβ1 deficiency can achieve prolonged clinical remission after antibiotics and IFN-γ are discontinued. Relapses may occur years after the initial episode. Treatment with antibiotics and IFN-γ should be prolonged, even after clinical remission is obtained.

In contrast, children with complete IFN-γR deficiency achieve full clinical remission less often and mycobacterial infections often relapse weeks to months after antibiotics are discontinued. Therefore, successful antibiotic therapy should not be discontinued. Because of the lack of specific receptors, IFN-γ therapy is not indicated. The role for other cytokines such as IFN-α, granulocyte-macrophage colony–stimulating factor (GM-CSF), or IL-12 is undefined. The only curative treatment available for patients with complete IFN-γR deficiency is BMT (Reuter et al., 2002). An international survey identified eight unrelated patients with complete IFN-γR1 deficiency who underwent BMT (Roesler et al., 2004). The results were disappointing; BMT in complete IFN-γR1 deficiency is associated with high morbidity and mortality. The only child receiving a human leukocyte antigen (HLA)-haploidentical transplant died after the second transplant (HLA identical) of EBV-induced lymphoproliferative disease. Of the seven patients transplanted with an HLA-identical intrafamilial graft, despite an initial full engraftment in most cases four are alive, but only two have a functional graft and are free of infection. There appears to be a selective advantage of IFN-γR-deficient over wild-type hemopoietic progenitors in IFN-γR-deficient children (which makes gene therapy for patients with IFN-γR deficiency challenging). Moreover, chronic EM/MAC infection before and during stem cell transplantation carries an unfavorable outcome. Prevention of infection is desirable, although many pathogens to which these individuals are susceptible are ubiquitous in the environment. BCG should be avoided and mycobacterial infection (both primary and secondary) may be prevented by the use of a macrolide such as clarithromycin or azithromycin. In patients with mild MSMD, prophylactic antibiotics are not absolutely required, as infectious episodes are relatively infrequent and can be controlled by IFN-γ and antibiotics if treated promptly. However, physicians and patients should weigh carefully the risks and benefits of recurrence of infection, especially if it recurs in bone, as is often the case with the dominant form of IFN-γR1 deficiency. In these patients recurrence of infection can have serious consequences, despite curative therapy.

In patients with complete IFN-γR deficiency, antibiotics should be continued indefinitely after therapy for acute infections. There is considerable diversity of pathogenic EM (particularly rapidly growing species), making absolute recommendations difficult. Most EM are susceptible to macrolides, and these should be strongly considered for long-term prophylaxis regardless of cure of other acute infections. Immunosupressive agents such as corticosteroids should be avoided as a rule, particularly in children with complete IFN-γR deficiency, although in some circumstances they may be helpful. Children with MSMD should be treated on an individual basis, and treatment should be undertaken in close collaboration with a center specialized in the care of such patients.

Animal Models

The study of gene-disrupted mice has greatly enhanced our understanding of the IL-12–IFN-γ pathway. Although not completely concordant, the phenotypic similarities between these animal models and patients with mutations in this axis are striking (Jouanguy et al., 1999a). Mice lacking *Ifngr1* are highly susceptible to BCG infection, with poorly defined granuloma formation and death (Kamijo et al., 1993). Mice lacking Ifn-γ also fail to control BCG, *M. avium*, or *M. tuberculosis* growth (Cooper et al., 1993; Dalton et al., 1993). More recently, *Ifngr2* knockout mice were shown to have defective Ifn-γ production and susceptiblity to *L. monocytogenes* infection (Lu et al., 1998). *Il12b* (il-12p40) knockout mice are more susceptible to *M. tuberculosis* infection than normal mice, leading to higher bacterial loads and disseminated disease (Cooper et al., 1997). Granulomata were poorly formed and multibacillary. *Il12rb1* knockout mice have defective Ifn-γ responses to mitogens and LPS (Wu et al., 1997). Disruption of *Ifng* in mice also leads to lethal infection with an attenuated strain of *S. typhimurium*, whereas wild-type mice clear infection within 4 weeks (Hess et al., 1996; Bao et al., 2000). However, comparisons between mice and humans are limited in several ways: most of the infections in MSMD patients are naturally occurring, whereas those in mice are experimental and often administered intravenously, and the strain and dose of pathogen are controlled. There are certain infections, such as *Toxoplasma gondii* and *Cryptococcus neoformans*, to which *Ifng*/Il-12 knockout mice have increased susceptibility that have not been observed in humans (Decken et al., 1998; Yap et al., 2000). This may reflect lack of exposure, experimental design, or the fact that knockout mice are generated in highly inbred strains. Genetic variation at other immunity-modifying loci is low in inbred mice whereas humans are outbred, even in the setting of consanguinity. Experimental infections in mice probably highlight even minor effects of the Il-12–Ifn-γ axis. Alternatively, mice and humans may differ in their handling of some of these nonmycobacterial infections.

Concluding Remarks and Future Challenges

Mutations in five genes involved in the IL-12–IFN-γ axis have been associated with the syndrome of MSMD, which encompasses a range of clinical phenotypes. The severity of the clinical phenotype depends primarily on the gene involved and the specific mutation. IFN-γ-mediated immunity appears to be a genetically controlled quantitative trait that determines the outcome of mycobacterial invasion (Dupuis et al., 2000). IFN-γ immunity to mycobacteria is dependent on IL-12 stimulation, and mediated by STAT1 and its homodimeric complex GAF. These defects are most pronounced with respect to mycobacteria and, to a lesser extent, salmonella and viruses. (Casanova and Abel, 2002). The investigation of more patients is necessary to broaden our knowledge of these genotype–phenotype correlations. Clinically, molecular diagnosis guides rational treatment based on pathophysiology.

Are There Other MSMD Genes?

There remain patients with the clinical syndrome of MSMD who do not have mutations in *IFNGR1*, *IFNGR2*, *STAT1*, *IL12B*, or *IL12RB1* (approximately 50% at our centers, S. Holland, M. Levin, and J.-L. Casanova, unpublished results). Characterization of the molecular defects in these patients will help in the identification of other MSMD genes and contribute further to our understanding of human mycobacterial immunity. Relevant genes upstream of IL-12 and downstream of STAT1 are expected to expand and define the limits of the IL-12–IFN-γ axis, especially the inducer and effector mechanisms of immunity to mycobacteria.

Definition of Clinical Boundaries of MSMD

The genetic defects of the IL-12–IFN-γ axis were found by investigating patients with disseminated, often lethal, BCG/EM disease. Subsequently, it was found that some affected individuals have recurrent local disease, whereas others are asymptomatic. The clinical boundaries of IL-12Rβ1 deficiency (Fieschi et al., 2003) and IFN-γR1 deficiency (Dorman et al., 2004) were made possible thanks to international collaberation. Other international surveys are currently under way to define the clinical features of each inherited disorder on the basis of clinical history of the patients identified. The question arises as to whether patients with unexplained local BCG/EM disease may suffer from these or related genetic defects. For example, EM pneumonitis in the elderly and EM adenitis in childhood are currently unexplained. Because of these considerations, patients with various forms of BCG/EM disease need to be studied in terms of the IL-12–IFN-γ axis to define the clinical frontiers of each genetic defect.

Role of MSMD Genes in Susceptibility to Tuberculosis and Leprosy

It is estimated that approximately 2 billion individuals worldwide are infected with *M. tuberculosis* (Dolin et al., 1994). The World Health Organization estimates that there were 8 million new cases of tuberculosis (TB) and 1.9 million deaths from the disease in 1998. The fact that only 10% of individuals infected with *M. tuberculosis* go on to develop clinical disease suggests that exposure to virulent mycobacteria alone is not sufficient and that the host immune response is an important determinant of susceptibility (or resistance) to disease (Murray et al., 1990). Several studies demonstrate a role for host genetic factors as determinants of susceptibility to TB (Casanova and Abel, 2002, 2004). However, the identification of specific genes involved in susceptibility to infectious diseases in outbred human populations is difficult. Complex interactions among the pathogen, which also has a genome, the environment, and host factors determine whether an individual is resistant or susceptible to disease. It is likely that a number of genes are involved, but it is not known exactly how many or how they interact. Population-based studies have reported associations between candidate genes and TB, but the effects have been modest and the functional relevance of these findings is yet to be established (Newport and Levin, 1999; Wilkinson et al., 1999; Abel and Casanova, 2000; Casanova and Abel 2002, 2004).

There is a spectrum of disease within the MSMD syndrome ranging from severe disease that is fatal in early childhood (complete IFN-γR deficiency) to moderate disease in individuals with partial IFN-γR1 deficiency (Jouanguy et al., 1997). The IL-12p40/IL-12Rβ1 mutations have a less severe clinical course. Mutations in *IL12RB1* and *IL12B* have been identified as a susceptibility factor for the development of abdominal *M. tuberculosis* infection (Altare et al., 2001) and tuberculous adenitis (Picard et al., 2002). Furthermore, two families have been observed whose affected members lacked IL-12β1 and suffered from disseminated tuberculosis; however, none of them had a history of clinical disease caused by BCG/EM (Caragol et al., 2003; Özbeck et al., 2005). Disorders of the IL-12–IFN-γ axis should thus be considered in selected children with severe tuberculosis, even in the absence of infection with poorly virulent mycobactreia or salmonella. Partial deficiency of either IL-12p40 or IL-12Rβ1 would be expected to have a less severe phenotype than complete deficiency and to show susceptibility to only the most virulent pathogens. More subtle polymorphisms in the MSMD genes identified thus far could result in impaired expression of a normal protein or normal expression of a slightly altered, less efficient protein. It is also likely that mutations or polymorphisms will be identified in other genes known to be involved in mycobacterial immunity that may play a different role and cause a different immune defect. Such individuals may retain immunity to organisms of low virulence while remaining susceptible to more virulent species.

References

Abel L, Casanova J-L. Genetic predisposition to clinical tuberculosis: bridging the gap between simple and complex inheritance. Am J Hum Genet 67:274–277, 2000.

Aksu G, Tirpan C, Cavusoglu C, Soydan S, Altare F, Casanova JL, Kutukculer N. *Mycobacterium fortuitum-chelonae* complex infection in a child with complete interleukin-12 receptor beta 1 deficiency. Pediatr Infect Dis J 20:551–553, 2001.

Allende LM, Lopez-Goyanes A, Paz-Artal E, Corell A, Garcia-Perez MA, Varela P, Scarpellini A, Negreira S, Palenque E, Arnaiz-Villena A. A point mutation in a domain of gamma interferon receptor 1 provokes severe immunodeficiency. Clin Diagn Lab Immunol 8:133–137, 2001.

Altare F, Durandy A, Lammas D, Emile J-F, Lamhamedi S, Le Deist F, Drysdale P, Jouanguy E, Doffinger R, Bernaudin F, Jeppsonn O, Gollob JA, Meinl E, Segal AW, Fischer A, Kumarante D, Casanova JL. Impairment of mycobacterial immunity in human interleukin-12 receptor deficiency. Science 280:1432–1435, 1998a.

Altare F, Ensser A, Breiman A, Reichenbach J, Baghdadi JE, Fischer A, Emile JF, Gaillard JL, Meinl E, Casanova JL. Interleukin-12 receptor beta 1 deficiency in a patient with abdominal tuberculosis. J Infect Dis 184:231–236, 2001.

Altare F, Jouanguy E, Lamhamedi S, Fondaneche MC, Merlin G, Dembic Z, Schreiber RD, Lisowska-Grospierre B, Fischer A, Seboun E, Casanova JL. A causative relationship between mutant *IFNgR1* alleles and impaired response to IFN-γ in a compound heterozygous child. Am J Hum Genet 62:723–726, 1998b.

Altare F, Lammas D, Revy P, Jouanguy E, Doffinger R, Lamhamedi S, Drysdale P, Scheel-Toellner D, Girdlestone J, Darbyshire P, Wadhwa M, Dockrell H, Salmon M, Fischer A, Durandy A, Casanova JL, Kumararante D. Inherited interleukin 12 deficiency in a child with bacille Calmette-Guerin and *Salmonella enteritidis* disseminated infection. J Clin Invest 102:2035–2040, 1998c.

Bach EA, Aguet M, Schreiber RD. The IFN-γ receptor: a paradigm for cytokine receptor signalling. Annu Rev Immunol 15:563–591, 1997.

Bach EA, Szabo SJ, Dighe AS, Ashkenazi A, Aguet M, Murphy KM, Schreiber RD. Ligand-induced autoregulation of IFN-γ receptor β chain expression in T helper cell subsets. Science 270:1215–1218, 1995.

Bao S, Beagley KW, France MP, Shen J, Husband AJ. Interferon-gamma plays a critical role in intestinal immunity against salmonella typhimurium infection. Immunology 99:464–472, 2000.

Buhler VB, Pollack A. Human infection with atypical acid-fast organisms. Am J Clin Pathol 23:363–374, 1953.

Camcioglu Y, Picard C, Lacoste V, Dupuis S, Akcakaya N, Cokura H, Kaner G, Demirkesen C, Plancoulaine S, Emile JF, Gessain A, Casanova JL. HHV-8-associated Kaposi sarcoma in a child with IFNγR deficiency. J Pediatr 144:519–523, 2004.

Caragol I, Raspall M, Fieschi C, Feinberg J, Hernadez M, Larrosa MN, Figueras C, Bertran J-M, Casanova J-L, Espanol T. Clinical tuberculosis in two of three siblings with interleukin-12 receptor β1 deficiency. Clin Infect Dis 37:302–306, 2003.

Casanova J-L, Abel L. Genetic dissection of immunity to mycobacteria: the human model. Annu Rev Immunol 20:581–620, 2002.

Casanova JL, Abel L. The human model: a genetic dissection of immunity to infection in natural conditions. Nat Rev Immunol 4:55–66, 2004.

Casanova J-L, Blanche S, Emile J-F, Stephan J-L, Bernaudin F, Jouanguy E, Lamhamedi S, Bordigoni P, Turck D, Albertini M, Dommergues J-P, Rybojad M, Pocidalo M-A, Le Deist F, Griscelli C, Fischer A. Idiopathic disseminated bacille Calmette-Guerin infection: a French national retrospective study. Pediatrics 98:774–778, 1996.

Casanova JL, Jouanguy E, Lamhamedi S, Blanche S, Fischer A. Immunological conditions of children with BCG disseminated infection. Lancet 346:581, 1995.

Cooper AM, Dalton DK, Stewart TA, Griffin JP, Russell DG, Orme IM. Disseminated tuberculosis in IFN-γ gene disrupted mice. J Exp Med 178:2243–2247, 1993.

Cooper AM, Magram J, Ferrante J, Orme IM. Interleukin-12 (IL-12) is crucial to the development of protective immunity in mice intravenously infected with *Mycobacterium tuberculosis*. J Exp Med 186:39–45, 1997.

Cunningham JA, Kellner JD, Bridge PJ, Trevenen CL, Mcleod DR, Davies HD. Disseminated bacille Calmette-Guerin infection in an infant with a novel deletion in the interferon-gamma receptor gene. Int J Tuberc Lung Dis 4:791–794, 2000.

Dalton D, Pitts-Meek S, Keshav S, Figari IS, Bradley A, Stewart TA. Multiple defects of immune cell function in mice with disrupted interferon-γ genes. Science 259:1739–1742, 1993.

Decken K, Kohler G, Palmer-Lehmann K, Wunderlin A, Mattner F, Magram J, Gately MK, Alber G. Interleukin-12 is essential for a protective Th1 response in mice infected with *Cryptococcus neoformans*. Infect Immun 66:4994–5000, 1998.

de Jong R, Altare F, Haagen I-A, Elferink DG, de Boer T, van Breda Vriesman PJC, Kabel PJ, Draaisma JMT, van Dissel JT, Kroon FP, Casanova J-L, Ottenhoff THM. Severe mycobacterial and *Salmonella* infections in interleukin-12 receptor–deficient patients. Science 280:1435–1438, 1998.

Doffinger R, Jouanguy E, Dupuis S, Fondaneche MC, Stephan JL, Emile JF, Lamhamedi-Cherradi S, Altare F, Pallier A, Barcenas-Morales G, Meinl E, Krause C, Pestka S, Schreiber RD, Novelli F, Casanova JL. Partial interferon-gamma receptor signaling chain deficiency in a patient with bacille Calmette-Guerin and *Mycobacterium abscessus* infection. J Infect Dis 181:379–384, 2000.

Doleckova V, Viklicky J, Sula L, Kubecova D. Fatal generalized BCG histiocytosis. Tubercle 58:13–18, 1977.

Dolin PJ, Raviglione MC, Kochi A. Global tuberculosis incidence and mortality during 1990–2000. Bull World Health Organ 72:213–220, 1994.

Dorman SE, Holland SM. Mutation in the signal transducing chain of the interferon-γ receptor and susceptibility to mycobacterial infection. J Clin Invest 101:2364–2369, 1998.

Dorman SE, Holland SM. Interferon-γ and interleukin-12 pathway defects and human disease. Cytokine Growth Factor Rev 11:321–333, 2000.

Dorman SE, Picard C, Lammas D, Heyne K, van Dissel JT, Baretto R, Rosenzweig SD, Newport M, Levin M, Roesler J, Kumararante D, Casanova JL, Holland SM. Clinical features of dominant and recessive interferon γ receptor 1 deficiencies. Lancet 364:2113–2121, 2004.

Dorman SE, Uzel G, Roesler J, Bradley JS, Bastian J, Billman G, King S, Filie A, Schermerhorn J, Holland SM. Viral infections in interferon-gamma receptor deficiency. J Pediatr 135:640–643, 1999.

D'Souza S, Levin M, Faith A, Yssel H, Bennett B, Lake RA, Brown IN, Lamb JR. Defective antigen processing associated with familial disseminated mycobacteriosis. Clin Exp Immunol 103:35–39, 1996.

Dupuis S, Dargemont C, Fieschi C, Thomassin N, Rosenzweig S, Harris J, Holland SM, Schreiber RD, Casanova JL. Impairment of mycobacterial but not viral immunity by a germline human *STAT1* mutation. Science 293:300–303, 2001.

Dupuis S, Doffinger R, Picard C, Fieschi C, Altare F, Jouanguy E, Abel L, Casanova JL. Human interferon-gamma-mediated immunity is a genetically controlled continuous trait that determines the outcome of mycobacterial invasion. Immunol Rev 178:129–137, 2000.

Dupuis S, Jouangy E, Al-Hajjar S, Fieschi C, Al-Mohsen IZ, Al-Jumaah S, Yang K, Chapgier A, Eidenschenk C, Eid P, Ghonaium A, Tufenkenkeji H, Schreiber RD, Gresser I, Casanova JL. Impaired responses to interferon-alpha/beta and lethal viral disease in human *STAT1* deficiency. Nat Genet 33:388–391, 2003.

Dvoracek C, Mores A, Neoral L. Generalized lymphadenopathy following BCG vaccination. Rozhledy v Tuberculose a v Nemocech Plicnich 19:107–114, 1959.

Edgar JD, Smyth AE, Pritchard J, Lammas D, Jouanguy E, Hague R, Novelli V, Dempsey S, Sweeney L, Taggart AJ, O'Hara D, Casanova JL, Kumararatne DS. Interferon-gamma receptor deficiency mimicking Langerhans' cell histiocytosis. J Pediatr 139:600–603, 2001.

Emile J-F, Patey N, Altare F, Lamhamedi S, Jouanguy E, Boman F, Quillard J, Lecomte-Houcke M, Verola O, Mousnier J-F, Dijoud F, Blanche S, Fischer A, Brousse N, Casanova JL. Correlation of granuloma structure with clinical outcome defines two types of idiopathic disseminated BCG infection. J Pathol 181:25–30, 1997.

Engbaek HC. Three cases in the same family of fatal infection with *M. avium*. Acta Tuberc Scand 45:105–117, 1964.

Fedak S. Testverpar rikta, BCG-oltasi reactioja. Gyermekgyogyaszat 25: 386–389, 1974.

Feinberg J, Fieschi C, Doffinger R, Feinberg M, Leclerc T, Boisson-Dupuis S, Picard C, Bustamante J, Chapgier A, Filipe-Santos O, Ku CL, de Beaucoudrey L, Reichenbach J, Antoni G, Balde R, Alcais A, Casanova JL. Bacillus Calmette Guerin triggers the IL-12/IFN-gamma axis by an IRAK-4- and NEMO-dependent, non-cognate interaction between monocytes, NK, and T lymphocytes. Eur J Immunol 34:3276–3284, 2004.

Fieschi C, Bosticardo M, de Beaucoudrey L, Boisson-Dupuis S, Feinberg J, Santos OF, Bustamante J, Levy J, Candotti F, Casanova JL. A novel form of complete IL-12/IL-23 receptor β1 deficiency with cell surface–expressed nonfunctional receptors. Blood 104:2095–2101, 2004.

Fieschi C, Casanova JL. The role of interleukin-12 in human infectious diseases: only a faint signature. Eur J Immunol 33:1461–1464, 2003.

Fieschi C, Dupuis S, Catherinot E, Feinberg J, Bustamante J, Breiman A, Altare F, Baretto R, Le Deist F, Kayal S, Koch H, Richter D, Brezina M, Aksu G, Wood P, Al-Jumaah S, Raspall M, Da Silva Duarte AJ, Tuerlinckx D, Virelizier JL, Fischer A, Enright A, Bernhoft J, Cleary AM, Vermylen C, Rodriguez-Gallego C, Davies G, Blutters-Sawatzki R, Siegrist CA, Ehlayel MS, Novelli V, Haas WH, Levy J, Freihorst J, Al-Hajjar S, Nadal D, De Moraes Vasconcelos D, Jeppsson O, Kutukculer N, Frecerova K, Caragol I, Lammas D, Kumararatne DS, Abel L, Casanova JL. Low penetrance, broad resistance and favourable outcome of interleukin 12 receptor β1 deficiency: medical and immunological implications. J Exp Med 197:527–535, 2003.

Fieschi C, Dupuis S, Picard C, Edvard Smith CI, Holland SM, Casanova JL. High levels of interferon gamma in the plasma of children with complete interferon gamma receptor deficiency. Pediatrics 107:e48, 2001.

Fleischer TA, Dorman SE, Anderson JA, Vail M, Brown MR, Holland SM. Detection of intracellular phosphorylted STAT-1 by flow cytometry. Clin Immunol 90:425–430, 1999.

Frucht DM, Holland SM. Defective monocyte costimulation for interferon gamma production in familial disseminated *Mycobacterium avium* complex infection. J Immunol 157:411–416, 1996.

Frucht DM, Sandberg DI, Brown MR, Gerstberger SM, Holland SM. IL-12-independent costimulation pathways for interferon-gamma production in familial disseminated mycobacterium avium complex infection. Clin Immunol 91:234–241, 1999.

Genin E, Tullio-Pelet A, Begeot F, Lyonnet S, Abel L. Estimating the age of rare disease mutations: the example of triple-A syndrome. J Med Genet 41:445–449, 2004.

Hess J, Ladel C, Miko D, Kaufmann SHE. *Salmonella typhimurium* aroA-infection in gene targetted immunodeficient mice. J Immunol 156: 3321–3326, 1996.

Heyne K. Generalized familial semi-benign BCG infections. *Salmonella* osteomyelitis and intestinal pseudotuberculosis due to a familial defect of the macrophage system. Eur J Pediatr 121:179–189, 1976.

Holland SM. Cytokine therapy of mycobacterial infection. Adv Intern Med 45:431–451, 2000a.

Holland SM. Treatment of infections in the patient with Mendelian susceptibility ot mycobacterial infection. Microbes Infect 2:1579–1590, 2000b.

Holland SM, Dorman SE, Kwon A, Pitha-Rowe IF, Frucht DM, Gerstberger SM, Noel GJ, Vesterhus P, Brown MR, Fleischer TA. Abnormal regulation of interferon gamma, interleukin-12, and tumor necrsosis factor alpha in interferon gamma receptor 1 deficiency. J Infect Dis 178:1095–1104, 1998.

Holland SM, Eisenstein EM, Kuhns DB, Turner ML, Fleischer TA, Strober W, Gallin JI. Treatment of refractory disseminated nontuberculous mycobacterial infection with interferon gamma. N Engl J Med 330:1348–1355, 1994.

Jouanguy E, Altare F, Lamhamedi S, Revy P, Newport M, Levin M, Blanche S, Fischer A, Casanova JL. Interferon-gamma-receptor deficiency in an infant with fatal bacille Calmette-Guerin infection. N Engl J Med 335:1956–1959, 1996.

Jouanguy E, Doffinger R, Dupuis S, Pallier A, Altare F, Casanova JL. IL-12 and IFN-γ in host defense against mycobacteria and salmonella in mice and men. Curr Opin Immunol 11:346–351, 1999a.

Jouanguy E, Dupuis S, Pallier A, Doffinger R, Fondaneche MC, Fieschi C, Lamhamedi-Cherradi S, Altare F, Emile J-F, Lutz P, Bordigoni P, Cokugras H, Akcakaya N, Landman-Parker J, Donnadieu J, Camciogllu Y, Casanova J-L. In a novel form of IFN-γ receptor 1 deficiency, cell surface receptors fail to bind IFN-γ. J Clin Invest 105:1429–1436, 2000.

Jouanguy E, Lamamedi-Cherradi S, Altare F, Fondaneche M-C, Tuerlinckx D, Blanche S, Emile J-F, Gaillard J-L, Schreiber R, Levin M, Fischer A, Hivroz C, Casanova JL. Partial interferon-γ receptor 1 deficiency in a

child with tuberculoid bacillus Calmette-Guérin infection and a sibling with clinical tuberculosis. J Clin Invest 100:2658–2664, 1997.

Jouanguy E, Lamhamedi-Cherradi S, Lammas D, Dorman SE, Fondaneche MC, Dupuis S, Doffinger R, Altare F, Girdlestone J, Emile J-F, Ducoulombier H, Edgar D, Clarke J, Oxelius V-A, Brai M, Novelli V, Heyne K, Fischer A, Holland SM, Kumararatne D, Schreiber RD, Casanova JL. A human *IFNGR1* small deletion hot spot associated with dominant susceptibility to mycobacterial infection. Nat Genet 21:370–378, 1999b.

Kamijo R, Le J, Shapiro D, Havell EA, Huang S, Aguet M, Bosland M, Vilcek J. Mice that lack the interferon-gamma receptor have profoundly altered responses to infection with bacillus Calmette-Guerin and subsequent challenge with lipopolysaccharide. J Exp Med 178:1435–1440, 1993.

Kaufman HL, Roden M, Nathanson D, Basso TM, Schwartzentruber DJ, Holland SM. Splenectomy in a child with chronic *Mycobacterium avium* complex infection and splenic sequestration. J Pediatr Surg 33:761–763, 1998.

Koscielniak E, de Boer T, Dupuis S, Naumann L, Casanova JL, Ottenhoff TH. Disseminated *Mycobacterium peregrinum* infection in a child with complete interferon-gamma receptor-1 deficiency. Pediatr Infect Dis J 22: 378–380, 2003.

Lammas DA, Casanova J-L, Kumararatne DS. Clinical consequences of defects in the IL-12-dependent interferon-gamma (IFN-γ) pathway. Clin Exp Immunol 121:417–425, 2000.

Levin M, Newport MJ, D'Souza S, Kalabalikis P, Brown I, Lenicker H, Vassallo Agius P, Davies EG, Thrasher A, Blackwell JM. Familial disseminated atypical mycobacterial infection in early childhood: a human mycobacterial susceptibility gene? Lancet 345:79–83, 1995.

Lu B, Ebensperger C, Dembic Z, Wang Y, Kvatyuk M, Lu T, Coffman RL, Pestka S, Rothman PB. Targeted disruption of the interferon-gamma receptor 2 gene results in severe immune defects in mice. Proc Natl Acad Sci USA 95:8233–8238, 1998.

MacLennan C, Fieschi C, Lammas DA, Picard C, Dorman SE, Sanal O, MacLennan JM, Holland SM, Ottenhoff TH, Casanova JL, Kumararatne DS. Interleukin (IL)-12 and IL-23 are key cytokines for immunity against *Salmonella* in humans. J Infect Dis 190:1755–1757, 2004.

Mimouni J. Notre experience de trois annees de vaccination BCGS au centre de IOPHS de Constantine. Etude de cas observes (25 becegites). Algier Med 55:1138–1147, 1951.

Murray GDL, Styblo K, Rouillon A. Tuberculosis in developing countries: burden, intervention and cost. Bull IUATLD 65:6–24, 1990.

Newport MJ, Huxley CM, Huston S, Hawrylowicz CM, Oostra BA, Williamson R, Levin M. A mutation in the interferon-gamma receptor gene and susceptibility to mycobacterial infections in man. N Engl J Med 335:1941–1949, 1996.

Newport MJ, Levin M. Genetic susceptibility to tuberculosis. J Infect 139: 117–121, 1999.

Novelli F, Casanova JL. The role of IL-12, IL-23 and IFN-gamma in immunity to viruses. Cytokine Growth Factor Rev 15:367–377, 2004.

Özbeck N, Fieschi C, Yilmaz BT, de Beaucoudrey L, Bikmaz YE, Casanova JL. Inerleukin-12 receptor β1 chain deficiency in a child with disseminated tuberculosis. Clin Infect Dis 40:e55–58, 2005.

Picard C, Fieschi C, Altare F, Al-Jumaah S, Al-Hajjar S, Feinberg J, Dupuis S, Soudais C, Al-Mohsen IZ, Genin E, Lammas D, Kumararatne DS, Leclerc T, Rafii A, Fraya H, Murugasu B, Wah LB, Sinniah R, Loubser M, Okamoto E, Al-Ghonaium A, Tufenkeji H, Abel L, Casanova JL. Inherited interleukin-12 deficiency: *IL12B* genotype and clinical phenotype of 13 patients from six kindreds. Am J Hum Genet 70:336–348, 2002.

Pierre-Audigier C, Jouanguy E, Lamhamedi S, Altare F, Rauzier J, Vincent V, Canioni D, Emile J-F, Fischer A, Blanche S, Gaillard JL, Casanova JL. Fatal dissemniated *Mycobacterium smegmatis* infection in a child with inherited interferon γ receptor deficiency. Clin Infect Dis 24:982–984, 1997.

Remus N, Reichenbach J, Picard C, Rietschel C, Wood P, Lammas D, Kumararatne DS, Casanova JL. Impaired interferon gamma-mediated immunity and susceptibility to mycobacterial infection in childhood. Pediatr Res 50:8–13, 2001.

Reuter U, Roesler J, Thiede C, Schulz A, Classen CF, Oelschlagel U, Debatin KM, Holland S, Casanova JL, Friedrich W. Correction of complete interferon-gamma receptor 1 deficiency by bone marrow transplantation. Blood 100:4234–4235, 2002.

Roesler J, Horwitz ME, Picard C, Bordigoni P, Davies G, Koscielniak E, Levin M, Veys P, Reuter U, Schulz A, Thiede C, Klingebiel T, Fischer A, Holland SM, Casanova JL, Friedrich W. Hematopoietic stem cell transplantation for complete IFN-gamma receptor 1 deficiency: a multi-institutional survey. J Pediatr 145:806–812, 2004.

Roesler J, Kofink B, Wendisch J, Heyden S, Paul D, Friedrich W, Casanova JL, Leupold W, Gahr M, Rosen-Wolff A. *Listeria* monocytogenes and recurrent mycobacterial infections in a child with complete interferon-gamma-receptor (IFNγR1) deficiency: mutational analysis and evaluation of therapeutic options. Exp Hematol 27:1368–1374, 1999.

Rosenzweig S, Dorman SE, Roesler J, Palacios J, Zelasko M, Holland SM. A novel autosomal recessive mutation defines a second mutational hotspot in the interferon gamma receptor 1 (*IFNGR1*) chain. Clin Immunol 102: 25–27, 2002.

Sakai T, Matsuoka M, Aoki M, Nosaka K, Mitsuya H. Missense mutation of the interleukin-12 receptor β1 chain encoding gene is associated with impaired immunity against *Mycobacterium avium* complex infection. Blood 97:2688–2694, 2001.

Sasaki Y, Nomura A, Kusuhara K, Takada H, Ahmed S, Takahata Y, Obinata K, Hamada K, Hara T. Genetic basis of patients with bacille Calmette-Guerin osteomyelitis in Japan: identification of dominant partial interferon-γ receptor 1 deficiency as a predominant type. J Infect Dis 185:706–709, 2002.

Sicevic S. Generalized BCG tuberculosis with fatal course in two sisters. Acta Paediatr Scand 61:178–184, 1972.

Staretz-Haham O, Melamed R, Lifshitz M, Porat N, Fieschi C, Casanova JL, Levy J. Interleukin-12 receptor β1 deficiency presenting as recurrent *Salmonella* infections. Clin Infect Dis 37:137–149, 2003.

Trinchieri G. Interleukin-12: a cytokine at the interface of inflammation and immunity. Adv Immunol 70:83–243, 1998.

Uchiyama N, Greene GR, Warren BJ, Morozumi PA, Spear GS, Galant SP. Possible monocyte killing defect in familial atypical mycobacteriosis. J Pediatr 98:785–788, 1981.

Ulgenalp I, Yalcin C, Cetiner M, Ozgen N, Koseli I. Olumle sonuclanan jeneralize BCG enfeksiyonu. Tuberculoz ve Toraks 21:11–19, 1973.

Uzel G, Frucht DM, Fleischer TA, Holland SM. Detection of intracellular phosphorylated STAT-4 by flow cytometry. Clin Immunol 100:270–273, 2001.

Uzel G, Premkumar A, Malech HL, Holland SM. Respiratory syncytial virus infection in patients with phagocyte defects. Pediatrics 106:835–837, 2000.

van der Hoeven LH, Rutten FJ, van der Sar A. An unusual acid-fast bacillus causing systemic disease and death in a child. Am J Clin Pathol 29:433–454, 1958.

Verhagen CE, de Boer T, Smits HH, Verreck FAW, Wierenga EA, Kurimoto M, Lammas DA, Kumararatne DS, Sanal O, Kroon FP, van Dissel JT, Sinigaglia F, Ottenhoff THM. Residual type 1 immunity in patients genetically deficient for interleukin 12 receptor β1 (IL-12Rβ1): evidence for an IL-12Rβ1-independent pathway of IL-12 responsiveness in human T cells. J Exp Med 192:517–528, 2000.

Vesterhus P, Holland SM, Abrahamsen TG, Bjerknes R. Familial disseminated infection due to atypical mycobacteria with childhood onset. Clin Infect Dis 27:822–825, 1998.

Villella A, Picard C, Jouanguy E, Dupuis S, Popko S, Abughali N, Meyerson H, Casanova J, Hostoffer R. Recurrent *Mycobacterium avium* osteomyelitis associated with a novel dominant interferon gamma receptor mutation. Pediatrics 107:E47, 2001.

Wilkinson RJ, Patel P, Llewelyn M, Hirsch CS, Pasvol G, Snounou G, Davidson RN, Toossi Z. Influence of polymorphism in the genes for the interleukin (IL)-1 receptor antagonist and IL-1β on tuberculosis. J Exp Med 189:1863–1874, 1999.

Wu C, Ferrante J, Gately MK, Magram J. Characterization of IL-12 receptor β1 chain (IL-12Rβ1)-deficient mice: IL-12Rβ1 is an essential component of the functional mouse IL-12 receptor. J Immunol 159:1658–1665, 1997.

Yap G, Pesin M, Sher A. Cutting edge: IL-12 is required for the maintenance of IFN-γ production in T cells mediating chronic resistance to the intracellular pathogen, *Toxoplasma gondii*. J Immunol 165:628–631, 2000.

29

Ataxia-Telangiectasia

MARTIN F. LAVIN and YOSEF SHILOH

Ataxia-telangiectasia (A-T) is a complex multisystem disorder characterized by progressive neurological impairment, variable immunodeficiency, and ocular and cutaneous telangiectasia. A-T has proven a fascinating but elusive subject of investigation since its first description 80 years ago (Syllaba and Henner, 1926). Only three reports of this syndrome were made between 1926 and its establishment as a disease entity 30 years later by Boder and Sedgwick (1957). While these physicians noted absence of the thymus, A-T was not recognized as an immunodeficiency syndrome until 6 years later (Peterson et al., 1963). Recurrent sinopulmonary infections and variable degrees of immunodeficiency, both cellular and humoral, were shown to be hallmarks of this disease during the 1960s and 1970s.

An adverse response to radiotherapy was reported by several groups in the same decade (Gotoff et al., 1967; Morgan et al., 1968), and hypersensitivity to X-rays and γ-rays was later established for A-T cells in culture (Taylor et al., 1975; Chen et al., 1978). These observations played a dominant role in determining the research direction into the nature of the defect in this syndrome for the following 20 years.

Gatti et al. (1988) used linkage analysis to map the A-T gene to chromosome 11q22–23, and the gene was eventually identified by positional cloning by Savitsky et al. (1995a). During that 7-year period, a scarcity of suitable microsatellite markers and unavailability of more recently described gene-hunting techniques were responsible for what appeared to be an inordinately long time between mapping and cloning of the gene. The identification of the gene *ATM* (Ataxia-*T*elangiectasia *M*utated) as a member of a family of phosphatidylinositol-3-kinase (PI3K)-related genes involved in cellular responses to DNA damage, cell cycle control, and intracellular protein transport, together with the myriad of data accumulated on cell and molecular biology studies over the previous 20 years, provided a basis for initial understanding of the pleiotropic nature of A-T.

The disease A-T has been assigned MIM #208900 and is inherited as an autosomal recessive trait with full penetrance (Tadjoedin and Fraser, 1965; McKusik and Cross, 1966; Ferak et al., 1968). The gene *ATM* has MIM number *607585. The disease has been reported in all races throughout the world, and, as expected from the type of inheritance, it is represented equally in males and females. The first estimate of disease prevalence was provided by Boder and Sedgwick (1970) at 1 in 40,000 live births. This estimate, derived from the number of children with A-T in schools for the physically handicapped as a proportion of the total school enrollment in the Los Angeles School District, appears to be too high. A more comprehensive case-finding study in Michigan by Swift et al. (1986) produced a maximum incidence of A-T of 1 case per 88,000 births. The incidence from studies conducted in 1970–1972 and 1980–1984 was fourfold lower, closer to 3 per 10^6 live births. This estimate is in good agreement with that calculated in a later study (Woods et al., 1990).

In this chapter we will provide insight into the clinical and cellular abnormalities associated with A-T, an overview of the function of the product of the *ATM* gene, the ATM protein, and our current understanding of how a defect in this function leads to the clinical manifestations. Some attention is also paid to hereditary aspects of A-T and methods of diagnosis, past and potential. Finally, we will outline some of the experimentation in human cells and animal models being used to address the pathogenesis of the disease.

Clinical and Pathological Manifestations

In the initial report of A-T, Syllaba and Henner (1926) observed progressive choreoathetosis and ocular telangiectasia in three

Table 29.1. Clinical Features in Ataxia-Telangectasia

Clinical Feature	Cases With Feature (No.)	Cases With Data Available (No.)	Cases With Feature (%)
I. Neurologic abnormalities			
Cerebellar ataxia, infantile or childhood onset	101	101	100
Diminished or absent deep reflexes	54	61	89
Flexor or equivocal plantar response	60	61	98
Negative Romberg sign	28	36	78
Intact deep and superficial sensation	51	52	98
Choreoathetosis	61	67	91
Oculomotor signs			
Apraxia of eye movements	47	56	84
Fixation of gaze nystagmus	48	58	83
Strabismus	7	15	47
Dysarthric speech	70	70	100
Drooling	43	49	88
Characteristic facies and postural attitudes	60	61	98
II. Telangiectasia, oculocutaneous	101	101	100
III. Frequent sinopulmonary infection	60	72	83
IV. Familial occurrence	43	96	45
V. Reported mental deficiency	22	66	33
VI. Equable disposition	34	34	100
VII. Retardation of somatic growth	42	58	72
VIII. Progeric changes of hair and skin	46	52	88

Source: From Boder (1985).

members of a single family. There was a gap of some 15 years before the next report, by Louis-Bar (1941), who described progressive cerebellar ataxia and cutaneous telangiectasia in a Belgian child. The syndrome subsequently bore the name of Louis-Bar. A-T was not described as a distinct clinical entity for a further 16 years, until Boder and Sedgwick (1957) and Biemond (1957), with the aid of autopsies, reported organ developmental abnormalities, neurological manifestations, and a third major characteristic of the disease, recurrent sinopulmonary infection. Several additional reports confirmed the major manifestations of this syndrome (Wells and Sly, 1957; Centerwall and Miller, 1958; Boder and Sedgwick, 1958; Sedgwick and Boder, 1960). The main clinical features of the disease are outlined in Table 29.1 (Boder, 1985; Boder and Sedgwick, 1963).

Cerebellar Ataxia

It is evident from the earliest reports that neurological features figure prominently in this syndrome. According to Boder (1985), A-T is stereotyped in its neurological symptomatology in contrast to the variable immunological characteristics of the disease. Ataxia, generally the presenting symptom in this syndrome, becomes evident when a child begins to walk at the end of the first year of life, manifesting ataxic gait and truncal movements. As with other major characteristics of A-T, ataxia is progressive, spreading to affect the extremities and then to speech. Eventually, involuntary movements become evident, and the child may require a wheelchair by the end of the first decade of life.

The underlying pathology appears to be primarily progressive cerebellar cortical degeneration. The neuropathological features of A-T have been comprehensively detailed in two reviews by Boder (1985) and Sedgwick and Boder (1991). Cortical cerebellar degeneration involves primarily Purkinje and granular cells, but basket cells are also affected. While degenerative changes in the brain are seen predominantly in the cerebellum, it is clear from an increasing number of autopsies that changes to the central

nervous system (CNS) in A-T are more widespread. Degenerative changes in the dentate and olivary nuclei were noted in early studies, and these observations were extended to include changes in the spinal cord and spinal ganglia, the cerebrum, the basal ganglia, and the brain stem, especially in older patients. Amromin et al. (1979) have described distinctive gliovascular abnormalities in the cerebral white matter and also in the brain stem and spinal cord. These consist of dilated capillary loops, many with fibrin thrombi, with perivascular hemorrhages and hemosiderosis, surrounded by demyelinated white matter, reactive gliosis, and numerous atypical astrocytes (Boder, 1985). These vascular changes are seldom seen in the basal ganglia or cerebral cortex and have not been reported in the cerebellum. Since they are seen only in older patients, it is unlikely that they are a primary cause of cerebellar or spinal cord degeneration.

Telangiectasia

A second major clinical manifestation of the disease is telangiectasia. It usually has a later onset than ataxia, between 2 and 8 years of age (McFarlin et al., 1972; Boder, 1985). However, telangiectasia can be observed considerably earlier, particularly if the clinician suspects A-T, such as in children with a prior family history. Telangiectasia represents a dilation of blood vessels, primarily in the ocular sclerae, and often gives the impression of bloodshot eyes (Color Plate 29.I). The telangiectasias are not confined to the eyes but may also appear in the butterfly area of the face and as hairline telangiectasias on the ears. Patches of telangiectasia elsewhere in the skin are less common. Ocular telangectasias may be mistaken for conjunctivitis but can be readily distinguished because they are characterized by dilated vessels against a white background, whereas in conjunctivitis the background is pink. It is not clear how the defect in an enzyme involved in intracellular cell signaling (ATM protein, see below) would give rise to telangiectasia, but it has been suggested that the blood vessel abnormality represents a progeric change, as it mimics telangectasias in normal aged individuals (Boder, 1985). The occurrence of telangiectasias in tissue of normal individuals undergoing radiotherapy may also be related to the telangiectasia in A-T. A-T is characterized by hypersensitivity to radiation and to compounds capable of generating active oxygen radicals. A decreased ability to cope with endogenously generated damage from oxygen radicals may contribute to the development of telangectasias in A-T. Indeed, there is now good evidence that A-T cells are in a state of oxidative stress (Barlow et al., 1999; Watters et al., 1999; Gatei et al., 2001a; Kamsler et al., 2001). However, telangiectasias in the eyes and on the skin might also be due to light or sun damage.

Predisposition to Sinopulmonary Infection

The third major feature of A-T is abnormal susceptibility to infections. Recurrent infections have been described in up to 80% of patients in some studies (Waldmann, 1982). Increased infections become evident by the age of 3, and the major sites are sinopulmonary (Centerwall and Miller, 1958; Andrews et al., 1960; McFarlin et al., 1972). These include otitis and sinusitis as well as recurrent pneumonia, which may progress to bronchiectasis and pulmonary fibrosis severe enough to cause clubbing of fingers and toes, and, eventually, to respiratory insufficiency and death (Sedgwick and Boder, 1991). Boder and Sedgwick (1963) have reported frequent respiratory infections in 83% of cases and chronic bronchitis with or without bronchiectasis in 52% of cases. Patients with A-T are particularly susceptible to common bacterial pathogens and viruses, but do not appear to be subject to generalized or persistent fungal or protozoan infections (Peterson and Good, 1968; McFarlin et al., 1972).

McFarlin et al. (1972) demonstrated a correlation between the severity of the respiratory infections and reduced immune responses. The observation of Boder and Sedgwick (1957) that the thymus is absent or poorly developed in A-T, together with reports of hypogammaglobulinemia (Williams et al., 1960; Gutmannn and Lemli, 1963), suggested a basis for the predisposition to infection. It is now obvious that there is a more generalized defect in multiple aspects of the immune response in A-T patients (Waldmann, 1982).

Cancer Predisposition

The fourth of the major hallmarks of A-T is the predisposition to develop a range of lymphoid malignancies (Boder and Sedgwick, 1963). The association between a defective thymus, immunodeficiency, and the high frequency of lymphoid malignancy became evident early (Peterson et al., 1964a; Leveque et al., 1966; Miller, 1967). Chromosome instability as an explanation for the increased incidence of malignancy was suggested by the observation that leukemic cells from an A-T patient had a translocation involving chromosomes 12 and 14 (Hecht et al., 1966). Regular monitoring of this patient revealed a progressive increase in translocation-bearing, abnormal lymphocytes to 78% of the total lymphocytes before the patient succumbed to infection (Hecht et al., 1973). However, while translocations involving chromosome 14 have been associated with malignancy in Burkitt's lymphoma (Klein, 1981), patients with A-T but with no signs of leukemia or lymphoma may have clonal expansion of cells with chromosome 14/14 translocations to as much as 80% of the total lymphocytes (Al Saadi et al., 1980; Beatty et al., 1986).

Lymphoid malignancies in A-T are of both B cell and T cell origin and include non-Hodgkin lymphoma, Hodgkin lymphoma,

and several forms of leukemia (Spector et al., 1982; Hecht and Hecht, 1990). At autopsy, non-Hodgkin lymphoma accounted for approximately 40% of neoplasms detected, leukemias about 20%, and Hodgkin lymphomas 10%. The increased frequency of lymphoid tumors in A-T could be accounted for by a defect in immune surveillance as part of the underlying immunodeficiency; but the picture is more complex, as malignancies are not confined to the lymphoid system. In an analysis of 108 A-T patients with 119 neoplasms, Hecht and Hecht (1990) reported that 31 of these (26%) were solid tumors varying in type and location. Determination of subsequent risk in A-T patients diagnosed with one type of neoplasm revealed that approximately 25% of patients with solid tumors subsequently developed non-Hodgkin lymphoma or leukemia. A very low risk of subsequent neoplasms existed when the first tumor was lymphoid in origin. In a retrospective study in the United States, mortality from all causes in A-T was 50-fold and 147-fold higher for white and black A-T patients, respectively, than expected, based on overall U.S. mortality rates (Morrell et al., 1986). Among 263 A-T patients there were 52 primary cancers—a 61-fold cancer excess for white probands and a 184-fold excess for black probands. Morrell et al. (1986) also found that the cancer excess was most pronounced for lymphoma, with 252-fold and 750-fold excesses observed for whites and blacks, respectively. As a cause of death in A-T, neoplasia is the second-most frequent after pulmonary disease. Of 62 complete autopsy reports (Sedgwick and Boder, 1991), 29 deaths (47%) were caused by pulmonary complications, 14 (22%) by malignancy, and 16 (26%) by a combination of both. The lifetime cancer risk among A-T patients has been estimated to be between 10% and 38% (Spector et al., 1982; Morrell et al., 1990).

Immunodeficiency

A-T is a highly variable primary immunodeficiency involving both cellular and humoral immunity (Peterson et al., 1963; McFarlin et al., 1972). Some patients have a history of chronic sinopulmonary infections, others have repeated infections, and yet another group shows no higher incidence of infections than their unaffected siblings (McFarlin et al., 1972). The major sites of infection are the upper and lower respiratory system, including the nasal sinuses and the middle ear. In the more persistent cases, progressive destructive changes in the lung, such as bronchiectasis, are common and eventually lead to fatal respiratory failure.

Humoral immunity

The presence of hypogammaglobulinemia has been equated with the high frequency of infections in A-T (Centerwall and Miller, 1958; Andrews et al., 1960; Williams et al., 1960; Gutmann and Lemli, 1963). The first insight into the nature of the immune defect was provided by Thieffry et al. (1961), who showed that IgA was absent in a number of patients with A-T. It was subsequently found that up to 80 of patients had low or absent IgA (Epstein et al., 1966; McFarlin et al., 1972; Boder, 1975). IgE deficiency has been reported in approximately the same frequency (Ammann et al., 1969; McFarlin et al., 1972). In a smaller percentage of patients, IgG, especially IgG2, is reduced. The presence of low–molecular weight IgM has also been reported in up to 80% of patients (Stobo and Tomasi, 1967; McFarlin et al., 1972). The disturbances in immunoglobulin levels in A-T are not due to reduced B cell numbers but appear to result from a defect in B cell differentiation (Lawton et al., 1972; Gail-Peczaska et al., 1973). A spectrum of responsiveness to bacterial antigens, from normal to severely reduced, is observed among A-T patients (McFarlin et al., 1972; Sedgwick and Boder, 1972). On the other hand, natural antibody and antibody responses to challenges with viral antigens are dramatically depressed compared to those of controls (Waldmann, 1982). Circulating autoimmune antibodies against immunoglobulin, muscle, and mitochondria are seen in A-T patients (Ammann and Hong, 1971). The deficiency in IgA and IgE is due primarily to a reduced rate of synthesis, but autoimmune antibodies against these molecules may increase their destruction rates (Strober et al., 1968; Waldmann, 1982). The defect in humoral immunity in A-T is best explained by either an intrinsic defect in the maturation of B cells into IgA and IgE plasma cells or by reduced T cell helper activity or both. Since two of the chromosomes that contain the immunoglobulin and T cell receptor genes, chromosomes 7 and 14, show frequent breaks, rearrangements, and translocations in lymphocytes from A-T patients, it has been suggested that the defect may also be due to disorders in gene regulation or in the recombination mechanisms required to generate mature T and B cell receptor genes (Hecht et al., 1973; Cohen et al., 1975; Taylor et al., 1976).

Cellular immunity

Faulty development of the thymus is very characteristic of A-T (Fireman et al., 1964; Peterson et al., 1964b; McFarlin et al., 1972). The thymus often cannot be identified grossly at autopsy, but only recognized microscopically as a scattered collection of thymic reticular elements with a marked paucity of thymocytes and absence of Hassell's corpuscles and corticomedullary demarcations. These abnormalities reflect a developmental defect rather than atrophy of the thymus (Peterson et al., 1964b). Approximately one-third of patients display unequivocal lymphocytopenia, but this is usually mild in degree. Roifman and Gelfand (1985) described severe and persistent lymphopenia in 1 patient and moderate lymphopenia in 5 others out of a total of 25 patients studied. The proportion of lymphocytes bearing T cell markers is reduced, and cells with receptors for IgM are also diminished in number (Waldmann, 1982). The in vivo and in vitro functional activity of T cells is variable; but when considered as a group, A-T patients are deficient in their responses (McFarlin et al., 1972). Variability is also evident in responses to skin test antigens such as mumps, tuberculin purified protein derivative (PPD), and dinitrochlorobenzene (Fireman et al., 1964; Epstein et al., 1966; McFarlin et al., 1972). Delayed rejection of a skin graft from a donor differing in human leukocyte antigen (HLA) type has been described in up to 80% of A-T patients (Waldmann, 1982). The poor in vivo immune responses of A-T patients are reflected in their depressed in vitro lymphocyte proliferation to several mitogens. McFarlin et al. (1972) reported reduced responses to phyto-hemagglutinin (PHA) in 80% and to pokeweed mitogen in 70% of patients. Because of the variability in responses to mitogens even in the same individual, McFarlin et al. (1972) suggested that a plasma inhibitor could be dampening the response. An alternative explanation for the defective blastogenesis was provided by O'Connor and Scott-Linthicum (1980), who demonstrated that bound PHA could be efficiently internalized by A-T lymphocytes, but that a defect existed at the level of intracellular signaling. This explanation was quite prophetic, now that we know the identity of the gene product defective in A-T.

Disruption of the *Atm* gene in mice gives rise to a phenotype that largely reflects that seen in the human disease (Barlow et al., 1996; Elson et al., 1996; Xu et al., 1996). Immune defects observed in Atm$^{-/-}$ mice include a smaller size of lymphoid tissues, a reduction of CD4 and CD8 single-positive T lymphocytes, an increase in premature double-positive mature T lymphocytes, greatly reduced peripheral T cells, and defective T cell responses. There is evidence that a productively rearranged TCR β-chain gene is required for thymocyte proliferation and TCRαβ rearrangement for the transition of double-positive to single-positive T cells (Shinaki et al., 1993; von Boehmer, 1994). Since Atm$^{-/-}$ mice were defective in both processes, Chao et al. (2000) introduced a functional TCRαβ transgene into these mutant mice to delineate the basis of the T cell developmental defect. This approach led to the rescue of defective T cell differentiation and partial rescue of thymus hypoplasia, indicating that positive selection of thymocytes is normal in Atm$^{-/-}$ mice (Chao et al., 2000). However, normal T cell–independent antibody responses suggested that B cells are functionally normal in Atm$^{-/-}$ mice. The overall conclusion was that the defective T cell–dependent immune response in Atm$^{-/-}$ mice must be secondary to reduced T cell numbers. It is also of interest that when quiescent mature T cells are exposed to DNA intercalating agents they readily undergo apoptosis in an Atm-dependent manner (Bhandoola et al., 2000). Immature thymocytes, by contrast, are resistant to apoptosis induced by this DNA damage signaling pathway, even though double-strand breaks (DSBs) are present in DNA. This resistance may be due to down-regulation of this pathway in immature cells, consistent with the observation that freshly prepared peripheral blood mononuclear cells from humans have low levels of ATM protein and a low basal level of ATM kinase (Fukao et al., 1999).

The availability of monoclonal antibodies specific for cell surface markers together with flow cytometry has allowed for the identification of subpopulations of T cells. With this information it was shown that the CD4/CD8 ratio in A-T patients is reversed compared to controls because of a decrease in the total number of CD4 T cells (Fiorilli et al., 1983). Furthermore, A-T patients have a relative increase in T cells bearing γ/δ antigen receptors compared to those with α/β receptors, unlike T cell populations in most other immunodeficiency syndromes. Carbonari et al. (1990) suggested that a defect in recombination may explain the defects in both T cell and B cell differentiation. Such a defect could also account for the high incidence of chromosomal rearrangements involving primarily chromosomes 7 and 14 (Aurias et al., 1980). Four common sites of chromosome breakage have been described in A-T patients: 7p14, 7q35, 14q11.2, and 14q32. The T cell receptor genes and the Ig heavy-chain genes map to these sites (Hedrick et al., 1984; Sim et al., 1984). Thus, a defect in DNA recombination could explain the immunodeficiency, the hypersensitivity to radiation, and the lymphoid malignancies seen in A-T. In support of this concept, Meyn et al. (1993) demonstrated spontaneous intrachromosomal recombination rates 30–200 times higher in A-T fibroblasts than in fibroblasts from controls. However, extrachromosomal test DNA substrates were recombined in normal fashion in A-T fibroblasts. Hsieh et al. (1993), also using extrachromosomal DNA substrates to analyze V(D)J recombination, failed to observe abnormalities in the signal and coding joint formation in an A-T complementation group D cell line. Taken together, these studies suggest that a defect in intrachromosomal recombination could contribute to genetic instability and predispose to cancer as well as cellular immunodeficiency in A-T.

Phenotypic Heterogeneity

Phenotypic heterogeneity has long been recognized in both the laboratory and clinical features of A-T. Susceptibility to pulmonary infection, presence and degree of mental retardation, and

Table 29.2. Comparison of Ataxia-Telangiectasia, Nijmegen Breakage Syndrome, and Ataxia-Telangiectasia–Like Disorder

Ataxia Telangiectasia	A-TLD	Nijmegen Breakage Syndrome
ATM-null mutations	MREII hypomorphic mutations	NBS1 hypomorphic mutations
Immunodeficiency	Immunodeficiency	Immunodeficiency
Neurodegeneration	Neurodegeneration	Neurodegeneration
Telangiectasia	—	Telangiectasia
—	—	Microcephaly
—	No evidence	Mental retardation
Radiosensitivity	Radiosensitivity	Radiosensitivity
Chromosomal translocations	Chromosomal translocations (+/−)	Chromosomal translocations
Radiosensitivity	Radiosensitivity (intermediate)	Radiosensitivity
Defective cell cycle checkpoints	Intermediate defect in cell cycle checkpoints	Defective cell cycle checkpoints
Defective DSB repair	?	Defective DSB repair
No ATM activity	Normal ATM basal activity, defective ATM activation	Normal basal ATM activity, defective ATM activation?
Genomic instability	Genomic instability	Genomic instability
Cancer predisposition	?	Cancer predisposition

A-TLD, ataxia-telangiectasia–like disorder; DSB, double-strand break.

predisposition to leukemia were used as a tentative classification of subgroups (Hecht and Kaiser-McCaw, 1982). Cellular biology techniques pointed in the early 1980s to a possible genetic heterogeneity underlying this phenotypic variability, with the description of four cellular complementation groups (Jaspers and Bootsma, 1982; Murnane and Painter, 1982; Chen et al., 1984). However, the identification of a single gene, ATM, which is mutated in A-T patients (Savitsky et al., 1995a), made it clear that all complementation groups with a classical A-T phenotype represented mutations in the same gene.

Two separate genetic disorders resulting from defects in a DNA damage response pathway that is functionally linked to ATM share phenotypic features with classical A-T. The first, Nijmegen breakage syndrome (NBS) (see Chapter 30 and Table 29.2), shares the radiosensitivity, immunodeficiency, and cancer predisposition of A-T; but unlike A-T, NBS involves microcephaly with various degrees of mental deficiency, and patients do not have ataxia or telangiectasias (Jaspers et al., 1988a, 1988b; Curry et al., 1989; Digweed et al., 1999; Digweed and Sperling, 2004). As discussed in more detail in Chapter 30, the link between A-T and NBS became more clear with the identification of NBS1 (nibrin), the product of the gene defective in NBS that is functionally linked to ATM (Carney et al., 1998; Matsuura et al., 1998; Varon et al., 1998).

The second disease, A-T-like disorder (ATLD), was first described by Taylor et al. (1993) in a family in which two first cousins presented with some of the features of A-T. The gene defect in this family did not map to the chromosomal location for A-T (11q23), and the clinical course of the disease was mild. Unlike classical A-T patients, these cousins were still ambulatory in their third decade of life. Both had progressive unsteadiness in walking, dysarthria, drooling, vertical nystagmus, and intention tremors, all characteristic of A-T, but there was no evidence of telangiectasia, and immunoglobulin and α-fetoprotein (AFP) levels were normal. Stewart et al. (1999) identified the gene responsible for ATLD as MRE11 that encodes the Mre11 protein, which is part of the hMrell/hRad50/Nbsl complex that senses DSBs in DNA (Nelms et al 1998; Stracker et al., 2004). The MRE11 gene locus is near the ATM locus on human chromosome 11q21, and only detailed linkage analysis allows separation of these loci, necessitating analysis of the MRE11 and ATM genes to distinguish between A-T and ATLD. Mutations in the

MRE11 gene lead to many of the characteristics observed in both A-T and NBS. These results provide evidence for a common involvement of both ATM and members of the Mre11/Rad50/Nbs1 in the cellular response to DSBs in DNA. Ataxia without telangiectasia has also been reported by Aicardi et al. (1988), Maserati et al. (1988), and Chessa et al. (1992).

Even in classical A-T with ataxia and telangiectasia the onset of clinical symptoms and rate of progression are variable. Several reports describe differences in the age of presentation and rates of progression (Sedgwick and Boder, 1991; Hernandez et al., 1993). In a study of 70 A-T patients, the incidence of onset of symptoms of ataxia was 20% prior to 1 year of age, 65% before 2 years, and 85% by 4 years of age (Woods and Taylor, 1992; Taylor et al., 1993). Variability in the appearance of telangiectasias has also been reported and is evident even between affected siblings (Sedgwick and Boder, 1991). Sanal et al. (1993) have identified 30 A-T patients with variant characteristics, including severity of the ataxia, presence of telangiectasia, degree of growth retardation, mental ability, facial appearance, and immunological abnormalities.

The types and frequencies of spontaneous chromosome aberrations including translocations and inversions, largely involving chromosomes 7 and 14, are remarkably consistent in A-T patients (Taylor and Edwards, 1982). These translocations are also observed in lymphocytes from normal individuals, but at a much lower frequency. Exposure of A-T cells to ionizing radiation gives rise to increased levels of chromatid damage compared to controls (Taylor et al., 1976; Kidson et al., 1982). Comparison of lymphocytes from different A-T patients indicates that heterogeneity exists in the extent of induced damage. This is also observed when cell survival is the end point (Cox et al., 1978; Fiorilli et al., 1985; Jaspers et al., 1988b; Ziv et al., 1989). Chessa et al. (1992) designated 14 A-T patients from several studies as being intermediate in their response to ionizing radiation. In 13 of the 14 cases, there was a correlation between radiosensitivity as determined by chromosomal breakage and cell survival. On the other hand, radioresistant DNA synthesis ranged from normal to equally defective as in classical A-T, indicating that this parameter is less significant in causing the radiosensitivity in A-T. Twelve of the 14 patients in this study had definite ataxia and either frank telangiectasia or an increase in conjunctival vascularity.

In summary, there is considerable phenotypic heterogeneity in A-T. Even among classical A-T patients there is some variability in clinical symptoms. Some patients are intermediate in their radiosensitivity, and others have normal radiosensitivity. How do we explain this heterogeneity in light of the identification of the *ATM* gene? Several studies on *ATM* mutations predict that 70%–80% give rise to truncated proteins, while the remainder represent small to large in-frame deletions and missense mutations (Savitsky et al., 1995a; Byrd et al., 1996; Gilad et al., 1996a, 1996b; Telatar et al., 1996; Wright et al., 1996; Chun and Gatti, 2004; Lavin et al., 2004). Most patients are compound heterozygotes with different mutations in the two *ATM* alleles. This information has been useful in accounting for milder forms of the disease in some A-T patients. A missense mutation in *ATM* that activates a cryptic splice/donor acceptor site resulting in the insertion of 137 nucleotides of intronic sequence (5762ins137) was present in the heterozygous state in 15% of A-T patients in the United Kingdom with a milder phenotype (McConville et al., 1996). A second missense mutation 7271T-G is also associated with a mild-variant A-T phenotype (Stankovic et al., 1998). Thus, allelic diversity might explain much of the heterogeneity in clinical severity in A-T. When sufficient mutations have been mapped, it will be possible to compare genotypes with the clinical, cellular, and molecular abnormalities found in this disease.

Other Clinical Characteristics

In addition to the major clinical hallmarks, a variety of other features characterize A-T (Table 29.1). Retardation of somatic growth was reported for about 70%, particularly evident in adolescents and older patients, whose heights were often below the third percentile. Stunting of growth may be due to the pulmonary complications, hypogonadism, and/or thymic dysplasia (Good et al., 1964; Boder, 1985). Female hypogonadism is quite common in A-T, evident at autopsy as absence or hypoplasia of the ovaries. This form of dysplasia is usually associated with infantile uterus and fallopian tubes (Boder and Sedgwick, 1957; Bowden et al., 1963). Its appearance in A-T may be due to an underlying mesenchymal abnormality (Dunn et al., 1964; Miller and Chatten, 1967). Hypogonadism is also observed in male A-T patients, but to a lesser extent than in females (Boder and Sedgwick, 1958). Puberty is delayed, there is abnormal testicular histology, and spermatogenesis is impaired (Strich, 1966; Aguilar et al., 1968).

An unusual type of diabetes mellitus has been described in patients with A-T, with marked hyperinsulinism, hyperglycemia without glycosuria or ketosis, and peripheral resistance to insulin action (Barlow et al., 1965; Schlach et al., 1970). Resistance to insulin could be explained by abnormalities in the number and affinity of insulin receptors in A-T (Bar et al., 1978). Furthermore, as discussed below, the product of the gene mutated in A-T, *ATM*, is related to phosphatidylinositol 3-kinase (Jackson and Jeggo, 1995; Lavin et al., 1995; Savitsky et al., 1995a; Zakian, 1995), an enzyme involved in signal transduction and glucose transport. Recent data demonstrate that the kinase activity of ATM is activated by insulin through a non–DNA-damage signaling pathway to phosphorylate 4E-BP1 (PHAS-1), a regulator of protein synthesis (Yang and Kastan, 2000). Thus a loss of ATM function in A-T patients could disrupt insulin signaling, thereby contributing to insulin resistance and glucose intolerance.

Mild hepatic dysfunction, as evidenced by abnormalities of serum alkaline phosphatase, serum glutamic oxalacetic transaminase (SGOT), serum glutamic pyruvic transaminase (SGPT), and lactate dehydrogenase (LDH), is also seen in A-T (McFarlin et al., 1972). Diffuse fatty infiltration of hepatic parenchymal cells, round cell infiltration in portal regions, and parenchymal cells with nuclear swelling and vacuolation are characteristic changes. It seems likely that the hepatic dysfunction is related to the generalized metabolic changes in A-T rather than to the immunodeficiency or infection. Elevated serum levels of AFP and carcinoembryonic antigen (CEA) in A-T patients are common and thought to be indicative of some form of abnormal development in the liver (Waldmann and McIntyre, 1972; Sugimoto et al., 1978). A widespread cellular histological abnormality, nucleocytomegaly, manifested as large, bizarre, hyperchromatic nuclei (Boder and Sedgwick, 1958; Aguilar et al., 1968; Amromin et al., 1979) occurs in most organs including the central nervous system, anterior pituitary, thyroid, adrenal glands, liver, kidney, lung, heart, and thymus, in smooth muscle cells, and in capsular cells of the spinal ganglia.

Laboratory Findings and Cellular Characteristics

Cellular Radiosensitivity and Chromosomal Instability

A number of cellular and molecular features characterize A-T (Lavin, 1992) (Table 29.3). Frequent chromosome breakage was described four decades ago (Hecht et al., 1966; Miller, 1967). Other reports led to the classification of A-T as a chromosomal instability syndrome together with Bloom's syndrome and Fanconi's anemia (Gropp and Flatz, 1967; Hecht et al., 1973; Higurashi and Conen, 1973; Cohen et al., 1975). Clinical radiosensitivity in A-T became evident about the same time (Gotoff et al., 1967; Morgan et al., 1968; Feigin et al., 1970) as adverse reactions in patients treated with X-rays were noted (Table 29.1). This adverse response was also demonstrated in A-T cells in vitro. Higurashi and Conen (1973) reported a higher level of radiation-induced chromosomal changes in lymphocytes from A-T patients than in controls, and a greater increase in chromosomal aberrations after G2 irradiation was also demonstrated (Rary et al., 1975). Taylor et al. (1975) found that A-T fibroblasts were three to four times more sensitive to ionizing radiation than control fibroblasts. These observations were confirmed and extended by others for radiation (Paterson et al., 1976; Chen et al., 1978; Edwards and Taylor, 1981; Lehmann et al., 1982), bleomycin (Cohen and Simpson, 1982; Morris et al., 1983), and treatment with neocarzinostatin (Cohen and Simpson, 1982; Shiloh et al., 1982a, 1982b, 1983).

While A-T cells were hypersensitive to ionizing radiation and radiomimetic chemicals, early studies failed to detect a defect in DNA single-strand break repair. It became evident later that A-T cells did not have a gross defect in DNA strand break repair, but rather residual DSBs were evident in these cells up to 72 hours post-irradiation (Table 29.3). Approximately 10% of breaks remained unrepaired. A number of other cellular and molecular abnormalities have been reported in A-T cells exposed to radiation (Table 29.3). A specific DNA binding protein, induced by ionizing radiation in control cells to translocate from the cytoplasm to the nucleus, was shown to be constituitively present in the nucleus in several A-T cell lines (Singh and Lavin, 1990; Teale et al., 1992, 1993). As discussed below, specific molecular tests, including mutation analysis of *ATM*, immunoblotting to detect the ATM protein, and specific ATM kinase assays have all been added to laboratory tests for A-T.

Cell Cycle Anomalies

Eukaryotic cells progress through the cell cycle in an ordered series of events called G1, S (DNA synthesis), G2, and M (mitosis).

Table 29.3. Cellular and Molecular Features of Ataxia-Telangiectasia Related to Radiation Response

Characteristic	Assay	Reference
Adverse clinical response to radiotherapy	Clinical assessment	Gotoff et al., 1967
		Morgan et al., 1968
		Feigin et al., 1970
Radiation-induced chromosome breaks	Cytogenetics	Higurashi and Conen, 1973
		Rary et al., 1975
Cell death post-irradiation	Colony survival	Taylor et al., 1975
	Cell viability	Chen et al., 1978
Cell death with neocarzinostatin,	Colony survival	Cohen and Simpson, 1982
bleomycin (radiomimetic drugs)	Cell viability	Shiloh et al., 1982a, 1982b
		Morris et al., 1983
Residual DNA double-strand breaks	Premature chromosome condensation	Cornforth and Bedford, 1985
		Pandita and Hittelman, 1992
	Pulsed-field gel electrophoresis	Foray et al., 1997
Abnormalities in DNA topoisomerase II	DNA unwinding	Mohamed et al., 1987
		Davies et al., 1989
Covalent modification of deoxyribose phosphate in DNA	HPLC analysis	Karam et al., 1990
Constitutive presence of DNA-binding protein in nucleus	Gel retardation	Singh et al., 1990
		Teale et al., 1992, 1993

Events occurring later in the cycle depend on the completion of earlier events, with control maintained through a series of checkpoints (Hoyt et al., 1991; Kastan et al., 1991; Weinert et al., 1994). Checkpoints introduce pauses to ensure the integrity of the genome by allowing for correction of episodic DNA damage or replication delays (Lukas et al., 2004). A series of yeast checkpoint null mutants have been described that lose chromosomes spontaneously and are hypersensitive to ionizing radiation (Weinert and Hartwell, 1990; Li and Murray, 1991; Al-Khodairy and Carr, 1992; Jimenez et al., 1992). These mutants fail to undergo arrest at either the G1/S or G2/M checkpoints in response to radiation damage and/or they fail to maintain the dependence of mitosis upon completion of DNA synthesis.

There are obvious parallels between the data for these yeast mutants and some of the early observations with A-T cells. However, unlike yeast, defective checkpoints do not account for the radiosensitivity in A-T cells, which is more likely due to failure to repair damage in DNA while allowing subsequent passage through the cycle. The first evidence for an abnormality in cell cycle control in A-T cells came from the observation that DNA synthesis continued after irradiation (radioresistant DNA synthesis), allowing cells to proceed through S phase unchecked (Houldsworth and Lavin, 1980; Painter and Young, 1980; de Wit et al., 1981; Edwards and Taylor, 1981). It is still not clear why A-T cells exhibit radioresistant DNA synthesis, but a defect in a signaling pathway from ATM through the checkpoint kinase Chk2 and Cdc25A phosphatase may be responsible. Falck et al. (2001) have shown that ionizing radiation exposure normally leads to the loss of Cdc25A, preventing dephosphorylation of Cdk2 kinase and producing a transient blockade in DNA replication. This blockade is defective in A-T cells, allowing DNA replication to proceed. A delay in radiation-induced phosphorylation of replication protein A, a component of the single-strand DNA binding protein complex, has also been implicated (Liu and Weaver, 1993). Furthermore, ultraviolet (UV)-induced hyperphosphorylation of RPA (p34 subunit) depends on expression of ATM (Oakley et al., 2001).

The physiologic transitory delay in DNA synthesis post-irradiation also appears to be mediated through a calmodulin-dependent regulatory cascade (Mirzayans et al., 1995), and this pathway is defective in A-T. A reduction of radiation suppression of mitotic index in A-T fibroblasts resulted from a failure to prevent cells irradiated in G2 phase from proceeding into mitosis (Scott and Zampetti-Bosseler, 1982). This finding appeared at first to contradict evidence that A-T lymphoblastoid cells and SV40-transformed fibroblasts experienced more prolonged delay in G2/M at longer times after irradiation (Ford et al., 1984; Bates et al., 1985; Smith et al., 1985). However, it is now evident that A-T cells that are in G2 phase at the time of irradiation undergo less delay in proceeding into mitosis at short times after irradiation, but cells irradiated at other phases of the cycle proceed through to G2 phase where they are for the most part irreversibly blocked (Beamish and Lavin, 1994). A-T cells also fail to undergo normal delay in progression from G1 to S phase post-irradiation (Imray and Kidson, 1983; Nagasawa and Little, 1983). The overall picture that emerges for A-T is a failure of cell cycle checkpoints at G1/S, during DNA synthesis, and at G2/M to respond to radiation damage (Beamish and Lavin, 1994).

An understanding of the molecular defect in A-T at the level of cell cycle checkpoints was enabled by recent advances in cell cycle control in yeast and mammalian cells (Hartwell and Smith, 1985; Nurse, 1985; Lukas et al., 2004). Passage of cells through the cycle is controlled by cyclin-dependent kinases (Pines and Hunter, 1991; Xiong et al., 1991), cyclin-kinase inhibitors (El-Deiry et al., 1993; Gu et al., 1993; Harper et al., 1993), other kinases and phosphatases, and a variety of other proteins, including the retinoblastoma protein and the transcription factor E2F (Hinds et al., 1992; Hall et al., 1993). The best-described disruption of this intricate pattern of control is the inhibition of DNA synthesis and slowing of cell division in response to radiation damage (Painter, 1985; Weinert and Hartwell, 1988). Kastan et al. (1991) provided an explanation for this inhibition when they demonstrated that the normal product of the tumor suppressor gene *p53* is induced by radiation and brings about delay in the passage of cells from G1 to S phase. These investigators subsequently showed that the G1/S checkpoint in A-T cells was impaired because of a defect in the p53 radiation signal transduction pathway at the level of p53 (Kastan et al., 1992). Khanna and Lavin (1993) then found that the defect in p53 induction by radiation extended to all four complementation groups of A-T, but there was normal induction of p53 in A-T cells in response to UV damage. In addition, inhibitors of protein kinase C and serine/threonine phosphatases interfered with the pathway.

Failure to observe a correlation between absence of p53 or mutated p53 and radiosensitivity (Clarke et al., 1993; Lee and Bernstein, 1993; Lowe et al., 1993; Slichenmyer et al., 1993) suggested that the A-T gene product operates in more than one pathway affecting cell cycle control and perhaps at other levels of cellular control. Sensitivity to ionizing radiation might be explained by a defect at the level of the G2/M checkpoint, since A-T cells accumulate at this checkpoint with time after exposure to radiation (Beamish and Lavin, 1994; Hong et al., 1994). In recent years the molecular basis for the cell cycle checkpoint defects in A-T have been further elucidated. ATM-dependent stabilization and activation of p53 are of central importance to the operation of the G1/S checkpoint in response to radiation damage to DNA. Radiation induces phosphorylation, dephosphorylation, and acetylation of p53 (Meek, 2004). Some of these modifications are ATM-dependent (Banin et al., 1998; Canman et al., 1998; Saito et al., 2002). ATM is responsible for the rapid phosphorylation of human p53 at serine 15 post-irradiation, and serine 20 phosphorylation is carried out by Chk2 in an ATM-dependent manner (Chehab et al., 1999). Serine 20 phosphorylation interferes with p53's binding to its inhibitor, Mdm2, which plays a major role in its degradation. ATM also phosphorylates Mdm2 itself, to inhibit the nuclear export of the p53Mdm2 complex, thus ensuring the stabilization of p53 after irradiation (Khosravi et al., 1999; Maya et al., 2001). Thus it is evident that ATM controls G1/S checkpoint through multiple interactions.

Stabilization of p53 by radiation and other DNA-damaging agents leads to the induction of a cyclin kinase (Cdk) inhibitor, WAF1 (p21, Cip1) (El-Deiry et al., 1993; Gu et al., 1993; Harper et al., 1993; Xiong et al., 1993). WAF1 binds to cyclin E/cdk2 and cyclin A/cdk2 kinase complexes and by inhibiting their activities prevents the progress of cells from G1 to S phase (Dulic et al., 1994; Waga et al., 1994). In keeping with the defective p53 response in A-T cells, Canman et al. (1994) showed a defective induction of WAF1, and the induction of Mdm2, another downstream effector of p53, was also shown to be defective (Price and Park, 1994). Khanna et al. (1995) subsequently demonstrated that the radiation signal transduction pathway operating through p53, its target gene *WAF1*, cyclin-dependent kinases, and the retinoblastoma protein (Rb) are all defective in A-T cells. Correction of the defect at the G1/S checkpoint was observed when wild-type p53 was constitutively expressed in A-T cells (Khanna et al., 1995). As expected, the WAF1 response in irradiated control cells resulted in an inhibition of cyclin-dependent kinase activity including cyclin E/cdk2, which plays an important role in the transition from G1 to S phase. No inhibition of cyclin-dependent kinase activity was observed in A-T cells, correlating with the delayed WAF1 response. An accumulation of the hypophosphorylated form of Rb protein occurred in irradiated control cells compatible with the G1/S–phase delay observed in these cells after exposure to radiation. In unirradiated A-T cells the amount of Rb protein was much higher than that in controls, and it was mainly in the hyperphosphorylated (inactive) form.

The discovery of the *ATM* gene and its protein product suggested that there might be a common defect in cell cycle control in A-T operating through the cyclin-dependent kinases that control multiple checkpoints (Savitsky et al., 1995a). In agreement with this, Beamish et al. (1996) demonstrated that several cyclin-dependent kinases in A-T cells are not inhibited by ionizing radiation, associated with insufficient induction of WAF1. Exposure

of control lymphoblastoid cells to radiation during S and G2 caused rapid inhibition of cyclin A/cdc2 and cyclin B/cdc2 activities, respectively. Irradiation led to a 5- to 20-fold increase in cdk-associated WAF1 in these cells, accounting at least in part for the decrease in cyclin-dependent kinase activity. In contrast, radiation did not inhibit any of the cyclin-dependent kinase activities in A-T cells at short times after irradiation, nor was there any significant change in the level of cdk-associated WAF1 compared to unirradiated cells (Beamish et al., 1996). These results were similar to those reported previously for the G1 checkpoint and provided additional evidence for the involvement of ATM at multiple points in cell cycle regulation. In relation to the abnormality in S phase, Mirzayans et al. (1995) had indirect evidence that radiation-induced cessation of DNA synthesis is mediated through a calmodulin-dependent signal transduction pathway, independent of protein kinase C (PKC) and p53; in addition to the p53 pathway, this signaling system is also defective in A-T cells.

As referred to above, A-T cells exhibit radioresistant DNA synthesis and defective S-phase checkpoint activation (Houldsworth and Lavin, 1980; Painter and Young, 1980). Falck et al. (2001) provided a functional link between ATM, the checkpoint signaling kinase Chk2, and the Cdc25A phosphatase that activates the cyclin kinase Cdk2 and control of the S-phase checkpoint. Exposure of cells to radiation leads to the activation of ATM kinase, which in turn activates Chk2 to phosphorylate Cdc25A phosphatase. This leads to the degradation of Cdc25A and thus Cdk2 remains phosphorylated and inactive, giving rise to a transient block in DNA replication. In cells with absent or mutated ATM this pathway does not function, Cdc25A remains stable, and cells continue to replicate DNA in the presence of damage (radioresistant DNA synthesis).

While considerably less is known about activation of the G2/M checkpoint, maintenance of inhibitory phosphorylations on Cdc2 leads to arrest of cells in G2 (Jin et al., 1996). In response to DNA damage Cdc25C phosphatase is phosphorylated and inactivated, again in this case preventing the dephosphorylation of Cdc2 kinase, which is required for passage of cells through G2 phase (Nilsson and Hoffmann, 2000). It is not established which kinase phosphorylates Cdc25C, but both Chk1 and Chk2 can phosphorylate this protein at serine 216 in vitro (Sanchez et al., 1997; Matsuoku et al., 1998). Phosphorylation creates a binding site for 14-3-3 protein, which results in inactivation of the phosphatase (Peng et al., 1997). Since ATM phosphorylates and activates Chk2 in response to DNA damage, it is likely that this is the pathway operating to activate the G2/M checkpoint (Blasina al., 1999; Brown et al., 1999).

To account for the defective radiation response in A-T cells, a "damage surveillance network" model has been proposed in which certain types of DNA damage trigger a signal transduction network with resulting activation of a group of pathways to promote genetic stability by temporarily arresting the cell cycle and enhancing DNA repair (Meyn et al., 1994; Meyn, 1995). It appears likely that ATM is recruited to sites of DSBs in DNA and subsequently signals via downstream substrates such as p53 and Chk2 to the cell cycle machinery to delay the passage of cells between the various phases prior to completion of DNA repair. Evidence for recruitment of ATM to DNA breaks was provided by Smith et al. (1999a), who showed that ATM binds preferentially to DNA ends in both monomeric and tetrameric forms. In addition, a combination of single-strand and sheared DNA is capable of stimulating ATM kinase activity for RPA substrate (Gately et al., 1998; Chan et al., 2000). Resistance to detergent extraction of a fraction of the ATM pool post-irradiation, together with colocalization of this ATM with the phosphorylated form of histone H2AX and with Nbs1 foci, suggests further that ATM associates with sites of DSBs (Andegeko et al., 2001).

The ATM Gene and A-T Mutations

The placement of an A-T locus by Gatti et al. (1988) on chromosome 11q22–23 spurred extensive positional cloning efforts (McConville et al., 1994; Rotman et al., 1994; Lange et al., 1995; Vanagaite et al., 1995), which culminated in identification of *ATM*, the gene mutated in A-T patients (Savitsky et al., 1995a, 1995b). *ATM*, occupies 150 kb of genomic DNA and encodes a large transcript of about 13 kb representing 66 exons (Savitsky et al., 1995b, 1996; Uziel et al., 1996; Platzer et al., 1997). There is no evidence of alternative splicing within the open reading frame of the *ATM* transcript. However, extensive variability has been detected in the untranslated regions (UTRs) of the transcript, creating multiple species of ATM mRNA. Several 3′ UTRs are formed via polyadenylation of alternative sites, while at least 12 5′ UTRs are obtained via alternative splicing of the first four exons of the gene (Savitsky et al., 1997). This complex pattern suggests that synthesis of the ATM protein might be subject to post-transcriptional regulation.

Several experiments confirmed that the deficiency of the ATM protein is indeed responsible for the A-T cellular phenotype. Thus, ectopic expression of recombinant ATM protein in A-T cells complemented various features of this phenotype (Zhang et al., 1997; Ziv et al., 1997), while down-regulation of ATM by means of antisense strategies conferred A-T features to various cell lines (Zhang et al., 1998; Uhrhammer et al., 1999; Fan et al., 2000). Furthermore, expression of ATM fragments containing the leucine zipper of this protein abrogated the S-phase checkpoint and increased the radiosensitivity of the human tumor cell line RKO (Morgan et al., 1997). Such protein fragments appear to act in a dominant-negative fashion, possibly by competing with ATM for specific interactor(s).

Extensive screening of the *ATM* transcript for mutations in A-T cells has been performed using a variety of methods (Savitsky et al., 1995a; Bryd et al., 1996; Gilad et al., 1996a, 1996b, 1998a, 1998b; McConville et al., 1996; Telatar et al., 1996; Wright et al., 1996; Concannon and Gatti, 1997; Watters et al., 1997; Broeks et al., 1998; Fukao et al., 1998; Laake et al., 1998, 2000; Sasaki et al., 1998; Sandoval et al., 1999; Teraoka et al., 1999; Becker-Catania et al., 2000; Pagani et al., 2002; Angele et al., 2003; Saviozzi et al., 2003). To date, over 400 separate mutations have been described and these have been compiled by Concannon and Gatti (http://www.benaroyaresearch.org/investigators/concannon_patrick/atm.htm). These mutations are distributed along the length of the gene with the majority predicted to cause premature truncations (70%–80%) and others causing small deletions, in-frame deletions, and missense changes (Stankovic et al., 1998). Thus *ATM* gene mutations in patients with classical A-T are expected to inactivate the ATM protein by truncating it or by deleting large segments from it. This mutation profile points to predominance of null alleles in classical A-T. Hence, mutations with milder effects on the protein might lead to non–A-T phenotypes. Most A-T mutations are unique to single families, and the majority of patients in Europe and North America are compound heterozygotes. Interestingly, a founder effect was observed among patients of Moroccan Jewish origin, in whom one mutation is predominant (Gilad et al., 1996b). Evidence for founder mutations has also been reported for patients in Japanese (Ejima and Sasaki, 1998),

Norwegian (Laake et al., 1998) and other populations (Teletar et al., 1998).

Compared to the predominance of null alleles among patients with classical A-T, a different mutation profile is emerging in "A-T variants," which show a milder phenotype, usually with later age of onset and less pronounced radiosensitivity. These patients may have leaky splicing mutations giving rise to a mixture of normal and aberrant transcripts, small in-frame deletions, or truncations of just the last few carboxy-terminal amino acids or in the *Mre11* gene (McConville et al., 1996; Gilad et al., 1998a; Teraoka et al., 1999; Stewart et al., 2001; Saviozzi et al., 2002; Dörk et al., 2004; Eng et al., 2004; Sutton et al., 2004).

Function of the ATM Protein

The open reading frame of *ATM* transcripts predicts a large protein of 3056 amino acids (Savitsky et al., 1995b). The predominant domain of this protein is the carboxy-terminal region of about 350 residues, which contains sequence signatures similar to those of the catalytic subunit of phosphatidylinositol 3-kinases (PI3Ks). These motifs, shared with the lipid kinases that play major roles in various signaling pathways, suggest a signaling role for ATM. They also place it within a multibranched family of large proteins with the carboxy-terminal PI3K signatures (PIK-related kinases [PIKKs]), which is represented in all eukaryotes (Abraham, 2004b). Most members of the PIKK family possess a protein kinase activity directed at serine/threonine residues. These kinases function at the top of various signaling cascades that sense specific types of stresses or stimuli related to cellular growth and are critical for the activation of cellular responses to these stimuli. Importantly, most of the PIK-related kinases are involved in sensing and responding to DNA damage and in maintaining genomic stability (Table 29.4).

The ATM ortholog in the budding yeast *Saccharomyces cerevisiae* is Tel1p, whose ectopic expression in human A-T cells partially complements their phenotype (Fritz et al., 2000). Tel1p and another PIK-related protein kinase in the budding yeast, Mec1p (see below), closely collaborate in maintaining telomere length and mediating cellular responses to DNA damage. Tel1p, which has protein kinase activity (Mallory and Petes, 2000), has been studied mainly with regard to its role in maintaining telomere length (Greenwell et al., 1995; Morrow et al., 1995; Ritchie et al., 1999). *TEL1* mutations lead to shortened telomeres, a typical characteristic of human A-T cells. Interestingly, in this function Tel1p cooperates with the double-strand breakage repair complex Mre11/Rad50p/Xrs (Ritchie and Petes, 2000), whereas in human cells ATM functionally interacts with the orthologous protein complex in the DNA damage response. The synergism between Tel1p and Mec1p in both telomere maintenance and cellular responses to DNA damage has been clearly documented in double-mutant *tel1/mec1* yeast, which are extremely sensitive to DNA damage and senesce prematurely (Greenwell et al., 1995; Vialard et al., 1998; Ritchie et al., 1999). While *tel1* mutants are not hypersensitive to DNA damaging agents, an extra copy of *TEL1* can largely complement such sensitivity in *mec1* mutants (Morrow et al., 1995).

The closest human ATM homolog is the ATR (homolog of *ATM* and *R*ad3) protein, which represents a separate branch of the PIK-related kinase family. ATR is a protein kinase that shares many substrates with ATM and acts in partial redundancy with ATM in a number of damage response pathways (Shechter et al., 2004). Recent evidence suggests that ATR and ATR-interacting protein (ATRIP) control S-phase progression in response to DNA

Table 29.4. ATM-Related Proteins Containing a PI3-kinase–Like Domain

Protein	Organism	Size (a.a.)	Mutant Phenotype	Predicted Function (Enzymatic Activity)	References
Te11p	Budding yeast	2789	Telomere shortening	Regulation of telomere length	Greenwell et al., 1995 Morrow et al., 1995
Mec1p	Budding yeast	2368	Sensitivity to DNA-damaging agents; mitotic instability; defects in meiotic recombination and cell cycle checkpoints	Regulates cell cycle checkpoints responding to DNA damage	Kato and Ogawa, 1994 Weinert et al., 1994 Allen et al., 1994 Paulovich and Hartwell, 1995
Rad3p	Fission yeast	2386	Sensitivity of DNA-damaging agents; mitotic instability; defective DNA repair and cell cycle checkpoints	Regulates cell cycle checkpoints responding to DNA damage	Al-Khodairy et al., 1994 Jimenez et al., 1992 A. Carr, personal communication
Mei-41	Fruit fly	2356	Sensitivity to DNA-damaging agents; mitotic instability; defective DNA repair and cell cycle checkpoints	Regulates cell cycle checkpoints responding to DNA damage	Boyd et al., 1976 Banga et al., 1986 Hari et al., 1995
Tor1p	Budding yeast	2470	Rapamycin resistance; perturbation of G1 cell cycle progression	Binds rapamycin, FKBP12; involved in G1/S transition	Heitman et al., 1991 Kunz et al., 1993
Tor2p	Budding yeast	2473	Rapamycin resistance; perturbation of G1 cell cycle progression	Binds rapamycin, FKBP12; involved in G1/S transition	
MTOR (FRAP)	Mammalian	2549	Rapamycin resistance; perturbation of G1 cell cycle progression	Binds rapamycin, FKBP12	Sabatini et al., 1994
RAFT1	Mammalian	2550		Involved in G1/S transition; activates p70^{S6} kinase (autophosphorylation on Ser)	Sabers et al., 1995 Brown et al., 1994 Brown et al., 1995
FRP1/ATR	Mammalian	2644	Embryonic lethal in mice; no known human syndrome	Protein kinase responding to UV, hydroxyurea	Cimprich et al., 1996 Canman, 2001 Bentley et al., 1996
DNA-PKcs	Humans	4096	SCID phenotype in mice; radiation sensitivity; immunodeficiency; defective repair of double-strand breaks and V(D)J recombination	Signals presence of DNA damage to cellular regulatory systems (Ser/Thr protein kinase)	Anderson, 1993 Gottlieb and Jackson, 1994 Hartley et al., 1995
TRAPP	Mammalian	3828	DNA repair; recruits histone acelylases, oncogene activation	No kinase activity	

a.a., amino acids.

damage and replication fork stalling, ultimately resulting in the downstream inhibition of the S-phase kinases that function to initiate DNA replication at origins of replication (Shechter et al., 2004).

Importantly, disruption of the *ATR* gene in mice leads to early embryonic lethality before embryonic day 8.5 (Brown and Baltimore, 2000; de Klein et al., 2000). While the embryonic lethal effect of complete ATR deficiency is indisputable, a hypomoprphic mutation (A2101G) in the human *ATR* gene was found to cause a rare form of Seckel syndrome (O'Driscoll et al., 2003) designated ATR-Seckel (Alderton et al., 2004; O'Driscoll et al., 2004). Genetically and clinically Seckel syndrome is a heterogenous disorder characterized by severe intrauterine growth retardation, proportionate dwarfism, and microcephaly, with skeletal and brain abnormalities (OMIM # 210600) (reviewed by O'Driscoll et al., 2004). Although lymphoma has been reported in some Seckel patients, they tend not to have ataxia or immunodeficiency. Patients with Seckel syndrome display features including microcephaly and dysmorphic facies that are commonly found in other syndromes associated with impaired responses to DNA damage. Alderton et al. (2004) found that ATR-Seckel cells exhibit a range of aberrant responses to agents that cause replication stalling. They also exhibit supernumery centrosomes in mitotic cells, demonstrating a novel role for ATR in the maintenance of centrosome stability.

Overexpression of a "kinase-dead" form of ATR gives rise to a dominant-negative effect leading to increased sensitization to

DNA damaging agents and defective cell cycle checkpoint activation (Cliby et al., 1998; Wright et al., 1998). ATR-deficient cells are hypersensitive to UV and hydroxyurea (HU), in contrast to A-T cells, in which γ-radiation causes hypersensitivity. Indeed, the phosphorylation of Rad17 induced by UV and HU is dependent on ATR, whereas that induced by γ-rays is dependent on ATM (Bao et al., 2001). Evidence has also been provided that ATR lies directly upstream from the checkpoint protein Chk1, which it activates in response to DNA replication blockage and agents that cause genotoxic stress to delay cells at the G2 checkpoint (Zhao and Piwnica-Worms, 2001).

In contrast to ATM, whose intrinsic kinase activity is contained in a single protein molecule, ATR is consitutively complexed and dependent on an accessory protein, ATRIP (Cortez et al., 2001). ATRIP is phosphorylated by ATR, regulates ATR expression, and is essential for proper ATR activity. ATR and ATRIP both localize to intranuclear foci after DNA damage or inhibition of replication. Small, interfering RNA directed against ATRIP caused the loss of both ATRIP and ATR expression and the loss of checkpoint responses to DNA damage, indicating the mutual dependence of these two proteins (Cortez et al., 2001). Replication protein A (RPA), a protein complex that associates with single-stranded DNA (ssDNA), is required for the recruitment of ATR to sites of DNA damage and for ATR-mediated Chk1 activation in human cells. In vitro, RPA stimulates the binding of ATRIP to ssDNA. The binding of ATRIP to RPA-coated ssDNA enables the ATR/ATRIP complex to associate with DNA and stimulates phosphorylation of the Rad17 protein that is bound to DNA (Zou and Elledge, 2003).

ATR orthologs are typically involved in maintaining genome stability and responding to DNA damage. The yeast ATR orthologs, Mec1p in the budding yeast and Rad3p in the fission yeast, maintain genomic stability and activate DNA damage responses by phosphorylating key proteins in these pathways (reviewed in Zhou and Elledge, 2000; Humphrey, 2000). As mentioned above, Mec1p collaborates with the ATM ortholog, Tel1p, in the damage response pathway and telomere maintenance in *S. cerevisiae* (Neecke et al., 1999; Longhese et al., 2000). Notably, Mec1p-dependent processes include cell cycle checkpoints induced by DNA damage or replication arrest (Santocanale and Diffley, 1998; Clarke et al., 1999; Vallen and Cross, 1999), redistribution of the Sir3 silencing protein from telomeres to DSBs (Mills et al., 1999); meiotic recombination (Grushcov et al., 1999); and silencing of gene expression at telomeres (Craven and Petes, 2000). The Rad3p of *S. pombe* is critical for the immediate activation of cell cycle checkpoints following DNA damage and for the activation and maintenance of responses to replication arrest. The mechanisms in each response are different and carried out by different effectors (Martinho et al., 1998). Many of the relevant pathways are conserved through evolution; hence, in mammalian cells, ATM and ATR phosphorylate orthologs of Mec1p and Rad3p substrates. In *Drosophila melanogaster* mutants in the ATR ortholog *mei-41* exhibit chromosomal instability, radiation sensitivity, and defective activation of cell cycle checkpoints by ionizing radiation (Hari et al., 1995). Recombination-defective lines of flies reveal a role for Mei-41 protein in meiotic precocious anaphase in females (McKim et al., 2000). The catalytic subunit of the DNA-dependent protein kinase (DNA-PKcs) is another major member of the PIK-related kinase family (reviewed by Burma and Chen, 2004). DNA-PKcs is recruited to DSB sites by the Ku70/Ku80 heterodimer and appears to play a central role in the rejoining process, in V(D)J recombination, and in triggering apoptosis in response to severe DNA damage or critically shortened telomeres. DNA-PK also appears to be involved in mounting an innate immune response to bacterial DNA and to viral infection. Because DNA-PK localizes very rapidly to DNA breaks and phosphorylates itself and other damage-responsive proteins, it appears that DNA-PK serves as both a sensor and a transducer of DNA-damage signals. ATM- and ATR-dependent pathways appear to be independent of DNA-PK (Araki et al., 1999; Khosravi et al., 1999). However, the critical role of DNA-PK in DSB response is underscored by the *scid* phenotype of DNA-PK–deficient mice, which includes radiosensitivity, chromosomal instability, immunodeficiency, and cancer predisposition (Jhappan et al., 1997).

The TOR subfamily of the PIK-related kinases represents a group of proteins whose role is to convey, via their kinase activity, extracellular signals rather than deal with DNA damage (Proud, 2004). The TOR proteins signal nutrient availability (e.g., amino acids levels) and pass on certain mitogenic stimuli to the mRNA translation machinery. One known mechanism is TOR-dependent phosphorylation of the $p70^{S6k}$ kinase. The pathways controlled by the mammalian homolog in this group, mTOR/FRAP/RAFT, may end up regulating both protein translation and transcription of rRNA and tRNA. Importantly, TOR-mediated pathways appear to intersect with certain PI3K pathways.

A recent newcomer to the PI3K-related protein kinase family is the hSMG1 protein (Abraham, 2004a). The protein kinase activity of hSMG-1 resembles that of ATM, both in terms of substrate specificity and its sensitivity to inhibition by the fungal metabolite wortmannin. hSMG-1 is the ortholog of a *Caenorhabditis elegans* protein, CeSMG-1, which has been genetically linked to a critical mRNA surveillance pathway termed *nonsense-mediated decay* (NMD). The function of NMD is to mark for rapid degradation mRNAs that bear a premature termination codon. Compelling evidence now indicates that hSMG-1 is also a central player in the NMD pathway in human cells. In addition, hSMG-1, like ATM, appears to be involved in the recognition and/or repair of damaged DNA in these cells.

Finally, members of the TRRAP branch of the PIK-related kinase superfamily are devoid of kinase activity because of inactivating sequence alterations in their kinase domains. The mammalian (TRRAP/PAF400) and yeast (Tra1p) homologs are part of large protein complexes involved in transcriptional regulation and chromatin remodeling via their histone actetyltransferase activity (Grant et al., 1998; Saleh et al., 1998; Vassilev et al., 1998). TRRAP/PAF400 is a co-activator of the c-Myc and E2F transcription factors and recruits the histone acetyltransferase GCN5 to c-Myc (McMahon et al., 1998, 2000). The existence of the TRRAP group in the PIK-related kinase family raises the possibility that members residing in other branches of the PIK-related kinase phylogenetic tree are involved in gene regulation and shaping of chromatin. In general, despite the apparently diverse functions of the different branches of this important protein family, they may share more functions than meet the eye.

ATM Functions

ATM activation

ATM is a predominantly nuclear protein with a strong serine/threonine kinase activity. Similar to DNA-PK and ATR, ATM's kinase activity appears to be directed at serine or threonine residues that are immediately followed by a glutamine (Kim et al., 1999; O'Neil et al., 2000). ATM's major function is to play a crucial role in the early response to the induction of DSBs in the DNA (Shiloh, 2003; Kurz and Lees-Miller, 2004). Immediately after the formation of DSBs in the DNA, ATM's kinase activity is enhanced (Banin et al., 1998; Canman et al., 1998; Khanna et al., 1998). The activated ATM then phosphorylates an extensive array of target proteins, each of which is a key player in a specific damage response pathway (Fig. 29.1). Bakkenist and Kastan (2003) found that ATM molecules are inactive in undamaged cells, being held as dimers or higher-order multimers. In this configuration, the kinase domain of each molecule is blocked by a region called the *FAT domain* of the other. Following DNA damage, each ATM molecule phosphorylates the other on a serine residue at position 1981 within the FAT domain, a phosphorylation that releases the two molecules from each other's grip, turning them into fully active monomers. Within minutes after the infliction of as few as several DSBs per genome, most ATM molecules become vigorously active. Another immediate step in ATM activation following DNA damage is rapid adherence of a portion of activated ATM to DSB sites (Andegeko et al., 2001). Both chromatin-bound and free ATM are autophosphorylated on serine 1981 (Uziel et al., 2003). So, following DSB induction, activated ATM seems to divide between two fractions: one is chromatin bound and the other is free to move throughout the nucleus. Importantly, many ATM substrates are phosphorylated by the chromatin-bound fraction of ATM, at the damaged sites (Lukas et al., 2003).

The early events in the DSB response are usually depicted by a linear scheme beginning with sensor proteins that sense the

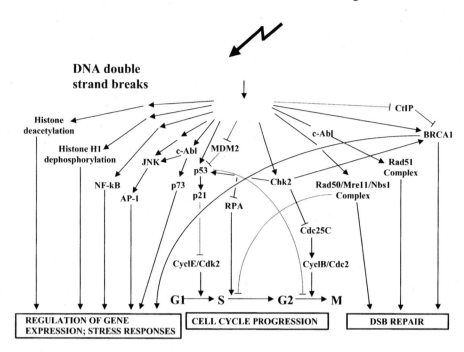

Figure 29.1. Scheme of ATM-dependent pathways in the double-strand break (DSB) response network, highlighting ATM effectors. Arrows indicate stimulation, while T-shaped lines represent inhibition. The transition from inactive ATM homodimers into active monomers and the role of the Rad50/ Mre11/Nbs1 (MRN) complex upstream of this process are indicated. ATR phosphorylates at least some of ATM's substrates in response to these DNA lesions at later time points and slower kinetics. (Reproduced from Shiloh et al., 2004, with permission.)

damage and convey it to the transducers, such as ATM and ATR. Growing evidence suggests, however, that the DSB signal may be initially amplified via a cyclic process rather than by a series of steps with a linear hierarchy. One of the first processes initiated by DSBs is the massive phosphorylation of the tail of a histone protein variant called *H2AX* (Fernandez-Capetillo et al., 2004). Foci of phosphorylated H2AX are rapidly formed at the DSB sites and are thought to be essential for further recruitment of repair factors such as the Mre11/Rad50/Nbs1 (MRN) complex (see below), Rad51, and Brca1 (Celeste et al., 2002). H2AX phosphorylation, a very early event in the cascade induced by DSBs, was reported to be ATM-dependent following DSB induction (Burma et al., 2001), and ATR-dependent following replicative stress (Ward and Chen, 2001). This process could thus serve as a rapid and powerful mechanism for amplification of the damage signal via repeated cycles of H2AX phosphorylation and recruitment of processing factors that facilitate further recruitment of damage transducers to the damaged sites, along with repair proteins.

Other cyclic processes of signal amplification may characterize ATM activation and subsequent phosphorylation of ATM substrates. An important player in this cycle is the Mre11/rad50/Nbs1 (MRN) complex (Stracker et al., 2004). The MRN complex serves as a sensor of DSBs caused by damaging agents. It is involved in the initial processing of such DSBs by virtue of the nuclease activity of one of its component—the Mre11 protein. MRN is also involved in processing DSBs that are formed during meiotic recombination and in telomere maintenance. The Nbs1 protein is a direct substrate of ATM (see below), but also seems to serve as an adaptor in the phosphorylation of other ATM substrates such as Chk2 (Buscemi et al., 2001; Girard et al., 2002) and Smc1 (Kim et al., 2002b; Yazdi et al., 2002), particularly at low damage levels. Similarly, the Brca1 protein, itself an ATM substrate, is an adaptor in the phosphorylation of other ATM substrates (Foray et al., 2003). So, in this interesting pathway, the phosphorylation of one substrate is required for the phosphorylation of others. A molecular explanation for the adaptor role of the MRN complex was provided by Lee and Paull (2004), who showed that MRN facilitates in vitro the binding between ATM and some of its

substrates. However, this is not the complete story of the complex, intimate relationships between ATM and the MRN complex. It turns out that MRN also plays a role in the actual activation of ATM. The presence of a functional MRN complex is required for full activation of ATM, particularly at low damage levels (Carson et al., 2003; Uziel et al., 2003; Horejsi et al., 2004) and for recruitment of ATM to the damaged sites (Kitagawa et al., 2004). A molecular explanation for these observations was provided by Costanzo et al. (2004), who showed that in *Xenopus* extracts, ATM, MRN, and broken DNA fragments assemble into an "activation complex" whose formation is required for full activation of ATM.

Another protein that appears to facilitate the phosphorylation of certain ATM substrates is 53BP1 (Mochan et al., 2004). Like Nbs1, 53BP1 contains a BRCT (breast cancer C-terminus) domain, is recruited to DSB-induced nuclear foci, is required for proper activation of certain cell cycle checkpoints, and is itself an ATM substrate (DiTullio et al., 2002; Fernandez-Capetillo et al., 2002; Wang et al., 2002). Another newly discovered, BRCT-containing protein, Nfbd1/Mdc1, may have similar characteristics (Stucki and Jackson, 2004). The emerging complex relationships between ATM, the MRN complex, and these BRCT proteins are drawing new flow charts for the DNA damage signal that deviate from the traditional linear ones and assign to several proteins more than one role "upstream" and "downstream" of the transducers of the DNA damage alarm.

ATM substrates and downstream pathways

The list of published ATM substrates is far from complete, and the study of the pathways associated with ATM targets is gradually disclosing a remarkably broad cellular response to DSBs that is meticulously orchestrated by ATM. The network of ATM-mediated pathways (Fig. 29.1) uses several sophisticated strategies. The first strategy is to approach the same effector from several different directions. A prime example is the G1/S checkpoint (reviewed by Shiloh, 2003; Kurz and Lees-Miller, 2004). A main component in this cell cycle checkpoint is activation and stabilization of p53, which in turn activates transcription of the gene that encodes the CDK2–cyclin-E inhibitor WAF1 (also known as p21 and CIP1) (Oren, 2003; Meek, 2004). p53 is phosphorylated by ATM on Ser15 (Banin et al., 1998; Canman et al., 1998). This contributes primarily to enhancing p53's activity as a transcription factor (Ashcroft et al., 1999; Dumaz and Meek, 1999; Khosravi et al., 1999). ATM also phosphorylates and activates Chk2 (Ahn et al., 2004), which phosphorylates p53 on Ser20. This process interferes with the p53–MDM2 interaction. The oncogenic protein Mdm2 is both a direct and indirect inhibitor of p53, as it serves as a ubiquitin ligase in p53 ubiquitylation, which mediates its proteasome-mediated degradation (Alarcon-Vargas and Ronai, 2002; Brooks and Gu, 2004). ATM also directly phosphorylates Mdm2 on Ser395, which interferes with nuclear export of the p53Mdm2 complex and hence the degradation of p53 (Khosravi et al., 1999; Maya et al., 2001). Finally, it has been reported that phosphorylations of p53 on Ser9 and Ser46 (Saito et al., 2002) and dephosphorylation of Ser376 (Waterman et al., 1998) are ATM-dependent as well, although the function of these changes is unclear.

This series of ATM-dependent modifications that activate and stabilize p53, although perhaps not complete, illustrates the elaborate way in which ATM handles a single effector, and indicates that ATM might regulate several effectors within the same pathway. This principle is also seen in ATM-mediated activation of the Brca1 tumor suppressor protein following DNA damage. Brca1 is involved in the early stage of the DNA damage response as well as in activating downstream pathways (Ting and Lee, 2004). Brca1 was found to be associated with large protein complexes that contain DSB repair and mismatch repair enzymes as well as ATM (Wang et al., 2000b). It also activates the expression of certain damage-responsive genes and is involved in the S-phase and G2–M checkpoints (El-Deiry, 2002; Jasin, 2002; Venkitaraman, 2002; Yarden et al., 2002). ATM phosphorylates Brca1 on several sites (Cortez et al., 1999; Gatei et al., 2000a, 2001b). Importantly, whereas ATM-mediated phosphorylation of Brca1 on Ser1387 activates Brca1 as a regulator of the intra-S-phase checkpoint (Xu et al., 2002), its phosphorylation by ATM on Ser1423 spurs its involvement in the G2–M checkpoint (Xu et al., 2001). Thus, phosphorylation on different sites may direct an effector to act in different pathways. The Chk2 kinase, which is activated by ATM, adds yet another phosphorylation on the Brca1 molecule (Lee et al., 2000), while at the same time ATM phosphorylates CtIP, an inhibitor of Brca1, on two residues, inhibiting its function and further stimulating Brca1 (Li et al., 2000).

ATM's hold on downstream pathways is demonstrated by not only its multipronged grip of specific pathways but also its ability to approach the same end point from several different directions. A notable example is, again, the intra-S checkpoint: several ATM-controlled pathways converge to regulate this crucial cellular response to DSBs (Fig. 29.1). At least five ATM-mediated pathways seem to be involved in this checkpoint. In addition to Brca1, ATM phosphorylates Nbs1 (Gatei et al., 2000b; Lim et al., 2000; Wu et al., 2000; Zhao et al., 2000), a component of the multifunctional Mre11Rad50Nbs1 (MRN) complex involved in DSB sensing (Stracker et al., 2004). Of several ATM phosphorylation sites on Nbs1, Ser343 and Ser278 seem to be particularly important for its unknown role in this checkpoint (Lim et al., 2000; Zhao et al., 2000). Another ATM substrate in the intra-S checkpoint pathway is the Smc1 (structural maintenance of chromosomes 1) protein. This protein, known primarily for its involvement in sister chromatid cohesion, is phosphorylated by ATM on two serine residues; interference with this phosphorylation abrogates the S-phase checkpoint (Kim et al., 2002b; Yazdi et al., 2002). Im-

portantly, cells from mice in which ATM phosphorylation sites on Smc1 had been abolished had an S-phase checkpoint defect, decreased survival, and increased chromosomal aberrations after DNA damage (Kitagawa et al., 2004). A recently identified effector of ATM in the intra-S checkpoint is the FancD2 protein, which is phosphorylated by ATM on Ser222 following DSB induction and undergoes Brca1-mediated mono-ubiquitylation (Taniguchi et al., 2002). FancD2 is a member of a multiprotein complex, defects of which lead to another genomic instability syndrome, Fanconi's anemia (see Chapter 30). At the same time, Chk2 and another ATM/ATR-activated kinase, Chk1, take care of several checkpoints. Both of them phosphorylate the checkpoint phosphatase Cdc25A, which marks it for degradation (Mailand et al., 2000, 2002; Falck et al., 2001, 2002; Zhao et al., 2002). Cdc25A's duty is to dephosphorylate—and hence maintain the activity of—the cyclin-dependent kinases Cdk2 and Cdk1. Cdk2 drives both the G1/S transition and S phase, and Cdk1 mobilizes the G2 phase onto mitosis. Therefore, the destruction of Cdc25A contributes to the G1/S, intra-S, and G2/M checkpoints (Fig. 29.1). Of interest is the observation that the Cdc25A-mediated component of the G1-S checkpoint is rapid and, unlike the p53-mediated component, is not dependent on gene activation and protein synthesis (Falck et al., 2002).

Notably, in addition to ATM's versatility as a protein kinase with numerous substrates, the ATM web contains protein kinases that are themselves capable of targeting several downstream effectors simultaneously, and so concomitantly control subsets of pathways. Chk2 is known to phosphorylate p53, BrcA1, Cdc25A, and Cdc25C (Bartek et al., 2001; McGowan, 2002) (Fig. 29.1). The Chk2–Cdc25C pathway is similar to the previously mentioned Chk2–Cdc25A pathway, but may act instead at the G2/M transition. Here, phosphorylation of Cdc25C by activated Chk2 is thought to lead to cytoplasmic sequestration of Cdc25C, which prevents activation of Cdk1.

Most of these pathways have not been completely characterized, and the involvement of ATM substrates in them has been inferred from defective activation of specific checkpoints following abrogation of ATM-mediated phosphorylation of these proteins. An interesting pathway is mediated by phosphorylation of hRad17, the human orthologue of Rad17 from the fission yeast *Schizosaccharomyces pombe*. hRad17 is phosphorylated in an ATM/ATR-mediated manner on two serine residues, and this phosphorylation is important for proper G1/S and G2/M checkpoint functions (Bao et al., 2001; Post et al., 2001). hRad17 is involved in a very early event in the DSB response: it loads a trimolecular complex onto the DNA that consists of the human orthologues of the fission yeast proteins Rad9, Hus1, and Rad1 ("the 9-1-1 complex"). This complex acts as a sliding clamp, probably a damage sensor (Parrilla-Castellar et al., 2004). Although this process may be upstream of the transducer recruitment, two essential proteins in this process, hRad17 and hRad9, are also phosphorylated in an ATM/ATR-dependent manner and participate in downstream checkpoint pathways (Bao et al., 2001; Chen et al., 2001; Post et al., 2001).

ATM and gene transcription

Many damage responses end up modulating gene expression. Indeed, a major ATM target, p53, is a transcription factor. Another transcription factor with a central role in cell cycle control, E2F1, has been reported to be phosphorylated and stabilized in an ATM-dependent manner (Lin et al., 2001). In addition, it is becoming evident that stress–response pathways that are best known for responding to other triggers in an ATM-independent manner, such as those mediated by the mitogen-activated protein kinases or the transcription factor NF-κB, also contain a DNA damage-responsive component (Pearce and Humphrey, 2001). Interestingly, when these pathways are activated by DSBs, their response becomes ATM-dependent (Wang et al., 2000a; Li et al., 2001; Bar-Shira et al., 2002). The direct targets of ATM in these pathways have not been elucidated, but these observations expand the ATM-dependent network considerably.

ATM and damage-independent genomic stability

ATM helps maintain genomic stability through mechanisms other than responding to DSBs caused by damaging agents. T cells from A-T patients have abnormally shortened telomeres, abnormal association of chromosome ends, telomere clustering, and altered interaction between the telomeres and the nuclear matrix (Pandita, 2001). Evidence is accumulating that ATM is functionally linked to telomere maintenance, a process crucial to aging and cancer (Pandita, 2001; Chan and Blackburn, 2002; Kim et al., 2002a; Maser and DePinho, 2002). Here, ATM may be responding continuously to an ongoing process rather than abruptly and vigorously to an acute insult (Karlseder et al., 1999). The functional relationships between ATM and the telomere maintenance machinery have been illuminated by a study that generated mice doubly null for Atm and the telomerase RNA component Terc (Wong et al., 2003). These animals showed increased genomic instability, enhanced aging, and premature death, with a general proliferation defect extending into stem and progenitor cell compartments. Interestingly, the rate of T cell malignancies in these mice was reduced rather than enhanced.

A substrate of ATM-dependent phosphorylation in the telomere maintenance system is TRF1, which negatively regulates telomere elongation. Phosphorylation of TRF1 seems to suppresses TRF1-mediated apoptosis following DNA damage (Kishi et al., 2001). Interestingly, inhibition of TRF1 in A-T cells rescues telomere shortening and decreases the radiosensitivity of these cells, providing further evidence of the link between telomere metabolism and the DNA damage response (Kishi and Lu, 2002).

Further evidence of ongoing activity of ATM at sites of normally occurring breakage and reunion of DNA was provided by its presence at sites of V(D)J recombination (Perkins et al., 2004). At those sites, p53 phosphorylated at the ATM target residue was also present, indicating that ATM continuously surveys the V(D)J recombination process and can induce a damage response if DSBs are not sealed in a timely manner. Indeed, A-T patients often show clonal translocations involving the sites of the T cell receptor and immunoglobulin genes, demonstrating the consequences of absence of this surveillance. These translocations often herald the onset of lymphoid malignancy (Xu, 1999).

ATM-Deficient Mice: An Animal Model of A-T

Mouse models of A-T were established in several laboratories by forming null alleles of the mouse homologue, Atm (Barlow et al., 1996; Elson et al., 1996; Herzog et al., 1996; Xu et al., 1996; Borghesari et al., 2000). Atm$^{-/-}$ mice share many clinical features of human A-T and highlight several features that have not received sufficient attention in humans and might be essential to understanding the functions of ATM. The reduced number and abnormal function of B and T cells, radiosensitivity, and a strong predisposition to cancer are similar between humans and mice. However, Atm$^{-/-}$ animals die almost exclusively from thymic lymphomas,

whereas human patients develop leukaemias, lymphomas, and solid tumors. Growth retardation is much more pronounced in Atm$^{-/-}$ mice than in human A-T patients. Fibroblasts from Atm$^{-/-}$ mice grow slowly and exhibit inefficient progression from G1 to S phase following serum stimulation (Xu and Baltimore, 1996). Atm-deficient mouse fibroblasts manifest radiosensitivity, genome instability, and defective radiation-induced cell cycle checkpoints. An Atm knock-in mutant mouse harbors a 9 nucleotide in-frame deletion (7666del9) corresponding to a common human mutation (7636del9) and producing near full-length Atm protein (Spring et al., 2001). The overall phenotype is similar to Atm$^{-/-}$ mice except for longer life span in nonspecific pathogen-free conditions, a lower incidence of thymic lymphomas, and more varied tumor types in older animals.

The neurologic deficit in Atm$^{-/-}$ mice is much less pronounced than in humans and can be elicited only by special testing. Moreover, the cerebella of these animals appear normal upon histopathological examination. The use of electron microscopy has provided evidence for degeneration of several different neuronal cell types in the cerebral cortex in 25% of neuronal profiles of 2-month-old Atm$^{-/-}$ mice (Kuljis et al., 1997). Degenerating Purkinje cells had abnormalities in nucleoplasm and cytoplasm as well as crenated cell membranes from which filiform appendages originated. Degeneration was also observed in other types of neurons and glial cells. Replacement of the Rad3 homology domain of Atm with a neol^r gene generated an Atm$^{-/-}$ mouse with ectopic and abnormally differentiated Purkinje cells (Borghesani et al., 2000). Although gross neurological abnormalities were found, none of the other Atm$^{-/-}$ mice exhibited such changes. However, Atm$^{-/-}$ mice show age-dependent defects in Ca^{2+} spike bursts and calcium currents (Chiesa et al., 2000), and cerebellar Purkinje cells from Atm$^{-/-}$ animals are in a state of oxidative stress (Barlow et al., 1999; Watters et al., 1999; Kamsler et al., 2001).

Male and female sterility due to absence of mature gametes is another striking feature that has not received special attention in human patients. Atm is clearly essential for mouse germ cell development. Xu et al. (1996) noticed that meiosis is arrested in these mice at the zygotene/pachytene stage of the first meiotic prophase as a result of abnormal chromosomal synapsis and subsequent fragmentation. Using electron microscopy, Barlow et al. (1998) showed that male and female gametogenesis is disrupted in Atm$^{-/-}$ mice as early as leptonema of prophase 1, resulting in apoptotic degeneration. These results are corroborated by the observation that Atm is physically associated with synapsed chromosomal axes at meiosis (Keegan et al., 1996; Plug et al., 1997). These findings provide direct evidence of the role of Atm in recognizing specific DNA structures formed during meiotic recombination.

In summary, observations in mouse knockout models highlight the role of Atm in normal somatic cell growth and chromosomal recombination in meiosis, in addition to its recognized function in radiation-induced signal transduction. Further genetic manipulation of Atm$^{-/-}$ mice will enable the elucidation of additional features of A-T previously undisclosed in the human disease (Barlow et al., 1996; Elson et al., 1996; Xu and Baltimore, 1996; Xu et al., 1996).

Diagnosis of Ataxia Telangiectasia

Diagnosis of A-T remains chiefly clinical and depends on age of presentation. Where no family history is present, the disease is usually detected by a pediatric neurologist on the basis of anomalies in station and gait accompanied by telangiectasias. However, before the telangiectasias appear (between 2 and 8 years of age), diagnosis may be difficult. Ataxia could be part of another syndrome, for example, Friedreich's ataxia, or due to a cerebral neoplasm or hematoma. The differential diagnosis includes infectious encephalitis, postinfectious encephalomyelitis, progressive rubella panencephalitis, and subacute sclerotising panencephalitis. Ataxia may also occur in a number of metabolic diseases of infancy and childhood, such as Gaucher disease, Niemann-Pick disease, GM1 and GM2 gangliosidoses, metachromatic leukodystrophy, and Krabbe leukodystrophy. However, metabolic diseases can be diagnosed with the assistance of laboratory assays. Careful history and physical examination allow discrimination between A-T and two other metabolic disorders, Hartnup disease (an aminoaciduria) and maple syrup urine disease; in both of these diseases ataxia is episodic rather than progressive, as in A-T. Friedreich's ataxia typically has later onset and pes cavus and kyphoscoliosis, which are unusual in A-T.

A-T can also be readily distinguished from the hereditary motosensory neuropathies Charcot-Marie-Tooth disease (distal weakness, pes cavus, hyporeflexia, and mild to moderate sensory loss), type III disease (distal weakness, nerve hypertrophy, and electromyographic abnormalities), and Refsum disease (polyneuropathy and ataxia). Other syndromes exhibiting ataxia include Joseph disease, dentatorubral degeneration of Ramsay Hunt, and olivopontocerebellar atrophy, but each of these differs from A-T in having a different pattern of inheritance or age of onset. Perhaps the closest to A-T is ataxia/ocular-motor apraxia, a syndrome characterized by progressive ataxia, choreoathetosis, and oculomotor apraxia (Aicardi et al., 1988). However, these patients do not have the immunodeficiency seen in A-T, nor the other laboratory markers.

Prior to the cloning of the *ATM* gene there were a host of laboratory tests to support the clinical diagnosis of A-T (Table 29.5). Reduced or absent IgA and elevated AFP were nonspecific but supportive of the clinical diagnosis. The description of a frequent chromosome breakage by Hecht et al. (1966) and demonstration that A-T cells in culture were hypersensitive to ionizing radiation provided the basis for tests developed in several laboratories to aid in the diagnosis of A-T.

Table 29.5. Laboratory Tests to Support Diagnosis of A-T

Assay	A-T Phenotype	Reference
Antibodies		
Serum IgA, IgE	Reduced	Thieffry et al. (1961)
Serum IgM	Monomeric form	Peterson et al. (1963)
Serum Proteins		
α-fetoprotein	Elevated	Waldmann and McIntire (1972)
Carcinoembryonic antigen	Elevated	Sugimoto et al. (1978)
Radiosensitivity		
Cell survival	Reduced	Taylor et al. (1976)
Chromosome aberrations	Elevated	Hecht et al. (1965) Higurashi and Conon (1973)
G2 phase delay	Exaggerated	Ford et al. (1984) Beamish and Lavin (1994)
p53 induction	Reduced/delayed	Kastan et al. (1992) Khanna and Lavin (1993)
Radioresistant DNA synthesis	Present	Houldsworth and Lavin (1980)

None of these assays has been successful in identifying family members at risk, with the occasional exception of their application to prenatal diagnosis. When mammalian cells are exposed to radiation, a biphasic pattern of inhibition of DNA synthesis is observed. The extent of this inhibition is markedly reduced in A-T cells and has been referred to as radioresistant DNA synthesis (Houldsworth and Lavin, 1980; Painter and Young, 1980; Lavin and Schroeder, 1988). Assay for radioresistant DNA synthesis has been used for prenatal diagnosis in A-T (Jaspers et al., 1981).

Once the *ATM* gene was identified, mutation diagnosis became theoretically possible. However, a large number of mutations have been found, distributed along most of the length of the cDNA. Unless specific mutations in a family are known, mutation detection for carrier and prenatal diagnosis remains a research tool. As an alternative to mutation detection, it is possible to carry out immunoblotting to detect ATM protein. Since most mutations in ATM are truncating and some missense mutations also destabilize the protein, ATM protein is either undetectable or reduced in amount in most A-T patients. In cases where mutant ATM protein is detectable by immunoblotting, it should have no ATM kinase activity. This is determined by immunoprecipitation of ATM and assay using a substrate such as p53 and ^{32}P-ATP (Banin et al., 1998; Canman et al., 1998).

A-T Heterozygotes and Elevated Cancer Risk

Although A-T heterozygotes do not exhibit symptoms of the disease, they do have radiosensitivity to a lesser extent than homozygotes, a finding first reported by Chen et al. (1978). A number of other assays have been used to confirm this finding (Paterson et al., 1985; Roisin and Ochs, 1986; Shiloh et al., 1986; Rudolph et al., 1989; Chen et al., 1994). However, there is considerable variation among heterozygotes, and none of the assays is sufficiently reliable for A-T carrier diagnosis without reference to a known homozygote relative.

A Hardy-Weinberg estimate for heterozygote using the early data of Boder and Sedgwick (1970) predicts a frequency of 1 in 100 individuals, whereas that of Swift et al. (1986) would give a value between 0.3 and 0.4 per 100. Because A-T is autosomal recessive, it would be expected that heterozygotes would show no symptoms. However, mortality from cancer among blood relatives of A-T patients is higher than expected. Swift et al. (1991) found an increased cancer risk in 1599 adult blood relatives of A-T patients from 161 A-T families, compared to 821 of their spouses as controls. A subgroup of 294 obligate heterozygotes had relative risks of 3.8-fold above controls for men and 3.5-fold for women for all types of cancer. The relative risk for breast cancer in women was 5.1-fold. Several other epidemiological studies also support an increased risk of breast cancer in A-T heterozygotes but with smaller relative risk (Pippard et al., 1988; Janin et al., 1999; Inskip et al., 1999; Geoffroy-Perez et al., 2001; Olsen et al., 2001). Molecular genotyping and mutation analysis have produced apparently conflicting data on the incidence of *ATM* mutations in different cohorts of breast cancer patients. In A-T family studies, Athma et al. (1996) detected 25 heterozygotes among 33 women with breast cancer where only 15 were expected by chance alone. Fitzgerald et al. (1997) detected heterozygous mutations in 2 of 202 healthy women with no history of cancer, whereas the figure was 2 of 410 for women with early-onset breast cancer. Other smaller studies support these observations (Chen et al., 1998; Bay et al., 1998; Bebb et al., 1999). However, Broeks et al. (2000) detected 7 germ-line *ATM* mutations in 82 breast cancer patients with either early-onset disease or bilateral breast cancer. In most of these studies truncating mutations were screened for, since they represent the bulk of mutations seen in A-T patients. One explanation for the disparate findings might reside in possible differences between truncating and missense mutations in *ATM*. Indeed, Gatti et al. (1999) proposed a model to explain the relationship between ATM mutations and cancer susceptibility discriminating between missense and truncating mutations. They envisaged that an *ATM* missense mutant expressing mutant protein could act in a dominant negative capacity to interfere with normal ATM function. There is evidence that missense mutations in the kinase domain of *ATM* have a dominant interfering effect (Lim et al., 2000). Recent evidence for an increased frequency of *ATM* missense mutations in breast cancer patients adds support for this model (Izatt et al., 1999; Broeks et al., 2000; Dörk et al., 2001; Teraoka et al., 2001).

Swift et al. (1991) asked whether diagnostic or occupational exposure to ionizing radiation increases the risk of breast cancer in women heterozygous for A-T. However, Norman and Withers (1993), estimating that annual mammography for 35 years would give a woman a total exposure of only 10 cGy, argued that on the basis of an increased sensitivity to radiation on the order of 30% (Cole et al., 1988), the lifetime risk for breast cancer from mammography would be 2 cases per 100 women. This would not significantly add to the natural lifetime risk of 1 in 9 in the general population. Additional studies of cancer and heterozygous *ATM* mutation are needed that also address the potential combined effects of mutations in the breast cancer susceptibility genes *BRCA1* and *BRCA2* as well as better-defined environmental risk factors.

Future Directions and Treatments

Progress in our understanding of the role of ATM has been rapid since the gene was cloned. More than 40 substrates have been identified for ATM, including the proteins shown to be defective in other genome instability syndromes such as A-T-like syndrome, Nijmegen breakage syndrome, Fanconi's anaemia, and Bloom's syndrome (Chapter 30). Clearly ATM is involved in many different signaling pathways. Challenges ahead include identifying additional substrates, establishing the physiological importance of specific ATM-mdiated phosphorylations, and assembling these events into signaling pathways. The overlap of A-T with other genomic instability syndromes promises to shed light on cellular processes associated with maintaining the integrity of the genome and preventing the development of tumors.

To date, only the kinase domain has been identified as a functional domain in ATM. This represents only a small part of the total protein and it is likely that other important functions will be assigned to other regions of the molecule. A proline-rich region binding to c-Abl has been described that is likely to be important in radiation-induced signaling. The N terminus of ATM binds substrates such as p53, BRCA1, BLM, and Nbsl. It remains to be determined whether this binding facilitates the kinase activity of ATM. Further mapping of the region of binding is required, as well as demonstration of its importance for ATM function. A particularly important mission is understanding the structural aspects of ATM activation. Since full-length ATM cDNA has been cloned and used to correct the A-T cellular phenotype, it is now also possible to introduce changes into this cDNA for investigations into the importance of individual sites on the molecule (e.g., sites of phosphorylation) for structural and functional studies (Lavin et al., 2004). This cDNA resource will also be instrumental in distinguishing between genomic missense mutations in

ATM and rare allelic variants that do not interfere with ATM function. In this context, it will be possible to use the methodology to address the issue of mutations and cancer predisposition in non-A-T families. Production of mutant ATM mice with knock-in missense mutations will also assist in investigations into the role of ATM mutations in breast cancer.

The progressive neurodegeneration that represents the most debilitating aspect of A-T has been more difficult to address. Most mouse models fail to recapitulate the neurodegeneration, but mouse models show abnormalities indicative of oxidative stress in the cerebellum. Treatment with antioxidants in an attempt to slow the progression of neurodegeneration has had mixed results in limited clinical trials. The advent of stem cell technology, with prospects for efficient delivery of genes to the brain, and the possibility of using other animal models (e.g., monkeys) provide greater hope of developing approaches that may prevent neurodegeneration.

Recent thoughts about drug screening for A-T treatments are based on new insights into the molecular basis of this disease. The crucial role of ATM in the DNA damage response calls for a laboratory assay for drug screening based on this response. The redundancy between ATM and other transducers provides hope that drugs that will stimulate enzymes partially redundant with ATM may alleviate some of the symptoms of A-T or at least slow its relentless progression. The available clear readouts for this response (e.g., the phosphorylation and activation of ATM effectors) could lead to a high-throughput drug screen for A-T. This kind of search would be conducted for small molecules that allow ATM-deficient cells to mount at least a partial DSB response despite ATM's absence (Shiloh et al., 2004). Drug screening attempts based on this rationale are expected in view of our growing understanding of the function and mode of activation of the ATM protein.

Acknowledgments

We wish to thank many colleagues for helpful discussion and critical reading of the manuscript. We apologize for inadvertently overlooking relevant work on this subject, being aware of the rapid rate of accumulation of knowledge in this area. This work was supported by the National Health and Medical Research Council of Australia, the Queensland Cancer Fund, the National Institute of Neurological Disorders and Stroke, The A-T Medical Research Foundation, the A-T Children's Project, and the A-T Medical Research Trust. We thank Tracey Laing and Ian Dillon for typing the manuscript.

References

Abraham RT. PI 3-kinase related kinases: "big" players in stress-induced signaling pathways. DNA Repair (Amst) 3:883–887, 2004a.
Abraham RT. The ATM-related kinase, hSMG-1, bridges genome and RNA surveillance pathways. DNA Repair (Amst) 3:919–925, 2004b.
Aguilar MJ, Kamoshita S, Landing BH, Boder E, Sedgwick RP. Pathological observations in ataxia-telangiectasia: a report on 5 cases. J Neuropathol Exp Neurol 27:659–676, 1968.
Ahn JY, Urist M, Prives C. The Chk2 protein kinase. DNA Repair (Amst) 3:1039–1047, 2004.
Aicardi J, Barbosa C, Andermann E, Andermann F, Morcos R, Ghanem Q, et al. Ataxia-ocular motor apraxia: a syndrome mimicking ataxia-telangiectasia. Ann Neurol 24:497–502, 1988.
Alarcon-Vargas D, Ronai Z. p53-Mdm2—the affair that never ends. Carcinogenesis 23:541–547, 2002.
Alderton GK, Joenje H, Varon R, Borglum AD, Jeggo PA, O'Driscoll M. Seckel syndrome exhibits cellular features demonstrating defects in the ATR signalling pathway. Hum Mol Genet 13:3127–3138, 2004.
Al-Khodairy F, Carr AM. DNA repair mutants defining G2 checkpoint pathways in *Schizosaccharoymces pombe*. EMBO J 11:1343–1350, 1992.
Al-Khodairy F, Fotou E, Sheldrick KS, Griffiths DJ, Lehmann AR, Carr AM. Identification and characterisation of new elements involved in checkpoints and feedback controls in fission yeast. Mol Biol Cell 5:147–160, 1994.

Allen JB, Zhou Z, Siede W, Friedberg EC, Elledge SJ. The SAD1/RAD53 protein kinase controls multiple checkpoints and DNA damage-induced transcription in yeast. Genes Dev 8:2401–2415, 1994.

Al Saadi A, Palutka M, Kumar GK. Evolution of chromosomal abnormalities in sequential cytogenetic studies of ataxia-telangiectasia. Hum Genet 5:23–29, 1980.

Ammann AJ, Cain WA, Ischizaka K, Hong R, Good RA. Immunoglobulin E deficiency in ataxia-telangiectasia. N Engl J Med 281:469–504, 1969.

Ammann AJ, Hong R. Autoimmune phenomena in ataxia-telangiectasia. J Pediatr 78:821–826, 1971.

Amromin GD, Boder E, Tepelits R. Ataxia-telangiectasia with a 32-year survival. A clinicopathological report. J Neuropathol Exp Neurol 38:621–643, 1979.

Andegeko Y, Moyal L, Mitelman L, Tsarfaty I, Shiloh Y, Rotman G. Nuclear retention of ATM at sites of DNA double-strand breaks. J Biol Chem 276:38224–38230, 2001.

Anderson CW. DNA damage and the DNA-activated protein kinase. Trends Biochem Sci 18:433–437, 1993.

Andrews BF, Kopack FM, Bruton OC. A syndrome of ataxia, oculocutaneous telangiectasia, and sinopulmonary infection. US Armed Forces Med J 11:587–592, 1960.

Angele S, Lauge A, Fernet M, Moullan N, Beauvais P, Couturier J, Stoppa-Lyonnet D, Hall J. Phenotypic cellular characterization of an ataxia-telangiectasia patient carrying a causal homozygous missense mutation. Hum Mutat 21:169–170, 2003.

Araki R, Fukumura R, Fujimori A, Taya Y, Shiloh Y, Kurimasa A, et al. Enhanced phosphorylation of p53 serine 18 following DNA damage in DNA-dependent protein kinase catalytic subunit-deficient cells. Cancer Res 59:3543–3546, 1999.

Ashcroft M, Kubbutat MH, Vousden KH. Regulation of p53 function and stability by phosphorylation. Mol Cell Biol 19:1751–1758, 1999.

Athma P, Rappaport R, Swift M. Molecular genotyping shows that ataxia-telangiectasia heterozygotes are predisposed to breast cancer. Cancer Genet Cytogenet 92:130–134, 1996.

Aurias AB, Dutrillaux DB, Lejeune J. High frequencies of inversions and translocations of chromosomes 7 and 14 in ataxia-telangiectasia. Mutat Res 69:369–374, 1980.

Bakkenist CJ, Kastan MB. DNA damage activates ATM through intermolecular autophosphorylation and dimer dissociation. Nature 421:499–506, 2003.

Banga SS, Shenkar R, Boyd JB. Hypersensitivity of Drosophila mei-41 mutants to hydroxyurea is associated with reduced mitotic chromosome stability. Mutat Res 163:157–165, 1986.

Banin S, Moyal L, Shieh S, Taya Y, Anderson CW, Chessa L, et al. Enhanced phosphorylation of p53 by ATM in response to DNA damage. Science 281:1674–1677, 1998.

Bao S, Tibbetts RS, Brumbaugh KM, Fang Y, Richardson DA, Ali A, et al. ATR/ATM-mediated phosphorylation of human Rad17 is required for general stress responses. Nature 411:969–974, 2001.

Bar RS, Levis WR, Rechler MM, Harrison LC, Siebert C, Podskalny J, et al. Extreme insulin resistance in ataxia-telangiectasia: defect in affinity of insulin receptors. N Engl J Med 298:1164–1171, 1978.

Barlow C, Dennery PA, Shigenaga MK, Smith MA, Morrow JD, Roberts LJ 2nd, et al. Loss of the ataxia-telangiectasia gene product causes oxidative damage in organs. Proc Natl Acad Sci USA 96:9915–9919, 1999.

Barlow C, Hirotsune S, Paylor R, Liyanage M, Eckhaus M, Collins FS, et al. Atm-deficient mice: a paradigm of ataxia-telangiectasia. Cell 86:159–171, 1996.

Barlow C, Liyanage M, Moens PB, Tarsounas M, Nagashima K, Brown K, et al. Atm deficiency results in severe meiotic disruption as early as leptonema of prophase I. Development 125:4007–4017, 1998.

Barlow MH, McFarlin DE, Schalch DS. An unusual type of diabetes mellitus with marked hyperinsulinism in patients with ataxia-telangiectasia. Clin Res 13:530, 1965.

Bar-Shira A, Rashi-Elkeles S, Zlochover L, Moyal L, Smorodinsky NI, Seger R, Shiloh Y. ATM-dependent activation of the gene encoding MAP kinase phosphatase 5 by radiomimetic DNA damage. Oncogene 21:849–855, 2002.

Bartek J, Falck J, Lukas J. CHK2 kinase—a busy messenger. Nat Rev Mol Cell Biol 2:877–886, 2001.

Bates PR, Imray FP, Lavin MF. Effect of caffeine on γ-ray–induced G2 delay in ataxia-telangiectasia. Int J Radiat Biol 47:713–722, 1985.

Bay JO, Grancho M, Pernin D, Presneau N, Rio P, Tchirkov A, et al. No evidence for constitutional ATM mutation in breast/gastric cancer families. Int J Oncol 12:1385–1390, 1998.

Beamish H, Lavin MF. Radiosensitivity in ataxia-telangiectasia: anomalies in radiation-induced cell cycle delay. Int J Radiat Biol 65:175–184, 1994.

Beamish H, Williams R, Chen P, Lavin MF. Defect in multiple cell cycle checkpoints in ataxia-telangiectasia post-irradiation. J Biol Chem 271:20486–20493, 1996.

Beatty DW, Arens LJ, Nelson MN. Ataxia-telangiectasia. X, 14 translocation, progressive deterioration of lymphocyte numbers and function, and abnormal in vitro immunoglobulin production. S Afr Med J 69:115–118, 1986.

Bebb DG, Yu Z, Chen J, Telatar M, Gelmon K, Phillips N, et al. Absence of mutations in the ATM gene in forty-seven cases of sporadic breast cancer. Br J Cancer 80:1979–1981, 1999.

Becker-Catania SG, Chen G, Hwang MJ, Wang Z, Sun X, Sanal O, Bernatowska-Matuszkiewicz E, Chessa L, Lee EY, Gatti RA. Ataxia-telangiectasia: phenotype/genotype studies of ATM protein expression, mutations, and radiosensitivity. Mol Genet Metab 70:122–133, 2000.

Bentley P, Pepper C, Hoy T. Regulation of clinical chemoresistance by bcl-2 and bax oncoprotein in B-cell chronic lymphocytic leukaemia. Br J Haematol 95:513–517, 1996.

Bhandoola A, Dolnick B, Fayad N, Nussenzweig A, Singer A. Immature thymocytes undergoing receptor rearrangements are resistant to ATM-dependent death pathway activated in mature T cells by double-strand DNA breaks. J Exp Med 192:891–897, 2000.

Biemond A. A Palaeocerebellar atrophy with extra-pyramidal manifestations in association with bronchiectasis and telangiectasis of the conjunctiva. In: Proceedings of the 1st International Congress of Neurological Sciences, Brussels, July 1957. London: Pergamon Press 4:206, 1957.

Blasina A, de Weyer IV, Laus MC, Luyten WH, Parker AE, McGowan CH. A human homologue of the checkpoint kinase Cds1 directly inhibits Cdc2 phosphatase. Curr Biol 9:1–10, 1999.

Boder E. Ataxia-telangiectasia: some historic, clinical and pathological observations. In: Bergsma D, Good RA, Finstad J, Paul NW, eds. Sunderland, MA: Sinauer, pp. 255–270, 1975.

Boder E. Ataxia-telangiectasia: an overview. In: Gatti RA, Swift M, eds. Ataxia-Telangiectasia. New York: Alan R. Liss, Kroc Foundation Series 19, pp. 1–63, 1985.

Boder E, Sedgwick RP. Ataxia-telangiectasia. A familial syndrome of progressive cerebellar ataxia, oculocutaneous telangiectasia and frequent pulmonary infection. A preliminary report on 7 children, an autopsy, and a case history. Univ S Calif Med Bull 9:15–28, 1957.

Boder E, Sedgwick RP. Ataxia-telangiectasia. A familial syndrome of progressive cerebellar ataxia, oculocutaneous telangiectasia and frequent pulmonary infection. Pediatrics 21:526–554, 1958.

Boder E, Sedgwick RP. Ataxia-telangiectasia. A review of 101 cases. In: Walsh G, ed. Little Club Clinics in Developmental Medicine No. 8. London: Heinemann Medical Books, pp. 110–118, 1963.

Boder E, Sedgwick RP. Ataxia-telangiectasia. Psychiatr Neurol Med Psychol Beitr 13–14:8–16, 1970.

Borghesani PR, Alt FW, Bottaro A, Davidson L, Aksoy S, Rathbun GA, et al. Abnormal development of Purkinje cells and lymphocytes in Atm mutant mice. Proc Natl Acad Sci USA 97:3336–3341, 2000.

Bowden DH, Danis PG, Sommers SC. Ataxia-telangiectasia. A case with lesions of ovaries and adenohypophysis. J Neuropathol Exp Neurol 22:549–554, 1963.

Boyd JB, Golino MD, Nguyen TD, Green MM. Isolation and characterization of X-linked mutants of Drosophila melanogaster which are sensitive to mutagens. Genetics 84:485–506, 1976.

Broeks A, de Klein A, Floore AN, Muijtjens M, Kleijer WJ, Jaspers NG, van't Veer LJ. ATM germline mutations in classical ataxia-telangiectasia patients in the Dutch population. Hum Mutat 12:330–337, 1998.

Broeks A, Urbanus JH, Floore AN, Dahler EC, Klijn JG, Rutgers EJ, et al. ATM-heterozygous germline mutations contribute to breast cancer susceptibility. Am J Hum Genet 66:494–500, 2000.

Brooks CL, Gu W. Dynamics in the p53-Mdm2 ubiquitination pathway. Cell Cycle 3:895–899, 2004.

Brown AL, Lee CH, Schwarz JK, Mitiku N, Piwnica-Worms H, Chung JH. A human Cds1-related kinase that functions downstream of ATM protein cellular response to DNA damage. Proc Natl Acad Sci USA 96:3745–3750, 1999.

Brown EJ, Albers MW, Shin TB, Ichikawa K, Keith CT, Lane WS, et al. A mammalian protein targeted by G1-arresting rapamycin receptor complex. Nature 369:756–758, 1994.

Brown EJ, Baltimore D. ATR disruption leads to chromosomal fragmentation and early embryonic lethality. Genes Dev 14:397–402, 2000.

Brown EJ, Beal PA, Keith CT, Chen J, Shin TB, Schreiber SL. Control of p70 S6 kinase by kinase activity of FRAP in vivo. Nature 377:441–446, 1995.

Burma S, Chen BP, Murphy M, Kurimasa A, Chen DJ. ATM phosphorylates histone H2AX in response to DNA double-strand breaks. J Biol Chem 276:42462–42467, 2001.

Burma S, Chen DJ. Role of DNA-PK in the cellular response to DNA double-strand breaks. DNA Repair (Amst) 3:909–918, 2004.

Buscemi G, Savio C, Zannini L, Micciche F, Masnada D, Nakanishi M, Tauchi H, Komatsu K, Mizutani S, Khanna K, Chen P, Concannon P, Chessa L, Delia D. Chk2 activation dependence on Nbs1 after DNA damage. Mol Cell Biol 21:5214–5222, 2001.

Byrd PJ, McConville CM, Cooper P, Parkhill J, Stankovic T, McGuire GM, et al. Mutations revealed by sequencing the 5 half of the gene for ataxia-telangiectasia. Hum Mol Genet 5:145–149, 1996.

Canman CE. Replication checkpoint: preventing mitotic catastrophe. Curr Biol 11:R121–124, 2001.

Canman CE, Lim DS, Cimprich KA, Taya Y, Tamai K, Sakaguchi K, Appella E, Kastan MB, Siliciano JD. Activation of the ATM kinase by ionizing radiation and phosphorylation of p53. Science 281:1677–1679, 1998.

Canman CE, Wolff AC, Chen CY, Fornace AJ Jr, Kastan MB. The p53-dependent G1 cell cycle checkpoint pathway and ataxia-telangiectasia. Cancer Res 54:5054–5058, 1994.

Carbonari M, Cherchi M, Paganelli R, Giannini G, Galli E, Gaetan C, et al. Relative increase of T cells expressing the gamma/delta rather than the alpha/beta receptor in ataxia-telangiectasia. N Engl J Med 322:73–76, 1990.

Carney JP, Maser RS, Olivares H, Davis EM, Le Beau M, Yates JR 3rd, et al. The hMre11/hRad50 protein complex and Nijmegen breakage syndrome: linkage of double-strand break repair to the cellular DNA damage response. Cell 93:477–486, 1998.

Carson CT, Schwartz RA, Stracker TH, Lilley CE, Lee DV, Weitzman MD. The Mre11 complex is required for ATM activation and the G2/M checkpoint. EMBO J 22:6610–6620, 2003.

Centerwall WR, Miller MM. Ataxia telangiectasia and sionpulmonary infections. A syndrome of slowly progressive deterioration in childhood. Am J Dis Child 95:385–396, 1958.

Celeste A, Petersen S, Romanienko PJ, Fernandez-Capetillo O, Chen HT, Sedelnikova OA, Reina-San-Martin B, Coppola V, Meffre E, Difilippantonio MJ, Redon C, Pilch DR, Olaru A, Eckhaus M, Camerini-Otero RD, Tessarollo L, Livak F, Manova K, Bonner WM, Nussenzweig MC, Nussenzweig A. Genomic instability in mice lacking histone H2AX. Science 296:922–927, 2002.

Chan DW, Son SC, Block W, Ye R, Khanna KK, Wold MS, et al. Purification and characterization of ATM from human placenta. A manganese-dependent, wortmannin-sensitive serine/threonine protein kinase. J Biol Chem 275:7803–7810, 2000.

Chan SW, Blackburn EH. New ways not to make ends meet: telomerase, DNA damage proteins and heterochromatin. Oncogene 21:553–563, 2002.

Chao C, Yang EM, Xu Y. Rescue of defective T cell development and function in Atm$^{-/-}$ mice by a functional TCR $\alpha\beta$ transgene. J Immunol 64:345–349, 2000.

Chehab NH, Malikzay A, Stavridi ES, Halazonetis TD. Phosphorylation of Ser-20 mediates stabilization of human p53 in response to DNA damage. Proc Natl Acad Sci USA 96:13777–13782, 1999.

Chen J, Birkholtz GG, Lindblom P, Rubio C, Lindblom A. The role of ataxia-telangiectasia heterozygotes in familial breast cancer. Cancer Res 58:1376–1379, 1998.

Chen MJ, Lin YT, Lieberman HB, Chen G, Lee EY. ATM-dependent phosphorylation of human Rad9 is required for ionizing radiation-induced checkpoint activation. J Biol Chem 276:16580–16586, 2001.

Chen P, Farrell A, Hobson K, Girjes A, Lavin MF. Comparative study of radiation-induced G2 phase delay and chromatid damage in families with ataxia-telangiectasia. Cancer Genet Cytogenet 76:43–46, 1994.

Chen P, Imray FP, Kidson C. Gene dosage and complementation analysis of ataxia-telangiectasia lymphoblastoid cell lines assayed by induced chromosome aberrations. Mutat Res 129:165–172, 1984.

Chen PC, Lavin MF, Kidson C, Moss D. Identification of ataxia telangiectasia heterozygotes, a cancer-prone population. Nature 274:484–486, 1978.

Chessa L, Petrinelli P, Antonelli A, Fiorelli M, Elli R, Marcucci L, et al. Heterogeneity in ataxia-telangiectasia: classical phenotype associated with intermediate cellular radiosensitivity. Am J Med Genet 42:741–746, 1992.

Chiesa N, Barlow C, Wynshaw-Boris A, Strata P, Tempia F. Atm-deficient mice Purkinje cells show age-dependent defects in calcium spike bursts and calcium currents. Neuroscience 96:575–583, 2000.

Chun HH, Gatti RA. Ataxia-telangiectasia, an evolving phenotype. DNA Repair (Amst) 3:1187–1196, 2004.

Cimprich KA, Shin TB, Keith CT, Schreiber SL. cDNA cloning and gene mapping of a candidate human cell cycle checkpoint protein. Proc Natl Acad Sci USA 93:2850–2855, 1996.

Clarke AR, Purdie CA, Harrison DJ, Morris RG, Bird CC, Hooper ML, Wylie AH. Thymocyte apoptosis induced by p53-dependent and independent pathways. Nature 362:849–852, 1993.

Clarke DJ, Segal M, Mondesert G, Reed SI. The Pds1 anaphase inhibitor and Mec1 kinase define distinct checkpoints coupling S phase with mitosis in budding yeast. Curr Biol 9:365–368, 1999.

Cliby WA, Roberts CJ, Cimprich KA, Stringer CM, Lamb JR, Schreiber SL, Friend SH. Overexpression of a kinase-inactive ATR protein causes sensitivity to DNA-damaging agents and defects in cell cycle checkpoints. EMBO J 17:159–169, 1998.

Cohen MM, Shaham M, Dagan JRK, Shmueli E, Kohn G. Cytogenetic investigations in families with ataxia-telangiectasia. Cytogenet Cell Genet 15:338–356, 1975.

Cohen MM, Simpson SJ. The effect of bleomycin on DNA synthesis in ataxia-telangiectasia lymphoid cells. Environ Mutagen 4:27–36, 1982.

Cole J, Arlett CF, Green MHL, Harcourt SA, Priestley A, Henderson L, et al. Comparative human cellular radiosensitivity: II. The survival following gamma-irradiation of unstimulated (G_o) T-lymphocytes, T-lymphocyte lines, lymphoblastoid cell lines and fibroblasts from normal donors, from ataxia-telangiectasia patients and from ataxia-telangiectasia heterozygotes. Int J Radiat Biol 54:929–942, 1988.

Concannon P, Gatti RA. Diversity of *ATM* gene mutations detected in patients with ataxia-telangiectasia. Hum Mutat 10:100–107, 1997.

Cornforth MN, Bedford JS. On the nature of a defect in cells from individuals with ataxia-telangiectasia. Science 227(4694):1589–1591, 1985.

Cortez D, Guntuku S, Qin J, Elledge SJ. ATR and ATRIP: partners in checkpoint signaling. Science 294:1713–1716, 2001.

Cortez D, Wang Y, Qin J, Elledge SJ. Requirement of ATM-dependent phosphorylation of Brca1 in the DNA damage response to double-strand breaks. Science 286:1162–1166, 1999.

Costanzo V, Paull T, Gottesman M, Gautier J. Mre11 assembles linear DNA fragments into DNA damage signaling complexes. PLoS Biol 2:E110, 2004.

Cox R, Hosking GP, Wilson J. Ataxia-telangiectasia: evaluation of radiosensitivity in cultured skin fibroblasts as a diagnostic test. Arch Dis Child 53:386–390, 1978.

Craven RJ, Petes TD. Involvement of the checkpoint protein Mec1p in silencing of gene expression at telomeres in *Saccharomyces cerevisiae*. Mol Cell Biol 20:2378–2384, 2000.

Crompton NE, Miralbell R, Rutz HP, Ersoy F, Sanal O, Wellmann D, et al. Altered apoptotic profiles in irradiated patients with increased toxicity. Int J Radiat Oncol Biol Phys 45:707–714, 1999.

Curry CJ, Tsai J, Hutchinson HT, Jaspers NG, Wara D, Gatti RA. A-T Fresno: a phenotype linking ataxia-telangiectasia with the Nijmegen breakage syndrome. Am J Hum Genet 45:270–275, 1989.

Davies SM, Harris AL, Hickson ID. Overproduction of topoisomerase II in an ataxia telangiectasia fibroblast cell line: comparison with a topoisomerase II-overproducing hamster cell mutant. Nucleic Acids Res. 17(4):1337–1351, 1989.

de Klein A, Muijtjens M, van Os R, Verhoeven Y, Smit B, Carr AM, Lehmann AR, Hoeijmakers JH. Targeted disruption of the cell-cycle checkpoint gene ATR leads to early embryonic lethality in mice. Curr Biol 10:479–482, 2000.

de Wit J, Jaspers NGJ, Bootsma D. The rate of DNA synthesis in normal and ataxia-telangiectasia cells after exposure to X-irradiation. Mutat Res 80:221–226, 1981.

Digweed M, Reis A, Sperling K. Nijmegen breakage syndrome: consequences of defective DNA double-strand break repair. Bioessays 21:649–656, 1999.

Digweed M, Sperling K. Nijmegen breakage syndrome: clinical manifestation of defective response to DNA double-strand breaks. DNA Repair (Amst) 3:1207–1217, 2004.

DiTullio RA Jr, Mochan TA, Venere M, Bartkova J, Sehested M, Bartek J, Halazonetis TD. 53BP1 functions in an ATM-dependent checkpoint pathway that is constitutively activated in human cancer. Nat Cell Biol 4:998–1002, 2002.

Dörk T, Bendix R, Bremer M, Rades D, Klöpper K, Nicke M, et al. Spectrum of *ATM* gene mutations in a hospital-based series of unselected breast cancer patients. Cancer Res 61:7608–7615, 2001.

Dörk T, Bendix-Waltes R, Wegner RD, Stumm M. Slow progression of ataxia-telangiectasia with double missense and in frame splice mutations. Am J Med Genet 126A:272–277, 2004.

Dulic V, Kaufmann WK, Wilson SJ, Tisty TD, Lees E, Harper JW, et al. p53-dependent inhibition of cyclin-dependent kinase activities in human fibroblasts during radiation-induced G_1 arrest. Cell 76:1013–1023, 1994.

Dumaz N, Meek DW. Serine15 phosphorylation stimulates p53 transactivation but does not directly influence interaction with HDM2. EMBO J 18:7002–7010, 1999.

Dunn HG, Meuwissen H, Livingstone CS, Pump KK. Ataxia-telangiectasia. CMAJ 91:1106–1118, 1964.

Edwards MJ, Taylor AMR. Unusual levels of (ADP-ribose) and DNA synthesis in ataxia telangiectasia cells following γ-ray irradiation. Nature 287: 745–747, 1981.

Ejima Y, Sasaki MS. Mutations of the ATM gene detected in Japanese ataxia-telangiectasia patients: possible preponderance of the two founder mutations 4612del165 and 7883del5. Hum Genet 102:403–408, 1998.

El-Deiry WS. Transactivation of repair genes by BRCA1. Cancer Biol Ther 1:490–491, 2002.

El-Deiry WS, Tokino T, Velculescu VE, Levy DB, Parsons R, Trent JM, et al. WAF1, a potential mediator of p53 tumor suppression. Cell 75:817–825, 1993.

Elson A, Wang Y, Daugherty CJ, Morton CC, Zhou F, Campos Torres J, Leder P. Pleiotropic defects in ataxia-telangiectasia (Atm-deficient) mice. Proc Natl Acad Sci USA 93:13084–13089, 1996.

Eng L, Coutinho G, Nahas S, Yeo G, Tanouye R, Babaei M, Dork T, Burge C, Gatti RA. Nonclassical splicing mutations in the coding and noncoding regions of the ATM gene: maximum entropy estimates of splice junction strengths. Hum Mutat 23:67–76, 2004.

Epstein WL, Fudenberg HH, Reed WB. Immunologic studies in ataxia-telangiectasia. Int Arch Allergy Appl Immunol 30:15–29, 1966.

Falck J, Mailand N, Syljuasen RG, Bartek J, Lukas J. The ATM-Chk2-Cdc25A checkpoint pathway guards against radioresistant synthesis. Nature 410:842–847, 2001.

Falck J, Petrini JH, Williams BR, Lukas J, Bartek J. The DNA damage-dependent intra-S phase checkpoint is regulated by parallel pathways. Nat Genet 30:290–294, 2002.

Fan Z, Chakravarty P, Alfieri A, Pandita TK, Vikram B, Guha C. Adenovirus-mediated antisense ATM gene transfer sensitizes prostate cancer cells to radiation. Cancer Gene Ther 7:1307–1314, 2000.

Feigin RD, Vietti TJ, Wyatt RG, Kaufmann DG, Smith CH Jr. Ataxia telangiectasia with granulocytopenia. J Pediatr 77:431–438, 1970.

Ferak V, Benko J, Cajkova E. Genetic aspects of Louis-Bar syndrome (ataxia-telangiectasia). Cs Neurol 5:319–327, 1968.

Fernandez-Capetillo O, Chen HT, Celeste A, Ward I, Romanienko PJ, Morales JC, Naka K, Xia Z, Camerini-Otero RD, Motoyama N, Carpenter PB, Bonner WM, Chen J, Nussenzweig A. DNA damage–induced G2-M checkpoint activation by histone H2AX and 53BP1. Nat Cell Biol 4: 993–997, 2002.

Fernandez-Capetillo O, Lee A, Nussenzweig M, Nussenzweig A. H2AX: the histone guardian of the genome. DNA Repair (Amst) 3:959–967, 2004.

Fiorilli M, Antonelli A, Russo G, Crescenzi M, Carbonary M, Petrinelli P. Variant of ataxia-telangiectasia with low-level radiosensitivity. Hum Genet 70:274–277, 1985.

Fiorilli M, Businol L, Pandolfi F, Paganelli R, Russ G, Aiuti F. Heterogeneity of immunological abnormalities in ataxia-telangiectasia. J Clin Immunol 3:135–141, 1983.

Fireman P, Boesman M, Gitlin D. Ataxia-telangiectasia. A dysgammaglobulinemia with deficient gamma IA (B2A)-globulin. Lancet 1:1193–1195, 1964.

Fitzgerald MG, Bean JM, Hegde SR, Unsal H, MacDonald DJ, Harkin DP, et al. Heterozygous ATM mutations do not contribute to early-onset breast cancer. Nature 15:307–310, 1997.

Foray N, Priestley A, Alsbeih G, Badie C, Capulas EP, Arlett CF, Malaise EP. Hypersensitivity of ataxia-telangiectasia fibroblasts to ionizing radiation is associated with a repair deficiency of DNA double-strand breaks. Int J Radiat Biol 72(3):271–283, 1997.

Foray N, Marot D, Gabriel A, Randrianarison V, Carr AM, Perricaudet M, Ashworth A, Jeggo P. A subset of ATM- and ATR-dependent phosphorylation events requires the BRCA1 protein. EMBO J 22:2860–2871, 2003.

Ford MD, Martin L, Lavin MF. The effects of ionizing radiation on cell cycle progression in ataxia telangiectasia. Mutat Res 125:115–122, 1984.

Fritz E, Friedl AA, Zwacka RM, Eckardt-Schupp F, Meyn MS. The yeast TEL1 gene partially substitutes for human ATM in suppressing hyperrecombination, radiation-induced apoptosis and telomere shortening in A-T cells. Mol Biol Cell 11:2605–2616, 2000.

Fukao T, Kaneko H, Birrell G, Gatei M, Tashita H, Yoshita T, et al. ATM is upregulated during the mitogenic response in peripheral blood mononuclear cells. Blood 94:1998–2006, 1999.

Fukao T, Tashita H, Teramoto T, Inoue R, Kaneko H, Komiyama K, et al. Novel exonic mutation (5319 G to A) resulting in two aberrantly spliced transcripts of the ATM gene in a Japanese patient with ataxia-telangiectasia. Hum Mutat (Suppl 1):S223–S225, 1998.

Gajl-Peczaska KJ, Park BH, Biggar WD, Good RH. B and T lymphocytes in primary immunodeficiency disease in man. J Clin Invest 52:919–928, 1973.

Gatei M, Scott SP, Filippovitch I, Soronika N, Lavin MF, Weber B, Khanna KK. Role for ATM in DNA damage-induced phosphorylation of BRCA1. Cancer Res 60:3299–3304, 2000a.

Gatei M, Shkedy D, Khanna KK, Uziel T, Shiloh Y, Pandita TK, et al. Ataxia-telangiectasia: chronic activation of damage-responsive functions is reduced by alpha-lipoic acid. Oncogene 20:289–294, 2001a.

Gatei M, Young D, Cerosaletti KM, Desai-Mehta A, Spring K, Kozlov S, Lavin MF, Gatti RA, Concannon P, Khanna K. ATM-dependent phosphorylation of nibrin in response to radiation exposure. Nat Genet 25:115–119, 2000b.

Gatei M, Zhou BB, Hobson K, Scott S, Young D, Khanna KK. Ataxia-telangiectasia mutated (ATM) kinase and ATM and Rad3 related kinase mediate phosphorylation of Brca1 at distinct and overlapping sites. In vivo assessment using phospho-specific antibodies. J Biol Chem 276: 17276–17280, 2001b.

Gately DP, Hittle JC, Chan GK, Yen TJ. Characterization of ATM expression, localization and associated DNA-dependent protein kinase activity. Mol Biol Cell 9:361–374, 1998.

Gatti RA, Berkel I, Boder E, Braedt G, Charmley P, Concannon P, et al. Localization of an ataxia-telangiectasia gene to chromosome 11q22–23. Nature 336:577–580, 1988.

Gatti RA, Tward A, Concannon P. Cancer risk in ATM heterozygotes: a model of phenotypic and mechanistic differences between missense and truncating mutations. Mol Genet Metab 68(4):419–423, 1999.

Geoffroy-Perez B, Janin N, Ossian K, Lauge A, Croquette MF, Griscelli C, et al. Cancer risk in heterozygotes for ataxia-telangiectasia. Int J Cancer 93:288–293, 2001.

Gilad S, Bar-Shira A, Harnik R, Shkedy D, Ziv Y, Khosravi R, et al. Ataxia-telangiectasia: founder effect among North African Jews. Hum Mol Genet 5:2033–2037, 1996a.

Gilad S, Chessa L, Khosravi R, Russell P, Galanty Y, Piane M, Gatti RA, Jorgensen TJ, Shiloh Y, Bar-Shira A. Genotype–phenotype relationships in ataxia-telangiectasia and variants. Am J Hum Genet 62:551–561, 1998a.

Gilad S, Khosravi R, Harnik R, Ziv Y, Shkedy D, Galanty Y, et al. Identification of ATM mutations using extended RT-PCR and restriction endonuclease fingerprinting, and elucidation of the repertoire of A-T mutations in Israel. Hum Mutat 11:69–75, 1998b.

Gilad S, Khosravi R, Shkedy D, Uziel T, Ziv Y, Savitsky K, et al. Predominance of null mutations in ataxia-telangiectasia. Hum Mol Genet 5: 433–439, 1996b.

Girard PM, Riballo E, Begg AC, Waugh A, Jeggo PA. Nbs1 promotes ATM-dependent phosphorylation events including those required for G1/S arrest. Oncogene 21:4191–4199, 2002.

Good RA, Martinez C, Gabrielson AE. Clinical considerations of the thymus in immunology. In: Good RA, Gabrielsen AE, eds. The Thymus in Immunology. New York: Paul B Hoeber, pp. 30–32, 1964.

Gotoff SP, Amirmokri E, Liebner EJ. Ataxia-telangiectasia. Neoplasia, untoward response to X-irradiation, and tuberous sclerosis. Am J Dis Child 114:617–625, 1967.

Gottlieb TM, Jackson SP. Protein kinases and DNA damage. Trends Biochem Sci 19:500–503, 1994.

Grant PA, Schieltz D, Pray-Grant MG, Yates YR 3rd, Workman JL. The ATM-related cofactor Tra1 is a component of the purified SAGA complex. Mol Cell 2:863–867, 1998.

Greenwell PW, Kronmal SL, Porter SE, Gassenhuber J, Obermaier B, Petes TD. TEL1, a gene involved in controlling telomere length in Saccharomyces cerevisiae, is homologous to the human ataxia-telangiectasia (ATM) gene. Cell 82:823–829, 1995.

Gropp A, Flatz G. Chromosome breakage and blastic transformation of lymphocytes in ataxia-telangiectasia. Hum Genet 5:77–79, 1967.

Gruschcow JM, Holzen TM, Park KJ, Weinert T, Lichten M, Bishop DK. Saccharomyces cerevisiae checkpoint genes MEC1, RAD17 and RAD24 are required for normal meiotic recombination partner choice. Genetics 153:607–620, 1999.

Gu Y, Turck CW, Morgan DO. Inhibition of Cdk2 activity in vivo by an associated 20K regulatory subunit. Nature 366:707–710, 1993.

Gutmann L, Lemli L. Ataxia-telangiectasia associated with hypogammaglobulinemia. Arch Neurol 8:318–327, 1963.

Hall FL, Williams RT, Wu L, Wu F, Carbonaro-Hall DA, Harper JW, Warburton D. Two potentially oncogenic cyclins, cyclin A and cyclin D1, share common properties of subunit configuration, tyrosine phosphorylation and physical association with the Rb protein. Oncogene 8:1377–1384, 1993.

Hari KL, Santerre A, Sekelsky JJ, McKim KS, Boyd JB, Hawley RS. The mei-41 gene of Drosophila melanogaster is functionally homologous to the human ataxia-telangiectasia gene. Cell 82:815–821, 1995.

Harper WJ, Adami GR, Wei N, Keyomarsi K, Elledge SJ. The p21 Cdk-interacting protein Cip1 is a potent inhibitor of G1 cyclin-dependent kinases. Cell 75:805–816, 1993.

Hartley KO, Gell D, Smith GCM, Zhang H, Divecha N, Connelly MA, et al. DNA-dependent protein kinase catalytic subunit: a relative of phosphatidylinositol 3-kinase and the ataxia-telangiectasia gene product. Cell 82:849–856, 1995.

Hartwell LH, Smith D. Altered fidelity of mitotic chromosome transmission in cell cycle mutants of *S. cerevisiae*. Genetics 110:381–395, 1985.

Hecht F, Hecht BK. Cancer in ataxia-telangiectasia patients. Cancer Genet Cytogenet 46:9–19, 1990.

Hecht F, Koler RD, Rigas DA, Dahnke GS, Cae MP, Tisdale V, Miller RW. Leukaemia and lymphoctyes in ataxia-telangiectasia. Lancet 2:1193, 1966.

Hecht F, Kaiser-McCaw B. Ataxia-telangiectasia: genetics and heterogeneity. In: Bridges BA, Harnden DG, eds. Ataxia-Telangiectasia. New York: Wiley, pp. 197–201, 1982.

Hecht F, McCaw BK, Koler RD. Ataxia-telangiectasia—clonal growth of translocation lymphocytes. N Engl J Med 289:286–291, 1973.

Hedrick SM, Cohen DI, Neilsen EA, Davis MM. Isolation of cDNA clones encoding T cell–specific membrane associated proteins. Nature 308:149–153, 1984.

Heitman J, Movva NR, Hall MN. Targets for cell cycle arrest by the immunosuppressant rapamycin in yeast. Science 253:905–909, 1991.

Hernandez D, McConville CM, Stacey M, Woods CG, Brown MM, Shutt P, et al. A family showing no evidence of linkage between the ataxia-telangiectasia gene and chromosome 11q22–23. J Med Genet 30:135–140, 1993.

Herzog KH, Chong MJ, Kapsetaki M, Morgan JI, McKinnon PJ. Requirement for ATM in ionizing radiation–induced cell death in the developing central nervous system. Science 280(5366):1089–1091, 1998.

Higurashi M, Conen PE. In vitro chromosomal radiosensitivity in "chromosomal breakage syndromes". Cancer 32:380–383, 1973.

Hinds PW, Mittnacht S, Dulic V, Arnold A, Reed SI, Weinberg RA. Regulation of retinoblastoma protein functions by ectopic expression of human cyclins. Cell 70:993–1006, 1992.

Hong JH, Gatti RA, Huo YK, Chiang CS, McBride WH. G2/M-phase arrest and release in ataxia-telangiectasia and normal cells after exposure to ionizing radiation. Radiat Res 140:17–23, 1994.

Horejsi Z, Falck J, Bakkenist CJ, Kastan MB, Lukas J, Bartek J. Distinct functional domains of Nbs1 modulate the timing and magnitude of ATM activation after low doses of ionizing radiation. Oncogene 23:3122–3127, 2004.

Houldsworth J, Lavin MF. Effect of ionizing radiation on DNA synthesis in ataxia telangiectasia cells. Nucl Acids Res 8:3709–3720, 1980.

Hoyt MA, Tolis L, Robert BT. *S. cerevisiae* genes required for cell cycle arrest in response to loss of microtubule function. Cell 66:507–517, 1991.

Humphrey T. DNA damage and cell cycle control in *Schizosaccharomyces pombe*. Mutat Res 451:211–226, 2000.

Imray F, Kidson C. Perturbations of cell-cycle progression in γ-irradiated ataxia telangiectasia and Huntington's disease cells detected by DNA flow cytometric analysis. Mutat Res 112:369–382, 1983.

Inskip HM, Kinlen LJ, Taylor AM, Woods CG, Arlett CF. Risk of breast cancer and other cancers in heterozygotes for ataxia-telangiectasia. Br J Cancer 79:1304–1307, 1999.

Izatt L, Greenman J, Hodgson S, Ellis D, Watts S, Scott G, et al. Identification of germline missense mutations and rare allelic variants in the ATM gene in early-onset breast cancer. Genes Chromosomes Cancer 26:286–294, 1999.

Jackson SP, Jeggo PA. DNA double-strand break repair and V(D)J recombination: involvement of DNA-PK. Trends Biochem Sci 20:412–415, 1995.

Janin N, Andrieu N, Ossian K, Lauge A, Croquette MF, Griscelli C, et al. Breast cancer risk in ataxia telangiectasia (AT) heterozygotes: haplotype study in French AT families. Br J Cancer 80:1042–1045, 1999.

Jasin M. Homologous repair of DNA damage and tumorigenesis: the BRCA connection. Oncogene 21:8981–8993, 2002.

Jaspers NG, Bootsma D. Genetic heterogeneity in ataxia-telangiectasia studied by cell fusion. Proc Natl Acad Sci USA 79:2641–2644, 1982.

Jaspers NG, Gatti RA, Baan C, Linssen PC, Bootsma D. Genetic complementation analysis of ataxia-telangiectasia and Nijmegen breakage syndrome: a survey of 50 patients. Cytogenet Cell Genet 49:259–263, 1988a.

Jaspers NG, Scheres JM, Dewit J, Bootsma D. Rapid diagnostic test for ataxia-telangiectasia [letter]. Lancet 2:473, 1981.

Jaspers NG, Taalman RD, Baan C. Patients with an inherited syndrome characterized by immunodeficiency, microcephaly, and chromosomal instability: genetic relationship to ataxia telangiectasia. Am J Hum Genet 42:66–73, 1988b.

Jhappan C, Morse HC, Fleischmann RD, Gottesman MM, Merlino G. DNA-PKcs: a T-cell tumour suppressor encoded at the mouse *Scid* locus. Nat Genet 17:483–486, 1997.

Jimenez G, Yucel J, Rowley R, Subramani S. The rad3+ gene of *Schizosaccharomyces pombe* is involved in multiple checkpoint functions and in DNA repair. Proc Natl Acad Sci USA 89:4952–4956, 1992.

Jin P, Gu Y, Morgan DO. Role of inhibitory CDC2 phosphorylation in radiation-indcued G2 arrest in human cells. J Cell Biol 134:963–970, 1996.

Kamsler A, Daily D, Hochman A, Stern N, Shiloh Y, Rotman G, Barzilai A. Increased oxidative stress in ataxia telangiectasia evidenced by alterations in redox state of brains from Atm-deficient mice. Cancer Res 61:1849–1854, 2001.

Karam LR, Calsou P, Franklin WA, Painter RB, Olsson M, Lindahl T. Modification of deoxyribose-phosphate residues by extracts of ataxia-telangiectasia cells. Mutat Res 236(1):19–26, 1990.

Karlseder J, Broccoli D, Dai Y, Hardy S, de Lange T. p53- and ATM-dependent apoptosis induced by telomeres lacking TRF2. Science 283:1321–1325, 1999.

Kastan MB, Onyekwere O, Sidransky D, Vogelstein B, Craig RW. Participation of p53 protein in the cellular response to DNA damage. Cancer Res 51:6304–6311, 1991.

Kastan MB, Zhan O, El-Deiry WS, Carrier F, Jacks T, Walsh WV, et al. A mammalian cell cycle checkpoint pathway utilizing p53 and GADD45 is defective in ataxia-telangiectasia. Cell 71:587–597, 1992.

Kato R, Ogawa H. An essential gene, *ESRI*, is required for mitotic cell growth. DNA repair and meiotic recombination in *Saccharomyces cerevisiae*. Nucl Acids Res 22:3104–3112, 1994.

Keegan KS, Holtzman DA, Plug AW, Christenson FR, Brainerd EE, Flaggs G, et al. The Atr and Atm protein kinases associate with different sites along meiotically pairing chromosomes. Genes Dev 10:2478–2490, 1996.

Khanna KK, Beamish H, Yan J, Hobson K, Williams R, Dunn I, Lavin MF. Nature of GS/1 cell cycle checkpoint defect in ataxia-telangiectasia. Oncogene 11:609–618, 1995.

Khanna KK, Keating KE, Kozlov S, Scott S, Gatei M, Hobson K, et al. ATM associates with and phosphorylates p53: mapping the region of interaction. Nat Genet 20:398–400, 1998.

Khanna KK, Lavin MF. Ionizing radiation and UV induction of p53 protein by different pathways in ataxia-telangiectasia cells. Oncogene 8:3307–3312, 1993.

Khosravi R, Maya R, Gottlieb T, Oren M, Shiloh Y, Shkedy D. Rapid ATM-dependent phosphorylation of MDM2 precedes p53 accumulation in response to DNA damage. Proc Natl Acad Sci USA 96:14973–14997, 1999.

Kidson C, Chen P, Imray P. Ataxia-telangiectasia heterozygotes: dominant expression of ionizing radiation sensitive mutants. In: Bridges BA, Harnden DG, eds. Neuropathology and Immune Deficiency. Chichester: John Wiley and Sons, pp. 363–372, 1982.

Kim SH, Kaminker P, Campisi J. Telomeres, aging and cancer: in search of a happy ending. Oncogene 21:503–511, 2002a.

Kim S-T, Lim D-S, Canman, CE, Kastan MB. Substrate specificities and identification of putative substrates of ATM kinase family members. J Biol Chem 274:37538–37543, 1999.

Kim ST, Xu B, Kastan MB. Involvement of the cohesin protein, Smc1, in Atm-dependent and independent responses to DNA damage. Genes Dev 16:560–570, 2002b.

Kirsch IR. V(D)J recombination and ataxia-telangiectasia: a review. Int J Radiat Biol 66:S97–S108, 1994.

Kishi S, Lu KP. A critical role for Pin2/TRF1 in ATM-dependent regulation. Inhibition of Pin2/TRF1 function complements telomere shortening, radiosensitivity, and the G(2)/M checkpoint defect of ataxia-telangiectasia cells. J Biol Chem 277:7420–7429, 2002.

Kishi S, Zhou XZ, Ziv Y, Khoo C, Hill DE, Shiloh Y, Lu KP. Telomeric protein Pin2/TRF1 as an important ATM target in response to double-strand DNA breaks. J Biol Chem 276:29282–29291, 2001.

Kitagawa R, Bakkenist CJ, McKinnon PJ, Kastan MB. Phosphorylation of SMC1 is a critical downstream event in the ATM–NBS1–BRCA1 pathway. Genes Dev 18:1423–1438, 2004.

Klein G. The role of gene dosage and genetic transpositions in carcinogenesis. Nature 294:313–318, 1981.

Kuljis RO, Xu Y, Aguila MC, Baltimore D. Degeneration of neurons, synapses, and neurophil and glial activation in a murine Atm knockout model of ataxia-telangiectasia. Proc Natl Acad Sci USA 94:12688–12693, 1997.

Kunz J, Henriquez R, Schneider U, Deuter-Reinhard M, Movva NR, Hall MN. Target of rapamycin in yeast, TOR2, is an essential phosphatidylinositol kinase homolog required for G1 progression. Cell 73:585–596, 1993.

Kurz EU, Lees-Miller SP. DNA damage-induced activation of ATM and ATM-dependent signaling pathways. DNA Repair (Amst) 3:889–900, 2004.

Laake K, Jansen L, Hahnemann JM, Brondum-Nielsen K, Lonnqvist T, Kaariainen H, Sankila R, Lahdesmaki A, Hammarstrom L, Yuen J, Tretli S, Heiberg A, Olsen JH, Tucker M, Kleinerman R, Borresen-Dale AL. Characterization of ATM mutations in 41 Nordic families with ataxia telangiectasia. Hum Mutat 16:232–246, 2000.

Laake K, Telatar M, Geitvik GA, Hansen RO, Heiberg A, Andresen AM, et al. Identical mutation in 55% of the ATM alleles in 11 Norwegian AT families: evidence for a founder effect. Eur J Hum Genet 6:235–244, 1998.

Lange E, Borreson A-L, Chen X, Chessa L, Chiplunkar S, Concannon P, et al. Localization of an ataxia-telangiectasia gene to a 850 kb interval on chromosome 11q23.1 by linkage analysis of 176 families in an international consortium. Am J Hum Genet 57:112–119, 1995.

Lavin MF. Biochemical defects in ataxia-telangiectasia. In: Gatti RA, Painter RB, eds. Ataxia-Telangiectasia NATO ISI Series H. Berlin: Springer-Verlag, pp. 235–255, 1992.

Lavin MF, Khanna KK, Beamish H, Spring K, Watters D, Shiloh Y. Relationship of the ataxia-telangiectasia protein ATM to phosphoinositide 3-kinase. Trends Biochem Sci 20:382–383, 1995.

Lavin MF, Schroeder AL. Damage-resistant DNA synthesis in eukaryotes. Mutat Res 193:193–206, 1988.

Lavin MF, Scott S, Gueven N, Kozlov S, Peng C, Chen P. Functional consequences of sequence alterations in the *ATM* gene. DNA Repair (Amst) 3:1197–1205, 2004.

Lawton AR, Royal SA, Self KS, Cooper MD. IgA determinants on B-lymphocytes in patients with deficiency of circulating IgA. J Lab Clin Med 80:26–33, 1972.

Lee JH, Bernstein A. p53 mutation increases resistance to ionizing radiation. Proc Natl Acad Sci USA 90:5742–5746, 1993.

Lee JH, Paull TT. Direct activation of the ATM protein kinase by the Mre11/Rad50/Nbs1 complex. Science 304:93–96, 2004.

Lee JS, Collins KM, Brown AL, Lee CH, Chung JH. hCds1-mediated phosphorylation of BRCA1 regulates the DNA damage response. Nature 404:201–204, 2000.

Lehmann AR, James MR, Stevens S. Miscellaneous observations on DNA repair in ataxia-telangiectasia. In: Bridges BA, Harnden DG, eds. A Cellular and Molecular Link with Cancer. New York: John Wiley and Sons, pp. 347–353, 1982.

Leveque B, Debauchez CL, Desbois JC, Feingold J, Barret J, Marie J. Les anomalies immunologiques et lymphocytaires dans le syndrome d'ataxie-teleniectasie: analyse des observations personnells. Ann Pediatr 13:2710–2725, 1966.

Li N, Banin S, Ouyang H, Li GC, Courtois G, Shiloh Y, Karin M, Rotman G. ATM is required for IκB kinase (IKKk) activation in response to DNA double-strand breaks. J Biol Chem 276:8898–8903, 2001.

Li R, Murray AW. Feedback control of mitosis in budding yeast. Cell 66:519–531, 1991.

Li S, Ting NSY, Zheng L, Chen P-L, Ziv L, Shiloh Y, Lee EYHP, Lee W-H. Functional link of BRCA1 and ataxia-telangiectasia gene product in DNA damage response. Nature 406:210–215, 2000.

Lim DS, Kim ST, Xu B, Maser RS, Lin J, Petrini JH, Kastan MB. ATM phosphorylates p95/nbs1 in an S-phase checkpoint pathway. Nature 404:613–617, 2000.

Lin WC, Lin FT, Nevins JR. Selective induction of E2F1 in response to DNA damage, mediated by ATM-dependent phosphorylation. Genes Dev 15:1833–1844, 2001.

Liu VF, Weaver DT. The ionizing radiation-induced replication protein A phosphorylation response differs between ataxia-telangiectasia and normal human cells. Mol Cell Biol 13:7222–7231, 1993.

Longhese MP, Paciotti V, Neecke H, Lucchini G. Checkpoint proteins influence telomeric silencing and length maintenance in budding yeast. Genetics 155:1577–1591, 2000.

Louis-Bar D. Sur un syndrome progressif comprenant des telegiectasies capillaires cutanees et conjonctivales symetriques, a disposition naevode et de troubles cerebelleux. Confin Neurol (Basel) 4:32–42, 1941.

Lowe S, Schmitt E, Smith S, Osborne B, Jacks T. p53 is required for radiation-induced apoptosis in mouse thymocytes. Nature 362:847–849, 1993.

Lukas C, Falck J, Bartkova J, Bartek J, Lukas J. Distinct spatiotemporal dynamics of mammalian checkpoint regulators induced by DNA damage. Nat Cell Biol 5:255–260, 2003.

Lukas J, Lukas C, Bartek J. Mammalian cell cycle checkpoints: signalling pathways and their organization in space and time. DNA Repair (Amst) 3:997–1007, 2004.

Mailand N, Falck J, Lukas C, Syljuasen RG, Welcker M, Bartek J, Lukas J. Rapid destruction of human Cdc25A in response to DNA damage. Science 288:1425–1429, 2000.

Mailand N, Podtelejnikov AV, Groth A, Mann M, Bartek J, Lukas J. Regulation of G(2)/M events by Cdc25A through phosphorylation-dependent modulation of its stability. EMBO J 21:5911–5920, 2002.

Mallory JC, Petes TD. *Aromyces cerevisiae* proteins related to the human ATM protein kinase. Proc Natl Acad Sci USA 97:13749–13754, 2000.

Martinho RG, Lindsay HD, Flaggs G, DeMaggio AJ, Hoekstra MF, Carr AM, Bentley NJ. Analysis of Rad3 and Chk1 protein kinases defines different checkpoint responses. EMBO J 17:7239–7249, 1998.

Maser RS, DePinho RA. Connecting chromosomes, crisis, and cancer. Science 297:565–569, 2002.

Maserati E, Ottolini A, Veggiotti P, Lanzi G, Pasquali F. Ataxia-without-telangiectasia in two sisters with rearrangements of chromosomes 7 and 14. Clin Genet 34:283–287, 1988.

Matsuoka S, Huang M, Elledge SJ. Linkage of ATM to cell cycle regulation by the Chk2 protein kinase. Science 282:1893–1897, 1998.

Matsuura S, Tauchi H, Nakamura A, Kondo N, Sakamoto S, Endo S, et al. Positional cloning of the gene for Nijmegen breakage syndrome. Nat Genet 19:179–181, 1998.

Maya R, Balass M, Kim ST, Shkedy D, Leal JF, Shifman O, et al. ATM-dependent phosphorylation of Mdm2 on serine 395: role in p53 activation by DNA damage. Genes Dev 15:1067–1077, 2001.

McConville CM, Byrd PJ, Ambrose HJ, Taylor AMR. Genetic and physical mapping of the ataxia-telangiectasia locus on chromosome 11q22-23. Int J Radiat Biol 66:S45–S56, 1994.

McConville CM, Stankovic T, Byrd PJ, McGuire GM, Yao Q-Y, Lennox GG, Taylor AMR. Mutations associated with variant phenotypes in ataxia-telangiectasia. Am J Hum Genet 59:320–330, 1996.

McFarlin DE, Strober W, Waldmann TA. Ataxia-telangiectasia. Medicine 51:281–314, 1972.

McGowan CH. Checking in on Cds1 (Chk2): a checkpoint kinase and tumor suppressor. Bioessays 24:502–511, 2002.

McKim KS, Jang JK, Sekelsky J, Laurencon A, Hawley RS. Mei-41 is required for precocious anaphase in *Drosophila* females. Chromosoma 109:44–49, 2000.

McKusick VA, Cross HE. Ataxia-telangiectasia and Swiss-type agamma gblobulinemia. JAMA 195:739–745, 1966.

McMahon SB, Van Buskirk HA, Dugan KA, Copeland TD, Cole MD. The novel ATM-related protein TRRAP is an essential cofactor for the c-Myc and E2F oncoproteins. Cell 94:363–374, 1998.

McMahon SB, Wood, MA, Cole, MD. The essential cofactor TRRAP recruits the histone acetyltransferase hGCN5 to c-Myc. Mol Cell Biol 20:556–562, 2000.

Meek DW. The p53 response to DNA damage. DNA Repair (Amst) 3:1049–1056, 2004.

Meyn MS. Ataxia-telangiectasia and cellular responses to DNA damage. Cancer Res 55:5591–6001, 1995.

Meyn MS, Lu-Kuo JM, Herzing LBK. Expression cloning of multiple human cDNAs that complement the phenotypic defects of ataxia-telangiectasia group D fibroblasts. Am J Hum Genet 53:1206–1216, 1993.

Meyn MS, Strasfeld L, Allen C. Testing the role of p53 in the expression of genetic instability and apoptosis in ataxia-telangiectasia. Int J Radiat Biol 66:S141–S149, 1994.

Miller ME, Chatten J. Ovarian changes in ataxia-telangiectasia. Acta Paediatr Scand 56:559–561, 1967.

Miller RW. Person with exceptionally high risk of leukaemia. Cancer Res 27:2420–2423, 1967.

Mills KD, Sinclair DA, Guarente L. MEC1-dependent redistribution of the Sir3 silencing protein from telomeres to DNA double-strand breaks. Cell 97:609–620, 1999.

Mirzayans R, Famulski KS, Enns L, Fraser M, Paterson MC. Characterization of the signal transduction pathway mediating gamma ray–induced inhibition of DNA synthesis in human cells: indirect evidence for involvement of calmodulin but not protein kinase C or p53. Oncogene 11:1597–605, 1995.

Mochan TA, Venere M, DiTullio RA Jr, Halazonetis TD. 53BP1, an activator of ATM in response to DNA damage. DNA Repair (Amst) 3:945–952, 2004.

Mohamed R, Pal Singh S, Kumar S, Lavin MF. A defect in DNA topoisomerase II activity in ataxia-telangiectasia cells. Biochem Biophys Res Common 149(1):233–238, 1987.

Morgan JL, Holcomb TM, Morrissey RW. Radiation reaction in ataxia-telangiectasia. Am J Dis Child 116:557–558, 1968.

Morgan SE, Lovly C, Pandita TK, Shiloh Y, Kastan MB. Fragments of ATM which have dominant-negative or complementing activity. Mol Cell Biol 17:2020–2029, 1997.

Morrell D, Chase CL, Kupper LL, Swift M. Diabetes mellitus in ataxia-telangiectasia, Fanconis anemia, xeroderma pigmentosum, common variable immune deficiency, and severe combined immune deficiency families. Diabetes 35:143–147, 1986.

Morrell D, Chase CL, Swift M. Cancers in 44 families with ataxia-telangiectasia. Cancer Genet Cytogenet 50:119–123, 1990.

Morris C, Mohamed R, Lavin MF. DNA replication and repair in ataxia-telangiectasia cells exposed to bleomycin. Mutat Res 112:67–74, 1983.

Morrow DM, Tagle DA, Shiloh Y, Collins FS, Hieter P. TEL1, a *Saccharormyces cerevisiae* homologue of the human gene mutated in ataxia-telangiectasia, is functionally related to the yeast checkpoint gene *MEC1/ESR1*. Cell 82:831–840, 1995.

Murname JP, Painter RB. Complementation of the defects of DNA synthesis in irradiated and unirradiated ataxia-telangiectasia cells. Proc Natl Acad Sci USA 79:1960–1963, 1982.

Nagasawa H, Little JB. Comparison of kinetics of X-ray-induced cell killing in normal, ataxia-telangiectasia and hereditary retinoblastoma fibroblasts. Mutat Res 109:297–308, 1983.

Neecke H, Lucchini G, Longhese MP. Cell cycle progression in the presence of irreparable DNA damage is controlled by a Mec1- and Rad53-dependent checkpoint in budding yeast. EMBO J 18:4485–4497, 1999.

Nelms BE, Maser RS, MacKay JF, Lagally MG, Petrini JH. In situ visualization of DNA double-strand break repair in human fibroblasts. Science 280:590–592, 1998.

Nilsson I, Hoffmann I. Cell cycle regulation by the Cdc25 phosphatase family. Prog Cell Cycle Res 4:107–114, 2000.

Norman A, Withers HR. Mammography screening for A-T heterozygotes. In: Gatti RA, Painter RB, eds. Ataxia-Telangiectasia: Nato ASI Series, Vol. 77. Berlin: Springer-Verlag, pp. 137–140, 1993.

Nurse P. Universal control mechanism regulating onset of M-phase. Nature 344:503–508, 1985.

Oakley GG, Loberg LI, Yao J, Risinger MA, Yunker RL, Zernik-Kobak M, Khanna KK, Lavin MF, Carty Dixon K. UV-induced hyperphosphorylation of replication protein a depends on DNA replication and expression of ATM protein. Mol Biol Cell 12:199–1213, 2001.

O'Connor RD, Scott-Linthicum D. Mitogen receptor redistribution defects and concomitant absence of blastogenesis in ataxia-telangiectasia T lymphocytes. Clin Immun Immunopathol 15:66–75, 1980.

O'Driscoll M, Gennery AR, Seidel J, Concannon P, Jeggo PA. An overview of three new disorders associated with genetic instability: LIG4 syndrome, RS-SCID and ATR-Seckel syndrome. DNA Repair (Amst) 3:1227–1235, 2004.

O'Driscoll M, Ruiz-Perez VL, Woods CG, Jeggo PA, Goodship JA. A splicing mutation affecting expression of ataxia-telangiectasia and Rad3-related protein (ATR) results in Seckel syndrome. Nat Genet 33:497–501, 2003.

Olsen JH, Hahnemann JM, Borresen-Dale AL, Brondum-Nielsen K, Hammarstrom L, Kleinerman R, Kaariainen H, Lonnqvist T, Sankila R, Seersholm N, Tretli S, Yuen J, Boice JD Jr, Tucker M. Cancer in patients with ataxia-telangiectasia and in their relatives in the Nordic countries. J Natl Cancer Inst 93:121–127, 2001.

O'Neill T, Dwyer AJ, Ziv Y, Chan DW, Lees-Miller SP, Abraham RH, Lai JH, Hill D, Shiloh Y, Cantley LC, Rathbun GA. Utilization of oriented peptide libraries to identify substrate motifs selected by ATM. J Biol Chem 275:22719–22727, 2000.

Oren M. Decision making by p53: life, death and cancer. Cell Death Differ 10:431–442, 2003.

Pagani F, Buratti E, Stuani C, Bendix R, Dork T, Baralle FE. A new type of mutation causes a splicing defect in ATM. Nat Genet 30:426–429, 2002.

Painter RB. Radiation sensitivity and cancer in ataxia-telangiectasia. Ann NY Acad Sci 459:382–386, 1985.

Painter RB, Young BR. Radiosensitivity in ataxia-telangiectasia: a new explanation. Proc Natl Acad Sci USA 77:7315–7317, 1980.

Pandita TK. The role of ATM in telomere structure and function. Radiat Res 156:642–647, 2001.

Pandita TK, Hittelman WN. The contribution of DNA and chromosome repair deficiencies to the radiosensitivity of ataxia-telangiectasia. Radiat Res 131(2):214–223, 1992.

Pandita TK, Pathak S, Geard C. Chromosome end associations, telomeres and telomerase activity in ataxia-telangiectasia cells. Cytogenet Cell Genet 71:86–93, 1995.

Parrilla-Castellar ER, Arlander SJ, Karnitz L. Dial 9-1-1 for DNA damage: the Rad9-Hus1-Rad1 (9-1-1) clamp complex. DNA Repair (Amst) 3:1009–1014, 2004.

Paterson MC, MacFarlane SJ, Gentner NE, Smith BP. Cellular hypersensitivity to chronic gamma-radiation in cultured fibroblasts from ataxia-telangiectasia heterozygotes. In: Gatti RA, Swift M, eds. Ataxia-Telangiectasia: Genetics, Neuropathology and Immunology of a Degenerative Disease of Childhood, Kroc Found Ser. 19. New York: Alan R. Liss, pp. 73–87, 1985.

Paterson MC, Smith BP, Lohman PH, Andrews AK, Fishman I. Defective excision repair of gamma ray–damaged DNA in human (ataxia-telangiectasia) fibroblasts. Nature 260:444–447, 1976.

Paulovich AG, Hartwell LH. A checkpoint regulates the rate of progression through S phase in *S. cerevisiae* in response to DNA damage. Cell 82:841–847, 1995.

Pearce AK, Humphrey TC. Integrating stress-response and cell-cycle checkpoint pathways. Trends Cell Biol 11:426–433, 2001.

Peng CY, Graves PR, Thoma RS, Wu Z, Shaw AS, Piwnica-Worms H. Mitotic and G2 checkpoint control: regulation of 14-3-3 protein binding by phosphorylation of Cdc25C on serine 216. Science 277:501–505, 1997.

Perkins EJ, Nair A, Cowley DO, Van Dyke T, Chang Y, Ramsden DA. Sensing of intermediates in V(D)J recombination by ATM. Genes Dev 16:159–164, 2004.

Peterson RDA, Blaw M, Good RA. Ataxia-telangiectasia: a possible clinical counterpart of the animals rendered immunologically incompetent by thymectomy. J Pediatr 63:701–703, 1963.

Peterson RDA, Good RA. Ataxia-telangiectasia. In: Bergsma D, Good RA, eds. Birth Defects—Immunological Deficiency Disease in Man, Vol. 4. New York: National Foundation, March of Dimes, pp. 370–377, 1968.

Peterson RD, Kelly WD, Good RA. Ataxia-telangiectasia: its association with a defective thymus, immunological-defective thymus, immunological-deficiency disease, and malignancy. Lancet 1:1189–1193, 1964a.

Peterson RDA, Kelly WD, Good RA. Ataxia-telangiectasia. Consideraciones a proposito de dos casos familiares. Rev Esp Otoneurooftal 23:166–178, 1964b.

Pines J, Hunter T. Isolation of a human cyclin cDNA: evidence for cyclin mRNA and protein regulation in the cell cycle and for interaction with p34 cdc2. Cell 58:833–846, 1991.

Pippard EC, Hall AJ, Barker DJ, Bridges BA. Cancer in homozygotes and heterozygotes of ataxia-telangiectasia and xeroderma pigmentosum in Britain. Cancer Res 48:2929–2932, 1988.

Platzer M, Rotman G, Bauer D, Uziel T, Savitsky K, Bar-Shira A, Gilad S, Shiloh Y, Rosenthal A. Ataxia-telangiectasia locus: sequence analysis of 184 kb of human genomic DNA containing the entire *ATM* gene. Genome Res 7:592–605, 1997.

Plug AW, Peters AH, Xu Y, Keegan KS, Hoekstra MF, Baltimore D, de Boer P, Ashley T. ATM and RPA in meiotic chromosome synapsis and recombination. Nat Genet 17:457–461, 1997.

Post S, Weng YC, Cimprich K, Chen LB, Xu Y, Lee EY. Phosphorylation of serines 635 and 645 of human Rad17 is cell cycle regulated and is required for G(1)/S checkpoint activation in response to DNA damage. Proc Natl Acad Sci USA 98:13102–13107, 2001.

Price BD, Park SJ. DNA damage increases the levels of MDM2 messenger RNA with wtp63 human cells. Cancer Res 54:896–899, 1994.

Proud CG. The multifaceted role of mTOR in cellular stress responses. DNA Repair (Amst) 3:927–934, 2004.

Rary JM, Bender MA, Kelly TE. A 14/14 marker chromosome lympoctye clone in ataxia-telangiectasia. J Hered 66:33–35, 1975.

Ritchie KB, Mallory JC, Petes TD. Interactions of *TLC1* (which encodes the RNA subunit of telomerase), *TEL1*, and *MEC1* in regulating telomere length in the yeast *Saccharomyces cerevisiae*. Mol Cell Biol 19:6065–6075, 1999.

Ritchie KB, Petes TD. The Mre11p/Rad50p/Xrs2p complex and the Tel1p function in a single pathway for telomere maintenance in yeast. Genetics 155:475–479, 2000.

Roifman CM, Gelfand EW. Heterogeneity of the immunological deficiency in ataxia-telangiectasia: absence of a clinical–pathological correlation. In: Gatti RA, Swift M, eds. Ataxia-Telangiectasia, Vol. 19. New York: Alan R. Liss, Kroc Foundation Series, pp. 273–285, 1985.

Rosin MP, Ochs HD. In vivo chromosomal instability in ataxia-telangiectasia homozygotes and heterozygotes. Hum Genet 74:335–340, 1986.

Rotman G, Savitsky K, Ziv Y, Cole CG, Higgins MJ, Bar-Am I, Dunham I, Bar-Shira A, Vanagaite L, Qin S, et al. A YAC contig spanning the ataxia-telangiectasia locus (groups A and C) at 11q22–q23. Genomics 24:234–242, 1994.

Rudolph NS, Nagasawa H, Little JB, Latt SA. Identification of ataxia-telangiectasia heterozygotes by flow cytometric analysis of X-ray damage. Mutat Res 211:19–29, 1989.

Sabatini DM, Erdjument-Bromage H, Lui M, Tempst P, Snyder SH. RAFT1. A mammalian protein that binds to FKBP12 in a rapamycin dependent fashion and is homologous to yeast TORs. Cell 78:35–43, 1994.

Sabers CJ, Martin MM, Brunn GJ, Williams JM, Dumont FJ, Wiederrecht G, Abraham RT. Isolation of a protein target of the FKBP12 rapamycin complex in mammalian cells. J Biol Chem 270:815–822, 1995.

Saito S, Goodarzi AA, Higashimoto Y, Noda Y, Lees-Miller SP, Appella E, Anderson CW. ATM mediates phosphorylation at multiple p53 sites, including Ser(46), in response to ionizing radiation. J Biol Chem 277: 12491–12494, 2002.

Saleh A, Schieltz D, Ting N, McMahon SB, Litchfield DW, Yates JR III, Lees-Miller SP, Cole MD, Brandl CJ. Tra1p is a component of the yeast Ada Spt transcriptional regulatory complexes. J Biol Chem 273:26559–26565, 1998.

Sanal O, Berkel AI, Ersoy F, Tezcan I, Topaloglu H. Clinical variants of ataxia-telangiectasia. In: Gatti RA, Painter RB, eds. Ataxia-Telangiectasia. NATO ASI Series. Berlin: Springer-Verlag, pp. 183–189, 1993.

Sanchez Y, Wong C, Thoma RS, Richman R, Wu Z, Piwnica-Worms H, Elledge SJ. Conservation of the Chk1 checkpoint pathway in mammals: linkage of DNA damage to Cdk regulation through Cdc25. Science 277: 1497–1501, 1997.

Sandoval N, Platzer M, Rosenthal A, Dork T, Bendix R, Skawran B, Stuhrmann M, Wegner RD, Sperling K, Banin S, Shiloh Y, Baumer A, Bernthaler U, Sennefelder H, Brohm M, Weber BH, Schindler D. Characterization of *ATM* gene mutations in 66 ataxia telangiectasia families. Hum Mol Genet 8:69–79, 1999.

Santocanale C, Diffley, JF. A Mec1- and Rad53-dependent checkpoint controls late-firing origins of DNA replication. Nature 395:615–618, 1998.

Sasaki T, Tian H, Kukita Y, Inazuka M, Tahira T, Imai T, Yamauchi M, Saito T, Hori T, Hashimoto-Tamaoki T, Komatsu K, Nikaido O, Hayashi K. *ATM* mutations in patients with ataxia-telangiectasia screened by a hierarchical strategy. Hum Mutat 12:186–195, 1998.

Saviozzi S, Saluto A, Piane M, Prudente S, Migone N, DeMarchi M, Brusco A, Chessa L. Six novel *ATM* mutations in Italian patients with classical ataxia-telangiectasia. Hum Mutat 21:450, 2003.

Saviozzi S, Saluto A, Taylor AM, Last JI, Trebini F, Paradiso MC, Grosso E, Funaro A, Ponzio G, Migone N, Brusco A. A late-onset variant of ataxia-telangiectasia with a compound heterozygous genotype, A8030G/7481insA. J Med Genet 39:57–61, 2002.

Savitsky K, Bar-Shira A, Gilad S, Rotman G, Ziv Y, Vanagaite L, Tagle DA, Smith S, Uziel T, Sfez S, Ashkenazi M, Pecker I, Frydman M, Harnik R, Patanjali SR, Simmons A, Clines GA, Sartiel A, Gatti RA, Chessa L, Sanal O, Lavin MF, Jaspers NGJ, Taylor AMR, Arlett CF, Miki T, Weissman SM, Lovett M, Collins FS, Shiloh Y. A single ataxia-telangiectasia gene with a product similar to PI-3 kinase. Science 268:1749–1753, 1995a.

Savitsky K, Platzer M, Uziel T, Gilad S, Sartiel A, Rosenthal A, Elroy-Stein O, Shiloh Y, Rotman G. Ataxia-telangiectasia: structural diversity of untranslated sequences suggests complex posttranscriptional regulation of *ATM* gene expression. Nucl Acids Res 25:1678–1684, 1997.

Savitsky K, Sfez S, Tagle D, Ziv Y, Sartiel A, Collins FS, Shiloh Y, Rotman G. The complete sequence of the coding region of the *ATM* gene reveals similarity to cell cycle regulators in different species. Hum Mol Genet 4: 2025–2032, 1995b.

Schlach DS, McFarlin DE, Barlow MH. An unsual form of diabetes mellitus in ataxia-telangiectasia. N Engl J Med 282:1396–1402, 1970.

Scott D, Zampetti-Bosseler F. Cell cycle dependence of mitotic delay in X-irradiated normal and ataxia-telangiectasia fibroblasts. Int J Radiat Biol 42:679–683, 1982.

Scully R, Livingston DM. In search of the tumour-suppressor functions of BRCA1 and BRCA2. Nature 408:429–432, 2000.

Sedgwick RP, Boder E. Progressive ataxia in childhood with particular reference to ataxia-telangiectasia. Neurology 10:705–715, 1960.

Sedgwick RP, Boder E. Ataxia-telangiectasia. In: Vinken PJ, Bruyn GW, eds. Handbook of Clinical Neurology, Vol. 14. Amsterdam: North Holland, pp. 267–339, 1972.

Sedgwick RP, Boder E. Ataxia-telangiectasia (208900; 208910; 208920). In: Vianney De Jong JMB, ed. Hereditary Neuropathies and Spinocerebellar Atrophies. Amsterdam: Elsevier Science, pp. 347–423, 1991.

Shechter D, Costanzo V, Gautier J. Regulation of DNA replication by ATR: signaling in response to DNA intermediates. DNA Repair (Amst) 3:901–908, 2004.

Shiloh Y. ATM and related protein kinases: safeguarding genome integrity. Nat Rev Cancer 3:155–168, 2003.

Shiloh Y, Andegeko Y, Tsarfaty I. In search of drug treatment for genetic defects in the DNA damage response: the example of ataxia-telangiectasia. Semin Cancer Biol 14:295–305, 2004.

Shiloh Y, Parshad R, Sanford KK, Jones GM. Carrier detection in ataxia-telangiectasia. Lancet 1:689–690, 1986.

Shiloh Y, Tabor E, Becker Y. Colony-forming ability of ataxia-telangiectasia skin fibroblasts is an indicator of their early senescence and increased demand for growth factors. Exp Cell Res 140:191–199, 1982a.

Shiloh Y, Tabor E, Becker Y. The response of ataxia-telangiectasia homozygous skin fibroblasts to neocarzinostatin. Carcinogenesis 3:815–820, 1982b.

Shiloh Y, Tabor E, Becker Y. Abnormal response of ataxia-telangiectasia cells to agents that break the deoxyribose moiety of DNA via a targeted free radical mechanism. Carcinogenesis 4:1317–1322, 1983.

Shinkai Y, Koyasu S, Nakayama K, Murphy KM, Loh DY, Reinherz EL, Alt FW. Restoration of T cell development in RAG-2-deficient mice by functional TCR transgenes. Science 259:822, 1993.

Sim GK, Yague J, Nelson J, Marrack P, Palmer E, Augustine A, Kappler J. Primary structure of human T cell receptor alpha chain. Nature 312:771–775, 1984.

Singh SP, Lavin MF. DNA-binding protein activated by γ-radiation in human cells. Mol Cell Biol 10:5279–5285, 1990.

Slichenmyer WJ, Nelson WG, Slebos RJ, Kastan MB. Loss of a p53-associated G1 checkpoint does not decrease cell survival following DNA damage. Cancer Res 53:4164–4168, 1993.

Smith GC, Cary RB, Lakin ND, Hann BC, Teo SH, Chen DJ, Jackson SP. Purification and DNA binding properties of the ataxia-telangiectasia gene product ATM. Proc Natl Acad Sci USA 96:11134–11139, 1999a.

Smith GC, di Fagagna F, Lakin ND, Jackson SP. Cleavage and inactivation of ATM during apoptosis. Mol Cell Biol 19:6076–6084, 1999b.

Smith PJ, Anderson CO, Watson JV. Abnormal retention of X-irradiated ataxia-telangiectasia fibroblasts in G2 phase of the cell cycle: cellular RNA content, chromatin stability and the effects of 3-aminobenzamide. Int J Radiat Biol 47:701–712, 1985.

Spector BD, Filipovich AH, Perry GS III, Kersey JH. Epidemiology of cancer in ataxia-telangiectasia. In: Bridges BA, Harnden DG, eds. Ataxia-Telangiectasia. Chichester: Wiley, p. 103, 1982.

Spring K, Cross S, Li C, Watters D, Ben-Senior L, Waring P, Ahangari F, Lu SL, Chen P, Misko I, Paterson C, Kay G, Smorodinsky NI, Shiloh Y, Lavin MF. Atm knock-in mice harboring an in-frame deletion corresponding to the human ATM 7636del9 common mutation exhibit a variant phenotype. Cancer Res 61:4561–4568, 2001.

Stankovic T, Kidd AM, Sutcliffe A, McGuire GM, Robinson P, Weber P, Bedenham T, Bradwell AR, Easton DF, Lennox GG, Haites N, Byrd PJ, Taylor AM. ATM mutations and phenotypes in ataxia-telangiectasia families in the British Isles: expression of mutant ATM and the risk of leukaemia, lyphoma, and cancer. Am J Hum Genet 62:334–345, 1998.

Stewart GS, Last JI, Stankovic T, Haites N, Kidd AM, Byrd PJ, Taylor AM. Residual ataxia telangiectasia mutated protein function in cells from ataxia telangiectasia patients, with 5762ins137 and 7271t → g mutations, showing a less severe phenotype. J Biol Chem 276:30133–30141, 2001.

Stewart GS, Maser RS, Stankovic T, Bressan DA, Kaplan MI, Jaspers NG, Raams A, Byrd PJ, Petrini JH, Taylor AM. The DNA double-strand break repair gene *hMRE11* is mutated in individuals with an ataxia-telangiectasia-like disorder. Cell 99:577–587, 1999.

Stobo JD, Tomaisi TB Jr. A low molecular weight immunoglobulin antigenically related to 19S IgM. J Clin Invest 46:1329–1337, 1967.

Stracker TH, Theunissen JW, Morales M, Petrini JH. The Mre11 complex and the metabolism of chromosome breaks: the importance of communicating and holding things together. DNA Repair (Amst) 3:845–854, 2004.

Strich S. Pathological findings in 3 cases of ataxia-telangiectasia. J Neurol Neurosurg Psychiatry 29:489–499, 1966.

Strober W, Wochner RD, Barlow MH, McFarlin DF, Waldmann T. Immunoglobulin metabolism in ataxia-telangiectasia. J Clin Invest 47:1905–1915, 1968.

Stucki M, Jackson SP. MDC1/NFBD1: a key regulator of the DNA damage response in higher eukaryotes. DNA Repair (Amst) 3:953–957, 2004.

Sugimoto T, Sawada T, Tozawa M, Kidowaki T, Kusonoki T, Yamaguchi N. Plasma levels of carcinoembryonic antigen in patients with ataxia-telangiectasia. J Pediatr 92:436–439, 1978.

Sutton IJ, Last JI, Ritchie SJ, Harrington HJ, Byrd PJ, Taylor AM. Adult-onset ataxia telangiectasia due to ATM 5762ins137 mutation homozygosity. Ann Neurol 55:891–895, 2004.

Swift M, Morrell D, Cromartie E, Chamberlin AR, Skolnick MH, Bishop DT. The incidence and gene frequency of ataxia-telangiectasia in the United States. Am J Hum Genet 39:573–583, 1986.

Swift M, Morrell D, Massey RB, Chase CL. Incidence of cancer in 161 families affected by ataxia-telangiectasia. N Engl J Med 325:1831–1836, 1991.

Syllaba K, Henner K. Contribution a l'independence de l'athetose double idiopathique et congenitale. Atteinte familiale, syndrome dystrophique, signe de reseau vasculaire conjonctival, integrite psychique. Rev Neurol 1:541–562, 1926.

Tadjoedin MK, Fraser FC. Heredity of ataxia-telangiectasia (Louis-Bar syndrome). Am J Dis Child 110:64–68, 1965.

Taniguchi T, Garcia-Higuera I, Xu B, Andreassen PR, Gregory RC, Kim ST, Lane WS, Kastan MB, D'Andrea AD. Convergence of the fanconi anemia and ataxia-telangiectasia signaling pathways. Cell 109:459–472, 2002.

Taylor AM, Edwards MJ. Malignancy, DNA damage and chromosomal aberrations in ataxia-telangiectasia. IARC Sci Publ 39:119–126, 1982.

Taylor AM, Harnden DG, Arlett CF, Harcourt SA, Lehmann AR, Stevens S, Bridges BA. Ataxia-telangiectasia: a human mutation with abnormal radiation sensitivity. Nature 4:427–429, 1975.

Taylor AM, Metcalfe JR, Oxford JM, Harden DG. Is chromatid-type damage in ataxia-telangiectasia after irradiation at GO a consequence of defective repair? Nature 260:441–443, 1976.

Taylor AMR, McConville CM, Woods CG, Byrd DJ, Hernandez D. Clinical and cellular heterogeneity in ataxia-telangiectasia. In: Gatti RA, Painter RB, eds. Ataxia-Telangiectasia. NATO ASI Series. Berlin: Springer-Verlag, pp. 209–234, 1993.

Teale B, Khanna KK, Singh SP, Lavin MF. Radiation-activated DNA-binding protein constitutively present in ataxia-telangiectasia nuclei. J Biol Chem 268:22455–22455, 1993.

Teale B, Singh S, Khanna KK, Findik D, Lavin MF. Purification and characterization of a DNA-binding protein activated by ionizing radiation. J Biol Chem 267:10295–10301, 1992.

Telatar M, Wang S, Castellvi-Bel S, Tai LQ, Sheikhavandi S, Regueiro JR, Porras O, Gatti RA. A model for ATM heterozygote identification in a large population: four founder-effect *ATM* mutations identify most of Costa Rican patients with telengiectasia. Mol Genet Metab 64:36–43, 1998.

Telatar M, Wang Z, Udar W, Liang T, Concannon P, Bernatowska-Matuscklewicz E, Lavin MF, Sholoh Y, Good RA, Gatti RA. Ataxia-telangiectasia: mutations in cDNA detected by protein truncation screening. Am J Hum Genet 59:40–44, 1996.

Teraoka SN, Malone KE, Doody DR, Suter NM, Ostrander EA, Daling JR, Concannon P. Increased frequency of ATM mutations in breast carcinoma patients with early-onset disease and positive family history. Cancer 92:479–487, 2001.

Teraoka SN, Telatar M, Becker-Catania S, Liang T, Onengut S, Tolun A, Chessa L, Sanal O, Bernatowska E, Gatti RA, Concannon P. Splicing defects in the ataxia-telangiectasia gene, *ATM*: underlying mutations and consequences. Am J Hum Genet 64:1617–1631, 1999.

Thieffry S, Arthuis M, Aicardi J, Lyon G. L'ataxie-telangiectasies. Rev Neurol 105:390–405, 1961.

Ting NS, Lee WH. The DNA double-strand break response pathway: becoming more BRCAish than ever. DNA Repair (Amst) 3:935–944, 2004.

Uhrhammer N, Fritz E, Boyden L, Meyn MS. Human fibroblasts transfected with an ATM antisense vector respond abnormally to ionizing radiation. Int J Mol Med 4:43–47, 1999.

Uziel T, Lerenthal Y, Moyal L, Andegeko Y, Mittelman L, Shiloh Y. Requirement of the MRN complex for ATM activation by DNA damage. EMBO J 22:5612–5621, 2003.

Uziel T, Savitsky K, Platzer M, Ziv Y, Helbitz T, Nehls M, Boehm T, Rosenthal A, Shiloh Y, Rotman G. Genomic organization of the *ATM* gene. Genomics 33:317–320, 1996.

Vallen EA, Cross FR. Interaction between the MEC1-dependent DNA synthesis checkpoint and G_1 cyclin function in *Saccharomyces cerevisiae*. Genetics 151:459–471, 1999.

Vanagaite L, James MR, Rotman G, Savitsky K, Bar-Shira A, Gilad S, Ziv Y, Uchenik V, Sartiel A, Collins FS, Sheffield VC, Weissenbach J, Shiloh Y. A high-density microsatellite map of the ataxia-telangiectasia locus. Hum Genet 95:451–455, 1995.

Varon R, Vissinga C, Platzer M, Cerosaletti KM, Chrzanowska KH, Saar K, Beckmann G, Seemanova E, Cooper PR, Nowak NJ, Stumm M, Weemaes CM, Gatti RA, Wilson RK, Digweed M, Rosenthal A, Sperling K, Concannon P, Reis A. Nibrin, a novel DNA double-strand break repair protein, is mutated in Nijmegen breakage syndrome. Cell 93:467–476, 1998.

Vassilev A, Yamauchi J, Kotani T, Prives C, Avantaggiati ML, Qin J, Nakatani Y. The 400 kDa subunit of the PCAF histone acetylase complex belongs to the ATM superfamily. Mol Cell 2:869–875, 1998.

Venkitaraman AR. Cancer susceptibility and the functions of BRCA1 and BRCA2. Cell 108:171–182, 2002.

Vialard JE, Gilbert CS, Green CM, Lowndes NF. The budding yeast Rad9 checkpoint protein is subjected to Mec1/Tel1-dependent hyperphosphorylation and interacts with Rad53 after DNA damage. EMBO J 17:5679–5688, 1998.

von Boehmer H. Positive selection of lymphocytes. Cell 76:219–228, 1994.

Waga S, Hannon GJ, Beach D, Stillman B. The p21 inhibitor of cyclin-dependent kinases controls DNA replication by interaction with PCNA. Nature 369:574–578, 1994.

Waldmann TA. Immunological abnormalities in ataxia-telangiectasia. In: Bridges BA, Harnden DG, eds. Ataxia-Telangiectasia: A Cellular and Molecular Link Between Cancer Neuropathology and Immune Deficiency. New York: Wiley, pp. 37–51, 1982.

Waldmann TA, McIntyre KR. Serum-alpha-feto-protein levels in patients with ataxia-telangiectasia. Lancet 25:1112–1115, 1972.

Wang B, Matsuoka S, Carpenter PB, Elledge SJ. 53BP1, a mediator of the DNA damage checkpoint. Science 298:1435–1438, 2002.

Wang JY. Regulation of cell death by the Abl tyrosine kinase. Oncogene 19:5643–5650, 2000.

Wang X, McGowan CH, Zhao M, He L, Downey JS, Fearns C, Wang Y, Huang S, Han J. Involvement of the MKK6-p38γ cascade in gamma-radiation–induced cell cycle arrest. Mol Cell Biol 20:4543–4552, 2000a.

Wang Y, Cortez D, Yazdi P, Neff N, Elledge SJ, Qin J. BASC, a super complex of BRCA1-associated proteins involved in the recognition and repair of aberrant DNA structures. Genes Dev 14:927–939, 2000b.

Ward IM, Chen J. Histone H2AX is phosphorylated in an ATR-dependent manner in response to replicational stress. J Biol Chem 276:47759–47762, 2001.

Waterman MJ, Stavridi ES, Waterman JL, Halazonetis TD. ATM-dependent activation of p53 involves dephosphorylation and association with 14-3-3 proteins. Nat Genet 19:175–178, 1998.

Watters D, Kedar P, Spring K, Bjorkman J, Chen P, Gatei M, Birrell G, Garrone B, Srinivasa P, Crane DI, Lavin MF. Localization of a portion of extranuclear ATM to peroxisomes. J Biol Chem 274:34277–34782, 1999.

Watters D, Khanna KK, Beamish H, Birrell G, Spring K, Kedar P, Gatei M, Stenzel D, Hobson K, Kozlov S, Farrell A, Ramsay J, Gatti R, Lavin MF. Cellular localisation of the ataxia-telangiectasia (ATM) gene proteins and discrimination between mutated and normal forms. Oncogene 14:1911–1921, 1997.

Weinert TA, Hartwell LH. The *RAD9* gene controls the cell cycle response to DNA damage in *Saccharomyces cervesiae*. Science 241:317–322, 1988.

Weinert TA, Hartwell LH. Characterization of *RAD9* of *Saccharomyces cerevisiae* and evidence that its function acts post-translationally in cell cycle arrest after DNA damagae. Mol Cell Biol 10:6554–6564, 1990.

Weinert TA, Kiser GL, Hartwell LH. Mitotic checkpoint genes in budding yeast and the dependence of mitosis replication and repair. Genes Dev 15:652–656, 1994.

Wells CE, Sly GM. Progressive familial choreoathetosis with cutaneous telangiectasia. J Neurol Neurosurg Psychiatry 20:98–104, 1957.

Williams HE, Denis DJ, Higdon RS. Ataxia-telangiectasia. A syndrome with characteristic cutaneous manifestations. Arch Dermatol 82:937–942, 1960.

Wong KK, Maser RS, Bachoo RM, Menon J, Carrasco DR, Gu Y, Alt FW, DePinho RA. Telomere dysfunction and Atm deficiency compromises organ homeostasis and accelerates ageing. Nature 241:643–648, 2003.

Woods CG, Bundey SE, Taylor AMR. Unusual features in the inheritance of ataxia-telangiectasia. Hum Genet 84:555–562, 1990.

Woods CG, Taylor AMR. Ataxia-telangiectasia in the British Isles. The clinical and laboratory features of 70 affected individuals. Q J Med 82:169–179, 1992.

Wright J, Keegan KS, Herendeen DR, Bentley NJ, Carr AM, Hoekstra MF, Concannon P. Protein kinase mutants of human ATR increase sensitivity to UV and ionizing radiation and abrogate cell cycle checkpoint control. Proc Natl Acad Sci USA 95:7445–7450, 1998.

Wright J, Teraoka S, Onegut S, Tolun A, Gatti RA, Ochs HD, Concannon P. A high frequency of distinct *ATM* gene mutations in ataxia-telangiectasia. Am J Hum Genet 59:839–846, 1996.

Wu X, Ranganathan V, Weisman DS, Heine WF, Ciccone DN, O'Neill TB, Crick KE, Pierce KA, Lane WS, Rathbun G, Livingston DM, Weaver DT. ATM phosphorylation of Nijmegen breakage syndrome protein is required in a DNA damage response. Nature 405:477–482, 2000.

Xiong Y, Connolly T, Futcher B, Beach D. Human D-type cyclin. Cell 65:691–699, 1991.

Xiong Y, Zhang H, Beach D. Subunit rearrangement of the cyclin-dependent kinases is associated with cellular transformation. Genes Dev 7:1572–1583, 1993.

Xu B, Kim S, Kastan MB. Involvement of Brca1 in S-phase and G(2)-phase checkpoints after ionizing irradiation. Mol Cell Biol 21:3445–3450, 2001.

Xu B, O'Donnell AH, Kim ST, Kastan MB. Phosphorylation of serine 1387 in Brca1 is specifically required for the Atm-mediated S-phase checkpoint after ionizing irradiation. Cancer Res 62:4588–4591, 2002.

Xu Y. ATM in lymphoid development and tumorigenesis. Adv Immunol 72:179–189, 1999.

Xu Y, Ashley T, Brainerd EE, Bronson RT, Meyn SM, Baltimore D. Targeted disruption of ATM leads to growth retardation, chromosomal fragmentation during meiosis, immune defects and thymic lymphomas. Genes Dev 10:2411–2422, 1996.

Xu Y, Baltimore D. Dual roles of ATM in the cellular response to radiation and cell growth control. Genes Dev 10:2401–2410, 1996.

Yang DQ, Kastan MB. Participation of ATM in insulin signalling through phosphorylation of eIF-4E-binding protein 1. Nat Cell Biol 2:893–898, 2000.

Yarden RI, Pardo-Reoyo S, Sgagias M, Cowan KH, Brody LC. BRCA1 regulates the G2/M checkpoint by activating Chk1 kinase upon DNA damage. Nat Genet 30:285–289, 2002.

Yazdi PT, Wang Y, Zhao S, Patel N, Lee EY, Qin J. SMC1 is a downstream effector in the ATM/NBS1 branch of the human S-phase checkpoint. Genes Dev 16:571–582, 2002.

Zakian VA. ATM-related genes: what do they tell us about functions of the human gene? Cell 82:685–687, 1995.

Zhang N, Chen P, Gatei M, Scott S, Khanna KK, Lavin MF. An anti-sense construct of full-length ATM cDNA imposes a radiosensitive phenotype on normal cells. Oncogene 17:811–818, 1998.

Zhang N, Chen P, Khanna KK, Scott S, Gatei M, Kozlov S, Watters D, Spring K, Yen T, Lavin MF. Isolation of full-length ATM cDNA and correction of the ataxia-telangiectasia cellular phenotype. Proc Natl Acad Sci USA 94:8021–8026, 1997.

Zhao H, Piwnica-Worms H. ATR-mediated checkpoint pathways regulate phosphorylation and activation of human Chk1. Mol Cell Biol 21: 4129–4139, 2001.

Zhao H, Watkins JL, Piwnica-Worms H. Disruption of the checkpoint kinase 1/cell division cycle 25A pathway abrogates ionizing radiation-induced S and G2 checkpoints. Proc Natl Acad Sci USA 99:14795–800, 2002.

Zhao S, Weng Y-C, Yuan S-SF, Lin Y-T, Hsu, H-C, Lin S-CJ, Gerbino E, Song M-H, Zdzlenicka, MZ, Gatti RA, Shay JW, Ziv Y, Shiloh Y, Lee EYHP. Functional link between ataxia-telangiectasia and Nijmegen breakage syndrome gene products. Nature 405:473–477, 2000.

Zhou B-BS, Elledge SJ. The DNA damage response: putting checkpoints in perspective. Nature 408:433–439, 2000.

Ziv Y, Amiel A, Jaspers NG, Berkel AI, Shiloh Y. Ataxia-telangiectasia: a variant with altered in vitro phenotype of fibroblast cells. Mutat Res 210: 211–219, 1989.

Ziv Y, Bar-Shira A, Pecker I, Russell P, Jorgensen TJ, Tsarfati I, Shiloh Y. Recombinant ATM protein complements the cellular A-T phenotype. Oncogene 15:159–167, 1997.

Zou L, Elledge SJ. Sensing DNA damage through ATRIP recognition of RPA-ssDNA complexes. Science 300:1542–1548, 2003.

30

Chromosomal Instability Syndromes Other Than Ataxia-Telangiectasia

ROLF-DIETER WEGNER, JAMES J. GERMAN, KRYSTYNA H. CHRZANOWSKA, MARTIN DIGWEED, and MARKUS STUMM

A number of syndromes exist in which an increased incidence of spontaneous and/or induced chromosomal aberrations is the unifying diagnostic criterion. These disorders, called *chromosomal instability syndromes*, include the classical chromosomal instability syndromes—namely, ataxia-telangiectasia (A-T), Fanconi anemia (FA), and Bloom syndrome (BS). On the basis of this definition, Nijmegen breakage syndrome (NBS) and A-T-like disorder (A-TLD) must also be added to this group. More recently, case reports of patients with ligase I (LIG1) deficiency, ligase IV (LIG4) deficiency, NHEJ1, and RAD50 deficiency have provided evidence for the existence of a long list of diseases belonging to this group.

There is growing evidence that the following genes mutated in chromosomal instability syndromes are involved in protecting—directly or indirectly—human genome integrity by contributing to the complex regulation of double-strand break (DSB) repair: *ATM* in A-T, *NBS1* in NBS, *BLM* in BS, *MRE11* in A-TLD, *Lig1* in ligase I deficiency, *Lig4* in ligase IV deficiencies, NHEJ1 in Cernunnos deficiency, *RAD50* (in *rad50*-deficient mice) (Luo et al., 1999), and the group of at least 12 genes known to be affected in the heterogenous disorder of FA. Recent studies of protein–protein interactions suggest that the normal gene products associated with most of these syndromes are in fact involved in forming or regulating a huge protein complex active in the surveillance and maintenance of genomic integrity. Results from these studies indicate that the gene products of *ATM, BLM, NBS1, MRE11*, and *RAD50* are all members of a complex named *BASC* (*BRCA1*-associated genome surveillance complex). They might appear as a single protein subunit or as a stable subcomplex such as nibrin, MRE11, and RAD50 (Wang et al., 2000). As described below, most of the known FA genes may be also linked indirectly or even directly to the BASC complex (Ahmad et al., 2002).

Most of these syndromes exhibit features of immunodeficiency or at least hematological symptoms resulting from a clinically relevant deficiency of cells in the immune system. In this chapter, the term *immunodeficiency* is used in this broader sense. The triad immunodeficiency, neoplasia, and infertility is typical for most of the syndromes associated with chromosomal instability. This observation can best be explained by defects in the complex system of DSB repair, affecting either nonhomologous end joining (NHEJ) or homologous rejoining (HR). Thus tumor development in these syndromes is a direct consequence of defective DNA repair, which leads to mutations of cancer susceptibility genes acting as gatekeepers or caretakers (Kinzler and Vogelstein, 1997; Duker, 2002). Since meiotic recombination requires the production and repair of DSBs, the high incidence of infertility observed in patients with chromosomal instability syndromes is not surprising. Because the production of immunoglobulins relies on the network of proteins supporting the process of NHEJ (reviewed in van Gent et al., 2001), failure of a member of this group of proteins could lead to immunodeficiency. Thus, although primary immunodeficiency is not a typical symptom of chromosomal instability syndromes, these disorders may further our understanding of the relationship between DSB induction, DSB repair, and immunglobulin production.

In this chapter, we will focus on three clinically defined syndromes—Fanconi anemia, Nijmegen breakage syndrome, and Bloom syndrome, followed by a short presentation of more recently discovered chromosomal instability syndromes that show A-T-like or NBS-like phenotypes due to specific gene mutations (*Mre11, Rad50, Lig1, Lig4, NHEJ1*). Other diseases, for example, Rothmund-Thompsen syndrome (MIM 268400) and Werner syndrome (MIM 277700), listed in Table 30.1, will either be briefly described or are beyond the scope of this text because the clinical presentation does not suggest a defect of

427

Table 30.1. Features of Chromosomal Instability Syndromes

	A-T	ATLD	NBS	NHEJ1	LIG4	RAD50	LIG1	Bloom	WRNS	FA	RS-SCID
General Data											
OMIM No.	208900	604391	251260	–	606593	604040	126391	210900	277700	227650	605988
Gene	ATM	MRE11	NBS1	NHEJ1	LIG4	RAD50	LIG1	BLM	WRN	>11 genes	DCLRE1C
Gene product	ATM	Mre11	Nibrin	DNA repair factor Cernunnos	Ligase IV	Rad50	Ligase I	RECQL2-helicase	RECQL3-helicase		Artemis
Gene Locus	11q23	11q21	8q21	2q35	13q22–q34	5q31	19q13.2–13.3	15q26.1	8p12		10p
Clinical Manifestations											
Growth retardation	+	+	+	+	+	+	+	+	+	+	+
Microcephaly	–	–	+	+	+	+		+		+	
Facial anomalies	–	–	+	+	+	+		+			
Receding forehead			+	+		+					
Receding mandible			+	+		+		+			
Disturbances of hair growth			+								
Scleral telangiectasia	+	–	(+)		–	–	+				
Cataract									+		
Skin abnormalities	+	–	+		+	+	+	+	+		
Photosensitivity	+	–	+		+		+	+			
Cutaneous telangiectasias	+	–	+		+		+	+	+		
Pigmentation defects			+			+		+		+	
Neurological abnormalities	+	+	–		–	+					
Cerebellar ataxia	+	+	–			–					
Oculomotor apraxia	+	+	–			–					
Choreathetosis	+	+	–			–					
Mental retardation	–	–	(+)	(+)	+	–				(–)	
Other manifestations	+	–	+	+	+	–					
Infertility	+		+	?	+		+	+		+	
Skeletal anomalies			+	+	+					+	
Renal anomalies			+	+						+	
Infections	+	–	+	+	+	–	+				+
Malignancies	+	–	+		+	?	+	+	+	+	+
Lymphoma			+				+	+	+		+
Leukemia			+		+			+	+	+	
Osteosarcoma	+								+		
Laboratory Manifestations											
Immunodeficiency	+	–	+	+	+		–	+			+
Pancytopenia			+	+	+			+		+	
Humoral immunodeficiency	+		+	+						–	
Cellular immunodeficiency	(+)		+	+						–	
Elevated AFP	+	–	–	–		–				–	
Cytogenetic Abnormalities	+	+	+		+	+	+	+	+	+	+
Spontaneous chromosomal instability	+	+	+		?	+		+		+	
Chromosome 7 and 14 rearrangements	+	+	+			(+)		–		–	
Increased translocation frequencies	+		+	+		+		+	+	+	
Hypersensitivity to ionizing radiation/bleomycin	+	+	+	+	+	+	+				+
Hypersensitivity to UV light							+				
Hypersensitivity to alkylating agents	+		+			+	+		–	+	
Radioresistant DNA synthesis	+		+			+				–	
Increased SCE frequency	–	–	–	–	(+)	–		+		–	

AFP, α-fetoprotein; A-T, ataxia-telangiectasia; A-TLD, ataxia-telangiectasia–like disease; Bloom, Bloom syndrome; FA, Fanconi anemia; LIG1, ligase I deficiency; LIG4, ligase IV deficiency; NBS, Nijmegen breakage syndrome; NHEJ1, non-homologous end-joining factor 1 (NHEJ1) responsible for SCID with microcephaly and chromosomal instability; RAD50, RAD50-deficiency; RS-SCID, radiosensitive severe combined immunodeficiency syndrome; UV, ultraviolet; WRNS, Werner Syndrome.

the immune system or published data are insufficient to classify them as immunodeficiency diseases. The preceding chapter is dedicated to ataxia-telangiectasia, a chromosomal instability syndrome with specific expression of immunodeficiency. Moreover, subgroups of patients with severe combined immunodeficiency (SCID) expressing radiosensitivity, and most probably also chromosomal instability, are excluded from this chapter. This subgroup of SCID is presented in greater detail in Chapter 11.

Fanconi Anemia

Fanconi anemia (MIM 227650) is an autosomal recessive chromosome instability syndrome characterized by bone marrow

A

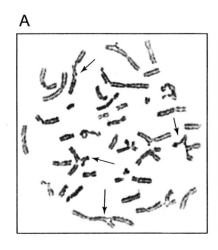

B

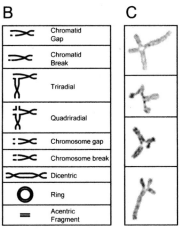

:✕	Chromatid Gap
─✕	Chromatid Break
Y	Triradial
─Ӿ	Quadriradial
:✕	Chromosome gap
═✕	Chromosome break
✕○✕	Dicentric
O	Ring
═	Acentric Fragment

C

Figure 30.1. Chromosomal instability in Fanconi anemia (FA). (A) Lymphocyte chromosomes of a patient with Fanconi anemia. Only some of the chromatid breaks in this massively damaged metaphase are indicated. (B) Schematic representation of the chromosome aberrations seen in lymphocyte chromosomes from patients with chromosomal instability syndromes. (C) Examples of characteristic chromosome reunion figures seen in FA patients.

failure and an increased risk of neoplasia, particularly leukemia. In addition, a range of congenital abnormalities, such as growth retardation, radius aplasia, and hyperpigmentation of the skin, are observed in some patients.

The clinical presentation of FA is highly variable. As is often the case, the more severe phenotypes have been overemphasized and one-third of FA patients have no congenital abnormalities (Glanz and Fraser, 1982; Giampietro et al., 1997). The generally accepted critical diagnostic criterion for FA is an increase in chromosome breakage after in vitro treatment of patient cells, usually peripheral blood lymphocytes, with bifunctional alkylating agents such as mitomycin C (MMC) (Sasaki and Tonomura, 1973).

Clinical and Pathological Manifestations

Hematological complications

The bone marrow of FA patients deteriorates, usually within the first decade of life, although this aspect also varies considerably. Thrombocytopenia and macrocytosis, for example increased erythrocyte volume (mean cell volume >100 fl) associated with increased fetal hemoglobin levels, are followed by granulocytopenia, leukopenia, and eventually pancytopenia. Although aplastic anemia is accompanied by recurrent infections, FA is clearly a genetic hematological disorder rather than a primary immunodeficiency. Pancytopenia, however, results in a clinically relevant deficiency of cells attributed to the immune system.

Acute myeloblastic leukemia occurs 15,000 times more frequently in FA patients than in the general population. In addition, squamous cell carcinoma of the skin and gastrointestinal tract are frequent. The true cancer risk cannot be estimated, since some patients have died prematurely from infections or during bone marrow transplantation; at least 15% of FA patients develop neoplasia (Alter, 1996).

Cytogenetics

The involvement of the FA gene(s) in the "metabolism and mechanics of the chromosome" was postulated by Schroeder and German (1974) on the basis of characteristic chromosome breaks observed in lymphocytes of FA patients (Fig. 30.1). These breaks are particularly chromatid breaks and translocations in-

volving nonhomologous chromosomes leading to triradial and quadriradial forms. This increased mutation rate in lymphocytes of FA patients is thought to explain the predisposition to acute myelogenic leukemia and other malignancies. A highly specific feature is a hypersensitivity to cross-linking agents. This phenomenon is still used as the diagnostic marker when a gene mutation cannot be proven. Detailed protocols describing common cytogenetic techniques are provided by Wegner and Stumm (1999).

The observation that peripheral blood lymphocytes of some FA patients apparently contain two populations of cells was first reported in 1983 by Kwee et al. Increasing doses of MMC shift one population to higher levels of chromosome damage while a second population remains as unaffected as wild-type cells. Although chromosome breakage analysis probably does not detect low-level mosaicism, such cases can be revealed by the isolation of MMC-resistant Epstein-Barr virus (EBV)-immortalized lymphoblasts. On the basis of this criterion, up to 25% of all FA patients are likely to be mosaic (Lo Ten Foe et al., 1997). In all mosaic patients analyzed, skin fibroblasts show the characteristic chromosome instability suggesting that the reversion events leading to a wild-type cell population are specific for lymphocyte progenitors (Waisfisz et al., 1999a; Gregory et al., 2001). The high incidence of mosaics may require cytogenetic analysis of fibroblasts from patients suspected of having FA but no increased breakage in standard lymphocyte cultures.

Cell Cycle

Analysis of the cell cycle in FA has consistently shown increased numbers of cells in G2 phase (Seyschab et al., 1993), where they are presumably arrested to repair DNA lesions. Treating FA cells with cross-linkers increases the proportion of cells in G2 and has become an alternative and/or substantiating diagnostic criterion for FA. This disturbance of the cell cycle explains the poor growth of FA cells in vitro.

Interestingly, the slow growth of FA cells and their accumulation in G2 can be normalized by keeping the cell cultures at reduced oxygen tension (Schindler and Hoehn, 1988). Even the spontaneous chromosomal breakage is lost at 5% O_2 (Joenje et al., 1981). These and other findings have led to the suggestion that the primary defect in FA is related to the avoidance of oxygen radicals or to repair of the DNA lesions caused by these highly reactive molecules.

Table 30.2. Fanconi Anemia (FA) Complementation Groups and Genes

Group	Prevalence (%)	FANCD2 monoubiquitinylation?	Gene	Chromosome	Exons	Protein Size (kDa)
FA-A	60	no	FANCA	16q24.3	43	163
FA-B	rare	no	FANCB	Xp22.31	10	95
FA-C	15	no	FANCC	9q22.3	14	65
FA-D1	5	yes	FANCD1/BRCA2	13q12–13	27	384
FA-D2	5	no	FANCD2	3p25.3	44	155
FA-E	rare	no	FANCE	6p21–22	10	59
FA-F	rare	no	FANCF	11p15	1	42
FA-G	10	no	FANCG/XRCC9	9p13	14	68
FA-I	rare	no				
FA-J	rare	no	FANCJ/BRIP1	17q23.2	20	130
FA-L	rare	yes	FANCL	2p16.1	14	52
FA-M	rare	no	FANCM	14q21.2	23	250

Genetics

Fanconi anemia is genetically heterogeneous and this heterogeneity can be assessed by somatic cell fusion and analysis of cross-linker sensitivity in the cell hybrids. Currently 12 complementation groups are known, these are denoted by the abbreviation *FA* followed by a letter—for example, FA-A, FA-B. FA-A is the largest group (approximately 60%) followed by FA-G (approximately 10%), and FA-C (approximately 10%). Identification of the underlying gene has been achieved for 11 of the groups, mostly by the technique of functional cloning by selecting cDNAs that enable patient cells to survive an otherwise lethal dose of MMC. The genes are denoted by the abbreviation *FANC*, followed by a letter—for example, *FANCA, FANCG*. In some cases a chromosomal localization for the gene had been previously established by linkage analysis in families (Pronk et al., 1995; Saar et al., 1998; Waisfisz et al., 1999a). After the demonstration by Garcia-Higuera et al. (2001) that FANCD2 interacts with BRCA1, *BRCA2* was identified as an FA gene after analysis of FA-B and FA-D1 patients for mutations in this gene (Howlett et al., 2002). *FANCL* (Meetei et al., 2003), *FANCM* (Meetei et al., 2005), and the X-chromosomal gene *FANCB* (Meetei et al., 2004) were identified through the finding that many FA proteins interact to form a stable complex. *FANCJ* was identified by a candidate gene approach as the BRCA1 binding protein BRIP1 (Levran et al., 2005). The current status of gene identification is given in Table 30.2 together with some details of the known FA genes.

While many FA genes were novel when they were identified, some were previously known or showed significant homology to known genes. *FANCG* (de Winter et al., 1998) proved to be identical to the gene *XRCC9*, which had been isolated through its ability to correct (or cross-complement) an X-ray sensitive hamster cell mutant from complementation group 9 (Liu et al., 1997a). *FANCD1* is identical to *BRCA2* and *FANCJ* is a BRCA1 binding protein. *FANCM* shows homology to the archaeal *Hef* gene that has ATP-dependent helicase activities and is involved in DNA repair (Meetei et al., 2005). *FANCD2* shows homology with sequences in lower organisms, such as *Drosophila* (Timmers et al., 2001). The protein product of the *FANCD2* gene is rather unique among FA proteins, as discussed below. Other functional motifs have so far not been identified in FA proteins.

Despite repeated efforts, a correlation between complementation group and clinical features or course of the disease has not generally been possible. Patients with and without congenital abnormalities are found in all groups with sufficient numbers of patients for analysis. Leukemia seems to occur earlier in FA-G patients than in FA-A or FA-C patients (Faivre et al., 2000).

Mutation Analysis

The FA genes have been extensively analyzed for mutations. Most patients are compound heterozygotes with private mutations, but there are also founder mutations in the three largest groups, FA-A, FA-C, and FA-G. Whereas particular deletions of *FANCA* exons are common in the Afrikaner population in South Africa (Tipping et al., 2001), a nonsense mutation, E105X, accounts for 44% of mutant *FANCG* alleles in Germany (Demuth et al., 2000). In *FANCC*, the mutation IVS4 + 4a > t is homozygous in the majority of Ashkenazi Jewish FA patients and is associated with a particularly severe disease in terms of both congenital abnormalities and hematopoietic failure (Whitney et al., 1993). In contrast, Japanese patients with the same mutation are not severely affected (Futaki et al., 2000). This finding indicates the strong influence of genetic background on disease manifestation and explains the difficulties in establishing a genotype–phenotype correlation, even within one complementation group. On the whole, truncation mutations strongly outweigh missense mutations in the FA genes. *FANCA* in particular has many deletions due to the Alu-repeat elements in and around the gene (Levran et al., 1998).

The biallelic mutations in the *BRCA2/FANCD1* gene found in FA-D1 patients are hypomorphic (Howlett et al., 2002). Presumably the amorphic mutations are embryonically lethal in the homozygous state, as in *Brca2* null-mutant mice (Ludwig et al., 1997).

For diagnostic purposes, the complementation group can be established by fusion of patient cells to reference cell lines or by retroviral transfer of the known FA genes, followed by examination of cross-linker sensitivity. DNA from patients assigned to a complementation group can be analyzed for mutations, and this information is then available for further diagnoses in the family, including prenatal diagnosis. The ongoing collection of clinical data and mutation analyses in Europe and the United States is facilitating attempts at a genotype–phenotype correlation (Gillio et al., 1997; Faivre et al., 2000).

Fanconi Anemia Mosaics

The molecular basis of reversion has been elucidated for at least six mosaic cases (Lo Ten Foe et al., 1997; Waisfisz et al.,

1999a). In one case, mitotic recombination with a break point within the *FANCC* gene placed both mutations on one allele and generated a heterozygous cell. In another patient, one mutation was lost in the reverted cells; retention of heterozygosity indicated that gene conversion was probably responsible for this reversion. The same mechanism was responsible for reversion in cells of this patient's affected brother. In three additional cases, all homozygous for *FANCA* or *FANCC* mutations, reversion was due to additional de novo mutations in *cis*. Thus a single base deletion was corrected by two further single base deletions that restored the reading frame. Similarly, a 5 bp insertion corrected the effects of an inherited single base insertion. Finally, a C>T transition corrected a missense mutation. This latter correction was found independently in two affected mosaic siblings, suggesting a specific molecular mechanism, whereas the other reversions are presumably due to random insertion or deletion events and selection.

Although reversions have been shown to occur in lymphohematopoietic stem cells and may be associated with a seemingly milder hematological disease, bone marrow failure and leukemia have been reported for several patients with revertant mosaicism (Gregory et al., 2001).

Molecular Biology of Fanconi Anemia

The chromosome breakage observed in FA is specific for agents like MMC, which are capable of intercalating into a DNA double helix and forming covalent cross-links between the two strands. Thus the DNA lesion to which FA cells are particularly sensitive is the interstrand cross-link. The hypothesis based on this observation postulates that FA cells are deficient in the repair of DNA cross-links.

This hypothesis has been difficult to prove, however; there are few biochemical demonstrations of a failure to repair DNA cross-links in FA cells. Thus a number of other primary defects have been suggested: regulation of the cell cycle, regulation of DNA synthesis, apoptosis, and the avoidance of DNA damage caused by active oxygen radicals. The similarity in the cellular and clinical phenotype within the complementation groups was taken as evidence for involvement of the FA proteins in a common pathway. Indeed, association of the FA proteins in multimeric complexes has been proven by immunoprecipitation studies and by yeast two-hybrid analyses (Medhurst et al., 2001). The currently understood order of events is that the FANCA protein binds to the FANCC and FANCG proteins in the cytoplasm and then moves as a complex to the nucleus; FANCA is at some point modified by phosphorylation. In the nucleus, the FANCB, FANCE, FANCF, and FANCL proteins join to form the FA core complex (Fig. 30.2) (de Winter et al., 2000; Meetei et al., 2003, 2004).

A direct link to DNA repair processes in the cell was not made until the cloning of *FANCG*, which was found to be identical to the gene mutated in UV40, a hamster cell DNA-repair mutant, and implicated in post-replicational repair (Busch et al., 1996; Liu et al., 1997a). Further and even stronger evidence for a role in DNA repair was provided by the cloning of the *FANCD2* gene and the discovery that its protein is monoubiquitinated as a response to DNA damage and relocates to discrete nuclear foci, where it associates with BRCA1 (Garcia-Higuera et al., 2001). These nuclear foci are almost certainly sites where DNA lesions (e.g., double-strand breaks, cross-links) are being actively repaired (see also the section on NBS, below).

BRCA1 is a binding partner of BRCA2/FANCD1, and both of these are required for the recruitment of RAD51, the RecA

homologue, to the sites of DSBs for error-free repair by HR and gene conversion. BRCA2/FANCD1-deficient cells have been shown to be inefficient in the formation of RAD51 foci (Yuan et al., 1999). This finding correlates with a loss of repair by gene conversion, an increase in repair by alternative error-prone pathways, and extreme cross-linker-induced chromosomal instability (Tutt et al., 2001).

The finding that the FA protein complex of FANCA, FANCB, FANCC, FANCG, FANCE, FANCF, and FANCL is required for modification of the FANCD2 protein (Fig. 30.2) has linked these proteins nicely into the same pathway (Garcia-Higuera et al., 2001; Pace et al., 2002; Meetei et al., 2003, 2004). The recent finding that RAD51 foci formation is reduced in FA cells from all complementation groups suggests that FANCD2-L (L, long isoform; derived by monoubiquination of the short [S] isoform), like BRCA1 and BRCA2/FANCD1, is involved in RAD51-mediated DNA repair (Digweed et al., 2002b). Furthermore, FANCD2 has been shown to interact directly with BRCA2/FANCD1 (Hussain et al., 2004). Figure 30.2 shows a model for these protein interactions.

The reliance on error-prone DNA repair pathways in the other FA complementation groups, may lead to the characteristic chromosomal instability of FA and be a direct result of the inability to modify FANCD2-S to FANCD2-L and efficiently recruit RAD51 for repair by gene conversion. Convincing data have been presented showing reduced homologous recombination in chicken DT40 cells mutated in *FANCG* (Yamamoto et al., 2003) and *FANCC* (Niedowitz et al., 2004). Similarly, using sophisticated plasmid reporters, defects in homologous recombination have been demonstrated in human and mouse cells with mutations in *FANCA*, *FANCD2*, and *FANCG* (Nakanishi et al., 2005; Yang et al., 2005). In contrast to previous studies, in the mutant mouse and human cells the error-prone repair pathway of single

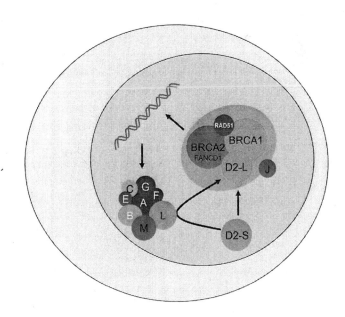

Figure 30.2. Network of Fanconi anemia (FA) proteins. A highly simplified schematic representation of interactions of the FA gene products. A core complex of eight of the FA proteins (FANCA, FANCB, FANCC, FANCE, FANCF, FANCG, FANCL, and FANCM) is required for monoubiquitination of a further FA protein, FANCD2, in response to DNA damage. Modified FANCD2 then relocates to the sites of DNA damage where it associates with BRCA1 and BRCA2, which is identical to FANCD1. BRCA1 and BRCA2 bind the important effector of homologous recombination, RAD51.

strand annealing (SSA) was also affected suggesting further roles for the monoubiquitinated FANCD2 protein. It is possible, even likely, that the individual FA proteins are involved in further interactions and that these may influence their activity in monoubiquitination of FANCD2. Thus the demonstrated oxygen sensitivity and cell cycle disturbance described in FA cells have yet to be incorporated logically into the FA pathway or, perhaps more appropriately, into the FA network. Interestingly, a functional link between FANCD2 and the NBS1/MRE11/RAD50 pathway has been indicated by several reports (Digweed et al., 2002a; Nakanishi et al., 2002; Pichierri et al., 2002).

Animal Models

Knockout mice for the *Fanca, Fancc,* and *Fancg* genes have been produced but show few of the disease symptoms observed in patients (Whitney et al., 1996; Cheng et al., 2000; Yang et al., 2001). They do not have skeletal malformations, nor, surprisingly, do they show anemia or increased neoplasia. Although cells from these animals show the characteristic chromosomal breakage and cross-linker sensitivity, the animals are hematologically healthy unless treated with cross-linkers, in which case they suffer bone marrow failure. The only feature that is similar to the human clinical phenotype is reduced fertility. Perhaps not surprisingly, double-knockout *Fanca/Fancc* mice are not more severely affected than the single-knockout animals, indicating that these genes probably do not have further functions over and above those of the protein core complex (Noll et al., 2002).

Spontaneous defective hematopoiesis has been reported in double-knockout mice, with disruptions in both *Fancc* and in the Cu/Zn superoxide dismutase genes (Hadjur et al., 2001). These results provide evidence that abnormal regulation of the cellular redox state in FA may be involved in the bone marrow failure of patients. Increased tumorigenesis was reported for a *Fancc/p53* double-knockout mouse with a spectrum of malignancies similar to those of FA patients (Freie et al., 2003). Increased frequencies of epithelial tumors were reported for the *Fancd2* knockout mouse, suggesting perhaps a phenotypic overlap with hypomorphic *Brca2/Fancd1* mice (Houghtaling et al., 2003).

Treatment and Prognosis

Several treatment possibilities are available for patients with FA. Erythrocyte and thrombocyte transfusions can compensate for bone marrow failure, although hemosiderosis is a concern. The bone marrow abnormalities of many patients respond to androgen and cytokine therapy, even if only temporarily. Allogeneic bone marrow transplantation from a histocompatible sibling can cure the bone marrow failure. Transplantations from matched unrelated donors have poor outcomes in FA (MacMillan et al., 2000). Bone marrow transplantation is complicated by the increased sensitivity of FA patients to pretransplant conditioning treatment. However, new cytoreductive regimens, particularly those including fludarabine, are encouraging (Kapelushnik et al., 1997; McCloy et al., 2001). The occurrence of expanding clonal aberrations in bone marrow, particularly those involving chromosome 3q, has been shown to correlate with a poor prognosis (Tönnies et al., 2003).

The relative accessibility of hematopoietic stem cells made FA an obvious candidate disorder for gene therapy, and the first trials were conducted in 1997 (Liu et al., 1997b, 1999). The expectation was that corrected stem cells would have a strong selective advantage in the hypoplastic bone marrow of FA patients, as suggested by the finding of mosaic patients in whom total hematopoiesis is driven by a reverted clone. Gene transfer experiments with the knockout *Fancc* mouse have shown that positive selection can indeed be achieved (Gush et al., 2000). Currently the main obstacle to the development of gene therapy in FA is the poor efficiency of gene transfer into hematopoietic stem cells.

Future Directions

The cloning of most of the FA genes and the final demonstration of a link to DNA repair have changed the course of current FA research. It is realistic to expect that much more detailed information on this novel network for DNA repair will be forthcoming. The availability of mouse models will enable the evaluation of treatment proposals including gene therapy, when gene transfer methodology is advanced enough to make this an alternative therapy for FA patients. In the meantime, the considerable improvement in bone marrow transplantation from unrelated donors must be extrapolated to the treatment of FA patients and new therapies for the treatment of squamous cell carcinoma in FA patients have to be developed. The finding that modification of the FANCD2-S protein does not occur in cells from most FA patients after DNA damage may be exploited in the future as a biochemical assay for diagnosis of the disease. Finally, the role of FA genes in the occurrence of malignancy in the general population will have to be addressed, in view of reports that indicate a role for *FANCF* silencing in acute myeloid leukemia (Tischkowitz et al., 2003) and cervical cancer (Narayan et al., 2004).

Nijmegen Breakage Syndrome

The Nijmegen breakage syndrome (NBS) (MIM 251260), a rare autosomal recessive disorder belonging to the group of chromosomal instability syndromes, was first described 26 years ago (Hustinx et al., 1979). The clinical hallmarks of NBS patients are severe microcephaly, growth retardation, typical facial appearance, combined immunodeficiency, radiosensitivity, and an increased cancer risk. On the cellular level, the NBS abnormalities are closely related to those observed in A-T patients. Cells of both syndromes reveal chromosomal instability, a marked sensitivity to ionizing irradiation (IR) and radiomimetic agents, a radioresistant DNA synthesis (RDS), and additional defects in cellular checkpoint control. Nevertheless, on the molecular genetic level, both syndromes are clearly distinguishable from each other. Whereas A-T is caused by mutations in the *ATM* gene located on chromosome 11q23 (Savitsky et al., 1995), NBS is typically caused by mutations in the *NBS1* gene localized on chromosome 8q21 (Varon et al., 1998). The *NBS1* gene product, nibrin, is part of the hRAD50/hMRE11/nibrin complex (Carney et al., 1998), which seems to function in concert with ATM in a damage response pathway that affects a DNA repair process as well as cell cycle checkpoint control (Girard et al., 2000).

Demographics

Whereas in the first edition of this text the number of diagnosed NBS patients amounted to 58, this figure has increased to approximately 170 patients at the end of 2004. Detailed clinical data on 55 patients collected in the NBS Registry in Nijmegen are included in the report of an international study group (International Nijmegen Breakage Syndrome Study Group, 2000). Among the remaining patients, not yet entered into the registry, there are 52 Polish (K. Chrzanowska, personal observation), 17

Czech (E. Seemanova, personal communication.), 21 German (R. Varon, personal communication), 8 Russian (Resnick et al., 2002), several American (Cerosaletti et al., 1998; Bakhshi et al., 2003), and single patients originating from Chile (Pincheira et al., 1998), Bosnia (Kleier et al., 2000), Argentina (Rosenzweig et al., 2001), Marocco (Maraschio et al., 2001), Turkey (Tekin et al., 2002), Yugoslavia (Pasic, 2002), and Italy (Barth et al., 2003). Thus, the majority of NBS patients known thus far are of Slavic origin (particularly of Polish and Czech descent, with 83 and 35 patients identified to date, respectively) and carry a common founder mutation 657del5 in exon 6 of the *NBS1* gene (Varon et al., 1998). The prevalence of this founder mutation was estimated by Varon et al. (2000) in the Czech Republic, Poland, and the Ukraine by the screening of Guthrie cards. A mean prevalence of 1:177 for NBS heterozygotes was found in these three populations. The highest prevalence was found in the Czech population (1:154), followed by the Ukraine (1:182) and Poland (1:198). However, marked regional differences were observed in Poland, ranging from 1:90 to 1:314. Further studies performed recently on populations of three large regions in Poland established a mean prevalence of 1:166 for the 657del5 mutation in Poland (Cybulski et al., 2004; Steffen et al., 2004; M. Mosor, personal communication). All of these frequencies were much higher than the prevalence of 1:866 reported for the same mutation in Germany (Carlomagno et al., 1999). On the basis of these data, the prevalence for NBS homozygotes in the Czech Republic can be estimated at 1 per 95,000. Interestingly, the actual frequency of 1 per 271,000 is much lower than expected. The most likely explanation for this discrepancy is the underdiagnosis of NBS patients because of the rarity of NBS and its relatively mild phenotype. This assumption is corroborated by two observations: (1) the late diagnosis of many NBS patients, often in cases where a malignancy requires examinations that finally disclose the presence of NBS; (2) detection of 3 new NBS patients in a cohort of 23 Czech patients with primary microcephaly tested for the major Czech mutation, the 657del5, in the *NBS1* gene (Seeman et al., 2004). This underdiagnosis is likely a general problem worldwide, thus more attention should be spent on the correct diagnosis of this disease.

Clinical and Pathological Manifestations

Since the first reports on two siblings from Nijmegen (Hustinx et al., 1979; Weemaes et al., 1981), NBS is recognized as a multisystem disorder similar to A-T. The main clinical manifestations (Table 30.3) indicate that various tissues and organs are affected, including brain, skin, blood, and gonads.

Growth and development

Growth. Microcephaly, the most striking symptom of the disorder, has been observed in the great majority of children at birth (van der Burgt et al., 1996). Those who are born with a normal head circumference (OFC) will develop progressive and severe microcephaly during the first months of life. The primary cause of small head size in NBS patients is the genetically determined stunted growth of the brain (see Pathologic Findings, below). Thus, the observed premature closing of the sutures and fontanels can be considered a developmental sequence (no increased intracranial pressure was noted, except in the two cases with coexisting hydrocephalus). Among the observed Polish patients, the decrease in OFC ranged from −9.0 SDS to −4.4 SDS, whereas the proportions among the diminished head measurements, i.e., length and breadth, were retained. Only one case with a normal OFC has

Table 30.3. Clinical Features of Nijmegen Breakage Syndrome

Microcephaly—severe and progressive
Characteristic face
    Sloping forehead and receding mandible
    Prominent midface
Retardation of statural growth
Ovarian failure
Immunodeficiency
Predisposition to malignancies
Intelligence level
    Normal or borderline in early childhood
    Progressive deficiency of IQ scores in later life

been described (Chrzanowska et al., 2001). Growth retardation may occur prenatally in some NBS patients, but in most cases birth weight and length correlate to gestational age. After an initial period of distinct growth retardation lasting from birth to about the second year of life, a slight improvement of growth rate (body height and weight, but not head circumference) is usually observed. Most affected individuals show growth below or around the third percentile whereas a few patients achieve a height around the 10th or even 25th percentile (International Nijmegen Breakage Syndrome Study Group, 2000; Chrzanowska et al., 2001). Intestinal malabsorption, cardiac defects, or hormonal abnormalities related to thyroid or pituitary gland functions have all been excluded as a cause of the growth retardation.

Sexual maturation. Longitudinal studies of growth and development of Polish patients, of whom three females and six males reached puberty, drew attention to the lack of development of secondary sexual characteristics in teenage girls. They presented with primary amenorrhea, absent breast development, and scanty pubic or axillary hair. In two of the three girls, all older than 18 years, repeated pelvic ultrasonography revealed small ovaries, resembling streak gonads, and infantile uteri. All three had markedly elevated plasma concentrations of follicle-stimulating hormone (FSH) and luteinizing hormone (LH) and very low estradiol levels indicating primary ovarian failure (Chrzanowska et al., 1996). A study of the pituitary–gonadal axis performed on a large group of Polish patients including 25 females confirmed the preliminary findings predicting a very high incidence of ovarian failure in this syndrome. Markedly elevated plasma concentrations of FSH, in relation to age, and very low estradiol levels (hypergonadotropic hypogonadism) were found in all but one of the tested females. Serum FSH concentrations exceeding 30 IU/l, a value indicative of ovarian failure, were documented in the majority (76% of those tested), both at pubertal and prepubertal ages (Chrzanowska, 1999; Chrzanowska et al., 2000). Single cases of hypergonadotropic hypogonadism had been reported earlier, including a 21-year-old female with NBS phenotype (Conley at al., 1986) and a now 24-year-old woman described earlier (Wegner et al., 1988) who subsequently developed primary amenorrhea. In males there was only a slight delay in onset of puberty and the levels of gonadotropins and testosterone corresponded to Tanner's classification of sexual maturity stages (Chrzanowska, 1999). Offspring from affected subjects have never been reported, and firm conclusions on fertility are hampered by the young age of the patients and their short life span. Thus, hypergonadotropic hypogonadism in females, indicative of either ovarian dysgenesis or hypoplasia, must be included in the clinical spectrum of NBS.

Psychomotor development and behavior. In general, developmental milestones are reached at expected times during the first years of life. Patients with normal intelligence (Seemanová et al., 1985; Wegner et al., 1988; Barbi et al., 1991; Green et al., 1995) or mental retardation of variable degree (Weemaes et al., 1981; Conley et al., 1986; Stoppa-Lyonnet et al., 1992; Chrzanowska et al., 1995a) have been reported. Follow-up studies of Polish patients showed that the level of intellectual function decreases with age. Most of the children tested in infancy and early childhood had IQ scores indicating a normal or borderline intelligence with striking psychomotor hyperactivity. When tested or retested after the age of 7, difficulties in concentration became more pronounced. At school age, lower levels of intellectual function were observed and became more evident in subjects over 14 years of age when all tested patients were mildly or moderately retarded (Chrzanowska, 1999). Most of the mentally retarded patients need educational support and should attend special education classes or schools. All of the children have a gentle and cheerful personality and, despite being shy, are usually capable of good social interactions.

Craniofacial manifestations. The craniofacial characteristics become more obvious with age because of the severe and progressive microcephaly. The facial appearance is very similar among NBS patients and is characterized by a sloping forehead and receding mandible, prominent midface with a relatively long nose (slightly beaked in most patients or upturned in some), and upward slanting of palpebral fissures (Fig. 30.3). In some individuals the ears seem to be relatively large and dysplastic.

Other manifestations

Central nervous system malformations. Developmental abnormalities of the brain are relatively frequent and appear to be more common than expected. Partial agenesis of the corpus callosum was documented in one-third (6/18) of Polish patients who underwent cranial magnetic resonance imaging (MRI) (Bekiesińska-Figatowska et al., 2000; 2004 Chrzanowska et al., 2001) as well as in at least three others (Maraschio et al., 2001; Resnick et al., 2002; Nortrop, personal communication). Agenesis of the corpus callosum was associated developmentally with colpocephaly—i.e., disproportionate enlargement of the trigones, occipital horns, and usually temporal horns of the lateral ventricles. Large collections of cerebrospinal fluid (arachnoid cysts) in the pari-etooccipital and/or occipitotemporal regions were found in four patients (Stoppa-Lyonnet et al., 1992; Bekiesińska-Figatowska et al., 2000; Chrzanowska et al., 2001; Nortrop, personal communication). The cysts resulted from an anomalous splitting of the arachnoid membrane and are a congenital anomaly of the developing subarachnoid system. Both defects, callosal hypoplasia and arachnoid cysts, may frequently be underdiagnosed in NBS patients because they are asymptomatic. Hydrocephalus was reported in several patients, including one pair of sibs (Taalman et al., 1989; Bekiesińska-Figatowska et al., 2000; Muschke et al., 2004). Neuronal migration disorder in the form of schizencephaly and focal pachygyria has been diagnosed each in a single patient (Der Kaloustian et al., 1996; Bekiesińska-Figatowska et al., 2000).

Skin and vascular anomalies. Skin pigmentation abnormalities expressed as café-au-lait–like spots (rather irregular in shape) and/or depigmented spots can be seen in most patients; in three Polish patients, progressive vitiligo was observed at the age of adolescence. Sun sensitivity of the eyelids is less frequent. Multiple pigmented nevi and cavernous or flat hemangiomae occur in a proportion of patients (Peréz-Vera et al., 1997; Chrzanowska, 1999; International Nijmegen Breakage Syndrome Study Group, 2000).

Skeletal anomalies. Minor skeletal defects such as clinodactyly of the fifth fingers and/or partial syndactyly of the second and third toes is encountered in about half of the patients (International Nijmegen Breakage Syndrome Study Group, 2000); less common is hip dysplasia (~15%) (Chrzanowska, 1999; unpublished observation). Uni- or bilateral preaxial polydactyly was observed in four patients (Chrzanowska et al., 1995a; Maraschio et al., 2001) and sacral agenesis was found in one (K. Chrzanowska, unpublished observation).

Urogenital, anal, and miscellaneous malformations. Anal atresia or stenosis was noted in six cases (Wegner et al., 1988; Chrzanowska, 1999; Tekin et al., 2002; Nortrop, personal communication). Among the urogenital anomalies, ectopic single kidney or dystopic kidneys were diagnosed in eight patients (Chrzanowska, 1999; International Nijmegen Breakage Syndrome Study Group, 2000; Muschke et al., 2004) and hydronephrosis in three additional patients (Seemanová et al., 1985; Taalman et al., 1989). Congenital cardiovacular or heart defect were noted in two cases (Chrzanowska et al., 2001; Tekin et al., 2002). Hypospadias (Der Kaloustian et al., 1996), cryptorchism (Pincheira et al., 1998), and genitourinary fistula (Chrzanowska, 1999) were observed each in only a single patient, as were other miscellaneous congenital anomalies such as cleft lip/palate (Seemanová et al., 1985), choanal atresia (Seemanová et al., 1985), and tracheal hypoplasia (Chrzanowska, 1999). Ultrasonographic evaluation of a large group of Polish patients revealed a high frequency of polysplenia (20%), a peculiarity with no clinical significance (Chrzanowska, 1999).

Infections and autoimmune disorders

As in A-T (see Chapter 29), the extent of immunodeficiency or proneness to infection in NBS patients showed striking intra- and interfamiliar variability. Respiratory tract infections were present in most children. Recurrent pneumonia and bronchitis may result in bronchiectasis, respiratory insufficiency, and premature death from respiratory failure (Weemaes et al., 1981; Seemanová et al., 1985). Meningitis, sinusitis, and otitis media with draining ears and mastoiditis were observed in some children, as were gastrointestinal infections with diarrhea and urinary tract infections. Opportunistic infections are very rare, as in A-T (International Nijmegen Breakage Syndrome Study Group, 2000). Other diseases, probably caused by a defective immune system, have been observed in single cases: autoimmune hemolytic anemia, hemolytic anemia followed by thrombocytopenia, childhood sarcoidosis with ocular and cutaneous manifestations (Chrzanowska, 1999), and a juvenile rheumatoid arthritis–like polyarthritis (Rosenzweig et al., 2001). In two unrelated Polish patients, coexistance of NBS and Gilbert syndrome (familial idiopathic unconjugated hyperbilirubinemia associated with a partial reduction of hepatic glucuronyl transferase activity) has been noted (Chrzanowska, 1999).

Predisposition to malignancies

Both the immunodeficiency and the chromosome instability may predispose NBS patients to tumor development at an early age. In A-T, approximately 10% to 15% of the homozygotes develop

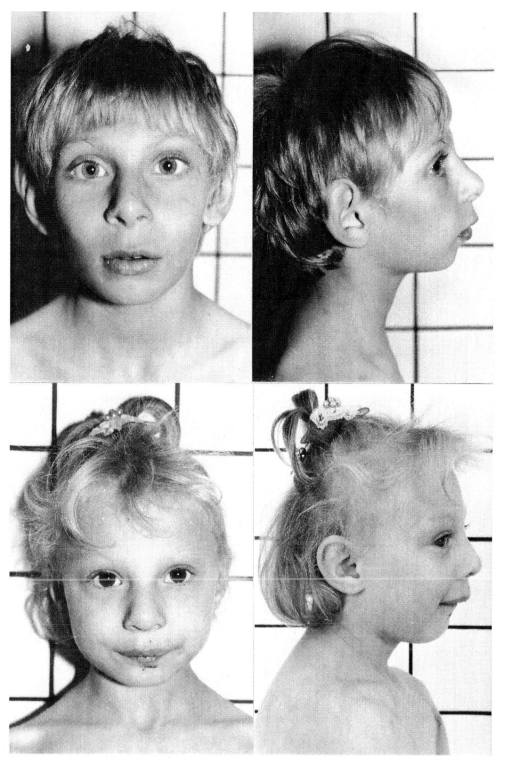

Figure 30.3. Characteristic facial features of a 7-year-old male patient with Nijmegen breakage syndrome (upper row) and his 5-year-old sister. Note microcephaly, microgenia, sloping forehead, slightly upward slanting of palpebral fissures, and prominent midface.

malignancy in early adulthood (Taylor et al., 1996). The rate is even higher in NBS. Cancer before the age of 21 years was noted in 40% (22/55) of the patients included in the NBS Registry in Nijmegen (International Nijmegen Breakage Syndrome Study Group, 2000). Updates from the two largest national NBS registries, the Polish registry (K. Chrzanowska, unpublished data) and the Czech registry (Seemanová et al., reported at the International Workshop on NBS, Prague, Czech Republic, 2002) indicated cancer development in 54% (45/83) and 65% (19/29) of

patients, respectively. The great majority of malignancies were of lymphoid origin, found in 41 and 15 patients, respectively. In the Polish series, the most frequent malignancies were non-Hodgkin lymphomas (NHL): in 30 patients (those of B cell origin slightly exceeded those of T cell origin), followed by lymphoblastic leukemia/lymphoma in 8 patients (T-LBL/ALL, T-ALL, pre-B-ALL) and Hodgkin disease in 3 patients (Gładkowska-Dura et al., 2000). Acute myeloblastic leukemia (AML) has been diagnosed in two NBS patients (Resnick et al., 2002; K. Chrzanowska, unpublished observation). Moreover, Michallet et al. (2003) described the first case of T cell prolymphocytic leukemia (T-PLL) in NBS.

At least seven patients are known to have developed a second malignancy. One German patient (Rischewski et al., 2000) and two Polish patients had two consecutive lymphomas of the same type, with complete remission of 5–7 years in between (Gład-kowska-Dura et al., 2000, 2005). Two additional Polish patients developed a different type of lymphoma as a second event (Gład-kowska-Dura et al., 2005), and two other patients (Dutch and Czech) developed a different type of tumor after 10 and 4 years of remission, respectively (Weemaes et al., 2002). One Polish patient was recently diagnosed to have a third consecutive lymphoma of the same type (time interval between the two relapses, 7 and 6 years, respectively; Gładkowska-Dura et al., 2005). Both concordance of tumor type in a pair of NBS siblings (Wegner, 1991) and discordance in another pair (Wegner et al., 1999) have been reported.

Solid tumors have been less frequently noted, probably because the tumors usually develop at an older age. Five patients have developed a medulloblastoma (Chrzanowska et al., 1997; Bakskhi et al., 2003; Distel et al., 2003; E. Seemanová, personal communication; F. Tzortzatou-Stathopoulou, personal communication) and two have a rhabdomyosarcoma (Der Kaloustian et al., 1996; Tekin et al., 2002). Other tumors are represented only in single cases and include malignant meningioma, gonadoblastoma, Ewing sarcoma (E. Seemanova, personal communication), and ganglioneuroblastoma (K. Chrzanowska, unpublished observation).

At least three patients who had medulloblastoma and received radiation therapy before being diagnosed with NBS were fatally injured and eventually died from complications of the therapy (Chrzanowska et al., 1997; Bakskhi et al., 2003; Distel et al., 2003). Alopecia was a side effect observed in a Polish patient with AML given an 18 Gy dose of cranial irradiation for central nervous system (CNS) prophylaxis. However, another Polish patient with T cell acute lymphoblastic leukemia (T-ALL) tolerated well an identical dose of prophylactic cranial irradiation. Both patients were treated for malignancy before the diagnosis of NBS was established (K. Chrzanowska, unpublished observation).

Most malignancies develop before the age of 20 years (median age, 9 years; range, 1 to 34 years), and in about 20% to 30% of patients cancer appears prior to the diagnosis of NBS (Varon et al., 2000). On the basis of available records, an approximately 50-fold risk of early onset of cancer and a >1000-fold risk of lymphoma are estimated for patients with NBS.

The precise mechanism(s) leading to the increased cancer prevalence in NBS is (are) still unclear. Thus it is an open question as to whether the *NBS1* gene has a general function as a tumor supressor gene. Molecular investigation of the frequency of the most common *NBS1* mutation, 657del5, in two NHL cohorts with 109 and 62 German children, respectively, failed to detect this mutation in the *NBS1* gene (Rischewski et al., 2000; Stanulla et al., 2000). Furthermore, a fluorescence in situ hybridization (FISH) analysis of tumor samples from 16 German NHL patients detected no deletions of the *NBS1* gene (Stumm et al., 2001b). Sequencing studies on 20 Japanese lymphomas (Hama et al., 2000) and tumor samples from 91 NHL patients in the United States (Cerosaletti et al., 2002) provided no evidence that *NBS1* mutations play a major role in the development of NHL. These studies demonstrate that neither a NBS heterozygote status nor mutations or deletions of the *NBS1* gene in the tumor itself are frequent events in patients with B and T cell lymphomas. However, a Polish study of 456 children with lymphoid malignancies (208 with NHL and 248 with ALL) revealed five heterozygous carriers of a germ-line 657del5 mutation, in contrast to the expected incidence of 2.75 (Chrzanowska et al., 2004). This study has been expanded showing similar results and suggesting that *NBS1* gene heterozygosity is not a major factor in lymphoid malignancies in childhood and adolescence (Chrzanowska et al., 2005).

In contrast to NHL, Varon et al. (2001) detected mutations in *NBS1* in 15% of cases of childhood ALL, whereas none was observed in controls, a finding indicating a possible involvement of the *NBS1* gene in development of ALL. There is evidence that heterozygotes for NBS also show a significantly increased rate of malignancies (Seemanová et al., 1990). Recently performed studies on 1683 nonselected Polish patients with malignant tumors detected increased germ-line mutation frequencies for the 657del5 mutation and increased frequencies for the R215W amino acid exchange variant, indicating that heterozygous carriers of NBS mutations may indeed have an increased risk of developing tumors, especially in breast cancer and melanoma (Steffen et al., 2004). These data have been corroborated by recent findings of increased translocation frequencies in NBS heterozygotes (Stumm et al., 2001a; see Cytogenetics, below). Recently Shimada et al. (2004) reported the first case of aplastic anemia with a homozygous missense mutation in the *NBS1* gene (I171V) and hypothesized that the *NBS1* gene may play an important role in the pathogenesis of this complication.

Pathologic findings

Premature death of more than 70 NBS patients has been ascertained. Less than 10 died from infections that led to fatal respiratory failure, and two from renal insufficiency due to amyloidosis. Two others died as a result of bone marrow aplasia (Resnick et al., 2002), a hallmark of another chromosomal instability syndrome, FA. All the remaining patients died from malignancies. The oldest survivors were a 33-year-old Polish patient and a 31-year-old Dutch patient, both males.

Autopsies performed on several patients showed a reduced brain weight of more than 50% in all patients examined and internal hydrocephalus in some (Seemanová et al., 1985; van de Kaa et al., 1994; Muschke et al., 2004). A clear neuropathologic difference from A-T has been demonstrated with a cerebellum of normal size and development in NBS (van de Kaa et al., 1994).

A simplified gyral pattern, especially in the frontal lobes, with a severely diminished number of neocortical neurons was recently documented (Lammens et al., 2003). Marked hypoplasia of the thymus, absent thymus, or thymus replacement by fibrous tissues was reported in several other cases (Seemanová et al., 1985; van de Kaa et al., 1994; Muschke et al., 2004).

Suspicion of a lymphoproliferative disorder is the most frequent indication for lymph node biopsy, but only a few reports have appeared on the histologic and immunophenotypic features of lymphomas (van de Kaa et al., 1994; Elenitoba-Johnson and Jaffe, 1997; Paulli et al., 2000). A detailed description of 10 cases of NHL and one of Hodgkin disease revealed morphologic and immunotypic diversity of these NBS-linked lymphomas, ranging from immature, precursor-type lymphoid malignancies to mature T cell lymphomas to immunoglobulin-producing, large B cell phenotypes (DLBCL), a spectrum that appears to be more characteristic for adult rather than pediatric patients (Gład-kowska-Dura et al., 2000, 2002, 2005). Further immunophenotypic and rearrangement studies have revealed clonal *IgH* gene

Table 30.4. Immune Defects in Patients with Ataxia-Telangiectasia Variant or Nijmegen Breakage Syndrome

Lymphopenia, T and B cells
Humoral immunity
    Absent or low serum levels of IgA, IgG, IgM, or IgE
    Abnormal IgG subclass distribution (deficient in IgG2, IgG4)
Cellular immunity
    Low numbers of CD4$^+$ subset
    Decreased CD4$^+$/CD8$^+$ ratio
    High number of NK cells
Impaired proliferative response to mitogens in vitro

rearrangements in all but one DLBCL case, clonal *IgK* gene rearrangements in all cases, and *IgL* gene rearrangements in two (Gladkowska-Dura et al., 2002). None of the cases showed a Bcl-2/IgH translocation.

Laboratory Findings

Laboratory tests helpful in the diagnosis of NBS include evaluation of humoral and cellular immunity, quantitation of serum α-fetoprotein (AFP) levels, karyotyping, and radiosensitivity assays. Molecular analysis is possible in most cases (see Genetics, below).

Immunological data

The immune deficiency in NBS patients is very heterogenic and concerns the humoral and cellular immune systems (Table 30.4).

A longitudinal follow-up study of 40 NBS patients, diagnosed and monitored at a single medical center, the Children's Memorial Health Institute (CMHI) in Warsaw, offered a unique opportunity to gather clinical and laboratory data on a large series of patients (Gregorek et al., 2002). This study extends and supplements data collected earlier to assess the immune system in individuals with NBS (Chrzanowska et al., 1995b; International Nijmegen Breakage Syndrome Study Group, 2000).

The most important observation is the considerable variability in immunodeficiency seen among different patients and in the same individual over the course of time (Gregorek et al., 2002). At diagnosis, severe hypogammaglobulinemia with IgG concentrations below 2.0 g/l, low or undetectable IgA, and decreased IgM was observed in approximately 21% of patients, while an additional 20% had normal concentrations of all three major immunoglobulin classes. The most common finding was a combined deficit of IgG and IgA (31%), followed by isolated IgG deficiency (28%). IgG subclass distribution was abnormal in most patients, affecting predominatly IgG4 (74%), followed by IgG2 (66%) and IgG1 (63%). It is worth noting that in about 37% of NBS patients, normal levels of total serum IgG can mask deficiency of IgG subclasses. This phenomenon points to the importance of determining IgG subclasses, especially in those NBS patients who suffer from frequent infections. The concentrations of IgM and IgG3 are rarely affected; in fact, IgM levels may be elevated (Wegner et al., 1988; Chrzanowska et al., 1995b; Gregorek et al., 2002). These observations suggest that the process of class switching to C$_H$ genes downstream of γ3 (γ1, α1, γ2, γ4, ϵ, and α2) is frequently blocked in NBS. Recently, Pan et al. (2002) provided the first evidence linking ATM and nibrin to class switch recombination (CSR). Lahdesmaki et al. (2004) have suggested that MRE11, nibrin, and ATM might play both common and independent roles in CSR.

Similar to A-T patients, both normal (Green et al., 1995; Der Kaloustian et al., 1996) and disturbed (Wegner et al., 1988; Weemaes et al., 1991) antibody responses to diphtheria and tetanus vaccination have been reported. One NBS patient failed to mount a primary antibody response to *Helix pommatia* hemocyanin (Weemaes et al., 1991). Naturally acquired IgG-specific antibodies to most invasive pneumococcal polysaccharides (e.g., serotypes 3, 19, 23) were not detectable or were found in very low titers in 75% of patients investigated at CMHI. Morover, only 25% of patients vaccinated against hepatitis B virus (HBV) developed antibodies to hepatitis B surface antigen of the protective IgG isotype, which are restricted to two IgG subclasses: IgG1 (present in all positive samples) and IgG3 (found in one patient only). In 65% of the individuals, only IgM antibodies to hepatitis B surface antigens were found; in the remaining 10%, no specific antibodies were detectable, despite normal or only moderately decreased levels of total IgG (Gregorek et al., 2002). Systematic longitudinal observations of 17 available NBS patients at CMHI showed a progressive deterioration of the immune system in 9 of 17 patients (53%). There was no correlation between immunodeficiency profile (or its severity) and duration of the disease, age or gender of the patients studied.

T cell immunity is abnormal in most tested patients. The most evident defects are reduced numbers of CD3$^+$ T cells observed in 93%, a reduced number of CD4$^+$ T cells in 95%, and a reduction in CD8$^+$ T cells in 80%. A decreased CD4/CD8 ratio is also a characteristic feature of this syndrome (Chrzanowska et al., 1995b; van der Burgt et al., 1996; International Nijmegen Breakage Syndrome Study Group, 2000). The number of B cells is reduced in most patients (~75%), but may also be normal or even elevated in some patients despite marked deficiency of serum immunoglobulins, suggesting an intrinsic B cell defect affecting class switch recombination (Gregorek et al., 2002). Detailed characteristics of lymphocyte surface receptors have been reported in a large group ($n = 42$) of NBS patients (Michałkiewicz et al., 2003).

A deficiency of CD4$^+$,CD45RA$^+$ (naive) cells and an excess of CD4$^+$,CD45RO$^+$ (memory) T cells has been observed in all patients tested (Chrzanowska et al., 1995b). A relatively high number of natural killer (NK) cells was noted in the majority of NBS patients (Green et al., 1995; Der Kaloustian et al., 1996). In vitro lymphocyte proliferation in response to mitogens (phytohemagglutinin [PHA], concanavalin A [Con A], pokeweed mitogen [PWM]) is defective in most patients (Weemaes et al., 1981; Seemanová et al., 1985; Conley et al., 1986; Der Kaloustian et al., 1986; Wegner et al., 1988; Chrzanowska et al., 1995b; International Nijmegen Breakage Syndrome Study Group, 2000). In one case lymphocyte proliferation in the presence of specific antigens (tetanus, tuberculin, candidin) was absent, in spite of normal response to PHA (Stoppa-Lyonnet et al., 1992). Recall antigens (Merieux) given intradermally produced no delayed-type hypersensitivity reactions (Wegner et al., 1988).

α-Fetoprotein level

Serum AFP concentration is within the normal range in NBS (van der Burgt et al., 1996), in contrast to A-T, where elevated levels are found in >90% of patients (Woods and Taylor, 1992).

Cytogenetics

In most cases, the diagnosis of NBS is entertained on clinical findings and confirmed by cytogenetic and/or molecular analysis of the *NBS1* gene. T lymphocytes of NBS patients often show a poor response to mitogens, consequently, cultures exhibit a low mitotic index. This limitation to cytogenetic characterization of patient's cells, particularly when testing for mutagenic sensitivity, can be overcome in most cases by using EBV-transformed lymphoblastoid cell lines.

Table 30.5. Cytogenetic and Cellular Features of Nijmegen Breakage Syndrome Cells

Normal constitutive karyotype
Increased spontaneous chromosomal instability
Open chromatid and chromosome breaks
Rearrangements of chromosomes 7 and 14
Telomere fusions
Radioresistant DNA synthesis
Hypersensitivity to ionizing radiation and radiomimetic agents
Increased sensitivity to alkylating agents

NBS cells express the typical cytogenetic features of a chromosomal instability syndrome (Table 30.5). In general, NBS patients have a normal karyotype, but chromosomal instability, as in A-T patients, is a consistent finding. One of the most striking features of NBS is the high level of chromosome rearrangements in cultured T lymphocytes involving chromosomes 7 and 14. Most of these rearrangements occur in chromosome bands 7p13, 7q35, 14q11, and 14q32 (as in A-T), which are the location of the human immunoglobulin and T cell receptor genes (Aurias et al., 1980; Aurias and Dutrillaux, 1986). Generally, translocations are detectable in 10% to 35% of NBS cells and in 5%–10% of A-T cells (van der Burgt et al., 1996). The most frequently detected aberration in T lymphocytes is inv(7)(p13q35), followed by other rearrangements such as t(7;14)(p13;q11), t(7;14)(q35;q11), t(7;7)(p13;q35), and t(14;14)(q11;q32) (van der Burgt et al., 1996; Hiel et al., 2001). Other less frequently reported NBS breakpoints, for example, t(X;14)(q27–28;q11–13), have also been found in A-T cells (Wegner, 1991).

Open chromosomal aberrations, such as chromatid breaks, chromosome breaks, and acentric fragments, as well as marker chromosomes and unspecific chromatid exchanges have been frequently found in lymphocytes and fibroblasts of NBS patients (Weemaes et al., 1981; Seemanová et al., 1985; Conley et al., 1986; Wegner et al., 1988; Taalman et al., 1989; Barbi et al., 1991; Stoppa-Lyonnet et al., 1992; Chrzanowska et al., 1995a; Der Kaloustian et al., 1996; Pérez-Vera et al, 1997; Tupler et al., 1997; Kleier et al., 2000; Chrzanowska et al., 2001; Maraschio et al., 2001). In contrast, chromosomal instability has not been observed in NBS bone marrow cells (Weemaes et al., 1981). An additional uncommon chromosomal abnormality has been described in a 5-year-old NBS patient who showed in addition to the typical 7/14 translocations monosomies of nearly all chromosomes in 64% of the analyzed lymphocyte metaphases (Der Kaloustian et al., 1996). This finding points to deficiencies in the fidelity of mitotic chromosome separation. Whether nibrin, the product of *NBS1*, is involved in chromosome segregations remains unclear. An elevated rate of spontaneous chromosomal instability has been observed in EBV-positive immortalized B lymphoblasts from many NBS patients (Conley et al., 1986; Tupler et al., 1997; Maraschio et al., 2001).

However, there are some NBS cell lines that have a low frequency of chromosomal aberrations or no chromosomal instability at all (Wegner, 1991; Stumm et al., 1997; Chrzanowska et al., 2001). In contrast to primary T lymphocytes, the spontaneous instability in lymphoblastoid cell lines (LCLs) is expressed as unspecific chromosomal aberrations, including a tendency of chromosomes to form telomeric associations resulting in dicentric chromosomes. Recent molecular and cellular data on NBS suggest that this cytogenetic phenomenon is a direct consequence of a functional deficiency of nibrin, a protein found at telomeres, where it associates with the telomeric repeat binding factor TRF2

(Lombard and Guarente, 2000; Zhu et al., 2000). Chromosomes from NBS patients have shortened telomeres that can be corrected by reintroduction of nibrin into patient fibroblasts (Ranganathan et al., 2001). Thus, the absence of nibrin might interfere with telomere metabolism, resulting in illegitimate fusion of telomeres between different chromosomes. Siwicki et al. (2003) have provided evidence that telomere length maintenance is intact in T lymphocytes in the absence of full-length nibrin, presumably because of an alternatively spliced NBS protein of 70 kDa.

All of the cytogenetic aberrations discussed above were obtained by standard microscopic analysis of Giemsa-stained and/or GTG-banded chromosomes. Very recently, more distinct insight into the chromosomal instability of NBS cells was obtained by use of FISH with a three-color whole-chromosome painting assay (WCP 1, 2, 4) (Color Plate 30.I). Through use of this technique, an increased frequency of spontaneous translocations was detected (Stumm et al., 2001a). The presence of chromosomal aberrations, which might escape detection by conventional cytogenetic techniques, demonstrates that the degree of spontaneous genomic instability in NBS might be even higher than previously thought and may be an important risk factor for tumor development. The WCP 1, 2, 4 assay is also suitable for the detection of radiation induced chromosomal instability in NBS and A-T patients (Neubauer et al., 2002).

Sister chromatid exchange (SCE) frequencies were found to be normal in lymphocytes (Weemaes et al., 1981; Conley et al., 1986; Wegner et al., 1988; Barbi et al., 1991; Der Kaloustian et al., 1996), fibroblasts, and LCLs (Conley et al., 1986) from all NBS patients investigated to date. The induction of chromosomal breakage in NBS lymphocytes and fibroblasts by irradiation proves a strong hypersensitivity to ionizing irradiation (IR) as well as to radiomimetic agents, such as bleomycin (Wegner et al., 1988; Taalman et al., 1989; Green et al., 1995; Hiel et al., 2001). These characteristics clearly separate NBS cells from normal cells (Fig. 30.4) and has been used in our laboratories to confirm the diagnosis. A metaphase with a typical spectrum of lesions is shown in Figure 30.5. Increased radiosensitivity of NBS cells is also apparent from a decrease in colony-forming ability following exposure to IR (Taalman et al., 1983; Jaspers et al., 1988a). Controversial results have been published concerning the hypersensitivity of NBS cells to alkylating agents. Seemanová et al. (1985) found weak evidence for increased chromosomal sensitivity to the bifunctional alkylating agent diepoxybutane (DEB) in one of two analyzed patients; Der Kaloustian et al. (1996) found normal DEB sensitivity in a third NBS patient. However, a clearly increased response to Trenimon was reported in siblings with NBS as early as 1991 (Wegner, 1991). Results obtained from these patients, now proven to carry the typical Slavic mutation 657del5, are shown in Figure 30.6. The speculation that the functionally deficient nibrin plays a central role in the aberrant repair processes of different types of DNA damage in NBS cells has been proven correct. Nakanishi et al. (2002) provided evidence for cooperation between the FA gene product FANCD2 and nibrin in the DNA cross-linking response (see Fanconi Anemia, above and Molecular Interactions Between Nibrin and Other Proteins, below). Extensive studies of a cohort of NBS and a group of typical A-T patients corroborated the finding of marked sensitivity to the trifunctional alkylating agent Trenimon (Wegner et al., 1994). At doses of 10^{-8} M Trenimon, the chromosomal breakage rates of some NBS cell lines exceeded the control rate by more than 10 times (Wegner, 1991; Wegner et al., 1994; Stumm et al., 1997) (Fig. 30.6). A moderate sensitivity to MMC has been observed in one NBS patient (Chrzanowska et al.,

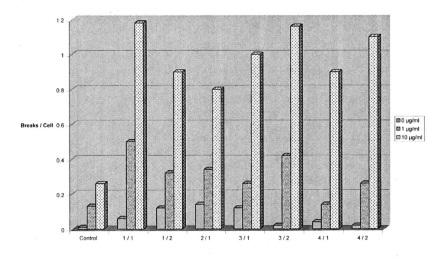

Figure 30.4. Spontaneous and bleomycin-induced chromosomal breakage rates in lymphoblastoid cell line metaphases from Nijmegen breakage syndrome (NBS) patients and a control, respectively. Bleomycin was added 1 hour before harvesting: 50 cells/column were counted in each situation. Note that there is an unequivocal discrimination between affected and control individuals at the higher bleomycin concentration. Patients are identified by family number (first digit) and individual number (second digit).

2001). This moderate sensitivity to MMC is lower than in FA patients but has also been found in cell lines from other NBS patients (Kraakman–van der Zwet et al., 1999; Nakanishi et al., 2002; M. Stumm and R. Wegner, unpublished observation). These findings are of significance with respect to chemotherapy for NBS patients: the intensity of the treatment should be adjusted to the patient's individual risk factors and tolerance (Seidemann et al., 2000). Therefore, testing cells for their response to cytostatic agents should be considered and might reduce the risk of therapeutic side effects in sensitive patients.

Cell cycle

Although the function of nibrin in cell cycle control is far from fully understood, its involvement in cell cycle checkpoints is supported by cellular, molecular, and cytogenetic data. Unlike in normal cells, DNA synthesis after IR or bleomycin treatment is not inhibited in NBS cells (Jaspers et al., 1988a; Wegner et al., 1988; Chrzanowska et al., 1995a). This feature, called *radioresistant DNA synthesis* (RDS), was initially described in A-T cells (Cramer and Painter, 1981; deWit et al., 1981). RDS in NBS cells seems to be linked to a pathway involving the interaction of nibrin and SMC1. The inhibition of DNA synthesis after IR seems to depend on phosphorylation of SMC1, a member of the cohesion proteins. Efficient phosphorylation of SMC1 by ATM requires nibrin (reviewed by Digweed and Sperling, 2004). In addition to this highly characteristic defect in an S-phase-dependent cell cycle checkpoint, there are further disturbances in cell cycle progression in some NBS cell lines. The role of *NBS1*

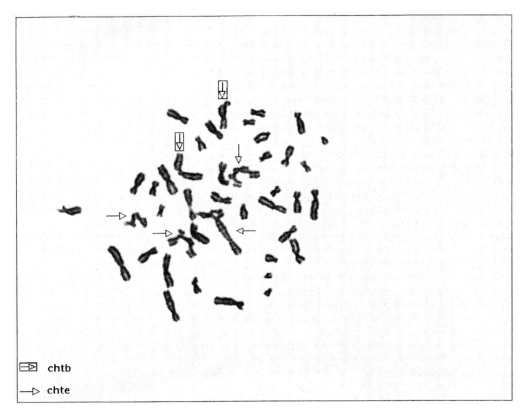

Figure 30.5. Lymphoblastoid cell line metaphase of a bleomycin-treated Nijmegen breakage syndrome cell showing chromatid breaks (chtb) and chromatid exchanges (chte).

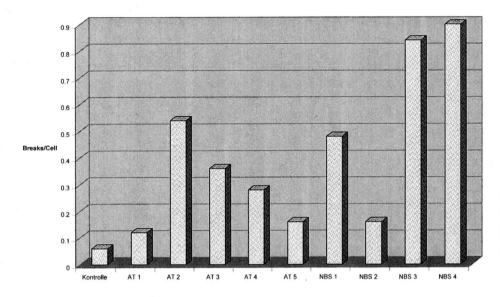

Figure 30.6. Trenimon-induced chromosomal breakage in lymphoblastoid cell line metaphases from Nijmegen breakage syndrome (NBS) and ataxia-telangiectasia (AT) patients. Trenimon exposure (10^{-8} M) lasted 24 hours. At least 50 cells/column were analyzed.

in G1/S checkpoint control is controversial, because the extent of p53 accumulation and strength of expression of G1/S arrest after irradiation differ substantially in individual NBS cell lines (Jongmans et al., 1997; Sullivan et al., 1997; Matsuura et al., 1998; Yamazaki et al., 1998; Antoccia et al., 1999; Girard et al., 2000). An explanation for these variations might be dose-dependent differences in the response, as Girard et al. (2002) showed G1/S arrest in NBS cells at 1 Gy that was abolished at 5 Gy. Irrespective of differences in p53 induction and G1/S checkpoint control, NBS and A-T cells show comparable chromosome aberrations, both in quantity and in quality. This means that there is no simple correlation between checkpoint control and radiation-induced chromosomal instability. Therefore, factors other than those related directly to G1/S cell cycle checkpoint control seem to be involved mainly in radiation sensitivity and chromosomal instability in NBS cells (Antoccia et al., 1999). The role of NBS1 in G2 checkpoint control is also controversial, because the G2/M-phase transition appears to be extremely variable among different NBS cell lines. Some NBS cells, like A-T cells, fail to stop entry into mitosis after irradiation, a finding suggesting that NBS1 deficiency may disturb the G2/M checkpoint (Pincheira et al., 1998; Buscemi et al., 2001; Maraschio et al., 2001). In contrast, other NBS cells show a normal G2/M transition (Antoccia et al., 1997, 2002; Yamazaki et al., 1998; Girard et al., 2000). Because recent reports suggest an impaired ability of NBS cell lines to phosphorylate checkpoint kinase 2 (CHK2) (Buscemi et al., 2001; Girard et al., 2002), it is reasonable to expect effects of nibrin mutations on G2/M checkpoint control (see Molecular Interactions Between Nibrin and Other Proteins, below).

The expression of checkpoint impairment in NBS cells appears to vary considerably and be dose-dependent. Therefore, checkpoint disturbance is likely not the main reason for the strong radiation sensitivity in these cells over a broad range of doses.

Genetics

Identification of the *NBS1* gene

Despite clear differences in the clinical characteristics of NBS and A-T, cells from patients with these diseases express nearly identical cytogenetic and cellular features. This phenomenon led to the suggestion that NBS and A-T are two disorders due to al-

lelic mutations (Curry et al., 1989). In contrast to this proposal, linkage analysis in six NBS families, formerly called ataxia-telangiectasia variant (AT-V) families, with at least two affected siblings proved unequivocally that the underlying *NBS* gene was not localized in the *ATM* region at 11q23.1 (Stumm et al., 1995). In agreement with this linkage exclusion, chromosome 11 could not complement the NBS phenotype on the cellular level in chromosome transfer studies (Komatsu et al., 1996). In 1988 it was postulated that NBS is a heterogeneous disease and that NBS patients fall into two complementation groups, AT-V1 (Nijmegen breakage syndrome) and AT-V2 (Berlin breakage syndrome) (Jaspers et al., 1988a, 1988b; Wegner et al., 1988). This conclusion was based on complementation studies using differentially labeled parental fibroblast cell lines in fusion experiments and comparing the rate of DNA synthesis in homokaryons with that in heterokaryons after irradiation or bleomycin treatment. Doubts about the reliability of this assay came with the report that A-T patients assigned to four complementation groups by employing the same assay actually all carried allelic mutations in the same gene, the *ATM* gene (Savitsky et al., 1995). Subsequent cell fusion studies between AT-V1 and AT-V2 LCLs failed to achieve complementation, although there was clear normalization in the rate of chromosomal aberrations after fusion with normal cells (Stumm et al., 1997).

Finally, mapping of the *NBS* gene was initiated using two approaches. One was a whole-genome scan by polymerase chain reaction (PCR)-based microsatellite markers, the other followed the concept of unmasking heterozygosity. The latter study involved linkage studies in NBS families with markers spanning the potential gene loci at the breakpoints of a constitutional translocation t(3;7)(q12;q31.3) in a NBS patient, where the derivative chromosomes were transmitted from the unaffected father to the affected daughter. Both linkage and haplotype analysis with markers spanning both translocation breakpoints on chromosomes 3 and 7 in 12 NBS families allowed the clear exclusion of an AT-V gene from the translocation breakpoints (Chrzanowska et al., 1997) but failed to identify the gene location. In contrast, the whole-genome scan was successful in localizing the gene. The analysis of 20 NBS patients from 14 families proved linkage to a 1 cM interval between markers D8S171 and D8S170 on chromosome 8q21 in all families. Furthermore, these results indicate that there is only one single *NBS* gene (Saar et al., 1997).

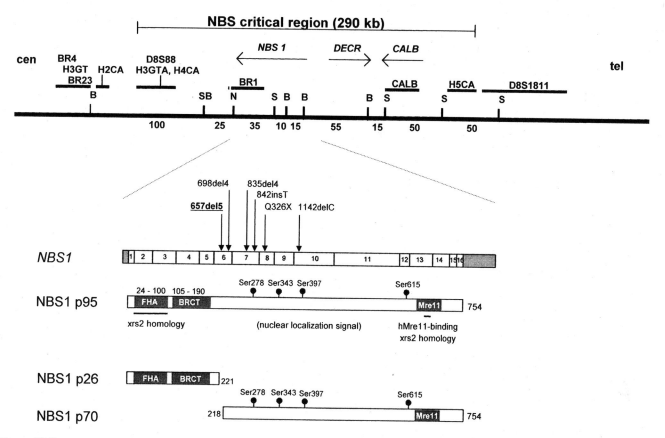

Figure 30.7. The *NBS1* gene and protein(s). Shown here is a physical map of the NBS1 region as defined by haplotype analyses of Nijmegen breakage syndrome (NBS) patients of Slavic origin. The positions of genes and genetic markers are indicated. The numbers below the line representing the DNA indicate the distances in kb between restriction enzyme sites (S, SalI; N, NotI; B, BamHI). Below the physical map, the exon structure of the *NBS1* gene is shown expanded. The position of mutations and the location of forkhead-associated (FHA) and breast cancer carboxy-terminal (BRCT) protein domains within the 754 residue p95 sequence are indicated. Serine residues that are phosphorylation targets are shown together with regions demonstrating similarity to yeast Xrs2 or implicated in binding to MRE11. Two protein fragments, p26 and p70, are found in NBS patient cells carrying the 657del5 mutation because of premature termination of translation and alternative translation, respectively.

The *NBS1* gene

The gene underlying NBS, designated *NBS1*, was identified independently by two groups. Varon et al. (1998) employed the positional cloning strategy, whereas Carney et al. (1998) studied the hMre11/hRad50 double-strand repair complex and identified a third member of this complex, p95, as being the product of the *NBS1* gene, now called *nibrin*. As shown in Figure 30.7, the *NBS* gene spans about 50 kb of genomic DNA, has 16 exons, codes for a protein with 754 amino acids, and has a calculated molecular weight of 85 kDa. The mRNA is polyadenylated at two alternative sites, leading to mRNAs of 4.4 and 2.4 kb in all tissues examined thus far. Altogether, nine different mutations have been identified so far in NBS patients (Varon et al., 1998; Hiel et al., 2001; Maraschio et al., 2001; Resnick et al., 2002; Digweed and Sperling, 2004; P.J. Concannon and R.A. Gatti, www.geneclinics .org). The 657del5 mutation is the most widespread Slavic founder mutation, which results in a frameshift causing the largest truncation of nibrin. Seven additional truncation mutations were identified in exons 6, 7, 8, and 10, all downstream of the FHA/BRCT domains (Fig. 30.7). Therefore, all NBS patients studied to date have large sequence losses on the C-terminal portion of the protein. Nevertheless, all patients express a truncated protein containing the N-terminal domains, a finding suggesting

that these sequences may be essential during embryonic development and that *NBS1* null mutants would result in fetal death. In 2001, Maser et al. reported that NBS cells with the common 657del5 mutation produce a 70 kDa protein fragment (NBS1^{p70}) lacking the native N terminus, which associates with the hRAD50/hMRE11 complex. This NBS1^{p70} fragment is produced by internal translation initiation within the *NBS1* mRNA using an open reading frame generated by the 657del5 frameshift. Therefore, the common *NBS1* 657del5 mutation seems to be a hypomorphic mutation, encoding a partially functional protein that diminishes the severity of the NBS phenotype. This hypomorphic mutation might be essential for fetal development in humans and other mammals, because null mutations have not been found in humans, and mouse null mutants are nonviable (Zhu et al., 2001, Dumon-Jones et al., 2003). Interestingly, null mutations in *MRE11* and *RAD50* are also lethal in mammals (Xiao and Weaver, 1997; Luo et al., 1999). Although the amino acid sequence of nibrin shows no global homology to other known proteins, there are two domains within the N-terminal 200 residues that can be found in other proteins: a breast cancer carboxy-terminal (BCRT) domain, first described in the *BRCA1* gene, and a fork-head–associated (FHA) domain, named after the transcription factor family in which it was initially found (Fig. 30.7). Both of these domains are expected to be involved in protein–protein interaction. Two members of the NHEJ repair pathway of DNA DSBs, hMRE11 and hRAD50, were identified as molecular partners of nibrin (Carney et al., 1998). Nibrin shows a weak similarity (46%) to the yeast protein XRS2, restricted only to the first 115 amino acids. In contrast, the entire amino acid sequences of the MRE11 and RAD50 proteins are widely conserved from yeast to mammals.

Molecular Biology of Nibrin

Nibrin appears to exert multifunctional activity. The identification of nibrin as a member of the human NHEJ repair complex of DSB suggests that defective DSB repair may be the central problem in NBS. The impass involving p53 activation and cell cycle arrest indicate that nibrin may also be involved in signal transduction. Another possible role of nibrin involves its interaction with histone γ-H2AX, forming a complex that associates with irradiation-induced DSBs (Kobayashi et al., 2002). However, nibrin seems to have a much more important role in the processing of DSB. Within 30 minutes of irradiation, discrete nuclear foci can be visualized in the irradiated nuclei of cells by staining with antibodies to the repair proteins hMRE11 or hRAD50. Staining with antibodies to nibrin produces exactly the same pattern, demonstrating that nibrin remains in the nuclei for more than 8 hours post-irradiation. The formation of nuclear foci is fully abrogated in NBS cells (Color Plate 30.II). Even the diffuse nuclear staining found in unirradiated normal cells is lacking in NBS cells, and considerable proportions of hRAD50 and hMRE11 are localized in the cytoplasm rather than in the nucleus. Since hRAD50 and hMRE11 are still found as a complex in NBS cells, a functional nibrin is clearly responsible for the location of these repair enzymes to the sites of DNA damage (Carney et al., 1998; Ito et al., 1999). In addition, nibrin is essential for the phosphorylation of hMRE11 after DNA damage (Dong et al., 1999) and it potentiates the ATP-driven DNA unwinding and endonuclease activity by the hRAD50/hMRE11 complex (Paull and Gellert, 1999). The hRAD50/hMRE11/nibrin complex has manganese-dependent, single-stranded DNA endonuclease and 3′ to 5′ exonuclease activities, thus it may be directly responsible for preparation of DNA ends for rejoining (Trujillo et al., 1998). Taken together, these findings indicate that nibrin plays an important regulatory role in the hRAD50/hMRE11/nibrin complex that responds to irradiation-induced DNA damage. The whole complex may act as a key factor in signaling and processing of DSB to initiate NHEJ and possibly homologous recombination as well.

Molecular interactions between nibrin and other proteins

Considering the strong similarities in the cellular phenotypes of A-T and NBS, an important finding was the discovery that ATM and the hRAD50/hMRE11/nibrin complex function in the same network. Four laboratories reported that ATM modifies the hRAD50/hMRE11/nibrin complex by phosphorylation of nibrin (Gatei et al., 2000; Lim et al., 2000; Wu et al., 2000; Zhao et al., 2000). Following exposure to IR, rapid phosphorylation of at least two serine residues of nibrin occurs. It is possible that the phosphorylation of distinct residues could modify the hRAD50/hMRE11/nibrin complex in different ways and therefore play a concerted regulatory role. This function is disturbed in NBS cells, because cells expressing mutant nibrin cannot be phosphorylated by ATM. ATM-dependent activation of CHK2, a key protein in cell cycle control in response to DNA

damage, requires functional nibrin (Buscemi et al., 2001). Thus, apart from the function in DSB repair, the hRAD50/hMRE11/nibrin complex appears to be specifically required to activate checkpoint control pathways following the formation of DSBs (reviewed in D'Amours and Jackson, 2002).

Nibrin physically interacts with histone by direct binding to γ-H2AX, which is phophorylated in response to the introduction of DSB and may therefore act as a very early responder to the DNA repair machinery. The FHA/BRCT domain of nibrin is essential for physical interaction with γ-H2AX and seems to play a crucial role in the binding to histone and in localization of the hMRE11/hRAD50 repair complex to damaged DNA (Kobayashi et al., 2002). Additionally, as Nakanishi et al. (2002) were able to show, nibrin and the FA subtype D2 protein (FANCD2) cooperate in two distinct cellular functions, one involved in the response to DNA cross-links and another involved in the S-phase checkpoint control. Therefore, nibrin functions at the intersection of two main signaling pathways. In response to the DNA cross-linking agent MMC, nibrin assembles in subnuclear foci with hMRE11/hRAD50 and FANCD2. Ionizing radiation activates an S-phase checkpoint through the ATM- and NBS1-dependent phosphorylation of FANCD2. Thus the involvement of nibrin in the pathway of DNA cross-linking repair, as shown by molecular and cellular analysis, fits with earlier cytogenetic results of a significant increase in chromosomal aberrations above normal levels in NBS cells exposed to Trenimon (Wegner, 1991; Stumm et al., 1997) or other cross-linkers as discussed above (in Cytogenetics).

Moreover, there is evidence that the hMRE complex also plays an important role in prevention of DSB formation during the normal replicative process. It has been shown that certain helicases, for example, proteins mutated in Werner syndrome (WRN) (Cheng et al., 2004) and in Bloom syndrome (BLM) (Franchitto and Pichierri, 2002a, 2002b), associate with the hMRE complex via binding to NBS1 in vitro, and in vivo after IR or MMC exposure, preventing the accumulation of DSB during chromosomal DNA replication (Costanzo et al., 2001). These observations provide convincing evidence for a functional link of multiple proteins that are mutated in many of the known chromosomal instability syndromes, including FA, NBS, BS, Werner syndrome, and A-T (see Chapter 29).

Heterogeneity of Nijmegen Breakage Syndrome

Some patients indistinguishable from NBS by clinical and cellular criteria do not carry mutations in the *NBS1* gene (Cerosaletti et al., 1998; Hiel et al., 2001, Maraschio et al., 2003). These observations strongly suggest mutations in one or more other genes that may cause NBS-like phenotypes. Indeed, a novel non-homologous end-joining factor, NHEJ1, also called Cernunnos protein, has recently been identified and found to be mutated in patients with an NBS-like phenotype characterized by microcephaly, SCID, and chromosomal instability (Ahnesorg et al., 2006; Buck et al., 2006).

Prenatal Diagnosis

Prenatal diagnosis of NBS is based on molecular methods whenever the underlying gene mutations in the index patient or parents are known. When no informative molecular data are available, RDS analysis in cultured chorionic villi or amniotic fluid cells is a reliable method for identifying NBS in a fetus (Jaspers et al., 1990; Kleijer et al., 1994; Der Kaloustian at al., 1996). Heterozygotes cannot be diagnosed by cytogenetic means (Wegner, 1991). Detailed protocols for cytogenetic analysis of NBS and other chromosomal instability syndromes are provided by Wegner and Stumm (1999).

Treatment and Prognosis

There is no specific therapy for NBS. All treatments are symptomatic and must be individualized. Intravenous administration of immunoglobulins (IVIG) and antibiotic prophylaxis may be an effective treatment in patients with significant immune deficiency and recurrent infections. One should also keep in mind that immunodeficiency mandates avoidance of live vaccines. Because cellular susceptibility to radiation and chemotherapy is increased in NBS patients, as in those with A-T, diagnostic irradiation should be reduced as much as possible and management of cancer therapy must be modified (Hart et al., 1987; Busch, 1994; Seidemann et al., 2000; Barth et al., 2003). NBS females presenting with hypergonadotropic hypogonadism require hormonal replacement therapy to induce and complete puberty and to avoid osteoporosis (Pozo and Argente, 2003). The overall prognosis for patients with NBS is unfavorable as compared to normal individuals, with premature death occurring due to either overwhelming infection or malignancies.

Bloom Syndrome

Bloom syndrome (BS) (MIM 210900) is an autosomal recessive chromosomal instability syndrome. The most consistant physical feature of BS is a strikingly small but well-proportioned body size and predisposition to the early development of a variety of cancers (German, 1993; German and Ellis, 2002). BS is the consequence of either homozygosity or compound heterozygosity of mutations in *BLM*, a gene that encodes the phylogenetically highly conserved nuclear RECQL2-helicase.

Clinical and Pathological Manifestations

Bloom syndrome was first recognized as a clinical entity by a dermatologist (Bloom, 1954). The most striking clinical feature, besides the small body size, is a sun-sensitive erythematous skin lesion in the butterfly area of the face, a feature that diagnostically sets the smallness of BS apart from other growth deficiencies (Color Plate 30.III). The full spectrum of BS has been defined by collecting clinical data through the Bloom Syndrome Registry (German and Passarge, 1989), in which a cohort of 169 patients diagnosed before 1991 has been enrolled and a second cohort of 60 additional cases added after January 1991. The clinical features and complications that constitute the phenotype BS, based on the Registry data, are summarized in Table 30.6 (German 1993; German and Ellis, 2002; unpublished registry data). Following Bloom's original report (1954) of a sun-sensitive "telangiectatic erythema resembling lupus erythematosus in dwarfs," additional classic features of BS were reported: (1) a striking sparcity of adipose tissue throughout infancy and childhood, (2) serious gastrointestinal problems during infancy, (3) susceptibility to respiratory tract and middle ear infections, and (4) sub- or infertility and an unusually early menopause. Nevertheless, at least five women with BS have become pregnant (Chisholm et al., 2001). Major complications of BS, subsequently observed and confirmed by findings from the registry, include chronic lung disease, which developed in at least 9 of the 169 individuals from cohort I, causing premature death in 5 at a mean age of 24.6 years. Although

Table 30.6. Clinical Phenotype, Immunodeficiency, and Chromosomal Abnormalities of Bloom Syndrome

Growth and Development

Abnormally small body size
Sparseness of subcutaneous fat
Slightly disproportional microcephaly
Characteristic facial and head configuration
Minor anatomical malformations

Skin Lesions

Sun-sensitive erythema limited almost exclusively to the face and dorsa of hands and forearms
Non–sun-sensitive hyper- and hypopigmented areas

Gastrointestinal Symptoms

Most consistent during infancy
Gastroesophageal reflux, vomiting
Anorexia
Diarrhea

Infertility

Lack of sperm production
Premature menopause

Complications

Chronic lung disease
Diabetes mellitus, type II
Neoplasia

Immunodeficiency

Hypogammaglobulinemia
Depressed delayed type hypersensitivity
Susceptibility to infections, mostly bacterial
    Upper and lower respiratory tract
    Otitis media

Genomic Instability in Somatic Cells

Aberrant DNA replication
Increased chromosomal interchanges
    Sister chromatid exchange
    Quadriradials, telomeric association

considered to be a consequence of recurrent lung infections, an alternative etiology, gastroesophageal reflux, has been proposed as cause of the chronic lung pathology. Diabetes mellitus, diagnosed at the mean age of 25.7 years, developed in 31 individuals of cohort I. A total of 143 episodes of cancer have been diagnosed in 90 of the 169 patients with BS. This remarkable predisposition to the early development of cancer is a hallmark of BS (German et al., 1997) and of the other chromosomal instability syndromes described in this chapter and in Chapter 29. By age 25, approximatley half of the patients with BS will have developed a malignacy, many of them more than one type. In the first two decades of life, the predominant types are leukemia and NHL. Later, carcinoma affecting predominantly the colon, skin, and breast are common. An increased risk of colorectal cancer in BLM heterocygosity has been observed in one study of Ashkenazi Jews (Gruber et al., 2002), but not in another (Cleary et al., 2003).

Laboratory Findings

Cytogenetics

Once BS is suspected, the diagnosis can be confirmed by kariotyping: the chromosomes of PHA-stimulated lymphocytes of an individual with BS exhibit an excessive number of sister-chromatid

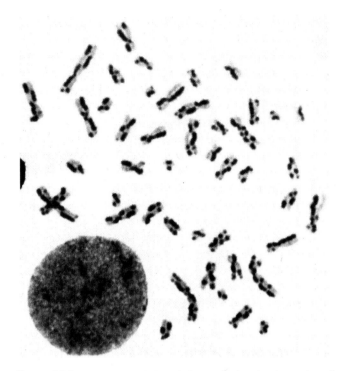

Figure 30.8. The characteristic and diagnostic elevation in number of sister chromatid exchanges (SCEs) in a cultured Bloom syndrome cell exposed to bromodeoxyuridine (BrdU) for two cell division cycles. Differentiation of the sister chromatids, dark or light, is accomplished by exposure of the BrdU-substituted chromosomes to the Hoechst dye 33258, then to light, and finally to Giemsa stain. The approximately 135 SCEs in this cell contrast with the fewer than 10 SCEs seen in similarly treated normal cells. A quadriradial chromosome is visible in the left field.

exchanges (SCE) (Fig. 30.8), a finding uniquely characteristic of BS (German et al., 1977).

In addition to the high numbers of SCEs, cultured B and T lymphocytes and skin fibroblasts from individuals with BS exhibit enhanced chromosome instability—"breakage"—as indicated by an increased number of chromatid gaps and breaks and structurally rearranged chromosomes. Approximately 1% of cultured lymphocytes in metaphase display a symmetrical four-armed configuration, designated as *quadriradial* (QR), composed of two homologous chromosomes. Opposite arms of the QR are of equal length, and the centromeres are positioned opposite one another (Fig. 30.8; see also Cytogenetics of Fanconi Anemia, above; Fig. 30.1). A QR of the type characteristic of BS is cytogenetic evidence that during the preceding S phase an interchange took place between chromatids of the members of a homologous chromosome pair, and the point of exchange apparently was at homologous sites. Historically, QRs constituted the first evidence that homologous recombination can occur in mammalian somatic cells in the form of somatic crossing-over.

Somatic cell mutability

Neither the SCEs nor the homologous chromatid interchanges exemplified by the QRs are necessarily mutagenic, although the interchanges would give rise to recombined chromosomes in half of the progeny of affected cells. However, the many gaps and breaks observed in metaphases do suggest that the excessive chromatid-exchange mechanism in BS cells is error prone. Direct evidence of increased spontaneous mutability of BS cells in vivo comes from studies that estimate the frequency of mutations affecting specific loci in human tissues. Coding loci that have been examined

cytogenetically (but not at the molecular level) include the enzyme hypoxanthine-guanine phosphoribosyltransferase (HGPRT) located on the X chromosome, the MN blood type (the glycophorin A locus on choromose 4), and the major histocompatibility complex (on chromosome 6). For all three loci studied, the frequency of mutations in BS cells is greatly increased, for example, up to eight-fold for HGPRT (Vijayalaxmi et al., 1983) and 50- to 100-fold for the glycophorin A locus (Langlois et al., 1989). Finally, noncoding repetitive loci examined by molecular techniques were found to be hypermutatable and molecular evidence confirming the cytogenic evidence for excessive somatic recombination has been obtained in proliferating cells from a patient with BS (Groden et al., 1990). Thus, BS has to be considered a "mutator phenotype" (German, 1992) with mutations of many types, arising from nucleotide substitutions, deletions, and homologous recombination, and presumably affecting any part of the genome, accumulating excessively in proliferating cells both in vivo and in vitro.

Hematologic studies

Standard hematologic parameters are normal except in those patients who have developed leukemia or preleukemia. Persistent anemia, usually mild and asymptomatic, is present in a subgroup of individuals with BS. Data submitted to the BS registry indicated that a myelodysplactic syndrome developed in 11 patients following cancer chemotherapy and spontaneously in one young adult BS patient.

Endocrine studies

Ten individuals with BS, 9 months to 28 years of age, underwent endocrine evaluation; three nondiabetic children were found to have glucose intolerance and insulin resistance; two young adults had unsuspected diabetes or prediabetes. Growth hormone production was normal in all 10 patients studied (M.I. New, unpublished results).

Semen from approximately a dozen men with BS lacked spermatozoa completely with one exception, an adolescent who had sperm of abnormal morphology (J. German, unpublished results). Men heterozygous for a BS-causing mutation (fathers of BS patients) produced an increased number of spermatozoa with multiple beaks and rearrangements (Martin et al., 1994), suggesting that the infertility in men with BS is the consequence of a disturbance in meiosis. Supporting this summation is the finding that in normal mouse testes the BS protein (BSM) (vide infra) colocalizes with the replication protein A in the meiotic bivalent at the time of crossing over (Walpita et al., 1999).

Immunologic studies

Abnormal immune function, a common finding in BS patients, is highly variable and usually not severe (Hutteroth et al., 1975; Weemaes et al., 1979, 1991; Taniguchi et al., 1982; Van Kerckhove et al., 1988; Etzioni et al., 1989; Kondo et al., 1992a, 1992b). Hypogammaglobulinemia has been present in 87% of patients entered in the BS registry and involves one or more serum immunoglobulin classes (IgM, IgA, and, less commonly, IgG). Although most BS patients have decreased in vitro production of immunoglobulin, the majority have normal in vitro antibody responses to vaccines. Delayed-type hypersensitivity skin tests are generally negative, but skin reactivity to DNCB has been induced. Absolute lymphocyte counts and percentages of CD4+ and CD8+ T cells, B cells, and NK cells are normal, and most BS patients have normal in vitro lymphocyte proliferation to mitogens. Abnormal NK cell function has been reported (Ueno et al., 1985).

It is unclear if the increased rate of infection is a direct consequence of usually mild and variable immune deficiency. Data from the BS registries indicate that 86% of individuals who develop serious infections have a deficiency of one or more serum immunoglobulin isotypes, but in 14% immunoglobulin concentrations are normal. Of those patients without a history of infections, however, 28% have abnormally low immunoglobulin levels. V(D)J recombination (Hsieh et al., 1993) and somatic hypermutation of immunoglobulin genes (Sack et al., 1998) are normal and in agreement with the observation that most patients with BS respond normally to vaccinations.

Genetics and Molecular Basis of Bloom Syndrome

Bloom syndrome had been recognized throughout the world as a very rare genetic disease, with the exception of the Ashkenazi Jewish population, in which approximately 1 in 110 individuals is a carrier of BS. Genetic analysis is consistent with autosomal recessive transmission: parents of BS patients are clinically unaffected; both sexes are equally affected; the ratio of affected to nonaffected siblings among those born after the index case are approximately 1:4; and, in non-Ashkenazi families, parental consanguinity is over 25%. The high parental consanguinity rate among non-Ashkenazi families with BS combined with the hypermutability of BS cells allowed for homozygosity mapping to localize the gene to chromosome band 15q26.1 (German et al., 1994). Subsequently, the gene responsible for BS was identified and found to be mutated in patients with BS (Ellis et al., 1995). The same group showed that 96% of patients whose parents were related were homozygous for a polymorphic marker in the proto-oncogene *FES*, strongly suggesting that the *BLM* gene is tightly linked to FES (Ellis et al., 1994). Ellis and associates (1995) observed that in some BS patients a minority of blood lymphocytes had normal SCE rates. Using lymphoblastoid cells established from patients with low SCE rates in peripheral blood lymphocytes, it was shown that polymorphic loci distal to the gene localization on 15q became homozygous, whereas markers proximal to the gene remained heterozygous. These findings were interpreted that low-SCE lymphocytes arose by recombination in patients who had inherited alleles from their (nonconsanguinous) parents that were mutated in different sites and thus had generated a functionally wild-type gene. On the basis of polymorphic markers used, the recombination must have occurred between the polymorphic loci D15S1108 and D15S127, a 250 kb region. Following the construction of a physical map of this region (Straughen et al., 1996), a candidate gene, designated *BLM*, was identified within the cDNA from this region (Ellis et al., 1995). Sequence analysis of this gene in BS patients revealed nonsense and missense mutations. The BLM cDNA consists of 4437 nucleotides and encodes a 1417–amino acid protein with homology to the RecQ family of helicases in *Escherichia coli*. The finding that the high SCE rate observed in BS cells could be reduced to control values if a normal *BLM* gene was transfected into cells obtained from BS patients further confirmed that *BLM* was indeed the gene responsible for BS. BLM, therefore, is a member of the same subfamily of helicases that includes the Sgs1 protein of *Saccharomyces cerevisiae* and the human proteins WRN and RECQ4, mutated, respectively, in Werner syndrome and some cases of Rothmund-Thomson syndrome. The fact that *BLM* is most closely related to the yeast proteins Rghlp and Sgs (Kusano et al., 1999) is of interest because *BLM* has been demonstrated to suppress premature aging and increased homologous recombination caused by mutations of the *Sgs1* gene (Heo et al., 1999). Studies of mutants for *Dmblm*, the *Drosophila* homolog of human *BLM*, suggests that this gene functions in DSB repair (Kusano

et al., 1999, 2001; Adams et al., 2003). BLM has been identified as a DNA binding protein with preference for DNA structures that resemble the presumed initial intermediate formed during homologous recombination; it can bind to and unwind such substrates in vitro, including holiday junctions and D loops (Van Brabant et al., 2000). These observations, together with the high rate of QR and SCE formation, support the hypothesis that *BLM* plays an antirecombinogenic function and that cells from BS patients, in which *BLM* function is lacking, are hyperrecombinogenic.

Western blot analysis and immunofluorescence microscopy demonstrate that cultured lymphblastoid cells from most BS patients lack BLM. In normal cells, BLM protein is localized within the nucleus, where its total amount, distribution, and colocalization with other nuclear proteins varies at different phases of the cell division cycle (Sanz et al., 2000).

BLM has been identified as a member of a group of proteins that associate with BRCA1 to form a large complex that has been named *BASC* (BRCA1-associated genome surveillance complex). This complex consists of tumor suppressors and DNA damage repair proteins including MSH2, MSH6, MLH1, ATM, BLM, and the RAD50/MRE11/NBS1 protein complex (Wang et al., 2000). These proteins colocalize to large nuclear foci when cells are treated with agents that interfere with DNA synthesis. All members of this complex play roles in the recognition of abnormal DNA structures or damaged DNA, suggesting that BASC may serve as a sensor for DNA damage. Thus, BLM is part of a protein complex that coordinates the activities required for maintenance and genome integrity during the process of DNA replication, activities suggesting a central role for BLM as well as NBS1 in DNA repair.

Transfection of a normal *BLM* gene into cultured SV40-transformed BS fibroblasts results in nuclear transfer of the BLM protein and reduction of the SCE rate, indicating that the helicase activity of BLM is required for its function (Ellis et al., 1999; Neff et al., 1999). The most common mutation of BLM is a 6 bp deletion/7 bp insertion in exon 10, which is the homozygous mutation causing BS in Ashkenazi Jews (Ellis et al., 1995). More than 60 unique mutations in the *BLM* gene have been identified in families with at least one affected individual. Homozygosity for a given BS mutation is found in most BS patients whose parents are known to be cousins. In non-Ashkenazi families, in which the parents are not related, compound heterozygosity is most common. There is no obvious genotype–phenotype correlation.

Other human genes in the RecQ family include *RECQ4*, mutated in Rothmund Thomson syndrome (Lindor et al., 2000); *RECQ3* (WRN), mutated in Werner syndrome (Yu et al., 1996); and *RECQL/RecQ1* and *RECQ5*, for which no syndromes have yet been identified.

Carrier Detection and Prenatal Diagnosis

Carrier females can be identified by DNA analysis if the mutation affecting the index case is known. A rapid method for detection of the Ashkenazi Jewish mutation is available (Straughen et al., 1998). Prenatal diagnosis of BS has been achieved by identifying a high rate of SCE in chorionic villi (Howell and Davies, 1994). Mutation analysis of fetal DNA is, however, the most reliable technique to establish the status of a fetus.

Treatment and Prognosis

Adequate nutrition is a common problem in infants and young children with BS, who typically show little interest in eating. This is compounded by frequent episodes of vomiting and diarrhea that may lead to life-threatening episodes of dehydration requiring hospitalization and may ultimately lead to the need for gastrostomy tube feeding. Infections require prompt diagnosis and adequate treatment with antibiotics. If hypogammaglobulinemia is documented and antibody deficiency demonstrated, the use of IVIG is recommended. In BS, as in patients with A-T, the extent of immune deficiency varies greatly.

Steps should be taken to protect the face of BS patients from sun exposure, especially during the early years of life. The diabetes mellitus observed in individuals with BS resembles that of the adult-onset condition, although it generally occurs earlier, usually in the 20s and 30s. Importantly, patients and their families should be informed about the high risk of developing cancer, so that appropriate surveillance mechanisms can be put into place. Because individuals with BS are hypersensitive to chemotherapeutic agents, use of these compounds may have to be adjusted. Interestingly, the tumors of BS patients seem to be more sensitive to these therapeutic agents and cures have been reported using approximately half the dose of standard protocols.

Measures to increase height in patients, including growth hormone administration, have been largely unsuccessful. It has been postulated that the absence of BLM from somatic cells places a restriction on cell number and size, possibly through the deregulation of the p53 tumor suppressor pathway, which may not be limited to malignant cells (Garkavtsev et al., 2001).

Animal Models

Disrupting *Blm* gene function in mice has created useful models for BS. Depending on the defect created by a targeted mutation of *Blm*, homozygous mutant animals may exhibit embryonic lethality while in other mice homozygosity may yield viable and fertile animals with a cancer predisposition. In one model, a site upstream of the Blm helicase homology domain was targeted for disruption by use of homologous recombination. Whereas heterozygous mice appear normal and are phenotypically identical to wild-type littermates, mouse embryos homozygous for this mutation appear developmentally delayed and die by embryonic day 13.5 (Chester et al., 1998). Blm$^{-/-}$ littermates were smaller in size by 50% at 9.5 days post-conception and remained smaller until death at 13.5 days post-conception. Interestingly, the Blm$^{-/-}$ embryos were normal in their own body proportion and without structural abnormalities.

This BS knockout mouse model recapitulates many aspects of the human disease, including small size of the embryos, increased numbers of micronuclei in embryo blood cells, slow growth of cultured embryo fibroblasts, and, finally, a high number of SCE in cultured embryo fibroblasts, characteristically also seen in cells from Bloom patients. These data suggest that mutation of *BLM* in humans is sufficient to cause most aspects of the human disorder.

In addition, studies of mouse embryos clearly demonstrate increased programed cell death, an observation not previously described in BS patients. There was also a marked reduction of the blood volume and the number of circulating red blood cells beginning at 9.5 days post-conception; the affected embryos had only 5% or 10% as much blood as their wild-type littermates. Furthermore, an increased number of macrocytes and an increased presence of nuclear fragments were present in mutant vs. wild-type erythrocytes (Chester et al., 1998).

Another knockout mouse model with a hypomorphic Blm protein produced a diminished quantity of normal mRNA and protein. These animals were viable and showed an inverse correlation between the quantity of Blm protein and the level of chromosome instability and a similar genotypic relationship for tumor predisposition, suggesting that Blm protein is rate limiting for maintaining genome stability and the avoidance of tumors (McDaniel et al., 2003). These viable knockout mice had an 18-fold increase in the rate of somatic loss of heterozygosity (LOH), indicating a marked elevation of the mitotic recombination rate in mutated cells (Luo et al., 2000). Cell lines from these mice show elevations in the rate of mitotic recombination. These mice are also prone to a wide variety of cancers.

A unique mouse model was generated using gene targeting by homologous recombination to disrupt the mouse *Blm* gene to simulate BLM^{Ash}, a BS-causing mutant allele of BLM carried by approximately 1% of Ashkenazi Jews (Li et al., 1998). This mutation causes a frameshift in exon 10 that results in premature translation termination. Homozygous disruption of Blm by this method resulted in embryonic lethality. Cell lysates from heterozygous animals (Blm$^{+/-}$) had an approximately 50% reduction in Blm compared to wild type. There was a twofold increase in the number of micronuclei in BrdU-treated cultures of heterozygous deficient cells, a result suggesting that heterozygous cells have a subtle increase in genomic instability presumably related to the reduced BLM level. There was a slight acceleration in the development of murine leukemia virus–induced metastatic T cell lymphoma and an increased incidence of intestinal adenomas in mice heterozygous for this Blm mutation (Goss et al., 2002). These results demonstrate that Blm haploinsufficiency is sufficient to affect tumor formation in susceptible mice and probably to alter genome stability. This increased susceptibility to cancer in heterozygous mice supports the finding in human carriers for BS that they have an increased risk of colorectal cancer (Gruber et al., 2002).

Rare Syndromes with Chromosomal Instability

Patients with the clinical and cytogenetic features of chromosomal instability syndromes, in particular NBS and AT, but without mutations in the respective genes are of particular interest because they may disclose clues about unknown gene products involved in the network of genome integrity surveillance. Ligase I (LIG1) deficiency (MIM 126391) was described in one female patient with typical features of a chromosomal instability syndrome: growth retardation, telangiectasia, immunodeficiency, and lymphoma, at the age of 19 years (Webster et al., 1992). Hypersensitivity to UV light, alkylating agents, and IR was observed at the clinical and cellular levels. Molecular analysis identified two missense mutations in the *LIG1* gene (Barnes et al., 1992). A link to the NHEJ repair network was suggested by the finding of a physical association of LIG1 with MRE11 (Petrini et al., 1995). Only one patient with LIG1 deficiency has been described thus far. This low number might be explained by the minor role of LIG1 in NHEJ, compared to that of ligase IV (LIG4) (see below), which can be substituted more easily. Another explanation might be the presence of undetected mutations in another gene involved in NHEJ.

More recently, mutations in the *LIG4* gene were shown to cause an NBS-like syndrome in four patients (O'Driscoll et al., 2001) (Table 30.1). On the cellular level, cell lines from LIG4-deficient patients show pronounced radiosensitivity similar to that in NBS. In contrast to NBS cells, LIG4-deficient cells show normal cell cycle checkpoint responses but impaired DSB rejoining. Since V(D)J recombination is also affected, immunodeficiency is part of the clinical phenotype. Thus, LIG4, if mutated,

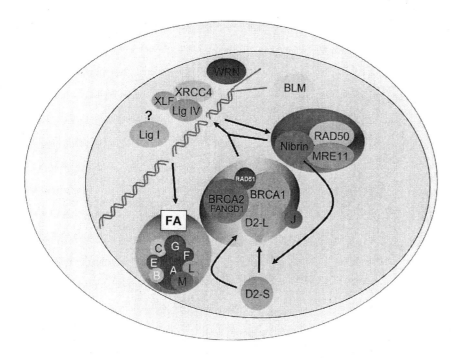

Figure 30.9. The network of proteins mutated in chromosomal instability syndromes. This highly simplified schematic drawing shows the proteins acting in the double-strand break network. Only proteins mutated in chromosomal instability syndromes presented in this chapter are shown. Four complexes are present: (1) the Fanconi anemia (FA) complex, (2) the MRE11/RAD50/nibrin complex, (3) the LIG4 complex, and (4) the complex consisting of BRCA 1/BRAC 2/RAD51/FA-D2-L. The BASC complex (Wang et al., 2000) includes BRCA1, BLM, and RAD50/MRE11/nibrin. Lig, ligase; WRN, Werner syndrome; XLF, XLF/NHEJ1/Cernunnos Protein.

is responsible for the defective DSB repair, resulting in a novel primary immunodeficiency syndrome (LIG4 syndrome, MIM *606593). By targeted disruption of both *LIG4* alleles in a human pre-B cell line studied for radiosensitivity, Grawunder et al. (1998) showed that LIG4 activity is responsible for the ligation step in nonhomologous DNA end joining and in V(D)J recombination.

It has been demonstrated that LIG4 forms a tight complex with the protein XRCC4 (Grawunder et al. 1998) to repair DSB by the NHEJ pathway. However, it took 8 more years to identify the third partner of this complex, which was suspected by Dai and colleagues (2003) while studying a patient with T⁻B⁻SCID whose cells showed dramatic radiosensitivity, decreased DSB rejoining, and reduced fidelity in signal and coding joint formation during V(D)J recombination. This patient (2BN), while sharing several characteristics of NBS and of LIG4 deficiency did not have mutations in the respective genes (Dai et al., 2003). Two groups recently reported independently mutations in a hitherto unknown gene through cDNA functional complementation cloning (Buck et al., 2006) and yeast two-hybrid screening for *XRCC4* interactors (Ahnesorg et al., 2006), respectively. This novel protein has been named Cernunnos (Buck et al., 2006) or XLF (Ahnesorg et al., 2006) and was officially designated as non-homologous end-joining factor 1 (NHEJ1). Mutations in this gene are responsible for the clinical phenotype mentioned above, including microcephaly, and for defective NHEJ and V(D)J recombination resulting in severe combined immune deficiency (Buck et al., 2006).

Bendix et al. reported (at the International Workshop on NBS, Prague, April 2002) a patient with a disorder resembling NBS who harbored different hypomorphic mutations, one in each allele of the *RAD50* gene. The girl, originally described in 1991 by Barbi et al., presented with many clinical characteristics of NBS, but not with immunodeficiency (Table 30.1). The Rad50 deficiency (MIM *604040) resulted in increased spontaneous chromosomal instability, radiosensitivity, RDS, impaired nibrin phosphorylation, and impaired nuclear foci formation after irradiation. Since hRAD50 is one of the three partners of the hMRE11/hRAD50/nibrin complex, it is not surprising to find the

NBS phenotype in a compound heterozygous individual. The link between RAD50 deficiency and increased radiosensitivity points to the importance of a fully functional hMRE11/hRAD50/nibrin complex for reliable NHEJ.

More surprising is the clinical picture of patients carrying mutations in the *hMRE11* gene (Stewart et al., 1999). Because these patients show many similarities to A-T, although with a milder phenotype and without mutations in the *ATM* gene, this syndrome has been called ataxia-telangiectasia–like disorder (A-TLD) (MIM #604391). The protein hMRE11 is engaged in forming the hMRE11/hRAD50/nibrin complex, which plays an early role in a signal transduction pathway responding to DSB induced by IR and radiomimetic chemicals (Taylor et al., 2004). Both these events activate DNA repair as well as cell cycle checkpoint controls. All *hMRE11* mutations observed in this recessive disorder result in the expression of proteins with some residual function that may be necessary for the survival of affected patients. Typically, this residual function results from a hypomorphic mutation of at least one *hMRE11* allele.

Concluding Remarks

The descriptive level of chromosomal instability syndromes of only one decade ago has been complemented by the discovery that the chromosomal instability syndromes not only form subgroups based on their descriptive features but are actually linked together at the molecular level. Most if not all genes mutated in the syndromes described in this chapter (including *ATM*) take part in the complex network of DSB sensing, signal transduction, and DNA repair. Although much more has to be done to determine specific functional aspects, the facts known to date allow a first glimpse into the complex network of genomic stability maintenance. A very simplified schema of this network is shown in Figure 30.9, which lists only those gene products mutated in chromosomal instability syndromes presented in this chapter. Their physiologic functions have been demonstrated by the analysis of gene mutations in relevant patients. The identification and investigation of additional pathological conditions are essential to a better understanding of these crucial cellular processes; for the benefit of our patients, it is even more important to generate new ideas that lead to more effective treatments of these devastating genetic disorders.

References

Adams MD, McVey ML, Sekelsky JJ. *Drosophila* BLM in double-strand break repair by synthesis-dependent strand annealing. Science 299:265–267, 2003.

Ahmad SI, Hanaoka F, Kirk SH. Molecular biology of Fanconi anaemia—an old problem, a new insight. Bioassays 24:439–448, 2002.

Ahnesorg P, Smith P, Jackson SP. XLF interacts with the XRCC4-DNA Ligase IV complex to promote DNA nonhomologous end-joining. Cell 124:301–313, 2006.

Alter BP. Fanconi's anemia and malignancies. Am J Hematol 53:99–110, 1996.

Antoccia A, di Masi A, Maraschio P, Stumm M, Ricordy R, Tanzarella C. G2-phase radiation response in lymphoblastoid cell lines from Nijmegen breakage syndrome. Cell Prolif 35:93–104, 2002.

Antoccia A, Ricordy R, Maraschio P, Prudente S, Tanzarella C. Chromosomal sensitivity to clastogenic agents and cell cycle perturbations in Nijmegen breakage syndrome lymphoblastoid cell lines. Int J Radiat Biol 71:41–49, 1997.

Antoccia A, Stumm M, Saar K Ricordy R, Maraschio P, Tanzarella C. Impaired p53-mediated DNA damage response, cell-cycle disturbance and chromosome aberrations in Nijmegen breakage syndrome lymphoblastoid cell lines. Int J Radiat Biol 75:583–591, 1999.

Aurias A, Dutrillaux B. Probable involvement of immunoglobin superfamily genes in most recurrent chromosomal rearrangements from ataxia telangiectasia. Hum Genet 72:210–214, 1986.

Aurias A, Dutrillaux B, Buriot D, Lejeune J. High frequency of inversions and translocations of chromosomes 7 and 14 in ataxia-telangiectasia. Mutat Res 69:369–374, 1980.

Bakhshi S, Cerosaletti KM, Concannon P, Bawle EV, Fontanesi J, Gatti R, Bharnabhani K. Medulloblastoma with adverse reaction to radiation therapy in Nijmegen breakage syndrome. J Pediatr Hematol Oncol, 25:248–251, 2003.

Barbi G, Scheres JM, Schindler D, Taalmann RD, Rodens K, Mehnert K, Müller M, Seyschab H. Chromosome instability and X-ray hypersensitivity in a microcephalic and growth-retarded child. Am J Med Genet 40:44–50, 1991.

Barnes DE, Tomkinson AE, Lehmann AR, Webster DB, Lindahl T. Mutations in the DNA ligase gene of an individual with immunodeficiencies and cellular hypersensitivity to DNA-damaging agents. Cell 69:495–503, 1992.

Barth E, Demori E, Pecile V, Zanazzo GA, Malorgio C, Tamaro P. Anthracyclines in Nijmegen breakage syndrome. Med Pediatr Oncol 40:122–124, 2003.

Bekiesinska-Figatowska M, Chrzanowska KH, Jurkiewicz E, Wakulinska A, Rysiewskis H, Gladkowska-Dura M, Walecki J. Magnetic resonance imaging of brain abnormalities in patients with the Nijmegen breakage syndrome. Acta Neurobiol Exp (Wars) 64:503–509, 2004.

Bekiesińska-Figatowska M, Chrzanowska KH, Sikorska J, Walecki J, Krajewska-Walasek M, Jóźwiak S, Kleijer WJ. Cranial MRI in the Nijmegen breakage syndrome. Neuroradiology 42:43–47, 2000.

Bloom D. Congenital telangiectatic erythema resembling lupus erythematosus in dwarfs. Am J Dis Child 88:754–758, 1954.

Buck D, Malivert L, de Chasseval R, Barraud A, Fondaneche MC, Sanal O, Plebani A, Stephan JL, Hufnagel M, le Deist F, Fischer A, Durandy A, de Villartay JP, Revy P. Cernunnos, a novel nonhomologous end-joining factor, is mutated in human immunodeficiency with microcephaly. Cell 124:287–299, 2006.

Buscemi G, Savio C, Zannini L, Micciche F, Masnada D, Nakanishi M, Tauchi H, Komatsu K, Mizutani S, Khanna K, Chen P, Concannon P, Chessa L, Delia D. Chk2 activation dependence on Nbs1 after DNA damage. Mol Cell Biol 21:5214–5222, 2001.

Busch D. Genetic susceptibility to radiation and chemotherapy injury: diagnosis and management. Int J Radiat Oncol Biol Phys 30:997–1002, 1994.

Busch DB, Zdzienicka MZ, Natarajan AT, Jones NJ, Overkamp WJ, Collins A, Mitchell DL, Stefanini M, Botta E, Albert RB, Liu N, White DA, van Gool AJ, Thompson LH. A CHO mutant, UV40, that is sensitive to diverse mutagens and represents a new complementation group of mitomycin C sensitivity. Mutat Res 363:209–221, 1996.

Carlomagno F, Chang-Claude J, Dunning AM, Ponder BA. Determination of the frequency of the common 657del5 Nijmegen breakage syndrome mutation in the German population. No association with risk of breast cancer. Genes Chrom Cancer 25:393–395, 1999.

Carney JP, Maser RS, Olivares H, Davis EM, Le Beau M, Yates JR 3rd, Hays L, Morgan WF, Petrini JH. The hMre11/hRad50 protein complex and Nijmegen breakage syndrome: linkage of double-strand break repair to the cellular DNA damage response. Cell 93:477–486, 1998.

Cerosaletti KM, Lange E, Stringham HM, Weemaes CM, Smeets D, Solder B, Belohradsky BH, Taylor AM, Karnes P, Elliott A, Komatsu K, Gatti RA, Boehnke M, Concannon P. Fine localization of the Nijmegen breakage syndrome gene to 8q21: evidence for a common founder haplotype. Am J Hum Genet 63:125–134, 1998.

Cerosaletti KM, Morrison VA, Sabath DE, Willerford DM, Concannon P. Mutations and molecular variants of the *NBS1* gene in non-Hodgkin lymphoma. Genes Chromosomes Cancer 35:282–286, 2002.

Cheng NC, van de Vrugt HJ, van der Valk MA, Oostra AB, Krimpenfort P, de Vries Y, Joenje H, Berns A, Arwert F. Mice with a targeted disruption of the Fanconi anemia homolog Fanca. Hum Mol Genet 9:1805–1811, 2000.

Cheng WH, von Kobbe C, Opresko PL, Arthur LM, Komatsu K, Seidman MM, Carney JP, Bohr VA. Linkage between Werner syndrome protein and the Mre11 complex via Nbs1. J Biol Chem 279:21169–21176, 2004.

Chester N, Kuo F, Kozak C, O'Hara CD, Leder P. Stage-specific apoptosis, developmental delay, and embryonic lethality in mice homozygous for a targeted disruption of the murine Bloom's syndrome gene. Genes Dev 12:3382–3393, 1998.

Chisholm C, Bray M, Karns L. Successful pregnancy in a woman with Bloom syndrome. Am J Med Genet 999:136–138, 2001.

Chrzanowska KH. The Nijmegen breakage syndrome: clinical and genetic analysis (dissertation). Children's Memorial Health Institute, Warsaw, 1999.

Chrzanowska KH, Kleijer WJ, Krajewska-Walasek M, Bialecka M, Gutkowska A, Goryluk-Kozakiewicz B, Michalkiewicz J, Stachowski J, Gregorek H, Lyson-Wojciechowska G, Janowicz W, Jozwiak S. Eleven Polish patients with microcephaly, immunodeficiency, and chromosomal instability: the Nijmegen breakage syndrome. Am J Med Genet 57:462–471, 1995a.

Chrzanowska KH, Krajewska-Walasek M, Bialecka M, Metera M, Pçdich M. Ovarian failure in female patients with the Nijmegen breakage syndrome. Eur J Hum Genet 4(Suppl 1):122, 1996.

Chrzanowska KH, Krajewska-Walasek M, Michalkiewicz J, Gregorek H, Stachowski J, Janowicz W, Bialecka M, Gutkowska A. A study of humoral and cellular immunity in the Nijmegen breakage syndrome. In: Caragol I, Espanol T, Fontan G, Matamoros N, eds. Progress in Immune Deficiency V. Barcelona: Springer-Iberica, pp. 145–146, 1995b.

Chrzanowska KH, Piekutowska-Abramczuk D, Gładkowska-Dura M, Małdyk J, Syczewska M, Popowska E, Krajewska-Walasek M, and the Polish Pediatric Leukemia/Lymphoma Study Group. Germline 657del5 in the NBS1 gene in lymphoma/leukemia of childhood and adolescence. In: Proceedings of the 18th Meeting of the European Association fro Cancer Research, Innsbruck (Austria), July 3–6, 2004.

Chrzanowska KH, Piekutowska-Abramczuk D, Popowska E, Gładkowska-Dura M, Małdyk J, Syczewska M, Krajewska-Walasek M, et al. Carrier frequency of mutation 657del5 in the NBS1 gene in a population of polish pediatric patients with sporadic lymphoid malignancies. Int J Cancer. 2005.

Chrzanowska KH, Romer T, Krajewska-Walasek M, Gajtko-Metera M, Szarras-Czapnik M, Abramczuk D, Varon R, Rysiewski H, Janas R, Syczewska M. Evidence for a high rate of gonadal failure in female patients with Nijmegen breakage syndrome. Eur J Hum Genet 8(Suppl 1):73, 2000.

Chrzanowska KH, Stumm M, Bekiesiska-Figatowska M, Varon R, Biaecka M, Gregorek H, Michakiewicz J, Krajewska-Walasek M, Jowiak S, Reis A. Atypical clinical picture of the Nijmegen breakage syndrome associated with developmental abnormalities of the brain. J Med Genet 38:E3, 2001.

Chrzanowska KH, Stumm M, Bialecka M, Saar K, Bernatowska-Matuszkiewicz E, Michalkiewicz J, Barszcz S, Reis A, Wegner RD. Linkage studies exclude the AT-V gene(s) from the translocation breakpoints in an AT-V patient. Clin Genet 51:309–313, 1997.

Cleary SP, Zhang W, Di Nicola N, Aronson M, Aube J, Steinman A, Haddad R, Redston M, Gallinger S, Narod SA, Gryfe R. Heterozygosity for the BLM(Ash) mutation and cancer risk. Cancer Res 63:1769–1771, 2003.

Conley ME, Spinner NB, Emanuel BS, Nowell PC, Nichols WW. A chromosomal breakage syndrome with profound immunodeficiency. Blood 67:1251–1256, 1986.

Costanzo V, Robertson K, Bibikova M, Kim E, Grieco D, Gottesman M, Carroll D, Gautier J. Mre11 protein complex prevents double-strand break accumulation during chromosomal DNA replication. Mol Cell 8:137–147, 2001.

Cramer P, Painter RB. Bleomycin-resistant DNA synthesis in ataxia telangiectasia cells. Nature 291:671–672, 1981.

Curry CJ, O'Lague P, Tsai J, Hutchison HT, Jaspers NG, Wara D, Gatti RA. AT$_{Fresno}$: a phenotype linking ataxia-telangiectasia with the Nijmegen breakage syndrome. Am J Hum Gent 45:270–275, 1989.

Cybulski C, Górski B, Dębniak T, Gliniewicz B, Mierzejewski M, Masojc B, Jakubowska A, Matyjasik J, Złowocka E, Sikorski A, Narod SA, Lubiński J. NBS1 is a prostate cancer susceptibility gene. Cancer Res 64:1215–1219, 2004.

Dai Y, Kysela B, Hanakahi LA, Manolis K, Riballo E, Stumm M, Harville TO, West SC, Oettinger MA, Jeggo PA. Non-homologous end joining and V(D)J recombination require an additional factor. Proc Natl Acad Sci USA 100:2462–2467, 2003.

D'Amours D, Jackson SP. The MRE11 complex: at the crossroads of DNA repair and checkpoint signaling. Nature Rev 3:317–327, 2002.

Demuth I, Wlodarski M, Tipping AJ, Morgan NV, de Winter JP, Thiel M, Grasl S, Schindler D, D'Andrea AD, Altay C, Kayserili H, Zatterale A, Kunze J, Ebell W, Mathew CG, Joenje H, Sperling K, Digweed M. Spectrum of mutations in the Fanconi anemia group G gene, FANCG/XRCC9. Eur J Hum Genet 8:861–868, 2000.

Der Kaloustian VM, Kleijer W, Booth A, Auerbach AD, Mazer B, Elliott AM, Abish S, Usher R, Watters G, Vekemans M, Eydoux P. Possible new variant of the Nijmegen breakage syndrome. Am J Hum Gen 65:21–26, 1996.

De Stefano P, Pasquali F, Pendroni E, Colombo A, Vitiello A. Rilievi sale anomalie citogenetiche e immunitarie nella syndrome di Bloom. Riv Ital Red 3:371–379, 1977.

de Winter JP, van der Weel L, de Groot J, Stone S, Waisfisz Q, Arwert F, Scheper RJ, Kruyt FA, Hoatlin ME, Joenje H. The Fanconi anemia protein FANCF forms a nuclear complex with FANCA, FANCC and FANCG. Hum Mol Genet 9:2665–2674, 2000.

de Winter JP, Waisfisz Q, Rooimans MA, van Berkel CG, Bosnoyan-Collins L, Alon N, Bender O, Demuth I, Schindler D, Pronk JC, Arwert F, Hoehn H, Digweed M, Buchwald M, Joenje H. The Fanconi anemia group G gene is identical with human XRCC9. Nat Genet 20:281–283, 1998.

deWit J, Jaspers NG, Bootsma D. The rate of DNA synthesis in normal human and ataxia telangiectasia cells after exposure to X-irradiation. Mutat Res 80:221–226, 1981.

Digweed M, Demuth I, Rothe S, Scholz R, Jordan A, Grotzinger C, Schindler D, Grompe M, Sperling K. SV40 large T-antigen disturbs the formation of nuclear DNA-repair foci containing MRE11. Oncogene 21:4873–4878. 2002a.

Digweed M, Rothe S, Demuth I, Scholz R, Schindler D, Stumm M, Grompe M, Jordan A, Sperling K. Attenuation of the formation of DNA-repair foci containing RAD51 in Fanconi anaemia. Carcinogenesis 23:1121–1126, 2002b.

Digweed M, Sperling K. Nijmegen breakage syndrome: clinical manifestation of defective response to DNA double-strand breaks. DNA Repair 3:1207–1217, 2004.

Distel L, Neubauer S, Varon R, Holter W, Grabenbauer G. Fatal toxicity following radio- and chemotherapy of medulloblastoma in a child with unrecognised Nijmegen breakage syndrome. Med Pediatr Oncol 41:44–48, 2003.

Dong Z, Zhong Q, Chen PL. The Nijmegen breakage syndrome protein is essential for Mre11 phosphorylation upon DNA damage. J Biol Chem 274: 19513–19516, 1999.

Duker NJ. Chromosome breakage syndromes and cancer. Am J Med Genet 115:125–129, 2002.

Dumon-Jones V, Frappart PO, Tong WM, Sajithlal G, Hulla W, Schmid G, Herceg Z, Digweed M, Wang ZQ. Nbn heterozygosity renders mice susceptible to tumor formation and ionising radiation-induced tumorigenesis. Cancer Res 63:7263–7269, 2003.

Elenitoba-Johnson KS, Jaffe ES. Lymphoproliferative disorders associated with congenital immunodeficiencies. Semin Diagn Pathol 14:35–47, 1997.

Ellis NA, Groden J, Ye TZ, Straughen J, Lennon DJ, Ciocci S, Proytcheva M, German J. The Bloom's syndrome gene product is homologous to RecQ helicases. Cell 83:655–666, 1995.

Ellis NA, Proytcheva M, Sanz MM, Ye TZ, German J. Transfection of BLM into cultured Bloom syndrome cells reduces the SCE rate toward normal. Am J Hum Genet 65:1368–1374, 1999.

Ellis NA, Roe AM, Kozloski J, Proytcheva M, Falk C, German J. Linkage disequilibrium between the FES, D15S127, and BLM loci in Ashkenazi Jews with Bloom syndrome. Am J Human Genet 55:453–460, 1994.

Etzioni A, Lahat N, Benderly A, Katz R, Pollack S. Humoral and cellular immune dysfunction in a patient with Bloom's syndrome and recurrent infections. J Clin Lab Immunol 28:151–154, 1989.

Faivre L, Guardiola P, Lewis C, Dokal I, Ebell W, Zatterale A, Altay C, Poole J, Stones D, Kwee ML, van Weel-Sipman M, Havenga C, Morgan N, de Winter J, Digweed M, Savoia A, Pronk J, de Ravel T, Jansen S, Joenje H, Gluckman E, Mathew CG. Association of complementation group and mutation type with clinical outcome in fanconi anemia. European Fanconi Anemia Research Group. Blood 96:4064–4070, 2000.

Franchitto A, Pichierri P. Bloom's syndrome protein is required for correct relocalization RAD50/MRE11/NBS1 complex after replication fork arrest. J Cell Biol 157:19–30, 2002a.

Franchitto A, Pichierri P. Protecting genomic integrity during DNA replication: correlation between Werner's and Bloom's syndrome gene products and the MRE11 complex. Hum Mol Genet 11:2447–2453, 2002b.

Freie B, Li X, Ciccone SL, Nawa K, Cooper S, Vogelweid C, Schantz L, Haneline LS, Orazi A, Broxmeyer HE, Lee SH, Clapp DW. Fanconi anemia type C and p53 cooperate in apoptosis and tumorigenesis. Blood 102:4146–4152, 2003.

Futaki M, Yamashita T, Yagasaki H, Toda T, Yabe M, Kato S, Asano S, Nakahata T. The IVS4 + 4 A to T mutation of the fanconi anemia gene FANCC is not associated with a severe phenotype in Japanese patients. Blood 95:1493–1498, 2000.

Garcia-Higuera I, Taniguchi T, Ganesan S, Meyn MS, Timmers C, Hejna J, Grompe M, D'Andrea AD. Interaction of the Fanconi anemia proteins and BRCA1 in a common pathway. Mol Cell 7:249–262, 2001.

Garkavtsev IV, Kley N, Grigorian IA, Gudkov AV. The Bloom syndrome protein interacts and cooperates with p53 regulation of transcription and cell growth control. Oncogene 20:8276–8280, 2001.

Gatei M, Young D, Cerosaletti KM, Desai-Mehta A, Spring K, Kozlov S, Lavin MF, Gatti RA, Concannon P, Khanna K. ATM-dependent phosphorylation of nibrin in response to radiation exposure. Nat Genet 25:115–119, 2000.

German J. Bloom's syndrome XVII. A genetic disorder that displays the consequences of excessive somatic mutation. In: Bonne-Tamir B, Adam A, eds. Genetic Diversity Among Jews. New York: Oxford University Press, pp.129–139, 1992.

German J. Bloom's syndrome: a mendelian prototype of somatic mutational disease. Medicine 72:393–406, 1993.

German J. Bloom syndrome. XX. The first 100 cancers. Cancer Genet Cytogenet 93:100–106, 1997.

German J, Ellis NA. Bloom syndrome. In: Vogelstein B, Kinzler KW, eds. The Genetic Basis of Human Cancer, 2nd Edition. New York: McGraw-Hill, pp. 267–288, 2002.

German J, Passarge E. Bloom's syndrome. XII. Report from the Registry for 1987. Clin Genet 35:57–69, 1989.

German J, Roe AM, Leppert MF, Ellis NA. Bloom syndrome: an analysis of consanguineous families assigns the locus mutated to chromosome band 15q26.1. Proc Natl Acad Sci USA 91:6669–6673, 1994.

German J, Schonberg S, Louie E, Chaganti RS. Bloom's syndrome. IV. Sister-chormatid exchanges in lymphocytes. Am J Hum Genet 29:248–255, 1977.

Giampietro PF, Verlander PC, Davis JG, Auerbach AD. Diagnosis of Fanconi anemia in patients without congenital malformations: an International Fanconi Anemia Registry study. Am J Med Genet 68:58–61, 1997.

Gillio AP, Verlander PC, Batish SD, Giampietro PF, Auerbach AD. Phenotypic consequences of mutations in the Fanconi anemia FAC gene: an International Fanconi Anemia Registry study. Blood 90:105–110, 1997.

Girard PM, Foray N, Stumm M, Waugh A, Riballo E, Maser RS, Phillips WP, Petrini J, Arlett CF, Jeggo PA. Radiosensitivity in Nijmegen Breakage Syndrome cells is attributable to a repair defect and not cell cycle checkpoint defects. Cancer Res 60:4881–4888, 2000.

Girard PM, Riballo E, Begg AC, Waugh A, Jeggo PA. Nbs1 promotes ATM-dependent phosphorylation events including those required for G1/S arrest. Oncogene 21:4191–4199, 2002.

Gładkowska-Dura M, Chrzanowska KH, Dura WT. Malignant lymphoma in Nijmegen breakage syndrome. Ann Pediatr Pathol 2:39–46, 2000.

Gładkowska-Dura M, Dzierżanowska-Fangrat K, Dura WT, Chrzanowska KH, Langerak AW, van Dongen JJ. Immunophenotype and immunogenotype of consecutive lymphomas in NBS patients. J Clin Pathol, 2005 (in press).

Gładkowska-Dura M, Dzierżanowska-Fangrat K, Langerak AW, van Dongen JJ, Chrzanowska KH. Immunophenotypic and immunogenotypic profile of NHL in Nijmegen breakage syndrome (NBS) with special emphasis on DLBCL. J Clin Pathol 55 (Suppl I):A15, 2002.

Glanz A, Fraser FC. Spectrum of anomalies in Fanconi anemia. J Med Genet 19:412–416, 1982.

Goss KH, Risinger MA, Kordich JJ, Sanz MM, Straughen JE, Slovek LE, Capobianco AJ, German J, Boivin GP, Groden J. Enhanced tumor formation in mice heterozygous for Blm mutation. Science 297:2051–2053, 2002.

Grawunder U, Zimmer D, Fugmann S, Schwarz K, Lieber MR. DNA ligase IV is essential for V(D)J recombination and DNA double-strand break repair in human precursor lymphocytes. Mol Cell 2:477–484, 1998.

Green AJ, Yates JR, Taylor AM, Biggs P, McGuire GM, McConville CM, Billing CJ, Barnes ND. Severe microcephaly with normal intellectual development: the Nijmegen breakage syndrome. Arch Dis Child 73:431–434, 1995.

Gregorek H, Chrzanowska KH, Michalkiewicz J, Syczewska M, Madalinski K. Heterogeneity of humoral immune abnormalities in children with Nijmegen breakage syndrome: an 8-year follow-up study in a single centre. Clin Exp Immunol 130:319–324, 2002.

Gregory JJ Jr, Wagner JE, Verlander PC, Levran O, Batish SD, Eide CR, Steffenhagen A, Hirsch B, Auerbach AD. Somatic mosaicism in Fanconi anemia: evidence of genotypic reversion in lymphohematopoietic stem cells. Proc Natl Acad Sci USA 98:2532–2537, 2001.

Groden J, Nakamura Y, German J. Molecular evidence that homologous recombination occurs in proliferating human somatic cells. Proc Natl Acad Sci USA 87:4315–4319, 1990.

Gruber SB, Ellis NA, Scott KK, Almog R, Kolachana P, Bonner JD, Kirchhoff T, Tomsho LP, Nafa K, Pierce H, Low M, Satagopan J, Rennert H, Huang H, Greenson JK, Groden J, Rapaport B, Shia J, Johnson S, Gregersen PK, Harris CC, Boyd J, Rennert G, Offit K. BLM heterozygosity and the risk of colorectal cancer. Science 297:2013, 2002.

Gush KA, Fu KL, Grompe M, Walsh CE. Phenotypic correction of Fanconi anemia group C knockout mice. Blood 95:700–704, 2000.

Hadjur S, Ung K, Wadsworth L, Dimmick J, Rajcan-Separovic E, Scott RW, Buchwald M, Jirik FR. Defective hematopoiesis and hepatic steatosis in mice with combined deficiencies of the genes encoding Fancc and Cu/Zn superoxide dismutase. Blood 98:1003–1011, 2001.

Hama S, Matsuura S, Tauchi H, Sawada J, Kato C, Yamasaki F, Yoshioka H, Sugiyama K, Arita K, Kurisu K, Kamada N, Heike Y, Komatsu K. Absence of mutations in the NBS1 gene in B-cell malignant lymphoma patients. Anticancer Res 20:1897–1900, 2000.

Hart RM, Kimler BF, Evans RG, Park CH. Radiotherapeutic management of medulloblastoma in a pediatric patient with ataxia telangiectasia. Int J Radiat Oncol Biol Phys 13:1237–1240, 1987.

Heo S, Tatebayashi K, Ohsugi I, Shimamoto A, Furuichi Y, Ikeda H. Bloom's syndrome gene suppresses premature ageing caused by Sgs1 deficiency in yeast. Genes Cells 4:619–625, 1999.

Hiel JA, Weemaes CM, van Engelen BG, Smeets D, Ligtenberg M, van Der Burgt I, van Den Heuvel LP, Cerosaletti KM, Gabreels FJ, Concannon P. Nijmegen breakage syndrome in a Dutch patient not resulting from a defect in NBS1. J Med Genet 38:E18, 2001.

Houghtaling S, Timmers C, Noll M, Finegold MJ, Jones SN, Meyn MS, Grompe M. Epithelial cancer in Fanconi anemia complementation group D2 (Fancd2) knockout mice. Genes Dev 17:2021–2035, 2003.

Howell RT, Davies T. Diagnosis of Bloom's syndrome by sister chromatid exchange evaluation in chorionic villus cultures. Prenat Diagn 14:1071–1073, 1994.

Howlett NG, Taniguchi T, Olson S, Cox B, Waisfisz Q, De Die-Smulders C, Persky N, Grompe M, Joenje H, Pals G, Ikeda H, Fox EA, D'Andrea AD. Biallelic inactivation of BRCA2 in Fanconi anemia. Science 297: 606–609, 2002.

Hsieh CL, Arlett F, Lieber MR. V(D)J recombination in ataxia telangiectasia, Bloom's syndrome, and a DNA ligase I–associated immunodeficiency disorder. J Biol Chem 268:20105–20109, 1993.

Hussain S, Wilson JB, Medhurst AL, Hejna J, Witt E, Ananth S, Davies A, Masson JY, Moses R, West SC, de Winter JP, Ashworth A, Jones NJ, Mathew CG. Direct interaction of FANCD2 with BRCA2 in DNA damage response pathways. Hum Mol Genet 13:1241–1248, 2004.

Hustinx TW, Scheres JM, Weemaes CM, ter Haar BG, Janssen AH. Karyotype instability with multiple 7/14 and 7/7 rearrangements. Hum Genet 49:199–208, 1979.

Hutteroth TH, Litwin SD, German J. Abnormal immune responses of Bloom's syndrome lymphocytes in vitro. J Clin Invest 56:1–7, 1975.

International Nijmegen Breakage Syndrome Study Group. Nijmegen breakage syndrome. Arch Dis Child 82:400–406, 2000.

Ito A, Tauchi H, Kobayashi J, Morishima K, Nakamura A, Hirokawa Y, Matsuura S, Ito K, Komatsu K. Expression of full-length NBS1 protein restores normal radiation responses in cells from Nijmegen breakage syndrome patients. Biochem Biophys Res Commun 265:716–721, 1999.

Jaspers NG, Gatti RA, Baan C, Linssen PC, Bootsma D. Genetic complementation analysis of ataxia telangiectasia and Nijmegen breakage syndrome: a survey of 50 patients. Cytogenet Cell Genet 49:259–263, 1988a.

Jaspers NG, Taalman RD, Baan C. Patients with an inherited syndrome characterized by immunodeficiency, microcephaly, and chromosomal instability: genetic relationship to ataxia telangiectasia and Nijmegen breakage syndrome. Am J Hum Genet 42:66–73, 1988b.

Jaspers NG, van der Kraan M, Linssen PC, Macek M, Seemanová E, Kleijer WJ. First-trimester prenatal diagnosis of the Nijmegen breakage syndrome and ataxia telangiectasia using an assay of radioresistant DNA synthesis. Prenat Diagn 10:667–674, 1990.

Joenje H, Arwert F, Eriksson AW, de Koning H, Oostra AB. Oxygen dependence of chromosomal aberrations in Fanconi's anemia. Nature 290: 142–143, 1981.

Jongmans W, Vuillaume M, Chrzanowska K, Smeets D, Sperling K, Hall J. Nijmegen breakage syndrome cells fail to induce the p53-mediated DNA damage response following exposure to ionizing radiation. Mol Cell Biol 17:5016–5022, 1997.

Kapelushnik J, Or R, Slavin S, Nagler A. A fludarabine-based protocol for bone marrow transplantation in Fanconi's anemia. Bone Marrow Transplant 20:1109–1110, 1997.

Kinzler KW, Vogelstein B. Gatekeepers and caretakers. Nature 386:761–762, 1997.

Kleijer WJ, van der Kraan M, Los FJ, Jaspers NG. Prenatal diagnosis of ataxia telangiectasia and Nijmegen breakage syndrome by the assay of radioresistant DNA synthesis. Int J Radiat Biol 66(Suppl 6):S167–S174, 1994.

Kleier S, Herrmann M, Wittwer B, Varon R, Reis A, Horst J. Clinical presentation and mutation identification in the NBS1 gene in a boy with Nijmegen breakage syndrome. Clin Genet 57:384–387, 2000.

Kobayashi J, Tauchi H, Sakamoto S, Nakamura A, Morishima K, Matsuura S, Kobayashi T, Tamai K, Tanimoto K, Komatsu K. NBS1 localizes to gamma-H2AX foci through interaction with the FHA/BRCT domain. Curr Biol 12:1846–1851, 2002.

Komatsu K, Matsuura S, Tauchi H, Endo S, Kodama S, Smeets D, Weemaes C, Oshimura M. The gene for Nijmegen breakage syndrome (V2) is not located on chromosome 11. Am J Hum Genet 58:885–888, 1996.

Kondo N, Motoyoshi F, Mori S, Kuwabara N, Orii T, German J. Long-term study of the immunodeficiency of Bloom's syndrome. Acta Paediatr 81: 86–90, 1992a.

Kondo N, Ozawa T, Kata Y, Motoyoshi F, Kasahara K, Kameyama T, Orii T. Reduced secreted mu mRNA synthesis in selective IgM deficiency of Bloom's syndrome. Clin Exp Immunol 88:35–40, 1992b.

Kraakman–van der Zwet M, Overkamp WJ, Friedl AA, Klein B, Verhaegh GW, Jaspers NG, Midro AT, Eckardt-Schupp F, Lohman PH, Zdzienicka MZ. Immortalization and characterization of Nijmegen breakage syndrome fibroblasts. Mutat Res 434:17–27, 1999.

Kusano K, Berres ME, Engels WR. Evolution of the RECQ family of helicases: a Drosophila homolog, Dmblm, is similar to the human Bloom syndrome gene. Genetics 157:1027–1039, 1999.

Kusano K, Johnson-Schlitz DM, Engels WR. Sterility in Drosophila with mutations in the Bloom syndrome gene. Science 291:2600–2602, 2001.

Kwee ML, Poll EH, van de Kamp JJ, de Koning H, Eriksson AW, Joenje H. Unusual response to bifunctional alkylating agents in a case of Fanconi anemia. Hum Genet 64:384–387, 1983.

Lahdesmaki A, Taylor AM, Chrzanowska KH, Pan-Hammarstrom Q. Delineation of the role of the Mre11 complex in class switch recombination. J Biol Chem 279:16479–16487, 2004.

Lammens M, Hiel JA, Gabreels FJ, van Engelen BG, van den Heuvel LP, Weemaes CM. Nijmegen breakage syndrome: a neuropathological study. Neuropediatrics 34:189–193, 2003.

Langlois RG, Bigbee WL, Jensen RH, German J. Evidence for increased in vivo mutation and somatic recombination in Bloom's syndrome. Proc Natl Acad Sci USA 86:670–674, 1989.

Levitus M, Rooimans MA, Steltenpool J, Cool NF, Oostra AB, Mathew CG, Hoatlin ME, Waisfisz Q, Arwert F, de Winter JP, Joenje H. Heterogeneity in Fanconi anemia: evidence for 2 new genetic subtypes. Blood 103: 2498–2503, 2004.

Levran O, Attwooll C, Henry RT, Milton KL, Neveling K, Rio P, Batish SD, Kalb R, Velleuer E, Barral S, Ott J, Petrini J, Schindler D, Hanenberg H, Auerbach AD. The BRCA1-interacting helicase BRIP1 is deficient in Fanconi anemia. Nat Genet 37:931–933, 2005.

Levran O, Doggett NA, Auerbach AD. Identification of Alu-mediated deletions in the Fanconi anemia gene FAA. Hum Mutat 12:145–152, 1998.

Li L, Eng C, Desnick RJ, German J, Ellis NA. Carrier frequency of the Bloom syndrome blmAsh mutation in the Ashkenazi Jewish population. Mol Genet Metab 64:286–290, 1998.

Lim DS, Kim ST, Xu B, Maser RS, Lin J, Petrini JH, Kastan MB. ATM phosphorylates p95/nbs1 in an S-phase checkpoint pathway. Nature 404:613–617, 2000.

Lindor N, Furuichi Y, Kitao S, Shimamoto A, Arndt C, Jalal S. Rothmund-Thomson syndrome due to RECQ4 helicase mutations: report and clinical and molecular comparisions with Bloom syndrome and Werner syndrome. Am J Med Genet 90:223–228, 2000.

Liu JM, Kim S, Read EJ, Futaki M, Dokal I, Carter CS, Leitman SF, Pensiero M, Young NS, Walsh CE. Engraftment of hematopoietic progenitor cells transduced with the Fanconi anemia group C gene (*FANCC*). Hum Gene Ther 10:2337–2346, 1999.

Liu N, Lamerdin JE, Tucker JD, Zhou ZQ, Walter CA, Albala JS, Busch DB, Thompson LH. The human *XRCC9* gene corrects chromosomal instability and mutagen sensitivities in CHO UV40 cells. Proc Natl Acad Sci USA 94:9232–9237, 1997a.

Liu JM, Young NS, Walsh CE, Cottler-Fox M, Carter C, Dunbar C, Barrett AJ, Emmons R. Retroviral mediated gene transfer of the Fanconi anemia complementation group C gene to hematopoietic progenitors of group C patients. Hum Gene Ther 8:1715–1730, 1997b.

Lombard DB, Guarente L. Nijmegen breakage syndrome disease protein and MRE11 at PML nuclear bodies and meiotic telomeres. Cancer Res 60: 2331–2334, 2000.

Lo Ten Foe JR, Kwee ML, Rooimans MA, Oostra AB, Veerman AJ, van Weel M, Pauli RM, Shahidi NT, Dokal I, Roberts I, Altay C, Gluckman E, Gibson RA, Mathew CG, Arwert F, Joenje H. Somatic mosaicism in Fanconi anemia: molecular basis and clinical significance. Eur J Hum Genet 5:137–148, 1997.

Ludwig T, Chapman DL, Papaioannou VE, Efstratiadis A. Targeted mutations of breast cancer susceptibility gene homologs in mice: lethal phenotypes of Brca1, Brca2, Brca1/Brca2, Brca1/p53, and Brca2/p53 nullizygous embryos. Genes Dev 11:1226–1241, 1997.

Luo G, Santoro IM, McDaniel LD, Nishijima I, Mills M, Youssoufian H, Vogel H, Schultz RA, Bradley A. Cancer predisposition caused by elevated mitotic recombination in Bloom mice. Nat Gene 26:424–429, 2000.

Luo G, Yao MS, Bender CF, Mills M, Bladl AR, Bradley A, Petrini JH. Disruption of mRad50 causes embryonic stem cell lethality, abnormal embryonic development, and sensitivity to ionizing radiation. Proc Natl Acad Sci USA 96:7376–7381, 1999.

MacMillan ML, Auerbach AD, Davies SM, Defor TE, Gillio A, Giller R, Harris R, Cairo M, Dusenbery K, Hirsch B, Ramsay NK, Weisdorf DJ, Wagner JE. Hematopoietic cell transplantation in patients with Fanconi anemia using alternate donors: results of a total body irradiation dose escalation trial. Br J Haematol 109:121–129, 2000.

Maraschio P, Danesino C, Antoccia A, Ricordy R, Tanzarella C, Varon R, Reis A, Besana D, Guala A, Tiepolo L. A novel mutation and novel features in Nijmegen breakage syndrome. J Med Genet 38:113–117, 2001.

Maraschio P, Spadoni E, Tanzarella C, Antoccia A, di Masi A, Maghnie, Varon R, Demuth I, Tiepolo L, Danesino C. Genetic heterogeneity for a Nijmegen breakage–like syndrome. Clin Genet 63:283–290, 2003.

Martin RM, Rademaker A, German J. Chromosomal breakage in human spermatozoa, a heterozygous effect of the Bloom syndrome mutation. Am J Hum Genet 55:1242–1246, 1994.

Maser RS, Zinkel R, Petrini JH. An alternative mode of translation permits production of a variant NBS1 protein from the common Nijmegen breakage syndrome allele. Nat Genet 27:417–421, 2001.

Matsuura K, Balmukhanov T, Tauchi H, Weemaes C, Smeets D, Chrzanowska K, Endou S, Matsuura S, Komatsu K. Radiation induction of p53 in cells from Nijmegen breakage syndrome is defective but not similar to ataxia-telangiectasia. Biochem Biophys Res Commun 242:602–607, 1998.

McCloy M, Almeida A, Daly P, Vulliamy T, Roberts IA, Dokal I. Fludarabine-based stem cell transplantation protocol for Fanconi's anemia in myelodysplastic transformation. Br J Haematol 112:427–429, 2001.

McDaniel LD, Chester N, Watson M, Borowsky AD, Leder P, Schultz R. Chromosome instability and tumor predisposition inversely correlate with BLM protein levels. DNA Repair (Amst) 2:1387–1404, 2003.

Medhurst AL, Huber PA, Waisfisz Q, de Winter JP, Mathew CG. Direct interactions of the five known Fanconi anemia proteins suggest a common functional pathway. Hum Mol Genet 10:423–429, 2001.

Meetei AR, de Winter JP, Medhurst AL, Wallisch M, Waisfisz Q, van de Vrugt HJ, Oostra AB, Yan Z, Ling C, Bishop CE, Hoatlin ME, Joenje H, Wang W. A novel ubiquitin ligase is deficient in Fanconi anemia. Nat Genet 35:165–170, 2003.

Meetei AR, Levitus M, Xue Y, Medhurst AL, Zwaan M, Ling C, Rooimans MA, Bier P, Hoatlin M, Pals G, de Winter JP, Wang W, Joenje H. X-linked inheritance of Fanconi anemia complementation group B. Nat Genet 36:1219–1224, 2004.

Meetei AR, Medhurst AL, Ling C, Xue Y, Singh TR, Bier P, Steltenpool J, Stone S, Dokal I, Mathew CG, Hoatlin M, Joenje H, de Winter JP, Wang W. A human ortholog of archaeal DNA repair protein Hef is defective in Fanconi anemia complementation group M. Nat Genet 37: 958–963, 2005.

Michallet A-S, Lesca G, Radford-Weiss I, Delarue R, Varet B, Buzyn A. T-cell prolymphocytic leukemia with autoimmune manifestations in Nijmegen breakage syndrome. Ann Hematol 82:515–517, 2003.

Michałkiewicz J, Barth C, Chrzanowska KH, Gregorek H, Syczewska M, Weemaes CM, Madaliński K, Stachowski J, Dzierżanowska D. Abnormalities in the T and NK lymphocyte phenotype in patients with Nijmegen breakage syndrome. Clin Exp Immunol 134:482–490, 2003.

Muschke P, Gola H, Varon R, Röpke A, Zumkeller W, Wieacker P, Stumm M. Retrospective diagnosis and subsequent prenatal diagnosis of Nijmegen breakage syndrome. Prenat Diagn 24:111–113, 2004.

Nakanishi K, Taniguchi T, Ranganathan V, New HV, Moreau LA, Stotsky M, Mathew CG, Kastan MB, Weaver DT, D'Andrea AD. Interaction of FANCD2 and NBS1 in the DNA damage response. Nat Cell Biol 4:913–920, 2002.

Nakanishi K, Yang YG, Pierce AJ, Taniguchi T, Digweed M, D'Andrea AD, Wang ZQ, Jasin M. Human Fanconi anemia monoubiquitination pathway promotes homologous DNA repair. Proc Natl Acad Sci USA 102: 1110–1115, 2005.

Narayan G, Arias-Pulido H, Nandula SV, Basso K, Sugirtharaj DD, Vargas H, Mansukhani M, Villella J, Meyer L, Schneider A, Gissmann L, Durst M, Pothuri B, Murty VV. Promoter hypermethylation of FANCF: disruption of Fanconi anemia–BRCA pathway in cervical cancer. Cancer Res 64:2994–2997, 2004.

Neff N, Ellis N, Ye T, Noonan J, Huang K, Sanz M, Proytcheva M. The DNA helicase activity of BLM is necessary for the correction of the genomic instability of Bloom syndrome cells. Mol Biol Cell 10:665–676, 1999.

Neubauer S, Arutyunyan R, Stumm M, Dork T, Bendix R, Bremer M, Varon R, Sauer R, Gebhart E. Radiosensitivity of ataxia telangiectasia and Nijmegen breakage syndrome homozygotes and heterozygotes as determined by three-color FISH chromosome painting. Radiat Res 157:312–321, 2002.

Niedzwiedz W, Mosedal G, Johnson M, Ong CY, Pace P, Patel KJ. The Fanconi anaemia gene *FANCC* promotes homologous recombination and error-prone DNA repair. Mol Cell 15:607–620, 2004.

Noll M, Battaile KP, Bateman R, Lax TP, Rathbun K, Reifsteck C, Bagby G, Finegold M, Olson S, Grompe M. Fanconi anemia group A and C double-mutant mice: functional evidence for a multi-protein Fanconi anemia complex. Exp Hematol 30:679–688, 2002.

O'Driscoll M, Cerosaletti KM, Girard PM, Dai Y, Stumm M, Kysela B, Hirsch B, Gennery A, Palmer SE, Seidel J, Gatti RA, Varon R, Oettinger MA, Neitzel H, Jeggo PA, Concannon P. DNA ligase IV mutations identified in patients exhibiting developmental delay and immunodeficiency. Mol Cell 8:1175–1185, 2001.

Pace P, Johnson M, Tan WM, Mosedale G, Sng C, Hoatlin M, de Winter J, Joenje H, Gergely F, Patel KJ. FANCE: the link between Fanconi anaemia complex assembly and activity. Embo J 21:3414–3423, 2002.

Pan Q, Petit-Frere C, Lahdesmaki A, Gregorek H, Chrzanowska KH, Hammarstrom L. Alternative end joining during switch recombination in patients with ataxia-telangiectasia. Eur J Immunol 32:1300–1308, 2002.

Pasic S. Aplastic anemia in Nijmegen breakage syndrome. J Pediatr 141:742, 2002.

Paull TT, Gellert M. Nbs1 potentiates ATP-driven DNA unwinding and endonuclease cleavage by the Mre11/Rad50 complex. Genes Dev 13: 1276–1288, 1999.

Paulli M, Viglio A, Boveri E, Pitino A, Lucioni M, Franco C, Riboni R, Rosso R, Magrini U, Marseglia GL, Marchi A. Nijmegen breakage syndrome–associated T-cell-rich B-cell lymphoma: case report. Pediatr Dev Pathol 3:264–270, 2000.

Perez-Vera P, Gonzalez-del Angel A, Molina B, Gomez L, Frias S, Gatti RA, Carnevale A. Chromosome instability with bleomycin and X-ray hypersensitivity in a boy with Nijmegen breakage syndrome. Am J Med Genet 70:24–27, 1997.

Petrini JH, Walsh ME, DiMare C, Chen XN, Korenberg JR, Weaver DT. Isolation and characterization of the human MRE11 homologue. Genomics 29:80–86, 1995.

Pichierri P, Averbeck D, Rosselli F. DNA cross-link-dependent RAD50/MRE11/NBS1 subnuclear assembly requires the Fanconi anemia C protein. Hum Mol Genet 11:2531–2546, 2002.

Pincheira J, Bravo M, Santos MJ. G2 repair in Nijmegen breakage syndrome: G2 duration and effect of caffeine and cycloheximide in control and X-ray irradiated lymphocytes. Clin Genet 53:262–267, 1998.

Pozo J, Argente J. Ascertainment and treatment of delayed puberty. Horm Res 60(Suppl 3):35–48, 2003.

Pronk JC, Gibson RA, Savoia A, Wijker M, Morgan NV, Melchionda S, Ford D, Temtamy S, Ortega JJ, Jansen S, et al. Localisation of the Fanconi anemia complementation group A gene to chromosome 16q24.3. Nat Genet 11:338–340, 1995.

Ranganathan V, Heine WF, Ciccone DN, Rudolph KL, Wu X, Chang S, Hai H, Ahearn IM, Livingston DM, Resnick I, Rosen F, Seemanova E, Jarolim P, DePinho RA, Weaver DT. Rescue of a telomere length defect of Nijmegen breakage syndrome cells requires NBS and telomerase catalytic subunit. Curr Biol 11:962–966, 2001.

Resnick IB, Kondratenk I, Togoev O, Vasserman N, Shagina I, Evgrafov O, Tverskaya S, Cerosaletti KM, Gatti RA, Concannon P. Nijmegen breakage syndrome: clinical characteristics and mutation analysis in eight unrelated Russion families. J Pediatr 140:355–361, 2002.

Rischewski J, Bismarck P, Kabisch H, Janka-Schaub G, Obser T, Schneppenheim R. The common deletion 657del5 in the Nibrin geneis not a major risk factor for B or T cell non-Hodgkin lymphoma in a pediatric population. Leukemia 14:1528–1529, 2000.

Rosenzweig SD, Russo RA, Galleo M, Zelazko M. Juvenile rheumatoid arthritis-like polyarthritis in Nijmegen breakage syndrome. J Rheumatol 28:2548–2550, 2001.

Saar K, Chrzanowska KH, Stumm M, Jung M, Nürnberg G, Wienker TF, Seemanová E, Wegner RD, Reis A, Sperling K. The gene for ataxia-telangiectasia-variant (Nijmegen breakage syndrome) maps to a 1 cM interval on chromosome 8q21. Am J Hum Genet 60:605–610, 1997.

Saar K, Schindler D, Wegner RD, Reis A, Wienker T, Hoehn H, Joenje H, Sperling K, Digweed M. Localisation of a Fanconi anemia gene to chromosome 9p. Eur J Hum Genet 6:501–508, 1998.

Sack SZ, Liu YX, German J, Green NS. Somatic hypermutation of immunoglobulin genes is independent of the Bloom's syndrome DNA helicase. Clin Exp Immunol 112:248–254, 1998.

Sanz MM, Proytcheva M, Ellis NA, Hollman WK, German J. BLM, the Bloom's syndrome protein, varies during the cell cycle in its amount, distribution, and co-localization with other nuclear proteins. Cytogenet Cell Genet 91:217–223, 2000.

Sasaki MS, Tonomura A. A high susceptiblity of Fanconi's anemia to chromosome breakage by DNA cross-linking agents. Cancer Res 33:1829–1836, 1973.

Savitsky K, Bar-Shira A, Gilad S, Rotmann G, Ziv Y, Vanagaite L, Tagle DA, Smith S, Uziel T, Sfez S, Ashkenazi M, Pecker I, Frydman M, Harnik R, Patanjali SR, Simmons A, Clines GA, Sartiel A, Gatti RA, Chessa L, Sanal O, Lavin MF, Jaspers NGJ, Taylor AMR, Arlett CF, Miki T, Weissman SM, Lovett M, Collins FS, Shiloh Y. A single ataxia-telangiectasia gene with a product similar to PI-3 kinase. Science 268:1749–1753, 1995.

Schindler D, Hoehn H. Fanconi anemia mutation causes cellular susceptibility to ambient oxygen. Am J Hum Genet 43:429–435, 1988.

Schroeder TM, German J. Bloom's syndrome and Fanconi's anemia: demonstration of two distinctive patterns of chromosome disruption and rearrangement. Humangenetik 25:299–306, 1974.

Seeman P, Gebertová K, Paděrová K, Sperling K, Seemanová E. Nijmegen breakage syndrome in 13% of age-matched Czech children with primary microcephaly. Pediatr Neurol 30:195–200, 2004.

Seemanová E. An increased risk for malignant neoplasms in heterozygotes for a syndrome of microcephaly, normal intelligence, growth retardation, remarkable facies, immunodeficiency and chromosomal instability. Mutat Res 238:321–324, 1990.

Seemanová E, Passarge E, Benesova J, Houstek J, Kasal P, Sevcikova M. Familial micocephaly with normal intelligence, immunodeficiency and risk for lymphoreticuler malignancies: a new autosomal recessive disorder. Am J Med Genet 20:639–648, 1985.

Seidemann K, Henze G, Beck JD, Sauerbrey A, Kühl J, Mann G, Reiter A. Non-Hodgkin's lymphoma in pediatric patients with chromosomal breakage syndrome genealogies (AT and NBS). Experience from the BFM trials. Ann Oncol 11:S141–S451, 2000.

Seyschab H, Sun Y, Friedl R, Schindler D, Hoehn H. G2 phase cell cycle disturbance as a manifestation of genetic cell damage. Hum Genet 92: 61–68, 1993.

Shimada H, Shimizu K, Mimaki S, Sakiyama T, Mori T, Shimasaki N, Yokota J, Nakachi K, Ohta T, Ohki M. First case of aplastic anemia in a Japanese child with a homozygous mutation in the NBS1 gene (I171V) associated with genomic instability. Hum Genet 115:372–376, 2004.

Siwicki JK, Degerman S, Chrzanowska KH, Roos G. Telomere maintenance and cell cycle regulation in spontaneously immortalized T-cell lines from Nijmegen breakage syndrome patients. Exp Cell Res 287:178–189, 2003.

Stanulla M, Stumm M, Dieckvoss BO, Seidemann K, Schemmel V, Muller Brechlin A, Schrappe M, Welte K, Reiter A. No evidence for a major role of heterozygous deletion 657del5 within the NBS1 gene in the pathogenesis of non-Hodgkin's lymphoma of childhood and adolescence. Br J Haematol 109:117–120, 2000.

Steffen J, Varon R, Mosor M, Maneva G, Maurer M, Stumm M, Nowakowska D, Rubach M, Kosakowska E, Ruka W, Nowecki Z, Rutkowski P, Demkow T, Sadowska M, Bidziński T, Gawrychowski K, Sperling K. In-

creased cancer risk of heterozygotes with NBS1 germline mutations in Poland. Int J Cancer 111:67–71, 2004.

Stewart GS, Maser RS, Stankovic T, Bressan DA, Kaplan MI, Jaspers NG, Raams A, Byrd PJ, Petrini JH, Tayler AM. The DNA double-strand break repair gene hMRE11 is mutated in individuals with an ataxia-telangiectasia–like disorder. Cell 99:577–587, 1999.

Stoppa-Lyonnet D, Girault D, LeDeist F, Aurias A. Unusual T cell clones in a patient with Nijmegen breakage syndrome. J Med Genet 29:136–137, 1992.

Straughen J, Ciocci S, Ye TZ, Lennon DJ, Proytcheva M, Alhadeff B, Goodfellow P, German J, Ellis NA, Gordon J. Physical mapping of the Bloom's syndrome region by the identification of YAC and P1 clones from human chromosome 15 band q26.1. Genomics 33:118–128, 1996.

Straughen JE, Johnson J, McLaren D, Proytcheva M, Ellis N, German J, Groden J. A rapid method for detecting the predominant Ashkenazi Jewish mutation in the Bloom's syndrome gene. Hum Mutat 11:175–178, 1998.

Stumm M, Gatti RA, Reis A, Udar N, Chrzanowska K, Seemanová E, Sperling K, Wegner RD. The ataxia-telangiectasia-variant genes 1 and 2 are distinct from the ataxia-telangiectasia gene on chromosome 11q23.1. Am J Hum Genet 57:960–962. 1995.

Stumm M, Neubauer S, Keindorff S, Wegner RD, Wieacker P, Sauer R. High frequency of spontaneous translocations revealed by FISH in cells from patients with the cancer-prone syndromes ataxia telangiectasia and Nijmegen breakage syndrome. Cytogenet Cell Genet 92:186–191, 2001a.

Stumm M, Sperling K, Wegner RD. Noncomplementation of radiation-induced chromosome aberrations in ataxia-telangiectasia/ataxia-telangiectasia-variant heterodikaryons. Am J Hum Genet 60:1246–1251, 1997.

Stumm M, von Ruskowsky A, Siebert R, Harder S, Varon R, Wieacker P, Schlegelberger B. No evidence for deletions of the NBS1 gene in lymphomas. Cancer Genet Cytogenet 126:60–62, 2001b.

Sullivan KE, Veksler E, Lederman H, Lees-Miller SP. Cell cycle checkpoints and DNA repair in Nijmegen breakage syndrome. Clin Immunol Immunopathol 82:43–48, 1997.

Taalmann RD, Hustinx TW, Weemaes CM, Seemanová E, Schmidt A, Passarge E, Scheres JM. Further delineation of the Nijmegen breakage syndrome. Am J Med Genet 32:425–431, 1989.

Taalmann RD, Jaspers NG, Scheres JM, de Wit, Hustinx TW. Hypersensitivity in vitro in a new chromosomal instability syndrome, the Nijmegen breakage syndrome. Mutat Res 112:23–32, 1983.

Taniguchi N, Mukai M, Nagaoki T, Miyawaki T, Moriya N, Takahashi H, Kondo N. Impaired B-cell differentiation and T-cell regulatory function in four patients with Bloom's syndrome. Clin Immunol Immunopathol 22: 247–258, 1982.

Taylor AM, Groom A, Byrd PJ. Ataxia-telangiectasia-like disorder (ATLD)—its clinical presentation and molecular basis. DNA Repair 3:1219–1225, 2004.

Taylor AM, Metcalfe JA, Thick J, Mak YF. Leukemia and lymphoma in ataxia telangiectasia. Blood 87:423–438, 1996.

Tekin M, Dogu F, Tacyildiz N, Akar E, Ikinciogullari A, Ogur G, Yavuz G, Babacan E, Akar N. 657del5 mutation in the NBS1 gene is associated with Nijmegen breakage syndrome in a Turkish family. Clin Genet 62: 84–88, 2002.

Timmers C, Taniguchi T, Hejna J, Reifsteck C, Lucas L, Bruun D, Thayer M, Cox B, Olson S, D'Andrea AD, Moses R, Grompe M. Positional cloning of a novel Fanconi anemia gene, FANCD2. Mol Cell 7:241–248, 2001.

Tipping AJ, Pearson T, Morgan NV, Gibson RA, Kuyt LP, Havenga C, Gluckman E, Joenje H, de Ravel T, Jansen S, Mathew CG. Molecular and genealogical evidence for a founder effect in Fanconi anemia families of the Afrikaner population of South Africa. Proc Natl Acad Sci USA 98: 5734–5739, 2001.

Tischkowitz M, Ameziane N, Waisfisz Q, De Winter JP, Harris R, Taniguchi T, D'Andrea A, Hodgson SV, Mathew CG, Joenje H. Bi-allelic silencing of the Fanconi anaemia gene FANCF in acute myeloid leukaemia. Br J Haematol 123:469–471, 2003.

Tönnies H, Huber S, Kuhl JS, Gerlach A, Ebell W, Neitzel H. Clonal chromosomal aberrations in bone marrow cells of Fanconi anemia patients: gains of the chromosomal segment 3q26q29 as an adverse risk factor. Blood 101:3872–3874, 2003.

Trujillo KM, Yuan SS, Lee EY, Sung P. Nuclease activities in a complex of human recombination and DNA repair factors Rad50, Mre11, and p95. J Biol Chem 273:21447–21450, 1998.

Tupler R, Marseglia GL, Stefanini M, Prosperi E, Chessa L, Nardo T, Marchi A, Maraschio P. A variant of the Nijmegen breakage syndrome with unusual cytogenetic features and intermediate cellular radiosensitivity. J Med Genet 34:196–202, 1997.

Tutt A, Bertwistle D, Valentine J, Gabriel A, Swift S, Ross G, Griffin C, Thacker J, Ashworth A. Mutation in Brca2 stimulates error-prone homology-directed repair of DNA double-strand breaks occurring between repeated sequences. EMBO J 20:4704–4716, 2001.

Ueno Y, Miyawaki T, Seki H, Hara K, Sato T, Taniguchi N, Takahashi H, Kondo N. Impaired natural killer cell activity in Bloom's syndrome could be restored by human recombinant IL-2 in vitro. Clin Immunol Immunopathol 35:226–233, 1985.

Van Brabant AJ, Ye T, Sanz M, German JL, Ellis, NA, Holloman WK. Binding and melting of D-loops by the Bloom syndrome helicase. Biochemistry 39:14617–14619, 2000.

van de Kaa CA, Weemaes CM, Wesseling P, Schaafsma HE, Haraldsson A, De Weger RA. Postmortem findings in the Nijmegen breakage syndrome. Pediatr Pathol 14:787–796, 1994.

van der Burgt I, Chrzanowska KH, Smeets D, Weemaes C. Nijmegen breakage syndrome. J Med Genet 33:153–156, 1996.

van Gent DC, Hoeijmakers JH, Kanaar R. Chromosomal stability and the DNA double-stranded break connection. Nat Rev Genet 2:196–206, 2001.

Van Kerckhove CW, Ceuppens JL, Vanderschueren-Lodeweyckx M, Eggermont E, Vertessen S, Stevens EA. Bloom's syndrome, clinical features and immunologic abnormalities of four patients. Am J Dis Child 142: 1089–1093, 1988.

Varon R, Reis A, Henze G, von Einsiedel HG, Sperling K, Seeger K. Mutations in the Nijmegen breakage syndrome gene (NBS1) in childhood acute lymphoblastic leukemia (ALL). Cancer Res 61:3570–3572, 2001.

Varon R, Seemanova E, Chrzanowska K, Hnateyko O, Piekutowska-Abramczuk D, Krajewska-Walasek M, Sykut-Cegielska J, Sperling K, Reis A. Clinical ascertainment of Nijmegen breakage syndrome (NBS) and prevalence of the major mutation, 657del5, in three Slav populations. Eur J Hum Genet 8:900–902, 2000.

Varon R, Vissinga C, Platzer M, Cerosaletti KM, Chrzanowska KH, Saar K, Beckmann G, Seemanova E, Cooper PR, Nowak NJ, Stumm M, Weemaes CM, Gatti RA, Wilson RK, Digweed M, Rosenthal A, Sperling K, Concannon P, Reis A. Nibrin, a novel DNA double-strand break repair protein, is mutated in Nijmegen breakage syndrome. Cell 93:467–476, 1998.

Vijayalaxmi, Evans HJ, Ray JH, German J. Bloom's syndrome: evidence for an increased mutation frequency in vivo. Science 221:851–853, 1983.

Waisfisz Q, Morgan NV, Savino M, de Winter JP, van Berkel CG, Hoatlin ME, Ianzano L, Gibson RA, Arwert F, Savoia A, Mathew CG, Pronk JC, Joenje H. Spontaneous functional correction of homozygous Fanconi anaemia alleles reveals novel mechanistic basis for reverse mosaicism. Nat Genet 22:379–383, 1999a.

Waisfisz Q, Saar K, Morgan NV, Altay C, Leegwater PA, de Winter JP, Komatsu K, Evans GR, Wegner RD, Reis A, Joenje H, Arwert F, Mathew CG, Pronk JC, Digweed M. The Fanconi anemia group E gene, FANCE, maps to chromosome 6p. Am J Hum Genet 64:1400–1405, 1999b.

Walpita D, Plug AW, Neff N, German J, Ashley T. Bloom's syndrome protein, BLM, colocalizes with replication protein A in meiotic prophase nuclei of mammalian spermatocytes. Proc Natl Acad Sci USA 96:5622–5627, 1999.

Wang Y, Cortez D, Yazdi P, Neff N, Elledge SJ, Qin J. BASC, a super complex of BRCA1-associated proteins involved in the recognition and repair of aberrant DNA structures. Genes Dev 14:927–939, 2000.

Webster AD, Barnes DE, Arlett CF, Lehmann AR, Lindahl T. Growth retardation and immunodeficiency in a patient with mutations in the DNA ligase I gene. Lancet 339:1508–1509, 1992.

Weemaes C and the International Nijmegen Breakage Syndrome Study Group. Malignancy in Nijmegen breakage syndrome. Časopis Lék Čes 141:IV, 2002.

Weemaes CM, Bakkeren JA, Haraldsson A, Smeets DF. Immunological studies in Bloom's syndrome. A follow-up report. Ann Genet 34:201–205, 1991.

Weemaes CM, Bakkeren JA, ter Haar BG, Hustinx TW, van Munster PJ. Immune responses in four patients with Bloom syndrome. Clin Immunol Immunopathol 12:12–19, 1979.

Weemaes CM, Hustinx TW, Scheres JM, van Munster PJ, Bakkeren JA, Taalman RD. A new chromosomal instability disorder: the Nijmegen breakage syndrome. Acta Paediat Scand 70:557–564, 1981.

Weemaes CM, van de Kaa C, Wesseling P, Haraldson A, Bakkeren J, Seemanová E, Schmidt A, Paasarge E. Nijmegen breakage syndrome: clinical, immunological and pathological findings. In: Chapel HM, Levinsky

RJ, Webster AD, eds. Progress in Immune Deficiency III. London: Royal Society of Medicine Services, pp. 191–193, 1991.

Wegner RD. Chromosomal instability syndromes in man. In: Obe G, ed. Advances in Mutagenesis Research 3. Heidelberg: Springer-Verlag, pp. 81–117, 1991.

Wegner RD, Chrzanowska K, Sperling K, Stumm M. Ataxia telangiectasia variants (Nijmegen breakage syndrome). In: Ochs HD, Smith CI, Puck JM, eds. Primary Immunodeficiency Diseases—A Molecular and Genetic Approach. New York: Oxford University Press, pp. 324–334, 1999.

Wegner RD, Metzger M, Hanefeld F, Jaspers NG, Baan C, Magdorf K, Kunze J, Sperling K. A new chromosomal instability disorder confirmed by complementation studies. Clin Genet 33:20–32, 1988.

Wegner RD, Reis A, Digweed M. Cytogenetic and molecular investigations in chromosomal instability syndromes. In: Obe G, Natarajan AT, eds. Chromosomal Alterations. Heidelberg: Springer-Verlag, pp. 269–281, 1994.

Wegner RD, Stumm M. Diagnosis of chromosomal instability syndromes. In: Wegner RD, ed. Diagnostic Cytogenetics. Berlin: Springer-Verlag, pp. 251–268, 1999.

Whitney MA, Royle G, Low MJ, Kelly MA, Axthelm MK, Reifsteck C, Olson S, Braun RE, Heinrich MC, Rathbun RK, Bagby GC, Grompe M. Germ cell defects and hematopoietic hypersensitivity to gamma-interferon in mice with a targeted disruption of the Fanconi anemia C gene. Blood 88:49–58, 1996.

Whitney MA, Saito H, Jakobs PM, Gibson RA, Moses RE, Grompe M. A common mutation in the FACC gene causes Fanconi anemia in Ashkenazi Jews. Nature Genet 4:202–205, 1993.

Woods CG, Taylor MR. Ataxia telangiectasia in the British Isles: the clinical and laboratory features of 70 affected individuals. Q J Med 82:169–179, 1992.

Wu X, Ranganathan V, Weisman DS, Heine WF, Ciccone DN, O'Neill TB, Crick KE, Pierce KA, Lane WS, Rathbun G, Livingston DM, Weaver DT. ATM phosphorylation of Nijmegen breakage syndrome protein is required in a DNA damage response. Nature 405:477–482, 2000.

Xiao YH, Weaver DT. Conditional gene targeted deletion by Cre recombinase demonstrates the requirement for the double-strand repair Mre11 protein in murine embryonic stem cells. Nucl Acids Res 25:2985–2991, 1997.

Yamamoto K, Ishiai M, Matsushita N, Arakawa H, Lamerdin JE, Buerstedde JM, Tanimoto M, Harada M, Thompson LH, Takata M. Fanconi anemia FANCG protein in mitigating radiation- and enzyme-induced DNA double-strand breaks by homologous recombination in vertebrate cells. Mol Cell Biol 23:5421–5430, 2003.

Yamazaki V, Wegner RD, Kirchgessner CU. Characterization of cell cycle checkpoint responses after ionizing radiation in Nijmegen breakage syndrome cells. Cancer Res 58:2316–2322, 1998.

Yang YG, Herceg Z, Nakanishi K, Demuth I, Piccoli C, Michelon J, Hildebrand G, Jasin M, Digweed M, Wang ZQ. The Fanconi anemia group A protein modulates homologous repair of DNA double-strand breaks in mammalian cells. Carcinogenesis 26:1731–1740, 2005.

Yang Y, Kuang Y, De Oca RM, Hays T, Moreau L, Lu N, Seed B, D'Andrea AD. Targeted disruption of the murine Fanconi anemia gene, Fancg/Xrcc9. Blood 98:3435–3440, 2001.

Yu C, Oshima J, Fu Y, Wijsman E, Hisama F, Alisch R, Matthews S, Nakura J, Miki T, Ouasis S, Martin G, Mulligan JK, Schellenberg G. Positional cloning of the Werner's syndrome gene. Science 272:258–262, 1996.

Yuan SS, Lee SY, Chen G, Song M, Tomlinson GE, Lee EY. BRCA2 is required for ionizing radiation-induced assembly of Rad51 complex in vivo. Cancer Res 59:3547–3551, 1999.

Zhao S, Weng YC, Yuan SS, Lin YT, Hsu HC, Lin SC, Gerbino E, Song MH, Zdzienicka MZ, Gatti RA, Shay JW, Ziv Y, Shiloh Y, Lee EY. Functional link between ataxia-telangiectasia and Nijmegen breakage syndrome gene products. Nature 405:473–477, 2000.

Zhu J, Petersen S, Tessarollo L, Nussenzweig A. Targeted disruption of the Nijmegen breakage syndrome gene NBS1 leads to early embryonic lethality in mice. Curr Biol 11:105–109, 2001.

Zhu XD, Kuster B, Mann M, Petrini JH, Lange T. Cell-cycle-regulated association of RAD50/MRE11/NBS1 with TRF2 and human telomeres. Nat Genet 25:347–352, 2000.

31

Wiskott-Aldrich Syndrome

HANS D. OCHS and FRED S. ROSEN

The first description of the Wiskott-Aldrich syndrome (WAS), published in 1937, defined accurately the clinical phenotype: three brothers, but not their sisters, presented shortly after birth with thrombocytopenia, bloody diarrhea, eczema, and recurrent ear infections (Wiskott, 1937). On the basis of this symptomatology, the early onset, and the predominance of male infants, Wiskott differentiated this entity from Morbus Werlhofii, a synonym for idiopathic thrombocytopenia. Seventeen years later, Aldrich described a large family with multiple affected males, clearly demonstrating X-linked inheritance (Aldrich et al., 1954). In 1957, additional cases were described (Huntley and Dees, 1957), including members of an African American family (Wolff and Bertucio, 1957).

Following these early clinical reports, the immunologic abnormalities characteristic of WAS were recognized, including progressive lymphopenia, absence of delayed-type hypersensitivity, and abnormal in vivo antibody production (Blaese et al., 1968; Cooper et al., 1968; Ochs et al, 1980; Sullivan et al., 1994). Most studies implicated a predominant T cell defect (Molina et al., 1993; Sullivan et al., 1994; Gallego et al., 1997). This idea was reinforced by the discovery that WAS protein (WASP), the protein mutated in this syndrome, plays a crucial role in cytoskeletal remodeling downstream of T cell receptor (TCR) engagement (Barda-Saad et al., 2005) and contributes to the immune synapse formation between T lymphocytes and antigen-presenting cells (Dupre et al., 2002). However, impaired maturation, decreased motility, reduced migration, and abnormal morphology of B cells from WAS patients have recently been recognized (Park et al., 2005; Westerberg et al., 2005). Abnormal natural killer (NK) cell function (Orange et al., 2002; Gismondi et al., 2004; Huang et al., 2005) and impaired migration of dendritic cells (Binks et al., 1998; de Noronha et al., 2004) indicate that innate immunity is also affected. In addition to the consistent microplatelet thrombocytopenia, characteristic functional and morphologic abnormalities of

WAS platelets were also recognized (Gröttum et al., 1969; Kuramoto et al., 1970; Ochs et al., 1980; Semple et al., 1997). The finding of eosinophilia, multiple food allergies (Huntley and Dees 1957), and elevated IgE levels suggested an allergic basis for the eczema (Berglund et al., 1968). An increased risk of malignancies, including lymphoma, malignant reticuloendotheliosis, and leukemia, was reported as early as 1961 (Kildeberg, 1961; ten-Bensel et al., 1966; Cotelingam et al., 1985; Sullivan et al., 1994).

Distinguishable from the classic WAS phenotype (MIM 301000) is a milder form designated *hereditary X-linked thrombocytopenia* (XLT, MIM 313900) (Canales and Mauer, 1967; Chiaro et al., 1972; Notarangelo et al., 1991; Stormorken et al., 1991). In patients with XLT, eczema, if present, is mild; immune functions are less disturbed or normal, autoimmune disorders are rare, and the incidence of malignancies appear to be less frequent. The thrombocytopenia may be present intermittently (Notarangelo et al., 2002).

The gene responsible for both WAS and XLT was initially mapped to Xp11.22 (Donnér et al., 1988; Kwan et al., 1991); it was subsequently identified by positional cloning and named *WASP* (Derry et al., 1994). WASP is composed of 12 exons containing 1823 base pairs and encodes a 502–amino acid protein with a predicted molecular weight of 54 kDa. WASP is constitutively expressed in all hematopoietic stem cell–derived lineages and is located predominantly in the cytoplasm with the highest protein density being toward the cell membrane (Riveo-Lezcano et al., 1995; Zhu et al., 1997). WASP belongs to a family of cytoskeleton regulatory proteins that include N-WASP and the Scar/WAVE proteins 1–3 (Oda et al., 2005). Several functional domains based on the genomic structure of WASP have been identified, including the N-terminal EVH1 (Ena/VASP homology 1) domain followed by a basic region (BR), a GTPase-binding domain (GBD), a polyproline-rich region, and a C-terminal *Verprolin*

454

homology/Central region/Acid region (VCA) domain (Burns et al., 2004).

One of the essential roles of WASP is the regulation of actin polymerization by actin-related protein (Arp) 2/3, as illustrated by the findings that WAS macrophages fail to organize the Arp2/3 complex in podosomes (Linder et al., 1999). In this model, WASP is present in two configurations: the active form, in which the C terminus of WASP is free to interact with the Arp2/3 complex, and the inactive form, in which the C terminus forms an autoinhibitory contact with the BR of the GBD (Kim et al., 2000).

The distinct domains of WASP form the basis for its multiple functions, which include self-regulation, cytoplasmic signaling, and, through the interaction with Arp2/3, actin polymerization. The identification of the WASP gene has not only provided new insight into the critical role played by this complex molecule in cell movement and cell–cell interaction but also has had an impact on establishing a genotype–phenotype correlation (Imai et al., 2004; Jin et al., 2004), carrier detection, and prenatal diagnosis. Early diagnosis is crucial for optimal therapy, which includes antibiotics and intravenous immunoglobulin (IVIG) substitution, and stem cell transplantation to cure this devastating disease.

Clinical and Pathologic Manifestations

Incidence, Onset of Symptoms, and Age at Diagnosis

The incidence of the classic WAS phenotype has been estimated to be between 1 and 10 in one million individuals (Ryser et al., 1988; Stray-Pederson et al., 2000). With broader awareness of the classic syndrome and the much milder XLT phenotype, along with the availability of reliable diagnostic tools, the true incidence is expected to be even higher.

Early manifestations of WAS and XLT are often present at birth and consist of petechiae, bruises, and bloody diarrhea (Wiskott, 1937). Because of the increased risk of intracranial bleeding during vaginal delivery, birth by cesarean section is an option if the diagnosis is known prenatally. Excessive hemorrhage following circumcision is an early diagnostic clue. Eczema, either mild and localized or severe and generalized, is a consistent early manifestation of classic WAS. The most persistent findings at diagnosis, both in classic WAS and in XLT, are thrombocytopenia and small platelets. Infections, including otitis media with drainage of mucoid purulent material, are frequent complaints during the first 6 months of life. In a retrospective study carried out in the United States, the average age at diagnosis was 21 months, with a range from birth to 25 years (Sullivan et al., 1994). The diagnosis was established earlier in patients with known affected family members (mean age at diagnosis 10 months) than in patients without a family history (24 months). Patients presenting with the XLT phenotype are often diagnosed as having idiopathic thrombocytopenia (ITP), considerably delaying the actual diagnosis, sometimes until adulthood.

Infections

Because of the profound cellular and humoral immune deficiency, infections are common manifestations of classic WAS. Upper and lower respiratory infections, often caused by common bacteria, are frequent and include otitis media (reported by 78% of WAS patients), sinusitis (24%), and pneumonia (45%) (Sullivan et al., 1994). In the same retrospective study, sepsis was observed in 24%, meningitis in 7%, and "infectious" diarrhea in 13%. Severe viral infections do occur, but less frequently, and include varicella

with systemic complications that may require treatment with acyclovir and high-dose IVIG or varicella-zoster immunoglobulin (VZIG). Recurrent herpes simplex infections are observed in 12% of WAS patients. *Pneumocystis carinii* pneumonia (PCP), reported to affect 9% of WAS patients, is less prevalent than in patients with severe combined immune deficiency (SCID) or X-linked hyper-IgM syndrome (X-HIM) (Sullivan et al., 1994). Fungal infections, caused predominantly by *Candida* species, are relatively rare (10% of WAS patients) but may become more extensive during treatment with antibiotics. Patients with the XLT phenotype often lack a history of severe and frequent infections (Villa et al., 1995; de Saint-Basile et al., 1996; Imai et al., 2004; Jin et al., 2004).

Defects of the Immune System

Cognate immunity

The extent of the immune deficiency varies from family to family and depends largely on the mutation and its effect on WASP expression (Imai et al., 2004; Jin et al., 2004). Both T and B lymphocyte functions are affected. During infancy, the number of circulating lymphocytes may be normal or moderately decreased (Ochs et al., 1980; Park et al., 2004). By 6 years of age, lymphopenia due to loss of T lymphocytes is a common finding in patients with classic WAS (Ochs et al., 1980). This may be in part due to accelerated cell death observed in peripheral blood lymphocytes from patients with WAS but not from those with XLT (Rawlings et al., 1999; Rengan et al., 2000). Serum IgG levels are usually normal, IgM levels are depressed, and IgA and IgE are frequently elevated. The fact that serum immunoglobulin levels are normal or elevated suggests increased production, considering that the catabolism of immunoglobulin and albumin are twice that of normal controls (Blaese et al., 1971). The absolute number of B cells may be normal or moderately depressed (Park et al., 2005). Isohemagglutinin titers are frequently low (Ochs et al., 1980; Sullivan et al., 1994).

Antibody responses are normal to some antigens and insufficient to others. A consistent finding is a markedly depressed response to polysaccharide antigens (Cooper et al., 1968; Ochs et al., 1980). This characteristic pattern of antibody deficiency is further illustrated by the observation that antibody responses to staphylococcal proteins are often normal, whereas antibody responses to streptococcal polysaccharides are consistently abnormal in WAS patients (Ayoub et al., 1968). In a multicenter retrospective review, abnormal antibody responses to a variety of protein antigens, including diphtheria and tetanus toxoid and to Hib vaccine (conjugated and unconjugated), were reported to be abnormal in more than 50% of WAS patients; in contrast, antibody responses to live virus vaccines were normal (Sullivan et al., 1994). Antibody responses to intravenous immunization with bacteriophage ΦX174 are severely depressed in patients with classic WAS (i.e., patients lacking the WAS protein in lymphocytes), characterized by lack of amplification and failure to switch from IgM to IgG (Fig. 31.1). These findings suggest abnormal class switch recombination and lack of somatic hypermutation. In contrast, patients with XLT mount a more robust response with amplification and isotype switching that may reach responses comparable to those of normal controls.

Abnormal T cell function is suggested by diminished but not absent lymphocyte responses to mitogens (Cooper et al., 1968), depressed proliferative responses to allogenic cells (Ochs et al., 1980) and immobilized anti-CD3 monoclonal antibody (Molina et al., 1993), and complete lack of proliferation in response to pe-

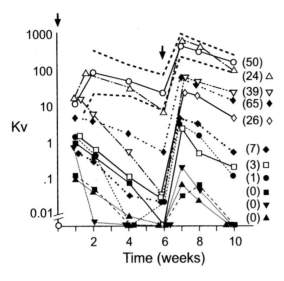

Figure 31.1. Antibody responses to the T cell–dependent neoantigen, bacteriophage φX174 (phage), in patients with WAS/XLT. Phage was injected intravenously twice, 6 weeks apart (primary and secondary immunization) at a dose of 2×10^9 PFU/kg body weight (↓), and the production of phage-specific antibody determined. Antibody titers were measured by a neutralizing assay expressed as rate of phage inactivation (Kv). The geometric mean antibody titers of normal males, following phage immunization, are indicated (0); ±1 SD is indicated by broken lines. Percent IgG (in parentheses) was determined for serum samples obtained 2 weeks after secondary immunization by treatment with 2-mercaptoethanol (2-ME). Patients characterized by ◆, ◆ and ▲, ▼ are two pairs of cousins from two unrelated families with severe classic WAS (scores 4 and 5). The two patients indicated by the symbols ■ and ● are unrelated and also have classic WAS (score 3 and 4). The symbols △, ▽, □, ◇ indicate patients with XLT (n = 3).

riodate (Siminovitch et al., 1995). In a retrospective study of 154 patients, Sullivan et al. (1994) reported depressed proliferative responses to mitogens and allogenic cells in approximately 50% of the patients. Skin tests for delayed-type hypersensitivity were abnormal in 90% of the patients studied. Partial chimerism due to the engraftment of only donor T lymphocytes corrected the immune defect, including antibody responses to polysaccharides, which suggests that the abnormal antibody production observed in WAS patients is largely caused by defective T lymphocyte function (Parkman et al., 1978). The increased incidence of *Pneumocystis carinii* pneumonia also points to a significant T cell defect in classic WAS. More recent studies suggest, however, that B cell function is equally affected. Epstein-Barr virus (EBV)-transformed B lymphoblasts derived from WAS patients have reduced levels of filamentous (F) actin (Facchetti et al., 1998). B cells from WAS patients with mutations that lead to a complete absence of WASP, compared with normal B cells, have a defect in cell motility in response to CXCL13, and decreased ability to adhere homotypically and form long cytoplasmic protrusions after stimulation with anti-CD40 and interleukin (IL)-4 (Westerberg et al., 2005). By extending these studies to Wasp-deficient murine B cells, a reduced and delayed antibody response to not only T cell–dependent but also T cell–independent antigens was discovered, a finding suggesting an intrinsic functional B cell defect. It is possible, however, that this B cell deficiency is secondary to the abnormal migration, impaired homing of B cells, and reduced germinal-center formation observed in Wasp knockout mice (Westerberg et al., 2005). Additional experimental evidence is required to determine if the observed B cell deficiency is at least in part due to defective macrophage/dendritic or T cell function.

Innate immunity

The susceptibility of WAS patients to viral infections and to malignancies may be the consequence of cytolytic or cytotoxic dysfunction. In normal NK cells, WAS can easily be detected in the immunologic synapse, together with F-actin. NK cells from patients with classic WAS lack WASP and show a markedly reduced accumulation of F-actin in the immunologic synapse. As a direct result, patients with WASP mutations have defective cytolytic NK cell function (Orange et al., 2002). These findings were confirmed and expanded in a recent study of NK cell cytotoxicity in both classic WAS and XLT patients (Gismondi et al., 2004). Although the percentage of NK cells was normal or increased, NK cell cytotoxicity was inhibited in all patients with classic WAS and in most patients carrying mutations associated with the XLT phenotype. This inhibition of NK cell–mediated cytotoxicity was associated with a reduced ability of WAS/XLT-NK cells to form conjugates with susceptible target cells and to accumulate F-actin on binding.

The involvement of the cytoskeleton in cell migration, active phagocytosis, and cell trafficking of myeloid cells, macrophages, dendritic cells, and Langerhans cells makes these cells vulnerable to WASP mutations. A large number of studies, some performed as early as 30 years ago (Altman et al., 1974), have investigated the functionality of WASP-deficient monocytes, macrophages, and dendritic cells. In both WAS and XLT patients and in Wasp$^{-/-}$ mice, a substantial defect in cell trafficking, pathogen clearance, and uptake of particulate antigen has been observed. Phagocytic cup formation and IgG-mediated and apoptotic cell phagocytosis are impaired in WASP-deficient macrophages (Lorenzi et al., 2000; Leverrier et al., 2001). A striking deficiency is the complete failure to assemble podosomes in monocytes or macrophages and dendritic cells, which results in a severe defect of adhesion and motility (Calle et al., 2004a). WASP-deficient macrophages have an abnormal, elongated shape, lack a clear lamellipodium front, and show impaired chemotactic responses (Calle et al., 2004a). Abnormalities are likely caused by defective filopodia formation, since filopodia are involved in sensing the immediate microenvironment of the cell. Transfection of full-length WASP cDNA into WASP-deficient macrophages restores chemotaxis in response to CSF-1 (Jones et al., 2002).

WASP is also involved in osteoclast function. In normal osteoclasts, during bone resorption, multiple podosomes are aggregated in actin rings, forming a sealing zone. Osteoclasts derived from Wasp$^{-/-}$ mice show abnormal morphology. The abnormalities observed in Wasp$^{-/-}$ osteoclasts result in defective bone absorption when these mice are exposed to resorption challenge (Calle et al., 2004b).

The number of circulating neutrophils, the efficiency of neutrophil migration into the tissue, phagocytosis, and bactericidal activity are normal. However, in vitro chemotaxis of WAS neutrophils in response to various chemoattractants is insufficient, an abnormality that is most pronounced in the early phase of chemotaxis (Ochs et al., 1980).

Platelet Abnormalities

The platelet defect, thrombocytopenia and small platelet volume, is a consistent finding in patients with mutations of the *WASP* gene. Platelet counts vary from patient to patient and within individual patients; platelet counts may be as low as 5000/mm³ or as high as 50,000/mm³. Higher counts, observed transiently, are often associated with inflammation or bacterial infections (Odda and Ochs, 2000). Families with intermittent thrombocytopenia associated with unique amino acid substitutions in the *WASP* gene have been described (Notarangelo et al., 2002). In most patients, the mean platelet volume (MPV) is half that of normal control subjects (MPV = 3.8–5.0 fl; compared with 7.1–10.5 fl), resulting in a thrombocrit of approximately 0.01%, compared with a normal range of 0.14% to 0.31% (Ochs et al., 1980). After splenectomy, platelet counts and platelet volume increase but are still less than that of normal controls (Litzman et al., 1996; Haddad et al., 1999). Partial but significant recovery of platelet counts following splenectomy suggests that the development of thrombocytopenia is at least in part due to the destruction of platelets in the spleen or other reticular endothelial organs of patients with WAS or XLT (Gröttum et al., 1969; Baldini, 1972; Murphy et al., 1972). This interpretation is supported by the observation that platelet and macrophages colocalize in spleen sections from WAS patients, a finding strongly suggesting that damaged platelets are ingested by macrophages in the spleen (Shcherbina et al., 1999). Increased expression of phosphatidylserine (PS) on circulating platelets from WAS patients has been interpreted as one of the reasons for the increased phagocytosis of PS-positive platelets in WAS and XLT (Shcherbina et al., 1999). An alternative explanation is a decrease in platelet production. This possibility was suggested by the observation that autologous platelet survival in WAS and XLT patients was only reduced to half that of normal (5 days ±1.3 days SD) (Ochs et al., 1980). A persistent finding was a decrease in platelet turnover, which was approximately 30% of the value found in normal subjects, indicating a significant platelet production defect. Because the marrow megakaryocyte mass is normal or increased in WAS and XLT patients (Ochs et al., 1980; Haddad et al., 1999), it has been suggested that ineffective thrombocytopoiesis is at least in part responsible for the low platelet count. The discrepancy between a normal to increased marrow substrate available for platelet production (megakaryocyte cytoplasmic mass) and the low rate at which platelets actually appear in the circulation (platelet turnover) characterizes the platelet production defect known as ineffective thrombocytopoiesis (Slichter and Harker, 1978). It was hypothesized that this abnormality was due to a defect in platelet demarcation and platelet release from megakaryocytes, possibly a direct consequence of the interaction of WASP with the cytoskeleton. This mechanism is supported by the observation of Kajiwara et al. (1999), who reported that in semi-solid culture assays, bone marrow CD34+ cells from WAS patients failed to form efficiently megakaryocyte colonies and to mature fully into platelet-releasing megakaryocytes. Using a megakaryoblastic cell line (MEG-01), Miki and coworkers (1997) showed that WASP is indispensable for actin filament reorganization to microvesicles during megakaryocyte differentiation. In contrast, Haddad and coworkers (1999), studying megakaryocytes derived in vitro from CD34+ cells, found normal megakaryocyte differentiation and proplatelet formation in both WAS and XLT patients. Interestingly, the in vitro–produced platelets were of normal size, whereas peripheral blood platelets from the same patient exhibited an abnormally small size. Moreover, F-actin distribution was abnormal in cultured megakaryocytes from WAS patients. In spite of these abnormalities, megakaryocytes from WAS patients migrated normally in response to stroma-derived factor-1 (SDF-1) α. At this point, it is unclear if transendothelial migration of megakaryocytes is important for enhanced platelet formation, or if megakaryocyte movements would be abnormal if other chemotactic active factors were used. The observation that WASP is tyrosine phosphorylated after stimulation of platelets by collagen (Oda et al., 1998) may be relevant to megakaryocyte migration since collagen seems to be involved in the interaction between megakaryocytes and endothelial cells. It is possible that abnormal interaction between

WAS megakaryocytes and endothelial cells through adhesion signals other than SDF-1α might have a direct impact on platelet formation. Several investigators have reported abnormal structure, function, and metabolism of WAS platelets (Kuramoto et al., 1970; Baldini, 1972). Because it is generally difficult to examine the function of platelets from thrombocytopenic patients, the data obtained may merely reflect the reduced size or damage of platelets. Platelet aggregation defects, as determined by abnormal responses to ADP, collagen, and epinephrine, have been reported (Gröttum et al., 1969; Kuramoto et al., 1970). These findings have been interpreted as platelet functional defects, but the severe thrombocytopenia compromises interpretation. One splenectomized XLT patient who had enough platelets for aggregation studies showed normal aggregation (Ochs et al., 1980). However, Tsuboi and colleagues have recently discovered that WASP binds to the calcium and integrin-binding (CIB) protein in platelets and that WASP altered by missssense mutations affecting exons 1–3 show lower affinity for CIB than wild type WASP. This impaired complex formation between mutant WASP and CIB reduces αIIbβ3-mediated cell adhesion and causes defective platelet aggregation, contributing to the hemorrhagic diathesis of WAS/XLT patients (Tsuboi et al., 2006). Furthermore, the incidence of severe, life-threatening bleeding is relatively small, in spite of platelet numbers being as low as 5000/mm³, suggesting that WAS platelets function normally in vivo. Nevertheless, a pronounced bleeding tendency is often the first sign of WAS or XLT and may be the only clinically relevant symptom in XLT patients. The presence of petechiae or prolonged bleeding after circumcision in newborns may alert the physician and lead to early diagnosis. In a large retrospective study, the clinical manifestation of bleeding was present in 84% of WAS patients and consisted of petechiae and/or purpura (78%), hematemesis and melena (28%), epistaxis (16%), and oral bleeding (6%). Life-threatening bleeding, including oral, gastrointestinal, and intracranial hemorrhage, occurred in 30% of WAS patients, with intracranial hemorrhage being observed in only 2% (Sullivan et al., 1994).

Carrier females with mutations leading to classic WAS have normal platelet numbers, size, function, and survival time. This finding is explained by the nonrandom X chromosome inactivation in T cells, B cells, and platelets (Gealy et al., 1980; Fearon et al., 1988; Greer et al., 1989; Puck et al., 1990). However, carrier females in families with a mild XLT phenotype may have random X chromosome inactivation in hematopoietic cells, with occasional skewing in favor of the X chromosome with the mutation. In these rare situations, carrier females may present with the XLT phenotype, which is often confused with ITP (Inoue et al., 2002; Lutskiy et al., 2002; Zhu et al., 2002).

Eczema and Other Atopic Manifestations

Eczema is another characteristic finding that differentiates WAS from ITP (Wiskott, 1937). The typical skin lesions resemble acute or chronic eczema in nature and distribution. A history of eczema, mild or severe, transient or consistent, was reported by 81% of a cohort of WAS patients (Sullivan et al., 1994). In the most severe cases, eczema is resistant to therapy and may persist into adulthood. *Molluscum contagiosum*, herpes simplex, or bacterial infections may develop in areas of the skin affected with eczema, often posing a therapeutic challenge. Patients with the XLT phenotype have either mild and transient eczema or none at all (Imai et al., 2004; Jin et al., 2004). Bacterial antigens appear to play an important role in the persistence of chronic eczema, because the skin lesions of WAS patients often respond promptly to treatment with systemic antibiotics. It has been hypothesized that defective chemotaxis of dendritic and Langerhans cells may play a role in generating T cells responsible for the development of atopic diathesis (Thrasher et al., 1998). This mechanism is further supported by the observation that eczema disappears during conditioning but before the infusion of donor bone marrow stem cells has occurred. The eczema tends to be worse in families with atopic diathesis, a finding suggesting that other genes responsible for allergies may have a modifying effect.

Some WAS patients develop allergies to certain foods or drugs. Exposure to these antigens may result in anaphylactic shock.

Autoimmune Manifestations

Autoimmune diseases are frequent and have been reported in 40% of a large cohort of WAS patients (Sullivan et al., 1994). The most common autoimmune manifestation reported has been hemolytic anemia, followed by vasculitis involving both small and large vessels, renal disease, Henoch-Schönlein-like purpura, and inflammatory bowel disease. Other less frequent autoimmune diseases include neutropenia, dermatomyositis, recurrent angioedema, uveitis, and cerebral vasculitis. Although the incidence of autoimmune diseases in XLT patients seems to be less frequent than in classic WAS (Sullivan et al., 1994), a recent report from Japan suggests that autoimmune diseases are equally frequent in patients with a low clinical score, representing XLT, as in those with a high score, representing WAS (Imai et al., 2004). IgA nephropathy, with or without Henoch-Schönlein purpura, often causing chronic renal failure requiring dialysis or renal transplantation, was a frequent complication in Japanese patients with the XLT phenotype (Imai et al., 2004). A recent report of risk factors, clinical features, and outcome of autoimmune complications from a single center in France further underlines the importance of this problem (Dupuis-Girod et al., 2003). Of 55 WAS patients, 40 had at least one autoimmune or inflammatory complication. Autoimmune hemolytic anemia was detected in 20 patients with onset before the age of 5 years. Arthritis was present in 29%, neutropenia in 25%, vasculitis including cerebral vasculitis in 29%, inflammatory bowel disease in 9%, and renal disease in 3%. A high serum IgM concentration was a significant risk factor for the development of autoimmune disease or early death. Of 15 patients with high serum IgM levels, 14 developed autoimmune hemolytic anemia. In contrast, low serum IgM concentration (a frequently observed finding in WAS/XLT) was a marker of a favorable prognosis. In an unpublished study by the European bone marrow transplantation/ESID working party, autoimmune diseases were observed in 21 of 97 long term survivors following hematopoietic stem cell transplantation. Of those with partial (mixed) chimerism, the incidence was 67% compaired with only 14% in those with full chimerism (H. Ozsahin, personal communication).

Malignancies

Malignancies can occur during childhood but are more frequent in adolescents and young adults with the classic WAS phenotype (Kildeberg, 1961; ten Bensel et al., 1966; Brand and Marinkovich, 1969; Cotelingam et al., 1985; Sullivan et al., 1994). In a large North American cohort, malignancies were present in 13% (Sullivan et al., 1994). The average age at onset of malignancies was 9.5 years. Considering the increasing life expectancy of patients, it is reasonable to assume that the incidence of malignancies will further increase as WAS patients get older. The most frequent malignancy reported is lymphoma, usually an EBV-positive B cell lymphoma, which suggests a direct relationship with a defective immune system. Only 3 of 21 tumors—1 glioma, 1 acoustic neu-

roma, and 1 testicular carcinoma—were not of lymphoreticular origin (Sullivan et al., 1994). WAS-associated malignancies have a poor prognosis, as illustrated by the fact that only 1 of the 21 patients who developed a malignancy was alive more than 2 years after establishing the diagnosis. Bone marrow transplantation was attempted in five WAS patients with malignancies, but none survived more than 6 months (Sullivan et al., 1994). To our knowledge, no patient who underwent successful transplantation has subsequently developed a malignancy. The incidence of malignancies in patients with the XLT phenotype is unknown but is less than in classic WAS. In a series of 25 patients with XLT, age 30 years or older, two developed malignancies—one, a 43-year-old man, who died of a B cell lymphoma; and one who presented with acute lymphocytic leukemia at 37 years of age (H.D. Ochs, unpublished observation).

Laboratory Findings

Blood Cell Abnormalities

The finding that WASP is expressed in CD34+ stem cells (Wengler et al., 1995) is compatible with the observation that in WAS all hematopoietic stem cell–derived lineages are functionally abnormal, including lymphocytes, platelets, neutrophils, and macrophages.

The most consistent laboratory abnormalities for WAS and XLT are thrombocytopenia, associated with small platelets. The other two findings of the classic triad of thrombocytopenia, immunodeficiency, and eczema are often absent at the initial evaluation, even in those developing a classic WAS phenotype later in life (Sullivan et al., 1994). Laboratory evidence to establish the diagnosis is therefore of prime necessity. Abnormal T and B lymphocyte functions are generally associated with classic WAS. Absence or a reduced quantity of WAS protein in lymphocytes of WAS patients is the best confirmatory test (short of mutation analysis), allowing rapid diagnosis by a simple flow-cytometric technique (Yamada et al., 1999).

Lymphopenia is a consistent finding in patients with classic WAS (Ochs et al., 1980) and may be present at an early age (Park et al., 2004).

Iron deficiency anemia is common in infants and children with WAS because of the constant loss of red blood cells. This can be corrected with increased dietary intake of iron. Chronic infection may further impair the production of red cells. Autoimmune Coombs-positive hemolytic anemia is a frequent complication and needs to be recognized early for proper therapy.

The thrombocytopenia and small platelet size are present at birth, are persistent, and do not respond to prednisone or high-dose IVIG. Platelet counts may vary and are usually between 10,000 and 40,000 platelets/mm^3. During infection or acute autoimmune disease, the number of platelets may temporarily increase, without increasing in size. Thrombocytopenia may be intermittent in patients with characteristic missense mutations (Notarangelo et al., 2002) or absent as in boys with X-linked neutropenia due to mutations within the Cdc42-binding site (Devriendt et al., 2001; Burns et al., 2004, A.J. Thrasher and P.Y. Ancliff, unpublished observation).

Other Laboratory Abnormalities

Patients with WAS respond to infections or to autoimmune diseases with increased sedimentation rates and elevated C-reactive protein (CRP). Vasculitis is a common complication affecting small and large arteries; deposits of IgA-containing immune complexes have been found in purpuric skin lesions and in the small bowel of a WAS patient with a Henoch-Schönlein purpura-like vasculities (H.D. Ochs, unpublished observation). Hemolytic anemia is often due to a warm autoantibody to red blood cell surface antigens that can be demonstrated by direct or indirect Coombs' test.

Radiologic Findings

X-ray films may reveal chronic lung disease, sinusitis, or mastoiditis. Subperiostal hemorrhage is seen occasionally. Brain scans are used if cerebral hemorrhage is expected.

Histopathology

The lymphoid tissue and thymus are prime targets for pathologic changes in patients with *WASP* mutations, although the degree of involvement varies considerably. A gradual loss of cellular elements occurs in the thymus and lymphoid organs (Cooper et al., 1968). The pathologic findings in lymph nodes and spleens from WAS patients consistently reveal depletion of small lymphocytes from T cell areas, prominence of the reticulum cell stroma, the presence of atypical plasma cells with and without plasmacytosis, and extramedullary hematopoiesis (Snover et al., 1981). Progressive depletion of germinal centers is also observed (Color Plate 31.I). In a study of spleens obtained from XLT and WAS patients undergoing splenectomy, a significant depletion of the white pulp was noticed. This depletion was not limited to the T cell–dependent area but also involved the B cell compartment. Specifically, a remarkable depletion of the marginal zone (MZ) was observed in WAS patients, an abnormality that may be directly responsible for the defective antibody response to polysaccharide and selected protein antigens. There was a strong correlation between morphologic abnormalities in the splenic tissue and the clinical severity of the disease (Vermi et al., 1999). Patients with severe disease (scores of 4 and 5) had more severe depletion of the white pulp, including the T cell area, B cell area, and MZ thickness, than patients with lower scores (2–3). The lymphoid tissues and follicles of the gastrointestinal (GI) tract are usually normal (Cooper et al., 1968), although GI lymphoid depletion may occur (Wolff and Bertucio, 1957).

A variable degree of thymic hypoplasia has been observed. Cooper et al. (1968) described normal thymic architecture, normal corticomedullary differentiation, and intact Hassall's corpuscles despite a small thymus. Wolff (1967) reported two patients with thymic pathology, one with thymic hypoplasia and the other with thymic atrophy. The surface of peripheral blood lymphocytes from WAS patients, when scanned by electron microscopy, is devoid of microvillous projections, compared with normal lymphocytes (Fig. 31.2) (Kenney at al., 1986). However, more recent studies indicate that WASP deficiency allows an intact microvilli organization, strongly suggesting that WASP is dispensable for lymphocyte microvilli formation (Majstoravich et al., 2004). This finding is in keeping with the notion that WASP-mediated Arp2/3 activation results in the formation of a network of short-acting filaments bound in an end-to-side manner, as observed in macrophage and dendritic cell ruffles, whereas microvilli are composed of parallel bundles of side-to-side linked actin filaments.

Molecular Basis

Through study of DNA from WAS families with multiple affected members, the *WASP* gene was mapped to the region Xp11.22–Xp11.3 (Kwan et al., 1991). On the basis of these mapping data, Derry and colleagues (1994) isolated the *WASP* gene

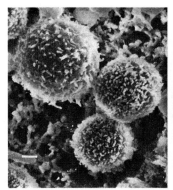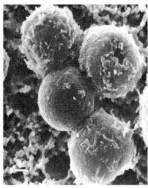

Figure 31.2. Scanning electron micrographs of normal T cells (left), and WAS T cells (right). The abundant microvilli covering the surface of the normal T cells are absent or sparse on the WAS T cells (from Kenney et al., 1986).

by positional cloning and demonstrated different mutations in lymphoblastoid cell lines derived from WAS and XLT patients.

Structure of *WASP*

The *WASP* gene consists of 12 exons spanning 9 kb of genomic DNA (Fig. 31.3). The 1821 base pair cDNA generates a protein of 502 amino acids with a predicted molecular weight of 54 kDa. WASP is constitutively expressed in all hematopoietic stem cell–derived lineages and located predominantly in the cytoplasmic compartment, with the highest protein density being along the cell membrane (Rivero-Lezcano et al., 1995; Zhu et al., 1997). WASP is a key member of a family of proteins that link signaling pathways to actin cytoskeleton reorganization by activating Arp2/3-medicated actin polymerization. Several functional domains based on the genomic structure of *WASP* have been identified (Fig. 31.3), including the N-terminal pleckstrin homology (PH) domain, the Ena/VASP homology 1 (EVH1) domain overlapping the PH domain, a basic region (BR), a GTPase binding domain (GBD)/Cdc42 or Rc-interactive binding (CRIB) motif, a proline-rich region (PPPP), and a verprolin (V) homology domain, a cofilin (C) homology domain, and an acidic (A) region (VCA) (Miki et al., 1996; Symons et al., 1996; Thrasher, 2002; Burns et al., 2004).

Pleckstrin homology domain

The PH-like domain is located close to the N-terminal region of WASP and N-WASP (a neurotissue homologue of WASP) and spans amino acids 6–105. Functionally, the PH domain is considered important for the localization of proteins through interactions with other proteins or lipids and may play a role in the binding of cytoplasmic proteins to membranes (Lemmon et al., 1996). Ligands for PH domains reported to date include phosphatidylinositol 4,5 biphosphate (PIP_2), which was shown to bind to the PH domain of N-WASP, resulting in actin polymerization in a PIP_2-dependent manner (Miki et al., 1996). PIP_2 is also bound by the BR that is N-terminal to the CRIB domain (Prehoda et al., 2000; Rohatgi et al., 2000). There is evidence that PIP_2 synergizes with Cdc42 to fully activate WASP/N-WASP in vitro (Higgs and Pollard, 2000; Rohatgi et al., 2000).

WASP interactive protein binding domain

The EVH1 domain at the N-terminal region of WASP allows recruitment of WASP-interacting protein (WIP) (Ramesh et al., 1997). In resting lymphocytes, WASP/N-WASP constitutively

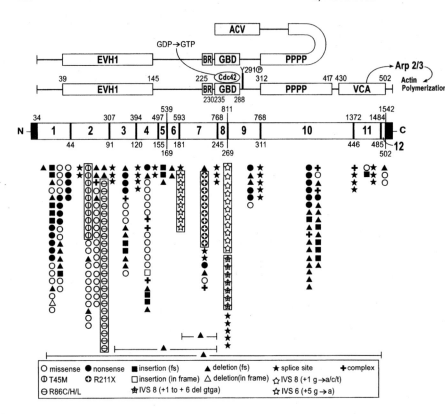

Figure 31.3. Schematic representation of WAS protein, representing 12 exons and the major functional WASP domains (center). The top panels illustrate autoinhibition of WASP. The VCA domain interacts with a region from residues 242 to 310, which include the C-terminal part of the GBD (Kim et al., 2000). If Cdc42 is activated (GDP→GTP), WASP assumes the active form, allowing the C-terminal VCA domain to freely interact with Arp2/3 to initiate actin polymerization (see text for details). The mutations of WASP identified in WASP families cared for in three Centers (Seattle, Brescia, and Tokyo) are visualized according to their location in the exons and the exon–intron junctions. Each symbol represents a single family with WASP mutation. Missense mutations are located mostly in exons 1–4; deletions and insertions are distributed throughout the *WASP* gene and splice site mutations are formed predominantly in introns 6, 8, 9, and 10. Arp2/3, actin-related protein 2/3; Br, basic region; EVH1, Ena/VASP homology 1 domain; GBD, GTPase binding domain; PPPP, proline-rich region; VCA, verpolin/cofilin homology domains/acidic region.

associates with WIP, stabilizing the inactive conformation of WASP (Martinez-Quiles et al., 2001; Sasahara et al., 2002; Volkman et al., 2002). Following engagement of the T cell antigen receptor, WIP also binds to the adaptor Crkl, which is part of a multimolecular complex that includes Crkl, WIP, and WASP and is recruited by ZAP-70 to lipid rafts and the immunologic synapse. TCR ligation causes protein kinase Cθ (PKCθ)-dependent WIP phosphorylation and disengagement of WASP from the WIP/WASP complex, thus allowing WASP activation by Cdc42 (Moreau et al., 2000; Sasahara et al., 2002). This leads to actin polymerization and stabilization of actin filaments (Volkman et al., 2002).

Cdc42 binding domain

The CBD or CRIB motif (amino acids 236–253) is located in exons 7 and 8 of the *WASP* gene (Aspenström et al., 1996; Kolluri et al., 1996; Symons et al., 1996; Abdul-Manan et al., 1999). Cdc42 is a member of the Rho family of GTPases and regulates the formation of filopodia and controls cell polarity and chemotaxis (Hall, 1998). Like other proteins containing a CRIB motif, WASP recognizes the GTP-bound but not the GDP-bound form of Cdc42 and binds to Cdc42-GTP with a 500-fold greater affinity than to Cdc42-GDP (Rudolph et al., 1998).

Computer modeling and binding experiments strongly suggest an autoinhibitory contact between the GBD and the carboxy-terminal region of WASP, which can be released by the activated (GTP) form of Cdc42 (Kim et al., 2000). Rho-like GTPases such as Cdc42 and Rac are key elements in the dynamic organization of the actin cytoskeleton (Lamarche et al., 1996). Thus, the GBD may have a direct effect on actin polymerization and an indirect effect on the interaction of the C terminus of WASP with the Arp2/3 actin nucleating complex (Fig. 31.3).

Toca-1 protein (transducer of Cdc42-dependent actin assembly) has recently been recognized as a crucial intermediate required for Cdc42/N-WASP/Arp2/3 complex–induced actin

polymerization (Ho et al., 2004). In order to mediate Cdc42-induced activation of purified N-WASP by toca-1, N-WASP must be complexed with WIP, thus demonstrating the importance of the WASP/N-WASP–WIP interaction in the regulation of actin polymerization.

SH3-Binding domain

A proline-rich region in exon 10 contains the PXXP binding consensus for SH3 binding domains. WASP was shown to interact with SH3 domains of selected signaling molecules, including the cytosolic adaptor prtoeins, Grb2, P47[nck], Fyn, cFgr, Lck, c-Src, and p[47phox]. WASP also interacts with the Tec family cytoplasmic tyrosin kinases, Btk, Tec, PLC-γ1, and Itk. This interaction may influence the localization of WASP and its contribution to the conformational changes of WASP by regulating its phosphorylation. These observations suggest that WASP, through its interaction with the SH3 domain of multiple but selected molecules, plays an important role in cytoplasmic signaling of hematopoietic cells (reviewed in Imai et al., 2003).

The proline-rich region is also required for the optimal actin polymerization activity of WASP (Castellano et al., 2001; Yarar et al., 2002) and for the recruitment of WASP to the immune synapse formed between T cells and antigen-presenting cells (Cannon et al., 2001; Badour et al., 2003; Barda-Saad et al., 2005).

Verprolin/Cofilin/Acidic region domain

The VCA domain, located in the C-terminus of WASP, plays a key role in the regulation of actin polymerization (Miki et al., 1996; Snapper and Rosen, 2003; Notarangelo and Ochs, 2003). If WASP is activated by GTP-Cdc42, the C-terminal region binds to Arp2 and Arp3 and to five unique polypeptides. The actin monomer that binds to the VC homology domain of WASP appears to be added to the Arp2/3 complex, thus promoting nucleation of the new daughter filament (Weaver et al., 2003).

Function and Regulation of WASP

WASP, with its multifunctional domains, is responsible for key tasks of hematopoietic cells. The progress made over the last 10 years in understanding the biologic functions of this complex protein has provided new insight into the pathogenesis and clinical presentation of WAS and XLT patients. WASP is expressed in CD34[+] hematopoietic precursors and in all lineage-committed cells, which suggests a role in hematopoiesis and differentiation. However, the finding that hematopoietic stem cell migration is defective in Wasp-deficient mice (Lacout et al., 2003) suggests that the nonrandom X chromosome inactivation in CD34[+] precursors and in all subsequent blood cell lineages of WASP carriers (Wengler et al., 1995) is a direct result of the failure of mutated stem cells to transit successfully from the fetal liver to the bone marrow.

Cytoskeleton and actin polymerization

WASP is a key member of a family of proteins that link signaling pathways to actin cytoskeleton reorganization by activating Arp2/3-mediated actin polymerization. This concept was suggested by Facchetti et al. (1998), who observed that the distribution of F-actin in EBV-transformed B lymphoblastoid cell lines from patients with classic WAS who lacked WASP was markedly reduced or completely absent compared with XLT subjects, who expressed reduced amounts of mutated WASP, and normal controls. In addition, cytoplasmic projections containing F-actin, recognizable as microvilli, were reduced in patients with WAS but not in patients with XLT.

Actin polymerization is initiated by the actin-related proteins (Arp), a group of proteins involved in the regulation of the actin cytoskeleton. WASP interacts directly with two of these proteins, Arp2 and Arp3, which form the Arp2/3 complex, leading to actin nucleation and formation of actin filaments (Carlier et al., 1999).

The binding of WASP to the Arp2/3 complex is mediated by the C-terminal acidic (A) region, which is preceded by the VC homology domain. This process is regulated by conformational changes in N-WASP (Rohatgi et al., 1999) and in WASP (Kim et al., 2000) by activated Cdc42 and PIP$_2$. As discussed earlier, WASP is present in two configurations. In the active form, the C terminus of WASP is free to interact with the Arp2/3 complex; in the inactive form the VCA domains interact with the hydrophobic core of the GBD. This binding is reinforced by the interaction of the acidic region (A) with a BR located N-terminal to the GBD (Kim et al., 2000). To revert to the active form, GTP-bound Cdc42 and PIP$_2$ cooperatively disrupt this autoinhibitory loop and release the C-terminal region for binding to the Arp2/3 complex (Fig. 31.3).

The importance of this cell-inhibitory mechanism is exemplified by the observation that point mutations within the GBD of WASP can cause congenital X-linked neutropenia; these mutations will interfere with the autoinhibitory contact of the C terminus of WASP with the GBD, resulting in a permanently "active" configuration of WASP (Devriendt et al., 2001; Burns et al., 2004; A.J. Thrasher and P.Y. Ancliff, unpublished results). This unregulated activation of the actin cytoskeleton promotes hematopoietic cell death by enhanced apoptosis affecting mainly myeloid progenitors (Burns et al., 2004).

Intracellular signaling

The proline-rich domain of WASP interacts with SH3 domains of selected cytoplasmic proteins, a finding suggesting that WASP is involved in intracellular signaling of hematopoietic cells.

Phosphorylation by tyrosine kinases regulates signal transduction by connecting upstream cell surface receptors to downstream pathways. WASP itself undergoes tyrosine phosphorylation following adherence of platelets to collagen (Oda et al., 1998). Baba and colleagues (1999) identified WASP as one of the major phosphoproteins associated with Btk. Together with Lyn and Btk, Hck has been shown to mediate phosphorylation of WASP Tyr291 (Scott et al., 2002). Tyr291 is conserved in N-WASP and is positioned adjacent to the Cdc42 binding site. Phosphorylation of Tyr291 stabilizes the active conformation of WASP and exposes the VCA domain, allowing them to interact with the Arp2/3 complex and to enhance cytoskeletal reorganization, which is required for the formation of the podosomes and filapodia (Cory et al., 2002). It is intriguing to speculate that the phosphorylation of Tyr291 modulates the affinity of WASP for its target, Cdc42. Dephosphorylation of Tyr291 by the tyrosine phosphatase PTP-PEST, by contrast, favors the formation of the autoinhibitory structure of WASP (Cote et al., 2002). The proline-rich region of WASP allows interaction with the SH3 domain of the linker protein, PSTPIP, which in turn binds PTP-PEST, thus establishing a physical link between WASP and PTP-PEST. This interaction results in the formation of a macromolecular complex that is recruited to the immunological synapse, where it initiates actin polymerization (Badour et al., 2003; Sasahara et al., 2002).

T cell antigen receptor engagement is crucial for the cytoplasmic signaling events that lead to cytoskeletal reorganization through actin polymerization. This process is essential for cellular shape change, cellular movement, and immune synapse formation. Recruitment of WASP to the site of actin polymerization depends on a series of biochemical events that follow TCR engagement. In mature T lymphocytes, activation of the TCR results in the phosphorylation of multiple tyrosine residues of LAT (linker for activation of T cells) and SLP-76, which leads to the migration of Nck and WASP to the cell periphery, where these molecules accumulate at an actin-rich circumferential ring. This process assures that the actin polymerization machinery is carried to the plasma membrane in the vicinity of the activated TCR. These events have recently been confirmed by direct visualization of the dynamic complexity of molecular recruitment, molecular interactions, and actin polymerization in single-living cells in time and space (Barda-Saad al., 2005).

Chemotaxes and phagocytosis

Podosomes are highly dynamic adhesion structures and are mainly found in monocytes, macrophages, osteoclasts, and dendritic cells. WAS macrophages are completely devoid of podosomes (Linder et al., 1999), resulting in defective adhesion and orientation in a chemotactic gradient (Badolato et al., 1998). Wasp-deficient murine dendritic cells fail to establish a leading edge, show defective attachment and detachment on fibronectin-coated surfaces, and display lack of chemokinesis to the chemokine CCL21 (de Noronha et al., 2005). Consequently, migration of Langerhans cells from the skin to the draining lymph node (Snapper et al., 2005) and accumulation of dendritic cells in the T cell area of the spleen following immunization are impaired in Wasp-deficient mice. Involvement of WASP in IgG-mediated phagocytosis has been demonstrated by the observation that this FcγR-dependent process is impaired in WASP-deficient peripheral blood macrophages (Lorenzi et al., 2000). In normal macrophages, WASP itself is actively recruited to the "actin cup"; in WASP-deficient macrophages, formation of the actin-cup and local recruitment of tyrosine-phosphorylated proteins are markedly reduced. These findings suggest that the cytoskeletal structure responsible for phagocytosis is dependent on WASP expression.

Clearance of apoptotic cells by macrophages and dendritic cells requires recruitment of WASP to the phagocytic cup. Lack of WASP results in delayed phagocytosis, both in vitro and in vivo (Leverrier et al., 2001).

Reduced chemotaxis of WASP-deficient neutrophils was reported in WAS patients (Ochs et al., 1980) and in Wasp-knockout mice, both in vitro and in vivo (Snapper et al., 2005). Deficiency of WASP also leads to abnormal migration of T lymphocytes. Wasp$^{-/-}$ murine T cells respond with reduced migration when exposed to the chemokine CCL19. This defect leads to impaired homing of T cells into the Payer's patches (Snapper et al., 2005).

Accelerated apoptosis

A correlation between actin cytoskeletal function, mutations of WASP, and programmed cell death has been suggested (Kothakota et al., 1997; Melamed and Gelfand, 1999; Rawlings et al., 1999; Rengan et al., 2000). The morphologic changes that occur during apoptosis require actin cytoskeletal remodeling, a process necessary for the execution of programed cell death. Defective actin polymerization may explain the accelerated in vitro cell death of lymphocytes and the progressive cellular and humoral immunodeficiency observed in individuals with classic WAS.

The precise role of WASP in apoptosis is not clearly defined. The down-regulation of a cell survival pathway or, conversely, the up-regulation of a cell death pathway in WAS lymphocytes has been considered. Accordingly, reduced Bcl-2 expression (Rawlings et al., 1999) and increased expression of caspase-3 and the cell death receptor CD95 (Fas) (Rengan et al., 2000) by WAS lymphocytes, compared with that in XLT and control lymphocytes, have been reported.

Mutation Analysis

The cloning and sequencing of the gene responsible for WAS and XLT have provided a tool for confirming the diagnosis in affected males, identifying carrier females, and performing prenatal diagnosis. Techniques are available to screen peripheral blood lymphocytes for the presence or absence of WASP, sequence cDNA and/or genomic DNA for mutations of the WASP gene, and estimate the quantity of WASP by Western blot analysis or flow cytometry.

Spectrum of WASP Mutations

Following the discovery of the gene responsible for WAS and XLT, large series of WASP mutations were published from clinical centers of Europe, North America, and Asia (Schwarz, 1996; Jin et al., 2004; Imai et al., 2004; see WASPbase at: http://homepage.mac.com/kohsukeimai/wasp/waspbase.html). Figure 31.3 summarizes the results of sequencing studies computed from three centers: Brescia, Italy; Seattle, USA; and Tokyo, Japan. Of the 312 patients from 270 families included in this analysis, 184 (from 159 families) were studied molecularly at the University of Washington, Seattle; 78 patients (from 68 families) were studied at the University of Brescia, Italy; and 50 patients (from 43 families) were investigated at the Medical and Dental University, Tokyo (Imai et al., 2004; Jin et al., 2004). Participants in these studies included natives of North, Central, and South America, Western and Eastern Europe, the Middle East, South East Asia,

Table 31.1. Distribution of Mutations in 270 Families with Wiskott-Aldrich Syndrome or X-Linked Thrombocytopenia

Mutation Type	Families Affected n (%)
Missense	93 (34.5)
Splice	59 (22)
Deletion	46 (17)
Nonsense	39 (14.5)
Insertion	19 (7)
Complex + large deletions	14 (5)
Total	270 (100)

and Japan. As expected, the incidence and type of mutations are similar in all parts of the globe. In this cohort of 270 families with WAS or XLT, 158 unique WASP mutations where identified. As shown in Table 31.1, the most common mutations observed were missense mutations ($n = 93$ families), followed by splice site mutations ($n = 59$), short deletions ($n = 46$), and nonsense mutations ($n = 39$). Insertions, complex mutations, and large deletions made up 12% of the mutations identified. Most deletions and insertions result in frameshift and early termination of transcription.

As was observed in smaller series reported previously (Derry et al., 1994; Kwan et al., 1995; Villa et al., 1995; Wengler et al., 1995; Zhu et al., 1995; Greer et al., 1996; Schindelhauer et al., 1996; Schwarz, 1996; Schwartz et al., 1996; Remold-O'Donnell et al., 1997; Zhu et al., 1997; Lemahieu et al., 1999; Itoh et al., 2000; Fillat et al., 2001), the predominant mutations of WASP, amino acid substitutions, were typically located in exons 1–4. Only four missense mutations, one each in exons 7, 9, 10, and 11, were observed downstream of exon 4. One of those, P361T in exon 10, is the only missense mutation identified to date affecting a proline in the polyproline region of WASP. In addition, two unrelated families, both with the XLT phenotype, had a point mutation affecting the termination codon of exon 12 (503 X > S), resulting in the absence of WASP.

The second-most common WASP mutations, splice site alterations, occurred predominantly in the downstream half (introns 6–11) of the WASP gene, as has been reported by others (Wengler et al., 1995; Schwarz, 1996; Zhu et al., 1997; Lemahieu et al., 1999). Of 31 unique splice site mutations, 22 affected a donor site and 9 an acceptor site. Mutations affecting variant splice sites resulted in multiple splicing products that often included small amounts of normal WASP cDNA. Insertions and short deletions typically involving less than 10 nucleotides resulted in most instances in frameshift and premature stop of translation. Complex mutations were rare and involved double missense mutations, point mutations followed by a deletion, or a combination of deletions and insertions. Four large deletions were observed, resulting in the loss of several exons. In one case, the entire WASP coding region was deleted. Of all deletions and insertions, 58% were due to "slippage" caused by the deletion or insertion of an extra nucleotide within a stretch of identical basis.

Mutational Hot Spots

In the 270 unrelated families studied, we found six mutational hot spots, defined as occurring in seven or more unrelated families (> 2.5%) (Table 31.2). Three were point mutations within the coding region; all three involved CpG dinucleotides (C > T or G > A) caused by methylation and deamination of a cytosine to

Table 31.2. *WASP* Hot-Spot Mutations and Clinical Phenotype

Mutation	Affected Families (Patients)	% of Total Families	Patients with Scores of 1–2.5*	Patients with Scores of 3–5
168C > T (T45M)	10 (11[†])	3.7	10	1**
290C > N/291G > N (R86S/G/C/H/L)	23 (25)	8.5	23	2**
IVS6 + 5g > a, fs stop aa 190/normal	8 (14)	3.0	11	3**
665C > T (R211X)	10 (11)	3.7	1	10
IVS8 + 1g > a/c/t, fs stop aa246	11 (14[†])	4.1	5	7
IVS8 +1 to +6 del gtga, fs stop aa246	7 (7)	2.6	1	6
Total	69 (82)	25.6	51	29

*A score of 2–3 is listed as a score of 2.5. Scores 1–2.5 are considered XLT; scores 3–5 represent the WAS phenotype.

[†]One patient with the T45M missense mutation and two patients with the IVS8 + 1g > a splice site mutation could not be scored because of insufficient clinical data.

**Of the six patients with high scores, four developed autoimmune diseases and one died of lymphoma at age 44 years.

Three of the hot-spot mutations (T45M; R86N; IVS6 + 5g > a) are associated with low scores and three hot-spot mutations (R211X; IVS8 + 1g > a; IVS8 +1 to +6 del gtga) are associated with high scores ($p < 0.001$). fs = frameshift

a thymidine in a sense or antisense strand. The other three hot-spot mutations involved splice sites.

The 168 C > T mutation, found in 10 families, results in the substitution of threonine with methionine at position 45; the 290 C > N/291G > N mutations, observed in 23 unrelated families, result in the substitution of arginine at position 86 with either a serine, glycine, cystidine, histidine, or leucine. The 665 C > T mutation, which converts arginine at position 211 to a stop codon, was found in 10 families. The IVS 6 + 5 g > a mutation, present in eight unrelated families, results in both abnormal and normal splicing products. The IVS 8 + 1 g > n mutation, identified in 11 families, results in the deletion of exon 8, leading to frameshift and premature stop of translation. The IVS8 + 1 to + 6 del gtga, resulting in the deletion of exon 8, frameshift, and early termination, was found in seven unrelated families. These six mutations account for 25.6% of all families included in this study. Three of these six mutations (168 C > T, 290 C > N/291 G > N, and IVSG + 5g > a) were consistently found in WASP-positive patients with a mild phenotype (XLT) who had a low score, whereas the three other mutations (665C > T, IVS8 + 1g > n-N, and IVS8 + 1to + 6 del gtga) were predominantly WASP negative and had a high score ($p < 0.001$) (Table 31.2).

Spontaneous Reversion of Mutations

Several recent studies reported somatic mosaicism due to spontaneous reversion of mutations or second-site mutations that restored WASP function (Ariga et al., 1998, 2001; Wada et al., 2001, 2003; Jin et al., 2004). These reversions have been found molecularly in both T and B cell lineages, but only revertant T cells were detected in significant numbers in the peripheral blood. This finding demonstrates that a normal copy of the *WASP* allele provides advantage of growth and survival to T cells but not to B cells. T lymphocytes that underwent reversion responded normally to CD3 stimulation and demonstrated normal actin rearrangement. Some patients seemed to improve clinically (Wada et al., 2001). The recent report of an 8-year-old WAS patient with a single nucleotide insertion in exon 4, who presented with a reversion limited to his NK cells, suggests a selective growth advantage of WAS-positive NK cells (Lutskiy et al., 2005). Although it is unclear in which precursor cells the reversions originated, these observations suggest that gene therapy (if it is possible to safely insert a normal gene into hematopoietic stem cells) could result in normalization of T and NK cells. These results also underline the key role WASP plays

in T cell proliferation and in the survival and function of both T and NK cells in vivo.

Genotype-Phenotype Correlation

Mutations of the *WASP* gene result in three distinct phenotypes: (1) the classic WAS triad of thrombocytopenia and microplatelets, recurrent infections as a result of immunodeficiency, and eczema (Wiskott, 1937; Sullivan et al., 1994); (2) the milder XLT variant, characterized predominantly by thrombocytopenia and small platelets (Villa et al., 1995; Zhu et al., 1995), which can be intermittent (Notarangelo et al., 2002); and (3) congenital neutropenia without the clinical findings characteristic of WAS and XLT (Devriendt et al., 2001). To clearly distinguish these clinical phenotypes, a scoring system, listed in Table 31.3, has been designed. The most consistent phenotype–genotype correlation was observed when the patients were divided into two categories: WASP positive if the mutated protein was of normal size, and WASP negative if the protein was absent or truncated. Patients with mutations that allowed the expression of normal-sized mutated

Table 31.3. Scoring System* to Define Phenotypes of *WASP* Mutations

	IXLT	XLT		WAS Classic		XLN
Score	<1	1	2	3	4	5	0
Thrombocytopenia	(+)	+	+	+	+	+	–
Small platelets	+	+	+	+	+	+	–
Eczema	–	–	(+)	+	++	(+)/+/++	–
Immunodeficiency	–	–/(+)	(+)	+	+	(+)/+	–
Infections	–	–	(+)	+	+/++	(+)/+/++	–
Autoimmunity and/or malignancy	–	–	–	–	–	+	–
Congenital neutropenia	–	–	–	–	–	–	+

IXLT, intermittent X-linked thrombocytopenia; WAS, Wiskott-Aldrich syndrome; WASP, Wiskott-Aldrich syndrome protein; XLN, X-linked neutropenia; XLT, X-linked thrombocytopenia.

*Scoring system: –/(+), absent or mild; (+), mild, transient eczema or mild, infrequent infections, not resulting in sequelae; +, persistent but therapy-responsive eczema and recurrent infections requiring antibiotics and often intravenous immunoglobulin prophylaxis; ++, eczema that is difficult to control and severe, life-threatening infections. Because patients with XLT may develop autoimmune disorders or lymphoma, although at a lower rate than those with classic WAS, a progression from a score of 1 or 2 to a score of 5 is possible for XLT.

From Stiehm ER, Ochs HD, Winkelstein JA, editors. Immunologic disorders in infants and children. Fifth edn. Philadelphia: Elsevier Saunders, 2004, with permission.

protein, often in reduced quantity, developed the XLT phenotype, whereas those patients whose lymphocytes could not express WASP or expressed only truncated WASP were more likely to have the WAS phenotype ($p < 0.001$, Table 31.4). When patients within one of the six hot spots were analyzed there was a highly significant concurrence of the phenotype within each group (Table 31.2). Progression to a score of 5 due to either autoimmune disease or malignancy was observed in both groups but was far more frequent in WASP-negative patients with an initial score of 3–4.

When the Japanese patients were analyzed separately (Imai et al., 2004), autoimmune diseases were equally frequent in patients with a low symptom score, representing XLT, and in those with a high score, representing WAS; this result was predominantly due to the high incidence of IgA nephropathy in the Japanese patients. There were other exceptions to the rule, as is evident from data shown in Table 31.4, a clear indication that it may be difficult in individual cases to accurately predict the clinical course based solely on the type of mutations of the WASP gene.

It is important to consider the complexity of the disease, the differences in lifestyle and medical care, chance exposure to unusual microorganisms, and the influence of genes that affect allergic predisposition, autoimmunity, and malignancies. Splice site mutations, especially if affecting variant intronic nucleotide positions, often allow the generation of multiple splicing products, including the generation of normally spliced mRNA and the production of variable quantities of normal WASP. For example, the hot-spot mutation IVS6 + 5 g > a causes the insertion of 38 nucleotides from the proximal end of intron 6, which results in frameshift and early termination of transcription, but also in the production of a small amount of normal WASP mRNA. Somatic mosaicism due to reversion is another possibility for a more favorable phenotype than that expected from the type of mutation (Wada et al., 2001). Genes that determine an individual's probability of developing atopic disease, such as allergies and eczema, or genes that control the effectiveness of host defense against infections may modify the WAS/XLT phenotype. Similarly, environmental factors, such as exposure to common or uncommon infectious agents, failure to establish the diagnosis at an early age, or less than optimal care, may affect the severity of the clinical presentation. Phenotype scoring before the age of 2 years is unreliable because it often suggests a phenotype that is milder than expected from the type of WASP mutation identified (Jin et al., 2004).

Table 31.4. Effect of Mutations on Expression of WASP*

Mutation Type	WASP+ Families Affected n (%)	WASP− Families Affected n (%)
Missense	64 (73.6)	10 (8.9)[†]
Splice	12 [I = 3, V = 9] (13.8)	30 [I = 25, V = 5] (26.8)[†]
Complex	4 (4.6)	4 (3.6)
Deletion** or insertion	5 (5.7)	32 (35.1)[†]
Nonsense	2 (2.3)	25 (22.3)[†]
Total[‡]	87 (100)	112 (100)

I, invariant sites; V, variant sites.

*Distribution of mutations in WASP-positive and WASP-negative families.

[†]Distribution of mutations observed in WASP+ and WASP− families is significantly different ($p < 0.001$).

**Including large deletions.

[‡]Not all patients analyzed were studied for expression of WASP.

Strategies for Diagnosis

Because of the wide spectrum of clinical findings, the diagnoses of WAS or XLT should be considered in any boy presenting with petechiae, bruises, and congenital or early-onset thrombocytopenia associated with small platelet size (Color Plate 31.II). The presence of transient, mild, or severe eczema supports the diagnosis of WAS or XLT. It is important to note that infections and immunologic abnormalities may be absent, mild, or severe and autoimmune disease may develop, more often in WAS than in XLT. Lymphopenia, characteristic for classic WAS, may be present during infancy but will develop invariably during childhood. Abnormal antibody response to bacteriophage Ø174 seems to be a consistent finding, even in patients with a mild phenotype (Fig. 31.1). Screening for WASP mutations can be successfully performed by flow cytometry, but patients with a substanial expression of mutated WASP may be missed. In atypical cases, mutation analysis of the WASP gene is essential for diagnosis; it may also assist in estimating the severity of the disease (with caution), and in performing carrier detection and prenatal diagnosis. It is vital to differentiate XLT from ITP patients because of the vulnerability of XLT patients to splenectomy, the need for different therapeutic approaches, and genetic implications.

Females with Wiskott-Aldrich Syndrome

Sporadic cases of females with clinical and laboratory findings compatible with the diagnosis of WAS have been described (Evans and Holzel, 1970; Lin and Hsu, 1984; Conley et al., 1992). Two sisters, born to healthy parents, who presented with recurrent infections, thrombocytopenia, petechiae, and eczema had low serum IgM, normal IgG, and elevated IgA and IgE. They had decreased T lymphocyte subsets and absent isohemagglutinins (Kondoh et al., 1995). Autosomal inheritance was also suspected in a second family with multiple affected female members, displaying clinical and laboratory findings resembling classic WAS (Rocca et al., 1996).

Several symptomatic female patients have been identified as being heterozygous for mutations of WASP. They presented with either a classic WAS phenotype (Parolini et al., 1998) or an XLT phenotype (Inoue et al., 2002; Lutskiy et al., 2002; Zhu et al., 2002). In each case, the symptomatic females were found to have markedly skewed X chromosome inactivation in favor of the X chromosome with the WASP mutation.

Carrier Detection and Prenatal Diagnosis

X-inactivation studies in WAS carrier females have shown that the normal X chromosome is preferentially used as the active X chromosome in all hematopoietic lineages, including CD34+ cells (Wengler et al., 1995). Exceptions to this rule are families with a very mild form of XLT, in which X chromosome inactivation may be random (Inoue et al., 2002; Lutskiy et al., 2002; Zhu et al., 2002).

If the WASP mutation is known in a given family, carrier females can be identified by mutation analysis. Similarly, prenatal diagnosis of a male fetus at risk for WAS or XLT can be performed by DNA analysis with chorionic villi sampling or cultured amniocytes as the source of genomic DNA (Giliani et al., 1999).

Treatment

Progress in nutrition, improved antimicrobial therapy including antiviral and antifungal drugs, and the prophylactic use of IVIG have contributed to the prolonged expectancy and quality of life of WAS patients. Early diagnosis is most important for effective prophylaxis and treatment. If an infection is suspected, careful evaluation for bacterial, viral, or fungal causes followed by appropriate antimicrobial therapy is of crucial importance. Infants with *WASP* mutations and lymphopenia are candidates for PCP prophylactics. If antibody responses to protein and/or polysaccharide antigens are defective, which is most often the case in patients with the classic WAS phenotype, prophylactic IVIG infusions at a full therapeutic dose should be initiated. The dose of IVIG may have to be increased during infections, which may aggravate the already accelerated IgG catabolism. Continuous antibiotic therapy should be considered if infections are occurring despite IVIG therapy.

Killed vaccines can be given, including pneumococcal polysaccharides and protein-conjugated vaccines; the response, however, may be abnormal and should be determined. Live-virus vaccines are not recommended. Varicella-zoster immunoglobulin or high-dose IVIG (which has high antivaricella antibody titers) and acyclovir are indicated following exposure to chickenpox. Antiviral drugs are also successfully used to treat recurrent herpes simplex infections.

Eczema, if severe, requires aggressive therapy including local steroids and, if indicated, short-term systemic use of steroids. Cutaneous infections are common and may necessitate local or systemic antibiotics. Lymphadenopathy is frequently observed and is often the consequence of infected eczema. Whether the newly approved tacrolimus ointment (Protopic 0.03%) or primecrolimuis cream (Elidel 1%) will be an alternative to steroid cream in the treatment of WAS-associated eczema remains to be seen. An appropriately restricted diet based on specific food allergies has to be selected for each patient.

Platelet transfusions are restricted to serious bleeding—for example, central nervous system hemorrhages or gastrointestinal bleeding. Blood products are best irradiated and should be cytomegalovirus negative. Aspirin, which interferes with platelet function, is contraindicated.

Splenectomy, sometimes recommended for XLT patients, effectively stops the bleeding tendency by increasing the number of circulating platelets. However, splenectomy increases the risk of septicemia and, if performed, requires continuous antibiotic prophylaxis. Data collected at the National Institutes of Health support the clinical experience that splenectomy does not effect the development of autoimmune diseases or malignancies (M. Blaese, personal communication). High-dose IVIG and systemic steroids may be considered for the treatment of autoimmune complications. Long-term immunosuppressive therapy, however, may cause the activation of viruses or increase the risk of fungal infections.

Because of poor dietary intake and constant loss of red cells, prophylactic treatment with iron is necessary to prevent chronic anemia.

Transplantation

Hematopoietic stem cell transplantation, using as source bone marrow, peripherial blood, stem cells, or cord blood, is the only curative therapy for WAS patients (Filipovich et al., 2001). To prevent rejection, a conditioning regimen with cyclophosphamide, busulfan, and antithymocyte globulin with or without irradiation is necessary. Fully matched siblings are preferred donors; their use results in highly successful stem cell transplantation, even in older patients. Matched unrelated donors are safe if the recipient is less than 5–8 years of age. In older WAS patients, matched

unrelated donor transplants are less successful and not recommended (Filipovich et al., 2001). Court blood stem cells, fully or partially matched, are excellent alternatives for boys with WAS who weigh < 25 kg, if a fully matched bone marrow donor is not available. Haploidentical bone marrow transplants have had disappointing results and are generally not recommended (Brochstein et al., 1991; Hong, 1996; Ozsahin et al., 1996), although a recent report describes successful engraftment of an unmanipulated HLA-haploidentical bone marrow transplantation from the patient's mother, resulting in stable chimerism 2 years after transplantation (Inagaki et al., 2005).

Gene Therapy

The observation that a few WAS patients spontaneously underwent in vivo reversion of an inherited mutation of the *WASP* gene in T lymphocytes (Ariga et al., 2001; Wada et al., 2001, 2003), B lymphocytes (Konno et al., 2004) and NK cells (Lutskiy et al., 2005) supports the hypothesis that, in this syndrome, genetically corrected stem cells have an in vivo advantage of developing into T cells and possibly NK cells, a prerequisite for gene therapy. On the basis of these reports, experiments are being performed with WASP-deficient human cell lines and Wasp knockout mice.

Primary T lymphocytes or herpesvirus saimiri–immortalized cell lines derived from WAS patients have been successfully transduced with lentiviral vectors expressing the human *WASP* gene. Following transduction, the cells demonstrated a substantial growth advantage; responded to TCR signaling, including down-regulation of CD3 surface expression; formed stable B and T cell conjugates; and secreted normal amounts of Il-2 upon appropriate stimulation (Dupre et al., 2004; Miao et al., 2004; Martin et al., 2005).

In experiments with Wasp knockout mice and either oncoretroviral or lentiviral vectors, the irradiated recipients showed stable expression of WASP and correction of the immune defect and cytoskeletal abnormalities (Strom et al., 2002, 2003; Charrier et al., 2005; Humblet-Baron et al., 2005).

These in vivo experiments provide proof of the principal that the WAS-associated T cell signaling defect can be improved or corrected by transplanting retrovirally transduced hematopoietic stem cells. At this time it is unclear if this technique can be used successfully in correcting other hematopoietic cell lineages—for example, the defect in megakaryocytes and platelets, macrophages and dentritic cells, or B lymphocytes, which do not show a growth advantage following transduction of the *WASP* gene.

Animal Models

Two mouse strains with Wasp deficiency have been generated by gene knockout technology (Snapper et al., 1998; Zhang et al., 1999). Hemizygous deficient male animals of both strains exhibit poor T cell proliferation and cytokine secretion in response to TCR activation by cross-linking of CD3. Wasp knockout mice have mild lymphopenia and moderate thrombocytopenia, which can be normalized by transplantation (Strom et al., 2002). However, Wasp$^{-/-}$ mice do not develop eczema or autoimmune diseases and susceptibility to infections is debatable and may not be clinically relevant (Strom et al., 2003; Andreansky et al., 2005). Importantly, these murine models have been used successfully to explore different techniques of gene therapy, including the evaluation of newly designed vectors and various conditioning regiments. However, to have access to a more relevant model of human disease, an outbred model, for instance, canine WAS/XLT, is necessary.

Conclusion and Future Directions

The clinical phenotype associated with mutations of *WASP* is as complex as the gene itself. By studying WAS, XLT, and XLN patients and their multiple *WASP* mutations, we have learned how a single gene defect can cause multiple and unique clinical symptoms. These investigations have provided new insight into the functions of WASP which facilitate not only TCR-initiated cytoplasmic signaling but also cytoskeletal reorganization and actin polymerization. The structure of WASP is responsible for two configurations of the molecule—the active form, in which the C-terminal end interacts with Arp2/3 to initiate actin polymerization, and the inactive form, in which the C-terminal end forms an autoinhibitory contact with the GBD. In the final analysis, WASP is required for efficient thrombocytopoiesis and platelet survival, T cell activation, T and B cell interaction and NK cell function, and function of the innate immune system. Since mutations of WASP interfere with the homing of hematopoietic stem cells, and thus affect all hematopoietic cell lineages, stem cell transplantation is the treatment of choice for curing this disease. For the same reason, gene therapy may work, and is one of the challenges for future *WAS* or XLT research.

Acknowledgments

The work presented here was supported by grants from the National Institutes of Health (HD17427), the Jeffrey Modell Foundation, and the Immunodeficiency Foundation.

References

Abdul-Manan N, Aghazadeh B, Liu GA, Majumdar A, Ouerfelli O, Siminovitch KA, Rosen MK. Structure of Cdc42 in complex with the GTPase-binding domain of the Wiskott-Aldrich syndrome protein. Nature 399: 379–383, 1999.

Aldrich RA, Steinberg AG, Campbell DC. Pedigree demonstrating a sex-linked recessive condition characterized by draining ears, eczematoid dermatitis and bloody diarrhea. Pediatrics 13:133–139, 1954.

Altman LC, Snyderman R, Blaese RM. Abnormalities of chemotactic lymphokine synthesis and mononuclear leukocyte chemotaxis in Wiskott-Aldrich syndrome. J Clin Invest 54:486–493, 1974.

Andreansky S, Liu H, Turner S, McCullers JA, Lang R, Rutschman R, Doherty PC, Murray PJ, Nienhuis AW, Strom TS. WASP-mice exhibit defective immune responses to influenza A virus, *Streptococcus pneumoniae*, and *Mycobacterium bovis* BDG. Exp Hematol 33:443–451, 2005.

Ariga T, Kondoh T, Yamaguchi K, Yamada M, Sasaki S, Nelson DL, Ikeda H, Kobayashi K, Moriuchi H, Sakiyama Y. Spontaneous in vivo reversion of an inherited mutation in the Wiskott-Aldrich syndrome. J Immunol 166: 5245–5249, 2001.

Ariga T, Yamada M, Sakiyama Y, Tatsuzawa O. A case of Wiskott-Aldrich syndrome with dual mutations in exon 10 of the *WASP* gene: an additional de novo one-base insertion, which restores frame shift due to an inherent one-base deletion, detected in the major population of the patient's peripheral blood lymphocytes. Blood 92:699–701, 1998.

Aspenström P, Lindberg U, Hall A. Two GTPases, Cdc42 and Rac, bind directly to a protein implicated in the immunodeficiency disorder Wiskott-Aldrich syndrome. Curr Biol 6:70–75, 1996.

Ayoub EM, Dudding BA, Cooper MD. Dichotomy of antibody response to group A streptococcal antigens in Wiskott-Aldrich syndrome. J Lab Clin Med 72:971–979, 1968.

Baba Y, Nonoyama S, Matsushita M, Yamadori T, Hashimoto S, Imai K, Arai S, Kunikata T, Kurimoto M, Kurosaki T, Ochs HD, Yata J, Kishimoto T, Tsukada S. Involvement of Wiskott-Aldrich syndrome protein in B-cell cytoplasmic tyrosine kinase pathway. Blood 93:2003–2012, 1999.

Badolato R, Sozzani S, Malacarne F, Bresciani S, Fiorini M, Borsatti A, Albertini A, Mantovani A, Ugazio AG, Notarangelo LD. Monocytes from Wiskott-Aldrich patients display reduced chemotaxis and lack of cell polarization in response to monocyte chemoattractant protein-1 and formyl-methionyl-leucyl-phenylalanine. J Immunol 161:1026–1033, 1998.

Badour K, Zhang J, Shi F, McGavin MK, Rampersad V, Hardy LA, Field D, Siminovitch KA. The Wiskott-Aldrich syndrome protein acts downstream of CD2 and the CD2AP and PSTPIP1 adaptors to promote formation of the immunological synapse. Immunity 18:141–154, 2003.

Baldini MG. Nature of the platelet defect in the Wiskott-Aldrich syndrome. Ann NY Acad Sci 201:437–444, 1972.

Barda-Saad M, Braiman A, Titerence R, Bunnell SC, Barr VA, Samelson LE. Dynamic molecular interactions linking the T cell antigen receptor to the actin cytoskeleton. Nat Immunol 6:80–89, 2005.

Berglund G, Finnström O, Johansson SGO, Möller K-L. Wiskott-Aldrich syndrome. A study of 6 cases with determination of the immunoglobulins A, D, G, M and ND. Acta Paediatr Scand 57:89–97, 1968.

Binks M, Jones GE, Brickell PM, Kinnon C, Katz DR, Thrasher AJ. Intrinsic dendritic cell abnormalities in Wiskott-Aldrich syndrome. Eur J Immunol 28:3259–3267, 1998.

Blaese RM, Strober W, Brown RS, Waldmann TA. The Wiskott-Aldrich syndrome. A disorder with a possible defect in antigen processing or recognition. Lancet 1:1056–1061, 1968.

Blaese RM, Strober W, Levy AL, Waldmann TA. Hypercatabolism of IgG, IgA, IgM, and albumin in the Wiskott-Aldrich syndrome. A unique disorder of serum protein metabolism. J Clin Invest 50:2331–2338, 1971.

Brand MM, Marinkovich VA. Primary malignant reticulosis of the brain in Wiskott-Aldrich syndrome. Report of a case. Arch Dis Child 44:546–542, 1969.

Brochstein JA, Gillio AP, Ruggiero M, Kernan NA, Emanuel D, Laver J, Small T, O'Reilly RJ. Marrow transplantation from human leukocyte antigen–identical or haploidentical donors for correction of Wiskott-Aldrich syndrome. J Pediatr 119:907–912, 1991.

Burns S, Cory GO, Vainchenker W, Thrasher AJ. Mechanisms of WASp-mediated hematologic and immunologic disease. Blood 104:3454–3462, 2004.

Calle Y, Chou HC, Thrasher AJ, Jones GE. Wiskott-Aldrich syndrome protein and the cytoskeletal dynamics of dendritic cells. J Pathol 204:460–469, 2004a.

Calle Y, Jones GE, Jagger C, Fuller K, Blundell MP, Chow J, Chambers T, Thrasher AJ. WASP deficiency in mice results in failure to form osteoclast sealing zones and defects in bone resorption. Blood 103:3552–3561, 2004b.

Canales L, Mauer AM. Sex-linked hereditary thrombocytopenia as a variant of Wiskott-Aldrich syndrome. N Engl J Med 277:899–901, 1967.

Cannon JL, Labno CM, Bosco G, Seth A, McGavin MH, Siminovitch KA, Rosen MK, Burkhardt JK. Wasp recruitment to the T cell:APC contact site occurs independently of Cdc42 activation. Immunity 15:249–259, 2001.

Carlier MF, Ducruix A, Pantaloni D. Signalling to actin: the Cdc42-N-WASP-Arp2/3 connection. Chem Biol 6:R235–240, 1999.

Castellano F, Le Clainche C, Patin D, Carlier MF, Chavrier P. A WASP-VASP complex regulates actin polymerization at the plasma membrane. EMBO J 20:5603–5614, 2001.

Charrier S, Stockholm D, Seye K, Opolon P, Taveau M, Gross DA, Bucher-Laurent S, Delenda C, Vainchenker W, Danos O, Galy A. A lentiviral vector encoding the human Wiskott-Aldrich syndrome protein corrects immune and cytoskeletal defects in WASP knockout mice. Gene Ther 12:597–606, 2005.

Chiaro JJ, Dharmkrong-at A, Bloom GE. X-linked thrombocytopenic purpura. I. Clinical and genetic studies of a kindred. Am J Dis Child 123: 565–568, 1972.

Cooper MD, Chase HP, Lowman JT, Krivit W, Good RA. Wiskott-Aldrich syndrome. An immunologic deficiency disease involving the afferent limb of immunity. Am J Med 44:499–513, 1968.

Conley ME, Wang WC, Parolini O, Shapiro DN, Campana D, Siminovitch KA. Atypical Wiskott-Aldrich syndrome in a girl. Blood 80:1264–1269, 1992.

Cory GO, Garg R, Cramer R, Ridley AJ. Phosphorylation of tyrosine 291 enhances the ability of WASP to stimulate actin polymerization and filopodium formation. Wiskott-Aldrich syndrome protein. J Biol Chem 277:45115–45121, 2002.

Cote JF, Chung PL, Theberge JF, Halle M, Spencer S, Lasky LA, Tremblay ML. PSTPIP is a substrate of PTP-PEST and serves as a scaffold guiding PTP-PEST toward a specific dephosphorylation of WASP. J Biol Chem 277:2973–2986, 2002.

Cotelingam JD, Witebsky FG, Hsu SM, Blaese RM, Jaffe ES. Malignant lymphoma in patients with the Wiskott-Aldrich syndrome. Cancer Invest 3:515–522, 1985.

de Noronha S, Hardy S, Sinclair J, Blundell MP, Strid J, Schulz O, Zwirner J, Jones GE, Katz DR, Kinnon C, Thrasher AJ. Impaired dendritic-cell homing in vivo in the absence of Wiskott-Aldrich syndrome protein. Blood 105:1590–1597, 2005.

Derry JMJ, Ochs HD, Francke U. Isolation of a novel gene mutated in Wiskott-Aldrich syndrome [published erratum appears in Cell 79(5): following 922, 1994]. Cell 78:635–644, 1994.

De Sainte-Basile G, Lagelouse RD, Lambert N, Schwarz K, Le Mareck B, Odent S, Schlegel N, Fischer A. Isolated X-linked thrombocytopenia in two unrelated families is associated with point mutations in the Wiskott-Aldrich syndrome protein gene. J Pediatr 129:56–62, 1996.

Devriendt K, Kim AS, Mathijs G, Frints SG, Schwartz M, Van Den Oord JJ, Verhoef GE, Boogaerts MA, Fryns JP, You D, Rosen MK, Vandenberghe P. Constitutively activating mutation in WASP causes X-linked severe congenital neutropenia. Nat Genet 27:313–317, 2001.

Donnér M, Schwartz M, Carlsson KU, Holmberg L. Hereditary X-linked thrombocytopenia maps to the same chromosomal region as the Wiskott-Aldrich syndrome. Blood 72:1849–1853, 1988.

Dupre L, Aiuti A, Trifari A, Martino S, Saracco P, Bordignon C, Roncarolo MG. Wiskott-Aldrich syndrome protein regulates lipid raft dynamics during immunological synapse formation. Immunity 17:157–166, 2002.

Dupre L, Trifari S, Follenzi A, Marangoni F, Lain de Lera T, Bernad A, Martino S, Tsuchiya S, Bordignon C, Naldini L, Aiuti A, Roncarolo MG. Lentiviral vector-mediated gene transfer in T cells from Wiskott-Aldrich syndrome patients leads to functional correction. Mol Ther 10:903–915, 2004.

Dupuis-Girod S, Medioni J, Haddad E, Quartier P, Cavazzana-Calvo M, Le Deist F, de Saint Basile G, Delaunay J, Schwarz K, Casanova JL, Blanche S, Fischer A. Autoimmunity in Wiskott-Aldrich syndrome: risk factors, clinical features, and outcome in a single-center cohort of 55 patients. Pediatrics 111:622–627, 2003.

Evans DI, Holzel A. Immune deficiency state in a girl with eczema and low serum IgM. Possible female variant of Wiskott-Aldrich syndrome. Arch Dis Child 45:527–533, 1970.

Facchetti F, Blanzuoli L, Vermi W, Notarangelo LD, Giliani S, Fiorini M, Fasth A, Stewart DM, Nelson DL. Defective actin polymerization in EBV-transformed B-cell lines from patients with the Wiskott-Aldrich syndrome. J Pathol 185:99–107, 1998.

Fearon ER, Kohn DB, Winkelstein JA, Vogelstein B, Blaese RM. Carrier detection in the Wiskott Aldrich syndrome. Blood 72:1735–1739, 1988.

Filipovich AH, Stone JV, Tomany SC, Ireland M, Kollman C, Pelz CJ, Casper JT, Cowan MJ, Edwards JR, Fasth A, Gale RP, Junker A, Kamani NR, Loechelt BJ, Pietryga DW, Ringden O, Vowels M, Hegland J, Williams AV, Klein JP, Sobocinski KA, Rowlings PA, Horowitz MM. Impact of donor type on outcome of bone marrow transplantation for Wiskott-Aldrich syndrome: collaborative study of the International Bone Marrow Transplant Registry and the National Marrow Donor Program. Blood 97:1598–1603, 2001.

Fillat C, Espanol T, Oset M, Ferrando M, Estivill X, Volpini V. Identification of WASP mutations in 14 Spanish families with Wiskott-Aldrich syndrome. Am J Med Genet 100:116–121, 2001.

Gallego M, Santamaria M, Pena J, Molina I. Defective actin reorganization and polymerization of Wiskott-Aldrich T cells in response to CD3-mediated stimulation. Blood 90:3089–3097, 1997.

Gealy WJ, Dwyer JM, Harley JB. Allelic exclusion of glucose-6-phosphate dehydrogenase in platelets and T lymphocytes from a Wiskott-Aldrich syndrome carrier. Lancet 1:63–65, 1980.

Giliani S, Fiorini M, Mella P, Candotti F, Schumacher RF, Wengler GS, Lalatta F, Fasth A, Badolato R, Ugazio AG, Albertini A, Notarangelo LD. Prenatal molecular diagnosis of Wiskott-Aldrich syndrome by direct mutation analysis. Prenat Diagn 19:36–40, 1999.

Gismondi A, Cifaldi L, Mazza C, Giliani S, Parolini S, Morrone S, Jacobelli J, Bandiera E, Notarangelo L, Santoni A. Impaired natural and CD16-mediated NK cell cytotoxicity in patients with WAS and XLT: ability of IL-2 to correct NK cell functional defect. Blood 104:436–443, 2004.

Greer WL, Kwong PC, Peacocke M, Ip P, Rubin LA, Siminovitch KA. X-chromosome inactivation in the Wiskott-Aldrich syndrome: a marker for detection of the carrier state and identification of cell lineages expressing the gene defect. Genomics 4:60–67, 1989.

Greer WL, Shehabeldin A, Schulman J, Junker A, Siminovitch KA. Identification of WASP mutations, mutation hotspots and genotype–phenotype disparities in 24 patients with the Wiskott-Aldrich syndrome. Hum Genet 98:685–690, 1996.

Gröttum KA, Hovig T, Holmsen H, Abrahamsen AF, Jeremic M, Seip M. Wiskott-Aldrich syndrome: qualitative platelet defects and short platelet survival. Br J Haematol 17:373–388, 1969.

Haddad E, Cramer E, Riviere C, Rameau P, Louache F, Guichard J, Nelson DL, Fischer A, Vainchenker W, Debili N. The thrombocytopenia of Wiskott-Aldrich syndrome is not related to a defect in proplatelet formation. Blood 94:509–518, 1999.

Hall A. Rho GTPases and the actin cytoskeleton. Science 279:509–514, 1998.

Higgs HN, Pollard TD. Activation by Cdc42 and PIP(2) of Wiskott-Aldrich syndrome protein (WASp) stimulates actin nucleation by Arp2/3 complex. J Cell Biol 150:1311–1320, 2000.

Ho HY, Rohatgi R, Lebensohn AM, Le Ma, Li J, Gygi SP, Kirschner MW. Toca-1 mediates Cdc42-dependent actin nucleation by activating the N-WASP-WIP complex. Cell 118:203–216, 2004.

Hong RT. Disorders of the T cell system. In: Stiehm ER, ed. Immunologic Disorders in Infants and Children, 4th edition. Philadelphia: WA Saunders, pp. 339–408, 1996.

Huang W, Ochs HD, Dupont B, Vyas YM. The Wiskott-Aldrich syndrome protein regulates nuclear translocation of NFAT2 and NF-κB (RelA) independently of its role in filamentous actin polymerization and actin cytoskeletal rearrangement. J Immunol 174:2602–2611, 2005.

Humblet-Baron S, Anover S, Kipp K, Zhu Q, Ye P, Zhang W, Ovechkina Y, Khim S, Astrakhan A, Strom TS, Kohn DB, Candotti F, Vyas Y, Ochs HD, Miao C, Rawlings D. Lentiviral vector–mediated gene therapy as treatment for Wiskott-Aldrich syndrome (WAS): preclinical studies in human cell lines and WASp−/− mice [abstract 341]. Presented at the American Society of Gene Therapy, 8th Annual Meeting, St Louis, Missouri, 2005.

Huntley CC, Dees SC. Eczema associated with thrombocytopenic purpura and purulent otitis media: report of five fatal cases. Pediatrics 19:351–361, 1957.

Imai K, Morio T, Zhu Y, Jin Y, Itoh S, Kajiwara M, Yata J, Mizutani S, Ochs HD, Nonoyama S. Clinical course of patients with WASP gene mutations. Blood 103:456–464, 2004.

Imai K, Nonoyama S, Ochs HD. WASP (Wiskott-Aldrich syndrome protein) gene mutations and phenotype. Curr Opin Allergy Clin Immunol 3:427–436, 2003.

Inagaki J, Park YD, Kishimoto T, Yoshioka A. Successful unmanipulated haploidentical bone marrow transplantation from an HLA 2-locus-mismatched mother for Wiskott-Aldrich syndrome after unrelated cord blood stem cell transplantation. J Pediatr Hemotol Oncol 27:229–231, 2005.

Inoue H, Kurosawa H, Nonoyama S, Imai K, Kumazaki H, Matsunaga T, Sato Y, Sugita K, Eguchi M. X-linked thrombocytopenia in a girl. Br J Haematol 118:1163–1165, 2002.

Itoh S, Nonoyama S, Moria T, Imai K, Okawa H, Ochs HD, Shimadzu M, Yata J. Mutations of the WASP gene in 10 Japanese patients with Wiskott-Adrich syndrome and X-linked thrombocytopenia. Int J Hematol 71:79–83, 2000.

Jin Y, Mazza C, Christie JR, Giliani S, Fiorini M, Mella P, Gandellini F, Stewart DM, Zhu Q, Nelson DL, Notarangelo LD, Ochs HD. Mutations of the Wiskott-Aldrich syndrome protein (WASP): hotspots, effect on transcription and translation and phenotype/genotype correlation. Blood 104:4010–4019, 2004.

Jones GE, Zicha D, Dunn GA, Blundell M, Thrasher A. Restoration of podosomes and chemotaxis in Wiskott-Aldrich syndrome macrophages following induced expression of WASp. Int J Biochem Cell Biol 34:806–815, 2002.

Kajiwara M, Nonoyama S, Eguchi M, Morio T, Imai K, Okawa H, Kaneko M, Sako M, Ohga S, Maeda M, Hibi S, Hashimito H, Shibuya A, Ochs HD, Nakahata T, Yata JI. WASP is involved in proliferation and differentiation of human haemopoietic progenitors in vitro. Br J Haematol 107:254–262, 1999.

Kenney DM, Cairns L, Remold-O'Donnell E, Peterson J, Rosen FS, Parkman R. Morphological abnormalities in the lymphocytes of patients with the Wiskott-Aldrich syndrome. Blood 68:1329–1332, 1986.

Kildeberg P. The Aldrich syndrome. Report of a case and discussion of pathogenesis. Pediatrics 27:362–369, 1961.

Kim AS, Kakalis LT, Abdul-Manan N, Liu GA, Rosen MK. Autoinhibition and activation mechanisms of the Wiskott-Aldrich syndrome protein. Nature 404:151–158, 2000.

Kolluri R, Tolias KF, Carpenter CL, Rosen FS, Kirchhausen T. Direct interaction of the Wiskott-Aldrich syndrome protein with the GTPase Cdc42. Proc Natl Acad Sci USA 93:5615–5618, 1996.

Kondoh T, Hayashi K, Matsumoto T, Yoshimoto M, Morio T, Yata J, Tsuji Y. Two sisters with clinical diagnosis of Wiskott-Aldrich syndrome: is the condition in the family autosomal recessive? Am J Med Genet 60: 364–369, 1995.

Konno A, Wada T, Schurman SH, Garabedian EK, Kirby M, Anderson SM, Candotti F. Differential contribution of Wiskott-Aldrich syndrome protein to selective advantage in T- and B-cell lineages. Blood 103:676–678, 2004.

Kothakota S, Azuma T, Reinhard C, Klippel A, Tang J, Chu K, McGarry TJ, Kirschner MW, Koths K, Kwiatkowski DJ, Williams LT. Caspase-3-generated fragment of gelsolin: effector of morphological change in apoptosis. Science 278:294–298, 1997.

Kuramoto A, Steiner M, Baldini MG. Lack of platelet response to stimulation in the Wiskott-Aldrich syndrome. N Engl J Med 282:475–479, 1970.

Kwan SP, Hagemann TL, Blaese RM, Knutsen A, Rosen FS. Scanning of the Wiskott-Aldrich syndrome (WAS) gene: identification of 18 novel alterations including a possible mutation hotspot at Arg86 resulting in thrombocytopenia, a mild WAS phenotype. Hum Mol Genet 10:1995–1998, 1995.

Kwan SP, Lehner T, Hagemann T, Lu B, Blaese M, Ochs H, Wedgwood R, Ott J, Craig IW, Rosen FS. Localization of the gene for the Wiskott-Aldrich syndrome between two flanking markers, TIMP and DXS255, on Xp11.22–Xp11.3. Genomics 10:29–33, 1991.

Lacout C, Haddad E, Sabri S, Svinarchouk F, Garcon L, Capron C, Foudi A, Mzali R, Snapper SB, Louache F, Vainchenker W, Dumenil D. A defect in hematopoietic stem cell migration explains the nonrandom X-chromosome inactiviation in carriers of Wiskott-Aldrich syndrome. Blood 102:1282–1289, 2003.

Lamarche N, Tapon N, Stowers L, Burbelo PD, Aspenström P, Bridges T, Chant J, Hall A. Rac and Cdc42 induce actin polymerization and G1 cell cycle progression independently of p65PAK and the JNK/SAPK MAP kinase cascade.Cell 87:519–529, 1996.

Lemahieu V, Gastier JM, Francke U. Novel mutations in the Wiskott-Aldrich syndrome protein gene and their effects on transcriptional, translational, and clinical phenotypes.Hum Mutat 14:54–66, 1999.

Lemmon MA, Ferguson KM, Schlessinger J. PH domains: diverse sequences with a common fold recruit signaling molecules to the cell surface. Cell 85:621–624, 1996.

Leverrier Y, Lorenzi R, Blundell MP, Brickell P, Kinnon C, Ridley AJ, Thrasher AJ. Cutting edge: the Wiskott-Aldrich syndrome protein is required for efficient phagocytosis of apoptotic cells. J Immunol 166:4831–4834, 2001.

Lin CY, Hsu HC. Acute immune complex mediated glomerulonephritis in a Chinese girl with Wiskott-Aldrich syndrome variant. Ann Allergy 53:74–78, 1984.

Linder S, Nelson D, Weiss M, Aepfelbacher M. Wiskott-Aldrich syndrome protein regulates podosomes in primary human macrophages. Proc Natl Acad Sci USA 96:9648–9653, 1999.

Litzman J, Jones A, Hann I, Chapel H, Strobel S, Morgan G. Intravenous immunoglobulin, splenectomy, and antibiotic prophylaxis in Wiskott-Aldrich syndrome. Arch Dis Child 75:436–439, 1996.

Lorenzi R, Brickell PM, Katz DR, Kinnon C, Thrasher AJ. Wiskott-Aldrich syndrome protein is necessary for efficient IgG-mediated phagocytosis. Blood 95:2943–2946, 2000.

Lutskiy MI, Beardsley DS, Rosen FS, Remold-O'Donnell E. Mosaicism of NK cells in a patient with Wiskott-Aldrich syndrome. Blood 106:2815–2817, 2005.

Lutskiy MI, Sasahara Y, Kenney DM, Rosen FS, Remold-O'Donnell E. Wiskott-Aldrich syndrome in a female. Blood 100:2763–2768, 2002.

Majstoravich S, Zhang J, Nicholson-Dykstra S, Linder S, Friedrich W, Siminovitch KA, Higgs HN. Lymphocyte microvilli are dynamic, actin-dependent structures that do not require Wiskott-Aldrich syndrome protein (WASp) for their morphology. Blood 104:1396–1403, 2004.

Martin F, Toscano MG, Blundell M, Frecha C, Srivastava GK, Santamaria M, Thrasher AJ, Molina IJ. Lentiviral vectors transcriptionally targeted to hematopoietic cells by WASP gene proximal promoter sequences. Gene Ther 12:715–723, 2005.

Martinez-Quiles N, Rohatgi R, Anton IM, Medina M, Saville SP, Miki H, Yamaguchi H, Takenawa T, Hartwig JH, Geha RS, Ramesh N. WIP regulates N-WASP–mediated actin polymerization and filopodium formation. Nat Cell Biol 3:484–491, 2001.

Melamed I, Gelfand EW. Microfilament assembly is involved in B-cell apoptosis.Cell Immunol 194:136–142, 1999.

Miao CH, Zhu Q, Zhou L, Humblet-Baron S, Lin D, Kohn DB, Candotti F, Ochs HD, Rawlings DJ. Lentiviral transduction of Wiskott-Aldrich syndrome protein (WASP) deficient T cells leads to long-term and progressive WASP expression and functional reconstitution [abstract 904]. Presented at the American Society of Gene Therapy, 7th Annual Meeting, Minneapolis, Minnesota 2004.

Miki H, Miura K, Takenawa T. N-WASP, a novel actin-depolymerizing protein, regulates the cortical cytoskeletal rearrangement in a PIP2-dependent manner downstream of tyrosine kinases. EMBO J 15:5326–5335, 1996.

Miki H, Nonoyama S, Zhu Q, Aruffo A, Ochs HD, Takenawa T. Tyrosine kinase signaling regulates Wiskott-Aldrich syndrome protein function, which is essential for megakaryocyte differentiation. Cell Growth Differ 8:195–202, 1997.

Molina IJ, Sancho J, Terhorst C, Rosen FS, Remold-O'Donnell E. T cells of patients with the Wiskott-Aldrich syndrome have a restricted defect in proliferative responses. J Immunol 151:4383–4390, 1993.

Moreau V, Frischknecht F, Reckmann I, Vincentelli R, Rabut G, Stewart D, Way M. A complex of N-WASP and WIP integrates signalling cascades that lead to actin polymerization. Nat Cell Biol 2:441–448, 2000.

Murphy S, Oski FA, Naiman JL, Lusch CJ, Goldberg S, Gardner FH. Platelet size and kinetics in hereditary and acquired thrombocytopenia. N Engl J Med 286:499–504, 1972.

Notarangelo LD, Mazza C, Giliani S, D'Aria C, Gandellini F, Ravelli C, Locatelli MG, Nelson DL, Ochs HD, Notarangelo LD. Missense mutations of the WASP gene cause intermittent X-linked thrombocytopenia. Blood 99:2268–2269, 2002.

Notarangelo LD, Ochs HD. Wiskott-Aldrich syndrome: a model for defective actin reorganization, cell trafficking and synapse formation. Curr Opin Immunol 15:585–591, 2003.

Notarangelo LD, Parolini O, Faustini R, Porteri V, Albertini A. Presentation of Wiskott-Aldrich syndromes as isolated thrombocytopenia. Blood 77:1125–1126, 1991.

Ochs HD, Slichter SJ, Harker LA, Von Behrens WE, Clark RA, Wedgwood RJ. The Wiskott-Aldrich syndrome: studies of lymphocytes, granulocytes, and platelets. Blood 55:243–252, 1980.

Oda A, Miki H, Wada I, Yamaguchi H, Yamazaki D, Suetsugu S, Nakajima M, Nakayama A, Okawa K, Miyazaki H, Matsuno K, Ochs HD, Machesky LM, Fujita H, Takenawa T. WAVE/Scars in platelets. Blood 105:3141–3148, 2005.

Oda A, Ochs HD. Wiskott-Aldrich syndrome protein and platelets [review]. Immunol Rev 178:111–7, 2000.

Oda A, Ochs HD, Druker BJ, Ozaki K, Watanabe C, Handa M, Miyakawa Y, Ikeda Y. Collagen induces tyrosine phosphorylation of Wiskott-Aldrich syndrome protein in human platelets. Blood 92:1852–1858, 1998.

Orange JS, Ramesh N, Remold-O'Donnell E, Sasahara Y, Koopman L, Byrne M, Bonilla FA, Rosen FS, Geha RS, Strominger JL. Wiskott-Aldrich syndrome protein is required for NK cell cytotoxicity and colocalizes with actin to NK cell–activating immunologic synapses. Proc Natl Acad Sci USA 99:11351–11356, 2002.

Ozsahin H, Le Deist F, Benkerrou M, Cavazzana-Calvo M, Gomez L, Griscelli C, Blanche S, Fischer A. Bone marrow transplantation in 26 patients with Wiskott-Aldrich syndrome from a single center. J Pediatr 129:238–244, 1996.

Park JY, Kob M, Prodeus AP, Rosen FS, Shcherbina A, Remold-O'Donnell E. Early deficit of lymphocytes in Wiskott-Aldrich syndrome: possible role of WASP in human lymphocyte maturation. Clin Exp Immunol 136:104–110, 2004.

Park JY, Shcherbina A, Rosen FS, Prodeus AP, Remold-O'Donnell E. Phenotypic perturbation of B cells in the Wiskott-Aldrich syndrome. Clin Exp Immunol 139:297–305, 2005.

Parkman R, Rappeport J, Geha R, Belli J, Cassady R, Levey R, Nathan DG, Rosen FS. Complete correction of the Wiskott-Aldrich syndrome by allogeneic bone-marrow transplantation. N Engl J Med 298:921–927, 1978.

Parolini O, Ressmann G, Haas OA, Pawlowsky J, Gadner H, Knapp W, Holter W. X-linked Wiskott-Aldrich syndrome in a girl. N Engl J Med 338:291–295, 1998.

Prehoda KE, Scott JA, Dyche MR, Lim WA. Integration of multiple signals through cooperative regulation of the N-WASP-Arp2/3 complex. Science 290:801–806, 2000.

Puck JM, Siminovitch KA, Poncz M, Greenberg CR, Rottem M, Conley ME. Atypical presentation of Wiskott-Aldrich syndrome: diagnosis in two unrelated males based on studies of maternal T cell X chromosome inactivation [see comments]. Blood 75:2369–2374, 1990.

Ramesh N, Anton IM, Hartwig JH, Geha RS. WIP, a protein associated with Wiskott-Aldrich syndrome protein, induces actin polymerization and redistribution in lymphoid cells. Proc Natl Acad Sci USA 94:14671–14676, 1997.

Rawlings SL, Crooks GM, Bockstoce D, Barsky LW, Parkman R, Weinberg KI. Spontaneous apoptosis in lymphocytes from patients with Wiskott-Aldrich syndrome: correlation of accelerated cell death and attenuated bcl-2 expression. Blood 94:3872–3882, 1999.

Remold-O'Donnell E, Cooley J, Shcherbina A, Hagemann TL, Kwan SP, Kenney DM, Rosen FS. Variable expression of WASP in B cell lines of Wiskott-Aldrich syndrome patients. J Immunology 158:4021–4025, 1997.

Rengan R, Ochs HD, Sweet LI, Keil ML, Gunning WT, Lachant NA, Boxer LA, Omann GM. Actin cytoskeletal function is spared, but apoptosis is increased, in WAS patient hematopoietic cells. Blood 95:1283–1292, 2000.

Rivero-Lezcano OM, Marcilla A, Sameshima JH, Robbins KC. Wiskott-Aldrich syndrome protein physically associates with Nck through Src homology 3 domains. Mol Cell Biol 15:5725–5731, 1995.

Rocca B, Bellacosa A, De Cristofaro R, Neri G, Della Ventura M, Maggiano N, Rumi C, Landolfi R. Wiskott-Aldrich syndrome: report of an autosomal dominant variant. Blood 87:4538–4543, 1996.

Rohatgi R, Ho HY, Kirschner MW. Mechanism of N-WASP activation by CDC42 and phosphatidylinositol 4, 5-bisphosphate. J Cell Biol 150:1299–1310, 2000.

Rohatgi R, Ma L, Miki H, Lopez M, Kirchhausen T, Takenawa T, Kirschner MW. The interaction between N-WASP and the Arp2/3 complex links Cdc42-dependent signals to actin assembly. Cell 97:221–231, 1999.

Rudolph MG, Bayer P, Abo A, Kuhlmann J, Vetter IR, Wittinghofer A. The Cdc42/Rac interactive binding region motif of the Wiskott Aldrich syndrome protein (WASP) is necessary but not sufficient for tight binding to Cdc42 and structure formation. Biol Chem 273:18067–18076, 1998.

Ryser O, Morell A, Hitzig WH. Primary immunodeficiencies in Switzerland: first report of the national registry in adults and children. J Clin Immunol 8:479–485, 1988.

Sasahara Y, Rachid R, Byrne MJ, de la Fuente MA, Abraham RT, Ramesh N, Geha RS. Mechanism of recruitment of WASP to the immunological synapse and of its activation following TCR ligation. Mol Cell 10:1269–1281, 2002.

Scott MP, Zappacosta F, Kim EY, Annan RS, Miller WT. Identification of novel SH3 domain ligands for the Src family kinase Hck. J Biol Chem 277:28238–28246, 2002.

Schindelhauser D, Weiss M, Hellebrand H, Golla A, Hergersberg M, Seger R, Belohradsky BH, Meindl A. Wiskott-Aldrich syrndrome: no strict genotype–phenotype correlations but clustering of missense mutations in the amino-terminal part of the WASP gene product. Hum Gent 98:68–76, 1996.

Schwartz M, Bekassy A, Donner M, Hertel T, Hreidarson S, Kerndrup G, Stormorken H, Stokland T, Tranebjaerg L, Orstavik KH, Skovby F. Mutation spectrum in patients with Wiskott-Aldrich syndrome and X-linked thrombocytopenia: identification of twelve different mutations in the WASP gene. Thromb Haemost 75:546–550, 1996.

Schwarz K. WASPbase: a database of WAS-and XLT-causing mutations. Immunol Today 11:496–502, 1996.

Semple JW, Siminovitch KA, Mody M, Milev Y, Lazarus AH, Wright JF, Freedman J. Flow cytometric analysis of platelets from children with the Wiskott-Aldrich syndrome reveals defects in platelet development, activation, and structure. Br J Haematol 97:747–754, 1997.

Shcherbina A, Rosen FS, Remold-O'Donnell E. Pathological events in platelets of Wiskott-Aldrich syndrome patients. Br J Haematol 106:875–883, 1999.

Siminovitch KA, Greer WL, Novogrodsky A, Axelsson B, Somani AK, Peacocke M. A diagnostic assay for the Wiskott-Aldrich syndrome and its variant forms. J Invest Med 43:159–169, 1995.

Slichter SJ, Harker LA. Thrombocytopenia: mechanisms and management of defects in platelet production. Clin Haematol 7:523–539, 1978.

Snapper SB, Meelu P, Nguyen D, Stockton BM, Bozza P, Alt FW, Rosen FS, von Andrian UH, Klein C. WASP deficiency leads to global defects of directed leukocyte migration in vitro and in vivo. J Leuk Biol 77:993–998, 2005.

Snapper SB, Rosen FS. A family of WASPs. N Engl J Med 348:350–351, 2003.

Snapper SB, Rosen FS, Mizoguchi E, Cohen P, Khan W, Liu CH, Hagemann TL, Kwan SP, Ferrini R, Davidson L, Bhan AK, Alt FW. Wiskott-Aldrich syndrome protein–deficient mice reveal a role for WASP in T but not B cell activation. Immunity 9:81–91, 1998.

Snover DC, Frizzera G, Spector BD, Perry GS, Kersey JH. Wiskott-Aldrich syndrome: histopathologic findings in the lymph nodes and spleens of 15 patients. Hum Pathol 12:821–831, 1981.

Stormorken H, Hellum B, Egeland T, Abrahamsen TG, Hovig T. X-linked thrombocytopenia and thrombocytopathia: attenuated Wiskott-Aldrich syndrome. Functional and morphological studies of platelets and lymphocytes. Thromb Haemost 65:300–305, 1991.

Stray-Pedersen A, Abrahamsen TG, Froland SS. Primary immunodeficiency diseases in Norway. J Clin Immunol 20:477–485, 2000.

Strom TS, Li X, Cunningham JM, Nienhuis AW. Correction of the murine Wiskott-Aldrich syndrome phenotype by hematopoietic stem cell transplantation. Blood 99:4626–4628, 2002.

Strom TS, Turner SJ, Andreansky S, Liu H, Doherty PC, Srivastava DK, Cunningham JM, Nienhuis AW. Defects in T-cell–mediated immunity to influenza virus in murine Wiskott-Aldrich syndrome are corrected by oncoretroviral vector–mediated gene transfer into repopulating hematopoietic cells. Blood 102:3108–3116, 2003.

Sullivan KE, Mullen CA, Blaese RM, Winkelstein JA. A multi-institutional survey of the Wiskott-Aldrich syndrome. J Pediatr 125:876–885, 1994.

Symons M, Derry JM, Karlak B, Jiang S, Lemahieu V, Mccormick F, Francke U, Abo A. Wiskott-Aldrich syndrome protein, a novel effector for the GTPase CDC42Hs, is implicated in actin polymerization. Cell 84:723–734, 1996.

Ten Bensel RW, Stadlan EM, Krivit W. The development of malignancies in the course of the Aldrich syndrome. J Pediatr 68:761–767, 1966.

Thrasher AJ. WASp in immune-system organization and function. Nat Rev Immunol 2:635–646, 2002.

Thrasher AJ, Jones GE, Kinnon C, Brickell PM, Katz DR. Is Wiskott-Aldrich syndrome a cell trafficking disorder? Immunol Today 19:537–539, 1998.

Tsuboi S, Nonoyama S, Ochs HD. Wiskott-Aldrich syndrome protein is involved in alphaIIbbeta3-mediated cell adhesion. EMBO Rep. 2006, in press.

Vermi W, Blanzuoli L, Kraus ND, Grigolato P, Donato F, Loffredo G, Marino CE, Alberti D, Notarangelo LD, Facchetti F. The spleen in the Wiskott-Aldrich syndrome. Histopathologic abnormalities of the white pulp correlate with the clinical phenotype of the disease. Am J Surg Pathol 23:182–191, 1999.

Villa A, Notarangelo L, Macchi P, Mantuano E, Cavagni G, Brugnoni D, Strina D, Patrosso MC, Ramenghi U, Sacco MG, Ugazio A, Vezzoni P. X-linked thrombocytopenia and Wiskott-Aldrich syndrome are allelic diseases with mutations in the WASP gene. Nat Genet 9:414–417, 1995.

Volkman BF, Prehoda KE, Scott JA, Peterson FC, Lim WA. Structure of the N-WASP EVH1 domain-WIP complex: insight into the molecular basis of Wiskott-Aldrich syndrome. Cell 111:565–576, 2002.

Wada T, Konno A, Schurman SH, Garabedian EK, Anderson SM, Kirby M, Nelson DL, Candotti F. Second-site mutation in the Wiskott-Aldrich syndrome (WAS) protein gene causes somatic mosaicism in two WAS siblings. J Clin Invest. 111:1389–1397, 2003.

Wada T, Schurman SH, Otsu M, Garabedian EK, Ochs HD, Nelson DL, Candotti F. Somatic mosaicism in Wiskott-Aldrich syndrome suggests in vivo reversion by a DNA slippage mechanism. Proc Natl Acad Sci USA 15:8697–8702, 2001.

Weaver AM, Young ME, Lee WL, Cooper JA. Integration of signals to the Arp2/3 complex. Curr Opin Cell Biol 15:23–30, 2003.

Wengler G, Gorlin JB, Williamson JM, Rosen FS, Bing DH. Nonrandom inactivation of the X chromosome in early lineage hematopoietic cells in carriers of Wiskott-Aldrich syndrome. Blood 85:2471–2477, 1995.

Westerberg L, Larsson M, Hardy SJ, Fernandez C, Thrasher AJ, Severinson E. Wiskott-Aldrich syndrome protein deficiency leads to reduced B-cell adhesion, migration, and homing, and a delayed humoral immune response. Blood 105:1144–1152, 2005.

Wiskott A. Familiärer, angeborener Morbus Werlhofii? Monatsschr Kinderheilkd 68:212–216, 1937.

Wolff JA. Wiskott-Aldrich syndrome: clinical, immunologic, and pathologic observations. J Pediatr 70:221–232, 1967.

Wolff JA, Bertucio M. A sex-linked genetic syndrome in a Negro family manifested by thrombocytopenia, eczema, bloody diarrhea, recurrent infection, anemia, and epistaxis. Am J Dis Child 93:74, 1957.

Yamada M, Ohtsu M, Kobayashi I, Kawamura N, Kobayashi K, Ariga T, Sakiyama Y, Nelson DL, Tsuruta S, Anakura M, Ishikawa N. Flow cytometric analysis of Wiskott-Aldrich syndrome (WAS) protein in lymphocytes from WAS patients and their familial carriers. Blood 93:756–757, 1999.

Yarar D, D'Alessio JA, Jeng RL, Welch MD. Motility determinants in WASP family proteins. Mol Biol Cell 13:4045–4059, 2002.

Zhang J, Shehabeldin A, da Cruz LA, Butler J, Somani AK, McGavin M, Kozieradzki I, dos Santos AO, Nagy A, Grinstein S, Penninger JM, Siminovitch KA. Antigen receptor–induced activation and cytoskeletal rearrangement are impaired in Wiskott-Aldrich syndrome protein–deficient lymphocytes. J Exp Med 90:1329–1342, 1999.

Zhu Q, Christie JR, Tyler EO, Watanabe M, Sibly B, Ochs HD. X-chromosome inactivation in symptomatic carrier females of X-linked thrombocytopenia. Clin Immunol 103:S129–S130, 2002.

Zhu Q, Watanabe C, Liu T, Hollenbaugh D, Blaese RM, Kanner SB, Aruffo A, Ochs H D. Wiskott-Aldrich syndrome/X-linked thrombocytopenia: WASP mutations, protein expression, and phenotype. Blood 90:2680–2689, 1997.

Zhu Q, Zhang M, Blaese RM, Derry JM, Junker A, Francke U, Chen SH, Ochs HD. The Wiskott-Aldrich syndrome and X-linked congenital thrombocytopenia are caused by mutations of the same gene. Blood 86:3797–3804, 1995.

32

X-Linked Lymphoproliferative Disease Due to Defects of *SH2D1A*

VOLKER SCHUSTER and COX TERHORST

X-linked lymphoproliferative disease (XLP; MIM 308240) is an inherited immunodeficiency involving primarily T, natural killer (NK) and natural killer T (NKT) cells that in most cases is exacerbated following exposure to Epstein-Barr virus (EBV). In older children and adults, EBV, one of the eight known human herpesviruses, is the causative agent of infectious mononucleosis (Henle and Henle, 1979). This is usually a self-limiting polyclonal lymphoproliferative disease with an excellent prognosis. In immunosuppressed individuals, EBV infection may lead to life-threatening lymphoproliferative disorders and lymphoma (Hanto et al., 1985). Moreover, EBV has been associated with certain malignancies, such as endemic Burkitt lymphoma, nasopharyngeal carcinoma, certain B and T cell lymphomas, and approximately 50% of Hodgkin disease (Zur Hausen et al., 1970; Ott et al., 1992; Weiss et al., 1989). In 1969 a family was described with two brothers suffering from hypogammaglobulinemia and malignant lymphoma following infectious mononucleosis (Hambleton and Cottom, 1969). This was the first report of XLP in the medical literature. In 1975, Purtilo et al. reported a large family, the Duncan kindred, in which multiple male members had died from fulminant infectious mononucleosis in early life, whereas others developed hypogammaglobulinemia after infectious mononucleosis or extranodal ileocecal malignant lymphoma during the next years of life. This apparently X-chromosomally inherited syndrome with a high vulnerability to EBV infection was classified as Duncan disease (in reference to the first described XLP family). Subsequently, when more families with similar signs and symptoms had been identified, and it became clear that only one XLP gene locus exists at Xq25 in all XLP families studied, the condition was named X-linked lymphoproliferative disease (Purtilo et al., 1991b). In 1978, an XLP registry was established for the collection of clinical and laboratory data to facilitate basic research on the pathogenesis of XLP and to develop new diagnostic and therapeutic tools for XLP patients (Hamilton et al., 1980). As of the year 2000, 309 males with one or more XLP phenotype(s) from 89 unrelated families had been registered (Seemayer et al., 1995; Sumegi et al., 2000). The disease has been shown to occur worldwide with an estimated incidence of 1 to 3 per million in males (Purtilo and Grierson, 1991). Primary EBV infection in XLP males may lead to severe and frequently fatal infectious mononucleosis, lymphoproliferative disorders usually of B cell origin, dysgammaglobulinemia, and other less frequent manifestations (Seemayer et al., 1995). However, XLP manifestations such as dysgammaglobulinemia or malignant lymphoma may develop in a similar frequency during the life of XLP males who have never been exposed to EBV (Gross et al., 1994, 1995; Strahm et al., 2000; Sumegi et al., 2000), indicating that clinical manifestations of XLP are not EBV-specific and that EBV may only act as a potent trigger of the earliest and most serious clinical manifestation of XLP—i.e., fatal infectious mononucleosis.

In general, XLP has an unfavorable prognosis. However, transplantation of hematopoietic stem cells from a suitable donor may cure this immunodeficiency.

The gene responsible for XLP, named *SH2D1A* (SH2 domain–containing gene 1A) or *SAP* (SLAM-associated protein) has been identified and characterized (Coffey et al., 1998; Nichols et al., 1998; Sayos et al., 1998). The gene encodes a protein of 128 amino acids containing a single SH2 domain. SH2D1A is thought to play an important role in signal transduction. Through use of in vitro experiments and Sh2d1a-deficient mice, SH2D1A has been shown to interfere with the signaling pathways in T lymphocytes, NK and NKT cells.

Clinical Phenotypes and Pathologic Manifestations

Prior to EBV infection, most boys carrying the defective XLP gene are clinically healthy. Some of them exhibit subtle immunological abnormalities before EBV infection (see Laboratory Findings, below).

Exposure to EBV may result in three clinical phenotypes in males carrying the defective XLP gene: fulminant and often fatal infectious mononucleosis occurs in more than half, lymphoproliferative disorders including malignant lymphoma develop in approximately one-third of affected males, and dysgammaglobulinemia is found in one-quarter of the patients (Table 32.1) (Seemayer et al., 1995; Sumegi et al., 2000). Less frequent manifestations are aplastic anemia, vasculitis, and lymphoid granulomatosis (each approximately 3% of cases), a hemophagocytic lymphohistiocytosis (HLH)-like clinical picture, and bronchiectasis (Seemayer et al., 1995; Schuster and Kreth, 2000; Strahm et al., 2000; Arico et al., 2001; Halasa et al., 2003). Several phenotypes (hypogammaglobulinemia, lymphoma, aplastic anemia) may manifest within the same XLP patient over time. Moreover, considerable intra- and interfamilial variations in XLP phenotypes exist.

XLP has an unfavorable prognosis: by 10 years of age more than 70% of affected boys are dead; only 2 XLP patients from the registered population of 272 males are older than 40 years of age (Seemayer et al., 1995). Only one man with XLP, who is not in the registry, is known to have survived for more than 60 years. He has a nonsense mutation of *SH2D1A* and a history of intestinal lymphoma at 21 years, and had hypogammaglobulinemia diagnosed at age 36 years (H.D. Ochs, unpublished observation, 2005). Survival rates for fulminant infectious mononucleosis, lymphoproliferative disorders, dysgammaglobulinemia, and aplastic anemia are 4%, 35%, 55%, and 50%, respectively (Seemayer et al., 1995).

Fulminant Infectious Mononucleosis

This is the most serious form of acute infectious mononucleosis. The median age of onset of illness is 2.5–3 years (range, 0.5–40 years) (Mroczek et al., 1987b; Sumegi et al., 2000); the median survival after onset of symptoms is 32 days (Mroczek et al., 1987b; Purtilo and Grierson, 1991). Signs and symptoms of disease are similar although more severe than those of infectious mononucleosis in older children and adults (Markin et al., 1987). Meningoencephalitis is common (Mroczek et al., 1987b; Sullivan and Woda, 1989; Schuster et al., 1993). During the course of fulminant mononucleosis, 89% of affected boys develop hepatic dysfunction, 81% have anemia, and 93% have thrombocytopenia (Mroczek et al., 1987b). Typically, polyclonal EBV-transformed B cells as well as CD4+ and CD8+ T cells (at approximately a 1:1 ratio of B to T cells) invade numerous organs, leading to infiltration and marked destruction of hematopoietic organs, liver, thymus, brain, heart, and other tissues (Markin et al., 1987; Mroczek et al., 1987a, 1987b; Sullivan and Woda, 1989).

The extensive destruction of liver and bone marrow often leads to fulminant hepatitis and virus-associated hemophagocytic syndrome (VAHS). In severe hepatitis, an intense periportal infiltration of EBV-positive B cells is typically found, surrounded by T cells, mainly of the CD8 phenotype (Markin et al., 1987). Liver failure with hepatic encephalopathy or hemorrhage involving the central nervous system, the gastrointestinal tract, or the lungs is the most frequent cause of death in these patients (Grierson and Purtilo, 1987).

Table 32.1. Common Manifestations of X-Linked Lymphoproliferative Disease*

Manifestation	Patients (%)
Fulminant infectious mononucleosis	58
Lymphoma (mostly of B cell origin)	30
Dysgammaglobulinemia (mostly low IgG; increased IgM)	31[†]

*$n = 272$ XLP boys from 80 families (Seemeyer et al., 1995). Since XLP males may exhibit more than one phenotype, the sum of percentage values exceeds 100.

[†]This percentage may have been calculated too high, since verification of the diagnosis XLP by genotyping was done in only 35 families (Sumegi et al., 2000). In these 35 families, only 22% of 152 males affected by XLP showed dysgammaglobulinemia (17% of 114 EBV-positive XLP males, 39% of 38 EBV-negative XLP males; $p = 0.3$) (Sumegi et al., 2000).

VAHS, occurring in 90% of boys with fatal mononucleosis (Mroczek et al., 1987b; Seemayer et al., 1995), is characterized by the appearance of numerous highly activated histiocytes and macrophages in different compartments (bone marrow, liver, lymph nodes). The development of VAHS in bone marrow leading to pancytopenia has been shown to progress in three phases. Initially, moderate pancytopenia and a myeloid hyperplastic marrow develop, followed at 2–3 weeks by the appearance of numerous activated histiocytes and macrophages with erythrophagocytosis (Color Plate 32.I). Later, lymphoid infiltration associated with necrosis and hemorrhage develops (Mroczek et al., 1987b). The pathogenesis of VAHS in XLP is not clear. The overwhelming activation of histiocytes and macrophages may be due to an uncontrolled release of tumor necrosis factor (TNF)-α or other cytokines by activated T cells (Su et al., 1995; Lay et al., 1997).

Dysgammaglobulinemia

This phenotype occurs in approximately 22%–31% of XLP males after EBV exposure. Median age at onset is 6 to 9 years of age (Grierson and Purtilo, 1987; Seemayer et al., 1995; Sumegi et al., 2000). Affected males exhibit varying degrees of hypogammaglobulinemia, and some may have increased serum IgM levels. Histologically, these patients present with extensive necrotic lesions in lymph nodes, thymus, bone marrow, and spleen. Long-term survivors have an inverted ratio of helper/cytotoxic T cell subpopulations (CD4/CD8) in their peripheral blood (Grierson and Purtilo, 1987; Hügle et al., 2004; Malbran et al., 2004). Patients with hypogammaglobulinemia have a relatively favorable prognosis, particularly if they are treated with monthly intravenous immunoglobulin (IVIG) infusions.

Common variable immunodeficiency (CVID) is a heterogeneous disorder characterized by a decrease in all or some immunoglobulin isotypes and an impaired antibody response leading to increased susceptibility to infection (see Chapter 23). Two recent studies have reported mutations affecting the *SH2D1A* gene in patients with a CVID-like phenotype (Gilmour et al., 2000; Morra et al., 2001c; Nistala et al., 2001).

Lymphoproliferative Disorders

Malignant lymphomas occur in approximately 30% of XLP patients, often associated with dysgammaglobulinemia and/or fulminant mononucleosis. The median age of affected males at the time of diagnosis of lymphoma is 4 to 6 years (Grierson and Purtilo, 1987; Harrington et al., 1987; Seemayer et al., 1995; Sumegi et al., 2000). Presenting symptoms are fever, nausea, vomiting, lymphadenopathy, weight loss, and abdominal pain (Harrington et al., 1987).

Most lymphomas studied so far occurred at extranodal sites; in approximately 75% the ileocecal region was primarily affected (Harrington et al., 1987). Other common sites of these tumors are the central nervous system, liver, and kidneys. Over 90% of malignant lymphomas are of B cell origin. These can be histologically subclassified as Burkitt lymphomas (small noncleaved; 53% of B cell lymphomas), immunoblastic lymphomas (18%), large noncleaved lymphomas (12%), small cleaved or mixed-cell lymphomas (12%), and unclassifiable lymphomas (5%) (Harrington et al., 1987). Only five cases have been classified as T cell lymphomas (6% of all lymphomas in XLP patients studied to date). Three brothers of one XLP family developed Hodgkin disease following EBV infection (approximately 3% of all lymphomas in XLP patients studied to date) (Donhuijsen-Ant et al., 1988). Malignant lymphomas with different histological subclassification may occur within the same family (Donhuijsen-Ant et al., 1988; Schuster et al., 1994). In at least four cases of Burkitt lymphomas, the characteristic 8;14 translocation (Egeler et al., 1992; Williams et al., 1993; Strahm et al., 2000) and in one case the 8;22 translocation (Turner et al., 1992) were demonstrated.

The prevalence of malignant lymphomas in XLP males is higher than in patients with other inherited immunodeficiencies such as the Wiskott-Aldrich syndrome, and the risk of developing a lymphoma has been estimated to be approximately 200 times greater than that in the general population (Grierson and Purtilo, 1987). In the case of Burkitt lymphoma, by using a mathematical model simulating lymphomagenesis, the cumulative lymphoma prevalence has been estimated to be 0.002% by chronological age of 18 years in the general population, 0.15% by chronological age of 6 years for endemic Burkitt lymphoma, 3% by chronological age of 10 years for Burkitt lymphoma in children with AIDS, and 25% by chronological age of 7 years for Burkitt lymphoma in boys with XLP (Ellwein and Purtilo, 1992). This markedly increased risk in XLP males, theoretically predicted and later statistically confirmed, may indirectly reflect the enhanced proliferation of B cells, which may be due to impaired immunosurveillance by T cells.

Characteristics that may distinguish malignant lymphomas in XLP patients from other malignant lymphomas include a family history of XLP, the early age of clinical manifestation (infectious mononucleosis), the ileocecal localization of the majority of XLP-associated lymphomas, and additional XLP phenotypes in the same affected male (such as dysgammaglobulinemia and severe or fulminant infectious mononucleosis). Approximately 30%–35% of XLP patients with malignant lymphoma survive for longer periods (>10 years) (Purtilo and Grierson, 1991; Seemayer et al., 1995).

Other Rare XLP Phenotypes

A small number of XLP patients (approximately 3% of cases) develop isolated bone marrow aplasia (either pancytopenia or pure red cell aplasia) in the absence of any evidence for VAHS. A similar percentage of affected patients may develop necrotizing lymphoid vasculitis or lymphoid granulomatosis of the lung or the central nervous system leading to extensive tissue damage (Loeffel et al., 1985; Seemayer et al., 1995; Dutz et al., 2001; Kanejone et al., 2005). Another rare clinical manifestation of XLP is bronchiectasis, which has been found in association with (Metha et al., 1999; Dutz et al., 2001; Hügle et al., 2004) and without (Strahm et al., 2000) dysgammaglobulinemia. In certain

cases, HLH may be the only clinical manifestation in males with XLP (Arico et al., 2001).

Clinical Manifestations and Immunological Findings in XLP Males with no Evidence of Previous Exposure to Epstein-Barr Virus

Thirty-eight (symptomatic) males with XLP, representing 12.5% of 304 registered males with clinical manifestations of XLP, had no evidence of prior EBV exposure (Sumegi et al., 2000). The number and percentage may be even higher, since the exact number of asymptomatic XLP males is not known.

Interestingly, EBV-negative XLP patients developed dysgammaglobulinemia and/or malignant lymphoma in a similar percentage to that of the EBV-positive group (Sumegi et al., 2000). In the EBV-negative group, median age at the onset of dysgammaglobulinemia was 4.5 years; for lymphoproliferative disease it was 8 years, which is not statistically different from the EBV-positive group. Infectious mononucleosis, which may be also caused by other herpesviruses such as cytomegalovirus (CMV), human herpes virus type 6 (HHV-6), and HHV-7 or by *Toxoplasma*, was never observed in the EBV-negative group. Survival for the EBV-negative group as a whole was significantly better, but this result is entirely accounted for by the poor suvival of fulminant infectious mononucleosis in the EBV-positive group (Sumegi et al., 2000).

Thirty-two EBV-negative males carrying the defective XLP gene as shown by restriction fragment length polymorphism (RFLP) analysis have been further immunologically investigated (Grierson et al., 1991; Gross et al., 1994; Seemayer et al., 1995). Among these, only five males were clinically healthy and had normal serum immunoglobulin levels. The remaining 27 males showed, prior to EBV exposure, one or both of the following XLP phenotypes: 17 subjects had elevated serum IgA or IgM and/or variable deficiency of IgG, IgG1, or IgG3, and 18 males developed lymphoproliferative disease (15 of B cell origin, three of T cell origin) without serologic and/or genomic evidence of previous EBV infection (22% of all lymphomas in XLP studied thus far). Eight of these 27 males (30%) had both dysgammaglobulinemia and lymphoma. These phenotypes resemble that of late-onset CVID. The findings clearly show that the immunodeficiency in XLP is not strictly EBV related.

In the few XLP males without evidence of prior EBV infection studied thus far, the number of peripheral T, B, and NK cells; the expression of CD3, CD4, CD8, and CD28; the CD4/CD8 ratio; the proliferative response to phytohemagglutinin (PHA), concanavalin A (ConA), and pokeweed mitogen (PWM); and NK cell activity seem to be normal (Sullivan and Woda, 1989; Gilleece et al., 2000; Strahm et al., 2000). In one XLP patient interferon-γ (IFN-γ) secretion by peripheral blood mononuclear cells was shown to be increased (ELISPOT assay) following stimulation with phorbol myristate acetate (PMA) but was decreased after stimulation with anti-CD3 and/or anti-2B4 (Sharifi et al., 2004).

The pattern of dysgammaglobulinemia appears to be due to a partial failure of the patient's B cells to undergo isotype switching from IgM to IgG. Moreover, EBV-seronegative (as well as EBV-seropositive) XLP patients exhibit a deficient switch to IgG antibody production following secondary challenge with bacteriophage φX174, a finding that has been used in the past for diagnostic evaluation of males at risk for XLP (Purtilo et al., 1989). However, for various reasons this test possesses only limited diagnostic validity and reliability, and may lead to false-positive and false-negative results (Purtilo, 1991). Therefore, the diagnosis of XLP in EBV-negative asymptomatic males depends on direct mutation analysis of the *SH2D1A* gene or indirect genotype analysis by RFLP. The finding of abnormal immunoglobulin and IgG subclass concentrations (vide supra) in serum of males at risk for XLP is suggestive, but not diagnostic. Because of the high prevalence of EBV in the general population, most males with XLP will be infected with EBV in childhood. About 58% of them will develop the most severe XLP phenotype, i.e., fatal infectious mononucleosis.

Laboratory Findings in XLP Males During Acute Epstein-Barr Virus Infection

During fulminant infectious mononucleosis a triphasic process develops along a continuum for several weeks within the blood and bone marrow (Purtilo, 1991). Initially (for 1–2 weeks), the leukocyte count is elevated, mostly because of increased numbers of atypical lymphoid cells, most of which are activated T cells. This abnormality is similar to but more extensive than that of immunocompetent children with uncomplicated infectious mononucleosis. At this time the bone marrow is hyperplastic with granulocytic hyperplasia with a left shift of maturation (Mroczek et al., 1987b). Later, severe pancytopenia develops (median leukocyte count, 1.5×10^9/l; median platelet count, 35.5×10^9/l; median hemoglobin level, 8.5 g/dl). The bone marrow shows extensive infiltration by lymphoid cells consisting of activated T cells, immunoblasts, and plasma cells. This is associated with cellular necrosis and VAHS (Color Plate 32.I) (Mroczek et al., 1987b). Terminally, the marrow shows massive necrosis with severe cellular depletion and marked histiocytic hemophagocytosis (Purtilo, 1991).

Elevation of serum transaminases, lactic dehydrogenase, and bilirubin, reflecting hepatic involvement, is found in all affected boys with fulminant mononucleosis. Hepatic encephalopathy or severe hemorrhages (central nervous system, gastrointestinal tract, lungs) due to liver failure are the most frequent cause of death in XLP boys with fatal mononucleosis (Grierson and Purtilo, 1987).

The age range of XLP males with fulminant mononucleosis is 5 months to 17–40 years (Mroczek et al., 1987b; Sumegi et al., 2000); the median age is 2.5–3 years. In most cases there is direct evidence of EBV infection as shown by the presence of heterophile antibodies and/or positive EBV-specific serology and/or the presence of EBV antigens or DNA in lymphoid tissues (positive in 100% of cases) (Mroczek et al., 1987b; Falk et al., 1990). Demonstration of EBV genomes in serum by polymerase chain reaction (PCR) analysis is also an indication of EBV infection (Sumazaki et al., 2001).

Immunological Studies of XLP Patients After Epstein-Barr Virus Infection

Subjects with XLP surviving EBV infection exhibit, as a rule, combined T and B cell defects. Most XLP patients have normal numbers of peripheral blood B and T cells. The proliferative responses of lymphocytes to B and T cell mitogens such as PHA, ConA, and PWM and to anti-IgM antibody were shown to be abnormally low during and after primary EBV infection in four of four XLP patients (Sullivan and Woda, 1989). In contrast, others have found normal lymphocyte proliferation in response to PHA, PWM, EBV, and *Staphylococcus aureus* strain Cowan (SAC) in 9/9 XLP patients (Lindsten et al., 1982; Arkwright et al., 1998). A decreased ratio of CD4$^+$ to CD8$^+$ T cells with a predominance of CD8$^+$ cells has been observed in most XLP patients (Lindsten et al., 1982; Hügle et al., 2004). The in vitro production of immunoglobulins by peripheral blood lymphocytes in response to PWM, EBV, and SAC was markedly decreased compared with

healthy controls (Lindsten et al., 1982). Furthermore, in XLP patients with hypogammaglobulinemia, the in vitro synthesis of IgG, IgM, and IgA by B lymphoblastoid cell lines in the presence of autologous T cells was markedly decreased (Lai et al., 1987; Yasuda et al., 1991). The degree of this T cell–mediated "suppression" of immunoglobulin synthesis correlated with the decreased serum levels of IgM and IgG in these patients (Yasuda et al., 1991).

XLP patients have a marked reduction in the number of circulating CD27$^+$ memory B cells, which undergo normal somatic hyper mutations, and a complete absence of switched memory B cells (Malbran et al., 2004; Ma et al., 2005; Ma et al., 2006). CD4$^+$ T cells from XLP patients do not efficiently differentiate in vitro into IL-10 secreting T helper cells and show reduced expression of inducible costimulator (ICOS) (Ma et al., 2005). These data suggest that in XLP the B cell defects are mainly extrinsic. It was recently reported that XLP patients have increased numbers of functionally immature CD24^{high}CD38^{high} B cells, which may further contribute to the humoral immunodeficient state (Cuss et al., 2006).

T cells from XLP patients failed to secrete normal amounts of IFN-γ following stimulation with autologous B lymphoblastoid cell lines or via the NK cell activation receptor 2B4 (Yasuda et al., 1991; Sharifi et al., 2004). In contrast, in three unrelated XLP patients the frequency of IFN-γ-producing CD3$^+$ T cells (measured intracytoplasmatically by FACS analysis after stimulation of the cells with PMA and ionomycin) was markedly increased (Ehl et al., 2002; Hügle et al., 2004). Furthermore, mononuclear cells from other XLP patients spontaneously produced normal or elevated levels of IFN-γ during EBV infection (Sullivan, 1983; Okano et al., 1990). It is therefore not clear if deficient IFN-γ production in XLP is a primary defect or only secondary to EBV infection. Skin tests with various antigens (purified protein derivative [PPD], tetanus toxoid, candida, and mumps) are frequently negative in XLP patients (Sullivan, 1983; Donhuijsen-Ant et al., 1988). A direct role of SH2D1A in early T cell antigen receptor-mediated signaling via CD3 was suggested by defective upregulation of IL-2 and IFN-γ production by herpesvirus saimiri-immortalized CD4$^+$ T cell, (Nakamura et al., 2001) and by defective IL-2 production, CD25 expression and homotypic cell aggregation (Sanzone et al., 2003).

NK cell activity of XLP males was found to be normal before, high at the time of, and low after EBV primary infection, results suggesting that this defect might be acquired during EBV infection (Sullivan et al., 1980; Sullivan, 1983; Argov et al., 1986; Rousset et al., 1986; Sullivan and Woda, 1989; Okano et al., 1990). Recent studies, however, have shown that in XLP patients NK cell cytotoxicity mediated by the NK cell activating receptor 2B4 seems to be selectively impaired, whereas NK cell activation mediated by NKp46, NKp44, NKp30, CD2, or CD16 as well as natural cytotoxicity against K562 cells and major histocompatibility complex (MHC) class I–deficient cells seem not to be affected (Benoit et al., 2000; Nakajima et al., 2000; Parolini et al., 2000; Tangye et al., 2000b).

Patients with XLP have a nearly complete absence of CD1d-restricted natural NKT cells (Chung et al., 2005; Pasquier et al., 2005; Nichols et al., 2005), which are important for Ag-specific T cell responses such as the regulation of EBV-specific lymphocyte expansions (Ho et al., 2004) and for bridging innate and adoptive responses by activating NK cells and by fostering dendritic cell maturation (Chung et al., 2005).

EBV-specific T cell immune function has been studied in only a few XLP patients. Three of eight XLP patients (Harada et al., 1982) were shown to exhibit EBV-specific memory T cell activity as measured by an outgrowth inhibition assay (regression assay).

In two XLP patients with hypogammaglobulinemia, EBV-specific, HLA-restricted cytotoxicity was demonstrated (Rousset et al., 1986). In recent studies, EBV-specific CD8+ T cells from XLP patients exhibited markedly decreased cytotoxic activity against autologous B cell lines (Sharifi et al., 2004; Dupre et al., 2005). The deficient EBV-specific cytotoxicity could be fully reconstituted by retroviral gene transfer of the *SH2D1A* gene into the T cell lines. These findings suggest that in XLP patients the lack of SH2D1A may result in severe disruption of cytotoxic T lymphocyte (CTL) function. XLP patients have normal numbers of EBV-specific CD8+ T cells that are extremely differentiated as defined by loss of CCR7 and CD27, low telomerase activity, and very short telomeres (Plunkett et al., 2005). These observations suggest that excessive proliferation of CD8+ T cells may lead to end-stage differentiation and loss of EBV-specific CD8+ T cells through replicative senescence. Lack of cytotoxic T cells may contribute to the development of EBV-associated B cell lymphomas.

Interestingly, some of these pathological findings in XLP patients can also be found transitorily and for a short period in patients with uncomplicated acute infectious mononucleosis. T lymphocytes obtained during acute infectious mononucleosis proliferate poorly in response to various mitogens such as PHA, ConA, and PWM as well as to antigens such as tetanus toxoid and *Candida albicans* (Tosato, 1989). Moreover, patients with acute infectious mononucleosis show low or absent delayed-type hypersensitivity reactions when challenged with recall antigens (Tosato, 1989) and respond poorly to the T cell–dependent neoantigen bacteriophage ΦX174, both in vivo and in vitro (Junker et al., 1986).

T cell activation during acute infectious mononucleosis leads to the amplification of CD8+ cytotoxic T cells, of which only a fraction is EBV-specific and HLA restricted (Tomkinson et al., 1989; Callan et al., 1996). It also leads to the proliferation of CD8+ T cells, which seem to be able to inhibit proliferation and immunoglobulin production by B cells as well as to inhibit nonactivated T cells in a probably virus-nonspecific, HLA-nonrestricted manner (Tosato, 1989; Tosato et al., 1982; Wang et al., 1987). In healthy immunocompetent individuals, both cytotoxic and suppressor functions, displayed by CD8+ T cells during infectious mononucleosis, appear to modulate and finally self-limit the course and severity of EBV infection. In XLP patients, the regulation of these interactions may be significantly disturbed possibly due to the lack of NKT cells. As a consequence, aberrant self-destructive killer cell populations and/or suppressor cells are not down-regulated or eliminated and may therefore proliferate in an uncontrolled manner leading to tissue and organ destruction (as found in fatal mononucleosis) and later on to hypogammaglobulinemia and diminished immunosurveillance against EBV-infected B cells, with an enhanced risk of B cell lymphomas.

Epstein-Barr Virus–Host Interaction in X-Linked Lymphoproliferative Disease

Males with XLP show a range of abnormal antibody responses after primary EBV infection. Antibody titers to the Epstein-Barr virus nuclear antigen (EBNA) are decreased or absent, which may indirectly reflect a T cell immunodeficiency, as this is also seen in other inherited or acquired immunodeficiencies (Purtilo et al., 1985; Okano et al., 1992). Antibodies against the EBV capsid antigen (VCA) are variable in XLP males. In rare instances, XLP patients may not be able to produce any EBV-specific antibodies (anti-VCA-IgM, anti–VCA-IgA, anti–VCA-IgG, or anti-EBNA) despite overwhelming infection with EBV (Hayoz et al., 1988; Turner et al., 1992; Dutz et al., 2001). In these cases the detection

of EBV genomes by PCR or the demonstration of EBNA by immunohistochemical staining in lymphoid tissue will document EBV infection in spite of seronegativity. In a large study of patients with sporadic or XLP-associated fatal mononucleosis, it was shown that 13 of 15 patients had histologic changes that were characteristic for polyclonal proliferation of B cells which expressed—in most cases, all EBV nuclear antigens (EBNA1-6), an expression pattern as seen also in lymphoblastoid B cell lines from healthy controls. In two cases, the B cells were of monoclonal origin and expressed only EBNA1, a pattern also found in Burkitt lymphoma (Falk et al., 1990).

In one patient with a nonsense mutation in *SH2D1A* (Hügle et al., 2004), EBV DNA and proteins could be detected in most of his peripheral T cells during the acute phase of infectious mononucleosis (Baumgarten et al., 1994). In general, B cells are the primary target of EBV in patients with infectious mononucleosis and other EBV-associated disorders (Kurth et al., 2000). EBV-infected T cells have been found in only one case of fatal acute mononucleosis (Mori et al., 1992) and in patients with severe chronic active EBV (CAEBV) infection (Quintanilla-Martinez et al., 2000; Ohga et al., 2001). Whether XLP is associated with an increased rate of EBV infection of T cells is unknown, but this seems unlikely, since only 6% of XLP-associated lymphoma are of T cell origin (90% B cell lymphoma, 4% Hodgkin disease) (Seemayer et al., 1995; Schuster and Kreth, 2000).

Normally, EBV type 1 is found predominantly in immunocompetent subjects after EBV infection. In immunodeficient individuals (HIV infection, organ transplantation), increased infection rates with EBV type 2 have been observed (Sculley et al., 1990). EBV strains isolated from XLP patients have not yet been genotyped systematically. In at least two unrelated XLP patients, EBV type 2 could be identified in lymphoid tissues (Mulley et al., 1992; Vowels et al., 1993). In two brothers with XLP and in one unrelated male with XLP we have detected EBV type 1 in lymphoma biopsy or peripheral blood (Schuster et al., 1996). More patients need to be examined to determine if one of these two EBV types is predominant in XLP.

Patients with XLP are vulnerable only to EBV, whereas the immune response to other herpes viruses, such as CMV, herpes simplex virus (HSV), HHV-6, HHV-7, and HHV-8, does not seem to be impaired.

Molecular Basis

In 1987 the XLP gene locus was mapped to the long arm of the X chromosome at Xq25 through RFLP analysis with polymorphic DNA markers from Xq24 to Xq26 (Skare et al., 1987, 1989a, 1989b, 1989c; Sylla et al., 1989). In several families with XLP, different partly overlapping deletions in the Xq25 region were identified and further characterized (Wyandt et al., 1989; Sanger et al., 1990; Skare et al., 1993; Wu et al., 1993, Lamartine et al., 1996; Lanyi et al., 1997; Porta et al., 1997; Coffey et al., 1998). In 1998, three groups independently identified the gene defective in XLP by positional cloning (Coffey et al., 1998; Nichols et al., 1998) or through a functional approach (Sayos et al., 1998). The gene (and its encoded protein) was originally designated *SH2D1A* (Coffey et al., 1998), *SAP* (Sayos et al., 1998), or *DSHP* (Nichols et al., 1998). The gene name approved by the Human Gene Nomenclature Commitee (HGNC) is *SH2D1A*. The human, monkey, and mouse *SH2D1A* genes consist of four exons and three introns spanning 25 kb (Coffey et al., 1998; Wu et al., 2000; Morra et al., 2001a, 2001d). The human *SH2D1A* gene encodes a small cytoplasmic protein of 128 amino acid residues consisting of a 5– amino acid amino-terminal sequence, a single

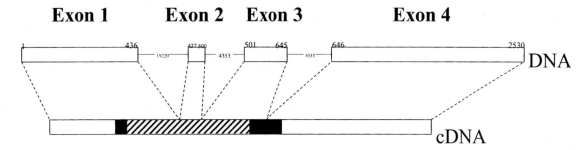

Figure 32.1. Organization of the *SH2D1A* gene. Black regions: coding sequences; portion with diagonal pattern: SH2 domain (adapted from Coffey et al., 1998).

SH2 domain, and a 25– amino acid carboxy-terminal tail (Coffey et al., 1998; Nichols et al., 1998; Sayos et al., 1998) (Fig. 32.1). Two SH2D1A mRNA species with a size of 2.5 kb and 0.9 kb are transcribed (Sayos et al., 1998).

The highest level of human SH2D1A mRNA expression has been found in the thymus. It has been found to a lesser extent in spleen, liver, lymph nodes, and other lymphoid organs as well as in peripheral blood lymphocytes (Coffey et al., 1998; Nichols et al., 1998; Sayos et al., 1998). SH2D1A is expressed in all major subsets of human T cells, with activated cells expressing the highest amounts, as well as in CD56$^+$CD3$^-$ NK cells (Coffey et al., 1998; Nichols et al., 1998; Sayos et al., 1998; Nagy et al., 2000, 2002). SH2D1A mRNA and/or protein expression has been reported to occur in different B and T cell lymphomas and Hodgkin disease as well as in different T cell lines, but not in EBV-immortalized B lymphoblastoid cell lines (Nichols et al., 1998; Sayos et al., 1998; Nagy et al., 2000, 2002; Kis et al., 2003). Similarly, in mice, SH2D1A expression is predominatly found in T cells and NK cells (Sayos et al., 2000; Wu et al., 2000). In mice and in humans, SH2D1A expression is down-regulated in CD4$^+$ and CD8$^+$ T cells upon anti-CD3 stimulation (Wu et al., 2000; D. Howie, unpublished data).

Function of the SH2D1A Protein

The SH2D1A protein, consisting of a single SH2 domain with a five–amino acid N-terminal tail, has been demonstrated to interfere, as a negative blocker, with the signaling pathways through the coreceptors SLAM (signaling lymphocyte activation molecule; CD150) (Sayos et al., 1998) and 2B4 (CD244), which is expressed on NK cells (Tangye et al., 1999; Benoit et al., 2000; Parolini et al., 2000; Sayos et al., 2001), CD8$^+$ T cells, and monocytes (Sayos et al., 2001). In both cases the SH2 domain of SH2D1A binds to the Thr-Ile-pTyr-x-x-Val/Ile (x = any amino acid; pTyr = phosphorylated Tyr residue) motif of phosphorylated SLAM or 2B4 and thus prevents recruitment of SHP-2 (SH2 domain–bearing tyrosine phosphatase-2) (Sayos et al., 1998; Poy et al., 1999). SHP-2 is involved in coupling signals from receptor tyrosine kinases and cytokine receptors (IL-3 receptor and others). SHP-2 is required for the activation of the Ras-mitogen-activated protein (MAP) kinase cascade and for the activation of cytokine-induced immediate to early gene expression (Huyer and Alexander, 1999). In agreement with these findings, it has been shown that 2B4-mediated NK cell cytotoxicity is selectively impaired in XLP patients, whereas NK cell activity against K562 target cells is not diminished (Benoit et al., 2000; Nakajima et al., 2000; Parolini et al., 2000; Tangye et al., 2000b). It was also shown that binding of SH2D1A to 2B4 depends on prior association of 2B4 with phosphoinositide 3-kinase (PI3K) (Aoukaty and Tan, 2002).

The Thr-Ile-pTyr-x-x-Val/Ile motif is also present in other members of the CD2 subgroup of the immunoglobulin superfamily (CD229 [Ly-9], CD84) (Li et al., 1999; Nakajima et al., 2000; Tangye et al., 2000a; Sayos et al., 2001) and SF2000 (Fraser et al., 2002), all of which have two such consensus sites in their cytoplasmic tails. Recently it was shown that SH2D1A binds to phosphorylated CD229 and CD84 (Sayos et al., 2001; Tangye et al., 2002).

SH2D1A also binds to nonphosphorylated SLAM (but not to nonphosphorylated 2B4) at Tyr281 (Sayos et al., 1998; Poy et al., 1999; Morra et al., 2001b; Howie et al., 2002b). Moreover, data derived from an SH2D1A crystal structure model suggest that interactions of SH2D1A with certain amino-terminal residues in SLAM are likely to further contribute to the high affinity of SH2D1A binding to SLAM (Li et al., 1999; Poy et al., 1999; Morra et al., 2001d; Howie et al., 2002b).

SH2D1A also binds to a phosphorylated site (tyrosine residue 449) in Dok1 (p62^{dok}), a 481–amino acid adaptor protein that associates with p120 Ras-GTPase-activating protein (GAP), Src C-terminal kinase (Csk), and the adaptor protein Nck (Sylla et al., 2000). Furthermore, signaling via the SLAM-SH2D1A pathway involves a protein complex that includes SH2 domain–containing inositol phosphatase (SHIP) and the adaptor molecule Dok2. SH2D1A also binds to the SH3 domain and the kinase domain of the Src-related protein tyrosine kinase FYN and directly couples FYN to SLAM (Latour et al., 2001, 2003; Chan et al., 2003; Engel et al., 2003; Li et al., 2003b) (Fig. 32.2). Therefore, *SH2D1A* appears to have (at least) dual functional roles by acting both as an adaptor for FYN and an inhibitor to SHIP-2 binding (Li et al., 2003b).

SLAM-SH2D1A signaling selectively inhibits in vitro IFN-γ production by a SLAM and SH2D1A cotransfected murine T cell line (which is normally SLAM$^-$/SH2D1A$^-$; Latour et al., 2001). In contrast, if SH2D1A-deficient T cells are similarly activated, IFN-γ production is increased compared with that of normal cells (Wu et al., 2001; Howie et al., 2002a). SH2D1A is required to attenuate Th1 immune responses in mice (Wu et al., 2001). It has been hypothesized that lack of SH2D1A in XLP patients results in the inability to mount an appropriate Th2 response after EBV infection, which leads to an uncontrolled Th1 response (Seemayer et al., 1995). In addition, overexpression of SH2D1A has been found to activate the transcription factor NF-κB in vitro (Sylla et al., 2000).

Taken together, SH2D1A appears to be a natural inhibitor of SH2 domain–dependent interactions between T and NK cells after immune activation that may affect multiple intracellular signaling pathways.

The role of SH2D1A in B cell activation has been investigated even less intensively. SH2D1A seems to act in B cells as a regulator of alternative interactions of CD150 with either SHP-2

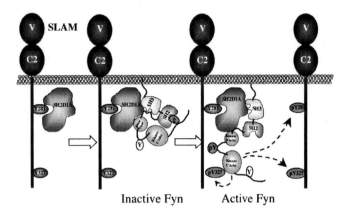

Inactive Fyn   Active Fyn

Figure 32.2. A model of FYN activation and recruitment by *SH2D1A*. During formation of the immunological synapse between T cells and antigen-presenting cells, clustering of signaling lymphocytic activation molecule (SLAM) receptors through homophilic binding brings SH2D1A and SLAM together. The binding of SH2D1A to SLAM promotes association with FYN (SH3 domain and kinase N lobe) and induces its activation. Subsequently, receptor-associated FYN can phosphorylate tyrosine residues in the cytoplasmic tail of the SLAM receptor (adapted from Engel et al., 2003). Alternatively, SH2D1A can also recruit already activated FYN (not shown).

or SHIP via the Thr-Ile-pTyr-x-x-Val/Ile motif (Shlapatska et al., 2001).

SH2D1A Gene Mutations in XLP Patients

Various *SH2D1A* gene mutations have been identified in XLP patients, including missense (M1I, M1T, Y7C, H8D, A22P, G27S, S28R, L31P, R32Q, R32T, D33Y, S34G, G39V, C42W, G49V, T53I, Y54C, R55L, R55P, S57P, E67D, E67G, T68I, I84T, F87S, E88P, G93D, Q99P, P101L, V102G), nonsense (R55X, Q58X, W64X, Y76X, Y100X, V102X, R129X), splice site mutations, and micro- and macrodeletions (Coffey et al., 1998; Nichols et al., 1998; Sayos et al., 1998; Brandau et al., 1999; Yin et al., 1999a; Benoit et al., 2000; Gilmour et al., 2000; Honda et al., 2000; Lappalainen et al., 2000; Parolini et al., 2000; Sumegi et al., 2000; Arico et al., 2001; Lewis et al., 2001; Morra et al., 2001a, 2001c; Nakamura et al., 2001; Nistala et al., 2001; Soresina et al., 2002; Halasa et al., 2003; Latour and Veilette, 2003; Hügle et al., 2004; Malbran et al., 2004; Nichols et al., 2005; Pasquier et al., 2005). At present, the R55X mutation has been identified in 20 unrelated XLP patients and seems to be the most prevalent mutation causing XLP (Coffey et al., 1998; Brandau et al., 1999; Lappalainen et al., 2000; Nakajima et al., 2000; Parolini et al., 2000, 2002; Sumegi et al., 2000; Arico et al., 2001; Bottino et al., 2001; Lewis et al., 2001; Morra et al., 2001c; Sumazaki et al., 2001; Hügle et al., 2004). An *SH2D1A* gene mutation registry (*SH2D1A*base) has been established, which is freely accessible through the Internet at http://www.uta.fi/imt/bioinfo/SH2D1A base/ (Lappalainen et al., 2000).

So far, no correlation between *SH2D1A* gene mutations and the clinical phenotype has been found. Identical mutations (for example, the R55X mutation) may manifest different clinical phenotypes even within the same family (Coffey et al., 1998; Sayos et al., 1998; Brandau et al., 1999; Lappalainen et al., 2000; Sumegi et al., 2000; Morra et al., 2001a).

Detectable mutations in the *SH2D1A* gene have been demonstrated in only 50%–70% of patients with the XLP phenotype (Coffey et al., 1998; Nichols et al., 1998; Sayos et al., 1998; Brandau et al., 1999; Sumegi et al., 2000). Therefore, the possi-

bility of a mutation in a *cis*-regulatory element distal from the *SH2D1A* gene or in one of its three introns, or the existence of a second gene in the proximity of the *SH2D1A* gene, which, if mutated, may also predispose for XLP, cannot be excluded.

Morra et al. (2001d) analyzed the effect of missense mutations identified in 10 XLP families on the interaction of SH2D1A with its binding proteins. Two sets of mutants were found: (1) those with a marked decrease in protein half-life, and (2) those resulting in structural changes that affect interaction with the SLAM-related cell surface receptors SLAM, Ly-9, 2B4, and CD84 in a distinct fashion. In the latter group, mutations that disrupt the interaction between the hydrophobic cleft of SH2D1A and Val in position +3 from the pTyr (Val +3) of its binding motif (e.g., mutant T68I), or mutations interfering with the SH2D1A phosphotyrosine pocket (e.g., mutants R32Q and C42W) abrogate SH2D1A binding to all four membrane receptors. Surprisingly, a mutation in SH2D1A known to interfere with Thr −2 (two amino acids N-terminal to the pTyr of the CD150 [SLAM] binding motif) (mutant T53I) severely impaired the nonphosphotyrosine interaction while preserving unaffected the binding of SH2D1A to CD150 (Hwang et al., 2002). Mutant T53I, however, did not bind to Ly-9 (CD229) or 2B4 (CD224), a finding supporting the notion that SH2D1A controls several distinct signal transduction pathways in T and NK cells. Furthermore, most SH2D1A mutants caused by amino acid substitutions studied thus far—i.e., Y7C, S28R, L31P, R32Q, T53I, Y54C, R55L, E67D, T68I, F87S, G93D, Q99P, P101L, V102G—exhibited significantly reduced binding to the FynT SH3 domain (Li et al., 2003a, 2003b).

SH2D1A gene mutations have not been detected in any of 62 cell lines derived from sporadic Burkitt lymphoma or in the peripheral blood of male patients with sporadic Burkitt lymphoma or Hodgkin disease, thus demonstrating that the *SH2D1A* gene does not play an important role in the development of (sporadic) Burkitt lymphoma (Yin et al., 1999b; Parolini et al., 2002).

Animal Models

The XLP SCID-Hu Mouse Model

Severe combined immunodeficient (SCID) mice engrafted with peripheral blood lymphocytes (PBL) from XLP patients as well as from healthy seropositive controls readily developed EBV-induced oligo- or polyclonal lymphoproliferative disease regardless of the immunocompetence of the donors (Purtilo et al., 1991a). These lesions expressed all EBV-latent antigens (EBNA1-6, LMP), regardless of whether the SCID mice had been engrafted with PBL from XLP patients or from healthy controls. Engrafted PBL of both groups also did not differ in their immunoglobulin production (IgG, IgA, and IgM). These findings suggest that the B cells of XLP patients are functionally normal and exhibit no primary defect.

Graft-vs.-host disease (GVHD) developed in 6 of 10 SCID mice engrafted with PBL from five normal donors (EBV seropositive, *n* = 2; EBV seronegative, *n* = 3), but in none of 9 mice engrafted with PBL from three XLP males (EBV seropositive, *n* = 2; EBV seronegative, *n* = 1). These findings may be taken as tentative evidence for a primary T cell deficiency in XLP.

The SH2D1A-Deficient Mouse

To examine the effect of an *SH2D1A* mutation on T cell functions, a mouse with a targeted disruption of the first exon of the *SH2D1A* gene (Wu et al., 2001) or with the T68I *SH2D1A* gene mutation (Czar et al., 2001; Crotty et al., 2003) was generated by homologous recombination in embryonic stem cells. Mice deficient in SH2D1A and wild-type littermates were infected with lymphocytic choriomeningitis virus (LCMV), a virus that elicits strong and well-defined immune responses. In the primary response, dramatically increased numbers of $CD8^+$ and $CD4^+$ IFN-γ-producing cells were found in the spleen of SH2D1A-deficient animals in comparison to wild-type littermates. In the liver of SH2D1A-deficient mice, five times more $CD8^+$, $CD4^+$ T cells, and LCMV-specific T cells were detected than in the wild-type mice after infection. IFN-γ production by LCMV-infected SH2D1A-deficient liver T cells was dramatically higher than that by wild-type liver T cells as measured in an in vitro culture system in the presence of anti-CD3. The increased production of IFN-γ by splenic and hepatic T cells was also apparent during a recall response to LCMV. Thus, SH2D1A-deficient mice mount more vigorous IFN-γ^+ $CD8^+$ and $CD4^+$ Th1 responses to infection with LCMV than their wild-type littermates, but their CTL and NK cells responses are intact.

SH2D1A-deficient T cells on the Balb/C background produced very low levels of IL-4, IL-10, and IL-13 when activated in vitro by anti-CD3 and anti-CD28 (Wu et al., 2001). The observation of impaired in vitro IL-4 production by SH2D1A-deficient $CD4^+$ T cells was confirmed in vivo during infection with the parasite *Leishmania major* (Wu et al., 2001). In agreement with these results and the well-known critical role played by IL-4 and IL-10 in immunoglobulin heavy-chain isotype switching were the significantly lower levels of total IgE in the *Leishmania major*–infected SH2D1A-deficient-mice. The aberrant immune responses in SH2D1A-deficient mice demonstrate that SH2D1A controls several distinct key T signal transduction pathways, which explain part of the underlying principles of the pathogenesis of the XLP.

SH2D1A operates as a natural inhibitor of the networking to signal transduction pathways by the cytoplasmic tail of at least five members of the SLAM family. SLAM (CD150), CD84, CD229 (Ly-9), CD244 (2B4), and SF2000, which are expressed on the surface of T cells, NK cells, and antigen-presenting cells, recruit the tyrosine phosphatases SHP-1 or SHP-2 to specific docking sites that are phosphorylated upon activation of T cells or NK cells. The concept of SH2D1A as an inhibitor is supported by its high affinity for the binding sites in the cytoplasmic tails of these cell surface receptors as well as by studies of SH2D1A missense mutations found in XLP patients. Whereas all four proteins are expressed on the surface of $CD8^+$ cells, $CD4^+$ cells lack 2B4 expression. The altered functions of SH2D1A-deficient T cells are therefore the sum of the interferences with the individual pathways.

Recently it was shown that SH2D1A-deficient mice also have a defect in $CD4^+$ helper T cells, as these animals generate only a short-lived IgG antibody response after LCMV infection, whereas the production of LCMV-specific, long-lived plasma cells and memory B cells was nearly absent (Crotty et al., 2003). These findings resemble the inability of XLP patients to mount a sustained anti-EBV humoral immune response. However, whereas XLP patients may exhibit deficient isotype switching (dysgammaglobulinemia with high IgM and low IgG), adoptive transfer experiments in SH2D1A-deficient mice show normal isotype switching (Crotty et al., 2003). In contrast, in vitro experiments indicate that B cells from SH2D1A-deficient mice fail to undergo class switch recombination, suggesting that B cells are directly affected in the absence of SAP (Al-Alem et al., 2006). The studies of SH2D1A-deficient mice supports the concept that the small cytoplasmic protein SH2D1A negatively interferes with the final

stages of Th1 and $CD8^+$ cell responses, but provides a positive signal for the development of Th2 cells during an infection.

Yin et al. (2003) generated SH2D1A-deficient mice with a partial deletion of intron 1 and exon 2. Infection of these animals with murine gammaherpesvirus-68, which is homologous to human EBV, led to marked tissue damage and hemophagocytosis, similar to findings observed in XLP patients. All 16 SH2D1A-deficient mice exhibited hypogammaglobulinemia, which was more pronounced following infection with murine gammaherpesvirus-68.

Recent data indicated that SH2D1A-deficient mice, similarly to XLP patients, completely lack NKT cells (Chung et al., 2005; Pasquier et al., 2005; Nichols et al., 2005). The phenotype of SH2D1A-deficient mice resembles in some aspects that of $Cd1d^{-/-}$ mice and of $Fyn^{-/-}$ mice, which both lack NKT cells (Nichols et al., 2005).

A recent study demonstrated that SH2D1A-deficient mice are protected from experimentally induced lupus and glomerulonephritis (Hron et al., 2004). They did not develop hypergammaglobulinemia, nor did they produce any autoantibodies (e.g., ANA, anti-DNA). It is not clear at present whether XLP patients are also protected from certain autoimmune diseases such as systemic lupus erythematosus.

Speculations about the Pathogenesis of X-Linked Lymphoproliferative Disease

The pathognomonic response to EBV infection observed in patients with XLP is characterized by an uncontrolled $CD8^+$ T cell proliferation leading to parenchymal damage, particularly in the liver and bone marrow. This is likely caused by increased production of IFN-γ and the absence of NKT cells. It has been hypothesized that the defect in XLP results from the inability to mount an appropriate Th2 response following EBV infection, leading to an uncontrolled Th1 response. The in vivo and in vitro studies of SH2D1A-deficient mice are conceptually in agreement with these aspects of XLP, for they demonstrate that absence of SH2D1A causes two distinct T cell defects in mice: (1) hyperproliferation of IFN-γ-producing $CD8^+$ and $CD4^+$ cells in parallel with excessive IFN-γ secretion, and (2) a defect in activation of the IL-4 gene upon T cell triggering, which causes an aberrant Th2 polarization that may lead to abnormal immunoglobulin class switching.

Infection with two LCMV strains, which are unrelated to EBV, induces more vigorous T cell responses in SH2D1A-deficient mice than those in wild-type mice. This is consistent with the observations that acquired hypogammaglobulinemia may also occur in EBV-negative XLP patients, possibly because of multiple infections with other viruses. We predict that SH2D1A-deficient mice will make a useful tool for dissecting the complex XLP phenotypes and will lead to additional studies to explore further the aberrant immune status of XLP patients. The *SH2D1A* gene knockout mouse model will also permit experiments that aid in our understanding of the fundamental role of a free SH2 domain in regulating T cell activation and terminal differentiation.

Diagnostic Considerations

Diagnosis of X-Linked Lymphoproliferative Disease

The diagnosis of XLP is based on clinical, immunological, and molecular findings and is confirmed by mutation analysis (Table 32.2). Prenatal diagnosis or the evaluation of a heterozygous status in (clinically healthy) women is possible by direct mutation analysis of the *SH2D1A* gene and/or its RNA or protein expression (Shinozaki et al., 2002; Hügle et al., 2004), or indirectly (in informative families) by RFLP analysis with X chromosomal markers flanking the *SH2D1A* gene proximally and distally (Fig. 32.3) (Mulley et al., 1992; Skare et al., 1992; Schuster et al., 1993, 1994, 1995). In the absence of a potential stem cell donor, prenatal diagnosis of an affected male may raise difficult ethical questions when the affected boy is initially healthy. In sporadic cases, a definite diagnosis of XLP can be verified only by mutation analysis of the *SH2D1A* gene. Because NKT cells are nearly absent in XLP patients, regardless of SH2D1A genotype, age, prior exposure to EBV, history of lymphoma or presence of dysgammaglobulinemia (Nichols et al., 2005) the quantification of NKT cells, together with clinical data and family history, may facilitate the diagnosis of XLP.

Differential Diagnosis

The clinical phenotypes of XLP share similarities with other disorders that need to be excluded. These are discussed below.

Sporadic fatal infectious mononucleosis (SFIM) occurs in approximately 1 in 3000 cases of infectious mononucleosis (Purtilo et al., 1992). The median age of patients is 5.5 years (FIM in XLP: 2.5 years), the male/female ratio is approximately 1:1 (Mroczek et al., 1987b). Presenting signs and symptoms are similar to those seen in XLP patients with fatal mononucleosis. Other XLP phenotypes (dysgammaglobulinemia, lymphoma) are absent. In 25 males with SFIM studied thus far, no mutations within the *SH2D1A* gene have been found (Sumegi et al., 2000).

A non-X-linked syndrome with susceptibility to severe EBV infections can be easily differentiated from XLP by its autosomal inheritance pattern. Common findings in this rare disorder are a decreased NK cell activity and a history of recurrent bacterial infections prior to EBV exposure (Fleisher et al., 1982).

Chronic active EBV (CAEBV) infection involving mostly T or NK cells is characterized by a perstistent severe mononucleosis-like illness (lasting for months or years) with additional unusual clinical features such as hypersensitivity to mosquito bites (43%), calcifications in basal ganglia (18%), hydroa vacciniforme (14%), hemophagocytic syndrome (21%), coronary artery aneurisms (21%), and malignant lymphoma (16%) (Kimura et al., 2001). Patients with CAEBV have a high EBV load in their peripheral blood (>$10^{2.5}$ copies/µg DNA).

Table 32.2. Criteria for Diagnosis of X-Linked Lymphoproliferative Disease

Definitive Diagnosis of XLP

Male patient with one or more XLP phenotypes plus SH2D1A deficiency (i.e., mutations in the *SH2D1A* gene, absent mRNA and/or absent protein expression (Gilmour et al., 2000; Shinozaki et al., 2002; Hügle et al., 2004; Tabata et al., 2005) of the *SH2D1A* gene in lymphocytes)*

Probable Diagnosis of XLP

One or more XLP phenotypes in a male patient plus one or more XLP phenotypes in at least one of his brothers, maternal cousins, uncles, or nephrews (*SH2D1A* gene status not known)

Diagnosis Suggestive of XLP

One or more XLP phenotypes in a single male family member (*SH2D1A* gene status not known)

*Presymptomatic diagnosis of XLP is also definitive in an (initially) healthy male carrying an *SH2D1A* gene mutation, which is known to cause XLP.
Source: Adapted and modified from Sullivan, 1999; Schuster and Kreth, 2000.

EBV infects predominantly T and/or NK cells (Kasahara et al., 2001; Kimura et al., 2001). In 18 male CAEBV patients studied, no mutations of the *SH2D1A* gene were found (Kimura et al., 2001; Sumazaki et al., 2001). One CAEBV patient exhibited a mutated perforin gene (Katano et al., 2004).

Males with X-linked agammaglobulinemia (XLA) have low or absent numbers of B cells, low concentrations of all serum immunoglobulin isotypes, and a severe defect in antibody production leading to recurrent bacterial infections. The molecular defect responsible for XLA is the mutation of a tyrosine kinase (Bruton tyrosine kinase, BTK). Neither any of the XLP phenotypes nor an increased vulnerability to EBV is observed in these patients (see Chapter 21).

X-linked hyper-IgM syndrome (XHIM, CD40 ligand deficiency) is caused by expression of a defective CD40 ligand (*CD40L*, CD154) by activated T lymphocytes due to mutations of the *CD40L* gene, resulting in the inability of B cells to undergo class switch recombination. Affected boys have normal or elevated IgM levels and decreased serum concentrations of IgG, IgE, and IgA. The disease is characterized by severe bacterial and opportunistic infections as well as an increased susceptibility to autoimmunity and neoplasms. Affected males do not exhibit an increased susceptibility to severe EBV infections (see Chapter 19).

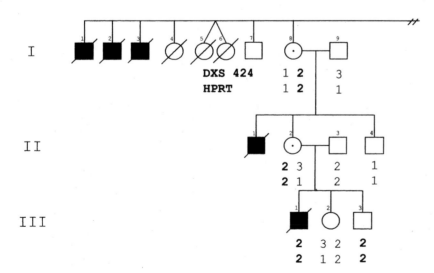

Figure 32.3. Pedigree of a Spanish XLP family with haplotypes of polymorphic markers DXS424 (proximal to *SH2D1A*) and HPRT (distal to *SH2D1A*). Male subjects I-1 to I-3, II-1, and III-1 (black symbols) suffered and died from fulminant infectious mononucleosis during early infancy. Haplotype 2-2 cosegregated with XLP (Brandau et al., 1999). In the index patient (III-1) but also in his healthy brother a nonsense mutation of the *SH2D1A* gene (Y100X) was identified (Brandau et al., 1999). Subjects I-8 and II-2, but not III-2, were shown to be heterozygous carriers for the Y100X mutation.

X-linked hyper-IgM syndrome associated with hypohydrotic ectodermal dysplasia (XHM-ED, NEMO), a rare disorder, is caused by mutations in the gene that encodes NF-κB essential modulator (*NEMO*, also known as IKKγ), which is required for activation of the transcription factor NF-κB (Doffinger et al., 2001; Jain et al., 2001). B cells from XHM-ED patients are unable to undergo immunoglobulin class-switch recombination, and antigen-presenting cells are unable to synthesize the NF-κB-regulated cytokines IL-12 or TNF-α when stimulated with CD40L (see Chapter 36).

Other genetically determined hyper-IgM syndromes also need to be included in the differential diagnosis of XLP. Mutations in the activation-induced cytidine deaminase (*AICD*) gene causes hyper-IgM syndrome with autosomal recessive inheritance (Revy et al., 2000) (see Chapter 20). Mutations in the gene *CD40*, the natural receptor of CD40L, results in a clinical phenotype similar to CD40L deficiency (Chapter 19). Mutations in the uridine-DNA-glycosylase (*UNG*) gene results in an HIGM phenotype due to abnormal class switch recombination and somatic hypermutation (Imai et al., 2003) (see Chapter 20).

Autoimmune lymphoproliferative syndrome (ALPS), also known as Canale-Smith syndrome, is caused by mutations within the Fas (CD95, *TNFRSF6*) or Fas ligand (FasL, CD95L, CD178, *TNFSF6*) genes (ALPS type I) (Fisher et al., 1995; Rieux-Laucat et al., 1995; Drappa et al., 1996; Le Deist et al., 1996) or within the caspase 10 gene (ALPS type II) (Wang et al., 1999). ALPS is characterized by massive nonmalignant lymphadenopathy, hepatosplenomegaly, autoimmune phenomena, hypergammaglobulinemia, and increased numbers of CD3⁺CD4⁻CD8⁻ double-negative lymphocytes. Clinical manifestations occur during early infancy (see Chapter 24). In some patients with an ALPS-like syndrome but with additional immunodeficiency characterized by recurrent sinopulmonary and HSV infections and poor responses to immunization, mutations within the caspase 8 gene have been demonstrated (Chun et al., 2002).

Common variable immunodeficiency (CVID) should also be considered in the differential diagnosis. The characteristic feature of this rather heterogeneous group of patients is a decrease in all or at least two major immunoglobulin isotypes and an impaired antibody response. In the majority of CVIC patients B cells are present in normal numbers. However, these cells are unable to differentiate into antibody-producing plasma cells, possibly due to a primary T cell abnormality. The clinical manifestation is similar to that of XLA. In a small subset of CVID patients, mutations in the *ICOS* (Grimbacher et al., 2003) or *TACI* genes (Castigli et al., 2005; Salzer et al., 2005) have been identified. In general, CVID occurs in a sporadic manner. Other than the antibody deficiency, there is little similarity to XLP (see Chapter 23). However, a subset of male XLP patients may present with a CVID-like disease (Gilmour et al., 2000; Morra et al., 2001c; Nistala et al., 2001; Soresina et al., 2002).

Hemophagocytic lymphohistiocytosis (HLH) is a heterogeneous group of disorders characterized by dysregulated activation of T cells and macrophages. Affected children may present with fever, splenomegaly, hepatomegaly, pancytopenia, coagulation abnormalities, neurological abnormalities, and high serum concentrations of IFN-γ and TNF-α. Patients with HLH subtype 2 harbor mutations in *PRF1*, the gene encoding perforin (Stepp et al., 1999). Patients with HLH subtype 3 have a mutated Munc13-4 gene (Feldmann et al., 2003). Patients with HLH subtype 4 have a mutated syntaxin 11 gene (Zur Stadt et al., 2005). A few male patients with an HLH-like disease were found to have

mutations in the *SH2D1A* gene (Arico et al., 2001; Halasa et al., 2003).

Laboratory Findings in XLP Female Carriers

None of the female carriers of the XLP gene studied thus far developed any of the XLP phenotypes. Subtle immunological abnormalities such as hypogammaglobulinemia and elevated IgA and/or IgM have been found in a few carrier females (Sakamoto et al., 1982; Grierson and Purtilo, 1987; Morra et al., 2001c). Forty-five of 56 female carriers (80%) have been shown to exhibit an abnormal serological response to EBV infection (Grierson and Purtilo, 1987).

However, EBV serology alone is not a reliable diagnostic finding in the predictive evaluation of female carriers, since transiently elevated serum antibodies against VCA and EA of the IgM, IgG, or IgA class are also found in normal subjects with a recent primary EBV infection. Carrier females have a random X-chromosome inactivation pattern in their B and T cells (Conley et al., 1990, Nichols et al., 2005). However, X-chromosome inactivation pattern in NKT cells of female XLP carriers is skewed (Nichols et al., 2005).

At present, direct mutation analysis of the *SH2D1A* gene or indirect genotype analysis (in informative families) is the only reliable means to determine if a female at risk is a carrier for XLP or not.

Treatment and Prognosis

Prophylactic Treatment of Males at Risk Prior to Epstein-Barr Virus Infection

There is evidence that maternal EBV-neutralizing antibodies may protect the newborn infant, including XLP males, from primary EBV infection for 4–6 months (Biggar et al., 1978; Mroczek et al., 1987b). Regular intravenous infusions with immunoglobulins rich in EBV-neutralizing antibodies were therefore started males at risk to prevent or lessen the effects of EBV infection. However, some boys succumbed to fulminant mononucleosis despite this therapy (Okano et al., 1990, 1991; Seemayer et al., 1995). In any case, all EBV-negative XLP males with hypogammaglobulinemia should receive regular immunoglobulin substitutions to prevent severe bacterial or viral infections.

Vaccination against EBV is potentially another strategy to protect males at risk for XLP. Such a vaccine may well be able to induce a solid immunity against natural-occurring EBV infections in immunocompetent subjects. Its use in males at risk for XLP may be dangerous and even contraindicated, however, since it is not known whether this vaccine may be able to trigger an uncontrolled and potentially fatal activation of T cells with disastrous consequences for the patient.

Currently, the only means of preventing EBV- and non-EBV–related complications in later life is early transplantation of allogeneic hematopoietic stem cells (cord blood, bone marrow) (Vowels et al., 1993; Williams et al., 1993; Pracher et al., 1994; Gross et al., 1996; Arkwright et al., 1998; Hoffmann et al., 1998; Ziegner et al., 2001; Lankester et al., 2005). The age of the patient at time of transplantation appears to be critical. Out of eight XLP patients who underwent stem cell transplantation, four boys less than 15 years of age were alive and well for more than 2 years post-transplantation, whereas all four boys older than 15 years of age at the time of transplantation died within 90 days of the occurrence of complications (Seemayer et al., 1995; Gross et al., 1996). Gene therapy may become an option in the future.

Treatment of XLP Males During or After Epstein-Barr Virus Infection

During fulminant mononucleosis, treatment attempts with high-dose immunoglobulins, antiviral drugs such as aciclovir, immunosuppressive agents, and IFN-α and IFN-γ have been rather diappointing (Okano et al., 1990, 1991).

Etoposide (VP-16), which has been effective in the treatment of lymphoma, leukemia, and hemophagocytic syndromes, has been shown to induce remissions in some XLP males with fulminant mononucleosis, VAHS, or aplastic crisis (Migliorati et al., 1994; Seemayer et al., 1995; Okano and Gross, 1996). One such patient showed rapid improvement of his clinical symptoms of fulminant mononucleosis for a short period after treatment with etoposide. Subsequently, after relapse and clinical deterioration, the boy underwent successful stem cell transplantation following conditioning with etoposide, busulfan, and cyclophosphamide (Pracher et al., 1994). In view of the unfavorable prognosis, a controlled clinical trial with etoposide, with or without stem cell transplantation, in patients with acute exacerbations of XLP is warranted.

Males with XLP who develop hypogammaglobulinemia in response to EBV infection require regular IVIG infusions to prevent recurrent bacterial and viral infections. Despite IVIG therapy, other XLP phenotypes such as aplastic anemia or lymphoma may develop in subsequent years (Purtilo, 1991).

XLP patients suffering from malignant lymphomas may enter remissions of short duration after undergoing standard chemotherapy protocols (Seemayer et al., 1995). However, relapses of the lymphomas are frequent and development of other XLP phenotypes may occur. XLP patients with active EBV infection and lymphoproliferative complications may be successfully treated with anti-CD20 monoclonal antibody (rituximab) in combination with prednisone, acyclovir and IVIG infusions (Malbran et al., 2004; Milone et al., 2006). Eventually, this procedure may also be useful in the treatment of B cell lymphoma in XLP patients.

Acknowledgments

This work was supported by grants from the Deutsche Forschungsgemeinschaft (Schu 560/4-3 to V.S.), the Medical Faculty of Leipzig University (grant 78261 101 to V.S.), and the National Institutes of Health (AI-35714 to C.T.).

References

Al-Alem U, Li C, Forey N, Relouzat F, Fondaneche MC, Tavtigian SV, Wang ZQ, Latour S, Yin L. Impaired Ig class switch in mice deficient for the X-linked lymphoproliferative disease gene Sap. Blood 106:2069–2075, 2005.

Aoukaty A, Tan R. Association of the X-linked lymphoproliferative disease gene product SAP/SH2D1A with 2B4, a natural killer cell-activating molecule, is dependent on phosphoinositide 3-kinase. J Biol Chem 277: 13331–13337, 2002.

Argov S, Johnson DR, Collins M, Koren HS, Lipscomb H, Purtilo DT. Defective natural killing activity but retention of lymphocyte-mediated antibody-dependent cellular cytotoxicity in patients with the X-linked lymphoproliferative syndrome. Cell Immunol 100:1–9, 1986.

Arico M, Imashuku S, Clementi R, Hibi S, Teramura T, Danesino C, Haber DA, Nichols KE. Hemophagocytic lymphohistiocytosis due to germline mutations in SH2D1A, the X-linked lymphoproliferative disease gene. Blood 97:1131–1133, 2001.

Arkwright PD, Makin G, Will AM, Ayres M, Gokhale DA, Fergusson WD, Taylor GM. X-linked lymphoproliferative disease in a United Kingdom family. Arch Dis Child 79:52–55, 1998.

Baumgarten E, Herbst H, Schmitt M, Seeger KH, Schulte-Overberg U, Henze G. Life-threatening infectious mononucleosis: is it correlated with virus-induced T cell proliferation? Clin Infect Dis 19:152–156, 1994.

Benoit L, Wang X, Pabst HF, Dutz J, Tan R. Defective NK cell activation in X-linked lymphoproliferative disease. J Immunol 165:3549–3553, 2000.

Biggar RJ, Henle W, Fleisher G, Bocker J, Lennette ET, Henle G. Primary Epstein-Barr virus infections in African infants. I. Decline of maternal antibodies and time of infection. Int J Cancer 22:239–243, 1978.

Bottino C, Falco M, Parolini S, Marcenaro E, Augugliaro R, Sivori S, Landi E, Biassoni R, Notarangelo LD, Moretta L, Moretta A. NTB-A, a novel SH2D1A-associated surface molecule contributing to the inability of natural killer cells to kill Epstein-Barr virus–infected B cells in X-linked lymphoproliferative disease. J Exp Med 194:235–246, 2001.

Brandau O, Schuster V, Weiss M, Hellebrand H, Fink FM, Kreczy A, Friedrich W, Strahm B, Niemeyer C, Belohradsky BH, Meindl A. Epstein-Barr virus–negative boys with non-Hodgkin lymphoma are mutated in the SH2D1A gene, as are patients with X-linked lymphoproliferative disease (XLP). Hum Mol Genet 8:2407–2413, 1999.

Callan MF, Steven N, Krausa P, Wilson JD, Moss PA, Gillespie GM, Bell JI, Rickinson AB, McMichael AJ. Large clonal expansions of CD8+ T cells in acute infectious mononucleosis. Nat Med 2:906–911, 1996.

Castigli E, Wilson SA, Garibyan L, Rachid R, Bonilla F, Schneider L, Geha RS. TACI is mutant in common variable immunodeficiency and IgA deficiency. Nat Genet 37:829–834, 2005.

Chan B, Lanyi A, Song HK, Griesbach J, Simarro-Grande M, Poy F, Howie D, Sumegi J, Terhorst C, Eck MJ. SAP couples Fyn to SLAM immune receptors. Nat Cell Biol 5:155–160, 2003.

Chun HJ, Zheng L, Ahmad M, Wang J, Speirs CK, Siegel RM, Dale JK, Puck J, Davis J, Hall CG, Skoda-Smith S, Atkinson TP, Straus SE, Lenardo MJ. Pleiotropic defects in lymphocyte activation caused by caspase-8 mutations lead to human immunodeficiency. Nature 419:395–399, 2002.

Chung B, Aoukaty A, Dutz J, Terhorst C, Tan R. Signaling lymphocytic activation molecule-associated protein controls NKT cell functions. J Immunol 174:3153–3157, 2005.

Coffey AJ, Brooksbank RA, Brandau O, Oohashi T, Howell GR, Bye JM, Cahn AP, Durham J, Heath P, Wray P, Pavitt R, Wilkinson J, Leversha M, Huckle E, Shaw-Smith CJ, Dunham A, Rhodes S, Schuster V, Porta G, Yin L, Serafini P, Sylla B, Zollo M, Franco B, Bolino A, Seri M, Lanyi A, Davis JR, Webster D, Harris A, Lenoir G, de St Basile GD, Jones A, Belohradsky BH, Achatz H, Murken J, Fässler R, Sumegi J, Romeo G, Vaudin M, Ross MT, Meindl A, Bentley R. Host response to EBV infection in X-linked lymphoproliferative disease results from mutations in an SH2-domain encoding gene. Nat Genet 20:129–135, 1998.

Conley ME, Sullivan JL, Neidich JA, Puck JM. X chromosome inactivation patterns in obligate carriers of X-linked lymphoproliferative syndrome. Clin Immunol Immunopathol 55:486–491, 1990.

Crotty S, Kersh EN, Cannons J, Schwartzberg PL, Ahmed R. SAP is required for generating long-term humoral immunity. Nature 421:282–287, 2003.

Cuss AK, Avery DT, Cannons JL, Yu LJ, Nichols KE, Shaw PJ, Tangye SG. Expansion of functionally immature transitional B cells is associated with human-immunodeficient states characterized by impaired humoral immunity. J Immunol 176:1506–1516, 2006.

Czar MJ, Kersh EN, Mijares LA, Lanier G, Lewis J, Yap G, Chen A, Sher A, Duckett CS, Ahmed R, Schwartzberg PL. Altered lymphocyte responses and cytokine production in mice deficient in the X-linked lymphoproliferative disease gene SH2D1A/DSHP/SAP. Proc Natl Acad Sci USA 98: 7449–7454, 2001.

Doffinger R, Smahi A, Bessia C, Geissmann F, Feinberg J, Durandy A, Bodemer C, Kenwrick S, Dupuis-Girod S, Blanche S, Wood P, Rabia SH, Headon DJ, Overbeek PA, Le Deist F, Holland SM, Belani K, Kumararatne DS, Fischer A, Shapiro R, Conley ME, Reimund E, Kalhoff H, Abinun M, Munnich A, Israel A, Courtois G, Casanova JL. X-linked anhidrotic ectodermal dysplasia with immunodeficiency is caused by impaired NF-κB signaling. Nat Genet 27:277–285, 2001.

Donhuijsen-Ant R, Abken H, Bornkamm G, Donhuijsen K, Grosse-Wilde H, Neumann-Haefelin D, Westerhausen M, Wiegand H. Fatal Hodgkin and non-Hodgkin lymphoma associated with persistent Epstein-Barr virus in four brothers. Ann Intern Med 109:946–952, 1988.

Drappa J, Vaishnaw A, Sullivan KE, Chu J-L, Elkon KB. Fas gene mutations in the Canale-Smith syndrome, an inherited lymphoproliferative disorder associated with autoimmunity. N Engl J Med 335:1643–1649, 1996.

Dupre L, Andolfi G, Tangye SG, Clementi R, Locatelli F, Arico M, Aiuti A, Roncarolo MG. SAP controls the cytolytic activity of CD8+ T cells against EBV-infected cells. Blood 105:4383–4389, 2005.

Dutz JP, Benoit L, Wang X, Demetrick DJ, Junker A, de Sa D, Tan R. Lymphocytic vasculitis in X-linked lymphoproliferative disease. Blood 97: 95–100, 2001.

Egeler RM, de Kraker J, Slater R, Purtilo DT. Documentation of Burkitt lymphoma with t(8)(q24,q32) in X-linked lymphoproliferative disease. Cancer 70:683–687, 1992.

Ehl S, Peters A, Strahm B, Schlesier M, Orlowska-Volk M, Kopp M, Gilmour KC, Gaspar HB, Niemeyer CM. Detailed immunological characterization of a boy with atypical Purtilo syndrome. Presented at the 10th Meeing of the European Society for Immunodeficiencies ESID, Weimar, October 17–20, 2002. ESID Newsletter 2002 (Suppl) S62, 2002.

Ellwein LB, Purtilo DT. Cellular proliferation and genetic events involved in the genesis of Burkitt lymphoma (BL) in immune compromised patients. Cancer Genet Cytogenet 64:42–48, 1992.

Engel P, Eck MJ, Terhorst C. The SAP and SLAM families in immune responses and X-linked lymphoproliferative disease. Nat Rev Immunol 3: 813–821, 2003.

Falk K, Ernberg I, Sakthivel R, Davis J, Christensson B, Luka J, Okano M, Grierson HL, Klein G, Purtilo DT. Expression of Epstein-Barr virus–encoded proteins and B-cell markers in fatal infectious mononucleosis. Int J Cancer 46:976–984, 1990.

Feldmann J, Callebaut I, Raposo G, Certain S, Bacq D, Dumont C, Lambert N, Ouachee-Chardin M, Chedeville G, Tamary H, Minard-Colin V, Vilmer E, Blanche S, Le Deist F, Fischer A, de Saint Basile G. Munc13-4 is essential for cytolytic granules fusion and is mutated in a form of familial hemophagocytic lymphohistiocytosis (FHL3). Cell 115:461–473, 2003.

Fisher GH, Rosenberg FJ, Straus SE, Dale JK, Middelton LA, Lin AY, Strober W, Lenardo MJ, Puck J. Dominant interfering Fas gene mutations impair apoptosis in a human autoimmune lymphoproliferative syndrome. Cell 81:935–946, 1995.

Fleisher G, Starr S, Koven N, Kamiya H, Douglas SD, Henle W. A non-X-linked syndrome with susceptibility to severe Epstein-Barr virus infections. J Pediatr 100:727–730, 1982.

Fraser CC, Howie D, Morra M, Qiu Y, Murphy C, Shen Q, Gutierrez-Ramos JC, Coyle A, Kingsbury GA, Terhorst C. Identification and characterization of SF2000 and SF2001, two new members of the immune receptor SLAM/CD2 family. Immunogenetics 53:843–850, 2002.

Gilleece MH, Boussiotis VA, Tangye S, Haber DA, Nadler LM, Nichols KE. Perturbed CD28 costimulation and activation-induced death in X-linked lymphoproliferative syndrome. Blood 94 (Suppl.1):435a (Abstract 1931), 1999.

Gilmour KC, Cranston T, Jones A, Davies EG, Goldblatt D, Thrasher A, Kinnon C, Nichols K E, Gaspar HB. Diagnosis of X-linked lymphoproliferative disease by analysis of SLAM-associated protein expression. Eur J Immunol 30:1691–1697, 2000.

Grierson H, Purtilo DT. Epstein-Barr virus infections in males with the X-linked lymphoproliferative syndrome. Ann Intern Med 106:538–545, 1987.

Grierson HL, Skare J, Hawk J, Pauza M, Purtilo DT. Immunoglobulin class and subclass deficiencies prior to Epstein-Barr virus infection in males with X-linked lymphoproliferative disease. Am J Med Genet 40:294–297, 1991.

Grimbacher B, Hutloff A, Schlesier M, Glocker E, Warnatz K, Drager R, Eibel H, Fischer B, Schaffer AA, Mages HW, Kroczek RA, Peter HH. Homozygous loss of ICOS is associated with adult-onset common variable immunodeficiency. Nat Immunol 4:261–268, 2003.

Gross TG, Filipovich AH, Conley ME, Pracher E, Schmiegelow K, Verdirame JD, Vowels M, Williams LL, Seemayer TA. Cure of X-linked lymphoproliferative disease (XLP) with allogeneic hematopoietic stem cell transplantation (HSCT)—report from the XLP registry. Bone Marrow Transplant 17:741–744, 1996.

Gross TG, Kelly CM, Davis JR, Pirruccello SJ, Sumegi J, Seemayer TA. Manifestation of X-linked lymphoproliferative disease (XLP) without evidence of Epstein-Barr virus (EBV) infection. Clin Immunol Immunopathol 75:281, 1995.

Gross TG, Patton DF, Davis JR, Sumegi J, Pirruccello SJ, Kelly CM, Seemayer TA. X-linked lymphoproliferative disease (XLP) manifested without apparent EBV infection [abstract]. Presented at the Cold Spring Harbor Meeting on Cancer Cells: Epstein-Barr Virus and Associated Diseases. Cold Spring Harbor, NY, 1994.

Halasa NB, Whitlock JA, McCurley TL, Smith JA, Zhu Q, Ochs HD, Dermody TS, Crowe JE. Fatal hemophagocytic lymphohistiocytosis associated with Epstein-Barr virus infection in a patient with a novel mutation in the SLAM-associated protein. Clin Infect Dis 37:e136–141, 2003.

Hambleton G, Cottom D G. Familial lymphoma. Proc R Soc Med 62:1095, 1969.

Hamilton JK, Paquin LA, Sullivan JL, Maurer HS, Cruzi FG, Provisor AJ, Steuber CP, Hawkins E, Yawn D, Cornet JA, Clausen K, Finkelstein GZ, Landing B, Grunnet M, Purtilo DT. X-linked lymphoproliferative syndrome registry report. J Pediatr 96:669–673, 1980.

Hanto DW, Frizzera G, Gajl-Peczalska KJ, Simmons RL. Epstein-Barr virus, immunodeficiency, and B cell lymphoproliferation. Transplantation 39: 461–472, 1985.

Harada S, Sakamoto K, Seeley JK, Lindsten T, Bechtold T, Yetz J, Rogers G, Pearson G, Purtilo DT. Immune deficiency in the X-linked lymphoproliferative syndrome. I. Epstein-Barr virus–specific defects. J Immunol 129: 2532–2535, 1982.

Harrington DS, Weisenburger DD, Purtilo DT. Malignant lymphoma in the X-linked lymphoproliferative syndrome. Cancer 59:1419–1429, 1987.

Hayoz D, Lenoir GM, Nicole A, Pugin P, Regamey C. X-linked lymphoproliferative syndrome. Identification of a large family in Switzerland. Am J Med 84:529–534, 1988.

Henle G, Henle W. The virus as the etiologic agent of infectious mononucleosis. In: Epstein MA, Achong BG, eds. The Epstein-Barr Virus. Berlin: Springer, pp. 297–320, 1979.

Ho LP, Urban BC, Jones L, Ogg GS, McMichael AJ. CD4(-)CD8alphaalpha subset of CD1d restricted NKT cells controls T cell expansion. J Immunol 172:7350–7358, 2004.

Hoffmann T, Heilmann C, Madsen HO, Vindelov L, Schmiegelow K. Matched unrelated allogeneic bone marrow transplantation for recurrent malignant lymphoma in a patient with X-linked lymphoproliferative disease (XLP). Bone Marrow Transplant 22:603–604, 1998.

Honda K, Kanegane H, Eguchi M, Kimura H, Morishima T, Masaki K, Tosato G, Miyawaki T, Ishii E. Large deletion of the X-linked lymphoproliferative disease gene detected by fluorescence in situ hybridization. Am J Hematol 64:128–132, 2000.

Howie D, Okamoto S, Rietdijk S, Clarke K, Wang N, Gullo C, Bruggeman JP, Manning S, AJ Coyle, Greenfield E, Kuchroo V, Terhorst C. Antibodies directed at murine CD150 (SLAM) mediate T cell co-stimulation in both a SAP-dependent and SAP-independen fashion. Blood 100:2899–2907, 2002a.

Howie D, Simarro M, Sayos J, Guirado M, Sancho J, Terhorst C. Molecular dissection of the signaling and costimulatory functions of CD150 (SLAM): CD150/SAP binding and CD150-mediated costimulation. Blood 99:957–965, 2002b.

Hron J, Caplan L, Gerth A, Schwartzberg P, Peng S. SH1D1A regulates T-dependent humoral autoimmunity. J Exp Med 200:261–266, 2004.

Hügle B, Suchowerskyj P, Hellebrand H, Adler B, Borte M, Sack U, Schulte Overberg-Schmidt U, Strnad N, Otto J, Meindl A,. Schuster B. Persistent hypogammaglobulinemia following mononucleosis in boys is highly suggestive of X-linked lymphoproliferative disease—report of three cases. J Clin Immunol 24:515–522, 2004.

Huyer G, Alexander DR. Immune signalling: SHP-2 docks at multiple ports. Curr Biol 9:R129–R132, 1999.

Hwang PM, Li C, Morra M, Lillywhite J, Muhandiram DR, Gertler F, Terhorst C, Kay LE, Pawson T, Forman-Kay JD, Li SC. A "three-pronged" binding mechanism for the SAP/SH2D1A SH2 domain: structural basis and relevance to the XLP syndrome. EMBO J 21:314–323, 2002.

Imai K, Slupphaug G, Lee WI, Revy P, Nonoyama S, Catalan N, Yel L, Forveille M, Kavli B, Krokan HE, Ochs HD, Fischer A, Durandy A. Human uracil-DNA glycosylase deficiency associated with profoundly impaired immunoglobulin class-switch recombination. Nat Immunol 4:1023–1028, 2003.

Jain A, Ma CA, Liu S, Brown M, Cohen J, Strober W. Specific missense mutations in NEMO result in hyper-IgM syndrome with hypohydrotic ectodermal dysplasia. Nat Immunol 2:223–228, 2001.

Junker AK, Ochs HD, Clark EA, Puterman ML, Wedgwood RJ. Transient immune deficiency in patients with acute Epstein-Barr virus infection. Clin Immunol Immunopathol 40:436–446, 1986.

Kanegane H, Ito Y, Ohshima K, Shichijo T, Tomimasu K, Nomura K, Futatani T, Sumazaki R, Miyawaki T. X-linked lymphoproliferative syndrome presenting with systemic lymphocytic vasculitis. Am J Hematol 78:130–133, 2005.

Kasahara Y, Yachie A, Takei K, Kanegane C, Okada K, Ohta K, Seki H, Igarashi N, Maruhashi K, Katayama K, Katoh E, Terao G, Sakiyama Y, Koizumi S. Differential cellular targets of Epstein-Barr virus (EBV) infection between acute EBV-associated hemophagocytic lymphohistiocytosis and chronic active EBV infection. Blood 98:1882–1888, 2001.

Katano H, Ali MA, Patera AC, Catalfamo M, Jaffe ES, Kimura H, Dale JK, Straus SE, Cohen JI. Chronic active Epstein-Barr virus infection associated with mutations in perforin that impair its maturation. Blood 103: 1244–1252, 2004.

Kimura H, Hoshino Y, Kanegane H, Tsuge I, Okamura T, Kawa K, Morishima T. Clinical and virologic characteristics of chronic active Epstein-Barr virus infection. Blood 98:280–286, 2001.

Kis LL, Nagy N, Klein G, Klein E. Expression of SH2D1A in five classical Hodgkin's disease–derived cell lines. Int J Cancer 104:658–661, 2003.

Kurth J, Spieker T, Wustrow J, Strickler GJ, Hansmann LM, Rajewsky K, Kuppers R. EBV-infected B cells in infectious mononucleosis: viral strategies for spreading in the B cell compartment and establishing latency. Immunity 13:485–495, 2000.

Lai PK, Yasuda N, Purtilo DT. Immunoregulatory T cells in males vulnerable to Epstein-Barr virus with the X-linked lymphoproliferative syndrome. Am J Pediatr Hematol Oncol 9:179–182, 1987.

Lamartine J, Nichols KE, Yin L, Krainer M, Heitzmann F, Bernard A, Gaudi S, Lenoir GM, Sullivan JL, Ikeda JE, Porta G, Schlessinger D, Romeo G, Haber DA, Sylla BS, Harkin DP. Physical map and cosmid contig encompassing a new interstitial deletion of the X-linked lymphoproliferative syndrome region. Eur J Hum Genet 4:342–351, 1996.

Lankester AC, Visser LF, Hartwig NG, Bredius RG, Gaspar HB, van der Burg M, van Tol MJ, Gross TG, Egeler RM. Allogeneic stem cell transplantation in X-linked lymphoproliferative disease: two cases in one family and review of the literature. Bone Marrow Transplant 36:99–105, 2005.

Lanyi A, Li B, Li S, Talmadge CB, Brichacek B, Davis JR, Kozel BA, Trask B, van den Engh G, Uzvolgyi E, Stanbridge EJ, Nelson DL, Chinault C, Heslop H, Gross TG, Seemayer TA, Klein G, Purtilo DT, Sumegi J. A yeast artificial chromosome (YAC) contig encompassing the critical region of the X-linked lymphoproliferative disease (XLP) locus. Genomics 39:55–65, 1997.

Lappalainen I, Giliani S, Franceschini R, Bonnefoy JY, Duckett C, Notarangelo LD, Vihinen M. Structural basis for SH2D1A mutations in X-linked lymphoproliferative disease. Biochem Biophys Res Commun 269:124–130, 2000.

Latour S, Gish G, Helgason CD, Humphries RK, Pawson T, Veillette A. Regulation of SLAM-mediated signal transduction by SAP, the X-linked lymphoproliferative gene product. Nat Immunol 2:681–690, 2001.

Latour S, Roncagalli R, Chen R, Bakinowski M, Shi X, Schwartzberg PL, Davidson D, Veillette A. Binding of SAP SH2 domain to FynT SH3 domain reveals a novel mechanism of receptor signalling in immune regulation. Nat Cell Biol 5:149–154, 2003.

Latour S, Veillette A. Molecular and immunological basis of X-linked lymphoproliferative disease. Immunol Rev 192:212–224, 2003.

Lay JD, Tsao CJ, Chen JY, Kadin ME, Su IJ. Upregulation of tumor necrosis factor-alpha gene by Epstein-Barr virus and activation of macrophages in Epstein-Barr virus–infected T cells in the pathogenesis of hemophagocytic syndrome. J Clin Invest 100:1969–1979, 1997.

Le Deist F, Emile JF, Rieux-Laucat F, Benkerrou M, Roberts I, Brousse N, Fischer A. Clinical, immunological, and pathological consequences of Fas-deficient conditions. Lancet 348:719–723, 1996.

Lewis J, Eiben LJ, Nelson DL, Cohen JI, Nichols KE, Ochs HD, Notarangelo LD, Duckett CS. Distinct interactions of the X-linked lymphoproliferative syndrome gene product SAP with cytoplasmic domains of members of the CD2 receptor family. Clin Immunol 100:15–23, 2001.

Li SC, Gish G, Yang D, Coffey AJ, Forman-Kay JD, Ernberg I, Kay LE, Pawson T. Novel mode of ligand binding by the SH2 domain of the human XLP disease gene product SAP/SH2D1A. Curr Biol 9:1355–1362, 1999.

Li C, Iosef C, Jia CY, Gkourasas T, Han VK, Shun-Cheng Li S. Disease-causing SAP mutants are defective in ligand binding and protein folding. Biochemistry 42:14885–14892, 2003a.

Li C, Iosef C, Jia CY, Han VK, Li SS. Dual functional roles for the X-linked lymphoproliferative syndrome gene product SAP/SH2D1A in signaling through the signaling lymphocyte activation molecule (SLAM) family of immune receptors. J Biol Chem 278:3852–3859, 2003b.

Lindsten T, Seeley JK, Ballow M, Sakamoto K, Onge SS, Yetz J, Aman P, Purtilo DT. Immune deficiency in the X-linked lymphoproliferative syndrome. II. Immunoregulatory T cell defects. J Immunol 129:2536–2540, 1982.

Loeffel S, Chang CH, Heyn R, Harada S, Lipscomb H, Sinangil F, Volsky DJ, McClain K, Ochs H, Purtilo DT. Necrotizing lymphoid vasculitis in X-linked lymphoproliferative syndrome. Arch Pathol Lab Med 109:546–550, 1985.

Ma CS, Hare NJ, Nichols KE, Dupre L, Andolfi G, Roncarolo MG, Adelstein S, Hodgkin PD, Tangye SG. Impaired humoral immunity in X-linked lymphoproliferative disease is associated with defective IL-10 production by CD4+ T cells. J Clin Invest 115:1049–1059, 2005.

Ma CS, Pittaluga S, Avery DT, Hare NJ, Maric I, Klion AD, Nichols KE, Tangye SG. Selective generation of functional somatically mutated IgM+CD27+, but not Ig isotype-switched, memory B cells in X-linked lymphoproliferative disease. J Clin Invest 116:322–333, 2006.

Malbran A, Belmonte L, Ruibal-Ares B, Bare P, Massud I, Parodi C, Felippo M, Hodinka R, Haines K, Nichols KE, de Bracco MM. Loss of circulating CD27+ memory B cells and CCR4+ T cells occurring in association with elevated EBV loads in XLP patients surviving primary EBV infection. Blood 103:1625–1631, 2004.

Markin RS, Linder J, Zuerlein K, Mroczek E, Grierson HL, Brichacek B, Purtilo DT. Hepatitis in fatal infectious mononucleosis. Gastroenterology 93:1210–1217, 1987.

Mehta VK, Massad MG, Tripathi SP, Koshy M, Geha AS. Immune-deficient bronchiectasis associated with X-linked lymphoproliferative disease. Ann Thorac Surg 68:578–580, 1999.

Migliorati R, Castaldo A, Russo S, Porta F, Fiorillo A, Guida S, Poggi V, Guarino A. Treatment of EBV-induced lymphoproliferative disorder with epipodophyllotoxin VP16-213. Acta Paediatr 83:1322–1325, 1994.

Milone M, Tsai DE, Hodinka RL, Silverman LB, Malbran A, Wasik MA, Nichols KE. Treatment of primary Epstein-Barr virus infection in patients with X-linked lymphoproliferative disease using B-cell directed therapy. Blood 105:994–996, 2005.

Mori M, Kurozumi H, Akagi K, Tanaka Y, Imai S, Osato T. Monoclonal proliferation of T cells containing Epstein-Barr virus in fatal mononucleosis. N Engl J Med 327:58, 1992.

Morra M, Howie D, Grande MS, Sayos J, Wang N, Wu C, Engel P, Terhorst C. X-linked lymphoproliferative disease: a progressive immunodeficiency. Annu Rev Immunol 19:657–682, 2001a.

Morra M, Lu J, Poy F, Martin M, Sayos J, Calpe S, Gullo C, Howie D, Rietdijk S, Thompson A, Coyle AJ, Denny C, Yaffe MB, Engel P, Eck MJ, Terhorst C. Structural basis for the interaction of the free SH2 domain EAT-2 with SLAM receptors in hematopoietic cells. EMBO J 20:5840–5852, 2001b.

Morra M, Silander O, Calpe S, Choi M, Oettgen H, Myers L, Etzioni A, Buckley R, Terhorst C. Alterations of the X-linked lymphoproliferative disease gene SH2D1A in common variable immunodeficiency syndrome. Blood 98:1321–1325, 2001c.

Morra M, Simarro-Grande M, Martin M, Chen AS, Lanyi A, Silander O, Calpe S, Davis J, Pawson T, Eck MJ, Sumegi J, Engel P, Li SC, Terhorst C. Characterization of SH2D1A missense mutations identified in X-linked lymphoproliferative disease patients. J Biol Chem 276:36809–36816, 2001d.

Mroczek EC, Seemayer TA, Grierson HL, Markin RS, Linder J, Brichacek B, Purtilo DT. Thymic lesions in fatal infectious mononucleosis. Clin Immunol Immunopathol 43:243–255, 1987a.

Mroczek EC, Weisenburger DD, Grierson HL, Markin R, Purtilo DT. Fatal infectious mononucleosis and virus-associated hemophagocytic syndrome. Arch Pathol Lab Med 111:530–535, 1987b.

Mulley JC, Turner AM, Gedeon AK, Berdoukas VA, Huang THM, Ledbetter DH, Grierson H, Purtilo DT. X-linked lymphoproliferative disease: prenatal detection of an unaffected histocompatible male. Clin Genet 42:76–79, 1992.

Nagy N, Cerboni C, Mattsson K, Maeda A, Gogolak P, Sumegi J, Lanyi A, Szekely L, Carbone E, Klein G, Klein E. SH2D1A and SLAM protein expression in human lymphocytes and derived cell lines. Int J Cancer 88:439–447, 2000.

Nagy N, Maeda A, Bandobashi K, Kis LL, Nishikawa J, Trivedi P, Faggioni A, Klein G, Klein E. SH2D1A expression in Burkitt lymphoma cells is restricted to EBV-positive group I lines and is downregulated in parallel with immunoblastic transformation. Int J Cancer 100:433–440, 2002.

Nakajima H, Cella M, Bouchon A, Grierson HL, Lewis J, Duckett CS, Cohen JI, Colonna M. Patients with X-linked lymphoproliferative disease have a defect in 2B4 receptor–mediated NK cell cytotoxicity. Eur J Immunol 30:3309–3318, 2000.

Nakamura H, Zarycki J, Sullivan JL, Jung JU. Abnormal T cell receptor signal transduction of CD4 Th cells in X-linked lymphoproliferative syndrome. J Immunol 167:2657–2665, 2001.

Nichols KE, Harkin DP, Levitz S, Krainer M, Koquist K A, Genovese C, Bernard A, Ferguson M, Zuo L, Snyder E, Buckler AJ, Wise C, Ashley J, Lovett M, Valentine MB, Look AT, Gerald W, Housman DE, Haber DA. Inactivating mutations in an SH2 domain-encoding gene in X-linked lymphoproliferative syndrome. Proc Natl Acad Sci USA 95:13765–13779, 1998.

Nichols KE, Hom J, Gong SY, Ganguly A, Ma CS, Cannons JL, Tangye SG, Schwartzberg PL, Koretzky GA, Stein PL. Regulation of NKT cell development by SAP, the protein defective in XLP. Nat Med 11:340–345, 2005.

Nistala K, Gilmour KC, Cranston T, Davies EG, Goldblatt D, Gaspar HB, Jones AM. X-linked lymphoproliferative disease: three atypical cases. Clin Exp Immunol 126:126–130, 2001.

Ohga S, Nomura A, Takada H, Ihara K, Kawakami K, Yanai F, Takahata Y, Tanaka T, Kasuga N, Hara T. Epstein-Barr virus (EBV) load and cytokine gene expression in activated T cells of chronic active EBV infection. J Infect Dis 183:1–7, 2001.

Okano M, Bashir RM, Davis JR, Purtilo DT. Detection of primary Epstein-Barr virus infection in a patient with X-linked lymphoproliferative disease receiving immunoglobulin prophylaxis. Am J Hematol 36:294–296, 1991.

Okano M, Gross TG. Epstein-Barr virus–associated hemophagocytic syndrome and fatal infectious mononucleosis. Am J Hematol 53:111–115, 1996.

Okano M, Nakanishi M, Taguchi Y, Sakiyama Y, Matsumoto S. Primary immunodeficiency diseases and Epstein-Barr virus–induced lymphoproliferative disorders. Acta Paediatr Jpn 34:385–392, 1992.

Okano M, Pirruccello SJ, Grierson HL, Johnson DR, Thiele GM, Purtilo DT. Immunovirological studies of fatal infectious mononucleosis in a patient with X-linked lymphoproliferative syndrome treated with intravenous immunoglobulin and interferon-alpha. Clin Immunol Immunopathol 54:410–418, 1990.

Ott G, Ott MM, Feller AC, Seidl S, Muller-Hermelink HK. Prevalence of Epstein-Barr virus DNA in different T-cell lymphoma entities in a European population. Int J Cancer 51:562–567, 1992.

Parolini O, Kagerbauer B, Simonitsch-Klupp I, Ambros P, Jaeger U, Mann G, Haas OA, Morra M, Gadner H, Terhorst C, Knapp W, Holter W. Analysis of *SH2D1A* mutations in patients with severe Epstein-Barr virus infections, Burkitt's lymphoma, and Hodgkin's lymphoma. Ann Hematol 81:441–447, 2002.

Parolini S, Bottino C, Falco M, Augugliaro R, Giliani S, Franceschini R, Ochs HD, Wolf H, Bonnefoy JY, Biassoni R, Moretta L, Notarangelo LD, Moretta A. X-linked lymphoproliferative disease: 2B4 molecules displaying inhibitory rather than activating function are responsible for the inability of natural killer cells to kill Epstein-Barr virus–infected cells. J Exp Med 192:337–346, 2000.

Pasquier B, Yin L, Fondaneche MC, Relouzat F, Bloch-Queyrat C, Lambert N, Fischer A, de Saint-Basile G, Latour S. Defective NKT cell development in mice and humans lacking the adapter SAP, the X-linked lymphoproliferative syndrome gene product. J Exp Med 201:695–701, 2005.

Plunkett FJ, Franzese O, Belaramani LL, Fletcher JM, Gilmour KC, Sharifi R, Khan N, Hislop AD, Cara A, Salmon M, Gaspar HB, Rustin MH, Webster D, Akbar AN. The impact of telomere erosion on memory CD8⁺ T cells in patients with X-linked lymphoproliferative syndrome. Mech Ageing Dev 126:855–865, 2005.

Porta G, MacMillan S, Najaraja R, Mumm S, Zucchi I, Pilia G, Maio S, Featherstone T, Schlessinger D. 4.5-Mb YAC STS contig at 50-kb resolution, spanning Xg25 deletions in two patients with lymphoproliferative syndrome. Genome Res 7:27–36, 1997.

Poy F, Yaffe M B, Sayos J, Saxena K, Morra M, Sumegi J, Cantley LC, Terhorst C, Eck MJ. Crystal structures of the XLP protein SAP reveal a class of SH2 domains with extended, phosphotyrosine-independent sequence recognition. Mol Cell 4:555–561, 1999.

Pracher E, Grumayer-Panzer ER, Zoubek A, Peters C, Gadner H. Bone marrow transplantation in a boy with X-linked lymphoproliferative syndrome and acute severe infectious mononucleosis. Bone Marrow Transplant 13:655–658, 1994.

Purtilo DT. X-linked lymphoproliferative disease (XLP) as a model of Epstein-Barr virus–induced immunopathology. Springer Semin Immunopathol 13:181–197, 1991.

Purtilo DT, Cassel CK, Yang JP, Harper R. X-linked recessive progressive combined variable immunodeficiency (Duncan's disease). Lancet I:935–940, 1975.

Purtilo DT, Falk K, Pirruccello SJ, Nakamine H, Kleveland K, Davis JR, Okano M, Taguchi Y, Sanger WG, Beisel KW. SCID mouse model of Epstein-Barr virus–induced lymphomagenesis of immunodeficient humans. Int J Cancer 47:510–517, 1991a.

Purtilo DT, Grierson HL. Methods of detection of new families with X-linked lymphoproliferative disease. Cancer Genet Cytogenet 51:143–153, 1991.

Purtilo DT, Grierson HL, Davis JR, Okano M. The X-linked lymphoproliferative disease: from autopsy toward cloning the gene 1975–1990. Pediatr Pathol 11:685–710, 1991b.

Purtilo DT, Grierson HL, Skare J, Ochs H. Detection of X-linked lymphoproliferative disease (XLP) using molecular and immunovirological markers. Am J Med 87:421–424, 1989.

Purtilo DT, Strobach RS, Okano M, Davis JR. Epstein-Barr virus–associated lymphoproliferative disorders. Lab Invest 67:5–23, 1992.

Purtilo DT, Tatsumi E, Manolov G, Manolova Y, Harada S, Lipskomb H, Krueger G. Epstein-Barr virus as an etiological agent in the pathogenesis of lymphoproliferative and aproliferative diseases in immune deficient patients. Int Rev Exp Pathol 27:113–183, 1985.

Quintanilla-Martinez L, Kumar S, Fend F, Reyes E, Teruya-Feldstein J, Kingma DW, Sorbara L, Raffeld M, Straus SE, Jaffe ES. Fulminant EBV(+) T-cell lymphoproliferative disorder following acute/chronic EBV infection: a distinct clinicopathologic syndrome. Blood 96:443–514, 2000.

Revy P, Muto T, Levy Y, Geissmann F, Plebani A, Sanal O, Catalan N, Forveille M, Dufourcq-Labelouse R, Gennery A, Tezcan I, Ersoy F, Kayserili H, Ugazio AG, Brousse N, Muramatsu M, Notarangelo LD, Kinoshita K, Honjo T, Fischer A, Durandy A. Activation-induced cytidine deaminase (AID) deficiency causes the autosomal recessive form of the Hyper-IgM syndrome (HIGM2). Cell 102:565–575, 2000.

Rieux-Laucat F, Le Deist F, Hivroz C, Roberts IA, Debatin KM, Fischer A, de Villartay JP. Mutations in Fas associated with human lymphoproliferative syndrome and autoimmunity. Science 268:1347–1349, 1995.

Rousset F, Souillet G, Roncarolo MG, Lamelin JP. Studies of EBV-lymphoid cell interactions in two patients with the X-linked lymphoproliferative syndrome: normal EBV-specific HLA-restricted cytotoxicity. Clin Exp Immunol 63:280–289, 1986.

Sakamoto K, Seeley JK, Lindsten J, Yetz J, Ballow M, Purtilo DT. Abnormal anti-Epstein Barr virus antibodies in carriers of the X-linked lymphoproliferative syndrome and in females at risk. J Immunol 128:904–907, 1982.

Salzer U, Chapel HM, Webster ADB, Pan-Hammarström Q, Schmitt-Graeff A, Schlesier M, Peter HH, Rockstroh JK, Schneider P, Schäffer AA, Hammarström L, Grimbacher B. Mutations in TNFRSF13B encoding TACI are associated with common variable immunodeficiency in humans. Nat Genet 37:820–828, 2005.

Sanger WG, Grierson HL, Skare J, Wyandt H, Pirruccello S, Fordyce R, Purtilo DT. Partial Xq25 deletion in a family with the X-linked lymphoproliferative syndrome (XLP). Cancer Genet Cytogenet 47:163–169, 1990.

Sanzone S, Zeyda M, Saemann MD, Soncini M, Holter W, Fritsch G, Knapp W, Candotti F, Stulnig TM, Parolini O. SLAM-associated protein deficiency causes imbalanced early signal transduction and blocks downstream activation in T cells from X-linked lymphoproliferative disease patients. J Biol Chem 278:29593–29599, 2003.

Sayos J, Martin M, Chen A, Simarro M, Howie D, Morra M, Engel P, Terhorst C. Cell surface receptors Ly-9 and CD84 recruit the X-linked lymphoproliferative disease gene product SAP. Blood 97:3867–3874, 2001.

Sayos J, Nguyen KB, Wu C, Stepp SE, Howie D, Schatzle JD, Kumar V, Biron CA, Terhorst C. Potential pathways for regulation of NK and T cell responses: differential X-linked lymphoproliferative syndrome gene product SAP interactions with SLAM and 2B4. Int Immunol 12:1749–1757, 2000.

Sayos J, Wu C, Morra M, Wang N, Zhang X, Allen D, van Schaik S, Notarangelo L, Geha R, Roncarolo M, Oettgen H, De Vries JE, Aversall G, Terhorst C. The X-linked lymphoproliferative-disease gene product SAP regulates signals induced through the co-receptor SLAM. Nature 395:462–469, 1998.

Schuster V, Kress W, Friedrich W, Grimm T, Kreth HW. X-linked lymphoproliferative disease: detection of a paternally inherited mutation in a German family using haplotype analysis. Am J Dis Child 147:1303–1305, 1993.

Schuster V, Kreth HW. X-linked lymphoproliferative disease is caused by deficiency of a novel SH2 domain-containing signal transduction adaptor protein. Immunol Rev 178:21–28, 2000.

Schuster V, Ott G, Seidenspinner S, Kreth HW. Common EBV type 1 variant strains in both malignant and benign EBV-associated disorders. Blood 87:1579–1585, 1996.

Schuster V, Seidenspinner S, Grimm T, Kress W, Zielen S, Bock M, Kreth HW. Molecular genetic haplotype segregation studies in three families with X-linked lymphoproliferative disease. Eur J Pediatr 153:432–437, 1994.

Schuster V, Seidenspinner S, Kreth HW. Prenatal diagnosis of X-linked lymphoproliferative disease using multiplex polymerase chain reaction. J Med Genet 32:756–757, 1995.

Sculley TB, Apolloni A, Hurren L, Moss DJ, Cooper DA. Coinfection with A- and B-type Epstein-Barr virus in human immunodeficiency virus-positive subjects. J Infect Dis 162:643–648, 1990.

Seemayer TA, Gross TG, Egeler RM, Pirruccello SJ, Davis JR, Kelly CM, Okano M, Lanyi A, Sumegi J. X-linked lymphoproliferative disease: twenty-five years after the discovery. Pediatr Res 38:471–477, 1995.

Sharifi R, Sinclair JC, Gilmour KC, Arkwright PD, Kinnon C, Thrasher AJ, Gaspar HB. SAP mediates specific cytotoxic T-cell functions in X-linked lymphoproliferative disease. Blood 103:3821–3827, 2004.

Shinozaki K, Kanegane H, Matsukura H, Sumazaki R, Tsuchida M, Makita M, Kimoto Y, Kanai R, Tsumura K, Kondoh T, Moriuchi H, Miyawaki T. Activation-dependent T cell expression of the X-linked lymphoproliferative disease gene product SLAM-associated protein and its assessment for patient detection. Int Immunol 14:1215–1223, 2002.

Shlapatska LM, Mikhalap SV, Berdova AG, Zelensky OM, Yun TJ, Nichols KE, Clark EA, Sidorenko SP. CD150 association with either the SH2-containing inositol phosphatase or the SH2-containing protein tyrosine phosphatase is regulated by the adaptor protein SH2D1A. J Immunol 166:5480–5487, 2001.

Skare JC, Grierson HL, Sullivan JL, Nussbaum RL, Purtilo DT, Sylla B, Lenoir J, Reilly DS, White BN, Milunsky A. Linkage analysis of seven kindreds with the X-linked lymphoproliferative syndrome (XLP) confirms that the XLP locus is near DXS42 and DXS37. Hum Genet 82: 354–358, 1989a.

Skare J, Grierson HJ, Wyandt H, Sanger W, Milunsky J, Purtilo D, Sullivan J, Milunsky A. Genetics of the X-linked lymphoproliferative syndrome. Am J Hum Genet 45:A161, 1989b.

Skare J, Madan S, Glaser J, Purtilo D, Nitowsky H, Pulijaal V, Milunsky A. First prenatal diagnosis of X-linked lymphoproliferative disease. Am J Med Genet 44:79–81, 1992.

Skare JC, Milunsky A, Byron KS, Sullivan JL. Mapping the X-linked lymphoproliferative syndrome. Proc Natl Acad Sci USA 84:2015–2018, 1987.

Skare JC, Sullivan JL, Milunsky A. Mapping the mutation causing the X-linked lymphoproliferative syndrome in relation to restriction fragment length polymorphism on Xq. Hum Genet 82:349–353, 1989c.

Skare J, Wu B-L, Madan S, Pulijaal V, Purtilo D, Haber D, Nelson D, Sylla B, Grierson H, Nitowsky H, Glaser J, Wissink J, White B, Holden J, Housman D, Lenoir G, Wyandt H, Milunsky A. Characterization of three overlapping deletions causing X-linked lymphoproliferative disease. Genomics 16:254–255, 1993.

Soresina A, Lougaris V, Giliani S, Cardinale F, Armenio L, Cattalini M, Notarangelo LD, Plebani A. Mutations of the X-linked lymphoproliferative disease gene SH2D1A mimicking common variable immunodeficiency. Eur J Pediatr 161:656–659, 2002.

Stepp SE, Dufourcq-Lagelouse R, Le Deist F, Bhawan S, Certain S, Mathew PA, Henter JI, Bennett M, Fischer A, de Saint Basile G, Kumar V. Perforin gene defects in familial hemophagocytic lymphohistiocytosis. Science 286:1957–1959, 1999.

Strahm B, Rittweiler K, Duffner U, Brandau O, Orlowska-Volk M, Karajannis MA, Zur Stadt U, Tiemann M, Reiter A, Brandis M, Meindl A, Niemeyer CM. Recurrent B-cell non-Hodgkin's lymphoma in two brothers with X-linked lymphoproliferative disease without evidence for Epstein-Barr virus infection. Br J Haematol 108:377–382, 2000.

Su I-J, Wang C-H, Cheng A-L, Chen R-L. Hemophagocytic syndrome in Epstein-Barr virus–associated T-lymphoproliferative disorders: disease spectrum, pathogenesis, and management. Leuk Lymphoma 19:401–406, 1995.

Sullivan JL. Epstein-Barr virus and the X-linked lymphoproliferative syndrome. In: Barness LA, ed. Advances in Pediatrics, Vol. 30. Chicago: Year Book Medical, pp. 365–399, 1983.

Sullivan JL. The abnormal gene in X-linked lymphoproliferative syndrome. Curr Opin Immunol 11:431–434, 1999.

Sullivan JL, Byron KS, Brewster FE, Purtilo DT. Deficient natural killer cell activity in the X-linked lymphoproliferative syndrome. Science 210:543–545, 1980.

Sullivan JL, Woda BA. X-linked lymphoproliferative syndrome. Immunodefic Rev 1:325–347, 1989.

Sumazaki R, Kanegane H, Osaki M, Fukushima T, Tsuchida M, Matsukura H, Shinozaki K, Kimura H, Matsui A, Miyawaki T. SH2D1A mutations in Japanese males with severe Epstein-Barr virus–associated illnesses. Blood 98:1268–1270, 2001.

Sumegi J, Huang D, Lanyi A, Davis JD, Seemayer TA, Maeda A, Klein G, Seri M, Wakiguchi H, Purtilo DT, Gross TG. Correlation of mutations of the SH2D1A gene and Epstein-barr virus infection with clinical phenotype and outcome in X-linked lymphoproliferative disease. Blood 96:3118–3125, 2000.

Sylla BS, Murphy K, Cahir-McFarland E, Lane WS, Mosialos G, Kieff E. The X-linked lymphoproliferative syndrome gene product SH2D1A associates with p62dok (Dok1) and activates NF-kappa B. Proc Natl Acad Sci USA 97:7470–7475, 2000.

Sylla BS, Wang Q, Hayoz D, Lathrop GM, Lenoir GM. Multipoint linkage mapping of the Xq25–q26 region in a family affected by the X-linked lymphoproliferative syndrome. Clin Genet 36:459–462, 1989.

Tabata Y, Villanueva J, Lee SM, Zhang K, Kanegane H, Miyawaki T, Sumegi J, Filipovich AH. Rapid detection of intracellular SH2D1A protein in cytotoxic lymphocytes from patients with X-linked lymphoproliferative disease and their family members. Blood 105:3066–3071, 2005.

Tangye SG, Lazetic S, Woollatt E, Sutherland GR, Lanier LL, Phillips JH. Cutting edge: human 2B4, an activating NK cell receptor, recruits the protein tyrosine phosphatase SHP-2 and the adaptor signaling protein SAP. J Immunol 162:6981–6985, 1999.

Tangye SG, Phillips JH, Lanier LL. The CD2-subset of the Ig superfamily of cell surface molecules: receptor–ligand pairs expressed by NK cells and other immune cells. Semin Immunol 12:149–157, 2000a.

Tangye SG, Phillips JH, Lanier LL, Nichols KE. Functional requirement for SAP in 2B4-mediated activation of human natural killer cells as revealed by the X-linked lymphoproliferative syndrome. J Immunol 165:2932–2936, 2000b.

Tangye SG, van de Weerdt BC, Avery DT, Hodgkin PD. CD84 is upregulated on a major population of human memory B cells and recruits the SH2-domain containing proteins SAP and EAT-2. Eur J Immunol 32:1640–1649, 2002.

Tomkinson BE, Maziarz R, Sullivan JL. Characterization of the T cell–mediated cellular cytotoxicity during acute infectious mononucleosis. J Immunol 143:660–670, 1989.

Tosato G. Cell-mediated immunity. In: Schlossberg D, ed. Infectious Mononucleosis. New York: Springer-Verlag, pp. 100–116, 1989.

Tosato G, Magrath IT, Blaese RM. T cell–mediated immunoregulation of Epstein-Barr virus (EBV)-induced B lymphocyte activation in EBV-seropositive and EBV-negative individuals. J Immunol 128:575–579, 1982.

Turner AM, Berdoukas VA, Tobias VH, Ziegler JB, Toogood IR, Mulley JC, Skare J, Purtilo DT. Report on the X-linked lymphoproliferative disease in an Australian family. J Paediatr Child Health 28:184–189, 1992.

Vowels MR, Lam-Po-Tang R, Berdoukas V, Ford D, Thierry D, Purtilo D, Gluckman E. Correction of X-linked lymphoproliferative disease by transplantation of cord-blood stem cells. N Engl J Med 329:1623–1625, 1993.

Wang F, Blaese RM, Zoon KC, Tosato G. Suppressor T cell clones from patients with Epstein-Barr virus–induced infectious mononucleosis. J Clin Invest 79:7–14, 1987.

Wang J, Zheng L, Lobito A, Chan FK, Dale J, Sneller M, Yao X, Puck JM, Straus SE, Lenardo MJ. Inherited human caspase 10 mutations underlie defective lymphocyte and dendritic cell apoptosis in autoimmune lymphoproliferative syndrome type II. Cell 98:47–58, 1999.

Weiss LM, Movahed LA, Warnke RA, Sklar J. Detection of Epstein-Barr viral genomes in Reed-Sternberg cells of Hodgkin's's disease. N Engl J Med 320:502–506, 1989.

Williams LL, Rooney CM, Conley ME, Brenner MK, Krance RA, Heslop HE. Correction of Duncan's syndrome by allogeneic bone marrow transplantation. Lancet II:587–588, 1993.

Wu B-L, Milunsky A, Nelson D, Schmeckpeper B, Porta G, Schlessinger D, Skare J. High-resolution mapping of probes near the X-linked lymphoproliferative disease (XLP) locus. Genomics 17:163–170, 1993.

Wu C, Nguyen KB, Pien GC, Wang N, Gullo C, Howie D, Sosa MR, Edwards MJ, Borrow P, Satoskar AR, Sharpe AH, Biron CA, Terhorst C. SAP controls T cell responses to virus and terminal differentiation of TH2 cells. Nat Immunol 2:410–414, 2001.

Wu C, Sayos J, Wang N, Howie D, Coyle A, Terhorst C. Genomic organization and characterization of mouse SAP, the gene that is altered in X-linked lymphoproliferative disease. Immunogenetics 51:805–815, 2000.

Wyandt HE, Grierson HL, Sanger WG, Skare JC, Milunsky A, Purtilo DT. Chromosome deletion of Xq25 in an individual with X-linked lymphoproliferative disease. Am J Med Genet 33:426–430, 1989.

Yasuda N, Lai PK, Rogers J, Purtilo DT. Defective control of Epstein-Barr virus–infected B cell growth in patients with X-linked lymphoproliferative disease. Clin Exp Immunol 83:10–16, 1991.

Yin L, Al-Alem U, Liang J, Tong WM, Li C, Badiali M, Medard JJ, Sumegi J, Wang ZQ, Romeo G. Mice deficient in the X-linked lymphoproliferative disease gene SAP exhibit increased susceptibility to murine γherpesvirus-68 and hypo-gammaglobulinemia. J Med Virol 71:446–455, 2003.

Yin L, Ferrand V, Lavoué MF, Hayoz D, Philippe N, Souillet G, Seri M, Giacchino R, Castagnola E, Hodgson S, Sylla BS, Romeo G. SH2D1A mutation analysis for diagnosis of XLP in typical and atypical patients. Hum Genet 105:501–505, 1999a.

Yin L, Tocco T, Pauly S, Lenoir GM, Romeo G. Absence of SH2D1A point mutations in 62 Burkitts lymphoma cell lines. Am J Hum Genet 65(Suppl.):A331 [abstract 1868], 1999b.

Ziegner UH, Ochs HD, Schanen C, Feig SA, Seyama K, Futatani T, Gross T, Wakim M, Roberts RL, Rawlings DJ, Dovat S, Fraser JK, Stiehm ER. Unrelated umbilical cord stem cell transplantation for X-linked immunodeficiencies. J Pediatr 138:570–573, 2001.

Zur Hausen H, Schulte-Holthausen T, Klein G, Henle W, Henle G, Clifford P, Santesson, L. EBV DNA in biopsies of Burkitt tumors and anaplastic carcinomas of the nasopharynx. Nature 228:1056–1058, 1970.

zur Stadt U, Schmidt S, Kasper B, Beutel K, Diler AS, Henter JI, Kabisch H, Schneppenheim R, Nurnberg P, Janka G, Hennies HC. Linkage of familial hemophagocytic lymphohistiocytosis (FHL) type-4 to chromosome 6q24 and identification of mutations in syntaxin 11. Hum Mol Genet 14:827–834, 2005.

33

DiGeorge Syndrome: A Chromosome 22q11.2 Deletion Syndrome

DEBORAH A. DRISCOLL and KATHLEEN E. SULLIVAN

The association of thymic aplasia with congenital hypoparathyroidism was initially noted by Lobdell in 1959 but wasn't recognized as a syndrome until 1965 when Dr. Angelo DiGeorge described a group of infants with congenital absence of the thymus and parathyroid glands (DiGeorge, 1965). Subsequently, facial dysmorphia and cardiac defects, specifically conotruncal malformations, were included in the spectrum of DiGeorge syndrome (DGS) (Conley et al., 1979). DGS (MIM 188400) is a heterogeneous disorder. However, cytogenetic and molecular studies have shown that deletion of chromosomal region 22q11.2 is the leading cause of DGS. In rare instances, DGS is seen in association with other chromosomal rearrangements, with exposure to teratogens such as retinoic acid, and with maternal diabetes (Lammer and Opitz, 1986; Wilson et al., 1993b).

DGS is a developmental disorder that occurs as a result of abnormal cephalic neural crest cell migration, differentiation, or signaling in the third and fourth pharyngeal arches during the fourth week of embryonic development. Kirby et al. (1983) demonstrated that removal of the premigratory cardiac neural crest cells in the chick embryo results in cardiac outflow tract anomalies similar to those seen in DGS. The cardiac neural crest cells have also been shown to be important in supporting the development of the glandular derivatives of the pharyngeal arches (Kirby and Bockman, 1984). The aortic arch anomalies have been duplicated in transgenic mice with haploinsufficiency due to a deletion of a region of mouse chromosome 16 (*Df1*) that is homologous to human chromosome 22q11.2 and contains the *Tbx1* gene encoding a transcription factor with "T-box" DNA-binding domain (Lindsay et al., 2001; Merscher et al., 2001). Jerome and Papaioannou (2001) produced a mouse knockout with a null mutation of *Tbx1*. The heterozygotes have cardiovascular anomalies seen in DGS, whereas the homozygotes are nonviable but display a DGS phenotype as embryos. In fact, the dose

of T-box1 transcription factor during embryonic development is critical for the phenotypic manifestations (Liao et al., 2004).

Confirming the importance of the human gene *TBX1* in human DGS, a few patients with classical features of DGS have now been identified with point mutations in *TBX1*. Mutations were also identified in patients with less classical manifestations (Yagi et al., 2003). A further consideration is that gene expression in the gene-rich DGS region of 22q11.2 may be influenced by a long-range regulatory element (Botta et al., 2001).

DGS was initially considered a rare sporadic disorder; however, recent studies suggest that the 22q11 deletion, seen in approximately 90% of DGS patients, may occur as frequently as once in 4000–6000 live births, affecting both sexes equally. Furthermore, acknowledgment of the phenotypic overlap with other genetic disorders that share the 22q11.2 deletion such as velocardiofacial syndrome (VCFS, MIM 192430) and conotruncal anomaly face syndrome (CTAFS) has led to further expansion of the phenotype and a better understanding of the immune, endocrine, cognitive, neurologic, and psychiatric problems arising in DGS patients. While most early studies evaluated patients with the classic features of DGS, recent studies have attempted to ascertain all patients with the deletion to better define the clinical spectrum. The immunodeficiency is comparable in all patients with the deletion regardless of the other clinical manifestations (Sullivan et al., 1998). Therefore, we will discuss all patients who carry the deletion under the nomenclature of DGS. It is important to remember that the nomenclature is still evolving, with the term *chromosome 22q11.2 deletion syndrome* being appropriately applied to patients in whom the deletion has been confirmed. DGS is still commonly used for both patients with 22q11.2 deletion and patients with the classical clinical triad of cardiac defects, immunodeficiency, and hypocalemia, but without a demonstrable deletion. Approximately 10% of patients with

Table 33.1. Diagnostic Criteria for DiGeorge Syndrome*

Diagnostic Category	Description
Definitive	<500 CD3 T cells/mm³ and two of the three following characteristics: Conotruncal cardiac defect; Hypocalcemia requiring therapy for >3 weeks; Deletion of chromosome 22q11.2
Probable	<1500 CD3 T cells/mm³ and deletion of chromosome 22q11.2
Possible	<1500 CD3 T cells/mm³ and at least one of the following: Cardiac defect; Hypocalcemia requiring therapy for >3 weeks; Dysmorphic facies or palatal anomaly

*Source: From the European Society for Immunodeficiencies.

DGS will not have chromosome 22q11.2 deletion, thus the deletion is not absolutely required for the diagnosis of DGS. One scheme for categorizing patients with DGS is given in Table 33.1. However, one problem with this strategy is that patients who have deletion of 22q11.2 but do not have reduced T cell numbers do not receive a separate diagnostic label.

Clinical Features

DiGeorge syndrome has classically been characterized as a triad of clinical features: congenital cardiac defects, immune deficiencies secondary to aplasia or hypoplasia of the thymus, and hypocalcemia due to small or absent parathyroid glands. We now recognize that the phenotypic features seen in patients with DGS are much more variable and extensive than previously recognized (Ryan et al., 1997; McDonald-McGinn et al., 1999; Vantrappen et al., 1999; Botto et al., 2003) (Table 33.2). The acknowledgment of similarities and phenotypic overlap with other disorders, including VCFS and CTAFS, as well as the association of all of these disorders with genetic defects in 22q11 has led to an expanded phenotype that includes palatal and speech abnormalities and cognitive, neurologic, and psychiatric difficulties.

Immune Deficiency

Most DGS patients have a mild to moderate immunodeficiency characterized by impaired production and function of T cells with occasional secondary abnormalities in B cell function (Barrett et al., 1981; Bastian et al., 1989; Mayumi et al., 1989; Schubert and Moss, 1992; Junker and Driscoll, 1995). The most obvious abnormality is the impaired production of T cells. T cell counts are typically in the range of 500 to 1500 cells/mm³ for the first months of life (Bastian et al., 1989; Junker and Driscoll, 1995). This defect in T cell production is due to an anatomical thymus gland deficiency. Studies have demonstrated that most patients have either a very small anterior mediastinal thymus or small rests of thymic tissue scattered throughout the neck and submandibular areas (Lischner and Huff, 1975; Bale and Sotelo-Avila, 1993). This tissue consists of normal thymic components and is apparently sufficient to support normal T cell maturation. Although decreased numbers of mature T cells are produced, the orderly sequence of maturation appears to be preserved.

The spectrum of immunodeficiency is broad. While the typical patient demonstrates impaired T cell production in the first months of life, some DGS patients have normal or near-normal T cell production, whereas a minority have almost no detectable

Table 33.2. Clinical Features of the 22q11 Deletion Syndrome

Conotruncal cardiac defects (49%–83%)
Immune deficiency (80%)
Hypocalcemia (17%–60%)
Palatal abnormalities (69%–100%)
  Cleft palate (9%–11%)
  Submucous cleft palate (5%–16%)
  Velopharyngeal insufficiency (27%–32%)
  Feeding and swallowing difficulties (30%)
Dysmorphic facies
  Prominent nasal root
  Narrow nasal alae with bulbous nasal tip
  Hooded eyelids
  Protruberant ears
  Cup-shaped or thick, overfolded helices
  Small mouth
Learning difficulties
Hearing loss (39%)
Renal anomalies (37%)

Less frequent

Thyroid disease
Microcephaly
Short stature
Slender hands and digits
Umbilical hernia
Inguinal hernia
Scoliosis
Skeletal anomalies
Hypospadias
Hematologic abnormalities
Neuropsychiatric disorders

T cell production. In general, the T cell deficit improves during the first year of life, and 35% of DGS patients produce normal numbers of total T cells by the end of the first year of life (Jawad et al., 2001). There is some suggestion that DGS patients with a normal-appearing thymus are unlikely to have substantial persistent immunodeficiency (Bastian et al., 1989). In contrast, complete anatomical absence of a thymus does not preclude the ultimate development of normal immunologic function.

Although all T cell subsets are reduced, CD8 T cells are diminished the most. In early infancy the average CD8 count is approximately 300/mm³ and the average CD4 count is approximately 850/mm³ (Bastian et al., 1989; Junker and Driscoll, 1995). In an effort to understand whether peripheral blood T cells in patients with DGS develop aberrantly as a result of insufficient thymic epithelium, patient cells have been stained with markers specific for different stages of thymic maturation (Reinherz et al., 1981; Sirianni et al., 1983a, 1983b; Muller et al., 1989). On the basis of these studies, it appears that T cells use the usual developmental pathways; however, DGS patients are simply not able to produce as many T cells during the first months of life. It is not known why CD8 T cells are more profoundly affected than CD4 T cells.

T cell function is usually grossly normal as measured by responses to T cell mitogens (Barrett et al., 1981; Bastian et al., 1989; Muller et al., 1989; Junker and Driscoll, 1995). However, a small minority of patients have markedly diminished T cell responses. In the past, this distinction has led to confusing nomenclature. Patients with minimal T cell mitogen responses were said to have complete DGS and patients with normal or near-normal T cell mitogen responses were said to have partial DGS. In fact, there is a spectrum of severity for all of the phenotypic features of this disorder. Some of the patients with markedly impaired T cell function will not improve with time and will require either a bone marrow transplant or thymus transplant whereas others will improve, although improvement becomes less likely after the first few months.

The consequences of T cell deficiency in DGS patients are an increased susceptibility to infections, particularly viral infections, and an increased risk of autoimmune disease. Specifically, parainfluenza, adenovirus, and rotavirus have been shown to cause severe morbidity in DGS patients (Beard et al., 1980; Tuvia et al., 1988; Wood et al., 1988; Gilger et al., 1992). Most viral illnesses are more prolonged in DGS patients with compromised T cell function. It is not known if decreased T cell numbers are an independent risk factor for prolonged viral diseases in the absence of T cell dysfunction. Two studies demonstrated that DGS patients have an impaired T cell repertoire, suggesting that markedly diminished T cell numbers do contribute to infectious morbidity (Pierdominici et al., 2000, Piliero et al., 2004). DGS patients with severely diminished T cells are also at risk from the same opportunistic infections as patients with severe combined immunodeficiency.

Juvenile rheumatoid arthritis, immune-mediated thrombocytopenia (ITP), and autoimmune hemolytic anemia occur with increased incidence in patients with DGS (Pinchas-Hamiel et al., 1994; Duke et al., 2000; Jawad et al., 2001). In addition, individual cases of autoimmune thyroiditis have been described, suggesting that there is a generalized increased frequency of autoimmune disease in DGS patients (Ham Pong et al., 1985). The delayed formation and maturation of T cell regulatory functions might allow for the development and proliferation of autoreactive T cells (Sullivan et al., 2002).

The natural killer (NK) cell compartment often comprises a large fraction of the total peripheral blood lymphocytes. In some cases, this reflects genuine expansion of this cell lineage. NK cell function has been examined in DGS patients and found to correlate poorly with NK cell number or T cell studies (Muller et al., 1989).

In contrast to the quantitative deficiency of T cells, the B cell compartment is typically normal or expanded. The B cells often comprise a larger fraction of the total lymphocyte pool than in normal infants and the absolute numbers of B cells may be expanded as well. Markedly increased B cell numbers may correlate with poorer T cell function (Muller et al., 1989; Jawad et al., 2001). This is thought to be due to aberrant regulation of B cells by the deficient T cells. There is evidence that there is defective T cell suppression of B cell immunoglobulin production in infants with DGS (Durandy et al., 1986) and it is not uncommon for infants with DGS to have hypergammaglobulinemia (Muller et al., 1988). On the other hand, hypogammaglobulinemia, IgA deficiency, and delayed acquisition of appropriate antitetanus and antidiphtheria antibody titers have been described in DGS patients (Mayumi et al., 1989; Junker and Driscoll, 1995; Smith et al., 1998). This is also thought to result from the relative deficiency of appropriate T cell help for immunoglobulin production. A DGS kindred with persistently impaired T cell production, normal T cell function, and defective ability to form some antipolysaccharide antibodies has been described. The occurrence of similar humoral dysfunction in the same kindred suggests that modifier genes may play a significant role in the ultimate level of humoral function. In general, however, it is not possible to predict the level of immunologic function of an affected child on the basis of previously diagnosed siblings or parents. Recognition that T cell dysfunction could alter immunoglobulin production prompted a study of immunoglobulin diversity in DGS patients. The immunoglobulin repertoire was normal in a patient with severe T cell deficits as well as in a patient with mild T cell compromise. However, somatic mutation was found to be markedly deficient in the patient with significant T cell dysfunction compared to the more mildly affected patient and normal controls (Haire et al., 1993).

Other Features

Congenital abnormalities

The most common cardiovascular malformations include interrupted aortic arch type B (14%–15%), truncus arteriosus (7%–9%), and tetralogy of Fallot (17%–22%). Although neonatal hypocalcemia is not uncommon in DGS, recent studies suggest that patients are at risk for a spectrum of parathyroid gland abnormalities including latent hypoparathyroidism, which may evolve to hypocalcemic hypoparathyroidism during adolescence or early adulthood (Cuneo et al., 1997). One study demonstrated that chromosome 22q11.2 deletions were seen in 10 of 14 neonates with hypocalcemia (Adachi et al., 1998).

Newborns and infants with DGS may have dysmorphic facial features such as widely spaced eyes (hypertelorism); low-set, prominent ears; and micrognathia. Later in childhood, adolescence, and adulthood their facial features become more characteristic of patients with VCFS (Fig. 33.1). The characteristic facial features of VCFS include a long face; a prominent nose with a bulbous nasal tip and narrow alar base; almond-shaped or narrow palpebral fissures; malar flattening; recessed chin; and malformed, prominent ears (Shprintzen et al., 1981). In addition, a spectrum of palatal abnormalities may be seen in DGS, such as cleft palate, submucous cleft palate, velopharyngeal insufficiency (VPI), bifid uvula, and cleft lip with or without cleft palate. Feeding difficulties and gastroesophageal reflux are common and can require tube-feeding or a gastrostomy tube (Eicher et al., 2000). Renal anomalies such as single kidney, multicystic dysplastic kidney, horseshoe kidney, and duplicated collecting system occur in approximately one-third of DGS patients. Hearing loss in one or both ears is not uncommon. Other features seen less frequently include microcephaly, short stature, hypospadias, ocular abnormalities, inguinal and umbilical hernias, hematologic abnormalities, and skeletal anomalies (Ryan et al., 1997; McDonald-McGinn et al., 1999).

Neurologic abnormalities

Neurologic manifestations may also be seen in DGS. Neural tube defects have been described in three patients (Nickel et al., 1994). Structural brain abnormalities including a small vermis, small posterior fossa, and small cysts adjacent to the anterior horns have been identified by magnetic resonance imaging (MRI); however, these findings did not appear to correlate with developmental, cognitive, or personality disorders (Mitnick et al., 1994). Enlarged Sylvian fissures on MRI have been reported in infants with the 22q11.2 deletion. However, prospective studies will be necessary to determine the significance of these findings (Bingham et al., 1997). Cerebellar atrophy was diagnosed by MRI in a 34-year-old DGS patient with progressive gait difficulties, muscle stiffness, dysarthria, and dysmetria suggestive of a neurodegenerative disorder (Lynch et al., 1995).

Advances in medical and surgical management of newborns and children with DGS have led to increased survival. Hence, prospective evaluations of these children have enabled us to understand the range of cognitive and neuropsychological problems

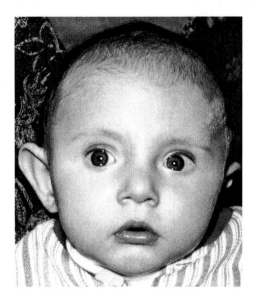 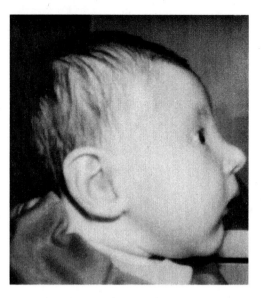

Figure 33.1. Frontal and side views of a 4-month-old male with DiGeorge syndrome and a 22q11.2 deletion. Note the prominent ears, bulbous nasal tip, mild micrognathia, and sloping forehead.

they are at risk to develop. In children of preschool age, developmental delay, mild hypotonia, and language and speech delays, especially for expressive language, are common. Behavioral problems observed include attention deficit–hyperactivity disorder (ADHD), inhibition, and shyness (Goldring-Kushner et al., 1985; Swillen et al., 1997; Gerdes et al., 1999; Solot et al., 2000). Psychoeducational and neurodevelopmental studies of children ages 4–20 with the 22q11 deletion demonstrated full-scale IQ scores in the normal to moderately retarded range, with significantly higher verbal than quantitative IQ scores. Math scores were lower than reading and spelling. These studies are consistent with nonverbal learning disabilities (Moss et al., 1999). Language difficulties persisted in approximately 50% of the children of school age (Solot et al., 2000). Recent studies also suggest an increased frequency of behavioral and psychiatric disorders. ADHD, specific phobias, schizophrenia, anxiety, and depressive disorders have been observed in adolescents and adults with the 22q11 deletion syndrome (Pulver et al., 1994; Sugama et al., 1999). Whether these conditions are primary consequences of 22q11 deletion or secondary to the nonverbal learning disability remains to be determined.

Other Disorders Associated with the 22q11 Deletion

In addition to the overlap between DGS and VCFS, there are striking similarities between patients with DGS and those with conotruncal anomaly face syndrome (CTAFS), a disorder predominantly described among the Japanese. CTAFS is characterized by conotruncal cardiac defects in association with a characteristic facial appearance. The facial features include ocular hypertelorism, lateral displacement of the inner canthi, flat nasal bridge, small mouth, narrow palpebral fissures, bloated eyelids, and malformed ears (Kinouchi et al., 1976). Some patients have a history of neonatal tetany, absent or hypoplastic thymus, and partial depression of T cell–mediated immune responses. The finding of 22q11 deletions in CTAFS patients confirmed an earlier suggestion that CTAFS, VCFS, and DGS are the same entity (Burn et al., 1993; Matsuoka et al., 1994).

Recent cytogenetic and linkage studies of patients diagnosed with Opitz/GBBB syndrome, suggest that there is at least one autosomal dominant locus for this disorder on chromosome 22q11 and a second on the X chromosome (Robin et al., 1995a). Opitz/GBBB syndrome (MIM 145410) is characterized by hypospadias, laryngotracheal anomalies, and hypertelorism (Opitz et al., 1965). Patients may have other features including cleft lip and palate, cardiac defects, umbilical and inguinal hernias, cryptorchidism, imperforate anus, and facial dysmorphia such as telecanthus, prominent nasal bridge, or depressed nasal root with anteverted nares. Four patients with Opitz/GBBB syndrome, including a father and son, have 22q11 deletions, which suggests that in some instances deletions within 22q11 are causally related to Opitz/GBBB syndrome (McDonald-McGinn et al., 1995). While there are some phenotypic similarities between these disorders, additional studies will be necessary to determine if Opitz/GBBB syndrome is a genetically distinct disorder from DGS and VCFS.

The DiGeorge anomaly has been observed in several other disorders, including CHARGE association (coloboma, heart defects, atresia of the choanae, retarded growth, genital hypoplasia, ear anomalies), Cayler cardiofacial syndrome, Kallman syndrome, and Noonan syndrome (Lammer and Opitz, 1986; Wilson et al., 1993a; Robin et al., 1995b; Bawle et al., 1998). However, the 22q11 deletion has not been found to be causally related to these disorders in a significant number of cases.

Phenotypic Variability of DiGeorge Syndrome and Velocardiofacial Syndrome

Although DGS and VCFS were previously recognized as two distinct disorders, there is significant phenotypic overlap and they share a common etiology; hence, we and others consider deletion-positive DGS and VCFS patients as having the same disorder, the 22q11 deletion syndrome. There is a wide range of phenotypic variability associated with the 22q11 deletion. While some individuals present with classic findings of DGS, others have relatively subtle features such as minor dysmorphic facial features or mild cognitive impairment. Furthermore, the observed differences between patients with DGS and VCFS probably reflect an ascertainment bias. Newborns with complex congenital cardiac defects associated with hypocalcemia and immune deficiencies are much more likely to be diagnosed with DGS. In contrast, school-age children with palatal abnormalities and speech and learning difficulties are usually diagnosed with VCFS by specialists in cleft palate or craniofacial abnormalities. Prospective studies of newborns and children with conotruncal defects initially believed to be isolated indicate that those patients who have the 22q11 deletion often eventually manifest other features of the syndrome, such as mild facial dysmorphism, velopharyngeal insufficiency, and learning difficulties (McDonald-McGinn et al., 1997). Such studies suggest that all deletion positive patients should receive comprehensive medical evaluations and follow-up as well as neuropsychological and educational assessments.

Cytogenetic and Molecular Studies

Cytogenetic studies of patients with DGS provided the initial evidence linking chromosome 22 to DGS (reviewed in Greenberg et al., 1988). Early reports of DGS patients with unbalanced translocations resulting in the loss of 22pter to q11 and two patients with interstitial deletions of 22q11 suggested that this region of chromosome 22 was important in the etiology of DGS. Subsequently, restriction fragment length polymorphism (RFLP) analysis and DNA dosage studies demonstrated that cytogenetically normal DGS patients had submicroscopic deletions within 22q11. Delineation of the DiGeorge chromosomal region (DGCR) was initially based on the finding of a consistently deleted region within 22q11 in the first 14 DGS patients described with 22q11 microdeletions (Driscoll et al., 1992a).

The presence of features common to DGS in patients diagnosed with VCFS prompted investigators to study VCFS patients for evidence of a 22q11 deletion. Cytogenetic studies using high-resolution banding techniques detected interstitial deletions (del 22q11.21–q11.23) in 20% of VCFS patients (Driscoll et al., 1992b). Molecular studies with chromosome 22 probes previously shown to be deleted in patients with DGS demonstrated that the majority of individuals with VCFS have similar deletions of 22q11 (Driscoll et al., 1992b, 1993; Kelley et al., 1993). These studies coincided with the increasing utilization of fluorescence in situ hybridization (FISH) for the detection of microdeletions and subtle translocations. FISH of metaphase chromosomes by use of DNA probes from the DGCR led to a dramatic increase in the detection of 22q11 deletions in patients with features of DGS, VCFS, CTAFS, and conotruncal cardiac malformations (Color Plates 33.I and 33.II).

Mechanism of the 22q11 Deletion

Most DGS patients have a large deletion (3 Mb) within 22q11.2 (Fig. 33.2). Approximately 10%–12% have a smaller deletion nested within the commonly deleted region (Shaikh et al., 2000; Emanuel et al., 2001). A few DGS patients have been identified with deletions outside this region (Rausch et al., 1999; Saitta et al., 1999). Significant progress has been made in our understanding of the mechanism of the 22q11.2 deletion. Numerous DGS-associated translocations within the commonly deleted region and identification of unstable DNA sequences near the recurrent constitutional t(11;22) translocation breakpoints, suggest that 22q11.2 is an unstable region (Kurahashi et al., 2000). The four low copy number repeats (LCRs) near the deletion boundaries are associated with aberrant interchromosomal exchanges (Shaikh et al., 2000, 2001; Saitta et al., 2004). Analysis of the sequence of these LCRs indicates that they are large, highly homologous, and complex.

Gene Identification

At least 40 genes have been identified within the 3 Mb commonly deleted region of 22q11.2. This entire gene-rich region of chromosome 22 has been sequenced and is now available in the public domain (Dunham et al., 1999). On the basis of reports of DGS patients with different nonoverlapping deletions and recent evidence from the mouse, it is possible that more than one gene could contribute to the phenotype. Several of the genes in the commonly deleted region that are in part responsible for some of the phenotypic features in DGS are described in this section.

The most likely single candidate gene for DGS is *TBX1*. The human *TBX1* gene was identified in the commonly deleted region and with rare exceptions is deleted in the majority of DGS patients (Chieffo et al., 1997). *TBX1* is a member of a conserved family of genes that share a "T-box" DNA-binding domain and function as transcription factors involved in the regulation of developmental processes. Animal models strongly suggest a dominant role for TBX1 protein in the DGS phenotype. The recent demonstration of point mutations in TBX1 leading to the full phenotype of DGS argues strongly for this being the major contributor to the phenotype (Yagi et al., 2003).

Several additional genes described in the common DGS deleted region may also contribute to the phenotype, given their expression patterns and potential role in cardiac and neural crest cell migration and differentiation. In 1995, *DGCR2/LAN/IDD*, a gene expressed in a variety of human adult and fetal tissues, was identified by several investigators (Budarf et al., 1995a; Demczuk et al., 1995; Wadey et al., 1995). This gene encodes a potential adhesion receptor that might mediate specific adhesive interactions between cells resulting in abnormal migration or interaction of the neural crest cells with the branchial arches.

The novel gene *DGCR6* is located in the proximal DGCR and shares homology with the *Drosophilia melanogaster* gonadal protein (gdl) and laminin g-1 (*LAMC1*) chain (Demczuk et al., 1996). Although *DGCR6* is present in all adult tissues except placenta, it appears to be most abundant in heart and skeletal muscle. Because of its homology with laminin, which, through its interactions with a receptor plays a role in cell attachment, migration, and tissue organization during embryonic development, it is possible that *DGCR6* may play a role in neural crest cell migration. A goosecoid-like homeobox gene, *GSCL* or *GSC2*, has also been identified within the DGS region (Funke et al., 1997; Gottlieb et al., 1997). *GSCL* is expressed during early human development in the derivatives of the cephalic neural crest cells.

Catechol-*O*-methyltransferase (*COMT*), also within the commonly deleted region (Grossman et al., 1992), is important in the metabolism of catecholamines such as noradrenaline, adrenaline, and dopamine. A polymorphism has been identified in *COMT* (*COMT* 158^{met}) that results in decreased enzyme activity and appears to be associated with the development of psychiatric disease, particularly bipolar spectrum disorder, in patients with the 22q11 deletion syndrome (Lachman et al., 1996; Graf et al., 2001). Thus *COMT* defects may play a role in the development of the psychiatric disorders in some DGS patients.

Glycoprotein Ibβ, encoded by the gene *GP1BB* in 22q11.2, is a component of the major platelet receptor for von Willebrand factor (Budarf et al., 1995b). Defects in this receptor result in

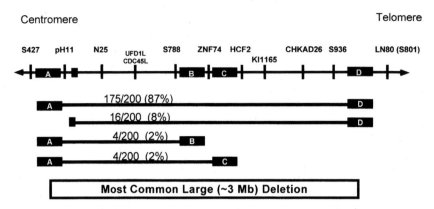

Figure 33.2. DiGeorge chromosomal region illustrating the size and location of the 22q11.2 deletions in 200 patients. Deletion size and boundaries (A–D) were determined by fluorescence in situ hybridization (FISH), using as probes cosmids containing the genes and markers listed on the map of 22q11.2. The duplicated blocks of sequence or low copy repeats, designated A, B, C, D, coincide with observed deletion end-points in patients. The extent and frequency of the four recurrent deletions are shown as lines below the map. Eighty-seven percent of DGS patients have a 3 Mb deletion extending from A to D. (Modified figure courtesy of B.S. Emanuel.)

a rare autosomal recessive bleeding disorder, Bernard-Soulier syndrome (BSS), which is characterized by excessive bleeding, thrombocytopenia, and very large platelets. A single patient with features of BSS and VCFS with a 22q11 deletion has been de-scribed (Budarf et al., 1995b). Haploinsufficiency for this region of chromosome 22 unmasked a mutation in the promotor region of the remaining *GP1BB* allele, resulting in manifestations of BSS (Ludlow et al., 1996). Haplosufficiency for *GPIBB* is likely to be responsible for the mild thrombocytopenia seen commonly in patients with deletions of 22q11.2 (Lawrence et al., 2003).

Animal Models

The creation of mouse models has enhanced our understanding of the molecular basis of DGS. Initially, maps and sequence of the region of mouse chromosome 16 that is homologous to the DGS chromosomal region on 22q11 were constructed (Puech et al., 1997; Sutherland et al., 1998; Lund et al., 1999). Targeted mutations of single genes and deletions of the homologous region of 16 have been developed to elucidate the role of individual genes or sets of genes in DGS. Most of the initial attempts failed to recapitulate the DGS phenotype. Eventually, using Cre-loxP chromosome engineering, Lindsay et al. (1999) success-fully created a mouse with cardiac defects similar to those seen in DGS. The mice had a 1.2 Mb deletion, designated *Df1*, of chro-mosome 16 containing at least 20 genes that are most often deleted in DGS patients. Most of the mice heterozygotes for this deletion were viable; 18%–26% had abnormalities of the fourth aortic arch arteries but no other manifestions of DGS. Subse-quently, through chromosome engineering and P1 artificial chro-mosome transgenesis, these investigators identified *Tbx1* as the gene in the *Df1* mouse responsible for the cardiac defects (Lind-say et al., 2001). A second group also used the Cre-loxP stategy to generate a slightly larger 1.5 Mb deletion in mouse chromo-some 16 that results in conotruncal cardiac anomalies (inter-rupted aortic arch type B, vascular ring, right aortic arch) and absent parathyroid glands (Mersher et al., 2001). They also used a rescue transgenesis technique and concluded that *Tbx1* was the critical gene for cardiac defects in mice with both deletions. In addition to the cardiac defects, the transgenic mice had a smaller than normal thymus, occasionally with small ectopic thymic lob-ules, along with a reduced number of CD4 and CD8 cells. How-ever, the parathyroids were normal. Similar to humans, the cardiac

defects in heterozygous *Df1* mice are not fully penetrant. This mouse model has provided insight into the pathogenesis of the cardiac defects and the basis for reduced penetrance. The aortic arch defects appear to correlate with a delay and occasional fail-ure of the differentiation of vascular smooth muscle from neural crest cell mesenchyme. Migration of the neural crest into the fourth arch and initial formation of the fourth pharyngeal arch arteries proceeds normally in the *Df1* mice but the affected ves-sels are impaired in their growth and do not acquire smooth mus-cle (Lindsay and Baldini, 2001). Many of the heterozygous *Df1* embryos were capable of overcoming this vascular defect and developed normally. These studies suggest that, contrary to pre-vious beliefs, the cardiac defects in DGS are secondary to de-layed growth and responsiveness to developmental signals for remodeling of the vasculature. This finding illustrates how the animal model has altered our understanding of DGS as a devel-opmental disorder.

At the same time, Jerome and Papaioannou (2001) reported on the production of a null mutation in mouse *Tbx1*. The heterozy-gotes were viable, but in 19%–45% of them, depending on the parental strain of mouse, the fourth aortic arches were absent or reduced in thickness. There were no differences in the weight of the thymus, absolute number of thymocytes, or cell surface mark-ers CD3, CD4, and CD8 in *Tbx1* heterozygote vs. wild-type mice. However, the *Tbx1* homozygous mutants were nonviable. Em-bryos that were recovered displayed a range of phenotypic find-ings similar to DGS, including short neck, abnormal facial structure, low-set or abnormally folded ears, single cardiac out-flow tract, right aortic arch or a double aortic arch, absent thymus, and absent parathyroids. Other investigators have confirmed the cardiac defects in *Tbx1* mutants (Lindsay et al., 2001; Merscher et al., 2001). In the mouse, a *Tbx1* mutation is sufficient to produce a DGS phenotype. The anomalies in the *Tbx1* knockout mouse model correlate with the expression pattern of *Tbx1* in the embryonic mouse head mesenchyme, pharyngeal arches and pouches, and the otic vesicle. This study provides further evidence that in humans the *TBX1* gene is a key gene in DGS (Jerome and Papaioannou, 2001).

The *Ckrol* mouse mutant developed by Guris et al. (2001) suggests that other genes may contribute to the classical features of DGS. *Crkol* is highly expressed in the branchial arches during mouse embryogenesis and maps to mouse chromosome 16 out-side the *Df1* deletion. Homozygous mice with a null mutation in

Crkol have cardiac defects including double-outlet right ventricle and VSD with an overriding aorta due to abnormal alignment of the outflow tract. Approximately 40% of the mutant embryos also had an abnormal thymus, parathyroid, and thyroid glands, and mild skeletal anomalies of the head. The similarities to DGS suggest that this gene may contribute to the development of at least some of the clinical features.

Clinical and Laboratory Diagnosis

DGS patients with the 22q11 deletion are ascertained through a variety of medical specialty clinics on the basis of presenting features. Recognition of the 22q11 deletion syndrome is important so that the medical community and schools can meet their diverse needs. Furthermore, identification of a 22q11 deletion enables the clinician to provide the affected patient and his or her family with a more accurate assessment of their recurrence risk. Deletions of 22q11 may be detected in 20%–25% of DGS patients by means of high-resolution cytogenetic analysis (Wilson et al., 1992). However, several studies have clearly shown that FISH of metaphase chromosomes with DNA probes from the DGCR is the most efficient method for detecting 22q11 deletions (Desmaze et al., 1993; Driscoll et al., 1993). Routine cytogenetic analysis continues to be important for the detection of other chromosomal rearrangements, such as translocations, which may involve chromosomes other than 22. Hence, it is recommended that FISH be used as an adjunct to routine cytogenetic analysis for the diagnosis of DGS. At the present time, many commercial and hospital-based laboratories are using FISH with the probes from the DGCR for the clinical and prenatal detection of the 22q11 deletion (Color Plate 33.I). Because of the recent recognition of the DGS phenotype in patients with intragenic single nucleotide mutations in *TBX1* (Yagi et al., 2003), gene sequencing may be considered in patients strongly suspected of having DGS in whom FISH is normal.

Carrier Detection and Prenatal Diagnosis

The majority of the 22q11 deletions are sporadic events, occurring only in the affected individual. The incidence of familial cases of DGS is approximately 10% (McDonald-McGinn et al., 2001). Hence, it is important to closely examine the parents of an affected child for subtle features, such as mild facial dysmorphia, hypernasal speech, and history of poor school performance, that are suggestive of a 22q11 deletion. Deletion testing of the parents is recommended. A parent or proband with a 22q11 deletion has a 50% chance of transmitting the deletion-bearing chromosome to his or her offspring. Parents with a 22q11 deletion benefit from preconception and antenatal genetic counseling to review their risk of having affected offspring and to discuss their reproductive options, including prenatal testing and preimplantation genetic diagnosis (Iwarsson et al., 1998; Driscoll, 2001).

Antenatal detection of the 22q11 deletion by FISH has been successfully performed on cultured amniocytes and chorionic villi obtained from at-risk pregnancies (Driscoll et al., 1993; Driscoll, 2001). Pregnancies considered at high risk include those of deletion-positive parents or parents with mosaicism for the 22q11 deletion, and those in which ultrasound or echocardiography demonstrates a fetal conotruncal cardiac malformation. Although the recurrence risk for normal parents with a previous affected child is low, parents often request prenatal testing for the deletion to exclude the small possibility of germ-line mosaicism.

Although testing for the deletion is highly accurate, it is impossible to predict the phenotype. The size and extent of the deletion have not shown correlation with the penetrance and severity of features of DGS (Lindsay et al., 1995). There is significant intrafamilial variability and the parental phenotype is not a reliable predictor of outcome for the fetus (McDonald-McGinn et al., 2001). Fetal imaging techniques such as ultrasonography and fetal echocardiography are recommended to evaluate the fetus for the presence of a cleft palate, renal anomaly, or cardiac defect. Subtle congenital anomalies such as a submucous cleft palate and dysmorphic features cannot be appreciated by sonography (Driscoll, 2001).

At the present time, it remains difficult to counsel families with children with nondeleted DGS unless an etiology such as a cytogenetic translocation or maternal diabetes has been identified. These individuals may have intragenic mutation of *TBX1* or a small deletion of chromosome 22 that cannot be detected with the probes currently used by clinical cytogenetic laboratories (Kurahashi et al., 1996; O'Donnell et al., 1997; McQuade et al., 1999; Rauch et al., 1999; Saitta et al., 1999). Currently, screening for smaller deletions within 22q11 and gene mutations is only available on a research basis.

A minority of DGS patients may have other cytogenetic abnormalities such as deletions of the short arm of chromosome 10, and FISH may be used to evaluate these patients for microdeletions of chromosome 10p (Daw et al., 1996; Gottlieb et al., 1998). For now, fetal sonography and echocardiography are the only available prenatal tests that are helpful when evaluating at-risk pregnancies that are not causally related to an abnormality of 22q11 or other recognizable chromosomal abnormality.

Management and Treatment of the Immunodeficiency

The clinical management of infants and children with DGS depends on their degree of immunocompromise. Most infants with the classic features of DGS are diagnosed in the first weeks of life through their characteristic cardiac anomalies and hypocalcemia, whereas older children may not be recognized until they develop speech and/or learning problems. As soon as the diagnosis of DGS or the 22q11.2 deletion syndrome is established, the individual should have an initial immunologic evaluation. It is important to specifically evaluate immunologic function regardless of the severity of the other phenotypic features. Depending on the age of the child, this could include T and B cell subset analyses, T cell mitogen and antigen responses, immunoglobulin production, and tests of specific antibody formation.

Newborns should be evaluated for T cell production and function by analyzing lymphocyte subsets and responses to mitogens. Very young infants with markedly diminished T cell numbers and function may be followed for a period of time to determine whether the immunodeficiency persists. During this time, they are at risk for opportunistic infections and should receive prophylaxis for *Pneumocystis lirovecii* pneumonia, reverse isolation, irradiated blood products, and careful monitoring. They should not receive live viral immunizations. Persistence of a SCID-like phenotype requires either a bone marrow or thymus transplant (Markert et al., 1999, 2003) to restore immunologic function. Because both interventions carry significant risk and the immunodeficiency of DGS is developmentally expressed, it seems wise to delay intervention for 1 to 2 months when possible.

Most infants with DGS or a 22q11 deletion will have a mild immunodeficiency with an excellent long-term prognosis. T cell

Table 33.3. Suggested Immunologic Evaluations of Newborns and Infants with DiGeorge Syndrome

Immunologic Evaluations	Time of Diagnosis	Age 4 Months	Age 8 Months	Age 12 Months
Lymphocyte subsets	X	X	X	X*
Mitogen responses	X*			
Antigen responses				X*
Humoral function				X*

*Requires reevaluation if abnormal.

production is usually moderately impaired and T cell mitogen responses are often normal or near normal. Strategies such as PCP prophylaxis and use of killed vaccines for the patient and family contacts may be considered. Most DGS infants will develop normal or near-normal immunologic function over time. However, the first year of life represents a vulnerable time during which they require careful monitoring. Although there are limited data to support specific management strategies, a reasonable approach to minimize risk to the affected infant is to withhold live viral vaccines until T cell function is normal and the child has demonstrated an ability to form functional antibodies. Using the criteria of normal T cell mitogen responses, normal T cell antigen recall responses, a CD8 count of at least 250/mm³, and normal antibody responses to diphtheria and tetanus, we and others have not observed any serious side effects with OPV (oral polio vaccine), MMR (measles, mumps, and rubella vaccine), or varicella vaccine administration (Perez et al., 2003; Moylett et al., 2004). The recent widespread use of inactivated poliovirus vaccine (IPV) has limited early infant exposure to live viral vaccines. PCP prophylaxis is required only for extremely low T cell counts. Sequential follow-up studies are important because the pace of immunologic recovery is very unpredictable. Furthermore, there are no laboratory studies or phenotypic markers that predict ultimate immunologic outcome. A typical strategy would be to measure lymphocyte subsets and mitogen responses at the time of diagnosis. If the mitogen responses are normal and the T cell production is moderately impaired, the lymphocyte subsets should be repeated every 4–12 months until they have normalized or stabilized (Table 33.3). At 8–12 months of age, T cell responses to antigen should be evaluated and an analysis of humoral function should be performed. Mitogen and antigen responses should be followed sequentially if abnormal on the first evaluation. More severely affected infants require more careful follow-up, while less severely affected infants may require somewhat less frequent follow-up.

Early management of DGS patients often revolves around their cardiac anomaly, and it may be difficult to adequately assess the patient's immunologic function. Blood transfusions and hemodynamic instability may require that the evaluation be limited or delayed. Although only a minority of patients (<2%) will have severe immunodeficiency, it is prudent to consider the patient as severely immunodeficient until such time as appropriate studies can be done. Because several cases of graft-versus-host disease due to blood transfusions have been recorded in DGS and because early infancy is the most vulnerable time for DGS infants, only irradiated and cytomegalovirus (CMV)-negative blood products should be given (Brouard et al., 1985; Muller et al., 1989; Wintergerst et al., 1989; Washington et al., 1993, 1994).

In older children it is possible to examine immunologic function thoroughly at the first evaluation. Patients with normal or near-normal T cell production, normal T cell mitogen and anti-

gen responses, and a demonstrated ability to form functional antibody do not require special treatment or restrictions. Some patients have persistent mild T cell abnormalities. These patients require individualized management depending on the degree of T cell compromise and the extent to which they develop significant infections. These patients also require follow-up studies because the immunologic changes in DGS can be unpredictable. Most immunologic improvement occurs in the first year of life, but additional T cell function and improved T cell production can occur later. Furthermore, patients with DGS experience thymic involution as they get older and have a decline in peripheral blood T cell counts (Piliero et al., 2004).

In spite of laboratory evidence of normal immunologic function, many DGS patients have recurrent upper respiratory infections due to abnormal palatal anatomy. These patients benefit from the same surgical interventions as other children, and prophylactic antibiotics as adjunct therapy may be considered.

Since the majority of DGS patients will ultimately have normal or near-normal immunologic function, most research efforts have been directed at improved management of the severely affected infants. Bone marrow transplantation from an HLA-matched sibling donor has been efficacious (Goldsobel et al., 1987; Borzy et al., 1989). It may provide sufficient numbers of mature T cells to allow adequate T cell function even in the absence of thymic tissue. Early therapeutic efforts were directed at replacing the missing thymic tissue and used fetal thymic grafts (Thong et al., 1978; Touranine, 1979). Although a minority of these grafts succeeded, the limitations imposed by the use of fetal tissue have compromised their practical application. Recently, success has been reported using partially HLA-matched, discarded postnatal thymic tissue obtained during cardiac surgery grafts (Markert et al., 1995, 1999, 2003, 2004). Four months after placement of a thymic graft, mature functional host T cells were identified in peripheral blood. Antigen-specific T cell responses developed and B cell function normalized. This management strategy appears to offer many advantages over fetal thymus or bone marrow transplantation for severely affected DGS patients, although involution of the thymic graft may be a long-term issue.

Future Challenges

DGS is characterized by a wide range of congenital malformations, facial dysmorphia, endocrine and immune disorders, cognitive impairment, and neurologic and psychiatric abnormalities. Cytogenetic and molecular studies have contributed greatly to our understanding of the genetic basis of this disorder. These studies have shown that deletions of chromosomal region 22q11 are the leading cause of DGS. More recently, *TBX1* was identified as a major contributor to the phenotype. Other genes within or outside the critical region may mold the phenotypic manifestations. Within the next several years we can expect to have a much clearer understanding of how these genes function and what their roles are in the pathogenesis of the complex and variable phenotype of the 22q11 deletion syndrome in humans.

Prospective studies of DGS patients with 22q11 deletions continue to further delineate the range and severity of the medical, cognitive, and neuropsychological problems for which these patients are at risk. The wide range of phenotypic variability remains poorly understood. Neither the size of the deletion nor the parental origin, a factor in some genetic syndromes because of differences in chromosomal imprinting, appear to explain the penetrance or severity of the phenotype. Murine studies suggest that genetic background is an important influence on the phenotype. Therefore, we hypothesize that the severity and phenotypic variability in DGS may be due to modifier genes. Genetic studies of potential modifying genes in both humans and animal models may further our understanding of this complex disorder, and eventually lead to more accurate prediction of the outcome and need for specific therapeutics and intervention. In the meantime, we urge clinicians to pursue comprehensive evaluations by a team of medical professionals in genetics, cardiology, immunology, endocrinology, plastic surgery, speech and hearing, and developmental pediatrics who have the expertise in caring for individuals with DGS.

Acknowledgments

The authors thank B.S. Emanuel, E.H. Zackai, M.L. Budarf, D.M. McDonald-McGinn, and the 22q11 families for their support and collaboration. This work was supported in part by grants from the National Institute of Deafness and Communication Disorders (DC02027), the National Heart, Lung and Blood Institute (HL074731), the General Clinical Research Center (M1-RR00240), and the Wallace Chair of Pediatrics.

References

Adachi, M, Tachibana, K, Masuno, M, et al. Clinical characteristics of children with hypoparathyroidism due to 22q11.2 microdeletion. Eur J Pediatr 157:34–38, 1998.

Bale PM, Sotelo-Avila C. Maldescent of the thymus: 34 necropsy and 10 surgical cases, including 7 thymuses medial to the mandible. Pediatr Pathol 13:181–190, 1993.

Barrett DJ, Ammann AJ, Wara DW, Cowan MJ, Fisher TJ, Stiehm ER. Clinical and immunologic spectrum of the DiGeorge syndrome. J Clin Lab Immunol 6:1–6, 1981.

Bastian J, Law S, Vogler L, Lawton A, Herrod H, Anderson S, Horowitz S, Hong R. Prediction of persistent immunodeficiency in the DiGeorge anomaly. J Pediatr 115:391–396, 1989.

Bawle EV, Conard J, Van Dyke DL, Czarnecki P, Driscoll D. Seven new cases of Cayler cardiofacial syndrome with chromosome 22q11.2 deletion, including a familial case. Am J Med Genet 79:406–410, 1998.

Beard LJ, Robertson EF, Thong YH. Para-influenza pneumonia in DiGeorge syndrome two years after thymic epithelial transplantation. Acta Paediatr Scand 69:403–406, 1980.

Bingham PM, Zimmerman RA, McDonald-McGinn D, Driscoll D, Emanuel BS, Zackai E. Enlarged sylvian fissures in infants with interstitial deletion of chromosome 22q11. Am J Med Genet 74:538–543, 1997.

Borzy MS, Ridgway D, Noya FJ, Shearer WT. Successful bone marrow transplantation with split lymphoid chimerism in DiGeorge syndrome. J Clin Immunol 9:386–392, 1989.

Botta A, Amati F, Novelli G. Causes of the phenotype–genotype dissociation in DiGeorge syndrome: clues from mouse models. Trends Genet 17: 551–554, 2001.

Botto LD, May K, Fernhoff PM, Correa A, Coleman K, Rasmussen SA, Merrit RK, O'Leary LA, Wong LY, Elixson EM, Mahle WT, Campbell RM. A population-based study of the 22q11.2 deletion: phenotype, incidence, and contribution to major birth defects in the population. Pediatrics 112:101–107, 2003.

Brouard J, Morin M, Borel B, Laloum D, Mandard JC, Duhamel JF, Venezia R. Syndrome de Di George complique d'une reaction du greffon contre l'hote. Arch Fr Pediatr 42:853–855, 1985.

Budarf ML, Collins J, Gong W, Roe B, Wang Z, Bailey LC, Sellinger B, Michaud D, Driscoll DA, Emanuel BS. Cloning a balanced translocation associated with DiGeorge syndrome and identification of a disrupted candidate gene. Nat Genet 10:269–278, 1995a.

Budarf ML, Konkle BA, Ludlow LB, Michaud D, Li M, Yamashiro DJ, McDonald-McGinn D, Zackai EH, Driscoll DA. Identification of a patient with Bernard-Soulier syndrome and a deletion in the DiGeorge/velo-cardio-facial chromosomal region in 22q11.2. Hum Mol Genet 4: 763–766, 1995b.

Burn J, Takao A, Wilson D, Cross I, Momma K, Wadey R, Scambler P, Goodship J. Conotruncal anomaly face syndrome is associated with a deletion within chromosome 22. J Med Genet 30:822–824, 1993.

Chieffo C, Garvey N, Roe B, Zhang G, Silver L, Emanuel BS, Budarf ML. Isolation and characterization of a gene from the DiGeorge chromosomal

region (DGCR) homologous to the mouse *Tbx1* gene. Genomics 43: 267–277, 1997.

Conley ME, Beckwith JB, Mancer JFK, Tenckhoff L. The spectrum of the DiGeorge syndrome. J Pediatr 94:883–890, 1979.

Cuneo BF, Driscoll DA, Gidding SS, Langman CB. The evolution of multigenerational latent hypoparathyroidism in familial 22q11 deletion syndrome. Am J Med Genet 69:50–55, 1997.

Daw SCM, Taylor C, Kraman M, Call K, Mao J, Schuffenhauer S, Meitinger T, Lipson T, Goodship J, Scambler PJ. A common region of 10p deleted in DiGeorge and velocardiofacial syndromes. Nat Genet 13:458–460, 1996.

Demczuk S, Aledo R, Zucman J, Delattre O, Desmaze C, Dauphinot L, Jalbert P, Rouleau GA, Thomas G, Aurias A. Cloning of a balanced translocation breakpoint in the DiGeorge syndrome critical region and isolation of a novel potential adhesion receptor gene in its vicinity. Hum Mol Genet 4:551–558, 1995.

Demczuk S, Thomas G, Aurias A. Isolation of a novel gene from the DiGeorge syndrome critical region with homology to *Drosphilia gdl* and to human *LAMC1* genes. Hum Mol Genet 5:633–638, 1996.

Desmaze C, Scambler P, Prieur M, Halford S, Sidi D, Le Deist F, Aurias A. Routine diagnosis of DiGeorge syndrome by fluorescent in situ hybridization. Hum Genet 90:663–665, 1993.

DiGeorge AM. Discussions on a new concept of the cellular basis of immunology. J Pediatr 67:907, 1965.

Driscoll DA. Prenatal diagnosis of the 22q11.2 deletion syndrome. Genet in Med 3:14–18, 2001.

Driscoll DA, Budarf ML, Emanuel BS. A genetic etiology for DiGeorge syndrome: consistent deletions and microdeletions of 22q11. Am J Hum Genet 50:924–933, 1992a.

Driscoll DA, Salvin J, Sellinger B, Budarf ML, McDonald-McGinn DM, Zackai EH, Emanuel BS. Prevalence of 22q11 microdeletions in DiGeorge and velocardiofacial syndromes: implications for genetic counseling and prenatal diagnosis. J Med Genet 30:813–817, 1993.

Driscoll DA, Spinner NB, Budarf ML, McDonald-McGinn DM, Zackai EH, Goldberg RB, Shprintzen RJ, Saal HM, Zonana J, Jones MC, Mascarello JT, Emanuel BS. Deletions and microdeletions of 22q11.2 in velo-cardio-facial syndrome. Am J Med Genet 44:261–268, 1992b.

Duke SG, McGuirt WF Jr, Jewett T, Fasano MB. Velocardiofacial syndrome: incidence of immune cytopenias. Arch Otolaryngol Head Neck Surg 126:1141–1145, 2000.

Dunham I and the International Chromosome 22 Sequencing Consortium. The DNA sequence of human chromosome 22. Nature 402:489–495, 1999.

Durandy A, Le Deist F, Fischer A, Griscelli C. Impaired T8 lymphocyte-mediated suppressive activity in patients with partial Di George syndrome. J Clin Immunol 6:265–270, 1986.

Eicher PS, McDonald-McGinn DM, Fox CA, Driscoll DA, Emanuel BS, Zackai EH. Dysphagia in children with 22q11.2 deletion: unusual pattern found on modified barium swallow. J Pediatr 137:158–164, 2000.

Emanuel BS, McDonald-McGinn D, Saitta SC, Zackai EH. The 22q11.2 deletion syndrome. Adv Pediatr 48:38–73, 2001.

Funke B, Saint-Jore B, Puech A, Sirotkin H, Edelmann L, Carlson C, Raft S, Pandita RK, Kucherlapati R, Skoultchi A, Morrow BE. Characterization of and mutation analysis of goosecoid-like (GSCL), a homeodomain-containing gene that maps to the critical region for VCFS/DGS on 22q 11. Genomics 46:364–372, 1997.

Gerdes M, Solot C, Wang PP, Moss E, LaRossa D, et al. Cognitive and behavior profile of preschool children with chromosome 22q11.2 deletion. Am J Med Genet 85:127–133, 1999.

Gilger MA, Matson DO, Conner ME, Rosenblatt HM, Finegold MJ, Estes MK. Extraintestinal rotavirus infections in children with immunodeficiency. J Pediatr 120:912–917, 1992.

Golding-Kushner KJ, Weller G, Shprintzen RJ. Velo-cardio-facial syndrome: language and psychological profiles. J Craniofacial Genet Dev Biol 5: 259–266, 1985.

Goldsobel AB, Haas A, Stiehm ER. Bone marrow transplantation in DiGeorge syndrome. J Pediatr 111:40–44, 1987.

Gong W, Gottlieb S, Collins J, Blescia A, Dietz H, Goldmuntz E, McDonald-McGuinn DM, Zackei EH, Emanuel BS, Driscoll DA, Budarf ML. Mutation analysis of *TBX1* in non-deleted patients with features of DGS/VCFS or isolated conotruncal cardiac defects. J Med Genet 38(12):E45, 2001.

Gottlieb S, Driscoll DA, Punnett H, Sellinger B, Emanuel BS, Budarf ML. Characterization of chromosome 10p deletions associated with DiGeorge syndrome suggests two non-overlapping regions contribute to phenotype. Am J Hum Genet 62:495–498, 1998.

Gottlieb S, Emanuel BS, Driscoll DA, Sellinger B, Wang Z, Roe B, Budarf ML. The DiGeorge syndrome minimal critical region contains a goosecoid-like homeobox gene which is expressed early in human development. Am J Hum Genet 60:1194–1201, 1997.

Graf WD, Unis AS, Yates CM, Sulzbacher S, Dinulos MB, Jack RM, Dugaw KA, Paddock MN, Parson WW. Catecholamines in patients with 22q11.2 deletion syndrome and the low-activity COMT polymorphism. Neurology 57:1–6, 2001.

Greenberg F, Elder FFB, Haffner P, Northrup M, Ledbetter DH. Cytogenetic findings in a prospective series of patients with DiGeorge anomaly. Am J Hum Genet 43:605–611, 1988.

Grossman MH, Emanuel BS, Budarf ML. Chromosomal mapping of the human catechol-O-methyl-transferase gene to Z2q11.1 q11.2. Genomics 12:822–825, 1992.

Guris DL, Fantes J, Tara D, et al. Mice lacking the homologue of the human 22q11.2 gene CRKL phenocopy neurocristopathies of DiGeorge syndrome. Nat Genet 27:293–298, 2001.

Haire RN, Buell RD, Litman RT, Ohta Y, Fu SM, Honjo T, Matsuda F, de la Morina M, Carro J, Good RA. Diversification, not use, of the immunoglobulin VH gene repertoire is restricted in DiGeorge syndrome. J Exp Med 178:825–834, 1993.

Ham Pong AJ, Cavallo A, Holman GH, Goldman AS. DiGeorge syndrome: long-term survival complicated by Graves disease. J Pediatr 106:619–620, 1985.

Iwarsson E, Ahrlund-Richter L, Inzunza J, Fridstrom M, Rosenlund B, Hillensjo T, Sjoblom P, Nordenskjold M, Blennow E. Preimplantation genetic diagnosis of DiGeorge syndrome. Mol Hum Reprod 4(9):871–875, 1998.

Jawad AF, McDonald-McGinn DM, Zackai E, Sullivan K. Immunologic features of chromosome 22q11.2 deletion syndrome (DiGeorge syndrome/velocardiofacial syndrome). J Pediatr 139:715–723, 2001.

Jerome LA, Papaioannou VE. DiGeorge syndrome phenotype in mice mutant for the T-box gene, Tbx1. Nat Genet 27:286–291, 2001.

Junker AK, Driscoll DA. Humoral immunity in DiGeorge syndrome. J Pediatr 127:231–237, 1995.

Kelley D, Goldberg R, Wilson D, Lindsay E, Carey A, Goodship J, Burn J, Cross I, Shprintzen RJ, Scambler PJ. Confirmation that the velocardiofacial syndrome is associated with haplo-insufficiency of genes at chromosome 22. Am J Med Genet 45:308–312, 1993.

Kinouchi A, Mori K, Ando M, Takao A. Facial appearance of patients with conotruncal anomalies. Pediatr Jpn 17:84, 1976.

Kirby ML, Bockman DL. Neural crest and normal development: a new perspective. Anat Rev 209:1–6, 1984.

Kirby ML, Gale TF, Stewart DE. Neural crest cells contribute to aorticopulmonary septation. Science 220:1059–1061, 1983.

Kurahashi H, Nakayama T, Osugi Y, Tsuda E, Masuno M, Imaizumi K, Kamiya T, Sano T, Okada S, Nishisho I. Deletion mapping of 22q11 in CATCH22 syndrome: identification of a second critical region. Am J Hum Genet 58:1377–1381, 1996.

Kurahashi H, Shaikh TH, Hu P, Roe BA, Emanuel BS, Budarf ML. Regions of genomic instability on 22q11 and 11q23 as the etiology for the recurrent constitutional t(11;22). Hum Mol Genet 9:1665–1670, 2000.

Lachman HM, Morrow B, Shprintzen R, Veit S, Parsia SS, Gaedda G, Goldber R, Kucherlapati R, Papolos DF. Association of codon 108/158 catechol-O-methyltransferase gene polymorphism with the psychiatric manisfestations of velo-cardio-facial syndrome. Am J Med Gene 67:468–472, 1996.

Lammer EJ, Optiz JM. The DiGeorge anomaly as a developmental field defect. Am J Med Genet 29:113–127, 1986.

Lawrence S, McDonald-McGinn D, Zackai E, Sullivan KE. Thrombocytopenia in patients with chromosome 22q11.2 deletion syndrome. J Pediatr 143:277–278, 2003.

Liao J, Kochilas L, Noroski LM, Shearer WT. Full spectrum of malformations in velocardiofacial syndrome/DiGeroge syndrome mouse models by altering TBx1 dosage. Hum Mol Genet 13:1577–1585, 2004.

Lindsay EA, Baldini A. Recovery from arterial growth delay reduces penetrance of cardiovascular defects in mice deleted for the DiGeorge syndrome region. Hum Mol Genet 10:997–1002, 2001.

Lindsay EA, Botta A, Jurecic V, Carattini-Rivera S, Cheah YC, Rosenblatt HM, Bradley A, Baldini A. Congenital heart disease in mice deficient for the DiGeorge syndrome region. Nature 401(6751):379–383, 1999.

Lindsay EA, Greenberg F, Shaffer LG, Shapira SK, Scambler PJ, Baldini A. Submicroscopic deletions at 22q11.2: variability of the clinical picture and delineation of a commonly deleted region. Am J Med Genet 56: 191–197, 1995.

Lindsay EA, Vitellio F, Su H, Morishima M, Huynh T, Pramparo T, Jurecic V, Ogunrino G, Sutherland HF, Scambler PJ, Bradley A, Baldini A. Tbx1 haploinsufficiency in the DiGeorge syndrome region causes aortic arch defects in mice. Nature 410:97–101, 2001.

Lischner HW, Huff DS. T-cell deficiency in DiGeorge syndrome. Birth Defects 10:16–21, 1975.

Ludlow LB, Schick BP, Budarf ML, Driscoll DA, Konkle BA. Identification of a mutation in a GATA binding domain of the glycoprotein Ib promoter resulting in the Bernard-Soulier syndrome. J Biol Chem 271:22076–22080, 1996.

Lund J, Roe B, Chen F, Budarf M, Galili N, Riblet R, Miller RD, Emanuel BS, Reeves RH. Sequence-ready physical map of the mouse chromosome 16 region with conserved synteny to the human velocardiofacial syndrome region on 22q11.2. Mamm Genet 10:438–443, 1999.

Lynch DR, McDonald-McGinn DM, Zackai EH, Emanuel BS, Driscoll DA, Whitaker LA, Fischbeck KH. Cerebellar atrophy in a patient with velocardiofacial syndrome. J Med Genet 32:562–563, 1995.

Markert ML, Alexieff MJ, Li J, Sarzotti M, Ozaki DA, Devlin BH, Sedlak DA, Sempowski GD, Hale LP, Rice HE, Mahaffey SM, Skinner MA. Postnatal thymus transplantation with immunosuppression as treatment for DiGeorge syndrome. Blood 104:2574–2582, 2004.

Markert ML, Boeck A, Hale LP, et al. Transplantation of thymus tissue in complete DiGeorge syndrome. N Engl J Med 341:1180–1189, 1999.

Markert ML, Sarzotti M, Ozaki DA, Sempowski GD, Rhein ME, Hale LP, LeDiest F, Alexieff MJ, Li J, Hauser ER, Haynes BF, Rice HE, Skinner MA, Mahaffey SM, Jaggers J, Stein LD, Mill MR. Thymus transplantation in complete DiGeorge syndrome: immunologic and safety evaluations in 12 patients. Blood 102:1121–1130, 2003.

Markert ML, Watson TJ, McLaughlin TM, McGuire CA, Ward FE, Kostyu D, Hale LP, Buckley RH, Schiff SE, Bleesing JJH, Broome CB, Ungerleider RM, Mahaffey SM, Oldman CT, Haynes BF. Development of T-cell function after post-natal thymic transplantation for DiGeorge syndrome. Am J Hum Genet 57:A14, 1995.

Matsuoka R, Takao A, Kimura M, Imamura S-I, Kondo C, Joh-o K, Ikeda K, Nishibatake M, Ando M, Momma K. Confirmation that the conotruncal anomaly face syndrome is associated with a deletion within 22q11.2. Am J Med Genet 53:285–289, 1994.

Mayumi M, Kimata H, Suehiro Y, Hosoi S, Ito S, Kuge Y, Shinomiya K, et al. DiGeorge syndrome with hypogammaglobulinemia: a patient with excess suppressor T cell activity treated with fetal thymus transplantation. Eur J Pediatr 148:518–522, 1989.

McDonald-McGinn DM, Driscoll DA, Bason L, Christensen K, Lynch D, Sullivan K, Canning D, Zacod W, Quinn N, Rome J, Paris Y, Weinberg P, Clark BJ, Emanuel BS, Zackai EH. Autosomal dominant "Opitz" GBBB syndrome due to a 22q11.2 deletion. Am J Med Genet 59:103–113, 1995.

McDonald-McGinn DM, Driscoll DA, Emanuel BS, Goldmuntz E, Clark BJ, Cohen M, Solot C, Schultz P, LaRossa D, Randall P, Zackai EH. Detection of 22q11.2 deletion in cardiac patients suggests a risk for velopharyngeal incompetence. Pediatrics 99:1–5, 1997.

McDonald-McGinn DM, Kirschner R, Goldmuntz E, Sullivan K, et al. The Philadelphia story: the 22q11.2 deletion: report on 250 patients. Genet Counsel 10:11–24, 1999.

McDonald-McGinn DM, Tonnesen ML, Laufer-Cahana A, Finucane B, Driscoll DA, Emanuel BS, Zackai EH. Phenotype of the 22q11.2 deletion in individuals identified through an affected relative: cast a wide FISHing net! Genet Med 3:23–29, 2001.

McQuade L, Christodoulou J, Budarf M, Sachdev R, Wilson M, Emanuel B, Colley A. Patient with a 22q11.2 deletion with no overlap of the minimal DiGeorge critical region (MDGCR). Am J Med Genet 86:27–33, 1999.

Merscher S, Funke B, Epstein JA, et al. TBX1 is responsible for cardiovascular defects in velo-cardio- facial/DiGeorge syndrome. Cell 104:619–629, 2001.

Mitnick RJ, Bello JA, Shprintzen RJ. Brain anomalies in velo-cardio-facial syndrome. Am J Med Genet (Neuropsychiatr Genet) 54:100–106, 1994.

Moss EM, Batshaw ML, Solot CB, Gerdes M, McDonald-McGinn DM, Driscoll DA, Emanuel BS, Zackai EH, Wang PP. Pyschoeducational profile of 22q11.2 microdeletion: a complex pattern. J Pediatr 134:193–198, 1999.

Moylett EH, Wasan AN, Noroski LM, Shearer WT. Live viral vaccines in patients with partial DiGeorge syndrome. Clin Immunol 112:106–112, 2004.

Muller W, Peter HH, Kallfelz HC, Franz A, Rieger CH. The DiGeorge sequence. II. Immunologic findings in partial and complete forms of the disorder. Eur J Pediatr 149:96–103, 1989.

Muller W, Peter HH, Wilken M, Juppner H, Kallfelz HC, Krohn HP, Miller K, Rieger CH. The DiGeorge syndrome. I. Clinical evaluation and course of partial and complete forms of the syndrome [review]. Eur J Pediatr 147:496–502, 1988.

Nickel RE, Pillers D-A, Merkens M, Magenis RE, Driscoll DA, Emanuel BS, Zonana J. Velo-cardio-facial syndrome and DiGeorge sequence with meningomyelocele and deletions of the 22q11 region. Am J Med Genet 52:445–449, 1994.

O'Donnell H, McKeown C, Gould C, Morrow B, Scampbler P. Detection of an atypical 22q11 deletion that has no overlap with the DiGeorge syndrome critical region. Am J Hum Genet 60:1544–1548, 1997.

Opitz JM, Summitt RL, Smith DW. Hypertelorism and hypospadias. A newly recognized hereditary malformation syndrome. J Pediatr 67:968, 1965.

Perez EE, Bokszczanin A, McDonald-McGinn D, Zackai E, Sullivan KE. Safety of live viral vaccines in patients with chromosome 22q11.2 deletion syndrome (DiGeorge syndrome/velocardiofacial syndrome). Pediatrics 112:277–278, 2003.

Pierdominici M, Marziali M, Giovannetti A, et al. T cell receptor repertoire and function in patients with DiGeorge syndrome and velocardiofacial syndrome. Clin Exp Immunol 121:127–132, 2000.

Piliero LM, Sanford AN, McDonald-McGinn DM, Zackai EH, Sullivan KE. T cell homeostasis in humans with thymic hypoplasia due to chromosome 22q11.2 deletion syndrome. Blood 103:1020–1025, 2004.

Pinchas-Hamiel O, Engelberg S, Mandel M, Passwell JH. Immune hemolytic anemia, thrombocytopenia and liver disease in a patient with DiGeorge syndrome. Isr J Med Sci 30:530–532, 1994.

Puech A, Saint-Jore B, Merscher S, Russell RG, Cherif D, Sirotkin H, Xu H, Factor S, Kucherlapati R, Skoultchi AI. Normal cardiovascular development in mice deficient for 16 genes in 550 kb of the velocardiofacial/DiGeorge syndrome region. Proc Natl Acad Sci USA 97:10090–10095, 2000.

Pulver AE, Nestadt G, Goldberg R, Shprintzen RJ, Lamacz M, Wolyniech PS, Morrow B, Karayiorgou M, Antonarakis SE, Housman D, Kucherlapati R. Psychotic illness in patients diagnosed with velo-cardio-facial syndrome and their relatives. J Nerv Ment Disord 182:476–478, 1994.

Rausch A, Pfeiffer RA, Leipold G, Singer H, Tigges M, Hofbeck M. A novel 22q11.2 microdeletion in DiGeorge syndrome. Am J Hum Genet 64:658–666, 1999.

Reinherz EL, Cooper MD, Schlossman SF. Abnormalities of T cell maturation and regulation in human beings with immunodeficiency disorders. J Clin Invest 68:699–705, 1981.

Robin NH, Feldman GJ, Aronson AL, Mitchell HF, Weksberg R, Leonard CO, Burton BK, Josephson KD, Laxova R, Aleck KA, Allanson JE. Opitz syndrome is genetically heterogeneous, with one locus on Xp22, and a second locus on 22q11.2. Nat Genet 11:459–461, 1995a.

Robin NH, Sellinger B, McDonald-McGinn D, Zackai EH, Emanuel BS, Driscoll DA. Classical Noonan syndrome is not associated with deletions of 22q11. Am J Med Genet 56:94–96, 1995b.

Ryan AK, Goodship JA, Wilson DI, Philip N, Levy A, Seidel J, et al. Spectrum of clinical features associated with interstitial chromosome 22q11 deletions: a European collaborative study. J Med Genet 34:798–804, 1997.

Saitta S, McGrath JM, Mensch H, Shaikh TH, Zackai EH, Emanuel BS. A 22q11.2 deletion that excludes UFD1L and CDC45L in a patient with conotruncal and craniofacial defects [letter]. Am J Hum Genet 65:562–566, 1999.

Saitta SC, Harris SE, Gaeth AP, Driscoll DA, McDonald-McGinn DM, Maisenbacher MK, Yersak JM, Chakraborty PK, Hacker AM, Zackai EH, Ashley T, Emanuel BS. Aberrant interchromosomal exchanges are the predominant cause of the 22q11.2 deletion. Hum Mol Genet 13:417–428, 2004.

Schubert MS, Moss RB. Selective polysaccharide antibody deficiency in familial DiGeorge syndrome. Ann Allergy 69:231–238, 1992.

Shaikh TH, Kurahashi H, Saitta SC, Mizrahy O'Hare A, Hu P, Roe BA, Driscoll DA, McDonald-McGinn DM, Zackai EH, Budarf ML, Emanuel BS. Chromosome 22-specific low copy repeats and the 22q11.2 deletion syndrome: genomic organization and deletion endpoint analysis. Hum Mol Genet 9:489–501, 2000.

Shaikh TH, Kurahashi H, Emanuel BS. Evolutionarily conserved low copy repeats (LCRs) in 22q11 mediate deletions, duplications, translocations, and genomic instability: an update and literature review. Genet Med 3:6–13, 2001.

Shprintzen RJ, Goldberg RB, Young D, Wolford L. The velo-cardio-facial syndrome: a clinical and genetic analysis. Pediatrics 67:167–172, 1981.

Sirianni MC, Businco L, Fiore L, Seminara R, Aiuti F. T-cell subsets and natural killer cells in DiGeorge and SCID patients. Birth Defects 19:107–108, 1983a.

Sirianni MC, Businco L, Seminara R, Aiuti F. Severe combined immunodeficiencies, primary T-cell defects and DiGeorge syndrome in humans: characterization by monoclonal antibodies and natural killer cell activity. Clin Immunol Immunopathol 28:361–370, 1983b.

Smith CA, Driscoll DA, Emanuel BS, et al. Increased prevalence of immunoglobulin A deficiency in patients with the chromosome 22q11.2 deletion syndrome (DiGeorge syndrome/velocardiofacial syndrome). Clin Diagn Lab Immunol 5:415–417, 1998.

Solot CB, Knightly C, Handler SD, Gerdes M, McDonald-McGinn DM, Moss E, Wang P, Cohen M, Randall P, LaRossa D, Driscoll DA. Communication disorders in the 22q11.2 microdeletion syndrome. J Commun Disord 33:187–204, 2000.

Sugama S, Namihira T, Matsuoka R, et al. Psychiatric inpatients and chromosome deletions within 22q11.2. Neurol Neurosurg Psychiatry 67:803–806, 1999.

Sullivan KE, Jawad AF, Randall P, et al. Lack of correlation between impaired T cell production, immunodeficiency and other phenotypic features in chromosome 22q11.2 deletions syndrome (DiGeorge syndrome/velocardiofacial syndrome). Clin Immunol Immunopathol 84:141–146, 1998.

Sullivan KE, McDonald-McGinn D, Driscoll D, Zmijewski CM, Ellabban AS, Reed L, Emanuel BS, Zackai E, Athreya BH, Keenan G. Juvenile rheumatoid arthritis in chromosome 22 deletion syndrome (DiGeorge anomalad/velocardiofacial syndrome/conotruncal anomaly face syndrome). Arthritis Rheum 40:430–436, 1997.

Sullivan KE, McDonald-McGinn DM, Zackai EH. CD4 CD25 T cell production in healthy humans and in patients with thymic hypoplasia. Clin Diagn Lab Immunol 9:1129–1131, 2002.

Sutherland HF, Kim UJ, Scambler PJ. Cloning and comparative mapping of the DiGeorge syndrome critical region in the mouse. Genomics 52:37–43, 1998.

Swillen A, Devriendt K, Legius E, Eyskens B, Dumoulin M, Gellis M, Fryns JP. Intelligence and psychosocial adjustment in velocardiofacial syndrome: a study of 37 children and adolescents with VCFS. J Med Genet 34:453–458, 1997.

Thong YH, Robertson EF, Rischbieth HG, Smith GF, Chetney K, Pollard AC. Successful restoration of immunity in the DiGeorge syndrome with fetal thymic epithelial transplant. Arch Dis Child 53:580–584,1978.

Touranine JL. Human T-lymphocyte differentiation in immunodeficiency diseases and after reconstitution by bone marrow or fetal thymus transplanation. Clin Immunol Immunopathol 12:228–237, 1979.

Tuvia J, Weisselberg B, Shif I, Keren G. Aplastic anaemia complicating adenovirus infection in DiGeorge syndrome. Eur J Pediatr 147:643–644, 1988.

Vantrappen G, Deviendt K, Swillen A, Rommel N, Cogels A, Eyskens B, et al. Presenting symptoms and clinical features in 130 patients with the velo-cardio-facial syndrome: the Leuven experience. Genet Counsel 10:3–9, 1999.

Wadey R, Daw S, Taylor C, Atif U, Kamath S, Halford S, O'Donnell H, Wilson D, Goodship J, Burn J, Scambler P. Isolation of a gene encoding an integral membrane protein from the vicinity of a balanced translocation breakpoint associated with DiGeorge syndrome. Hum Mol Genet 4:1027–1033, 1995.

Washington K, Gossage DL, Gottfried MR. Pathology of the liver in severe combined immunodeficiency and DiGeorge syndrome. Pediatr Pathol 13:485–504, 1993.

Washington K, Gossage DL, Gottfried MR. Pathology of the pancreas in severe combined immunodeficiency and DiGeorge syndrome: acute graft-versus-host disease and unusual viral infections. Hum Pathol 25:908–914, 1994.

Wilson DI, Britton SB, McKeown C, Kelly D, Cross IE, Strobel S, Scambler PJ. Noonan's and DiGeorge syndromes with monosomy 22q11. Arch Dis Child 68:187–189, 1993a.

Wilson DI, Cross IE, Goodship JA, Brown J, Scambler PJ, Bain HH, Taylor JF, Walsh JC, Bankier A, Burn J, Wolsten Holme J. A prospective cytogenetic study of 36 cases of DiGeorge syndrome. Am J Hum Genet 51:957–963, 1992.

Wilson TA, Blethen SL, Vallone A, Alenick SC, Nolan P, Katz A, Amorillo TP, Goldmuntz E, Emanuel BS, Driscoll DA. DiGeorge anomaly with renal agenesis in infants of mothers with diabetes. Am J Med Genet 47:1078–1082, 1993b.

Wintergerst U, Meyer U, Remberger K, Belohradsky BH. Graft versus host reaction in an infant with DiGeorge syndrome [in German]. Monatsschr Kinderheilkd 137:345–347, 1989.

Wood DJ, David TJ, Chrystie IL, Totterdell B. Chronic enteric virus infection in two T-cell immunodeficient children. J Med Virol 24:435–444, 1988.

Yagi H, Furutani Y, Hamada H, Sasaki T, Asakawa S, Minoshima S, Ichida F, Joo K, Kimura M, Imamura S, Kamatani N, Momma K, Takao A, Nakazawa M, Shimizu N, Matsuoka R. Role of TBX1 in human del22q11.2 syndrome. Lancet 362:1366–1373, 2003.

34

Hyper-IgE Recurrent Infection Syndromes

BODO GRIMBACHER, JENNIFER M. PUCK, and STEVEN M. HOLLAND

Hyper-IgE recurrent infection syndrome (MIM %147060, #243700) is a primary immunodeficiency characterized by recurrent staphylococcal skin abscesses, pneumonias with pneumatocele formation, extreme elevations of serum IgE, eosinophilia, and distinct abnormalities of the connective tissue, skeleton, and dentition (Davis et al., 1966; Buckley et al., 1972; Hill and Quie, 1974; Donabedian and Gallin, 1983a; Belohradsky et al., 1987; Grimbacher et al., 1999a; Erlewyn-Lajeunesse, 2000).

History

"So went Satan forth from the presence of the Lord, and smote Job with sore boils from the sole of his foot unto his crown." With this citation from Job II:7, Davis, Schaller, and Wedgewood coined the term *Job syndrome* in 1966 (Davis et al., 1966). They reported two red-haired, fair-skinned girls who had frequent sinopulmonary infections, severe dermatitis, and recurrent staphylococcal skin infections that were remarkable for their lack of surrounding warmth, erythema, or tenderness. The syndrome was further defined and clarified by Buckley et al. (1972), who noted similar infectious problems in two boys with severe dermatitis, distinctive facial appearance, and elevated IgE levels, leading to the term *Buckley syndrome*. Following this report, elevated levels of IgE and a defect in neutrophil chemotaxis were reported in the two girls from the initial report (Hill and Quie, 1974), showing that Job syndrome and Buckley syndrome represented the same condition. To avoid further confusion, the name *hyper-immunoglobulin E recurrent infection syndrome* (HIES) is now widely used. In 1999 a group at the U.S. National Institutes of Health (NIH) undertook to define further the phenotype of HIES. The incidence of 19 clinical features associated with HIES was published, based on a cohort of 30 patients with the disease (Table 34.1) (Grimbacher et al., 1999a).

Clinical Presentation

The clinical features of HIES include the immune system, the skeleton, and dentition. However, the expressivity of each finding in HIES varies with age and among individuals. Table 34.1 shows the frequency of the 19 most consistent clinical and laboratory findings in HIES.

Immune System

Eczema, abscesses, pneumonia, mucocutaneous candidiasis, elevated serum IgE, and eosinophilia are the most common features of immunodeficiency and immune dysregulation in HIES patients. Some degree of eczema is present in almost all HIES patients, although persistent moderate to severe eczema is seen in only 80%. A newborn rash occurs in roughly three-quarters of HIES patients (Color Plate 34.I). Eczema with pruritis and lichenification usually appears in the first days to weeks of life (Color Plate 34.II), in a distribution somewhat atypical for atopic dermatitis (involving the posterior auricular areas, back, buttocks, and scalp). Skin infections typically include staphylococcal furunculosis and cellulitis. The abscesses may occur anywhere on the body but are most common around the face and trunk. A "cold" abscess may be either a large fluctuant mass or may feel like a tumor. It is typically neither hot nor tender and is usually not associated with fever or signs of local or generalized inflammation (Erlewyn-Lajeunesse, 2000). In most cases the abscesses are well walled off, filled with pus and almost always grow *Staphylococcus aureus*. Surgical drainage of these lesions is commonly required, and they typically resolve without spreading through the dermis and fascia. Although cold abscesses have been said to be pathognomonic of HIES, they are not essential to the diagnosis. Following institution of almost any prophylactic

Table 34.1. Incidence of Clinical Findings Associated with Hyper-IgE Recurrent Infection Syndrome in 30 Patients with Diagnosis of Hyper-IgE Syndrome

Findings Related to Infections and Immune System	%
Moderate to severe eczema	100
Serum IgE >2000 IU/ml	97
Eosinophilia (>2 SD above normal mean)	93
Recurrent (≥2) pneumonia, X-ray proven	87
Recurrent (>4) skin abscesses	87
Recurrent (>3 per year) upper respiratory infections	84
Mucocutaneous candidiasis	83
Pneumatoceles	77
Newborn rash	74
Other serious infections	52
Lymphoma, other cancer	3
Findings Related to Bones, Teeth, and Connective Tissue	
Characteristic face	83
Retained primary teeth (more than 4)	72
Hyperextensibility of joints	68
Increased nasal width (interalar distance) (>1 SD above normal value for age, race)	65
Scoliosis >10°	63
Recurrent fractures following minor trauma	57
High palate	48
Congenital skeletal anomalies	10

antistaphylococcal antibiotics, recurrent cutaneous abscesses are rare. In some patients abscesses are frequent early in life; but recently, with the institution of prophylactic antibiotics, we have seen mostly impetiginized eczema. In our cohort, 87% of HIES patients had recurrent skin abscesses, and over half had a history of more than four abscesses.

Upper respiratory infections such as sinusitis, bronchitis, otitis media, otitis externa, and mastoiditis are frequent in HIES. Seventy-two percent of patients reported four or more episodes per year. A clinical hallmark of HIES is recurrent pneumonia. The great majority of patients have had at least one bout of pneumonia in their lifetime, but more than half have had three or more. The most common pathogens of acute pneumonia in HIES are *Staphylococcus aureus* and *Haemophilus influenzae*. For reasons still unclear, pneumonias in HIES are frequently complicated. About three-quarters (77%) of HIES patients develop long-term pulmonary complications including bronchiectasis and pneumatoceles (Fig. 34.1). The cycle of infection and lung destruction is further exacerbated by superinfection of the cavities and bronchiectatic lung with *Pseudomonas aeruginosa* and *Aspergillus fumigatus*. Pulmonary infections less commonly seen in HIES include *Pneumocystis jiroveci* (Freeman et al., 2006) and nontuberculous mycobacteria.

Chronic candidiasis of mucosal sites and the nail beds affects 83% of HIES patients, including children (Color Plate 34.III). Although primary invasive fungal infections are relatively uncommon in HIES, cryptococcal infections of the genitourinary tract and colon have been reported (Jacobs et al., 1984; Hutto et al., 1988).

Skeletal Anomalies

Skeletal and facial abnormalities associated with HIES were recognized in the original reports by Davis et al. (1966) and Buckley et al. (1972). They noted characteristic facies and hyperextensibility of the joints. The facies in HIES are often asymmetric with a prominent forehead and mild prognathism, increased interalar

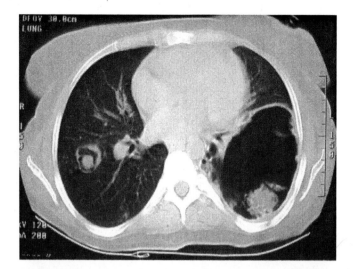

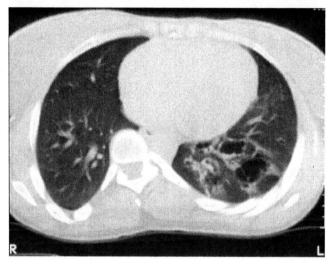

Figure 34.1. Pulmonary complications of hyper-IgE syndrome. (A) Postinflammatory cysts containing aspergillomas. (B) Scoliosis evident in angle of vertebra.

width of the nose, wide-set eyes, thickening of the soft tissue of ears and nose, and a high-arched palate (Borges et al., 1998; Grimbacher et al., 1999a). Although only 83% of HIES patients of all ages in our cohort showed the characteristic facies, the facial features progressively develop and become almost universal by late adolescence (Color Plate 34.IV). Sixty percent have an increased interalar distance (width across the bottom of the nose) and almost half have a high arched palate (Color Plate 34.V, top right). Craniosynostosis has also been reported in a few cases of HIES (Smithwick et al., 1978; Höger et al., 1985; Gahr et al., 1987).

Recurrent pathologic fractures occur in 57% of patients, confirming the multisystem nature of HIES. Fractures occur most commonly in the long bones and ribs (Fig. 34.2A). Although osteopenia is common in HIES and may be cytokine or immune driven (Leung et al., 1988; Cohen-Solal et al., 1995), the fractures that occur are not at the same sites typical of osteoporosis in postmenopausal females. Scoliosis has been seen in 63% of patients: over half had a curvature >15°, and one-third had >20° (Fig 34.2A). Although many cases of scoliosis are idiopathic, diverse contributing factors have been noted, such as leg length discrepancy, prior thoracotomy (e.g., for lung cyst removal), and

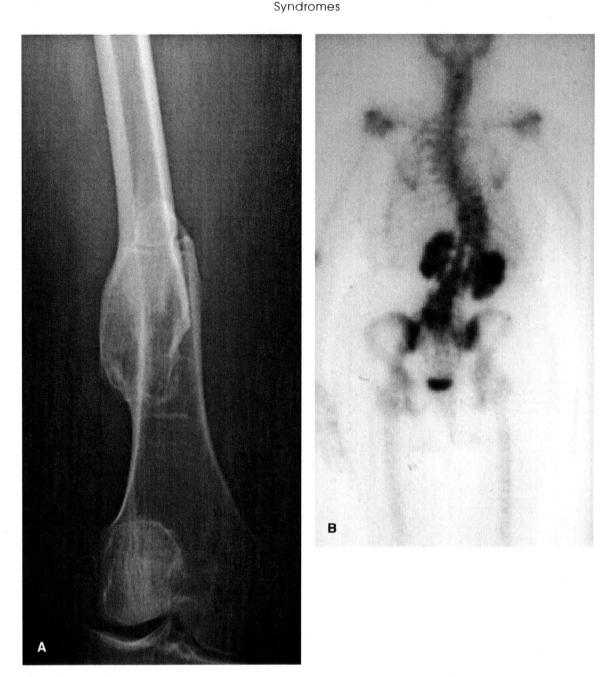

Figure 34.2. Skeletal manifestations of Job's syndrome. (A) Healed pathologic distal femoral fracture suffered while wading in the ocean. (B) Bone scan showing marked scoliosis.

vertebral body anomalies. Hyperextensibility of the joints was noted in the initial reports and was found in 68% of our patients.

Dental System

Impaired shedding of primary teeth in HIES patients was only recently recognized and appears to be quite a consistent finding. Reduced resorption of primary tooth roots may lead to prolonged retention of the primary teeth, which in turn prevents the appropriate eruption of the permanent successors (O'Connell et al., 2000). The mechanism underlying this unique developmental abnormality is unknown. In our cohort of HIES patients older than age 6, 72% had delayed shedding of primary teeth (Color Plate 34.V). We currently recommend that, after checking by radiography for the existence and developmental age of the sec-

ondary teeth, children with HIES undergo extraction of retained primary teeth. This procedure is usually followed by normal eruption of the permanent teeth.

Other Associated Clinical Findings

Several malignancies have been reported in HIES, which suggests that these patients may be at increased risk (Bale et al., 1977; Buckley and Sampson, 1981; Gorin et al., 1989; Einsele et al., 1990; Kowalchuk, 1996; Takimoto et al., 1996; Nester et al., 1998; Huber et al., 1987). In the NIH cohort, two patients developed non-Hodgkin lymphoma and both were successfully treated; another was successfully treated for nodular sclerosing Hodgkin disease. One patient developed metastatic squamous cell carcinoma of the tongue. To date, none of our patients have

Table 34.2. Hyper-IgE Syndrome Scoring Sheet

Clinical Findings	Points									
	0	1	2	3	4	5	6	7	8	10
Highest IgE (IU/ml)	<200	200–500			501–1000				1001–2000	>2000
Skin abscesses (total)	None		1–2		3–4				>4	
Pneumonias (X-ray proven, total)	None		1		2		3		>3	
Parenchymal lung abnormalities	Absent						Bronchiectasis		Pneumatocele	
Other serious infection	None				Severe					
Fatal infection	Absent				Present					
Highest eosinophils/µl	<700			700–800			>800			
Newborn rash	Absent				Present					
Eczema (worst stage)	Absent	Mild	Moderate		Severe					
Sinusitis, otitis (no. of times in worst year)	1–2	3	4–6		>6					
Candidiasis	None	Oral, vaginal	Fingernail		Systemic					
Retained primary teeth	None	1	2		3				>3	
Scoliosis, maximum curvature	<10°		10°–14°		15°–20°				>20°	
Fractures with little trauma	None				1–2				>2	
Hyperextensibility	Absent				Present					
Characteristic face	Absent		Mild			Present				
Increased nose width (interalar distance)	<1 SD	1–2 SD		>2 SD						
High palate	Absent		Present							
Congenital anomaly	Absent					Present				
Lymphoma	Absent				Present					

developed systemic lupus erythematosus, another condition previously reported associated with HIES (Schopfer et al., 1983; Leyh et al., 1986; North et al., 1997; Brugnoni et al., 1998). Autoimmune vasculitis (Kimata, 1995), dermatomyositis (Min et al., 1999), and membranoproliferative glomerulonephritis (Tanji et al., 1999) have also been reported in HIES but have not occurred in the NIH cohort.

Diagnostic Criteria

An HIES scoring system (Table 34.2) was developed at the NIH to help estimate the likelihood that a relative of an affected subject might carry an autosomal dominant HIES gene, based on his or her clinical and laboratory phenotype. The scores were shown to be in agreement with the diagnostic opinions of five physicians familiar with HIES who examined the same patients without knowledge of the score. This scoring system was then used to make phenotype assignments for linkage studies (see below). For each clinical finding associated with HIES a point scale was developed. The more specific and more objective findings were assigned higher point scores. This scoring is age sensitive, since older patients are likely to have collected more points. Moreover, some clinical features, such as shedding of primary teeth, cannot be evaluated in very young patients; therefore an age correction is included. In HIES families, an HIES genotype was considered highly likely if the HIES score (based on numbers and severity of HIES characteristics exhibited) exceeded 40 points, and unlikely if the score was less than 20 points. Between 20 and 40 points is an indeterminate zone; patients with these scores may be suspected of having HIES and should be followed over time to gather more conclusive data. We suggest using at least 40 points as a cutoff for a diagnosis of HIES, and more certainty is

afforded if the points are derived from both immune and nonimmune features. Patients with certain conditions such as severe atopic disease may occasionally have very high IgE levels and scores in the HIES range without having HIES. We prefer a multicomponent scoring system for the diagnosis of HIES because no definitive diagnostic laboratory tests, either immunologic or genetic, are currently available.

Laboratory Findings

The syndrome takes its name from marked polyclonal elevations of IgE in serum. An IgE of >2000 IU/ml often has been used as an arbitrary diagnostic level. However, because IgE levels are very low in utero and climb only after birth in normal infants, infants affected with HIES may not achieve a diagnostic level of 2000 IU/ml early in life. In affected infants the IgE is consistently elevated over the age-adjusted value. For these cases, 10 times the age-appropriate level has been a reasonable guide. IgE levels of >10,000 IU/ml are characteristic of HIES and levels of >50,000 IU/ml have been reported (Buckley and Becker, 1978; Grimbacher et al., 1999a). However, serum IgE levels are not static. Substantial fluctuations in serum IgE concentrations have been noted over time without any obvious change in the clinical status. IgE levels fell below 2000 IU/ml, even close to or into the normal range, in 5 of 30 patients followed at the NIH (Grimbacher et al., 1999a). Therefore, although a high IgE level is part of the diagnostic criteria for HIES, authentic cases may lack this particular feature at some point in their course. The level of serum IgE apparently is not correlated with disease activity or severity. IgE production is thought to be elevated in HIES because of an increased number of B cells making subnormal levels of IgE (Garraud et al., 1999). The driving force for this abnormality is still unclear, but it is not especially cytokine responsive in vivo (King et al., 1989). IgE catabolism is also impaired in HIES, contributing to the elevation (Dreskin et al., 1987a). In addition to IgE elevation, eosinophilia is seen in >90% of HIES patients. This eosinophilia is at least 2 standard deviations above normal, usually above 700 cells/μl, but it is not correlated with the extent of IgE elevation. The tropism of the elevated IgE in HIES is still unclear. A high proportion of the IgE in HIES binds to *S. aureus* and *C. albicans* (Berger et al., 1980). Similar binding activity was not seen in IgE from other patients infected frequently with *S. aureus*, indicating that this abnormality may be host driven, and not organism driven. Anti–*Staphylococcus aureus* and anti–*Candida albicans* IgE titers have been noted to be raised in HIES, but any relationship to the severity of the disease is not known. Unfortunately, raised antistaphylococcal titers are also seen in atopic patients and are therefore not helpful in the diagnosis of HIES (Walsh et al., 1981).

White blood cell counts are typically in the normal range, but have been reported to range from 1700 to 60,000/μl (Buckley and Becker, 1978; Donabedian and Gallin, 1983a). Chronic leukopenia with borderline neutropenia has been observed in several patients (Donabedian and Gallin, 1983a).

Complement levels have been normal when studied. Elevated levels of urinary histamine have been reported in some patients and correlate with the extent of the eczematoid dermatitis (Dreskin et al., 1987).

Etiology

The underlying cause of HIES is still unknown. Many studies have focused on the immune aspects of the disease, such as detection of eosinophilia in blood, sputum, and abscesses (Belohradsky et al., 1987; Gahr et al., 1987; Buckley, 1996); defective granulocyte chemotaxis (Buckley et al., 1972; Hill and Quie, 1974; Hill et al., 1974; Van Scoy et al., 1975; Van Epps et al., 1983); abnormal T lymphocyte subsets (Geha et al., 1981; Gahr et al., 1987; Buckley et al., 1991); defective antibody production (Buckley and Becker, 1978; Geha et al., 1981; Dreskin et al., 1985, 1987a); and decreased production of or responsiveness to cytokines such as interleukin-4 (IL-4) and interferon-γ (IFN-γ) (King et al., 1989; Vercelli et al., 1990; Paganelli et al., 1991; Rousset et al., 1991; Borges et al., 2000). Originally, HIES was considered to be due to a defect in neutrophil function, because chemotaxis was abnormal at least some of the time in most of the patients (Hill et al., 1974). However, the failure to demonstrate a consistent chemotactic defect, even in the same patient over time, suggested that the chemotactic defects were not central and reproducible aspects of HIES. Even when present, the impaired chemotaxis was not marked in the in vitro assays, compared to syndromes with more profound, primary chemotaxis defects. The 61 kDa protein inhibitor of chemotactic activity described from HIES patients by Donabedian and Gallin (1982, 1983b) is still not completely defined. In summary, no specific immune defect has been found to be present consistently in all patients with HIES.

Several features of HIES have been considered central enough to be of potential etiologic significance. IgE is greatly elevated at most points in the life of patients with HIES (Buckley and Becker, 1978; Donabedian and Gallin, 1983a; Grimbacher et al., 1999a). An infant daughter of a mother with HIES subsequently developed HIES herself and was noted to have elevated cord blood IgE (Dreskin and Gallin, 1987). Since IgE does not cross the placenta, cord blood elevation reflected endogenous fetal synthesis of IgE and suggests that IgE dysregulation is a primary feature of HIES. Although these findings suggest an important role for extremely elevated IgE in the genesis of HIES, 17% of patients were observed to have IgE levels drop below 2000 IU/ml over long-term follow-up (Grimbacher et al., 1999a), yet retained their increased susceptibility to infection.

The role of IFN in HIES has been investigated because of its participation in IgE responses. IFN-γ specifically inhibited the IgE-enhancing activity of a concanavalin–A–stimulated T helper cell line supernatant (Coffman and Carty, 1986) and inhibited the effect of IL-4 on cell expansion and induction of DNA synthesis (Rabin et al., 1986). In HIES patients, there appears to be a reduction in lymphocytes producing either IFN-γ or tumor necrosis factor-α (TNF-α) (DelPrete et al., 1989). However, synthesis of IL-2 and IL-4 appears to be normal. A correlation between elevated in vitro IgE synthesis and diminished IFN-γ production in T cells has been reported in HIES patients (DelPrete et al., 1989). Vercelli et al. (1990) did not find in vitro modulation of IgE synthesis by IFN-γ, but suggested that T cell–independent mechanisms of IgE regulation were possible.

King et al. (1989) examined effects of IFN-γ on HIES peripheral blood mononuclear cell IgE production in vitro and in vivo. They used subcutaneous IFN-γ to treat five patients with HIES for 2 to 6 weeks. IFN-γ suppressed spontaneous IgE production in vitro and in vivo in most of their patients, as was seen when peripheral blood mononuclear cells were assayed for spontaneous IgE production before and after IFN-γ administration. However, serum IgE levels fell in only two of the five patients treated (one received 0.05 mg/m^2, the other received 0.1 mg/m^2 IFN-γ). After the study, serum IgE levels rebounded to their pretreatment levels in both patients. No patient had any clinical change from the brief course of IFN-γ administration.

Garraud et al. (1999) showed that although both IFN-γ and IL-12 reduced IgE synthesis, neither cytokine could totally shut it off in HIES cells in vitro. Blocking antibodies to IL-4 or IL-13 reduced in vitro IgE, whereas neutralization of both IL-4 and IL-13 completely suppressed IgE production in cells from subjects with HIES. Interestingly, addition of IL-8 or blockade of IL-6 and TNF-α completely inhibited IgE production in HIES cells in vitro.

Borges et al. (2000) described decreased in vitro IFN-γ production in HIES, especially when patient cells were activated with staphylococcal antigen. They postulated that there is a shift toward a T helper-2 type cytokine response, which may result in deficient IFN-γ production and promote IL-4, IL-5, IL-13, and, ultimately, IgE production. However, we have not seen decreased IFN-γ production in vitro in response to phytohemagglutinin (PHA); if this abnormality exists it may be antigen-specific (D.M. Frucht and S.M. Holland, unpublished observations). Recent studies in patients with sporadic HIES indicated that cytokines and chemokines may be dysregulated in HIES (elevation of IL-12, but decrease of ENA-78, MCP-3, and eotaxin), although it is not clear whether these abnormalities are primary or are secondary to intercurrent infection and inflammation (Chehimi et al., 2001).

Despite the interesting in vitro abnormalities centered around IgE and neutrophil function, the complex multisystem nature of this disease and its effects on skin, bone, teeth, lung, immunity, and infection susceptibility suggest aberrant regulation of some cell or molecular pathway common to all these tissues.

Genetics

Autosomal Dominant Hyper-IgE Recurrent Infection Syndrome

Although HIES is thought to be rare, the exact incidence is unknown. Over 200 cases have been published. Although first described in Caucasians with red hair, HIES occurs in all racial and ethnic groups with apparently equal frequency. In one current collected global series there are 68 males and 61 females, suggesting an equal gender distribution in HIES. This is in contrast to earlier reports that suggested a female predominance.

Most pedigrees of multiplex HIES families are consistent with autosomal dominant inheritance (Van Scoy et al., 1975; Blum et al., 1977; Donabedian and Gallin 1983a; Leung und Geha, 1988; Buckley, 1996). Grimbacher et al. (1999a) confirmed autosomal dominant transmission in seven families extending over multiple generations with variable expressivity of the disease phenotype. In a previous collection of HIES families by Grimbacher et al. (1999b), 16 of 19 pedigrees demonstrated parent-to-child transmission, most consistent with dominant inheritance. In six families, transmission from father to son excluded linkage to the X chromosome. Assuming a simple autosomal dominant mode of inheritance, the index patients of the 16 families with apparent dominant transmission had 56 offspring, who would all be at a 50% risk of having HIES. In fact, 29 of them (51%) actually were affected, supporting a Mendelian autosomal dominant trait with high penetrance.

Linkage analysis of a large cohort of 19 multiplex HIES families with 57 affecteds (Grimbacher et al., 1999b) demonstrated linkage to the centromeric region and proximal long arm of chromosome 4. Attention was directed to this region of the genome by a sporadic patient with HIES plus autism and mental retardation, who was found to have a supernumerary marker chromosome derived from a 15–20 cM interstitial deletion from chromosome 4q21 (Grimbacher et al., 1999c). Interestingly, among those 19 families with apparent autosomal dominant transmission of HIES, at least 6 families had an HIES trait that was not linked to chromosome 4, a finding suggesting that at least one additional genetic locus could be responsible for autosomal dominant HIES (AD-HIES). There were no clinical or laboratory features that distinguished HIES linked to chromosome 4 from HIES not linked to 4.

Hershey et al. (1997) identified a polymorphism in the IL-4 receptor (Q576R) linked to atopic eczema and suggested a link to HIES. However, analysis of 25 controls and 20 HIES patients from the NIH cohort showed that Q576R is a polymorphism within the IL-4 receptor unassociated with the HIES phenotype (Grimbacher et al., 1998). Moreover, a pilot linkage study with seven autosomal dominant multiplex families was inconsistent with linkage to the IL-4 receptor locus on chromosome 16 (Grimbacher et al., 1998).

Autosomal Recessive Hyper-IgE Recurrent Infection Syndrome

In 2004, 13 HIES patients from six consanguineous families with severe recurring infections (pneumonia and abscesses), eczema, high IgE, and eosinophilia were described who fulfilled the criteria for diagnosis of HIES (Renner et al., 2004). Because affected individuals were siblings with consanguineous parents, the mode of inheritance was concluded to be autosomal recessive (AR-HIES). This cohort of patients with AR-HIES, in addition to the recurrent bacterial infections characteristic of sporadic and dominant HIES (*Staphylococcus aureus, Haemophilus influenzae, Proteus mirabilis, Pseudomonas aeruginosa,* and *Cryptococcus*), also had severe chronic therapy-resistant *Molluscum contagiosum* infections. Furthermore, 7 of 13 patients suffered recurring herpes simplex infections, which caused mouth ulcerations and also keratitis. One patient suffered recurrent *Varicella zoster*. These patients with AR-HIES demonstrate an increased susceptibility to viral infections. A defect in T cells is thus possible in this cohort, especially given the occurrence of recurrent fungal infections in 10 of 13 patients.

Whereas post-pneumonia pneumatocele formation is pathognomonic in dominant or sporadic HIES, no pneumatoceles occurred in patients with AR-HIES, although pneumonia was equally frequent. This observation differentiates the two types of HIES clinically and may be of use as a differential diagnostic parameter. Autoimmune hemolytic anemia was seen in two patients with AR-HIES, and one patient had a pericardial effusion, possibly an indication of autoimmunity. In the AR-HIES cohort, 7 of 13 patients had neurological symptoms, which varied from partial facial paralysis to hemiplegia. Of these patients, four died of neurologic complications, although the etiology is still not clear. AR-HIES patients did not have the skeletal abnormalities, fractures, dental abnormalities, or dysmorphic faces as seen in dominant or sporadic cases of HIES, further differentiating the AR-HIES variant.

All AR-HIES patients had elevated IgE serum levels and eosinophilia. IgE levels were comparable to those in AD-HIES patients. Furthermore, serum levels of the other immunolglobulin isotypes were also raised, indicating a nonspecific stimulation of the humoral response. The eosinophilia was more severe in AR-HIES patients than in AD-HIES patients; values up to 17,500/µl (normal <700) were reached.

Lymphocyte phenotyping of patients with AR-HIES revealed normal lymphocyte subpopulations, including a normal CD4/CD8 ratio. However, in vitro stimulation of lymphocytes by T cell mitogens and the Cowan strain of *S. aureus* strain (SAC), a T cell–independent mitogen, revealed reduced lymphocyte proliferation. This finding indicates that the cellular defect in AR-HIES is qualitative in nature, a hypothesis supported by the occurrence of viral and fungal infections in AR-HIES. In contrast, granulocyte function seems to be normal in AR-HIES.

Linkage analysis of AR-HIES has been complicated by a high mortality rate in early childhood. The only linkage information available thus far is that more than one genetic locus seems to be responsible for this phenotype.

Hyper-IgE Overlap Syndromes

Interestingly, in rare cases of other defined genetic diseases, the classical triad of HIES with recurrent skin abscesses, recurrent pneumonia, and extreme elevations of IgE is also fulfilled. Antoniades et al. (1996), reported the coexistence of HIES and Dubowitz syndrome, defined by postnatal growth retardation, microcephaly, and characteristic facial appearance. Boeck et al. (1999) reported the coexistence of pentasomy X and HIES. Boeck et al. (2001) further reported the coexistence of HIES and Saethre-Chotzen syndrome (defined by acrocephalosyndactyly, hypertelorism, and ptosis), caused by mutations in the *TWIST* gene. The relationships of these patients to those discussed above is unknown.

Table 34.3. Treatment Alternatives in Hyper-IgE Recurrent Infection Syndromes

Treatment	Number of HIES Patients	Desired Outcome	Results and Remarks	Reference
Cimetidine	8	Reduce eczema	Modest benefit; at least one clinical relapse after discontinuation	Mawhinney et al., 1980; Thompson and Kumararatne, 1989
Interferon-γ	5	Reduce IgE	IgE reduction in 2/5; rapid rebound after treatment; thrombocytopenia	King et al., 1989
Cyclosporin A	3	Control eczema	Transient benefit; relapse after discontinuation	Wolach et al., 1996; Etzioni et al., 1997
Cromoglycate	1	Reduce inflammation	Benefit	Yokota et al., 1990
Isotretionin	1	Reduce dermatitis	Improvement in dermatitis	Shuttleworth et al., 1988
I.V. immunoglobulin	8	Reduce infections	Difficult to assess effect	Kimata, 1995; Espanol and Matamoros, personal communication
Plasmapheresis	3?	Control keratoconjunctivitis	Short-lived improvement	Ishikawa et al., 1982; Dau, 1988; Leung et al., 1988

Therefore, HIES is a complex autosomal disorder with several possible genotypes producing a common phenotype of immunodeficiency, eczema, and elevated IgE. Inspection of different pedigrees suggests that HIES may be caused by mutation of a single gene, mutations in different genes in different families (genetic heterogeneity), or deletion of contiguous genes in a short chromosomal region. Because the genetic backgrounds of our patients are diverse and because survival to reproductive age before the advent of antibiotics has previously been unusual, multiple newly arising mutations are expected.

Treatment

Aggressive skin care and prompt treatment of infections are the main pillars of HIES management. The dermatitis is heavily dependent on ongoing infection, typically with *Staphylococcus aureus*. Therefore, antibiotic treatment is often an essential part of management of HIES eczema, in association with topical moisturizing creams and topical steroids. We have also used topical antiseptic treatments such as bathing in a dilute bleach solution to reduce the bacterial burden in the skin. Skin abscesses are a common complication of HIES and may require incision and drainage. Interestingly, after the introduction of prophylactic antibiotics, skin abscesses are unusual. The role of prophylactic antibiotics has not been rigorously investigated in this setting, but there is general consensus in favor of their use. Most physicians cover *S. aureus* with a semisynthetic penicillin such as dicloxacillin.

The other major recurrent infectious problem in HIES is mucocutaneous candidiasis. This typically manifests as onychomycosis, vaginal candidiasis, and/or thrush. Candida rarely disseminates, and these infections are typically highly responsive to oral triazole antifungals. The use of oral antifungals, such as the triazoles, has made an enormous difference in the prevalence and severity of mucocutaneous candidiasis in HIES. Overuse of antibiotics and antifungals is currently discouraged in general practice because of concerns about selection for resistant organisms. However, there is no clear demonstration of increasingly resistant organisms in HIES patients on prolonged prophylactic and suppressive antibiotic therapy, and the benefits of this approach are readily appreciated.

One remarkable feature of HIES is the enormous infectious burden with which patients often present. By the time the patient or parent is aware of illness, there is usually nothing subtle about

the diagnosis. One of the most difficult problems in the management of HIES is that even in the presence of obvious auscultatory and radiographic evidence of pneumonia, patients do not feel unwell and may be unwilling to submit to invasive diagnostic testing or prolonged courses of therapy. In addition, the hesitance of physicians to believe that patients who appear no different from their baseline are really on the verge of collapse is difficult to overcome.

As in most of medicine, the firm establishment of a microbiologic diagnosis cannot be overemphasized. Bronchoscopy may help in both obtaining the specimen and mobilizing secretions. Thick inspissated secretions typically plug ectatic bronchi and are tenacious and difficult to clear. Lung abscesses may require thoracotomy for adequate drainage or resection. However, thoracotomy and lung resection are more difficult in HIES than in other pulmonary infections because of the common failure of remaining HIES lobes to expand and fill the chest cavity. Surgery often results in a need for very prolonged chest tube drainage, thoracoplasty, or pneumonectomy, along with intensive parenteral antibiotic treatment. Therefore, pulmonary surgery in HIES should not be undertaken lightly, and should be performed at a center with experience with the disease where possible.

High-dose intravenous antibiotics for a prolonged course are required for eradication of infection and to prevent bronchopleural fistula formation and bronchiectasis. Empirical acute coverage should consider *S. aureus*, *H. influenzae*, and *S. pneumoniae*. The former two organisms account for the majority of acute infections. One of the typical features of HIES is that following the resolution of acute pneumonias, pulmonary cysts form. These pneumatoceles then serve as the focus for colonization with *Pseudomonas aeruginosa*, *Aspergillus*, and other fungal species. These superinfections are the most difficult aspect of long-term management of HIES. Potential management strategies include prophylactic itraconazole or voriconazole, aerosolized colistin, or aerosolized aminoglycosides.

The role for immune modulators in HIES is unproven (Table 34.3). Levamisole was tried in a double-blind, placebo-controlled trial, and caused an increase in infectious complications in the treatment arm (Donabedian et al., 1982). This is the only published double-blind, placebo-controlled trial of any management intervention in HIES.

It has been previously supposed that since immunodeficiency is a central part of HIES, the underlying defect in HIES must reside in the leukocytes; thus bone marrow transplantation has been suggestive as a curative treatment. Two cases of bone marrow transplantation in HIES have been reported (Nester et al., 1998; Gennery et al., 2000). The first was a 46-year-old man with HIES who had experienced many pneumonias from childhood onward. Two of his four children were also affected. He developed a B cell lymphoma that was treated with a peripheral stem cell transplant from his HLA-identical sister, preceded by total body irradiation. He was maintained on prednisolone and cyclosporine A post-transplant. Serum IgE fell to normal values following transplant and no infections were reported. However, he died 6 months later from interstitial pneumonitis.

The second patient was a 7-year-old girl who was transplanted in an effort to treat her severe HIES. She received marrow from a matched unrelated donor after cytoreductive therapy. Cyclosporine A was used for prophylaxis of graft-versus-host disease. Engraftment appeared eventually to be complete by study of peripheral blood markers. Initially, the skin lesions cleared, but 4 years after transplant, she developed recurrent staphylococcal and pseudomonal skin infections. Interestingly, the IgE level also returned to pretransplant elevated levels. This result is particularly surprising in view of the reported full engraftment of the B cell compartment.

This case suggests that the features that led to IgE elevation in this patient may have been somatic, and that the features that made her susceptible to infection may not have been confined to the hematopoietic system. The possible somatic components that might lead to this syndrome are unknown; however, this case reinforces the multisystem nature of the disease and suggests that the cardinal IgE elevation and infectious features that have given the syndrome its name may not be intrinsically immune.

Acknowledgments

We are indebted to all physicians who contributed data and/or DNA from their patients to facilitate better diagnosis and patient management in HIES and eventually unravel the genetic cause of this enigmatic disease. B.G. was a fellow of the Immune Deficiency Foundation in 1999 and was supported by a grant of the Deutsche Forschungsgemeinschaft (GR1617/2).

References

Antoniades K, Hatzistilianou M, Pitsavas G, Agouridaki C, Athanassiadou F. Co-existence of Dubowitz and hyper-IgE syndromes: a case report. Eur J Pediatr 155:390–392, 1996.

Bale JF, Wilson JF, Hill HR. Fatal histiocytic lymphoma of the brain associated with hyperimmunoglobulinemia-E and recurrent infections. Cancer 39:2386–2390, 1977.

Belohradsky BH, Daeumling S, Kiess W, Griscelli C. Das Hyper-IgE-Syndrom (Buckley-oder Hiob-Syndrom). In: Ergebnisse der Inneren Medizin und Kinderheilkunde, Bd. 55. Berlin: Springer-Verlag, pp. 1–39, 1987.

Berger M, Kirkpatrick CH, Goldsmith PK, Gallin JI. IgE antibodies to Staphylococcus aureus and Candida albicans in patients with the syndrome of hyperimmunoglobulin E and recurrent infections. J Immunol 125:2437–2443, 1980.

Blum R, Geller G, Fish LA. Recurrent severe staphylococcal infections, eczematoid rash, extreme elevations of IgE, eosinophilia, and divergent chemotactic responses in two generations. J Pediatr 90:607–609, 1977.

Boeck A, Gfatter R, Braun F, Fritz B. Pentasomy X and hyper IgE syndrome: co-existence of two distinct genetic disorders. Eur J Pediatr 158:723–726, 1999.

Boeck A, Kosan C, Ciznar P, Kunz J. Saethre-Chotzen syndrome and hyper IgE syndrome in a patient with a novel 11 bp deletion of the TWIST gene. Am J Med Genet 104:53–56, 2001.

Borges WG, Hensley T, Carey JC, Petrak BA, Hill HR. The face of Job. J Pediatr 133:303–305, 1998.

Borges WG, Augustine NH, Hill HR. Defective IL-12/interferon–gamma pathway in patients with hyperimmunoglobulinemia E syndrome. J Pediatr 136:176–180, 2000.

Brugnoni D, Franceschini F, Airo P, Cattaneo R. Discordance for systemic lupus erythematosus and hyper-IgE syndrome in a pair of monozygotic twins. Br J Rheumatol 37:807–808, 1998.

Buckley RH. Disorders of the IgE system; the hyper IgE syndrome. In: Stiehm ER, ed. Immunologic Disorders in Infants and Children, 4th edition. Philadelphia: WB Saunders, pp. 413–422, 1996.

Buckley RH, Becker WG. Abnormalities in the regulation of human IgE synthesis. Immunol Rev 41:288, 1978.

Buckley RH, Sampson HA. The hyperimmunoglobulinemia E syndrome. In: Franklin EC, ed. Clinical Immunology Update. New York: Elsevier North-Holland, pp. 147–167, 1981.

Buckley RH, Schiff SE, Hayward AR. Reduced frequency of CD45RO+ T lymphocytes in blood of hyper-IgE syndrome patients. J Allergy Clin Immunol 87:313, 1991.

Buckley RH, Wray BB, Belmaker EZ. Extreme hyperimmunoglobulin E and undue susceptibility to infection. Pediatrics 49:59, 1972.

Chehimi J, Elder M, Greene J, Noroski L, Stiehm ER, Winkelstein JA, Sullivan KE. Cytokine and chemokine dysregulation in hyper-IgE syndrome. Clin Immunol 100:49–56, 2001.

Claassen JJ, Levine AD, Schiff SE, Buckley RH. Mononuclear cells from patients with the hyper-IgE syndrome produce little IgE when they are stimulated with recombinant human interleukin-4. J Allergy Clin Immunol 88:713–721, 1991.

Coffman RL, Carty J. A T cell activity that enhances polyclonal IgE production and its inhibition by interferon gamma. J Immunol 136:949, 1986.

Cohen-Solal M, Prieur AM, Prin L, Denne MA, Launay JM, Graulet AM, Brazier M, Griscelli C, de Vernejoul MC. Cytokine-mediated bone resorption in patients with the hyperimmunoglobulin E syndrome. Clin Immunol Immunopathol 76:75–81, 1995.

Dau PC. Remission of hyper-IgE syndrome treated with plasmapheresis and cytotoxic immunosuppression. J Clin Apheresis 4:8–12, 1988.

Davis SD, Schaller J, Wedgewood RJ. Job's syndrome. Recurrent, "cold," staphylococcal abscesses. Lancet 1:1013, 1966.

Del Prete G, Tiri A, Maggi E, et al. Defective in vitro production of gamma interferon and tumor necrosis factor alpha by circulating T cells from patients with hyper-immuno globulin E syndrome. J Clin Invest 84:1830–1835, 1989.

Donabedian H, Alling DW, Gallin JI. Levamisole is inferior to placebo in the hyperimmunoglobulin E recurrent-infection (Job's) syndrome. N Engl J Med 307:290–292, 1982.

Donabedian H, Gallin JI. Mononuclear cells from patients with the hyperimmunoglobulin E–recurrent infection syndrome produce an inhibitor of leukocyte chemotaxis. J Clin Invest 69:1155–1163, 1982.

Donabedian H, Gallin JI. The hyperimmunoglobulin E recurrent infection (Job's) syndrome: a review of the NIH experience and the literature. Medicine (Baltimore) 62:195–208, 1983a.

Donabedian H, Gallin JI. Two inhibitors of neutrophil chemotaxis are produced by hyperimmunoglobulin E recurrent infection syndrome mononuclear cells exposed to heat-killed staphylococci. Infect Immun 40:1030–1037, 1983b.

Dreskin SC, Goldsmith PK, Gallin JI. Immunoglobulins in the hyperimmunoglobulin E and recurrent infection (Job's) syndrome. Deficiency of anti–Staphylococcus aureus immunoglobulin A. J Clin Invest 75:26–34, 1985.

Dreskin SC, Goldsmith PK, Strober W, Zech LA, Gallin JI. Metabolism of immunoglobulin E in patients with markedly elevated serum immunoglobulin E levels. J Clin Invest 79:1764–1772, 1987a.

Dreskin SC, Kaliner MA, Gallin JI. Elevated urinary histamine in the hyperimmunoglobulin E and recurrent infection (Job's) syndrome: association with eczematoid dermatitis and not with infection. J Allergy Clin Immunol 79:515–522, 1987b.

Dreskin SC, Gallin JI. Evolution of hyperimmunoglobulin E and recurrent infection (HIE, Job's) syndrome in a young girl. J Allergy Clin Immunol 80:746–751, 1987.

Einsele H, Saal JG, Dopfer R, Niethammer D, Waller HD, Mueller CA. Hochmalignes Non-Hodgkin-Lymphom bei Hyper-IgE Syndrom. Dtsch Med Wochenschr 115:1141–1144, 1990.

Erlewyn-Lajeunesse MD. Hyperimmunoglobulin-E syndrome with recurrent infection: a review of current opinion and treatment. Pediatr Allergy Immunol 11:133–141, 2000.

Etzioni A, Shehadeh N, Brecher A, Yorman S, Pollack S. Cyclosporin A in hyperimmunoglobulin E syndrome. Ann Allergy Asthma Immunol 78:413–414, 1997.

Farkas LG. Anthropometry of the Head and Face in Medicine, 2nd edition. New York: Raven Press, 1994.

Freeman AF, Barson W, Davis J, Puck JM, Holland SM. *Pneumocystis jiroveci* infection in patients with hyper-immunoglobulin E syndrome. Pediatrics, In press, 2006.

Gahr M, Mueller W, Allgeier B, Speer CP. A boy with recurrent infections, impared PMN-chemotaxis, increased IgE concentrations and cranial synostosis—a variant of the hyper-IgE syndrome? Helv Paediatr Acta 42: 185–190, 1987.

Garraud O, Mollis SN, Holland SM, Sneller MC, Malech HL, Gallin JI, Nutman TB. Regulation of immunoglobulin production in hyper-IgE (Job's) syndrome. J Allergy Clin Immunol 103:333–340, 1999.

Geha RS, Leung DYM. Hyper-immunoglobulin E syndrome. Immunodefic Rev 1:155–172, 1989.

Geha RS, Reinherz E, Leung D, McKee JT, Schlossmann S, Rosen FS. Deficiency of supressor T cells in the hyperimmunoglobulin E syndrome. J Clin Invest 68:783–791, 1981.

Gennery AR, Flood TJ, Abinun M, Cant AJ. Bone marrow transplantation does not correct the hyper IgE syndrome. Bone Marrow Transplant 25: 1303–1305, 2000.

Gorin LJ, Jeha SC, Sullivan MP, Rosenblatt HM, Shearer WT. Burkitt's lymphoma developing in a 7-year-old boy with hyper-IgE syndrome. J Allergy Clin Immunol 83:5–10, 1989.

Grimbacher B, Holland SM, Gallin JI, Greenberg F, Hill SC, Malech HL, Miller JA, O'Connell AC, Puck JM. Hyper-IgE syndrome with recurrent infections—an autosomal dominant multisystem disorder. N Engl J Med 340:692–702, 1999a.

Grimbacher B, Holland SM, Puck JM. The interleukin-4 receptor variant Q576R in hyper-IgE syndrome. N Engl J Med 338:1073–1074, 1998.

Grimbacher B, Schaffer AA, Holland SM, Davis J, Gallin JI, Malech HL, Atkinson TP, Belohradsky BH, Buckley RH, Cossu F, Espanol T, Garty BZ, Matamoros N, Myers LA, Nelson RP, Ochs HD, Renner ED, Wellinghausen N, Puck JM. Genetic linkage of hyper-IgE syndrome to chromosome 4. Am J Hum Genet 65:735–744, 1999b.

Grimbacher B, Dutra AS, Holland SM, Fisher RE, Páo M, Gallin JI, Puck JM. Analphoid marker chromosome in a patient with hyper-IgE syndrome, autism, and mild mental retardation. Genet Med 1:213–218, 1999c.

Hershey GKK, Friedrich MF, Esswein LA, Thomas ML, Chatila TA. The association of atopy with a gain-of-function mutation in the alpha subunit of the interleukin-4 receptor. N Engl J Med 337:1720–1725, 1997.

Hill HR, Ochs HD, Quie PG, et al. Defect in neutrophil granulocyte chemotaxis in Job's syndrome of recurrent 'cold' staphylococcal abscesses. Lancet 2:617–619, 1974.

Hill HR, Quie PG. Raised serum IgE levels and defective neutrophil chemotaxis in three children with exzema and recurrent bacterial infections. Lancet 1:183–187, 1974.

Höger PH, Boltshauser E, Hitzig WH. Craniosynostosis in hyper-IgE syndrome. Eur J Pediatr 144:414–417, 1985.

Huber A, Mietens C. Recurrent staphyloderma in marked IgE elevation: the hyper-IgE syndrome. Klin Paediatr 199:445–446, 1987 [In German].

Hutto JO, Bryan CS, Greene FL, White CJ, Gallin JI. Cryptococcosis of the colon resembling Crohn's disease in a patient with the hyperimmunoglobulinemia E-recurrent infection (Job's) syndrome. Gastroenterology 94: 808–812, 1988.

Ishikawa I, Fukuda Y, Kitada H, et al. Plasma exchange in a patient with hyper-IgE syndrome. Ann Allergy 49:295–297, 1982.

Jacobs DH, Macher AM, Handler R, et al. Esophageal cryptococcosis in a patient with the hyperimmunoglobulin E-recurrent infection (Job's) syndrome. Gastroenterology 87:201–203, 1984.

Kimata H. High-dose intravenous gammaglobulin treatment for hyperimmunoglobulinemia E syndrome. J Allergy Clin Immunol 95:771–774, 1995.

King CL, Gallin JI, Malech HL, Abramson SL, Nutman TB. Regulation of immunoglobulin production in hyperimmunoglobulin E recurrent-infection syndrome by interferon-γ. Proc Natl Acad Sci USA 86: 10085–10089, 1989.

Kowalchuk RM. Case of the season. Job's syndrome with superimposedlymphoma. Semin Roentgenol 31:254–256, 1996.

Leung DY, Geha RS. Clinical and immunologic aspects of the hyperimmunoglobulin aspects of the hyperimmunoglobulin E syndrome. Hematol Oncol Clin North Am 2:81–100, 1988.

Leung DY, Key L, Steinberg JJ, Young MC, Von Deck M, Wilkinson R, Geha RS. Increased in vitro bone resorption by monocytes in the hyper-immunoglobulin E syndrome. J Immunol 140:84–88, 1988.

Leyh F, Wendt V, Scherer R. Systemic lupus erythematosus and hyper-IgE syndrome in a 13-year-old child. Z Hautk 61:611–614, 1986 [in German].

Mawhinney H, Killen M, Fleming WA, Roy AD. The hyperimmunoglobulin E syndrome—a neutrophil chemotactic defect reversible by histamine H2 receptor blockade? Clin Immunol Immunopathol 17:483–491, 1980.

Min JK, Cho ML, Kim SC, et al. Hyperimmunoglobulin E–recurrent infection syndrome in a patient with juvenile dermatomyositis. Korean J Intern Med 14:95–98, 1999.

Nelson RP, Ochs HD, Renner ED, Wellinghausen N, Puck JM. Genetic linkage of hyper-IgE syndrome to chromosome 4 Am J Hum Genet 65:735–744, 1999.

Nester TA, Wagnon AH, Reilly WF, Spitzer G, Kjeldsberg CR, Hill HR. Effects of allogeneic peripheral stem cell transplantation in a patient with job syndrome of hyperimmunoglobulinemia E and recurrent infections. Am J Med 105:162–164, 1998.

North J, Kotecha S, Houtman P, Whaley K. Systemic lupus erythematosus complicating hyper IgE syndrome. Br J Rheumatol 36:297–298, 1997.

O'Connell AC, Puck JM, Grimbacher B, Facchetti F, Majorana A, Gallin JI, Malech HL, Holland SM. Delayed eruption of permanent teeth in hyperimmunoglobulinemia E recurrent infection syndrome. Oral Surg Oral Med Oral Pathol Oral Radiol Endod 89:177–185, 2000.

Paganelli R, Scala E, Capobianchi MR, et al. Selective deficiency of interferon-gamma production in the hyper-IgE syndrome. Relationship to in vitro synthesis. Clin Exp Immunol 84:28–33, 1991.

Rabin EM, Mond JJ, Ohara J, Paul WE. Interferon gamma inhibits the action of B cell stimulatory factor (BSF-1) on resting B cells. J Immunol 137:1573–1576, 1986.

Renner ED, Puck JM, Holland SM, Schmitt M, Weiss M, Frosch M, Bergmann M, Davis J, Belohradsky BH, Grimbacher B. Autosomal recessive hyperimmunoglobulinemia E syndrome: a distinct disease entity. J Pediatr 144:93–99, 2004.

Rousset F, Robert J, Andary M, et al. Shifts in interleukin-4 and interferon-γ production by T cells of patients with elevated serum IgE levels and the modulatory effects of these lymphokines on spontaneous IgE synthesis. J Allergy Clin Immunol 87:58–69, 1991.

Schopfer K, Feldges A, Baerlocher K, Parisot RF, Wilhelm JA, Matter L. Systemic lupus erythematosus in staphylococcal aureus hyperimmunoglobulinemia E syndrome. BMJ 287:524–526, 1983.

Shuttleworth D, Holt PJ, Mathews N. Hyperimmunoglobulin E syndrome: treatment with isotretinoin. Br J Dermatol 119:93–99, 1988.

Smithwick EM, Finelt M, Pahwa S, et al. Cranial synostosis in Job's syndrome. Lancet 1:826, 1978.

Takimoto Y, Imanaka F, Nanba K. Mantle cell lymphoma associated with hyper-IgE syndrome. Rinsho Ketsueki 37:1400–1404, 1996.

Tanji C, Yorioka N, Kanahara K, Naito T, Oda H, Ishikawa K, Taguchi T. Hyperimmunoglobulin E syndrome associated with nephrotic syndrome. Intern Med 38:491–494, 1999.

Thompson RA, Kumararatne DS. Hyper-IgE syndrome and H2-receptor blockade. Lancet 9;2(8663):630, 1989.

Van Epps DE, El-Naggar A, Ochs HD. Abnormalities of lymphocyte locomotion in immunodeficiency disease. Clin Exp Immunol 53:678–688, 1983.

Van Scoy RE, Hill HR, Ritts RE, Quie PG. Familial neutrophil chemotaxis defect, recurrent bacterial infections, mucocutaneous candidiasis, and hyperimmunoglobulinemia E. Ann Intern Med 82:766–771, 1975.

Vercelli D, Jabara HH, Cunningham-Rundles C, et al. Regulation of Immunoglobulin (Ig) E synthesis in the hyper-IgE syndrome. J Clin Invest 85:1666–1671, 1990.

Walsh GA, Richards KL, Douglas SD, Blumenthal MN. Immunoglobulin E anti-*Staphylococcus aureus* antibodies in atopic patients. J Clin Microbiol 13:1046–1048, 1981.

Wolach B, Eliakim A, Pomeranz A, Cohen AH, Nusbacher J, Metzker A. Cyclosporin treatment of hyperimmunoglobulin E syndrome. Lancet 6;347(8993):67, 1996.

Yokota S, Mitsuda T, Shimizu H, Ibe M, Matsuyama S. Cromoglycate treatment of patient with hyperimmunoglobulinaemia E syndrome. Lancet 7;335(8693):857–858, 1990.

35

Immunodeficiency with Centromere Instability and Facial Anomalies

R. SCOTT HANSEN, CORRY WEEMAES, and CISCA WIJMENGA

Immunodeficiency with centromere instability and facial anomalies (ICF syndrome) (MIM 242860) is a rare autosomal recessive disease characterized by a variable immunodeficiency, mild facial anomalies, and chromosome instability involving the pericentromeric regions of chromosomes 1, 9, and 16. This disease was reported for the first time in the late 1970s by two groups independently (Hultén, 1978; Tiepolo et al., 1978, 1979). The patient described earlier by Østergaard (1973) also appears to have had ICF syndrome, based on the clinical symptoms and chromosomal abnormalities reported. The acronym *ICF* was suggested in accordance with the characteristic features of the syndrome: *I*mmunodeficiency, *C*entromeric instability, and *F*acial anomalies (Maraschio et al., 1988). Only about 30 ICF patients have been described in the literature thus far, but underdiagnosis of the syndrome is quite possible because of phenotypic variability and infrequent chromosome analysis. Here we summarize the common clinical features of this limited set of patients as well as the molecular defects associated with ICF.

Clinical and Pathological Manifestations

Although ICF patients have been found all over the world, they are particularly concentrated in the Mediterranean area, including Italy (Tiepolo et al., 1979; Maraschio et al., 1988; Gimelli et al., 1993; Franceschini et al., 1995), Turkey (Wijmenga et al., 2000), Algeria (Fasth et al., 1990), and Lebanon (Björck et al., 2000). Inheritance is autosomal recessive and consanguinity has been found in several ICF families (Østergaard, 1973; Fasth et al., 1990; Bauld et al., 1991; Wijmenga et al., 1998; Björck et al., 2000). Males and females appear to be equally affected and present with similar phenotypes.

Facial Anomalies

Mild facial dysmorphic features are found in most ICF patients (Color Plate 35.I). In 1978, Hultén described a boy with a peculiar facial appearance characterized by bilateral epicanthus and slight protrusion of the right external ear. The patient of Tiepolo et al. had an epicanthus and low nasal bridge (Tiepolo et al., 1978, 1979; Maraschio et al., 1988). Later on, several dysmorphisms were described, namely macroglossia (Fryns et al., 1981), micrognathia (Howard et al., 1985), and hypertelorism (Carpenter et al., 1988). The characteristic features in ICF syndrome that are currently considered part of the phenotype may include a round face with epicanthus, telecanthus, flat nasal bridge, hypertelorism, up-turned nose, macroglossia, micrognathia, and low-set ears. Many of these features become more obvious during childhood. Dysmorphic features are not always present in adult ICF patients. Turleau et al. (1989) noted facial anomalies and macroglossia in an ICF patient immediately after birth, but such characteristic features can be absent at birth. For example, the brother of the patient described by Smeets et al. (1994) did not show dysmorphic features until the age of 1 year when he presented with a round face and telecanthus (Color Plate 35.I).

Growth and Development

Most ICF patients have normal birth weight, although some patients have been significantly smaller than normal. Growth retardation occurred in some patients because of a failure to thrive following infections or gastrointestinal problems. Most ICF patients have shown a delay in walking as well as in initial speech. In addition, hypotonia was demonstrated in several patients

Table 35.1. Summary of Clinical Features

Facial Anomalies

Round face
Epicanthus
Telecanthus
Hypertelorism
Macroglossia
Flat nasal bridge
Micrognathia
Low-set ears
Up-turned nose

Infections

Lower respiratory tract infections
Otitis media
Failure to thrive
Opportunistic infections
Sepsis

Neurological Problems

Hypotonia
Delay in walking
Delay in initial speech
Intelligence: normal, subnormal, mentally retarded

Gastrointestinal Problems

Malabsorption
Ileus, motility disorder
Vomiting

(Carpenter et al., 1988; Schuffenhauer et al., 1995; Petit et al., 1997). Some ICF children need physiotherapy and/or speech therapy to learn to walk or talk.

The intelligence of ICF patients is quite variable. A few patients have been moderately or severely mentally retarded (Tiepolo et al., 1979; Howard et al., 1985; Gimelli et al., 1993; Schuffenhauer et al., 1995). The initial cytogenetic analysis for some of these patients, however, was performed because they presented with mental retardation and dysmorphisms rather than immunodeficiency. Because the cytogenetic abnormalities associated with ICF are characteristic (see below), the number of mentally retarded and/or dysmorphic ICF children may be overrepresented because of ascertainment bias. Because many patients succumb to infections at an early age, little is known about sexual development in ICF individuals. Puberty generally appears to be normal in the few cases followed. A pregnancy has been reported, for example, in one adult female patient, although her older affected brother is azoospermic (G. Gimelli, personal communication).

Infections

Infections are a prominent clinical feature in ICF syndrome, especially respiratory tract infections, which occur in nearly all cases (Table 35.1). Pneumonia, most often caused by *Haemophilus influenzae* or *Streptococcus pneumoniae* (Østergaard, 1973; Howard et al., 1985), is a common disease among ICF children. Bacterial sepsis, due to infection with *Klebsiella*, *Pseudomonas*, or *Staphyloccus aureus*, has occurred in several patients. In addition, opportunistic infections such as *Pneumocystis carinii* (Bauld et al., 1991), cytomegalovirus (CMV) (Fasth et al., 1990), and *Candida albicans* (Valkova et al., 1987; Fasth et al., 1990) frequently occur in ICF patients. One English ICF patient developed poliomyelitis after vaccination with an oral polio vaccine (G. Davies, personal communication). Despite substitution therapy with immunoglobulin, many ICF patients die from infection at a very young age.

Gastrointestinal Problems

Protruding abdomen has been described in several ICF patients (Fryns et al., 1981; Turleau et al., 1989; Smeets et al., 1994). Failure to thrive is common. Many patients suffer from diarrhea (Valkova et al., 1987; Maraschio et al., 1988; Turleau et al., 1989; Fasth et al., 1990; Smeets et al., 1994) and extended, total parenteral feeding was necessary in three children (Turleau et al., 1989; Smeets et al., 1994). Microorganisms such as *Cryptosporidium* or *Giardia lambliae* were not identified in these patients. Malabsorption was reported for several patients (Fryns et al., 1981; Turleau et al., 1989; Smeets et al., 1994; Petit et al., 1997), and villous atrophy has been demonstrated in some patients (Fryns et al., 1981; Carpenter et al., 1988; Turleau et al., 1989).

Laboratory Findings

Immune Function

One of the characteristic abnormalities in the ICF syndrome is immunodeficiency (Table 35.2). Agammaglobulinemia with normal number of B cells is the most common finding in ICF patients. The immune defect is quite variable, ranging from severe immunodeficiency to a nearly normal immune system. Microarray expression analysis of lymphoblastoid cell lines from ICF patients and controls suggests that mutations of *DNMT3B*, the gene responsible for ICF, cause lymphogenesis associated gene dysregulation by indirectly affecting gene expression; this may interfere with normal lymphocyte signaling, maturation and migration (Ehrlich et al., 2001). From the few families known to have more than one ICF patient, it has been suggested that siblings share a similar immunodeficiency phenotype (Fasth et al., 1990; C. Weemaes, unpublished observations). Immunodeficiency has been found in all but one ICF patient, who was reported to have only a slightly decreased number of CD4 cells (Gimelli et al., 1993). The first ICF patient reported (Hultén, 1978) was originally considered to have common variable immunodeficiency (CVID) with low IgG, IgA, and IgM, reduced numbers of T and B cells, and poor lymphocyte transformation with either phytohemagglutinin (PHA) or pokeweed mitogen (PWM). The ICF patient described the same year by Tiepolo et al. (1978, 1979) had IgA and IgE deficiency. Agammaglobulinemia, a decreased percentage of T cells, and low to normal in vitro lymphocyte proliferation to mitogens was found in others (Fryns et al., 1981; Fasth et al., 1990). Additional patients with agammaglobulinemia and normal B and T cells have subsequently been described (Howard et al., 1985; Smeets et al., 1994; Sawyer et al., 1995).

Table 35.2. Summary of Immunologic Features

Humoral Immunity

Absent or low levels of one or more of the immunglobulins IgG, IgA,
    and IgM
Disturbance in antibody synthesis

Cellular Immunity

Decreased number of CD3, CD4, and CD8 cells
Impaired lymphoproliferation by PHA, PWM, and antigens

PHA, phytohemagglutinin; PWM, pokeweed mitogen.

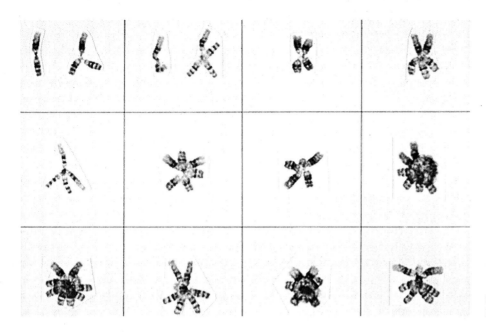

Figure 35.1. Cytogenetic abnormalities in ICF syndrome.

Lymphopenia with or without inverted CD4/CD8 ratio was reported in some individuals (Gimelli et al., 1993; Franceschini et al., 1995; Pezzolo et al., 2002). Hypogammaglobulinemia and abnormal antibody production to vaccinations and absence of isohemagglutinin were found in two boys with ICF (Franceschini et al., 1995). IgM deficiency, failure to produce antibodies to polysaccharide antigens, but a normal response to protein antigens such as tetanus toxoid and diphtheria toxoid was initially observed in a patient with ICF who subsequently was found to have normal IgM levels and normal isohemagglutinin titers; antibodies to *H. influenzae*, however, remained absent (Østergaard, 1973, 1977).

Cytogenetic Abnormalities

Aberrations of chromosomes 1 and/or 16 involving their heterochromatic pericentromeric blocks can be observed at high frequency in cultures of peripheral blood lymphocytes from ICF patients (Fig. 35.1). These aberrations can be recognized as gaps, breaks, deletions, isochromosomes, multiradial figures, interchanges between pericentromeric regions, and multiradial configurations. Two short arms of chromosomes 1 and 16 are present in all aberrant cells, with a varying number of long arms. These findings suggest that breaks occurred just below the centromere within the heterochromatic region on the proximal long arm (Haas, 1990). Similar aberrations involving chromosome 9 (Tiepolo et al., 1979; Fryns et al., 1981; Valkova et al., 1987) and, rarely, chromosomes 2 (Valkova et al., 1987) and 10 (Turleau et al., 1989) have also been reported.

The overall frequency of ICF cells with chromosomal aberrations increases with culture time (Tiepolo et al., 1979; Maraschio et al., 1988; Smeets et al., 1994), although the opposite has also been reported (Turleau et al., 1989). Moreover, aberrations become more complex with increasing time in culture (Hultén, 1978; Tiepolo et al., 1979; Howard et al., 1985; Smeets et al., 1994). Interphase nuclei consistently show an increased number of micronuclei and/or nuclear protrusions (Fasth et al., 1990; Maraschio et al., 1992). Fluorescence in situ hybridization (FISH) studies have clearly demonstrated that portions of chromosomes 1 and 16 are present in these micronuclei (Maraschio et al., 1992;

Smeets et al., 1994). Cultured peripheral blood lymphocytes always display numerous aberrations, whereas other tissues, such as cultured fibroblasts, Epstein-Barr virus (EBV)-transformed B cells, and bone marrow cells, usually show much fewer, if any, aberrant cells. When aberrations are present in such cells, they are usually reduced in complexity compared to those seen in lymphocytes (Howard et al., 1985; Maraschio et al., 1989; Turleau et al., 1989; Fasth et al., 1990; Gimelli et al., 1993).

Hypomethylation

Another diagnostic feature of ICF syndrome is hypomethylation of classical satellite repeats. The cytogenetic abnormalities seen in lymphocytes are quite similar to those found in normal cells treated with DNA demethylation agents such as 5-azacytidine (Viegas-Pequignot and Dutrillaux, 1976; Schmid et al., 1984). A defect in DNA methylation in ICF patients was therefore proposed (Maraschio et al., 1988). It has since been demonstrated by Southern blot analysis that the pericentromeric classical satellites involved in the 5-azacytidine–induced abnormalities in normal cells are indeed abnormally hypomethylated in ICF cells (Jeanpierre et al., 1993; Hassan et al., 2001). The pericentromeric satellite regions on chromosomes 1q and 16q are large heterochromatic regions comprised mainly of satellite 2 repeats. The analogous region on chromosome 9q contains a large concentration of satellite 3 repeats. The frequency of CpG dinucleotides at these loci is higher than that for most of the genome and they are normally hypermethylated in somatic cells, as evidenced by their resistance to digestion with methylation-sensitive restriction enzymes such as HpaII and BstBI. In ICF cells, however, these sequences are extensively digested with such enzymes, suggesting extreme undermethylation. These restriction enzyme–based data are largely supported by bisulfite methylation analysis of satellite 2 sequences, although hypomethylation of these sequences is not complete in ICF cells (Hassan et al., 2001).

The methylation status of other regions of the genome has also been examined in ICF cells. Genome-wide methylation is generally unaffected (Ji et al., 1997; Kondo et al., 2000), whereas undermethylation of other heterochromatic regions such as the

CpG islands of the inactive X (Miniou et al., 1994; Bourc'his et al., 1999; Hansen et al., 2000) and certain other CpG-rich repetitive elements (Kondo et al., 2000) is frequently observed.

Molecular Basis

Localization of the Defective Gene

Several ICF families have been described with multiple affected siblings, a finding suggesting a strong genetic basis for the syndrome (Valkova et al., 1987). That some of the ICF patients came from consanguineous marriages is consistent with autosomal recessive transmission (Valkova et al., 1987). The extremely rare occurrence of the ICF syndrome and the existence of affected inbred individuals made the localization of the ICF gene a suitable target for homozygosity mapping. This mapping approach is based on the inheritance of two identical copies of the disease locus by the affected inbred child from a common ancestor—i.e., homozygosity by descent (Lander and Botstein, 1987). Wijmenga et al. (1998) performed homozygosity mapping in three consanguineous ICF families: one of Dutch ancestry, and two that were Turkish. The Dutch ICF family included two affected brothers whose parents had common ancestors five generations previously; an initial genome-wide scan of this family was used to find regions that were homozygous and shared between the two affected sibs. Inclusion of the other two consanguineous families confirmed and delimited a 9 cM region on chromosome 20q11–q13 that was homozygous in all four affected inbred individuals (Wijmenga et al., 1998).

The chromosomal localization of the ICF gene to chromosome 20 was the first step in the positional cloning approach. Traditionally, the candidate region had to be narrowed down by analysis of additional ICF families, followed by cloning the region into workable pieces that would allow the isolation of genes and subsequent mutation analysis. A function-based, candidate gene approach, however, has increasingly become more attractive since chromosome-specific sequence data have become available from the Human Genome Project, including those from chromosome 20.

Identification of DNMT3B as the ICF Gene

Although the etiology of ICF syndrome was initially not clear, the hypomethylation observed in ICF patients suggested a role for DNA methylation in this disorder (Jeanpierre et al., 1993). This hypothesis was further substantiated by the observation that the cytogenetic abnormalities in ICF syndrome could be complemented by fusion of ICF cells to normal cells (Schuffenhauer et al., 1995). Cell fusion also led to a partial restoration of the de novo methylation of ICF satellite 2 and 3 sequences (Hansen et al., 1999), presumably through the activity of a functional de novo DNA methyltransferase from the non-ICF cell. Although there were no de novo DNA methyltransferase genes known to exist in the human genome at that time, two DNA methyltransferases (MT3α, encoded by Dnmt3a, and MT3β, encoded by Dnmt3b) with de novo activity had been identified in the mouse (Okano et al., 1998). Because of the strong evolutionary conservation between humans and mice, it was tempting to speculate that these genes would also exist in the human genome. A search of the raw sequence data from human chromosome 20 for the presence of a DNA methyltransferase gene led to the identification of a gene highly homologous to murine Dnmt3b. The DNMT3B gene was localized to 20q11 (by FISH and radiation hybrid mapping) within the 9 cM region to which the ICF gene had been localized previously. Mutations of this gene in ICF patients confirmed that DNMT3B was indeed a gene responsible for ICF syndrome (Hansen et al., 1999; Okano et al., 1999a; Xu et al., 1999).

Gene Structure and Mutational Analysis

The DNMT3B gene spans a region of about 50 kb and encodes a transcript of 4.3 kb representing 22 coding exons (Xie et al., 1999). Alternative splicing of the gene leads to at least five isoforms: DNMT3B1, DNMT3B2, DNMT3B3, DNMT3B4, and DNMT3B5 (Hansen et al., 1999; Robertson et al., 1999). DNMT3B expression can be detected in several tissues, but occurs at much higher levels in testis and thymus. The C-terminal region of the protein contains five highly conserved DNA methyltransferase motifs (I, IV, VI, IX, and X) (Xie et al., 1999) and a motif (VIII) with a much weaker similarity (Hansen et al., 1999). Functions for these motifs in the transmethylation reaction, such as cofactor binding, is inferred from crystallography data for other methyltransferases. The N-terminal region of MT3β contains a cysteine-rich domain that shows homology to the zinc finger helicase region found in the ATRX protein (Picketts et al., 1996) that might mediate protein–protein or protein–DNA interactions. Closer to the N terminus of MT3β is a PWWP domain that may also be involved in protein–protein interactions (Stec et al., 2000) but has subsequently been shown to bind DNA (Qiu et al., 2002). Recent reports suggest that DNMT3B binds nonspecifically to DNA via the PWWP domain (Chen et al., 2004) and that the PWWP domain is essential for targeting methyltransferase to pericentric heterochromatin in mammalian cells (Chen et al., 2004; Ge et al., 2004).

From the limited number of ICF patients who have been subjected to mutation analysis, 19 different mutations have been discovered in 17 ICF patients from 15 families (Fig. 35.2) (Hansen et al., 1999; Okano et al., 1999a; Xu et al., 1999; Wijmenga et al., 2000; Shirohzu et al., 2002). ICF mutations can be divided into three classes: (1) nonsense mutations that occur early in the transcript, (2) missense and splice site mutations in the methyltransferase catalytic domain, and (3) a missense mutation near the PWWP domain. While the nonsense mutations are not expected to result in protein, the second class of mutations leads to proteins with compromised catalytic activity (Xu et al., 1999; Gowher and Jeltsch, 2002). The missense mutation found within the PWWP domain in a Japanese ICF family (Shirohzu et al., 2002) suggests an important role for this motif in MT3β function. This prediction was confirmed experimentally by demonstrating that the protein with the naturally occurring mutation (S270P), located in the PWWP domain, completely loses its chromatin targeting capacity (Ge et al., 2004). Studies in mice (Okano et al., 1999b) have shown that complete MT3β deficiency is embryonically lethal; such lethality might also apply to humans. Consistent with the retention of some essential MT3β activity in ICF patients, all three predicted null mutations described thus far are accompanied by a missense mutation in the other allele (Xu et al., 1999; Wijmenga et al., 2000). Bisulfite methylation studies of ICF cells also support residual methyltransferase activity for missense mutant enzymes (Hassan et al., 2001). Furthermore, some of the missense mutations have been shown to produce proteins with significant methyltransferase activity in vitro (Gowher and Jeltsch, 2002).

Given the rarity of the disease and the finding of consanguinity in some ICF families, the early prediction was that most ICF

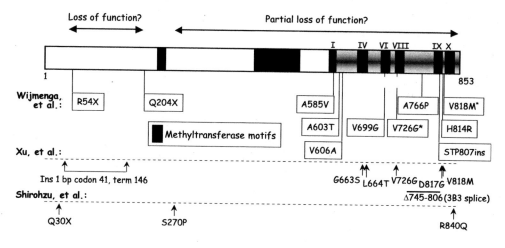

Figure 35.2. The *DNMT3B* gene and known ICF mutations. (Codon numbers for mutations refer to the largest isoform, 3B1 (genBank assession no. AF156488) (Hansen et al., 1999). Data presented are from Wijmenga et al. (2000), Xu et al. (1999), and Shirohzu et al. (2002).

cases would involve homozygous mutations derived from a limited number of founders. We now know, however, that only 8 of 17 ICF patients had homozygous mutations and that these all differed from each other, thus the majority of *DNMT3B* mutations may have arisen from several unique events. Alternatively, it is possible that the number of gene carriers—and, in turn, the number of potential ICF patients—is much larger than expected; some mutations may be incompatible with life in certain heterozygous combinations, while others may lead to extremely mild phenotypes that have not been connected to the ICF syndrome. Phenotype–genotype relationships have not been determined yet because of the limited set of patients with known mutations, many of which are compound heterozygotes. In addition, phenotypic variability is likely for any given mutation because the corresponding molecular defects are predicted to derive from epigenetic abnormalities that are intrinsically quite variable.

Genetic Heterogeneity

There are at least six ICF patients in which no *DNMT3B* mutation has been found (Wijmenga et al., 2000). Interestingly, at least two of these ICF2 patients are from consanguineous families but do not show homozygosity for the *DNMT3B* gene region on chromosome 20. This observation raises the intriguing possibility that the ICF syndrome is a genetically heterogeneous disorder in which more than one gene is involved in the disease etiology. It is now clear that the spectrum of hypomethylation defects is different in non-*DNMT3B* ICF cases. Although classical satellites are hypomethylated in both types of ICF, other regions, such as α satellites (Jiang et al., 2004), are only hypomethylated in ICF2 cases. Hypomethylation of the inactive X is more pronounced in *DNMT3B* cases (R.S. Hansen, unpublished observations). Localization of the ICF2 gene will probably require additional mapping studies. One complication is that non-*DNMT3B* ICF may also be heterogeneous because satellite 2 methylation levels differ among such cases (Hassan et al., 2001; Kubota et al., 2004).

Functional Aspects of the *DNMT3B* Gene

Genetic information, encoded by DNA sequences, is modulated by "epigenetic modification," which includes DNA methylation, demethylation, methyl-CpG-recognition, histone modification, and chromatin remodeling (Fitzpatrick and Wilson, 2003; Teitell and Richardson, 2003). Although we know that DNA methylation

plays important roles in vertebrate genome structure and expression, our understanding of how genomic methylation patterns are established and maintained is limited (Colot and Rossignol, 1999). The selective hypomethylation of heterochromatic regions in ICF cells may provide a model to explain these phenomena and guide us to the genes affected by this undermethylation that are involved in the ICF phenotype.

The primary defects leading to phenotypic consequences in ICF are predicted to result from abnormal escape from transcriptional silencing due to lack of methylation by MT3β. Hypomethylation and escape from silencing in ICF cells have been demonstrated for certain genes on the inactive X chromosome (Hansen et al., 2000; Gartler and Hansen, 2002; Tao et al., 2002; Hansen, 2003), the Y chromosome (Hansen et al., 2000), an autosomal repetitive element (Kondo et al., 2000), and an autosomal cancer-testis gene (Tao et al., 2002). In many cases hypomethylation in the promoter region is not sufficient for escape to occur because silencing is maintained by inactive histone modification, unless accompanied by advanced replication (Hansen et al., 2000; Gartler et al., 2004). Although it is not clear how these particular genes could be responsible for the ICF phenotype, it is likely that a similar mechanism is responsible for genes that do play key roles in facial development and the immune system. Abnormal gene regulation could also result from hypomethylation at pericentromeric regions or other repetitive, CpG-rich regions by a mechanism similar to the phenomenon of position-effect variegation found in yeast, *Drosophila*, and mammalian systems (Kleinjan and van Heyningen, 1998; Wakimoto, 1998). Genes of this type would be affected in *cis* because they are within or near repetitive regions that are normally hypermethylated and late replicating. In addition to transcriptional regulation abnormalities, immunoglobulin deficiency in ICF could potentially result from a failure to achieve productive germ-line rearrangements critical to B and T cell development because of hypomethylation within the rearrangement loci (Engler et al., 1993; Mostoslavsky et al., 1998; Whitehurst et al., 2000). This could lead to defective B cell differentiation, lack of memory B cells, and impaired B cell negative selection (Blanco-Betancourt et al., 2004).

In the immune system alone, the list of potential candidate genes for misregulation with ICF-like consequences is quite long (Fitzpatrick and Wilson, 2003; Teitell and Richardson, 2003). One hope for finding key genes involved in ICF is the cDNA microarray approach for large-scale studies of gene expression in normal and ICF cells. Such data may help to identify key pathways affected in ICF that might be targeted for therapeutic intervention. A similar problem exists for understanding the bases of phenotypic abnormalities associated with Rett syndrome; the gene defective in these patients codes for a protein, MECP2, that recognizes methylated DNA and acts as a transcriptional repressor (Amir et al., 1999).

Animal Model

Additional evidence that MT3α and MT3β do, indeed, have de novo methyltransferase activity came from studies in mice in which both genes were inactivated by homologous recombination (Okano et al., 1999a). The expression level of *Dnmt3a* and *Dnmt3b* are extremely high in undifferentiated embryonic stem cells but are rapidly down-regulated after differentiation and found at much lower levels in adult somatic tissues. Both *Dnmt3a* and *Dnmt3b* appear to be essential for mouse development, as the Dnmt3b$^{-/-}$ mice die before postconception day 11.5 and the Dnmt3a$^{-/-}$ mice die perinatally. The *Dnmt3a* and *Dnmt3b* genes exhibit some overlapping methylation target sites, but *Dnmt3b* deficiency specifically decreases methylation at pericentromeric minor satellite repeats, similar to the hypomethylation seen in ICF syndrome patients at analogous satellite repeats. Further studies of this model and of future conditional mutations and "knock-in" or transgene ICF mutations should help to elucidate the mechanisms underlying the ICF phenotype.

Strategies for Diagnosis

Without chromosome studies, most patients with ICF syndrome would be classified as suffering from CVID, according to the World Health Organization (WHO) classification for primary immunodeficiencies. ICF syndrome should be considered, therefore, for all patients with B cell–positive agammaglobulinemia or CVID without a known gene defect, even when facial anomalies are absent. A history of delayed milestones, such as walking and speech, is also suggestive of ICF syndrome. Diagnosis of ICF syndrome can be made by cytogenetic analysis and Southern blot analysis of satellite methylation. Direct confirmation of ICF can be expected to be obtained in about 70% of cases by performing mutation analysis of the *DNMT3B* gene (Wijmenga et al., 2000).

Prenatal Diagnosis

Prenatal diagnosis of ICF syndrome by linkage analysis has recently been performed in a Lebanese family that already had an ICF syndrome child. The family structure contained two consanguineous marriages and the proband was found to be homozygous for the ICF gene region. The fetus was heterozygous, and the couple was counseled that there was a more than 90% probability that the fetus would be unaffected, the uncertainty being due to the possibility of genetic heterogeneity (Björck et al., 2000). The couple decided to continue the pregnancy and a healthy boy was born. A homozygous *DNMT3B* mutation was demonstrated in the proband (Wijmenga et al., 2000), thus confirming the prenatal linkage analysis. In the future, the identification of *DNMT3B* mutations in ICF patients through direct mutational analysis will enable more accurate genetic counseling for their families.

Treatment and Prognosis

Nearly all ICF patients receive regular infusions of immunoglobulins. This treatment reduces the severity and frequency of infec-

tions in most patients. In spite of treatment, however, at least 10 patients have died in infancy or in childhood because of infections (Fryns et al., 1981; Valkova et al., 1987; Fasth et al., 1990; C. Weemaes, unpublished observations). Most of these patients suffered from agammaglobulinemia with some T cell defect, but a patient with only IgA deficiency also died at a young age (11 years) (Tiepolo et al., 1979).

Opportunistic infections with *Pneumocystis carinii* resulting in interstitial pneumonia (PCP), CMV, and *Candida* have been described (Valkova et al., 1987; Fasth et al., 1990; Bauld et al., 1991). Prophylactic use of trimethoprim-sulfamethoxazole to prevent PCP may be indicated, even when a T cell defect has not been demonstrated.

Bone marrow transplantation (BMT) should be considered in patients suffering from infections and failure to thrive. BMT was successful in two ICF patients with agammaglobulinemia (Gennery et al., 2004). The first patient had agammaglobulinemia, recurrent respiratory chest infections, and persistent norovirus diarrhea and poliovirus type 2 excretion associated with failure to thrive. Following partial conditioning with Alemtuzumab, Fludarabine, and Melphalan, she received marrow from an unrelated donor. At 18 months follow-up, the viruses had cleared, her weight had increased from below the first to the 25th percentile, T cell numbers were normal, B cell counts were low, and she remained on IVIG. The second patient presented with agammaglobulinemia and developed persistent diarrhea and intestinal ileus following *Campylobacter* infection at the age of 2 years. He received bone marrow from an HLA-identical sibling after a conditioning regimen consisting of busulfan and cyclophosphamide. He had normal T and B cell reconstitution and produced immunoglobulins 6 months after BMT. He is doing well without infections or intestinal problems. Because B cells are defective in ICF syndrome (Blanco-Betancourt et al., 2004), it is important to consider an extensive conditioning regimen to achieve not only T cell but also B cell reconstitution. Further investigation with mouse models should help to evaluate the efficacy of potential therapies.

Concluding Remarks

On the basis of our current knowledge, it is likely that a compromised MT3β methyltransferase leads to hypomethylation of specific chromosomal loci, de-heterochromatinization, advanced replication, and transcriptional activation of key genes whose misregulation affects facial and lymphocyte development. Discovery of such genes should further our understanding of the ICF phenotype and of the normal role of MT3β in methylation-dependent transcriptional regulation. Examination of the molecular properties of MT3β and its potential interacting proteins will help explain its apparent specificity for methylating heterochromatic regions and provide candidate genes that might be mutated in non-*DNMT3B*, ICF2 patients. Although the syndrome appears to be quite rare, increased ascertainment may develop as awareness of ICF increases and diagnosis of immunodeficiency includes more cytogenetic and/or methylation studies. Rare or not, the ICF syndrome provides one of the first examples of a human disease whose major defect alters the epigenetic structure and regulation of the genome and thus provides us with an excellent model system for study. Because proper epigenetic regulation is crucial for development and differentiation, explication of the epigenetic alterations in ICF and their functional consequences should have implications for a large spectrum of human disease.

References

Amir RE, Van Den Veyver IB, Wan M, Tran CQ, Francke U, Zoghbi HY. Rett syndrome is caused by mutations in X-linked MECP2, encoding methyl-CpG-binding protein 2. Nat Genet 23:185–188, 1999.

Bauld R, Grace E, Richards N, Ellis PM. The ICF syndrome: a rare chromosome instability syndrome. J Med Genet 28:63a, 1991.

Björck EJ, Bui TH, Wijmenga C, Grandell U, Nordenskjöld M. Early prenatal diagnosis of the ICF syndrome. Prenat Diagn 20:828–831, 2000.

Blanco-Betancourt CE, Moncla A, Milili M, Jiang YL, Viegas-Pequignot EM, Roquelaure B, Thuret I, Schiff C. Defective B-cell-negative selection and terminal differentiation in the ICF syndrome. Blood 103:2683–2690, 2004.

Bourc'his D, Miniou P, Jeanpierre M, Molina Gomes D, Dupont J, De Saint-Basile G, Maraschio P, Tiepolo L, Viegas-Pequignot E. Abnormal methylation does not prevent X inactivation in ICF patients. Cytogenet Cell Genet 84:245–252, 1999.

Carpenter NJ, Filipovich A, Blaese RM, Carey TL, Berkel AI. Variable immunodeficiency with abnormal condensation of the heterochromatin of chromosomes 1, 9, and 16. J Pediatr 112:757–760, 1988.

Chen T, Tsujimoto N, Li E. The PWWP domain of Dnmt3a and Dnmt3b is required for directing DNA methylation to the major satellite repeats at pericentric heterochromatin. Mol Cell Bol 24:9048–9058, 2004.

Colot V, Rossignol JL. Eukaryotic DNA methylation as an evolutionary device. Bioessays 21:402–411, 1999.

Ehrlich M, Buchanan KL, Tsien F, Jiang G, Sun B, Uicker W, Weemaes CMR, Smeets D, Sperling K, Belohradsky BH, Tommerup N, Misek DE, Rouillard J-M, Kuick R, Hanash SM. DNA methyltransferase 3B mutations linked to the ICF syndrome cause dysregulation of lymphogenesis genes. Hum Mol Genet 10:2917–2931, 2001.

Engler P, Weng A, Storb U. Influence of CpG methylation and target spacing on V(D)J recombination in a transgenic substrate. Mol Cell Biol 13:571–577, 1993.

Fasth A, Forestier E, Holmberg E, Holmgren G, Nordenson I, Soderstrom T, Wahlstrom J. Fragility of the centromeric region of chromosome 1 associated with combined immunodeficiency in siblings. A recessively inherited entity? Acta Paediatr Scand 79:605–612, 1990.

Fitzpatrick DR, Wilson CB. Methylation and demethylation in the regulation of genes, cells, and responses in the immune system. Clin Immunol 109:37–45, 2003.

Franceschini P, Martino S, Ciocchini M, Ciuti E, Vardeu MP, Guala A, Signorile F, Camerano P, Franceschini D, Tovo PA. Variability of clinical and immunological phenotype in immunodeficiency–centromeric instability–facial anomalies syndrome. Report of two new patients and review of the literature. Eur J Pediatr 154:840–846, 1995.

Fryns JP, Azou M, Jaeken J, Eggermont E, Pedersen JC, Van den Berghe H. Centromeric instability of chromosomes 1, 9, and 16 associated with combined immunodeficiency. Hum Genet 57:108–110, 1981.

Gartler SM, Hansen RS. ICF syndrome cells as a model system for studying X chromosome inactivation. Cytogenet Genome Res 99:25–29, 2002.

Gartler SM, Varadarajan KR, Luo P, Canfield TK, Traynor J, Francke U, Hansen RS. Normal histone modifications on the inactive X chromosome in ICF and Rett syndrome cells: implications for methyl-CpG binding proteins. BMC Biol 2:21, 2004.

Ge YZ, Pu MT, Gowher H, Wu HP, Ding JP, Jeltsch A, Xu GL. Chromatin targeting of de novo DNA methyltransferases by the PWWP domain. J Biol Chem 279:25447–25454, 2004.

Gennery AR, Lankester AC, Slatter MA, Bredius RG, Flood TJ, Breese GJ, Cant AJ, Weemaes C. Successful bone marrow transplantation for immunodeficiency, centromeric instability and facial anomalies (ICF) syndrome. In: Proceedings from the 11th Meeting for the European Society for Immunodeficiencies, pp. 94–95, 2004.

Gimelli G, Varone P, Pezzolo A, Lerone M, Pistoia V. ICF syndrome with variable expression in sibs. J Med Genet 30:429–432, 1993.

Gowher H, Jeltsch A. Molecular enzymology of the catalytic domains of the Dnmt3a and Dnmt3b DNA methyltransferases. J Biol Chem 277:20409–20414, 2002.

Haas OA. Centromeric heterochromatin instability of chromosomes 1, 9, and 16 in variable immunodeficiency syndrome—a virus-induced phenomenon? Hum Genet 85:244–246, 1990.

Hansen RS. X inactivation–specific methylation of LINE-1 elements by DNMT3B: implications for the Lyon repeat hypothesis. Hum Mol Genet 12:2559–2567, 2003.

Hansen RS, Stoger R, Wijmenga C, Stanek AM, Canfield TK, Luo P, Matarazzo MR, D'Esposito M, Feil R, Gimelli G, Weemaes CM, Laird CD, Gartler SM. Escape from gene silencing in ICF syndrome: evidence

for advanced replication time as a major determinant. Hum Mol Genet 9:2575–2587, 2000.

Hansen RS, Wijmenga C, Luo P, Stanek AM, Canfield TK, Weemaes CMR, Gartler SM. The DNMT3B DNA methyltransferase gene is mutated in the ICF immunodeficiency syndrome. Proc Natl Acad Sci USA 96:14412–14417, 1999.

Hassan KM, Norwood T, Gimelli G, Gartler SM, Hansen RS. Satellite 2 methylation patterns in normal and ICF syndrome cells and association of hypomethylation with advanced replication. Hum Genet 109:452–462, 2001.

Howard PJ, Lewis IJ, Harris F, Walker S. Centromeric instability of chromosomes 1 and 16 with variable immune deficiency: a new syndrome. Clin Genet 27:501–505, 1985.

Hultén M. Selective somatic pairing and fragility at 1q12 in a boy with common variable immunodeficiency. Clin Genet 14:294, 1978.

Jeanpierre M, Turleau C, Aurias A, Prieur M, Ledeist F, Fischer A, Viegas-Pequignot E. An embryonic-like methylation pattern of classical satellite DNA is observed in ICF syndrome. Hum Mol Genet 2:731–735, 1993.

Ji W, Hernandez R, Zhang XY, Qu GZ, Frady A, Varela M, Ehrlich M. DNA demethylation and pericentromeric rearrangements of chromosome 1. Mutat Res 379:33–41, 1997.

Jiang YL, Rigolet M, Bourc'his D, Nigon F, Bokesoy I, Fryns JP, Hulten M, Jonveaux P, Maraschio P, Megarbane A, Moncla A, Viegas-Pequignot E. DNMT3B mutations and DNA methylation defect define two types of ICF syndrome. Hum Mutat 25:56–63, 2004.

Kleinjan DJ, van Heyningen V. Position effect in human genetic disease. Hum Mol Genet 7:1611–1618, 1998.

Kondo T, Bobek MP, Kuick R, Lamb B, Zhu X, Narayan A, Bourc'his D, Viegas-Pequignot E, Ehrlich M, Hanash SM. Whole-genome methylation scan in ICF syndrome: hypomethylation of non-satellite DNA repeats D4Z4 and NBL2. Hum Mol Genet 9:597–604, 2000.

Kubota T, Furuumi H, Kamoda T, Iwasaki N, Tobita N, Fujiwara N, Goto Y, Matsui A, Sasaki H, Kajii T. ICF syndrome in a girl with DNA hypomethylation but without detectable DNMT3B mutation. Am J Med Genet 129:290–293, 2004.

Lander ES, Botstein D. Homozygosity mapping: a way to map human recessive traits with the DNA of inbred children. Science 236:1567–1570, 1987.

Maraschio P, Cortinovis M, Dainotti E, Tupler R, Tiepolo L. Interphase cytogenetics of the ICF syndrome. Ann Hum Genet 56:273–278, 1992.

Maraschio P, Tupler R, Dainotti E, Piantanida M, Cazzola G, Tiepolo L. Differential expression of the ICF (immunodeficiency, centromeric heterochromatin, facial anomalies) mutation in lymphocytes and fibroblasts. J Med Genet 26:452–456, 1989.

Maraschio P, Zuffardi O, Dalla Fior T, Tiepolo L. Immunodeficiency, centromeric heterochromatin instability of chromosomes 1, 9, and 16, and facial anomalies: the ICF syndrome. J Med Genet 25:173–180, 1988.

Miniou P, Jeanpierre M, Blanquet V, Sibella V, Bonneau D, Herbelin C, Fischer A, Niveleau A, Viegas-Pequignot E. Abnormal methylation pattern in constitutive and facultative (X inactive chromosome) heterochromatin of ICF patients. Hum Mol Genet 3:2093–2102, 1994.

Mostoslavsky R, Singh N, Kirillov A, Pelanda R, Cedar H, Chess A, Bergman Y. Kappa chain monoallelic demethylation and the establishment of allelic exclusion. Genes Dev 12:1801–1811, 1998.

Okano M, Bell DW, Haber DA, Li E. DNA methyltransferases Dnmt3a and Dnmt3b are essential for de novo methylation and mammalian development. Cell 99:247–257, 1999a.

Okano M, Takebayashi S, Okumura K, Li E. Assignment of cytosine-5 DNA methyltransferases Dnmt3a and Dnmt3b to mouse chromosome bands 12A2-A3 and 2H1 by in situ hybridization. Cytogenet Cell Genet 86:333–334, 1999b.

Okano M, Xie S, Li E. Cloning and characterization of a family of novel mammalian DNA (cytosine-5) methyltransferases. Nat Genet 19:219–220, 1998.

Østergaard PA. A girl with recurrent infections, low IgM and an abnormal chromosome number 1. Acta Paediatr Scand 62:211–215, 1973.

Østergaard PA. Clinical aspects of transient immunoglobulin deficiency in children. Dan Med Bull 24:206–209, 1977.

Petit P, Alliët P, Gillis P, Fryns JP. ICF syndrome (immunodeficiency–centromeric instability–facial anomalies syndrome): delineation of the clinical syndrome. Genet Couns 8:67, 1997.

Pezzolo A, Prigione I, Chiesa S, Castellano E, Gimelli G, Pistoia V. A novel case of immunodeficiency, centromeric instability, and facial anomalies (the ICF syndrome): immunologic and cytogenetic studies. Haematologica 87:329–331, 2002.

Picketts DJ, Higgs DR, Bachoo S, Blake DJ, Quarrell OW, Gibbons RJ. ATRX encodes a novel member of the SNF2 family of proteins: mutations point to a common mechanism underlying the ATR-X syndrome. Hum Mol Genet 5:1899–1907, 1996.

Qiu C, Sawada K, Zhang X, Cheng X. The PWWP domain of mammalian DNA methyltransferase Dnmt3b defines a new family of DNA-binding folds. Nat Struct Biol 9:217–224, 2002.

Robertson KD, Uzvolgyi E, Liang G, Talmadge C, Sumegi J, Gonzales FA, Jones PA. The human DNA methyltransferases (DNMTs) 1, 3a and 3b: coordinate mRNA expression in normal tissues and overexpression in tumors. Nucl Acids Res 27:2291–2298, 1999.

Sawyer JR, Swanson CM, Wheeler G, Cunniff C. Chromosome instability in ICF syndrome: formation of micronuclei from multibranched chromosomes 1 demonstrated by fluorescence in situ hybridization. Am J Med Genet 56:203–209, 1995.

Schmid M, Haaf T, Grunert D. 5-Azacytidine-induced undercondensations in human chromosomes. Hum Genet 67:257–263, 1984.

Schuffenhauer S, Bartsch O, Stumm M, Buchholz T, Petropoulou T, Kraft S, Belohradsky B, Hinkel GK, Meitinger T, Wegner RD. DNA, FISH and complementation studies in ICF syndrome: DNA hypomethylation of repetitive and single copy loci and evidence for a trans acting factor. Hum Genet 96:562–571, 1995.

Shirohzu H, Kubota T, Kumazawa A, Sado T, Chijiwa T, Inagaki K, Suetake I, Tajima S, Wakui K, Miki Y, Hayashi M, Fukushima Y, Sasaki H. Three novel *DNMT3B* mutations in Japanese patients with ICF syndrome. Am J Med Genet 112:31–37, 2002.

Smeets DF, Moog U, Weemaes CM, Vaes-Peeters G, Merkx GF, Niehof JP, Hamers G. ICF syndrome: a new case and review of the literature. Hum Genet 94:240–246, 1994.

Stec I, Nagl SB, van Ommen GJ, den Dunnen JT. The PWWP domain: a potential protein–protein interaction domain in nuclear proteins influencing differentiation? FEBS Lett 473:1–5, 2000.

Tao Q, Huang H, Geiman TM, Lim CY, Fu L, Qiu GH, Robertson KD. Defective de novo methylation of viral and cellular DNA sequences in ICF syndrome cells. Hum Mol Genet 11:2091–2102, 2002.

Teitell M, Richardson B. DNA methylation in the immune system. Clin Immunol 109:2–5, 2003.

Tiepolo L, Maraschio P, Gimelli G, Cuoco C, Gargani GF, Romano C. Concurrent instability at specific sites of chromosomes 1, 9 and 16 resulting in multibranched structures. Clin Genet 14:313–314, 1978.

Tiepolo L, Maraschio P, Gimelli G, Cuoco C, Gargani GF, Romano C. Multibranched chromosomes 1, 9, and 16 in a patient with combined IgA and IgE deficiency. Hum Genet 51:127–137, 1979.

Turleau C, Cabanis MO, Girault D, Ledeist F, Mettey R, Puissant H, Prieur M, de Grouchy J. Multibranched chromosomes in the ICF syndrome: immunodeficiency, centromeric instability, and facial anomalies. Am J Med Genet 32:420–424, 1989.

Valkova G, Ghenev E, Tzancheva M. Centromeric instability of chromosomes 1, 9 and 16 with variable immune deficiency. Support of a new syndrome. Clin Genet 31:119–124, 1987.

Viegas-Pequignot E, Dutrillaux B. Segmentation of human chromosomes induced by 5-ACR (5-azacytidine). Hum Genet 34:247–254, 1976.

Wakimoto BT. Beyond the nucleosome: epigenetic aspects of position-effect variegation in *Drosophila*. Cell 93:321–324, 1998.

Whitehurst CE, Schlissel MS, Chen J. Deletion of germline promoter PD beta 1 from the TCR beta locus causes hypermethylation that impairs D beta 1 recombination by multiple mechanisms. Immunity 13:703–714, 2000.

Wijmenga C, Hansen RS, Gimelli G, Björck EJ, Davies G, Valentine D, Belohradsky BH, van Dongen JJ, Smeets DFCM, van den Heuvel LPWJ, Luyten JAFM, Strengman E, Weemaes C, Pearson PL. Genetic variation in ICF syndrome: evidence for genetic heterogeneity. Hum Mutat 16: 509–517, 2000.

Wijmenga C, van den Heuvel LP, Strengman E, Luyten JA, van der Burgt IJ, de Groot R, Smeets DF, Draaisma JM, van Dongen JJ, De Abreu RA, Pearson PL, Sandkuijl LA, Weemaes CM. Localization of the ICF syndrome to chromosome 20 by homozygosity mapping. Am J Hum Genet 63:803–809, 1998.

Xie S, Wang Z, Okano M, Nogami M, Li Y, He WW, Okumura K, Li E. Cloning, expression and chromosome locations of the human *DNMT3* gene family. Gene 236:87–95, 1999.

Xu GL, Bestor TH, Bourc'his D, Hsieh CL, Tommerup N, Bugge M, Hulten M, Qu X, Russo JJ, Viegas-Pequignot E. Chromosome instability and immunodeficiency syndrome caused by mutations in a DNA methyltransferase gene. Nature 402:187–191, 1999.

36

Immunodeficiencies with Associated Manifestations of Skin, Hair, Teeth, and Skeleton

MARIO ABINUN, ILKKA KAITILA, and JEAN-LAURENT CASANOVA

In several complex syndromes associated with immunodeficiency (reviewed by Ming et al., 1996, 1999), immunological defects are combined with abnormalities of the skin, hair, and teeth. Most of these conditions, such as the Chediak-Higashi syndrome, Griscelli syndrome, Kotzot syndrome, Wiskott-Aldrich syndrome, Omenn syndrome, and dyskeratosis congenita, have been reviewed (Ming et al., 1996, 1999; Pignata et al., 2001) and are discussed in other chapters in this book (see Chapters 12, 29, 33–35, 40, and 41). A mutation in the human ortholog of the *nude/whn* gene (Frank et al., 1999; Pignata et al., 2001) has been identified in only one family and thus will not be reviewed here. We will focus on two syndromes associated with skin, hair, dental, and skeletal anomalies: anhidrotic ectodermal dysplasia with immunodeficiency (EDA-ID), and cartilage-hair hypoplasia (CHH).

Anhidrotic (Hypohidrotic) Ectodermal Dysplasia with Immune Deficiency

Description and Historical Overview

The main clinical features of anhidrotic (hypohidrotic) ectodermal dysplasia (EDA) include hypo- or anodontia with conical-shaped maxillary incisors, dry skin with hypo- or anhidrosis, and hypo- or atrichosis. In addition, most patients suffer from recurrent but mainly benign respiratory tract infections (Clarke et al., 1987). Historically, the most common immunological abnormality reported in these patients has been dysgammaglobulinaemia with low immunoglobulin (Ig) G and low or elevated IgM levels (Franken, 1966; Davis et al., 1976; Huntley and Ross, 1981; Clarke, et al., 1987). Although some patients have been described with unusually severe infections due to different microorganisms, including pseudomonas and mycobacteria (Frix and Bronson, 1986; Sitton and Reimund, 1992; Smythe et al., 2000), the syn-

drome *immunodeficiency associated with ectodermal dysplasia* was classified only recently as an independent primary immunodeficiency (World Health Organization, 1999). However, without consistent humoral or cellular immune functional defects and no clear mode of inheritance, this syndrome has not always been recognized as an autonomous disorder (Abinun, 1995). For instance, it was still not recognized in the 12th edition of Mc Kusick's *Catalog of Mendelian Inheritance of Man* in 1998.

A small number of male patients with classical features of EDA have been reported with severe, life-threatening infections with pyogenic bacteria such as *Streptococcus pneumoniae* and *Staphylococcus aureus* (Abinun et al., 1996; Schweizer et al., 1999). All had associated specific polysaccharide antibody deficiency, pointing toward the possibility of a distinct recessive X-linked entity resulting in EDA with impaired antibody response to polysaccharides (XL-EDA-ID). The nature of this association is not clear and a transient maturational delay or a persistent selective impaired response to polysaccharide antigens could be the explanation, as had been proposed for children without features of EDA who suffer from recurrent respiratory infections (Rijkers et al., 1993; Sanders et al., 1993). Progressive immunoglobulin deficiency may develop in some of these patients, however, and recently a mutation in *Btk* (Bruton's tyrosine kinase) has been reported as one of the underlying causes (Wood et al., 2001).

Recent progress has been made in our understanding of the molecular basis of the related syndromes of EDA without immune deficiency (ID) (Priolo and Lagana, 2001). Mutations in *EDA*, the gene encoding for ectodysplasin-A (Eda), a transmembrane protein required for development of ectodermal appendages, cause the X-linked form of EDA (MIM *305100) (Kere et al., 1996; Monreal et al., 1998). This protein is a member of the tumor necrosis factor (TNF) family of proteins (Copley, 1999; Ezer et al., 1999). Both the autosomal dominant (MIM 129490) and the autosomal recessive (MIM 224900) forms of EDA, by contrast, are caused by mutations in the *EDAR* gene (MIM *604095) (originally *DL* corresponds to the mouse downless [*dl*] phenotype) on chromosome 2 (Monreal et al., 1999). The protein encoded by this gene acts as a receptor for Eda (EDAR) and is a member of TNF receptor (TNFR) family of proteins, so these two proteins function as receptor and ligand in a common signaling pathway (Kumar et al., 2001).

The breakthrough in our understanding of the association of EDA and immunodeficiency came with the recent description of a surviving male patient from a family affected by X-linked incontinentia pigmenti (IP) (MIM 308300) due to a mutation in the *NEMO* (*NF-κB Essential MOdulator*) or *IKBG* (Inhibitor of *Kappa* light polypeptide gene enhancer in *B* cells, kinase, *Gamma*) gene (MIM 300248) (Smahi et al., 2000). This gene is essential for intact NF-κB activation, which plays a central role in the inhibition of apoptosis, host defense, and inflammatory responses (Karin and Lin, 2002). The germ-line loss-of-function mutations in *NEMO* are lethal in male fetuses affected by familial IP, an X-linked dominant syndrome. This surviving male, however, and subsequently described male patients (Smahi et al., 2000; Zonana et al., 2000; Aradhya et al., 2001; Doffinger et al., 2001; Jain et al., 2001; Mansour et al., 2001; Dupuis-Girod et al., 2002), have milder *NEMO* mutations that impair but do not abolish NF-κB signaling. Different hypomorphic mutations of *NEMO* cause two distinct XL allelic syndromes of IP: missense mutations in the coding region are associated with the EDA-ID phenotype (MIM 300291), whereas stop codon mutations cause a clinically more severe syndrome that includes features of osteopetrosis and/or lymphoedema (OL-EDA-ID) (MIM 300301). Here we will review the syndromes of XL-EDA-ID and XL-OL-EDA-ID, associated with *NEMO* mutations, excluding other forms of EDA-ID of unknown molecular basis.

Clinical and Pathological Manifestations

The main developmental features are those of EDA, although they are somewhat milder than those in children with "classical" EDA without immunodeficiency, and most patients have normal or sparse scalp hair. Of 33 patients from 23 kindreds reported to date (Table 36.1), 2 unrelated children manifested a more severe phenotype with features including osteopetrosis and lymphedema—i.e., OL-EDA-ID (Smahi et al., 2000; Doffinger et al., 2001; Mansour et al., 2001; Dupuis-Girod et al., 2002). Two related

children from another kindred have been described with EDA-ID and increased bone density (Zonana et al., 2000), a finding suggesting that osteopetrosis could be a variable clinical part of this syndrome. Only in a few of the reported mothers of affected boys in EDA-ID kindreds had variable features of EDA or IP (dry and/or hyperpigmented skin, hypodontia, conical teeth) and elevated IgA levels, whereas mothers of both children with the OL-EDA-ID phenotype showed mild features of IP.

Affected boys suffer in early childhood from unusually severe, life-threatening, and recurrent bacterial infections of the lower respiratory tract, skin and soft tissues, bones, and gastrointestinal tract; meningitis; and septicemia. The causative pathogens have most often been gram-positive bacteria (*Streptococcus pneumoniae, Staphylococcus aureus*), followed by gram-negative bacteria (*Pseudomonas* species, *Haemophilus influenzae*) and mycobacteria (Table 36.1). Interestingly, two children had *Pneumocystis jiroveci* infection and two others had severe adenovirus and cytomegalovirus (CMV) infections, which suggest a more profound and combined immunodeficiency. The two children with XL-OL-EDA-ID had a particularly severe phenotype, as they acquired *Mycobacterium* infections in the first year of life and died. A comprehensive description of the clinical features of children with XL-EDA-ID and XL-OL-EDA-ID is not yet available, but an international survey has been undertaken. Data in Table 36.1 are based exclusively on material published by authors cited above.

Laboratory Findings

An international survey has been undertaken to describe the immunologic abnormalities of patients carrying mutations in *NEMO*. Data in Table 36.2 are based on the available literature. B cell abnormalities are the predominant feature of the routine immunologic work-up. Most patients have hypogammaglobulinemia with a low IgG (and IgG2) level in serum, while the levels of other immunoglobulin isotypes (IgA, IgM, and IgE) vary. Occasionally, patients with EDA-ID may have markedly elevated serum IgA levels, possibly as a consequence of recurrent respiratory infections. A number of patients with EDA-ID have been described with elevated serum IgM levels (the hyper-IgM phenotype) (Zonana et al., 2000; Doffinger et al., 2001; Jain et al., 2001). However, despite normal CD40 ligand (CD154) expression on

Table 36.1. Clinical Features of Anhidrotic Ectodermal Dysplasia with Immune Deficiency

Features of Anhidrotic Ectoderma Dysplasia	Reccurent Severe Bacterial Infections*
Inability to sweat and dry skin	Pneumonia
Delayed dentition and conical teeth	Cellulitis, abscesses
Sparse scalp hair (variable)	Meningitis
Family history of EDA or IP (mothers, variable)	Septicemia
	Gastroenteritis
Other Features	*Complications*
Osteopetrosis	Bronchiectasis and chronic lung disease
Lymphoedema	Intractable diarrhea and failure to thrive

*Bacteria include *Streptococcus pneumoniae*, *Staphylococcus aureus*, *Pseudomonas* species, *Haemophilus influenzae*, and mycobacteria.

Table 36.2. Laboratory Findings (Routine Immunology Tests) of Anhidrotic Ectodermal Dysplasia with Immune Deficiency

Usually Found

Hypogammaglobulinemia (IgG, IgG2; occasionally IgA, IgM, IgE)
Elevated levels of IgM (often)
Elevated levels of IgA (often)
Absent or low isohemagglutinin titers
Absent or low specific antibody levels to polysaccharide antigens (after naturally occurring *S. pneumoniae* infection or post-Pneumovax)
Deficient NK cell cytotoxicity (K562 killing) (in some patients)

Normal

Peripheral blood lymphocyte numbers and subpopulations (CD3+, CD3/4+, CD3/8+, CD19+, CD3−/16+/56+)
CD40 ligand expression
T cell function (mitogen- and antigen-induced proliferation)
Neutrophil and complement function
Specific antibody levels to protein antigens
Antibody-dependent cell cytotoxicity (ADCC)

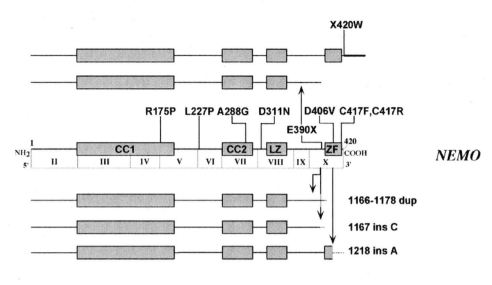

Figure 36.1. *NEMO* mutations associated with XL-OL-EDA-ID and XL-EDA-ID. The human NEMO protein is shown with the mutations identified in kindreds with EDA-ID and OL-EDA-ID. X420W leads to a predicted 27–amino acid elongated protein. Frameshift insertions, such as 1167insC and 1218insA, cause premature stops. The predicted out-of-frame protein sequence is shown by a dotted line. The structural domains of NEMO are indicated: coiled coil (CC1 and CC2), leucine zipper (LZ), and zinc finger (ZF).

their activated T cells and CD40 expression on B cells, their B cells were not able to proliferate (Doffinger et al., 2001), express surface CD27, or up-regulate CD54 expression when stimulated with trimeric CD40 ligand (Jain et al., 2001). They were capable of IgE production and expression of CD23 (Doffinger et al., 2001). These experiments show that some but not all CD40-mediated signals are NEMO-dependent in B cells. B cells have kept an intrinsic ability to switch in response to CD40L, but impairment of proliferation and activation results in a hyper-IgM–like phenotype in some patients. The impaired antibody response to polysaccharide antigens, with low specific antibodies after infection caused by *S. pneumoniae* or post immunization with polyvalent pneumococcal polysaccharide vaccine, and low isohemagglutinin titers are the most consistent laboratory features (Table 36.2).

In contrast to these B cell abnormalities, patients with XL-EDA-ID and XL-OL-EDA-ID have normal T cell proliferation to mitogens and antigens. Recently, three new patients with XL-EDA-ID and deficient CD40 signaling were described with deficient natural killer (NK) cell cytotoxicity (deficient K562 killing); however, their peripheral blood NK cell numbers and antibody-dependent cell cytotoxicity (ADCC) were normal (Orange et al., 2002).

Molecular Basis

Because not all investigated families with the X-linked form of EDA have mutations of *EDA* and no immunodeficiency has been seen in most families with known *EDA* mutations (Monreal et al., 1998), different mechanisms may be involved in development of skin and the immune system to be involved in. Indeed, the importance of NF-κB activation has been shown to be linked with the EDA/EDAR pathway. Whereas EDAR binds the EDA-1 isoform of the ectodysplastin receptor protein, an X-linked form of the receptor (XEDAR; MIM *300276) binds EDA-2 isoform and causes activation of NF-κB through binding of TNF receptor–associated factor-6 (TRAF6) (Yan et al., 2000). Final evidence of the role of NF-κB activation in the pathogenesis of this syndrome was shown when the International Incontinentia Pigmenti Consortium (IIPC) demonstrated that loss-of function mutations in *NEMO* cause X-linked dominant IP and that the most common one (~80% of new mutations) is a genomic rearrangement resulting in deletion of part of the gene (exons 4–10). The conse-

quence is loss of NEMO (IKBKG) function (vide infra) and lack of NF-κB activation (Aradhya and Nelson, 2001; Courtois et al., 2001). These features in turn result in extreme susceptibility to apoptosis and lead to embryonic death in males. The clinical features and extremely skewed X inactivation seen in females with IP are also explained by these deficiencies (Smahi et al., 2000). The finding of another, different mutation of *NEMO* affecting the stop codon in a surviving male (Table 36.1 and Fig. 36.1) raised the question of whether this milder phenotype is the result of partial loss of NEMO function.

Indeed, several groups have subsequently reported different mutations in both previously described (Sitton and Reimund, 1992; Abinun et al., 1996; Schweizer et al., 1999; Doffinger et al., 2001) and newly diagnosed patients (Zonana et al., 2000; Aradhya et al., 2001; Doffinger et al., 2001; Jain et al., 2001) with association of EDA and immunodeficiency (Table 36.1). Both the original patient (Doffinger et al., 2001; Smahi et al., 2000; Mansour et al., 2001), now diagnosed as allelic OL-EDA-ID phenotype rather than IP, and another unrelated patient (Doffinger et al., 2001; Dupuis-Girod et al., 2002) had the hypomorphic X420W stop codon mutation. Sequence analysis in four families (Zonana et al., 2000) revealed mutations in exon 10 (MIM 300248.0007-300248.0010) affecting the C terminus of the NEMO protein, a domain believed to connect the IκB kinase (IKK) signaling complex to upstream activators. In this group, two boys from the same kindred had features of subclinical osteopetrosis, but not lymphedema, associated with EDA-ID. The frameshift mutation in exon 10 at codon 390 (1167–1168insC) resulted in a premature stop at codon 394. However, another described patient with the same mutation had no features of osteopetrosis (Doffinger et al., 2001). The nonsense mutation at codon 391 (E391X), resulting in truncated protein and 1218insA frameshift mutation, both in exon 10, as well as the previous two mutations, leads to prevention of translation (Doffinger et al., 2001) or deletion (Zonana et al., 2000) of the *NEMO* C-terminal zinc-finger domain. A number of other missense mutations have been reported (Doffinger et al., 2001; Orange et al., 2002), but the vast majority occurred in exon 10 and almost half of these affect cysteine 417, a key residue of the C-terminal zinc-finger domain of *NEMO* (Zonana et al., 2000; Doffinger et al., 2001).

Similar mutations C417R and N406V in the putative zinc-finger motif of *NEMO*, a potentially shared intracellular signaling component for DL (EDAR) and CD40L, were reported in two patients with the hyper-IgM phenotype (the XHM-ED syndrome) (Jain et al., 2001). Two families with atypical IP type II were reported with duplications of 13 bp at a cytosine tract in exon 10 and intron 3 to exon 6 (Aradhya et al., 2001; Nishikomori et al., 2004). These duplication mutations allowed males to survive and affected females to have random or slightly skewed X inactivation. These findings suggest that these hypomorphic mutations are not deleterious enough to cause lethality in cells with an active mutant X chromosome and are consistent with the survival to term of affected males in these families. Rather than VOIMIE syndrome (Vascular anomalies, Osteopetrosis, Immune dysfunction in Males with IP or ED), as suggested by Aradhya and Nelson (2001), we propose that XHM-ED and atypical IP type II be designated XL-EDA-ID, as they are all caused by hypomorphic mutations in the coding region of NEMO. In males, there is a correlation between the type of NEMO mutation and the clinical phenotype, since loss-of-function mutations cause IP and stop-codon hypomorphic mutations found in two patients cause the allelic XL-OL-EDA-ID syndrome. Whether there is a further form of correlation between specific NEMO coding region hypomorphic mutations and cellular and clinical phenotypes is currently being investigated (Puel et al., 2006).

Functional Aspects of the Protein, and Pathophysiology

Activation of NF-κB (i.e., nuclear translocation) requires the phosphorylation of inhibitors of NF-κB (such as IκB-α), which are constitutively bound to NF-κB and retain the complex in the cytoplasm. NEMO interacts with the α and β subunits of a complex kinase, known as IκB kinase (IKK), and is required for activation of the kinase complex in response to extracellular or intracellular stimuli (Rothwarf et al., 1998; Yamaoka et al., 1998). NEMO (IKK-γ or IKBKG, inhibitor of κB kinase-γ) is the essential regulatory subunit of IKK required for NF-κB activation and resistance to TNF-induced apoptosis, and it is central to many immune and inflammatory pathways. Its absence results in a complete inhibition of NF-κB activation. Whether different mutations in NEMO have a different impact on NF-κB activation in response to certain stimuli remains to be determined. A structure–function characterization of NEMO may be facilitated by the investigation of patients with XL-EDA-ID.

What mechanisms underlie the developmental clinical features of patients with XL-EDA-ID and XL-OL-EDA-ID? NEMO-dependent NF-κB activation has been shown to be an essential step in the developmental pathway engaged by ectodysplastin and its receptor (Yan et al., 2000; Doffinger et al., 2001; Kumar et al., 2001). The mild clinical features of EDA and the overlap in phenotype with IP seen in these patients are probably accounted for by residual EDAR signaling. NF-κB has a role in endothelial cell survival, and a role for NEMO in capillary architecture is supported by the fact that retinal vascular abnormalities are an important complication in affected females with IP (Mansour et al., 2001). Most patients with EDA-ID do not manifest retinal vessel abnormalities, but an occasional patient has been described with hematopoietic or vascular development problems (Roberts et al., 1998; Aradhya et al., 2001). The vascular anomalies in the OL-EDA-ID phenotype (Mansour et al., 2001; Dupuis-Girod et al., 2002) show a resemblance to primary lymphedema, an autosomal dominant developmental disorder caused by mutations of vascular endothelial growth factor receptor-3 (VEGFR-3) (Karkkainent et al., 2000). These anomalies are very likely due to disruption of the signaling between VEGFR-3 and NF-κB

mediated via NEMO. NF-κB-mediated signaling is important in the differentiation and function of osteoclasts (Franzoso et al., 1997), and mice deficient in the receptor activator of NF-κB (RANK) suffer from severe osteopetrosis due to a block in osteoclast differentiation (Dougall et al., 1999). Osteopetrosis in the OL-IDA-ED phenotype is therefore probably due to impaired RANK signaling. Residual NF-κB signaling may vary and account for the milder phenotype seen in some EDA-ID patients.

What accounts for the infectious diseases seen in the patients? In-depth investigations following the identification of NEMO mutations have shown impaired cellular responses of peripheral blood lymphocytes to lipopolysaccharide (LPS), interleukin-1β (IL-1β), IL-18, TNF-α, and CD40 ligand in OL-EDA-ID patients bearing the X420W mutation (Doffinger et al., 2001). NEMO-dependent NF-κB activation is important to the signaling pathways downstream of Toll receptors (Tlr) (O'Neill and Dinarello, 2000). These germ-line–encoded receptors recognize conserved molecular patterns shared by large groups of microorganisms and have a crucial role in inducing an appropriate inflammatory and antimicrobial process (Janeway and Medzhitov, 2002). LPS/Tlr-4 mediated signaling was impaired in one of these patients, a finding suggesting that impaired recognition of pathogens, rather than of antigen, appears to be an important immunopathogenic mechanism (Doffinger et al., 2001). These patients exhibit very poor inflammatory response, both clinically and biologically, because of impaired cellular responses to proinflammatory cytokines (IL-1β, IL-18, TNF-α) (Doffinger et al., 2001). An impaired response to LPS and partially impaired CD40 signaling could explain the susceptibility of these patients to infections with gram-negative bacteria and PCP, respectively (Doffinger et al., 2001). Infections by gram-positive bacteria may result from impaired responses to IL-1β, IL-18, or other NF-κB-dependent signaling pathways (Doffinger et al., 2001). It is known that S. pneumoniae activates NF-κB mainly but not exclusively through Tlr-2 mediated signaling (Yoshimura et al., 1999). The occurrence of severe mycobacterial disease in these patients is not due to the impairment of essential antimicrobacterial pathways mediated by IL-12 and IFN-γ (Underhill et al., 1999). However, it could be due to impaired IL-1β- and IL-18-dependent induction of IFN-γ, impaired cellular responses to IFN-γ-inducible TNF-α, or to impaired signaling through Tlr-2 or Tlr-4 (Doffinger et al., 2001). M. tuberculosis activates NF-κB through Tlr-2 and Tlr-4 (Means et al., 1999) and induces TNF-α by a Tlr-2 dependent pathway (Underhill et al., 1999).

The immunological pathways in patients with XL-EDA-ID have not been investigated, and the pathogenesis of their susceptibility to bacterial infections is unknown. These patients suffer almost exclusively from gram-positive, gram-negative, and acid-fast bacterial infection. The links between hypomorphic mutations in the NEMO coding region, impaired NF-κB activation, the various stimuli that trigger NF-κB, the various immune cell subsets, the genes induced by NF-κB, and these bacterial infections remain to be established. In any case, NEMO-dependent NF-κB activation seems to be particularly important for the control of extracellular and intracellular bacteria, even though the association of more severe mutations of NEMO (such as X420W) with fungal disease suggests that the role of NF-κB in host defense may be broader (Uzel, 2005).

Mutation Analysis and Strategies for Diagnosis

Many boys with "classical" EDA have problems as infants with feeding and episodes of fevers associated with respiratory infections, mainly pneumonia, along with high reported mortality at 30% (Clarke et al., 1987). Although a number of these patients will remain susceptible to recurrent upper respiratory infections, bouts of fever, eczema, and asthma or chronic obstructive airway disease believed to be related to the abnormal mucosa of the gastrointestinal and respiratory tracts, most of these patients are unlikely to fall seriously ill. In contrast, boys with EDA-ID suffer from recurrent, severe, life-threatening infections caused mainly by encapsulated bacteria and, particularly in those with the OL-EDA-ID phenotype, mycobacteria. As mentioned above, they manifest less obvious clinical features of EDA (Table 36.1).

Laboratory investigations will reveal different types of dysgammaglobulinemia, but the most striking finding is failure to respond by specific antibody synthesis to either naturally occurring infection or to immunization with *S. pneumoniae* polysaccharide (Table 36.2). Boys in whom the diagnosis of XL-EDA-ID is suspected on the basis of infections and/or impaired humoral immunity should be tested for NF-κB activation with fibroblast cell lines and stimuli such as IL-1β and TNF-α. If there is impaired NF-κB activation, *NEMO* mutations can be sought by sequence analysis.

Mode of Inheritance, Carrier Detection, and Prenatal Diagnosis

XL-EDA-ID is inherited as an X-linked recessive trait; It has thus been assumed that only males have EDA-ID. However, a female patient with features of EDA-ID and a heterozygous hypomorphic *NEMO* mutation has been reported (Kosaki et al., 2001), widening further the phenotypic spectrum of this gene mutation in females and opening the question of the type of genetic counseling these families should be given. The clinical status of mothers and sisters of males with EDA-ID, who are heterozygotes for such coding region *NEMO* mutations, have never been carefully analyzed. An international survey is in progress to address this important question.

Females who are carriers of stop codon mutations (and male patients with XL-OL-EDA-ID) may show variable features of IP, such as dry and hyperpigmented skin, hypodontia, and conical teeth, and some will have elevated serum IgA levels (Smahi et al., 2000; Zonana et al., 2000; Aradhya et al., 2001; Doffinger et al., 2001; Jain et al., 2001; Mansour et al., 2001; Dupuis-Girod et al., 2002). Interestingly, some female carriers are reported to have random or only slightly skewed X inactivation, which suggests that these hypomorphic (milder) *NEMO* mutations may not cause lethality in cells with an active mutant X chromosome (Aradhya et al., 2001). In contrast, loss-of-function *NEMO* mutation results in extreme susceptibility to apoptosis leading to embryonic death in males and extremely skewed X inactivation in females (Smahi et al., 2000). It is also important to note that the same mutation causing OL-EDA-ID in hemizygous males may cause IP in heterozygous females (Mansour et al., 2001; Dupuis-Girod et al., 2002). It turns out that the two mothers carrying X420W had mild IP, but it is unpredictable whether this will be the case in all affected females in a kindred. Although very rare and unique, cases of fully manifesting females with X-linked recessive disorders have been reported (Kosaki et al., 2001). Hence, genetic counseling regarding the status of a female baby should remain cautious at this time.

As with other single-gene mutations, presuming the mutation in the affected family is known, there are possibilities for prenatal diagnosis (Roberts et al., 1998). Given the severity of XL-OL-EDA-ID and, to a lesser extent, of XL-EDA-ID, a prenatal diagnosis in males can probably be offered to the family irrespective of the type of *NEMO* mutation. In females, a prenatal diagnosis may be offered to families in which OL-EDA-ID, but not EDA-ID, is diagnosed.

Treatment and Prognosis

The two children with OL-EDA-ID died in their second year of life of overwhelming mycobacterial disease after they had experienced a variety of fungal and bacterial infections. Bone marrow transplantation was attempted in one patient, who died 2 weeks after transplant of massive hepatic veno-occlusive disease (Dupuis-Girod et al., 2002).

EDA-ID is also a syndrome of severe immunodeficiency with significant morbidity and mortality. Recurrent infections lead to repeated hospitalizations and cause serious complications, such as bronchiectasis, chronic lung disease, intractable diarrhea, and failure to thrive (Table 36.1). The mortality is as high at 50% in childhood; at least 15 of 33 reported patients from 23 kindreds died at ages ranging from birth to 17 years (Smahi et al., 2000; Smythe et al., 2000; Zonana et al., 2000; Aradhya et al., 2001; Doffinger et al., 2001; Jain et al., 2001; Kosaki et al., 2001; Mansour et al., 2001; Dupuis-Girod et al., 2002; Orange et al., 2002). Four of these children died with disseminated mycobacterial infections.

As with other humoral immunodeficiencies with specific antibody production failure, regular intravenous immunoglobulin (IVIG) substitution is the mainstay of treatment. However, even though the majority of patients were on regular IVIG after the diagnosis was established, this treatment was not always protective against recurrent infections by *S. pneumoniae* and development of bronchiectasis. This finding, together with the increased susceptibility of patients to infections caused by gram-negative bacteria and mycobacteria, may suggest existence of additional immunological defects. Antibiotic prophylaxis should be determined on a case-by-case basis, as there is significant clinical heterogeneity between patients. As a rule, live vaccines such as BCG should be avoided.

Animal Models

There are no mouse models of hypomorhic *NEMO* mutations. In NEMO-deficient mouse models for IP (Makris et al., 2000; Schmidt-Supprian et al., 2000), as in human males bearing loss-of-function *NEMO* mutations (Smahi et al., 2000), the pro-apoptotic effects of TNF result in embryonic lethality in males. In heterozygous females, the skewing of X-inactivation in blood results from progressive apoptotic elimination of cells bearing mutated *NEMO* on the active X chromosome. Female mice heterozygous for *NEMO* mutations exhibit a severe but self-limiting dermatopathy, or *genodermatosis* and transient growth retardation (Makris et al., 2000; Schmidt-Supprian et al., 2000), traits almost identical to the human X-linked genodermatosis IP caused by loss-of-function *NEMO* mutations (Smahi et al., 2000). In contrast to humans, these mice exhibit increased apoptosis in both thymus and spleen (Rudolph et al., 2000).

Concluding Remarks and Future Challenges

XL-EDA-ID and XL-OL-EDA-ID are severe immunodeficiencies and developmental defects caused by hypomorphic mutations in *NEMO*. The milder developmental and immunological phenotype of EDA-ID, compared with that of OL-EDA-ID, is probably due to higher levels of residual NF-κB signaling, at least in certain tissues at certain developmental stages. Abnormal immunity in the OL-EDA-ID phenotype results from impaired cellular responses to at least LPS, IL-1β, IL-18, TNF-α, and CD154, whereas the immunological signaling pathways affected in patients with EDA-ID phenotype remain to be determined. Patients with EDA-ID show phenotypic heterogeneity, as some have overwhelming clinical diseases caused by several microorganisms whereas others seem to be susceptible to a limited number of species. Encapsulated bacteria are the leading pathogens in EDA-ID and all patients tested have impaired antibody response to polysaccharide antigens, with low specific antibodies to *S. pneumoniae* and low isohemagglutinin titers. A detailed comparison of the cellular and clinical phenotypes of patients with known genotypes is required to better define the genotype–phenotype correlation and to further improve our understanding of the pathophysiology of EDA-ID. Finally, it will be important to unravel the molecular basis of other forms of EDA-ID that are not associated with mutations in *NEMO*.

Cartilage-Hair Hypoplasia

Description and Historical Review

Cartilage-hair hypoplasia (CHH), or metaphyseal chondrodysplasia, McKusick type (MIM 250250), is an autosomal recessive form of skeletal dysplasia in which immunodeficiency is a constant feature (McKusick et al., 1965). There are more than 250 genetic human diseases of the skeleton or osteochondrodysplasias. The metaphyseal chondrodysplasias constitute a subgroup of bone dysplasias with eight distinct and well-defined disorders in the recent international classification (Hall, 2002). The molecular defects have been detected in four metaphyseal dysplasias: Schmid type (OMIM 156500), Jansen type (OMIM 156400), adenosine deaminase (ADA) deficiency (SCID) (OMIM 102700), and, recently, CHH and a third metaphyseal dysplasia associated with hematopoietic abnormalities, Shwachman-Diamond syndrome (OMIM 260400). The association of immunodeficiency and/or aplastic anemia with growth failure and other skeletal disease has been observed relatively often (Hong, 1989). Well-defined examples are Schimke immunoosseous dysplasia (OMIM 242900) and Nijmegen breakage syndrome (OMIM 251260) (see Chapter 30).

CHH shows a high incidence among the Amish in the United States and among the Finns in Europe. Families with affected offspring have also been observed in most Caucasian and Asian populations, whereas there are no reports from black populations (Makitie et al., 1998, 2000b). CHH is a pleiotropic condition, as indicated in the original description and confirmed in investigations on the Finnish patients (McKusick et al., 1965; Makitie and Kaitila, 1993; Makitie et al., 1995). In the original description on CHH, McKusick and coworkers observed an increased propensity to infections, caused by viruses in particular. Since then the defective immunity in CHH has been repeatedly confirmed by clinical and laboratory studies (Makitie et al., 1998, 2000b). The disease-causing gene, *RMRP*, has recently been identified following a positional cloning approach, and a number of mutations have been found (Makitie et al., 1992a, 2000b, 2001c). However, the pathogenic mechanisms of the pleiotropic features, including the immunodeficiency syndrome, have remained elusive.

Table 36.3. Phenotypic Findings in Cartilage-Hair Hypoplasia

Finding	Frequency (%)
Disportionately short limbed-short stature	100
Short fingers and toes	100
Increased lumbar lordosis	85
Marked	20
Moderate	65
Extension limitation in the elbow joints	92
>25°	28
5–25°	64
Laxity in finger joints and knees	95
Marked	58
Mild	38
Curved lower extremities	63
Marked	20
Mild	43
Chest deformity	68
Harrison's grooves	38
Prominent sternum	33
Narrow chest	40
Asymmetry	6
Scoliosis	21
Thin and sparse hair	93
Severe	55
Mild	38

Source: Modified from Makitie and Kaitila (1993).

Clinical and Pathological Manifestations

Nonimmunological features

The clinical phenotypic findings and their frequencies in CHH are listed in Table 36.3 (see also Color Plate 36.1). The pleiotropic features include growth failure (Makitie and Kaitila, 1993; Makitie et al., 1995), hair hypoplasia (Makitie and Kaitila, 1993; Makitie et al., 1995), refractory anemia in childhood (Makitie et al., 1992b), intestinal neurocristopathy or Hirschsprung disease (HD) (Makitie et al., 2001a), and risk of malignancies (Makitie et al., 1999) (Table 36.4). Recently, defective spermatogenesis was added to the features (Makitie et al., 2001c).

Table 36.4. Pleiotropic Features in Cartilage-Hair Hypoplasia

Feature	Frequency (%)
Short stature, −4 SD or <5th percentile	100
Hair hypoplasia	93
Immunodeficiency	56
Propensity to infections	56
In vitro immunodeficiency	88
Hypoplastic childhood anemia	79
Gastrointestinal dysfunction	18
Hirschsprung disease	9
Defective spermatogenesis	100
Metaphyseal chondrodysplasia on childhood skeletal radiographs	100
Overall risk of malignancies (SIR)	6.9
Non-Hodgkin lymphoma	90
Basal cell carcinoma	35

SIR, standardized incidence ratio.

Source: Modified from Makitie and Kaitila (1993) and Makitie et al. (1999, 2001b).

The marked disproportionately short-limbed, short stature is due to metaphyseal dysplasia (Makitie and Kaitila, 1993; Makitie et al., 1995). The CHH-specific growth curves based on Finnish patients indicated a progressive retardation of growth, with mean birth length of 45.8 cm (range, 38–50 cm) for boys and 44.9 cm (range, 38–51 cm) for girls. The median height was 131.2 cm (range, 110.7–158 cm) for adult males and 122.5 cm (range, 103.7–137.4 cm) for females, which was −7.9 SD for the Finnish normal males and females (Makitie et al., 1992; I. Kaitila, unpublished observations). In spite of normal or slightly delayed pubertal development, there was no pubertal growth spurt in boys and girls. The relative weight was around 20% less for both girls and boys. However, there is a substantial risk for being overweight after puberty in both genders (Makitie et al., 1992a).

The radiographic skeletal abnormalities are short and thick tubular bones with splaying and irregular metaphyseal border of the growth plate (Fig. 36.2). The costochondral junctions are similarly splayed and irregular, whereas the vertebrae are normal or slightly tall. These findings develop and are diagnostic by the age of 6 to 9 months. In adults the spine and skull are about normal, whereas the tubular bones of the extremities remain short and thick but are otherwise unspecific (Makitie and Kaitila, 1993; Makitie et al., 1995).

The characteristic hair hypoplasia in CHH presents as fair, thin, and sparse hair growth from the newborn. However, there is

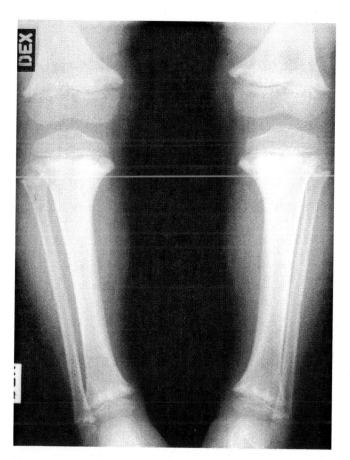

Figure 36.2. Radiograph of the lower extremities of a 6-years 9-months–old child with cartilage-hair hypoplasia. The tubular bones are short and thick, and there is remarkable generalized splaying and irregularities at the metaphyses.

a marked variation and individuals with normal hair have been observed (Table 36.3) (Verloes et al., 1990; Makitie and Kaitila, 1993; Makitie et al., 1995; Bonafe et al., 2002).

Gastrointestinal problems, such as intestinal neurocristopathy or neuronal dysplasia of the intestine, are common in CHH. In a recent study, congenital HD was found in 13 of 147 Finnish patients with CHH (9%), all of whom had an overall severe form (Makitie et al., 2001a). Eight patients had the classic form with rectosigmoid involvement, two had long-segment colonic disease, and three had total colonic aganglionosis. Six of the patients had episodes of enterocolitis, two with colonic perforations prior the first surgery. Eleven patients had postoperative enterocolitis and some died of enterocolitis-related septicemia. The bacterial etiology was nonspecific with *Clostridium difficile* mentioned (I. Kaitila, unpublished data).

In another recent study, defective quantitative and qualitative spermatogenesis was observed in all 11 patients studied (Makitie et al., 2001c), although whether this finding was associated with male infertility was not studied.

Defective erythrogenesis in early childhood presenting as hypoplastic anemia is a common feature in CHH and was found in 54 of 74 Finnish patients (73%). Three children died of anemia and four additional patients were treated with repeated erythrocyte transfusions at up to 2–3 years of age. Macrocytosis often remained into adulthood (Makitie et al., 1992b, 2000a). In a study of colony formation of myeloid lineages from blood and bone marrow in vitro, all patients with CHH showed defective erythroid and granulocyte-macrophage colony formation, which was not caused by a decreased number of progenitors (Juvonen et al., 1995). Anemia is related to body growth and to the insulin-like growth factor system (Makitie et al., 2000a).

Immunodeficiency

In the original description of CHH there was an increased propensity to infections, including viral diseases (McKusick et al., 1965). A peculiar feature was that varicella occasionally resulted in a prolonged and severe disease with hemorrhagic vesicles, high fever, and even fatality. Since then a number of patients with chronic, severe, and even fatal infections due to viruses, bacteria, and fungi have been reported (Lux et al., 1970; Saulsbury et al., 1975; Steele et al., 1976; Polmar and Pierce, 1986; Hong, 1989; Castigli et al., 1995; Berthet et al., 1996). A classical presentation is that of a child with a history of recurrent respiratory infections and chronic diarrhea from 6 months of age. She had multiple episodes of sepsis caused by *Klebsiella pneumoniae, Streptococcus fecalis, and Staphylococcus epidermidis* and had stool cultures positive for *Clostridium difficile*, rotavirus, and adenovirus. She also had recurrent vesicular eruptions due to varicella and needed continuous acyclovir therapy (Castigli et al., 1995). Such severe clinical presentations reflect impaired cellular immunity and are rare; however, most CHH patients do relatively well and have only mild impairment of humoral immunity (Makitie et al., 1998, 2000b). Trojak et al. (1981) studied 18 CHH patients with no history of infections and found consistent defective immunity by laboratory studies. In a recent retrospective questionnaire study of 35 Finnish patients, the parents reported 31% increased respiratory and other infection rates during the preceding year for their CHH children, compared to rates for the unaffected siblings (Makitie et al., 1998, 2000b). Chronic progressive lung disease, such as bronchitis and bronchiectasis, was the cause of death in three adolescents (I. Kaitila, personal experience). Thrombocytopenia and autoimmune hemolytic anemia have also been reported as an association with

CHH (Ashby and Evans, 1986; Berthet et al., 1996; Matsumoto et al., 2000; authors' personal experience).

Children with CHH have usually been vaccinated with routine regimens with BCG, diphtheria, tetanus, polio, and mumps, etc. without reported complications (I. Kaitila, personal experience). However, two patients developed severe disease following live poliovirus vaccine (Saulsbury et al., 1975; Ashby and Evans, 1986).

Variability

There is some variability of adult height, from <100 cm up to 158 cm (Makitie and Kaitila, 1993; I. Kaitila, personal observations). Most patients present with marked hair hypoplasia. However, there are case reports describing normal hair (Verloes et al., 1990; Bonafe et al., 2002), and among the Finnish patients 7% had normal hair and only 55% severe hair hypoplasia (Makitie and Kaitila, 1993). The clinical presentation of the immunodeficiency syndrome itself varies from lethal septicemic infections in early childhood to no infection in adults (Makitie et al., 1998, Makitie 2000b). In a recent study the mortality in CHH was increased, mainly but not exclusively because of defective immunity in childhood. The major causes of mortality in adulthood have been chronic pulmonary infections related to the immunodeficiency, and lymphomas (Makitie et al., 1999, 2001; I. Kaitila, personal experience). As a result, the variability of the clinical outcome in CHH is quite extensive, ranging from lethality in the newborn period to normal life span. The global morbidity also varies from case to case.

Laboratory Findings

McKusick and coworkers demonstrated in 1970 that two Amish patients had mild to moderate lymphopenia, decreased delayed hypersensitivity, and impaired leukocyte responses to mitogens whereas the immunoglobulin concentrations and antibody synthesis were normal (Lux et al., 1970). Similar results were subsequently confirmed in other Amish patients (Trojak et al., 1981; Pierce and Polmar, 1982; Pierce et al., 1983; Polmar and Pierce, 1986). The proportions of the major T lymphocyte subpopulations were normal. The results of allogeneic stimulations indicated an intrinsic T cell defect, whereas antigen-presenting cells were not affected. Furthermore, they showed that the IL-2 production by CHH lymphocytes was reduced, but exogeneous IL-2 did not correct the defect in proliferation (Pierce and Polmar, 1982; Pierce et al., 1983; Polmar and Pierce, 1986). The NK cell activity was normal or even above normal. There was an impaired proliferation of B lymphocytes in response to stimulation in vitro, despite the lack of detectable antibody deficiency.

In studying the Finnish CHH patients we also found depressed or absent delayed skin hypersensitivity reactions and decreased lymphocyte proliferative responses to mitogens in vitro (Ranki et al., 1978; Virolainen et al., 1978). The absolute lymphocyte count was about half that of normal controls. Again, the serum immunoglobulin concentrations and antibody synthesis were normal. In the Finnish patients, a reduction of 50% in CD4+ cell count and a reduction of 30% in CD4+/CD8+ cell ratio have been reported. The B lymphocyte count was usually normal, whereas the NK cell count was often elevated (Makitie et al., 1998). Unexpectedly, we found that one-third of the Finnish CHH patients also had partially defective humoral immunity presenting as isolated IgA and IgG subclass deficiencies (Makitie et al., 2000b).

Other patients have also been investigated to determine the immunological basis of infections in CHH. The decreased prolifera-

tive response of T cells to phytohemagglutin (PHA) could not be restored by addition of rIL-2 (Kooijman et al., 1997). On the basis of increased expression of Fas (CD95), CD95L, and Bax, and decreased expression of Bcl-2 and inhibitor of apoptosis protein (IAP) in both CD4+ and CD8+ cells, it has been suggested that the lymphopenia might be due to increased apoptosis of these cells (Yel et al., 1999). In another study, the levels of mRNA encoding c-myc, IL-2Rα, IL-2, and IFN-γ were decreased in the stimulated CHH lymphocytes, whereas those of other early activation gene products, such as c-fos and c-jun, were not impaired, findings suggesting a lymphocyte intracellular signaling defect (Castigli et al., 1995). One child with CHH had severe combined immunodeficiency (SCID) with severe T lymphopenia but normal numbers of B cells (Berthet et al., 1996).

Molecular Basis

On the basis of molecular linkage studies on Finnish multiplex CHH families, the disease-causing gene was mapped to 9p12 in 1993, and the homogeneity of the condition was confirmed in the Finnish and Amish populations by haplotype analyses of the nearby molecular markers (Sulisalo et al., 1993, 1994, 1995b). The location was refined by disequilibrium analysis; finally, the mutated gene, *RMRP*, was detected through physical mapping and sequencing (Ridanpaa et al., 2001). Several dozen *RMRP* mutations have been detected (Fig. 36.3A) (Makitie et al., 2000b, 2001c; Bonafé et al., 2005).

Three types of mutations of *RMRP* are associated with CHH (Fig. 36.3A,B). Most are base substitutions, insertions, or short duplications that alter conserved nucleotide sequences in the transcribed region. The second set of mutations consists of insertions or duplications in the promoter region between the TATA box and the site of initiation of transcription. The third set includes insertions and duplications in the 5' end of the transcribed region. All patients with insertion or duplication in the promoter region on one allele carry a mutation in the transcribed region on their second allele. This finding suggests that if two allelic mutations in the promoter region would have a lethal outcome.

Recently, we have shown that the most common CHH-causing mutation is 70A > G, found in 92% of Finnish CHH patients and probably all Amish patients. The same mutation accounts for 48% of the mutations among patients from other parts of Europe, North and South America, the Near East, and Australia (Makitie et al., 2000b). In the non-Finnish families the same major mutation segregates with the same major haplotype as in most of the Finnish families. Thus all the chromosomes with the 70A > G mutation probably arose from a solitary founder many thousand years ago. A minor common mutation, 262G > T, accounts for 7% of the Finnish patients, always in compound heterozygosity with the 70A > G mutation. Compound heterozygosity for the 70A > G mutation and for a private mutation was also common in the non-Finnish, non-Amish patients, and several patients presented as homozygotes for a private mutation in *RMRP* gene (Makitie et al., 2000b). The sites for the different types of mutation in the transcribed region are evolutionarily conserved (Schmitt et al., 1993; Sbisa et al., 1996; Shadel et al., 2000).

Functional Aspects of the Gene Product

The human *RMRP* gene encodes the 267 bp RNA molecule of the RNase MRP complex, which consists of protein components and the RNA molecule. Thus, exceptional to most of the known disease-associated genes, the *RMRP* is an untranslated gene. It is

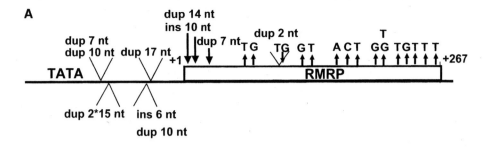

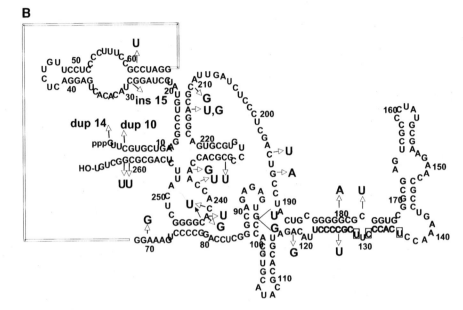

Figure 36.3 (A) *RMRP* gene mutations in cartilage-hair hypoplasia. There are three duplications and one insertion, and 15 base pair substitutions in the transcript, which is only 267 base pairs in length. Between the TATA box and the initiation site of the the transcription—i.e., in the promoter—there are five duplications and one insertion of varying length. A, adenine; C, cytosine; G, guanine; T, thymidine (B) Schematic presentation of the RNA molecule encoded by *RMRP*. Base pair substitutions and the sites of duplications are indicated by arrows. A, adenine; C, cytosine; G, guanine; U, uridine.

found in mammals, *C. elegans*, yeast, and bacteria (van Eenennaam et al., 2000). The RNase MRP is a ribonucleoprotein endoribonuclease involved in the processing of precursor ribosomal RNA and in priming of the RNA for mitochondrial DNA replication. It has been suggested that the RNase MRP also carries other important biological functions, such as control of cell proliferation (Clayton, 2001). In situ hybridization experiments have indicated the presence of RNase MRP in both mitochondria and nucleoli, the majority being localized to the latter. The central region of the RNA molecule is important for its mitochondrial localization, whereas the 5′-terminal region is required for nucleolar localization, which suggests that these domains determine the transportation to these subcellular compartments. In yeast, the RNase MRP cleaves the pre-rRNA to two forms of 5.8S rRNA, the long and short forms. Experimental mutations in yeast RNase MRP RNA result in lethal, temperature-conditional lethal and nutrient preferent, and altered growth phenotypes; the growth defect was proportional to the severity of the 5.8S rRNA processing phenotype (Shadel et al., 2000). The pathogenetic mechanisms of the *RMRP* mutations in human health and disease are still unknown.

Mutation Analysis

DNA samples are screened for insertions and deletions in the promoter region by use of two polymerase chain reaction (PCR) primers, RM3IF 5′-CTTAGAAAGTTATGCCCGAAAAC-3′ and RM3IR 5′-GAAAGGGGAGGAACAGAGTC-3′, for amplification, and 5% Sequagel (National Diagnostics) gels for separation. In case of changes in the length, this region is amplified with RM3F 5′-GGCCAGACCATATTTGCATAAG-3′ and RM3R 5′-CGGACTTTGGAGTGGGAAG-3′ primers and then sequenced.

The major mutation (70A > G) is amplified with PCR primers RM70F 5′-GTGCTGAAGGCCTGTATCCT-3′ and RM70R 5′-CTAGGGGAGCTGACGGATG-3′. Single-strand conformation polymorphism (SSCP) analyses are performed in 0.7 × MDE (FMC BioProducts) gels at room temperature using 5W overnight. For sequencing of the whole RNA coding region of *RMRP*, PCR primers RMF 5′-CCAACTTTCTCACCCTAACCA-3′ and RMR 5′-AAGGCCAAGAACAGCGTAAA-3′ are used. The 3′ region can be separately amplified for sequencing with RM4F 5′-AGA GAGTGCCACGTGCATAC-3′ and RM4R 5′-CTTCATAGCAAG GCCAAGAAC-3′. All PAGE and SSCP gels are detected through silver staining (Ridanpaa et al., 2001).

Strategies for Diagnosis

The diagnosis of CHH is based on the clinical phenotype, family history and radiographic phenotypes; it can be confirmed by mutation analysis of the *RMRP* gene. The clinical variability in CHH is marked but well analyzed (Makitie and Kaitila, 1993; Makitie et al., 1995; Ridanpaa et al., 2001). However, with the detection of the defective *RMRP* gene, enlarged phenotypic variation has emerged. The essential features are short birth length for gestational age, and delayed growth in height ranging from −3 to −8 SD of the mean in the population and for the patient's gender. The extremities are usually disproportionately short. With the exception of elbow joints, the hyperextensibility of the joints is marked. The lower extremities are often curved, and the lumbar lordosis is increased. The physical handicap is usually a minor problem, and patients do not have early osteoarthrosis.

Most patients have sparse, thin, fair hair. About one-third present with hypoplastic anemia in infancy and early childhood, and erythrocyte macrocytosis may prevail throughout their lives. Lymphopenia is common, hypogammalobulinemia with low IgA and/or low IgG2 is relatively rare, and SCID is exceedingly rare. Immunodeficiency in CHH is often associated with chronic sinusitis and respiratory disease. A minority of the patients present with chronic constipation, and newborns occasionally have HD.

A consistent diagnostic feature is the generalized metaphyseal irregularity of the tubular bones on childhood skeletal radiographs. The characteristic radiographic features cannot be observed in the newborn, but they do develop by the age of 6 to 9 months. Detection of mutations in the *RMRP* gene will confirm the suspected diagnosis.

Mode of Inheritance, Carrier Detection, and Prenatal Diagnosis

The mode of inheritance is autosomal recessive. Thus, it is typical to find one or more affected siblings whose healthy carrier parents may be consanguineous. Two epidemiological studies have indicated a lower than expected number of affected siblings (McKusick et al., 1965; Makitie et al., 1992a). Two cases of maternal isodisomy were observed among approximately 100 Finnish families (Sulisalo et al., 1997).

Carrier detection is feasible for individuals at risk for affected offspring through direct mutation analysis. For prenatal diagnosis, the fetal ultrasound in the first and second trimester should be regarded as unreliable, and it should be replaced by molecular studies for the *RMRP* gene on either chorionic biopsy material or amniotic fluid cells taken at the tenth week or later of pregnancy (Sulisalo et al., 1995a).

Treatment and Prognosis

For patients with CHH, the standardized mortality ratio is 9.3 compared to normal parents and healthy siblings, according to Finnish population figures. This increased mortality is confined to young age-groups and associated with defective immunity (Makitie et al., 2001b). The standardized incidence ratio for overall cancer is also higher, at 6.9, the main cancer type being non-Hodgkin lymphoma, with a ratio of 90 (Makitie et al., 1999).

Most patients with CHH present with a relatively mild phenotype; however, careful annual follow-up for growth and psychomotor development is indicated. Hypoplastic anemia must be carefully evaluated and patients should be followed with appropriate hematological studies. Regular erythrocyte transfusions may be needed during the first 2 to 3 years of life. Autoimmune hemolytic anaemia is probably rare and may or may not respond to prednisone treatment (Ashby and Evans, 1986). Erythropoetin treatment has been shown to be ineffective (I. Kaitila, personal experience). Bone marrow transplantation (BMT) has cured the immunodeficiency and autoimmune hemolytic anemia but not the skeletal disease: a 16-month-old child with unusually severe CHH and SCID had a complete reconstitution of cellular immunity at 4 months and humoral immunity at 15 months after BMT from an HLA-identical sister (Berthet et al., 1996).

Children with CHH should not be vaccinated with live or attenuated bacteria or viruses. Antibiotic and antiviral treatment of infections, as well as prophylactic antibiotics, should be recommended on a case-by-case basis. The HD of the newborn requires immediate operative treatment. Rarely, long-segment intestinal neurocristopathy occurs that is associated with severe functional (constipation or diarrhea) and inflammatory bowel disease and thus major nutritional problems (Makitie et al., 2001a). The

skeletal growth failure cannot be corrected with growth-hormone or other hormonal therapy (I. Kaitila, personal experience). The only effective means to achieve more height is bone-lengthening procedures of the lower extremities. However, this treatment has been associated with a variety of complications (I. Kaitila, unpublished observations).

Animal Models

There are presently no animal models for CHH.

Concluding Remarks and Future Challenges

Pleiotropic, autosomal recessive CHH is caused by mutations in an untranslated gene, *RMRP*, which encodes the RNA component of an endoribonuclease, RNase MRP. There is no observed genotype–phenotype correlation between the mutations and clinical manifestations, which vary from a lethal, infantile condition of severe growth failure, immunodeficiency, hypoplastic anemia, and HD to a mild condition with disproportionately short stature with normal life span. Until now, immunological studies have confirmed complex and variable deficiencies in both cell-mediated and humoral immunity. The pathogenetic mechanisms involved are still unknown. Future research should be directed toward understanding the mechanisms of suppressed cellular differentiation and proliferation as a result of the mutated *RMRP* gene in multiple human tissues and organs, and in other organisms, including bacteria, yeast, fish, amphibians, and mammals.

References

Abinun M. Ectodermal dysplasia and immunodeficiency. Arch Dis Child 73: 185, 1995.

Abinun M, Spickett G, Appleton AL, Flood T, Cant AJ. Anhidrotic ectodermal dysplasia associated with specific antibody deficiency. Eur J Pediatr 155:146–147, 1996.

Aradhya S, Courtois G, Rajkovic A, et al. Atypical forms of incontinentia pigmenti in male individuals result from mutations of a cytosine tract in exon 10 of NEMO (IKK-γ). Am J Hum Genet 68:765–771, 2001.

Aradhya S, Nelson DL. NF-κB signaling and human disease. Curr Opin Genet Dev 11:300–306, 2001.

Ashby GH, Evans DI. Cartilage hair hypoplasia with thrombocytopenic purpura, autoimmune haemolytic anaemia and cell-mediated immunodeficiency. J R Soc Med 79:113–114, 1986.

Berthet F, Siegrist CA, Ozsahin H, et al. Bone marrow transplantation in cartilage-hair hypoplasia: correction of the immunodeficiency but not of the chondrodysplasia. Eur J Pediatr 155:286–290, 1996.

Bonafé L, Dermitzakis LT, Unger S, Greenberg CR, Campos-Xavier BA, Zankl A, Ulca C, Antonarakis SE, Superti-Furga A, Reymond A. Evolutionary comparison provides evidence for pathogenicity of RMRP mutations. PLoS genet 1(4): e47, 2005.

Bonafé L, Schmitt K, Eich G, Giedion A, Superti-Furga A. *RMRP* gene sequence analysis confirms a cartilage-hair hypoplasia variant with only skeletal manifestations and reveals a high density of single-nucleotide polymorphisms. Clin Genet 61:146–151, 2002.

Castigli E, Irani AM, Geha RS, Chatila T. Defective expression of early activation genes in cartilage-hair hypoplasia (CHH) with severe combined immunodeficiency (SCID). Clin Exp Immunol 102:6–10, 1995.

Clarke A, Phillips DI, Brown R, Harper PS. Clinical aspects of X-linked hypohidrotic ectodermal dysplasia. Arch Dis Child 62:989–996, 1987.

Clayton DA. A big development for a small RNA. Nature 410:29–31, 2001.

Copley RR. The gene for X-linked anhidrotic ectodermal dysplasia encodes a TNF-like domain. J Mol Med 77:361–363, 1999.

Courtois G, Smahi A, Israel A. NEMO/IKK-γ: linking NF-κ B to human disease. Trends Mol Med 7:427–430, 2001.

Davis JR, Solomon LM. Cellular immunodeficiency in anhidrotic ectodermal dysplasia. Acta Derm Venereol 56:115–120, 1976.

Doffinger R, Smahi A, Bessia C, et al. X-linked anhidrotic ectodermal dysplasia with immunodeficiency is caused by impaired NF-κB signaling. Nat Genet 27:277–285, 2001.

Dougall WC, Glaccum M, Charrier K, et al. RANK is essential for osteoclast and lymph node development. Genes Dev 13:2412–2424, 1999.

Dupuis-Girod S, Corradini N, Hadj-Rabia S, Fournet JC, Faivre L, Le Deist F, Durand P, Doeffinger R, Smahi A, Courtois G, Israel A, Brousse N, Blanche S, Munnich A, Fischer A, Casanova JL, Bodemer C. Osteopetrosis, lymphedema, anhydrotic ectodermal dysplasia, and immunodeficiency in a boy and incontinentia pigmenti in his mother. Pediatrics 109(6):e97, 2002.

Ezer S, Bayes M, Elomaa O, Schlessinger D, Kere J. Ectodysplasin is a collagenous trimeric type II membrane protein with a tumor necrosis factor–like domain and co-localizes with cytoskeletal structures at lateral and apical surfaces of cells. Hum Mol Genet 8:2079–2086, 1999.

Frank J, Pignata C, Panteleyev AA, et al. Exposing the human nude phenotype. Nature 398:473–474, 1999.

Franken E. [Anhidrotic form of ectodermal dysplasia with hypogammaglobulinemia and properdin deficiency]. Dermatol Wochenschr 152:841–845, 1996.

Franzoso G, Carlson L, Xing L, et al. Requirement for NF-κB in osteoclast and B-cell development. Genes Dev 11:3482–3496, 1997.

Frix CD 3rd, Bronson DM. Acute miliary tuberculosis in a child with anhidrotic ectodermal dysplasia. Pediatr Dermatol 3:464–467, 1986.

Hall CM. International nosology and classification of constitutional disorders of bone (2001). Am J Med Genet 113:65–77, 2002.

Hong R. Associations of the skeletal and immune systems. Am J Med Genet 34:55–59, 1989.

Huntley CC, Ross RM. Anhidrotic ectodermal dysplasia with transient hypogammaglobulinemia. Cutis 28:417–419, 1981.

Jain A, Ma CA, Liu S, Brown M, Cohen J, Strober W. Specific missense mutations in NEMO result in hyper-IgM syndrome with hypohydrotic ectodermal dysplasia. Nat Immunol 2:223–228, 2001.

Janeway CA Jr, Medzhitov R. Innate immune recognition. Annu Rev Immunol 20:197–216, 2002.

Juvonen E, Makitie O, Makipernaa A, Ruutu T, Kaitila I, Rajantie J. Defective in-vitro colony formation of haematopoietic progenitors in patients with cartilage-hair hypoplasia and history of anaemia. Eur J Pediatr 154: 30–34, 1995.

Karin M, Lin A. NF-κB at the crossroads of life and death. Nat Immunol 3: 221–227, 2002.

Karkkainen MJ, Ferrell RE, Lawrence EC, et al. Missense mutations interfere with VEGFR-3 signalling in primary lymphoedema. Nat Genet 25: 153–159, 2000.

Kere J, Srivastava AK, Montonen O, et al. X-linked anhidrotic (hypohidrotic) ectodermal dysplasia is caused by mutation in a novel transmembrane protein. Nat Genet 13:409–416, 1996.

Kooijman R, van der Burgt CJ, Weemaes CM, Haraldsson A, Scholtens EJ, Zegers BJ. T cell subsets and T cell function in cartilage-hair hypoplasia. Scand J Immunol 46:209–215, 1997.

Kosaki K, Shimasaki N, Fukushima H, Hara M, Ogata T, Matsuo N. Female patient showing hypohidrotic ectodermal dysplasia and immunodeficiency (HED-ID). Am J Hum Genet 69:664–666, 2001.

Kumar A, Eby MT, Sinha S, Jasmin A, Chaudhary PM. The ectodermal dysplasia receptor activates the nuclear factor-κB, JNK, and cell death pathways and binds to ectodysplasin A. J Biol Chem 276:2668–2677, 2001.

Lux SE, Johnston RB Jr, August CS, et al. Chronic neutropenia and abnormal cellular immunity in cartilage-hair hypoplasia. N Engl J Med 282:231–236, 1970.

Makitie O, Juvonen E, Dunkel L, Kaitila I, Siimes MA. Anemia in children with cartilage-hair hypoplasia is related to body growth and to the insulin-like growth factor system. J Clin Endocrinol Metab 85:563–568, 2000a.

Makitie O, Kaitila I. Cartilage-hair hypoplasia—clinical manifestations in 108 Finnish patients. Eur J Pediatr 152:211–217, 1993.

Makitie O, Kaitila I, Rintala R. Hirschsprung disease associated with severe cartilage-hair hypoplasia. J Pediatr 138:929–931, 2001a.

Makitie O, Kaitila I, Savilahti E. Susceptibility to infections and in vitro immune functions in cartilage-hair hypoplasia. Eur J Pediatr 157:816–820, 1998.

Makitie O, Kaitila I, Savilahti E. Deficiency of humoral immunity in cartilage-hair hypoplasia. J Pediatr 137:487–492, 2000b.

Makitie O, Perheentupa J, Kaitila I. Growth in cartilage-hair hypoplasia. Pediatr Res 31:176–180, 1992a.

Makitie O, Pukkala E, Kaitila I. Increased mortality in cartilage-hair hypoplasia. Arch Dis Child 84:65–67, 2001b.

Makitie O, Pukkala E, Teppo L, Kaitila I. Increased incidence of cancer in patients with cartilage-hair hypoplasia. J Pediatr 134:315–318, 1999.

Makitie O, Rajantie J, Kaitila I. Anaemia and macrocytosis—unrecognized features in cartilage-hair hypoplasia. Acta Paediatr 81:1026–1029, 1992b.

Makitie O, Sulisalo T, de la Chapelle A, Kaitila I. Cartilage-hair hypoplasia. J Med Genet 32:39–43, 1995.

Makitie OM, Tapanainen PJ, Dunkel L, Siimes MA. Impaired spermatogenesis: an unrecognized feature of cartilage-hair hypoplasia. Ann Med 33: 201–205, 2001c.

Makris C, Godfrey VL, Krahn-Senftleben G, et al. Female mice heterozygous for IKK-γ/NEMO deficiencies develop a dermatopathy similar to the human X-linked disorder incontinentia pigmenti. Mol Cell 5:969–979, 2000.

Mansour S, Woffendin H, Mitton S, et al. Incontinentia pigmenti in a surviving male is accompanied by hypohidrotic ectodermal dysplasia and recurrent infection. Am J Med Genet 99:172–177, 2001.

Matsumoto S, Ozono K, Yamamoto T, et al. Treatment with recombinant IL-2 for recurrent respiratory infection in a case of cartilage-hair hypoplasia with autoimmune hemolytic anemia. J Bone Miner Metab 18:36–40, 2000.

McKusick VA. Mendelian Inheritance in Man. Catalogs of Human Genes and Genetic Disorders. Baltimore: Johns Hopkins University Press, 1998.

McKusick VA, Eldridge R, Hostetler JA, Ruangwit U, Egeland JA. Dwarfism in the Amish. II. Cartilage-hair hypoplasia. Bull Johns Hopkins Hosp 116: 231–272, 1965.

Means TK, Wang S, Lien E, Yoshimura A, Golenbock DT, Fenton MJ. Human toll-like receptors mediate cellular activation by Mycobacterium tuberculosis. J Immunol 163:3920–3927, 1999.

Ming JE, Stiehm ER, Graham JM Jr. Immunodeficiency as a component of recognizable syndromes. Am J Med Genet 66:378–398, 1996.

Ming JE, Stiehm ER, Graham JM Jr. Syndromes associated with immunodeficiency. Adv Pediatr 46:271–351, 1999.

Monreal AW, Ferguson BM, Headon DJ, Street SL, Overbeek PA, Zonana J. Mutations in the human homologue of mouse dl cause autosomal recessive and dominant hypohidrotic ectodermal dysplasia. Nat Genet 22:366–369, 1999.

Monreal AW, Zonana J, Ferguson B. Identification of a new splice form of the EDA1 gene permits detection of nearly all X-linked hypohidrotic ectodermal dysplasia mutations. Am J Hum Genet 63:380–389, 1998.

Nishikomori R, Akutagawa H, Maruyama K, Nakata-Hizume M, Ohmori K, Mizuno K, Yachie A, Yasumi T, Kusonoki T, Heike T, Nakahata T. X-linked ectodermal dysplasia and immunodeficiency caused by a reversion mosaicism of NEMO reveals a critical role for NEMO in human T-cell development and/or survival. Blood 103:4565–4572, 2004.

O'Neill LA, Dinarello CA. The IL-1 receptor/toll-like receptor superfamily: crucial receptors for inflammation and host defense. Immunol Today 21: 206–209, 2000.

Orange JS, Brodeur SR, Jain A, et al. Deficient natural killer cell cytotoxicity in patients with IKK-λ/NEMO mutations. J Clin Invest 109:1501–1509, 2002.

Pierce GF, Brovall C, Schacter BZ, Polmar SH. Impaired culture generated cytotoxicity with preservation of spontaneous natural killer-cell activity in cartilage-hair hypoplasia. J Clin Invest 71:1737–1743, 1983.

Pierce GF, Polmar SH. Lymphocyte dysfunction in cartilage hair hypoplasia. II. Evidence for a cell cycle–specific defect in T cell growth. Clin Exp Immunol 50:621–628, 1982.

Pignata C, Gaetaniello L, Masci AM, et al. Human equivalent of the mouse Nude/SCID phenotype: long-term evaluation of immunologic reconstitution after bone marrow transplantation. Blood 97:880–885, 2001.

Polmar SH, Pierce GF. Cartilage hair hypoplasia: immunological aspects and their clinical implications. Clin Immunol Immunopathol 40:87–93, 1986.

Priolo M, Lagana C. Ectodermal dysplasias: a new clinical-genetic classification. J Med Genet 38:579–585, 2001.

Puel A, Reichenbach J, Bustamante J, et al. The NEMO mutation creating the most-upstream premature stop codon is hypomorhic because of a reinitiation of translation. Am J Hum Genet 78:691–701, 2006.

Ranki A, Perheentupa J, Andersson LC, Hayry P. In vitro T- and B-cell reactivity in cartilage hair hypoplasia. Clin Exp Immunol 32:352–360, 1978.

Ridanpaa M, van Eenennaam H, Pelin K, et al. Mutations in the RNA component of RNase MRP cause a pleiotropic human disease, cartilage-hair hypoplasia. Cell 104:195–203, 2001.

Rijkers GT, Sanders LA, Zegers BJ. Anti-capsular polysaccharide antibody deficiency states. Immunodeficiency 5:1–21, 1993.

Roberts JL, Morrow B, Vega-Rich C, Salafia CM, Nitowsky HM. Incontinentia pigmenti in a newborn male infant with DNA confirmation. Am J Med Genet 75:159–163, 1998.

Rothwarf DM, Zandi E, Natoli G, Karin M. IKK-γ is an essential regulatory subunit of the IκB kinase complex. Nature 395:297–300, 1998.

Rudolph D, Yeh WC, Wakeham A, et al. Severe liver degeneration and lack of NF-κB activation in NEMO/IKK-γ–deficient mice. Genes Dev 14: 854–862, 2000.

Sanders LA, Rijkers GT, Kuis W, et al. Defective antipneumococcal polysaccharide antibody response in children with recurrent respiratory tract infections. J Allergy Clin Immunol 91:110–119, 1993.

Saulsbury FT, Winkelstein JA, Davis LE, et al. Combined immunodeficiency and vaccine-related poliomyelitis in a child with cartilage-hair hypoplasia. J Pediatr 86:868–872, 1975.

Sbisa E, Pesole G, Tullo A, Saccone C. The evolution of the RNase P- and RNase MRP-associated RNAs: phylogenetic analysis and nucleotide substitution rate. J Mol Evol 43:46–57, 1996.

Schmidt-Supprian M, Bloch W, Courtois G, et al. NEMO/IKK-γ-deficient mice model incontinentia pigmenti. Mol Cell 5:981–992, 2000.

Schmitt ME, Bennett JL, Dairaghi DJ, Clayton DA. Secondary structure of RNase MRP RNA as predicted by phylogenetic comparison. FASEB J 7:208–213, 1993.

Schweizer P, Kalhoff H, Horneff G, Wahn V, Diekmann L. [Polysaccharide-specific humoral immunodeficiency in ectodermal dysplasia. Case report of a boy with two affected brothers]. Klin Padiatr 211:459–461, 1999.

Shadel GS, Buckenmeyer GA, Clayton DA, Schmitt ME. Mutational analysis of the RNA component of *Saccharomyces cerevisiae* RNase MRP reveals distinct nuclear phenotypes. Gene 245:175–184, 2000.

Sitton JE, Reimund EL. Extramedullary hematopoiesis of the cranial dura and anhidrotic ectodermal dysplasia. Neuropediatrics 23:108–110, 1992.

Smahi A, Courtois G, Vabres P, et al. Genomic rearrangement in NEMO impairs NF-κB activation and is a cause of incontinentia pigmenti. The International Incontinentia Pigmenti (IP) Consortium. Nature 405:466–472, 2000.

Smythe WR, Bridges ND, Gaynor JW, Nicolson S, Clark BJ, Spray TL. Bilateral sequential lung transplant for ectodermal dysplasia. Ann Thorac Surg 70:654–656, 2000.

Steele RW, Britton HA, Anderson CT, Kniker WT. Severe combined immunodeficiency with cartilage-hair hypoplasa: in vitro response to thymosin and attempted reconstitution. Pediatr Res 10:1003–1005, 1976.

Sulisalo T, Francomano CA, Sistonen P, et al. High-resolution genetic mapping of the cartilage-hair hypoplasia (CHH) gene in Amish and Finnish families. Genomics 20:347–353, 1994.

Sulisalo T, Sillence D, Wilson M, Ryynanen M, Kaitila I. Early prenatal diagnosis of cartilage-hair hypoplasia (CHH) with polymorphic DNA markers. Prenat Diagn 15:135–140, 1995a.

Sulisalo T, Sistonen P, Hastbacka J, et al. Cartilage-hair hypoplasia gene assigned to chromosome 9 by linkage analysis. Nat Genet 3:338–341, 1993.

Sulisalo T, van der Burgt I, Rimoin DL, et al. Genetic homogeneity of cartilage-hair hypoplasia. Hum Genet 95:157–160, 1995b.

Trojak JE, Polmar SH, Winkelstein JA, et al. Immunologic studies of cartilage-hair hypoplasia in the Amish. Johns Hopkins Med J 148:157–164, 1984.

Underhill DM, Ozinsky A, Smith KD, Aderem A. Toll-like receptor-2 mediates mycobacteria-induced proinflammatory signaling in macrophages. Proc Natl Acad Sci USA 96:14459–14463, 1999.

Uzel G. The range of defects associated with nuclear factor kappa-B essential modulator. Curr Opin Allergy Clin Immunol 5:513–518, 2005.

van Eenennaam H, Jarrous N, van Venrooij WJ, Pruijn GJ. Architecture and function of the human endonucleases RNase P and RNase MRP. IUBMB Life 49:265–272, 2000.

Verloes A, Pierard GE, Le Merrer M, Maroteaux P. Recessive metaphyseal dysplasia without hypotrichosis. A syndrome clinically distinct from McKusick cartilage-hair hypoplasia. J Med Genet 27:693–696, 1990.

Virolainen M, Savilahti E, Kaitila I, Perheentupa J. Cellular and humoral immunity in cartilage-hair hypoplasia. Pediatr Res 12:961–966, 1970.

Wood PM, Mayne A, Joyce H, Smith CI, Granoff DM, Kumararatne DS. A mutation in Bruton's tyrosine kinase as a cause of selective anti-polysaccharide antibody deficiency. J Pediatr 139:148–151, 2001.

World Health Organizarion (WHO). Primary immunodeficiency diseases. Report of an IUIS Scientific Committee. International Union of Immunological Societies. Clin Exp Immunol 118(Suppl 1):1–28, 1999.

Yamaoka S, Courtois G, Bessia C, et al. Complementation cloning of NEMO, a component of the IκB kinase complex essential for NF-κB activation. Cell 93:1231–1240, 1998.

Yan M, Wang LC, Hymowitz SG, et al. Two–amino acid molecular switch in an epithelial morphogen that regulates binding to two distinct receptors. Science 290:523–537, 2000.

Yel L, Aggarwal S, Gupta S. Cartilage-hair hypoplasia syndrome: increased apoptosis of T lymphocytes is associated with altered expression of Fas (CD95), FasL (CD95L), IAP, Bax, and Bcl2. J Clin Immunol 19:428–434, 1999.

Yoshimura A, Lien E, Ingalls RR, Tuomanen E, Dziarski R, Golenbock D. Cutting edge: recognition of gram-positive bacterial cell wall components by the innate immune system occurs via Toll-like receptor 2. J Immunol 163:1–5, 1999.

Zonana J, Elder ME, Schneider LC, et al. A novel X-linked disorder of immune deficiency and hypohidrotic ectodermal dysplasia is allelic to incontinentia pigmenti and due to mutations in IKK-γ (*NEMO*). Am J Hum Genet 67:1555–1562, 2000.

37

Chronic Granulomatous Disease

DIRK ROOS, TACO W. KUIJPERS, and JOHN T. CURNUTTE

Chronic granulomatous disease (CGD) is an uncommon congenital immunodeficiency seen in approximately 1 in 250,000 individuals. It is caused by a profound defect in a burst of oxygen consumption that normally accompanies phagocytosis in all myeloid cells (neutrophils, eosinophils, monocytes, and macrophages). This "respiratory burst" involves the catalytic conversion of molecular oxygen to the oxygen free-radical superoxide (O_2^-), which in turn gives rise to hydrogen peroxide (H_2O_2), hypochlorous acid (HOCl), and hydroxyl radical ($\cdot$OH). These oxygen derivatives play a critical role in the killing of pathogenic bacteria and fungi. As a result of the failure to activate the respiratory burst in their phagocytes, the majority of CGD patients suffer from severe recurrent infections, the most common of which are pneumonia, lymphadenitis, cutaneous and hepatic abscesses, osteomyelitis, and septicemia. These severe infections usually become apparent during the first year of life and are caused predominantly by *Staphylococcus aureus*, *Aspergillus* species, enteric gram-negative bacteria, *Serratia marcescens*, and *Burkholderia (Pseudomonas) cepacia*. In addition, CGD patients have diffuse granulomas (presumably caused by microbes) that can become sufficiently large to cause obstructive or painful symptoms in the esophagus, stomach, biliary system, ureters, or urinary bladder.

While all CGD patients share the severe defect in the respiratory burst, there is substantial heterogeneity in the molecular mechanisms responsible. The enzyme that catalyzes the respiratory burst, NADPH oxidase, consists of at least four subunits (designated *phox* for *ph*agocyte *ox*idase): gp91^{phox} and p22^{phox} (the two membrane-bound subunits of a low-potential flavocytochrome *b*, termed flavocytochrome b_{558}, that is the redox center of the oxidase) as well as two cytosolic oxidase components, p47^{phox} and p67^{phox}. CGD is caused by a defect in any one of these four components. Mutations in the gp91^{phox} gene (*CYBB* on chromosome Xp21.1) cause the X-linked recessive form of

the disease that affects about 70% of all CGD patients. As expected from the genetics, the overwhelming majority of X-linked patients are males. The remaining 30% of cases are inherited in an autosomal recessive manner in which males and females are equally affected. These patients have mutations in the genes encoding p47^{phox} (*NCF1* on chromosome 7q11.23; about 25% of cases), p67^{phox} (*NCF2* on chromosome 1q25; about 2% of cases), or p22^{phox} (*CYBA* on chromosome 16q24; about 3% of cases). Deletions, insertions, splice site defects, nonsense mutations, missense mutations, and, in rare cases, regulatory mutations have been identified in the four types of CGD at the molecular genetic level. With the exception of p47^{phox}-deficient patients, who are usually homozygous for a GT deletion at the beginning of exon 2 in *NCF1*, most CGD patients have mutations unique to their families. The diversity of these mutations and the multiple genes affected provide an explanation for the genetic, biochemical, and clinical heterogeneity of CGD.

In two separate reports in 1957, Landing and Shirkey as well as Good and colleagues described a new syndrome of recurrent bacterial infections in male children that were associated with pigmented lipid-laden histiocytes in visceral organs, diffuse granulomas, and normal immunoglobulin levels (Berendes et al., 1957; Landing and Shirkey, 1957). The syndrome was originally referred to as "fatal granulomatous disease of childhood," because most patients succumbed to death at early ages from severe infections that responded poorly to even the most aggressive therapy (Berendes et al., 1957; Bridges et al., 1959). Over the ensuing several decades, the prognosis for children afflicted with this rare disorder has steadily improved because of an increasing understanding of its molecular and clinical features. Fatal granulomatous disease is now known by its more upbeat appellation, *chronic granulomatous disease* (CGD). What is remarkable about the early reports on CGD is the extent to which the clinical and genetic observations in a relatively small number of patients have held true; since then over 2000 additional patients have been identified and, in numerous cases, reported in the literature.

Because the most striking hallmark of the early cases of CGD was unresolved bacterial and fungal infections, investigators were drawn to study the function of granulocytes from these patients. Indeed, patient neutrophils demonstrated markedly abnormal killing of organisms such as *S. aureus* and *Escherichia coli* in in vitro assays (Quie et al., 1967). This defect was not due to an immunoglobulin or complement deficiency in patient serum, nor to an abnormality in neutrophil chemotaxis, ingestion, or degranulation. (Patient neutrophils also contained normal levels of lysosomal proteins and degradative enzymes.) The first clue to the underlying molecular defect came in 1959 in a seminal report by Sbarra and Karnovsky. It had been known since 1933 that neutrophils substantially increase their consumption of oxygen concomitant with phagocytosis of microbes (Baldridge and Gerard, 1933), and it had been assumed that this was due to increased energy metabolism. Sbarra and Karnovsky demonstrated, however, that the oxygen was not used for mitochondrial respiration but was instead utilized for the production of potentially microbicidal molecules such as hydrogen peroxide. This set the stage for the report in 1967 that CGD neutrophils did not undergo this respiratory burst when bacteria were ingested (Holmes et al., 1967). A subsequent report in 1973 identified the oxygen radical, superoxide (O_2^-), as the initial product formed from the oxygen consumed in the respiratory burst and the precursor of the other microbicidal oxygen derivatives (Babior et al., 1973). CGD neutrophils were found not to generate superoxide (Curnutte et al., 1974). The absence of the respiratory burst and its various products (such as superoxide and hydrogen peroxide) was then used as the defining characteristic of CGD and remains the cornerstone for its diagnosis today. Interestingly, one of the earliest assays used to measure respiratory burst activity in phagocytes, the nitroblue tetrozolium (NBT) test, is still one of the most widely used tests for detecting CGD (Baehner and Nathan, 1968).

The NBT test also proved to be a powerful tool in defining the genetics of CGD. When used to stain neutrophils adherent to a microscope slide, the NBT "slide" test revealed that many of the mothers of affected males had two populations of cells: one that underwent a respiratory burst and stained positive, and another that failed to stain with the dye and therefore resembled the defective cells in the patient. While this finding indicated that CGD could be inherited in an X-linked recessive fashion, an autosomal recessive mode of inheritance was also suggested by pedigrees with females suffering from a nearly identical syndrome of recurrent infections and absent respiratory burst but normal respiratory burst in neutrophils from patients' mothers (Azimi et al., 1968; Quie et al., 1968). It was hypothesized that X-linked CGD involved a defect in the enzyme that catalyzed the respiratory burst whereas the autosomal form was due to defects in other aspects of phagocyte metabolism (such as glutathione peroxidase activity) that indirectly affected the respiratory burst (Holmes et al., 1970).

Before this confusing genetic picture could be clarified, it was first necessary for the field to identify the enzyme responsible for the respiratory burst. A debate raged for over a decade as to whether the "respiratory burst oxidase" was a soluble NADH oxidase or a membrane-bound NADPH oxidase (Rossi, 1986; Curnutte and Babior, 1987). Finally, the ability of the two candidate enzymes to produce superoxide was used as one of the defining properties of the respiratory burst oxidase, and it eventually became clear that NADPH oxidase was the enzyme responsible for the burst in human neutrophils (Curnutte et al., 1975). An additional important breakthrough occurred in 1978 when Segal and colleagues found that a low-potential cytochrome *b* was undetectable in the neutrophils from four CGD patients (Segal et al., 1978). A multicenter European study of the prevalence of cytochrome *b* deficiency in a group of 27 CGD patients revealed that the cytochrome was undetectable in all 19 males who had X-linked CGD whereas it was present in normal levels in all 8 patients (7 females and 1 male) who appeared to have autosomal recessive inheritance (Segal et al., 1983). It thus appeared that cytochrome *b* (termed cytochrome b_{-245} or b_{558} to reflect its -245 mV midpoint potential or its 558 nm absorption peak, respectively) was an important component of NADPH oxidase and that X-linked CGD could be explained by its deficiency. The defect in autosomal recessive CGD remained unknown, and the picture was complicated by the identification of patients with this form of the disease who had undetectable levels of cytochrome b_{558} (Weening et al., 1985b). Thus, at least three distinct forms of CGD appeared to exist: X-linked, cytochrome *b*-negative (X^0); autosomal recessive, cytochrome *b*-positive (A^+); and autosomal recessive, cytochrome *b*-negative (A^0). That these three types of CGD are genetically distinct was conclusively demonstrated by complementation studies in which monocytes from pairs of these three groups of patients were fused with each other to form heterokaryons. Complementation (measured as acquisition of NBT staining) was observed in the X^0/A^0, X^0/A^+, and A^0/A^+ fusions, indicating three distinct complementation groups in CGD (Hamers et al., 1984; Weening et al., 1985b).

One of the other major breakthroughs in unraveling the mystery of the genetic heterogeneity of CGD was the discovery in several laboratories of a cell-free system for activating NADPH oxidase (Bromberg and Pick, 1984; Heyneman and Vercauteren, 1984; Curnutte, 1985; McPhail et al., 1985). Studies with this system revealed that both the plasma membrane and cytosol fractions were required for oxidase activity. In both the X-linked and autosomal recessive forms of cytochrome b_{558} deficiency, it was the membrane fraction that was defective in the cell-free system (Curnutte, 1985; Curnutte et al., 1987) whereas in the autosomal recessive, cytochrome b_{558}–positive patients the cytosol was devoid of activity (Curnutte et al., 1988). The identities of the missing or defective proteins came to light in parallel with these findings through the convergence of several lines of investigation. First, Orkin and colleagues identified the gene affected in X-linked CGD, without knowledge of its protein product, through restriction fragment length polymorphism (RFLP) studies that localized the gene to Xp21 and the study of two patients with X-linked CGD who had small interstitial deletions within this region of the X chromosome (Baehner et al., 1986; Royer-Pokora et al., 1986). Second, Jesaitis, Parkos, and colleagues (Parkos et al., 1987) and Segal (1987) found that cytochrome b_{558} is a heterodimer composed of a heavily glycosylated 91 kDa subunit (termed β) and a nonglycosylated 22 kDa component (termed α). The 91 kDa subunit was found to be identical with the product of the X-CGD gene identified by Orkin et al. (termed *CYBB*) (Dinauer et al., 1987; Teahan et al., 1987) whereas the α subunit gene (termed *CYBA*) was localized to chromosome 16q24 and found to be defective in autosomal recessive, cytochrome b_{558}–negative patients (Parkos et al., 1988; Dinauer et al., 1990). Finally, selected pairs of defective cytosols from patients with autosomal recessive, cytochrome b_{558}–positive CGD were found to complement each other in the cell-free activation system and restore near normal activity (Nunoi et al., 1988; Curnutte et al., 1989). Two cytosolic complementation groups were thus defined by this method, and the deficient proteins were identified as two novel myeloid-specific polypeptides—one that was 47 kDa in mass and the other that was 67 kDa (Nunoi et al., 1988; Volpp et al., 1988; Leto et al., 1990). In one major cooperative study, the 47 kDa protein was undetectable in 22 of 25 CGD patients with defective cytosols whereas the 67 kDa polypeptide was absent in the remaining three patients (Clark et al., 1989). The gene encoding the 47 kDa component (termed *NCF1*) maps to 7q11.23 and the 67 kDa gene (termed *NCF2*) localizes to 1q25, findings consistent with the autosomal recessive mode of inheritance for each of these deficiencies in CGD (Francke et al., 1990).

A CGD-like syndrome caused by a defect in the activation mechanism of the NADPH oxidase (Rac2 deficiency) or by a shortage of substrate supply for the oxidase (glucose 6-phosphate dehydrogenase [G6PD] deficiency) has to be considered for differential diagnosis.

Clinical and Pathological Manifestations

Given the key role the products of the respiratory burst play in host defense, it is not surprising that patients with CGD suffer from a variety of recurrent bacterial and fungal infections. These infections occur most commonly in those organs in contact with the outside world—the lungs, gastrointestinal tract, and skin, as well as the lymph nodes that drain these structures. Because of both contiguous and hematogenous spread of infection, a wide range of other organs can be affected, most notably the liver, bones, kidneys, and brain. In approximately two-thirds of patients, the first symptoms of CGD appear during the first year of life in the form of infections (lymphadenitis, pneumonia, rectal abscesses, and osteomyelitis), dermatitis (sometimes seen at birth), and gastro-

intestinal complications (vomiting secondary to granulomatous obstruction of the gastric antrum; intermittent bloody diarrhea due to CGD colitis) (Johnston and Newman, 1977). On physical exam, CGD infants are often underweight and anemic, particularly the X-linked males. It is worth noting that this clinical picture can be quite variable, with some infants suffering from several or more of these complications whereas others appear far less ill. In some cases, the presenting symptoms of CGD can be mistaken for pyloric stenosis, food or milk allergy, or iron-deficiency anemia. In general, infants with X-linked CGD tend to present earlier and with more dramatic symptoms than infants with the autosomal recessive forms of the disease, especially p47phox deficiency (Weening et al., 1985a; Margolis et al., 1990; Gallin et al., 1991; Winkelstein et al., 2000). In a small but noteworthy subset of patients, the diagnosis of CGD is not made until the teenage or adult years because of the mildness of the symptoms (Liese et al., 1996). The underlying reasons for this somewhat surprising clinical variability will be discussed below.

The full spectrum of CGD is summarized in Table 37.1. Despite the rarity of CGD, a number of investigators have either reviewed or assembled large series of patients from the United States, Europe, and Japan (Johnston and Newman, 1977; Cohen et al., 1981; Gallin et al., 1983; Hitzig and Seger, 1983; Tauber et al., 1983; Hayakawa et al., 1985; Forrest et al., 1988; Mouy et al., 1989; Winkelstein et al., 2000). The approximately 750 patients represented by these studies provide a striking picture of the multiple manifestations of the disease. As shown in Table 37.1, *Staphylococcus aureus, Aspergillus* species, enteric gram-negative bacteria (including *Serratia marcescens* and various *Salmonella* species), and *Burkholderia cepacia* (previously termed *Pseudomonas cepacia*) are the most frequently encountered pathogens. Most CGD pathogens share the property of containing

Table 37.1. Infections, Chronic Conditions, and Organisms Associated with Chronic Granulomatous Disease*

Infections	Percent of Infections	Condition	Percent of Cases	Infecting Organisms	Percent of Isolates
Pneumonia	70–80	Lymphadenopathy	98	*Staphylococcus aureus*	30–50
Lymphadenitis[†]	60–80	Hypergammaglobulinemia	60–90	*Escherichia coli*	5–10
Cutaneous infections/impetigo[†]	60–70	Hepatosplenomegaly	50–90	*Aspergillus* species	10–20
Hepatic/perihepatic abscesses[†]	30–40	Splenomegaly	60–80	*Salmonella* species	5–10
Osteomyelitis	15–30	Anemia of chronic disease	Common[‡]	*Klebsiella* species	5–10
Septicemia	10–20	Underweight	70	*Burkholderia cepacia*	5–10
Otitis media[†]	15–20	Chronic diarrhea	20–60	*Staphylococcus epidermidis*	5
Conjunctivitis	10–20	Short stature	50	*Serratia marcescens*	5–10
Enteric infections	5–15	Gingivitis	50	*Enterobacter* species	3
Urinary tract infections/pyelonephritis	5–15	Dermatitis	35	*Streptococcus* species	4
Sinusitis	<10	Chorioretinitis	20–35	*Proteus* species	3
Renal/perinephric abscesses	<10	Hydronephrosis	10–25	*Candida albicans*	3
Brain abscesses	<5	Ulcerative stomatitis	5–25	*Nocardia* species	2
Pericarditis	<5	Pulmonary fibrosis	<10	*Haemophilus influenzae*	1
Meningitis	<5	Esophagitis	<10	*Pneumocystis* carinii	<1
		Gastric antral narrowing	<10	*Mycobacterium fortuitum*	<1
		Granulomatous ileocolitis	<10	*Chromobacterium violaceum*	<1
		Granulomatous cystitis	<10	*Chromobacterium violaceum*	<1
		Glomerulonephritis	<10	*Francisella philomiragia*	<1
		Discoid lupus erythematosus	<10	*Torulopsis glabrata*	<1

*The relative frequencies of different types of infection in CGD are estimated from data pooled from several large series of patients in the United States, Europe, and Japan (Johnston and Newman, 1977; Cohen et al., 1981; Gallin et al., 1983; Hitzig and Seger, 1983; Tauber et al., 1983; Hayakawa et al., 1985; Forrest et al., 1988; Mouy et al., 1989; Winkelstein et al., 2000). These series encompass approximately 550 CGD patients after accounting for overlap between reports. The list of infecting organisms is also arranged according to data in these reports and is not paired with the entries in the first column

[†]These infections are most frequently seen at the time of presentation.

[‡]In some instances, the incidence is estimated from the 100 cases of CGD followed at Scripps Clinic (unpublished data).

Reproduced with permission (Curnutte, 1992).

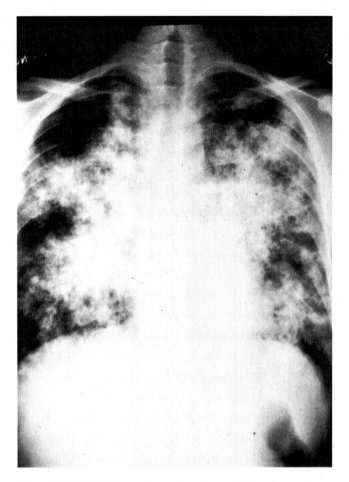

Figure 37.1. Chest X-ray of a male patient with chronic granulomatous disease (CGD) and fatal *Aspergillus* infection.

catalase; as such, they are unable to "lend" hydrogen peroxide generated metabolically within the microbes to the peroxide-starved CGD phagocytes. For catalase-negative organisms, the CGD phagocytes use bacteria-generated peroxide (once converted to hypochlorous acid by neutrophil myeloperoxidase) to kill the microbes (Mandell and Hook, 1969). Catalase production may thus be a microbial pathogenicity factor in CGD. However, this view has been questioned (Chang et al., 1998; Messina et al., 2002).

Pneumonia is the most common type of infection encountered in CGD in all age groups and is typically caused by *Staphylococcus aureus, Aspergillus* species, *Burkholderia cepacia*, and enteric gram-negative bacteria (Fig. 37.1). In cases where the pneumonia is already severe or where the patient fails to respond promptly to the empiric regimen, more invasive approaches are warranted to establish the diagnosis, such as bronchoscopy, needle biopsy, and open lung biopsy. Rarer pathogens requiring special types of treatment (for example, *Nocardia* infections) are usually only identified by this more aggressive approach. One of the more problematic pulmonary pathogens is *B. cepacia* (and the closely related organisms *B. gladioli, B. mallei, B. pseudomallei,* and *B. pickettii*). These bacteria are unusually virulent in CGD patients and have come to be identified as one of the predominant causes of fatal pneumonias in these patients (Speert et al., 1994). Contributing to this mortality is the fact that many strains of *Burkholderia* are not adequately treated with the antibiotics used for the empiric treatment of CGD infections because most are resistant to aminoglycosides and many strains are resistant to cef-

tazidime. Moreover, cultures from patients infected with *Burkholderia* often grow slowly. The virulence of these organisms is compounded by their ubiquitous presence in the environment. *Aspergillus* and other fungal infections of the lung also pose difficult challenges because they typically require prolonged treatment (4–6 months). If possible, it is important to determine the source of the *Aspergillus* in the patient's environment so that the risk of reexposure can be minimized.

Cutaneous abscesses and lymphadenitis represent the next most common types of infection in CGD and are typically caused by *S. aureus* followed by various gram-negative organisms, including *B. cepacia* and *Serratia marcescens* (Color Plate 37.I). These infections may respond slowly to antimicrobial therapy and require incision and drainage for resolution. Recurrent impetigo, frequently in the perinasal area and caused by *S. aureus,* usually requires prolonged courses of oral antibiotics to clear. Hepatic (and perihepatic) abscesses are also quite common in CGD and are typically caused by *S. aureus.* Patients usually present with fever, malaise, and weight loss. Liver function laboratory tests are often normal. Resolution may require surgical drainage or excision of the lesion as well as several months of parenteral antibiotics. Osteomyelitis is another important infection in CGD and can arise from hematogenous spread of organisms (*S. aureus, Salmonella* spp., *Serratia marcescens*) or contiguous invasion of bone, typically seen with *Aspergillus* pneumonia spreading to the ribs or vertebral bodies. Perirectal abscesses are also common in CGD patients and once formed can persist for years despite aggressive antimicrobial therapy and fastidious local care. Other important but less commonly seen infections in CGD are summarized in Table 37.1.

Not all encounters with microorganisms in CGD result in overt pyogenic infections, as stalemates may develop between the pathogen and the patient's leukocytes. In these cases, chronic inflammatory cell reactions consisting of lymphocytes and histiocytes develop, which can then organize to form granulomas, one of the hallmarks of CGD. As discussed above and noted in Table 37.1, esophageal and gastric granulomas can cause dysphagia, stomach pain, and even recurrent vomiting if they partially block the pylorus (Renner et al., 1991; Danziger et al., 1993). Similarly, granulomas in the urinary bladder can present with dysuria, decreased urine volume, and penile pain (Aliabadi et al., 1989; Walther et al., 1992). Hydronephrosis can develop if these lesions are in the vicinity of the ureters and do not resolve. Another important type of chronic inflammation in CGD is a form of inflammatory bowel disease that closely resembles Crohn's disease and affects approximately 10% of patients. While the colon is typically involved, the ileum and other parts of the gastrointestinal tract can be affected. The symptoms can range from mild diarrhea to a debilitating syndrome of bloody diarrhea and malabsorption that can necessitate a colectomy (Ament and Ochs, 1973). Other types of chronic inflammation include gingivitis, chorioretinitis, glomerulonephritis, and destructive white matter lesions in the brain (Table 37.1) (Martyn et al., 1972; Frifelt et al., 1985; Hadfield et al., 1991). In rare cases, patients may develop either discoid or (even more rarely) systemic lupus erythematosus (Sillevis Smitt et al., 1990a; Manzi et al., 1991).

Patients with CGD can suffer from a variety of other chronic complications outlined in Table 37.1. One of the more striking is short stature, seen most commonly in X-linked males, in which the children grow at or below the fifth percentile until adolescence, when some catch-up growth can occur. Lymphadenopathy, hepatosplenomegaly, and eczematoid dermatitis are also common features of CGD and are most frequently encountered in infants and children. Children with CGD are typically anemic with hemoglobin levels in the 8–10 g/dl range with microcytic erythrocyte indices. The anemia is most likely due to the chronic disease state and, not surprisingly, responds poorly to iron therapy. Interestingly, this anemia tends to spontaneously resolve near the end of the first decade of life. A few X-linked CGD patients have McLeod syndrome, a mild hemolytic anemia characterized by acanthocytosis and weak Kell antigens (Marsh and Redman, 1987). This anemia is caused by a deletion in the X chromosome that affects both the gene for gp91^phox (*CYBB*) and the nearby *Xk* gene that encodes a 37 kDa erythrocyte membrane protein necessary for expression of Kell antigens.

Carriers of CGD, whether of the X-linked form or any of the three autosomal recessive forms, are usually asymptomatic, with three important exceptions. First, roughly half of X-linked carriers have either recurrent stomatitis or moderately severe gingivitis or both. Second, in a small percentage of X-linked carriers, there can be an unusually high degree of inactivation of the normal X chromosome in their myeloid cells. If the circulating neutrophil population is skewed to the point that fewer than 10% of the cells function, then the carrier has an increased risk of infection (usually mild) (Mills et al., 1980; Curnutte et al., 1992). Third, approximately one-quarter of X-linked carriers develop discoid lupus erythematosus characterized by discoid skin lesions on the face, shoulders, arms, and upper chest and back that can be induced or exacerbated by sun exposure. This syndrome typically becomes apparent in the second decade of life, can range from mild (common) to fairly intense, and does not appear to progress to systemic lupus erythematosus either clinically or serologically (Schaller, 1972; Brandrup et al., 1981; Sillevis Smitt et al., 1990b; Manzi et al., 1991; Yeaman et al., 1992). Severe cases usually respond well to hydroxychloroquine. Discoid lupus erythematosus has not been associated with the carrier state in any of the autosomal recessive forms of CGD. The underlying mechanism responsible for discoid lupus in X-linked CGD carriers is not known, although it has been hypothesized that autoantibodies to antigens from incompletely destroyed microbes (derived from the defective subpopulation of neutrophils) may be responsible (Manzi et al., 1991).

Composition, Activation, and Function of the NADPH Oxidase

Composition of the NADPH Oxidase

The phagocyte NADPH oxidase consists of a membrane-bound catalytic subunit and a number of activity-regulating components that reside in the cytosol of resting phagocytes but translocate to the membrane upon cell activation (Fig. 37.2). In this way, the activity of this potent enzyme is restricted to the time when and the site where it is needed. The membrane-bound catalytic subunit is the flavohemeprotein gp91^phox, which is stabilized in a 1:1 complex with the transmembrane p22^phox protein (Table 37.2) (Huang et al., 1995; Wallach and Segal, 1996). The complex together is called flavocytochrome b_{558}. The N-terminal half of gp91^phox contains six hydrophobic regions that may serve as membrane-spanning domains and three N-linked glycosylation sites (Wallach and Segal, 1997) (Fig. 37.3). This part of gp91^phox contains two heme moieties, each located between two histidines in transmembrane domains of the protein (Fig. 37.3) (Cross et al., 1995; Finegold et al., 1996; Yu et al., 1998). The location of the heme binding domain has been deduced from sequence homology

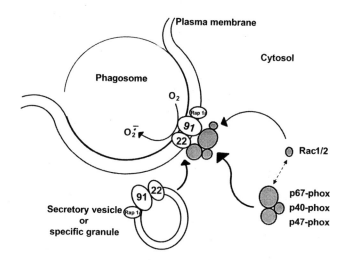

Figure 37.2. Activation of the NADPH oxidase. The membrane-bound NADPH-oxidase components gp91^phox and p22^phox and the small GTP-binding protein Rap1A are located in resting neutrophils in the membranes of specific granules and secretory vesicles. During cell activation (e.g., after binding of opsonized microorganisms to surface receptors on the neutrophils), these organelles fuse with the plasma membrane, thus leading to up-regulation of the expression of these components on the neutrophil surface, especially in plasma membrane areas surrounding phagocytosed material (phagosomes). Concomitantly, the cytosolic NADPH-oxidase components p40^phox, p47^phox, and p67^phox translocate to the cytochrome b_{558} subunits (gp91^phox and p22^phox) and induce a conformational change in gp91^phox that allows NADPH to bind to gp91^phox and donate its electrons to the FAD moiety in this subunit. The cytosolic small GTP-binding proteins Rac1 (in macrophages) and Rac2 (in neutrophils) regulate the translocation process by binding to p67^phox, to gp91^phox, and to the plasma membrane.

between the N-terminal half of gp91^phox and the FRE1 protein of the iron reductase in *Saccharomyces cerevisiae* (Finegold et al., 1996). This part of gp91^phox also appears to be involved in the interaction with p22^phox. The C-terminal part of gp91^phox is hydrophilic, probably cytosolic, and contains one FAD group. The location of the putative FAD binding domain has been deduced from sequence homology between the C-terminal half of gp91^phox and the ferridoxin NADP reductase flavoenzyme family (Rotrosen et al., 1992; Segal et al., 1992; Sumimoto et al., 1992; Leusen et al., 2000). In a similar way, the position of the putative NADPH binding domain has been mapped on gp91^phox (Fig. 37.3). Like gp91^phox, the N-terminal half of p22^phox contains hydrophobic helices that may be transmembrane domains, and the C-terminal half is more hydrophilic.

The cytosolic NADPH oxidase components p47^phox and p67^phox each contain two src homology region 3 (SH3) motifs, known to interact with proline-rich regions in the same or in other proteins (Table 37.2). Both of these cytosolic components also contain at least one such proline-rich region. The SH3–proline interactions may be involved both in keeping p47^phox and p67^phox in an inactive conformation in resting cells (by mutual interaction) and activating the NADPH oxidase enzyme by promoting interactions between the cytosolic components and flavocytochrome b_{558} (De Mendez et al., 1994; Finan et al., 1994; Leto et al., 1994; Leusen et al., 1994a, 1994b, 1995; Sumimoto et al., 1994). The p67^phox protein also contains four tetratricopepide (TTP) regions in its C terminus, which form binding regions for the small GTPases Rac1 or Rac2; this constitutes another activation mechanism of the phagocyte NADPH oxidase

Table 37.2. Properties of Phagocyte Respiratory Burst Oxidase (*phox*) Components

	gp91*phox*	p22*phox*	p47*phox*	p67*phox*	p40*phox*
Synonyms	α-chain Heavy chain Nox-2	β-chain Light chain	NCF-1	NCF-2	NCF-4
Amino acids	570	195	390	526	339
Molecular weight (kDa)					
Predicted	65.0	20.9	44.6	60.9	39.0
By PAGE	70–91	22	47	67	40
Glycosylation	Yes (N-linked)	No	No	No	No
Phosphorylation	No	Yes	Yes	Low level	Low level
PI	9.7	10.0	9.5	5.8	6.4
mRNA(kb)	4.7	0.8	1.4	2.4	1.4
Gene locus	CYBB Xp21.1	CYBA 16q24	NCF1 7q11.23	NCF2 1q25	NCF4 22q13.1
Exons/span	13/30 kb	6/8.5 kb	11/15 kb	16/40 kb	10/18 kb
Cellular location in resting neutrophils	Specific granule membrane; plasma membrane	Specific granule membrane; plasma membrane	Cytosol; cytoskeleton	Cytosol; cytoskeleton	Cytosol; cytoskeleton
Level in neutrophils (pmols/10^6 cells)	3.3–5.3	3.3–5.3	3.3	1.2	1.2
Tissue specificity	Myeloid, low levels in mesangial cells, endothelial cells, and B lymphocytes	mRNA in all cells tested, protein only in myeloid and endothelial cells	Myeloid cells and B lymphocytes	Myeloid cells and B lymphocytes	Myeloid and other hematopoietic cells
Functional domains	Binding sites for cytosolic oxidase components; heme, FAD, and NADPH binding domains	Pro-rich domain that binds p47*phox*	Nine Ser-P sites; 2 SH3 domains; Pro-rich domains; 1 PX domain	Two SH3 domains; 4 TTP regions; 1 PB1 domain; Pro-rich domains	One SH3 domain, 1 PX domain, 1 OPR domain
Homologies	Ferredoxin-NADP+ reductase (FNR)* (weak homology)	Polypeptide I of cytochrome *c* oxidase	SH3 domain of *src*, p47*phox*, and p67*phox*; PX domain of many proteins[†]; homology to p40*phox* N terminus	SH3 domain of *src*, p40*phox*, and p47*phox*; TTP regions of many proteins[‡]; PBI domain of budding yeast protein Bem1p	SH3 domains of *src* and p67*phox*; OPR domain of Cdc24p, MEK5, and Zip; PX domain of many proteins[†]; homology to p47*phox* N terminus
GenBank Accession No.	X04011**	M21186, J03774	M25665, M26193	M32011	U50720–U50729

Abbreviations used: *CYBA*, cytochrome-*b* alpha; *CYBB*, cytochrome-*b* beta; FNR, ferredoxin-NADP reductase; *NCF*, neutrophil cytosol factor; OPR, octicosa peptide repeat; PAGE, polyacrylamide gel electrophoresis; PB1, *P*hox and *B*em-1 domain; phox, *p*hagocyte *ox*idase component; Pro, proline; PX, phox homology; Ser-P, serine phosphorylation; SH3, *src* homology domain 3; TTP, tetratricopeptide.

*Weak homology to both the NADPH and FAD-binding domains in the FNR family.

[†]PX domain homology with kinesins, phospholipases, PI3-kinases, protein kinases, SNAREs, and sorting nexins.

[‡]TTP region homology with subunits of anaphase-promoting complex, hsp90-binding immunophilins, transcription factors, PKR protein kinase inhibitor, and peroxisomal and mitochondrial import proteins.

**This GenBank accession number refers to the sequence as originally published. The complete corrected sequence (encoding an additional 64 amino acids) has not been deposited in GenBank.

Adapted with permission (Curnutte, 1992b).

(Nisimoto et al., 1997; Koga et al., 1999). A third cytosolic component, called p40*phox*, with N-terminal homology to p47*phox* and one SH3 domain resembling that of p67*phox*, is possibly involved in stabilization of the p47*phox*/p67*phox* complex in resting cells and in facilitating membrane recruitment of this complex during oxidase activation (Table 37.2) (Fuchs et al., 1995; Kuribayashi et al., 2002). Both p47*phox* and p40*phox* contain a so-called PX (phox homology) region that can bind to phosphatidyl phosphoinositides in the plasma membrane as yet another interaction to stabilize the active NADPH oxidase complex (Ellson et al., 2001; Kanai et al., 2001). P40*phox* also contains in its C terminus an octicosa peptide repeat (OPR), also

called PC (Phox Cdc24p) domain, which is involved in binding to a so-called PB1 (Phox and Bem-1) domain in p67*phox* (Ponting, 1996; Nakamura et al., 1998; Ito et al., 2001). The regions within the cytoplasmic oxidase components that interact with each other or with flavocytochrome b_{558} are partially known from studying natural mutations (Dinauer et al., 1991; Leusen et al., 1994a, 1994b; 2000; Leto et al., 1994; Sumimoto et al., 1994). More detailed information in this respect has been gained from analyzing peptides in the two-hybrid system (Fuchs et al., 1995) or in a phage display system (DeLeo et al., 1995a, 1995b), or from peptide walking (Joseph and Pick, 1995; Morozov et al., 1998).

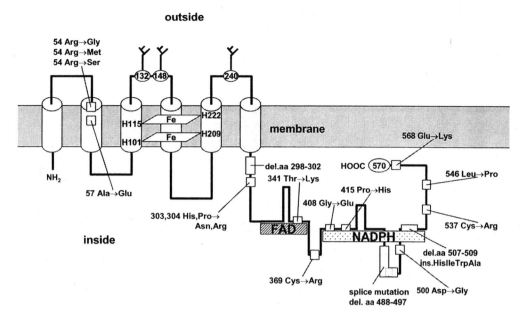

Figure 37.3. Schematic picture of gp91^{phox} and X91$^+$ CGD mutations. The hydrophobic regions of gp91^{phox} that may serve as membrane-spanning domains are shown as cylinders, while the asparagines that are N-glycosylated are indicated by the codon number and a carbohydrate tree. The heme-binding histidines are located in the third and fifth trans-membrane regions. The putative FAD and NADPH binding regions are also indicated, as are the mutations that lead to the X91$^+$ phenotype of CGD. The loop of 20 amino acids that covers the cleft of the NADPH binding region in resting cells is indicated in the lower right corner of the picture.

Activation of the NADPH Oxidase

It is possible to construct a provisional model for the mechanism of NADPH oxidase activation based on a synthesis of multiple reports. In the inactive state of the enzyme in quiescent phagocytes, the flavohemeprotein gp91^{phox} is inaccessible for its substrate NADPH because a stretch of 20 amino acids (residues 484–504) lies over the nucleotide-binding cleft (Fig. 37.4) (Taylor et al., 1993). Interaction of p47^{phox} and p67^{phox} with flavocytochrome b_{558} results in movement of this 20–amino acid loop and hence provides NADPH with access to its binding site in gp91^{phox}. Some evidence suggests that binding of p67^{phox} to flavocytochrome b_{558} suffices for electron flow from NADPH via FAD and the heme groups to oxygen, thus generating superoxide; the function of p47^{phox} may be to tighten the binding of the cytosolic oxidase components to the assembled oxidase complex (Freeman et al., 1996; Koshkin et al., 1996). One of the heme goups is probably attached to histidine-115, located in the middle of an H-X-X-X-H-X-X-X-H motif that may be involved in proton translocation for charge compensation of superoxide release outside the cells or in the phagosomes (Henderson, 1998; Henderson and Meech, 1999). Whether the hemes participate in this proton conductance is not known. However, the concept of gp91^{phox} itself acting as a proton channel is contradicted by the findings of DeCoursey (2003).

The translocation of the cytosolic NADPH oxidase components to the flavocytochrome is initiated by serine phosphorylation of p47^{phox} (and of p67^{phox} and p40^{phox}) during phagocyte activation (Segal et al., 1985; Okamura et al., 1988; Bolscher et al., 1989; Dusi and Rossi, 1993; Bouin et al., 1998; Forbes et al., 1999). This phosphorylation may cause exposure of SH3 and proline-rich domains in these proteins that are inaccessible in the p40^{phox}/p47^{phox}/p67^{phox} complex in the cytosol of resting cells (Leto et al., 1994; Fuchs et al., 1995). One proline-rich region in p22^{phox} involved in binding an SH3 region in p47^{phox} has been identified from the mutation in this proline-rich region in a CGD patient (Leto et al., 1994; Leusen et al., 1994a; Sumimoto et al., 1994). The phosphorylation of several serines in p47^{phox} appears to be critical for the translocation of this protein and for the activation of the NADPH oxidase (Faust et al., 1995; Johnson et al., 1998; Price et al., 2002b). In addition, phosphorylation of p22^{phox} also correlates with NADPH oxidase activation (Regier et al., 2000). It is not yet known which protein kinases are responsible for the phosphorylation of these oxidase components, nor how these kinases are activated. Possibly, protein kinase C β plays an important role in this respect (El Benna et al., 1996; Korchak et al., 1998; Reeves et al., 1999). Positioning of the cytosolic oxidase components in the membrane is facilitated by the formation of phosphatidylinositol (PtdIns) species phosphorylated at the inositol-3 position in the membrane by phosphoinositide-3-OH kinase [PI(3)K] during neutrophil activation. The PX domain of p40^{phox} binds to PtdIns(3)P and the PX domain of p47^{phox} binds to PtdIns(3,4)P$_2$ (Kanai et al., 2001). Charge interactions between gp91^{phox} and the cytosolic components may play a role in the formation of the oxidase complex, because several substitutions of amino acids in gp91^{phox} for amino acids with a different charge lead to stable expression of mutant gp91^{phox} molecules that no longer support translocation of cytosolic components (Leusen et al., 1994b, 2000). The proper positioning and stabilization of the oxidase complex may also depend on binding of the cytosolic components to cytoskeletal proteins, such as coronin, actin, moesin, and the calcium-binding protein S100A8/A9 (Grogan et al., 1997; Tamura et al., 2000; Wientjes et al., 2001; Doussière et al., 2002). In addition, the myeloid-related proteins MRP8 and MRP14 appear to be involved in the conformational change induced in gp91^{phox} during phagocyte activation, in synergy with p47^{phox} and p67^{phox} (Berthier et al., 2003). Finally, cPLA2-generated arachidonic

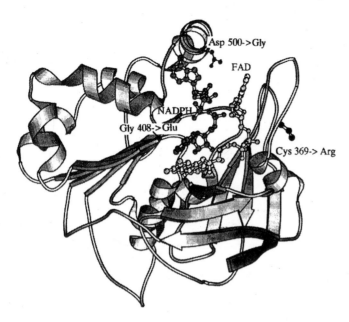

Asp 500->Gly

FAD

NADPH

Gly 408->Glu

Cys 369-> Arg

Figure 37.4. Three-dimensional model of the C-terminal, cytosolic part of gp91[phox]. This figure shows a model of the cytosolic portion of gp91[phox] based on that for spinach ferridoxin NADP reductase (Karplus et al., 1991), as described by Taylor et al. (1993). The figure was kindly provided by Dr. Nicholas Keep from Prof. Segal's group (London, U.K.). The protein is shown in the activated, NADPH-bound state. The 20–amino acid coil covering the cleft over the NADPH binding region in the active protein is now drawn aside (on top of the picture). In this coil, the position of Asp-500 is indicated. Cys-369 is located in another protein loop exposed to the cytosol, but Gly-408 is buried in the protein between these two loops. Mutations Asp500Gly, Cys369Arg, and Gly408Glu lead to the X91[+] CGD phenotype with defective translocation of cytosolic NADPH oxidase components.

acid is an essential cofactor in NADPH oxidase activation in intact or permeabilized cells, but the mechanism of this phenomenon is unknown (Dana et al., 1998).

Several low–molecular weight GTP-binding proteins are involved in the NADPH oxidase activation (Table 37.3) (Knaus et al., 1991; Abo et al., 1991). One of these is p21rac, of which two subtypes exist in phagocytes—Rac1 (mainly in macrophages) and Rac2 (mainly in neutrophils) (Dusi et al., 1995). During neutrophil activation, these GTP-binding proteins change from an inactive, GDP-bound state into an active, GTP-bound state, a process that is regulated by guanine-nucleotide exchange factors (GEFs) and GTPase-activating proteins (GAPs). Two Rac-activating GEFs have been identified in phagocytes: P-Rex1 and Vav1. P-Rex1 is synergistically activated by PtdIns(3,4,5)P$_3$ and the $\beta\gamma$ subunits of trimeric G proteins associated with seven-span membrane receptors (Welch et al., 2002). This indicates that P-Rex1 in neutrophils is under direct control of ligand binding to these receptors, but this was proven only for C5a. Vav1 is activated by tyrosine phosphorylation in its acidic region, a process downstream of receptor-linked tyrosine kinases. Vav1 appears to activate Rac1 and Rac2 in phagocytes in response to formyl-methionyl-leucyl-phenylalanine (fMLP), C5a, IgG complexes, lipopolysaccharide (LPS), or Ca^{2+} ionophore, but not to interleukin-8 (IL-8) or leukotriene B$_4$ (LTB$_4$) (Price et al., 2002a; Vilhardt et al., 2002; Kim et al., 2003; Zhao et al., 2003). Several GAPs are known in these cells, both in the cytosol and in the membrane (Geiszt et al., 2001). By inactivating Rac, these proteins may be involved in termination of the respiratory burst

(Szaszi et al., 1999). The inactive form of Rac is kept in a complex with Rho GDP-dissociation inhibitor (RhoGDI), which shields the geranylgeranyl moiety of Rac (Abo et al., 1991; Mizuno et al., 1992; Kwong et al., 1993). The activated, GTP-bound Rac, liberated from RhoGDI, binds to p67[phox] and associates with its fatty-acid tail into the phospholipids of the plasma membrane (Diekmann et al., 1994). However, p47[phox] and p67[phox] are drawn to the membrane and can form a complex with the flavocytochrome independent of the translocation of Rac (Heyworth et al., 1994; Dorseuil et al., 1995; Zhao et al., 2003). Probably, Rac also interacts with gp91[phox] itself, to facilitate electron flux through this protein (Diebold and Bokoch, 2001). Another low–molecular weight GTP-binding protein called Rap1A is associated with flavocytochrome b_{558} in the membrane (Table 37.3) (Quinn et al., 1992). This association is decreased upon protein kinase A–mediated phosphorylation of Rap1A, which suggests that Rap1A may modulate NADPH oxidase activity in response to agents that elevate cAMP in the cells (Bokoch et al., 1991).

Function of the NADPH Oxidase

It is clear that the functional defects of CGD phagocytes result from the inability of these cells to generate superoxide, hydrogen peroxide, hypochlorous acid, and other products derived from superoxide. However, the bactericidal potency of superoxide and hydrogen peroxide is low, and cells with myeloperoxidase deficiency, which are unable to generate hypochlorous acid, show almost normal bactericidal activity. By contrast, CGD cells incubated with bacteria together with beads covered with glucose oxidase, which generate hydrogen peroxide in the presence of glucose, show clearly improved killing of the bacteria (Johnston and Baehner, 1970). Similar results have been obtained with liposomes filled with glucose oxidase (Gerber et al., 2001). This would indicate that the reactive oxygen compounds themselves are the prime bactericidal agents. An alternative hypothesis has been formulated by the group of Segal (Reeves et al., 2002). These investigators found that mice deficient in leukocyte elastase and cathepsin G have a similar defect in bacterial killing to that of gp91[phox] knockout mice. They also found that these proteases are liberated from their carbohydrate matrix in the granules by cations, and that this process takes place in neutrophil phagosomes containing ingested bacteria because of an influx of potassium. This influx is induced together with the influx of protons by the accumulation of superoxide, with its negative charge, generated in the phagosomes. In CGD phagocytes, this process does not take place, resulting in decreased protease activity in these organelles and hence decreased bacterial killing. Recently, the potassium channel involved was identified as a large-conductance Ca^{2+}-activated K$^+$ channel (Ahluwalia et al., 2004). However, the idea expressed in this article, that the K$^+$ influx into the phagosome is responsible for most or all of the charge compensation needed to neutralize the superoxide generated in this compartment, has met strong criticism (DeCoursey, 2004). In addition, recent evidence from the group of Ligeti indicates that both direct and indirect bactericidal activity of the reactive oxygen species play an important role in the antimicrobial defense of phagocytes (Rada et al., 2004).

Another hallmark of CGD is the occurrence of diffuse granulomas. Some recent articles indicate that this too may be caused by the failure of the leukocyte NADPH oxidase in these patients to generate reactive oxygen species, in particular H$_2$O$_2$ (Hampton et al., 2002; Kobayashi et al., 2004). Phagocytosis of bacteria by

Table 37.3. Properties of Low–Molecular Mass GTP-Binding Proteins and Rac Regulatory Proteins Implicated in Phagocyte NADPH Oxidase Activation

Property	GTP Binding Proteins			Regulatory Proteins		
	Rac1	Rac2	Rap1A	RhoGDI	P-Rex1	Vav1*
Amino acids	192	192	184	204	1659	877/790
Molecular weight (kDa)						
Predicted	21.4	21.4	20.9	23.4	185	101.4/91.9
By PAGE	22	22	22	26	197	?
PI†	8.5	7.6	6.5	4.9	6.2	6.5/6.2
mRNA (kb)	1.1	1.45	1.6	1.9	6	2.9/2.7
	2.4					
Cellular location‡	Cytosol	Cytosol	Membrane	Cytosol	Cytosol	Cytosol
Tissue specificity	Myeloid and other	Myeloid	Widespread	Widespread	Leukocytes and brain	Hematopoietic system
Covalent modification	Isoprenylation	Isoprenylation	Isoprenylation Phosphorylation			Phosphorylation
Homology	92% with Rac2 58% with Rho ~30% with Ras	92% with Rac1 58% with Rho ~30% with Ras	<30% with Rac1/2 <30% with Rho ~50% with Ras	Weak with RasGAP	Tandem PH/DH domain with Rho GEFs 2 DEP and 2 PDZ domains C-terminal - Ins-poly-P 4-phosphatase	Tandem PH/DH domain with Rho GEFs CH domain Ac region ZF domain 2 SH3 domains 1 SH2 domain Pro-rich region

*Vav1 has several alternative splice variants.

†Calculated from the amino acid sequences.

‡For resting cells; subcellular localization may vary with activation state of the cell and method of cellular disruption.

Abbreviations used: Ac, acidic; CH, calponin homology; DEP, domain found in dishevelled, Egl-10, and pleckstrin; DH, diffuse B cell lymphoma (DBL) homology; GAP, GTPase-activating protein; GEF, guanine-nucleotide exchange factor; Ins, inositol; PDZ, Domain found in PSD-95, Dlg, and ZO-1/2; PH, pleckstrin homology; P-Rex1, PtdIns(3,4,5)P₃-dependent Rac exchanger; Pro, proline; RhoGDI, GDP dissociation inhibitor for Rho proteins; SH, *src* homology; ZF, zink finger.

Adapted with permission (Heyworth et al., 1992).

neutrophils leads to externalization of phosphatidylserine (PS) in the plasma membrane and to other apoptosis-related changes in these cells (Kobayashi et al., 2003), and this PS exposure labels these cells for removal by macrophages. Both PS exposure and uptake by macrophages appear to be dependent on the formation of hydrogen peroxide by the neutrophils (Hampton et al., 2002). Thus, clearance of stimulated neutrophils might be delayed in CGD, a concept that was proven in gp91phox knockout mice. This defect may well relate to the formation of granulomas in CGD patients. Gene expression profiling has shown that CGD neutrophils have constitutively up-regulated expression of genes encoding mediators of inflammation and host defense. In contrast, during phagocytosis-induced apoptosis, CGD neutrophils did not display increased Bax expression, as do normal neutrophils (Kobayashi et al., 2004). Thus, granuloma formation in CGD patients may reflect increased proinflammatory activity and defective apotosis of CGD neutrophils. This aberrant gene expression profile may be a direct effect of diminished reactive oxygen species (ROS) production or ROS-sensitive gene expression. Also, the diminished production of anti-inflammatory mediators by CGD neutrophils and macrophages during phagocytosis of bacteria or apoptotic cells (Brown et al., 2003) may contribute to the persistence of inflammation in CGD.

Nonphagocyte NADPH Oxidases

Recently, several homologues of gp91phox have been identified in cells other than phagocytes. These homologues have conserved the overall structure of six transmembrane domains with four heme-coordinating histidines in the N-terminal part of the mole-

cule, followed by a cytosolic C-terminus that contains highly conserved binding sites for FAD and NADPH. In a new nomenclature, these proteins are now called Nox (NADPH oxidase) proteins, including gp91phox (Nox2). Mox1 (or Nox1) mRNA is expressed in colon, uterus, and vascular smooth muscle cells (Suh et al., 1999). Reactive oxygen species produced by this enzyme seem to be generated intracellularly, in contrast to the situation with the phagocyte NADPH oxidase. Overexpression of Nox1 results in increased cell growth, suggesting a role for these oxygen species in signal transduction for cell growth regulation. Another gp91phox homologue, called Renox or Nox4, has been detected by in situ RNA hybridization and immunohistochemistry in the renal cortex, predominantly in proximal convoluted tubule epithelial cells (Geiszt et al., 2000; Shiose et al., 2001). It has been suggested that Nox4 may participate in the oxygen-sensing mechanism that regulates the production of erythropoietin. Transfection of Nox4 into 3T3 fibroblasts resulted in enhanced superoxide production; however, these modified cells displayed substantially diminished cell growth. Nox 3 is highly expressed in the inner ear, especially in the vestibular and cochlear sensory epithelia, but its function there is unknown. Nox5 is distinguished from the other family members by its longer N terminus, which contains four EF hand Ca²⁺-binding motifs. It is found in B and T lymphocytes. Some of these alternative NADPH oxidases, in particular Nox1, Nox 3, and Nox4, may interact with specific cytosolic partners for activity regulation and localization—i.e. with the recently discovered alternative members of the p47 and p67 protein families (Bánfi et al., 2003; Geiszt et al., 2003; Takeya et al., 2003).

Finally, two similar homologues have been discovered that are characterized by an N-terminal extension containing a peroxidase homology domain, a calmodulin-like calcium-binding motif, and an additional transmembrane domain (De Deken et al., 2000). RNA for these proteins, called ThOX-1 and ThOX-2 (or Duox1 and Duox2), is expressed specifically in the thyroid gland, at the apical membrane of the thyrocytes. Duox2, and perhaps also Duox1, is involved in the iodination of the thyroid hormone, because nonsense mutations in the gene for Duox2 have been identified in patients with congenital hypothyroidism (Moreno et al., 2002).

Molecular Basis

Deficiency of the phagocyte NADPH oxidase, as seen in CGD, can be the result of any of a number of defects. First, one of the structural components of the enzyme can be deficient, which is the case when mutations occur in the genes encoding gp91^{phox}, p22^{phox}, p47^{phox}, or p67^{phox}. Mutations in the gene for p40^{phox} have not been described. Together, mutations in these four genes account for the overwhelming majority of CGD cases, with defects in the X chromosome–encoded gp91^{phox} found in about 70% of the cases and in p47^{phox} in about 25%. Defects in p22^{phox} or p67^{phox} are rare. Even more rare are defects in the activation process of the NADPH oxidase. In particular, one patient has been described with a mutation in Rac2, leading to CGD-like symptoms in combination with defects in chemotaxis and in degranulation (Ambruso et al., 2000; Williams et al., 2000). This finding indicates that Rac2 is involved not only in the activation of superoxide production but also in the activation of other neutrophil functions. Finally, defects may occur in the process that provides the cell with the substrate for the oxidase, i.e., NADPH. This compound is generated in phagocytes for the largest part in the hexose monophosphate pathway, in the successive G6PD and the 6-phosphogluconate dehydrogenase (6PGD) reactions. Occasionally, patients are found with a deficiency of G6PD in not only the erythrocytes but also the leukocytes (Baehner et al., 1972; Gray et al., 1973; Roos et al., 1999). These patients suffer from a mild form of CGD.

The *CYBB* gene for gp91^{phox} has a size of 30 kb, with 13 exons (Table 37.2). It is located on the X chromosome, at Xp21.1. Its promoter region has been clarified in some detail. In transgenic mice, 450 bp of the 5′ flanking region of *CYBB* suffices for expression of reporter genes in a subset of mononuclear phagocytes, but not in all myelomonocytic cells (Skalnik et al., 1991a). The same investigators have identified a repressor region around the CCAAT box motif at about 160 and 170 bp 5′ from the *CYBB* initiation codon (Skalnik et al., 1991b) and a high-mobility group (HMG) chromosomal protein binding to the same region and supposedly acting as a transcriptional activator (Skalnik and Neufeld, 1992). Another transcription factor involved in *CYBB* activity regulation is YY1, which binds at five places within the first 412 bp of its promoter region (Jacobsen and Skalnik, 1999). Six CGD families are known with mutations in the promoter region of *CYBB* that interfere with binding of Elf-1 and PU.1 (Newburger et al., 1994; Woodman et al., 1995; Suzuki et al., 1998; Voo and Skalnik, 1999; Weening et al., 2000; Stasia et al., 2003). In addition, the transcription of *CYBB* and *NCF1* is enhanced by interferon-γ (IFN-γ) (Cassatella et al., 1990; Weening et al., 1996).

The *CYBA* gene for p22^{phox} has a size of 8.5 kb, with six exons (Table 37.2). It is located on chromosome 16, at 16q24. Its promoter region has been partly characterized (Moreno et al., 2003). The *NCF1* gene for p47^{phox} has a size of 15 kb, with 11 exons, and the *NCF2* gene of p67^{phox} measures 40 kb, with 16 exons (Table 37.2). These genes are located on chromosomes

7 and 1, respectively, at 7q11.23 and 1q25. Finally, the *NCF4* gene for p40^{phox} has a size of 18 kb, with 10 exons, and is located on chromosome 22, at 22q13.1. Detailed information on the promoter regions of these *NCF* genes has been collected (Li et al., 1997, 1999, 2001, 2002). In none of the NADPH oxidase genes do the exon organizations coincide with the various functional regions of the proteins they encode.

The *RAC2* gene is located on chromosome 22, at 22q13. It has a size of 18 kb, with at least seven exons. The promoter region of this gene has not yet been studied in detail. The Rac2 protein has a molecular weight of 22,000 and consists of 192 amino acids. The *G6PD* gene is located on the X chromosome, at Xq28. It has a size of 18 kb, with 13 exons. The first exon is not translated. Comparison of the promoter region of *G6PD* with 10 other housekeeping enzyme genes confirmed the presence of common features. In particular, in eight of these genes in which a TATA box was present, a conserved region of 25 bp is found immediately downstream. The G6PD protein has a molecular weight of 58,000 and consists of 531 amino acids. By binding NADP$^+$, the protein forms catalytically active dimers.

Laboratory Findings

Diagnosis

As mentioned above, CGD is caused by dysfunction of the NADPH oxidase enzyme in phagocytic leukocytes (neutrophils, eosinophils, monocytes, and macrophages). This enzyme generates superoxide, the one-electron reduction product of molecular oxygen. Superoxide is subsequently converted into hydrogen peroxide, either spontaneously or catalyzed by superoxide dismutase. Hydrogen peroxide is further metabolized through the action of myeloperoxidase into hypochlorous acid and other microbicidal metabolites. In CGD, the activated phagocytes fail to generate superoxide and as a result also fail to generate the other reactive oxygen products. As a consequence, phagocytosed microorganisms are less efficiently killed by CGD leukocytes.

Patients suspected of suffering from CGD can therefore be diagnosed by the inability of their blood phagocytes to kill catalase-positive bacteria (e.g., *Staphylococcus aureus* or *Escherichia coli*) in vitro or by their inability to generate reactive oxygen species. The respiratory burst can be measured by oxygen consumption (with an oxygen electrode), by superoxide generation (reduction of ferricytochrome *c* or nitroblue tetrazolium), or by hydrogen peroxide production (oxidation of homovanillic acid or Amplex red). Chemiluminescence with luminol or lucigenin is often used as a very sensitive test of NADPH oxidase activity. Flow-cytometric detection of this activity combines the advantage of sensitivity with the possibility of using nonpurified leukocyte suspensions rapidly derived from whole blood. One such assay, using dihydrorhodamine-1,2,3 (DHR) as the fluorescent detector of hydrogen peroxide production, has proven to be highly reliable and sensitive, even on blood that is 24–48 hours old. This assay has therefore replaced superoxide measurements and the NBT slide test as the primary screening assay for CGD in many laboratories (Emmendorffer et al., 1994; van Pelt et al., 1996; Vowells et al., 1996).

Chronic Granulomatous Disease Subgroup Identification

Because the NADPH oxidase is composed of multiple subunits, four of which may be affected by mutations leading to CGD (see above, Table 37.2), further differentiation of the diagnosis is needed before mutation analysis can be performed. CGD subgroup investigation starts with immunoblot analysis of neutrophil fractions or intracellular staining in permeabilized neutrophils with antibodies against these four NADPH oxidase components. In cases where one of the cytosolic components (p47phox or p67phox) is missing, one can be confident that the gene carrying the mutation has been identified. However, if one of the membrane-bound components (gp91phox or p22phox) is missing, the other is always undetectable as well (Parkos et al., 1989; Verhoeven et al., 1989), because the subunits stabilize each other for full maturation and expression (Porter et al., 1994; Yu et al., 1997). In that case, distinction can usually be made by searching for a mosaic pattern of NADPH oxidase activity or gp91phox/p22phox expression in the neutrophils of female relatives of the patient, because the gene for gp91phox is located on the X chromosome. Convenient assays for this purpose are the NBT slide test, which scores the NADPH oxidase activity per cell on a semiquantitative basis (Meerhof and Roos, 1986), or the DHR flow-cytometric assay (Roesler et al., 1991; Vowells et al., 1996). Alternatively, one can perform flow cytometry to detect gp91phox/p22phox on the neutrophil surface with certain anti-flavocytochrome b_{558} antibodies (Mizuno et al., 1988). However, it must be kept in mind that up to one-third of all X-linked defects may arise from new mutations in germ-line cells and will therefore not always be present in the somatic cells from the mother. Thus failure to define the mother as an X-linked carrier does not disprove the X-linked origin of the disease.

If all four subunits of the NADPH oxidase are detectable, even though the activity of this enzyme is absent or strongly decreased, the possibility of so-called (+) variants must be considered (Table 37.4). These are caused by mutations in any of the four subunits that leave the protein expression intact but destroy the enzymatic activity of the assembled oxidase complex. In that case, a cell-free oxidase assay may be used to distinguish a defect in a cytosolic component (p47phox or p67phox) from a defect in a membrane-bound component (gp91phox or p22phox). For this assay, neutrophil membranes from the patient are mixed with neutrophil cytosol from a healthy donor (or vice versa), incubated with NADPH, and activated with an amphiphilic agent (low concentrations of sodium dodecyl sulfate [SDS] or arachidonic acid). The resulting oxidase activity can be measured by superoxide formation or oxygen consumption and used to localize the defect to either the cytosol or membrane fraction (Curnutte et al., 1987). Identification of the mutated gene that causes the defect in NADPH oxidase activity can also be made if transfection of the patient's Epstein Barr virus (EBV)-transformed B lymphocytes with retroviral vectors that contain the wild-type cDNA restores this activity (Malech et al., 1997).

Patients with variant forms of X-linked CGD are characterized by a partial loss of gp91phox expression and a proportional loss of NADPH oxidase activity (so-called X− variants) (Table 37.4). For an exact idea of gp91phox expression, it can be useful to measure the heme content of flavocytochrome b_{558} (Cross and Curnutte, 1995).

Finally, some patients with CGD-like symptoms are known with defects in either G6PD or Rac2. The first type can easily be recognized by measuring the activity of the G6PD enzyme in the red blood cells and confirming the diagnosis by repeating the assay with a leukocyte preparation (Roos et al., 1999; Van Bruggen et al., 2002). Moreover, one will usually find a mosaic of normally and faintly stained cells in the NBT slide test or DHR assay with purified neutrophils of the mother, because the G6PD

Table 37.4. Mutations in *CYBB* (gp91phox)

	No. of Kindreds	Frequency (%)	Phenotype*
Deletions	92	22.1	X91⁰
Insertions	38	9.1	X91⁰
Splice site mutations	81	19.5	X91⁰
Missense mutations	103	24.8	X91⁰, X91−, X91+
Nonsense mutations	102	24.5	X91⁰

*In this nomenclature, the first letter (X) represents the mode of inheritance, while the number (91) indicates the phox component that is genetically affected. The superscript symbols indicate whether the level of protein of the affected component is undetectable (⁰), diminished (−), or normal (+) as measured by immunoblot analysis.

Data from a multicenter database (Vihinen et al., 2001).

gene is localized on the X chromosome. Rac2 deficiency can be recognized by the defect in NADPH oxidase activity in combination with defects in chemotaxis toward complement fragment C5a, IL-8, fMLP, LTB$_4$, and platelet-activating factor (PAF). A defect in the release of proteins from the azurophilic granules but not from the specific granules or secretory vesicles is also apparent (Roos et al., 1993; Ambruso et al., 2000). The Rac2 deficiency can only be diagnosed with certainty when the oxidase activity in the cell-free assay is restored by addition of purified Rac.

Carrier Detection

Carrier detection of X-CGD is usually performed by searching for a mosaic pattern of oxidase-positive and -negative neutrophils in the NBT slide test, in the DHR flow-cytometric assay, or in a flow-cytometric assay of gp91phox/p22phox protein expression. However, because of the random process of X chromosome inactivation, X-CGD carriers may show a near-normal or a near-pathological pattern in these tests. Once the family-specific mutation is known, it is more reliable to perform carrier detection at the DNA level. This is best performed by polymerase chain reaction (PCR) amplification of the relevant region of genomic DNA, followed by sequencing or allele-specific restriction enzyme analysis. Alternatively, single-strand conformation polymorphism (SSCP) can be informative if the mutation leads to an abnormal band pattern. If the mutation involves a large deletion, simple RFLP analysis of genomic DNA may reveal the carriers.

Carriers of autosomal (A) CGD subtypes are difficult to detect. The NADPH oxidase activity of phagocytes from obligate carriers (parents of patients) is normal unless phorbol-myristate acetate is used to activate these cells (Verhoeven et al., 1988; de Boer et al., 1994). However, this is a rather insensitive assay, and it has not been tested with A22 CGD carriers. Also, the expression of p47phox and p67phox proteins appears normal in obligate carriers of A47 and A67 CGD, respectively. Hence, detection of carriers of autosomal CGD is much better performed at the DNA level. Unfortunately, for A47 CGD, this is difficult (see Mutation Analysis).

Mutation Analysis

Mutation Analysis in X-Linked Chronic Granulomatous Disease

In our laboratories, the mutations in more than 400 families with X-CGD (MIM 306400) have been characterized (Hopkins et al., 1992; Roos et al., 1996a, 1996b; Rae et al., 1998; Cross et al.,

2000; Heyworth et al., 2001). In addition, about 100 X-CGD mutations have been identified and some of these have been published by other investigators; updates of all mutations known to us can be found in Heyworth et al. (2001) and at the Internet address http://www.uta.fi/imt/bioinfo/CYBBbase/. The results show that CGD is a very heterogeneous disease, not only clinically and cell biologically but also at the molecular level, even within one subgroup. All possible mutations, except gene conversions, have been found in the *CYBB* gene. These different categories will be briefly mentioned, followed by a more detailed description of a few mutations that have given us insight into the structure–function relation of gp91^{phox}.

Deletions and/or insertions in *CYBB* are encountered in about 31% of all X-CGD patients; single nucleotide substitutions are seen in the remaining 69%. This last category can be subdivided into splice site mutations leading to aberrant mRNA processing (19%), missense mutations causing single amino acid substitutions (25%), and nonsense mutations inducing premature termination of protein synthesis (25%) (Heyworth, Roos in: Vihinen et al., 2001). Table 37.4 provides an overview.

Deletions range in size from about 5,000,000 to one single nucleotide. When the deletions are very large, not only the *CYBB* gene is affected but neighboring genes as well. Such patients suffer from other clinical syndromes in addition to CGD—for example, Duchenne muscular dystrophy, retinitis pigmentosa, and, as mentioned above, McLeod syndrome (a mild hemolytic anemia with decreased levels of Kell erythrocyte antigens due to defects in the K^x system). In two families, affected brothers were detected who each carried different deletions in their *CYBB* genes (de Boer et al., 1998). Only in one patient has an in-frame partial exon deletion been reported to lead to expression of the truncated (inactive) gp91^{phox} protein (Schapiro et al., 1991).

Insertions in *CYBB* are usually small in size and, like small deletions, may be caused by slipped mispairing at the DNA replication fork. A few larger tandem duplications of 24, 31, and 40 base pairs, respectively, have been detected, apparently due to unequal crossing-over during meiosis or misalignment during DNA repair (Rabbani et al., 1993; Bu-Ghanim et al., 1995; Roos et al., unpublished findings). Several combinations of small deletions and insertions have been found (Ariga et al., 1995; Rae et al., 1998; Heyworth et al., 2001; Roos et al., unpublished findings), in one of them predicting substitution of three amino acids by four others near the C terminus of gp91^{phox} (Azuma et al., 1995). This mutation leads to a stable mutant protein and thus to the X91$^+$ CGD phenotype. The lack of oxidase activity in this patient may be due to decreased binding of NADPH to flavocytochrome b_{558}, because the mutation is in the putative NADPH binding region of gp91^{phox}, but this possibility was not investigated. Finally, two large fragments of LINE-1 transposable elements have recently been identified within *CYBB*. The first one is a 1 kb fragment within intron 5, causing a complicated pattern of misspliced mRNA (Meischl et al., 2000). The second is a 2.1 kb fragment within exon 4, causing a frameshift (Brouha et al., 2002). In both families, the insertion was a recent event because it was not found in the somatic cell DNA from the patients' mothers. The 2.1 kb fragment was identified as part of an active LINE-1 element on chromosome 2 of the patient's mother.

Single nucleotide substitutions at exon–intron boundaries lead to aberrations in mRNA splicing, usually causing skipping of an entire exon. However, this phenomenon was proven in only about half of the cases (in the other half, only genomic DNA was investigated). The percentage of splice site mutations found in CGD is similar to that found in other diseases (Krawczak et al., 1992).

Single nucleotide changes in the middle of exon 6 and in the middle of introns 5 and 6 have created new splice sites, causing a partial exon deletion or insertions, respectively, in the mRNA (de Boer et al., 1992a; Noack et al., 1999, 2001a).

Missense and nonsense mutations constitute the most frequently encountered cause of many genetic diseases. A hot spot for such mutations is the CpG sequence, especially in the CGA codon for arginine, leading to the stop codon TGA. Nonsense mutations in *CYBB* affect the level of mRNA for gp91^{phox} to a variable degree but have not been seen in CGD to produce stable truncated proteins. Similarly, deletions, insertions, and splice site mutations in general also lead to the X91^0 phenotype (no gp91^{phox} protein expression, no NADPH oxidase activity). In contrast, missense mutations do not influence the level of mRNA and may give rise to any of three phenotypes. Single amino acid replacements due to missense mutations can lead to intrinsically unstable gp91^{phox} or to gp91^{phox} unable to be stabilized by interaction with p22^{phox} (X91^0 phenotype), to partial deficiencies in this respect (X91$^-$ phenotype: decreased expression, decreased oxidase activity), or to stable but inactive gp91^{phox} (X91$^+$ phenotype) (Table 37.4). Small in-frame deletions and a few splice site mutations with residual normal mRNA splicing have also been found associated with the X91$^-$ phenotype.

The X91$^+$ mutations can be very informative for our understanding of the properties of the different domains in gp91^{phox}. At present, 13 X91$^+$ patients are known with missense mutations in *CYBB*. (Two additional X91$^+$ patients carry deletions that remove 5 or 10 amino acids while another has a 3–amino acid deletion/4–amino acid insertion.) Four X91$^+$ patients have amino acid substitutions in the N-terminal half of gp91^{phox} (Fig. 37.3). The first one is an Ala57Glu substitution; this mutant protein has not been studied in detail (Ariga et al., 1993). The other three are Arg54 substitutions; one of these (Arg54Ser) has been studied in detail. This substitution affects the function of one of the heme groups in flavocytochrome b_{558}, as evidenced by a slight shift in the optical absorbance and a decrease in the midpoint potential (Cross et al., 1995). Superoxide production was completely inhibited and both heme groups were nonfunctional, suggesting that the electron flow from FAD to oxygen requires sequential involvement of the two heme groups (Cross et al., 1995; Cross and Curnutte, 1995). The investigators speculate that Arg54 may interact with one of the propionate side chains of a heme group.

The other X91$^+$ patients have amino acid substitutions in the C-terminal half of gp91^{phox} (Fig. 37.3). In four of these, the translocation of p47^{phox} and p67^{phox} to cytochrome b_{558} upon neutrophil activation was found to be strongly diminished (Leusen et al., 1994b, 2000). This was seen with Cys369Arg, Gly408Glu, Asp500Gly, and Glu568Lys, residues located (respectively) in a loop between the putative FAD and NADPH binding regions, on the edge of the NADPH binding region, in the 20–amino acid loop over the NADPH cleft, and in the extreme C-terminal region of the gp91^{phox} protein. Apparently, not only the loop over the NADPH cleft is of importance as a docking site for the cytosolic oxidase components, but other regions surrounding this area as well (Fig. 37.4). All together, these results provide strong support of the three-dimensional model of the C-terminal half of gp91^{phox} as constructed by Taylor et al. (1993). Support for the putative NADPH binding region of gp91^{phox} comes from the decreased binding of NADPH observed in a mutant gp91^{phox} containing a Pro415His substitution, a residue believed to be part of the NADPH binding domain (Segal et al., 1992).

Some X91$^-$ mutations have also proven to be informative. Tsuda et al. (1998) have described a patient with a His101Tyr mutation, causing 90% loss of gp91^{phox} protein expression but total loss of heme incorporation. This indicates that His101 of gp91^{phox} may be involved in heme binding, in accordance with the prediction based on the FRE1 protein (Finegold et al., 1996) and with the need of heme incorporation for maturation and stability of the gp91^{phox}/p22^{phox} complex (Yu et al., 1997). A mutation of His338Tyr led to about 80% decreased heme levels but almost complete loss of FAD incorporation, in accordance with the His-Pro-Phe-Thr 338-341 motif being involved in FAD binding (Yoshida et al., 1998). This is probably also the explanation for the loss of activity in an X91^{+} CGD patient with a Thr341Lys mutation in gp91^{phox} (Leusen et al., 2000).

Finally, four different single nucleotide substitutions have been identified in the 5′ promoter region of *CYBB* (Newburger et al., 1994; Woodman et al., 1995; Suzuki et al., 1998; Weening et al., 2000; Stasia et al., 2003). Mutations at −52 and −53 were found to be located in a binding element for the nuclear transcription factor PU.1 and to suppress the binding of PU.1 and the subsequent promoter activity. Remarkably, these mutations abolished NADPH oxidase activity in the neutrophils, monocytes, and transformed B lymphocytes of the patients, but not in their eosinophils (Suzuki et al., 1998). This finding probably explains the mild clinical phenotype of these patients (Weening et al., 2000). Apparently, eosinophils have an additional *CYBB* activation mechanism, which has been identified as the eosinophil-specific transcription factor GATA-1 (Yang et al., 2000). The patients with mutations at −55 and −57 had small subsets of neutrophils (approximately 5%) with normal NADPH oxidase activity. These mutations strongly reduced the association of Elf-1 and PU.1 and also reduced the ability of these factors to *trans*-activate the promoter (Voo and Skalnik, 1999). The investigators speculate that different DNA binding proteins are used in different neutrophil subsets for the initiation, enhancement, and repression of *CYBB* transcription.

On the basis of a multicenter review of the mutations identified in 416 X-linked CGD kindreds (Heyworth, Roos, in Vihinen et al., 2001), 69% of them are family-specific. Only four polymorphisms in *CYBB* have been detected to date, two of which predict an amino acid substitution, thus pointing to an extreme sensitivity of this protein for mutations (Heyworth et al., 2001).

Mutation Analysis in Autosomal Chronic Granulomatous Disease

The number of well-characterized mutations in autosomal CGD is much lower than that in X-linked CGD, owing to the lower incidence of these forms of the disease. Thirty-three A22 families, about 100 A47 families, and 23 A67 families have been investigated in this respect. The results indicate that the molecular genetic basis of A22 and A67 CGD is as heterogeneous as that of X91 CGD, but A47 CGD is much more homogeneous in origin.

In the 33 A22 CGD families with mutations of p22^{phox} (MIM 233690), 27 different mutations have been found in the 66 alleles, including deletions, insertions, splice site mutations, nonsense, and missense mutations (for a detailed overview see Cross et al., 2000, and the Internet address http://www.uta.fi/imt/bio info/CYBAbase/). In 26 families, the patients carried homozygous deficiencies; in 7 families, the patients were compound heterozygotes. Ten mutations were found in more than one unrelated family, with a hot spot of a missense mutation at 354C → A, changing the AGC codon for Ser118 into the AGA codon for Arg, in three families (six alleles). Only seven polymorphisms

are known in the p22^{phox} protein. Thus, small changes in the composition of this protein appear to lead to intrinsic instability and/or instability due to decreased interaction with gp91^{phox}. Only one A22^{+} patient has been found, with a Pro156Glu substitution (Dinauer et al., 1991). Pro156 is in a proline-rich region of p22^{phox} that serves as a binding region for an SH3 domain in p47^{phox}. Apparently, the Pro156Glu substitution destroys the interaction between these proteins and hence the activation of the NADPH oxidase (Leto et al., 1994; Leusen et al., 1994a; Sumimoto et al., 1994). This substitution is the first recognized mutation that disturbs an SH3–proline interaction and leads to a genetic disease.

The mutations that cause A47 CGD have long puzzled investigators. In more than 100 unrelated patients with p47^{phox} deficiency (MIM 233700), a dinucleotide deletion has been found at a GTGT tandem repeat corresponding to the first four bases of exon 2 in the *NCF1* gene (Casimir et al., 1991; Volpp and Lin, 1993; Iwata et al., 1994; Roos et al., 1996a; Roesler et al., 2000; Noack et al., 2001b; Vazquez et al., 2001). In all but 13 of these reported families, the GT deletion appeared to be homozygous. In these 13 exceptions, 9 patients were heterozygotes for the GT deletion and one additional mutation, and 4 had mutations other than ΔGT on both alleles of *NCF1*. Of these last four patients, three were homozygotes for a mutation and one was a compound heterozygote. For an overview of these mutations see Cross et al. (2000) and the Internet address http://www.uta.fi/imt/bioinfo/NCF1base/. The spectrum of these non-ΔGT mutations is as diverse as that in the other CGD genes (Noack et al., 2001b; de Boer et al., 2002; Roos et al., unpublished findings). Obviously, the ΔGT-bearing allele of *NCF1* is the most common CGD-causing allele in the population, carried by approximately 1 in 500 individuals. The reason for this predominance is that most normal individuals have on each chromosome 7 two p47^{phox} pseudogenes, which colocalize with the functional *NCF1* gene to 7q11.23. These pseudogenes are >99% homologous to *NCF1* but carry the GT deletion, which renders them inactive because the predicted protein from these pseudogenes contains a premature stopcodon. Recombination events between *NCF1* and the pseudogenes lead to the incorporation of ΔGT into *NCF1*, and thus to CGD (Goerlach et al., 1997; Roesler et al., 2000; Vazquez et al., 2001). To date, only one polymorphism has been recognized in *NCF1*, but the identification of these variations is complicated by the presence of the pseudogenes. All mutations in *NCF1* identified thus far lead to absence of p47^{phox} protein.

Unfortunately, this complicated genetic background of A47 CGD renders reliable carrier testing difficult, because normal individuals appear to be "heterozygous" for the GT deletion by virtue of containing the pseudogenes. Allele-specific PCR amplification can be used to solve this problem but is not easily applicable (Noack et al., 2001b). A screening method for the GT deletion with the restriction enzyme *Dra*III, which cuts only the GTGT-containing sequence, distinguishes homozygous GT deletion patients from healthy donors (no reaction with patients, 33% reaction with healthy donors), but it is too insensitive to discriminate between a normal individual and either an A47 patient who is a compound heterozygote for the GT deletion or a carrier for the GT deletion. Recently, a gene-scan method has been developed for determining the relative number of *NCF1* and pseudogenes in genomic DNA. With this test, patients and carriers with the GT deletion can be distinguished from normal individuals and from each other (Dekker et al., 2001). However, it is not yet clear whether the compound protein with the GTGT sequence from *NCF1* followed by the 3′ sequence of the pseudogenes is expressed and has oxidase-promoting activity (Heyworth et al., 2002). In all A47 CGD patients analyzed thus far, the mRNA levels for p47^{phox} were normal, but the amount of p47^{phox} protein in each was undetectable. Thus, only A47^0 patients have been identified to date.

In the 23 characterized A67 CGD families with abnormal p67^{phox} (MIM 233710), the patients carry 22 different (and 2 unidentified) mutations among the 46 total alleles affected. These include missense mutations, splice site mutations, nonsense mutations, a dinucleotide insertion, and a variety of deletions ranging from one nucleotide to 11–13 kb (for a detailed review see Cross et al., 2000, and the Internet address http://www.uta.fi/imt/bioinfo/NCF2base/). In 16 families, the patients are homozygous for one mutation, in 7 they are compound heterozygotes. Four mutations were found in more than one unrelated family, with a hot spot of a gt → at splice site mutation at the start of intron 4 in four families. Twelve polymorphisms in NCF2 are known (including the 5′ untranslated region), six of which predict amino acid substitutions. In some of the A67 CGD patients, the level of mRNA for p67^{phox} is normal, but in most the p67^{phox} protein is undetectable. However, in one of the patients, with a trinucleotide deletion (170–172) on one allele (the other allele carried a large deletion), about half the normal amount of protein was found. In this patient, the mutation predicts an in-frame deletion of Lys58 from the protein and apparently results in the expression of a nonfunctional p67^{phox} that fails to translocate to the plasma membrane because of the inability of this protein to bind Rac (Leusen et al., 1996). Hence, A67$^+$ patients may exist.

Mutation Analysis in Rac2 Deficiency

Rac2 deficiency has been described in one patient only (MIM 602049) (Ambruso et al., 2000; Williams et al., 2000), although the cellular deficiencies exactly match those described in another patient with neutrophil defects of unknown etiology (Roos et al., 1993). The patient with proven Rac2 deficiency suffered from severe bacterial infections and poor wound healing, symptoms that, together with late separation of the umbilical stump, leukocytosis, and absence of pus in infected areas, also observed in the patient, are reminiscent of leukocyte adhesion deficiency (LAD). Indeed, neutrophil studies indicated a defect in chemotaxis toward C5a, fMLP, and IL-8, but in contrast to LAD1, normal expression of β_2 integrins (CD18) on the leukocytes (see Chapter 38). Moreover, despite a normal content of enzymes of the azurophil granules, strongly decreased release of these enzymes after neutrophil activation with either fMLP or phorbol myristate acetate (PMA) was found. In contrast, the release of lactoferrin from the specific granules induced by these agents was normal. Neutrophil polarization and actin polymerization in response to fMLP was also deficient, as was transient adhesion to the L-selectin ligand GlyCAM-1 and stable adhesion to fibronectin. Finally, the neutrophils from this patient failed to respond with superoxide production after activation with fMLP or C5a, but responded normally with PMA. Thus, this syndrome combined defects seen in LAD with those observed in CGD and in addition included defects in degranulation and actin-dependent functions. However, in contrast to CGD, the NADPH oxidase defect was selective for certain stimuli. A common defect in intracellular signaling for activation of the various neutrophil functions seemed plausible. Indeed, in the cell-free NADPH oxidase assay, the defect was localized in the cytosol fraction, and the activity was restored by addition of recombinant, GTP-activated Rac1, which

can substitute for Rac2 in this assay system. A possible defect in Rac2 activity was corroborated by half-normal expression of this protein in the patient's neutrophils. Mutation analysis of the patient's Rac2 gene showed a heterozygous 169G → A transition, predicting a substitution of Asp57 for Asn. This Asp57 is in a conserved D-X-X-G motif involved in GTP binding to Ras GTPases. Recombinant Rac2^{D57N} bound GDP normally but failed to bind GTP.

The involvement of Rac2 in multiple neutrophil functions had already been deduced from studies with Rac2 knockout mice (Roberts et al., 1999). However, in these studies it was shown that both Rac2 alleles had to be disrupted for defects to become apparent. The fact that the patient was heterozygous for the Rac2 mutation and expressed both normal and mutant mRNA for Rac2 but nevertheless exhibited strong neutrophil defects indicates that Rac2^{D57N} has a dominant negative effect on the function of wild-type Rac2. This was proven in the cell-free NADPH oxidase assay with recombinant proteins (Ambruso et al., 2000) and in normal human bone marrow cells transduced with Rac2^{D57N} or patient bone marrow cells transduced with wild-type Rac2 (Williams et al., 2000). The mechanism of this dominant negative effect of Rac2^{D57N} was clarified by Gu et al. (2001), who found that Rac2^{D57N} binds the guanine nucleotide exchange factor (GEF) TrioN normally, but that this binding had no effect on the exchange of GDP for GTP, in contrast to the increased exchange seen with wild-type Rac2. These results suggest that Rac2^{D57N} sequesters GEFs in neutrophils by binding these factors but, because of the impaired binding of GTP, do not release these factors, resulting in decreased turnover rates of Rac2 and possibly other Rho-like GTPases that use these GEFs.

Mutation Analysis in Glucose-6-Phosphate Dehydrogenase Deficiency

Deficiency of G6PD is one of the most common genetic defects in humans (MIM 305900), probably because of the protection of G6PD-deficient erythrocytes against proliferation of malaria parasites. The clinical expression of G6PD deficiency varies from mild hemolytic anemia induced by infections or drugs (World Health Organization [WHO] class 3) to chronic nonspherocytic hemolytic anemia with attacks of severe anemia induced by infections and drugs (WHO class 1). The clinical symptoms are often restricted to the erythrocytes, for several reasons. One is that G6PD and the next enzyme in the hexose monophosphate pathway (6-PGD) catalyze the only NADPH-generating reactions in cells that lack mitochondria, i.e., erythrocytes. These cells need NADPH for protection against oxidative stress. Other reasons for G6PD deficiency effects in erythrocytes are the long survival time of these cells in the circulation and their lack of protein synthesis. G6PD mutant enzymes often have decreased protein stability, causing a decline in enzyme activity, especially in long-living cells that cannot generate new proteins. A total lack of G6PD activity is probably incompatible with life, because mutations in G6PD concern missense mutations or small in-frame deletions, but not frameshift mutations, gross deletions, or nonsense mutations (with one exception near the end of the protein) (Beutler et al., 1996).

Occasionally, patients with G6PD deficiency have been described with a decreased neutrophil respiratory burst after activation with opsonized particles, as well as an increased susceptibility of patients to bacterial or fungal infections (Baehner et al., 1972; Cooper et al., 1972; Gray et al., 1973; Vives Corrons et al., 1982; Mamlok et al., 1987; Roos et al., 1999; Van Bruggen et al.,

2002). In general, the G6PD activity in these cells needs to be below 5% of normal for such impairment to occur (Baehner et al., 1972). This situation might arise if mutations in G6PD severely decrease the enzyme activity even in newly synthesized protein. To date, information about mutations that give rise to these CGD-like symptoms is restricted to a few families. In one of these, we found replacement of Pro172 by Ser, leading to a thermolabile variant G6PD with about 15% of normal activity (Roos et al., 1999). Interestingly, the only patient in the family was a female, with somatic cells that contained only the mutant mRNA. This phenomenon was explained by the failure of paternal X chromosome inactivation, a trend in the female line in this family. Recently, we analyzed two additional families with mild CGD and G6PD deficiency. Both were found to carry a triplet nucleotide deletion that predicted deletion of Leu61 from the protein. G6PD protein expression and enzyme activity in all blood cells were extremely low, being detectable only in actively dividing lymphocytes (Van Bruggen et al., 2002).

Phenotype–Genotype Correlation

In general, the A22 and A67 subgroups of CGD appear to be as severe as X91^0 CGD. Clinical comparisons between X-CGD and A47 CGD patients have been made by several investigators, with the general contention that X-CGD patients follow a more severe clinical course than that of A47 CGD patients (Weening et al., 1985a; Margolis et al., 1990; Gallin et al., 1991; Winkelstein et al., 2000). The milder disease course may be due to residual superoxide or hydrogen peroxide formation by p47^{phox}-deficient neutrophils (Bemiller et al., 1991; Cross et al., 1994; Cross and Curnutte, 1995).

It might be expected that patients with the X91$^-$ phenotype, with 3%–30% of residual NADPH oxidase activity in their phagocytes (Roos et al., 1992), would follow a more benign clinical course than that of patients with the X91^0 or X91$^+$ phenotype. This generally appears to be the case, but it is not universally true (Roos et al., 1992). Female carriers of X-CGD mutations may occasionally present with clinical manifestations of the disease similar to those of hemizygous patients. In general, this concerns only carriers with less than 10% of normal phagocytes (Roos et al., 1996a), but healthy carriers with less than 10% of normal phagocytes are also known (Roos et al., 1986).

Functional polymorphisms in the oxygen-independent antimicrobial systems or other host defense elements play an important role in this respect. Foster et al. (1998) have found that in a cohort of 129 clinically well-defined CGD patients (104 X-linked, 25 autosomal recessive), an increased risk for abnormal granulomatous or inflammatory processes leading to gastrointestinal or urogenital complications was strongly associated with a polymorphism in the promoter region of myeloperoxidase that increases transcriptional activity and with the NA2 allele of the Fcγ receptor IIIb, which reacts less efficiently with IgG$_1$-opsonized microorganisms than does the NA1 allotype. Autoimmune and rheumatologic disorders were seen more frequently in CGD patients with variant alleles of mannose-binding lectin and Fcγ receptor IIa.

Another disease-modifying gene in CGD may be nitric oxide (NO) synthase-2, which catalyzes the production of NO radicals and subsequently formed reactive nitrogen intermediates. Recent data reveal an important functional difference between CGD and either normal or myeloperoxidase (MPO)-deficient neutrophils in their ability to metabolize NO (Clark et al., 2002). This difference may have bearing on the formation of granulomas in CGD

patients, but not in normal or MPO-deficient individuals. In addition, the presence of cation transporters, such as Nramp1, may exacerbate the effects of these toxic nitrogen intermediates on invading microbes. The question as to how oxidative and nonoxidative mechanisms cooperate in intraphagosomal killing has recently been addressed by the work of Reeves et al. (2002), who found that charge compensation for superoxide generation not only leads to potassium influx, thus liberating proteases from the proteoglycan matrix in the azurophil granules that have fused with the phagosome, but also to increased pH needed for optimal functioning of these proteases. While some of these antimicrobial systems may operate independently, the combination of their activities is synergistic in the successful containment of the invading pathogens. Such gene modifiers may explain the variability in the infectious burden in CGD. Also the prevalence of specific pathogens in certain patients, such as *Nocardia* or atypical mycobacterial strains, may depend on these nonoxidative systems (Weening et al., 2000; Winkelstein et al., 2000; Dorman et al., 2002). In addition, weak nonoxidative defense systems may allow also catalase-negative microorganisms to infect CGD patients. Finally, this variability of non-oxidative defense systems may explain the beneficial effects of rhIFN-γ in vivo in CGD patients (see below), despite its lack of effect on NADPH oxidase activity; many of the nonoxidative systems are activated and modulated by microbial products and a series of temporally expressed cytokines such as IFN-γ.

Prenatal Diagnosis

Prenatal diagnosis of CGD can be performed by analysis of the NADPH oxidase activity of fetal blood neutrophils (Newburger et al., 1979), but fetal blood sampling cannot be undertaken before 16–18 weeks of gestation. Instead, analysis of DNA from amniotic fluid cells or chorionic villi now provides an earlier and more reliable diagnosis for families at risk. In cases where the family-specific mutation is known, this analysis can be performed as indicated above. Between our laboratories and that of Heyworth and Cross at Scripps, we have analyzed more than 80 pregnancies at risk for X-CGD of the fetus (de Boer et al., 1992b). In all cases, the fetal origin of the DNA was checked in a genetic center with markers for X and Y chromosomes. The sequence of the fetal PCR product was always compared on one gel with that of the indicator patient in the family, the mother of the fetus, and a healthy control individual. The same strategy can be used for prenatal diagnosis of other CGD subtypes, although this may be more complicated if the parents carry different mutations. Recently, we have performed prenatal diagnosis in two families with a p67^{phox}-deficient CGD patient and in two families with p47^{phox}-deficient CGD patients. In the latter two families, the deficiency proved to be due to mutations other than the GT deletion at the start of exon 2 in *NCF1*, which was proven by sequencing of *NCF1*-specific PCR products (de Boer et al., 2002).

In cases where the family-specific mutations are not known, different methods must be applied. Partial or complete gene deletions can be recognized by RFLP analysis of genomic DNA, but more subtle abnormalities require the use of allele-specific markers. Within the *CYBB* gene, two *Nsi*I-specific RFLPs have been detected (Battat and Francke, 1989; Mühlebach et al., 1990; Pelham et al., 1990), as well as several highly polymorphic (GT/AC)$_n$ repeats (Hardwick et al., 1993; Gorlin, 1998) and single-nucleotide polymorphisms (Heyworth et al., 2001). Within the *NCF2* gene, a *Hin*dIII-specific RFLP exists (Kenney et al.,

1993); single-nucleotide polymorphisms in the *CYBA, NCF1,* and *NCF2* genes are listed in Cross et al. (2000). These markers offer a more than 50% reliable method for prenatal diagnosis of CGD.

Animal Models, Comparison with Human Disease

Natural animal models of CGD are not known. However, Dinauer's group succeeded in constructing a mouse model of X-linked CGD through *Cybb* gene targeting of murine embryonic stem cells (Pollock et al., 1995). With a similar technique, p47^{phox} knockout mice have been constructed (Jackson et al., 1995; Reeves et al., 2002). Such models are of great value for testing the safety and efficacy of correction of the genetic defect by gene transfer technologies (see Future Directions, below). In addition, the clinical differences between the various subgroups of CGD and new therapeutic strategies are studied in detail with these models. By comparison with elastase knockout mice, cathepsin-G knockout mice, and elastase/cathepsin-G double-knockout mice, the importance of the oxidative and nonoxidative microbicidal mechanisms can be studied in vivo (Tkalcevic et al., 2000). The mice deficient in NADPH oxidase components have also been used to study the involvement of this enzyme system in oxygen sensing, blood pressure regulation, and pathogenesis of atherosclerosis (Archer et al., 1999; Fu et al., 2000; Hsich et al., 2000; Kirk et al., 2000; O'Kelly et al., 2000; Wang et al., 2001; Brandes et al., 2002). For instance, a gp91^{phox}-containing NADPH oxidase seems to play an important role in the development of angiotensin II–induced cardiac hypertrophy, independent of changes in blood pressure (Bendall et al., 2002). However, a role for one or more of the classical phox proteins in human vascular disease cannot be deduced from the clinical symptoms of CGD patients thus far. Finally, the Rac2 knockout mouse has been used to study the role of this signal transduction protein in the activation of the various neutrophil functions (Roberts et al., 1999).

Treatment Options

The prognosis for patients with CGD has dramatically improved since the disorder was first described in the 1950s as fatal granulomatous disease. The grim prognosis in these earlier times was borne out in retrospective epidemiological studies. In one such review of 31 patients followed between 1964 and 1989, actuarial analysis shows 50% survival through the third decade of life (Finn et al., 1990). In another retrospective study of 48 patients followed between 1969 and 1985 in Paris, the survival rate was 50% at 10 years of age with substantially fewer deaths thereafter (Mouy et al., 1989). This latter point is noteworthy in that CGD patients of all genetic types appear to suffer from fewer serious infections after they reach adolescence. While there are no large recent series examining the impact of newer treatment approaches on prognosis, there is a general consensus that a majority of patients should survive well into their adult years, particularly those individuals with CGD caused by p47^{phox} deficiency. One important factor in the improving prognosis for CGD patients is the emergence of several centers in the world that have concentrated on the study and care of scores of patients with CGD (e.g., the National Institutes of Health, Scripps Clinic/Stanford University, the Pediatric Clinics of the Universities of Amsterdam, Munich, and Zürich). Many insights have been gained from the coordi-

nated treatment of these large groups of patients, and this information has been widely disseminated through the literature and through personal communications.

The cornerstones of treatment of CGD are as follows: (1) prevention of infections through immunizations and avoidance of certain sources of pathogens; (2) use of prophylactic trimethoprim-sulfamethoxazole or dicloxacillin; (3) use of prophylactic recombinant human interferon-γ (rhIFN-γ); (4) early and aggressive use of parenteral antibiotics; and (5) surgical drainage or resection of recalcitrant infections. Of these five components, the most important is early intervention in infections before they have the potential to overwhelm the compromised immune system of the CGD patient.

There are multiple ways in which CGD patients can minimize their risk of infection. They should receive all routine immunizations (including live-virus vaccines) on schedule as well as influenza vaccine yearly. Lacerations and skin abrasions should be promptly washed with soap and water and rinsed with an antiseptic agent such as 2% hydrogen peroxide or a Betadine solution. The risk of developing perirectal abscesses can be lessened by careful attention to hygiene, avoidance of constipation, and frequent soaking in warm, soapy baths. The frequency of pulmonary infections can be reduced by refraining from smoking, not using bedside humidifiers, and avoiding sources of *Aspergillus* spores (e.g., hay, straw, mulch, decaying plant material, rotting wood/sawdust, and compost piles). Professional dental cleaning, flossing, and antibacterial mouthwashes can help prevent gingivitis and periodontitis.

Chronic prophylaxis with trimethoprim-sulfamethoxazole (5 mg/kg per day of trimethoprim given orally in one or two doses up to a maximum dose of 160 mg trimethoprim per day) can decrease the number of bacterial infections in CGD patients— by more than half in one series of 36 patients (Margolis et al., 1990). Similar conclusions were reached in a review of 48 European patients (Mouy et al., 1989). In sulfa-allergic patients, dicloxacillin can be used (25–50 mg/kg per day), although there is less documentation of the efficacy of this antibiotic in the prophylactic setting. At one point, there was concern that the sustained use of prophylactic antibiotics could lead to an increased risk of fungal infections. Fortunately, the data do not warrant this concern (Margolis et al., 1990). The effectiveness of antifungal prophylaxis is far less clear. Itraconazole, a newer orally active triazole antifungal antibiotic, has been reported to be an effective prophylactic agent in one study (Mouy et al., 1994). The long-term safety of this drug, however, has not been fully investigated in the CGD setting.

The efficacy of rIFN-γ as a prophylactic agent in CGD was evaluated in a phase III multicenter, double-blind, randomized, placebo-controlled study involving 128 patients. The results, published in 1991, showed a 70% reduction in the risk of developing a serious infection in the rIFN-γ-treated group compared to placebo (Gallin et al., 1991). This benefit is maintained in patients treated for longer periods of time, as reported in two phase IV studies (Bemiller et al., 1995; Weening et al., 1995). Side effects are generally minimal, even with prolonged therapy, and are mainly mild headaches and low-grade fevers within a few hours after administration. The recommended dose is 0.05 mg/m^2 given subcutaneously three times per week. (For infants <0.5 m^2, the recommended dose is 0.0015 mg/kg given subcutaneously three times per week.) The significant clinical improvements in the phase III patients were not accompanied by improvements in superoxide production, a finding confirmed in subsequent studies

(Mühlebach et al., 1992; Woodman et al., 1992; Davis et al., 1995). It now appears that rIFN-γ augments host defense in the vast majority of CGD patients, regardless of genetic subtype, by means other than reversing the respiratory burst defect.

One of the most serious errors in the management of CGD patients is the failure to treat potentially serious infections promptly with appropriate parenteral antibiotics and to continue therapy long enough to eradicate them. Once bacterial and fungal infections become well established and gain the upper hand in a CGD patient, even the best-chosen antibiotics may be relatively ineffective. Therefore, early intervention can be of critical importance. It is usually necessary to begin antibiotic therapy empirically before culture results are available; in these cases, the antibiotics should be chosen to provide strong coverage for *S. aureus* and gram-negative bacteria, including *B. cepacia* (e.g., a combination of nafcillin and ceftazidime). If the infection fails to respond within 24–48 hours, then more aggressive diagnostic procedures should be instituted to identify the responsible microorganism. Additional empirical changes in antibiotic coverage may be warranted, such as adding high-dose intravenous trimethoprim-sulfamethoxazole to cover ceftazidime-resistant *B. cepacia*. If fungus is identified or strongly suspected, amphotericin B is the drug of choice. *Aspergillus* infections of the lung and bone are the most common fungal infections and require 5–6 months of treatment, 2–3 months of which should be given on a daily basis before switching to alternate-day therapy. Amphotericin B treatment should be continued even longer if necessary depending on radiographic, clinical, and culture data (and the return of the erythrocyte sedimentation rate to its "normal" baseline for the patient). Once it is discontinued, most patients should be treated for at least several years with oral itraconazole to prevent recurrence or reactivation of the fungal infection. Caspofungin, a new echinocandin antifungal, has now been approved by the U.S. Food and Drug Administration for the treatment of invasive *Aspergillus* infections in patients unresponsive or unable to receive amphotericin B. New triazole antifungals for intravenous and oral use, itraconazole and voriconazole, have already shown promise in clinical trials in patients with refractory fungal infections. Fungal infection may progress under amphotericin B therapy in CGD, depite the addition of rhIFN-γ, filgrastim, and transfusions with donor granulocytes. Early treatment with additional intravenous antifungals and surgical resection of infected tissues must be given (Jabado et al., 1998; Van 't Hek et al., 1998; Walsh et al., 2002).

Surgery plays an important role in the management of CGD patients. As noted above, surgical drainage (and sometimes excision) of infected lymph nodes and abscesses involving the liver, skin, rectum, kidney, and brain is often necessary for healing, particularly for the visceral abscesses. In cases of highly aggressive fungal or bacterial infections that fail to respond to the medical and surgical approaches outlined above, granulocyte transfusions may be helpful.

Special caution must be exercised in CGD patients regarding transfusions, whether they be granulocytes, erythrocytes, or platelets. Some CGD patients have McLeod syndrome, as discussed earlier. Since the K^x protein is absent and other Kell antigens are only weakly expressed on the erythrocytes of these patients, they will become quickly sensitized to the Kell antigens that are ubiquitous in the population if they are not transfused with K^x-negative McLeod blood products. Unless the molecular genetic basis of a patient's CGD is known not to involve a deletion of the Xp21.1 region, erythrocyte antigen phenotyping should be done prior to a CGD patient's first blood product transfusion.

Clinically significant or symptomatic complications of granuloma formation are best treated with corticosteroids, as these lesions respond quickly to relatively low doses of these agents (e.g., 0.5–1.0 mg/kg per day of prednisone) (Chin et al., 1987; Danziger et al., 1993). It is usually necessary to treat the granulomas for a few weeks before tapering the steroid dose to prevent a rapid relapse. Corticosteroid therapy (topical or by mouth) may also be required to control the symptoms of CGD inflammatory bowel disease. In general, however, corticosteroid therapy in CGD patients should be avoided whenever possible to minimize the inevitable immunosuppression caused by these agents.

Bone marrow transplantation in CGD (see Chapter 47) can be curative and has been successfully employed in several cases (Fischer et al., 1986; Kamani et al., 1988; Ho et al., 1996). However, the overall results have been mixed, as failure to engraft has been a major problem, at least in the earlier transplants. It appears that newer conditioning regimens employing higher doses of busulphan to achieve adequate myeloid suppression may have overcome this problem (Ho et al., 1996; Seger et al., 2002). A recent European study reports the outcome of 27 transplanted CGD patients in the period 1985–2000. Most of these were children, and most received a myeloablative busulphan-based regimen and had unmodified marrow allografts from HLA-identical sibling donors. After myeloablative conditioning all patients (23) were fully engrafted with donor cells, whereas after myelosuppressive regimens only 2 of 4 patients were engrafted (Seger et al., 2002). This latter result recalls a similar observation in the United States (Horwitz et al., 2001). In the European study, severe graft vs. host disease, exacerbation of infection during aplasia, and an inflammatory flare were seen in the subgroup of nine patients with preexisting infection. Overall survival was 85%, with 96% cured of CGD. Survival was excellent in patients without infection at the moment of transplantation. Preexisting infections and inflammatory lesions cleared in all engrafted survivors.

The future will indicate when and whether gene therapy offers the best cure (see below), but until that time the alternative of myeloablative conditioning followed by transplantation of unmodified hematopoietic stem cells is a valid option for children with CGD having an HLA-identical donor. The decision should be made early during childhood, preventing the hazards of severe disease or an ominous course during the procedure of bone marrow transplantation. Although secondary malignancies due to bone marrow conditioning will not be the biggest fear, cyclophosphamide-related infertility still has a dominant effect. Prognostic indicators such as disease-modifying genes associated with a severe course of CGD (see genotype phenotype correlation section) may be helpful in making relevant treatment decisions.

Future Directions

The improvement in the prognosis for patients with CGD over the past 10–15 years is remarkable. Patients diagnosed in infancy and treated with prophylactic antibiotics and rIFN-γ before a relentless cycle of serious infections begins have a fairly optimistic future. It is clear, however, that the prophylactic and therapeutic approaches currently employed are still imperfect, as even these very young, optimally treated children can develop disastrous infections and die. Moreover, all of the treatments developed to date (with the exception of bone marrow transplantation) are only supportive, not curative, and demand a lifetime of diligence and compliance. While further refinements in the medical and surgical management of CGD are likely in the years to come, the ultimate goal is the development of curative approaches for this immunodeficiency. Attention has appropriately been directed toward gene replacement therapy (see Chapter 48). Partial correction of the oxidase defect has been achieved in vitro by transduction of CD34-positive peripheral blood or bone marrow progenitor cells from patients with each of the four types of CGD, using retroviral vectors containing the correct cDNA for the missing NADPH oxidase component (Sekhsaria et al., 1993; Li et al., 1994; Porter et al., 1996; Weil et al., 1997). Substantial reconstitution of oxidase activity was also achieved in granulocyte/monocyte bone marrow progenitors from an X-CGD gp91phox knockout mouse using a retroviral vector system (Ding et al., 1996). This approach has been extended to the treatment of gene knockout CGD mice lacking either gp91phox or p47phox in which bone marrow progenitors were treated ex vivo and then transplanted into irradiated syngeneic CGD mice (Björgvinsdóttir et al., 1997; Mardiney et al., 1997). In both cases, the recipient mice showed increased resistance to bacterial or fungal infection. Levels and duration of expression of the transfected oxidase subunits have been sufficiently large to justify the initiation of early clinical trials for these two forms of CGD (Malech et al., 1997).

The results have been disappointing. In five p47phox-deficient CGD patients, the fraction of gene-corrected neutrophils in the circulation was never more than 0.05%, and corrected cells were no longer detectable after 6 months (Malech et al., 1997). Similar results were obtained in two X-CGD patients (Malech, 1999). Several problems are evident: the corrected bone marrow cells have no growth advantage over the uncorrected cells (so bone marrow conditioning may be necessary); the corrected gene may be silenced because of its linkage to an unnatural promoter (so vectors may be needed with the capacity to contain the original promoter sequence); and the retroviral vectors used integrate only in dividing cells, thus precluding correction of uncommitted stem cells (so lentiviral vectors are needed). Indeed, new viral vectors are now being tested, such as those that after insertion excise proviral sequences not required for gene expression (Grez and von Melchner, 1998), vectors that contain a selectable marker gene in addition to the disease-correcting gene (Grez et al., 2000; Sadat et al., 2003; Sugimoto et al., 2003), and lentivirus-based vectors (Demaison et al., 2002; Roesler et al., 2002; Scherr et al., 2002). A highly encouraging clinical trial with a monocistronic gp91phox retroviral vector was reported during the 2004 European Society for Immune Deficiency (ESID) meetings (by G.M. Ott for the groups of M. Grez and R. Seger). Both patients were conditioned with liposomal busulphan before reinfusion of the transduced (40%–45% transduction efficiency) granulocyte colony–stimulating factor (G-CSF)-mobilized CD34+ cells. A significant fraction of gene marked cells has been detected in peripheral blood of both patients since day +21. The patients have clinically improved: in one patient, a chronic liver abscess resolved, the other achieved resolution of a fungal lung infection. In addition, a new mouse model for testing the effects of gene therapy has been developed. When CD34+ peripheral blood stem cells from X-CGD patients were injected into NOD/SCID mice, these animals produced X-CGD neutrophils, which were corrected by pretreatment of the CD34+ cells with self-inactivating lentivector encoding gp91phox (Roesler et al., 2002). Impressive improvement of gene therapy in this mouse model was achieved by infusion of peripheral blood CD34+ stem cells from X-CGD patients transduced ex vivo with a retroviral vector (the same that

was used in the treatment of X-CGD patients [Malech, 1999] and A47⁰ CGD patients [Malech et al., 1997]) that expressed not only the missing gp91phox protein but also the feline endogenous virus (RD114) envelope. This envelope binds to neutral amino acid transporter (RDR), which is highly expressed on human CD34+CD38− hematopoietic stem cells (Brenner et al., 2003). Further improvement of gene therapy may perhaps be expected from targeted gene therapy in which a mutated gene can be repaired in vivo (Kren et al., 1998; Strauss, 1998). This would overcome the danger of unintentionally activating genes by the random insertion of viral vectors into the genome, which can induce malignant growth in the recipient cells (Hacein-Bey-Abina et al., 2003).

While these are early days in the field of gene therapy, there is some room for optimism in the case of CGD. The study of patients with variant forms of X-linked CGD has revealed that levels of oxidase activity as low as 3%–5% in all of the myeloid cells may be associated with a mild clinical phenotype. In addition, insights derived from X-linked CGD carriers indicate that as few as 5% fully functioning neutrophils can provide substantial protection against infection. It is thus clear that full correction of 100% of the circulating neutrophils in CGD patients will not be required to have an impact on the immune deficit. Even if corrected cells are only transiently generated, there is the potential for substantial benefits for CGD patients, as this therapeutic approach could be used to help treat stubborn, recalcitrant infections.

Acknowledgments

D.R. and T.W.K. thank Jan Dekker, Martin de Boer, Elsbeth van Koppen, Ron Weening, and Rob van Zwieten for their experimental and clinical investigations, and the Netherlands Foundation for Preventive Medicine (Praeventiefonds) and the CGD Research Trust (U.K.) for financial support.

References

Abo A, Pick E, Hall A, Totty N, Teahan CG, Segal AW. Activation of the NADPH oxidase involves the small GTP-binding protein p21rac1. Nature 353:668–670, 1991.

Ahluwalia J, Tinker A, Clapp LH, Duchen MR, Abramov AY, Pope S, Nobles M, Segal AW. The large-conductance Ca²⁺-activated K⁺ channel is essential for innate immunity. Nature 427:853–858, 2004.

Aliabadi H, Gonzalez R, Quie PG. Urinary tract disorders in patients with chronic granulomatous disease. N Engl J Med 321:706–708, 1989.

Ambruso DR, Knall C, Abell AN, Panepinto J, Kurkchubasche A, Thurman G, Gonzalez-Aller C, Hiester A, de Boer M, Harbeck RJ, Oyer R, Johnson GL, Roos D. Human neutrophil immunodeficiency syndrome is associated with an inhibitory Rac2 mutation. Proc Natl Acad Sci USA 97: 4654–4659, 2000.

Ament ME, Ochs HD. Gastrointestinal manifestations of chronic granulomatous disease. N Engl J Med 288:382–387, 1973.

Archer SL, Reeve HL, Michelakis E, Puttagunta L, Waite R, Nelson DP, Dinauer MC, Weir EK. O₂ sensing is preserved in mice lacking the gp91-phox subunit of NADPH oxidase. Proc Natl Acad Sci USA 96: 7944–7949, 1999.

Ariga T, Sakiyama Y, Matsumoto S. A 15-base pair (bp) palindromic insertion associated with a 3-bp deletion in exon 10 of the gp91-phox gene, detected in two patients with X-linked chronic granulomatous disease. Hum Genet 96:6–8, 1995.

Ariga T, Sakiyama Y, Tomizawa K, Imajoh-Ohmi S, Kanegasaki S, Matsumoto S. A newly recognized point mutation in the cytochrome b₅₅₈ heavy chain gene replacing alanine-57 by glutamic acid, in a patient with cytochrome-b-positive X-linked chronic granulomatous disease. Eur J Pediatr 152:469–472, 1993.

Azimi PH, Bodenbender JG, Hintz RL, Kontras SB. Chronic granulomatous disease in three female siblings. JAMA 206:2865–2870, 1968.

Azuma H, Oomi H, Sasaki K, Kawabata I, Sakaino T, Koyano S, Suzutani T, Nunoi H, Okuno A. A new mutation in exon 12 of the gp91-phox gene leading to cytochrome b-positive X-linked chronic granulomatous disease. Blood 85:3274–3277, 1995.

Babior BM, Kipnes RS, Curnutte JT. Biological defense mechanisms: the production by leukocytes of superoxide, a potential bactericidal agent. J Clin Invest 52:741–744, 1973.

Baehner RL, Johnston RB Jr, Nathan DG. Comparative study of the metabolic and bactericidal characteristics of severely glucose-6-phosphate dehydrogenase–deficient polymorphonuclear leukocytes and leukocytes from children with chronic granulomatous disease. J Reticuloendothel Soc 12:150–69, 1972.

Baehner RL, Kunkel LM, Monaco AP, Haines JL, Conneally PM, Palmer C, Heerema N, Orkin SH. DNA linkage analysis of X chromosome–linked chronic granulomatous disease. Proc Natl Acad Sci USA 83:3398–340l, 1986.

Baehner RL, Nathan DG. Quantitative nitroblue tetrazolium test in chronic granulomatous disease. N Engl J Med 278:971–976, 1968.

Baldridge CW, Gerard RW. The extra respiration of phagocytosis. Am J Physiol 103:235–236, 1933.

Bánfi B, Clark RA, Steger K, Krause K-H. Two novel proteins activate superoxide generation by the NADPH oxidase NOX1. J Biol Chem 278:3510–3513, 2003.

Battat L, Francke U. *Nsi*I RFLP at the X-linked chronic granulomatous disease locus (*CYBB*). Nucl Acids Res 17:3619–3619, 1989.

Bemiller LS, Roberts DH, Starko KM, Curnutte JT. Safety and effectiveness of long-term interferon gamma therapy in patients with chronic granulomatous disease. Blood Cells Mol Dis 21:239–247, 1995.

Bemiller LS, Rost JR, Ku-Balai TL, Curnutte JT. The production of intracellular oxidants by stimulated neutrophils correlates with the clinical severity of chronic granulomatous disease (CGD) [abstract]. Blood 78:377a, 1991.

Bendall JK, Cave AC, Heymes C, Gall N, Shah AM. Pivotal role of a gp91-*phox*-containing NADPH oxidase in angiotensin II-induced cardiac hypertrophy in mice. Circulation 105:293–296, 2002.

Berendes H, Bridges RA, Good RA. Fatal granulomatous of childhood: clinical study of new syndrome. Minn Med 40:309–312, 1957.

Berthier S, Paclet M-H, Lerouge S, Roux F, Vergnaud S, Coleman AW, Morel F. Changing the conformation state of cytochrome *b*558 initiates NADPH oxidase activation. J Biol Chem 278:25499–25508, 2003.

Beutler E, Vulliamy T, Luzzatto L. Hematologically important mutations: glucose-6-phosphate dehydrogenase. Blood Cells Mol Dis 22:49–56, 1996.

Björgvinsdóttir H, Ding C, Pech N, Gifford MA, Li LL, Dinauer MC. Retroviral-mediated gene transfer of gp91-*phox* into bone marrow cells rescues defect in host defense against *Aspergillus fumigatus* in murine X-linked chronic granulomatous disease. Blood 89:41–48, 1997.

Bokoch GM, Quilliam LA, Bohl BP, Jesaitis AJ, Quinn MT. Inhibition of Rap1A binding to cytochrome *b*558 of NADPH oxidase by phosphorylation of Rap1A. Science 254:1794–1796, 1991.

Bolscher BGJM, van Zwieten R, Kramer IM, Weening RS, Verhoeven AJ, Roos D. A phosphoprotein of Mr 47,000, defective in autosomal chronic granulomatous disease, copurifies with one of two soluble components required for NADPH:O₂ oxidoreductase activity in human neutrophils. J Clin Invest 83:757–763, 1989.

Bouin AP, Grandvaux N, Vignais PV, Fuchs A. p40-*phox* is phosphorylated on threonine-154 and serine-315 during activation of the phagocyte NADPH oxidase. Implication of a protein kinase C–type kinase in the phosphorylation process. J Biol Chem 273:30097–30103, 1998.

Brandes RP, Miller FJ, Beer S, Haendeler J, Hoffmann J, Ha T, Holland SM, Goerlach A, Busse R. The vascular NADPH oxidase subunit p47-*phox* is involved in redox-mediated gene expression. Free Radic Biol Med 32:1116–1122, 2002.

Brandrup F, Koch C, Petri M, Schidt M, Johansen KS. Discoid lupus erythematosus–like lesions and stomatitis in female carriers of X-linked chronic granulomatous disease. Br J Dermatol 104:495–505, 1981.

Brenner S, Whiting-Theobald NL, Linton GF, Holmes KL, Anderson-Cohen M, Kelly PF, Vanin EF, Pilon AM, Bodine DM, Horwitz ME, Malech HL. Concentrated RD114-pseudotyped MFGS-gp91[phox] vector achieves high levels of functional correction of the chronic granulomatous disease oxidase defect in NOD/SCID/β2-microglobulin⁻/⁻ repopulating mobilized human peripheral blood CD34⁺ cells. Blood 102:2789–2797, 2003.

Bridges RA, Berendes H, Good RA. A fatal granulomatous disease of childhood. The clinical, pathological, and laboratory features of a new syndrome. Am J Dis Child 97:387–408, 1959.

Bromberg Y, Pick E. Unsaturated fatty acids stimulate NADPH-dependent superoxide production by cell-free system derived from macrophages. Cell Immunol 88:213–221, 1984.

Brouha B, Meischl C, Ostertag E, de Boer M, Zhang Y, Neijens H, Roos D, Kazazian HH Jr. Evidence consistent with human L1 retrotransposition in maternal meiosis I. Am J Hum Genet 71:327–336, 2002.

Brown JR, Goldblatt D, Buddle J, Morton, Thrasher AJ. Diminished production of anti-inflammatory mediators during neutrophil apoptosis in chronic granulomatous disease. J Leukoc Biol 73:591–599, 2003.

Bu-Ghanim HN, Segal AW, Keep NH, Casimir CM. Molecular analysis in three cases of X91-variant chronic granulomatous disease. Blood 86:3575–3582, 1995.

Casimir CM, Bu-Ghanim HN, Rodaway ARF, Bentley DL, Rowe P, Segal AW. Autosomal recessive chronic granulomatous disease caused by deletion at a dinucleotide repeat. Proc Natl Acad Sci USA 88:2753–2757, 1991.

Cassatella MA, Bazzoni F, Flynn RM, Dusi S, Trinchieri G, Rossi F. Molecular basis of interferon-gamma and lipopolysaccharide enhancement of phagocyte respiratory burst capability. Studies on the gene expression of several NADPH components. J Biol Chem 265:20241–20246, 1990.

Chang YC, Segal BH, Holland SM, Miller GF, Kwon-Chung KJ. Virulence of catalase-deficient *Aspergillus nidulans* in p47-*phox*⁻/⁻ mice. Implications for fungal pathogenicity and host defense in chronic granulomatous disease. J Clin Invest 101:1843–1850, 1998.

Chin TW, Stiehm ER, Falloon J, Gallin JI. Corticosteroids in treatment of obstructive lesions of chronic granulomatous disease. J Pediatr 111:349–352, 1987.

Clark RA, Malech HL, Gallin JI, Nunoi H, Volpp BD, Pearson DW, Nauseef WM, Curnutte JT. Genetic variants of chronic granulomatous disease: prevalence of deficiencies of two cytosolic components of the NADPH oxidase system. N Engl J Med 321:647–652, 1989.

Clark SR, Coffey MJ, Maclean RM, Collins PW, Lewis MJ, Cross AR, O'Donnell VB. Characterization of nitric oxide consumption pathways by normal, chronic granulomatous disease and myeloperoxidase-deficient human neutrophils. J Immunol 169:5889–5896, 2002.

Cohen MS, Isturiz RE, Malech HL, Root RK, Wilfert CM, Gutman L, Buckley RH. Fungal infection in chronic granulomatous disease. The importance of the phagocyte in defense against fungi. Am J Med 71:59–66, 1981.

Cooper MR, DeChatelet LR, McCall CE, LaVia MF, Spurr CL, Baehner RL. Complete deficiency of leukocyte glucose-6-phosphate dehydrogenase with defective bactericidal activity. J Clin Invest 51:769–778, 1972.

Cross AR, Curnutte JT. The cytosolic activating factors p47-*phox* and p67-*phox* have distinct roles in the regulation of electron flow in NADPH oxidase. J Biol Chem 270:6543–6548, 1995.

Cross AR, Noack D, Rae J, Curnutte JT, Heyworth PG. Hematologically important mutations: the autosomal recessive forms of chronic granulomatous disease (first update). Blood Cells Mol Dis 26:561–565, 2000.

Cross AR, Rae J, Curnutte JT. Cytochrome *b*₋₂₄₅ of the neutrophil superoxide-generating system contains two nonidentical hemes. J Biol Chem 270:17075–17077, 1995.

Cross AR, Yarchover JL, Curnutte JT. The superoxide-generating system of human neutrophils possesses a novel diaphorase activity. Evidence for distinct regulation of electron flow within NADPH oxidase by p67-*phox* and p47-*phox*. J Biol Chem 269:21448–21454, 1994.

Curnutte JT. Activation of human neutrophil nicotinamide adenine dinucleotide phosphate, reduced (triphosphopyridine nucleotide, reduced) oxidase by arachidonic acid in a cell-free system. J Clin Invest 75:1740–1743, 1985.

Curnutte JT. Disorders of granulocyte function and granulopoiesis. In: Nathan DG, Oski FA, eds. Hematology of Infancy and Childhood, 4th ed. Philadelphia: WB Saunders, pp. 904–977, 1992.

Curnutte JT, Babior BM. Chronic granulomatous disease. In: Harris H, Hirschhorn K, eds. Advances in Human Genetics. New York: Plenum, pp. 229–297, 1987.

Curnutte JT, Berkow RL, Roberts RL, Shurin SB, Scott PJ. Chronic granulomatous disease due to a defect in the cytosolic factor required for nicotinamide adenine dinucleotide phosphate oxidase activation. J Clin Invest 81:606–610, 1988.

Curnutte JT, Hopkins PJ, Kuhl W, Beutler E. Studying X inactivation. Lancet 339:749, 1992.

Curnutte JT, Kipnes RS, Babior BM. Defect in pyridine nucleotide dependent superoxide production by a particulate fraction from the granulocytes of patients with chronic granulomatous disease. N Engl J Med 293:628–632, 1975.

Curnutte JT, Kuver R, Scott PJ. Activation of neutrophil NADPH oxidase in a cell-free system. Partial purification of components and characterization of the activation process. J Biol Chem 262:5563–5569, 1987.

Curnutte JT, Scott PJ, Mayo LA. Cytosolic components of the respiratory burst oxidase: resolution of four components, two of which are missing in complementing types of chronic granulomatous disease. Proc Natl Acad Sci USA 86:825–829, 1989.

Curnutte JT, Whitten DM, Babior BM. Defective superoxide production by granulocytes from patients with chronic granulomatous disease. N Engl J Med 290:593–597, 1974.

Dana R, Leto TL, Malech HL, Levy R. Essential requirement of cytosolic phopholipase A2 for activation of the phagocyte NADPH oxidase. J Biol Chem 273:441–445, 1998.

Danziger RN, Goren AT, Becker J, Greene JM, Douglas SD. Outpatient management with oral corticosteroid therapy for obstructive conditions in chronic granulomatous disease. J Pediatr 122:303–305, 1993.

Davis BH, Bigelow NC, Curnutte JT, Ornvold K. Neutrophil CD64 expression: potential diagnostic indicator of acute inflammation and therapeutic monitor of interferon-gamma therapy. Lab Hematol 1:3–12, 1995.

de Boer M, Bakker E, Van Lierde S, Roos D. Somatic triple mosaicism in a carrier of X-linked chronic granulomatous disease. Blood 91:252–257, 1998.

de Boer M, Bolscher BGJM, Dinauer MC, Orkin SH, Smith CIE, Åhlin A, Weening RS, Roos D. Splice site mutations are a common cause of X-linked chronic granulomatous disease. Blood 80:1553–1558, 1992a.

de Boer M, Bolscher BGJM, Sijmons RH, Scheffer H, Weening RS, Roos D. Prenatal diagnosis in a family with X-linked chronic granulomatous disease with the use of the polymerase chain reaction. Prenat Diagn 12:773–777, 1992b.

de Boer M, Hilarius-Stokman PM, Hossle J-P, Verhoeven AJ, Graf N, Kenney RT, Seger R, Roos D. Autosomal recessive chronic granulomatous disease with absence of the 67-kD cytosolic NADPH oxidase components: identification of mutation and detection of carriers. Blood 83:531–536, 1994.

de Boer M, Singh V, Dekker J, Di Rocco M, Goldblatt D, Roos D. Prenatal diagnosis in two families with autosomal, p47-phox-deficient chronic granulomatous disease due to a novel point mutation in NCF1. Prenat Diagn 22:235–240, 2002.

DeCoursey TE. Voltage-gated proton channels and other proton transfer pathways. Physiol Rev 83:475–579, 2003.

DeCoursey TE. During the respiratory burst, do phagocytes need proton channels or potassium channels or both? Science 233:pe21, 2004.

De Deken X, Wang D, Many MC, Costagliola S, Libert F, Vassart G, Dumont JE, Miot F. Cloning of two human thyroid cDNAs encoding new members of the NADPH oxidase family. J Biol Chem 275:23227–23233, 2000.

Dekker J, de Boer M, Roos D. Gene-scan method for the recognition of carriers and patients with p47-phox-deficient autosomal recessive chronic granulomatous disease. Exp Hematol 29:1319–1325, 2001.

DeLeo FR, Nauseef WM, Jesaitis AJ, Burritt JB, Clark RA, Quinn MT. A domain of p47-phox that interacts with human neutrophil flavocytochrome b_{558}. J Biol Chem 270:26246–26251, 1995a.

DeLeo FR, Yu L, Burritt JB, Loetterle LR, Bon CW, Jesaitis AJ, Quinn MT. Mapping sites of interaction of p47-phox and flavocytochrome b with random-sequence peptide phage display libraries. Proc Natl Acad Sci USA 92:7110–7114, 1995b.

Demaison C, Parsley K, Brouns G, Scherr M, Battmer K, Kinnon C, Grez M, Thrasher AJ. High-level transduction and gene expression in hematopoietic repopulating cells using a human immunodeficiency virus type 1–based lentiviral vector containing an internal spleen focus–forming virus promoter. Hum Gene Ther 13:803–813, 2002.

De Mendez I, Garrett MC, Adams AG, Leto TL. Role of p67-phox SH3 domains in assembly of the NADPH oxidase system. J Biol Chem 269:16326–16332, 1994.

Diebold BA, Bokoch GM. Molecular basis for Rac2 regulation of phagocyte NADPH oxidase. Nat Immunol 2:211–215, 2001.

Diekmann D, Abo A, Johnston C, Segal AW, Hall A. Interaction of Rac with p67-phox and regulation of phagocytic NADPH oxidase activity. Science 267:531–533, 1994.

Dinauer MC, Orkin SH, Brown R, Jesaitis AJ, Parkos CA. The glycoprotein encoded by the X-linked chronic granulomatous disease locus is a component of the neutrophil cytochrome b complex. Nature 327:717–720, 1987.

Dinauer MC, Pierce EA, Bruns GAP, Curnutte JT, Orkin SH. Human neutrophil cytochrome b light chain (p22-phox): gene structure, chromosomal location, and mutations in cytochrome-b-negative autosomal recessive chronic granulomatous disease. J Clin Invest 86:1729–1737, 1990.

Dinauer MC, Pierce EA, Erickson RW, Muhlebach TJ, Messner H, Orkin SH, Seger RA, Curnutte JT. Point mutation in the cytoplasmic domain of the neutrophil p22-phox cytochrome b subunit is associated with a nonfunctional NADPH oxidase and chronic granulomatous disease. Proc Natl Acad Sci USA 88:11231–11235, 1991.

Ding C, Kume A, Björgvindottir H, Hawley RG, Pech N, Dinauer MC. High-level reconstitution of respiratory burst activity in human X-linked chronic granulomatous disease (X-CGD) cell line and correction of murine X-CGD bone marrow cells by retroviral-mediated gene transfer of human gp91-phox. Blood 88:1834–1840, 1996.

Dorman SE, Guide SV, Conville PS, DeCarlo ES, Malech HL, Gallin JI, Witebsky FG, Holland SM. Nocardia infection in chronic granulomatous disease. Clin Infect Dis 35:390–394, 2002.

Dorseuil O, Quinn MT, Bokoch GM. Dissociation of Rac translocation from p47phox/p67phox movement in human neutrophils by tyrosine kinase inhibitors. J Leukoc Biol 58:108–113, 1995.

Doussière J, Bouzidi F, Vignais PV. The S100A8/A9 protein as a partner for the cytosolic factors of NADPH oxidase activation in neutrophils. Eur J Biochem 269:3246–3255, 2002.

Dusi S, Donini M, Rossi F. Mechanisms of NADPH oxidase activation in human neutrophils: p67-phox is required for the translocation of rac-1 but not of rac-2 from cytosol to the membranes. Biochem J 308:991–994, 1995.

Dusi S, Rossi F. Activation of NADPH oxidase of human neutrophils involves the phosphorylation and the translocation of cytosolic p67-phox. Biochem J 296:367–371, 1993.

El Benna J, Faust RP, Johnson JL, Babior BM. Phosphorylation of the respiratory burst oxidase subunit p47-phox as determined by two-dimensional phosphopeptide mapping. Phosphorylation by protein kinase C, protein kinase A, and a mitogen-activated protein kinase. J Biol Chem 271:6374–6378, 1996.

Ellson CD, Gobert-Gosse S, Anderson KE, Davidson K, Erdjument-Bromage H, Tempst P, Thuring JW, Cooper MA, Lim ZY, Holmes AB, Gaffney PR, Coadwell J, Chilvers ER, Hawkins PT, Stephens LR. PtdIns(3)P regulates the neutrophil oxidase complex by binding to the PX domain of p40-phox. Nat Cell Biol 3:679–682, 2001.

Emmendorffer A, Nakamura M, Rothe G, Spiekermann K, Lohmann-Matthes M-L, Roesler J. Evaluation of flow cytometric methods for diagnosis of chronic granulomatous disease variants under routine laboratory conditions. Cytometry 18:147–155, 1994.

Faust LP, El Benna J, Babior BM, Chanock SJ. The phosphorylation targets of p47-phox, a subunit of the respiratory burst oxidase. J Clin Invest 96:1499–1505, 1995.

Finan P, Shimizu Y, Gout I, Hsuan J, Truong O, Butcher C, Bennet P, Waterfield MD, Kellie S. An SH3 domain and proline-rich sequence mediate an interaction between two components of the phagocyte NADPH oxidase complex. J Biol Chem 269:13752–13755, 1994.

Finegold AA, Shatwell KP, Segal AW, Klausner RD, Dancis A. Intramembrane bis-heme motif for transmembrane electron transport conserved in a yeast iron reductase and the human NADPH oxidase. J Biol Chem 271:31021–31024, 1996.

Finn A, Hadzic N, Morgan G, Strobel S, Levinsky RJ. Prognosis of chronic granulomatous disease. Arch Dis Child 65:942–945, 1990.

Fischer A, Friedrich W, Levinsky R, Vossen J, Griscelli C, Kubanek B, Morgan G, Wagemaker G, Landais P. Bone-marrow transplantation for immunodeficiencies and osteopetrosis: European survey, 1968–1985. Lancet 2:1080–1084, 1986.

Forbes LV, Truong O, Wientjes FB, Moss SJ, Segal AW. The major phosphorylation site of the NADPH oxidase component p67-phox is Thr233. Biochem J 338:99–105, 1999.

Forrest CB, Forehand JR, Axtell RA, Roberts RL, Johnston RB Jr. Clinical features and current management of chronic granulomatous disease. Hematol Oncol Clin North Am 2:253–266, 1988.

Foster CB, Lehrnbecher T, Mol F, Steinberg SM, Venzon DJ, Walsh TJ, Noack D, Rae J, Winkelstein JA, Curnutte JT, Chanock SJ. Host defense molecule polymorphisms influence the risk for immune-mediated complications in chronic granulomatous disease. J Clin Invest 102:2146–2155, 1998.

Francke U, Hsieh C-L, Foellmer BE, Lomax KJ, Malech HL, Leto TL. Genes for two autosomal recessive forms of chronic granulomatous disease assigned to 1q25 (NCF2) and 7q11.23 (NCF1). Am J Hum Genet 47:483–492, 1990.

Freeman JL, Abo A, Lambeth JD. Rac "insert region" is a novel effector region that is implicated in the activation of NADPH oxidase, but not PAK65. J Biol Chem 271:19794–19801, 1996.

Frifelt JJ, Schonheyder H, Valerius NH, Strate M, Starklint H. Chronic granulomatous disease associated with chronic glomerulonephritis. Acta Paediatr Scand 74:152, 1985.

Fu XW, Wang D, Nurse CA, Dinauer MC, Cutz E. NADPH oxidase is an O_2 sensor in airway chemoreceptors: evidence from K+ current modulation in wild-type and oxidase-deficient mice. Proc Natl Acad Sci USA 97:4374–4379, 2000.

Fuchs A, Dagher M-C, Vignais PV. Mapping the domains of interaction of p40-phox with both p47-phox and p67-phox of the neutrophil oxidase complex using the two-hybrid system. J Biol Chem 270:5695–5697, 1995.

Gallin JI, Buescher ES, Seligmann BE, Nath J, Gaither T, Katz P. Recent advances in chronic granulomatous disease. Ann Intern Med 99:657–674, 1983.

Gallin JI, Malech HL, Weening RS, Curnutte JT, Quie PG, Jaffe HS, Ezekowitz RAB, and the International Chronic Granulomatous Disease Cooperative Study Group. A controlled trial of interferon gamma to prevent infection in chronic granulomatous disease. N Engl J Med 324: 509–516, 1991.

Geiszt M, Dagher MC, Molnar G, Havasi A, Faure J, Paclet MH, Morel F, Ligeti E. Characterization of membrane-localized and cytosolic Rac-GTPase-activating proteins in human neutrophil granulocytes: contribution to the regulation of NADPH oxidase. Biochem J 355:851–858, 2001.

Geiszt M, Kopp JB, Varnai P, Leto TL. Identification of renox, an NAD(P)H oxidase in kidney. Proc Natl Acad Sci USA 97:8010–8014, 2000.

Geiszt M, Lekström K, Witta J, Leto TL. Proteins homologous to p47phox and p67phox support superoxide production by NAD(P)H oxidase 1 in colon epithelial cells. J Biol Chem 278:20006–20012, 2003.

Gerber CE, Bruchelt G, Falk UB, Kimpfler A, Hauschild O, Kuci C, Bachi T, Niethammer D, Schubert R. Reconstitution of bactericidal activity in chronic granulomatous disease cells by glucose-oxidase-containing liposomes. Blood 98:3097–3105, 2001.

Goerlach A, Lee P, Roesler J, Hopkins PJ, Christensen B, Green ED, Chanock SJ, Curnutte JT. A p47-phox pseudogene carries the most common mutation causing p47-phox deficient chronic granulomatous disease. J Clin Invest 100:1907–1918, 1997.

Gorlin J. Identification of (CA/GT)n polymorphisms within the X-linked chronic granulomatous disease (X-CGD) gene: utility for prenatal diagnosis. J Pediatr Hematol Oncol 20:112–119, 1998.

Gray GR, Stamatoyannopoulos G, Naiman SC, Kliman MR, Klebanoff SJ, Austin T, Yoshida A, Robinson GC. Neutrophil dysfunction, chronic granulomatous disease, and non-spherocytic haemolytic anaemia caused by complete deficiency of glucose-6-phosphate dehydrogenase. Lancet 2: 530–534, 1973.

Grez M, Becker S, Saulnier S, Knoss H, Ott MG, Maurer A, Dinauer MC, Hoelzer D, Seger R, Hossle JP. Gene therapy of chronic granulomatous disease. Bone Marrow Transplant 25 (Suppl 2):S99–104, 2000.

Grez M, von Melchner H. New vectors for gene therapy. Stem Cells 16 (Suppl 1):235–243, 1998.

Grogan A, Reeves E, Keep N, Wientjes F, Totty NF, Burlingame AL, Hsuan JJ, Segal AW. Cytosolic phox proteins interact with and regulate the assembly of coronin in neutrophils. J Cell Sci 110:3071–3081, 1997.

Gu Y, Jia B, Yang FC, D'Souza M, Harris CE, Derrow CW, Zheng Y, Williams DA. Biochemical and biological characterization of a human Rac2 GTPase mutant associated with phagocytic immunodeficiency. J Biol Chem 276:15929–15938, 2001.

Hacein-Bey-Abina S, Von Kalle C, Schmidt M, McCormack MP, Wulffraat N, et al. LMO2-associated clonal T cell proliferation in two patients after gene therapy for SCID-X1. Science 302:415–419, 2003.

Hadfield MG, Ghatak NR, Laine FJ, Myer EC, Massie FS, Kramer WM. Brain lesions in chronic granulomatous disease. Acta Neuropathol 81: 467–470, 1991.

Hamers MN, de Boer M, Meerhof LJ, Weening RS, Roos D. Complementation in monocyte hybrids revealing genetic heterogeneity in chronic granulomatous disease. Nature 307:553–555, 1984.

Hampton MB, Vissers MC, Keenan JI, Winterbourn CC. Oxidant-mediated phosphatidylserine exposure and macrophage uptake of activated neutrophils: possible impairment in chronic granulomatous disease. J Leukoc Biol 71:775–781, 2002.

Hardwick LJ, Brown J, Wright AF. An STR polymorphism at the CYBB locus. Hum Mol Genet 2:1755–1755, 1993.

Hayakawa H, Kobayashi N, Yata J. Chronic granulomatous disease in Japan: a summary of the clinical features of 84 registered patients. Acta Paediatr Jpn 27:501–510, 1985.

Henderson LM. Role of histidines identified by mutagenesis in the NADPH oxidase-associated H+ channel. J Biol Chem 273:33216–33223, 1998.

Henderson LM, Meech RW. Evidence that the product of the human X-linked CGD gene, gp91-phox, is a voltage-gated H+ pathway. J Gen Physiol 114:771–786, 1999.

Heyneman RA, Vercauteren RE. Activation of an NADPH oxidase from horse polymorphonuclear leukocytes in a cell-free system. J Leukoc Biol 36:751–759, 1984.

Heyworth PG, Bohl BP, Bokoch GM, Curnutte JT. Rac translocates independently of the neutrophil NADPH oxidase components p47phox and p67phox. Evidence for its interaction with flavocytochrome b558. J Biol Chem 269:30749–30752, 1994.

Heyworth PG, Curnutte JT, Rae J, Noack D, Roos D, van Koppen E, Cross AR. Hematologically important mutations: X-linked chronic granulomatous disease (second update). Blood Cells Mol Dis 27:16–26, 2001.

Heyworth PG, Noack D, Cross AR. Identification of a novel NCF-1 (p47-phox) pseudogene not containing the signature GT deletion: significance for A47° chronic granulomatous disease carrier detection. Blood 100: 1845–1851, 2002.

Heyworth PG, Peveri P, Curnutte JT. Cytosolic components of NADPH oxidase: identity, function and role in regulation of oxidase activity. In: Cochrane CG, Gimbrone MA Jr, eds. Cellular and Molecular Mechanisms of Inflammation. Vol. 4: Biological Oxidants: Generation and Injurious Consequences. San Diego: Academic Press, pp. 43–81, 1992.

Hitzig WH, Seger RA. Chronic granulomatous disease, a heterogeneous syndrome. Hum Genet 64:207–215, 1983.

Ho CML, Vowels MR, Lockwood L, Ziegler JB. Successful bone marrow transplantation in a child with X-linked chronic granulomatous disease. Bone Marrow Transpl 18:213–215, 1996.

Holmes B, Page AR, Good RA. Studies of the metabolic activity of leukocytes from patients with a genetic abnormality of phagocytic function. J Clin Invest 46:1422–1432, 1967.

Holmes B, Park BH, Malawista SE, Quie PG, Nelson DL, Good RA. Chronic granulomatous disease in females: a deficiency of leukocyte glutathione peroxidase. N Engl J Med 283:217–221, 1970.

Hopkins PJ, Bemiller LS, Curnutte JT. Chronic granulomatous disease: diagnosis and classification at the molecular level. Clin Lab Med 12:277–304, 1992.

Horwitz ME, Barrett AJ, Brown MR, Carter CS, Childs R, Gallin JI, Holland SM, Linton GF, Miller JA, Leitman SF, Read EJ, Malech HL. Treatment of chronic granulomatous disease with nonmyeloablative conditioning and a T-cell–depleted hematopoietic allograft. N Engl J Med 344:881–888, 2001.

Hsich E, Segal BH, Pagano PJ, Rey FE, Paigen B, Deleonardis J, Hoyt RF, Holland SM, Finkel T. Vascular effects following homozygous disruption of p47-phox: an essential component of NADPH oxidase. Circulation 101:1234–1236, 2000.

Huang J, Hitt ND, Kleinberg ME. Stoichiometry of p22-phox and gp91-phox in phagocyte cytochrome b558. Biochemistry 34:16753–16757, 1995.

Ito T, Matsui Y, Ago T, Ota K, Sumimoto H. Novel modular domain PB1 recognizes PC motif to mediate functional protein–protein interactions. EMBO J 20:3938–3946, 2001.

Iwata M, Nunoi H, Yamazaki H, Nakano T, Niwa H, Tsuruta S, Ohga S, Ohmi S, Kanegasaki S, Matsuda I. Homologous dinucleotide (GT or TG) deletion in Japanese patients with chronic granulomatous disease with p47-phox deficiency. Biochem Biophys Res Commun 3:1372–1377, 1994.

Jabado N, Casanova JL, Haddad E, Dulieu F, Fournet JC, Dupont B, Fischer A, Hennequin C, Blanche S. Invasive pulmonary infection due to Scedosporium apiospermum in two children with chronic granulomatous disease. Clin Infect Dis 27:1437–1441, 1998.

Jackson SH, Gallin JI, Holland SM. The p47-phox mouse knock-out model of chronic granulomatous disease. J Exp Med 182:751–758, 1995.

Jacobsen BM, Skalnik DG. YY1 binds five cis-elements and trans-activates the myeloid cell–restricted gp91-phox promoter. J Biol Chem 274: 29984–29993, 1999.

Johnson JL, Park JW, Benna JE, Faust LP, Inanami O, Babior BM. Activation of p47-phox, a cytosolic subunit of the leukocyte NADPH oxidase. Phosphorylation of Ser-359 or Ser-370 precedes phosphorylation at other sites and is required for activity. J Biol Chem 273:35147–35152, 1998.

Johnston RB Jr, Baehner RL. Improvement of leukocyte bactericidal activity in chronic granulomatous disease. Blood 35:350–355, 1970.

Johnston RB Jr, Newman SL. Chronic granulomatous disease. Pediatr Clin North Am 24:365–376, 1977.

Joseph G, Pick E. "Peptide walking" is a novel method for mapping functional domains in proteins. Its application to the Rac1-dependent activation of NADPH oxidase. J Biol Chem 270:29079–29082, 1995.

Kamani N, August CS, Campbell DE, Hassan NF, Douglas SD. Marrow transplantation in chronic granulomatous disease: an update, with 6-year follow-up. J Pediatr 113:697–700, 1988.

Kanai F, Liu H, Field SJ, Akbary H, Matsuo T, Brown GE, Cantley LC, Yaffe MB. The PX domains of p47-phox and p40-phox bind to lipid products of PI(3)K. Nat Cell Biol 3:675–678, 2001.

Karplus PA, Daniels MJ, Herriott JR. Atomic structure of ferredoxin-NADP reductase: prototype for a structurally novel flavoenzyme family. Science 251:60–66, 1991.

Kenney RT, Malech HL, Epstein ND, Roberts RL, Leto TL. Characterization of the p67-phox gene: genomic organization and restriction fragment length polymorphism analysis for prenatal diagnosis in chronic granulomatous disease. Blood 82:3739–3744, 1993.

Kim C, Marchal CC, Penninger J, Dinauer MC. The hemopoietic Rho/Rac nucleotide exchange factor Vav1 regulates N-formyl-methionyl-leucyl-phenylalanine-activated neutrophil functions. J Immunol 171:4425– 4430, 2003.

Kirk EA, Dinauer MC, Rosen H, Chait A, Heinecke JW, LeBoeuf RC. Impaired superoxide production due to a deficiency in phagocyte NADPH oxidase fails to inhibit atherosclerosis in mice. Arterioscler Thromb Vasc Biol 20:1529–1535, 2000.

Knaus UG, Heyworth PG, Evans T, Curnutte JT, Bokoch GM. Regulation of phagocyte oxygen radical production by the GTP-binding protein Rac 2. Science 254:1512–1515, 1991.

Kobayashi SD, Braughton KR, Whitney AR, Voyich JM, Schwan TG, Musser JM, DeLeo FR. Bacterial pathogens modulate an apoptosis differentiation program in human neutrophils. Proc Natl Acad Sci USA 10:10948–10953, 2003.

Kobayashi SD, Voyich JM, Braughton KR, Whitney AR, Nauseef WM, Malech HL, DeLeo FR. Gene expression profiling provides insight into the pathophysiology of chronic granulomatous disease. J Immunol 172: 636–643, 2004.

Koga H, Terasawa H, Nunoi H, Takeshige K, Inagaki F, Sumimoto H. Tetra-tricopeptide repeat (TPR) motifs of p67-phox participate in interaction with the small GTPase Rac and activation of the phagocyte NADPH oxidase. J Biol Chem 274:25051–25060, 1999.

Korchak HM, Rossi MW, Kilpatrick LE. Selective role for beta-protein kinase C in signaling for O_2^- generation but not degranulation or adherence in differentiated HL60 cells. J Biol Chem 273:27292–27299, 1998.

Koshkin V, Lotan O, Pick E. The cytosolic component p47-phox is not a sine qua non participant in the activation of NADPH oxidase but is required for optimal superoxide production. J Biol Chem 271:30326–30329, 1996.

Krawczak M, Reiss J, Cooper DN. The mutational spectrum of single base-pair substitutions in mRNA splice junctions of human genes: causes and consequences. Hum Genet 90:41–54, 1992.

Kren BT, Bandyopadhyay P, Steer CJ. In vivo site-directed mutagenesis of the factor IX gene by chimeric RNA/DNA oligonucleotides. Nat Med 4: 285–290, 1998.

Kuribayashi F, Nunoi H, Wakamatsu K, Tsunawaki S, Sato K, Ito T, Sumimoto H. The adaptor protein p40-phox as a positive regulator of the superoxide-producing phagocyte oxidase. EMBO J 21:6312–6320, 2002.

Kwong CH, Malech HL, Rotrosen D, Leto TL. Regulation of the human neutrophil NADPH oxidase by rho-related G-proteins. Biochemistry 32: 5711–5717, 1993.

Landing BH, Shirkey HS. A syndrome of recurrent infection and infiltration of viscera by pigmented lipid histiocytes. Pediatrics 20:431–438, 1957.

Leto TL, Adams AG, De Mendez I. Assembly of the phagocyte NADPH oxidase: binding of src homology 3 domains to proline-rich targets. Proc Natl Acad Sci USA 91:10650–10654, 1994.

Leto TL, Lomax KJ, Volpp BD, Nunoi H, Sechler JMG, Nauseef WM, Clark RA, Gallin JI, Malech HL. Cloning of a 67-kD neutrophil oxidase factor with similarity to a noncatalytic region of p60c-src. Science 248:727–730, 1990.

Leusen JHW, Bolscher BGJM, Hilarius PM, Weening RS, Kaulfersch W, Seger RA, Roos D, Verhoeven AJ. 156ProGln substitution in the light chain of cytochrome b_{558} of the human NADPH oxidase (p22-phox) leads to defective translocation of the cytosolic proteins p47-phox and p67-phox. J Exp Med 180:2329–2334, 1994a.

Leusen JHW, de Boer M, Bolscher BGJM, Hilarius PM, Weening RS, Ochs HD, Roos D, Verhoeven AJ. A point mutation in gp91-phox of cytochrome b_{558} of the human NADPH oxidase leading to defective translocation of the cytosolic proteins p47-phox and p67-phox. J Clin Invest 93:2120–2126, 1994b.

Leusen JHW, de Klein A, Hilarius PM, Åhlin A, Palmblad J, Smith CIE, Diekmann D, Hall A, Verhoeven AJ, Roos D. Disturbed interaction of p21-rac with mutated p67-phox causes chronic granulomatous disease. J Exp Med 184:1243–1249, 1996.

Leusen JHW, Fluiter K, Hilarius PM, Roos D, Verhoeven AJ, Bolscher BGJM. Interactions between the cytosolic components p47-phox and p67-phox of the human neutrophil NADPH oxidase that are not required for activation in the cell-free system. J Biol Chem 270:11216–11221, 1995.

Leusen JH, Meischl C, Eppink MH, Hilarius PM, de Boer M, Weening RS, Åhlin A, Sanders L, Goldblatt D, Skopczynska H, Bernatowska E, Palmblad J, Verhoeven AJ, van Berkel WJ, Roos D. Four novel mutations in the gene encoding gp91-phox of human NADPH oxidase: consequences for oxidase assembly. Blood 95:666–673, 2000.

Li F, Linton GF, Sekhsaria S, Whiting-Theobald N, Katin JP, Gallin JI, Malech HL. CD34 peripheral blood progenitors as a target for genetic correction of the two flavocytochrome b_{558} defective forms of chronic granulomatous disease. Blood 84:53–58, 1994.

Li SL, Schlegel W, Valente AJ, Clark RA. Critical flanking sequences of PU.1 binding sites in myeloid-specific promoters. J Biol Chem 274: 32453–32460, 1999.

Li SL, Valente AJ, Qiang M, Schlegel W, Gamez M, Clark RA. Multiple PU.1 sites cooperate in the regulation of p40-phox transcription during granulocytic differentiation of myeloid cells. Blood 99:4578–4587, 2002.

Li SL, Valente AJ, Wang L, Gamez MJ, Clark RA. Transcriptional regulation of the p67-phox gene: role of AP-1 in concert with myeloid-specific transcription factors. J Biol Chem 276:39368–39378, 2001.

Li SL, Valente AJ, Zhao SJ, Clark RA. PU.1 is essential for p47-phox promoter activity in myeloid cells. J Biol Chem 272:17802–17809, 1997.

Liese JG, Jendrossek V, Jansson A, Petropoulou T, Kloos S, Gahr M, Belohradsky BH. Chronic granulomatous disease in adults. Lancet 347: 220–223, 1996.

Malech HL. Progress in gene therapy for chronic granulomatous disease. J Infect Dis 179(Suppl 2):S318–325, 1999.

Malech HL, Maples PB, Whiting-Theobald N, Linton GF, Sekhsaria S, Vowells SJ, Li F, Miller JA, DeCarlo, E, Holland SM, Leitman SF, Carter CS, Butz RE, Read EJ, Fleisher TA, Schneiderman RD, Van Epps DE, Spratt SK, Maack CA, Rokovich JA, Cohen LK, Gallin JI. Prolonged production of NADPH oxidase–corrected granulocytes after gene therapy of chronic granulomatous disease. Proc Natl Acad Sci USA 94:12133– 12138, 1997.

Mamlok RJ, Mamlok V, Mills GC, Daeschner CW, Schmalstieg FC, Anderson DC. Glucose-6-phosphate dehydrogenase deficiency, neutrophil dysfunction and Chromobacterium violaceum sepsis. J Pediatr 111:852–854, 1987.

Mandell GL, Hook EW. Leukocyte bactericidal activity in chronic granulomatous disease: correlation of bacterial hydrogen peroxide production and susceptibility in intracellular killing. J Bacteriol 100:531–532, 1969.

Manzi S, Urbach AH, McCune AB, Altman HA, Kaplan SS, Medsger TA Jr, Ramsey-Goldman R. Systemic lupus erythematosus in a boy with chronic granulomatous disease: case report and review of the literature. Arthritis Rheum 34:101–105, 1991.

Mardiney M, Jackson SH, Spratt SK, Li F, Holland SM, Malech HL. Enhanced host defense after gene transfer in the murine p47-phox–deficient model of chronic granulomatous disease. Blood 89:2268–2275, 1997.

Margolis DM, Melnick DA, Alling DW, Gallin JI. Trimethoprim-sulfamethoxazole prophylaxis in the management of chronic granulomatous disease. J Infect Dis 162:723–726, 1990.

Marsh WL, Redman CM. Recent developments in the Kell blood group system. Trans Med Rev 1:4–20, 1987.

Martyn LJ, Lischner HW, Pileggi AJ, Harley RD. Chorioretinal lesions in familial chronic granulomatous disease of childhood. Am J Ophthalmol 73: 403–418, 1972.

McPhail LC, Shirley PS, Clayton CC, Snyderman R. Activation of the respiratory burst enzyme from human neutrophils in a cell-free system. J Clin Invest 75:1735–1739, 1985.

Meerhof LJ, Roos D. Heterogeneity in chronic granulomatous disease detected with an improved nitroblue tetrazolium slide test. J Leukoc Biol 39:699–711, 1986.

Meischl C, Boer M, Åhlin A, Roos D. A new exon created by intronic insertion of a rearranged LINE-1 element as the cause of chronic granulomatous disease. Eur J Hum Genet 8:697–703, 2000.

Messina CG, Reeves EP, Roes J, Segal AW. Catalase-negative Staphylococcus aureus retain virulence in mouse model of chronic granulomatous disease. FEBS Lett 518:107–110, 2002.

Mills EL, Rholl KS, Quie PG. X-linked inheritance in females with chronic granulomatous disease. J Clin Invest 66:332–340, 1980.

Mizuno T, Kaibuchi K, Ando S, Musha T, Hiraoka K, Takaishi K, Asada M, Nunoi H, Matsuda I, Takai Y. Regulation of the superoxide-generating NADPH oxidase by a small GTP-binding protein and its stimulatory and inhibitory GDP/GTP exchange proteins. J Biol Chem 267:10215–10218, 1992.

Mizuno Y, Hara T, Nakamura M, Ueda K, Minakami S, Take H. Classification of chronic granulomatous disease on the basis of monoclonal antibody–defined surface cytochrome b deficiency. J Pediatr 113:458–462, 1988.

Moreno JC, Bikker H, Kempers MJ, van Trotsenburg AS, Baas F, de Vijlder JJ, Vulsma T, Ris-Stalpers C. Inactivating mutations in the gene for thyroid oxidase 2 (THOX2) and congenital hypothyroidism. N Engl J Med 347:95–102, 2002.

Moreno MU, San Jose G, Orbe J, Paramo JA, Beloqui O, Diez J, Zalba G. Preliminary characterisation of the promoter of the human p22phox gene: identification of a new polymorphism associated with hypertension. FEBS Lett 542:27–31, 2003.

Morozov I, Lotan O, Joseph G, Gorzalczany Y, Pick E. Mapping of functional domains in p47-phox involved in the activation of NADPH oxidase by "peptide walking". J Biol Chem 273:15435–15444, 1998.

Mouy R, Fischer A, Vilmer E, Seger R, Griscelli C. Incidence, severity, and prevention of infections in chronic granulomatous disease. J Pediatr 114: 555–560, 1989.

Mouy R, Veber F, Blanche S, Donadieu J, Brauner R, Levron J-C, Griscelli C, Fischer A. Long-term itraconazole prophylaxis against *Aspergillus* infections in thirty-two patients with chronic granulomatous disease. J Pediatr 125:998–1003, 1994.

Mühlebach TJ, Gabay J, Nathan CF, Erny C, Dopfer G, Schroten H, Wahn V, Seger RA. Treatment of patients with chronic granulomatous disease with recombinant human interferon-gamma does not improve neutrophil oxidative metabolism, cytochrome b_{558} content or levels of four antimicrobial proteins. Clin Exp Immunol 88:203–206, 1992.

Mühlebach TJ, Robinson W, Seger RA, Machler M. A second *Nsi*I RFLP at the *CYBB* locus. Nucl Acids Res 18:4966–4966, 1990.

Nakamura R, Sumimoto H, Mizuki K, Hata K, Ago T, Kitajima S, Takeshige K, Sakaki Y, Ito T. The PC motif: a novel and evolutionarily conserved sequence involved in interaction between p40-*phox* and p67-*phox*, SH3 domain–containing cytosolic factors of the phagocyte NADPH oxidase. Eur J Biochem 251:583–589, 1998.

Newburger PE, Cohen HJ, Rothchild SB, Hobbins JC, Malawista SE, Mahoney MJ. Prenatal diagnosis of chronic granulomatous disease. N Engl J Med 300:178–181, 1979.

Newburger PE, Skalnik DG, Hopkins PJ, Eklund EA, Curnutte JT. Mutations in the promoter region of the gene for gp91-*phox* in X-linked chronic granulomatous disease with decreased expression of cytochrome b_{558}. J Clin Invest 94:1205–1211, 1994.

Nisimoto Y, Freeman JL, Motalebi SA, Hirshberg M, Lambeth JD. Rac binding to p67-*phox*. Structural basis for interactions of the Rac1 effector region and insert region with components of the respiratory burst oxidase. J Biol Chem 272:18834–18841, 1997.

Noack D, Heyworth PG, Curnutte JT, Rae J, Cross AR. A novel mutation in the *CYBB* gene resulting in an unexpected pattern of exon skipping and chronic granulomatous disease. Biochim Biophys Acta 1454:270–274, 1999.

Noack D, Heyworth PG, Newburger PE, Cross AR. An unusual intronic mutation in the *CYBB* gene giving rise to chronic granulomatous disease. Biochim Biophys Acta 1537:125–131, 2001a.

Noack D, Rae J, Cross AR, Ellis BA, Newburger PE, Curnutte JT, Heyworth PG. Autosomal recessive chronic granulomatous disease caused by defects in *NCF-1*, the gene encoding the phagocyte p47-*phox*: mutations not arising in the *NCF-1* pseudogenes. Blood 97:305–311, 2001b.

Nunoi H, Rotrosen D, Gallin JI, Malech HL. Two forms of autosomal chronic granulomatous disease lack distinct neutrophil cytosol factors. Science 242:1298–1301, 1988.

Okamura N, Curnutte JT, Roberts RL, Babior BM. Relationship of protein phosphorylation to the activation of the respiratory burst in human neutrophils. Defects in the phosphorylation of a group of closely related 48-kDa proteins in two forms of chronic granulomatous disease. J Biol Chem 263:6777–6782, 1988.

O'Kelly I, Lewis A, Peers C, Kemp PJ. O_2 sensing by airway chemoreceptor-derived cells. Protein kinase C activation reveals functional evidence for involvement of NADPH oxidase. J Biol Chem 275:7684–7692, 2000.

Parkos CA, Allen RA, Cochrane CG, Jesaitis AJ. Purified cytochrome *b* from human granulocyte plasma membrane is comprised of two polypeptides with relative molecular weights of 91,000 and 22,000. J Clin Invest 80: 732–742, 1987.

Parkos CA, Dinauer MC, Jesaitis AJ, Orkin SH, Curnutte JT. Absence of both the 91 kD and 22 kD subunits of human neutrophil cytochrome *b* in two genetic forms of chronic granulomatous disease. Blood 73:1416–1420, 1989.

Parkos CA, Dinauer MC, Walker LE, Allen RA, Jesaitis AJ, Orkin SH. Primary structure and unique expression of the 22-kilodalton light chain of human neutrophil cytochrome *b*. Proc Natl Acad Sci USA 85:3319–3323, 1988.

Pelham A, O'Reilly MJ, Malcolm S, Levinsky RJ, Kinnon C. RFLP and deletion analysis for X-linked chronic granulomatous disease using the cDNA probe: potential for improved prenatal diagnosis and carrier determination. Blood 76:820–824, 1990.

Pollock JD, Williams DA, Gifford MAC, Li LL, Du X, Fisherman J, Orkin SH, Doerschuk CM, Dinauer MC. Mouse model of X-linked chronic granulomatous disease, an inherited defect in phagocyte superoxide production. Nat Genet 9:202–209, 1995.

Ponting CP. Novel domains in NADPH oxidase subunits, sorting nexins, and PtdIns 3-kinases: binding partners of SH3 domains? Protein Sci 5:2353–2357, 1996.

Porter CD, Parkar MH, Collins MK, Levinsky RJ, Kinnon C. Efficient retroviral transduction of human bone marrow progenitor and long-term

culture-initiating cells: partial reconstitution of cells from patients with X-linked chronic granulomatous disease by gp91-*phox* expression. Blood 87:3722–3730, 1996.

Porter CD, Parkar MH, Verhoeven AJ, Levinsky RJ, Collins MKL, Kinnon C. P22-*phox* deficient chronic granulomatous disease: reconstitution by retrovirus-mediated expression and identification of a biosynthetic intermediate of gp91-*phox*. Blood 84:2767–2775, 1994.

Price MO, Atkinson SJ, Knaus UG, Dinauer MC. Rac activation induces NADPH oxidase activity in transgenic COSphox cells, and the level of superoxide production is exchange factor-dependent. J Biol Chem 277: 19220–19228, 2002a.

Price MO, McPhail LC, Lambeth JD, Han CH, Knaus UG, Dinauer MC. Creation of a genetic system for analysis of the phagocyte respiratory burst: high-level reconstitution of the NADPH oxidase in a nonhematopoietic system. Blood 99:2653–2661, 2002b.

Quie PG, Kaplan EL, Page AR, Gruskay FL, Malawista SE. Defective polymorphonuclear-leukocyte function and chronic granulomatous disease in two female children. N Engl J Med 278:976–980, 1968.

Quie PG, White JG, Holmes B, Good RA. In vitro bactericidal capacity of human polymorphonuclear leukocytes: diminished activity in chronic granulomatous disease of childhood. J Clin Invest 46:668–679, 1967.

Quinn MT, Mullen ML, Jesaitis AJ, Linner JG. Subcellular distribution of the Rap1A protein in human neutrophils: colocalization and cotranslocation with cytochrome b_{559}. Blood 79:1563–1573, 1992.

Rabbani H, de Boer M, Åhlin A, Sundin U, Elinder G, Hammarström L, Palmblad J, Smith CIE, Roos D. A 40-base-pair duplication in the gp91-*phox* gene leading to X-linked chronic granulomatous disease. Eur J Haematol 51:218–222, 1993.

Rada BK, Geiszt M, Kaldi K, Timar C, Ligeti E. Dual role of phagocytic NADPH oxidase in bacterial killing. Blood 104:2947–2953, 2004.

Rae J, Newburger PE, Dinauer MC, Noack D, Hopkins PJ, Kuruto R, Curnutte JT. X-linked chronic granulomatous disease: mutations in the *CYBB* gene encoding the gp91-*phox* component of respiratory burst oxidase. Am J Hum Genet 62:1320–1331, 1998.

Reeves EP, Dekker LV, Forbes LV, Wientjes FB, Grogan A, Pappin DJ, Segal AW. Direct interaction between p47-*phox* and protein kinase C: evidence for targeting of protein kinase C by p47-*phox* in neutrophils. Biochem J 344:859–866, 1999.

Reeves EP, Lu H, Jacobs HL, Messina CG, Bolsover S, Gabella G, Potma EO, Warley A, Roes J, Segal AW. Killing activity of neutrophils is mediated through activation of proteases by K^+ flux. Nature 416:291–297, 2002.

Regier DS, Greene DG, Sergeant S, Jesaitis AJ, McPhail LC. Phosphorylation of p22-*phox* is mediated by phospholipase D-dependent and -independent mechanisms. Correlation of NADPH oxidase activity and p22-*phox* phosphorylation. J Biol Chem 275:28406–28412, 2000.

Renner WR, Johnson JF, Lichtenstein JE, Kirks DR. Esophageal inflammation and stricture: complication of chronic granulomatous disease of childhood. Radiology 178:189–191, 1991.

Roberts AW, Kim C, Zhen L, Lowe JB, Kapur R, Petryniak B, Spaetti A, Pollock JD, Borneo JB, Bradford GB, Atkinson SJ, Dinauer MC, Williams DA. Deficiency of the hematopoietic cell–specific Rho family GTPase Rac2 is characterized by abnormalities in neutrophil function and host defense. Immunity 10:183–196, 1999.

Roesler J, Brenner S, Bukovsky AA, Whiting-Theobald N, Dull T, Kelly M, Civin CI, Malech HL. 3rd generation of self-inactivating gp91-*phox* lentivector corrects the oxidase defect in NOD/SCID mouse repopulating peripheral blood mobilized CD34+ cells from patients with X-linked chronic granulomatous disease. Blood 100:4381–4390, 2002.

Roesler J, Curnutte JT, Rae J, Barrett D, Patino P, Chanock SJ, Goerlach A. Recombination events between the p47-*phox* gene and its highly homologous pseudogenes are the main cause of autosomal recessive chronic granulomatous disease. Blood 95:2150–2156, 2000.

Roesler J, Hecht M, Freihorst J, Lohmann-Matthes ML, Emmendorffer A. Diagnosis of chronic granulomatous disease and of its mode of inheritance by dihydrorhodamine-1,2,3 and flow microcytofluorometry. Eur J Pediatr 150:161–165, 1991.

Roos D, Curnutte JT, Hossle JP, Lau YL, Ariga T, Nunoi H, Dinauer MC, Gahr M, Segal AW, Newburger PE, Giacca M, Keep NH, van Zwieten R. X-CGDbase: a database of X-CGD-causing mutations. Immunol Today 17:517–421, 1996b.

Roos D, de Boer M, Borregaard N, Bjerrum OW, Valerius NH, Seger RA, Mühlebach T, Belohradsky BH, Weening RS. Chronic granulomatous disease with partial deficiency of cytochrome b_{558} and incomplete respiratory burst: variants of the X-linked, cytochrome b_{558}–negative form of the disease. J Leukoc Biol 51:164–171, 1992.

Roos D, de Boer M, Kuribayashi F, Meischl C, Weening RS, Segal AW, Ahlin A, Nemet K, Hossle JP, Bernatowska-Matuszkiewicz E,

Middleton-Price H. Mutations in the X-linked and autosomal recessive forms of chronic granulomatous disease. Blood 87:1663–1681, 1996a.

Roos D, Kuijpers TW, Mascart-Lemone F, Koenderman L, de Boer M, van Zwieten R, Verhoeven AJ. A novel syndrome of severe neutrophil dysfunction: unresponsiveness confined to chemotaxin-induced functions. Blood 81:2735–2743, 1993.

Roos D, van Zwieten R, Wijnen JT, Gomez-Gallego F, de Boer M, Stevens D, Pronk-Admiraal CJ, de Rijk T, van Noorden CJ, Weening RS, Vulliamy TJ, Ploem JE, Mason PJ, Bautista JM, Khan PM, Beutler E. Molecular basis and enzymatic properties of glucose 6-phosphate dehydrogenase Volendam, leading to chronic nonspherocytic anemia, granulocyte dysfunction, and increased susceptibility to infections. Blood 94:2955–2962, 1999.

Roos D, Weening RS, de Boer M, Meerhof LJ. Heterogeneity in chronic granulomatous disease. In: Vossen J, Griscelli C, eds. Progress in Immunodeficiency Research and Therapy, 2nd ed. Amsterdam: Elsevier, pp. 139–146, 1986.

Rossi F. The O_2^--forming NADPH oxidase of the phagocytes: nature, mechanisms of activation and function. Biochim Biophys Acta 853:65–89, 1986.

Rotrosen D, Yeung CL, Leto TL, Malech HL, Kwong CH. Cytochrome b_{558}: the flavin-binding component of the phagocyte NADPH oxidase. Science 256:1459–1462, 1992.

Royer-Pokora B, Kunkel LM, Monaco AP, Goff SC, Newburger PE, Baehner RL, Cole FS, Curnutte JT, Orkin SH. Cloning the gene for an inherited human disorder—chronic granulomatous disease—on the basis of its chromosomal location. Nature 322:32–38, 1986.

Sadat MA, Pech N, Saulnier S, Leroy BA, Hossle JP, Grez M, Dinauer MC. Long-term high-level reconstitution of NADPH oxidase activity in murine X-linked chronic granulomatous disease using a bicistronic vector expressing gp91phox a Delta LNGFR surface marker. Hum Gene Ther 14:651–666, 2003.

Sbarra AJ, Karnovsky ML. The biochemical basis of phagocytosis. I. Metabolic changes during the ingestion of particles by polymorphonuclear leukocytes. J Biol Chem 234:1355–1362, 1959.

Schaller J. Illness resembling lupus erythematosus in mothers of boys with chronic granulomatous disease. Ann Intern Med 76:747–750, 1972.

Schapiro BL, Newburger PE, Klempner MS, Dinauer MC. Chronic granulomatous disease presenting in a 69-year-old man. N Engl J Med 325:1786–1790, 1991.

Scherr M, Battmer K, Blomer U, Schiedlmeier B, Ganser A, Grez M, Eder M. Lentiviral gene transfer into peripheral blood–derived CD34+ NOD/SCID-repopulating cells. Blood 99:709–712, 2002.

Segal AW. Absence of both cytochrome b_{-245} subunits from neutrophils in X-linked chronic granulomatous disease. Nature 326:88–92, 1987.

Segal AW, Cross AR, Garcia RC, Borregaard N, Valerius NH, Soothill JF, Jones OTG. Absence of cytochrome b_{-245} in chronic granulomatous disease: a multicenter European evaluation of its incidence and relevance. N Engl J Med 308:245–251, 1983.

Segal AW, Heyworth PG, Cockcroft S, Barrowman MM. Stimulated neutrophils from patients with autosomal recessive chronic granulomatous disease fail to phosphorylate a Mr-44,000 protein. Nature 316:547–549, 1985.

Segal AW, Jones OTG, Webster D, Allison AC. Absence of a newly described cytochrome b from neutrophils of patients with chronic granulomatous disease. Lancet 2:446–449, 1978.

Segal AW, West I, Wientjes F, Nugent JHA, Chavan AJ, Haley B, Garcia RC, Rosen H, Scrace G. Cytochrome b_{-245} is a flavocytochrome containing FAD and the NADPH-binding site of the microbicidal oxidase of phagocytes. Biochem J 284:781–788, 1992.

Seger RA, Gungor T, Belohradsky BH, Blanche S, Bordigoni P, Di Bartolomeo P, Flood T, Landais P, Mueller S, Ozsahin H, Passwell JH, Porta F, Slavin S, Wulffraat N, Zintl F, Nagler A, Cant A, Fischer A. Treatment of chronic granulomatous disease with myeloablative conditioning and an unmodified hematopoietic allograft: a survey of the European experience 1985–2000. Blood 100:4344–4350, 2002.

Sekhsaria S, Gallin JI, Linton GF, Mallory RM, Mulligan RC, Malech HL. Peripheral blood progenitors as a target for genetic correction of p47-phox-deficient chronic granulomatous disease. Proc Natl Acad Sci USA 90:7446–7450, 1993.

Shiose A, Kuroda J, Tsuruya K, Hirai M, Hirakata H, Naito S, Hattori M, Sakaki Y, Sumimoto H. A novel superoxide-producing NAD(P)H oxidase in kidney. J Biol Chem 276:1417–1423, 2001.

Sillevis Smitt JH, Bos JD, Weening RS, Krieg SR. Discoid lupus erythematosus–like skin changes in patients with autosomal recessive chronic granulomatous disease. Arch Dermatol 126:1656–1658, 1990a.

Sillevis Smitt JH, Weening RS, Krieg SR, Bos JD. Discoid lupus erythematosus–like lesions in carriers of X-linked chronic granulomatous disease. Br J Dermatol 122:643–650, 1990b.

Skalnik DG, Dorfman DM, Perkins AS, Jenkins NA, Copeland NG, Orkin SH. Targeting of transgene expression in monocyte/macrophages by the gp91-phox promoter and consequent histiocytic malignancies. Proc Natl Acad Sci USA 88:8505–8509, 1991a.

Skalnik DG, Neufeld EJ. Sequence-specific binding of HMG-I(Y) to the proximal promoter of the gp91-phox gene. Biochem Biophys Res Commun 16:563–569, 1992.

Skalnik DG, Strauss EC, Orkin SH. CCAAT displacement protein as a repressor of the myelomonocytic-specific gp91-phox gene promoter. J Biol Chem 266:16736–16744, 1991b.

Speert DP, Bond M, Woodman RC, Curnutte JT. Infection with Pseudomonas cepacia in chronic granulomatous disease: role of nonoxidative killing by neutrophils in host defense. J Infect Dis 170:1524–1531, 1994.

Stasia M-J, Brion JP, Boutonnat J, Morel F. Severe clinical forms of cytochrome b–negative chronic granulomatous disease (X91−) in 3 brothers with a point mutation in the promoter region of CYBB. J Infect Dis 188:1593–1604, 2003.

Strauss M. The site-specific correction of genetic defects. Nat Med 4:274–275, 1998.

Sugimoto Y, Tsukahara S, Sato S, Suzuki M, Nunoi H, Malech HL, Gottesman MM, Tsuruo T. Drug-selected co-expression of P-glycoprotein and gp91 in vivo from an MDR1-bicistronic retrovirus vector Ha-MDR-IRES-gp91. J Gene Med 5:366–376, 2003.

Suh YA, Arnold RS, Lassegue B, Shi J, Xu X, Sorescu D, Chung AB, Griendling KK, Lambeth JD. Cell transformation by the superoxide-generating oxidase Mox1. Nature 401:79–82, 1999.

Sumimoto H, Kage Y, Nunoi H, Sasaki H, Nose T, Fukumaki Y, Ohno M, Minakami S, Takeshige K. Role of src homology 3 domains in assembly and activation of the phagocyte NADPH oxidase. Proc Natl Acad Sci USA 91:5345–5349, 1994.

Sumimoto H, Sakamoto N, Nozaki M, Sakaki Y, Takeshige K, Minakami S. Cytochrome b_{558}, a component of the phagocyte NADPH oxidase, is a flavoprotein. Biochem Biophys Res Commun 186:1368–1375, 1992.

Suzuki S, Kumatori A, Haagen IA, Fujii Y, Sadat MA, Jun HL, Tsuji Y, Roos D, Nakamura M. PU.1 as an essential activator for the expression of gp91-phox gene in human peripheral neutrophils, monocytes, and B lymphocytes. Proc Natl Acad Sci USA 95:6085–6090, 1998.

Szaszi K, Korda A, Wolfl J, Paclet MH, Morel F, Ligeti E. Possible role of Rac-GTPase-activating protein in the termination of superoxide production in phagocytic cells. Free Radic Biol Med 27:764–772, 1999.

Takeya R, Ueno N, Kami K, Taura M, Kohjima M, Izaki T, Nunoi H, Sumimoto H. Novel human homologues of p47phox and p67phox participate in activation of superoxide-producing NADPH oxidases. J Biol Chem 278:25234–25246, 2003.

Tamura M, Kai T, Tsunawaki S, Lambeth JD, Kameda K. Direct interaction of actin with p47-phox of neutrophil NADPH oxidase. Biochem Biophys Res Commun 276:1186–1190, 2000.

Tauber AI, Borregaard N, Simons E, Wright J. Chronic granulomatous disease: a syndrome of phagocyte oxidase deficiencies. Medicine 62:286–309, 1983.

Taylor WR, Jones DT, Segal AW. A structural model for the nucleotide binding domains of the flavocytochrome b_{-245} β-chain. Protein Sci 2:1675–1685, 1993.

Teahan C, Rowe P, Parker P, Totty N, Segal AW. The X-linked chronic granulomatous disease gene codes for the beta-chain of cytochrome b_{-245}. Nature 327:720–721, 1987.

Tkalcevic J, Novelli M, Phylactides M, Iredale JP, Segal AW, Roes J. Impaired immunity and enhanced resistance to endotoxin in the absence of neutrophil elastase and cathepsin G. Immunity 12:201–210, 2000.

Tsuda M, Kaneda M, Sakiyama T, Inana I, Owada M, Kiryu C, Shiraishi T, Kakinuma K. A novel mutation at a probable heme-binding ligand in neutrophil cytochrome b_{558} in atypical X-linked chronic granulomatous disease. Hum Genet 103:377–381, 1998.

Van Bruggen R, Bautista JM, Petropoulou T, de Boer M, van Zwieten R, Gomez-Gallego F, Belohradsky BH, Hartwig NG, Stevens D, Mason PJ, Roos D. Deletion of leucine-61 in glucose-6-phosphate dehydrogenase leads to chronic nonspherocytic anemia, granulocyte dysfunction, and increased susceptibility to infections. Blood 100:1026–1030, 2002.

van Pelt LJ, van Zwieten R, Weening RS, Roos D, Verhoeven AJ, Bolscher BG. Limitations on the use of dihydrorhodamine-1,2,3 for flow cytometric analysis of the neutrophil respiratory burst. J Immunol Methods 191:187–196, 1996.

Van 't Hek LG, Verweij PE, Weemaes CM, van Dalen R, Yntema JB, Meis JF. Successful treatment with voriconazole of invasive aspergillosis in chronic granulomatous disease. Am J Respir Crit Care Med 157:1694–1696, 1998.

Vazquez N, Lehrnbecher T, Chen R, Christensen BL, Gallin JI, Malech H, Holland S, Zhu S, Chanock SJ. Mutational analysis of patients with p47-*phox*-deficient chronic granulomatous disease: The significance of recombination events between the p47-*phox* gene (*NCF1*) and its highly homologous pseudogenes. Exp Hematol 29:234–243, 2001.

Verhoeven AJ, Bolscher BGJM, Meerhof LJ, van Zwieten R, Keijer J, Weening RS, Roos D. Characterization of two monoclonal antibodies against cytochrome b_{558} of human neutrophils. Blood 73:1686–1694, 1989.

Verhoeven AJ, van Schaik MLJ, Roos D, Weening RS. Detection of carriers of the autosomal form of chronic granulomatous disease. Blood 71: 505–507, 1988.

Vihinen M, Arredondo-Vega FX, Casanova JL, Etzioni A, Giliani S, Hammarström L, Hershfield MS, Heyworth PG, Hsu AP, Lahdesmaki A, Lappalainen I, Notarangelo LD, Puck JM, Reith W, Roos D, Schumacher RF, Schwarz K, Vezzoni P, Villa A, Valiaho J, Smith CI. Primary immunodeficiency mutation databases. Adv Genet 43:103–188, 2001.

Vilhardt F, Plastre O, Sawada M, Suzuki K, Wiznerowicz M, Kiyokawa E, Trono D, Krause K-H. The HIV-1 NEF protein and phagocyte oxidase activation. J Biol Chem 277:42136–42143, 2002.

Vives Corrons JL, Feliu E, Pujades MA, Cardellach F, Rozman C, Carreras A, Jou JM, Vallespi MT, Zuazu FJ. Severe glucose-6-phosphate dehydrogenase (G6PD) deficiency associated with chronic hemolytic anemia, granulocyte dysfunction, and increased susceptibility to infections: description of a new molecular variant (G6PD Barcelona). Blood 59:428–434, 1982.

Volpp BD, Lin Y. In vitro molecular reconstitution of the respiratory burst in B lymphoblasts from p47-*phox*-deficient chronic granulomatous disease. J Clin Invest 91:201–207, 1993.

Volpp BD, Nauseef WM, Clark RA. Two cytosolic neutrophil oxidase components absent in autosomal chronic granulomatous disease. Science 242: 1295–1297, 1988.

Voo KS, Skalnik DG. Elf-1 and PU.1 induce expression of gp91-*phox* via a promoter element mutated in a subset of chronic granulomatous disease patients. Blood 93:3512–3520, 1999.

Vowells SJ, Fleisher TA, Sekhsaria S, Alling DW, Maguire TE, Malech HL. Genotype-dependent variability in flow cytometric evaluation of reduced nicotinamide adenine dinucleotide phosphate oxidase function in patients with chronic granulomatous disease. J Pediatr 128:104–107, 1996.

Wallach TM, Segal AW. Stoichiometry of the subunits of flavocytochrome b_{558} of the NADPH oxidase of phagocytes. Biochem J 320:33–38, 1996.

Wallach TM, Segal AW. Analysis of glycosylation sites on gp91-*phox*, the flavocytochrome of the NADPH oxidase, by site-directed mutagenesis and translation in vitro. Biochem J 321:583–585, 1997.

Walsh TJ, Lutsar I, Driscoll T, Dupont B, Roden M, Ghahramani P, Hodges M, Groll AH, Perfect JR. Voriconazole in the treatment of aspergillosis, scedosporiosis and other invasive fungal infections in children. Pediatr Infect Dis J 21:240–248, 2002.

Walther MM, Malech H, Berman A, Choyke P, Venzon DJ, Linehan WM, Gallin JI. The urological manifestations of chronic granulomatous disease. J Urol 147:1314–1318, 1992.

Wang HD, Xu S, Johns DG, Du Y, Quinn MT, Cayatte AJ, Cohen RA. Role of NADPH oxidase in the vascular hypertrophic and oxidative stress response to angiotensin II in mice. Circ Res 88:947–953, 2001.

Weening RS, Adriaansz LH, Weemaes CMR, Lutter R, Roos D. Clinical differences in chronic granulomatous disease in patients with cytochrome *b*–negative or cytochrome *b*–positive neutrophils. J Pediatr 107:102–104, 1985a.

Weening RS, Corbeel L, de Boer M, Lutter R, van Zwieten R, Hamers MN, Roos D. Cytochrome *b* deficiency in an autosomal form of chronic granulomatous disease. A third form of chronic granulomatous disease recognized by monocyte hybridization. J Clin Invest 75:915–920, 1985b.

Weening RS, de Boer M, Kuijpers TW, Neefjes VM, Hack WW, Roos D. Point mutations in the promoter region of the *CYBB* gene leading to mild chronic granulomatous disease. Clin Exp Immunol 122:410–417, 2000.

Weening RS, de Klein A, de Boer M, Roos D. Effect of interferon-γ, in vitro and in vivo, on mRNA levels of phagocyte oxidase components. J Leukoc Biol 60:716–720, 1996.

Weening RS, Leitz GJ, Seger RA. Recombinant human interferon-gamma in patients with chronic granulomatous disease—European follow-up study. Eur J Pediatr 154:295–298, 1995.

Weil WM, Linton GF, Whiting-Theobald N, Vowells SJ, Rafferty SP, Li F, Malech HL. Genetic correction of p67-*phox* deficient chronic granulomatous disease using peripheral blood progenitor cells as a target for retrovirus mediated gene transfer. Blood 89:1754–1761, 1997.

Welch HC, Coadwell WJ, Ellson CD, Ferguson GJ, Andrews SR, Erdjument-Bromage H, Tempst P, Hawkins PT, Stephens LR. P-Rex1, a Pt-dIns(3,4,5)P$_3$- and G$_{\beta\gamma}$-regulated guanine-nucleotide exchange factor for Rac. Cell 108:809–821, 2002.

Wientjes FB, Reeves EP, Soskic V, Furthmayr H, Segal AW. The NADPH oxidase components p47-*phox* and p40-*phox* bind to moesin through their PX domain. Biochem Biophys Res Commun 289:382–388, 2001.

Williams DA, Tao W, Yang F, Kim C, Gu Y, Mansfield P, Levine JE, Petryniak B, Derrow CW, Harris C, Jia B, Zheng Y, Ambruso DR, Lowe JB, Atkinson SJ, Dinauer MC, Boxer L. Dominant negative mutation of the hematopoietic-specific Rho GTPase, Rac2, is associated with a human phagocyte immunodeficiency. Blood 96:1646–1654, 2000.

Winkelstein JA, Marino MC, Johnston RB Jr, Boyle J, Curnutte J, Gallin JI, Malech HL, Holland SM, Ochs H, Quie P, Buckley RH, Foster CB, Chanock SJ, Dickler H. Chronic granulomatous disease. Report on a national registry of 368 patients. Medicine 79:155–169, 2000.

Woodman RC, Erickson RW, Rae J, Jaffe HS, Curnutte JT. Prolonged recombinant interferon-gamma therapy in chronic granulomatous disease: evidence against enhanced neutrophil oxidase activity. Blood 79:1558–1562, 1992.

Woodman RC, Newburger PE, Anklesaria P, Erickson RW, Rae J, Cohen MS, Curnutte JT. A new X-linked variant of chronic granulomatous disease characterized by the existence of a normal clone of respiratory burst-component phagocytic cells. Blood 85:231–241, 1995.

Yang D, Suzuki S, Hao LJ, Fujii Y, Yamauchi A, Yamamoto M, Nakamura M, Kumatori A. Eosinophil-specific regulation of gp91-*phox* gene expression by transcription factors GATA-1 and GATA-2. J Biol Chem 275: 9425–9432, 2000.

Yeaman GR, Froebel K, Galea G, Ormerod A, Urbaniak SJ. Discoid lupus erythematosus in an X-linked cytochrome-positive carrier of chronic granulomatous disease. Br J Dermatol 126:60, 1992.

Yoshida LS, Saruta F, Yoshikawa K, Tatsuzawa O, Tsunawaki S. Mutation at histidine-338 of gp91-*phox* depletes FAD and affects expression of cytochrome b_{558} of the human NADPH oxidase. J Biol Chem 273:27879–27886, 1998.

Yu L, Quinn MT, Cross AR, Dinauer MC. Gp91-*phox* is the heme binding subunit of the superoxide-generating NADPH oxidase. Proc Natl Acad Sci USA 95:7993–7998, 1998.

Yu L, Zhen L, Dinauer MC. Biosynthesis of the phagocyte NADPH oxidase cytochrome b_{558}. Role of heme incorporation and heterodimer formation in maturation and stability of gp91-*phox* and p22-*phox* subunits. J Biol Chem 272:27288–27294, 1997.

Zhao T, Benard V, Bohl BP, Bokoch GM. The molecular basis for adhesion-mediated suppression of reactive oxygen species generation by human neutrophils. J Clin Invest 112:1732–1740, 2003.

38

Cell Adhesion and Leukocyte Adhesion Defects

AMOS ETZIONI and JOHN M. HARLAN

Leukocyte trafficking from bloodstream to tissue is important for the continuous surveillance for foreign antigens and for rapid leukocyte accumulation at sites of inflammatory response or tissue injury. Leukocyte emigration to sites of inflammation is a dynamic process, involving multiple steps in an adhesion cascade. These steps must be precisely orchestrated to ensure a rapid response with only minimal damage to healthy tissue (Carlos and Harlan, 1994; Springer, 1994; von Andrian and Mackay, 2000). Leukocyte interaction with vascular endothelial cells is a pivotal event in the inflammatory response and is mediated by several families of leukocyte and endothelial adhesion molecules, including the integrins, the selectins, and members of the immunoglobulin gene superfamily (IgSF). Each is involved in a different phase of leukocyte adherence to and migration across the endothelium, and the synchronization of their surface expression and activation is crucial for the leukocyte trafficking.

While the importance of leukocyte movement toward sites of inflammation was well recognized more than a century ago, the molecular basis of leukocyte emigration from the bloodstream through the endothelium was only recently elucidated. The integrin family and several integrin ligands of the IgSF were described in the 1980s, whereas the selectins and their carbohydrate counterstructures were discovered in the 1990s. Several years after reporting the structure of the leukocyte integrin molecule, a genetic defect in the subunit of the molecule (ITGB2) was discovered. The resultant syndrome, now called leukocyte adhesion defect type I (LAD I; MIN 116920), has been described in more than 200 children and is characterized by delayed separation of the umbilical cord, recurrent soft tissue infections, chronic periodontitis, marked leukocytosis, and a high mortality rate at an early age. Currently, the only definite therapy is bone marrow transplantation. In vivo and in vitro studies have shown a marked defect in neutrophil motility.

In 1992 a second defect, LAD II (MIM 266265), was discovered in two children and was found to be due to a defect in the synthesis of selectin ligands (Frydman et al., 1992). Although several adhesive functions of LAD II leukocytes are markedly impaired in vitro, the clinical course with respect to infectious complications is milder than that in LAD I. However, patients with LAD II present with other abnormal features, such as growth and mental retardation, which are related to the primary defect in fucose metabolism and are not observed in LAD I.

Recently, a third rare LAD syndrome has been described (Alon et al., 2003; Alon and Etzioni, 2003). Patients with LAD III suffer from severe recurrent infections, similar to LAD I, but also have a bleeding tendency. Although integrin expression is normal and its structure is intact, a defect in integrin activation is the primary abnormality in LAD III.

In this chapter we will briefly review the various adhesion molecules involved in leukocyte–endothelial interactions and then focus on the clinical consequences of defects in these molecules.

Adhesion Molecules

Leukocyte Integrins

Integrins are transmembrane cell surface proteins that bind externally to matrix and membrane proteins and internally to cytoskeletal proteins and thereby communicate extracellular signals (Hynes, 1992). Each integrin consists of noncovalently linked, heterodimeric α and β subunits. Each subunit is composed of a large extracellular domain (1000 to 1150 amino acids for the α subunit and 700 to 740 for the β subunit), a single transmembrane domain of about 20 amino acids, and a short cytoplasmic domain of 40 to 50 amino acids (Humphries, 2000). The crystal structure of the integrin α-subunits containing a β-propeller domain has been described and elegant models of the domain structure of the other regions have been proposed (Springer, 1997). Specificity of receptor binding to various ligands appears to depend primarily on the extracellular portion of the α subunit, although both subunits are required for functional activity of the receptor.

Integrins have been arranged in subfamilies according to the β subunits, and each β subunit may have from 1 to 10 different α subunits associated with it. To date, there are 19 α- and 8 β-subunit genes identified in mammals, encoding polypeptides that combine to form up to 25 receptors. Within this large family of integrin receptors only four members have been clearly shown to be significantly involved in leukocyte adhesion to endothelium.

Two belong to the β_2 subfamily and one each to the β_1 and the β_7 subfamilies.

β_2 Integrins

This subfamily comprises four heterodimeric glycoproteins with a common β-subunit, designated β_2 (CD18) (Table 38.1). The first three heterodimers identified were lymphocyte function–associated antigen-1 (LFA-1), macrophage antigen-1 (Mac-1), and p150, 95; their α subunits are designated α_L (CD11a), α_M (CD11b), and α_X (CD11c), respectively. A fourth heterodimer, $\alpha D\beta_2$, was subsequently identified. The α_L, α_M, α_X, α_D, and β_2 polypeptides are initially assembled in the cytoplasm, and only then is the complete β_2 heterodimer expressed extracellularly. Both subunits are required for expression on the plasma membrane; if the

Table 38.1. Adhesion Molecules Involved in Leukocyte–Endothelial Interactions

Name	Distribution	Mediators (Induced by; Activated by)	Counterstructure(s)	Function(s)
Integrins				
LFA-1 ($\alpha_L\beta_2$, CD11a/CD18)	All leukocytes	Constitutively expressed; activated by crosslinking of other surface receptors, chemokines	ICAM-1, 2	Leukocyte firm adhesion and transmigration
Mac-1 ($\alpha_M\beta_2$, CD11b/CD18)	Neutrophils, monocytes, natural killer cells, eosinophils	Constitutively expressed; activated by cytokines, chemokines, chemoattractants	ICAM-1	Phagocyte firm adhesion and transmigration
$\alpha_4\beta_7$	Lymphocytes, eosinophils, natural killer cells	Constitutively expressed; activated by chemokines	MAdCAM-1, VCAM-1, fibronectin	Leukocyte rolling and firm adhesion
VLA-4 ($\alpha_4\beta_1$, CD49d/CD29)	All leukocytes except neutrophils	Constitutively expressed; activated by crosslinking of other surface receptors, chemokines, chemoattractants	VCAM-1, fibronectin	Leukocyte rolling, firm adhesion, and migration
Ig Superfamily				
ICAM-1 (CD54)	Endothelial cells, lymphocytes, other cell types	Constitutively expressed; upregulated by IL-1, LPS, TNF, IFN-γ	LFA-1, Mac-1	Leukocyte firm adhesion and transmigration
ICAM-2 (CD102)	Endothelial cells, leukocytes	Constitutively expressed	LFA-1	Leukocyte firm adhesion
VCAM-1 (CD106)	Endothelial cells, other cell types	Induced by TNF IL-1, LPS, etc.	VLA-4, $\alpha_4\beta_7$	Leukocyte rolling and firm adhesion
PECAM-1 (CD31)	Leukocytes, endothelial cells, platelets	Constitutively expressed	PECAM-1	Transmigration
MAdCAM-1	Mucosal HEV	Constitutively expressed	$\alpha_4\beta_7$, L-Selectin	Leukocyte rolling and firm adhesion
Selectins				
E-selectin (CD62E)	Endothelial cells	Induced by TNF, IL-1, LPS, etc.	Sialylated, fucosylated structures (e.g., SLeX) expressed on PSGL-1, ESL-1, other glycoproteins	Leukocyte rolling
P-selectin (CD62P)	Endothelial cells, platelets	Induced by histamine, thrombin, etc.	Sialylated, fucosylated, sulfated structures on PSGL-1	Leukocyte rolling
L-selectin (CD62L)	Most leukocytes	Constitutively expressed; shed by diverse activating agents	Sialyated, fucosylated (and often sulfated) structures expressed on CD34, MAdCAM-1, GlyCAM-1, PSGL-1, and other glycoproteins	Leukocyte rolling

ESL-1, E-selectin ligand-1; HEV, high endothelial venule; ICAM, intercellular adhesion molecule; IL-1, interleukin-1; LFA-1, lymphocyte function-associated antigen-1; LPS, lipopolysaccharide; Mac-1, macrophage antigen-1; MAdCAM-1, mucosal addressin cell adhesion molecule-1; PECAM-1, platelet-endothelial cell adhesion molecule-1; PSGL-1, P-selectin glycoprotein ligand-1; SLeX, sialyl Lewis X; TNF, tumor necrosis factor; VCAM-1, vascular cell adhesion molecule-1; VLA, very late antigen.

β_2 subunit is absent, α_L, α_M, and α_X are not detected on the cell surface, even if the synthesis of the α subunits is normal (Springer et al., 1984).

β_2 integrin expression is restricted to leukocytes, but among subsets of leukocytes the distribution of the CD11/CD18 heterodimers differs. LFA-1 ($\alpha_L\beta_2$, CD11a/CD18) is expressed by all leukocytes. Mac-1 ($\alpha_M\beta_2$, CD11b/CD18) and p150, 95 ($\alpha_X\beta_2$, CD11c/CD18) are expressed primarily by myeloid cells, although they are also expressed by some lymphocytes and natural killer (NK) cells. $\alpha_D\beta_2$ (CD11d/CD18) is expressed at moderate levels on myelomonocytic cell lines and subsets of peripheral blood leukocytes. Leukocyte adhesion to endothelium involves primarily LFA-1 and Mac-1. Importantly, the β_2 integrins participate in many adhesion-related functions in addition to adherence to endothelium, such as phagocytosis, killing of bacteria, antibody-dependent cell-mediated cytotoxicity, and homotypic and heterotypic aggregation.

An important characteristic of the leukocyte β_2 integrins is that under baseline conditions they exist in a relatively inactive conformation, rendering the leukocyte nonadhesive. One of the key events in leukocyte adhesion to endothelium is the activation and deactivation of these integrins at the appropriate time and place. Activation of leukocytes by a variety of mediators (e.g., for phagocytes C5a, platelet-activating factor, leukotriene B4, or interleukin-8) results in a transient increase in adhesion by CD11/CD18–dependent mechanisms. This increased adhesiveness occurs through qualitative changes, involving transformation of LFA-1 and Mac-1 from a low- to high-affinity state and clustering of receptors, which increases avidity. In phagocytes, there is also concurrent up-regulation of the surface expression of Mac-1 and p150, 95 (Carlos and Harlan, 1994). β_2 integrins mediate leukocyte adhesion to endothelium through binding to their ligands, members of the IgSF that are expressed on most cells, and this β_2 integrin–dependent adhesion promotes leukocyte interactions with all cells in the body, particularly during inflammatory conditions. Aside from its role in leukocyte adhesion, CD11/CD18 binding to its ligands may also induce intracellular signals. Thus ligand binding could affect cellular functions such as apoptosis, cytotoxicity, proliferation, and cytokine production (Lub et al., 1995).

α_4 Integrins

β_1 or very late antigen (VLA) integrins comprise the largest subfamily (Table 38.1). Most are receptors for extracellular matrix proteins, including fibronectin, collagen, and laminin. One member of this subfamily, $\alpha_4\beta_1$ (VLA-4; CD49d/CD29), has been shown to be involved in lymphocyte, eosinophil, basophil, NK cell, and monocyte adhesion to the CS-1 fragment of fibronectin and to the cytokine-induced endothelial cell surface protein, vascular cell adhesion molecule-1 (VCAM-1). Because circulating human neutrophils do not normally express significant levels of VLA-4, they do not normally use this pathway to adhere to activated endothelium.

The $\alpha_4\beta_7$ integrin is expressed on lymphocytes and eosinophils and functions as the homing receptor that binds to the mucosal vascular addressin cell adhesion molecule (MAdCAM-1) and, to a lesser extent, to VCAM-1 or fibronectin (Table 38.1).

Immunoglobulin Superfamily

Intercellular adhesion molecules

The intercellular adhesion molecules (ICAMs), of which five have been identified, were originally defined functionally as LFA-1 ligands (Springer, 1994) (Table 38.1). Only ICAM-1 and ICAM-2 are expressed on endothelium and participate in leukocyte adhesion to endothelium. The gene for ICAM-1 is located on chromosome 19. The molecule has five Ig-like domains, with a short hinge region separating the third and fourth Ig-like domain (Diamond et al., 1991). ICAM-1 is a ligand for both LFA-1 and Mac-1. The binding sites in ICAM-1 for the two integrins are distinct; LFA-1 binds to domains 1 and 2 and Mac-1 binds to domain 3. Human ICAM-2 is a single-copy gene located on chromosome 17. It has only two extracellular Ig-like domains, and the binding site for LFA-1 is located in these domains (Staunton et al., 1989). The other β_2 integrins do not bind ICAM-2.

ICAM-1 is expressed only at low levels on some endothelial cells, but it is dramatically up-regulated by lipopolysaccharides (LPS), interleukin-1 (IL-1), and tumor necrosis factor (TNF). This increased expression of ICAM-1 peaks at 4–6 hours and persists for days with continued exposure to cytokines. ICAM-2 expression, in contrast, is expressed constitutively, and is not regulated by cytokines.

Vascular cell adhesion molecule-1

VCAM-1 also belongs to the IgSF. A single VCAM-1 gene gives rise through alternative splicing to distinct isoforms that differ in the number of integrin binding sites (Pepinsky et al., 1992). In humans the predominant isoform contains seven Ig-like domains with binding sites for the integrin VLA-4 located within the first and fourth domains (Table 38.1). VCAM-1 is induced by cytokines on endothelial cells with a time course similar to that of ICAM-1.

Mucosal addressin cell adhesion molecule-1

MAdCAM-1 is a member of the IgSF that has a mucin-like domain, which functions as a ligand for L-selectin, as well as an Ig-like domain(s) that serves as a ligand for the $\alpha_4\beta_7$ integrin (Briskin et al., 1993). MAdCAM-1 may serve as a bridge between selectin- and β_2 integrin–dependent events (Bargatze et al., 1995).

Platelet–Endothelial cell adhesion molecule-1

Platelet–endothelial cell adhesion molecule-1 (PECAM-1; CD31) is a member of the IgSF that is expressed at low levels on most leukocytes and platelets but at high levels in endothelial cells where it is localized to intercellular junctions. PECAM-1 is involved in phagocyte transendothelial migration, primarily in migration through the subendothelial basement membrane (Duncan et al., 1999).

Selectins

This family of adhesion molecules was discovered in 1989, when the cDNA sequences for three distinct cell surface glycoproteins found on endothelium (E-selectin, CD62E), platelets (P-selectin, CD62P), and leukocytes (L-selectin, CD62L) were reported (Bevilacqua and Nelson, 1993). These molecules were initially designated ELAM-1; PADGEM or GMP-140; and MEL-14 or LECAM-1, respectively. The genes for the selectins are closely linked on chromosome 1, reflecting their common evolutionary origin. All three members have common structural features, most prominently an N-terminal lectin-like domain that is central to the carbohydrate binding properties of all three selectins (Kansas, 1996). The lectin domain is followed by a domain homologous to the epidermal growth factor (EGF) and then by a discrete number of domains similar to those found in certain complement binding proteins. The term *selectin* was proposed to highlight the amino-terminal lectin domain and to indicate the selective function and expression of these molecules.

All three selectins are involved in the recruitment of leukocytes to sites of tissue injury, but there are fundamental differences in their distribution, activation, and mode of expression (Tedder et al., 1995). For example, while all three selectins take part in the first step of the adhesion cascade, the rolling phase (vide infra), E-selectin participates somewhat later in the recruitment process (Ley and Tedder, 1995).

E-selectin

E-selectin is restricted to endothelial cells and its expression is induced when the cells are activated by LPS, IL-1, TNF, and other stimuli (Table 38.1). These substances activate the transcription and translation of E-selectin, resulting in peak cell surface expression at 4–6 hours, decreasing to near basal levels by 24 hours (Cotran et al., 1986). Although E-selectin expression in vitro is typically transient, it is expressed chronically in certain inflammatory conditions.

P-selectin

P-selectin is expressed on platelets as well as on endothelial cells (Table 38.1). Its expression does not necessarily require de novo synthesis because it is stored in the granules in platelets and in secretory granules (Weibel-Palade bodies) in endothelial cells. Thus, within minutes of activation of either cell type by thrombin or histamine, P-selectin is rapidly redistributed to the surface of the cells. Its expression in vitro is typically very short-lived—up to 15 minutes. However, studies in vivo suggest that endothelial P-selectin may also be regulated at the level of protein synthesis, providing a mechanism for more prolonged expression (Gotsch et al., 1994).

L-selectin

In contrast to the E- and P-selectins, L-selectin is not expressed on quiescent or activated endothelial cells but rather is constitutively expressed on leukocytes (Table 38.1). Although originally described as a lymphocyte homing receptor, it was subsequently shown to be expressed on most other leukocytes (Lewinsohn et al., 1987). After a transient increase of this selectin during activation, it is shed rapidly because of proteolytic cleavage near the membrane insertion. Cleavage of L-selectin may serve to limit further leukocyte recruitment at inflammatory sites.

Selectin ligands

Studies of the molecular basis of selectin adhesion have focused mainly on carbohydrate recognition by the lectin domains. Identification of the physiological ligands for the selectins has been challenging because, like many lectins, the selectins can bind a variety of carbohydrate structures in vitro (Kansas, 1996). These ligands are carbohydrate groups typically found as terminal structures on one or more glycoproteins and/or glycolipids. The EGF domain as well as the lectin domain contributes to selectin binding to glycoconjugates.

One major selectin ligand is a member of a class of sialylated and fucosylated tetrasaccharides related to the sialylated Lewis X blood group (SLeX, CD15s). SLeX is usually expressed at high levels on neutrophils and monocytes, whereas most peripheral lymphocytes express SLeX only after activation. Both the sialic acid and the fucose moieties are critical for efficient binding. Monoclonal antibodies against SLeX block the binding of neutrophils to activated endothelial cells. Cell lines that do not express this structure show no binding, but after induction of SLeX by transfection of appropriate fucosyltransferases, binding

is observed. Furthermore, infusion of SLeX blocks leukocyte rolling along inflamed venules (Asako et al., 1994). Although the detailed carbohydrate structures for the various physiological selectin ligands are not fully characterized, carbohydrate recognition is clearly critical for selectin-mediated adhesion.

While the selectins bind weakly to small sialylated, fucosylated oligosaccharides, they appear to bind with much higher avidity to carbohydrate determinants on a limited number of glycoproteins. L-selectin binds at least three different heavily glycosylated mucin-like proteins: GlyCAM-1X, CD34X, and MAdCAM-1. P-selectin and, to a lesser extent, E-selectin have been reported to selectively bind P-selectin glycoprotein ligand-1 (PSGL-1), which is expressed on most leukocytes (Sako et al., 1993). A monoclonal antibody specific for PSGL-1 completely inhibited P-selectin–mediated rolling of leukocytes under a range of physiologic shear stress (Moore et al., 1995).

The Adhesion Cascade

The migration of leukocytes from the bloodstream to the tissue occurs in several distinct steps (Butcher, 1991) (Fig. 38.1). First, under conditions of flow, loose adhesion to the vessel wall, primarily in postcapillary venules, causes the leukocytes to roll on the endothelium. This transient and reversible step is a prerequisite for the next stage, the activation of leukocytes. This is followed by firm adhesion, i.e., sticking, after which migration occurs. Each of these steps involves different adhesion molecules and can be differentially regulated.

Selectin-Mediated Rolling

Leukocytes in the circulation must resist shear forces to arrest along the vascular endothelium. Under normal conditions, leukocytes move rapidly in the laminar flow stream of blood and do not adhere to the endothelium. However, with activation of the

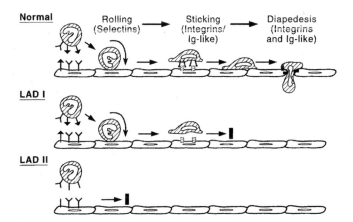

Figure 38.1. The adhesion cascade and leukocyte adhesion deficiency (LAD) syndromes. Under conditions of flow at sites of inflammation, normal leukocytes first roll along the venular wall via selectin–carbohydrate interactions. Following integrin activation by local chemoattractants or chemokines, the rolling cells then adhere firmly via binding of leukocyte integrins to endothelial immunoglobulin gene superfamily (IgSF) ligands. Subsequently, the adherent leukocytes diapedese between endothelial cells utilizing PECAM-1 and integrin–IgSF ligand interactions. Defects in selectin-mediated rolling or integrin-mediated sticking impair emigration. In LAD I, neutrophils deficient in β_2 integrin are able to roll along the endothelium but are unable to adhere firmly to transmigrate. In LAD II, neutrophils deficient in fucosylated carbohydrate ligands for selectins are unable to roll and thus cannot adhere and transmigrate.

endothelium due to local trauma or inflammation, leukocytes immediately begin to roll along the venular wall. This phenomenon of leukocyte rolling was observed for more than a century, but its molecular basis was delineated only recently. Several studies showed that although CD18 monoclonal antibodies block sticking, they do not prevent rolling (Arfors et al., 1987). Monoclonal antibodies to selectins, however, markedly reduced the rolling process in vivo and in vitro (Olofsson et al., 1994). Moreover, rolling is much diminished in both P- and L-selectin–deficient mice (Mayadas et al., 1993; Ley and Tedder, 1995). The endothelial selectins will bind to the leukocytes through their carbohydrate ligands. Patients who lack SLeX molecules and other fucosylated selectin ligands show defective in vivo rolling (von Andrian et al., 1993). The presentation of SLeX to E- and P-selectins may be partially mediated by L-selectin, which is expressed on microvilli of the leukocytes (von Andrian et al., 1995). L-selectin itself recognizes sialylated, fucosylated, counterstructures on glycoproteins such as CD34 on high endothelial venules (Baumheter et al., 1993) and as yet poorly characterized ligands on systemic vasculature (Spertini et al., 1991). The rolling phase is transient in part because L-selectin is shed quickly from the leukocytes and P-selectin on endothelial cells is internalized.

Activation of Integrins

The initial rolling interaction of leukocytes with endothelium is reversible unless the leukocytes are activated and become firmly adherent. Binding to the selectins tethers the leukocytes, exposing them to stimuli in the local microenvironment (Zimmerman et al., 1992). Chemoattractants released from endothelium or cells in the surrounding tissue can rapidly trigger the leukocyte integrins to proceed to activation-dependent sticking and arrest. The leukocyte chemoattractants include classical chemoattractants, such as C5a and leukotriene B4, and chemokines, which bind to the apical surface of endothelial cells (Mackay, 2001). The importance of chemotactic agents in mediating firm adhesion was illustrated in experiments using the flow chamber model. In this model leukocyte rolling stops immediately after a small amount of a chemotactic agent is added and the cells then start to spread (Lawrence and Springer, 1991). Increased adhesive capacity is mediated primarily through qualitative changes in integrin receptor affinity or avidity, although in phagocytes a rapid increase in surface expression of Mac-1 also occurs through translocation of $\alpha_M\beta_2$ heterodimers from cytoplasmic granules to the plasma membrane.

Adhesion and Transendothelial Migration Via Integrins and Immunoglobulin Superfamily Ligands

Activation of integrins results in increased binding to their Ig-like ligands on the endothelial cells. This ensures that adhesion is firm enough to withstand the continuous shear forces in the blood vessels. Monoclonal antibodies to both integrins and their IgSF ligands block the firm adhesion of leukocytes to endothelial cells. The final event, the transendothelial migration of the leukocytes to the site of inflammation, is in part dependent on integrin–IgSF interactions and can be blocked by monoclonal antibodies to these molecules. Another member of the endothelial IgSF, PECAM-1, was found to be important mainly in migration of phagocytes through the subendothelial basement membrane (Duncan et al., 1999).

Adhesion Molecule Deficiency Syndromes

Perhaps the best way to appreciate the in vivo importance of leukocyte and endothelial adhesion molecules in humans is to examine those rare "experiments of nature" in which a genetically determined defect in an adhesion molecule is associated with disease. Two such syndromes have been recognized (Table 38.2). In the first LAD syndrome (LAD I), the β_2-integrin family is deficient, whereas in the second, LAD II, the fucosylated carbohydrate ligands for selectins are absent (Etzioni, 1996). Most recently, a third leukocyte adhesion deficiency, LAD III, has been identified (Alon et al., 2003; Alon and Etzioni, 2003).

Leukocyte Adhesion Deficiency Type I

Before 1980, several reports documented a group of patients with recurrent bacterial and fungal infections, defective leukocyte motility and phagocytosis, impaired wound healing, and delayed separation of the umbilical cord (Boxer et al., 1974; Gallin et al., 1978; Hayward et al., 1979). In 1980, a seminal study suggested a possible molecular basis for this emerging syndrome (Crowley et al., 1980). Crowley and colleagues reported the absence of a high–molecular weight neutrophil membrane glycoprotein in a young boy with an inherited defect in neutrophil adhesion. This abnormality was manifested in vitro by failure to spread on surfaces and impaired chemotaxis. In 1982 the association of this syndrome with a missing membrane glycoprotein was confirmed in two other patients (Bowen et al., 1982).

At the same time as this clinical syndrome was being characterized, in separate studies other investigators were identifying a new leukocyte membrane glycoprotein complex involved in multiple adhesion-related functions. Mac-1 and LFA-1 were identified in 1979 and 1981, respectively (Anderson et al., 1995). A third complex belonging to this family, p150, 95, was described several years later. A relationship between the inherited defect of neutrophil adhesion and these glycoproteins was suggested by the fact that monoclonal antibodies to the α or β chains of this complex induced in vitro defects in chemotaxis and phagocytosis

Table 38.2. Leukocyte Adhesion Deficiency Syndromes

Features	LAD I	LAD II	LAD III
Clinical Manifestation			
Recurrent severe infections	+++	+	+++
Neutrophilia			
Basal	+	+++	++
With infection	+++	+++	+++
Periodontitis	++	++	?
Skin infection	++	+	++
Delayed separation of the umbilical cord	+++	−	+
Developmental abnormalities	−	+++	
Bleeding tendency	−	−	+++
Laboratory Findings			
CD18 expression	↓↓↓ or absent	NL	NL
SLeX expression	NL	Absent	NL
Neutrophil motility	↓↓↓	↓↓	↓↓
Neutrophil rolling	NL	↓↓↓	NL
Neutrophil adherence	↓↓↓	↓	↓↓↓
Opsonophagocytic activity	↓	NL	NL
T and B cell function	↓	NL	?

NL, normal.

similar to those observed in affected patients. Indeed, in 1984, using specific monoclonal antibodies, multiple groups reported that leukocytes of patients with this syndrome were deficient in both the common subunit as well as in the various subunits (Schwartz and Harlan, 1991). These findings led to the proposal that the primary defect in this syndrome is related to the β_2 subunit and that biosynthesis of the β_2 subunit is necessary for surface expression of the α subunits (Springer, 1985).

While many names had previously been given to this syndrome, in the interest of brevity and comprehensiveness, the term *leukocyte adhesion deficiency* (LAD) was proposed in 1987 (Anderson and Springer, 1987). LAD I is inherited in an autosomal recessive manner with heterozygotes exhibiting no significant clinical manifestations. More than 200 patients with this defect have now been described (Etzioni, 1999).

Clinical and pathologic manifestations

The prominent clinical feature of these patients is recurrent bacterial infections, primarily localized to skin and mucosal surfaces. These infections are indolent and necrotic and tend to recur. Sites of infection often progressively enlarge, and they may lead to systemic spread of the bacteria. Infections are usually apparent from birth onward, and a common presenting infection is omphalitis with delayed separation of the umbilical cord (Color Plate 38.I). The most frequently encountered bacteria are *Staphylococcus aureus* and gram-negative enteric organisms, but fungal infections are also common. The absence of pus formation at the sites of infection is one of the hallmarks of LAD I. Severe gingivitis and periodontitis are major features among all patients who survive infancy. Impaired healing of traumatic or surgical wounds is also characteristic of this syndrome.

The recurrent infections observed in affected patients result from a profound impairment of leukocyte mobilization into extravascular site of inflammation. Skin windows yield few, if any, leukocytes, and biopsies of infected tissues demonstrate inflammation totally devoid of neutrophils. These findings are particularly striking considering that marked peripheral blood leukocytosis (5 to 20 times normal values) is consistently observed during infections. Transfusions of normal leukocytes resulted in the appearance of donor cells in the skin of one LAD I patient (Bowen et al., 1982), indicating that the defect is intrinsic to the leukocyte. In contrast to the difficulties experienced in defense against bacterial and fungal microorganisms, LAD I patients do not exhibit a marked increase in susceptibility to viral infections.

The severity of clinical infectious complications among patients with LAD I appears to be directly related to the degree of CD18 deficiency. Two phenotypes, designated *severe deficiency* and *moderate deficiency*, have been defined (Fischer et al., 1988). Patients with less than 1% of the normal surface expression exhibited a severe form of disease with earlier, more frequent, and more serious episodes of infection, often leading to death in infancy, whereas patients with some surface expression of CD18 (2.5%–10%) manifested a moderate to mild phenotype with fewer serious infectious episodes and survival into adulthood.

The hallmark pathological finding in LAD I is the complete absence of neutrophils in sites of infection. The necrotic areas are devoid of pus. While this finding is typical for many tissues, in the lung, neutrophil migration to the site of infection may be normal and a normal inflammatory response has been observed (Hawkins et al., 1992). Lymphoid tissue is also severely depleted of lymphocytes, indicating a role for LFA-1 in lymphocyte homing.

Laboratory findings

The defective migration of neutrophils from patients with LAD I has been observed in studies in vivo as well as in vitro (Bowen et al., 1982; Schwartz and Harlan, 1991; Harlan, 1993). Neutrophils failed to mobilize to skin sites in the in vivo Rebuck skin-window test. In vitro studies demonstrated a marked defect in random migration as well as chemotaxis to various chemoattractant substances. Adhesion and transmigration through endothelial cells were found to be severely impaired (Harlan et al., 1985). With the use of an intravital microscopy assay it was found that fluorescein-labeled neutrophils from a LAD I boy rolled normally on inflamed rabbit venules, a finding suggesting that they were capable of initiating adhesive interactions with inflamed endothelial cells (von Andrian et al., 1993). However, these cells failed to perform activation-dependent, β_2 integrin–mediated adhesion steps and did not stick or emigrate when challenged with a chemotactic stimulus (Fig. 38.1).

Patients with LAD I exhibit mild to moderate neutrophilia in the absence of overt infection. Marked granulocytosis with neutrophil counts in peripheral blood reaching levels of up to 100,000/µl occurs during acute infections. Defects in other myeloid functions are also observed. Binding and phagocytosis of iC3b-opsonized particles is also deficient, in agreement with the function of Mac-1 as complement receptor 3 (CR3). Abnormalities of neutrophil-mediated, antibody-dependent cellular cytotoxicity have been reported in several patients (Kohl et al., 1986).

A wide variety of in vitro abnormalities of lymphocyte function have also been described in LAD I, but their in vivo relevance remains unclear. Although no humoral immune deficiency has been described in most of the patients, an impaired primary and secondary antibody response to a T-dependent neoantigen was found (Ochs et al., 1993).

Functional aspects

The CD11/CD18 integrin receptor is expressed on all normal leukocytes, and CD11/CD18 plays an important role in multiple leukocyte functions. However, the predominant clinical manifestation of LAD I—i.e., markedly impaired phagocyte emigration in response to pyogenic infections—can be attributed to the reduced adhesion to endothelium and impaired transendothelial migration observed in CD18-deficient neutrophils of patients with this syndrome.

Molecular basis

Early on, several lines of evidence supported an autosomal recessive pattern of inheritance. Equal numbers of male and female patients were described, and family studies showed heterozygous male and female carriers who expressed 50% of the normal amount of the β_2-integrin molecules on their neutrophils. Furthermore, a frequent history of consanguineous marriages strongly supported the concept that LAD I is inherited as an autosomal trait (Anderson et al., 1995). Early studies showed that patients with this disorder were uniformly deficient in the expression of all three leukocyte integrins (Mac-1, LFA-1, p150, 95), suggesting that the primary defect was in the common β_2 subunit, which is encoded by a gene located at the tip of the long arm of chromosome 21q22.3 (Solomon et al., 1988). To date, none of the reported affected individuals has demonstrated a selective deficiency of a single β_2-integrin heterodimer. Normal B cell lines synthesize α_L and β_2 precursors, which associate in the cytoplasm and then are transported to the cell surface as an $\alpha_L\beta_2$ heterodimer. In contrast, lymphoblasts of patients with LAD I synthesize only normal α_L subunit precursor, but it is never expressed on the cell surface and is apparently degraded in the absence of a normal β_2 subunit (Springer et al., 1984).

Heterogeneity among LAD I patients was first described with respect to the extent of β_2-integrin deficiency on the leukocyte surface as shown by flow cytometry. As previously discussed, the severity of the clinical features and the magnitude of the functional deficits observed are directly related to the degree of CD18 deficiency, but the underlying molecular basis for this heterogeneity remained largely undefined until the β_2-subunit gene (*ITGB2*) was cloned (Kishimoto et al., 1987).

Subsequently, several LAD I variants were reported in which there was a defect in β_2-integrin adhesive functions despite normal surface expression of CD18. A child with classical LAD I features with normal surface expression of CD18 was reported (Hogg et al., 1999) in whom a mutation in CD18 led to a nonfunctional molecule. Another child with a moderately severe form of LAD I was found to have a novel point mutation in CD18, leading to the expression of dysfunctional β_2 integrin (Mathew et al., 2000).

Mutation analysis

The molecular basis for CD18 deficiency varies (Vihinen et al., 2001). In some cases it is due to the lack of or diminished expression of CD18 mRNA. In other cases there is expression of mRNA or protein precursors of aberrant size with both larger and smaller CD18 subunits. In still other cases LAD I results from a failure to process normal-sized protein precursors to the mature normal product (Wright et al., 1995). Analysis at the gene level has revealed a degree of heterogeneity, which reflects this diversity. A number of point mutations have been reported, some of which lead to the biosynthesis of defective proteins with single amino acid substitutions, while others lead to splicing defects, resulting in the production of truncated and unstable proteins (Kishimoto et al., 1987). In one kindred a 90-nucleotide deletion in the CD18 mRNA produced an in-frame deletion of a 30–amino acid region. Analysis of the genomic DNA showed this 90bp region to be encoded by a single exon (exon 9) (Kishimoto et al., 1989). The 30–amino acid deletion is located in a 241–amino acid region of the extracellular domain of the CD18 molecule that is highly conserved in evolution. Notably, a high percentage of CD18 mutations identified in LAD I are contained in this highly conserved segment (Kishimoto et al., 1989) (Fig. 38.2). Domains within this segment are presumably required for association and biosynthesis of precursors and may represent critical contact sites between the α-subunit and β-subunit precursors.

Mutation analysis of other severe and moderate LAD I phenotypes has defined point mutations in the coding region of the

CD18 subunit mRNA. In one case, a normal-sized β_2-subunit precursor was present in the cytoplasm but was not expressed on the cell surface membrane. The mutations were found again in the same highly conserved extracellular domain (Sligh et al., 1992). Several splicing defects resulting in the production of abnormal proteins were reported. Other mutations were found in exons 7 and 13 (Back et al., 1992). Homozygosity for the mutation was described in some cases, whereas in others compound heterozygosity was observed. Thus far over 20 different mutations have been described (Fig. 38.2). In many cases no molecular analysis has been performed.

Thus, LAD I can be caused by a number of distinct mutational events, all resulting in the failure to produce a functional leukocyte β_2 subunit. In most cases a point mutation, small insertions, or deletions in the *CD18* (*ITGB2*) gene have been reported, although an infant with LAD I and gross abnormality in chromosome 21, representing a deletion of q22.1–3, has been described (Rivera-Matos et al., 1995).

Strategy for diagnosis

In any infant male or female with recurrent soft tissue infections and a very high leukocyte count, the diagnosis of LAD I should be considered. The diagnosis is even more suggestive if a history of delayed separation of the umbilical cord is present. To confirm the diagnosis, absence of the α and β subunits of the β_2-integrin complex must be demonstrated. This can be accomplished with the use of the appropriate CD11 and CD18 monoclonal antibodies and flow cytometry. Sequence analysis to define the exact molecular defect in the β_2 subunit is a further option. In rare cases functional assays must be performed to diagnose a LAD I variant.

Carrier detection and prenatal diagnosis

LAD I carriers have 40%–60% of normal CD18 and lack clinical symptoms. Sequence analysis shows one normal and one abnormal gene.

Because leukocytes express CD18 on their surface at 20 weeks of gestation, cordocentesis performed at this age can establish a prenatal diagnosis (Weening et al., 1991). In families in whom the exact molecular defect has been previously identified, an earlier prenatal diagnosis is possible by chorionic biopsy and mutation analysis.

Treatment and prognosis

Patients with the moderate LAD I phenotype usually respond to conservative therapy and the prompt use of antibiotics during acute infectious episodes. Prophylactic antibiotics may reduce the risk of infections. A trial of interferon-γ (IFN-γ), which can

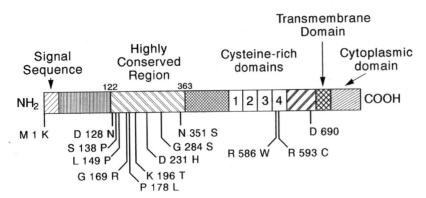

Figure 38.2. Representative mutations in the β_2-integrin subunit that have been identified in patients with LAD I syndrome.

enhance transcription of the β_2 subunit, was found to be ineffective in a single LAD I patient studied (Weening et al., 1992). Transfusion of granulocytes immediately after harvest by leukopheresis has been found to be useful in selected cases of infections that otherwise could not be controlled. Although granulocyte transfusions may be live saving, their use is limited because of difficulties in supply of daily donors and immune reactions to the allogeneic leukocytes.

At present, the only corrective treatment that should be offered to all cases with the severe phenotype is bone marrow transplantation (Le Deist et al., 1989; Thomas et al., 1995). The absence of host LFA-1 may be advantageous in these transplants because graft rejection appears to be in part dependent on the CD18 complex. Indeed, a higher rate of successful engraftment of transplants, even with only partially compatible HLA matching, was reported in patients with LAD I than that for patients with other forms of primary immunodeficiency syndromes (Fischer et al., 1994).

The introduction of a normal β_2-subunit gene (*ITGB2*) into hematopoietic stem cells has the potential to cure children with LAD I (Bauer and Hickstein, 2000). Retroviral-mediated transduction of the *CD18* gene was shown to reconstitute a functional CD11a/CD18 in lymphoblastoid cell lines derived from patients with LAD I (Back et al., 1990; Wilson et al., 1990; Krauss et al., 1991), and transduction of murine bone marrow cells with CD18 retroviral vector resulted in gene expression in a variable percentage of neutrophils at 2 weeks post-transduction (Wilson et al., 1993). Retroviral-mediated transfer of the *CD18* gene into primary LAD I bone marrow cells has also been reported (Yorifuji et al., 1993; Bauer et al., 1998). Expression of CD18 in a low percentage of neutrophils in two LAD I patients undergoing gene therapy without conditioning was observed (Bauer et al., 1998). With the future development of gene therapy techniques that allow efficient gene transfer into hematopoietic stem cells, severely deficient LAD I patients may be ideal candidates for this procedure.

Leukocyte Adhesion Deficiency Type II

LAD II syndrome results from a general defect in fucose metabolism, causing the absence of SLeX and other fucosylated ligands for the selectins. LAD II was first described in two unrelated Palestinian boys, each the offspring of consanguineous parents (Frydman et al., 1992). Subsequently, two additional unrelated Palestinian children and one Turkish child (Etzioni and Tonetti, 2000b) and a child of Brazilian origin whose parents were consanguinous (Hidalgo et al., 2003) have been reported, for a total of five LAD II patients.

Clinical and pathologic manifestations

Affected children are born after uneventful pregnancies with normal height and weight. No delay in the separation of the umbilical cord has been observed. Patients with LAD II have severe mental retardation, short stature, a distinctive facial appearance, and the rare Bombay (hh) blood phenotype (Table 38.2). They develop recurrent episodes of bacterial infections early in life, mainly pneumonia, periodontitis, otitis media, and localized cellulitis. Mild to moderate skin infections without obvious pus have also been observed. The infections are generally not life threatening and are usually treated in the outpatient clinic (Etzioni et al., 1998). Interestingly, after the age of 3 years, the frequency of infections decreases and the children no longer need prophylactic antibiotics.

At an older age their main infectious problem is severe periodontitis, which is also observed in patients with LAD I. During times of infections the neutrophil count increases up to 150,000/µl. It is of interest to note that from the first days of life there is marked neutrophilia, ranging between 25,000 and 30,000/µl, even when patients are free of infections.

Overall, the infections in LAD II appear to be comparable to the moderate rather than the severe phenotype of LAD I. It is possible that the ability of LAD II neutrophils to adhere and transmigrate via β_2 integrin under conditions of reduced shear forces (von Andrian et al., 1993) may permit some neutrophils to emigrate to sites of severe inflammation where flow may be impaired, thereby allowing some level of neutrophil defense against bacterial infections.

As is observed in LAD I, at the site of infection there is no pus formation, and there is a striking absence of neutrophils in the lesions. Lymphocytic infiltration, by contrast, is clearly present (see below).

Laboratory findings

The clinical picture of skin infections, pneumonia, and periodontitis associated with a very high blood neutrophil count initially suggested a neutrophil defect as the cause of this syndrome. Subsequently it was found that although the opsonophagocytic activity was normal, a marked defect in neutrophil motility was present in all LAD II patients (Etzioni et al., 1992). Both random migration and directed migration toward chemotactic factors were markedly decreased (10% of normal).

Furthermore, homotypic aggregation of patient neutrophils was found to be defective (Etzioni, 1994). These observations suggested that the problem was a defect in neutrophil adherence to surfaces; therefore, the possibility of a defect in adhesion molecules was investigated. Indeed, while patients' and their parents' neutrophils exhibited normal levels of integrin subunits, LAD II neutrophils were found to be deficient in expression of the SLeX antigen (Etzioni et al., 1992). In contrast to LAD I neutrophils, which failed to flatten and spread on phorbol ester–treated glass coverslips, the majority of LAD II neutrophils flattened and spread extensively in a pseudopod formation (Phillips et al., 1995). Interestingly, a small percentage of the LAD II cells exhibited an intermediate appearance and retained a more spherical shape. The poor migration toward chemoattractants in an under-agarose assay and the defective homotypic neutrophil adhesion could not be readily explained by the biochemical deficiency of SLeX and suggested a more global defect in cell activation or adhesion. Nevertheless, LAD II neutrophils could be activated normally with up-regulation of various adhesion molecules (Phillips et al., 1995).

Functional aspects

To examine further the significance of the fucosylation defect, both in vitro and in vivo functions of LAD II neutrophils were assessed. Neutrophils isolated from peripheral blood of one LAD II patient failed to bind to purified platelet-derived P-selectin and recombinant E-selectin in vitro (Phillips et al., 1995). To determine the effect of SLeX deficiency on neutrophil–endothelial interactions, neutrophil adherence to IL-1-, TNF-, histamine-, and phorbol ester–activated human umbilical vein endothelial cells was examined. No adhesion of LAD II neutrophils was observed when the endothelial cells were activated with IL-1β (Fig. 38.3) or TNF-α, both potent inducers of E-selectin, whereas normal neutrophils bound avidly. Similarly, endothelial cells activated

LAD II Neutrophil Adhesion to Endothelial Cells

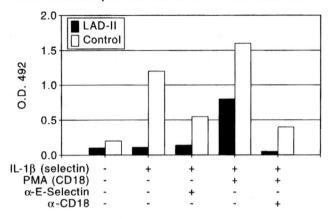

Figure 38.3. Selectin-dependent adhesion of LAD II neutrophils in vitro is impaired in LAD II syndrome. Purified neutrophils from a normal donor (open columns) or the LAD II patient (filled columns) were incubated for 5 minutes on human umbilical vein endothelial cell monolayers that had been treated with control medium or with recombinant human IL-1. In some wells neutrophil CD18 was activated by addition of phorbol myristate acetate (PMA). An anti–CD18 monoclonal antibody or an anti–E-selectin monoclonal antibody was added to some wells during incubation. The plates were washed and neutrophil adherence was quantitated by spectrophotometric analysis of the neutrophil-specific enzyme myeloperoxidase (Etzioni et al., 1992; Phillips et al., 1995).

LAD I and LAD II Neutrophil Rolling in Inflamed Rabbit Mesenteric Vessel

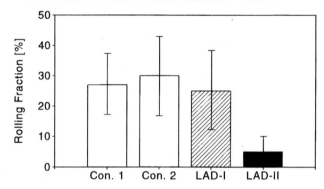

Figure 38.4. Selectin-dependent rolling of neutrophils in vivo is reduced in LAD II syndrome. Quantitation of neutrophil rolling from control subjects and patients with LAD I and LAD II was assessed in inflamed mesenteric venules in rabbits. Samples of fluorescent neutrophils were injected into the terminal mesentery artery blood stream 4 to 6 hours after intraperitoneal injection of IL-1. Cells passing through venules in the downstream segment were made visible by stroboscopic epi-illumination and were recorded on videotape. Tapes were analyzed for assessment of neutrophil rolling behavior. The rolling fraction was determined as the percentage of rolling neutrophils in the total flux of fluorescent cells passing a venule during an injection (Arbones et al., 1994). A total of 10 venules was analyzed, 5 vessels for each neutrophil sample in each rabbit. Means +/- SD are shown (von Andrian et al., 1993). Reproduced from the *Journal of Clinical Investigation* 1993; 191:2893–2897, by copyright permission of the American Society for Clinical Investigation.

by histamine to express P-selectin bound normal neutrophils but not LAD II neutrophils. By contrast, normal adhesion to endothelial cells was observed after activation with phorbol myristate acetate (PMA), an activating stimulus for β_2 integrins (Fig. 38.3). Furthermore, LAD II neutrophil migration across endothelial monolayers in response to f-Met-Leu-Phe (fMLP), a CD11/CD18–dependent function, was comparable to that of normal neutrophils (Phillips et al., 1995).

Rolling, the first step in neutrophil recruitment to the site of inflammation, is mediated primarily by the binding of the selectins to their fucosylated glycoconjugate ligands. Through intravital microscopy, the in vivo behavior of fluorescein-labeled neutrophils from a normal donor and from LAD I and LAD II patients was investigated during their passage through the inflamed microcirculation of rabbit mesentery (von Andrian et al., 1993). The rolling fraction of normal donor neutrophils in this assay was approximately 30%, and LAD I neutrophils behaved similarly. In contrast, LAD II neutrophils rolled poorly and failed to emigrate (Fig. 38.1). Their rolling fraction was only 5% (Fig. 38.4), and most of the cells that did interact with endothelial cells had a higher rolling velocity, rolled only over short distances, and frequently detached from the vessel wall. This marked inability to interact with inflamed vasculature was observed only in the presence of intravascular shear force: when the mesenteric blood flow was temporarily stopped and LAD II cells were injected into the nonperfused microvasculature, it was observed that numerous LAD II cells became stuck and did not detach when the blood flow was subsequently restored. These experiments indicate that the defect in LAD II is due to a shear-dependent inability of neutrophils to roll and slow down in inflamed venules and is not due to a dysfunction of the later shear-independent steps in the adhesion cascade.

To examine in vivo chemotaxis, the response of patient neutrophils to cutaneous inflammation was assessed by both skin-chamber and skin-window techniques. Neutrophil emigration was markedly diminished in both tests, the values being approximately 1.5% and 6% of normal in the skin-window and skin-chamber tests, respectively (Price et al., 1994). Monocyte migration to the skin-window site was reduced to a similar degree. Notably, neutrophils from a patient with LAD I, studied concurrently, showed the same magnitude of defect in these assays.

Adhesion molecules are known to participate in the immune reaction of T lymphocytes (Springer, 1995) and, as noted above, some lymphocyte functions are defective in LAD I (Beatty et al., 1984; Fischer et al., 1988; Ochs et al., 1993). In contrast, LAD II patients show a normal proportion and absolute numbers of T lymphocyte subpopulations. They also exhibit normal proliferative responses to various mitogens, normal NK cell activity, and normal immunoglobulin levels. Furthermore, in contrast to patients with LAD I, antibody production in response to immunization with bacteriophage 0X174 was found to be normal with appropriate switching from IgM to IgG (Price et al., 1994). However, delayed cutaneous hypersensitivity reactions were not observed upon intradermal injection of various antigens. This apparent anergy may be due to absence of the skin homing T cell antigen, CLA, which contains fucose in its structure (Picker, 1994). Therefore, the in vivo immune response to keyhole limpet hemocyanin (KLH) was investigated. Normal KLH-specific in vitro T cell proliferation and normal in vivo anti-KLH antibody titers were found, indicating normal T and B cell function and collaboration. However, skin testing with KLH failed to elicit a positive reaction (rubor, calor, edema) (Kuijpers et al., 1997a). A biopsy of the site of intradermal KLH injection revealed that the number and phenotype (CD3+) of infiltrating lymphocytes were identical to those of a positive control (except for the lack of CLA staining in the LAD II biopsy). Up-regulation of various

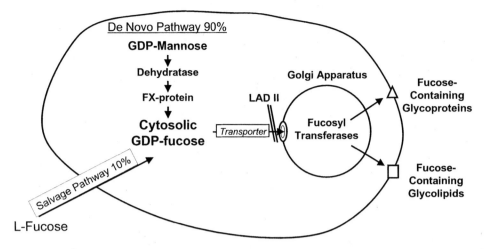

Figure 38.5. LAD II is a congenital disorder of glycosylation. GDP-l-fucose is synthesized in the cytosol and must be transported into the Golgi apparatus where fucosyl transferases are located. In the Golgi, fu-cosyl transferases add fucose to macromolecules. In LAD II, deficiency of the GDP-fucose transporter prevents fucosylation of membrane glycoproteins and glycolipids.

endothelial adhesion molecules was similar in the patient and control. The discrepancy between the almost normal histological findings and the absence of an intradermal reaction remains unexplained. Rather than mediating trafficking, CLA may be important in activating T cells to induce the inflammatory reaction and to initiate the classical signs of delayed-type hypersensitivity reaction in the skin.

Molecular basis

Because the first two LAD II patients identified were the offspring of first-degree relatives and the parents were clinically unaffected, autosomal recessive inheritance was assumed (Frydman et al., 1992). In addition to being of the Bombay phenotype (absence of the H antigen), the cells of LAD II patients were found to lack Lewis a and b antigens and the patients were nonsecretors. Therefore, the biochemical abnormality in LAD II is a general defect in fucosylation of macromolecules (Fig. 38.5). The three unique blood phenotypes (Bombay, Lewis a and b) have in common a lack of fucosylation of glycoconjugates. Because at least four different fucosyltransferases would have to be affected to produce negativity for SLeX, H, Lewis, and secretor and the genes in these molecules are not physically linked in the human genome (loci include chromosomes 11, 19p, and 19q), LAD II cannot result from abnormal fucosyltransferase(s). Furthermore, LAD II patients possess normal activity of α-2-fucosyltransferase (Shechter et al., 1995), which is needed for H antigen and is defective in individuals who carry the rare Bombay blood phenotype but do not have LAD II. These findings suggest that the primary defect in LAD II must instead be a general defect in fucose production.

After the observation was made that the defect in the Palestinian patients may affect the de novo GDP-1-fucose biosynthesis pathway (Karsan et al., 1998), the two enzymes involved in this pathway, GMD and FX protein, were assessed and found to be normal, without a mutation in cDNA isolated from LAD II patients. Subsequently, theTurkish child with LAD II was found to have decreased GDP-1-fucose transport into the Golgi vesicles (Lubke et al., 1999). Similar studies were performed in the Palestinian patients and indeed, the same general defect in fucose transport to the Golgi vesicles was found. Still, marked kinetic differences were observed between the Turkish and the Palestinian patients (Sturla et al., 2001). This finding may explain

the different response to fucose supplementation in the Turkish and the Arab children (see below). Recently, through use of the complementation cloning technique, the human gene encoding the fucose transporter was found to be located on chromosome 11 (Lubke et al., 2001). The Turkish child was homozygous for a mutation at amino acid 147, in which arginine is changed to cysteine (Lubke et al., 2001; Luhn et al., 2001), whereas the two Palestinian patients examined had a homozygous mutation in amino acid 308, in which threonine is changed to arginine (Lubke et al., 2001). Both mutations are located in highly conserved transmembrane domains. The Brazilian patient has a homozygous single nucleotide deletion (588delG) resulting in frameshift and premature stop codon 34 residuals after the mutation (Hidalgo et al., 2003). LAD II is thus one of the congenital disorders of glycosylation (CDG) and is classified as CDG-IIc (Lubke et al., 2001). Although only three unique mutations (in five affected patients) have been described thus far, there seems to be a genotype–phenotype correlation (Etzioni et al., 2002). Recently it was found that in some mutations the transporter is located in the Golgi apparatus, but it is nonfunctional, while in others the transporter cannot be localized to the Golgi (Helmus et al., 2006).

Strategies for diagnosis

LAD II is a very rare syndrome, described originally in four Palestinian children from two apparently unrelated families, one child from a Turkish family, and subsequently in a Brazilian child. Because the clinical phenotype is very striking, the diagnosis can be made based on the presence of recurrent, albeit mild, infections, marked leukocytosis, and the Bombay blood group, in association with mental and growth retardation.

Analysis of peripheral blood leukocytes by flow cytometry with an anti-CD15s monoclonal antibody will demonstrate the absence of SLeX expression. To confirm the diagnosis, sequence analysis of the gene encoding the GDP-fucose transporter is required.

Carrier detection and prenatal diagnosis

Prenatal diagnosis was carried out successfully through use of a cord blood sample obtained from a female fetus of one of the affected families. Because of the presence of the Bombay blood phenotype the pregnancy was aborted (Frydman et al., 1996).

Having cloned the gene causing LAD II, carrier detection is possible, and prenatal diagnosis can be performed earlier with chorionic villus samples for DNA analysis.

Treatment and prognosis

Each of the LAD II patients described to date suffered from recurrent episodes of infections that responded well to antibiotics. No serious consequences were observed, and prophylactic treatment was never considered in the Palestinian patients, whereas the Turkish child was placed on prophylactic antibiotics. A chronic problem for all patients has been periodontitis, a condition that is especially difficult to treat in children with severe mental retardation (Etzioni et al., 1998). The oldest LAD II patient is now 14 years old, has severe psychomotor retardation, but only mild infectious problems.

Because of the proposed defect in fucose production, supplemental administration of fucose through either addition to the diet or intravenous infusion has been suggested. Indeed, fucose supplementation caused dramatic improvement in the condition of the Turkish child (Marquardt et al., 1999). A marked decrease in leukocyte count with improved neutrophil adhesion was noted. Furthermore, improvement in developmental delay was observed and no episodes of infections occurred during fucose therapy. However, the same protocol produced no improvement in laboratory data or clinical features in two Palestinian children (Etzioni and Tonetti, 2000a). This difference may be due to the genetic defect in the Turkish child, which leads to decreased affinity of the transporter for fucose. An increase in cytosolic concentration of fucose would be expected to overcome, at least in part, the defect in fucose transport.

Leukocyte Adhesion Deficiency Type III

Recently, a rare, autosomal recessive LAD syndrome that is distinct from LAD I and LAD II has been reported (Alon et al., 2003; Alon and Etzioni, 2003). Although leukocyte integrin expression and intrinsic adhesion to endothelial integrin ligands have been found to be normal in LAD III, in situ activation of all major leukocyte integrins, including LFA-1, Mac-1, and VLA-4, by endothelial-displayed chemokines or chemoattractants is severely impaired in patient-derived lymphocytes and neutrophils. Whereas the rolling of LAD III leukocytes on endothelial surfaces is normal, they fail to arrest on endothelial integrin ligands in response to endothelial-displayed chemokines. G protein–coupled receptor (GPCR) signaling appears to be normal and the ability of leukocytes to migrate toward a chemotactic gradient is not impaired. The key defect in this syndrome has been attributed to a genetic loss of integrin activation by rapid chemoattractant-stimulated GPCR signaling (Alon et al., 2003). This novel LAD shows striking similarities to three cases previously referred to as LAD I variants (Kuijpers et al., 1997b; Harris et al., 2001; McDowall et al., 2003). All four cases had similar clinical symptoms, characterized by severe recurrent infections, a bleeding tendency, and marked leukocytosis (Table 38.2). In all cases tested, integrin expression and structure were intact with a defect in integrin activation by physiological stimuli. Because LAD I leukocytes have defects in integrin expression or structure, it was proposed that this group of integrin activation disorders be designated *LAD III* (Alon and Etzioni, 2003; Kinashi et al., 2004). The term *LAD I variant*, which was ascribed to this unique syndrome, is inaccurate because this syndrome does not evolve from structural defects in leukocyte or platelet integrins.

In all of the LAD III cases studied, defects in GPCR-mediated integrin activation are accompanied by variable defects in activation of leukocyte integrins by non–GPCR-mediated signals. A growing body of evidence implicates the Ras-related GTPase Rap-1 as a key regulator of integrin activation by multiple stimuli (Caron, 2003). Rap-1 is also implicated in the activation of platelet and megakaryocyte GpIIbIIIa integrin, which is defective in LAD III (Eto et al., 2002). It is thus highly attractive to hypothesize that at least some of the LAD III cases have either a direct or an indirect defect in the activation of integrins in leukocytes and platelets by Rap-1. Although lymphocytes from two patients expressed normal levels of Rap-1 (Kinashi et al., 2003; McDowall et al., 2003), in one case studied an abnormal pattern of Rap-1 activation was observed (Kinashi et al., 2004). However, the ubiquitous expression of Rap-1 in most tissues and its highly diverse functions in nonhematopoietic cells (Bos et al., 2001) make it unlikely that Rap-1 is structurally mutated in any of the LAD III cases. It is more likely that a hematopoietic-restricted effector of Rap-1 or a specific hematopoietic adaptor that links this GTPase to cytoskeletal partners involved in integrin activation is functionally defective in patients with LAD III syndrome.

E-selectin deficiency

Recently, another potentially inherited defect in the selectin system was described in a child with moderate neutropenia and severe recurrent infections (DeLisser et al., 1999). There was markedly reduced expression of E-selectin on blood vessels of inflamed tissue with increased levels of circulating soluble E-selectin, suggesting increased cleavage of surface E-selectin. Notably, the E-selectin gene sequence was normal.

Animals Models

CD18-Deficient Dogs and Cattle

A spontaneous mutation in the gene coding for the β_2 single integrin has been described in both dogs (Giger et al., 1987) and cattle (Shuster et al., 1992). Canine LAD (CLAD) occurs in Irish setters and results from a single missense mutation in the *CD18* gene, resulting in a change from cysteine to serine at amino acid 36 (Kijas et al., 1999). In bovine LAD (BLAD) there is a also a point mutation (Asp128Gly) in the *CD18* gene. Animals homozygous for this mutation exhibited persistent neutrophilia and suffered from recurrent infections associated with poor growth performance. The carrier frequency of the defective gene among Holstein cattle has been approximately 15% in bulls and 6% in cows (Shuster et al., 1992).

CD18-Deficient Mice

Multiple mice with targeted disruption of one or more leukocyte and endothelial adhesion molecules have been generated (Etzioni et al., 1999). Of particular interest are those knockouts that most closely mimic LAD I or LAD II.

Mutant mice lineages with complete deficiency of CD18 have defects similar to the severe clinical phenotype of LAD I (Mizgerd et al., 1997; Scharffetter-Kochanek et al., 1998). As in LAD I, these animals exhibit marked neutrophilia (11- to 30-fold increase over wild type). The granulocytosis observed in the CD18-deficient mice was due mainly to continuous stimulation of the bone marrow as a consequence of the defective antimicrobial functions leading to infections (Horwitz et al., 2001). Similar to LAD I, there was almost no emigration of neutrophils in the CD18-null animals into sites of inflammation in the skin. In contrast, the CD18-deficient mice exhibited comparable numbers of neutrophils in lavage fluid from inflamed peritoneum and increased emigration into inflamed lung when compared with wild type. The lack of neutrophil emigration to the skin with normal emigration to the lungs was also described in one patient with the severe phenotype of LAD I (Hawkins et al., 1992). The persistence of neutrophil emigration into the inflamed peritoneum in the CD18 animals may result from the marked increase in circulating neutrophils in the CD18-deficient animals. Because the number of emigrating neutrophils is in part dependent on the number of circulating neutrophils, the observation that the same absolute numbers of neutrophils emigrate in the CD18 animals as in the wild-type mice may reflect a significant inhibition. However, limited studies in one LAD I patient showed an absence of neutrophils in infected peritoneum (Hawkins et al., 1992). This discrepancy may reflect a biological difference between mice and humans, a sampling effect (peritoneal fluid in mice vs. tissue in humans), or a difference in the duration of the inflammatory response (4 hours in mice vs. days in the patient).

Selectin-Deficient Mice

The defective GDP-fucose transporter gene responsible for LAD II has only recently been identified, and studies of mice with targeted disruption of this gene have not been reported. Although the genetic deficiency in LAD II has no direct effect on the selectin genes themselves, the resulting defect in fucose metabolism produces a deficiency of fucosylated leukocyte ligands for endothelial E- and P-selectins. The endothelium in LAD II patients likely also exhibits reduced expression of fucosylated leukocyte L-selectin ligands (Karsan et al., 1998). Thus, with respect to leukocyte adhesion, LAD II patients are the human equivalent of mice with combined knockout of E-, P-, and L-selectin genes or mice with knockout of the genes that direct biosynthesis of fucose-containing selectin ligands.

Mice deficient in E- and P-selectin (E/P) and mice deficient in E-, P-, and L- selectin (E/P/L) show leukocytosis, dramatic reduction in leukocyte rolling, markedly reduced emigration into inflamed peritoneum, and increased susceptibility to mucocutaneous infections (Bullard et al., 1996; Frenette et al., 1996; Jung and Ley, 1999; Robinson et al., 1999). In contrast to the E/P- or E/P/L-deficient mice, the two older LAD II patients have had no increase in systemic infections, and the few episodes of localized infection have responded to conventional treatment as in any immunocompetent child. The phenotype of the multiple selectin-deficient animals thus appears to be much more severe than that observed in LAD II, perhaps reflecting differences between humans and mice in susceptibility to mucocutaneous infections. However, the possibility that nonfucosylated ligands participate in selectin interactions in vivo has not been completely excluded. If this were the case, then the absence of fucosylated ligands in LAD II would not impact all E-, P-, and L-selectin–dependent functions, whereas the selectin-null mice would be severely affected (Etzioni et al., 1999).

Mice deficient in biosynthesis of SLeX have also been generated. The gene encoding $\alpha(1,3)$ fucosyltransferase Fuc-TVII, an enzyme that controls synthesis of SLeX, was knocked out in mice, resulting in a phenotype reminiscent of the human LAD II, with defective adhesion and marked leukocytosis (Maly et al., 1996). The same phenotype was observed in mice deficient in core 2 β1-6 N-acetylglucosaminyltransferase, which is also important in the synthesis of SLeX (Ellies et al., 1998). However, neither murine models showed any gross abnormalities, confirming that the growth and mental retardation in LAD II is most likely due to the general defect in fucose metabolism and not to the adhesion deficiency.

Conclusion

The crucial role of the β_2-integrin subfamily in leukocyte emigration was convincingly demonstrated after LAD I was discovered. Patients with this disorder suffer from life-threatening bacterial infections. In its severe form, death usually occurs in early childhood unless bone marrow transplantation is performed.

The LAD II disorder clarifies the role of the selectin receptors and their fucosylated ligands such as SLeX. In vitro as well as in vivo studies establish that this family of adhesion molecules is essential for neutrophil rolling, the first step in neutrophil emigration through the blood vessel. Clinically, patients with LAD II suffer from a less severe form of disease, resembling the moderate phenotype of LAD I. This may be due in part to the ability of LAD II neutrophils to emigrate when blood flow rate is reduced and to the observed normal T and B lymphocyte function in LAD II as opposed to that in LAD I. The molecular defect responsible for LAD III is not yet known, but experimental evidence points toward a defect in integrin activation, resulting in severe recurrent infections, a bleeding tendency, and marked leukocytosis.

References

Alon R, Aker M, Feigelson S, Sokolovsky-Eisenberg M, Stauton D, Cinamon G, Grabovsky V, Shamri R, Etzioni A. A novel genetic leukocyte adhesion deficiency in sub-second triggering of integrin avidity by endothelial chemokines results in impaired leukocyte arrest on vascular endothelium under shear flow. Blood 101:4437–4445, 2003.

Alon R, Etzioni A. LAD III, a novel group of leukocyte integrin activation deficiencies. Trends Immunol 24:561–566, 2003.

Anderson DC, Kishimoto TK, Smith CW. Leukocyte adhesion deficiency and other disorders of leukocyte adherence and motility. In: Scriver CR, Beaudet AL, Sly WS, Valle D, eds. The Metabolic and Molecular Basis of Inherited Diseases, 7th ed. New York: McGraw-Hill, pp. 3955–3995, 1995.

Anderson DC, Springer TA. Leukocyte adhesion deficiency: an inherited defect in the Mac-1, LFA-1, and p150,95 glycoproteins. Annu Rev Med 38: 175–194, 1987.

Arbones ML, Ord DC, Ley K, Ratech H, Maynard-Curry C, Otten G, Capon DJ, Tedder TF. Lymphocyte homing and leukocyte rolling and migration are impaired in L-selectin–deficient mice. Cell Genesys 1:247–260, 1994.

Arfors KE, Lundberg C, Lindbom L, Lundberg K, Beatty PG, Harlan JM. A monoclonal antibody to the membrane glycoprotein complex CD18 inhibits polymorphonuclear leukocyte accumulation and plasma leakage in vivo. Blood 69:338–340, 1987.

Asako H, Kurose I, Wolf R, DeFrees S, Zheng ZL, Phillips ML, Paulson JC, Granger DN. Role of H1 receptors and P-selectin in histamine-induced leukocyte rolling and adhesion in postcapillary venules. J Clin Invest 93:1508–1515, 1994.

Back AL, Kwok WW, Adam M, Collins SJ, Hickstein DD. Retroviral-mediated gene transfer of the leukocyte integrin CD18 subunit. Biochem Biophys Res Commun 171:787–795, 1990.

Back AL, Kwok WW, Hickstein DD. Identification of two molecular defects in a child with leukocyte adherence deficiency. J Biol Chem 267: 5482–5487, 1992.

Bargatze RF, Jutila MA, Butcher EC. Distinct roles of L-selectin and integrins alpha 4 beta 7 and LFA-1 in lymphocyte homing to Peyer's patch-HEV in situ: the multistep model confirmed and refined. Immunity 3:99–108, 1995.

Bauer TR Jr, Hickstein DD. Gene therapy for leukocyte adhesion deficiency. Curr Opin Mol Ther 2:383–388, 2000.

Bauer TR, Schwartz BR, Liles WC, Ochs HD, Hickstein DD. Retroviral-mediated gene transfer of the leukocyte integrin CD18 into peripheral blood CD34+ cells derived from a patient with leukocyte adhesion deficiency type 1. Blood 91:1520–1526, 1998.

Baumheter S, Singer MS, Henzel W, Hemmerich S, Renz M, Rosen SD, Lasky LA. Binding of L-selectin to the vascular sialomucin CD34. Science 262:436–438, 1993.

Beatty PG, Ochs HD, Harlan JM, Price TH, Rosen H, Taylor RF, Hansen JA, Klebanoff SJ. Absence of monoclonal-antibody-defined protein complex in boy with abnormal leucocyte function. Lancet 1:535–537, 1984.

Bevilacqua MP, Nelson RM. Selectins. J Clin Invest 91:379–387, 1993.

Bos JL, de Rooij J, Reedquist KA. Rap1 signaling: adhering to new models. Nat Rev Mol Cell Biol 2:369–377, 2001.

Bowen TJ, Ochs HD, Altman LC, Price TH, Van Epps DE, Brautigan DL, Rosin RE, Perkins WD, Babior BM, Klebanoff SJ, Wedgwood RJ. Severe recurrent bacterial infections associated with defective adherence and chemotaxis in two patients with neutrophils deficient in a cell-associated glycoprotein. J Pediatr 101:932–940, 1982.

Boxer LA, Hedley-Whyte ET, Stossel TP. Neutrophil action dysfunction and abnormal neutrophil behavior. N Engl J Med 291:1093–1099, 1974.

Briskin MJ, McEvoy LM, Butcher EC. MAdCAM-1 has homology to immunoglobulin and mucin-like adhesion receptors and to IgA1. Nature 363:461–464, 1993.

Bullard DC, Kunkel EJ, Kubo H, Hicks MJ, Lorenzo I, Doyle NA, Doerschuk CM, Ley K, Beaudet AL. Infectious susceptibility and severe deficiency of leukocyte rolling and recruitment in E-selectin and P-selectin double-mutant mice. J Exp Med 183:2329–2336, 1996.

Butcher EC. Leukocyte–endothelial cell recognition: three (or more) steps to specificity and diversity. Cell 67:1033–1036, 1991.

Carlos TM, Harlan JM. Leukocyte–endothelial adhesion molecules. Blood 84:2068–2101, 1994.

Caron E. Cellular functions of the Rap1 GTP-binding protein: a pattern emerges. J Cell Sci 116:435–440, 2003.

Cotran RS, Gimbrone MA Jr, Bevilacqua MP, Mendrick DL, Pober JS. Induction and detection of a human endothelial activation antigen in vivo. J Exp Med 164:661–666, 1986.

Crowley CA, Curnutte JT, Rosin RE, Andre-Schwartz J, Gallin JI, Klempner M, Snyderman R, Southwick FS, Stossel TP, Babior BM. An inherited abnormality of neutrophil adhesion. Its genetic transmission and its association with a missing protein. N Engl J Med 302:1163–1168, 1980.

DeLisser HM, Christofidou-Solomidou M, Sun J, Nakada MT, Sullivan KE. Loss of endothelial surface expression of E-selectin in a patient with recurrent infections. Blood 94:884–894, 1999.

Diamond MS, Staunton DE, Marlin SD, Springer TA. Binding of the integrin Mac-1 (CD11b/CD18) to the third immunoglobulin-like domain of ICAM-1 (CD54) and its regulation by glycosylation. Cell 65:961–971, 1991.

Duncan GS, Andrew DP, Takimoto H, Kaufman SA, Yoshida H, Spellberg J, Luis de la Pompa J, Elia A, Wakeham A, Karan-Tamir B, Muller WA, Senaldi G, Zukowski MM, Mak TW. Genetic evidence for functional redundancy of platelet/endothelial cell adhesion molecule-1 (PECAM-1): CD31-deficient mice reveal PECAM-1-dependent and PECAM-1-independent functions. J Immunol 162:3022–3030, 1999.

Ellies LG, Tsuboi S, Petryniak B, Lowe JB, Fukuda M, Marth JD. Core 2 oligosaccharide biosynthesis distinguishes between selectin ligands essential for leukocyte homing and inflammation. Immunity 9:881–890, 1998.

Eto K, Murphy R, Kerrigan SW, Bertoni A, Stuhlmann H, Nakano T, Leavitt AD, Shattil SJ. Megakaryocytes derived from embryonic stem cells implicate CalDAG-GEFI in integrin signaling. Proc Nat Acad Sci USA 99:12819–12824, 2002.

Etzioni A. Adhesion molecule deficiencies and their clinical significance. Cell Adhes Commun 2:257–260, 1994.

Etzioni A. Adhesion molecules—their role in health and disease. Pediatr Res 39:191–196, 1996.

Etzioni A. Integrins—the glue of life. Lancet 353:341–343, 1999.

Etzioni A, Doerschuk CM, Harlan JM. Of man and mouse: leukocyte and endothelial adhesion molecule deficiencies. Blood 94:3281–3288, 1999.

Etzioni A, Frydman M, Pollack S, Avidor I, Phillips ML, Paulson JC, Gershoni-Baruch R. Brief report: recurrent severe infections caused by a novel leukocyte adhesion deficiency. N Engl J Med 327:1789–1792, 1992.

Etzioni A, Gershoni-Baruch R, Pollack S, Shehadeh N. Leukocyte adhesion deficiency type II: long-term follow-up. J Allergy Clin Immunol 102:323–324, 1998.

Etzioni A, Sturla L, Antonellis A, Green ED, Gershoni-Baruch R, Berninsone PM, Hirschberg CB, Tonetti M. Leukocyte adhesion deficiency (LAD) type II/carbohydrate deficient glycoprotein (CDG) IIc founder effect and genotype/phenotype correlation. Am J Med Genet. 110:131–135, 2002.

Etzioni A, Tonetti M. Fucose supplementation in leukocyte adhesion deficiency type II. Blood 95:3641–3643, 2000a.

Etzioni A, Tonetti M. Leukocyte adhesion deficiency II—from A to almost Z. Immunol Rev 178:138–147, 2000b.

Fischer A, Landais P, Friedrich W, Gerritsen B, Fasth A, Porta F, Vellodi A, Benkerrou M, Jais JP, Cavazzana-Calvo M, et al. Bone marrow transplantation (BMT) in Europe for primary immunodeficiencies other than severe combined immunodeficiency: a report from the European Group for BMT and the European Group for Immunodeficiency. Blood 83:1149–1154, 1994.

Fischer A, Lisowska-Grospierre B, Anderson DC, Springer TA. Leukocyte adhesion deficiency: molecular basis and functional consequences. Immunodefic Rev 1:39–54, 1988.

Frenette PS, Mayadas TN, Rayburn H, Hynes RO, Wagner DD. Susceptibility to infection and altered hematopoiesis in mice deficient in both P- and E-selectins. Cell 84:563–574, 1996.

Frydman M, Etzioni A, Eidlitz-Markus T, Avidor I, Varsano I, Shechter Y, Orlin JB, Gershoni-Baruch R. Rambam-Hasharon syndrome of psychomotor retardation, short stature, defective neutrophil motility, and Bombay phenotype. Am J Med Genet 44:297–302, 1992.

Frydman M, Vardimon D, Shalev E, Orlin JB. Prenatal diagnosis of Rambam-Hasharon syndrome. Prenat Diagn 16:266–269, 1996.

Gallin JI, Malech HL, Wright DG, Whisnant JK, Kirkpatrick CH. Recurrant severe infections in a child with abnormal leukocyte function: possible relationship to increased microtubule assembly. Blood 51:919–933, 1978.

Giger U, Boxer LA, Simpson PJ, Lucchesi BR, Todd RF 3rd. Deficiency of leukocyte surface glycoproteins Mo1, LFA-1, and Leu M5 in a dog with recurrent bacterial infections: an animal model. Blood 69:1622–1630, 1987.

Gotsch U, Jager U, Dominis M, Vestweber D. Expression of P-selectin on endothelial cells is upregulated by LPS and TNF-α in vivo. Cell Adhes Commun 2:7–14, 1994.

Harlan JM. Leukocyte adhesion deficiency syndrome: insights into the molecular basis of leukocyte emigration. Clin Immunol Immunopathol 67: S16–24, 1993.

Harlan JM, Senecal PD, Senecal FM, Schwartz BR, Yee EK, Taylor RF, Beatty PG, Price TH, Ochs HD. The role of neutrophil membrane glycoprotein GP-150 in neutrophil adherence to endothelium in vitro. Blood 66:167–178, 1985.

Harris ES, Shigeoka AO, Li W, Adams RH, Prescott SM, McIntyre TM, Zimmerman GA, Lorant DE. A novel syndrome of variant leukocyte adhesion deficiency involving defects in adhesion mediated by beta1 and beta2 integrins. Blood 97:767–776, 2001.

Hawkins HK, Heffelfinger SC, Anderson DC. Leukocyte adhesion deficiency: clinical and postmortem observations. Pediatr Pathol 12:119–130, 1992.

Hayward AR, Harvey BA, Leonard J, Greenwood MC, Wood CB, Soothill JF. Delayed separation of the umbilical cord, widespread infections, and defective neutrophil mobility. Lancet 1:1099–1101, 1979.

Helmus Y, Denecke J, Yakubenia S, Robinson P, Luhn K, Watson DL, McGrogan PJ, Vestweber D, Marquardt T, Wild MK. Leukocyte adhesion deficiency II patients with a dual defect of the GDP-fucose transporter. Blood, 2006 in press.

Hidalgo A, Ma S, Peired AJ, Weiss LA, Cunningham-Rundles C, Frenette PS. Insights into leukocyte adhesion deficiency type 2 from a novel mutation in the GDP-fucose transporter gene. Blood 101:1705–1712, 2003.

Hogg N, Stewart MP, Scarth SL, Newton R, Shaw JM, Law SK, Klein N. A novel leukocyte adhesion deficiency caused by expressed but nonfunctional beta2 integrins Mac-1 and LFA-1. J Clin Invest 103:97–106, 1999.

Horwitz BH, Mizgerd JP, Scott ML, Doerschuk CM. Mechanisms of granulocytosis in the absence of CD18. Blood 97:1578–1583, 2001.

Humphries MJ. Integrin structure. Biochem Soc Trans 28:311–339, 2000.

Hynes RO. Integrins: versatility, modulation, and signaling in cell adhesion. Cell 69:11–25, 1992.

Jung U, Ley K. Mice lacking two or all three selectins demonstrate overlapping and distinct functions for each selectin. J Immunol 162:6755–6762, 1999.

Kansas GS. Selectins and their ligands: current concepts and controversies. Blood 88:3259–3287, 1996.

Karsan A, Cornejo CJ, Winn RK, Schwartz BR, Way W, Lannir N, Gershoni-Baruch R, Etzioni A, Ochs HD, Harlan JM. Leukocyte adhesion deficiency type II is a generalized defect of de novo GDP-fucose biosynthesis. Endothelial cell fucosylation is not required for neutrophil rolling on human nonlymphoid endothelium. J Clin Invest 101:2438–2445, 1998.

Kijas JM, Bauer TR Jr, Gafvert S, Marklund S, Trowald-Wigh G, Johannisson A, Hedhammar A, Binns M, Juneja RK, Hickstein DD, Andersson L. A missense mutation in the beta-2 integrin gene (ITGB2) causes canine leukocyte adhesion deficiency. Genomics 61:101–107, 1999.

Kinashi T, Aker M, Sokolovsky-Eisenberg M, Grabovsky V, Tanaka C, Shamri R, Feigelson S, Etzioni A, Alon R. LAD-III, a leukocyte adhesion deficiency syndrome associated with defective Rap 1 activation and impaired stabilization of integrin bonds. Blood 103:1033–1036, 2004.

Kishimoto TK, Hollander N, Roberts TM, Anderson DC, Springer TA. Heterogeneous mutations in the beta subunit common to the LFA-1, Mac-1, and p150,95 glycoproteins cause leukocyte adhesion deficiency. Cell 50:193–202, 1987.

Kishimoto TK, O'Conner K, Springer TA. Leukocyte adhesion deficiency. Aberrant splicing of a conserved integrin sequence causes a moderate deficiency phenotype. J Biol Chem 264:3588–3595, 1989.

Kohl S, Loo LS, Schmalstieg FS, Anderson DC. The genetic deficiency of leukocyte surface glycoprotein Mac-1, LFA-1, p150,95 in humans is associated with defective antibody-dependent cellular cytotoxicity in vitro and defective protection against herpes simplex virus infection in vivo. J Immunol 137:1688–1694, 1986.

Krauss JC, Bond LM, Todd RF 3rd, Wilson JM. Expression of retroviral transduced human CD18 in murine cells: an in vitro model of gene therapy for leukocyte adhesion deficiency. Hum Gene Ther 2:221–228, 1991.

Kuijpers TW, Etzioni A, Pollack S, Pals ST. Antigen-specific immune responsiveness and lymphocyte recruitment in leukocyte adhesion deficiency type II. Int Immunol 9:607–613, 1997a.

Kuijpers TW, Van Lier RA, Hamann D, de Boer M, Thung LY, Weening RS, Verhoeven AJ, Roos D. Leukocyte adhesion deficiency type 1 (LAD-1)/variant. A novel immunodeficiency syndrome characterized by dysfunctional beta2 integrins. J Clin Invest 100:1725–1733, 1997b.

Lawrence MB, Springer TA. Leukocytes roll on a selectin at physiologic flow rates: distinction from and prerequisite for adhesion through integrins. Cell 65:859–873, 1991.

Le Deist F, Blanche S, Keable H, Gaud C, Pham H, Descamp-Latscha B, Wahn V, Griscelli C, Fischer A. Successful HLA nonidentical bone marrow transplantation in three patients with the leukocyte adhesion deficiency. Blood 74:512–516, 1989.

Lewinsohn DM, Bargatze RF, Butcher EC. Leukocyte–endothelial cell recognition: evidence of a common molecular mechanism shared by neutrophils, lymphocytes, and other leukocytes. J Immunol 138:4313–4321, 1987.

Ley K, Tedder TF. Leukocyte interactions with vascular endothelium. New insights into selectin-mediated attachment and rolling. J Immunol 155:525–528, 1995.

Lub M, van Kooyk Y, Figdor CG. Ins and outs of LFA-1. Immunol Today 16:479–483, 1995.

Lubke T, Marquardt T, Etzioni A, Hartmann E, von Figura K, Korner C. Complementation cloning identifies CDG-IIc, a new type of congenital disorders of glycosylation, as a GDP-fucose transporter deficiency. Nat Genet 28:73–76, 2001.

Lubke T, Marquardt T, von Figura K, Korner C. A new type of carbohydrate-deficient glycoprotein syndrome due to a decreased import of GDP-fucose into the Golgi. J Biol Chem 274:25986–25989, 1999.

Luhn K, Wild MK, Eckhardt M, Gerardy-Schahn R, Vestweber D. The gene defective in leukocyte adhesion deficiency II encodes a putative GDP-fucose transporter. Nat Genet 28:69–72, 2001.

Mackay CR. Chemokines: immunology's high-impact factors. Nat Immunol 2:95–101, 2001.

Maly P, Thall A, Petryniak B, Rogers CE, Smith PL, Marks RM, Kelly RJ, Gersten KM, Cheng G, Saunders TL, Camper SA, Camphausen RT, Sullivan FX, Isogai Y, Hindsgaul O, von Andrian UH, Lowe JB. The α(1,3)fucosyltransferase Fuc-TVII controls leukocyte trafficking through an essential role in L-, E-, and P-selectin ligand biosynthesis. Cell 86:643–653, 1996.

Marquardt T, Luhn K, Srikrishna G, Freeze HH, Harms E, Vestweber D. Correction of leukocyte adhesion deficiency type II with oral fucose. Blood 94:3976–3985, 1999.

Mathew EC, Shaw JM, Bonilla FA, Law SK, Wright DA. A novel point mutation in CD18 causing the expression of dysfunctional CD11/CD18 leukocyte integrins in a patient with leukocyte adhesion deficiency (LAD). Clin Exp Immunol 121:133–138, 2000.

Mayadas TN, Johnson RC, Rayburn H, Hynes RO, Wagner DD. Leukocyte rolling and extravasation are severely compromised in P selectin–deficient mice. Cell 74:541–554, 1993.

McDowall A, Inwald D, Leitinger B, Jones A, Liesner R, Klein N, Hogg N. A novel form of integrin dysfunction involving beta 1, beta 2 and beta 3 integrins. J Clin Invest 111:51–60, 2003.

Mizgerd JP, Kubo H, Kutkoski GJ, Bhagwan SD, Scharffetter-Kochanek K, Beaudet AL, Doerschuk CM. Neutrophil emigration in the skin, lungs, and peritoneum: different requirements for CD11/CD18 revealed by CD18-deficient mice. J Exp Med 186:1357–1364, 1997.

Moore KL, Patel KD, Bruehl RE, Li F, Johnson DA, Lichenstein HS, Cummings RD, Bainton DF, McEver RP. P-selectin glycoprotein ligand-1 mediates rolling of human neutrophils on P-selectin. J Cell Biol 128:661–671, 1995.

Ochs HD, Nonoyama S, Zhu Q, Farrington M, Wedgwood RJ. Regulation of antibody responses: the role of complement and adhesion molecules. Clin Immunol Immunopathol 67:S33–40, 1993.

Olofsson AM, Arfors KE, Ramezani L, Wolitzky BA, Butcher EC, von Andrian UH. E-selectin mediates leukocyte rolling in interleukin-1-treated rabbit mesentery venules. Blood 84:2749–2758, 1994.

Pepinsky B, Hession C, Chen LL, Moy P, Burkly L, Jakubowski A, Chow EP, Benjamin C, Chi-Rosso G, Luhowskyj S. Structure/function studies on vascular cell adhesion molecule-1. J Biol Chem 267:17820–17826, 1992.

Phillips ML, Schwartz BR, Etzioni A, Bayer R, Ochs HD, Paulson JC, Harlan JM. Neutrophil adhesion in leukocyte adhesion deficiency syndrome type 2. J Clin Invest 96:2898–2906, 1995.

Picker LJ. Control of lymphocyte homing. Curr Opin Immunol 6:394–406, 1994.

Price TH, Ochs HD, Gershoni-Baruch R, Harlan JM, Etzioni A. In vivo neutrophil and lymphocyte function studies in a patient with leukocyte adhesion deficiency type II. Blood 84:1635–1639, 1994.

Rivera-Matos IR, Rakita RM, Mariscalco MM, Elder FF, Dreyer SA, Cleary TG. Leukocyte adhesion deficiency mimicking Hirschsprung disease. J Pediatr 127:755–757, 1995.

Robinson SD, Frenette PS, Rayburn H, Cummiskey M, Ullman-Cullere M, Wagner DD, Hynes RO. Multiple, targeted deficiencies in selectins reveal a predominant role for P-selectin in leukocyte recruitment. Proc Natl Acad Sci USA 96:11452–11457, 1999.

Sako D, Chang XJ, Barone KM, Vachino G, White HM, Shaw G, Veldman GM, Bean KM, Ahern TJ, Furie B. Expression cloning of a functional glycoprotein ligand for P-selectin. Cell 75:1179–1186, 1993.

Scharffetter-Kochanek K, Lu H, Norman K, van Nood N, Munoz F, Grabbe S, McArthur M, Lorenzo I, Kaplan S, Ley K, Smith CW, Montgomery CA, Rich S, Beaudet AL. Spontaneous skin ulceration and defective T cell function in CD18 null mice. J Exp Med 188:119–131, 1998.

Schwartz BR, Harlan JM. Consequences of deficient granulocyte endothelium interaction. In Gordon JL, ed. Vascular Endothelium Interactions with Circulating Cells, ed. Amsterdam: Elsevier Science, B.V., pp. 231–252, 1991.

Shechter Y, Etzioni A, Levene C, Greenwell P. A Bombay individual lacking H and Le antigens but expressing normal levels of alpha-2- and alpha-4-fucosyltransferases. Transfusion 35:773–776, 1995.

Shuster DE, Kehrli ME Jr, Ackermann MR, Gilbert RO. Identification and prevalence of a genetic defect that causes leukocyte adhesion deficiency in Holstein cattle. Proc Natl Acad Sci USA 89:9225–9229, 1992.

Sligh JE Jr, Hurwitz MY, Zhu CM, Anderson DC, Beaudet AL. An initiation codon mutation in CD18 in association with the moderate phenotype of leukocyte adhesion deficiency. J Biol Chem 267:714–718, 1992.

Solomon E, Palmer RW, Hing S, Law SK. Regional localization of CD18, the beta-subunit of the cell surface adhesion molecule LFA-1, on human chromosome 21 by in situ hybridization. Ann Hum Genet 52:123–128, 1988.

Spertini O, Luscinskas FW, Kansas GS, Munro JM, Griffin JD, Gimbrone MA Jr, Tedder TF. Leukocyte adhesion molecule-1 (LAM-1, L-selectin) interacts with an inducible endothelial cell ligand to support leukocyte adhesion. J Immunol 147:2565–2573, 1991.

Springer TA. The LFA-1, Mac-1 glycoprotein family and its deficiency in an inherited disease. Fed Proc 44:2660–2663, 1985.

Springer TA. Traffic signals for lymphocyte recirculation and leukocyte emigration: the multistep paradigm. Cell 76:301–314, 1994.

Springer TA. Traffic signals on endothelium for lymphocyte recirculation and leukocyte emigration. Annu Rev Physiol 57:827–872, 1995.

Springer TA. Folding of the N-terminal, ligand-binding region of integrin alpha-subunits into a beta-propeller domain. Proc Natl Acad Sci USA 94:65–72, 1997.

Springer TA, Thompson WS, Miller LJ, Schmalstieg FC, Anderson DC. Inherited deficiency of the Mac-1, LFA-1, p150,95 glycoprotein family and its molecular basis. J Exp Med 160:1901–1918, 1984.

Staunton DE, Dustin ML, Springer TA. Functional cloning of ICAM-2, a cell adhesion ligand for LFA-1 homologous to ICAM-1. Nature 339:61–64, 1989.

Sturla L, Puglielli L, Tonetti M, Berninsone P, Hirschberg CB, De Flora A, Etzioni A. Impairment of the Golgi GDP-L-fucose transport and unresponsiveness to fucose replacement therapy in LAD II patients. Pediatr Res 49:537–542, 2001.

Tedder TF, Steeber DA, Chen A, Engel P. The selectins: vascular adhesion molecules. FASEB J 9:866–873, 1995.

Thomas C, Le Deist F, Cavazzana-Calvo M, Benkerrou M, Haddad E, Blanche S, Hartmann W, Friedrich W, Fischer A. Results of allogeneic bone marrow transplantation in patients with leukocyte adhesion deficiency. Blood 86:1629–1635, 1995.

Vihinen M, Arredondo-Vega FX, Casanova JL, Etzioni A, Giliani S, Hammarstrom L, Hershfield MS, Heyworth PG, Hsu AP, Lahdesmaki A, Lappalainen I, Notarangelo LD, Puck JM, Reith W, Roos D, Schumacher RF, Schwarz K, Vezzoni P, Villa A, Valiaho J, Smith CI. Primary immunodeficiency mutation databases. Adv Genet 43:103–188, 2001.

von Andrian UH, Berger EM, Ramezani L, Chambers JD, Ochs HD, Harlan JM, Paulson JC, Etzioni A, Arfors KE. In vivo behavior of neutrophils from two patients with distinct inherited leukocyte adhesion deficiency syndromes. J Clin Invest 91:2893–2897, 1993.

von Andrian UH, Hasslen SR, Nelson RD, Erlandsen SL, Butcher EC. A central role for microvillous receptor presentation in leukocyte adhesion under flow. Cell 82:989–999, 1995.

von Andrian UH, Mackay CR. T-cell function and migration. Two sides of the same coin. N Engl J Med 343:1020–1034, 2000.

Weening RS, Bredius RG, Vomberg PP, van der Schoot CE, Hoogerwerf M, Roos D. Recombinant human interferon-gamma treatment in severe leucocyte adhesion deficiency. Eur J Pediatr 151:103–107, 1992.

Weening RS, Bredius RG, Wolf H, van der Schoot CE. Prenatal diagnostic procedure for leukocyte adhesion deficiency. Prenat Diagn 11:193–197, 1991.

Wilson JM, Ping AJ, Krauss JC, Mayo-Bond L, Rogers CE, Anderson DC, Todd RF. Correction of CD18-deficient lymphocytes by retrovirus-mediated gene transfer. Science 248:1413–1416, 1990.

Wilson RW, Yorifuji T, Lorenzo I, Smith W, Anderson DC, Belmont JW, Beaudet AL. Expression of human CD18 in murine granulocytes and improved efficiency of infection of deficient human lymphoblasts. Hum Gene Ther 4:25–34, 1993.

Wright AH, Douglass WA, Taylor GM, Lau YL, Higgins D, Davies KA, Law SK. Molecular characterization of leukocyte adhesion deficiency in six patients. Eur J Immunol 25:717–722, 1995.

Yorifuji T, Wilson RW, Beaudet AL. Retroviral mediated expression of CD18 in normal and deficient human bone marrow progenitor cells. Hum Mol Genet 2:1443–1448, 1993.

Zimmerman GA, Prescott SM, McIntyre TM. Endothelial cell interactions with granulocytes: tethering and signaling molecules. Immunol Today 13:93–100, 1992.

39

Cyclic and Congenital Neutropenia Due to Defects in Neutrophil Elastase

DAVID C. DALE and ANDREW G. APRIKYAN

Severe neutropenia predisposes patients to recurrent bacterial infections (Boxer and Dale, 2002). These infections are usually caused by organisms that are resident on body surfaces—i.e., staphylococci, streptococci, and enteric organisms. In general, the susceptibility is inversely related to the neutrophil count. Infections of two general types occur: superficial infections of the skin and oropharyngeal areas and more serious infections involving the lung and gastrointestinal tract, which may be complicated by sepsis. In general, these infections are poorly responsive to antibiotics. Both cyclic and congenital neutropenias are now effectively treated with the hematopoietic growth factor, granulocyte colony–stimulating factor (G-CSF). Recent studies have shown that both of these diseases are attributable to mutations in the gene for neutrophil elastase, a protease made and packaged in the primary granules of neutrophils early in their differentiation from the hematopoietic stem cells.

Cyclic Neutropenia

Cyclic neutropenia (MIM 162800) was first described in 1910 in a child with recurrent mouth ulcers (Leale, 1910). The oscillations of blood neutrophils were reported again for this same patient in 1932, a finding illustrating the extremely consistent pattern of oscillations of blood counts characteristic for this disorder (Rutledge et al., 1930). In 1949, Reiman described a parent and child with cyclic neutropenia (Reiman and de Berardinis, 1949) and Morley later described five families with occurrence of disease in a classic autosomal dominant pattern (Morley et al., 1967). The estimated disease frequency is approximately 1 case per million population and most cases have occurred among Caucasians.

Clinical Features

The classic manifestations of cyclic neutropenia are oscillations of neutrophils and monocytes with a 21-day periodicity (Dale et al., 2002). At the nadir, neutrophils are usually less than $0.2 \times 10^9/l$, for 3 to 5 days, after which they rise rapidly to levels near the lower limits of normal, about $2 \times 10^9/l$. Neutrophil counts then remain at this approximate level for several days until neutropenia recurs (Fig. 39.1). Blood monocytes oscillate reciprocally with the peak levels occurring during the neutropenic period. Monocyte counts generally cycle from normal to above-normal levels. In many patients there are also detectable oscillations of reticulocytes and platelets and, in some cases, oscillations of other cells, such as eosinophils and lymphocytes. The term *cyclic hematopoiesis* is sometimes used because of the oscillations in so many blood cells (Guerry et al., 1973; Brandt et al., 1975). In some patients with strictly regular oscillations in childhood, quite commonly the oscillations become much less obvious in adulthood. Family studies also show that not all family members affected by this disease have easily detected neutrophil oscillations (Haurie et al., 1998). There also are rare cases of acquired cyclic neutropenia, in which patients are well throughout childhood with normal blood counts but have characteristic 21-day oscillations of their neutrophil counts later in life. Other periodicities, ranging from 15 to 35 days, have been reported in rare instances.

Serial bone marrow examinations done at 2 to 4 day intervals show waves of hematopoietic activity (Guerry et al., 1973; Brandt et al., 1975). At times, the marrow has only promyelocytes and some myelocytes in the neutrophil series, with a total absence of more mature neutrophil precursors. A few days later, when blood neutrophils have recovered, there is often a large proportion of

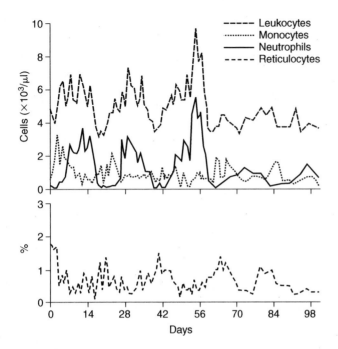

Figure 39.1. Serial blood cell counts in a patient with cyclic neutropenia.

mature neutrophils in the marrow. Electron-microscopic studies done during the cycle show cytoplasmic blebbing and nuclear condensation in neutrophils and their precursors at all phases of the cycle (Parmley et al., 1984; Aprikyan et al., 2001). Macrophages are laden with cellular debris (Aprikyan et al., 2001). Flow-cytometric analyses of myeloid progenitor cells demonstrate increased numbers of annexin V–staining cells. These findings suggest that the primary cellular abnormality in cyclic neutropenia is selective apoptotic death of neutrophil precursors with their removal by marrow macrophages (Aprikyan et al., 2001).

As a consequence of the recurrent severe neutropenia, patients usually have recurrent fever at 3-week intervals (Bar-Joseph et al., 1997; Wright et al., 1981). During neutropenia, patients may develop deep, painful aphthous ulcers, cervical adenopathy, pharyngitis, sinusitis, and cellulitis. Perirectal cellulitis is particularly common. Deep tissue abscesses occur less often. Abdominal pain and signs of peritonitis are alarm signals for the development of sepsis, often clostridial in origin, which may be fatal.

Pathophysiological, Molecular, and Genetic Studies

For many years, the cyclic oscillations in marrow cells and proliferative activity have been interpreted as suggesting that cyclic neutropenia occurs because of regular interruptions in neutrophil production (Wright et al., 1981). This concept was supported by investigations using tritiated thymidine administered in vivo at different phases of the cycle (Guerry et al., 1973). At the time of onset of neutropenia, very little of the injected thymidine is incorporated into neutrophils. During the proliferative phase, when neutrophils are abundant, normal incorporation occurs. Studies with radioisotopically labeled neutrophils show that the blood half-life of the mature neutrophils is normal, indicating that neutropenia is not attributable to a defect in the survival of the mature cells (Guerry et al., 1973). In vitro studies of colony-forming cells have shown that early precursors are present at all stages in the

cycle, but the number of these cells measured as colony-forming unit (CFU)-C/10^3 nucleated marrow cells oscillated with the same periodicity as that of the blood counts (Migliaccio et al., 1990). Recent studies have demonstrated marked differences in the formation of various types of CFU-C from CD34$^+$ marrow cells. High proliferative potential cell colonies (HPPC) appear to form normally, but more differentiated colonies—i.e., colony-forming units–granulocyte macrophage (CFU-GM)—are severely decreased (Aprikyan et al., 2001). These studies suggest that as the precursors mature, they lose their proliferative potential. These data, together with the electron-microscopic and annexin V studies, indicate that increased cell loss by apoptosis early in neutrophil development is the cellular basis for the cyclic neutropenia (Aprikyan et al., 2000b).

Linkage analysis studies of a series of 13 families with autosomal dominant cyclic neutropenia localized the genetic defect for this disorder to chromosome 19p13.3 (Horwitz et al., 1999). In this region of chromosome 19, there are three genes for well-characterized proteases found in neutrophil granules: protease 3, cathepsin G, and neutrophil elastase (ELA-2). Sequencing of these genes revealed that all patients with cyclic neutropenia have mutations in the gene for ELA2, occurring predominantly in exon 5, or at the junction of exon 4 and intron 4 (Fig. 39.2) (Horwitz et al., 1999; Aprikyan et al., 2000a; Dale et al., 2001). The presently favored hypothesis postulates that the mutations in one allele of the ELA2 gene result in a gain of function or an aberrant function of the product of this mutant gene that triggers the death of the developing cells at the promyelocyte stage (Dale et al., 2001). Studies are in progress to confirm this hypothesis and define its precise cellular mechanisms.

In 1978, Mackey hypothesized that oscillations in the hematopoietic system originate with abnormalities of hematopoietic stem cells. He developed a mathematical model in which oscillations of peripheral blood cells were attributable to irreversible loss of cells from an early proliferative compartment. In this model, the pattern of the peripheral counts varies according to the rate of early cell loss and the strength of the feedback signal from the periphery; this signal is presumed to be a specific or a combination of several hematopoietic growth factors (Haurie et al., 1999). Although other hypotheses have been advanced to explain cycling (von Schulthess and Mazer, 1982; Dunn, 1983; Wichmann et al., 1998), the recent data on accelerated apoptosis due to mutations in the gene for neutrophil elastase are most consistent with the Mackey hypothesis.

Treatment Responses

Recombinant human G-CSF is a very effective treatment for cyclic neutropenia, usually administered subcutaneously at doses of 2–3 μg/kg on a daily or alternate-day basis (Dale et al., 2003). This therapy increases the amplitude of oscillations of blood neutrophils and other cells and shortens the oscillations from 21 days to about 14 days, with a reduction in the duration of severe neutropenia, from 3–5 days to usually 1 day or less (Lund et al., 1967). With this shortening of neutropenia, the recurrent fevers, mouth ulcers, and other manifestations of the disease are eliminated or ameliorated substantially. Studies of marrow precursors show that treatment with G-CSF improves the survival properties of isolated CD34$^+$ cells (Aprikyan et al., 2001). The clinical improvement on G-CSF appears to be due to both increase in survival and proliferative activity of the marrow precursor cells.

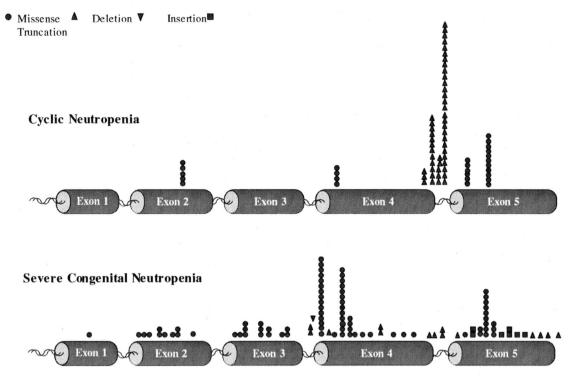

Figure 39.2. Mutations in the neutrophil elastase gene (*ELA-2*) and cyclic and congenital neutropenia.

Severe Congenital Neutropenia

In 1956, Kostmann described severe congenital neutropenia (MIM 202700), or congenital agranulocytosis, in a large kindred in northern Sweden as an autosomal recessive disorder. These patients had extremely low neutrophil counts and usually died of severe infections in early childhood. Typically, there are no other congenital abnormalities in this disorder. A number of patients with this syndrome have been identified with a familial pattern suggesting autosomal dominant inheritance, although most are sporadic cases. Cases of both congenital and cyclic neutropenia in the same family have also been recognized. The estimated frequency of congenital neutropenia is probably one to three cases per million population. Severe neutropenia is also associated with other congenital disorders, including Schwachman-Diamond syndrome, cartilage-hair hypoplasia syndrome (see Chapter 36), Gricelli syndrome (Chapter 41), Barth syndrome, X-linked agammaglobulinemia (Chapter 21), the X-linked hyper—IgM syndrome (Chapter 19), and the Wiskott-Aldrich syndrome associated with mutations affecting the Cdc42 binding domain (Chapter 31). The term *severe congenital neutropenia* is generally reserved, however, for patients with selective neutropenia of the Kostmann type.

Clinical Features

Serial blood counts usually reveal that untreated patients have blood neutrophil counts of less than $0.2 \times 10^9/l$. Carefully collected serial counts examined mathematically may show oscillatory patterns (Haurie et al., 1999; Bellanne-Chantelot et al., 2004). Characteristically, there is a marked monocytosis with levels often two to four times that of normal (Dale et al., 2000). Most patients have anemia and mild thrombocytosis attributable to chronic inflammation. Marrow examinations show the pres-

ence of early precursor cells but very few mature cells beyond the promyelocyte stage, or "promyelocytic arrest." As in cyclic neutropenia, electron-microscopic studies often show evidence of accelerated apoptosis in neutrophil precursors and cellular debris in marrow macrophages.

Patients with severe congenital neutropenia frequently have fever and abscesses in the subcutaneous tissues, liver, and lungs. Sinusitis, otitis, pharyngitis, and other infections are quite common, although sepsis occurs relatively infrequently. Children often grow and develop slowly, ultimately resulting in short stature in many cases.

Pathophysiological, Molecular, and Genetic Studies

In vitro marrow culture studies of colony-forming cells generally have shown that very few colonies are formed from precursor cells, even with the addition of a rich mix of colony-stimulating factors (Nakamura et al., 2000). The colonies that form are also small and appear to degenerate rapidly. CFU-C assays of isolated precursors show reduced formation of primitive precursors, the HPPC colonies, but formation of more mature colonies (CFU-GM, early and late) is even more severely decreased. Flow-cytometric analysis of the cycle for CD34+ cells suggests a block in the G_0/G_1 transition to S phase in congenital but not cyclic neutropenia (Aprikyan et al., 2003; Debatin, 2003). Annexin V staining shows that a high proportion of CD34+ precursors are in an apoptotic state (Debatin, 2003). An elevated degree of apoptosis was observed in the bone marrow of patients with congenital neutropenia and a selective decrease in B cell lymphoma-2 (Bcl-2) expression was seen in myeloid progenitor cells. In vitro apoptosis of bone marrow derived progenitor cells was increased, and mitochondrial release of cytochrome C was detected in CD34+ and CD33+ progenitors from neutropenic patients, but not in controls, suggesting a role for mitochondria-dependent apoptosis in the pathogenesis of Kostmann syndrome (Carlsson et al., 2004). Accelerated apoptosis of differentiating but not of proliferating cells was observed in vitro using the HL-60 promyolocytic cell line retrovirally transduced with the naturally occuring G185R neutrophil elastase mutant that is associated with severe congenital neutropenia (Massullo et al., 2005).

Because some patients with congenital neutropenia may have oscillations in their blood counts, a series of patients was examined for mutations of the gene for neutrophil elastase, based on the presumption that a molecular mechanism similar to that in patients with cyclic neutropenia could be the mechanism (Dale et al., 2000). This study reported that more than 80% of patients had mutations in the ELA-2 gene, with a greater diversity of mutations than that observed in patients with cyclic neutropenia (Fig. 39.2). Molecular modeling suggests that these mutations result in structural changes of the molecule remote from the active site of the enzyme and supports the idea that the mutations cause abnormalities in the packaging or storage of the enzyme in the primary neutrophil granules (Dale et al., 2000). Further studies are ongoing to examine this hypothesis and define more precisely the molecular mechanisms that connect mutations of neutrophil elastase and accelerated apoptosis of precursor cells observed in these patients.

Treatment and Complications

Severe congenital neutropenia responds to treatment with G-CSF, usually in doses of 5 to 10 μg/kg per day given subcutaneously; the dosage of G-CSF required to elevate neutrophils to $>1.0 \times 10^9/l$ varies substantially from patient to patient, but for individual patients the same dosage is effective for very long periods (Dale et al., 1993). More than 90% of patients respond to this therapy. With increases in neutrophils there is uniformly a reduction in infection-related events. With treatment, patients' elevated platelet counts decline toward normal and hematocrit levels gradually increase to normal. Other growth factors, such as granulocyte-macrophage colony-stimulating factor, are not of proven benefit for treatment of this condition. Patients with severe congenital neutropenia that are refractory to G-CSF treatment may have mutations of the G-CSF receptor (Druhan et al., 2005).

Before the availability of the hematopoietic growth factors, it was known that some patients with congenital neutropenia developed leukemia (Gilman et al., 1970; Rosen and Kang, 1979). Over the past decade, the Severe Chronic Neutropenia International Registry has accumulated data on more than 300 patients with congenital neutropenia. These data show that there is at least a 10% risk for evolution of severe congenital neutropenia to leukemia for patients treated with G-CSF (Freedman and Alter, 2002). Development of leukemia is often associated with acquired chromosomal abnormalities (most frequently monosomy 7) and mutations of the *Ras* oncogene and the gene for the G-CSF receptor. Sequential studies have suggested that these occur in a stepwise fashion and that evolution occurs slowly, usually over many months (Ancliff et al., 2003). Most but not all patients evolving to leukemia have preexisting mutations in the gene for neutrophil elastase (Freedman and Alter, 2002; Bellanne-Chantelot et al., 2004). It is now hypothesized that the neutrophil elastase gene mutations result in accelerated proliferative activity of very primitive precursors, which is the primary predisposing factor for the molecular events that lead to leukemia (Dale et al., 2001). It is not known if treatment with G-CSF contributes to this predisposition.

Animal Models

Collie dogs with a distinctive gray coat color can have autosomal recessive cyclic neutropenia that has many features of the human disease (Lund et al., 1967). In these dogs, the cycle length is approximately 13 days and involves all hematopoietic elements (Dale et al., 1972). Dogs respond to treatment with lithium (an agent that stimulates endogenous G-CSF production) (Hammond and Dale, 1980), daily injections of endotoxin (which also elevates production of endogenous G-CSF), and exogenous canine G-CSF (Hammond et al., 1979). Treatment, however, does not affect the coat color of these dogs. Canine cyclic neutropenia is attributable to mutations in the β subunit of adaptor protein complex 3 (AP3) that direct localizations of enzymes to the granules of neutrophils (Benson et al., 2003). This canine model suggests that the molecular basis of hereditary neutropenia involves the mistrafficking of neutrophil elastase and that an intact AP3 recognizes neutrophil elastase as a cargo protein (Horwitz et al., 2004).

Mouse models with knockouts of the gene for G-CSF (Lieschke et al., 1994) and its receptor (Liu et al., 1997) have been developed in an attempt to better understand the relationship between mutations in the G-CSF receptor and predisposition to the development of leukemia. Mice with homozygous deletions of the gene for neutrophil elastase or with knock-in mutations are not neutropenic (Belaaouaj et al., 1998). Studies are ongoing to determine if specific mutations in the neutrophil elastase gene may result in murine neutropenia or the risk of leukemia.

Acknowledgments

This work was supported by grants from the National Institutes of Health (NIH/NIHLB, RO1 HL65649; NIH/NIAMD, POI OK55820) NIH/NCI, R01CA089135; RSG105061-LIB, American Cancer Society, and Amgen, Inc., Thousand Oaks, CA.

References

Ancliff PJ, Gale RE, Liesner R, Hann I, Linch DC. Long-term follow-up of granulocyte colony–stimulating factor receptor mutations in patients with severe congenital neutropenia: implications for leukaemogenesis and therapy. Br J Haematol 120:685–690, 2003.

Aprikyan AA, Germeshausen M, Rodger E, Stein S, Zeidler C, Welte K, Dale DC. The diversity of neutrophil elastase mutations in congenital neutropenia. Blood (Suppl)96:706a, 2000a.

Aprikyan AA, Kutyavin T, Stein S, Aprikian P, Rodger E, Liles WC, Boxer LA, Dale DC. Cellular and molecular abnormalities in severe congenital neutropenia predisposing to leukemia. Exp Hematol 31:372–381, 2003.

Aprikyan AA, Liles WC, Dale DC. Emerging role of apoptosis in the pathogenesis of severe neutropenia. Curr Opin Hematol 7:131–132, 2000b.

Aprikyan AA, Liles WC, Rodger E, Jonas M, Chi EY, Dale DC. Impaired survival of bone marrow hematopoietic cells in cyclic neutropenia. Blood 97:147–153, 2001.

Bar-Joseph G, Halberthal M, Sweed Y, Bialik V, Shoshani O, Etzioni A. Clostridium septicum infection in children with cyclic neutropenia. J Pediatr 131:317–319, 1997.

Belaaouaj A, McCarthy R, Baumann M, Gao Z, Ley TJ, Abraham SN, Shapiro SD. Mice lacking neutrophil elastase reveal impaired host defense against gram negative bacterial sepsis. Nat Med 4:615–618, 1998.

Bellanne-Chantelot C, Clauin S, Leblanc T, Cassinat B, Rodrigues-Lima F, Beaufils S, Vaury C, Barkaoui M, Fenneteau O, Maier-Redelsperger M, Chomienne C, Donadieu J. Mutations in the ELA2 gene correlate with more severe expression of neutropenia: a study of 81 patients from the French Neutropenia Register. Blood 103:4119–4125, 2004.

Benson KF, Li FQ, Person RE, Albani D, Duan Z, Wechsler J, Meade-White K, Williams K, Acland GM, Niemeyer G, Lothrop CD, Horwitz M. Mutations associated with neutropenia in dogs and humans disrupt intracellular transport of neutrophil elastase. Nat Genet 35:90–96, 2003.

Boxer L, Dale DC. Neutropenia: causes and consequences. Semin Hematol 39:75–81, 2002.

Brandt L, Forssman O, Mitelman F, et al. Cell production and cell function in human cyclic neutropenia. Scand J Haematol 15:228–240, 1975.

Carlsson G, Aprikyan AA, Tehranchi R, Dale DC, Porwit A, Hellstrom-Lindberg E, Palmblad J, Henter JI, Fadeel B. Kostmann syndrome: severe congenital neutropenia associated with defective expression of Bcl-2, constitutive mitochondrial release of cytochrome c, and excessive apoptosis of myeloid progenitor cells. Blood 103:3355–3361, 2004.

Dale DC, Alling DW, Wolff SM. Cyclic hematopoiesis: the mechanism of cyclic neutropenia in grey collie dogs. J Clin Invest 51:2197–204, 1972.

Dale DC, Bolyard AA, Aprikyan AA. Cyclic neutropenia. Semin Hematol 39:89–94, 2002.

Dale DC, Bonilla MA, Davis MW, Nakanishi A, Hammond WP, Kurtzbert J, Wang W, Jakubowski A, Winton E, Lalezari P, Robinson W, Glaspy JA, Emerson S, Gabrilove J, Vincent M, Boxer LA. A randomized controlled phase III trial of recombinant human G-CSF for treatment of severe chronic neutropenia. Blood 181:2496–2502, 1993.

Dale DC, Cottle TE, Fier CJ, Bolyard AA, Bonilla, MA, Boxer LA, Cham B, Freedman MH, Kannourakis G, Kinsey SE, Davis R, Scarlata D, Schwinzer B, Zeidler C, Welte K. Severe chronic neutropenia: treatment and follow-up of patients in the Severe Chronic Neutropenia International Registry. Am J Hematol 72:82–93, 2003.

Dale DC, Liles WC, Garwicz D, Aprikyan AG. Clinical implications of mutations in neutrophil elastase in cyclic and severe congenital neutropenia. J Ped Hematol Oncol 23:208–210, 2001.

Dale DC, Person RE, Bolyard AA, Aprikyan AG, Bos CE, Bonilla MA, Boxer LA, Kannourakis G, Ziedler C, Wlete K, Benson KF, Horwitz M. Mutations in the gene encoding neutrophil elastase in congenital and cyclic neutropenia. Blood 96:2317–2322, 2000.

Debatin KM. Role of apoptosis in congenital hematological disorders and bone marrow failure. Rev Clin Exp Hematol 7:57–71, 2003.

Druhan LJ, Ai J, Massullo P, Kindwall-Keller T, Ranalli MA, Avalos BR. Novel mechanism of G-CSF refractoriness in patients with severe congenital nuetropenia. Blood 105:584–591, 2004.

Dunn CDR. Cyclic hematopoiesis: the biomathematics. Exp Hematol 11:779–791, 1983.

Freedman MH, Alter BP. Risk of myelodysplastic syndrome and acute myeloid leukemia in congenital neutropenias. Semin Hematol 39:128–133, 2002.

Gilman PA, Jackson DP, Guild HG. Congenital agranulocytosis: prolonged survival and terminal acute myeloid leukemia. Blood 36:576–585, 1970.

Guerry D, Dale DC, Omine M, et al. Periodic hematopoiesis in human cyclic neutropenia. J Clin Invest 52:3220–3230, 1973.

Hammond WP, Dale DC. Lithium therapy of canine cyclic hematopoiesis. Blood 55:26–28, 1980.

Hammond WP, Engelking ER, Dale DC. Cyclic hematopoiesis: the effect of endotoxin on colony-forming cells and colony stimulating activity in grey collie dogs. J Clin Invest 63:785–792, 1979.

Haurie C, Dale DC, Mackey MC. Cyclical neutropenia and other periodic hematological disorders: a review or mechanisms and mathematical models. Blood 92:2629–2640, 1998.

Haurie C, Dale DC, Mackey MC. Occurrence of periodic oscillations in the different blood counts of congenital, idiopathic, and cyclical neutropenic patients before and during treatment with G-CSF. Exp Hematol 27:401–409, 1999.

Horowitz M, Benson KF, Duan Z, Li FQ, Person RE. Hereditary neutropenia dogs explain human neutrophil elastase mutations. Trends Mol Med 10:163–170, 2004.

Horwitz M, Benson KF, Person RE, Aprikyan AG, Dale DC. Mutations in ELA2, encoding neutrophil elastase, define a 21-day biological clock in cyclic neutropenia. Nat Genet 23:433–436, 1999.

Kostmann R. Infantile genetic agranulocytosis. Acta Pediatr 45(Suppl):1–78, 1956.

Leale M. Recurrent furunculosis in an infant showing an unusual blood picture. JAMA 54:1854–1855, 1910.

Lieschke DJ, Grail D, Hodgson G, Metcalf D, et. al. Mice lacking the granulocyte colony stimulating factor have chronic neutropenia, granulocyte and macrophage progenitor deficiency, and impaired neutrophil mobilization. Blood 84:1737–1746, 1994.

Liu F, Pourcine-Laurent J, Link DC. The granulocyte colony stimulating factor receptor is required for the mobilization of murine hematopoietic progenitors into peripheral blood by cyclophosphamide or IL-8 but not flt-3 ligand. Blood 90:2522–2528, 1997.

Lund JE, Padgett GA, Oh RL. Cyclic neutropenia in grey collie dogs. Blood J Hematol 29:452–461. 1967.

Mackey MC. Unified hypothesis for the origin of aplastic anemia and periodic hematopoeisis. Blood 5:941–956, 1978.

Massullo P, Druhan LJ, Bunnell BA, Hunter MG, Robinson JM, Marsh CB, Avalos BR. Aberrant subcellular targeting of the G185R neutrophil elastase mutant associated with severe congenital neutropenia induces premature apoptosis of differentiating promyelocytes. Blood 105(9):3397–3404, 2005.

Migliaccio AR, Migliaccio G, Dale DC, Hammond WP. Hematopoietic progenitors in cyclic neutropenia: effect of granulocyte colony stimulating factor in vivo. Blood 75:1951–1959, 1990.

Morley AA, Carew JP, Baikie AG. Familial cyclical neutropenia. Br J Haematol 13:719–738, 1967.

Nakamura K, Kobayashi M, Konishi N, Kawaguchi H, Miyagawa S, Sato T, Toyoda H, Komada Y, Kojima S, Katoh O, Ueda K. Abnormalities of primitive myeloid progenitor cells expressing granulocyte colony–stimulating factor receptor in patients with severe congenital neutropenia. Blood 96:4366–4369, 2000.

Palmer SE, Stephens K, Dale DC. Genetics, phenotype, and natural history of autosomal dominant cyclic hematopoiesis. Am J Med Genet 66:413–422, 1996.

Parmley RT, Presbury GJ, Wang WC, Wilimas J. Cyclic ultrastructural abnormalities in human cyclic neutropenia. Am J Pathol 116:279–288, 1984.

Reiman HA, de Berardinis CT. Periodic (cyclic) neutropenia, an entity. A collection of sixteen cases. Blood 4:1109–1116, 1949.

Rosen RB, Kang SJ. Congenital agranulocytosis terminating in acute myelomonocytic leukemia. J Pediatr 94:406–408, 1979.

Rutledge BH, Hansen-Preiss OC, Thayer WS. Recurrent agranulocytosis. Bull Johns Hopkins Hosp 46:369–389, 1930.

von Schulthess GK, Mazer NA. Cyclic neutropenia (CN): a clue to the control of granulopoiesis. Blood 59:27–37, 1982.

Wichmann HE, Loeffler M, Schmitz S. A concept of hemopoietic regulation and its biomathematical realization. Blood Cells 14:411–429, 1998.

Wright DG, Dale DC, Fauci AS, Wolff SM. Human cyclic neutropenia: clinical review and long-term follow-up of patients. Medicine 60:1–13, 1981.

40

Chediak-Higashi Syndrome

RICHARD A. SPRITZ

Chediak-Higashi syndrome (CHS; MIM #214500) is a frequently fatal autosomal recessive genetic disorder characterized clinically by hypopigmentation or albinism, severe immunologic deficiency, mild bleeding tendency, neurologic abnormalities, and early death from a lymphoma-like syndrome, the so-called "accelerated phase" of the disorder. Striking abnormally large granules and even giant organelles are seen in peripheral blood leukocytes and many other cell types (Spritz, 1998; Shiflett et al., 2002; Ward et al., 2002). First reported by Beguez-Cesar (1943), a Cuban pediatrician, CHS was further described by Steinbrinck (1948), Chediak (1952), and Higashi (1954), the latter two of whose names then came to be associated with the disorder (Sato, 1955; Donohue and Bain, 1957). The incidence of CHS has been reported as 3 per 15,500 hospital admissions (Moran and Estevez, 1969), although the true frequency of the disorder appears to be far lower. CHS is very rare in almost all populations, although a cluster of cases has been described in a genetic isolate in Tachira State, high in the Venezuelan Andes (Ramirez-Duque et al., 1982).

Disorders similar to human CHS occur in many mammalian species, including mink (Leader et al., 1963; Padgett et al., 1964), cattle (Padgett et al., 1964), cats (Kramer et al., 1977), foxes (Nes et al., 1983, 1985), rats (Nishimura et al., 1989), and even killer whales (Taylor and Farrell, 1973)—could Moby Dick, the Great White Whale, have had CHS? Most important, though, is the beige (*bg*) mouse (Lutzner et al., 1966), which has been extensively studied as an animal model of human CHS. In recent years human CHS (Barbosa et al., 1996; Nagle et al., 1996), mouse beige (Barbosa et al., 1996; Perou et al., 1996b), rat beige (Mori et al., 1999), and cattle CHS (Kunieda et al., 1999; Yamakuchi et al., 2000) have all been found to result from mutations in the *LYST* gene (MIM *606897, also termed *CHS1*),

which encodes a novel protein of unknown function that appears to play a key role in organellar protein trafficking.

Clinical and Pathologic Manifestations

Dermatologic manifestations of CHS (Color Plate 40.I) range from mild pigmentary dilution of the skin and hair to severe hypopigmentation comparable to tyrosinase-positive oculocutaneous albinism (Pierini and Abulafia, 1958; Stegmaier and Schneider, 1965) with concomitant photophobia, nystagmus, and reduced visual acuity (Rescigno and Dinowitz, 2001) (Table 40.1). Patients generally have lighter hair than that of their unaffected family members, as illustrated in the Caucasian and the Japanese patients in Color Plate 40.I, frequently with an usual sheen. Hyperpigmentation in sun-exposed areas has been noted in several cases.

Immunologic and hematologic manifestations of CHS include neutropenia and lack of natural killer (NK) cell function, resulting in recurrent, sometimes fatal cutaneous and systemic pyogenic infections, most typically with staphylococci and streptococci. There is a mild bleeding diathesis, due to storage pool deficiency of platelets (Boxer et al., 1977; Buchanan and Handin, 1977), characterized clinically principally by bruisability, although hemorrhages may become severe during the accelerated phase of CHS. Hepatosplenomegaly and pancytopenia are frequently present.

Neurologic manifestations are frequent, including seizures, mental deficiency or progressive intellectual decline, cranial nerve palsies, and progressive peripheral neuropathy with tremor, muscle weakness, stiffness, clumsiness, abnormal gait, and foot drop (Lockman et al., 1967; Misra et al., 1991; Uyama et al., 1994).

Table 40.1. Clinical Findings in Chediak-Higashi Syndrome

System	Clinical Findings
Integument	Pigmentary dilution in skin and hair; may resemble oculocutaneous albinism
Ocular	Variably present reduced iris pigmentation, photophobia, decreased visual acuity, nystagmus, strabismus, macular hypoplasia
Neurologic	Seizures, mental deficiency, cranial nerve palsies, tremor; progressive peripheral neuropathy with muscle weakness (particularly lower extremities), clumsiness, foot drop, abnormal gait, decreased deep tendon reflexes
Hematologic	Bleeding diathesis, bruisability
Immunologic	Frequent pyogenic infections (staphylococcal and streptococcal); routine childhood immunizations are well tolerated
Accelerated phase (85% of patients)	Fever, jaundice, hepatosplenomegaly, lymphadenopathy, bleeding, gingivitis, pseudomembranous sloughing of buccal mucosa

About 85% of patients progress to an accelerated phase, characterized by an enigmatic lymphoproliferative syndrome, with generalized lymphohistiocytic infiltrates, fever, jaundice, hepatosplenomegaly, lymphadenopathy, pancytopenia, and bleeding (Page et al., 1962; Dent et al., 1966; Argyle et al., 1982; Rubin et al., 1985). Though somewhat resembling lymphoma, the accelerated phase of CHS does not appear to be a true malignancy (Dent et al., 1966) but more closely resembles familial erythrophagocytic lymphohistiocytosis and the virus-associated hemophagocytic syndrome (Spritz, 1985). There is widespread belief that the accelerated phase of CHS is caused by active Epstein-Barr virus (EBV) infection (Rubin et al., 1985; Okano and Gross, 2000), although there is little actual evidence that this is the case.

Many children with CHS die during the first decade of life from pyogenic infections, hemorrhage, or complications of the accelerated phase of the disorder. Nevertheless, 10% to 15% of patients have a relatively mild early clinical course and may survive to adulthood with few or even no severe infections and no sign of the accelerated phase. Some of these patients have chronic periodontal (Delcourt-Debruyne et al., 2000; Shibutani et al., 2000) and dermatologic infections, and most eventually develop progressively severe peripheral neuropathy and other neurologic manifestations that may become debilitating and even fatal (Misra et al., 1991; Uyama et al., 1994; Hauser et al., 2000). Many of these patients with the clinically milder adolescent or adult forms of CHS appear to have mutations of the *LYST* gene that allow some residual function of the CHS1 polypeptide (Karim et al., 2002).

The ultrastructural hallmark of CHS is giant organelles—inclusion bodies, lysosomes, and melanosomes (Color Plate 40.IIA). Giant inclusion bodies occur in virtually all granulated cells, and histochemical and electron-micrographic studies of these structures have indicated that they are derived from lysosomes in many cell types (White, 1966; Windhorst et al., 1966; Lockman et al., 1967; Jones et al., 1992; Burkhardt et al., 1993) and from secretory granules in others. CHS melanocytes are characterized by giant melanosomes (Windhorst et al., 1966; Zelickson et al., 1967; Bedoya, 1971). It seems likely that CHS, like Hermansky-Pudlak syndrome in humans and a number of other mutants of mice, involves a common step required for the

biogenesis, structure, or function of a variety of intracellular organelles—lysosomes, melanosomes, and some secretory granules (Windhorst et al., 1966)—and recent findings suggest that these disorders involve pathways of organellar protein trafficking shared among these otherwise quite different organelles (Spritz, 1999; Huizing et al., 2000; Starcevic et al., 2002).

The clinical presentation of CHS is sufficiently variable that the only invariant finding is the observation of giant intracellular granules, raising the question of whether all cases truly represent the same entity. The age at first diagnosis of 67 reported cases of CHS has ranged from 4 weeks to 39 years, with a mean of 5.6 years but with wide variation. The diagnosis is first suspected for many patients by the juxtaposition of significant hypopigmentation with the occurrence of frequent or even fatal pyogenic infections, or on the basis of a similarly affected sibling in whom the diagnosis had been made previously. However, in some patients the diagnosis of CHS may be considered only after observation of giant intracellular granules as an incidental finding on a peripheral blood smear. In general, the clinical presentations and clinical course of CHS tend to be similar among affected siblings, especially when the parents are consanguineous, or among patients in an inbred population (Ramirez-Duque et al., 1982; Leal et al., 1985). In particular, the clinically milder adolescent and adult forms of CHS, with slowly progressive or indolent clinical course with no accelerated phase and prolonged survival, tends to "breed true" within sibships, although even this is not always the case. Whereas much of the clinical heterogeneity among patients with CHS appears to result from a diversity of mutations in the *LYST* gene, resulting in an apparent genotype–phenotype correlation (Karim et al., 2002), it is likely that epistatic factors, perhaps even the involvement of other genes besides *LYST*, may also play some role.

Laboratory Findings

The classic laboratory finding in CHS (Table 40.2) is giant granules in all cells of the leukocytic series in peripheral blood and bone marrow (Donohue and Bain, 1957; White, 1966) (Color Plate 40.IIA). Those in neutrophils, eosinophils, and basophils are irregularly shaped, blue to slate gray, and PAS positive (Blume and Wolff, 1972), whereas lymphocytes typically contain at most one round or ovoid azurophilic giant granule. Platelets may also contain abnormal giant granules. Red blood cells generally appear normal. The bone marrow is usually normocellular, although granulocytic cells are extensively vacuolated, with PAS-positive, acid phosphatase–positive inclusions, occasional giant vacuoles, and abnormal granules (Blume et al., 1968; Blume and Wolff, 1972). In fact, enlarged cytoplasmic granules are found in all granulated cells, including granulocytes, lymphocytes, monocytes, erythroid precursors, histiocytes, mast cells, platelets, melanocytes, Schwann cells, neurons, renal tubular epithelium, and fibroblasts, and appear to represent structurally abnormal but histologically normal granular elements (Page et al., 1962; Kritzler et al., 1964; Windhorst et al., 1968; Kjeldsen et al., 1998).

The accelerated phase of CHS is characterized by diffuse lymphohistiocytic infiltrates of many tissues (Color Plate 40.IIB), particularly the bone marrow, spleen, lymph nodes, liver, and lungs. Erythrophagocytosis may be a prominent feature of the infiltrate. Hematologic analysis during the accelerated phase typically shows pancytopenia.

There are a variety of immunologic abnormalities in CHS, perhaps most importantly virtually absent NK and T cell cytotoxicity (Haliotis et al., 1980; Klein et al., 1980; Roder et al., 1980). The

Table 40.2. Laboratory Findings in Chediak-Higashi Syndrome

System	Laboratory Findings
Integument	Giant granules in skin fibroblasts; giant immature melanosomes in skin and hair melanocytes; large clumped melanin granules and vacuolization in skin histiocytes, endothelial cells, fibroblasts
Ocular	Visual evoked potentials showing misrouting characteristic of albinism; giant melanosomes in optic cup and neural crest–derived melanocytes
Neurologic	Diffuse brain and spinal cord atrophy seen by cranial imaging (CT and MRI scans); markedly delayed nerve conduction; variable neurogenic changes by electromyelography; giant granules in Schwann cells and muscle cells
Hematologic	Giant azurophilic, PAS-positive granular inclusions in leukocytes of peripheral blood; red cells and platelets usually do not, but may also contain inclusions; giant cytoplasmic inclusions in all granulated cells of bone marrow; cells frequently vacuolated
Immunologic	Decreased neutrophil and monocyte migration and chemotaxis; normal leukocyte phagocytosis, but delayed intracellular killing; absent NK cell and reduced antibody-dependent cellular cytotoxicity; normal B and T cell functions
Other	Giant granules in cells of many tissues
Accelerated phase	Generalized lymphohistiocytic infiltrates, pancytopenia, erythrophagocytosis

NK cell number appears to be normal, and NK cells bind their targets normally, but there is defective effector function (Katz et al., 1982). NK T cell cytotoxicity appears normal (Bannai et al., 2000). Loss of T cell cytotoxicity appears to result from inability to secrete cytolytic proteins stored in the giant granules, perhaps the result of defective secretion of these granules due to abnormal vesicular membrane fusion (Baetz et al., 1995; Stinchcombe et al., 2000). Antibody-dependent cellular cytotoxicity is also reduced (Merino et al., 1983), and the proportion of T cells bearing γδ T cell receptor antigens is increased (Holcombe et al., 1990). Neutrophil and monocyte migration and chemotactic responses are diminished (Clark and Kimball, 1971; Wolff et al., 1972; Yamazaki et al., 1985), perhaps due to mechanical impediment by giant granules (Clawson et al., 1978) or a primary defect in chemotactic response (Wilkinson, 1993). Nevertheless, leukocyte phagocytosis is normal (Root et al., 1972; Wolff et al., 1972), although intracellular killing of various microorganisms is de-

layed (Clark and Kimball, 1971; Root et al., 1972; Gallin et al., 1979). These chemotactic and cell-killing defects are improved in vitro by agents that increase cyclic GMP (Boxer et al., 1976; Oliver, 1976; Rister and Haneke, 1980), although effects in vivo are less clear. Defective cell surface expression of CTLA-4 after T cell activation may contribute to the lymphoproliferative accelerated phase of CHS (Barrat et al., 1999). B lymphocyte functions are usually entirely normal (Blume and Wolff, 1972; Deprez et al., 1978; Prieur et al., 1978; Klein et al., 1980; Merino et al., 1983), and routine childhood immunizations are well tolerated by patients with CHS.

Light and electron microscopy of skin (Stegmaier and Schneider, 1965; Windhorst et al., 1966, 1968; Zelickson et al., 1967; Bedoya, 1971; Deprez et al., 1978; Fukai et al., 1993; Zhao et al., 1994) and ocular (Valenzuela and Morningstar, 1981) melanocytes has shown giant, abnormal melanosomes, with an aberrant maturation pathway. Apparent inappropriate fusion of premelanosomes with lysosomes results in their premature destruction, likely accounting for the pigmentary dilution and oculocutaneous albinism in CHS.

Cranial computed tomography (CT) and magnetic resonance imaging (MRI) show diffuse atrophy of the brain and spinal cord (Ballard et al., 1994; Uyama et al., 1994). Electrophysiologic studies show markedly impaired transmission of action potentials along nerve fibers, but electromyography is either normal or shows only neurogenic changes (Lockman et al., 1967; Blume and Wolff, 1972; Uyama et al., 1994). Histochemistry and electron microscopy of peripheral nerve tissue shows characteristic giant granules in Schwann cells (Lockman et al., 1967; Blume and Wolff, 1972; Uyama et al., 1994) and in muscle shows neurogenic atrophy with unusual acid phosphatase–positive granules and autophagic vacuoles (Uchino et al., 1993).

Molecular Basis

The critical clues to identification of the *LYST* gene came from studies of the beige mouse. It was long thought that mouse beige might be homologous to human CHS (Lutzner et al., 1966; Windhorst and Padgett, 1973), and this hypothesis was supported by the failure of fusion of human CHS and beige mouse fibroblasts to complement the lysosomal structural defects (Perou and Kaplan, 1993). Further evidence of homology between mouse beige and human CHS came from gene mapping studies; the mouse *bg* gene is located on chromosome 13 (Holcombe et al., 1987, 1991; Jenkins et al., 1991), and the human *LYST* gene mapped to the homologous segment of chromosome 1q42–q43

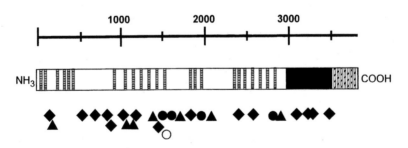

Figure 40.1. Molecular architecture of human 3801–amino acid CHS polypeptide. Amino acid residue numbers are indicated on the scale above the diagram. Positions of identified pathologic *LYST* gene mutations are indicated by diamonds (frameshifts), triangles (nonsense mutations), and filled circles (missense substitutions) (Barbosa et al., 1996; Nagle et al., 1996; Karim et al., 1997, 2002; Certain et al., 1999). Open circle indicates a common nonpathologic polymorphic amino acid substitution. Horizontal hatched columns, hydrophobic motifs analogous to HEAT and ARM repeats; filled black area, BEACH domain; diagonal hatched columns, WD40 repeats (after Nagle et al., 1996). The GenBank accession number for the human *LYST* cDNA sequence is U67615.

(Barrat et al., 1996; Fukai et al., 1996). The mouse *bg* gene was positionally cloned (Barbosa et al., 1996; Perou et al., 1996a, 1996b) and a mouse *bg* probe was then used to isolate the homologous human *LYST* gene (Nagle et al., 1996). Subsequent analyses of the human *LYST* gene in patients with CHS quickly demonstrated obvious pathologic mutations (Barbosa et al., 1996; Nagle et al., 1996) (Fig. 40.1), formally proving that the mouse beige and human CHS phenotypes are homologous.

The human *LYST* gene is enormous, consisting of 55 exons spanning more than 222 kb in chromosome 1q42 (Karim et al., 2002). The *LYST* cDNA is also enormous, 13.5 kb (Nagle et al., 1996), corresponding closely to a ~12 kb mRNA observed on Northern blot analysis of many tissues (Barbosa et al., 1996; Perou et al., 1996b). Several other minor mRNAs result from alternative splicing of *LYST* pre-mRNA, although it is not clear that the corresponding related proteins are of functional significance in vivo.

Functional Aspects

The human CHS polypeptide consists of 3801 amino acids with a molecular mass of 429,153 kDa (Fig. 40.1). The CHS protein does not have extensive sequence homology to any other known proteins, although CHS contains several peptide motifs: a number of so-called "ARM" (*ARM*adillo; Peifer et al., 1994) and "HEAT" (*H*untingtin, *E*F3, PP2A regulatory *A* subunit, *T*OR1; Andrade and Bork, 1995) repeats, and seven consecutive WD40 (Trp [*W*]-Asp [*D*]-X$_{40}$; Neer et al., 1994) motifs near the carboxyl terminus. One particularly interesting region of the human CHS protein shares extensive sequence homology with various anonymous proteins of many different species; thus, this region of sequence homology probably corresponds to a functional domain, named *BEACH* (*BE*ige *A*nd *C*hediak-*H*igashi; Nagle et al., 1996). Crystal structure analysis of the BEACH domain from neurobeachin, a BEACH domain protein that is otherwise unrelated to CHS, indicates that the BEACH domain assumes a novel and unusual protein fold and may mediate certain protein–protein interactions (Jogl et al., 2002).

The only protein known to contain helical HEAT and ARM motifs, C-terminal consecutive WD40 motifs, and a globular α/β domain in an arrangement similar to that of CHS is a yeast serine/threonine protein kinase, Vps15. Vps15 is a component of a membrane-associated protein complex that regulates intracellular trafficking of proteins to the yeast vacuole (Stack et al., 1993), one of more than 40 different Vps proteins involved in this process (Klionsky and Emr, 1990; Herman et al., 1991). Although Vps15 is not a direct homologue of CHS, the vacuolar protein-trafficking defects in yeast *Vps* mutants are similar to the defects of vesicular protein trafficking to and from the lysosome and late endosome and aberrant compartmentalization of lysosomal and granular enzymes in both human CHS (Zhao et al., 1994) and mouse beige (Brandt et al., 1975; Swank and Brandt, 1978). Recently, similar findings have come from the unicellular slime mold, *Dictyostelium*, whose genome contains BEACH protein genes (Wang et al., 2002), at least two of which, *LvsA* and *LvsB*, are involved in lysosomal protein trafficking (Cornillon et al., 2002). Indeed, null mutants of *LvsB* displayed enlarged vesicles, abnormal trafficking lysosomal enzymes, and other subcellular abnormalities very similar to those in human CHS (Harris et al., 2002).

The specific cell biological defect in CHS is not yet known. Lysosomes and melanosomes tend to be distributed in the perinuclear region, rather than more widely distributed throughout the cytoplasm, suggesting a defect in maturation of these organelles. Defective endosomal sorting of major histocompatibility complex (MHC) class II molecules and subcellular ultrastructural abnormalities suggests that CHS may involve a defect of sorting endosomal resident proteins into late multivesicular endosomes (Faigle et al., 1998). Tchnernev and coworkers (2002) demonstrated that the CHS protein interacts with components of the t-SNARE complex, which plays a key role in vesicle docking and fusion. These findings suggest that CHS might help mediate intracellular membrane fusion.

Mutation Analysis

Because of the very large size of the *LYST* gene and the large number of exons, molecular diagnostic testing for *LYST* mutations is currently available only on a research basis. At least 26 different pathologic mutations of the *LYST* gene have been reported in patients with CHS (Fig. 40.1) (Barbosa et al., 1996; Nagle et al., 1996; Karim et al., 1997, 2002; Certain et al., 2000). These mutations, shown in Figure 40.1, are instructive, as there appears to be a rough genotype–phenotype correlation. The great majority are nonsense mutations and frameshifts, predicted to result in functionally null alleles (Karim et al., 1997). Indeed, all patients with severe childhood CHS have these types of null mutations, although in some such cases it has not been possible to identify mutations of the *LYST* gene at all, which suggests that these cases might result from mutations in genes other than *LYST* (Karim et al., 2002). Surprisingly, some patients with relatively mild clinical courses have had *LYST* nonsense or frameshift mutations (Nagle et al., 1996; Certain et al., 2000; Karim et al., 2002), and in some instances both mild and severe cases of CHS have occurred in the same family (Certain et al., 2000). Clearly, factors other than *LYST* mutations alone may play roles in determining the ultimate clinical phenotype. Nevertheless, one important genotype–phenotype correlation has emerged. Only four patients have been described with *LYST* missense mutations resulting in amino acid substitutions (Karim et al., 2002). Two of these, with homozygous missense substitutions, had mild, adult-onset CHS. Two other patients, both compound heterozygotes for one missense mutant *LYST* allele and one null-mutant allele, had relatively mild disease, intermediate in severity between childhood and adult CHS, termed *adolescent CHS*. Overall, it appears that most although not all patients with null-mutant *LYST* alleles manifest a clinically severe course, whereas many or all patients with missense mutant alleles manifest a relatively mild clinical course. Thus, molecular diagnosis of *LYST* mutations may provide a useful prognostic indicator in counseling parents of young children with CHS.

One particularly interesting patient has been reported with a homozygous nonsense mutation of *LYST*. The patient's mother was found to be a carrier of this mutation, whereas no mutation of the gene was found in the father. Nonpaternity was excluded by analysis of microsatellite markers on chromosome 1, which instead demonstrated maternal uniparental isodisomy for the entire chromosome 1 (Dufourcq-Lagelouse et al., 1999).

Strategies for Diagnosis

The diagnosis of CHS must be considered in any child with hypopigmentation and abnormal susceptibility to infection, especially if accompanied by neurologic abnormalities or signs of the accelerated phase, such as hepatosplenomegaly, jaundice, and bleeding tendency. Histologic demonstration of giant azurophilic cytoplasmic inclusions, readily seen by routine microscopic examination of granulocytes on a peripheral blood smear (Color Plate 40.IIA), provides strong support for the diagnosis of CHS. Molecular confirmation can be provided by mutation analysis of the *LYST* gene in patient DNA, although this is not yet routinely available. Moreover, in at least some patients with clinically typical CHS, the disorder may not result from mutations in *LYST* but rather at an as yet unidentified locus (Karim et al., 2002).

Carrier Detection and Prenatal Diagnosis

Prenatal diagnosis of CHS has been accomplished in a number of cases by fetal blood sampling and demonstration of enlarged lysosomes and granules in polymorphonuclear leukocytes (Diukman et al., 1992; Durandy et al., 1993) and by light and electron microscopic demonstration of giant melanosomes in fetal hair shafts (Durandy et al., 1993). Retrospective studies have shown that lysosomes were also enlarged in cultured amniotic fluid cells and chorionic villus cells (Diukman et al., 1992), indicating that these cells might also be used for prenatal diagnosis of CHS.

Molecular analysis of the *LYST* gene permits direct mutation-based carrier detection and prenatal diagnosis in families with defined *LYST* gene mutations, although application of this technique has not yet been reported. While the demonstration of pathologic mutations in the *LYST* gene may be considered diagnostic, molecular diagnosis of CHS may be complicated by the fact that some cases of typical CHS may result from mutations in other genes (Karim et al., 2002). In particular, locus heterogeneity for CHS would greatly complicate any attempt to perform carrier detection and prenatal diagnosis by genetic linkage analysis alone in families in which pathologic *LYST* gene mutations have not been identified.

Treatment and Prognosis

The prognosis for long-term survival in CHS is relatively poor, with many patients not surviving the first decade. In a retrospective analysis of 56 reported patients with CHS, Blume and Wolff (1972) found that 66% had died, at a mean age of 3.1 years, usually from pyogenic infection, hemorrhage, or complications of the accelerated phase. Nevertheless, these data predated treatment by bone marrow transplantation, which has proved successful in many cases of CHS and can significantly improve survival and longevity.

There is no specific treatment for CHS. Diagnosis and treatment of infections and management of hemostasis are of great importance, following standard approaches. However, treatment during the accelerated phase is a particular problem. Chemotherapy can be of limited transient benefit during the accelerated phase (Bejaoui et al., 1989), but relapses are typical and bone marrow transplantation is eventually required in most cases (Kazmierowski et al., 1975; Virelizier et al., 1982; Filipovich et al., 1992; Haddad et al., 1995). In families in which no sibling donor is available, transplantation using an HLA-matched unrelated donor has proved successful (Liang et al., 2000). While immunologic reconstitution regularly accompanies successful bone marrow transplantation, this treatment does not alter the hypopigmentation of CHS. Similarly, long-term follow-up indicates that the development and progression of neurological symptoms is unfortunately not arrested by bone marrow transplantation.

Bone marrow transplantation does result in cure of the accelerated phase and of the immunologic defect, even in patients in whom transplantation results only in mixed hematopoietic chimerism (Haddad et al., 1995; Mottonen et al., 1995; Trigg and Schugar, 2001). A similar immunologic improvement with only mixed chimerism following bone marrow transplantation also occurs in familial hemophagocytic lymphohistiocytosis (Landman-Parker et al., 1993), which the accelerated phase of CHS somewhat resembles. Because the 429 kDa CHS polypeptide does not appear to be a soluble, circulating factor, functions supplied by even a relatively small fraction of donor cells are apparently sufficient to reconstitute the immune system and suppress or prevent the accelerated phase. These findings raise the intriguing prospect of relatively facile gene or stem cell therapy for CHS, since apparently even a small fraction of genetically corrected cells, derived from the patients themselves, might provide beneficial effects of significant degree.

As discussed above, 10%–15% of patients with CHS manifest the clinically milder adolescent and adult forms of the disease, surviving to over 30 years of age with few infections and requiring only minimal treatment. Granulocyte colony–stimulating factor (G-CSF) may be useful in managing acute infections in such patients (Baldus et al., 1999). Most of these patients eventually develop peripheral neuropathy or more severe neurologic symptoms. Treatment with oral prednisolone has proved helpful in treating the neuropathy in at least one case (Fukuda et al., 2000), a result suggesting that neurological deterioration in CHS might stem at least in part from chronic inflammation.

Animal Models

As mentioned above, disorders similar to human CHS have been described in many mammalian species, including mink (Leader et al., 1963; Padgett et al., 1964), cattle (Padgett et al., 1964), cats (Kramer et al., 1977), foxes (Nes et al., 1983, 1985), killer whales (Taylor and Farrell, 1973), rats (Nishimura et al., 1989; Ozaki et al., 1994), and mice (Lutzner et al., 1966). Of these models, the beige mouse is by far the most important. The mouse *beige* locus consists of a series of at least seven mutant alleles of the mouse *Lyst* gene homologue on chromosome 13 (Holcombe et al., 1987, 1991), three of which have been characterized in molecular terms (Barbosa et al., 1996; Nagle et al., 1996). The phenotype of the beige mouse corresponds to human CHS in virtually all respects, including diluted coat and eye pigmentation, reduced chemotactic and bacteriocidal activity of granulocytes (Gallin et al., 1974), greatly reduced NK cell function (Roder, 1979), deficient cytotoxic T cell and antibody-dependent cytotoxic responses (Saxena et al., 1982; Carlson et al., 1984), increased susceptibility to bacterial infections, enlarged melanosomes in pigment cells, enlarged lysosomes in many cell types (Oliver and Essner, 1973; Windhorst and Padgett, 1973), and platelet storage pool deficiency (Novak et al., 1984). Growth of syngeneic tumor cells is greater in beige mutant mice than in normal littermates, a phenomenon thought to result from deficient NK cell function (Karre et al., 1980; Talmadge et al., 1980), although beige mice ordinarily do not develop either tumors or signs of an accelerated phase, perhaps simply because mice do not live long enough. Like CHS, beige mice exhibit aberrant compartmentalization of lysosomal and granular enzymes (Brandt et al., 1975; Swank and Brandt, 1978; Holcombe et al., 1994).

Beige rats (Nishimura et al., 1989; Ozaki et al., 1998) and CHS cattle (Padgett et al., 1964; Ogawa et al., 1997; Shiraishi et al., 2002a, 2002b) also exhibit mutant phenotypes very similar to those of beige mice and humans with CHS. Like human CHS, both beige rats (Mori et al., 1999) and CHS cattle (Kunieda et al., 1999; Yamakuchi et al., 2000) have pathologic mutations in their respective *LYST* gene homologues. The many other animal CHS models have not been studied nearly as extensively, and none have yet been defined in molecular detail.

Concluding Remarks and Future Challenges

The past few years have seen great progress in understanding the molecular basis of the Chediak-Higashi and Griscelli syndromes. Similarly, there has been considerable progress in treatment, largely brought about by improved management of patients undergoing bone marrow transplantation. Nevertheless, considerable challenges remain in the diagnosis and treatment of patients with these disorders. Even though the genes are now known and numerous gene mutations associated with these diseases have been described, the rarity of these mutations and the large sizes and genomic complexity of these genes renders DNA-based diagnosis technically difficult and generally unavailable. As the result, improved molecular understanding has generally not yet been translated into improved diagnosis of these disorders. Likewise, discovery of the causal genes for these diseases has not yet resulted even in solid understanding of the cell biological or biochemical mechanisms of disease pathogenesis. The remarkably large sizes of the *LYST* cDNA and CHS protein, for example, make systematic laboratory investigation of CHS pathogenesis exceedingly difficult. Accordingly, the very substantial advances in understanding these disorders at the molecular level remain to be translated into meaningful advances in patient management and new approaches to treatment. The challenge for the future is to achieve these goals.

References

Andrade MA, Bork P. HEAT repeats in the Huntington's disease protein. Nature Genet 11:115–116, 1995.

Argyle JC, Kjeldsberg CR, Marty J, Shigeoka AO, Hill HR. T-cell lymphoma and the Chediak-Higashi syndrome. Blood 60:672–676, 1982.

Baetz K, Isaaz S, Griffiths GM. Loss of cytotoxic T lymphocyte function in Chediak-Higashi syndrome arises from a secretory defect that prevents lytic granule exocytosis. J Immunol 154:6122–6131, 1995.

Baldus M, Zunftmeister V, Geibel-Werle G, Claus B, Mewes D, Uppenkamp M, Nebe T. Chediak-Higashi-Steinbrinck syndrome (CHS) in a 27-year-old woman—effects of G-CSF treatment. Ann Hematol 78:321–327, 1999.

Ballard R, Tien RD, Nohria V, Juel V. The Chediak-Higashi syndrome: CT and MR findings. Pediatr Radiol 24:266–267, 1994.

Bannai M, Oya H, Kawamura T, Naito T, Shimizu T, Kawamura H, Miyaji C, Watanabe H, Hatakeyama K, Abo T. Disparate effect of *beige* mutation on cytotoxic function between natural killer and natural killer T cells. Immunology 100:165–169, 2000.

Barbosa MDFS, Nguyen QA, Tchernev VT, Ashley JA, Detter JC, Blaydes SM, Brandt SJ, Chotai D, Hodgman C, Solari RCE, Lovett M, Kingsmore SF. Identification of the homologous *beige* and Chediak-Higashi syndrome genes. Nature 382:262–265, 1996.

Barrat FJ, Auloge L, Pastural E, Lagelouse RD, Vilmer E, Cant AJ, Weissenbach J, Le Paslier D, Fischer A, de Saint Basile G. Genetic and physical mapping of the Chediak-Higashi syndrome on chromosome 1q42–q43. Am J Hum Genet 59:625–633, 1996.

Barrat FJ, Le Deist F, Benkerrou M, Bousso P, Feldmann J, Fischer A, de Sainte Basile G. Defective CTLA-4 cycling pathway in Chediak-Higashi syndrome: a possible mechanism for deregulation of T lymphocyte activation. Proc Natl Acad Sci USA 20:8645–8650, 1999.

Bedoya V. Pigmentary changes in Chediak-Higashi syndrome. Br J Dermatol 85:336–347, 1971.

Beguez-Cesar AB. Neutropenia cronica maligna familiar con granulaciones atipicas de los leucocitos. Bol Soc Cubana Pediatr 15:900–922, 1943.

Bejaoui M, Veber F, Girault D, Gaud C, Blanche S, Griscelli C, Fischer A. Phase acceleree de la maladie de Chediak-Higashi. Arch Fr Pediatr 46:733–736, 1989.

Blume RS, Bennett JM, Yankee RA, Wolff SM. Defective granulocyte regulation in the Chediak-Higashi syndrome. N Engl J Med 279:1009–1015, 1968.

Blume RS, Wolff SM. The Chediak-Higashi syndrome: studies in four patients and a review of the literature. Medicine 51:247–280, 1972.

Boxer GJ, Holmsen H, Robkin L, Bang NU, Boxer LA, Baehner RL. Abnormal platelet function in Chediak-Higashi syndrome. Br J Haematol 35:521–533, 1977.

Boxer L, Watanabe A, Rister M, Begh H, Allen J, Baehner R. Correction of leukocyte function in Chediak-Higashi syndrome by ascorbate. N Engl J Med 295:1041–1045, 1976.

Brandt EJ, Elliott RW, Swank RT. Defective lysosomal enzyme secretion in kidneys of Chediak-Higashi (*beige*) mice. J Cell Biol 67:774–788, 1975.

Buchanan GR, Handin RI. Platelet function in the Chediak-Higashi syndrome. Blood 47:941–948, 1977.

Burkhardt JK, Wiebel FA, Hester S, Aragon A. The giant organelles in *beige* and Chediak-Higashi fibroblasts are derived from late endosomes and mature lysosomes. J Exp Med 178:1845–1856, 1993.

Carlson GA, Marshall ST, Truesdale AT. Adaptive immune defects and delayed rejection of allogeneic tumor cells in beige mice. Cell Immunol 87:348–356, 1984.

Certain S, Barrat F, Pastural E, Le Deist F, Goyo-Rivas J, Jabado N, Benkerrou M, Seger R, Vilmer E, Beullier G, Schwarz K, Fischer A, de Saint Basile G. Protein truncation test of LYST reveals heterogeneous mutations in proteins with Chediak-Higashi syndrome. Blood 95:979–983, 2000.

Chediak M. Nouvelle anomalie leukocytaire de caractere constitutionnel et familiel. Rev Hematol 7:362–367, 1952.

Clark RA, Kimball HR. Defective granulocyte chemotaxis in the Chediak-Higashi syndrome. J Clin Invest 50:2645–2652, 1971.

Clawson CC, White JG, Repine JE. The Chediak-Higashi syndrome. Am J Pathol 92:745–753, 1978.

Cornillon S, Dubois A, Bruckert F, Lefkir Y, Marchetti A, Benghezal M, De Lozanne A, Letourneur F, Cosson P. Two members of the *beige*/CHS (BEACH) family are involved at different stages in the organization of the endocytic pathway in *Dictyostelium*. J Cell Sci 115:737–744, 2002.

Delcourt-Debruyne EM, Boutigny HR, Hildebrand HF. Features of severe periodontal disease in a teenager with Chediak-Higashi syndrome. J Periodontol 71:816–824, 2000.

Dent PB, Fish LA, White JG, Good RA. Chediak-Higashi syndrome: observations on the nature of the associated malignancy. Lab Invest 15:1634–1642, 1966.

Deprez P, Laurent R, Griscelli C, Buriot D, Agache P. La maladie de Chediak-Higashi. A propos d'une nouvelle observation. Ann Dermatol Venereol 105:841–849, 1978.

Diukman R, Tanigawara S, Cowan MJ, Golbus MS. Prenatal diagnosis of Chediak-Higashi syndrome. Prenat Diagn 12:877–885, 1992.

Donohue WL, Bain HW. Chediak-Higashi syndrome: a lethal familial disease with anomalous inclusions in the leukocytes and constitutional stigmata: report of a case with necropsy. Pediatrics 20:416–430, 1957.

Dufourcq-Lagelouse R, Lambert N, Duval M, Viot G, Vilmer E, Fischer A, Prieur M, de Saint Basile G. Chediak-Higashi syndrome associated with maternal uniparental isodisomy of chromosome 1. Eur J Hum Genet 7:633–637, 1999.

Durandy A, Breton-Gorius J, Guy-Grand D, Dumez C, Griscelli C. Prenatal diagnosis of syndromes associating albinism and immune deficiencies (Chediak-Higashi syndrome and variant). Prenat Diagn 13:13–20, 1993.

Faigle W, Raposo G, Tenza D, Pinet V, Vogt AB, Kropshofer H, Fischer A, de Saint-Basile G, Amigorena S. Deficient peptide loading and MHC class II endosomal sorting in a human genetic immunodeficiency disease: the Chediak-Higashi syndrome. J Cell Biol 141:1121–1134, 1998.

Filipovich AH, Shapiro RS, Ramsay NKC, Kim T, Blazar B, Kersey J, McGlave P. Unrelated donor bone marrow transplantation for correction of lethal congenital immnodeficiencies. Blood 80:270–276, 1992.

Fukai K, Ishii M, Kadoya A, Chanoki M, Hamada T. Chediak-Higashi syndrome: report of a case and review of the Japanese literature. J Dermatol 20:231–237, 1993.

Fukai K, Oh J, Karim MA, Moore KJ, Kandil HH, Ito H, Burger J, Spritz RA. Homozygosity mapping of the gene for Chediak-Higashi syndrome to chromosome 1q42–q44 in a segment of conserved synteny that includes the mouse *beige* locus (*bg*). Am J Hum Genet 59:620–624, 1996.

Fukuda M, Morimoto T, Ishida Y, Suzuki Y, Murakami Y, Kida K, Ohnishi A. Improvement of peripheral neuropathy with oral prednisolone in Chediak-Higashi syndrome. Eur J Pediatr 159:300–310, 2000.

Gallin JI, Bujak JS, Patten E, Wolff SM. Granulocyte function in the Chediak-Higashi syndrome of mice. Blood 43:201–206, 1974.

Gallin JI, Elin RJ, Hubert RT, Fauci AS, Kallner MA, Wolff SM. Efficiency of ascorbic acid in Chediak-Higashi syndrome (CHS): studies in humans and mice. Blood 53:226–234, 1979.

Haddad E, Le Deist F, Blanche S, Benkerrou M, Rohrlich P, Vilmer E, Griscelli C, Fischer A. Treatment of Chediak-Higashi syndrome by allogenic bone marrow transplantation. Blood 85:3328–3333, 1995.

Haliotis T, Roder J, Klein M, Ortaldo J, Fauci AS, Herberman RB. Chediak-Higashi gene in humans. I. Impairment of natural-killer function. J Exp Med 151:1039–1048, 1980.

Harris E, Wang N, Wu WI, Weatherfore A, De Lozanne A, Cardelli J. Dictyostelium LvsB mutants model the lysosomal defects associated with Chediak-Higashi syndrome. Mol Biol Cell 13:656–669, 2002.

Hauser RA, Friedlander J, Baker MJ, Zuckerman TJ. Adult Chediak-Higashi parkinsonian syndrome with dystonia. Mov Disord 15:705–708, 2000.

Herman PK, Stack JH, Emr SD. A genetic and structural analysis of the yeast Vps15 protein kinase: evidence for a direct role of VPS15p in vacuolar protein delivery. EMBO J 10:4049–4060, 1991.

Higashi O. Congenital gigantism of peroxidase granules. Tohoku J Exp Med 59:315–332, 1954.

Holcombe RF, Jones KL, Stewart RM. Lysosomal enzyme activities in Chediak-Higashi syndrome: evaluation of lymphoblastoid cell lines and review of the literature. Immunodeficiency 5:131–140, 1994.

Holcombe RF, Stephenson DA, Zweidler A, Stewart RM, Chapman VM, Seidman JG. Linkage of loci associated with two pigment mutations on mouse chromosome 13. Genet Res 58:41–50, 1991.

Holcombe RF, Strauss W, Owen FL, Boxer LA, Warren RW, Conley ME, Ferrara J, Leavitt RY, Fauci AS, Taylor BA, Seidman JG. Relationship of the genes for Chediak-Higashi syndrome (beige) and the T-cell receptor γ chain in mouse and man. Genomics 1:287–291, 1987.

Holcombe RF, van de Griend R, Ang S-L, Bolhuis RLH, Seidman JG. Gamma-delta T cells in Chediak-Higashi syndrome. Acta Haematol 83: 193–197, 1990.

Huizing M, Anikster Y, Gahl WA. Hermansky-Pudlak syndrome and related disorders of organelle formation. Traffic 1:823–835, 2000.

Jenkins NA, Justice MJ, Gilbert DJ, Chu M-L, Copeland NG. Nidogen/entactin (Nid) maps to the proximal end of mouse chromosome 13 linked to beige (bg) and identifies a new region of homology between mouse and human chromosomes. Genomics 9:401–403, 1991.

Jogl G, Shen Y, Bebauer D, Li J, Wiegmann K, Kashkar H, Kronke M, Tong L. Crystal structure of the BEACH domain reveals an unusual fold and extensive association with a novel PH domain. EMBO J 21:4785–4795, 2002.

Jones KL, Stewart RM, Fowler M, Fukuda M, Holcombe RF. Chediak-Higashi lymphoblastoid cell lines: granule characteristics and expression of lysosome-associated membrane proteins. Clin Immunol Immunopathol 65:219–226, 1992.

Karim MA, Nagle DL, Kandil HH, Bürger J, Moore KJ, Spritz RA. Mutations in the Chediak-Higashi syndrome gene (CHS1) indicate requirement for the complete 3801 amino acid CHS protein. Hum Mol Genet 6: 1087–1089, 1997.

Karim MA, Suzuki K, Fukai K, Oh J, Nagle DL, Moore KJ, Barbosa E, Falik-Borenstein T, Filipovich A, Ishida Y, Kivrikko S, Klein C, Kreuz F, Levin A, Miyajima H, Regueiro J, Russo C, Uyama E, Vierimaa O, Spritz RA. Apparent genotype–phenotype correlation in childhood, adolescent, and adult Chediak-Higashi syndrome. Am J Med Genet 108:16–22, 2002.

Karre K, Klein GO, Kiessling R, Klein G, Roder JC. Low natural in vivo resistance to syngeneic leukaemias in natural killer–deficient mice. Nature 284:624–626, 1980.

Katz P, Zaytoun AM, Fauci AS. Deficiency of active natural killer cells in the Chediak-Higashi syndrome: localization of the defect using a single cell cytotoxicity assay. J Clin Invest 69:1231–1238, 1982.

Kazmierowski JA, Elin RJ, Reynolds HY. Chediak-Higashi syndrome: reversal of increased susceptibility to infection by bone marrow transplantation. Blood 47:555–559, 1975.

Kjeldsen L, Calafat J, Borregaard N. Giant granules of neutrophils in Chediak-Higashi syndrome are derived from azurophil granules but not from specific and gelatinase granules. J Leukoc Biol 64:72–77, 1998.

Klein M, Roder J, Haliotis T, Korec S, Jett JR, Herberman RB, Katz P, Fauci AS. Chediak-Higashi gene in humans. II. The selectivity of the defect in natural-killer and antibody-dependent cell-mediated cytotoxicity function. J Exp Med 151:1049–1058, 1980.

Klionsky DJ, Emr SD. A new class of lysosomal/vacuolar protein sorting signals. J Biol Chem 265:5349–5352, 1990.

Kramer JW, Davis WC, Prieur DJ. The Chediak-Higashi syndrome of cats. Lab Invest 36:554–562, 1977.

Kritzler RA, Terner JY, Lindenbaum J, Magidson J, Williams R, Presig R, Phillips GB. Chediak-Higashi syndrome. Cytologic and serum lipid observations in a case and family. Am J Med 36:583–594, 1964.

Kunieda T, Nakagiri M, Takami M, Ide H, Ogawa H. Cloning of bovine LYST gene and identification of a missense mutation associated with Chediak-Higashi syndrome of cattle. Mamm Genome 10:1146–1149, 1999.

Landman-Parker J, Le Deist F, Blaise A, Brison O, Fischer A. Partial engraftment of donor bone marrow cells associated with long-term remission of hemophagocytic lymphohistiocytosis. Br J Haematol 85:37–41, 1993.

Leader RW, Padgett GA, Gorham JR. Studies of abnormal leukocyte bodies in the mink. Blood 22:477–484, 1963.

Leal I, Merino F, Soto H, Goihman-Yahr M, De Salvo L, Amesty C, Bretana A. Chediak-Higashi syndrome in a Venezuelan black child. J Am Acad Dermatol 13:337–342, 1985.

Liang JS, Lu MY, Tsai MJ, Lin DT, Lin KH. Bone marrow transplantation from an HLA-matched unrelated donor for treatment of Chediak-Higashi syndrome. J Formos Med Assoc 99:499–502, 2000.

Lockman LA, Kennedy WR, White JG. The Chediak-Higashi syndrome: electrophysiological and electron microscopic observations on the peripheral neuropathy. J Pediatr 70:942–951, 1967.

Lutzner MA, Lowrie CT, Jordan HW. Giant granules in leukocytes of the beige mouse. J Hered 58:299–300, 1966.

Merino F, Klein GO, Henle W, Ramirez-Duque P, Forsgren M, Amesty C. Elevated antibody titers to Epstein-Barr virus and low natural killer cell activity in patients with Chediak-Higashi syndrome. Clin Immunol Immunopathol 27:326–339, 1983.

Misra VP, King RHM, Harding AE, Muddle JR, Thomas PK. Peripheral neuropathy in the Chediak-Higashi syndrome. Acta Neuropathol 81:354–358, 1991.

Moran TJ, Estevez JM. Chediak-Higashi disease. Morphologic studies of a patient and her family. Arch Pathol 88:329–339, 1969.

Mori M, Nishikawa T, Higuchi K, Nishimura M. Deletion in the beige gene of the beige rat owing to recombination between LINE1s. Mamm Genome 10:692–695, 1999.

Mottonen M, Lanning M, Saarinen UM. Allogeneic bone marrow transplantation in Chediak-Higashi syndrome. Pediatr Hematol Oncol 12:55–59, 1995.

Nagle DL, Karim MA, Woolf EA, Holmgren L, Bork P, Misumi DJ, McGrail SH, Dussault BJ Jr, Perou CM, Boissy RE, Duyk GM, Spritz RA, Moore KJ. Identification and mutation analysis of the complete gene for Chediak-Higashi syndrome. Nature Genet 14:307–311, 1996.

Neer EJ, Schmidt CJ, Nambudripad R, Smith TF. The ancient regulatory-protein family of WD-repeat proteins. Nature 371:297–300, 1994.

Nes N, Lium B, Braend M, Sjaastad O. A Chediak-Higashi–like syndrome in Arctic blue foxes. Finsk Veterinaertidsskrift 89:313, 1983.

Nes N, Llium B, Sjaastad O, Blom A. Norsk perlerevmutant med Chediak-Higashi-liknende syndrom. Norsk Pelsdyrblad 59:325–328, 1985.

Nishimura M, Inoue M, Nakano T, Nishikawa T, Miyamoto M, Kobayashi Y, Kitamura Y. Beige rat: a new animal model of Chediak-Higashi syndrome. Blood 74:270–273, 1989.

Novak EK, Hui SW, Swank RT. Platelet storage pool deficiency in mouse pigment mutations associated with seven distinct genetic loci. Blood 63: 536–544, 1984.

Ogawa H, Tu CH, Kagamizono H, Soki K, Inoue Y, Akatsuka H, Nagata S, Wada T, Ikeya M, Makimura S, Uchida K, Yamaguchi R, Otsuka H. Clinical, morphologic, and biochemical characteristics of Chediak-Higashi syndrome in fifty-six Japanese black cattle. Am J Vet Res 58:1221–1226, 1997.

Okano M, Gross TG. A review of Epstein-Barr virus infection in patients with immunodeficiency disorders. Am J Med Sci 319:392–396, 2000.

Oliver C, Essner E. Distribution of anomalous lysosomes in the beige mouse: a homologue of the Chediak-Higashi syndrome. J Histochem Cytochem 21:218–228, 1973.

Oliver JM. Impaired microtubule function correctable by cyclic GMP and cholinergic agonists in the Chediak-Higashi syndrome. Am J Pathol 85: 395–418, 1976.

Ozaki K, Fujimori H, Nomura K, Nishikawa T, Nishimura M, PanHou H, Narama I. Morphologic and hematologic characteristics of storage pool deficiency in beige rats (Chediak-Higashi syndrome of rats). Lab Anim Sci 48:502–506, 1998.

Ozaki K, Maeda H, Nishikawa T, Nishimura M, Narama I. Chediak-Higashi syndrome in rats: light and electron microscopical characterization of abnormal granules in beige rats. J Comp Pathol 110:369–379, 1994.

Padgett GA, Leader RW, Gorham JR, O'Mary CC. The familial occurrence of Chediak-Higashi syndrome in mink and cattle. Genetics 49:505–512, 1964.

Page AR, Berendes H, Warner J, Good RA. The Chediak-Higashi syndrome. Blood 20:330–343, 1962.

Peifer M, Berg S, Reynolds AB. A repeating amino acid motif shared by proteins with diverse cellular roles. Cell 76:789–791, 1994.

Perou CM, Justice MJ, Pryor RJ, Kaplan J. Complementation of the *beige* mutation in cultured cells by episomally replicating murine yeast artificial chromosomes. Proc Natl Acad Sci USA 93:5905–5909, 1996a.

Perou CM, Kaplan J. Complementation analysis of Chediak-Higashi syndrome: the same gene may be responsible for the defect in all patients and species. Somat Cell Mol Genet 19:459–468, 1993.

Perou CM, Moore KJ, Nagle DL, Misumi DJ, Woolf EA, McGrail SH, Holmgren L, Brody TH, Dussault BJ Jr, Monroe CA, Duyk GM, Pryor RJ, Li L, Justice MJ, Kaplan J. Identification of the murine *beige* gene by YAC complementation and positional cloning. Nat Genet 13:303–307, 1996b.

Pierini DO, Abulafia J. Manifestaciones cutaneas del sindrome de Chediak-Higashi. Arch Argent Dermatol 8:23–31, 1958.

Prieur A-M, Griscelli C, Dasuillard F. Lymphotoxin (LT) production by lymphocytes from children with primary immunodeficiency disease. Clin Immunol Immunopathol 10:468–476, 1978.

Ramirez-Duque P, Arends T, Merino F. Chediak-Higashi syndrome: description of a cluster in a Venezuelan-Andean isolated region. J Med 13:431–451, 1982.

Rescigno R, Dinowitz M. Ophthalmic manifestations of immunodeficiency states. Clin Rev Allergy Immunol 20:163–181, 2001.

Rister M, Haneke C. Therapy of the Steinbrinck-Chediak-Higashi-Syndrom [in German]. Klin Pädiatiatr 192:19–24, 1980.

Roder JC. The *beige* mutation in the mouse. I. A stem cell predetermined impairment in natural killer cell function. J Immunol 123:2168–2173, 1979.

Roder JC, Haliotis T, Klein M, Korec S, Jett JR, Ortaldo J, Heberman RB, Katz P, Fauci AS. A new immunodeficiency disorder in humans involving NK cells. Nature 284:553–555, 1980.

Root RK, Rosenthal AS, Balestra DJ. Abnormal bactericidal, metabolic, and lysosomal functions of Chediak-Higashi syndrome leukocytes. J Clin Invest 51:649–665, 1972.

Rubin CM, Burke BA, McKenna RW, McClain KL, White JG, Nesbit ME Jr, Filipovich AH. The accelerated phase of Chediak-Higashi syndrome: an expression of the virus-associated hemophagocytic syndrome? Cancer 56:524–530, 1985.

Sato A. Chediak and Highashi's disease: probable identity of "a new leukocytal anomaly (Chediak)" and "congenital gigantism of peroxidase granules (Higashi)." Tohoku J Exp Med 61:201–210, 1955.

Saxena RK, Saxena QB, Adler WH. Defective T-cell response in *beige* mutant mice. Nature 295:240–241, 1982.

Shibutani T, Gen K, Shibata M, Horiguchi Y, Kondo N, Iwayama Y. Long-term follow-up of periodontitis in a patient with Chediak-Higashi syndrome. A case report. J Periodontol 71:1024–1028, 2000.

Shiflett SL, Kaplan J, Ward DM. Chediak-Higashi syndrome: a rare disorder of lysosomes and lysosome related organelles. Pigment Cell Res 15:251–157, 2002.

Shiraishi M, Kawashima S, Moroi M, Shin Y, Morita T, Horii Y, Ikeda M, Ito K. A defect in collagen receptor–Ca^{2+} signaling system in platelets from cattle with Chediak-Higashi syndrome. Thromb Haemost 87:334–341, 2002a.

Shiraishi M, Ogawa H, Ikeda M, Kawashima S, Ito K. Platelet dysfunction in Chediak-Higashi syndrome–affected cattle. J Vet Med Sci 64:751–760, 2002b.

Spritz RA. The familial histiocytoses. Pediatr Pathol 3:43–57, 1985.

Spritz RA. Genetic defects in Chediak-Higashi syndrome and the *beige* mouse. J Clin Immunol 18:97–105, 1998.

Spritz RA. Multi-organellar disorders of pigmentation. Trends Genet 15:337–340, 1999.

Stack JH, Herman PK, Schu PV, Emr SD. A membrane-associated complex containing the Vps15 protein kinase and the VPS34 PI 3-kinase is essential for protein sorting to the yeast lysosome-like vacuole. EMBO J 12:2195–2204, 1993.

Starcevic M, Nazarian R, Dell'Angelica E. The molecular machinery for the biogenesis of lysosome-related organelles: lessons from Hermansky-Pudlak syndrome. Semin Cell Dev Biol 13:271–278, 2002.

Stegmaier OC, Schneider LA. Chediak-Higashi syndrome. Arch Dermatol 1:1–9, 1965.

Steinbrinck W. Uber eine neue Granulationsanomalie der Leukocyten. Dtsch Arch Klin Med 193:577–581, 1948.

Stinchcombe JC, Page LJ, Griffiths GM. Secretory lysosome biogenesis in cytotoxic T lymphocytes from normal and Chediak-Higashi syndrome patients. Traffic 1:435–444, 2000.

Swank RT, Brandt EJ. Turnover of kidney β-glucuronidase in normal and Chediak-Higashi (*beige*) mice. Am J Pathol 92:755–771, 1978.

Talmadge JE, Meyers KM, Prieur DJ, Starkey JR. Role of NK cells in tumour growth and metastasis in *beige* mice. Nature 284:622–624, 1980.

Taylor RF, Farrell RK. Light and electron microscopy of peripheral blood neutrophils in a killer whale affected with Chediak-Higashi syndrome. Fed Proc 32:822a, 1973.

Tchernev VT, Mansfield TA, Giot L, Kumar AM Nandabalan K, Li Y, Mishra VS, Detter JC, Rothberg JM, Wallace MR, Southwick, FS, Kingsmore SF. The Chediak-Higashi protein interacts with SNARE complex and signal transduction proteins. Mol Med 8:56–64, 2002.

Trigg ME, Schugar R. Chediak-Higashi syndrome: hematopoietic chimerism corrects genetic defect. Bone Marrow Transplant 27:1211–1213, 2001.

Uchino M, Uyama E, Hirano T, Nakamura T, Fukushima T, Audo M. A histochemical and electron microscopic study of skeletal muscle in an adult case of Chediak-Higashi syndrome. Acta Neuropathol 86:521–524, 1993.

Uyama E, Hirano T, Ito K, Nakashima H, Sugimoto M, Naito M, Uchino M, Ando M. Adult Chediak-Higashi syndrome presenting as parkinsonism and dementia. Acta Neurol Scand 89:175–183, 1994.

Valenzuela R, Morningstar WA. The ocular pigmentary disturbance of human study and review of the literature. Am J Clin Pathol 75:591–596, 1981.

Virelizier JL, Lagrue A, Durandy A, Arenzana F, Oury C, Griscelli C, Reinert P. Reversal of natural killer defect in a patient with Chediak-Higashi syndrome after bone marrow transplantation. Lancet 306:1055–1056, 1982.

Wang N, Wu WI, De Lozanne A. BEACH family of proteins: phylogenetic and functional analysis of six Dictyostelium BEACH proteins. J Cell Biochem 86:561–570, 2002.

Ward DM, Shiflett SL, Kaplan J. Chediak-Higashi syndrome: a clinical and molecular view of a rare lysosomal storage disorder. Curr Mol Med 2:469–477, 2002.

White JG. The Chediak-Higashi syndrome: a possible lysosomal disease. Blood 28:143–156, 1966.

Wilkinson PC. Defects of leukocyte locomotion and chemotaxis: prospects, assays, and lessons from Chediak-Higashi neutrophils. Eur J Clin Invest 23:690–692, 1993.

Windhorst DB, Padgett B. The Chediak-Higashi syndrome and the homologous trait in animals. J Invest Dermatol 60:529–537, 1973.

Windhorst DB, White JG, Zelickson AS, Clawson CC, Dent PB, Pollara B, Good RA. The Chediak-Higashi anomaly and the aleutian trait of mink: homologous defects of lysosomal structure. Ann NY Acad Sci 155:818–846, 1968.

Windhorst DB, Zelickson AS, Good RA. Chediak-Higashi syndrome: hereditary gigantism of cytoplasmic organelles. Science 151:81–83, 1966.

Windhorst DB, Zelickson AS, Good RA. A human pigmentary dilution based on a heritable subcellular structural defect—the Chediak-Higashi syndrome. J Invest Dermatol 50:9–18, 1968.

Wolff SM, Dale DC, Clark RA, Root RK, Kimball HR. The Chediak-Higashi syndrome: studies of host defenses. Ann Intern Med 76:293–306, 1972.

Yamakuchi H, Agaba M, Hirano T, Hara K, Todoroki J, Mizoshita K, Kubota C, Tabara N, Sugimoto Y. Chediak-Higashi syndrome mutation and genetic testing in Japanese black cattle (Wagyu). Anim Genet 31:13–19, 2000.

Yamazaki M, Yamazaki T, Yasui K, Komiyama A, Akabane T. Monocyte chemotaxis in primary immunodeficiency syndrome. Acta Paediatr Jpn 27:535–542, 1985.

Zelickson AS, Windhorst DB, White JG, Good RA. The Chediak-Higashi syndrome: formation of giant melanosomes and the basis of hypopigmentation. J Invest Dermatol 49:575–581, 1967.

Zhao H, Boissy YL, Abdel-Malek Z, King RA, Nordlund JJ, Boissy RE. On the analysis of the pathophysiology of Chediak-Higashi syndrome. 71:25–34, 1994.

41

Inherited Hemophagocytic Syndromes

GENEVIÈVE DE SAINT BASILE

Several hereditary disorders of the immune system are characterized by the occurrence of a similar T lymphocyte and macrophage activation syndrome, also called hemophagocytic lymphohistiocytosis (HLH) syndrome or accelerated phase of the disease, which is generally fatal in the absence of treatment. Hemophagocytic syndrome is characterized by lymphoid organ and extranodal infiltration by polyclonal activated T cells and activated macrophages that phagocytose blood cells (Table 41.1). HLH is in most cases triggered by a viral infection, especially of the herpes group (Epstein-Barr virus [EBV], cytomegalovirus [CMV]). Four inherited disorders have been identified that lead to HLH syndrome (Dufourcq-Lagelouse et al., 1999b): the familial hemophagocytic lymphohistiocytosis (FHL) (MIM 267700), the Griscelli syndrome (GS) (MIM 214450), the Chediak-Higashi syndrome (CHS) (MIM 214500), and the X-linked lymphoproliferative syndrome (X-LP) (MIM 308240). Only FHL and GS will be discussed in this chapter, the two other disorders being addressed in other chapters (Chapters 19 and 31). The primary causes of HLH should be distinguished from lymphohistiocytic proliferation with hemophagocytosis, which develops secondary to severe infections in an immunocompromised host, or during the course of malignancies.

Familial Hemophagocytic Lymphohistiocytosis

Familial hemophagocytic lymphohistiocytosis is inherited as an autosomal recessive disease, with an incidence estimated at 0.12 per 100,000 per year, or 1 in 50,000 live births (Henter et al., 1991c). FHL was first reported by Farquhar and Claireaux in 1952 in two siblings as a rapidly fatal disease, which they termed *familial hemophagocytic reticulosis*. Both infants developed fever, diarrhea, vomiting, and irritability at the age of 9 weeks,

with enlargement of liver and spleen and pancytopenia. A remarkably widespread histiocytic infiltration in lymph nodes, spleen, liver, and kidney, with active phagocytosis mainly of the red cells, was revealed on autopsy. The term *hemophagocytosis* chosen by Farquhar and Claireaux underscores the importance of this feature in the diagnosis of this disease. *Reticulosis* was further modified to *lymphohistiocytosis* when the origin of the involved cells became better understood. Since 1952, many additional cases have been reported in various ethnic groups and from all continents (Arico et al., 1996).

Because secondary causes can lead to similar clinical and biological features, establishing the diagnosis of FHL remains a difficult task in families with a single affected case. Interestingly enough, however, almost all children with familial disease appear to have low or absent natural killer (NK) cell activity during the entire course of their disease (Arico et al., 1996; Egeler et al., 1996; Sullivan et al., 1998). In 1999, by means of homozygosity mapping, two loci for FHL were disclosed—on 9q21 (FHL1) (Ohadi et al., 1999) and 10q21 (FHL2) (Dufourcq-Lagelouse et al., 1999a). The mutation in the gene encoding perforin, at FHL2, was shown to cause FHL in about one-third of familial cases (Stepp et al., 1999; Goransdotter Ericson et al., 2001). More recently, a third locus was identified on 17q25 (FHL3) and mutation in a gene encoding hMunc13-4 was shown to account for a second third of FHL cases (Feldmann et al., 2003). This now makes feasible detection of presymptomatic affected patients as well as prenatal diagnosis in families in which FHL results from a perforin or hMunc13-4 deficiency. Several groups are working worldwide toward identification of the gene located on chromosome 9 region and on the other causative genes suggested by genetic heterogeneity studies (Dufourcq-Lagelouse et al., 1999b; Ohadi et al., 1999; G. de Saint Basile, unpublished data).

Table 41.1. Clinical and Biological Features of Hematophagocytic Lymphohistiocytosis Syndrome

Clinical Manifestations	Biological Manifestations
High fever	Cytopenia
Edema	Hypofibrinogenemia
Hepatomegaly	Hypertriglyceridemia
Splenomegaly	Elevated liver enzymes
Icterus, skin rash	Cerebrospinal fluid pleocytosis
Neurologic symptoms	Low natural killer cell activity
	Presence of activated T lymphocytes and macrophages infiltrating various organs Hemophagocytosis by activated macrophages

Clinical Phenotypes and Pathologic Manifestations of Familial Hemophagocytic Lymphohistiocytosis

Most patients develop the disease very early in life, within the first half year of life in two-thirds of the patients. A short period of normal development and absence of symptoms after birth is typical. In rare cases onset occurs earlier, *in utero* or at birth (Lipton et al., 2004). In contrast, familial forms have been reported with a later onset (Janka, 1983; Arico et al., 1996; Henter et al., 1998). Several studies suggest that within a family, a tendency toward a similar age at onset is observed.

The symptoms may vary widely. In nearly all patients, high fever, frequently undulant and protracted, is the first sign in association with hepatomegaly and splenomegaly. Pallor, anorexia, vomiting, and irritability are often noted. Transient uncharacteristic skin rash and moderate lymph node enlargement may occasionally be observed. Signs of central nervous system (CNS) involvement may be pronounced and early, but more commonly they develop later during disease progression. Neurological symptoms consist mostly of seizure, hypotonia, or hypertonia, ataxia, hemiplegia, or nonspecific signs of increased intracranial pressure. Nonspecific findings such as jaundice, edema, and failure to thrive as well as purpura and bleeding resulting from thrombocytopenia may be associated (Table 41.1).

Pathologic Features

The major histologic finding is infiltration of the various organs by a nonmalignant activated lymphocyte population, mainly of the CD8+ T cell phenotype, associated with macrophage/histiocyte cell infiltration (Farquhar and Claireaux, 1952; Janka, 1983; Henter et al., 1991a; Favara, 1992). The infiltrating lymphocytes and macrophages are most prominent in the interstitial and perivascular spaces of the organs. Active hemophagocytosis of red blood cells and occasionally of platelets or leukocytes is a frequent feature, although not constant. All the organs may be infiltrated, predominantly the spleen, liver, bone marrow, lymph nodes, and CNS (Filipovich, 1997; Haddad et al., 1997; Henter and Nennesmo, 1997).

When examined at an early stage, the white pulp of the spleen is often reduced in size and depleted of lymphocytes, whereas the red pulp is expanded as a result of the mononuclear cell infiltration. In the liver, portal tracts are the place of moderate to extensive lymphocytic infiltration; in the lymphe nodes, sinuses are frequently involved and dilated (Henter et al., 1998). Hemophagocytic cells are predominantly found in the T cell areas, frequently depleted of lymphocytes in the later stages of the disease.

CNS infiltration begins generally in the meninges, then perivascular changes occur, leading to diffuse infiltration of the tissue and multifocal necrosis at a later stage.

Laboratory Findings

Hematology

Viral infection, principally of the herpes group, can be identified at onset of the disease. However, in many cases viral, bacteriologic, and serologic investigations fail to implicate a known infectious agent.

At onset of the disease, most patients present with anemia, thrombocytopenia, and, to a lesser degree, neutropenia. Leukopenia at first presentation is less frequent and an initial leukocytosis is reported in 15% of patients. Nearly all patients become severely pancytopenic during disease progression.

In the cerebrospinal fluid, moderate pleocytosis ($5–50 \times 10^6/l$), consisting mostly of lymphocytes and occasionally monocytes as well as an increased protein level, is observed in about half of the patients early in the course of the disease (Janka, 1983; Arico et al., 1996; Haddad et al., 1997). However, spinal fluid may be normal even in children with encephalitis. Hyperdense areas, atrophy, and brain edema may be found by magnetic resonance (MR) imaging or computed tomography (CT) scan, particularly later during the prolonged course of the disease.

Chemistry

Signs of liver dysfunction or cytolysis are constant findings and include hypertriglyceridemia, hyperbilirubinemia, elevated serum transaminases, elevated ferritin, hyponatremia, and hypoproteinemia. Coagulation abnormalities are common during active disease, particularly hypofibrinogenemia.

Immunologic findings

Before onset of the disease, patients with FHL have normal numbers of T and B lymphocytes. The proliferative response of peripheral blood lymphocytes to phytohemagglutinin (PHA) and antigen is normal. However, markedly decreased NK cell activity and decreased T cell cytotoxic activity have been observed in many patients with FHL, a function that does not normalize during remission phase, in contrast to the decrease in cytotoxic activity of NK cells in patients with secondary HLH (Arico et al., 1996; Egeler et al., 1996; Janka et al., 1998; Sullivan et al., 1998). When observed, this decrease in cytotoxic activity may help in differentiation between these two diagnoses. Suppressed NK cytotoxic activity has also been reported in first-degree relatives (Sullivan et al., 1998). Activated CD8+ T cells and, to a lesser extent, CD4+ T cells are observed in FHL patients during the course of an active hemophagocytic syndrome. T cell count may be transiently increased but then decreased, as with the other hematopoietic lineages. High levels of soluble CD8 and CD25 molecules as well as hypercytokinemia with elevated serum levels of inflammatory cytokines, such as tumor necrosis factor-α (TNF-α), interferon-γ (IFN-γ), and interleukins IL-1 and IL-6, are striking features of FHL and reflect the T lymphocyte and macrophage activation (Henter et al., 1991b) (Table 41.2).

Molecular Basis of Familial Hemophagocytic Lymphohistiocytosis

Studies based on linkage analysis in several consanguineous and/or multiplex families with FHL identified three FHL loci, on

Table 41.2. T Lymphocyte and Macrophage Activation Markers During Hematophagocytic Lymphohistiocytosis Syndrome

Lymphocyte Activation	Macrophage Activation
Expression of HLA DR+, CD25+, Fas+	High serum level of IL-1, TNF-α, IL-6, neopterin
High serum level of soluble CD8 and CD25	Hemophagocytosis
High serum level of IFN-γ secretion	

chromosome 9q21.3–22 (FHL1) (Ohadi et al., 1999), 10q21–22 (FHL2) (Dufourcq-Lagelouse et al., 1999a), and 17q25 (FHL3) (Feldmann et al., 2003). Investigators have also found evidence for additional genetic heterogeneity (Graham et al., 2000; Goransdotter Ericson et al., 2001; G. de Saint Basile, unpublished data). On chromosome 9 q21–22, a 7.8 cM region between markers D9S1867 and D9S1790 was identified by homozygosity mapping in four inbred FHL families of Pakistani descent, although not all FHL cases in Pakistani families segregate with this locus (Feldmann et al., 2003). It is not known whether this genetic form is associated with lymphocyte cytotoxic defect.

FHL2, located on 10q21–22, results from mutation in the gene encoding perforin (PRF1) (Stepp et al., 1999), an important effector of cellular cytotoxicity. The perforin gene comprises three exons, of which only exons 2 and 3 are translated, encoding for the 555–amino acid polypeptide (Lichtenheld and Podack, 1989). Perforin defect accounts for approximately one-third of FHL cases (Stepp et al., 1999; Goransdotter Ericson et al., 2001). Patients whose disease is associated with FHL3 locus have typical features of FHL that are indistinguishable from those of patients with the perforin defect (FHL2) (Feldmann et al., 2003). However, impairment of lymphocyte cytotoxic function in these patients occurs independently of perforin, which is normally expressed in lymphocytes. FHL3 is associated with mutations in the gene *UnC13D* encoding for hMunc13-4, a member of the Munc13-UNC13 family (Feldmann et al., 2003). This gene contains 32 exons that encode a 123 kDa protein. Two calcium binding (C2) domains separated by long sequences containing two Munc13-homology domains (MHD1 and MHD2) structurally characterize hMunc13-4. The other causes of FHL remain unidentified.

Functional Aspects

Perforin and hMunc13-4 are two critical effectors of the granule-dependent cytotoxic pathway of lymphocytes. This process involves several steps, including recognition of the target cell by the cytotoxic cell, adhesion and formation of a synapse between both cells, polarization of the lytic granules of the cytotoxic T lymphocytes (CTLs) toward the target cell contact site, and granule contents secretion.

Perforin is a lytic protein synthesized by activated CTL and NK cells that is stored in the lytic granules before its secretion. Perforin is synthesized as a 70 kDa inactive precursor that is cleaved at the C terminus in an acidic compartment to yield a 60 kDa active form (Uellner et al., 1997). This proteolytic cleavage removes a linked glycan within the cleaved piece at the boundary of the C2 domain, allowing exposition and thus calcium-dependent binding of the C2 domain to membrane phospholopids. Following release from lytic granules, perforin is thought to oligomerize to form a pore-like structure in the target

cell membrane that is analogous to the C9 component of complement. This model has not be experimentally demonstrated, however (Henkart, 1985).

The function of Munc13-4 is required at a late stage of the lytic granule secretory pathway. Munc13-4–deficient lymphocytes have normal lytic granule formation. These granules are able to polarize and closely associate with the plasma membrane at the lymphocyte–target cell contact, but secretion of their contents is impaired. Therefore, Munc13-4 likely plays a role in the priming step of lytic granule secretion that follows granule docking and precedes plasma granule membrane fusion (Feldmann et al., 2003). That the granule release cytotoxic pathway is central to defense against viruses and intracellular bacteria had long been suspected and was definitively proven by the immune disregulation observed in perforin-deficient mice (Binder et al., 1998; Matloubian et al., 1999; Jordan et al., 2004).

How does this cytotoxic pathway regulate T cell proliferation?

Several hypotheses may be proposed involving *cis/trans* processes and different target cells. A *trans*-action of cytotoxic granules is highly supported by the observation that following allogenic stem cell transplantation, the presence of even a few donor cells in the recipient is usually sufficient to durably control FHL (Landman-Parker et al., 1993). The most likely explanation is that of a transcytolytic action exerted on antigen-presenting cells (APC) (Fig. 41.1). Although T cell–mediated recognition leads to T cell activation and clonal expansion, lymphocytes deficient in cytotoxic function fail to kill the infected cells and thus to remove the source of antigen stimulation. Persistent activated T cells, which produce high quantities of cytokines (e.g., INF-γ), leads to macrophage activation. The sustained macrophage activation results in tissue infiltration and the production of high levels of TNF-α, IL-1, and IL-6, which play a major role in the various clinical symptoms and in tissue damage (Binder et al., 1998; Kagi et al., 1999; Matloubian et al., 1999; Nansen et al., 1999). In fact, there is a striking resemblance between biologic changes induced by inflammatory cytokines and the clinical and laboratory findings that characterize FHL (Henter et al., 1991c).

A recent model of hemophagocytic syndrome induced in pfp−/− lymphocytic choriomeningitis virus (LCMV)-infected mice emphasizes the determinant role of INF-γ in this mechanism. In this model, increased IFN-γ production by CD8 lymphocytes appears to result from elevated or prolonged antigen presentation (Jordan et al., 2004). Prolonged contact between T cells and APCs occurring in the absence of cytolytic function may rescue activated T cells from activation-induced cell death (AICD). Alternatively, it may induce the formation of a mature activated synapse in place of an immature synapse restricted to lytic function, independent of antigen load (Faroudi et al., 2003), and further increase the secretion of IFN-γ and other mediators.

Expansion of CTLs can also be limited by a fratricide killing exerted against neighboring T cells. During the killing of target cells, CTLs transiently acquire into their own membrane peptide in association with major histocompatibility complex (MHC) class I molecules at the site of contact with the target cells (Huang et al., 1999; Hudrisier et al., 2001; Stinchcombe et al., 2001b), potentially becoming targets for other CTLs. These various mechanisms are not mutually exclusive and may participate in the considerable sustained expansion of CD8+ lymphocytes and, to a lesser extent, of CD4+ lymphocytes observed in cytotoxic-deficient conditions.

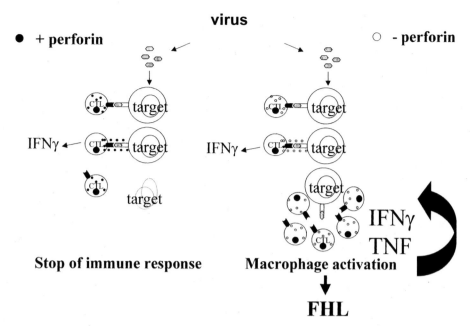

Figure 41.1. In response to a viral infection, antigen-specific cytotoxic T cells (CTL) will expand, secrete soluble mediators (IFN-γ) that enhance immunity and interfere with viral replication, and mediate lysis of infected cells. These various mechanisms participate in down-regulation of the immune response. In perforin-deficient cells (– perforin), uncontrolled increased expansion of antigen-specific effectors occurs. Activated lymphocytes secrete high levels of INF-γ and induce a feed-back loop on macrophage and T cells that continuously activate each others and expand. High levels of inflammatory cytokines are secreted including IFNγ, TNFα, and interleukins 1, 6, 18. Activated macrophages phagocytose bystander hematopoietic cells (hemophagocytosis). Activated lymphocytes and macrophages infiltrate various organs resulting in massive tissue necrosis and organ failure.

Mutation Analysis

Spectrum of mutations

Over 50 different mutations in the perforin gene have been found in FHL2 patients and consist of either microdeletion, nonsense, or missense mutations. These mutations are distributed all along the sequence. Some perforin mutations recur in the same ethnic populations, which suggests common ancestors. For example, the Trp374 stop (G1122A) appears to occur at high frequencies in Turkish families, the L364 frameshift (1090delCT) in the Japanese population, and the L17 frameshift (50delT) alteration in the African population. Some peculiar mutations of the perforin gene have been observed that specifically affect proteolytic cleavage and thus maturation of the protein (Katano et al., 2004) or its calcium binding ability (Voskoboinik et al., 2004; G. de Saint Basile, unpublished data). Most of these mutations result in undetectable expression of perforin in lytic granules. Mutations impairing only partially perforin expression are exceptional (Kogawa et al., 2002, unpublished data).

So far, the mutations identified in FHL patients, even those allowing some residual perforin expression, all lead to severe impairment of the in vitro cytotoxic activity of T and/or NK cells, provided that both alleles are mutated. This observation likely explains why clinical and biological analyses of FHL in 14 families could not differentiate between the patients carrying nonsense mutations and those with missense mutations (Feldmann et al., 2002). However, age at diagnosis, which tends to be similar within members of a same family, can be delayed in some patients with missense mutations (Clementi et al., 2001; Feldmann et al., 2002; Ueda et al., 2003). One hypothesis is that, in association with missense mutations, there is a residual in vivo perforin

function, allowing other factors such as the nature of the triggering infectious agent to influence the age of disease onset. Perforin gene mutations account for about 30% of FHL cases.

In about 30% of FHL families, disease results from mutation in the gene encoding for hMunc13-4. Six different hMunc13-4 mutations have been identified in FHL3 patients from seven different families. These mutations are predicted to result in major changes in the protein when there is a deletion, splice site mutation, or nonsense mutation within the first part of the protein. The role of hMunc13-4 in granule-dependent cytotoxic activity was unequivocally demonstrated by complementation of patients' lymphocyte defect transiently expressing the wild-type protein (Feldmann et al., 2003).

Strategies for Diagnosis

Establishing a diagnosis of FHL may indeed be very difficult. Diagnostic guidelines (Henter et al., 1991a) include the association of five criteria: fever, cytopenia (two or three lineages), splenomegaly, hypertriglyceridemia and/or hypofibrinogenemia, and hemophagocytosis. In addition, positive familial history and parental consanguinity are contributing factors. Defective cytotoxic activity makes the diagnosis of FHL very likely.

Diagnosis of FHL due to a perforin defect is highly suggested by defective perforin expression and confirmed by mutation analysis. In patients with normal perforin expression, markedly decreased NK activity and decreased T cell cytotoxic capacity strongly suggest a defect in hMunc13-4 that should be confirmed by mutation detection (Feldmann et al., 2003). The impairment of cell cytotoxic function during the course of the disease and resulting from yet-unknown molecular causes also exists. In contrast, the low NK cytotoxic activity, which may be observed in patients with secondary HLH, normalizes during the remission period (Janka et al., 1998). This parameter, although difficult to evaluate when immunotherapy is used, may become an important feature for differentiating primary disease (FHL) from secondary forms of HLH. Secondary forms may be associated with severe infections (also termed *virus-associated hemophagocytic syndrome*), autoimmune diseases, or malignancies.

Diagnosis of FHL also depends on the exclusion of the other inherited diseases, which are characterized by the occurrence of the same HLH (Dufourcq-Lagelouse et al., 1999b): the Chédiak-Higashi syndrome, the Griscelli syndrome, and the X-linked lymphoproliferative syndrome. In the two former syndromes, onset of HLH and defective cytotoxic activity are associated with characteristic partial albinism of the skin and the hair. Obviously, only males are affected with X-linked lymphoproliferative syndrome. In addition, cytotoxic activity of NK cells tested during a remission period was shown to be defective only when triggered through 2B4 molecules (Nakajima et al., 2000; Parolini et al., 2000; Tangye et al., 2000).

Diagnosis of FHL thus depends on the association of both positive and negative criteria, including early occurrence and severity of the hemophagocytic syndrome, relapse, evidence of autosomal recessive inheritance, defective cytotoxic activity, and absence of associated albinism. In the group of patients with perforin and hMunc13-4 defects, definitive diagnosis can be obtained.

Mode of Inheritance, Carrier Detection, and Prenatal Diagnosis

FHL is a typical autosomal recessive disease. Obligatory carriers are asymptomatic. In families with known mutations in the perforin or hMunc13-4 genes, unambiguous identification of carrier and affected subjects can be made. Through immunostaining, an absence of perforin expression was detected in the cell cytotoxic granules from most of the patients analyzed, regardless of mutation type (Stepp et al., 1999; G. de Saint Basile, unpublished result). Since polymorphisms have been observed in PRF1, even at the protein level, it is well advised that granule perforin detection be linked with mutation analysis of the gene. Prenatal diagnosis can be used only in those families in which a clear association with a perforin or hMunc13-4 defect has been demonstrated.

Treatment and Prognosis

Without treatment, FHL is usually rapidly fatal, with a median survival of about 2 months. A number of treatments including cytotoxic agents were initially tried with moderate or no effect, until the usage of the epipodophyllotoxin derivatives etoposide (VP-216) was introduced, which is effective in most cases (Ambruso et al., 1980; Delaney et al., 1984; Fischer et al., 1985; Ware et al., 1990; Blanche et al., 1991). More recently, immunotherapy with antithymocyte globulins (ATG) and cyclosporin A (CsA) have achieved remissions (Stephan et al., 1993; Jabado et al., 1997). The use of intrathecal methotrexate injections helps transiently to treat the neurocerebral involvement and to limit further relapse (Jabado et al., 1997). However, chemotherapy or immunosuppression is sometimes ineffective in treatment of the primary onset and frequently fails to control relapses. Allogenic bone marrow transplantation (BMT) remains the only curative treatment for this disease (Fischer et al., 1986). Partial engraftment is compatible with long-term remission, and only a small proportion of the donor cells in the patient is sufficient to pre-

vent HLH reactivation in most cases (Landman-Parker et al., 1993).

Clinical observations suggest that there may be some correlation between age of disease onset and prognosis (very early onset being more aggressive), although this has not been statistically proven (Arico et al., 1996). Children with late diagnosis often present with severe and irreversible brain damage.

Animal Models

No naturally occurring animal models for FHL are available. However, the perforin gene (*Pfp*) has been disrupted by homologous recombination in mice. The murine gene encoding perforin has approximately 84% homology with the human *PRF1* gene. Perforin knockout mice are generally healthy when maintained in a pathogen-free, controlled environment, although they do have defective granule-dependent cytotoxic activity (Kagi et al., 1994). When challenged with certain strains of viruses, such as LCMV, perforin knockout mice (pfp$^{-/-}$) develop an overreactive, virus-specific T cell response, and mice die within a few weeks as a consequence of immune damages mediated by CTLs, macrophages, IFN-γ, and TNF-α. Pathology in this case appears to be very similar or identical to that of human HLH (Jordan et al., 2004).

Several studies have shown that death of infected perforin-deficient mice results not from a defect in viral clearance but from persistence of the bulk of activated CD8$^+$ cells and the deleterious action of the cytokines they secrete (Rossi et al., 1998; Kagi et al., 1999; Matloubian et al., 1999; Nansen et al., 1999; White et al., 2000; Jordan et al., 2004). Depletion of the CD8$^+$ T cells or induction of thymic tolerance to viral epitope considerably reduces the reactive immunopathology in these mice (Binder et al., 1998; von Herrath et al., 1999; Jordan et al., 2004).

Griscelli Syndrome

Griscelli syndrome (GS; MIM 214450) is an autosomal recessive heterogeneous disorder characterized by pigmentary dilution, with silvery gray sheen of the hair and a typical pattern of uneven distribution of large pigment granules easily detectable by light-microscopic examination (Griscelli et al., 1978; Klein et al., 1994). Sun-exposed areas of patients' skin are often hyperpigmented, and microscopic dermoepidermis junction analysis detects accumulation of mature melanosomes in melanocytes contrasting with the hypopigmented surrounding keratinocytes (Griscelli et al., 1978). This typical pigmentary dilution is either associated with the occurrence of an HLH (GS2) or primary neurological feature (GS1) or can be isolated in rare patients (GS3), defining three genetic forms of the syndrome (GS1, GS2, and GS3).

Clinical and Pathological Manifestations

The single-most consistent cutaneous expression of partial albinism in patients with GS is a silvery gray sheen to their hair (Klein et al., 1994; Ménasché et al., 2000). This is more obvious in patients with black hair but is also visible in patients with blond hair. Patients generally have lighter hair than that of their unaffected family members. Hypopigmented spots on the retinas have been described in some patients (Klein et al., 1994) but is not a constant feature. In association with this characteristic pigmentary dilution, most patients develop a recurrent hemophagocytic syndrome (or accelerated phases) with features identical to those mentioned above in FHL patients (Table 41.1) or

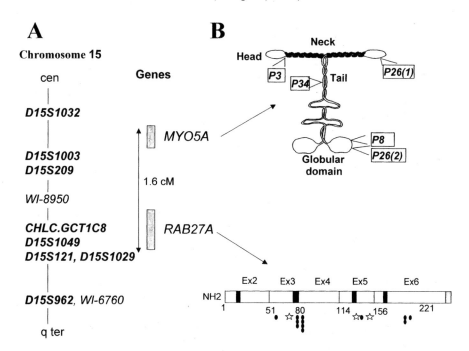

Figure 41.2. Schematic representation of Griscelli syndrome 1 and 2 gene localization, structure, and mutations. (A) Representation of the genetic map of human chromosome 15 q21–22 region encompassing the first two Griscelli syndrome loci; polymorphic markers are shown in bold. (B) From top to bottom: location of patient termination codons on the MyoVa protein, relative to the different domains identified; location of patient mutations in the Rab27A protein. The Rab consensus sequences for GTP-binding (black boxes) and C-terminal prenylation (gray box) motif, as well as the numbering of the coding exons (Ex), are indicated. An asterisk denotes a missense mutation and a filled oval a termination codon.

observed in Chédiak-Higashi syndrome and X-linked lymphoproliferative syndrome. Similarly, onset of HLH syndrome in this condition is frequently triggered by an infection (Klein et al., 1994; Wagner et al., 1997) and is characterized by hyperactivation and proliferation of T cells and macrophage, in association with fever, edema, hepatosplenomegaly, pancytopenia, coagulation abnormality, liver dysfunction, and features of hemophagocytosis. These patients have been defined as having GS type 2, which results from mutation in the Rab27a gene (*RAB27A*).

Neurological manifestations are frequently observed in association with HLH in GS2 patients, as a result of brain infiltration by activated lymphocytes and macrophages. However, in a few GS patients, severe and static neurological symptoms are noticeable since birth, without any sign of HLH, and consist of hypotonia, absence of coordinated voluntary movements, and severe psychomotor developmental delay (Sanal et al., 2002). These symptoms are similar to the neurological signs described by Elejalde et al. (1979). In this condition, CNS disorder is static and never improves with time.

Patients presenting with the typical hypopigmentation of GS in association with this isolated severe neurological manifestation have been shown to carry mutations in the myosine VA gene (*MYO5A*), which defines GS1 (Pastural et al., 1997). In addition, isolated hypopigmentation with typical hair and skin features of GS was recently observed in a subject, independent of *MYOVA* or *RAB27A* mutation. Hypopigmentation in this case resulted from mutation in the melanophilin gene (*MLPH*) (Ménasché et al., 2003b), defining a third form of Griscelli syndrome (GS3).

Molecular Basis of Griscelli Syndrome

Genetic linkage analysis performed in several GS1 and GS2 families has enabled localization of both disease loci on the same 15q21 chromosome region (Fig. 41.2). Mutations in either the *MYOVA* gene or *RAB27A* gene, two genes separated by less than 1.6 cM in this genetic region, account for the GS1 and GS2 phenotypes, respectively (Fig. 41.2) (Ménasché et al., 2000; Pastural et al., 2000).

The *dilute* mutant mice and the *ashen* mutant mice were shown to be the mouse counterparts of GS1 and GS2, although *ashen* mice do not develop a spontaneously accelerated phase of the disease (Wilson et al., 2000). In addition, the melanophilin gene, located on chromosome 2q37.3, leads to GS3 when mutated. In this condition, the GS phenotype is restricted to the characteristic hypopigmentation of this condition (Ménasché et al., 2003b). The *leaden* mutant is the mouse counterpart of GS3 (Matesic et al., 2001).

Functional Aspects

Myosin Va is an unconventional myosin heavy chain implicated in vesicle transport in cells and is particularly abundant in neurons and melanocytes. It has the expected structure for a member of this family—i.e., a globular head domain containing the ATP- and actin-binding sites; a "neck" domain, which is the site of calmodulin (or light-chain) binding; and a tail domain, which is thought to represent the cargo-binding domain (Fig. 41.2). Myosin VA acts as a dimer and moves cargo along actin filaments in a plus-end-directed manner, allowing their capture and accumulation at the periphery of the cells. In addition, there is recent evidence of a role for myosin Va in structural and functional cross-talk between the actin- and microtubule-based cytoskeletons. Myosin Va is required for melanosome transport in melanocytes (Wu et al., 1997) and likely synaptic vesicles in nerve terminals (Prekeris and Terrian, 1997). Study in *dilute* mice has shown that a defect in myosin Va leads to concentration of melanosomes in the center of the melanocytes; they are also concentrated in dendrites and dendritic tips in wild-type mouse melanocytes. This defect also impairs processing of presynaptic vesicles in the peripheral regions of neurons and the distribution of smooth endoplasmic reticulum in Purkinje cell neurons (Takagishi et al., 1996).

Rab27A is expressed in melanocytes, peripheral leukocytes, platelets, and many other cells and tissue types, except in the brain (Chen et al., 1997). Each member of the Rab protein family has a characteristic intracellular distribution pattern, suggesting their unique function in transport. Like myosin Va, Rab27A colocalizes in part with melanosomes in melanocytes and its defect leads to the abnormal melanosome distribution observed in GS (Bahadoran et al., 2001). In addition, Rab27A is necessary for cytotoxic granule exocytosis and thus cytotoxic activity of T and NK cells, which has been shown to be defective in this group of GS2 patients (Ménasché et al., 2000).

Melanophilin is an effector of Rab27a, which is specifically expressed in melanocytes (Fukuda, 2003). MLPH deficiency leads to the same defective transport of melanosomes as that resulting from MYO5A and RAB27A defects. Pigmentary dilution is indistinguishable among these three molecular defects. A specific role of the three proteins Rab27a, MyoVa, and Mlph in the capture and actin-based transport of melanosomes to the periphery of the dendrites has been demonstrated. Analyses in mouse mutant models determined that Rab27a first associates with the membrane of melanosomes, then interacts with melanophilin, which recruits myosin Va through its tail region (Wu et al., 2002). Binding of the head domain of myosin Va to actin filaments links melanososmes with the peripheral actin network.

Because of the role of myosin-Va in brain tissue, however, only patients with myosin-Va defect develop a primitive and severe neurological impairment with no immunological expression. In contrast, defective Rab27A expression is always associated with abnormal lymphocyte cytotoxic activity, which results in the occurrence of a lymphoproliferative syndrome, as observed in the case of the FHL caused by genetically determined perforin or hMunc13-4 deficiency (Stepp et al., 1999; Feldmann et al., 2003). When neurological signs are observed in GS2 patients, they are the consequence of an accelerated phase, and appear secondary to perivascular lymphohistiocytic organ infiltration.

Laboratory Findings

The light-microscopic examination and electron-microscopic findings of patients' hair and skin are characteristic. Hair shafts contain a typical pattern of uneven accumulation of large pigment granules, instead of the homogeneous distribution of small pigment granules in normal hair. Fontana-stained silver sections of the skin show hyperpigmented melanocytes, contrasting with poorly pigmented adjacent keratinocytes, instead of the homogeneous distribution of melanin granules observed in melanocytes and surrounding keratinocytes in normal epidermis. Electron microscopy shows that the cytoplasm of melanocytes is filled with numerous mature stage IV melanosomes, predominantly around the nucleus, but have normal dendritic processes (Griscelli et al., 1978; Klein et al., 1994; Takagishi et al., 1996; Chan et al., 1998). These findings are consistently observed and identical in the three groups of patients (with MYO5A, RAB27A, or MLPH mutations).

Immunological abnormalities are restricted to patients with the Rab27A defect. Biological features of the accelerated phase are not specific to GS; they are identical to those observed in FHL patients. The capacity of lymphocytes and NK cells of these

patients to lyse target cells is impaired or absent. This decrease in T and NK cell cytotoxicity, which results from an inability to secrete cytotoxic granules when Rab27a is not functional, is a constant feature in this group of patients (Ménasché et al., 2000; Stepp et al., 2000). Patients have normal numbers of T, B, and NK cells as well as normal B and neutrophil functions, although decreased chemiluminescence and chemotactic responses have been reported (Klein et al., 1994). In addition, impaired skin reactions to tuberculin, streptokinase-streptodornase antigen, and candida have been described in some cases. The lymphocytes proliferate in vitro in response to PHA, purified protein derivative (PPD), or candida, and in mixed lymphocyte reaction (MLR). No immunological abnormalities have been observed in GS patients with a myosin-Va or melanophilin defect. Myosin-Va and melanophilin defects do not affect cytotoxic granule secretion, and these patients never develop an accelerated phase (Ménasché et al., 2000, 2003b).

Mutation Analysis

Spectrum of mutations

RAB27A consists of seven exons, the first two being untranslated. It encodes a 221–amino acid polypeptide with a molecular mass of 25 kDa (Chen et al., 1997). Mutations in RAB27A have been characterized in about 50 independent patients (Ménasché et al., 2000, unpublished results). Only three single missense mutations have been reported: a W73G transition that lies within the conserved GTP-binding motif and affects interaction with a specific effector, and L130P and A152P transitions that disrupt protein folding by affecting residues that are highly conserved among Rab proteins (Menasche et al., 2003a). The other mutations are nonsense mutations, deletions, or splice site alterations, all predicting an early protein truncation. In each case, location of the stop codon predicts truncation of the consensus carboxyl-terminal motif of the protein, involved in Rab protein geranylgeranylation, and thus should leave Rab27a protein in an inactive state.

The MYO5A gene contains an open reading frame of 1855 codons that encodes a protein of 215 kDa (Mercer et al., 1991). MyosinVa is a member of the molecular motor molecules with structurally conserved heads followed by a neck domain, a tail region, and a globular C-terminal domain (Cheney et al., 1993). Alternatively spliced transcripts can be generated within the tail region of MyoVa. Four different mutations in MYO5A have been identified, each leading to a predicted truncated protein. One patient was homozygous for a C2332T transition in codon 779, resulting in a nonsense mutation that leads to a protein lacking the last 1078 residues. The second patient had a homozygous insertion of 47 bp at position 4634 (residue 1545), which resulted in a protein lacking most of the globular domain. The third patient was heterozygous for a 1 bp deletion at nucleotide 4950 as well as a C2893T transition affecting codons 1650 and 965 respectively, each leading to early protein truncation (Fig. 41.2) (G. de Saint Basile, unpublished result). Alternative splicing within the tail region of myosin Va produces different spliced isoforms with tissue-restricted expression: in melanocytes, the majority of myosin Va transcripts contain the longest isoform of myosin Va, whereas brain transcripts contain a shorter isoform lacking exon F (Huang et al., 1998; Lambert et al., 1998; Pastural et al., 2000). In one patient, homozygous intragenic deletion of myosin Va exon F led to a phenotype restricted to typical hypopigmentation of GS without neurological symptoms, demonstrating that exon

F of myosin Va is dispensable for neurological function (Ménasché et al., 2003b).

The *MLPH* gene comprises seven exons spaning 2403 bp and encodes for a protein of 66 kDa. A homozygous R35W substitution was identified in the synaptotagmin-like protein homology domain (SHD) of the protein in one patient, which completely blocked Mlph interaction with the active form of Rab27a (Ménasché et al., 2003a).

Genotype-Phenotype Correlation

As discussed above, there is a strict correlation between the type of gene affected (*RAB27A/MYO5A/MLPH*) and the phenotype displayed by patients with GS. Although pigmentary dilution is identical in these three groups of patients, only the patients with *RAB27A* mutations have decreased cytotoxic activity resulting in the development of a hemophagocytic syndrome, whereas primary, severe, and irreversible neurological impairment characterizes patients with *MYO5A* mutations (Ménasché et al., 2000).

Strategies for Diagnosis

The diagnosis of GS must be considered in any child with decreased pigmentation accompanied or not by neurological abnormalities or signs of the accelerated phase, such as hepatosplenomegaly, jaundice, or pancytopenia. Microscopic examination of the hair shaft provides strong support for the diagnosis of GS. The characteristic neurological symptoms and analysis of cytotoxic activity of patient lymphocytes tend to distinguish the three molecular causes. Confirmation can be provided by mutation analysis of patient DNA.

Prenatal diagnosis of GS was first accomplished by light-microscopic examination of the hair shaft (Durandy et al., 1993). With the recent identification of the GS genes, direct mutation-based carrier detection and prenatal diagnosis are now feasible in families with defined *MYO5A* or *RAB27A* gene mutations. In addition, given the proximity of these two genes causing the severe forms of GS, polymorphic markers linked to the GS locus region in 15q21 can be used for this purpose, even if the precise mutation has not been identified in a consanguineous family (Ménasché et al., 2000).

Several additional disorders exhibit clinical similarity to GS but can be clearly distinguished. Chédiak-Higashi syndrome (CHS), a disorder similar to GS, involves variable hypopigmentation of the skin and the hair, frequent pyogenic infections, and defective NK and T lymphocyte cytotoxicity; the recurrent accelerated phase is virtually identical to that of GS2 (Beguez-Cesar, 1943; Blume and Wolff, 1972; Baetz et al., 1995). However, light-microscopic examination of the hair enables distinction between these two disorders, as in CHS the clusters of the pigment are smaller than those in GS, although they remain abnormal. In addition, a hallmark of CHS is the presence of giant organelle inclusion bodies in virtually all granulated cells, including granulocytes, lymphocytes, monocytes, mast cells, melanocytes, Schwann cells, neurons, renal tubular epithelium, and fibroblasts. Studies of these bodies indicate that they are derived from lysosomes in many cell types and represent structurally abnormal but histologically normal granular elements (Windhorst and Padgett, 1973; Burkhardt et al., 1993). Thanks to CHS homology to the beige mutant mouse, CHS has been mapped to chromosome 1q42–43 and its gene, *CHS1*, identified (Barbosa et al., 1996; Barrat et al., 1996; Nagle et al., 1996). In patients with classical form of CHS, nonsense or frameshift mutations have been reported that lead to early truncation of the protein. In contrast, missense mutations were identified in the few patients described with a milder clinical course (Spritz, 1998; Certain et al., 2000; Karim et al., 2002). Studies of the CHS protein function suggest its role in lysosomal fission (Perou et al., 1997) as well as intracellular protein trafficking or sorting (Faigle et al., 1998; Barrat et al., 1999).

Partial albinism with immunodeficiency, termed *PAID syndrome*, is similar to GS, but with progressive demyelination of the white matter of the brain. This syndrome has been described in eight Saudi Arabian kindred (Harfi et al., 1992). Recent genetic analysis in one family with PAID syndrome from the same origin identified a mutation in the *RAB27A* gene, which indicates that PAID syndrome and GS most probably correspond to the same disorder (G. de Saint Basile, unpublished data). Similarly, Elejalde syndrome, or neuroectodermal melanolysosomal syndrome, was described with the same albinism features as those observed in GS associated with early onset of severe CNS disorder, without signs and symptoms of accelerated phase (Elejalde et al., 1979). This exact phenotype is displayed by the three unrelated GS patients with myosin Va defect (Pastural et al., 2000; Sanal et al., 2000; G. de Saint Basile, unpublished data). These findings strongly suggest that Elejalde syndrome and this form of GS are allelic.

In FHL, X-linked lymphoproliferative syndrome, and virus-associated hemaphagocytic syndrome, patients develop an accelerated phase identical to the one observed in GS, and NK cytotoxic activity is often decreased or absent (Dufourcq-Lagelouse et al., 1999b). However, these disorders do not involve partial albinism, and microscopic examination of the hair shaft allows easy differentiation of GS from these disorders.

Treatment and Prognosis

The prognosis for long-term survival in GS is relatively poor. In the form caused by the Rab27A defect, GS is usually rapidly fatal within 1 to 4 years. Treatment is similar to that described above for FHL patients. Allogenic bone marrow transplantation, the only curative treatment for this disease, can cure the cytotoxic defect and consequently prevent the occurrence of further accelerated phases. Even a low number of donor cells in the patient bone marrow is enough to control the disease, probably because of the ability of each cytotoxic cell to kill several targets. These findings indicate that successful transfer of a normal *RAB27A* gene, even in a small proportion of patient cells, should be sufficient to restore cytotoxic activity and control immune homeostasis in a gene therapy attempt.

No specific treatment can be proposed for myosin-Va deficiency. The severe neurological impairment and psychomotor delay do not improve with time. Recurrent infections presented by some of these patients have been improved with positional changes and antibiotic treatment.

Animals Models

Three naturally occurring mutants in mice—the dilute (*d*), ashen (*ash*), and *leaden* (*lead*) mice—are the ortholog for the three GS forms, which result from myosin-Va, Rab2A, and Mlph deficiency respectively. All murine mutants present with identical pigmentary dilution, normal pigment granule synthesis, but abnormal melanosome transport. The melanosomes are localized mainly in the perinuclear region of the melanocytes (Provance et al., 1996; Wu et al., 1997; Wilson et al., 2000).

Dilute null mice also show a neurological defect, characterized by opisthotonus and ataxia, which results in death of the animal 2–3 weeks after birth (Dekker Ohno et al., 1996; Takagishi et al., 1996). The neurological defect is thought to result from the failure to transport smooth endoplasmic reticulum from the dendritic shaft to the dendritic spines of cerebellar Purkinje cells, which probably affect the regulation of intracellular Ca^{2+} and postsynaptic signal transduction. Retroviral integration into the *d* gene in mice (*dv*) allowed its cloning and demonstrated that it encodes an unconventional myosin heavy chain, myosin Va, expressed in nearly all tissues in adults (Jenkins et al., 1981; Mercer et al., 1991). Neurological impairment and pigmentary dilution may vary, however, with the type of myo5a defect (Huang et al., 1998). Murine myosin-Va displays the same dimeric structure function and shares 93% homology with human myosin-Va.

In contrast, *ashen* mice exhibit the same pigmentary dilution as *dilute* mice, but in association with defective cytotoxic activity (Haddad et al., 2001; Stinchcombe et al., 2001a). Like in GS, this defective function results from the role of Rab27a in cytotoxic granule exocytosis. *Ashen* mice have also been described with increased bleeding times and a reduction in the number of platelet dense granules (Wilson et al., 2000), but this feature depends on the genetic background. Meiotic and physical linkage allowed mapping of the *ashen* critical region on murine chromosome 9, which is tightly associated with the *dilute* locus. A splicing defect resulting from a single transversion in exon 4 donor spice site, activation of a cryptic downstream site and abnormal Rab27a transcript was identified in these mice (Wilson et al., 2000). However, no signs of an accelerated phase have been observed in *ashen* mice, a condition that may require viral challenge. Isolated pigmentation dilution identical to that of the *dilute* and *ashen* mice characterizes the *leaden* mice and results from a deletion of seven residues in the SHD of the melanophilin gene (Matesic et al., 2001).

Acknowledgments

The author thanks Françoise Le Deist, Jérôme Feldmann, Gaël Ménashé, and Rémi Dufourcq-Lagelouse for their stimulating discussion and contribution to this work, and Alain Fischer for insightful advice and chapter review. This work was supported by INSERM, the Association "Vaincre les Maladies Lysosomiales" (V.M.L.), and l'Association de Recherche contre le Cancer (A.R.C.).

References

Ambruso DR, Hays T, Zwartes WJ, Turbegen DG, Favara BE. Successful treatment of lymphohistiocytic reticulosis with phagocytosis with epidophyllotoxin VP16-213. Cancer 45:2516–2520, 1980.

Arico M, Janka G, Fischer A. Hemophagocytic lymphohistiocytosis: diagnosis, treatment and pronostic factors. Report of 122 children from the International Registry. FHL Study Group of the Histiocyte Society. Leukemia 10:197–203, 1996.

Baetz K, Isaaz S, Griffiths GM. Loss of cytotoxic T lymphocyte function in Chediak-Higashi syndrome arise from a secretory defect that prevents lytic granule exocytosis. J Immunol 154:6122–6131, 1995.

Bahadoran P, Aberdam E, Mantoux F, Busca R, Bille K, Seabra M, Yalman N, de Saint Basile G, Casaroli R, Ortonne J-P, Ballotti R. Rab27A: a key to melanosome transport in human melanocytes. J Cell Biol 152:843–849, 2001.

Barbosa MDFS, Nguyen QA, Tchernev VT, Aschley JA, Detter JC, Blaydes SM, Brandt SJ, Chotai D, Hodgman C, Solari RCE, Lovett M, Kingsmore SF. Identification of the homologous beige and Chediak-Higashi genes. Nature 382:262–265, 1996.

Barrat F, Auloge L, Pastural E, Dufourcq-Lagelouse R, Vilmer E, Cant A, Weissenbach J, Le Paslier D, Fischer A, De Saint Basile G. Genetic and physical mapping of the Chédiak-Higashi syndrome on chromosome 1q42–43. Am J Hum Genet 59:625–632, 1996.

Barrat FJ, Le Deist F, Benkerrou M, Bousso P, Feldmann J, Fischer A, de Saint Basile G. Defective CTLA-4 cycling pathway in Chediak-Higashi syndrome: a possible mechanism for deregulation of T lymphocyte activation. Proc Natl Acad Sci USA 96:8645–8650, 1999.

Beguez-Cesar A. Neutropenia cronica maligna familiar con granulaciones atipicas de los leucocitos. Sociedad cubana de pediatr boletin 15:900–922, 1943.

Binder D, van den Broek MF, Kagi D, Bluethmann H, Fehr J, Hengartner H, Zinkernagel RM. Aplastic anemia rescued by exhaustion of cytokine-secreting CD8+ T cells in persistent infection with lymphocytic choriomeningitis virus. J Exp Med 187:1903–1920, 1998.

Blanche S, Caniglia M, Girault D, Landman J, Griscelli C, Fischer A. Treatment of hemophagocytic lymphohistiocytosis with chemotherapy and bone marrow transplantation: a single-center study of 22 cases. Blood 78: 51–54, 1991.

Blume R, Wolff S. The Chediak-Higashi syndrome: studies in four patients and a review of the literature. Medicine 51:247–280, 1972.

Burkhardt J, Wiebel F, Hester S, Argon Y. The giant organelles in beige and Chediak-Higashi fibroblasts are derived from late endosomes and mature lysosomes. J Exp Med 178:1845–1856, 1993.

Certain S, Barrat F, Pastural E, Le Deist F, Goyo-Rivas J, Jabado N, Benkerrou M, Seger R, Vilmer E, Beullier G, Schwarz K, Fischer A, de Saint Basile G. Protein truncation test of LYST reveals heterogenous mutations in patients with Chediak-Higashi syndrome. Blood 95:979–983, 2000.

Chan L, Lapiere J, Chen M, Traczyk T, Mancini A, Paller A, Woodley D, Marinkovich M. Partial albinism with immunodeficiency: Griscelli syndrome: report of a case and review of the literature. J Am Acad Dermatol 38:295–300, 1998.

Chen D, Guo J, Miki T, Tachibana M, Gahl W. Molecular cloning and characterization of rab27a and rab27b, novel human rab proteins shared by melanocytes and platelets. Biochem Mol Med 60:27–37, 1997.

Cheney RE, O'Shea MK, Heuser JE, Coelho MV, Nolensky JS, Forsher EM, Larson RE, Mooseker MS. Brain myosin-V is a two-headed unconventional myosin with motor activity. Cell 75:13–23, 1993.

Clementi R, zur Stadt U, Savoldi G, Varoitto S, Conter V, De Fusco C, Notarangelo LD, Schneider M, Klersy C, Janka G, Danesino C, Arico M. Six novel mutations in the PRF1 gene in children with haemophagocytic lymphohistiocytosis. J Med Genet 38:643–646, 2001.

Dekker Ohno K, Hayasaka S, Takagishi Y, Oda S, Wakasugi N, Mikoshiba K, Inouye M, Yamamura H. Endoplasmic reticulum is missing in dendritic spines of Purkinje cells of the ataxic mutant rat. Brain Res 714:226–230, 1996.

Delaney MM, Shafford EA, Al-Attar A, Pritchard J. Familial erythrophagocytic reticulosis. Complete response to combination chemotherapy. Arch Dis Child 59:173–175, 1984.

Dufourcq-Lagelouse R, Jabado N, Le Deist F, Stephan JL, Souillet G, Bruin M, Vilmer E, Schneider M, Janka G, Fischer A, de Saint Basile G. Linkage of familial hemophagocytic lymphohistiocytosis to 10q21–22 and evidence for heterogeneity. Am J Hum Genet 64:172–179, 1999a.

Dufourcq-Lagelouse R, Pastural E, Barrat F, Feldmann J, Le Deist F, Fischer A, De Saint Basile G. Genetic basis of hemophagocytic lymphohistiocytosis syndrome [review]. Int J Mol Med 4:127–133, 1999b.

Durandy A, Breton-Gorius J, Guy-Grand D, Dumez C, Griscelli C. Prenatal diagnosis of syndromes associating albinism and immune deficiencies (Chediak-Higashi syndrome and variant). Prenat Diagn 13:13–20, 1993.

Egeler RM, Shapiro R, Loechelt B, Filipovich A. Characteristic immune abnormalities in hemophagocytic lymphohistiocytosis. J Pediatr Hematol Oncol 18:340–345, 1996.

Elejalde BR, Holguin J, Valencia A, Gilbert EF, Molina J, Marin G, Arango LA. Mutations affecting pigmentation in man: I. Neuroectodermal melanolysosomal disease. Am J Med Genet 3:65–80, 1979.

Faigle W, Raposo G, Tenza D, Pinet V, Vogt AB, Kropshofer H, Fischer A, de Saint Basile G, Amigorena S. Deficient peptide loading and MHC class II endosomal sorting in a human genetic immunodeficiency disease: the Chediak-Higashi syndrome. J Cell Biol 141:1121–1134, 1998.

Faroudi M, Utzny C, Salio M, Cerundolo V, Guiraud M, Muller S, Valitutti S. Lytic versus stimulatory synapse in cytotoxic T lymphocyte/target cell interaction: manifestation of a dual activation threshold. Proc Natl Acad Sci USA 100:14145–14150, 2003.

Farquhar J, Claireaux A. Familial haemophagocytic reticulosis. Arch Dis Child 27:519–525, 1952.

Favara BE. Hemophagocytic lymphohistiocytosis: a hemophagocytic syndrome [review]. Semin Diagn Pathol 9:63–74, 1992.

Feldmann J, Callebaut I, Raposo G, Certain S, Bacq D, Dumont C, Lambert N, Ouachee-Chardin M, Chedeville G, Tamary H, Minard-Colin V,

Vilmer E, Blanche S, Le Deist F, Fischer A, de Saint Basile G. Munc13-4 is essential for cytolytic granules fusion and is mutated in a form of familial hemophagocytic lymphohistiocytosis (FHL3). Cell 115:461–473, 2003.

Feldmann J, Le Deist F, Ouachee-Chardin M, Certain S, Alexander S, Quartier P, Haddad E, Wulffraat N, Casanova JL, Blanche S, Fischer A, de Saint Basile G. Functional consequences of perforin gene mutations in 22 patients with familial haemophagocytic lymphohistiocytosis. Br J Haematol 117:965–972, 2002.

Filipovich AH. Hemophagocytic lymphohistiocytosis: a lethal disorder of immune regulation. J Pediatr 130:337–338, 1997.

Fischer A, Cerf-Bensussan N, Blanche S, Le Deist F, Bremard-Oury C, Leverger G, Schaison G, Durandy A, Griscelli C. Allogeneic bone marrow transplantation for erythrophagocytic lymphohistiocytosis. J Pediatr 108:267–270, 1986.

Fischer A, Virelizier JL, Arenzana-Seisdedos F, Perez N, Nezelof C, Griscelli C. Treatment of four patients with erythrophagocytic lymphohistiocytosis by a combination of VP16-213, steroids, intrathecal methotrexate and cranial irradiation. Pediatrics 76:263–268, 1985.

Fukuda M. Distinct Rab binding specificity of Rim1, Rim2, rabphilin, and Noc2. Identification of a critical determinant of Rab3A/Rab27A recognition by Rim2. J Biol Chem 278:15373–15380, 2003.

Goransdotter Ericson K, Fadeel B, Nilsson-Ardnor S, Soderhall C, Samuelsson A, Janka G, Schneider M, Gurgey A, Yalman N, Revesz T, Egeler R, Jahnukainen K, Storm-Mathiesen I, Haraldsson A, Poole J, de Saint Basile G, Nordenskjold M, Henter J. Spectrum of perforin gene mutations in familial hemophagocytic lymphohistiocytosis. Am J Hum Genet 68:590–597, 2001.

Graham GE, Graham LM, Bridge PJ, Maclaren LD, Wolff JEA, Coppes MJ, Egeler RM. Further evidence for genetic heterogeneity in familial hemophagocytic lymphohistiocytosis (FHLH). Pediatr Res 48:227–232, 2000.

Griscelli C, Durandy A, Guy-Grand D, Daguillard F, Herzog C, Prunieras M. A syndrome associating partial albinism and immunodeficiency. Am J Med 65:691–702, 1978.

Haddad E, Sulis ML, Jabado N, Blanche S, Fischer A, Tardieu M. Frequency and severity of central nervous system lesions in hemophagocytic lymphohistiocytosis. Blood 89:794–800, 1997.

Haddad EK, Wu X, Hammer JA, Henkart PA. Defective granule exocytosis in rab27a-deficient lymphocytes from ashen mice. J Cell Biol 152:835–842, 2001.

Harfi H, Brismar J, Hainau B, Sabbah R. Partial albinism, immunodeficiency, and progressive white matter disease: a new primary immunodeficiency. Allergy Proc 13:321–328, 1992.

Henkart PA. Mechanism of lymphocyte-mediated cytotoxicity. Annu Rev Immunol 3:31–58, 1985.

Henter JI, Arico M, Elinder G, Imashuku S, Janka G. Familial hemophagocytic lymphohistiocytosis. Primary hemophagocytic lymphohistiocytosis. Hematol Oncol Clin North Am 12:417–433, 1998.

Henter J-I, Elinder G, Öst A. Diagnostic guidelines for hemophagocytic lymphohistiocytosis, The FHL Study Group of the Histiocyte Society. Semin Oncol 18:29–33, 1991a.

Henter JI, Elinder G, Soder O, Hansson M, Andersson B, Andersson U. Hypercytokinemia in familial hemophagocytic lymphohistiocytosis. Blood 78:2918–2922, 1991b.

Henter J-I, Elinder G, Söder Q, Öst A. Incidence and clinical features of familial hemophagocytic lymphohistiocytosis in Sweden. Acta Pardiatr Scand 80:428–435, 1991c.

Henter JI, Nennesmo I. Neuropathologic findings and neurologic symptoms in twenty-three children with hemophagocytic lymphohistiocytosis. J Pediatr 130:358–365, 1997.

Huang JD, Mermall V, Strobel MC, Russell LB, Mooseker MS, Copeland NG, Jenkins NA. Molecular genetic dissection of mouse unconventional myosin-VA: tail region mutations. Genetics 148:1963–1972, 1998.

Huang JF, Yang Y, Sepulveda H, Shi W, Hwang I, Peterson PA, Jackson MR, Sprent J, Cai Z. TCR-mediated internalization of peptide-MHC complexes acquired by T cells. Science 286(5441):952–954, 1999.

Hudrisier D, Riond J, Mazarguil H, Gairin JE, Joly E. Cutting edge: CTLs rapidly capture membrane fragments from target cells in a TCR signaling-dependent manner. J Immunol 166:3645–3649, 2001.

Jabado N, Degraeffmeeder ER, Cavazzana-Calvo M, Haddad E, Le Deist F, Benkerrou M, Dufourcq R, Caillat S, Blanche S, Fischer A. Treatment of familial hemophagocytic lymphohistiocytosis with bone marrow transplantation from HLA genetically nonidentical donors. Blood 90:4743–4748, 1997.

Janka GE. Familial hemophagocytic lymphohistiocytosis. Eur J Pediatr 140:221–230, 1983.

Janka G, Imashuku S, Elinder G, Schneider M, Henter JI. Infection- and malignancy-associated hemophagocytic syndromes. Secondary hemophagocytic lymphohistiocytosis. Hematol Oncol Clin North Am 12:435–444, 1998.

Jenkins NA, Copeland NG, Taylor BA, Lee BK. Dilute (d) coat colour mutation of DBA/2J mice is associated with the site of integration of an ecotropic MuLV genome. Nature 293(5831):370–374, 1981.

Jordan MB, Hildeman D, Kappler J, Marrack P. An animal model of hemophagocytic lymphohistiocytosis (HLH): CD8+ T cells and interferon gamma are essential for the disorder. Blood 104:735–743, 2004.

Kagi D, Ledermann B, Burki K, Seiler P, Odermatt B, Olsen KJ, Podack ER, Zinkernagel RM, Hengartner H. Cytotoxicity mediated by T cells and natural killer cells is greatly impaired in perforin-deficient mice. Nature 369(6475):31–37, 1994.

Kagi D, Odermatt B, Mak TW. Homeostatic regulation of CD8+ T cells by perforin. Eur J Immunol 29:3262–3272, 1999.

Karim MA, Suzuki K, Fukai K, Oh J, Nagle DL, Moore KJ, Barbosa E, Falik-Borenstein T, Filipovich A, Ishida Y, Kivrikko S, Klein C, Kreuz F, Levin A, Miyajima H, Regueiro J, Russo C, Uyama E, Vierimaa O, Spritz RA. Apparent genotype–phenotype correlation in childhood, adolescent, and adult Chediak-Higashi syndrome. Am J Med Genet 108:16–22, 2002.

Katano H, Ali MA, Patera AC, Catalfamo M, Jaffe ES, Kimura H, Dale JK, Straus SE, Cohen JI. Chronic active Epstein-Barr virus infection associated with mutations in perforin that impair its maturation. Blood 103:1244–1252, 2004.

Klein C, Philippe N, Le Deist F, Fraitag S, Prost C, Durandy A, Fischer A, Griscelli C. Partial albinism with immunodeficiency (Griscelli syndrome). J Pediatr 125(6 Pt 1):886–895, 1994.

Kogawa K, Lee SM, Villanueva J, Marmer D, Sumegi J, Filipovich AH. Perforin expression in cytotoxic lymphocytes from patients with hemophagocytic lymphohistiocytosis and their family members. Blood 99:61–66, 2002.

Lambert J, Naeyaert J, Callens T, De Paepe A, Messiaen L. Human myosin V gene produces different transcripts in a cell type-specific manner. Biochem Biophys Res Commun 252:329–333, 1998.

Landman-Parker J, Le Deist F, Blaise A, Brison O, Fischer A. Partial engraftment of donor bone marrow cells associated with long-term remission of haemophagocytic lymphohistiocytosis. Br J Haematol 85:37–41, 1993.

Lichtenheld MG, Podack ER. Structure of the human perforin gene: a simple gene organization with interesting potential regulatory sequences. J Immunol 143:4267–4274, 1989.

Lipton JM, Westra S, Haverty CE, Roberts D, Harris NL. Case records of the Massachusetts General Hospital. Weekly clinicopathological exercises. Case 28-2004. Newborn twins with thrombocytopenia, coagulation defects, and hepatosplenomegaly. N Engl J Med 351:1120–1123, 2004.

Matesic LE, Yip R, Reuss AE, Swing DA, O'Sullivan TN, Fletcher CF, Copeland NG, Jenkins NA. Mutations in Mlph, encoding a member of the Rab effector family, cause the melanosome transport defects observed in leaden mice. Proc Natl Acad Sci USA 98:10238–10243, 2001.

Matloubian M, Suresh M, Glass A, Galvan M, Chow K, Whitmire JK, Walsh CM, Clark WR, Ahmed R. A role for perforin in downregulating T-cell responses during chronic viral infection. J Virol 73:2527–2536, 1999.

Ménasché G, Feldmann J, Houdusse A, Desaymard C, Fischer A, Goud B, de Saint Basile G. Biochemical and functional characterization of Rab27a mutations occurring in Griscelli syndrome patients. Blood 101:2736–2742, 2003a.

Ménasché G, Ho CH, Sanal O, Feldmann J, Tezcan I, Ersoy F, Houdusse A, Fischer A, de Saint Basile G. Griscelli syndrome restricted to hypopigmentation results from a melanophilin defect (GS3) or a MYO5A F-exon deletion (GS1). J Clin Invest 112:450–456, 2003b.

Ménasché G, Pastural E, Feldmann J, Certain S, Ersoy F, Dupuis S, Wulffraat N, Bianci D, Fischer A, Le Deist F, de Saint Basile G. Mutations in RAB27A cause Griscelli syndrome associated with hemophagocytic syndrome. Nat Genet 25:173–176, 2000.

Mercer JA, Sepenack PK, Strobel MC, Copeland NG, Jenkins NA. Novel myosin heavy chain encoded by murine dilute coat colour locus. Nature 349:709–713, 1991.

Nagle DL, Karim AM, Woolf EA, Holmgren L, Bork P, Misumi DJ, McGrail SH, Dussault BJ, Perou CM, Boissy RE, Duyk GM, Spritz RA, Moore KJ. Identification and mutation analysis of the complete gene for Chediak-Higashi syndrome. Nat Genet 14:307–311, 1996.

Nakajima H, Cella M, Bouchon A, Grierson HL, Lewis J, Duckett CS, Cohen JI, Colonna M. Patients with X-linked lymphoproliferative disease have a defect in 2B4 receptor-mediated NK cell cytotoxicity. Eur J Immunol 30:3309–3318, 2000.

Nansen A, Jensen T, Christensen JP, Andreasen SO, Ropke C, Marker O, Thomsen AR. Compromised virus control and augmented perforin-mediated immunopathology in IFN-gamma-deficient mice infected with lymphocytic choriomeningitis virus. J Immunol 163:6114–6122, 1999.

Ohadi M, Lalloz M, Sham P, Zhao J, Dearlove A, Shiach C, Kinsey S, Rhodes M, Layton D. Localization of a gene for familial hemophagocytic lymphohistiocytosis at chromosome 9q21.3–22 by homozygosity mapping. Am J Hum Genet 64:165–171, 1999.

Parolini S, Bottino C, Falco M, Aug̣ugliaro R, Giliani S, Franceschini R, Ochs HD, Wolf H, Bonnefoy JY, Biassoni R, Moretta L, Notarangelo LD, Moretta A. X-linked lymphoproliferative disease. 2B4 molecules displaying inhibitory rather than activating function are responsible for the inability of natural killer cells to kill Epstein-Barr virus–infected cells. J Exp Med 192:337–346, 2000.

Pastural E, Barrat FJ, Dufourcq-Lagelouse R, Certain S, Sanal O, Jabado N, Seger R, Griscelli C, Fischer A, de Saint Basile G. Griscelli disease maps to chromosome 15q21 and is associated with mutations in the myosin-Va gene. Nat Genet 16:289–292, 1997.

Pastural E, Ersoy F, Yalman N, Wulffraat N, Grillo E, Ozkinay F, Tezcan I, Gedikoğlu G, Philippe N, Fischer A, de Saint Basile G. Two genes are responsible for Griscelli syndrome at the same 15q21 locus. Genomics 63: 299–306, 2000.

Perou CM, Leslie JD, Green W, Li L, Ward DM, Kaplan J. The beige/Chediak-Higashi syndrome gene encodes a widely expressed cytosolic protein. J Biol Chem 272:29790–29794, 1997.

Prekeris R, Terrian D. Brain myosin V is a synaptic vesicle–associated motor protein: evidence for a Ca^{2+}-dependent interaction with the synaptobrevin-synaptophysin complex. J Cell Biol 137:1589–1601, 1997.

Provance DJ, Wei M, Ipe V, Mercer JA. Cultured melanocytes from dilute mutant mice exhibit dendritic morphology and altered melanosome distribution. Proc Natl Acad Sci USA 93:14554–14558, 1996.

Rossi CP, McAllister A, Tanguy M, Kagi D, Brahic M. Theiler's virus infection of perforin-deficient mice. J Virol 72:4515–4519, 1998.

Sanal O, Ersoy F, Tezcan I, Metin A, Yel L, Menasche G, Gurgey A, Berkel I, de Saint Basile G. Griscelli disease: genotype–phenotype correlation in an array of clinical heterogeneity. J Clin Immunol 22:237–243, 2002.

Sanal O, Yel L, Kucukali T, Gilbert-Barnes E, Tardieu M, Texcan I, Ersoy F, Metin A, de Saint Basile G. An allelic variant of Griscelli disease: presentation with severe hypotonia, mental-motor retardation, and hypopigmentation consistent with Elejalde syndrome (neuroectodermal melanolysosomal disorder). J Neurol 247:570–572, 2000.

Spritz RA. Genetic defects in Chediak-Higashi syndrome and the beige mouse. J Clin Immunol 18:97–105, 1998.

Stephan J, Donadieu J, Ledeist F, Blanche S, Griscelli C, Fischer A. Treatment of familial hemophagocytic lymphohistiocytosis with antithymocyte globulins, steroids, and cyclosporin A. Blood 82:2319–2323, 1993.

Stepp S, Dufourcq-Lagelouse R, Le Deist F, Bhawan S, Certain S, Mathew P, Henter J, Bennett M, Fischer A, de Saint Basile G, Kumar V. Perforin gene defects in familial hemophagocytic lymphohistiocytosis. Science 286:1957–1959, 1999.

Stepp SE, Mathew PA, Bennett M, de Saint Basile G, Kumar V. Perforin: more than just an effector molecule. Immunol Today 21:254–256, 2000.

Stinchcombe JC, Barral DC, Mules EH, Booth S, Hume AN, Machesky LM, Seabra MC, Griffiths GM. Rab27a is required for regulated secretion in cytotoxic T lymphocytes. J Cell Biol 152:825–834, 2001a.

Stinchcombe JC, Bossi G, Booth S, Griffiths GM. The immunological synapse of CTL contains a secretory domain and membrane bridges. Immunity 15:751–761, 2001b.

Sullivan KE, Delaat CA, Douglas SD, Filipovich AH. Defective natural killer cell function in patients with hemophagocytic lymphohistiocytosis and in first degree relatives. Pediatr Res 44:465–468, 1998.

Takagishi Y, Oda S, Hayasaka S, Dekker Ohno K, Shikata T, Inouye M, Yamamura H. The dilute-lethal (dl) gene attacks a Ca^{2+} store in the dendritic spine of Purkinje cells in mice. Neurosci Lett 215:169–172, 1996.

Tangye SG, Phillips JH, Lanier LL, Nichols KE. Functional requirement for SAP in 2B4-mediated activation of human natural killer cells as revealed by the X-linked lymphoproliferative syndrome. J Immunol 165:2932–2936, 2000.

Ueda I, Morimoto A, Inaba T, Yagi T, Hibi S, Sugimoto T, Sako M, Yanai F, Fukushima T, Nakayama M, Ishii E, Imashuku S. Characteristic perforin gene mutations of haemophagocytic lymphohistiocytosis patients in Japan. Br J Haematol 121:503–510, 2003.

Uellner R, Zvelebil MJ, Hopkins J, Jones J, MacDougall LK, Morgan BP, Podack E, Waterfield MD, Griffiths GM. Perforin is activated by a proteolytic cleavage during biosynthesis which reveals a phospholipid-binding C2 domain. EMBO J 16:7287–7296, 1997.

von Herrath M, Coon B, Homann D, Wolfe T, Guidotti LG. Thymic tolerance to only one viral protein reduces lymphocytic choriomeningitis virus-induced immunopathology and increases survival in perforin-deficient mice. J Virol 73:5918–5925, 1999.

Voskoboinik I, Thia MC, De Bono A, Browne K, Cretney E, Jackson JT, Darcy PK, Jane SM, Smyth MJ, Trapani JA. The functional basis for hemophagocytic lymphohistiocytosis in a patient with co-inherited missense mutations in the perforin (PFN1) gene. J Exp Med 200:811–816, 2004.

Wagner M, Muller-Berghaus J, Schroeder R, Sollbergh S, Luka J, Leyssens N, Schneider B, Krueger G. Human herpesvirus-6 (HHV-6)-associated necrotizing encephalitis in Griscelli's syndrome. J Med Virol 53:306–312, 1997.

Ware R, Friedman HS, Kinney TR, Kurtzberg J, Chaffee S, Falletta JM. Familial erythrophagocytic lymphohistiocytosis: late relapse despite continuous high-dose VP-16 chemotherapy. Med Pediatr Oncol 18:27–29, 1990.

White DW, Badovinac VP, Kollias G, Harty JT. Cutting edge: antilisterial activity of CD8+ T cells derived from TNF-deficient and TNF/perforin double-deficient mice. J Immunol 165:5–9, 2000.

Wilson SM, Yip R, Swing DA, O'Sullivan TN, Zhang Y, Novak EK, Swank RT, Russell LB, Copeland NG, Jenkins NA. A mutation in Rab27a causes the vesicle transport defects observed in ashen mice. Proc Natl Acad Sci USA 97:7933–7938, 2000.

Windhorst DB, Padgett G. The Chediak-Higashi syndrome and the homologous trait in animals. J Invest Dermatol 60:529–537, 1973.

Wu X, Bowers B, Wei Q, Kochner B, Hammer JA. Myosin V associates with melanosomes in mouse melanocytes: evidence that myosin V is an organelle motor. J Cell Sci 110:847–859, 1997.

Wu XS, Rao K, Zhang H, Wang F, Sellers JR, Matesic LE, Copeland NG, Jenkins NA, Hammer JA 3rd. Identification of an organelle receptor for myosin-Va. Nat Cell Biol 4:271–278, 2002.

42

Genetically Determined Deficiencies of the Complement System

KATHLEEN E. SULLIVAN and JERRY A. WINKELSTEIN

The complement system is composed of a series of plasma proteins that play a critical role in host defense and inflammation. The first patient with a genetically determined deficiency of an individual component of the complement system was described in 1960 (Silverstein, 1960). Since then, inherited deficiencies of nearly all of the individual components of complement have been identified (Ross and Densen, 1984; Figueroa and Densen, 1991). In this chapter, we review the biochemistry and biology of the normal complement system and relate them to the clinical presentation of complement deficiency diseases and their molecular genetic basis.

The Normal Complement System

Most of the biologic functions of the complement system are mediated by the third component (C3) and the terminal components (C5–C9) (Fig. 42.1). In order to subserve their defensive and inflammatory functions, however, C3 and C5–C9 must be activated. At least three pathways exist by which they may be activated: the classical pathway, the alternative pathway, and the lectin pathway.

The Classical Pathway

Activation of the classical pathway (Fig. 42.1) is usually initiated by antigen/antibody complexes (reviewed in Sullivan and Winkelstein, 2001). Antibodies of the appropriate class (IgG or IgM) and subclass (IgG1, IgG2, and IgG3) bind to the antigen, forming an immune complex which then is capable of binding and activating the first component of complement (C1). C1 is composed of three distinct subunits, C1q, C1r, and C1s, present in a molecular ratio of 2:2:1. It is the C1q that binds to the heavy chain of the immunoglobulin molecules and is responsible for

activating C1r, which in turn activates C1s. Activated C1s possesses serine protease activity and activates the fourth component (C4). Activation of C4 results in the cleavage of a small fragment (C4a) from the parent molecule, exposing an intrachain reactive thiolester in the larger cleavage product (C4b). The larger fragment (C4b) is then able to bind covalently to immunoglobulins of the immune complex, or to the surface of the cells that carry the immune complex (e.g., microbes), by esterification of hydroxyl groups of carbohydrates or amidation of amino groups of proteins by the acyl group of the thiolester. Activation of the classical pathway continues with the activation of the second component (C2) by C1s. The activation of C2 results in its cleavage into a small peptide (C2b), which is released into the fluid phase, and a larger fragment (C2a). The C2a remains complexed with the C4b to create a bimolecular enzyme, C4b,2a, which is capable of activating the third component (C3) and initiating the assembly of the terminal components (C5–C9) into the membrane attack complex (MAC).

If the activation of the classical pathway were to proceed uncontrolled, the phlogistic activities of C3 and the terminal components could be produced in excessive amounts, resulting in immunopathologic damage to the host. Fortunately, a number of factors control the assembly and expression of the C3-cleaving enzyme, C4b,2a. First, the C4b,2a enzyme is very labile and undergoes spontaneous decay with release of the C2a and loss of enzymatic activity. Second, the enzymatic activity of both C1r and C1s can be inhibited by C1 esterase inhibitor (C1INH). C1 esterase inhibitor is a serine protease inhibitor that binds covalently to activated C1r and C1s and inactivates them, leading to the dissociation of the C1 macromolecular complex. Third, another protein, C4 binding protein (C4bp), binds to C4b and exerts two regulatory effects. It increases the rate of dissociation of C2a from the C4b and also makes the C4b more susceptible to

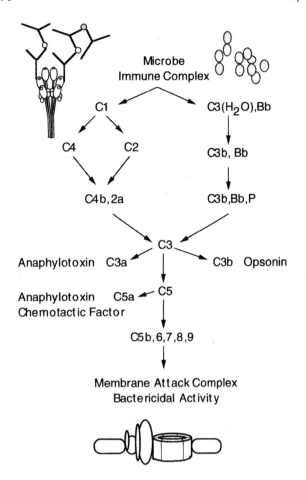

Figure 42.1. The complement system. The classical pathway is typically activated by immune complexes binding to C1q. The alternative pathway is activated directly by microorganisms. The actions of the two pathways converge on the C3 protein.

the action of yet another inhibitor, factor I. Finally, a fourth inhibitor, decay accelerating factor (DAF), also promotes the release of C2a from the C4b,2a enzyme.

The Alternative Pathway

Activation of the alternative pathway (Fig. 42. 1) can occur without the participation of antibody (Fearon, 1979). Native C3, like native C4, contains an internal thiolester that slowly undergoes spontaneous hydrolysis. This hydrolyzed C3, or $C3(H_2O)$, is capable of binding factor B, which allows its cleavage by factor D into two fragments. The larger fragment, Bb, remains attached to the $C3(H_2O)$, creating a low-grade C3-cleaving enzyme, $C3(H_2O)$,Bb. The cleavage of C3, like that of C4, exposes a reactive thiolester in the larger cleavage product, C3b, allowing covalent binding of the nascent C3b to suitable cell surfaces (such as microbial surfaces) through transacylation with hydroxyl or amino groups. The cell-bound C3b then can bind native factor B, allowing its cleavage by factor D to form a highly efficient C3-cleaving enzyme, C3b,Bb. It should be noted that since activation of the classical pathway results in the generation of nascent C3b, activation of the classical pathway can lead to activation of the alternative pathway. In addition, since C3b is both the product of the alternative pathway C3-cleaving enzyme and also is a component of the enzyme itself, the activation of C3 via the alternative pathway creates a positive amplification feedback loop (Fig. 42.1).

As is the case in the classical pathway, a number of factors act to modulate the activity of the alternative pathway. First, like C4b,2a, the C3b,Bb enzyme rapidly undergoes spontaneous decay as a result of dissociation of Bb. Properdin (P) stabilizes the binding of Bb to the C3b and thereby retards the enzyme's intrinsic decay. Another control protein, factor H, competes with factor B for binding to C3b but also displaces Bb from the enzyme complex. A third control protein, factor I, inhibits the alternative pathway C3-cleaving enzyme by inactivating the cell-bound C3b through proteolytic cleavage to create iC3b, a molecule that is unable to function in the C3bBb enzyme.

The Lectin Pathway

In recent years, evidence has accumulated that a third mechanism exists by which C3 can be activated. Mannose-binding lectin (MBL) is a member of the collectin family of proteins and is composed of identical subunits. The predominant circulating form is a 600,000 kDa multimer (Lipscombe et al., 1995). Although the binding of each carbohydrate recognition domain is relatively weak, the presence of multiple binding sites probably endows the molecule with significant avidity when it binds to microbial surfaces with repeating sugar groups. MBL is capable of binding to a variety of microorganisms, including bacteria such as *Haemophilus influenzae*, *Neisseria meningitidis*, and streptococci, fungi such as cryptococcus and candida, and several viruses, but the binding is significantly impaired by the presence of a capsule.

MBL is capable of activating C3 via the classical pathway without a requirement for C1q or immunoglobulin, thereby playing a role in so-called natural immunity. The multimer interacts with novel serine proteases, termed *MBL-associated serine proteases* (MASP1 and MASP2), proteins that share 39% homology with both human C1r and C1s. Like C1s, MASP1 and MASP2 can cleave both C4 and C2, thereby generating C4b,2a and its C3-cleaving activity. In addition, there is some evidence to support the ability of the MBL–MASP complex to activate C3 via the alternative pathway and directly.

Activation of C3 and the Terminal Components

The activation of C3 via either the classical or alternative pathway (Fig. 42.1) results in its cleavage into two fragments of unequal size (reviewed in Hostetter and Gordon, 1987). Cleavage of C3 releases a small peptide (C3a) from the parent molecule, exposing the reactive thiolester in the larger fragment (C3b), which in turn allows the covalent binding of the C3b to immune complexes or cell surfaces. The cell-bound C3b can then act as an opsonin (see below) or combine with either the classical pathway or alternative pathway C3-cleaving enzymes to create two new enzymes, the classical and alternative pathway C5-cleaving enzymes. The classical pathway C3-cleaving enzyme is composed of C4b,2a,3b, whereas the alternative pathway C3-cleaving enzyme is composed of $(C3b)_2$,Bb. Activation of C5 by either enzyme results in its cleavage into two fragments of unequal size. The smaller fragment, C5a, is released into the fluid phase where it can act as an anaphylatoxic or chemotactic fragment (see below). If the larger fragment, C5b, combines immediately with C6, it initiates formation of the MAC, a multimolecular complex of C5b, C6, C7, C8, and C9 that possesses cytolytic activity. A number of proteins regulate the formation of the MAC. Homologous restriction factor (HRF), also known as C8 binding protein (C8bp), is an integral membrane protein present on a wide variety of peripheral blood cells that impedes the formation and insertion of the MAC. A second protein, termed *HRF20* or *CD59*, inhibits the unfolding of C9 that is required for membrane insertion.

Biological Consequences of Complement Activation

Activation of C3 and C5–C9 results in the generation of a variety of biologic activities that play an important role in host defense and inflammation. The smaller cleavage products of C3 and C5 (C3a and C5a) possess anaphylatoxic activity, causing histamine release from basophils and mast cells, increased vascular permeability, and smooth muscle contraction (Hugli, 1981). On a mole-per-mole basis, C5a is significantly more potent as an anaphylatoxin than is C3a. C5a is also a potent chemotactic agent, attracting mobile phagocytic cells to sites of complement activation (Snyderman and Goetzl, 1981). In addition, it can cause degranulation of phagocytic cells with discharge of lysosomal enzymes, enhanced production of microbicidal oxygen products, and production of leukotrienes.

The larger cleavage product of C3 (C3b) is an important opsonin when fixed to the surface of an activating particle, such as a microorganism, and binding to the phagocytic cell through CR1 receptors (Johnston et al., 1969; Hostetter and Gordon, 1987). Particles bearing the C3b degradation product iC3b on their surface can interact in a similar fashion with another receptor on the phagocytic surface, CR3. Since iC3b is the major C3 cleavage product formed on most particles in the presence of serum, it is probably the most important C3-derived opsonin in vivo.

Bactericidal activity is generated by activation of the terminal components and assembly of C5b–C9 into the membrane attack complex. However, only gram-negative bacteria are susceptible to the bactericidal activity of the complement system because gram-positive bacteria have a thick protective cell wall.

The complement system also plays an important role in the clearance and processing of soluble immune complexes (Schifferli et al., 1986). A number of mechanisms exist by which the complement system can modify the structure of immune complexes, influence their biological properties, and enhance their clearance. First, C3b fixed to an immune complex can act as an opsonin, favoring their ingestion by phagocytic cells. Second, the binding of C3b to immune complexes retards their precipitation from serum (Schifferli et al., 1980, 1985) and their deposition in tissues, and also helps solubilize them once they have precipitated (Czop and Nussenzweig, 1976; Takahaski et al., 1978; Schifferli et al., 1985). Finally, the complement system in primates provides an additional mechanism for immune complex clearance. Primates possess CR1 receptors on their erythrocytes and circulating immune complexes bearing C3b will fix to them. The erythrocytes bearing immune complexes on their surface then pass through the liver and spleen, where Kupffer cells and other phagocytic cells strip the immune complexes from the erythrocytes and return the erythrocytes to the circulation (Cornacoff et al., 1983). In this manner, erythrocytes serve to capture immune complexes in the circulation, prevent them from depositing in organs such as the kidney, and enhance their clearance by the reticuloendothelial system.

The complement system also plays an important role in the production of a normal humoral immune response (Pepys, 1974; Ochs et al., 1983; O'Neil et al., 1988). Animals and humans deficient in C2, C3, or C4 exhibit impaired primary and secondary antibody production (Bottger et al., 1986; Ochs et al., 1983,

1993; O'Neil et al., 1988; Fischer et al., 1996; Ma et al., 1996). Mice deficient in CR1 and CR2 receptors are similarly impaired in functional humoral responses (Molina et al., 1996). The explanation for the impaired antibody responses relates to the loss of C3d stimulation of B cells through the CR2 receptor (CD21) (Dempsy et al., 1996). Antigen associated with C3d stimulates B cells more effectively than antigen alone. Signaling through the CD19–CD21 complex links the complement receptor to distal signaling effects mediated through the antigen receptor complex. Additionally, complement also aids in follicular dendritic cell trapping of antigen, thereby augmenting a humoral response (Ochs et al., 1983; Molina et al., 1996).

Pathophysiologic Basis of Clinical Manifestations of Complement Deficiencies

The clinical expression of genetically determined deficiencies of the complement system is variable and depends on the role of the deficient component in normal host defense and inflammation (Tables 42.1 and 42.2). Individuals with genetically determined deficiencies of complement components may have an increased susceptibility to infection, rheumatic disorders, or angioedema or may be asymptomatic.

Infection

A number of studies in experimental animals have established that the complement system plays a critical role in the host's defense against infection (Table 42.2). Complement is especially important during the first few hours of infection (Winkelstein et al., 1975) and in containing the infection at its initial site (Bakker-Wondenberg et al., 1979). If dissemination should occur, complement contributes to the clearance of microbes from the bloodstream (Hosea et al., 1980). Furthermore, complement plays an important role in resistance to infection in both the "immune" host with high levels of antibody and in the "nonimmune" host with little if any antibody.

Although studies in experimental animals have shown that the complement system has the potential to contribute to the host's defense against a wide variety of bacteria, fungi, and viruses, clinical experience would suggest that the greatest susceptibility of complement-deficient patients is to bacterial infections (Ross and Densen, 1984; Figueroa and Densen, 1991). The kinds of bacteria that most commonly cause infections in complement-deficient patients reflect the specific role of the missing component in normal host defense. For example, the major cleavage products of C3 (C3b and C3bi) are important opsonins. Therefore, patients with a deficiency of C3 have a marked increased susceptibility to infection with those bacteria for which opsonization is the primary mechanism of host defense (e.g., *Streptococcus pneumoniae*, *Streptococcus pyogenes*, and *Haemophilus influenzae*). Patients with a deficiency of C1, C4, or C2 also have an increased susceptibility to these same encapsulated bacteria, since these components are necessary for the activation of C3 via the classical pathway. However, they do not appear to be as susceptible as patients with C3 deficiency, since their alternative pathway is intact and able to activate C3.

Activation of the terminal components, C5–C9, results in the assembly of the membrane attack complex and the generation of bactericidal activity for gram-negative bacteria. Therefore, patients with deficiencies of one of the terminal components have an increased susceptibility to infection with those gram-negative bacteria, such as *Neisseria meningitidis*, that are most susceptible to the

Table 42.1. Complement Component Deficiencies: Genetic Basis

Component	Gene Name	Chromosomal Location	Size of Gene	Inheritance Pattern
C1q	C1QA, C1QB, C1QG	1p36.3–p34.1	3 kb	AR
C1r/C1s	C1R/C1S	12p13	<50 kb	AR
C4	C4A, C4B	6p21.3	C4A = 22 kb, C4B = 16–22 kb	AR
C2	C2	6p21.3	18 kb	AR
C3	C3	19q13	41 kb	AR
C5	C5	9q34.1	10 kb	AR
C6	C6	5p13	80 kb	AR
C7	C7	5p13	80 kb	AR
C8A/B	C8A/C8B	1p32	A = 70 kb	AR
C8G	C8G	9	1.8 kb	AR
C9	C9	5p13	80 kb	AR
Factor B	BF	6p21.3	6 kb	AR
Factor D	DF	19p13.3	4 kb	AR
Factor H	HFI	1q32	80–100 kb	AR and AD
Factor I	IF	4q25	63 kb	AR and AD
Properdin	PFC	Xp11.4–p11.23	6 kb	X-linked recessive
C4bp	C4BPA, C4BPB	1q32	C4bpA = 40 kb, C4bpB = 13 kb	Unknown
C1 inhibitor	C1NH	11q11–q13.1	17 kb	AD
DAF	DAF	1q32	35 kb	AR
CD59	CD59	11p13	20 kb	AR
MBL	MBL	10q11.2–q21	7 kb	AD and AR

AD, autosomal dominant; AR, autosomal recessive.

bactericidal activities of the complement system. As expected, infections with gram-positive bacteria, such as the pneumococcus, are not seen with any greater frequency in patients with deficiencies of a terminal component because these bacteria are not susceptible to the bactericidal activity of the complement system.

Although blood-borne, systemic infections such as bacteremia and meningitis are the most common bacterial infections reported in complement-deficient patients (Ross and Densen, 1984; Figueroa and Densen, 1991), localized infections such as sinusitis, otitis, and pneumonia have also been seen. Infections in complement-deficient individuals are usually caused by the common encapsulated bacteria to which normal hosts are also susceptible, such as the pneumococcus, streptococcus, and meningococcus. However, systemic infections with unencapsulated strains of pathogenic bacteria such as the meningococcus, which are extremely rare in normal individuals, have been described in a number of complement-deficient individuals (Hummel et al., 1987). Some clinical features of meningococcal infections are different in complement-deficient individuals from those of meningococcal infections in individuals with an intact complement system. Two studies suggest that meningococcal disease is less severe in complement-deficient individuals and is associated with a lower mortality rate (Figueroa and Densen, 1991; Platonov et al., 1993).

Rheumatic Disorders

The pathophysiologic basis for the occurrence of rheumatic disorders in patients with genetically determined complement deficiencies is not completely understood. There are a number of hypotheses to explain the association of rheumatic disorders and complement deficiencies. One of the more attractive explanations is based on the role of the complement system in the processing and clearance of immune complexes (Schifferli et al., 1986). Another attractive explanation relates to the recently dis-

covered role of the early components of the classical pathway, such as C1q, in the clearance of apoptotic cells (Botto et al., 1998; Navratil and Ahearn, 2000). As cells undergo apoptosis, intracellular constituents are reorganized and appear on the surface of the cell in blebs. Autoantigens targeted in patients with systemic lupus erythematosis (SLE), such as SSA and/or SSB, are often found on the surface in these blebs (Casciolo-Rosen et al., 1994), rendering a normally invisible antigen visible.

Although rheumatic disorders are a common clinical manifestation of genetically determined disorders of the complement system (Ross and Densen, 1984; Figueroa and Densen, 1991), they are seen more commonly in patients with deficiencies of the early components of the classical pathway than in deficiencies of terminal components (Table 42.2). For example, just over 30% of patients with C2 deficiency and nearly 80% of patients with either C4 or C3 deficiency have a rheumatic disease. In contrast, fewer than 10% of patients with deficiencies of C5, C6, C7, C8, or C9 have rheumatic disorders. The risk of developing a rheumatic disease for a given deficiency correlates with the inability of patients with that specific deficiency to process immune complexes. For example, serum from patients with genetically determined deficiencies of C1, C4, C2, and C3 fails to prevent the precipitation of immune complexes (Schifferli et al., 1980, 1985), does not resolubilize immune complexes once they have formed (Czop and Nussenzweig, 1976; Takahaski et al., 1978; Schifferli et al., 1985), and does not support the binding of immune complexes to CR1 receptors on human erythrocytes (Paccaud et al., 1987). Conversely, the sera of patients with deficiencies of terminal components are normal with respect to these activities.

A variety of rheumatic diseases, including SLE, discoid lupus, dermatomyositis, scleroderma, anaphylactoid purpura, vasculitis, and membranoproliferative glomerulonephritis, have been reported in patients with complement deficiencies (Ross and Densen, 1984; Figueroa and Densen, 1991). There are some clinical differences between the SLE seen in patients with C2

Table 42.2. Complement Component Deficiencies: Clinical Characteristics

Component	Patients/ Kindreds	Ethnic Predisposition	Clinical Manifestations
C1q	28/20	None	1. SLE 2. Recurrent infections
C1r/C1s	12/8	None	1. SLE 2. Recurrent infections
C4	21/17	None	1. SLE 2. Recurrent infections
C2	Hundreds	Caucasian	1. Recurrent infections 2. SLE
C3	22/15	None	1. Streptococcal infections 2. Neisserial infections 3. Glomerulonephritis
C5	27/17	None	Neisserial infections
C6	77/49	African	1. Neisserial infections 2. SLE
C7	73/50	None	1. Neisserial infections 2. Autoimmune disorders
C8	73/52	None	Neisserial infections
C9	18/15	Asian	Neisserial infections
Factor B	1/1	Unknown	Neisserial infections
Factor D	3/2	Unknown	Recurrent infections
Factor H	12/6	None	1. Renal disease 2. Neisserial infections 3. Atypical hemolytic uremic syndrome 4. A polymorphism of Factor H (Y402H) is responsible for a 50% of age related macular degeneration
Factor I	23/19	None	1. Neisserial infections 2. Streptococcal infections 3. A typical hemolytic uremic syndrome
Properdin	70/23	Caucasian	Neisserial infections
C4bp	3/1	Unknown	Angioedema and Behcet's syndrome
C1 inhibitor	Hundreds	None	1. Angioedema 2. SLE
MBL	Thousands	None	1. Recurrent infections 2. SLE
DAF	5/3	Unknown	None known
CD59	1/1	Unknown	Hemolysis

SLE, systemic lupus erythematosis.

deficiency and the SLE seen in individuals without inherited complement deficiencies. The SLE seen in C2-deficient patients often has its onset in childhood, is frequently characterized by a prominent annular photosensitive dermatitis, and may have relatively mild pleuropericardial and renal involvement. In addition, it is not uncommon for C2-deficient patients to have low (or absent) titers of antibodies to nuclear antigen and/or native DNA (Glass et al., 1976; Provost et al., 1983; Meyer et al., 1985). In contrast, the prevalence of anti-Ro antibodies is reported to be much higher than in non–C2-deficient patients with lupus (Provost et al., 1983; Meyer et al., 1985). The SLE seen in patients with C1q deficiency tends to have severe end-organ effects and is usually associated with positive titers to nuclear antigen (Bowness et al., 1994).

Epidemiology of Complement Deficiencies

Infections and rheumatic disorders are common clinical manifestations of genetically determined complement deficiencies. Accordingly, a number of studies have attempted to estimate the incidence of complement deficiencies in these disorders to determine how frequently complement deficiencies contribute to their pathogenesis and to evaluate the utility of screening certain groups of patients for complement deficiencies.

Infection

The prevalence of complement deficiencies is significantly higher in individuals with systemic meningococcal infections than in the general population. The frequency of complement deficiencies in sporadic cases of systemic meningococcal infections has been estimated to be between 1% and 15% (Ellison et al., 1983; Merino et al., 1983; Leggiadro and Winkelstein, 1987; Rasmussen et al., 1987; Platonov et al., 1993). In general, the prevalence is even greater in those patients who have had recurrent meningococcal disease (40%) (Nielsen et al., 1989; Platonov et al., 1993), a positive family history of meningococcal disease (10%) (Nielsen et al., 1989), or an unusual serotype of the meningococcus (20%–50%) (Fijen et al., 1989). On the basis of these studies, it appears reasonable to screen any patient with a systemic meningococcal infection for a complement deficiency. Since there is a relatively high risk for recurrence, early identification of complement deficiency in patients with systemic meningococcal infections may prevent subsequent meningococcal infections.

The evidence that screening patients with systemic pneumococcal, streptococcal, or *H. influenzae* infections for complement deficiencies is useful is less compelling (Rasmussen et al., 1987; Rowe et al., 1989; Densen et al., 1990; Ekdahl et al., 1995). Although sepsis and meningitis caused by these organisms are very common among patients with inherited complement deficiencies (Ross and Densen, 1984; Figueroa and Densen, 1991), one study demonstrated only a single complement-deficient patient in a series of 389 patients with bacteremia and/or meningitis caused by bacteria other than the meningococcus (Densen et al., 1990).

Rheumatic Disorders

The prevalence of homozygous C2 deficiency is significantly higher in patients with SLE than in the general population. Genetically determined C2 deficiency is found in approximately 1 in 10,000 (0.01%) individuals in the general population (Ruddy, 1986; Sullivan et al., 1994). In contrast, the prevalence of homozygous C2 deficiency in large series of patients with SLE has varied between 0.4 and 2.0 (Glass et al., 1976; Hartung et al., 1989; Sullivan et al., 1994). Although a number of patients with genetically determined C2 deficiency have also had other rheumatic diseases (Ross and Densen, 1984; Figueroa and Densen, 1991), there have been no studies that have documented a significantly increased prevalence of C2 deficiency in these disorders.

Specific Deficiencies

Deficiencies of all of the soluble complement components and many of the membrane-bound receptors and regulatory proteins have been described in humans (Tables 42.1 and 42.2). Most are inherited as autosomal recessive disorders, although C1 esterase deficiency is inherited as an autosomal dominant disorder and properdin deficiency is inherited as an X-linked recessive disorder.

C1q Deficiency

Molecular biology and pathophysiology

Native C1q is composed of three polypeptides, C1qA, C1qB, and C1qC, each of which is encoded by one of three highly homologous genes on chromosome 1 (Sellar et al., 1991). One of each of the three C1q polypeptides combines to form the C1q subunit, six of which combine to form C1q. Each of the six globular heads of C1q is capable of binding to the CH3 domain of IgM or the CH2 domain of IgG. When at least two of the globular heads of C1q are engaged, C1r becomes activated, which in turn cleaves C1s leading to activation C3 and C5–C9 through the classical pathway. Therefore, deficiency of C1q not only affects the patient's ability to generate those biologic activities related to C3 and C5–C9, such as opsonization, chemotaxis and bactericidal activity, but it also may affect the clearance of apoptotic cells.

In some patients there is no detectable C1q protein (Leyva-Cobian et al., 1981; Berkel and Nakakuma, 1993; Loos and Colomb, 1993). Other patients produce a dysfunctional C1q molecule, which can neither bind to immunoglobulin heavy chains nor activate C1r (Thompson et al., 1980; Chapius et al., 1982; Reid and Thompson, 1983; Hannema et al., 1984; Slingsby et al., 1996). Patients with C1q deficiency (MIM 120550, 120570, 120575) have markedly reduced serum hemolytic complement activity and C1 functional activity.

The molecular defects causing C1q deficiency are diverse, although there is a nonsense mutation at amino acid position 186 of C1qA that is common among C1q-deficient patients from Turkey (Petry et al., 1996; Berkel et al., 2000). C1q deficiency is not restricted to a specific ethnic heritage and has been identified in people of European, Asian, and Arabic heritage. Mutations in each of the three chains have been identified (McAdam et al., 1988; Petry et al., 1995; Slingsby et al., 1996; Stone et al., 2000). In one case with a premature termination codon and undetectable A chain, B and C polypeptide chains were also absent, which suggests that C1A must be present for formation and secretion of C1q (Petry et al., 1995). Because there are many mutations causing C1q deficiency, carrier detection and prenatal testing rely on the identification of each individual mutation in affected family members. Allele-specific polymerase chain reaction (PCR) has been used to identify carriers of the common Turkish mutation.

Clinical expression

The most common clinical presentation of C1q deficiency is SLE (Ross and Densen, 1984; Figueroa and Densen, 1991; Bowness et al., 1994). Approximately 30 patients with C1q deficiency have been described and all but 2 have developed SLE (Bowness et al., 1994). This deficiency is the strongest known genetic risk factor for SLE. The basis for this predisposition is believed to be the result of impaired immune complex clearance and/or impaired clearance of apoptotic cells. The manifestations of SLE in patients with C1q deficiency are not markedly different from those seen in complement-sufficient people; however, the age of onset is somewhat earlier and the disease can be very severe, with significant central nervous system (CNS) involvement and nephritis. The cutaneous manifestations are typically prominent, and skin biopsies demonstrate IgG, IgM, and C3 deposition, as is characteristic for SLE.

Patients with C1q deficiency also have an increased frequency of infections with pyogenic organisms, which reflects their inability to activate the classical pathway and efficiently opsonize bacteria.

Animal model

A C1q-deficient knockout mouse spontaneously develops proliferative glomerulonephritis with subendothelial deposits of C3 and immunoglobulin. These mice have also been noted to have defective immune complex clearance (Botto et al., 1996).

C1r and C1s Deficiency

Molecular biology and pathophysiology

The genes for C1r and C1s are highly homologous and lie closely linked on chromosome 12p13 in a tail-to-tail orientation (Kusumoto et al., 1988). Both proteins contain serine esterase motifs, epidermal growth factor motifs, and several short consensus repeat units. Like most other complement components, C1r and C1s are produced primarily in liver and macrophages.

Twelve individuals with C1r deficiency (MIM 216950) have been described (Ross and Densen, 1984; Figueroa and Densen, 1991; Loos and Colomb, 1993). Typically, C1r levels are markedly reduced (1% of normal) and C1s levels are 20%–50% that of normal (Lee et al., 1978; Loos and Colomb, 1993). A single patient has been described in which C1s has been markedly reduced, while C1r levels were 50% that of normal (Suzuki et al., 1992), a finding suggesting that neither monomer is stable in the absence of the other.

Three mutations have been identified in patients with C1s deficiency (MIM 12058). One patient had a 4 bp deletion in exon 10, and two others nonsense mutations in exon 12 (Inoue et al., 1998; Endo et al., 1999; Dragon-Durey et al., 2001). The mutations in patients with C1r deficiency have not been identified, but the fact that 7 of the first 12 patients identified with C1r deficiency have been of Puerto Rican descent suggests that there may be a founder effect.

Clinical expression

The most common clinical presentation of C1r/C1s deficiency is SLE, although bacterial infections and glomerulonephritis are also seen in these patients (Figueroa and Densen, 1991; Ross and Densen, 1984).

C4 Deficiency

Molecular biology and pathophysiology

The fourth component of complement (C4) is synthesized as a single polypeptide that is proteolytically processed into a mature protein composed of three disulfide linked chains. C4 is evolutionarily related to C3, C5, and β_2 macroglobulin. It exists as two isotypes encoded by two distinct loci, C4A and C4B, within the major histocompatibility complex (MHC) class III region on chromosome 6 (Carroll et al., 1984). The two isotypes are largely identical but differ with respect to electrophoretic mobility and their specific functional hemolytic activity (Hauptmann et al., 1988). The C4A isotype is more efficient at transacylating with amino groups of proteins, and C4B is more efficient at transacylating with hydroxyl groups of carbohydrates (Dodds et al., 1996). The basis for these functional differences between C4A and C4B is four amino acids located between positions 1101 and

1106 of the α chain. C4 is the most polymorphic of the complement components; each isotype has dozens of variants. C4 is produced primarily in liver and macrophages, and it is an acute-phase reactant.

Complete deficiency of C4 (MIM 120810, 120820) is the result of being homozygous deficient at both the *C4A* and *C4B* locus (*C4A*Q0,C4B*Q0*) and is uncommon, with only approximately 20 cases described (Ross and Densen, 1984; Hauptmann et al., 1988; Figueroa and Densen, 1991). Patients who have complete C4 deficiency have markedly reduced levels of total serum hemolytic activity and both functional and antigenic C4 in their serum. Those functions of the complement system that can be mediated by activation of the alternative pathway, such as serum opsonic, chemotactic, and bactericidal activity, are present although reduced, because the alternative pathway is less efficient at activating C3 than the classical pathway.

In contrast to the rarity of patients deficient in both isotypes, deficiencies of one or the other isotype are relatively common (Hauptmann et al., 1988). Individuals heterozygous for the *C4A*Q0* null allele are found in 12%–14% of the general population while approximately 15%–16% of individuals are heterozygous for *C4B*Q0*. The corresponding frequencies for individuals homozygous for each null allele are 1% for *C4A*Q0* and 3% for *C4B*Q0*. C4A deficiency in Caucasians is typically due to a large gene deletion and arises on the extended haplotype HLA-A1-Cw7-B8-C2C-BfS-C4A*Q0-C4B1-DR3 (Kemp et al., 1987). Additionally, a 2 bp insertion in exon 29 has been identified as the most common cause of nonexpression of an intact C4A gene in Caucasians and is usually linked to HLA-B60-DR6 (Barba et al., 1993). Gene conversion can cause either C4A or C4B deficiency and additional *C4B*Q0* alleles are the result of gene deletions (Braun et al., 1990). Most other causes of C4B deficiency have not yet been identified. C4 allotyping and isotyping have been performed in a number of kindreds to determine carrier status in siblings.

Clinical expression

Most C4-deficient patients have immune complex disorders such as SLE or glomerulonephritis (Fig. 42.2) (Hauptmann et al., 1988). In fact, the most common manifestation of complete C4 deficiency is SLE. The disease onset is somewhat earlier than for SLE in complement-sufficient patents, and cutaneous features, including Raynaud's phenomenon and vasculitic ulcers, are common. Anti-DNA titers are sometimes absent, as is also seen in C2-deficient SLE patients. Biopsies of inflammatory lesions from C4-deficient patients usually demonstrate the presence of immunoglobulin and C1q, consistent with immune complex deposition and complement activation. C3 deposition has also been identified in kidney and skin, suggesting that the alternative pathway can also play a role in the development of these lesions (Lhotta et al., 1993). Because these patients also have suboptimal functional antibody responses in addition to their defect in opsonization, bacterial infections are also a common cause of morbidity and mortality (Ross and Densen, 1984; Figueroa and Densen, 1991; Ochs et al., 1993).

There may also be some clinical manifestations of isolated C4A or C4B deficiency. For example, the prevalence of homozygous C4A deficiency is approximately 10 times higher in SLE patients than in normal individuals (Christiansen et al., 1983; Fiedler et al., 1983; Howard et al., 1986; Petri et al., 1993), a finding suggesting that loss of C4A functional activity significantly compromises immune complex clearance. SLE patients with C4A deficiency appear to have a lower prevalence of anti-

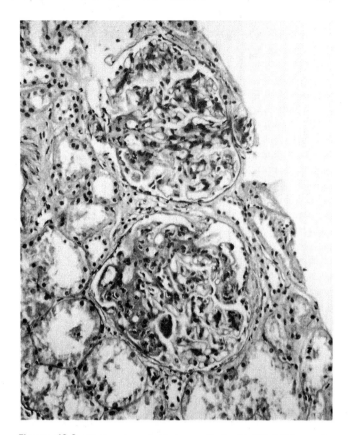

Figure 42.2. Glomerulonephritis in a patient with C4 deficiency. Inherited deficiencies of early complement components are associated with systemic lupus erythematosus and glomerulonephritis. This patient with C4 deficiency developed a malar rash and glomerulonephritis in early adolescence. A renal biopsy demonstrated an increase in mesangial matrix and cellularity. Immunofluorescence confirmed paramesangial deposits of IgG, C3, and C1q. (Courtesy of Thomas R. Welch, M.D.)

cardiolipin, anti-Ro, anti-dsDNA, and anti-Sm antibodies; less neurologic disease and renal disease; and more photosensitivity than other SLE patients (Petri et al., 1993; Welch et al., 1998). Homozygous C4B deficiency is associated with an increased risk of bacterial infection (Rowe et al., 1989; Biskof et al., 1990).

Animal model

There is a naturally occurring strain of guinea pigs completely deficient in C4 (Ellman et al., 1970). They exhibit an increased susceptibility to bacterial infections; however, they have no evidence of autoimmune disease. At the time of their initial description in 1970, these animals provided valuable evidence for the existence of an alternative pathway (Frank et al., 1971). They have also been useful in defining the relative roles of the classical and alternative pathways in a variety of complement-mediated biological activities (Ellman et al., 1971; Hosea et al., 1980, Ochs et al., 1983). A C4-deficient knockout mouse has confirmed the importance of C4 in humoral responses and the clearance of endotoxin (Fischer et al., 1996; Ma et al., 1996; Prodeus et al., 1996; Reid et al., 1996).

C2 Deficiency

Molecular biology and pathophysiology

The gene for C2 is closely linked to that for factor B within the class III region of the MHC complex (Carroll et al., 1984). C2 is a serine protease and is highly homologous to factor B. Both components contain multiple 60–amino acid short consensus repeat units believed to interact with C4 (Ishii et al., 1993). C2 is produced by hepatocytes, macrophages, and fibroblasts.

C2 deficiency (MIM 217000) is the most common of the complete complement deficiencies (Ruddy, 1986; Sullivan et al., 1994). C2-deficient individuals have markedly reduced total hemolytic complement activity and C2 functional activity. Complement-mediated serum activities, such as opsonization and chemotaxis, are present in patients with C2 deficiency and reflect the fact that their alternative pathway is intact (Johnson et al., 1971; Friend et al., 1975). However, they are not generated to the same degree or as quickly as in individuals with an intact classical pathway (Johnston et al., 1969; Friend et al., 1975; Geibink et al., 1977; Repine et al., 1977).

Over 95% of C2-deficient individuals are homozygous for a 28 bp deletion at the end of exon 6, which causes a splicing abnormality and premature termination of transcription (Johnson et al., 1992; Truedsson et al., 1993b; Sullivan et al., 1994). The 28 bp deletion is associated with a conserved MHC haplotype: *HLA-B18, BF*S, C2*Q0, C4A*4, C4B*2, DR2* (Johnson et al., 1992; Truedsson et al., 1993a; Sullivan et al., 1994). The gene frequency of this deletion has been found to be 0.005–0.007 in Caucasoid populations (Truedsson et al., 1993b; Sullivan et al., 1994), a frequency consistent with previous estimates of the prevalence of homozygous C2 deficiency of approximately 1 in 10,000 (Ruddy, 1986). In addition to the common 28 bp deletion, a 2 bp deletion has been found that results in a premature stop codon (Wang et al., 1998), and two different missense mutations have been identified that impair secretion of mature C2 (Wetzel et al 1996). Detection of the 28 bp deletion through PCR has been used for both carrier detection and prenatal diagnosis (Sullivan and Winkelstein, 1994).

Clinical expression

Approximately 40% of patients with C2 deficiency develop SLE or discoid lupus and approximately 50% develop recurrent infections (Ross and Densen, 1984; Ruddy, 1986; Figueroa and Densen, 1991). Some asymptomatic C2-deficient individuals have also been identified in studies of kindreds. The association of C2 deficiency with SLE is believed to be due to the compromise in immune complex clearance that results when any of the early complement components is deficient (Davies et al., 1993). SLE patients with C2 deficiency possess immune complexes that contain increased amounts of C4 but lack C3 (Garred et al., 1990). In the absence of C3, the immune complexes are not cleared efficiently. Direct identification of immune complex deposition in C2-deficient individuals has determined that splenic uptake is markedly impaired (Davies et al., 1993). Normalization of serum complement after the administration of fresh-frozen plasma returned the immune complex clearance to normal. For this reason, fresh-frozen plasma infusions have been advocated by some investigators for the treatment of SLE in complement-deficient individuals (Steinsson et al., 1989).

Although patients with C2 deficiency express many of the characteristic features of lupus, severe nephritis, cerebritis, and aggressive arthritis are less common than in complement-sufficient SLE patients. However, cutaneous lesions are common in C2-deficient patients with lupus, and many have a characteristic annular photosensitive rash. Patients with C2 deficiency and SLE have a lower incidence of anti-DNA and antinuclear antigen antibodies than do other SLE patients (Glass et al., 1976; Provost

et al., 1983; Meyer et al., 1985), but their incidence of anti-Ro antibodies is higher (Provost et al., 1983; Meyer et al., 1985). A variety of other rheumatic disorders have also been described in C2 deficiency, including glomerulonephritis, dermatomyositis, anaphylactoid purpura, and vasculitis (Ross and Densen, 1984; Figueroa and Densen, 1991).

The bacterial infections seen in patients with C2 deficiency are usually systemic infections (e.g., sepsis and meningitis) with encapsulated organisms (i.e., pneumococcus and *H. influenzae*) and are more common in childhood (Fasano et al., 1990). The infections are thought to result from impaired opsonization of the organism due to the absence of C2 cleavage of C3, although their impaired humoral immune response may also contribute (Ochs et al., 1983).

Animal model

C2-deficient guinea pigs were a valuable early model for investigating the role of complement in opsonization. Early gene mapping experiments demonstrated linkage of the mutant C2 in guinea pigs with MHC (Bitter-Suermann et al., 1981).

C3 Deficiency

Molecular biology and pathophysiology

The gene for C3 is located on chromosome 19 (Whitehead et al., 1982). It is produced as a single polypeptide precursor that is processed to yield two disulfide-linked chains. C3 is the most abundant of the complement components in plasma and plays a pivotal role in generating most of the biologically significant activities of the complement system. Most of serum C3 is produced by the liver (Alper et al., 1969), but C3 is also generated by endothelial cells, fibroblasts, renal tubular cells, endometrium, lymphocytes, and neutrophils (Colten, 1992).

Twenty patients with C3 deficiency (MIM 120700) have been described to date (Ross and Densen, 1984; Figueroa and Densen, 1991; Singer et al., 1994a). Total serum hemolytic complement activity and the levels of serum C3 antigen and hemolytic activity are markedly reduced. As a result, those serum activities that are directly related to C3 (e.g., opsonizing activity) or indirectly related to C3 because of its role in activating C5–C9 (e.g., anaphylatoxic, chemotactic, and bactericidal activity) are also markedly reduced. In a limited number of cases the molecular genetic defect has been identified. The first C3-deficient patient to be examined was found to have a mutation in the 5′ donor splice site of intron 18, resulting in partial deletion of exon 18, activation of a cryptic splice site in exon 18, frameshift, and a premature stop codon (Botto et al., 1990). The second C3-deficient patient has a donor splice site mutation in intron 10 (Huang and Lin, 1994). An interesting mutation affecting the maturation of proC3 to mature C3 (Singer et al. 1994b), due to a point mutation in exon 13, results in an amino acid substitution that blocks the maturation of intracellular C3. Finally, an Afrikaans-speaking patient was found to have an 800 bp deletion thought to be due to homologous recombination between two Alu repeats flanking the deletion (Botto et al., 1992). This 800 bp deletion has been found with a relatively high gene frequency (0.0057) in the Afrikaans-speaking South African population (Botto et al., 1992).

Clinical expression

Infection is the most significant clinical finding in C3-deficient individuals (Ross and Densen, 1984; Figueroa and Densen, 1991;

Singer et al., 1994a). Meningitis, osteomyelitis, sepsis, and pneumonia are all common. The typical organisms include encapsulated bacteria such as pneumococcus, *Haemophilus influenzae*, and *Neisseria* species. Patients tend to present early in life with recurrent severe infections. The severity of the infections emphasizes the important physiologic role of C3 as an opsonin, particularly in early childhood.

Approximately 25% of C3-deficient patients also have rheumatic diseases (Ross and Densen, 1984; Figueroa and Densen, 1991; Singer et al., 1994b). Some patients have had a syndrome involving multiple organs that closely resembles systemic lupus erythematosis. In other patients, the rheumatic disease has involved the kidney and most closely resembles membranoproliferative glomerulonephritis with mesangial cell proliferation, an increase in the mesangial matrix, and electron-dense deposits in both the subendothelium of capillary loops and the mesangium. Still other patients have had isolated vasculitic skin rashes. The predilection for rheumatic diseases may relate to the role of C3 in the clearance of immune complexes. In fact, circulating immune complexes have been found in some C3-deficient patients with rheumatic diseases, but not in all.

Animal model

Dogs with genetically determined C3 deficiency were discovered in 1981 (Winkelstein, 1981). Affected animals have both an increased susceptibility to infection and membranoproliferative glomerulonephritis, thereby resembling closely their human counterparts (Blum et al., 1985; Cork et al., 1991). The C3-deficient dog has been useful in demonstrating the role C3 plays in a variety of physiologic functions such as the generation of a normal antibody response (O'Neil et al., 1988) and in resistance to endotoxic shock and multiple organ failure (Quezado et al., 1994). C3-deficient guinea pigs produce normal intracellular C3 and approximately 5% of normal serum levels of C3. They have been useful in demonstrating the importance of C3 in bactericidal activity (Burger et al., 1986). A C3-deficient knockout mouse is most remarkable for impaired humoral responses but has also been noted to have increased mortality after endotoxin challenge (Fischer et al., 1996; Ma et al., 1996; Prodeus et al., 1996; Reid et al., 1996). Recently the role of complement in mast cell–dependent natural immunity was studied in C3-deficient knockout mice (Prodeus et al., 1997). C3-deficient mice were much more sensitive to cecal ligation and puncture than wild-type controls. C3-deficient mice also exhibited reductions in peritoneal mast cell degranulation, production of tumor necrosis factor (TNF), neutrophil infiltration, and clearance of bacteria.

C5 Deficiency

Molecular biology and pathophysiology

C5 consists of two disulfide-linked polypeptide chains transcribed from a single gene located on the long arm of chromosome 9. C5 is distantly related to C3, C4, and β2-macroglobulin, although C5 does not share the internal reactive thiolester bond (Carney et al., 1991). The liver is the major source of serum-derived C5, although macrophages, lung, intestine, and lymphocytes also produce it.

Approximately 30 patients with C5 deficiency (MIM 120900) have been described. Patients with C5 deficiency have decreased total hemolytic complement activity and very little C5 functional activity. Consequently, their serum is unable to generate any

chemotactic or bactericidal activity. In three African-American patients, the mutations in one allele have been identified. Two patients from unrelated kindreds had a nonsense mutation in exon 1, and the third patient had a nonsense mutation in exon 36 (Wang et al., 1995). The patients represent compound heterozygotes for C5 deficiency. None of these mutations were identified in four Caucasian C5-deficient patients. Therefore, it appears that diverse mutations are associated with C5 deficiency.

Clinical expression

The most common clinical manifestation of C5 deficiency has been an increased susceptibility to neisserial infections (Ross and Densen, 1984; Figueroa and Densen, 1991). Recurrent meningococcal infections are the most common, although systemic gonococcal infections are also seen. One C5-deficient patient developed SLE, but it is not clear that this represents a true association between C5 deficiency and lupus (Figueroa et al., 1993).

Animal model

A number of inbred strains of mice have been found to have a complete deficiency of C5 (Rosenberg and Tachibana, 1962). Mice deficient in C5 have been of value in defining the relative role of C5 in generating a local inflammatory response in a variety of organs (Snyderman et al., 1971).

C6 Deficiency

Molecular biology and pathophysiology

The genes for C6 and C7 lie in a tail–tail orientation at a distance apart of approximately 150 kb on chromosome 5 (Setien et al., 1993). C6 contains several thrombospondin repeat motifs that probably function in protein–protein and protein–phospholipid interactions during the assembly of the membrane attack complex and shares considerable homology with C7, C8, and C9 (Chakravarti et al., 1989). The liver produces most of the serum C6.

C6 deficiency (MIM 217050) is one of the more common complement deficiencies (Ross and Densen, 1984; Figueroa and Densen, 1991). Its prevalence among African Americans has been estimated to be as high as 1 in 1600 (Zhu et al., 2000), while its prevalence among Asians and Europeans is significantly less (Inai et al., 1999). The most common form of C6 deficiency is characterized by undetectable serum levels of C6 and absent serum bactericidal activity. The basis for complete C6 deficiency has been determined in three unrelated North American patients of African-American and Japanese ancestry (Nishizaka et al., 1996a; Zhu et al., 1996). One African-American patient was homozygous for a single base-pair deletion in exon 12 that results in a frameshift and premature termination. A second African-American patient was heterozygous for the same exon 12 deletion and a single base-pair deletion in exon 7. The third patient was a compound heterozygote with a deletion of four nucleotides on one chromosome and an undefined defect on the other chromosome. Complete C6 deficiency occurs most frequently in South Africa, where haplotype determinations of flanking genes have demonstrated that the majority of C6*Q0 alleles in this population arose from the same distant ancestor (Fernie et al., 1994, 1995). However, in a minority of cases, the C6*Q0 allele was found on a different haplotype, suggesting that there is some diversity even in this population. These haplotype determinations have been used to identify carriers in individual families.

Another form of C6 deficiency has also been described. Subtotal deficiency of C6 (C6SD for C6 subtotal deficiency) is characterized by 1%–2% of normal serum levels of C6 (Wurzner et al., 1995a). The molecular genetic basis for this deficiency is a loss of the splice donor site of intron 15 and premature termination (Wurzner et al., 1995a). Although the mutated C6 protein is truncated, it can be incorporated into the membrane attack complex, where it supports lytic activity to some degree. None of the C6SD patients have had recurrent infections. C6SD has also been seen in association with subtotal C7 deficiency (Fernie et al., 1995, 1996c) and is the result of two independent mutations.

Clinical expression

Individuals with genetically determined C6 deficiency most commonly present with systemic blood-borne meningococcal infections (Ross and Densen, 1984; Figueroa and Densen, 1991). Disseminated gonococcal infections have also been described. Although the terminal complement components do not appear to participate in the clearance of immune complexes, a few C6-deficient patients have been identified with SLE. Whether this is due to an ascertainment bias of complement-deficient individuals within populations of patients with SLE or to an association based on pathophysiology is not known.

Animal model

Genetically determined C6 deficiency has been described in rats (Leenarts et al., 1994) and rabbits (Rother et al., 1966). These animals have been especially valuable in demonstrating that extrahepatic synthesis of complement can contribute significantly to some of the biologic functions of the complement system (Brauer et al., 1995).

C7 Deficiency

Molecular biology and pathophysiology

The gene for C7 is linked to that for C6 and C9 on chromosome 5 (Setien et al., 1993). Like C6 and C9, it contains protein domains with homology to thrombospondin, low-density lipoprotein receptor, and the epidermal growth factor receptor (Hobart et al., 1995). Although the liver is the major site of synthesis of C7, a significant amount of serum C7 is derived from synthesis by bone marrow–derived cells (Naughton et al., 1996).

Patients with C7 deficiency (MIM 217070) have markedly diminished total hemolytic complement activity, little if any C7 in their serum, and markedly reduced serum bactericidal activity. A number of different mutations have been found to be responsible for complete C7 deficiency (Nishizaka et al., 1996b; Fernie et al., 1997; Fernie and Hobart, 1998; O'Hara et al., 1998; Horiuchi et al., 1999), although mutations consistent with two independent founders are present in the Irish and Sephardic Jews from Morocco (Fernie et al., 1996a, 1997; O'Hara et al., 1998). A second type of C7 deficiency has been described in which the quantity of C7 is diminished. This has also been seen in association with C6SD. This defect is due to a missense mutation in exon 11, which results in an arginine-to-serine change (Fernie et al., 1996b).

Clinical expression

Systemic neisserial infections are the most common clinical expression of C7-deficient individuals (Ross and Densen, 1984; Figueroa and Densen, 1991). However, patients with C7 deficiency have also had SLE, rheumatoid arthritis, pyoderma gan-

grenosum, and scleroderma. The relationship of autoimmune disease to C7 deficiency is not entirely clear.

C8 Deficiency

Molecular biology and pathophysiology

C8 is composed of three polypeptide chains (α, β, and γ), each encoded by distinct genes (*C8A, C8B,* and *C8G*). *C8A* and *C8B* are found on the short arm of chromosome 1 while *C8G* is located on the long arm of chromosome 9 (Kaufman et al., 1989). The α and β chains are covalently linked to form one subunit (C8α,β), which is joined by noncovalent bonds to the other subunit (C8γ).

Two types of C8 deficiency (MIM 120950, 120960) exist, and both result in loss of total hemolytic complement activity. C8β deficiency is more common in Caucasians and C8α-γ deficiency is more common in African Americans. In the case of C8β deficiency, C8 antigen can be detected in the patient's serum using standard immunochemical techniques, since these patients possess the C8α-γ subunit. In either form of C8 deficiency, serum C8 functional activity and bactericidal activity are markedly reduced. The overwhelming majority (86%) of *C8B*-null alleles are due to a C-T transition in exon 9, producing a direct premature stop codon (Saucedo et al., 1995). Three additional C-T transitions and two single base-pair deletions causing a frameshift and premature stop codons have also been identified in C8β deficiency (Saucedo et al., 1995). An allele-specific PCR system has been used to detect heterozygous carriers of the common C8β mutation. The molecular basis of C8-α-β deficiency has been identified in three patients. In five of the six alleles, a 10 bp insertion in C8A resulting in a premature stop codon occurs as a result of an intronic mutation that alters the splicing of exons 6 and 7 (Densen et al., 1996a).

Clinical expression

Meningococcal meningitis and disseminated gonococcal infections have been the predominant clinical expression of C8 deficiency (Fig. 42.3) (Ross and Densen, 1984; Figueroa and Densen, 1991), reflecting the inability of C8-deficient serum to generate cytolytic activity.

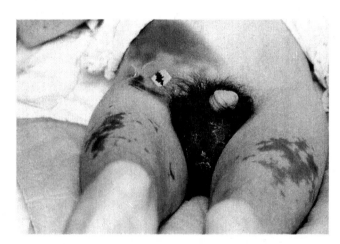

Figure 42.3. Meningococcal sepsis in a patient with C8 deficiency. Inherited deficiencies of terminal complement components are associated with an increased risk of meningococcal disease. This patient with C8 deficiency developed meningococcal meningitis and sepsis. (Courtesy of Peter Densen, M.D.)

C9 Deficiency

Molecular biology and pathophysiology

C9 is a 70 kDa glycoprotein that has sequence homology to C8α, C8β, C6, and perforin. The C9 gene lies approximately 2.5 megabase pairs (mbp) from the C6 and C7 genes on chromosome 5. C9 is produced by hepatocytes and is highly developmentally regulated (Lassiter et al., 1994).

Although C9 deficiency (MIM 120940) is relatively common among individuals of Japanese descent, with an estimated prevalence of 1 in 1000 (Horiuchi et al., 1998), it is relatively uncommon in Occidentals (Ross and Densen, 1984; Figueroa and Densen, 1991). Patients with C9 deficiency have markedly reduced levels of C9 in their serum. Because the complex of C5b, C6, C7, and C8 can form small unstable pores in biomembranes, patients with C9 deficiency possess some serum hemolytic and bactericidal activity, although less than in normal serum (Petersen et al., 1976); Inai et al., 1979; Lint et al., 1980; Harriman et al., 1981). The molecular genetic basis for C9 deficiency in individuals of Japanese descent is a nonsense mutation in exon 4 (Horiuchi et al., 1998). In addition, two different point mutations in exons 2 and 4 resulted in direct premature stop codons in a Swiss kindred (Witzel-Schlomp et al., 1997).

Clinical expression

C9-deficient patients are often asymptomatic, although some patients with C9 deficiency have presented with systemic meningococcal infections (Ross and Densen, 1984; Figueroa and Densen, 1991). A large epidemiologic study in Japan, where C9 deficiency is relatively common, firmly established that there is a relationship between C9 deficiency and systemic meningococcal infections (Nagata et al., 1989). However, the relationship between C9 deficiency and neisserial disease may not be as strong as it is with other terminal complement component deficiencies, reflecting the partial serum bactericidal activity in C9-deficient patients.

Factor B Deficiency

Molecular biology and pathophysiology

Factor B is a serine protease that is highly homologous to C2. The gene for factor B is part of the HLA class III region on chromosome 6. Factor B, like C2, carries the active enzymatic site for the subsequent cleavage of C3 and C5 and is expressed primarily in hepatocytes and monocytic cells. A single factor B–deficient patient has been described, and the basis for that patient's factor B deficiency is not yet understood (Densen et al., 1996b).

Clinical expression

The factor B–deficient patient presented with meningococcemia and was found to have a mildly decreased classical pathway activity and no detectable alternative pathway activity. No functional factor B was detected, and factor B protein had an abnormal molecular weight (Densen et al., 1996b). The association of factor B with meningococcemia is probably not coincidental since most alternative pathway deficiencies are associated with meningococcal disease.

Animal model

A factor B–deficient knockout mouse model has been developed (Matsumoto et al., 1996). Unlike mice deficient in classical path-

way components, this mouse model demonstrates normal humoral function, suggesting that the alternative pathway does not significantly augment humoral responses.

Factor D Deficiency

Molecular biology and pathophysiology

Factor D is identical to adipsin and, unlike other complement components, is not synthesized in the liver but rather in adipocytes, muscle cells, lung, and monocytes/macrophages (White et al., 1992). The precise genetic locus for factor D has not been identified but it maps to chromosome 19.

Only a few kindreds with factor D deficiency (MIM 134350) have been identified and its mode of inheritance has not been firmly established, although it is most consistent with an autosomal recessive trait. In one family, monozygous twins were found to have only 8% of the normal levels of factor D (Kluin-Nelemans et al., 1984), whereas in another family, factor D was undetectable in the proband and present at approximately 50% of normal in the mother (Hiemstra et al., 1989). In all patients identified to date, alternative pathway activity was absent while classical pathway complement activity was normal or near normal. The molecular genetic basis was determined in one family and has been found to be a mutation causing a premature stop codon (Biesma et al., 2001).

Clinical expression

The patients with factor D deficiency have presented with recurrent sinopulmonary infections or recurrent systemic meningococcal or pneumococcal infections (Kluin-Nelemans et al., 1984; Hiemstra et al., 1989; Weiss et al., 1998).

C1 Inhibitor Deficiency

Molecular biology and pathophysiology

C1 inhibitor (C1INH) is encoded by a 17 kb gene on chromosome 11. The primary sequence of C1INH has been determined and it is homologous with other serine protease inhibitors such as α1-proteinase inhibitor, α1-antichymotrypsin, and anti-thrombin III (Bock et al., 1986).

There are two forms of C1INH deficiency (MIM 106100) and both are inherited as autosomal dominant traits (Rosen et al., 1965, 1971). In the most common form (type I), accounting for approximately 85% of the patients, the serum of affected individuals is deficient in both C1INH protein (5%–30% of normal) and C1INH functional activity (Rosen et al., 1971; Frank et al., 1976; Cicardi et al., 1982). In the other, less common, form (type II), a dysfunctional protein is present in normal or elevated concentrations, but the functional activity of C1INH is markedly reduced (Donaldson and Evens, 1963; Rosen et al., 1965; Frank et al., 1976; Cicardi et al., 1982). The lower than expected levels of C1INH functional activity in heterozygotes is thought to be the result of increased catabolism of the normal protein, although some patients may also demonstrate decreased synthesis (Ernst et al., 1996). In patients with type I C1INH deficiency, the diagnosis can be established easily by demonstrating a decrease in serum C1INH protein when assessed by immunochemical techniques. However, in patients with type II C1INH deficiency, the diagnosis must rest on demonstrating a decrease in C1INH functional activity. In either case, C4 levels are usually reduced below the lower limit of normal both during and between attacks

(Austen and Sheffer, 1965; Pickering et al., 1968; Frank et al., 1976; Cicardi et al., 1982) because of their uncontrolled cleavage by C1s, thus making their measurement useful as a diagnostic clue (Pickering et al., 1968; Frank et al., 1976).

The mediators responsible for producing the edema are incompletely understood. When purified C1s is injected into normal skin or skin of patients with C1INH deficiency, angioedema is produced (Klemperer et al., 1968). The intradermal response to C1s in C2-deficient individuals is diminished, whereas it is preserved in C3-deficient individuals, a result suggesting the direct involvement of C2 in the production of the angioedema. Other evidence suggests that the plasma kallikrein system may also be involved in the generation of the edema. C1INH inhibits the ability of activated Hageman factor to initiate kinin generation, and it inhibits kallikrein activation of the kinin system directly. Blister fluids from C1INH-deficient patients contain active plasma kallikrein, and their serum has decreased amounts of prekallikrein and kininogen (Curd et al., 1980), which suggests activation of the kinin system during attacks of edema. Furthermore, treatment with drugs that inhibit the release of vasoactive mediators is effective prophylaxis (Frank et al., 1972; Sheffer et al., 1972).

This division of C1INH-deficient patients into two forms has no correlation with clinical phenotype and only limited correlation with genotype, as there are some examples of *C1INH* gene mutations in which a dysfunctional protein is produced but is degraded so rapidly that it is not detectable in the serum (Agostoni and Cicardi, 1992; Davis et al., 1993). Alu-mediated deletions and duplications account for the most common genotypes (Stoppa-Lyonnet et al., 1991; Davis et al., 1993). Four of the seven introns in the C1INH gene (*C1NH*) contain a total of 17 Alu-repetitive DNA elements. These Alu elements are responsible for most of the large deletions and duplications leading to C1INH deficiency. A variety of single base changes and smaller deletions and duplications have also been identified (Davis et al., 1993). Most patients with detectable but dysfunctional C1INH have a mutation that replaces the reactive center arginine residue. The other mutations identified in patients with dysfunctional protein are found in the hinge region and result in blockade of the reactive center loop, thereby inactivating the C1INH (Davis et al., 1993; Verpy et al., 1995).

Clinical expression

Patients with C1INH deficiency most commonly present with recurrent angioedema, which has led to the commonly accepted clinical term for the disorder, *hereditary angioedema* (HAE) (Donaldson and Rosen, 1966; Frank et al., 1976; Oltvai et al., 1991; Agostoni and Cicardi, 1992; Agostoni et al., 1993; Cicardi et al., 1993). The angioedema involves the submucosa of the airway or gastrointestinal tract or the subcutaneous area of the skin. Although most patients present clinically in the first two decades of life, a significant minority of patients do not have symptoms until well into adult life. Since the disease is inherited as an autosomal dominant characteristic, most C1INH-deficient individuals have a family history of angioedema, which assists in establishing the correct diagnosis.

When the angioedema involves the skin it is neither pruritic nor painful. Although the edema is usually pale, there may be a serpiginous rash that occurs with the angioedema. It should be noted that urticaria is not a manifestation of HAE. The edema may involve an extremity, the face, or the genitalia and usually progresses for 1–2 days and resolves in an additional 2–3 days.

Involvement of the gastrointestinal tract is very common, with nearly three-quarters of patients having a significant history of abdominal pain due to bowel wall edema (Frank et al., 1976). Additional clinical symptoms include anorexia and emesis and may occur in the absence of concurrent airway or cutaneous symptoms. Bowel wall edema is unusual in other forms of angioedema and is therefore very suggestive of C1INH deficiency.

The most feared complication in this disorder is edema of the upper airways (Color Plate 42.I). In one series, pharyngeal edema had occurred at least once in nearly two-thirds of the patients and tracheostomies had been performed in one out of every six patients (Frank et al., 1976). The patient may experience a feeling of tightness in the throat, followed by swelling of the tongue, buccal mucosa, and oropharynx. If the edema progresses to involve the larynx, there may be hoarseness and stridor followed by respiratory obstruction.

Although the biochemical mechanisms responsible for initiating attacks are not understood, many patients report that minor trauma or stress precipitates individual attacks. In addition, estrogens and angiotensin-converting enzyme inhibitors may precipitate attacks (Megerian et al., 1992; Agostoni et al., 1993). Exogenous estrogens reduce C1INH levels, as does pregnancy. Angiotensin-converting enzyme inhibitors reduce kinin metabolism and may facilitate angioedema. For therapy, see Management of Complement Deficiencies, below.

Decay Accelerating Factor

Molecular biology and pathophysiology

Decay accelerating factor (DAF), also known as CD55, is a control protein of the classical and alternative pathways. It is a glycosyl phosphatidylinositol (GPI)-anchored membrane protein found on erythrocytes, lymphocytes, granulocytes, endothelium, and epithelium. It is encoded by a 35 kb gene in the RCA region of chromosome 1 (Lublin et al., 1987). The main function of DAF appears to be the protection of cells from complement-mediated cytolysis; however, it also plays a role in T cell and macrophage activation (Shenoy-Scaria et al., 1992; Hammann et al., 1999).

Five patients from three kindreds with DAF deficiency have been reported. A patient from one kindred had no detectable DAF. A single nucleotide substitution affecting codon 53 and resulting in a direct premature stop codon was found to be responsible for the complete deficiency of DAF in this patient who was born to consanguineous parents (Lublin et al., 1994). Members of the other two kindreds had some detectable DAF on the surface of their erythrocytes. In a DAF-deficient individual from one of these two kindreds, a point mutation was identified in one allele that altered antigenicity, and a second mutation, which resulted in utilization of a cryptic splice site that then altered the reading frame, was identified (Lublin et al., 1994).

Clinical expression

DAF deficiency (MIM 125240) is associated with the Inab phenotype (absence of all blood group antigens of the Cromer complex) (Telen and Green, 1989). DAF deficiency is not associated with spontaneous hemolysis, although DAF-deficient erythrocytes are moderately more susceptible to hemolysis when complement is activated via the classical pathway (Telen and Green, 1989). Two patients with the Inab phenotype have had severe protein-losing enteropathies, which is of uncertain relationship to the DAF deficiency (Telen and Green, 1989). These patients were originally identified on the basis of blood typing, rather than a specific infectious or rheumatic disease. Although DAF plays an important role in the prevention of complement-mediated lysis of the individual's own cells, this function can also be served by CD59 and CR1 receptor. In fact, CD59 may play the more important role. Therefore, DAF deficiency may not be associated with any clinical consequences.

Factor I Deficiency

Molecular biology and pathophysiology

Factor I consists of two disulfide-linked polypeptides that act to regulate the alternative pathway-cleaving enzyme (C3b, Bb). One polypeptide carries serine protease activity that cleaves C3b to produce iC3b (inactive C3b), a C3-cleavage product that can not function in the C3-cleaving enzyme of the alternative pathway. Factor I is encoded by a gene on chromosome 4q.

Because patients with factor I deficiency (MIM 217030) are missing a major control protein of the alternative pathway, there is no control imposed on the assembly and expression of the alternative pathway C3-cleaving enzyme, C3b,Bb. As a result, there is continuous activation and cleavage of native C3 through the alternative pathway and the production of C3b (Alper et al., 1970a, 1970b; Abramson et al., 1971; Nicol and Lachmann 1973; Ziegler et al., 1975). Patients with factor I deficiency, therefore, have a secondary deficiency of C3 with markedly reduced levels of C3 in their serum, most of which is in the form of C3b (Alper et al., 1970b). Typically, total hemolytic activity of the serum, whether measured through the alternative or classical pathway, is very low or undetectable. Those serum activities that depend directly or indirectly on C3, such as opsonic, chemotactic, and bactericidal activities, are also markedly reduced (Alper et al., 1970b).

Factor I deficiency has been identified in a limited number of patients (Ross and Densen, 1984; Figueroa and Densen, 1991; Vyse et al., 1994). The genetic basis for factor I deficiency has been identified in four patients and found to be diverse (Vyse et al., 1994; Morley et al., 1996). In one patient, substitution of a histidine at position 400 to a leucine suggests that this amino acid is critical.

Clinical expression

The most consistent clinical feature of factor I deficiency is an increased susceptibility to infection, with neisserial infections reported in approximately half of the patients (Ross and Densen, 1984; Figueroa and Densen, 1991; Vyse et al., 1994). The defect in opsonization also makes these patients susceptible to the same recurrent pyogenic infections, caused by *Streptococcus pneumoniae* and *Haemophilus influenzae*, seen in patients with primary deficiency of C3. Only two of the patients have been asymptomatic. One patient has died of a fatal vasculitis and another suffered from transient serum sickness (Vyse et al., 1994). Heterozygous mutations in factor I have been associated with atypical hemolytic uremic syndrome (Kavanagh et al., 2005).

Factor H Deficiency

Molecular biology and pathophysiology

The gene for factor H lies within the RCA gene cluster on chromosome 1 (Holers et al., 1985). Factor H is synthesized in hepatocytes, macrophages, B cells, endothelial cells, and platelets. Factor H, like factor I, is an inhibitor of the alternative pathway. It competes with factor B for binding to C3b in the assembly of the alternative pathway C3-cleaving enzyme, C3b,Bb, and also displaces Bb once the enzyme has been assembled.

In some families, serum factor H has been undetectable (Brai et al., 1988; Nielsen et al., 1989) whereas in other families factor H has been present but markedly reduced (Levy et al., 1986; Nielsen et al., 1989). Since deficiency of factor H (like factor I) leads to uncontrolled activation of the alternative pathway and C3 consumption, serum levels of C3 are reduced, and total hemolytic complement activity and alternative pathway complement activity are usually significantly reduced.

There have only been a few cases of complete factor H deficiency (MIM 134370) described (Ross and Densen, 1984; Figueroa and Densen, 1991; Sim et al., 1993). In only one of the cases has a specific genetic defect been identified. That patient was a compound heterozygote for two missense mutations affecting conserved cysteine residues (Ault et al., 1997). In another patient, PCR amplification of factor H cDNA recovered from Epstein-Barr virus (EBV)-transformed lymphocytes suggested that a truncated mRNA was produced; however, a specific mutation was not identified (Wurzner et al., 1995b).

Clinical expression

Renal disease is the most common finding in complete factor H deficiency (Ross and Densen, 1984; Figueroa and Densen, 1991; Vyse et al., 1994). Glomerulonephritis, IgA nephropathy, and hemolytic uremic syndrome have been described in humans with factor H deficiency. Infections with neisserial species and encapsulated organisms are also common. In some kindreds, asymptomatic family members with factor H deficiency have been detected. Heterozygous mutations in factor H as is true for factor I and the transmembrane complement regulator membrane co-factor protein (MCP), are associated with atypical hemolytic uremic syndrome (Sanchez-Corral et al., 2002). A heterozygous or homozygous polymorphism of factor H (Y402H) is responsible for almost 50% of age-related macular degeneration (Edwards et al., 2005; Haines et al., 2005; Klein et al., 2005).

Animal model

A porcine strain with factor H deficiency spontaneously develops membranoproliferative renal disease (Hogasen et al., 1995). In the porcine model, deposition of complement components occurs along the capillary walls of the renal glomeruli, as is seen in human renal disease associated with factor H deficiency.

Properdin Deficiency

Molecular biology and pathophysiology

The gene for properdin is the only gene of the complement system that is located on the short arm X chromosome. It encodes a protein with six thrombospondin repeat units that circulates as cyclic oligomers of 53 kDa subunits (Nolan et al., 1991). Properdin is synthesized by monocytes, hepatocytes, and T cells, and it is a component of the secondary granule in neutrophils. Properdin acts to stabilize the alternative pathway enzymes that activate C3 and C5.

Properdin deficiency (MIM 312060) is inherited as an X-linked recessive trait. In some families, properdin is undetectable (Sjoholm et al., 1982; Densen et al., 1987), whereas in others, affected males may have levels as high as 10% of normal (Nielsen and Kock, 1987; Sjoholm et al., 1988b). In still other kindreds, serum levels of antigenic properdin are normal but the protein is dysfunctional (Sjoholm et al., 1988a). The serum of patients with properdin deficiency is unable to support the activation of C3 via the alternative pathway. Serum bactericidal activity for some strains of the meningococcus is reduced in properdin-deficient serum.

Mutations have been identified in five properdin-deficient patients. Three patients with no detectable serum properdin had mutations resulting in early stop codons (Westberg et al., 1995; Fredrikson et al., 1996; Spath et al., 1999). In kindreds in whom low levels of properdin were detected, different mutations were identified that resulted in amino acid substitutions (Westberg et al., 1995). One kindred with normal levels of dysfunctional properdin had a single base-pair mutation in exon 9 resulting in the substitution of aspartic acid for tyrosine, rendering the molecule unable to interact with C3b (Fredrikson et al., 1996).

Clinical expression

Approximately 50% of the patients with properdin deficiency have had meningococcal disease (Ross and Densen, 1984; Figueroa and Densen, 1991), emphasizing the importance of the alternative pathway in host defense against *Neisseria*. Isolated cases of SLE and discoid lupus have also been described.

CD59 Deficiency

Molecular biology and pathophysiology

CD59 (HRF 20, membrane inhibitor of reactive lysis) is a 20 kDa GPI-anchored glycoprotein that inhibits lysis by C8 and C9 in a species-specific fashion. It is widely expressed on erythrocytes, leukocytes, and endothelial cells, where it functions to prevent intravascular complement attack (Lehto and Meri, 1993).

A single patient with inherited CD59 deficiency (MIM 107271) has been described (Yamashina et al., 1990). He was homozygous for a CD59 gene bearing two mutations in codons 16 and 96 (Motoyama et al., 1992). This form of CD59 deficiency is distinct from paroxysmal nocturnal hemoglobinuria, which is an acquired deficiency of all GPI-anchored cell surface proteins.

Clinical expression

The CD59-deficient patient was the product of a consanguineous marriage. He presented with recurrent hemolytic anemia as a child and recurrent cerebral infarctions (Yamashina et al., 1990). Studies of four GPI-anchored proteins, which are typically lost in paroxysmal nocturnal hemoglobinuria, revealed normal levels of all except for CD59. CD59 was absent from the surface of his erythrocytes and fibroblasts. His mother and father expressed half-normal levels, a finding suggesting autosomal recessive inheritance. The recurrent hemolytic anemia reflects the important role of CD59 in the prevention of homologous complement attack.

Mannose Binding Lectin Deficiency

Molecular biology and pathophysiology

Mannose binding lectin (MBL), also sometimes referred to as mannose binding protein (MBP), is composed of a trimer, each chain of which contains a collagen-like region, cyteine repeats, and a lectin domain (Sastry et al., 1989). MBL binds to carbohydrates such as acetylglucosamine and mannose found on both gram-negative and gram-positive bacteria more avidly than to

other sugars. MBL circulates with MBL-associated serine proteases (MASP1 and MASP2) that activate C4 and C2 and ultimately C3.

There are five polymorphic bases in MBL that affect serum concentrations of MBL. Three of these polymorphic bases affect the collagen-like region of the molecule at codon 54 (structural allele *B*), codon 57 (structural allele *C*) and codon 52 (structural allele *D*) and are associated with markedly reduced serum levels of MBL because of decreased stability of the higher-order forms (Madsen et al., 1995). Two other polymorphic variants occur in the promoter region of the gene and are also associated with markedly reduced serum levels of MBL (Madsen et al., 1995). The gene frequency of each of these polymorphisms has recently been defined in several different populations, and four of the polymorphisms have been found with high frequency in at least one population. For example, the codon 54Asp polymorphism is found with a gene frequency of 0.13–0.19 in Caucasians, compared to 0.03 in West Africans, and the codon 57Glu variant is found with a gene frequency of 0.23–0.29 in West Africans, compared to 0.02 in Caucasians (Madsen et al., 1994, 1995; Babovic-Vuksanovic et al., 1999). The two polymorphic promoter variants are in linkage disequilibrium and exist as three haplotypes present in varying proportions in different populations. Because of the high frequency of these polymorphic variants in some populations, it is not uncommon to have homozygous deficient individuals. On the basis of studies that correlated serum levels of MBL with the genotype of the donor, it has been found that the structural variants have a dominant negative effect; however, the promoter variants are autosomal codominant.

Clinical expression

MBL deficiency (MIM 154545) is associated with an increased frequency of infection in both adults and children (Sumiya et al., 1991; Summerfield et al., 1995; Kakkanaiah et al., 1998). It has also been found with increased frequency in patients with SLE (Davies et al., 1995; Sullivan et al., 1996).

Diagnosis of Complement Deficiencies

Most of the deficiencies of the classical pathway (C1 through C9) can be detected by using a hemolytic assay that assesses the functional integrity of the pathway. The most common of these, the CH_{50} assay, determines the ability of the patient's serum to lyse antibody-sensitized sheep erythrocytes. Since lysis depends on the functional integrity of the complete cascade, patients who have severe deficiencies of any of the individual components of the classical pathway will usually have less than 5% of normal total serum hemolytic activity. One exception is C9 deficiency. Because lysis of antibody-sensitized erythrocytes can occur in the absence of C9 (Stolfi, 1968), albeit to a lesser degree, patients with C9 deficiency have some total serum hemolytic activity, but usually between 30% and 50% of the normal level.

Deficiencies of components of the alternative pathway (factors B, H, I, and properdin) can be detected by using a hemolytic assay that tests the functional activity of the alternative pathway (AH50). The most common of these use rabbit erythrocytes, which are potent activators of the human alternative pathway (Polhill et al., 1978). Thus, patients with deficiencies of components of the alternative pathway, as well as patients with deficiencies of C5–C9, will fail to lyse rabbit erythrocytes.

Identification of the specific component that is deficient usually depends on both functional and immunochemical tests. Highly specific functional assays are available for each component (Nelson et al., 1966). In each case, they depend on reagents that lack the specific component in question but provide the other components of the appropriate hemolytic pathway in excess. Monospecific antibodies are also available for each of the components and can be used in a variety of immunochemical assays to assess the presence or absence of the component in question. In most instances, the component will be deficient when assessed by both functional and immunochemical methods. However, there are some important exceptions. One form of C1 esterase inhibitor deficiency and one form of C1q deficiency are characterized by dysfunctional proteins that are present in immunochemical assays but are reduced in functional assays. In addition, patients with C8 deficiency lack the β chain but possess the α and γ chains and may therefore have some antigenic C8 while lacking C8 function.

Management of Complement Deficiencies

The management of complement deficiencies is usually limited to supportive care and relates to the clinical manifestations that are secondary to the specific deficiency.

Prevention of Infectious Diseases

Two strategies have been attempted to reduce complement-deficient patients' susceptibility to infections and/or modify the clinical course of the infections. One strategy is to immunize these patients against common bacterial pathogens such as *Streptococcus pneumoniae*, *Haemophilus influenzae*, and *Neisseria meningitidis*. Unfortunately, there are important factors that may limit the utility of immunizations in these patients in preventing infections. For example, when patients with C4 or C2 are immunized with neoantigens, such as ϕX 179, their primary response is limited and their secondary response is delayed with reduced isotype switching (Ochs et al., 1983). Other studies have shown that while initial responses to immunization against *Neisseria meningitidis* are normal in patients with deficiencies of C5–C9, their titers fall more dramatically than in complement-sufficient individuals (Andreoni et al., 1993; Biselli et al., 1993; Schlesinger et al., 1994, 2000). Therefore, it is possible that complement-deficient patients require more frequent immunization than a normal host (Fijen et al., 1998). Another limitation to the use of immunizations in complement-deficient patients is that the vaccines may not include all of the serotypes to which complement-deficient patients are susceptible. For example, the new pneumococcal conjugate vaccine is limited to seven serotypes and the meningococcal vaccine contains only serotypes A, C, Y and W.

A second strategy in the prevention of infection is the use of prophylactic antibiotics. Because patients with complement deficiencies have a high risk for recurrent episodes of blood-borne infections and because immunizations may not afford them complete protection, some patients have been placed on antibiotic prophylaxis. However, any recommendation for antibiotic prophylaxis must be viewed in the context of the emergence of antibiotic resistance among bacteria.

Management of Rheumatic Disorders

Regardless of the rheumatologic disorder, it is most often treated with the same immunosuppressive agents and anti-inflammatory medications as those used in a complement-sufficient patient. In a series of patients with C2 deficiency in Iceland and Great Britain, however, fresh-frozen plasma was used to treat the clinical signs of SLE (Steinsson et al., 1989; Hudson-Peacock et al.,

1997). There were concerns that the provision of additional complement components would accelerate deposition in end organs and exacerbate the inflammation. This was not the case in the two patients for whom this treatment has been attempted. In fact, nearly all clinical indicators improved on this regimen. Although it has only been used in a small number of patients, it is an attractive modality for those complement-deficient patients who are refractory to standard management or who have not done well on immunosuppression.

Management of Angioedema

Treatment of C1INH deficiency is different from that of other complement deficiencies in that there are specific measures available to ameliorate symptoms and prevent recurrences. In some patients, episodes of angioedema may occur frequently enough or be so difficult to manage as to justify long-term prophylaxis. Attenuated androgens such as stanozolol or danazol are highly effective (Gelfand et al., 1976) and act by increasing transcription of the normal allele of *C1INH* (Agostoni et al., 1993). Another class of agents used for long-term prophylaxis is the antifibrinolytics agents (Frank et al., 1972; Sheffer et al., 1972). Tranexamic acid and aminocaproic acid act by blocking plasmin generation. Although their efficacy is less than that of attenuated androgens, their incidence of side effects is also less than that of attenuated androgens. For this reason, these agents may be preferred in childhood.

In some instances, patients may require short-term prophylaxis for surgery or oral procedures. Attenuated androgens, fibrinolytic agents, fresh-frozen plasma, and C1 esterase concentrate have all been used successfully for short-term prophylaxis (Agostoni et al., 1993).

C1 esterase inhibitor concentrate is the most effective agent for the treatment of acute attacks (Agostoni et al., 1993; Waytes et al., 1996). However, it is not yet approved for use in the United States, and its use is usually restricted to life-threatening situations. Epinephrine, antihistamines, and corticosteriods are of no proven benefit in C1INH-deficient patients.

References

Abramson N, Alper CA, Lachmann PJ, Rosen FS, Jandl JH. Deficiency of C3 inactivator in man. J Immunol 107:19–25, 1971.

Agostoni A, Cicardi M. Hereditary and acquired C1-inhibitor deficiency: biological and clinical characteristics in 235 patients. Medicine 71:206–215, 1992.

Agostoni A, Cicardi M, Cugno M, Storti E. Clinical problems in the C1-inhibitor deficient patient. Behring Inst Mitt 93:306–312, 1993.

Alper CA, Abramson N, Johnston RB Jr, Jandl JH, Rosen FS. Increased susceptibility to infection associated with abnormalities of complement-mediated functions and of the third component of complement (C3). N Engl J Med 282:349–353, 1970a.

Alper CA, Abramson N, Johnston RB Jr, Jandl JH, Rosen FS. Studies in vivo and in vitro on an abnormality in the metabolism of C3 in a patient with increased susceptibility to infection. J Clin Invest 49:1975–1981, 1970b.

Alper CA, Johnson AM, Birtch AG, Moore RD. Human C3: evidence for the liver as the primary site of synthesis. Science 163:286–288, 1969.

Andreoni J, Kayhty H, Densen P, Ochonisky S, Intrator L, Wechsler J, et al. Vaccination and the role of capsular polysaccharide antibody in prevention of recurrent meningococcal disease in late complement component–deficient individuals. Acquired C1 inhibitor deficiency revealing systemic lupus erythematosus. J Infect Dis 168:227–231, 1993.

Ault BH, Schmidt BZ, Fowler NL, Kashtan CE, Ahmed AE, Vogt BA, Colten HR. Human factor H deficiency. Mutations in framework cysteine residues and block in H protein secretion and intracellular catabolism. J Biol Chem 272:25168–25175, 1997.

Austen KF, Sheffer AL. Detection of hereditary angioneurotic edema by demonstration of a reduction in the second component of human complement. N Engl J Med 272:649–653, 1965.

Babovic-Vuksanovic D, Snow K, Ten RM. Mannose-binding lectin (MBL) deficiency. Variant alleles in a midwestern population of the United States. Ann Allergy Asthma Immunol 82:134–138, 1999.

Bakker-Wondenberg IAJM, DeJong-Hoenderop YJT, Michel MF. Efficacy of antimicrobial therapy in experimental pneumococcal pneumonia: effects of impaired phagocytosis. Infect Immun 25:366–373, 1979.

Barba G, Rittner C, Schneider PM. Genetic basis of human complement C4A deficiency. J Clin Invest 91:1681–1686, 1993.

Berkel AI, Birben E, Oner C, Oner R, Loos M, Petry F. Molecular, genetic and epidemiologic studies on selective complete C1q deficiency in Turkey. Immunobiology 201:347–355, 2000.

Berkel AI, Nakakuma H. Studies of immune response in a patient with selective complete C1q deficiency. Turk J Pediatr 35:221–266, 1993.

Biesma D, Hannema AJ, Van Velzen-Biad H, Mulder L, Van Zwieten R, Kluijt I, Roos D. A family with complement factor D deficiency. J Clin Invest 108:233–240, 2001.

Biselli R, Casapollo I, D'Amelio R, Salvato S, Matricardi PM, Brai M. Antibody response to meningococcal polysaccharides A and C in patients with complement defects. Scand J Immunol 37:644–650. 1993.

Biskof NA, Welch TR, Beischel LS. C4B deficiency: a risk factor for bacteremia with encapsulated organisms. J Infect Dis 162:248–254, 1990.

Bitter-Suermann D, Hoffamn T, Burger R, Hadding U. Linkage of total deficiency of the second component (C2) of the complement system and genetic C2-polymorphism to the major histocompatibility complex of the guinea pig. J Immunol 127:608–612, 1981.

Blum JR, Cork LC, Morris JM, Olsen JL, Winkelstein JA. The clinical manifestations of a genetically determined deficiency of the third component of complement in the dog. Clin Immunol Immunopathol 34:304–310, 1985.

Bock SC, Skriver, K, Nielsen E, Thogersen H-C, Wiman B, Donaldson VH, Eddy RL, Marrinan J, Radziejewska E, Huber R, Shows TB, Magnusson S. Human C1 inhibitor: primary structure, cDNA cloning, and chromosomal location. Biochemistry 25:4292–4301, 1986.

Bottger EC, Metzger S, Bitter-Suermann D, Stevenson G, Kleindienst S, Burger R. Impaired humoral immune response in complement C3–deficient guinea pigs: absence of secondary antibody response. Eur J Immunol 16: 1231–1235, 1986.

Botto M, Dell'Agnola C, Bygrave AE, Thompson EM, Cook HT, Petry F, et al. Homozygous C1q deficiency causes glomerulonephritis associated with multiple apoptotic bodies. Nat Genet 19:56–59, 1998.

Botto M, Fong KY, So AK, Barlow R, Routier R, Morley BJ, Walport MJ. Homozygous hereditary C3 deficiency due to a partial gene deletion. Proc Natl Acad Sci USA 89: 4957–4961, 1992.

Botto M, Fong KY, So AK, Rudge A, Walport MJ. Molecular basis of hereditary C3 deficiency. J Clin Invest 86: 1158–1163, 1990.

Botto M, Nash J, Taylor P, Bygrave A, Pandolfi PP, Loos M, Davies KA, Walport MJ. Immune complex processing in a murine model of C1q deficiency. Mol Immunol 33(Suppl 1):71, 1996.

Bowness P, Davies KA, Norsworthy PJ, Athanassiou P, Taylor-Wiedeman J, Borysiewicz LK, Meyer PAR, Walport MJ. Hereditary C1q deficiency and systemic lupus erythematosus. Q J Med 87:455–464, 1994.

Brai M, Misiano G, Maringhini S, Cutaja I, Hauptmann G. Combined homozygous factor H and heterozygous C2 deficiency in an Italian family. J Clin Immunol 8:50–56, 1988.

Brauer RB, Lam TT, Wang D, Horwitz LR, Hess AD, Klein AS, Sanfilippo F, Baldwin WMR. Extrahepatic synthesis of C6 in the rat is sufficient for complement-mediated hyperacute rejection of a guinea pig cardiac xenograft. Transplantation 59:1073–1076, 1995.

Braun L, Schneider PM, Giles CM, Bertrams J, Rittner C. Null alleles of human complement C4. J Exp Med 171:129–140, 1990.

Burger R, Gordon J, Stevenson G, Ramadori G, Zanker B, Hadding U, Bitter-Suermann D. An inherited deficiency of the third component of complement, C3, in guinea pigs. Eur J Immunol 16:7–11, 1986.

Carney DF, Haviland DL, Noack D, Wetsel RA, Vik DP, Tack BF. Structural aspects of the human C5 gene. J Biol Chem 266:18786–18791, 1991.

Carroll MC, Campbell RD, Bently DR, Porter RR. A molecular map of the human major histocompatibility complex class III region linking complement genes C4, C2, and factor B. Nature 307:237–240, 1984.

Casciola-Rosen LA, Anhalt G, Rosen A. Autoantigens targeted in systemic lupus erythematosus are clustered in two populations of surface structures on apoptotic keratinocytes. J Exp Med 179:1317–1330, 1994.

Chakravarti DN, Chakravarti B, Parra CA, Muller-Eberhard HJ. Structural homology of complement protein C6 with other channel-forming proteins of complement. Proc Natl Acad Sci USA 86:2799–2803, 1989.

Chapius RM, Hauptmann G, Grosshans E, Isliker H. Structural and functional studies in C1q deficiency. J Immunol 129:1509–1515, 1982.

Christiansen FT, Dawkins RL, Uko G, McCluskey J, Kay PH, Zilko PJ. Complement allotyping in SLE: association with C4A null. Aust NZ J Med 13:483–488, 1983.

Cicardi M, Bergamaschini L, Marasini B, Boccassini G, Tucci A, Agostini A. Hereditary angioedema: an appraisal of 104 cases. Am J Med Sci 284: 2–9, 1982.

Cicardi M, Bisiani G, Cugno M, Spath P, Agostini A. Autoimmune C1 inhibitor deficiency: report of eight patients. Am J Med 95:169–175, 1993.

Colten HR. Tissue specific reglation of inflammation. J Appl Physiol 72:1–7, 1992.

Cork LC, Morris JM, Olson JL, Krakowka S, Swift AJ, Winkelstein JA. Membranoproliferative glomerulonephritis in dogs with a genetically determined deficiency of the third component of complement. Clin Immunol Immunopathol 60:455–470, 1991.

Cornacoff JB, Hebert LA, Smead WL, Van Amman ME, Birmingham DJ, Waxman FJ. Primate erythrocyte–immune complex–clearing mechanism. J Clin Invest 71:236–241, 1983.

Curd JG, Progais LJ Jr, Cochrane CG. Detection of active kallikrein in induced blister fluids ofhereditary angioedema patients. J Exp Med 152: 742–748, 1980.

Czop J, Nussenzweig V. Studies on the mechanisms of solubilization of immune precipitates by serum. J Exp Med 143:615–620, 1976.

Davies EJ, Snowden N, Hillarby MC, Carthy D, Grennan DM, Thomson W, Ollier WER. Mannose-binding protein gene polymorphism in systemic lupus erythematosus. Arthritis Rheum 38:110–114, 1995.

Davies KA, Erlendsson K, Beynon HLC, Peters AM, Steinsson K, Valdimarsson H, Walport MJ. Splenic uptake of immune complexes in man is complement dependent. J Immunol 151:3866–3873, 1993.

Davis AEI, Bissler JJ, Cicardi M. Mutations in the C1 inhibitor gene that result inhereditary angioneurotic edema. Behring Inst Mitt 93:313–320, 1993.

Dempsy PW, Allison MED, Akkaraju S, Goodnow CC, Fearon DT. C3d of complement as a molecular adjuvant: bridging innate and acquired immunity. Science 271:348–350, 1996.

Densen P, Ackerman L, Saucedo L, Figueroa J, Si Z-H, Stoltzfus C M. The genetic basis of C8α-γ deficiency. Mol Immunol 33(Suppl 1):68, 1996a.

Densen P, Sanford M, Burke T, Densen E, Wintermeyer L. Prospective study of the prevalence of complement deficiency in meningitis. 30th Interscience Conference on Antimicrobial Agents and Chemotherapy: Abstract 320, 1990.

Densen P, Weiler J, Ackermann L, Barson B, Zhu Z-B, Volanakis J. Functional and antigenic analysis of human factor B deficiency. Mol Immunol 33(Suppl 1):68, 1996b.

Densen P, Weiler JM, Griffss JM, Hoffmann LG. Familial properdin deficiency and fatal meningococcemia: correction of the bactericidal defect by vaccination. J Immunol Method 316:922–926, 1987.

Dodds AW, Ren X-D, Willis AC, Law SKA. The reaction mechanism of the internal thioester in the human complement component C4. Nature 379: 177–179, 1996.

Donaldson VH, Evans RR. A biochemical abnormality in hereditary angioedema: absence of serum inhibitor or C1-esterase inhibitor. Am J Med 35:37–42, 1963.

Donaldson VH, Rosen FS. Hereditary angioneurotic edema: a clinical survey. Pediatrics 37:1017–1023, 1966.

Dragon-Durey MA, Quartier P, Fremeaux-Bacchi V, Blouin J, de Barace C, Prieur A, Weiss L, Fridman WH. Molecular basis of a selective C1s deficiency associated with multiple autoimmune diseases. J Immunol 166: 7612–7616, 2001.

Edwards AO, Ritter R 3rd, Abel KJ, Manning A, Panhuysen C, Farrer LA. Complement factor H polymorphism and age-related macular degeneration. Science 308:421–424, 2005.

Ekdahl K, Truedsson L, Sjoholm AG, Braconier JH. Complement analysis in adult patients with a history of bacteremic pneumococcal infections or recurrent pneumonia. Scand J Infect Dis 27:111–117, 1995.

Ellison RT, Kohler PH, Curd JG, Judson FN, Reller LB. Prevalence of congenital and acquired complement deficiency in patients with sporadic meningococcal disease. N Engl J Med 308:913–916, 1983.

Ellman L, Green I, Frank MM. Genetically controlled deficiency of the fourth component of complement in the guinea pig. Science 170:74–81, 1970.

Ellman L, Green I, Judge F, Frank MM. In vivo studies in C4 deficient guinea pigs. J Exp Med 134:162–171, 1971.

Endo Y, Kanno K, Takahashi M, Yamaguchi K, Kohno Y, Fujita T. Molecular basis of human complement C1s deficiency. J Immunol 162:2180–2183, 1999.

Ernst SC, Circolo A, Davis AEI, Gheesling-Mullis K, Fleisler M, Strunk R. Impaired production of both normal and mutant C1 inhibitor proteins in type I hereditary angioedema with a duplication in exon 8. J Immunol 157:405–410, 1996.

Fasano MB, Hamosh A, Winkelstein JA. Recurrent systemic bacterial infections in homozygous C2 deficiency. Pediatr Allergy Immunol 1:46–49, 1990.

Fearon DT. Activation of the alternative complement pathway. CRC Crit Rev Immunol 1:1–3, 1979.

Fernie BA, Hobart MJ. Complement C7 deficiency: seven further molecular defects and their associated marker haplotypes. Hum Genet 103:513–519, 1998.

Fernie BA, Hobart MJ, Delbridge G, Potter PC, Orren A, Lachmann PJ. C6 haplotypes: associations of a Dde I site polymorphism to complement deficiency genes and the Msp I restriction fragment length polymorphism (RFLP). Clin Exp Immunol 95:351–356, 1994.

Fernie BA, Orren A, Sheehan G, Schlesinger M, Hobart MJ. Molecular bases of C7 deficiency. Three different defects. J Immunol 159:1019–1026, 1997.

Fernie BA, Orren A, Wurzner R, Jones AM, Potter PC, Lachman PJ, Hobart MJ. Complement component C6 and C7 haplotypes associated with deficiencies of C6. Ann Hum Genet 59:183–195, 1995.

Fernie BA, Price D, Chan E, Finlay A, Orren A, Joysey VC, Joysey KA, Schlesinger M, Hobart MJ. DNA markers in the C6 and C7 genes: biological anthropology and deficiency. Mol Immunol 33(Suppl 1):60, 1996a.

Fernie BA, Wurzner R, Morgan BP, Lachmann PJ, Hobart MJ. Molecular basis of combined C6 and C7 deficiency. Mol Immunol 33(Suppl 1):59, 1996b.

Fernie BA, Wurzner R, Orren A, Morgan BP, Potter PC, Platonov AE, et al. Molecular bases of combined subtotal deficiencies of C6 and C7: their effects in combination with other C6 and C7 deficiencies. J Immunol 157:3648–3657, 1996c.

Fiedler AHL, Walport MJ, Batchelor JR, Rynes RI, Black CM, Dodi IA, Hughes GRV. Family study of the major histocompatibility complex in patients with systemic lupus erythematosus: importance of null alleles of C4A and C4B in determining disease susceptibility. BMJ 286:425–428, 1983.

Figueroa J, Andreoni J, Densen P, Fredrikson GN, Truedsson L, Sjoholm AG. Complement deficiency states and meningococcal disease. New procedure for the detection of complement deficiency by ELISA. Analysis of activation pathways and circumvention of rheumatoid factor influence. Immunol Res 12:295–311, 1993.

Figueroa JE, Densen P. Infectious diseases associated with complement deficiencies. Clin Microbiol Rev 4:359–395, 1991.

Fijen CA, Juijper EJ, Hannema AJ, Sjohom AG, Van Putten JPM. Complement deficiencies in patients over ten years old with meningococcal disease due to uncommon serogroups. Lancet ii:585–588, 1989.

Fijen CA, Kuijper EJ, Drogari-Apiranthitou M, Van Leeuwen Y, Daha MR, Dankert J. Protection against meningococcal serogroup ACYW disease in complement-deficient individuals vaccinated with the tetravalent meningococcal capsular polysaccharide vaccine. Clin Exp Immunol 114:362–369, 1998.

Fischer MB, Ma M, Goerg S, Zhou X, Xia J, Finco O, Han S, Kelsoe G, Howard RG, Rothstein TL, Kremmer E, Rosen F, Carroll MC. Regulation of the B cell response to T-dependent antigens by classical pathway complement. J Immunol 157:549–556, 1996.

Frank MM, May J, Gaither T, Ellman L. In vitro studies of complement function in C4-deficient guinea pigs. J Exp Med 134:176–185, 1971.

Frank MM, Gelfand JA, Atkinson JP. Hereditary angioedema: the clinical syndrome and its management. Ann Intern Med 84:580–591, 1976.

Frank MM, Sergent JS, Kane MA, Alling DW. Epsilon aminocaproic acid therapy of hereditary angioneurotic edema: a double-blind study. N Engl J Med 286:808–812, 1972.

Fredrikson GN, Westburg J, Kuijper EJ, Tijssen CC, Sjoholm AG, Uhlen M, Truedsson L. Molecular genetic characterization of properdin deficiency type III: dysfunction due to a single point mutation in exon 9 of the structural gene causing a tyrosine to aspartic acid interchange. Mol Immunol 33(Suppl 1):1, 1996.

Friend P, Repine J, Kim Y, Clawson CC, Michael AF. Deficiency of the second component of complement (C2) with chronic vasculitis. Ann Intern Med 83:813–816, 1975.

Garred P, Mollnes TE, Thorsteinsson L, Erlendsson K, Steinsson K. Increased amounts of C4-containing immune complexes and inefficient activation of C3 and the terminal complement pathway in a patient with homozygous C2 deficiency and systemic lupus erythematosus. Scand J Immunol 31:59–64, 1990.

Geibink GS, Verhoef J, Peterson PK, Quie PG. Opsonic requirements for phagocytosis of Streptococcus pneumoniae types VI, XVIII, XXIII and XXV. Infect Immun 18:291–297, 1977.

Gelfand JA, Sherins RJ, Alling DW, Frank MM. Treatment of hereditary angioedema with danazol: reversal of clinical and biochemical abnormalities. N Engl J Med 295:1444–1450, 1976.

Glass D, Raum D, Gibson D, Stillman JS, Schur PH. Inherited deficiency of the second component of complement. Rheumatic Disease Association. J Clin Invest 58:853–861, 1976.

Haines JL, Hauser MA, Schmidt S, Scott WK, Olson LM, Gallins P, Spencer KL, Kwan SY, Noureddine M, Gilbert JR, Schnetz-Boutaud N, Agarwal A, Postel EA, Pericak-Vance MA. Complement factor H variant increases the risk of age-related macular degeneration. Science 308:419–421, 2005.

Hamann J, Wishaupt JO, van Lier RA, Smeets TJ, Breedveld FC, Tak PP. Expression of the activation antigen CD97 and its ligand CD55 in rheumatoid synovial tissue. Arthritis Rheum 42:650–658, 1999.

Hannema AJ, Kluin-Nelemans JC, Hack CE, Erenberg-Belmer AJM, Mallee C, Van Helden HPT. SLE-like syndromes and functional deficiency of C1q in members of a large family. Clin Exp Immunol 55:106–110, 1984.

Harriman GR, Esser AF, Podack ER, Wunderlich AC, Braude AI, Lint TF, Curd JG. The role of C9 in complement-mediated killing of Neisseria. J Immunol 127:2386–2390, 1981.

Hartung K, Fontana A, Klar M, Krippner H, Jorgens K, Lang B, Peter HH, Pichler WJ, Schendel D, Robin-Winn M, Deicher H. Association of class I, II, and III MHC gene products with systemic lupus erythematosus. Rheumatol Int 9:13–18, 1989.

Hauptmann G, Tappeiner G, Schifferli JA. Inherited deficiency of the fourth component of complement. Immunodefic Rev 1:3–22, 1988.

Hiemstra PS, Langeler E, Compier B, Keepers Y, Leijh PCJ, van den Barselaar MT, Overbosch D, Daha MR. Complete and partial deficiencies of complement factor D in a Dutch family. J Clin Invest 84:1957–1961, 1989.

Hobart MJ, Fernie BA, DiScipio RG. Structure of the human C7 gene and comparison with the C6, C8A, C8B, and C9 genes. J Immunol 154:5188–5194, 1995.

Hogasen K, Jansen JH, Mollnes TE, Hovdenes J, Harboe M. Hereditary porcine membranoproliferative glomerulonephritis type II is caused by factor H deficiency. J Clin Invest 95:1054–1061, 1995.

Holers VM, Cole JL, Lublin DM, Seya T, Atkinson JP. Human C3b- and C4b-regulatory proteins: a new multigene family. Immunol Today 6:188–192, 1985.

Horiuchi T, Ferrer JM, Serra P, Matamoros N, Lopez-Trascasa M, Hashimura C, et al. A novel nonsense mutation at Glu-631 in a Spanish family with complement component 7 deficiency. J Hum Genet 44:215–218, 1999.

Horiuchi T, Neshizaka H, Jojima T, Sawabe T, Niko Y, Schneider PM, Inaba S, Sakai K, Hayashi K, Hashimura C, Fukumori Y. A nonsense mutation at Arg 95 is predominant in C9 deficiency in Japanese. J Immunol 160:1509–1513, 1998.

Hosea SW, Brown EJ, Frank MM. The critical role of complement in experimental pneumococcal sepsis. J Infect Dis 142:903–908, 1980.

Hostetter MK, Gordon DL. Biochemistry of C3 and related thiolester proteins in infections and inflammation. Rev Infect Dis 9:97–102, 1987.

Howard PF, Hochberg MC, Bias WB, Arnett FC, McLean RH. Relationship between C4 null genes, HLA-D region antigens, and genetic susceptibility to systemic lupus erythematosus in Caucasian and black Americans. Am J Med 81:187–193, 1986.

Huang JL, Lin CY. A hereditary C3 deficiency due to aberrant splicing of exon 10. Clin Immunol Immunopathol 73:267–273, 1994.

Hudson-Peacock MJ, Joseph SA, Cox J, Munro CS, Simpson NB. Systemic lupus erythematosus complicating complement type 2 deficiency: successful treatment with fresh frozen plasma. Br J Dermatol 136:388–392, 1997.

Hugli TE. The structural basis for anaphylotoxin and chemotactic functions of C3a, C4a, and C5a. CRC Crit Rev Immunol 2:321–330, 1981.

Hummel DS, Mocca LF, Frasch CE, Winkelstein JA, Jean-Baptiste JHH, Canas JA, Leggiardro RJ. Meningitis caused by a nonencapsulated strain of Neisseria meningitidis in twin infants with C6 deficiency. J Infect Dis 155:815–819, 1987.

Inai S, Akagaki Y, Moriyama T, Fukumori Y, Yoshimura K, Ohnoki S, et al. Inherited deficiencies of the late-acting complement components other than C9 found among healthy blood donors. Int Arch Allergy Appl Immunol 90:274–279, 1999.

Inai S, Kitamura H, Hiramatsu S, Nagaki K. Deficiency of the ninth component of complement in man. J Clin Lab Immunol 2:85–87, 1979.

Inoue N, Saito T, Masuda R, Suzuki Y, Ohtomi M, Sakiyama H. Selective complement C1s deficiency caused by homozygous four-base deletion in the C1s gene. Hum Genet 103:415–418, 1998.

Ishii Y, Zhu Z-B, Macon K, Volanakis JE. Structure of the human C2 gene. J Immunol 151:170–174, 1993.

Johnson CA, Densen P, Hurford RK, Colten HR, Wetsel RA. Type I human complement C2 deficiency. J Biol Chem 267:9347–9353, 1992.

Johnson FR, Agnello V, Williams RC Jr. Opsonic activity in human serum deficient in C2. J Immunol 109:141–145, 1971.

Johnston RBJ, Klemperer MR, Alper CA, Rosen FS. The enhancement of bacterial phagocytosis by serum. The role of complement components. J Exp Med 129:1275–1281, 1969.

Kakkanaiah VN, Shen GQ, Ojo-Amaize EA, Peter JB. Association of low concentrations of serum mannose-binding protein with recurrent infections in adults. Clin Diagn Lab Immunol 5:319–321, 1998.

Kaufman KM, Snider JV, Spurr NK, Schwartz CE, Sodetz JM. Chromosomal assignment of genes encoding the α, β, and γ subunits of human complement protein C8: identification of a close physical linkage between the and β loci. Genomics 5:475–480, 1989.

Kavanagh D, Kemp EJ, Mayland E, Winney RJ, Duffield JS, Warwick G, Richards A, Ward R, Goodship JA, Goodship TH. Mutations in complement factor I predispose to development of atypical hemolytic uremic syndrome. J Am Soc Nephrol 16:2150–2155, 2005.

Kemp ME, Atkinson JP, Skanes VM, Levine RP, Chaplin D. Deletion of C4A genes in patients with systemic lupus erythematosus. Arthritis Rheum 30:1015–1022, 1987.

Klein RJ, Zeiss C, Chew EY, Tsai JY, Sackler RS, Haynes C, Henning AK, SanGiovanni JP, Mane SM, Mayne ST, Bracken MB, Ferris FL, Ott J, Barnstable C, Hoh J. Complement factor H polymorphism in age-related macular degeneration. Science 308:385–389, 2005.

Klemperer MR, Donaldson VH, Rosen FS. Effect of C1 esterase on vascular permeability in man: studies on normal and complement deficient individuals and in patients with hereditary angioneurotic edema. J Clin Invest 47:604–610, 1968.

Kluin-Nelemans HC, van Velzen-Blad H, van Helden HPT, Daha MR. Functional deficiency of complement factor D in a monozygous twin. Clin Exp Immunol 58:724–730, 1984.

Kusumoto H, Hirasawa S, Salier JP, Hagen FS, Kurachi K. Human genes for complement components C1r and C1s in a close tail-to-tail arrangement. Proc Natl Acad Sci USA 85:7307–7311, 1988.

Lassiter HA, Wilson JL, Feldhoff RC, Hoffpauir JM, Klueber KM. Supplemental complement component C9 enhances the capacity of neonatal serum to kill multiple isolates of pathogenic Escherichia coli. Pediatr Res 35:389–396, 1994.

Lee SL, Wallace SL, Barone R, Blum L, Chase PH. Familial deficiency of two subunits of the first component of complement: C1r and C1s associated with a lupus erythematosus–like disease. Arthritis Rheum 21:958–967, 1978.

Leenaerts PL, Stad RK, Hall BM, Van Damme BJ, Vanrenterghem Y, Daha MR. Hereditary C6 deficiency in a straw of PV6/c rats. Clin Exp Immunol 97:478–482, 1994.

Leggiadro RJ, Winkelstein JA. Prevalence of complement deficiencies in children with systemic meningococcal infections. Pediatr Infect Dis 6:75–79, 1987.

Lehto T, Meri S. Interactions of soluble CD59 with the terminal complement complexes. J Immunol 151:4941–4949, 1993.

Levy M, Halbwachs-Mecarelli L, Gubler MC, Kohout G, Bensenouci A, Niaudet P, Hauptmann G, Lesavre P. H deficiency in two brothers with atypical dense intramembranous deposit disease. Kidney Int 30:949–956, 1986.

Leyva-Cobian F, Moneo I, Mampaso R, Sanchez-Boyle M, Ecija JL. Familial C1q deficiency associated with renal and cutaneous disease. Clin Exp Immunol 44:173–176, 1981.

Lhotta K, Thoenes W, Glatzl J, Hintner H, Kronenberg F, Joannidis M, Konig P. Hereditary complete deficiency of the fourth component of complement: effects on the kidney. Clin Nephrol 39:117–124, 1993.

Lint TF, Zeitz HJ, Gewurz H. Inherited deficiency of the ninth component of complement in man. J Immunol 125:2252–2258, 1980.

Lipscombe RJ, Sumiya M, Summerfield JA, Turner MW. Distinct physicochemical characteristics of human mannose binding protein expressed by individuals of different genotypes. Immunology 85:660–667, 1995.

Loos M, Colomb M. C1, the first component of complement: structure-function relationship of C1q and collectins (MBP, SP-A, SP-D, conglutinin), C1-esterases (C1r and C1s), and C1-inhibitor in health and disease. Behring Inst Mitt 93:1–5, 1993.

Lublin DM, Lemons RS, LeBeau MM, Holers VM, Tykocinski ML, Medof ME, Atkinson JP. The gene encoding decay-accelerating factor (DAF) is located in the complement-regulatory locus on the long arm of chromosome 1. J Exp Med 165:1731–1736, 1987.

Lublin DM, Mallinson G, Poole J, Reid ME, Thompson S, Ferdman BR, Telen MJ, Anstee DJ, Tanner MJA. Molecular basis of reduced or absent expression of decay-accelerating factor in Cromer blood group phenotypes. Blood 84:1276–1282, 1994.

Ma M, Fischer MB, Goerg S, Han S, Kelsoe G, Carroll MC. Regulation of the B cell response to T-dependent antigens by classical pathway complement. Mol Immunol 33(Suppl 1):78, 1996.

Madsen HO, Garred P, Kurtzhals JAL, Lamm LU, Ryder LP, Thiel S, Svejgaard A. A new frequent allele is the missing link in the structural polymorphism of the human mannan-binding protein. Immunogenetics 40:37–44, 1994.

Madsen HO, Garred P, Thiel S, Kurtzhals JAL, Lamm LU, Ryder LP, Svejgaard A. Interplay between promoter and structural gene variants controls basal serum level of mannan-binding protein. J Immunol 155:3013–3020, 1995.

Matsumoto M, Fukuda W, Goellner J, Strauss-Schoenberger J, Huang G, Karr GW, Colten HR, Chaplin DD. Generation and characterization of mice deficient for factor B. Mol Immunol 33:63, 1996.

McAdam RA, Goundis D, Reid KBM. A homozygous point mutation results in a stop codon in the C1q B-chain of a C1q deficient individual. Immunogenetics 27:259–264, 1988.

Megerian CA, Arnold JE, Berger M. Angioedema: 5 years experience with a review of the disorder's presentation and treatment. Laryngoscope 102:256–260, 1992.

Merino J, Rodriguez-Valverde V, Lamelas JA. Prevalence of deficits of complement components in patients with recurrent meningococcal infections. J Infect Dis 148:331–336, 1983.

Meyer O, Hauptmann G, Tappeiner G, Ochs HD, Mascart-Lemove F. Genetic deficiency of C4, C2, or C1q and lupus syndromes. Association with anti-Ro (SS-A) antibodies. Clin Exp Immunol 62:678–682, 1985.

Molina H, Holers VM, Fang YF, Chaplin DD. Immune response abnormalities in mice deficient in complement receptor 1 and 2. Mol Immunol 33(Suppl 1):28, 1996.

Morley BJ, Vyse TJ, Bartok I, Spath PJ, Theodoridis E, Davies KA, Webster ADB, Walport MJ. Molecular basis of hereditary factor I deficiency. Mol Immunol 33(Suppl 1):71, 1996.

Motoyama N, Okada N, Yamashina M, Okada H. Paroxysmal nocturnal hemoglobinuria due to hereditary nucleotide deletion in the HRF20 (CD59) gene. Eur J Immunol 22:2669–2673, 1992.

Nagata M, Hara T, Aoki T, Mizuno Y, Akeda H, Inaba S, Tsumoto K, Veda K. Inherited deficiency of the ninth component of complement: an increased risk of meningococcal meningitis. J Pediatr 114:260–265, 1989.

Naughton MA, Walport MJ, Wurzner R, Carter MJ, Alexander GJ, Goldman JM, et al. Organ-specific contribution to circulating C7 levels by the bone marrow and liver in humans. Eur J Immunol 26:2108–2112, 1996.

Navratil JS, Ahearn JM. Apoptosis and autoimmunity. Complement deficiency and systemic lupus erythematosus revisited. Curr Rheumatol Rep 2:32–38, 2000.

Nelson RA Jr, Jensen J, Gigli I, Tamura N. Methods for the separation, purification and measurement of the nine components of the hemolytic complement in guinea pig serum. Immunochemistry 3:111–116, 1966.

Nicol PAE, Lachmann PJ. The alternative pathway of complement activation. The role of C3 and its inactivator (KAF). Immunology 24:259–265, 1973.

Nielsen HE, Koch C. Congenital properdin deficiency and meningococcal infection. Clin Immunol Immunopathol 44:134–138, 1987.

Nielsen HE, Koch C, Magnussesn P, Lind I. Complement deficiencies in selected groups of patients with meningococcal disease. Scand J Infect Dis 21:389–344, 1989.

Nishizaka H, Horiuchi T, Zhu Z-B, Fukumori Y, Nagasawa K, Hayashi K, Krumdieck R, Cobbs CG, Higuchi M, Yasunaga S, Niho Y, Volanakis JE. Molecular bases for inherited human complement component C6 deficiency in two unrelated individuals. J Immunol 156:2309–2315, 1996a.

Nishizaka H, Horiuchi T, Zhu Z-B, Fukumori Y, Volanakis JE. Genetic bases of human complement C7 deficiency. J Immunol 157:4239–4243, 1996b.

Nolan KF, Schwaeble W, Kaluz S, Dierich MP, Reid KBM. Molecular cloning of the cDNA coding for properdin, a positive regulator of the alternative pathway of human complement. Eur J Immunol 21:771–776, 1991.

Ochs HD, Nonoyama S, Zhu Q, Farrington M, Wedgwood RJ. Regulation of antibody responses: the role of complement and adhesion molecules. Clin Immunol Immunopathol 67:S33–40, 1993.

Ochs HD, Wedgwood RJ, Frank MM, Heller SR, Hosea SW. The role of complement in the induction of antibody responses. Clin Exp Immunol 53:208–213, 1983.

O'Hara AM, Fernie BA, Moran AP, Williams YE, Connaughton JJ, Orren A, et al. C7 deficiency in an Irish family: a deletion defect which is predominant in the Irish. Clin Exp Immunol 114:355–361, 1998.

Oltvai ZN, Wong ECC, Atkinson JP, Tung KSK. C1 inhibitor deficiency: molecular and immunologic basis of hereditary and acquired angioedema. Lab Invest 65:381–388, 1991.

O'Neil KM, Ochs HD, Heller SR, Cork LC, Morris JM, Winkelstein JA. Role of C3 in humoral immunity: defective antibody production in C3-deficient dogs. J Immunol 149:1939–1945, 1988.

Paccaud JP, Steiger G, Sjoholm AG, Spaeth PJ, Schifferli JA. Tetanus toxoid–anti-tetanus toxoid complexes: a potential model to study the complement transport system for immune complexes in humans. Clin Exp Immunol 69:468–472, 1987.

Pepys MB. The role of complement in induction of antibody production in vivo. J Exp Med 140:126–133, 1974.

Petersen BH, Graham JA, Brooks GF. Human deficiency of the eighth component of complement. The requirement of C8 for serum *Neisseria gonorrhoeae* bactericidal activity. J Clin Invest 57:283–290, 1976.

Petri M, McLean RH, Watson R, Winkelstein JA. Clinical expression of systemic lupus erythematosus in patients with C4A deficiency. Medicine 72:236–244, 1993.

Petry F, Berkel AI, Loos M. Repeated identification of a nonsense mutation in the C1qA-gene of deficient patients in southeast Europe. Mol Immunol 33(Suppl 1):9, 1996.

Petry F, Le DT, Kirschfink M, Loos M. Non-sense and missense mutations in the structural genes of complement component C1q A and C chains are linked with two different types of complete selective C1q deficiencies. J Immunol 155:4734–4738, 1995.

Pickering RJ, Gewurz H, Kelly JR, Good RA. The complement system in hereditary angioneurotic edema—a new perspective. Clin Exp Immunol 3:423–428, 1968.

Platonov AE, Beloborodov VB, Vershinina IV. Meningococcal disease in patients with late complement component deficiency: studies in the U.S.S.R. Medicine 72:374–392, 1993.

Polhill RB Jr, Pruitt KM, Johnson RB Jr. Kinetic assessment of alternative pathway activity in a hemolytic system. I. Experimental and kinetic analysis. J Immunol 121:363–369, 1978.

Prodeus AP, Fischer MB, Ma M, Murrow J, Reid R, Nicholson-Weller A, Warren H, Lage A, Carroll MC. Complement C3 and C4 deficient mice are highly susceptible to endotoxic shock. Mol Immunol 33(Suppl 1):79, 1996.

Prodeus AP, Zhou X, Maurer M, Galil SJ Carroll MC. Impaired mast cell–dependent natural immunity in C3-deficient mice. Nature 390:172–175, 1997.

Provost TT, Arnett FC, Reichlin M. Homozygous C2 deficiency, lupus erythematosus, and anti-Ro (SSA) antibodies. Arthritis Rheum 26:1279–1284, 1983.

Quezado ZMN, Hoffman WD, Winkelstein JA, Yatsiv I, Koev TCA, Cork LC, Elin RJ, Eichacker PQ, Natanson C. The third component of complement protects against endotoxin-induced shock and multiple organ failure. J Exp Med 179:569–168, 1994.

Rasmussen JM, Brandslund I, Teisner B, Isager H, Suehag S-E, Maarup L, Willumsen L, Ronne-Rasmussen JO, Permin H, Andesen PL, Svokmann O, Sorensen H. Screening for complement deficiencies in unselected patients with meningitis. Clin Exp Immunol 68:437–441, 1987.

Reid KBM, Thompson RA. Characterization of a non-functional form of C1q found in patients with a genetically linked deficiency of C1q activity. Mol Immunol 20:117–122, 1983.

Reid R, Prodeus AP, Khan W, Carroll MC. Natural antibody and complement are critical for endotoxin clearance from the circulation. Mol Immunol 33(Suppl 1):78, 1996.

Repine JE, Clawson CC, Friend PS. Influence of a deficiency of the second component of complement on the bactericidal activity of neutrophils in vitro. J Clin Invest 59:802–809, 1977.

Rosen FS, Alper CA, Pensky J, Klemperer MR, Donaldson VH. Genetically determined heterogeneity of the C1 esterase inhibitor in patients with hereditary angioneurotic edema. J Clin Invest 50:2143–2149, 1971.

Rosen FS, Charache P, Pensky J, Donaldson V. Hereditary angioneurotic edema: two genetic variants. Science 148:957–960, 1965.

Rosenberg LT, Tachibana DK. Activity of mouse complement. J Immunol 89:861–871, 1962.

Ross SC, Densen P. Complement deficiency states and infection: epidemiology pathogeneisis and consequences of neisserial and other infections in an immune deficiency. Medicine 63:243–273, 1984.

Rother RK, Rother U, Muller-Eberhard HJ, Nilsson U. Deficiency of the sixth component of complement in rabbits. J Exp Med 124:773–776, 1966.

Rowe PC, McLean RH, Wood RA, Leggiadro RJ, Winkelstein JA. Association of C4B deficiency with bacterial meningitis. J Infect Dis 160:448–451, 1989.

Ruddy S. Component deficiencies: the second component. Prog Allergy 39:250–260, 1986.

Sanchez-Corral P, Perez-Caballero D, Huarte O, Simckes AM, Goicoechea E, Lopez-Trascasa M, de Cordoba SR. Structural and functional characterization of factor H mutations associated with atypical hemolytic uremic syndrome. Am J Hum Genet 71:1285–1295, 2002.

Sastry K, Herman GA, Day L, Deignan E, Bruns G, Morton CC, Ezekowitz RAB. The human mannose binding protein gene. J Exp Med 170:1175–1189, 1989.

Saucedo L, Ackerman L, Platonov AE, Gewurz A, Rakita RM, Densen P. Delineation of additional genetic bases for C8 deficiency. J Immunol 155:5022–5028, 1995.

Schifferli JA, Bartolotti SR, Peters DK. Inhibition of immune precipitation by complement. Clin Exp Immunol 42:387–341, 1980.

Schifferli JA, Ng YC, Peters DK. The role of complement and its receptor in the elimination of immune complexes. N Engl J Med 315:488–491, 1986.

Schifferli JA, Steiger G, Hauptmann G, Spaeth PJ, Sjoholm AG. Formation of soluble immune complexes by complement in sera of patients with various hypocomplementemic states. J Clin Invest 76:2127–2131, 1985.

Schlesinger M, Greenberg R, Levy J, Kayhty H, Levy R. Killing of meningococci by neutrophils: effect of vaccination on patients with complement deficiency. J Infect Dis 170:449–453, 1994.

Schlesinger M, Kayhty H, Levy R, Bibi C, Meydan N, Levy J. Phagocytic killing and antibody response during the first year after tetravalent meningococcal vaccine in complement-deficient and in normal individuals. J Clin Immunol 20:46–53, 2000.

Sellar GC, Blake DJ, Reid KBM. Characterization and organization of the genes encoding the A-, B-, and C-chains of human complement subcomponent C1q. Biochem J 274:481–490, 1991.

Setien F, Alvarez V, Coto E, DiScipio RG, Lopez-Larrea C. A physical map of the human complement component C6, C7, and C9 genes. Immunogenetics 38:341–344, 1993.

Sheffer AL, Austen KF, Rosen FS. Tranexamic acid therapy inhereditary angioneurotic edema. N Engl J Med 287:452–459, 1972.

Shenoy-Scaria AM, Kwong J, Fujita T, Olszowy MW, Shaw AS, Lublin DM. Signal transduction through decay-accelerating factor. J Immunol 149:3535–3541, 1992.

Silverstein AM. Essential hypocomplementemia: report of a case. Blood 16:1338, 1960.

Sim RB, Kolble K, McAleer MA, Dominguez O, Dee VM. Genetics and deficiencies of the soluble regulatory proteins of the complement system. Int Rev Immunol 10:65–86, 1993.

Singer L, Colten HR, Wetsel RA. Complement C3 deficiency: human, animal, and experimental models. Pathobiology 62:14–28, 1994a.

Singer L, Whitehead WT, Akama H, Katz Y, Fishelson Z, Wetsel RA. Inherited human complement C3 deficiency. An amino acid substitution in the beta-chain (ASP549 to ASN) impairs C3 secretion. J Biol Chem 269:28484–28499, 1994b.

Sjoholm AG, Braconier JH, Soderstrom C. Properdin deficiency in a family with fulminant meningococcal infections. Clin Exp Immunol 50:291–297, 1982.

Sjoholm AG, Kuijper EJ, Tijssen CC, Jansz A, Bol P, Spanjaard L, Zanen H C. Dysfunctional properdin in a Dutch family with meningococcal disease. N Engl J Med 319:33–40, 1988a.

Sjoholm AG, Soderstrom C, Nilsson LA. A second variant of properdin deficiency: the detection of properdin at low concentrations in affected males. Complement 5:130–137, 1988b.

Slingsby JH, Norsworthy P, Pearce G, Vaishnaw AK, Issler H, Morley BJ, Walport MJ. Homozygous hereditary C1q deficiency and systemic lupus erythematosus. Arthritis Rheum 39:663–670, 1996.

Snyderman R, Goetzl EJ. Molecular and cellular mechanisms of leukocyte chemotaxins. Science 213:830–835, 1981.

Snyderman R, Phillips JK, Mergenhagen SE. Role of C5 in the accumulation of polymorphonuclear leukocytes in inflammatory exudates. J Exp Med 134:113–121, 1971.

Spath PJ, Sjoholm AG, Fredrikson GN, Misiano G, Scherz R, Schaad UB, et al. Properdin deficiency in a large Swiss family: identification of a stop codon in the properdin gene, and association of meningococcal disease with lack of the IgG2 allotype marker G2m(n). Clin Exp Immunol 118:278–284, 1999.

Steinsson K, Erlandsson K, Valdimarsson H. Successful plasma infusion treatment of a patient with C2 deficiency and systemic lupus erythematosus: clinical experience over forty-five months. Arthritis Rheum 32:906–913, 1989.

Stolfi RL. Immune lytic transformation. A state of irreversible damage as a result of the reaction of the eighth component in the guinea pig complement system. J Immunol 100:46–51, 1968.

Stone NM, Williams A, Wilkinson JD, Bird G. Systemic lupus erythematosus with C1q deficiency. Br J Dermatol 142:521–524, 2000.

Stoppa-Lyonnet D, Duponchel C, Meo T, Laurent J, Carter PE, Arala-Chaves M, Cohen JHM, Dewald G, Goetz J, Hauptmann G, Lagrue G, Lesavre P, Lopez-Trascasa M, Misiano G, Moraine C, Sobel A, Spath PJ, Tosi M.

Recombinational biases in the rearranged C1-inhibitor genes of hereditary angioedema patients. Am J Hum Genet 49:1055–1062, 1991.

Sullivan KE, Petri MA, Schmeckpeper BJ, McLean RH, Winkelstein JA. Prevalence of a mutation causing C2 deficiency in systemic lupus erythematosus. J Rheumatol 21:1128–1133, 1994.

Sullivan KE, Winkelstein JA. Prenatal diagnosis of heterozygous deficiency of the second component of complement. Clin Diagn Lab Immunol 1: 606–607, 1994.

Sullivan KE, Winkelstein JA. Genetically determined deficiencies of complement. In: Scriver CR, Beaudet AL, Sly WS, Valle DL, eds. Metabolic Basis of Inherited Disease, 8th Edition. New York: McGraw-Hill, pp. 4785–4815, 2001.

Sullivan KE, Wooten C, Goldman D, Petri M. Mannose binding protein genetic polymorphisms in black patients with systemic lupus erythematosus. Arthritis Rheum 39:2046–2051, 1996.

Sumiya M, Super M, Tabona P, Levinsky RJ, Arai T, Turner MW, Summerfield JA. Molecular basis of opsonic defect in immunodeficient children. Lancet 337:1569–1570, 1991.

Summerfield JA, Ryder S, Sumiya M, Thursz M, Gorchein A, Monteil MA, Turner MW. Mannose binding protein gene mutations associated with unusual and severe infections in adults. Lancet 345:886–889, 1995.

Suzuki Y, Ogura Y, Otsubo O, Akagi K, Fujita T. Selective deficiency of C1s associated with a systemic lupus erythematosus-like syndrome. Arthritis Rheum 35:576–579, 1992.

Takahaski M, Takahaski M, Bade V, Nussenzweig V. Requirements for solubilization of immune aggregates by complement. J Clin Invest 62:349–354, 1978.

Telen MJ, Green AM. The Inab phenotype: characterization of the membrane protein and complement regulatory defect. Blood 74:437–441, 1989.

Thompson RA, Haeney R, Reid KBM, Davies JG, White RHR, Cameron AH. A genetic defect of the C1q subcomponent of complement associated with childhood (immune complex) nephritis. N Engl J Med 303:22–24, 1980.

Truedsson L, Alper CA, Awdeh ZL, Johansen P, Sjoholm AG, Sturfelt C. Characterization of type I complement C2 deficiency MHC haplotypes. Strong conservation of the complotype/HLA-B-region and absence of disease association due to linked class II genes. J Immunol 151:5856–5863, 1993a.

Truedsson L, Sturfelt G, Nived O. Prevalence of the type I complement C2 deficiency gene in Swedish systemic lupus erythematosus patients. Lupus 2:325–327, 1993b.

Verpy E, Couture-Tosi E, Eldering E, Lopez-Trascasa M, Spath P, Meo T, Tosi M. Crucial residues in the carboxy-terminal end of C1-inhibitor revealed by pathogenic mutants impaired in secretion or function. J Clin Invest 95:350–359, 1995.

Vyse TJ, Spath PJ, Davies KA, Morley BJ, Philippe P, Athanassiou P, Giles CM, Walport MJ. Hereditary complement factor I deficiency. Q J Med 87:385–401, 1994.

Wang X, Circolo A, Lokki ML, Shackelford PG, Wetsel RA, Colten HR. Molecular heterogeneity in deficiency of complement protein C2 type I. Immunology 93:184–191, 1998.

Wang X, Fleischer DT, Whitehead WT, Haviland DL, Rosenfeld SI, Leddy JP, Snyderman R, Wetsel RA. Inherited human complement C5 deficiency. Nonsense mutations in exons 1 (Gln1 to Stop) and 36 (Arg1458 to Stop) and compound heterozygosity in three African-American families. J Immunol 154:5464–5471, 1995.

Waytes AT, Rosen FS, Frank MM. Treatment of hereditary angioedema with vapor-heated C1 inhibitor concentrate. N Engl J Med 334:1630–1634, 1996.

Weiss SJ, Ahmed AE, Bonagura VR. Complement factor D deficiency in an infant first seen with pneumococcal neonatal sepsis. J Allergy Clin Immunol 102:1043–1044, 1998.

Welch TR, Brickman C, Bishof N, Maringhini S, Rutkowski M, Frenzke M, Kantor N. The phenotype of SLE associated with complete deficiency of complement isotype C4A. J Clin Immunol 18:48–51, 1998.

Westberg J, Nordin G, Fredrikson N, Truedsson L, Sjoholm AG, Uhlen M. Sequence-based analysis of properdin deficiency: identification of point mutations in two phenotypic forms of an X-linked immunodeficiency. Genomics 29:1–8, 1995.

Wetsel RA, Kulics J, Lokki ML, Kiepiela P, Akama H, Johnson CA, Densen P, Colten HR. Type II human complement C2 deficiency. Allele-specific amino acid substitutions (Ser189 → Phe; Gly444 → Arg) cause impaired C2 secretion. J Biol Chem 271:5824–5831, 1996.

White RT, Damm D, Hancock N, Rosen BS, Lowell BB, Usher P, Flier JS, Spiegelman BM. Human adipsin is identical to complement factor D and is expressed at high levels in adipose tissue. J Biol Chem 267:9210–9213, 1992.

Whitehead AS, Solomon E, Chambers S, Bodmer WF, Povey S, Fey G. Assignment of the structural gene for the third component of complement to chromosome 19. Proc Natl Acad Sci USA 79:5021–5024, 1982.

Winkelstein JA. Genetically determined deficiency of the third component of complement in the dog. Science 215:1169–1170, 1981.

Winkelstein JA, Smith MR, Shin HS. The role of C3 as an opsonin in the early stages of infection. Proc Soc Exp Biol Med 149:397–402, 1975.

Witzel-Schlomp K, Spath PJ, Hobart MJ, Fernie BA, Rittner C, Kaufmann T, Schneider PM. The human complement C9 gene. Identification of two mutations causing deficiency and revision of the gene structure. J Immunol 158:5043–5049, 1997.

Wurzner R, Hobart MJ, Fernie BA, Mewar D, Potter PC, Orren P, Lachman PJ. Molecular basis of subtotal complement C6 deficiency. J Clin Invest 95:1877–1883, 1995a.

Wurzner R, Steinkasserer A, Hunter D, Dominguez O, Lopez-Larrea C, Sim RB. Complement factor H mRNA in Epstein-Barr virus transformed B lymphocytes of a factor H-deficient patient: detection by polymerase chain reaction. Exp Clin Immunogenet 12:82–87, 1995b.

Yamashina M, Ueda E, Kinoshita T, Takami T, Ojima A, Ono H, Tanaka H, Kondo N, Orii T, Okada N, Okada H, Inoue K, Kitani T. Inherited complete deficiency of 20-kilodalton homologous restriction factor (CD59) as a cause of paroxysmal nocturnal hemoglobinuria. N Engl J Med 323: 1184–1189, 1990.

Zhu Z, Atkinson TP, Hovanky KT, Boppana SB, Dai YL, Densen P, et al. High prevalence of complement component C6 deficiency among African-Americans in the southeastern USA. Clin Exp Immunol 119:305–310, 2000.

Zhu ZB, Totemchokchyakarn K, Atkinson TP, Whiteley RJ, Volanakis JE. Molecular defects leading to human complement component C6 deficiency. FASEB J 10:A1446, 1996.

Ziegler JB, Alper CA, Rosen FS, Lachmann PJ, Sherington L. Restoration by purified C3b inactivator of complement-mediated function in vivo in a patient with C3b inactivator deficiency. J Clin Invest 55:668–675, 1975.

III

Assessment and Treatment

43

Assessment of the Immune System

HELEN M. CHAPEL, SIRAJ MISBAH, and A. DAVID B. WEBSTER

Progress in clinical and molecular immunology has heightened the awareness of primary immune deficiency diseases (PIDD) and improved the diagnostic options and therapeutic choices available to physicians and clinical immunologists. Since many immunodeficiency syndromes can be treated or even cured, early diagnosis is of prime importance. As more physicians become familiar with the clinical and laboratory findings of these syndromes, PIDD patients will live longer and have better-quality lives. The most common reason for diagnostic delay is still lack of awareness of medical advisers and diagnostic centers; a widespread misconception is that PIDDs occur predominantly in children, whereas most of these syndromes present in individuals over 10 years of age. The presenting features, usually an excess of infections, are similar in patients of all ages.

Prime candidates for evaluation of the immune system are patients with recurrent or severe infections or those with infections that fail to respond appropriately to antibiotic therapy. Infants with failure to thrive and patients who develop fevers, suffer from diarrhea or malabsorption, or present with opportunistic infections are also candidates, as are those, especially adults, with chronic obstructive pulmonary disease often associated with bronchiectasis. Finally, patients with recurrent skin infections, poor wound healing, cold staphylococcal abscesses, or persistent or recurrent periodontitis; patients with recurrent neisserial infections; and those with clinical symptoms and findings of syndromes associated with abnormal immune functions—for example, thrombocytopenia and small platelets, albinism, or ataxia-telangiectasia—should also have their immune system evaluated. The diagnostic approach, from a practical point of view, is influenced not only by clinical criteria but also by other factors including age, gender, ethnic background, and consanguineous marriage. Molecular evaluation, if leading to a diagnosis, may allow the identification of carrier females and prenatal diagnosis. It is extremely important to test infants and children born to families known to have members with PIDD, including siblings or close relatives that fit the pattern of X-linked recessive, autosomal recessive, or autosomal dominant inheritance.

In this chapter, we will discuss the general principles of diagnosis of defects in different parts of the immune system. These are guided by the underlying etiology, involving antigen-specific immunity caused by defective B and T cell function or defects of the innate, non-antigen-specific immune system, such as defects of phagocyte and complement functions. We then go on to outline the diagnostic approach to the individual immune deficiency diseases. Both single-gene defects, which are covered in detail in preceding chapters, and disorders not well defined either phenotypically or genetically—for example, common variable immunodeficiency (see Chapter 23), IgG subclass deficiencies, and hyper-IgE syndrome (see Chapter 34)—are included in this chapter.

A rational approach is presented in Figure 43.1. The type of infectious agent(s) identified in a given patient gives a clue to the type of immune defect. Recurrent bacterial infections are associated with a B cell deficiency, as protection from gram-positive and gram-negative organisms depends on specific antibodies that act as opsonins. In such patients, B cell function and the ability to produce antibody are investigated first. If a patient presents with recurrent neisserial infections, assessment of the complement system is high on the list. Early-onset *Pneumocystis carinii* (recently renamed *jiraveci*) pneumonia (PCP) is a telltale sign of a severe T cell deficiency/abnormality, such as severe combined immune deficiency (SCID) or X-linked hyper-IgM syndrome (and, of course, HIV). Recurrent skin infections with staphylococci, *Serratia marcescens*, or candida suggest a neutrophil defect. The discovery of an unusual infectious agent, such as enterovirus-induced dermatomyositis or encephalitis, points to the diagnosis of X-linked agammaglobulinemia or one of the common variable

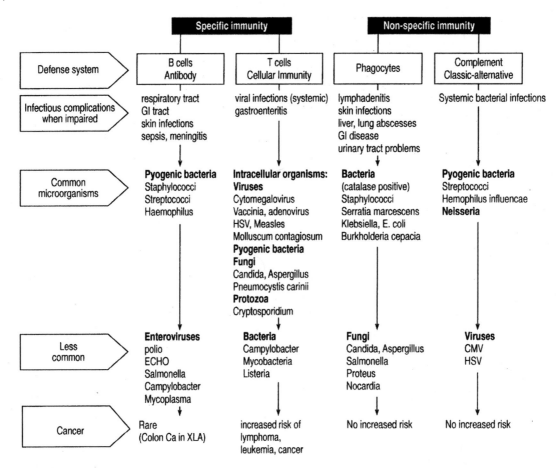

Figure 43.1. Types of infection and risks of malignancy in primary immune deficiencies affecting different defense systems

immunodeficiency disorders (CVID). As yet unrecognized but particular patterns of infections may prove to be associated with one of the newly recognized defects in innate immunity, such as Toll-like receptor pathway defects.

The age of presentation is also a helpful indicator for the likely diagnosis. Many primary immune deficiencies are caused by a single gene defect (see Chapter 1) and present in infancy or early childhood. However, certain genetic mutations may give rise to less severe disease, a so-called leaky phenotype, with presentation later in life. Others are "acquired" and probably depend on a combination of environmental factors and susceptibility genes, presenting in young adulthood or middle age. Adult patients should be tested for a range of PIDDs, including gene analysis for single gene defects known to have a particular clinical phenotype, as this will influence management and genetic counseling. The so-called acquired PIDDs are diagnoses of exclusion (Conley et al., 1999; Stiehm et al., 2004).

To provide a standard approach to diagnosis, criteria for each of the most common PIDDs have been devised on a collaborative basis between the European and Pan American groups for Primary Immunodeficiencies (see Table 43.1 and European Society for Immunodeficiencies [ESID] Web site provided at the end of the chapter). These criteria use a combination of clinical, laboratory, and molecular features to define a particular diagnosis as definite, probable, or possible.

Patients with a definitive diagnosis are assumed to have a >98% probability that in 20 years they will still be given the same diagnosis (Conley et al., 1999). Since a mutation does not change, there is an assumption that mutation detection is the most reliable method of making a definitive diagnosis. In patients with mutations that re-

sult in the absence of the specific mRNA or protein, the diagnosis can be established by appropriate testing; in others, the mRNA and/or protein may be transiently expressed, produced at very low levels, or be present and nonfunctional. For most diseases functional assays have not yet been developed. To guard against the inclusion of patients who have polymorphic variants in the genes associated with immunodeficiency, the patient must fulfill all the

Table 43.1. Primary Immunodeficiency Diseases for Which There Are Diagnostic Criteria

Definite*

Severe combined immunodeficiency (SCID) due to mutations of γc, Jak3, Rag1, Rag2, *Artemis*, IL-γR, CD45, CD38, ADA, ZAP-70
DiGeorge syndrome (due to 22q11.2 deletion)
MHC class II deficiency (due to mutations of *CIITA, RFxANK, RFx5, RfxAP*)
Leukocyte adhesion defects (LAD1, LAD2)
Chronic granulomatous disease (due to mutation of $gp91^{phox}$, $p22^{phox}$, $p47^{phox}$, $p67^{phox}$)
X-linked agammaglobulinemia due to mutation of *Btk*
X-linked hyper-IgM (XHIM) due to mutation of *CD40L*
Ataxia-telangiectasia (due to mutation of *ATM*)
Wiskott-Aldrich syndrome (due to mutation of *WASP*)
X-linked lymphoproliferative syndrome (due to mutation of *SH2D1A*)

Probable†

Common variable immunodeficiency (CVID)

---

*These are usually dependent on mutation detection with clinical and laboratory features (with or without a positive family history).

†Diagnosis of exclusion using clinical and laboratory features as well as exclusion criteria.

clinical and laboratory inclusion criteria characteristic of the disorder. The tests used to detect the most consistently abnormal findings in a particular disorder are discussed in the rest of this chapter. The diagnostic tools available range from simple, routine laboratory tests to complex immunologic and genetic procedures. Technical details for the assessment of the immune system can be found in *Current Protocols in Immunology* (Coligan et al., 1994), *Manual of Clinical Laboratory Immunology* (Rose et al., 1997).

General Assessment of Primary Immunodeficiency Diseases

History

Primary immunodeficiency disorders caused by a single gene defect often have a family history that points to either an X-linked or an autosomal recessive or dominant mode of inheritance (see

Chapters 2 and 44). A detailed family tree must consider premature deaths, the gender of affected individuals, paternity issues, and the possibility of consanguinity. However, about 50% of patients with an X-linked immunodeficiency, documented by mutation analysis, do not have a family history of immunodeficiency because they represent the first manifestation of a new mutation. The presence of consanguinity increases the possibility that a patient has a rare autosomal recessive immunodeficiency, but many patients with rare disorders are compound heterozygotes—i.e., they have different mutations on each of the pair of affected chromosomes because of mutations in both the maternal and paternal alleles. In a patient with atypical clinical or laboratory findings, the presence of a sibling with more typical disease can suggest a diagnosis, but this does not permit a definitive diagnosis in the absence of mutation detection.

A medical history (Table 43.2) should emphasize the age at onset of symptoms, the nature and etiology of infections, organs

Table 43.2. Historical and Physical Findings Suggestive of Primary Immunodeficiencies

Predominant T Cell Deficiency	*Phagocytic Defects*
Early onset, failure to thrive	Early onset
Oral candidiasis	Gram⁺, gram⁻ bacteria
Skin rashes, sparse hair	Catalase + organisms (CGD)
Protracted diarrhea	*Staphylococcus, Serratia marcescens, Klebsiella, Burkholderia cepacia*
Opportunistic Infections	*Candida, Aspergillus, Nocardia*
Pneumocystis carinii, CMV, EBV (lymphoproliferation)	Involvement of skin (seborrhoic dermatitis, impetigo)
Systemic BCG infection postvaccination	Cellulitis without pus (LAD)
Extensive candidiasis	Prolonged attachment of cord (LAD)
Graft vs. host disease (GVHD)	Lymph nodes (suppurative adenitis) (CGD; hyper-IgE)
Due to maternal engraftment	Respiratory tract: pneumonia, abscesses; pneumatoceles (hyper-IgE)
Due to nonirradiated blood transfusion	Oral cavity (periodontitis, ulcers, abscesses)
Bony abnormalities	Gastrointestinal
ADA deficiency, short-limb dwarfism	Crohn disease (CGD)
Hepatosplenomegaly (Omenn syndrome)	Gastric outlet obstruction (CGD)
Malignancies	Liver abscesses (CGD)
	Bones
Predominant B Cell Deficiency	Osteomyelitis (CGD)
Onset after maternal antibodies have disappeared	Urinary tract
Recurrent respiratory tract infections	Bladder outlet obstruction (CGD)
(gram⁺, gram⁻ bacteria; mycoplasma)	
Otitis media, mastoiditis	*Complement Defects*
Chronic sinusitis	Onset at any age
Broncho- and lobar pneumonia	Increased susceptibility to infections
Bronchiectasis	C1q, C1r/C1s, C4, C2, C3 (streptococcal, neisserial infections)
Pulmonary infiltrates/granulomas (CVI)	C5, C6, C7, C8, C9 (neisserial infections)
PCP (XHIM)	Factor D (recurrent infections)
Gastrointestinal symptoms, malabsorption	Factor B, factor I, properdin (neisserial infections)
Giardia, Cryptosporidia (XHIM), *Campylobacter*	Rheumatoid disorders (more often in early C-component deficiencies)
Cholangitis (XHIM)	SLE, discoid lupus, dermatomyositis, scleroderma, vasculitis,
Splenomegaly (CVI, XHIM)	membrane-proliferative glomerulonephritis
Nodular lymphoid hyperplasia, ileitis, colitis (CVI)	C1q, C1r/C1s, C4, C2; (rarely) C6 and C7 (SLE)
Skeletal, muscular	C3, factor F (glomerulonephritis)
Arthritis (bacterial, mycoplasma, noninfectious)	C1 esterase inhibitor (angioedema, SLE)
Dermatomyositis/fasciitis, due to enteroviruses (XLA)	
CNS	
Meningoencephalitis due to enteroviruses (XLA)	
Other findings	
Lymphadenopathy (abdominal, thoracic) (CVI)	
Neutropenia (XHIM, XLA)	
Anemia: hemolytic, parvovirus induced (XHIM)	
Lymphoma, thymoma (CVI)	
Bile duct, pancreatic duct malignancies (XHIM)	
Urinary tract mycoplasma (CVI)	

ADA, adenosine deaminase; BCG, bacillus Calmette Guérin; CGD, chronic granulomatous disease; CMV, cytomegalovirus; CVI, common variable immunodeficiency; EBV, Epstein-Barr virus; LAD, leukocyte adhesion deficiency; PCP, *Pneumocystis carinii* pneumonia; SLE, systemic lupus erythematosus; XHIM, X-linked hyper-IgM; XLA, X-linked agammaglobulinemia.

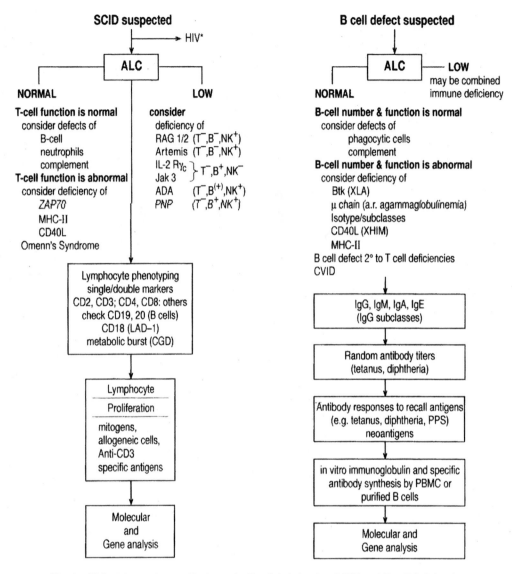

Figure 43.2. Diagnostic overall scheme for T cell deficiencies (SCID) and B cell deficiencies.

involved, the need for and response to antibiotics, as well as acute vs. chronic infections. Infants with T cell abnormalities often present with PCP and fungal infections in addition to bacterial infections, usually before the age of 3 months. Adults with T cell defects may have repeated viral infections, ranging from recurrent shingles to generalized chickenpox, or severe fungal infections. In contrast, most patients with a predominant B cell abnormality do not develop symptoms until maternal antibodies have disappeared in infants. Most adults and children with B cell defects are troubled by bacterial infections of the upper and lower airways. Patients with neutrophil defects may present at any age with skin infections, abscesses, and lymphadenopathy due to *Staphylococcus*, *Serratia marcescens*, *Klebsiella*, or *Aspergillus*. Late complement component deficiencies often cause generalized infections with encapsulated organisms. Older patients with PIDD may present with chronic lung disease, including bronchiectasis, and/or with chronic sinusitis and mastoiditis, diarrhea or other gastrointestinal complaints, or arthritis.

It is essential to have information about exposure to standard immunization antigens to interpret antibody titers. Full details of immunization and all childhood and adult infections are required.

The definite diagnosis of PIDD depends on laboratory evidence including assessment of humoral and cellular immunity and molecular analysis (Fig. 43.2, Tables 43.3 and 43.4), as physical findings are often absent, may be nonspecific, or very discreet. Occasionally, an immune deficiency is an incidental finding during investigation for an unrelated condition. These patients need full investigation to determine the clinical significance of the defect. To confirm the diagnosis of a primary immunodeficiency, secondary immunodeficiencies (e.g., HIV infection, lymphoid malignancies, antirheumatic or anticonvulsant drugs) have to be excluded and the relevant history must be taken.

Physical Examination

The physical examination (Table 43.2) may be totally negative, as, for instance, in patients with complement component deficiencies or in males with the XLP gene before being exposed to Epstein-Barr virus (EBV). Patients with SCID, by contrast, appear chronically ill; present with failure to thrive; are often pale, irritable, and wasted; and may have chronic nasal discharge and often diarrhea. The skin is frequently affected—erythroderma, eczema, pyoderma, or fungal lesions are common. Extensive

Table 43.3. Initial Laboratory Screening for Immune Deficiencies

CBC including granulocytes with differential, lymphocytes, platelets (with
　　size if available), hemoglobin
Quantitative serum immunoglobulins—IgG, IgA, IgM +/– IgE
Lymphocyte subset analysis by flow cytometry for
　　Quantitation of total T cells (CD3$^+$, CD2$^+$)
　　T cell subsets (CD4$^+$, CD8$^+$)
　　B cells (CD19$^+$, CD20$^+$)
　　NK cells (CD16$^+$, CD56$^+$)
　　HLA-DR to rule out MHC class II deficiency
　　Dihydrorhodamine to rule out CGD
Isohemagglutinin titers
IgG antibodies to
　　Known exposure (VZ)
　　Known immunizations (tetanus, diphtheria, Hib, meningococcus, polio,
　　　rubella)
CH50 and AP50
Sweat test to exclude cystic fibrosis
α_1 antitrypsin level

CBC, complete blood count; CGD, chronic granulomatous disease; MHC, major
histocompatibility complex; VZ, varicella-zoster.

warts of prolonged duration, persistent generalized molluscum
contagiosum, or other recurrent virus-induced skin lesions are
associated with T cell defects. Ectodermal dysplasia or severe
eczema is also a specific defect in the rare X-linked type of SCID
associated with an NF-κB signaling defect (Zonana et al., 2000;
Orange et al., 2002a; Smahi et al., 2002). Some features, such as
alopecia or sparse hair, are common in any individual who suf-
fers from chronic disease. But in rare cases these features may
represent specific syndromes, for example, the human equivalent
of the mouse Nude/SCID phenotype (Pignata et al., 2001) or
the rare and fatal X-linked condition associated with neonatal
polyendocrinopathy and enteropathy (IPEX) syndrome (Bennett
et al., 2002) (Chapter 26).

　　The presence of petechiae and bruises suggests a bleeding
problem (Cunningham-Rundles, 2002). Partial albinism in a child
with recurrent infections is typical of the Chediak-Higashi syndrome, although this can also be a feature of other genetic abnormalities. The absence of lymph nodes despite repeated infection
is a telling sign of a nonfunctional antigen-specific lymphoid
system. In patients with a neutrophil defect (such as chronic granulomatous disease), lymph nodes are usually enlarged and suppurative. Sometimes the immunodeficiency is a component of a
rare, generalized disorder of metabolism and/or development
(e.g., Nijmegen breakage syndrome, glycogen storage disease).

　　Examination of the oral cavity may provide important clues:
therapy-resistant candidiasis suggests a T cell or neutrophil defect and may involve the entire esophagus. Extensive periodontitis is a hallmark of leukocyte adhesion defects. Recurrent mouth
ulcers may indicate cyclic neutropenia or recurrent Herpes simplex infection associated with a T cell defect. Lack of tonsillar
tissue is a feature of total failure of B lymphocyte development,
as in X-linked agammaglobulinemia (see Chapter 26), in contrast
to hypertrophy and significant lymphadenopathy in patients with
activation-induced cytidine deaminase (AID) deficiency (see
Chapter 20).

　　Gross signs of structural damage are seen in patients with
long-standing undiagnosed or untreated PIDD. Persistent cough
at night or early morning suggests the presence of chronic lung
disease such as asthma or bronchiectasis; signs of restrictive lung
disease are often present during chest examination. Nasal polyps,

Table 43.4. Comprehensive Laboratory Evaluation for Immune
Deficiency

B Cell Deficiency

Quantitative IgG, IgM, IgA, IgE
IgG subclasses
B cell numbers in peripheral blood (CD19, CD20)
Antibody responses to test immunizations, e.g., D/T, Pneumovax
In vitro IgG synthesis by mitogen-stimulated PBL or purified B cells
　　cultured in the presence of anti-CD40 and lymphokines
In vitro proliferation of B cells in response to anti-CD40 and IL-4
Biopsies: rectal mucosa; lymph nodes (if appropriate)
Molecular and mutation analysis (e.g., Btk, μ heavy chain)

T Cell Deficiency

Absolute lymphocyte count
T cell, T subset, and NK cell enumeration (CD3, CD4, CD8; also CD16,
　　CD56)
Delayed-type hypersensitivity skin tests (only in older children and adults)
　　(candida, tetanus toxoid, mumps)
In vitro proliferation of lymphocytes to mitogens (PHA, ConA), allogeneic
　　cells, and specific antigens (candida, tetanus toxoid)
Production of cytokines by activated lymphocytes
Expression of activation markers (e.g., CD40L, CD69) and lymphokine
　　receptors (e.g., IL-2Rγ_c, IFN-γR) after mitogenic stimulation
Enumeration of MHCI and MHCII expressing lymphocytes
Chromosome analysis (probe for 22q11)
Enzyme assays (ADA, PNP)
Biopsies: skin, lymph node, thymus (if appropriate)
Molecular and mutation analysis (e.g., CD40L, γ_c chain, Jak3, ZAP-70)

Deficiency of Phagocytic System

Absolute neutrophil count (serially to rule out cyclic neutropenia)
WBC turnover
Antineutrophil antibody
Bone marrow biopsy
Chemotaxis, assessment of adhesion in vivo and in vitro
CD11/CD18 assessment (flow cytometry)
Bombay phenotype (LAD2)
Phagocytosis (baker's yeast)
NBT slide test; metabolic burst (flow cytometry); chemiluminescence;
　　bacterial assays
Enzyme assays
　　MPO, G6PD
　　Glutathione peroxidase
　　NADPH oxidase
Mutation analysis (e.g., gp91^{phox}; p22^{phox}; p47^{phox}; p67^{phox}; β integrin)

Complement Deficiencies

CH50, AH50
Analysis of quantity and function of C components
Chemotactic activity of complement split products, e.g., C3a, C5a

Other Diagnostic Tests

α_1-antitrypsin
Sweat Cl$^-$
Nasal mucosa biopsy (to rule out immotile cilia syndrome)
Rule out tracheoesophageal fistula (imaging)

ADA, adenosine deaminase; ConA, concanavalin A; G6PD, glucose-6-phosphate
dehydrogenase; LAD, leukocyte adhesion deficiency; MPO, myeloperoxidase;
NBT, nitroblue tetrazolium; PBL, peripheral blood lymphocytes; PHA, phytohemagglutinin; PNP, purine nucleoside phosphorylase.

tender sinuses, or damaged tympanic membranes suggest previous recurring upper respiratory tract infections. Since many
patients with PIDD present to ear–nose–throat (ENT) clinics initially, these symptoms may be of long duration (Cooney et al.,
2001). Nasal endoscopy and computed tomography (CT) of the

sinuses are indicated if there is persistent infection or if surgery is being considered. Endoscopically guided microswab culture obtained from the middle meatus or sinuses themselves correlate well (80%) with results from now-abandoned antral puncture (Osguthorpe, 2001).

Congenital malformation of the heart and large vessels, especially if associated with hypocalcemia in a newborn, makes DiGeorge syndrome the most likely diagnosis (see Chapter 33). Liver abscesses, suppurative lymphadenopathy, hepatosplenomegaly, and perirectal fistulas are often associated with chronic granulomatous disease (see Chapter 37). Progressive omphalitis, if associated with neutrophilia, suggests an adhesion molecule defect of neutrophils (see Chapter 38). Progressive cerebellar ataxia, in association with discreet or pronounced telangiectasia involving the conjunctiva, ears, and sometimes the face and shoulders are classic findings in ataxia-telangiectasia (see Chapter 29).

Laboratory Diagnosis

Initial screening for immune deficiencies

Initially, an attempt is made to establish the diagnosis of PIDD by screening the different defense systems and by ruling out rare nonimmunologic disorders, including cystic fibrosis, inhalation of a foreign body, congenital absence of the spleen, immobile cilia syndrome, or anatomic abnormalities, for example, tracheoesophageal fistula. A set of useful initial tests that can be performed in most general laboratories is listed in Table 43.3; such tests benefit from reliable quality assurance measures and are widely available.

A full blood count will reveal a neutropenia, lymphopenia, and thrombocytopenia. Lymphocyte counts are much ignored yet give vital information for the diagnosis of SCID (Gossage and Buckley, 1990). Quantitative determination of serum IgG, IgM, IgA, and IgE is also part of the initial screening. The interpretation of serum immunoglobulin levels may be difficult; not only patient age but also the possibility of protein loss or previous immunoglobulin substitution must be considered. The presence of hemolytic complement activity (CH50), even at reduced amounts, rules out most congenital complement deficiencies of the classic pathway (see Chapter 42). The normal ranges for lymphocytes and lymphocyte subset numbers as well as serum immunoglobulin levels are age-dependent (Erkeller-Yuksel et al., 1992; Melaranci et al., 1992; Stiehm et al., 2004) and comparison with age-matched controls is essential.

In the absence of steroid or immunosuppressive therapy, lymphopenia usually indicates a T cell deficiency, as >60% of circulating lymphocytes are normally T cells. The percentages and absolute numbers of T and B cell subsets are measured by means of flow cytometry (Fleisher and Oliveira, 2004), using monoclonal antibodies that recognize cell type–specific antigens (Tables 43.3 and 43.4). The proportions of these cells in peripheral blood are also age-dependent (Fig. 43.3) (Erkeller-Yuksel et al., 1992; Stiehm et al., 2004). Most patients with SCID or a predominant T cell deficiency have reduced numbers of cells with CD3, CD4, or CD8 antigens on their surface. Those with agammaglobulinemia and a subset of patients with SCID have low numbers of B cells with CD19, CD20, or CD21 expression. The widespread use of flow cytometry and standardization of commercially available monoclonal antibodies, coupled with excellent quality assurance schemes, make these assays reliable screening tests.

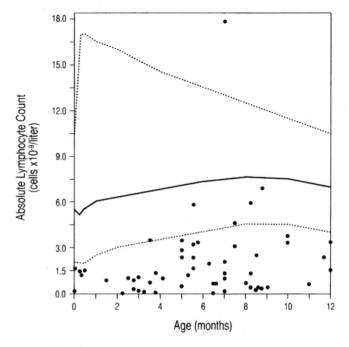

Figure 43.3. Absolute lymphocyte counts in normal infants and infants with severe combined immunodeficiency.

Comprehensive and Specific Evaluation for Immune Deficiencies

Tests for antibody deficiencies

Primary antibody deficiencies are more common than T cell or combined deficiencies. An approach to the diagnosis of the known types of primary antibody deficiency is shown in Figure 43.2 and Table 43.4. After measurement of the serum levels of the three major immunoglobulin isotypes, the most important investigation is the assessment of specific antibody activity. Failure to produce antibodies to immunizations or after known exposure to common pathogens forms part of the international criteria for primary antibody deficiencies (Conley et al., 1999; Stiehm et al., 2004).

Titers of naturally occurring IgM antibodies such as anti-A or anti-B isohemagglutinins can be determined in a bloodbank-associated laboratory. The presence of serum IgG antibodies to agents to which the individual is known to have been exposed (e.g., varicella, since chickenpox is a distinct clinical entity, or definite immunization) is also helpful. In the absence of such antibodies, the use of test immunizations to measure the kinetics of specific IgG antibody responses to defined antigens is most informative. Serum is collected before and 3–4 weeks after immunization and antibody titers are determined. Normal pre- and postvaccination values are available and assays can be quality assured (Gibb et al., 1995). The most widely used recall antigens are diphtheria/tetanus toxoid and conjugated *Haemophilus influenzae* B (Hib) vaccines; these proteins provoke T cell–dependent IgG responses. The use of protein neoantigens, such as keyhole limpet hemocyanin (KLH) (Kondratenko et al., 1997) and bacteriophage ØX174 (Stiehm et al., 2004), allows precise assessment of primary, secondary, and tertiary responses, including immunologic memory, class switch from IgM to IgG, and amplification following multiple exposures to antigen.

To measure antibodies to polysaccharides (short-lived, relatively T cell–independent responses), a polysaccharide vaccine

(Pneumovax) against 23 pneumococcal serotypes is still available. In most European countries, responses to the vaccine as a whole are determined for diagnosis of immune deficiencies; in the United States, responses to at least 12 serotypes are measured before and after immunization, and a positive response is taken as a significant rise in at least 8 of the 12 (less in children). With the development of an assay for the pure polysaccharide vaccine to *Salmonella typhi* (Typhum Vi) an alternative carbohydrate vaccine has become available, for which the assay has been published (Ferry et al., 2004). Children less than 2 years of age do not respond reliably to unconjugated polysaccharide vaccines.

IgG subclass levels should be measured only under certain circumstances. These include patients with normal or near-normal IgG concentrations and with demonstrable (though often partial) antibody deficiency, or abnormal responses to protein or polysaccharide antigens; patients with selective IgA deficiency who have shown an increased susceptibility to infection to rule out an associated IgG2/IgG4 deficiency; and adults with persistent sinusitis and upper respiratory tract infections and normal serum immunoglobulin levels who may have selective loss of IgG2 or IgG3. Assays are now standardized and quality assured, and age-matched, normal IgG-subclass concentrations are available (Stiehm et al., 2004).

The presence of circulating, mature B cells is determined by flow-cytometric analysis of whole blood. To execute an effective antibody response, B cells, CD4+ T helper cells, and antigen-presenting cells are colocalized in secondary immune organs, where they form characteristic structures (germinal centers, follicles). Biopsies of rectal mucosa, lymph nodes, and bone marrow may show characteristic structural abnormalities, and absence of a given cell type may be found if immunohistological techniques are used. Determination of the stage of B cell maturation arrest in the bone marrow may provide a clue to the genetic defect in patients with absent circulating B cells (see Chapters 21 and 22). However, these invasive procedures are performed infrequently.

If a single gene defect is suspected, it may be possible to identify the gene product (see Tables 43.5 and 43.6). An example is X-linked agammaglobulinemia (XLA), where Bruton tyrosine

kinase (Btk) deficiency can be detected in about 70%–80% of affected males through demonstration of lack of Btk protein in circulating monocytes and platelets (Futatani et al., 1998, 2001). The protein can also be detected by Western blotting, and mRNA by Northern blotting. Finally, genomic or complementary DNA must be examined by sequence analysis to detect nonfunctional but present protein.

In vitro assessment of immunoglobulin synthesis by stimulated peripheral blood B lymphocytes is used predominantly as a research tool. Purified B cells can be stimulated to produce and secrete immunoglobulins in a T cell–independent manner if directly activated through CD40 and in the presence of exogenous lymphokines. They then proliferate and secrete IgE if interleukin-4 (IL-4) is added to the culture, or secrete IgG and IgM if IL-10 is added (Nonoyama et al., 1993, 1994). These assays have been used to distinguish patients with intrinsic B cell defects from those in whom T cell help is inadequate. With the increased understanding of B cell activation and switched and unswitched memory markers, however, flow cytometry offers more promise (Agematsu et al., 1998, 2002; Warnatz et al., 2002; Piqueras et al., 2003), especially in view of the satisfactory use of whole blood rather than separated peripheral blood mononuclear cells (PBMC) (Ferry et al., 2005).

Tests for T cell deficiencies and severe combined immunodeficiencies

Significant and persistent lymphopenia is a hallmark of severe T cell deficiency (Figs. 43.2 and 43.3). Absolute lymphocyte counts and assessment of lymphocyte subsets, both by percentage and absolute number, are readily available and reliable. As for B cells, the method of choice for T cell subset enumeration is flow cytometry. The use of whole blood for analysis by flow cytometry is not only more accurate but is especially useful for pediatric patients because of the small sample volume required. An initial, standard analysis by flow cytometry is shown in Tables 43.3 and 43.4. Interpretation is based on the presence or absence of the three major types of cells involved: T, B, and natural killer (NK) cells (Fig. 43.2).

Total lymphocyte numbers and T lymphocyte subsets are age-dependent, being markedly increased in newborns and young

Table 43.5. Diagnostic Approach to X-Linked Inherited Immunodeficiencies

Disorder	Gene	Diagnostic Tests
X-linked agammaglobulinaemia (XLA)	Bruton tyrosine kinase (*Btk*)	Btk expression by immunoblotting or flow cytometry (monocytes or platelets)
		Mutation analysis
X-linked severe combined immunodeficiency (XSCID)	Common gamma chain (c) (*IL2RG*)	Gamma c (CD132) expression on activated T cells (flow cytometry)
		Mutation analysis
Wiskott-Aldrich syndrome (WAS/XLT)	WAS protein (*WASP*)	WASP expression (Western blot, flow cytometry)
		Mutation analysis
X-linked hyper-IgM syndrome (CD40 ligand deficiency)	CD40L (*CD154*)	CD40L expression on activated CD4+ T cells (flow cytometry)
		Mutation analysis
X-linked anhidrotic ectodermal dysplasia with immunodeficiency	IKKBG, NF-κB essential modulator (*NEMO*)	EMSA (NF-κB)
		Mutation analysis
X-linked lymphoproliferative syndrome (Duncan disease; XLP)	SH2D1A (*SAP*)	SAP expression
		Mutation analysis
Immune dysregulation, polyendocrinopathy, enteropathy, X-linked (IPEX)	*FOXP3*	Lack of regulatory T cells, FOXP3 absent
		Mutation analysis
X-linked chronic granulomatous disease (XCGD)	gp91phox	NBT slide test; dihydrorhodamine flow cytometry
		Mutation analysis
Properdin deficiency	Properdin factor C (*PFC*)	AP50, serum properdin levels, mutation analysis

Table 43.6. Diagnostic Approach to Autosomally Inherited Immunodeficiencies

Disorder	Gene Name	Diagnostic Tests
Severe Combined Immunodeficiencies (SCID)		
Recombinase-activating gene protein 1 and 2 (RAG1, RAG2) deficiency, Omenn syndrome	*RAG1, RAG2*	Mutation analysis
Artemis deficiency	*Artemis*	Radiation sensitivity, mutation analysis
JAK3 deficiency	*Jak3*	Jak3 protein absent (Western blot)
		Mutation analysis
T cell receptor deficiencies		
CD3γ	*CD3G*	Low CD3 expression
CD3ε	*CD3E*	Mutation analysis
CD3δ	*CD3D*	
IL-7 receptor deficiency	*ZAP70*	CD8$^+$ T cells reduced or absent, CD4$^+$ T cells nonfunctional
		Lack of ZAP-70 (Western blot)
		Mutation analysis
Deficiency of Purine Metabolism		
Adenosine deaminase (ADA) deficiency	*ADA*	ADA activity reduced in RBC; purine metabolites increased in RBC, plasma, urine
		Mutation analysis
Purine nucleoside phosphorylase (PNP) deficiency	*PNP*	PNP activity reduced in RBC; purine metabolites increased in RBC, plasma, urine
		Mutation analysis
Major Histocompatability Complex (MHC) Deficiency		
MHC class I deficiency (bare lymphocyte syndrome type I)	*TAP1*	HLA class I expression (flow cytometry)
	TAP2	Mutation analysis
MHC class II deficiency (bare lymphocyte syndrome type II)	*CIITA*	MHC class II (DR) expression absent on flow cytometry
	RFXANK	Mutation analysis
	RFX5	
	RFXAP	
Inherited Mycobacterial Susceptibility		
Interferon-γ receptor deficiencies	*IFNGR1/2*	IFN-γR1/2 decreased or absent
IL-12 deficiency	*IL12 p40*	IL-12 expression absents
IL-12 receptor deficiency	*IL12ReB1*	IL-12 receptor expression absent
		Mutation analysis
Hyper-IgM Syndromes (Autosomal Recessive)		
CD40 deficiency	*CD40*	B cells lack CD40 expression on flow cytometry
Activation-induced cytidine deaminase (AID) deficiency	*AICDA*	Very high serum levels of IgM, lymphadenopathy, mutation analysis
Uracil-DNA glycosylase (UNG) deficiency	*UNG*	High serum levels of IgM
		Mutation analysis
Common Variable Immunodeficiency (CVID) Subcategories		
ICOS (inducible costimulatory) deficiency	*ICOS*	CVID-like, mutation analysis
CD19 deficiency	*CD19*	CVID-like, lack of CD19 expression by B cells, mutation analysis
TACI (tumor necrosis factor receptor [TNFR] super family member 13B) deficiency	*TNFRSF13B*	CVID-like, mutation analysis
BAFF receptor (TNFR super family member 13C) deficiency	*TNFRSF13C*	CVID-like, mutation analysis
Autoimmune Lymphoproliferative Syndrome (ALPS)		
Type Ia (Fas/APO-1; CD95 deficiency)	*TNFRSF6*	>1% double-negative (α/β) T cells (CD4$^-$, CD8$^-$, CD3$^+$)
Type IIb (FasL, CD178 deficiency)	*TNFSF6*	Defective lymphocyte apoptosis
Type IIa (caspase 10 deficiency)	*CASP10*	Mutation analysis
Type IIb (caspase 8 deficiency)	*CASP8*	
Chromosome Breakage Syndromes		
Ataxia-telangiectasia (AT)	*ATM*	DNA radiation sensitivity, translocations
		Mutation analysis
Immunodeficiency, centromere instability, facial abnormalities syndrome (ICF)	*DNMT3B* (methyltransferase)	Multibranched chromosomal configurations, chromosomal breakage only in lymphocytes
		Mutation analysis
Nijmegen breakage syndrome (NBS)	*NBS1*	Radiation sensitivity, chromosome instability, mutation analysis
Bloom syndrome	*BLM* (α helicase)	Radiation sensitivity, sister chromatid exchange, mutation analysis

(continued)

Table 43.6. (*continued*)

Disorder	Gene Name	Diagnostic Tests
Phagocytic Defects		
Chronic granulomatous disease	*p47^{phox}*	p47^{phox}, p67^{phox}, p22^{phox} expression (Western blot)
(autosomal recessive genes)	*p67^{phox}*	Mutation analysis
	p22^{phox}	
Leucocyte adhesion deficiency type I (LAD1)	*CD18*	CD11/CD18 expression absent
Leukocyte adhesion deficiency type II (LAD2)	Fucose transporter	Sialyl-Lewis X absent (flow cytometry)
	(*NAALLAD2*)	Mutation analysis
Cyclic neutropenia and Kostman syndrome	Neutrophil elastase	Cyclic or congenital neutropenia, mutation analysis
Chediak-Higashi syndrome	*LYST*	Giant inclusions in granulocytes
		Mutation analysis
Griscelli syndrome		
Type 1	*M405A*	Mutation analysis
Type 2	*RAB27A*	Mutation analysis
Other Well-defined Immune Deficiency Syndromes		
APECED (autoimmune polyendocrinopathy, candidiasis,		
ectodermal dystophy)	*AIRE1*	Mutation analysis
WHIM (warts, hypogammaglobulinemia, recurrent		
bacterial infections, myelokathexis)	*CXCR4*	Mutation analysis

EMSA, electrophoresis mobility shift assay; NBT, nitroblue tetrazolium; RBC, red blood cells.

infants and decreasing with age (Fig. 43.3). In infants under 4 months of age, a CD4 count of <1000/mm^3 (in infants infected with HIV, a count of 1500/mm^3) is generally associated with impaired cellular immunity, whereas in children over age 2 years and in adult patients it is <500 CD4 cells/mm^3 (Melaranci et al., 1992). In these situations all transfused blood or blood cellular products should be pre-irradiated and live vaccines should be avoided. A CD4:CD8 ratio <1.0, in the absence of a gross CD8 lymphocytosis, may also indicate abnormal T cell function and a ratio of 0.3 is often associated with profound T cell deficiency.

In vitro lymphocyte proliferation to mitogens, including phytohemagglutinin (PHA), pokeweed mitogen (PWM), and concanavalin A (Con A), or to cross-linking of T cell surface antigens by monoclonal antibodies to CD3 provides a rough estimate of T cell function. These assays are difficult to perform, requiring sterile culture conditions for 3–6 days and, in the past, methods for incorporation and subsequent measurement of radiolabeled thymidine. Recently, nonradioactive methods such as expression of activation markers, cytokine production, or uptake of carboxyfluorescein succinimidyl ester (CFSE), detected by flow cytometry (Table 43.4), are used. A more sensitive way to measure T lymphocyte function in adults and older children is in vitro stimulation with specific antigens to which patients have been previously exposed, such as diphtheria or tetanus toxoid, purified protein derivative (PPD) (following bacillus Calmette Guérin [BCG] immunization), or candida antigen.

Cytokines can be measured in culture supernatants by ELISA or intracellularly by flow cytometry and may help identify a functional T cell defect in rare cases. Kits to quantitate mRNA are now commercially available to measure transcription of most lymphokines during lymphocyte activation on a research basis. However, only one specific cytokine deficiency—IL-12p40 deficiency—has been described to date. There has been a single case of SCID in which transcription of the IL-2 gene and other lymphokine genes were affected (Pahwa et al., 1989).

Mutations affecting interferon-γ (IFN-γ) receptors (IFN-γR$_1$ or IFN-γR$_2$), observed in infants with normal numbers of T cells and severe nontuberculous mycobacterial disease (see Chapter 28), result in defective IFN-γ signaling, such as failure of STAT1 phosphorylation following IFN-γ activation of patient monocytes (Fleisher et al., 1999) and impaired tumor necrosis factor-alpha (TNF-α) production by PBMC in response to a combination of lipopolysaccharide (LPS) and IFN-γ (Holland et al., 1998). This approach has been greatly facilitated by a new flow cytometry method for intracellular and nuclear staining of STAT1 and STAT4 in response to IFN-γ or IL-12 activation (Uzel et al., 2001). IL-12Rβ1 deficiency, observed in patients with disseminated nontuberculous mycobacterial and salmonella infections, is confirmed by lack of cell surface expression of IL-12Rβ1 on stimulated T and NK cells, resulting in depressed IFN-γ production by these cells (see Chapter 28).

If the diagnosis of autosomal recessive SCID is suspected, mutations of the purine metabolism enzymes, adenosine deaminase (ADA), or purine nucleoside phosphorylase (PNP) should be considered and the enzyme activities in red blood cells determined (Carlucci et al., 2003). Deficiencies of these enzymes result in intracellular accumulation of purine metabolites, which after release from the cytoplasm, can be demonstrated at high concentration in blood and urine (see Chapter 12). In the case of PNP deficiency, important clues are low serum and urinary levels of uric acid. It is important to determine that the patient has not been recently transfused, as the donor red cells will mask the defective erythrocytes.

Although traditionally skin tests to assess recall antigens (such as mumps, trichophyton, *Candida albicans*, and PPD) have been used to detect T cell function (delayed-type hypersensitivity), these are often unreliable and difficult to evaluate, especially in infants and young children. Except for PPD, antigens have not been standardized for this purpose, and the result at 72 hours (indicative of a cell-mediated reaction) may be obscured by a humoral (Arthus) reaction at 24 hours.

NK cell deficiency may be present as an isolated defect (Biron et al., 1989) or as part of a broad-based immune deficiency, as in patients with X-linked SCID, Chediak-Higashi syndrome, ecto-dermal dysplasia associated with *NEMO* mutations, or Wiskott-Aldrich syndrome (Orange, 2002; Orange et al., 2002a, 2002b). In most cases it is adequate to enumerate NK cells by flow cytometry (CD16, CD56); in some situations, functional cytotoxic assays are required to help reach a diagnosis (Bernard et al., 2004).

Evaluation of phagocytic defects

Evaluation for defects in the phagocytic system (Table 43.4) is indicated in patients with a history of early-onset suppurative staphylococcal skin infections, cellulitis without pus formation, lymphadenitis, liver abscesses, splenomegaly, or the presence of unusual organisms such as *Serratia marcescens*, *Klebsiella*, *Nocardia*, or invasive *Aspergillus* (Fig. 43.1). Neutrophil defects include congenital or acquired neutropenia, cyclic neutropenia (see Chapter 39), adhesion defects (see Chapter 38), and defective bactericidal function (see Chapter 37). Most of these molecularly defined defects can be screened for with relatively simple tests and then confirmed with appropriate functional assay systems and specific molecular techniques.

The absolute neutrophil count may be persistently low, as in Kostmann disease; intermittently low, as in cyclic neutropenia; or high, as in patients with a leukocyte adhesion defect (LAD1, LAD2, LAD3). Neutropenia is considered if the neutrophil count is <1500/mm³, but clinical symptoms may not occur until the neutrophil count is <300/mm³. To demonstrate cyclic neutropenia, often accompanied by short-term symptoms of fever, mouth ulcers, and infections, it is necessary to obtain neutrophil counts two to three times a week for at least 4 weeks, in conjunction with a symptoms diary. The diagnosis has to be confirmed by demonstrating a mutation in the nentrophil elastase gene (Horwitz et al., 1999). A bone marrow examination is required to determine whether the neutropenia is due to insufficient production or increased consumption.

Tests for defective locomotion and phagocytosis are difficult to perform, as there are nonspecific factors that can interfere with in vivo and in vitro chemotaxis, resulting in secondary failure. Primary diseases of chemotaxis or phagocytosis have not been identified. Most disorders of phagocytosis are the result of opsonic defects rather than intrinsic phagocytic defects (see below).

Flow cytometry is an important tool in the diagnosis of patients lacking adhesion molecules on their surface, such as it is the case in LAD1 and LAD2, for which the molecular defect is currently known (see Chapter 38). Patients with LAD1, lacking the common subunit CD18, are unable to form the heterodimer CD11/CD18. The absence of the subunit of the integrin molecule can be demonstrated by use of anti-CD18 monoclonal antibodies. Patients with LAD2 lack the fucosylated selectin ligand, sialyl-Lewis-X (CD15), on their neutrophils (Etzioni et al., 1999). LAD3, a leukocyte adhesion deficiency associated with impaired integrin rearrangement and a bleeding disorder, has not yet been molecularly defined and has normal CD18 and CD15 expression (see Chapter 38).

Neutrophils from patients with chronic granulomatous disease (CGD) fail to kill catalase-producing bacteria and fungi; during infections the neutrophil count is often abnormally high. The quantitative bacterial killing assay, originally designed to identify such patients, is no longer used for diagnostic purposes. During phagocytosis and killing, normal neutrophils show markedly increased metabolic activity, and several methods to measure the oxidative metabolic burst have been developed. Easy-to-perform laboratory tests to confirm the diagnosis depend on the reduction of a dye to detect the generation of superoxide. A flow-cytometric method employing dihydrorhodamine is widely used and is both reliable and sufficiently sensitive to pick up female carriers of the X-linked form (Carulli et al., 1996). The small amount of blood needed makes this a useful test for infants or for prenatal diagnosis, and quality assurance measures are available. Defective NADPH oxidase activity is the major cause of CGD and may be the result of mutations of one of several cytoplasmic or membrane-associated components of NADPH oxidase (see Chapter 37). Other screening methods include assessment of glucose metabolism, oxygen consumption, glucose monophosphate shunt activity, chemiluminescence, nitroblue tetrazolium (NBT) reduction, and hydrogen peroxide production by phagocytosing leukocytes, but these are no longer widely used.

A small group of patients presenting with clinical findings of CGD may have a complete absence of functional glucose-6-phosphate dehydrogenase (G6PD) in white cells, defective myeloperoxidase, or abnormal glutathione peroxidase. These metabolic defects can cause defective neutrophil bactericidal activity but are not always associated with symptoms (see Chapter 8).

Evaluation of complement defects

Patients with complement deficiencies (see Chapter 42) often have immune complex diseases or recurrent, serious infections (Fig. 43.1, Table 43.2). Patients having deficiencies in the early components of the classical pathway present with immune complex diseases and those having defects in the final lytic pathway with meningitis or septicemia due to encapsulated *Neisseria* species—for example, systemic meningococcal disease or generalized gonococcal infections.

Two assays are sufficient to screen for most complement deficiencies (Table 43.4). Function of the classical pathway in serum is measured by the rate of hemolysis of sheep red cells (CH50) and that of the alternative pathway by lysis of either rabbit or guinea pig red cells (AH50). The availability of simple-to-use and cheap kits has resulted in many laboratories undertaking these assays inappropriately; they are exquisitely sensitive to temperature and difficulties in quality assurance mean that they should only be done in laboratories with considerable experience.

Evaluation of chromosomal defects

Chromosomal abnormalities are pathognomonic for several immunodeficiency syndromes. Deletions within the long arm of chromosome 22, demonstrable with a specific DNA probe, confirm the diagnosis of the DiGeorge syndrome (Goldmuntz et al., 1993) (see Chapter 33), although few patients have evidence of a serious immune defect (Junker and Driskoll, 1995; Ryan et al., 1997). In the presence of clinical features of DiGeorge syndrome but failure to demonstrate a 22q11 defect, chromosome 10q13 should be examined (Markert et al., 2004). Lymphocytes and epithelial cells from patients with ataxia-telangiectasia (see Chapter 29), the Nijmegen breakage syndrome, and Bloom syndrome (both covered in Chapter 30) show chromosomal breaks and sister chromatid exchanges when cultured in vitro. These chromosomal breakage syndromes are caused by mutations of genes coding for proteins involved in DNA repair.

Analysis of Primary Immune Deficiency Disease at the Molecular Level

In recent years, the number of PIDD with a known single gene defect has increased from a handful to over 120 entities (see Table 1.1 in Chapter 1). If the gene product and its function are known, as in ADA deficiency, quantitation of the gene product (usually a protein), including assessment of function, may identify individuals that carry the defect. If the defective gene has been mapped to a specific site on a single chromosome and sufficient family members are available to identify haplotypes carrying the mutation, linkage analysis may identify carriers or affected fetuses even if the gene responsible for the disease has not yet been cloned and sequenced, as, for example, in a subgroup of the hyper-IgE syndrome.

In some families, the mutations result in impaired gene transcription and complete absence of the gene product; in others a nonfunctional gene product may be generated. Using standard protocols (see Tables 43.5 and 43.6), including Western blot analyses, flow cytometry, Northern blot analysis, polymerase chain reaction (PCR), reverse transcriptase (RT)-PCR, and sequence analysis, affected patients can be identified and carriers detected, and prenatal diagnosis can be performed.

For genetic and molecular considerations, carrier females of X-linked diseases can be divided into two categories. For example, in a carrier female of X-linked CGD, the affected neutrophils (as all hemopoetic cells) show random X chromosome inactivation. As a result, approximately 50% of a carrier female's activated neutrophils undergo a normal metabolic burst; this is easily demonstrated by dihydrorhodamine and flow cytometry. This is also true in CD40L deficiency, where the proportion of the activated T cells expressing CD40L will reflect the extent of the randomness of X chromosome inactivation. The second category of carrier females, exemplified by those heterozygous for mutations of Btk (responsible for XLA) or WASP (responsible for Wiskott-Aldrich syndrome, WAS), have nonrandom X chromosome inactivation in those cells that depend on the function of the mutated genes. Carrier women in this category exhibit selective use of the nonmutant, normal X chromosome as the active X chromosome in the relevant cell population, for example, B cells in XLA, all hematopoietic cell lines in Wiskott-Aldrich syndrome (Conley, 1992). X chromosome inactivation studies, although now superseded by molecular analysis for most PIDD, have been useful in the past and are still a useful tool for genetic assessment of X-linked disorders that are not molecularly characterized.

Prenatal diagnosis is now possible in most PIDD. If the syndrome is X-linked, sex determination by high-resolution ultrasound or by DNA analysis of material obtained through chorionic villi biopsy or amniocentesis will identify pregnancies at risk. If the mutation is known, sequence analysis of PCR-amplified fetal DNA is the method of choice for prenatal diagnosis. If the defective gene is unknown or if the mutation within a specific family is not yet determined, fetal blood samples can be obtained to study the characteristic peripheral blood abnormalities. For instance, thrombocytopenia and small platelets in the peripheral blood of a male fetus at risk for Wiskott-Aldrich syndrome will confirm the diagnosis. Similarly, fetuses with SCID and lymphopenia can be identified. For some disorders, such as ADA deficiency, the activity of the gene product in fetal cells can be measured. Protein studies are possible but have not yet been validated in prenatal diagnosis and may not be sufficiently reliable to use as potential indications for pregnancy termination.

Diagnostic Approaches in Specific Immunodeficiency Disorders

Severe Combined Immune Deficiency Diseases

Severe combined immunodeficiency diseases are rare diseases affecting both T and B lymphocytes, and may be inherited as an X-linked or autosomal recessive disorder, although as many as 70% of infants with SCID have a negative family history (Hague et al., 1994). At least 10 molecularly defined SCID disorders with characteristic phenotype and inheritance patterns can be distinguished (Fischer, 2000) (Fig. 43.4) (see Chapter 1, Table 1.1, and Chapters 9–15).

Patients with SCID typically present during the first few months of life with failure to thrive, skin rashes, sparse hair, diarrhea, weight loss, and bacterial, fungal, and viral infections. Absence of a thymic shadow is diagnostically useful only when the X-ray is taken early, before thymic involution has occurred from chronic infection. Primary and secondary lymphoid organs are hypoplastic but some T cell deficiencies may present with hepatosplenomegaly due to graft-versus-host disease (GVHD) following transfer of maternal cells across the placenta (Stephan et al., 1993; Hague et al., 1994) or due to histiocytic infiltrates as in Omenn syndrome. If immunized with BCG, SCID patients often develop lymphadenopathy and local or disseminated BCG-osis.

Once the diagnosis of SCID is suspected, it is vital to transfer the infant, before chronic infections have developed, to a tertiary care center with experience in the diagnosis and care of patients with SCID (Gennery and Cant, 2000). The vulnerability of the SCID infant to bacterial, viral, and fungal infections, to potentially lethal complications from live vaccines, and to GVHD caused by unirradiated blood transfusions makes SCID a legitimate pediatric emergency (Rosen, 1997). Early diagnosis improves the chance of survival by initiating timely transplantation of bone marrow or cord blood stem cells, intravenous immunoglobulin (IVIG) and PCP prophylaxis, polyethylene glycol–adenosine deaminase (PEG-ADA) treatment in ADA deficiency, or high-dose substitution with vitamin B_{12} in patients with transcobalamin II deficiency.

The most informative screening test is the absolute lymphocyte count (ALC). In most but not all SCID patients the ALC is

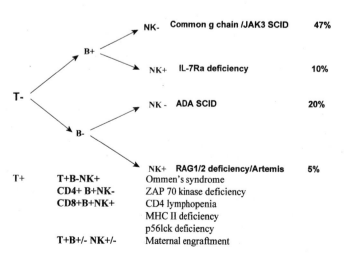

Figure 43.4. Type of severe combined immunodeficiency by lymphocyte lineage—i.e., SCID by flow markers.

low (Gossage and Buckley, 1990; Gennery and Cant, 2000). Since the normal range in infants is much higher than that in older children and adults, age-related control values are required for comparison (Fig. 43.3). Assessment of lymphocyte markers by flow cytometry allows the quantitation, in terms of absolute numbers, of T cells, T cell subsets, B cells, NK cells, and cells expressing major histocompatibility complex (MHC) II (Buckley et al., 1997). Age-matched normal values for these lymphocyte subpopulations are available (Erheller-Yuksel et al., 1992; Melaranci et al., 1992; Stiehm et al., 2004). The results of the lymphocyte count and the assessment of the types of lymphocytes present are interpreted together (Fig. 43.2).

Normal ALCs are found in individuals in whom T cell numbers and function are largely normal—namely, in patients with ZAP-70 deficiency (normal number of CD4, decreased number or absent CD8); MHC II deficiency (normal or decreased CD4); Omenn syndrome (often moderately decreased CD4 and CD8); and CD40L deficiency (normal numbers of CD4, CD8). A low ALC may indicate reticular dysgenesis (T^-, B^-, NK^-, neutropenia, decreased number of megakaryocytes); Rag1/Rag2 deficiency (T^-, B^-, NK^+); Artemis deficiency (T^-, B^-, NK^+); XSCID or Jak3 deficiency (T^-, B^+, NK^-); interleukin-7 receptor (IL-7R) deficiency (T^-, B^+, NK^+); ADA deficiency (T^-, B^-, $NK^{+/-}$); IL-$2R\alpha$ deficiency (T^-, B^+, NK^-); or CD3δ deficiency (T^-, B^+, NK^+) (Figs. 43.2 and 43.4).

As noted above, there may be normal numbers of T lymphocytes but with poor function; in those PIDD cases, assessment of proliferation in response to mitogens will indicate the severity of the T cell defect. Those patients whose lymphocytes are nonresponsive to mitogens may tolerate bone marrow or stem cell transplants without conditioning, whereas those responding with significant lymphocyte proliferation or those with substantial numbers of circulating NK cells need to undergo a conditioning regimen (see Chapter 47). Similarly, if maternal lymphocytes can be demonstrated as the cause of GVHD, conditioning is needed prior to marrow transplantation. MHC typing of the entire family is indicated as soon as the diagnosis of SCID has been established as part of the search for either a matched sibling, a matched unrelated donor, or a partially matched cord blood (see Chapter 47).

Patients with significant T cell deficiency should not receive live vaccines; especially dangerous are BCG, attenuated polio vaccine, and measles, mumps and rubella (MMR) vaccine. Blood products containing cellular elements have to be irradiated and blood products from cytomegalovirus (CMV)-positive donors should be avoided.

There are potential pitfalls in the procedures for the diagnosis of SCID (Table 43.7). Serum immunoglobulin levels are often

Table 43.7. Pitfalls in Diagnosis of Severe Combined Immunodeficiency

- Serum immunoglobulin levels may be normal in infants because of masking effect of
  Maternal IgG
  Paraproteins, underlying the need for serum electrophoresis in all suspected cases
- Presence of normal or increased numbers of oligoclonal T cells, as in Omenn syndrome
- Presentation in later life as "leaky" SCID
- Need for in vitro activation to detect maximal expression of lymphocyte markers, e.g., CD40L
- Compounding effect of blood transfusion or of maternofetal engraftment causing graft-vs.-host disease

difficult to interpret in very young infants. Most infants with SCID have low or absent IgM and IgA, and show persistently dropping IgG levels as the maternal antibodies disappear. Some patients, for example, those with Omenn syndrome, may have elevated serum IgE levels. It is essential to rule out congenital HIV infection by testing the mother's serum for HIV antibody and, if positive, the infant for HIV-RNA by PCR.

As illustrated in Table 1.1 (Chapter 1) and Chapters 9–15 of this book, a molecular diagnosis is now possible in >80% of SCID patients.

Primary T Cell Defects

DiGeorge syndrome

Affected patients present with some or all of the following findings: congenital cardiac malformation involving the large vessels, hypoplastic thymus, parathyroid deficiency, velopharyngeal insufficiency, cleft palate, dysmorphic features, and an increased risk of autoimmune diseases (see Chapter 33). These abnormalities can be explained by abnormal formation of the neural crest from which the third and fourth pharyngeal arches develop. Most patients with DiGeorge anomaly have microdeletions affecting q11 of chromosome 22, which is also associated with impairment of language and motor development, mild mental retardation, persistent coordination deficits, a high frequency of behavioral disorder with attention deficit during childhood, and a high frequency of psychotic disorders (bipolar disorder and schizophrenia [Pinquier et al., 2001]) during adolescence and young adulthood. The possibility of immune deficiency in those with primary psychotic disease and 22q11 deletion has not yet been investigated systematically.

The extent of immunodeficiency varies greatly, but all infants with tetralogy of Fallot, ventricular septal defects, interrupted aortic arch, pulmonary artery atresia, and truncus arteriosus, especially if associated with hypocalcemia and seizures, should be evaluated for DiGeorge syndrome. Most patients have normal T cell numbers and function or only moderate lymphopenia (Junker and Driscoll, 1995; Ryan et al., 1997). Less than 1% of patients with this syndrome present as having SCID (Goldsobel et al., 1987). However, it is important to measure the numbers of $CD4^+$ T cells because those infants of less than 4 months of age who have $<1000/mm^3$ $CD4^+$ T cells and older children with $<500/mm^3$ $CD4^+$ T cells may be at risk of developing PCP and so benefit from PCP prophylaxis. Absolute lymphocyte counts, T cells, and T cell subsets and mitogen responses at the time of diagnosis, at 6 months, and at 12 months of age are useful to follow those patients with reduced numbers of T cells, as the lymphopenia resolves in most patients by the age of 1 year. Patients with normal lymphocyte subsets and normal mitogen responses at 15 months of age can safely be immunized with live vaccines. Older infants (>15 months) with $<500/mm^3$ CD4 cells should not receive live vaccines or unirradiated blood until their $CD4^+$ T cell numbers are normal for their age (Pierdominici et al., 2000). The diagnosis is confirmed by FISH analysis of chromosome 22 and, if this is negative, by chromosome 10 analysis or, in a few cases, a mutation in the *TBX1* gene (Yagi et al., 2003).

CD8 deficiency

Familial CD8 deficiency due to a homozygous mutation in the CD8α gene has recently been described in a 25-year-old Spanish male from a consanguineous family (Chapter 16). The index case suffered recurrent bacterial sinopulmonary infections and a total absence of CD8+ T cells (de la Calle-Martin et al., 2001). Two of the patient's six sisters had an identical defect but where clinically asymptomatic.

Primary Antibody Defects

X-Linked agammaglobulinemia

The most characteristic finding in infants with X-linked agammaglobulinemia (XLA, see Chapter 21) is the severely decreased number of B lymphocytes in the peripheral blood (Fig. 43.2). If XLA is suspected at the time of birth (e.g., positive family history), cord blood should be collected and analyzed by flow cytometry. Whereas there are normal numbers of circulating CD4+ and CD8+ T cells, B lymphocytes are absent or markedly reduced in numbers. The diagnosis should then be confirmed by demonstrating absence of Btk in patient-derived monocytes or platelets and by sequence analysis. Immunoglobulin levels in cord blood or in serum from very young infants are not informative because the transfer of maternal IgG provides affected infants with normal IgG levels (temporarily), and IgM and IgA are physiologically low in normal infants less than 6 months of age. Because of the presence of maternal antibodies, the onset of symptoms is usually delayed, occurring between 6 and 12 months of age.

Patients with XLA fail to produce antibodies in response to routine childhood vaccines. Their lymph nodes lack germinal centers and plasma cells, and rectal mucosal biopsies are void of plasma cells (Ament et al., 1973). Invasive techniques are no longer necessary to reach a diagnosis.

Measurement of the Btk protein and its kinase activity in monocytes (Futatani et al., 1998; Gaspar et al., 1998) or in platelets (Futatani et al., 2001) is a useful screening test but has to be confirmed by identifying a mutation in the *Btk* gene. Some XLA patients with *Btk* mutations have a milder phenotype, with significant serum concentrations of IgG, IgM, and IgA (Ochs and Smith, 1996); these patients may be erroneously classified as having CVID (see below and Chapter 21). Conversely, *Btk* mutations account for only about 70%–80% of unselected males with panhypogammaglobulinemia and lack of B cells. As more molecular defects in B cell development are identified (Chapters 20–22), a wide range of disorders should be considered in the differential diagnosis (Figs. 43.2, 43.5).

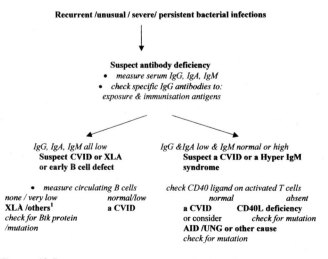

Figure 43.5. Approach to diagnosis of antibody deficiencies.

If not treated with sufficient IVIG substitution (see Chapters 21 and 46), XLA patients continue to suffer from recurrent upper and lower respiratory infections and many develop bronchiectasis. This is a common finding when the diagnosis has been delayed or when patients were treated inadequately for more than 10 years (Plebani et al., 2002). Patients with XLA are also susceptible to chronic mycoplasma and enteroviral infections, and exposure to attenuated oral polio vaccine can cause paralytic polio. Chronic infection with echovirus and Coxsackie virus causes meningoencephalitis and an unusual fasciitis-myositis, which is often lethal. Positive viral culture or PCR for enteroviruses confirms this complication.

X-Linked Hyper-IgM and other forms of Hyper-IgM syndromes

Since X-linked hyper IgM (XHIM) is a T cell deficiency (see Chapter 19), it is not surprising that half of the affected male infants present with PCP (Levy et al., 1997) or other infections related to a T cell defect such as cryptosporidium, cryptococcus, or persistent molluscum contagiosum. A high proportion of XHIM patients develop chronic cholangitis associated with cryptosporidia, and tumors of the bile ducts and surrounding tissues have been reported (Hayward et al., 1997). Cryptosporidia can be difficult to detect by microscopy in stools; monoclonal antibody–enhanced immunofluorescent microscopy and PCR can now be used to detect the presence of these organisms in stool and bile (Alles et al., 1995). Neutropenia, either persistent or transient, is common.

Affected patients have low levels of serum IgG and IgA and either normal or elevated IgM at presentation. Absolute numbers of circulating lymphocytes and lymphocyte subsets are normal. Peripheral blood lymphocytes respond to mitogens but often fail to proliferate in vitro in response to specific antigens such as candida and tetanus (Ameratunga et al., 1997). The diagnosis is confirmed by demonstrating that peripheral blood lymphocytes, activated in vitro with phorbol myristate acetate (PMA) and ionophore, fail to express a functional CD40 ligand (CD40L) due to mutations affecting the *CD40L* gene. CD40L can be identified on the surface of activated T cells by specific monoclonal antibodies or by the counter receptor, soluble CD40-Ig, and flow cytometry (Notarangelo and Hayward, 2000). It is worth noting that a subgroup of patients with CVID and all newborn infants express decreased amounts of CD40L. The diagnosis of XHIM is confirmed by sequence analysis of the *CD40L* gene.

Female patients or males with an autosomal recessive form of the hyper-IgM syndrome have a normal *CD40L* gene. Several molecular defects in this group of patients have been identified in recent years. The first group recognized had mutations in the activation–induced cytidine deaminase gene (*AID*) (Revy et al., 2000). AID is a key cytoplasmic enzyme restricted to germinal-center B cells and essential for both B cell isotype switching and somatic hypermutation (see Chapter 20). Lymphadenopathy and tonsillar hypertrophy are striking features of AID deficiency. Lymph nodes of patients with AID deficiency are enlarged and have characterized giant germinal centres, in contrast to the distinct lack of germinal centres in lymph nodes of XHIM patients.

Lack of CD40 expression on circulating B cells and monocytes due to mutations in the *CD40* gene also results in autosomal recessive hyper-IgM syndrome (Ferrari et al., 2001) (see Chapter 19). XHIM and CD40 deficiency appear to have the same clinical phenotype, which is not surprising since they share a defective CD40L–CD40 signaling pathway.

624 Assessment and Treatment

Most recently, mutations of uracil-DNA glucosylase (*UNG*) (Imai et al., 2003), an autosomal recessive disorder (see Chapter 20), and mutations of *NEMO* (X-linked) (Jain et al., 2001) were discovered to cause hyper-IgM syndrome (see Chapter 36). Sequence analysis of these genes is required to confirm these diagnoses.

Common variable immunodeficiency

CVID is a heterogenous group of "acquired" conditions of primary antibody failure. As in other acquired conditions, these may be associated with several susceptibility and/or disease-modifying genes (see Chapter 23). Thus CVID is a diagnosis of exclusion (Table 43.8). Diagnostic criteria define only probable (a >85% probability that in 20 years the diagnosis will be the same) or possible disease, and depend entirely on clinical and laboratory criteria (Table 43.9).

The CVIDs start usually during the second or third decade, although some CVID patients have a history of recurrent res-

Table 43.8. Differential Diagnosis of Hypogammaglobulinemia

Drug Induced

Antimalarial agents
Captopril
Carbamazepine
Glucocorticoids
Fenclofenac
Gold salts
Penicillamine
Phenytoin
Sulfasalazine

Genetic Disorders

Ataxia-telangiectasia
Autosomal forms of SCID
Hyper-IgM immunodeficiency
Transcobalamin II deficiency
X-linked agammaglobulinemia
X-linked lymphoproliferative disorder (EBV associated)
X-linked SCID
Some metabolic disorders
Chromosomal anomalies
Chromosome 18q-syndrome
Monosomy 22
Trisomy 8
Trisomy 21

Infectious Diseases

HIV (may be associated with hypergammaglobulinemia)
Congenital rubella
Congenital infection with CMV
Congenital infection with *Toxoplasma gondii*
Epstein-Barr virus

Malignancy

Chronic lymphocytic leukemia
Immunodeficiency with thymoma
Non-Hodgkin lymphoma
B cell malignancy

Systemic Disorders

Immunodeficiency caused by hypercatabolism of immunoglobulin
Immunodeficiency caused by excessive loss of immunoglobulins (nephrosis, severe burns, lymphangiectasia, severe diarrhea)

CMV, cytomegalovirus; EBV, Epstein-Barr virus.
Source: From Conley et al. (1999).

Table 43.9. Criteria for Diagnosis of Common Variable Immunodeficiency

Probable

Male or female patient who has a marked decrease (at least 2 SD below the mean for age) in two of the three major isotypes (IgM, IgG, and IgA) and fulfills all of the following criteria:
1. Onset of immunodeficiency at greater than 2 years of age
2. Absent isohemagglutinins and/or poor response to vaccines
3. Defined causes of hypogammaglobulinemia have been excluded (see Table 43.8)

Possible

Male or female patient who has a marked decrease (at least 2 SD below the mean for age) in one of the major isotypes (IgM, IgG, and IgA) and fulfills all of the following criteria:
1. Onset of immunodeficiency at greater than 2 years of age
2. Absent isohemagglutinins and/or poor response to vaccines
3. Defined causes of hypogammaglobulinemia have been excluded (see Table 43.8)

Source: From Conley et al. (1999).

piratory infections starting in early childhood (Cunningham-Rundles, 1989; Hermaszewski and Webster, 1993) and may form a separate subgroup. Symptoms of CVID may also first appear in patients who are 50 years of age or older and have no history of unusual infections at an earlier age.

About 80% of CVID patients have a negative family history except for an increased incidence of autoimmune diseases. Up to 20% of CVID patients may have first-degree relatives with CVID or IgA deficiency (Vorechovsky et al., 1995; Hammarstrom et al., 2000). The presence of unique allotypes within the MHC of chromosome 6 suggests that there is at least one locus of genetic susceptibility in this subgroup of patients. In a few families, an autosomal dominant mode of inheritance has been reported. There are reports of patients presenting first with selective IgA deficiency and then progressing to CVID, supporting the hypothesis that, in the main, these are not purely genetic disorders.

Thymoma with antibody deficiency appears to be a different disease, as it is rare in patients under the age of 40 years. This disorder may become more widely recognized because regular CT scanning is performed to monitor bronchiectasis in patients with primary antibody deficiencies.

Patients with CVID may present with, or develop during the course of the disease, acute or chronic gastrointestinal complaints of a sprue-like syndrome. Pathogens are rarely found on stool culture or microscopy, although patients are known to be susceptible to chronic *Giardia* infection (Ament et al., 1973). The most reliable method of its detection is the collection of multiple biopsies and demonstration of the trophozoites. Direct immunofluorescence (monoclonal antibody–enhanced) assays have increased the sensitivity of detection (Alles et al., 1995), and more recently enzyme immunoassays, which demonstrate *Giardia* antigen in stool specimen, have become available (Maraha and Buiting, 2000; Hanson and Cartwright, 2001). Eradication of the parasites by metronidazole or tinidazole results in disappearance of the gastrointestinal symptoms. Patients with CVID have a high incidence of nodular lymphoid hyperplasia, which can be demonstrated radiologically or by endoscopic examination of the small bowel. Plasma cells in the lamina propria are often absent or markedly reduced.

A subgroup of CVID patients develops severe granulomatous changes in the lungs resembling sarcoidosis. Others present with lymphadenopathy and hepatosplenomegaly caused by nonspecific lymphoid and/or granulomatous proliferation. Lymphoid interstitial pneumonitis is another complication that is unexplained (Davies et al., 2000). Splenomegaly is present in about 30% of CVID patients and hypersplenism may be severe enough to necessitate splenectomy, although this is best avoided. Lymphadenopathy, especially in the abdominal cavity and the mediastinum, is a frequent finding and may require an exploratory laparatomy to rule out a malignant process. There is an increased incidence of lymphoreticular and gastrointestinal malignancies in older patients with CVID, although this is less marked than originally thought (Mellemkjaer et al., 2002).

The laboratory findings of CVID are heterogeneous (Cunningham-Rundles and Bodian, 1999). By definition, CVID patients have low but demonstrable IgG and at least one other low Ig isotype. Serum IgA is undetectable in two-thirds of patients. IgM is low, in addition to reduced levels of IgG and IgA, in about a quarter of patients meeting the diagnostic criteria for CVID.

The diagnostic criteria require that antibody responses to proteins, polysaccharides, and neoantigens are abnormal. Some patients are able to amplify responses and switch from IgM to IgG; others fail to produce antibody other than IgM, and some patients make barely detectable antibodies (Stiehm et al., 2004). Most patients have normal numbers of lymphocytes and lymphocyte subsets, although a moderate CD4+ T cell lymphopenia with a reversed CD4:CD8 ratio occurs in about 25% of CVID patients (Spickett et al., 1997). Abnormal in vitro lymphokine production by cultured lymphocytes has been reported (Sneller and Strober, 1990). B cell numbers are often but not always normal, leading to the hypothesis that those with low numbers of circulating B cells form a (as-yet undefined) subgroup. The hypothesis of a T cell defect as one of the causes of another subgroup of CVID is supported by the fact that lymphocytes from some patients fail in vitro to respond to activation by recall antigens, and activated lymphocytes from some patients express only small amounts of CD40L (Farrington et al., 1994). Other studies have shown intrinsic B cell defects in at least 25% of patients (Levy et al., 1998; Schwartz et al., 1999).

In view of the heterogeneity of CVID, it is not surprising that some patients with a provisional diagnosis of CVID have been shown to have mutations in one of several genes known to cause PIDD, such as *Btk, CD40L, AID*, UNG, and *SH2D1A*. Recent reports suggest that XLP should always be considered when more than one male with CVID is encountered within the same family (Morra et al., 2001). Consequently, a strict diagnosis of CVID can only be made after the exclusion of mutations in these genes. A subgroup of CVID patients was recently found to lack expression of ICOS (inducible costimulator) on activated T cells because of a homozygous deletion within the *ICOS* gene. This is a rare event, however (Grimbacher et al., 2003; Salzer et al., 2004). Other genes found to be mutated in patients with CVID phenotypes include BAFF receptor, CD19, and TACI (Salzer et al., 2005). It is predictable that additional genes required for B cell activation will be identified to cause one of the CVID phenotypes.

Antibody deficiency with normal or elevated serum immunoglobulin levels

This entity, more often observed in adults than in children, resembles CVID. Affected patients often present with recurrent pulmonary disease, complicated by chronic lung disease and bronchiectasis. Serum immunoglobulin levels, by definition, are normal or elevated; this makes it difficult to establish the diagno-

sis. A mild T cell abnormality similar to that observed in a subgroup of CVID patients may be present. The most informative diagnostic procedure that effectively identifies these patients is in vivo antibody production to a battery of antigens that include proteins (e.g., diphtheria and tetanus toxoid), polysaccharide antigens (e.g., Pneumovax, Typhim Vi), and neoantigens (e.g., KLH, bacteriophage ØX174). Characteristically, patients with this disorder respond to some antigens but not to others, making it difficult to establish a reliable diagnosis. Replacement immunoglobulin therapy (usually after a failed trial of prophylactic antibiotics) must be monitored with great attention to clinical improvement and documented reduction of significant infections.

Isotype and IgG subclass deficiencies

This diagnosis is made by measuring serum immunoglobulin levels and IgG subclass levels. It is important to compare the results with normal age-matched controls (Stiehm et al., 2004). IgA deficiency is considered if serum IgA is <5 mg/dl (0.05 g/l); IgM deficiency, if the serum level is <20 mg/dl (0.2 g/l); and IgG subclass deficiency is considered if the levels are below 2 SD, or less than the fifth percentile of age-matched controls. Most patients with "selective IgA" deficiency are asymptomatic. Those with susceptibility to infections may have associated IgG2 and IgG4 deficiency, and some may respond poorly to antigenic stimulation, resembling CVID.

IgG subclass deficiencies are unlikely to be clinically significant if specific antibody production is intact. It is important, therefore, to determine specific antibody responses to immunizations with protein and polysaccharide antigens and to reserve the diagnosis and treatment to those with documented failure of specific antibody production.

The Wiskott-Aldrich Syndrome

Any male infant with petechiae and easy bruising, eczema, bloody diarrhea, and recurrent otitis media has the Wiskott-Aldrich syndrome (WAS) until proven otherwise (Chapter 31). The combination of thrombocytopenia and small platelets is considered diagnostic. There is a subgroup of male infants with congenital thrombocytopenia and small platelets without the other clinical symptoms characteristic for WAS; these patients have been categorized as having X-linked thrombocytopenia (XLT), atypical WAS, or WAS variant. In patients with a classic WAS phenotype, both humoral and cellular immunity are affected (Ochs et al., 1980; Thrasher and Kinnon, 2000). Serum immunoglobulin levels are normal or low for IgG (often with IgG2 deficiency), moderately depressed for IgM, and often elevated for IgA and IgE. Isohemagglutinin titers are very low and antibody responses to polysaccharides (e.g., Pneumovax) are consistently depressed. Antibody responses to diphtheria and tetanus toxoid are often but not always abnormal, and responses to bacteriophage X174 lack immunologic memory, amplification, and isotype switching. Lymphopenia often develops by the age of 6–8 years with a proportional decrease in all lymphocyte subsets. Absolute B lymphocytes remain usually within normal range. In vitro lymphocyte proliferation to mitogens is often diminished, but not absent, and responses to allogeneic cells or immobilized anti-CD3 monoclonal antibodies are markedly depressed.

The diagnosis of WAS or XLT is confirmed by demonstrating a mutation within the WAS protein (*WASP*) gene, located in Xp11.22–23. As a consequence, cytoplasmic WASP is absent or the amount is decreased (Jin et al., 2004).

X-linked Lymphoproliferative Disease

Patients carrying the XLP gene (*SH2D1A*) are usually clinically normal until they are exposed to EBV. Following exposure, affected males may develop fulminant infectious mononucleosis, agammaglobulinemia, or lymphoproliferative disorders and lymphoma. Before exposure to EBV, most affected individuals have normal immunologic parameters. The laboratory findings in males with a mutation of the *SH2D1A* gene during acute EBV infection are described in Chapter 32. Recent evidence suggests that patients may be susceptible to other herpes viruses that can provoke an erythrophagocytic picture.

After EBV infection, surviving XLP patients often show a combined T and B cell defect (Sullivan et al., 1983). Some but not all patients will develop a persistent decrease in lymphocyte proliferation to mitogens, a decreased CD4:CD8 ratio with a predominance of CD8 cells, and decreased in vitro immunoglobulin synthesis by B cells in the presence of autologous T cells. Stimulated lymphocytes show a decrease in lymphokine production. Antibody responses to a neoantigen (e.g., bacteriophage X174) are quantitatively normal, but antibody produced by XLP patients after EBV infection is often limited to the IgM isotype.

The diagnosis is confirmed by sequence analysis of *SH2D1A*, the gene responsible for XLP. Those males at risk for XLP, i.e., family members and all male siblings with the diagnosis CVID, should be studied for *SH2D1A* mutations.

Natural Killer Cell Defects

A novel syndrome characterized by severe prenatal and postnatal growth failure, mild skeletal and facial abnormalities, and primary immunodeficiency was described in two sisters (Bernard et al., 2004). The immune defect consisted of very low numbers of detectable natural killer cells ($CD16^+/CD56^+$), lack of NK cell function, and small numbers of $CD8^+$ T cells and neutrophils. This novel syndrome is probably caused by an autosomal recessive gene defect impairing both intrauterine growth and NK cell development.

Neutrophil Defects

Persistent neutropenia

Persistent neutropenia has multiple etiologies and may be associated with other disorders, including Shwachman syndrome, X-linked hyper-IgM syndrome, and X-linked agammaglobulinemia. Mutations of neutrophil elastase (Horwitz et al., 1999) can cause congenital neutropenia (Kostmann syndrome) or cyclic neutropenia (see Chapter 39). In small infants, neutropenia can be a sign of overwhelming infection and increased neutrophil consumption. A bone marrow examination is required to see if the neutropenia is due to insufficient production or increased consumption. Consumption due to an autoantibody is detected by the presence of antineutrophil antibodies. In alloimmune neutropenia these have NA1 and NA2 specificities; these can only be identified in a specialized laboratory (Lakshman and Finn, 2001).

Defective locomotion and phagocytosis

Defective locomotion and phagocytosis have been observed in a number of syndromes including leukocyte adhesion deficiency, "lazy leukocyte syndrome," Chediak-Higashi syndrome, hyper-IgE syndrome, and the Wiskott-Aldrich syndrome, through techniques available for directed (chemotaxis) and random movement of neutrophils (Kuijpers et al., 1999). Rebuck skin window or a collecting chamber can be used to measure in vivo adhesion and chemotaxis (Bowen et al., 1982). However, these tests are difficult to perform as there are nonspecific factors that can interfere with in vivo and in vitro chemotaxis, and primary diseases restricted to abnormalities of chemotaxis or phagocytosis are not known. Most disorders of phagocytosis are the result of opsonic defects rather than intrinsic phagocytic defects. If an opsonising defect is suspected, it is important to test phagocytosis by normal neutrophils in the presence of patient serum.

Leukocyte adhesion deficiency

Patients with leukocyte adhesion deficiency (LAD) (see Chapter 38) present in early infancy with characteristic clinical findings. Patients with LAD often present with delayed separation of the cord, omphalitis and cellulitis without pus formation, and neutrophilia that may reach $60,000–80,000/mm^3$ during active infection. In vivo and in vitro chemotaxis is abnormal. Patients with LAD1, lacking the common subunit CD18, are unable to form the heterodimer CD11/CD18, demonstrated by flow cytometry with anti-CD18 monoclonal antibodies. Their neutrophils fail to adhere to plastic, glass, or cultured endothelial cells. Sequence analysis of the subunit confirms the diagnosis of LAD1.

Variants of LAD1 deficiency associated with normally expressed but functionally defective β_2 integrins (CD11/CD18) as well as combined defects in β_1 and β_2 integrins have recently been described (Kuijpers et al., 1997; Hogg et al., 1999; Harris et al., 2001). The clinical phenotypes in these LAD variants have ranged from mild to severe. The more recent description of a novel form of integrin dysfunction involving β_1, β_2, and β_3 integrins in a patient with LAD1 and a rare bleeding tendency (termed *Glanzmann thrombasthenia*) due to mutations in the platelet integrin CD41/CD61 illustrates the expanding spectrum of adhesion molecule defects (McDowell et al., 2003).

Patients with LAD2 lack the fucosylated selectin ligand, sialyl Lewis X (SLeX, CD15) (without the demonstration of a mutation) on their neutrophils. They have the Bombay red cell phenotype, as they do not express the blood group antigen H. LAD2 neutrophils fail to roll along the endothelial wall. The defect of LAD2 is a mutation in the fucose transporter gene. The diagnosis is suspected by the combination of the clinical phenotype, the presence of the Bombay blood group, and the absence of SLeX on leukocytes on flow cytometry.

Lack of endothelial expression of E selectin has been described and produces a clinical picture similar to LAD deficiency, with the important exception of a mild neutropenia rather than a neutrophil leucocytosis (DeLisser et al., 1999).

Chronic granulomatous disease

Neutrophils from patients with chronic granulomatous disease (CGD) (see Chapter 37) ingest microorganisms but fail to kill catalase-producing bacteria and fungi. Patients present with recurrent abscesses involving lymphnodes, liver and spleen, brain, and bone. The infections are often due to staphylococci and fail to respond to antibiotics, or they are serious fungal infections, often pulmonary. Regional lymphadenopathy (sometimes suppurative), often associated with persistent hepatosplenomegaly, leads to a diagnostic lymph node biopsy, in which granulomata are a feature.

Although several methods to measure the oxidative metabolic burst have been developed, the most useful is the dihydrorhodamine (DHR) test using flow cytometry (Carulli, 1996; Jirapongsananuruk et al., 2003). Defective NADPH oxidase activity is the major cause of CGD and may be the result of mutations of one of several cytoplasmic or membrane-associated components of NADPH oxidase (see Chapter 37).

Complement Deficiencies

Complement component deficiencies may affect the early components of the classical complement pathway, or the alternative or the terminal pathway (see Chapter 42). Usually a single component is involved, and this is associated with a homozygous gene defect resulting in absence of that component. Even small amounts of a component allow adequate function of the total pathway; levels of most components are increased in an acute-phase response.

Screening is done with the CH50 (which tests classical and final lytic components except C9) and AP 50 (which tests alternative and final lytic pathways) assays. These tests should only be done in laboratories with considerable experience of these assays, usually specialized clinical immunology laboratories. To avoid misinterpretation due to the possible effects of complement consumption by immune complex formation, it is advisable that the assays be performed when the patient has completely recovered from immune complex disease or infection. Both tests require that blood be taken atraumatically and serum be separated within 1 hour and then stored at −70°C. Failure to achieve lysis can be due to inadequate storage, release of enzymes on venepuncture, aged red cells, and limited quality assurance.

If either of these screening tests identifies failure of a complement pathway on two occasions, the specific component defect should be determined. Fresh serum should be collected properly and shipped on dry ice to laboratories with expertise in complement assessment. It is preferable that both functional and immunochemical determinations be performed, as a protein may be present but dysfunctional. Enzyme-linked immunobsorbent assay (ELISA) techniques measure individual components and functional assays are available to detect present but nonfunctioning proteins. If dysfunctional or missing components cannot be identified, an inhibitor should be considered.

All first-degree family members should be screened with the appropriate hemolytic complement assay (CH50, AP50). Some affected individuals are asymptomatic. A careful family history with analysis of three or four generations may reveal a pattern of inheritance that is compatible with an X-linked, autosomal recessive, or autosomal dominant mode of inheritance. A family history of early death is more informative if it occurred after 1945 when penicillin had become widely available. Consanguinity, or being a member of a close-knit community based on religion or ethnicity, increases the possibility of an autosomal recessive disease. The occurrence of a new mutation in those complement component deficiencies with X-linked inheritance has to be considered, as in any X-linked disease.

Defects of Antigen-Presenting Cells

TAP deficiency syndromes

The TAP (transporter associated with antigen presentation) deficiency syndromes are variants of the bare lymphocyte syndrome type I, characterized by severe down-regulation of HLA class I molecules due to mutations or deletions of genes encoding either TAP1 or TAP2 proteins (Gadola et al., 2000) (see Chapter 18). Clinical features of affected patients vary from severe and ulti-

mately fatal recurrent bacterial, fungal, and parasitic infections beginning in infancy (group 1, only a few patients described) to those patients who develop necrotizing granulomatous skin lesions on a background of recurrent sinopulmonary bacterial infections (group 3, the largest number of cases but still rare). There have been two families with asymptomatic individuals (group 2). In patients with sinus and nasal involvement, the histology resembles that of Wegener's granulomatosis.

The unifying immunological feature in both groups is defective HLA class I expression on peripheral blood mononuclear cells. Patients in group 1 have also shown a complete lack of antibody production. Analysis of lymphocyte repertoire has shown low numbers of α-β CD8 T cells, with an expansion of NK and γ-δ T cells in most patients. These latter cell types are activated by bacterial infection and provoke a Th1 response resulting in granulomata.

Major histocompatibility complex Class II defiency

MHC class II deficiency is caused by the absence of MHC class II molecules on the surface of antigen-presenting cells (B cells, dentritic cells, macrophages, thymic epithelial cells, and activated T cells). In MHC class II deficiency, also called bare lymphocyte syndrome type II, the defect is caused by mutations affecting one of at least four transcription factors that control MHC class II gene expression (see Chapter 17). As a result of this defect, both cellular and humoral immune responses are affected and patients are highly susceptible to viral, bacterial, and fungal infections, primarily of the respiratory and gastrointestinal tract.

All antigen-presenting cells from affected patients completely lack MHC class II molecules, even following activation with IFN-γ. Affected patients have normal numbers of circulating T and B lymphocytes; however CD4+ T cells are reduced in number while CD8 T cell numbers are proportionately increased. The diagnosis of bare lymphocyte syndrome type II should be considered in all children with recurrent respiratory tract infections, diarrhea, and failure to thrive. The diagnosis is based on the absence of MHC class II molecules on the surface of B cells, monocytes, and dentritic cells, or IFN-γ activated T cells. Early diagnosis is important because the only effective treatment is timely stem cell transplantation.

Immunodeficiency Associated with Defects of DNA Repair

This group includes three well-described clinical syndromes discussed below and other less-characterized and rare conditions, such as DNA ligase defects, xeroderma pigmentosum, and unrecognized conditions that tend to show a mixture of features including radiosensitivity, antibody deficiency (and predictable consequences), and autoimmunity (Gennery et al., 2000).

Ataxia-Telangiectasia

Ataxia-telangiectasia (AT) (see Chapter 29) is an autosomal recessive disorder characterized by progressive cerebellar degeneration, cutaneous or ocular telangiectasia, and immunodeficiency affecting predominantly cellular immunity, sensitivity to ionizing radiation, and a high incidence of malignancies. There is considerable clinical heterogeneity. The characteristic ataxia develops during infancy and is initially difficult to recognize; occasionally, the onset of ataxia is delayed until 4 or 5 years of age. More than two-thirds of AT patients suffer from recurrent bacterial infections due to defective T and B lymphocyte function. Endocrine problems are common.

The most consistent laboratory abnormality, almost pathognomonic for AT, is an elevated α-fetoprotein level. Most (80%) patients have IgA and IgE deficiency, which is occasionally associated with IgG2 and IgG4 subclass deficiency. Serum IgM may be elevated. Antibody responses to viral and bacterial antigens are often but not always deficient and correlate with the frequency of respiratory infections. T cell abnormalities include depressed proliferative responses to mitogens and specific antigens. Lymphopenia may be present in some patients because of a loss of CD4+ cells, but in most AT patients lymphocyte subsets are normal. Excessive chromosomal breakage can be observed in lymphocytes and fibroblasts, with breakpoints at 14q32, 14q12, 7q35, and 7p12, corresponding with the sites of gene complexes coding for immunoglobulin heavy chains and the T cell receptor chains α, β, and γ, respectively. In culture, cells from AT patients display increased sensitivity to ionizing radiation and radiomimetic chemicals, and uninhibited postirradiation DNA synthesis.

The identification of the AT gene, designated *ATM* (AT, mutated), has allowed the molecular analysis of the defect in affected families and makes carrier detection and prenatal diagnosis possible. The clinical heterogeneity may be explained by the type of mutation; frameshifts are associated with the absence of protein whereas milder phenotypes have missense mutations and some intracellular protein is detected (Gilad et al., 1998).

Nijmegen breakage syndrome

Patients with Nijmegen breakage syndrome (see Chapter 30), often of Czech or Polish descent, share many clinical findings with AT patients. They characteristically have microcephaly and growth retardation but they do not develop ataxia nor telangiectasia, and α-fetoprotein is normal. They share with AT patients a tendency toward recurrent infections, predisposition to malignancies, chromosomal instability, and hypersensitivity to irradiation and alkylating agents, and they have uninhibited postirradiation DNA synthesis.

These patients often present with immunodeficiencies affecting both T and B cells and hypogammaglobulinemia, and they may have deficiency of IgG2 and IgG4 (Gregorek et al., 2002). Flow-cytometric analysis shows a decreased number of CD4+ T cells and decreased CD4:CD8 ratio. Affected patients often have increased numbers of NK cells. In vitro lymphocyte proliferation to mitogens is impaired.

The gene for the Nijmegen breakage syndrome, *NBS1*, has been localized to chromosome 8q21, and the defective protein, NBS1 (nibrin), shows functional homology to a DNA repair protein in yeast. However, not all patients with Nijmegen breakage syndrome have an NBS1 mutation and other proteins may be involved (see Chapter 30).

Bloom syndrome

Patients with Bloom syndrome (see Chapter 30) have characteristic features and may develop a sun-sensitive erythematous skin rash that often but not always occurs along with recurrent bacterial respiratory infections. These patients have a high risk of cancer and a tendency to develop endocrine problems. Lymphocytes and fibroblasts develop sister chromatid exchanges and show gaps and breaks and increased rearrangements.

The associated immune deficiency is characterized by great variability. Some patients have hypogammaglobulinemia; others have normal levels of all immunoglobulin isotypes. Antibody responses to various antigens are either normal or moderately depressed. In vitro lymphocyte proliferation in response to PHA is

generally normal, but some patients have decreased responses to PWM, ConA, and allogeneic cells. The numbers of circulating lymphocytes and lymphocyte subsets are normal.

The gene for Bloom syndrome, *BLM*, is located at 15q26.1 and has recently been cloned and sequenced. It encodes a nuclear protein, which is absent in Bloom syndrome patients. Bloom syndrome is a clinical diagnosis, and the availability of molecular techniques has made it possible to confirm the diagnosis, detect variants, identify carriers, and perform prenatal diagnosis.

Other Deficiencies to Be Considered

The hyper-IgE (Job) syndrome, characterized by coarse facial features, recurrent staphylococcal and candida infections, abscess formation, recurrent lung abscesses often resulting in pneumatoceles, and atopic disease, most often occurs sporadically, rarely as an autosomal dominant disorder (see Chapter 34). Affected patients have markedly elevated IgE levels that exceed 5000 IU/ml and may be as high as 50,000–100,000 IU/ml, and often have eosinophilia. The diagnosis is based on clinical presentation, a strikingly elevated IgE level, and presence of associated features (see Table 43.10). A single-locus autosomal dominant trait with variable expressivity has been linked to a proximal region on the long arm of chromosome 4 (Grimbacher et al., 1999a,1999b) in a subgroup of unrelated, ethnically diverse, familial cases, findings suggesting sporadic mutation. There is ongoing study to examine the variable expression and apparently greater severity in succeeding generations. Autosomal recessive inheritance has been reported in families of Turkish descent (Renner et al., 2004). Serum immunoglobulin levels and specific antibodies to immunization and exposure antigens should be measured, as a few patients have improved with therapeutic immunoglobulin (Bilora et al., 2000).

Chronic mucocutaneous candidiasis is characterized by candida infections at multiple sites affecting the skin and mucosa. The candida infections may spread into the esophagus and lungs. A subgroup of patients may develop autoimmune polyendocrinopathy–candidiasis–ectodermal dystrophy (APECED), an autosomal recessive condition (Ahonen et al., 1990) due to the mutation of AIRE, a recently identified DNA-binding protein expressed by thymic epithelial cells and containing two zinc-finger motifs (Aaltonen et al., 1997) (see Chapter 25). In contrast to patients with cellular immune deficiencies, most patients with this syndrome have normal T cell numbers and normal in vitro lymphocyte proliferation to mitogens. Responses to specific antigen, except to candida antigens, which are often depressed, are variable regardless of whether measured by cytokine production or lymphocyte transformation.

Interleukin 12 (IL-12) and the interferon pathway defects result in familial generalized atypical tuberculosis or generalized infection with BCG (see Chapter 28). Most patients identified to date belong to consanguineous families and are therefore homozygous for the defect and exhibit reduced antigen-induced IFN-γ production in vitro. Detection of intracellular phosphorylated STAT-4 by flow cytometry has facilitated the diagnosis of these conditions (Uzel et al., 2001). The precise location of the defect within the pathways is delineated by studies of cell surface expression of the IL-12 and IFN-γ receptors, assays of IL-12 and IFN-γ production, and mutation analysis of the relevant genes (Lammas et al., 2000). A reduction of TNF-α production is a common secondary feature in this group of patients.

Hereditary transcobalamin II (TCII) deficiency is a recessive disorder caused by a mutation of the TCII gene located on chro-

Table 43.10. Diagnostic Features of Hyper-IgE Syndrome*

Feature	Level Considered Significant	Prevalence in Hyper-IgE	Level of Diagnostic Usefulness[†]
Neonatal rash	Present	Approaches 100%	Useful
Eczema	Severe	100%	Present, nonspecific
Raised serum IgE level	>2000 IU/ml at highest	97%	Defining hallmark
Eosinophilia	>0.8 × 10⁹/l	93%	Useful
Recurrent abscesses	>4 separate sites or episodes	87%	Defining hallmark
Pneumonia	X-ray proven Any invasive organism[‡]	87%	2–3 = useful
Candidiasis in fingernails	Present	83%	Useful
Characteristic facies	Present in adolescence	83%	Useful
Interalar distance	>1 SD above mean for age, gender, ethnicity	80%	Useful
Pneumatocoeles	Present	77%	Defining hallmark
Scoliosis	>15°–20° in patients over 16 years of age	76%	Useful
Delay in shedding primary dentition	>3 primary teeth	72%	Defining hallmark
Hyperextensible joints		68%	Variable, nonspecific
Recurrent fractures or osteoporosis	>1–2 from minimal trauma	57%	Useful

*Diagnosis is probable if there are three or more defining hallmarks plus two useful criteria. Diaagnosis is possible if two defining hallmarks and three useful criteria are present (see below).

[†]Defining hallmark = scores of 7–10 on diagnostic score sheet; useful = scores of 4–6 on diagnostic score sheet; variable = scores of 0–3 on diagnostic score sheet.

[‡]For example, *Haemophilus influenza, Streptococcus pneumoniae, Staphylococcus, Pseudomonas, Pneumocystistis,* atypical mycobacteria, etc.

Source: From Grimbacher et al., 1999a and J. Puck (personal communication).

mosome 22. TCII is required for absorption and transport of vitamin B$_{12}$. Patients with TCII deficiency present in the first few months of life with failure to thrive, diarrhea, ulcers of the oral mucous membrane, irritability, lethargy, delayed neurologic development, severe macrocytic anaemia, and neutropenia. Affected patients often present with decreased serum IgG and defective antibody responses (Hitzig and Kenny, 1975). Since treatment with high-dose vitamin B$_{12}$ is highly efficient, establishing the diagnosis at an early age is vital. The human TCII gene has been cloned, and mutations have been identified (Li et al., 1994).

References

Aaltonen J, Horelli-Kuitunen N, Fan JB, Bjorses P, Perheentupa J, Myers R, Palotie A, Peltonen L. High-resolution physical and transcriptional mapping of the autoimmune polyendocrinopathy–candidiasis–ectodermal dystrophy locus on chromosome 21q22.3 by FISH. Genome Res 7:820–829, 1997.

Agematsu K, Futatani T, Hokibara S, Kobayashi N, Takamoto M, Tsukada S, Suzuki H, Koyasu S, Miyawaki T, Sugane K, Komiyama A, Ochs HD. Absence of memory B cells in patients with common variable immunodeficiency. Clin Immunol 103:34–42, 2002.

Agematsu K, Nagumo H, Shinozaki K, Hokibara S, Yasui K, Terada K, Kawamura K, Toba T, Nonoyama S, Ochs HD, Komiyama A. Absence of IgD- CD27+ memory B cell population in X-linked hyper-IgM syndrome. J Clin Invest 102:853–860, 1998.

Ahonen P, Myllarniemi S, Sipila I, Perheentupa J. Clinical variation of autoimmune polyendocrinopathy–candidiasis–ectodermal dystrophy (APECED) in a series of 68 patients. N Engl J Med 322:1829–1836, 1990.

Alles AJ, Waldron MA, Sierra LS, Mattia AR. Prospective comparison of direct immunofluorescence and conventional staining methods for the detection of *Giardia* and *Cryptosporidium* spp. in human faecal specimens. J Clin Microbiol 33:1632–1634, 1995.

Ament ME, Ochs HD, Davis SD. Structure and function of the gastrointestinal tract in primary immunodeficiency syndromes. A study of 39 patients. Medicine 52:227–248, 1973.

Ameratunga R, Lederman HM, Sullivan KE, Seyama K, French JK, Prestidge R, Marbrook J, Fanslow WC, Winkelstein JA. Defective antigen-induced lymphocyte proliferation in the X-linked hyper-IgM syndrome. J Pediatr 131:147–150, 1997.

Bennett CL, Christie J, Ramsdell F, Brunkow ME, Ferguson PJ, Whitesell L, Kelly TE, Saulsbury FT, Chance PF, Ochs HD. The immune dysregulation, polyendocrinopathy, enteropathy, X-linked syndrome (IPEX) is caused by mutations of FOXP3. Nat Genet 27:20–21, 2001.

Bernard F, Picard C, Cormier-Daire V, Eidenschenk C, Pinto G, Bustamante JC, Jouanguy E, Teillac-Hamel D, Colomb V, Funck-Brentano I, Pascal V, Vivier E, Fischer A, Le Deist F, Casanova JL. A novel developmental and immunodeficiency syndrome associated with intrauterine growth retardation and a lack of natural killer cells. Pediatrics 113:136–141, 2004.

Bilora F, Petrobelli F, Boccioletti V, Pomerri F. Moderate dose IVIG treatment of Job's syndrome: case report. Minerva Med 91:113–116, 2000.

Biron CA, Byron KS, Sullivan JL. Severe herpes virus infections in an adolescent without natural killer cells. N Engl J Med 320:1731–1735, 1989.

Bowen TJ, Ochs HD, Altman LC, Price TH, Van Epps DE, Brautigan DL, Rosin RE, Perkins WD, Babior BM, Klebanoff SJ, Wedgwood RJ. Severe recurrent bacterial infections associated with defective adherence and chemotaxis in two patients with neutrophils deficient in a cell-associated glycoprotein. J Pediatr 101:932–940, 1982.

Buckley RH, Schiff RI, Schiff SE, Markert ML, Williams LW, Harville TO, Roberts JL, Puck JM. Human severe combined immunodeficiency: genetic, phenotypic, and functional diversity in one hundred eight infants. J Pediatr 130:378–387, 1997.

Carlucci F, Tabucchi A, Aiuti A, Rosi F, Floccari F, Pagani R, Marinello E. Capillary electrophoresis in diagnosis and monitoring of adenosine deaminase deficiency. Clin Chem 49:1830–1838, 2003.

Carulli G. Applications of flow cytometry in the study of human neutrophil biology and pathology. Hematopathol Mol Hematol 10:39–61, 1996.

Coligan JE, Kruisbeek AM, Shevach EM, Strober W, eds. Current Protocols in Immunology, Vols. 1 and 2. New York: Green, Wiley-Interscience, 1994 [regularly updated].

Conley ME. Molecular approaches to analysis of X-linked immunodeficiencies. Annu Rev Immunol 10:215–238, 1992.

Conley ME, Larche M, Bonagura VR, Lawton AR, Buckley RH, Fu SM, Coustan-Smith E, Herrod HG, Campana D. Hyper IgM syndrome associated with defective CD40-mediated B cell activation. J Clin Invest 94:1404–1409, 1994.

Conley ME, Notarangelo LD, Etzioni A. Diagnostic criteria for primary immunodeficiencies. Representing PAGID (Pan-American Group for Immunodeficiency) and ESII (European Society for Immunodeficiencies). Clin Immunol 93:190–197, 1999.

Cooney TR, Huissoon AP, Powell RJ, Jones NS. Investigation for immunodeficiency in patients with recurrent ENT infections. Clin Otolaryngol 26:184–188, 2001.

Cunningham-Rundles C. Clinical and immunologic analysis of 103 patients with common variable immunodeficiency. J Clin Immunol 9:22–23, 1989.

Cunningham-Rundles C. Hematologic complications of primary immune deficiencies. Blood Rev 16:61–64, 2002.

Cunningham-Rundles C, Bodian C. Common variable immunodeficiency: clinical and immunologic features of 248 patients. Clin Immunol 92:34–48, 1999.

Davies CW, Juniper MC, Gray W, Gleeson FV, Chapel HM, Davies RJ. Lymphoid interstitial pneumonitis associated with common variable hypogammaglobulinaemia treated with cyclosporin A. Thorax 55:88–90, 2000.

de la Calle-Martin O, Hernandez M, Ordi J, Casamitjana N, Arostegui JI, Caragol I, Ferrando M, Labrador M, Rodriguez-Sanchez JL, Espanol T. Familial CD8 deficiency due to a mutation in the CD8 alpha gene. J Clin Invest 108:117–123, 2001.

DeLisser HM, Christofidou-Solomidou M, Sun J, Nakada MT, Sullivan KE. Loss of endothelial surface expression of E-selectin in a patient with recurrent infections. Blood 94:884–894, 1999.

Erkeller-Yuksel FM, Deneys V, Yuksel B, Hannet I, Hulstaert F, Hamilton C, Mackinnon H, Turner Stokes L, Munhyeshuli V, Vanlangendonck F, de Bruyere M, Bach B, Lydyard PM. Age-related changes in human blood lymphocyte subpopulations. J Pediatr 120:216–222, 1992.

Etzioni A, Doetschuk CM, Harlan JM. Of man and mouse: leukocyte and endothelial adhesion molecule deficiencies. Blood 94:3281–3288, 1999.

Farrington ML, Grosmaire LS, Nonoyama S, Fischer S, Hollenbaugh D, Ledbetter JA, Noelle RJ, Aruffo A, Ochs HD. CD40 ligand expression is defective in a subset of patients with common variable immunodeficiency. Proc Natl Acad Sci USA 91:1099–1103, 1994.

Ferrari S, Giliani S, Insalaco A, Al-Ghonaium A, Soresina AR, Loubser M, Avanzini MA, Marconi M, Badolato R, Ugazio AG, Levy Y, Catalan N, Durandy A, Tbakhi A, Notarangelo LD, Plebani A. Mutations of CD40 gene cause an autosomal recessive form of immunodeficiency with hyper IgM. Proc Natl Acad Sci USA 98:12614–12619, 2001.

Ferry BL, Jones J, Bateman EA, Woodham N, Warnatz K, Schlesier M, Misbah SA, Peter HH, Chapel HM. Measurement of peripheral B cell populations in common variable immunodeficiency (CVID) using a whole blood method. Clin Exp Immunol 140:532–539, 2005.

Ferry BL, Misbah SA, Stephens P, Sherrell Z, Lythgoe H, Bateman E, Banner C, Jones J, Groome N, Chapel HM. Development of an anti-Salmonella typhi Vi ELISA: assessment of immunocompetence in healthy donors. Clin Exp Immunol 136:297–303, 2004.

Fischer A. Severe combined immunodeficiencies. Clin Exp Immunol 122:143–149, 2000.

Fleisher TA, Dorman SE, Anderson JA, Vail M, Brown MR, Holland SM. Detection of intracellular phosphorylated STAT-1 by flow cytometry. Clin Immunol 90:425–430, 1999.

Fleisher TA, Oliveira JB. Functional and molecular evalutation of lymphocyyes. J Allergy Clin Immunol 114:227–234, 2004.

Futatani T, Miyawaki T, Tsukada S, Hashimoto S, Kunikata T, Arai S, Kurimoto M, Niida Y, Matsuoka H, Sakiyama Y, Iwata T, Tsuchiya S, Tatsuzawa O, Yoshizaki K, Kishimoto T. Deficient expression of Bruton's tyrosine kinase in monocytes from X-linked agammaglobulinemia as evaluated by a flow cytometric analysis and its clinical application to carrier detection. Blood 91:595–602, 1998.

Futatani T, Watanabe C, Baba Y, Tsukada S, Ochs HD. Bruton's tyrosine kinase is present in normal platelets and its absence identifies patients with X-linked agammaglobulinemia and carrier females. Br J Haematol 114:141–149, 2001.

Gadola SD, Moins-Teisserenc HT, Trowsdale J, Gross WL, Cerundolo V. TAP deficiency syndrome. Clin Exp Immunol 121:173–178, 2000.

Gaspar HB, Lester T, Levinsky RJ, Kinnon C. Bruton's tyrosine kinase expression and activity in X linked agammaglobulinaemia (XLA): the use of protein analysis as a diagnostic indicator of XLA. Clin Exp Immunol 111:334–338, 1998.

Gennery AR, Cant AJ. Diagnosis of severe combined immune deficiency. J Clin Pathol 54:191–195, 2000.

Gennery AR, Cant AJ, Jeggo PA. Immunodeficiency associated with DNA repair defects. Clin Exp Immunol 121:1–7, 2000.

Gibb D, Spoulou V, Giacomelli A, Griffiths H, Masters J, Misbah S, Nokes L, Pagliaro A, Giaquinto C, Kroll S, Goldblatt D. Antibody responses to Haemophilus influenzae type b and Streptococcus pneumoniae vaccines in children with HIV infection. Pediatr Infect Dis J 14:129–135, 1995.

Gilad S, Chessa L, Khosravi R, Russell P, Galanty Y, Piane M, Gatti RA, Jorgensen TJ, Shiloh Y, Bar-Shira A. Genotype–phenotype relationships in ataxia telangiectasia (A-T) and A-T variants. Am J Hum Genet 62:551–561, 1998.

Goldmuntz E, Driscoll D, Budarf ML, Zackai EH, McDonald-McGinn DM, Biegel JA, Emanuel BS. Microdeletions of chromosomal region 22q11 in patients with congenital conotruncal cardiac defects. J Med Genet 30:807–812, 1993.

Goldsobel AL, Haas A, Stiehm ER. Bone marrow transplantation in DiGeorge syndrome. J Pediatr 111:40–44, 1987.

Gossage DL, Buckley RH. Prevalence of lymphocytopenia in severe combined immunodeficiency. N Engl J Med 323:1422–1423, 1990.

Gregorek H, Chrzanowska KH, Michalkiewicz J, Syczewska M, Madalinski K. Heterogeneity of humoral immune abnormalities in children with Nijmegen breakage syndrome: an 8-year follow-up study in single centre. Clin Exp Immunol 130:319–324, 2002.

Grimbacher B, Holland SM, Gallin JI, Greenberg F, Hill SC, Malech HL, Miller JA, O'Connell AC, Puck JM. Hyper-IgE syndrome with recurrent infections—an autosomal dominant multi-system disorder. N Engl J Med 340:692–702, 1999a.

Grimbacher B, Hutloff A, Schlesier M, Glocker E, Warnatz K, Drager R, Eibel H, Fischer B, Schaffer AA, Mages HW, Kroczek RA, Peter HH. Homozygous loss of ICOS is associated with adult-onset common variable immunodeficiency. Nat Immunol 4:261–268, 2003.

Grimbacher B, Schaffer AA, Holland SM, et al. Genetic linkage of hyper-IgE syndrome to chromosome 4. Am J Hum Genet 65:735–744, 1999b.

Hague RA, Rassam S, Morgan G, Cant A. Early diagnosis of severe combined immunodeficiency syndrome. Arch Dis Child 70:260–263, 1994.

Hammarstrom L, Vorechovsky I, Webster ADB. Selective IgA deficiency and common variable immunodeficiency. Clin Exp Immunol 120:225–231, 2000.

Hanson KL, Cartwright CP. Use of an enzyme immunoassay does not eliminate the need to analyse multiple stool specimens for sensitive detection of Giardia lamblia. J Clin Microbiol 39:474–477, 2001.

Harris ES, Shigeoka AO, Li W, Adams RH, Prescott SM, McIntyre TM, Zimmerman GA, Lorant DE. A novel syndrome of variant leukocyte adhesion deficiency involving defects in adhesion mediated by β1 and β2 integrins. Blood 97:767–776, 2001.

Hayward AR, Levy J, Facchetti F, Notarangelo L, Ochs HD, Etzioni A, Bonnefoy JY, Cosyns M, Weinberg A. Cholangiopathy and tumours of the pancreas, liver, and biliary tree in boys with X-linked immunodeficiency with hyper-IgM. J Immunol 158:977–983, 1997.

Hermaszewski RA, Webster ADB. Primary hypogammaglobulinaemia: a survey of clinical manifestations and complications. Q J Med 86:31–42, 1993.

Hitzip WH, Kenny AB. The role of vitamin B12 and its transport globulins in the production of antibodies. Clin Exp Immunol 20:105–111, 1975.

Hogg N, Stewart MP, Scarth SL, Newton R, Shaw JM, Law SK, Klein N. A novel leukocyte adhesion deficiency caused by expressed but nonfunctional β2 integrins Mac-1 and LFA-1. J Clin Invest 103:97–106, 1999.

Holland SM, Dorman SE, Kwon A, Pitha-Rowe IF, Frucht DM, Gerstberger SM, Noel GJ, Vesterhus P, Brown MR, Fleisher TA. Abnormal regulation of interferon-γ, interleukin-12, and tumor necrosis factor-α in human interferon-γ receptor 1 deficiency. J Infect Dis 178:1095–1104, 1998.

Horwitz M, Benson KF, Person RE, Aprikyan AG, Dale DC. Mutations in ELA2, encoding neutrophil elastase, define a 21-Da biological clock in cyclic haematopoiesis. Nat Genet 23:433–446, 1999.

Imai K, Slupphaug G, Lee WI, Revy P, Nonoyama S, Catalan N, Yel L, Forveille M, Kavli B, Krokan HE, Ochs HD, Fischer A, Durandy A. Human uracil-DNA glycosylase deficiency associated with profoundly impaired immunoglobulin class-switch recombination. Nat Immunol 4:1023–1028, 2003.

Jain A, Ma CA, Liu S, Brown M, Cohen J, Strober W. Specific missense mutations in NEMO result in hyper-IgM syndrome with hypohydrotic ectodermal dysplasia. Nat Immunol 2:223–228, 2001.

Jin Y, Mazza C, Christie JR, Giliani S, Fiorini M, Mella P, Gandellini F, Stewart DM, Zhu Q, Nelson D, Notarangelo LD, Ochs HD. Mutations of the Wiskott-Aldrich syndrome protein (WASP): hotspots, effect on transcription, and translation and phenotype/genotype correlation. Blood 104:4010–4019, 2004.

Jirapongsananuruk O, Malech HL, Kuhns DB, Niemela JE, Brown MR, Anderson-Cohen M, Fleisher TA. Diagnostic paradigm for evaluation of male patients with chronic granulomatous disease, based on the dihydro rhodamine 123 assay. J Allergy Clin Immunol 111:374–379, 2003.

Junker AK, Driscoll DA. Humoral immunity in DiGeorge syndrome. J Pediatr 127:231–237, 1995.

Kondratenko I, Amlot PL, Webster AD, Farrant J. Lack of specific antibody response in common variable immunodeficiency (CVID) associated with failure in production of antigen-specific memory T cells. Clin Exp Immunol 108:9–13, 1997.

Kuijpers TW, Van Lier RA, Hamann D, de Boer M, Thung LY, Weenin RS, Verhoeven AJ, Roos D. Leukocyte adhesion deficiency type 1 (LAD-1)/variant. A novel immunodeficiency syndrome characterized by dysfunctional β2 integrins. J Clin Invest 100:1725–1733, 1997.

Kuijpers TW, Weening RS, Roos D. Clinical and laboratory work-up of patients with neutrophil shortage or dysfunction J Immunol Methods 232:211–229, 1999.

Lakshman R, Finn A. Neutrophil disorders and their management. J Clin Pathol 54:7–19, 2001.

Lammas DA, Drysdale P, Ben-Smith A, Girdlestone J, Edgar D, Kumararatne DS. Diagnosis of defects in the type 1 cytokine pathway. Microbes Infect 2:1567–1578, 2000.

Levy J, Espanol-Boren T, Thomas C, Fischer A, Tovo P, Bordigoni P, Resnick I, Fasth A, Baer M, Gomez L, Sanders EAM, Tabone M-D, Plantaz D, Etzioni A, Monafo V, Abinun M, Hammarstrom L, Abrahamsen T, Jones A, Finn A, Klemola T, DeVries E, Sanal O, Peitsch MC, Notarangelo LD. Clinical spectrum of X-linked hyper-IgM syndrome. J Pediatr 131:47–54, 1997.

Levy Y, Gupta N, Le Deist F, Garcia C, Fischer A, Weill JC, Reynaud CA. Defect in IgV gene somatic hypermutation in common variable immunodeficiency syndrome. Proc Natl Acad Sci USA 95:13135–13140, 1998.

Li N, Rosenblatt DS, Kamen BA, Seetharam S, Seetharam B. Identification of two mutant alleles of transcobalamin II in an affected family. Hum Mol Genet 3:1835–1840, 1994.

Maraha B, Buiting AG. Evaluation of four enzyme immunoassays for the detection of Giardia lamblia antigen in stool specimens. Eur J Clin Microbiol Infect Dis 19:485–487, 2000.

Markert ML, Alexieff MJ, Li J, Sarzotti M, Ozaki DA, Devlin BH, Sempowski GD, Rhein ME, Szaboles P, Hale LP, Buckley RH, Coyne KI, Rice HE, Mahaffey SM, Skinner MA. Complete DiGeorge syndrome: development of rash, lymphadenopathy, and oligoclonal T cells in 5 cases. J Allergy Clin Immunol 113:734–741, 2004.

McDowall A, Inwald D, Leitinger B, Jones A, Liesner R, Klein N, Hogg N. A novel form of integrin dysfunction involving β1, β2, and β3 integrins. J Clin Invest 111:51–60, 2003.

Melaranci C, Ciaffi P, Zerella A, Martinelli V, Cutrera R, Plebani A, Duse M, Ugazio GA. T cell subpopulations in paediatric healthy children: age-normal values. J Clin Lab Immunol 38:143–149, 1992.

Mellemkjaer L, Hammarstrom L, Andersen V, Yuen J, Heilmann C, Barington T, Bjorkander J, Olsen JH. Cancer risk among patients with IgA deficiency or common variable immunodeficiency and their relatives: a combined Danish and Swedish study. Clin Exp Immunol 130:495–500, 2002.

Morra M, Silander O, Calpe S, Choi M, Oettgen H, Myers L, Etzioni A, Buckley R, Terhorst C. Alterations of the X-linked lymphoproliferative disease gene SH2D1A in common variable immunodeficiency syndrome. Blood 98:1321–1325, 2001.

Nonoyama S, Farrington M, Ishida H, Howard M, Ochs HD. Activated B cells from patients with common variable immunodeficiency proliferate and synthesize immunoglobulin. J Clin Invest 92:1282–1287, 1993.

Nonoyama S, Farrington ML, Ochs HD. Effect of IL-2 on immunoglobulin production by anti–CD40-activated human B cells: synergistic effect with IL-10 and antagonistic effect with IL-4. Clin Immunol Immunopathol 72:373–379, 1994.

Notarangelo LD, Hayward AR. X-linked immunodeficiency with hyper-IgM (XHIM) Clin Exp Immunol 120:399–405, 2000.

Ochs HD, Slichter SJ, Harker LA, Von Behrens WE, Clark RA, Wedgwood RJ. The Wiskott-Aldrich syndrome: studies of lymphocytes, granulocytes, and platelets. Blood 55:243–252, 1980.

Ochs HD, Smith CIE. X-linked agammaglobulinemia: a clinical and molecular analysis. Medicine (Baltimore) 75:287–299, 1996.

Orange JS. Human natural killer cell deficiencies and susceptibility to infection. Microbes Infect 4:1545–1558, 2002.

Orange JS, Brodeur SR, Jain A, Bonilla FA, Schneider LC, Kretschmer R, Nurko S, Rasmussen WL, Kohler JR, Gellis SE, Ferguson BM, Strominger JL, Zonana J, Ramesh N, Ballas ZK, Geha RS. Deficient natural killer cell cytotoxicity in patients with IKK-γ/NEMO mutations. J Clin Invest 109:1501–1509, 2002a.

Orange JS, Ramesh N, Remold-O'Donnell E, Sasahara Y, Koopman L, Byrne M, Bonilla FA, Rosen FS, Geha RS, Strominger JL. Wiskott-Aldrich syndrome protein is required for NK cell cytotoxicity and colocalizes with actin to NK cell–activating immunologic synapses. Proc Natl Acad Sci USA 99:11351–11356, 2002b.

Osguthorpe JD. Adult rhinosinusitis: diagnosis and management. Am Fam Physician 63:69–76, 2001.

Pahwa R, Chatila T, Pahwa S, Paradise C, Day NK, Geha R, Schwartz S, Slade H, Oyaizu N, Good RA. Recombinant interleukin 2 therapy in severe combined immunodeficiency disease. Proc Natl Acad Sci USA 86: 5069–5073, 1989.

Pierdominici M, Marziali M, Giovannetti A, Oliva A, Rosso R, Marino B, Digilio MC, Giannotti A, Novelli G, Dallapiccola B, Aiuti F, Pandolfi F. T cell receptor repertoire and function in patients with DiGeorge syndrome and velocardiofacial syndrome. Clin Exp Immunol 121:127–132, 2000.

Pignata C, Gaetaniello L, Masci AM, Frank J, Christiano A, Matrecano E, Racioppi L. Human equivalent of the mouse Nude/SCID phenotype: long-term evaluation of immunologic reconstitution after bone marrow transplantation. Blood 97:880–885, 2001.

Pinquier C, Heron D, de-Carvalho, W, Lazar G, Mazet P, Cohen D. La microdeletion 22q11: a propos d'une observation de schizophrenie chez une adolescente. Encephale 27:45–50, 2001.

Piqueras B, Lavenu-Bombled C, Galicier L, Bergeron–van der Cruyssen Mouthon L, Chevret S, Debre P, Schmitt C, Oksenhendler E. Common variable immunodeficiency patient classification based on impaired B cell memory differentiation correlates with clinic aspects. J Clin Immunol 23: 385–400, 2003.

Plebani A, Soresina A, Rondelli R, Amato GM, Azzari C, Cardinale F, Cazzola G, Consolini R, De Mattia D, Dell'Erba G, Duse M, Fiorini M, Martino S, Martire B, Masi M, Monafo V, Moschese V, Notarangelo LD, Orlandi P, Panei P, Pession A, Pietrogrande MC, Pignata C, Quinti I, Ragno V, Rossi P, Sciotto A, Stabile A, Italian Pediatric Group for XLA AIEOP. Clinical, immunological, and molecular analysis in a large cohor of patients with X-linked agammaglobulinemia: an Italian multicenter study. Clin Immunol 104:201–203, 2002.

Puel A, Ziegler SF, Buckley RH, Leonard WLJ. Defective IL7R expression in T(−)B(+)NK(+) severe combined immunodeficiency. Nat Genet 20: 394–397, 1998.

Renner ED, Puck JM, Holland SM, Schmitt M, Weiss M, Frosch M, Bergmann M, Davis J, Belohradsky BH, Grimbacher B. Autosomal recessive hyperimmunoglobulin E syndrome: a distinct disease entity. J Pediatr 144(1):93–97, 2004.

Revy P, Muto T, Levy Y, Geissmann F, Plebani A, Sanal O, Catalan N, Forveille M, Dufoureq-Labelouse R, Gennery A, Tezcan I, Ersoy F, Kayserili H, Ugazio AG, Brousse N, Muramatsu M, Notarangelo LD, Kinoshita K, Honjo T, Fischer A, Durandy A. Activation-induced cytidine deaminase (AID) deficiency causes the autosomal recessive form of the hyper-IgM syndrome (HIGM2). Cell 102:565–575, 2000.

Rose NR, de Macario EC, Folds JD, Lane HC, Nakamura RM, eds. Manual of Clinical Laboratory Immunology. Washington, DC: ASM Press, 1997.

Rosen FS. Severe combined immunodeficiency: a pediatric emergency. J Pediatr 130:345–356, 1997.

Ryan AK, Goodship JA, Wilson DI, Philip N, Levy A, Seidel H, Schuffenhauer S, Oechsler H, Belohradsky B, Prieur M, Aurias A, Raymond FL, Clayton-Smith J, Hatchwell E, McKeown C, Beemer FA, Dallapiccola B, Novelli G, Hurst JA, Ignatius J, Green AJ, Winter RM, Brueton L, Brndum-Nielsen K, Stewart F, Van Essen T, Patton M, Paterson J, Scambler PJ. Spectrum of clinical features associated with interstitial chromosome 22q11 deletions: a European collaborative study. J Med Genet 34: 798–804, 1997.

Salzer U, Chapel HM, Webster AD, Pan-Hammarstrom Q, Schmitt-Graeff A, Schlesier M, Peter HH, Rockstroh JK, Schneider P, Schaffer AA, Hammarstrom L, Grimbacher B. Mutations in TNFRSF13B encoding TACI are associated with common variable immunodeficiency in humans. Nat Genet 37:820–828, 2005.

Salzer U, Maul-Pavicic A, Cunningham-Rundles C, Urschel S, Belohradsky BH, Litzman J, Holm A, Franco JL, Plebani A, Hammarstrom L, Skrabl A, Schwinger W, Grimbacher B. ICOS deficiency in patients with common variable immunodeficiency. Clin Immunol 113:234–240, 2004.

Schwartz R, Porat YB, Handzel Z, Sthoeger Z, Garty BZ, Confino-Cohen R, Levy J, Zan-Bar I. Identification of a subset of common variable immunodeficiency patients with impaired B-cell protein tyrosine phosphorylation. Clin Diagn Lab Immunol 6:856–860, 1999.

Smahi A, Courtois G, Rabia SH, Doffinger R, Bodemer C, Munnich A, Casanova JL, Israel A. The NF-κB signalling pathway in human diseases:

from incontinentia pigmenti to ectodermal dysplasias and immune-deficiency syndromes. Hum Mol Genet 11:2371–2375, 2002.

Sneller MC, Strober W. Abnormalities of lymphokine gene expression in patients with common variable immunodeficiency. J Immunol 144:3762–3769, 1990.

Spickett GP, Farrant J, North ME, Zhang JG, Morgan L, Webster AD. Common variable immunodeficiency: how many diseases? Immunol Today 18:325–328, 1997.

Stephan JL, Vlekova V, Le Deist F, Blanche S, Donadieu J, De Saint-Basile G, Durandy A, Griscelli C, Fischer A. Severe combined immunodeficiency. A retrospective single centre study of clinical presentation and outcome in 117 patients. J Pediatr 123:564–572, 1993.

Stiehm ER, Ochs HD, Winkelstein JA. Immunodeficiency disorders: general considerations. In: Stiehm ER, Ochs HD, Winkelstein JA, editors. Immunologic Disorders in Infants and Children, Fifth ed. Philadelphia: Elsevier Saunders, pp. 289–356, 2004.

Sullivan JL, Byron KS, Brewster FE, Baker SM, Ochs HD. X-linked lymphoproliferative syndrome: natural history of the immunodeficiency. J Clin Invest 71:1765–1778, 1983.

Thrasher AJ, Kinnon C. The Wiskott-Aldrich syndrome. Clin Exp Immunol 120:2–9, 2000.

Uzel G, Frucht DM, Fleisher TA, Holland SM. Detection of intracellular phosphorylated STAT-4 by flow cytometry. Clin Immunol 100:270–276, 2001.

Vorechovsky I, Zetterquist H, Paganelli R, Koskinen S, Webster ADB, Smith CIE, Hammarstrom L. Family and linkage study of selective IgA deficiency and common variable immunodeficiency. Clin Immunol Immunopathol 77:185–192, 1995.

Warnatz K, Denz A, Drager R, Braun M, Groth C, Wolff-Vorbeck G, Eibel H, Schlesier M, Peter HH. Severe deficiency of switched memory B cells (CD27(+)IgM(−)IgD(−)) in subgroups of patients with common variable immunodeficiency: a new approach to classify a heterogeneous disease. Blood 99:1544–1551, 2002.

Yagi H, Furutani Y, Hamada H, Sasaki T, Asakawa S, Minoshima S, Ichida F, Joo K, Kimura M, Imamura S, Kamatani N, Momma K, Takao A, Nakazawa M, and N. Shimizu, Matsuoka R. Role of TBX1 in human del22q11.2 syndrome. Lancet 362:1366–1373, 2003.

Web Sites

European Society for Immunodeficiencies, at: http://www.esid.org

Pan American Group for Immunodeficiencies, at: http://www.pagid.org

The ImmunoDeficiency Resource (IDR), a Web-accessible compendium of information on the immunodeficiencies. This resource includes tools for clinical, biochemical, genetic, structural, and computational analyses as well as links to related information maintained by others. Available at: http://www.uta.fi/imt/bioinfo/idr

44

Genetic Aspects of Primary Immunodeficiencies

JENNIFER M. PUCK

There are three reasons why evaluation of an immunological disorder in any patient should include consideration of potential underlying genetic determinants. First, genetic studies can confirm a suspected diagnosis of immunodeficiency; they can also help to pinpoint a specific genetic etiology even when other available data are unusual, incomplete, or inconclusive. Second, new understanding of the immunological basis and pathogenesis of immunodeficiencies can be gleaned as more disease genes are identified through the partnership between researchers in molecular genetics, clinicians, and affected patients. Finally, diagnosing a genetic disorder in an index patient, or proband, has profound implications for the patient's family members, both affected and unaffected, living and as yet unborn.

Disorders of the immune system may be due to defects in single genes, either already known or currently unidentified. Because we have now recognized frequent new mutations and variant phenotypes for many immunodeficiency genes, we know that even immunodeficient patients lacking a positive family history may have genetic mutations underlying their condition that pose a reproductive risk in their family members. More common in the population than single-gene disorders causing immunodeficiency are many as yet poorly understood immune dysfunctions with a complex etiology, but this complexity probably includes one or more genetic factors that may interact with environmental influences. As the field of genetics advances, the existence of genetic contributions to all categories of human disease, including immunodeficiencies, is becoming increasingly apparent. While this chapter emphasizes the available genetic tests for single gene diseases, the field is changing rapidly. Not only are additional disease genes being discovered, but technologies for finding mutations and determining carrier status are in constant evolution. The technical ability to determine the genetic constitution of an individual will in many instances exceed the capacity of our

medical and social systems to help individuals learn about their risks, to evaluate the potential harms and benefits of genetic testing, and to develop and provide new therapies made possible by genetic advances.

The reader is referred to Chapter 2 for a summary of genetic principles and technologies. This chapter will present an overview of genetic tests used to diagnose inherited immunodeficiencies, but these tests should be viewed in a broad context of evolving basic knowledge, technological advances, and social and regulatory issues. The physician specializing in the diagnosis and treatment of immunodeficiencies should stay in contact with patients and their families to be able to pass on relevant new information. Much can be gained through enlisting the involvement of clinical geneticists and genetic counselors, who specialize in helping individuals and families understand and manage their genetic risks.

Establishing a Genetic Etiology

Positive Family History

The first diagnostic measure when considering any heritable disorder is to obtain a full pedigree and family health history; heritable immunodeficiencies are no exception. Although most of the immunodeficiencies in this book have been identified at the gene level very recently, families can often provide details about potentially affected members in past generations whose presentation and course might be compatible with the disorder (see agammaglobulinemia pedigree and discussion in Chapter 1). Assembly and recall of complete information often require more than one session and interviews with more individuals than just the nuclear family of the proband. Retrieval and review of medical records from relatives can provide critical data and are well worth seeking. Ethnic and geographical ancestry should be recorded as part of every family history because they may suggest consanguinity or increased risks associated with particular populations.

The X chromosome harbors more recognized immunodeficiency genes than any other chromosome, and the X-linked immunodeficiency diseases occur in disproportionately high frequency (Table 44.1). This is because in males, mutations in genes on the sole copy of the X chromosome are uncompensated, and therefore a single mutation causes overt disease. The X-linked inheritance pattern of multiple affected males related through maternal lines, as discussed in Chapter 2, should be sought in all families with a male presenting with immunodeficiency.

Recessive diseases, in contrast, require defects in both alleles of a gene in order for a disease phenotype to be manifest. One way in which this occurs is through consanguinous marriages, such as with the interferon gamma (IFN-γ) receptor mutations causing susceptibility to mycobacterial infections (Chapter 28). Belonging to a genetically isolated population is another risk factor for homozygous recessive diseases in which the same mutation may be transmitted through both maternal and paternal lines to the patient because of inbreeding. This phenomenon is found in the ataxia-telangectasia of Jews of Moroccan origin (Chapter 29) and the severe combined immunodeficiency (SCID) of Native Americans of the southwestern United States (Chapter 11) (Li et al., 2002). In many recessive immunodeficiencies, however, such as adenosine deaminase (ADA)-deficient SCID (Chapter 12), most patients have a different mutation in each of their two alleles.

There are relatively few dominant immunodeficiency phenotypes. As a rule, they are characterized by incomplete penetrance (skipping generations in family pedigrees) and or variable expressivity (a large spectrum of severity among relatives with the same genetic mutation). Examples include DiGeorge syndrome (Chapter 33); autoimmune lymphoproliferative syndrome due to Fas deficiency (Chapter 24); some instances of hyper IgE-recurrent

infection syndrome, or Job's syndrome (Chapter 34); and, importantly, some instances of common variable immunodeficiency (CVID) and IgA deficiency (Chapter 23); and even atopy and allergic disorders (Holgate, 1997). These may turn out to be diseases in which a dominant gene mutation has a predisposing or contributory effect in a group of families, but in which genetic or environmental factors act as modifiers of the phenotype.

Several immunodeficiency syndromes, such as SCID or chronic granulomatous disease (CGD), can be caused by defects in any of several different genes; existence of autosomal phenocopies of the X-linked immune disorders are indicated in Table 44.1. Family history can be critical in differentiating the X-linked from autosomal forms.

Importance of Family History, Even If Negative

Documentation of a complete family pedigree is helpful even if it fails to reveal any sign of disease comparable to that of a proband affected with immunodeficiency. First, the structure of the pedigree determines the quantity of genetic information. A large kindred with many siblings of both sexes has had more opportunities to have affected relatives, whereas at the other extreme, there may be no information whatsoever about an adopted infant's heredity. Second, the absence of disease in many relatives who could potentially be at risk is useful. For example, if a male with SCID has many healthy maternal uncles, either a new occurrence of an *IL2RG* gene mutation (Table 44.1) or recessive disease is considerably more likely than an X-linked mutation inherited from the patient's grandmother. A third benefit of obtaining a family history is the insight it can provide into the way in which family members will approach a serious immunodeficiency disease. We can provide optimal care for patients and their families only if we understand what the disease means to them. In previous generations or when the initial diagnosis has

Table 44.1. X-linked Immunodeficiencies and Their Disease Genes

Immunodeficiency Disease	Gene Name	Protein	Location	Female Skewed X Inactivation	Autosomal Genocopy	Chapter in Book
X-linked chronic granulomatous disease (CGD)	CYBB	Cytochrome oxidase gp91phox that generates reactive oxygen species	Xp21.1	No	Yes	37
Properdin deficiency	PFC	Properdin activator of complement	Xp11.23	No	Yes	42
Immunodysregulation polyendocrinopathy enteropathy syndrome (IPEX)	FOXP3	Forkhead/winged-helix transcriptional regulator critical for regulatory T cells	Xp11.23	No	Not known	26
Wiskott-Aldrich syndrome (WAS)	WAS	WAS protein (WASP) activator of actin polymerization and signal transduction	Xp11.22	Yes: all hematopoietic cells	Probably	31
X-linked severe combined immunodeficiency (XSCID)	IL2RG	Common γ chain of cytokine receptors	Xq13.1	Yes: T, B, NK cells (not phagocytes)	Yes	9
X-linked agammaglobulinemia (XLA)	BTK	B cell tyrosine kinase	Xq21.3–q22	Yes: B cells (not T cells, phagocytes)	Yes	21
X-linked lymphoproliferative syndrome (XLP)	SAP, SH2D1A	Lymphocyte signaling activation molecule	Xq25	No	Not known	32
X-linked hyper-IgM syndrome	CD40L	CD40 ligand	Xq26.3–q27.1	No	Yes	19
G6PD deficiency	G6PD	Glucose-6-phosphate dehydrogenase	Xq28	No	No	38
X-linked ectodermal dysplasia with immunodeficiency (NEMO)	NEMO, IKBKG	Inhibitor of κ light polypeptide gene enhancer in B cells, kinase γ	Xq28	Sometimes; females have incontinentia pigmenti	Not known	36

been delayed and treatment was ineffective, children born with immunodeficiencies are likely to have died, leading to parental feelings of guilt, secrecy, and other family stresses. Important family events or beliefs unrelated to immunodeficiency also strongly influence the outlook of family members. Finally, the family history may bring to light facts that influence the type of genetic testing that may be indicated, such as multiple miscarriages (a risk factor for chromosomal rearrangements) or nonpaternity.

Genetic Testing for Abnormalities in Immune System Genes

Inherited immunodeficiencies are sufficiently rare that population-based screening has not been implemented to date. Genetic testing is therefore used to establish the diagnosis in an affected individual or to determine the status of relatives of a person already suspected to have a primary immunodeficiency. Individuals in a family with recognized immunodeficiency for whom genetic testing may be indicated include affected patients who are ill; individuals who may have inherited a defective immune system gene, but as yet show no symptoms (presymptomatic testing); and healthy relatives not at risk for becoming immunodeficient but who may be carriers of a defective copy a gene and are concerned about their reproductive risks. In addition, prenatal testing has been performed for many immunodeficiencies in pregnancies following the diagnosis of an affected child. No single testing modality is appropriate for all situations. The reader is referred to specific chapters for discussions of the available options for each disease.

Techniques That Do Not Rely on Isolation of Patient DNA or RNA

Biochemical Tests

The immunodeficiencies associated with enzyme abnormalities such as ADA deficiency can be diagnosed by detecting increased amounts of physiologic precursors, such as deoxyadenosine or dATP, or by direct measurement of enzyme activity in vitro (see Chapter 12). Similarly, glucose-6-phosphate dehydrogenase (G6PD) deficiency, associated with impaired intracellular killing by neutrophils, is best detected by enzyme assay (see Chapter 8) (Buetler et al., 1979; Luzzatto and Mehta, 1995). The advantage of this type of testing is that the functional consequences of the underlying gene mutation can be immediately demonstrated without the need for DNA sequencing. Moreover, gene defects that permit production of inactive or partially active protein will be distinguished from DNA sequence variants of no physiologic significance (genetic polymorphisms). A disadvantage, however, is that carrier testing, which relies on demonstrating enzyme activity intermediate between the normal and deficient ranges, may be imprecise because of overlap with the partial activity of some mutant proteins in affected individuals. Careful assay standards with positive and negative controls in every run are essential.

Immunologic Tests

Enumeration of leukocyte populations, measurement of their secreted products, such as immunoglobulins, and functional tests involving in vitro activation are necessary for definitive diagnosis of virtually all immunodeficiencies. Their use in diagnosis is discussed in Chapter 43. In only a few circumstances, however, have these immunologic tests been made specific for a particular

gene product so that they can be used to establish a specific gene diagnosis. One example is X-linked hyper-IgM syndrome due to CD40 ligand (CD40L) deficiency (Table 44.1 and Chapter 19). Stimulated T cells from normals express CD40L, which can be detected by binding to immunofluorescent-tagged soluble CD40 or anti-CD40L monoclonal antibodies (Conley et al., 1994). However, mutations that allow production and expression of defective protein at the cell surface may not all be detected by this test, nor can it be used for testing of female heterozygous carriers, or for prenatal testing early in pregnancy.

Another example of an immunodeficiency with a useful immunologic test is CGD (Chapter 37). Formerly diagnosed by counting cells able to reduce nitroblue tetrazolium (NBT) dye, the inability of CGD granulocytes to produce superoxide is now more accurately measured by flow-cytometric determination of neutrophil NADP oxidase activity (Jirapongsananuruk et al., 2002). Not only are patient cells readily shown to be defective in this test, but the results can be quantified to yield some predictive information about disease severity. Moreover, female carriers of the X-linked form of CGD can be identified because the Lyonization, or random X inactivation of their neutrophils, results in two distinct populations when their cells are analyzed (see below). Cells whose active X chromosome has intact CYBB have normal NADP oxidase, whereas those with an active X chromosome bearing mutated CYBB demonstrate very little or no activity.

A special use of immunologic tests is in the prenatal evaluation of fetal blood samples. By the middle of the second trimester of pregnancy it is possible to obtain blood from the fetal umbilical vein to determine whether functional T cells, B cells, or granulocytes are present in normal numbers (Lau and Levinski, 1988). Fetal blood sampling involves greater risk to the fetus than does either amniocentesis or chorionic villus biopsy and should be performed only in a center with extensive experience in the technique. It is possible for the sample to be contaminated with maternal blood. Only a small volume of fetal blood is collected, and it must be analyzed without delay by an immunology laboratory that has successfully tested normal fetal blood samples as controls. Despite these caveats, fetal blood sampling is sought by some pregnant couples who have had a previous affected child with immunodeficiency, but who lack a gene-specific diagnosis. For example, cell surface staining for T cells and lymphocyte mitogen responses can be tested in a fetal blood sample to rule in or rule out a diagnosis of SCID in a pregnancy at risk, even if the genotype of the SCID of the proband is not known.

Cytogenetic Studies

Cytogenetics studies involve the analysis of chromosome structure by microscopic examination, usually when the chromosomes are condensed during metaphase of mitosis. Giemsa banded karyotypes can reveal abnormal numbers of chromosomes or large structural changes, such as translocations, deletions, or duplications. The most common cytogenetic abnormality, trisomy 21, or Down syndrome, is associated with many qualitative immune defects, but is almost always diagnosed before immune dysfunction is recognized because of its many obvious physical stigmata. While chromosomal abnormalities should be suspected when immune dysfunction is accompanied by additional congenital anomalies, there are instances in which a cytogenetic abnormality has only an immune phenotype, such as in males with X-linked lymphoproliferative disease due to deletions within Xq25 (Chapter 32). Pursuit of cytogenetic abnormalities has led directly to the identification of at least one immunodeficiency gene, *CYBB*, in X-linked CGD (Orkin, 1989); a small minority of CGD patients have total *CYBB* deletions that can involve adjacent genes as well and cause a phenotype of CGD plus other abnormalities (Chapter 37). Balanced translocations can be clinically silent except for the disruption of particular genes at the chromosomal breakpoints. However, family history of multiple miscarriages should prompt cytogenetic investigation because offspring undergoing fetal demise may have received an unbalanced parental chromosomal complement. Thus, while the yield of karyotype analysis may be rather low in immunodeficiencies, this simple test is at times extraordinarily helpful in uncovering a genetic basis for a puzzling clinical syndrome and pinpointing the region of the genome involved.

The power of cytogenetics has been greatly extended by fluorescent in situ hybridization (FISH). In this technique, a cloned unique human DNA fragment is tagged with a fluorescent label and allowed to hybridize to its corresponding sequence within chromosomes spread on a microscope slide. Viewed with a fluorescence microscope, the two homologous chromosomes are marked with the fluorescent DNA probe. FISH can be used to localize and diagnose certain immune diseases. For example, DiGeorge syndrome (thymic hypoplasia, hypoparathyroidism, and conotruncal heart malformations) is associated with interstitial deletions on one copy of chromosome 22q11 (Chapter 33). Although some patients have a deletion large enough to be detected by simple karyotype analysis, FISH with fluorescent probes from 22q11 reveals only one signal in 90% of DiGeorge syndrome patients (Color Plate 33.II).

DNA- and RNA-Based Techniques

Molecular methods for mutation diagnosis are being applied to hundreds of genetic conditions today, and many more genetic tests will be performed in the future. Certain generalizations distinguish mutation detection in immunodeficiency disease genes from that in many other well-studied genetic disorders. In some disorders, such as sickle cell disease, a single mutation predominates (Kan, 1992). Even in the cystic fibrosis disease gene *CFTR*, about two-thirds of mutated chromosomes in Caucasians have the same Δ508 mutation (Zielenski and Tsui, 1995), and testing for a panel of 25 mutations can effectively diagnose the great majority of cases (Richards et al., 2002). In contrast, immunodeficiency gene mutations tend to be extremely diverse, with half or more of the mutations unique to a single family. Unlike the dystrophin gene, which is defective in Duchene muscular dystrophy and in which large deletions and duplications account for 66% of mutations (Worton, 1992), by far the most common immunodeficiency gene mutations are small changes on the order of one to a few nucleotides, occurring in both coding sequences and splice regions. An important new class of mutations described in human neurologic and muscular diseases is the expansion of triplet repeats either in coding regions or in regions near a gene that are subject to silencing by methylation (Everett and Wood, 2004). However, to date no immunodeficiency-causing gene mutation of this type has been described.

In other respects, gene mutations that cause inherited immune disorders are similar to those found in other genetic diseases (discussed in Chapter 2). These include a high proportion, approximately one-third, of newly arising mutations for X-linked disorders (Haldane, 1935). As previously noted for the hemoglobin locus, factor IX locus, and many other genes (Cooper and Krawczak, 1995), the occurrence of C-to-T mutations at CpG

dinucleotides in immunodeficiency genes is greatly increased above the number that would be expected if all nucleotide changes were completely random.

Linkage to PCR-Based Polymorphic Markers

Linkage analysis is discussed in some detail in Chapter 2. For immunodeficiency diseases mapped to a unique genomic region but not yet identified, linkage analysis can define which chromosome segments in a family carry mutated disease gene alleles, provided there are both affected and unaffected relatives available for testing. Linkage analysis can also be useful when the gene that is defective in a family is known but the specific mutation has not been determined. Linkage diagnosis can be used for carrier testing and for prenatal diagnosis. One should select tightly linked markers that flank the disease locus and are polymorphic in the required members of the family being tested. The alleles at each flanking marker locus are identified for both disease-bearing and normal chromosomes in the parents of the individual at risk. Then the alleles of the person at risk are determined. If the flanking alleles on both sides of the disease locus match parental alleles from an unaffected chromosome, the person is likely to have inherited the entire block of DNA including the normal copy of the disease gene. Similarly, flanking alleles co-inherited from a disease-bearing chromosome predict that a mutated copy of the disease gene has been inherited. The likelihood that such predictions are correct depends on the genetic distance between the markers (see Chapter 2). However, if a genetic crossover has occurred between the flanking markers, the linkage test is uninformative and no prediction can be made.

The first linkage markers to be used were restriction fragment length polymorphisms (RFLPs), nucleotide variations resulting in the presence or absence of a restriction enzyme site in a defined genomic DNA segment (Botstein et al., 1980; Drayna and White, 1985). RFLPs are defined by the variable presence of restriction sites in segments of DNA from different individuals; digestion with the relevant restriction endonuclease will demonstrate allelic variants with either shorter or longer DNA fragment sizes depending on whether the polymorphic restriction site is present or absent. Fragment lengths are assayed by Southern blotting (see below), or other means of visualization.

The discovery of the polymerase chain reaction (PCR) revolutionized linkage analysis. PCR depends on designing short synthetic oligonucleotides flanking a DNA segment to be amplified. These oligonucleotides, called *primers*, are added in excess to genomic DNA along with free nucleotides, magnesium salts, pH buffer, and a heat-stable DNA polymerase enzyme, such as *Taq* polymerase. First, the reaction mixture is denatured by heating to 95°C so that the DNA helices unwind and the DNA becomes single stranded. Next, the mixture is cooled to a moderate temperature, typically between 50° and 65°C, enabling the oligonucleotides to bind by complementary base pairing to the particular regions of template DNA that they exactly match. Finally, warming the mixture to 72°C allows the polymerase to synthesize new DNA by using the oligonucleotides as primers and adding free nucleotides to form new complementary strands. Each repetition of this sequence of denaturation, annealing, and extension produces a doubling of each template strand. This succession of temperatures constitutes one cycle of PCR. In each successive cycle the segment of DNA between the primers is exponentially amplified. Eventually the amount of product becomes large enough to be detected by either hybridization or direct visualization after gel electrophoresis and staining. More details about PCR protocols can be found in textbooks such as the one by Erlich (1992).

Segments of DNA that are polymorphic can be readily detected by PCR. If the primers flank a polymorphic restriction site, the product can be digested to assign the restriction site allele. Another type of polymorphism is called a microsatellite or short tandem repeat polymorphism (STRP). The most common repeated unit, occurring on average once every 50,000 nucleotides throughout the genome, is CA on one DNA strand, and TG on the opposite strand (Litt and Luty, 1989; Weber and May, 1989). Other repeats of units of two to five nucleotides also occur frequently. Very often, assorted numbers of repeated units are found in chromosomes from different individuals, and the number of repeats represents a stable polymorphism that is inherited from parents to offspring. PCR amplification of the DNA segment containing a series of simple repeated units followed by size separation by gel electrophoresis reveals the length differences between the polymorphic alleles. Each lane of the gel on the left of Figure 44.1 shows DNA from an unrelated male amplified with appropriate primers surrounding the CA repeat present at the STRP marker DXS441 in Xq13 very close to the X-linked SCID locus (Ram et al., 1992). Alleles of six distinct sizes are seen, indicating that the number of CA units can vary considerably between individual X chromosomes. The right side of Figure 44.1 shows a family linkage study using another X chromosome STRP, GATA182e04 in Xq28, for which the repeated unit is the tetranucleotide GATA. The maternal allele A1, with the smaller number of repeat units, has been inherited by two of her sons, while four other sons and her daughter have inherited her A2 allele. The daugher has also interited the A1 allele from the paternal X chromosome.

STRPs have several advantages over RFLPs, reflecting the power of PCR as a tool for molecular genetic analysis. Foremost is the very high frequency of these polymorphisms throughout the genome. For family linkage studies, useful STRPs can be found that flank any known immunodeficiency gene. STRPs are also very quickly and easily assayed by PCR, and high-throughput genotyping of STRPs makes possible genome-wide linkage scans to identify the locus of disease genes. Miniscule amounts of input DNA template can be successfully amplified, and DNA can be rescued for PCR from dried blood cards or formalin-fixed tissues and histologic slides, even if an affected patient has died without having had samples preserved specifically for molecular analysis. Finally, the multiplicity of commonly observed alleles means that it is very likely that a child's

alleles can be unambiguously traced to one or the other parent; or, in mathematical terms, the information content at each locus is high.

Even more common than STRPs are single nucleotide polymorphisms, or SNPs, which occur at a rate of around 1 per 1000 nucleotides of genomic DNA sequence. Unlike highly informative STRPs, SNPs have only two alleles, but the huge numbers of SNPs can make up for this inconvenience; an initial map of 1.42 million SNPs in the human genome was assembled in 2001 (Sachidanandam et al., 2001), and far more are now available in the database dbSNP at the National Center for Biotechnology Information (NCBI), at http://www.ncbi.nlm.nih.gov. Clusters of neighboring SNPs tend to be inherited together in haplotype blocks, sizable regions that have been maintained with little crossing over since ancestral origins of humans (Gabriel et al., 2002; The International HapMap Consortium, 2005). SNP tags will be able to identify haplotype blocks in humans of diverse ancestral origins, facilitating linkage analysis by automated technology. Furthermore, SNPs with functional importance that alter the expression or activity of gene products promise to shed light on genetic risks for diverse health outcomes and make possible tailoring of medical treatment to the genetic makeup of each individual.

Southern Blotting, Evaluation of Genomic DNA

Southern blotting, named for its inventor (Southern, 1975), is the prototypic technique for specific gene detection. A cloned segment of DNA is labeled by incorporation of radioactive nucleotides containing ^{32}P and used as a probe to hybridize to a complex mixture of DNA, such as genomic DNA prepared from the cells of a particular person. Now considered too labor-intensive for most clinical applications, this was the method historically used for evaluation of RFLP markers and changes in genomic DNA before the development of PCR. First the DNA to be probed is digested with a restriction enzyme, producing fragments varying in size. Because of the complexity of mammalian DNA, these fragments appear to form a continuous smear when they are separated by size using the technique of agarose gel electrophoresis. The size-separated lanes of DNA are denatured into single strands and transferred from the gel to a solid membrane where they are permanently stuck. Single-stranded probe DNA is then incubated with the filter under conditions that favor annealing of DNA complementary sequences. After washing off excess labeled probe, the only probe left sticking to the filter is located in

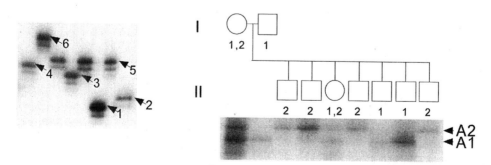

Figure 44.1. Short tandem repeat polymorphism (STRP). Left: DNA from eight unrelated males amplified with primers defining STRP locus DXS441 in Xq13 (Ram et al., 1992). Six alleles, numbered according to their increasing numbers of CA repeat units, were amplified using flank-ing PCR primers. Darker bands are the primary signal; lighter "shadow" bands seen below each primary band are typical artifacts in CA repeat STRPs. Right: DNA from family members in the illustrated pedigree, amplified with primers defining the STRP GATA182e04 at Xq28.

a band corresponding to the size of the genomic DNA fragment with the same nucleotide sequence as the probe (Sambrook et al., 1989; Ausubel et al., 1994).

Southern blotting can detect disease-causing mutations that involve either large DNA deletions or rearrangements in the disease gene of an affected individual; it can also detect single nucleotide changes that alter the restriction enzyme pattern produced. In such circumstances, a probe from the disease gene will fail to detect in affected patient DNA one or more bands seen in unaffected controls; alternatively, or in addition, the probe may hybridize to DNA fragments of unexpected size. Southern blot alterations have often provided the first clue that a candidate gene in fact harbors deleterious mutations in individuals affected with inherited immunodeficiencies or other genetic disorders. For example, they were used to find some of the first *BTK* mutations in patients with X-linked agammaglobulinemia (XLA) (Vetrie et al., 1993).

Because the great majority of immunodeficiency gene mutations are small changes at the level of one to a few nucleotides, Southern blot analysis is insensitive for finding suspected mutations in new patients. Moreover, finding altered Southern blot band patterns does not readily indicate the location or specific nature of a mutation. However, in families with a previously documented disease-associated Southern blot abnormality, this test can be successfully applied for carrier and prenatal diagnosis in relatives at risk of having inherited the same defect.

Northern Blotting and Reverse Transcription-PCR

Many mutations within or adjacent to exons of genes affect the quantity or size of the mRNA produced. These changes can be detected by Northern blot analysis, which is carried out in a manner similar to that of Southern blots (Sambrook et al., 1989; Ausubel et al., 1994). RNA is isolated from cells and electrophoresed through a gel so that all mRNA species are ordered by size. After transferring all the RNA to a membrane and allowing a labeled nucleic acid probe to hybridize to it, the mRNA with the specific nucleotide sequence of interest can be detected. Mutations can produce differences in the expected size or amount of RNA detected by Northern analysis.

As with DNA analysis, PCR has greatly enhanced our ability to analyze RNA through a process called reverse transcriptase PCR (RT-PCR). First, a complementary DNA strand (cDNA) is created by incubating mRNA with the enzyme reverse transcriptase and a DNA oligonucleotide primer. Even the nanogram quantities of RNA that can be purified from small numbers of cells can yield enough cDNA for successful amplification by PCR. Amplified cDNA can be sequenced, sized by gel electrophoresis, and even quantitated to reflect the amount of cellular mRNA originally present (provided carefully monitored conditions and appropriate controls are used).

Mutations that disrupt the 3' and 5' splice motifs prevent normal processing of newly made mRNA. These mutations are generally associated with low or undetectable levels of correctly spliced mRNA in the cytoplasm of cells. However, some aberrantly spliced mRNA species may be detected, such as molecules that fail to undergo intron removal, or that skip one or more exons adjacent to the mutation. Coding sequence missense or frameshift mutations that generate termination signals within exons in the 5' portions of genes also usually cause destabilization of mRNA (known as nonsense-mediated decay) or exon skipping.

Studies of mRNA are important in assessing the actual consequences of a mutation in DNA sequence. Nonetheless, investigation of mRNA quantity or sequence is often complex and therefore not well suited to clinical diagnostic testing for patients and relatives in families with immunodeficiency.

X Chromosome Inactivation Pattern in Potential Female Carriers

The high frequency of immunodeficiencies linked to the X chromosome and the special property of inactivation of one of the two X chromosome in females have been exploited for identification of carriers of immunodeficiency diseases (Table 44.1). A unique feature of the sex chromosomes is that males have one X and one Y, whereas females have two X chromosomes. As first hypothesized by Mary Lyon (1966), the problem of expression of double doses of genes from the female's X chromosomes is solved in mammals by inactivation of one X chromosome in all somatic tissues.

A random inactivation of either the maternally or the paternally derived X chromosome occurs before differentiation of specialized tissues in the early female embryo (but, interestingly, not in the placenta, where the paternal X is preferentially inactivated). The random X inactivation imprint of each embryonic cell is maintained throughout subsequent cellular proliferation and differentiation, so that the contribution of maternal and paternal active X chromosomes in all tissues statistically follows a normal distribution. Thus the blood cells of normal women show on average 50% maternal and 50% paternal active X chromosomes. In individual women, however, this ratio can vary substantially. The variance of the distribution (the broadness of the distribution curve) of X chromosome inactivation can be used to estimate the number of primordial embryonic cells that eventually develop into blood cells. For example, if only one cell in the embryo was fated to be the precursor of all blood cells, that one X chromosome would be active in all the blood cells. Estimates using several independent techniques predict a precursor pool size of around 10–20 embryonic cells that eventually become hematopoietic progenitor cells. As a result, some normal women by chance have X inactivation ratios quite different from 50:50 (Puck et al., 1992).

Carriers of certain X-linked immunodeficiencies have negative selection superimposed on the underlying inactivation pattern in the hematopoietic cells lineages affected by the gene defect they carry. If one of the X chromosomes bears a mutation in a gene that confers a survival advantage upon cells of a particular lineage, then cells of that lineage will have skewed X inactivation. As indicated in Table 44.1, this is the case for B cells of carriers of XLA (Fearon et al., 1987; Conley and Puck, 1988; Allen et al., 1994); T, B, and natural killer (NK) cells of carriers of X-linked SCID (Puck et al., 1987; Conley et al., 1988; Wengler et al., 1993); and all hematopoietic cells of carriers of Wiskott-Aldrich syndrome (WAS) (Prchal et al., 1980; Puck et al., 1990b). In contrast, there is no selective pressure on X inactivation in carriers of X-linked CGD. Thus, as discussed under immunologic assays for CGD above, two populations of granulocytes can be detected in female carriers—one with the mutated and one with the normal copy of the disease gene *CYBB*. In a rare circumstance of extreme, constitutional unbalanced X inactivation, a female carrier of a *CYBB* mutation whose normal X was inactive was diagnosed with severe CGD (Anderson-Cohen et al., 2003).

To assay X inactivation one must both distinguish the two X chromosomes from another and determine whether the chromosomes are active. This was first done by isolating the active X chromosomes of several cells from a female subject in a panel of

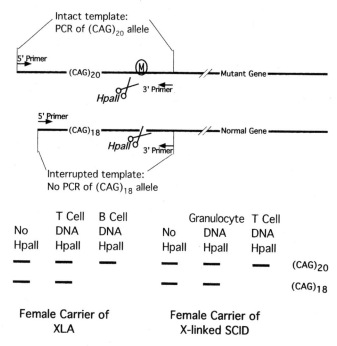

T Cell DNA HpaII   B Cell DNA HpaII   Granulocyte DNA HpaII   T Cell DNA HpaII

Figure 44.2. X inactivation testing for female carriers of selected X-linked immunodeficiencies. Top: Differential methylation of the HpaII recognition sequence near the $(CAG)_n$ polymorphism in the androgen receptor gene (*AR*). The upper chromosome with a $(CAG)_{20}$ allele bears the mutant immune disease gene and is inactive and therefore methylated (M). The lower X chromosome with $(CAG)_{18}$ has a normal copy of the disease gene and is active, unmethylated, and susceptible to cutting by the methylation-sensitive enzyme HpaII. After exposure of DNA from the test cell lineage to HpaII, only the template from the mutation-bearing X chromosome is intact and able to undergo amplification with *AR* 5′ and 3′ PCR primers. Bottom: Patterns of allele amplification visualized after separation of the two alleles by gel electrophoresis. In the test cell lineages of female carriers, only the inactive, mutation-bearing *AR* allele has been amplified by PCR. For these examples, women with *AR* alleles with $(CAG)_{18}$ and $(CAG)_{20}$ repeats are illustrated, but any other heterozygous allele combinations are assayed in the same manner.

human–rodent hybrid cell lines and using RFLPs, and later STRP polymorphisms and PCR, to count how many times each X chromosome was the active one (Puck et al., 1987). A more efficient method is to use a PCR-based STRP that includes cytosine (C) nucleotides that are methylated only on the inactive X (Fig. 44.2). The androgen receptor (*AR*) gene is an X-linked gene with a variable number of CAG glutamine codons in its first exon; 90% of women have two different lengths of CAG repeats on their two X chromosomes and can therefore be tested by this assay. A nearby HpaII restriction site has a C that is methylated and therefore not subject to digestion by HpaII when present on an inactive X chromosome. Primers have been designed to surround both the repeat and the methylation-sensitive restriction sites, as shown at the top of Figure 42.2 (Allen et al., 1994). In the most informative utilization of this test, DNA is isolated from a purified control cell lineage and test cell lineage of a suspected female carrier. As shown in the lower part of Figure 42.2, appropriate control and test lineages for XLA would be T cells (not dependent on Btk expression for their development and survival) and B cells, respectively. Similarly, for X-linked SCID, control and test lineages could be granulocytes (not dependent on the cytokine receptor common γ chain) and T cells. Restriction enzyme

digestion with the methylation-sensitive enzyme HpaII is followed by PCR and allele separation by gel electrophoresis. PCR of DNA from an affected cell lineage from a carrier will amplify only the allele from her inactive X chromosome, diagrammed in the lower portion of Figure 42.2. Samples not exposed to HpaII, samples from uninvolved cell lineages, and samples from all cell lineages of noncarriers will show PCR amplification of alleles from both X chromosomes.

X inactivation testing was an invaluable research tool for mapping SCIDX1, WAS, and XLA. Moreover, discovery of which hematopoietic lineages are targeted by each gene defect was accomplished before the disease genes were found by observing which lineages had skewed X inactivation in obligate carriers. Carrier diagnosis by X inactivation analysis can be clinically useful when a specific mutation, or even genotype (autosomal vs. X-linked recessive), is not known, such as in an affected male with no positive family history. Demonstration of maternal lineage–specific skewed X inactivation in a clinical setting of SCID, for example, has been used to prove that the inheritance pattern was X-linked, thus making possible genetic counseling and prenatal testing (Puck et al., 1990a). The technique has similarly been applied in XLA, comparing X inactivation of isolated B cells, the potentially affected lineage, to that of T cells in women at risk for being carriers (Allen et al., 1994). In WAS, there is no hematopoietic control lineage because of the selective disadvantage of all cells failing to express the normal gene product WASP. This is an important limitation of the test, because a small percentage of women who do not carry any X-linked immune disease gene have markedly unbalanced X inactivation ratios simply by chance or for other underlying reasons involving the X inactivation process itself (Naumova et al., 1996; Puck and Willard, 1998).

As alluded to in the context of CGD above, females can be encountered who demonstrate moderate or even severe phenotypes of X-linked genetic disorders because they have one mutated copy of a disease gene on an X chromosome that is active in most of their cells. X inactivation should be kept in mind when evaluating females affected with CGD, combined immunodeficiency, features of WAS, or other phenotypes usually seen in males with X-linked hemizygous gene defects. Specific mutation detection is a more accurate diagnostic approach than X inactivation analysis.

Mutation Detection

All of the newer mutation detection techniques begin with PCR amplification of genomic DNA or cDNA of individuals affected with immunodeficiencies or at-risk relatives. Cloning of these DNA segments into plasmids makes possible the preparation of larger amounts of DNA template for analysis and also separates DNA derived from each chromosomal allele of an individual, results of which can be potentially important for diagnosis of individuals with compound heterozygous mutations causing autosomal recessive disease as well as individuals with dominant disorders and carriers. However, direct analysis without cloning is rapid and accurate in many applications. Because even a single molecule of DNA can be amplified in the proper conditions, PCR is extremely sensitive to contamination. Strict attention to laboratory design and sample flow as well as extensive monitoring with positive and negative controls are needed to avoid contamination of test samples with cloned or already amplified DNA or even with normal DNA from the hands of laboratory workers. Mutation screening techniques are designed for detection of

P   M   C

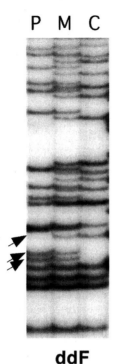

ddF

Figure 44.3. Dideoxyfingerprinting (ddF). Shown are dideoxy-T sequencing reactions of exon 5 of *IL2RG* in DNA from an X-linked SCID patient (P), his carrier mother (M), and an unrelated control (C). Multiple bands with altered mobility are seen in the patient's lane, starting with two extra bands and a missing band, marked by arrows. The band pattern in the lane of the heterozygous carrier mother is a composite of the patient's hemizygous mutated pattern and the control pattern.

single nucleotide changes or small insertions and deletions, the most commonly encountered mutations in immunodeficiency diseases. Elucidation of large disruptions, such as deletions or duplications of several kilobases of DNA, may require Southern blots or other methods.

The simplest technique for mutation screening is single-strand conformation polymorphism (SSCP) (Orita et al., 1989; Hyashi and Yandell, 1993; Sheffield et al., 1993; Puck et al., 1997a). In this method, amplified DNA segments of up to 300 nucleotides in length are denatured by heating and then quickly chilled so that they assume single-stranded conformation depending on their primary nucleotide sequence. The single-stranded segments are separated on nondenaturing acrylamide gels to preserve the secondary structure. Even single base changes can alter the mobility of one or both of the single strands. However, this method fails to detect about 10% of mutations, particularly those close to the primers at either end of the segment.

An improvement in sensitivity of mutation detection to nearly 100% can be achieved by using a dideoxy nucleotide mixture from a dideoxy terminator sequencing reaction instead of PCR of an entire fragment to make single strands of DNA for conformation testing. This method is called *dideoxy fingerprinting* (ddF) (Sarkar et al., 1992; Puck et al., 1997a). Increasing lengths of DNA from under 50 bases to 300 bases or more show more conformations than only a full-length fragment as in SSCP. The lanes of a ddF autoradiogram viewed from bottom to top, as in Figure 44.3, show abnormal bands from the level in the sequence ladder at which a mutation is introduced (bottom arrow); above this level, multiple band shifts are apparent in a hemizygous mutated X-linked SCID (XSCID) patient (P, left lane) compared to the control (C, right lane). The middle lane shows the DNA from the patient's heterozygous mother (M), revealing a composite of both sets of bands from her mutated and wild-type *IL2RG* alleles. In a study of 87 unrelated patients with XSCID, *IL2RG* mutations were detected in all cases by ddF (Puck et al., 1997b).

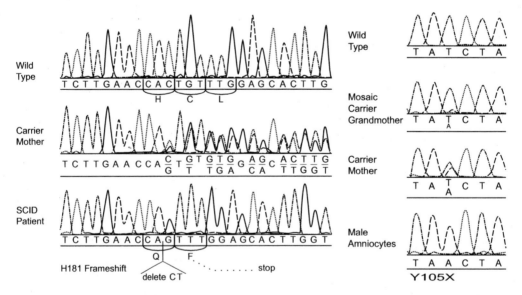

Figure 44.4. Fluorescence-based sequence determination. Left: Wild type (upper), carrier (middle), and X-linked SCID patient (lower) sequences from exon 3 of the *IL2RG* gene. The patient's deletion of two nucleotides in codon 181, normally specifying histidine (H), results in a frameshift specifying glutamine (Q) followed by several further missense codons and a premature termination. The mother's genomic sequence is a composite of wild type and mutant, reflecting the two *IL2RG* alleles on her two X chromosomes. Right: *IL2RG* gene sequence in exon 3 showing wild type and three generations of a kindred with XSCID. The second tracing shows minor mosaicism in the grandmother for the mutant TAA allele (encoding a termination signal instead of the wild-type tyrosine [Y] residue). Her daughter, the mother of the patient, is a carrier of this mutation with roughly equal wild-type and mutant signals, while her male fetus is hemizygous for the mutant allele.

Determination of the actual nucleotide sequence of mutant DNA is the gold standard for mutation detection. Regardless of whether prescreening with SSCP or ddF is used, sequence determination must be carried out to learn the exact nature of the mutational event. Nucleotide changes detected by any DNA-based evaluation must be interpreted in light of expression studies and functional data before concluding that they are pathogenic mutations.

Radioactive isotopes were initially used for sequencing, but fluorescent technologies now give superior length and quality of sequences from PCR-amplified genomic DNA. The left side of Figure 44.4 shows detection by fluorescent sequencing of a two-base deletion in *IL2RG*. The wild-type sequence and reading frame (upper tracing) and frame-shifted, deleted sequence of a patient with XSCID (lower tracing) can be seen superimposed in the central tracing from the patient's heterozygous mother. Sequence analysis of another XSCID kindred, shown in Figure 44.4 on the right, reveals the origin of the premature termination mutation in exon 3, V105X. The tracing of blood-derived DNA from the grandmother, whose son died of infections in infancy, shows only a minor admixture of an A base at the position that is a T in the wild type, indicating somatic mosaicism for this mutation in blood cells. The grandmother must also have had the new mutation in some of her egg cells, accounting for her affected son (not shown) and daughter, whose tracing in Figure 44.4 with equal amounts of mutant T and wild-type A is diagnostic of a heterozygous carrier state. Amniocyte DNA from the male fetus of this carrier demonstrates presence of the mutant allele, in which a TAT tyrosine codon has become an immediate TAA termination codon. This fetus was therefore predicted to be affected with XSCID.

In the future, detection of specific gene mutations may be further automated. Detection of mutations in cancer susceptibility genes, such as *BRCA1*, have used hybridization of PCR enriched DNA to chips containing microarrays of partially overlapping oligonucleotides that span the gene's normal coding sequence and include specific mutated oligonucleotides for known mutations (Hacia et al., 1996).

Genetic Counseling

Genetic testing has received increasing public attention because of the rapidly growing number of tests that can be performed for gene mutations associated with a wide variety of conditions. Testing is becoming publicly available in some cases before research has established its true ability to predict future development of a disease, such as breast cancer (Struewing et al., 1997). Our society is in the process of adjusting to increasing genetic information, but many issues, such as population screening, testing of minor children, protection of confidentiality, and insurability of persons carrying genetic mutations, remain to be resolved (Clarke et al., 1994; American Society of Human Genetics and American College of Medical Genetics Boards of Directors, 1995; Rowley et al., 1997). Unlike most other forms of medical evaluation, molecular genetic testing has implications not just for the proband but also for all of his or her relatives who share the same DNA. For all of these reasons, genetic counseling should precede genetic testing. Counseling should preferably be done by a geneticist or genetic counselor rather than the medical team primarily involved with treating an affected child who may be critically ill. A genetic diagnosis that becomes available while a child is in the hospital should be reviewed with the family at a later time when the information can be processed more fully, questions can be answered, and implications for each family member sorted out.

Molecular diagnostic testing is usually undertaken to establish a diagnosis in an affected individual. Parents of an affected child are likely to be concerned about the risk of recurrence in a future pregnancy. For autosomal recessive diseases it is assumed that the parents are both carriers and the recurrence rate is one in four for pregnancies of either sex. For X-linked diseases in which the mother of an affected child is demonstrated to be a carrier, there is a 50% chance that each subsequent male pregnancy will be affected and a 50% chance that each female pregnancy will carry the mutation but not be affected with immunodeficiency.

Risks for being affected with the disease in question or for having affected children of one's own can be calculated for other family members. For example, a sibling of a proband affected with an autosomal recessive disease may be a carrier, but unless his or her mate is also a carrier of a mutation in the same gene (which is very unlikely unless the members of the couple are related to each other), the risk of having affected offspring is exceedingly low. On the other hand, sisters of males with X-linked diseases are at 50% risk of being carriers, in which case their male offspring will be at risk of being affected with the disease.

Now that many males with X-linked immunodeficiency diseases have been successfully treated and are reaching adulthood, it is important to help them understand that their reproductive risks have not changed, even if their disease has been permanently treated, such as by bone marrow transplantation. Affected males will pass on their mutation-bearing X chromosome to all of their daughters, who will be carriers; however, none of their sons will be affected because they will inherit the Y chromosome, and not the X chromosome, from their father.

Prenatal testing is possible for a large number of immunodeficiencies, and the chapters in Part II of this volume outline specific considerations for prenatal evaluation of each disorder. However, bringing the findings and techniques of research laboratories into a clinical setting has lagged. Because of high costs and low numbers of DNA-based diagnostic tests for each immunodeficiency gene, many tests have not yet been offered by clinical laboratories certified by the Clinical Laboratory Improvement Amendments of 1988 (CLIA) Act (Regulations, 1992). Fetal cells can be sampled by chorionic villus biopsy as early as the ninth week of pregnancy, or amniotic fluid can be obtained some weeks later as a source of fetal DNA for molecular testing. Fetal blood sampling between 16 and 20 weeks of pregnancy has also been used to evaluate the number and function of leukocytes in pregnancies at risk for well-defined abnormalities.

Preimplantation diagnosis is another procedure for families in which the specific mutation(s) for the pregnancy at risk are known. This was first performed successfully in humans in the setting of cystic fibrosis in which the parents were both carriers of the common Δ F508 mutation in the *CFTR* gene (Ao et al., 1996). In vitro fertilization was carried out with superovulated eggs and sperm from the parents, embryos were grown to the eight-cell stage, and a single cell from each embryo was removed and genotyped by PCR. Embryos with an unaffected genotype were reimplanted into the mother. Of 22 couples in one early study, 5 had singleton pregnancies carried to term with the birth of healthy, unaffected infants.

Only limited information is available to indicate how parents with an at-risk pregnancy weigh the difficult choices that confront them. When a fetus is diagnosed as affected, pregnancy may be terminated, but neonatal and even prenatal treatment options are increasingly available. The parents' perceptions of the burden of the disease are undoubtedly distinct for each immunodeficiency and are colored by the particular experience each person has shared with his or her affected relatives. A series of families followed with pregnancies at risk for XSCID indicated that most couples wanted to have prenatal testing, but few affected pregnancies were terminated (Puck et al., 1997a). In this disease, the improving outlook over the past two decades of bone marrow transplantation therapy has given families hope. Couples anticipating delivery of affected infants took advantage of the information gained through counseling and prenatal testing to learn about options for treatments. Pediatric centers performing bone marrow transplantation for immunodeficiency were contacted and financial and care arrangements were made. In some cases, the prenatal sample was HLA typed to identify potential matched bone marrow donors, either among the parents' healthy children or in an unrelated donor registry. One family chose an experimental in utero bone marrow transplant; this treatment may become successful with a variety of immune disorders (Flake et al., 1996; Flake and Zanjani, 1997).

A further development is the harvesting of cord blood at delivery as a source of autologous hematopoietic stem cells in which the gene defect could be corrected by gene therapy. Retroviral gene transfer has proven effective for XSCID and ADA-deficient SCID (Chapter 48). However, the development of leukemia due to retroviral insertional mutagenesis in XSCID patients receiving this treatment has delayed the acceptance of gene therapy for this form of SCID until safety can be improved.

Population-Based Newborn Screening for Immunodeficiencies

Primary immunodeficiencies are underdiagnosed and frequently diagnosed late because of their low incidence and insufficient awareness on the part of physicians and the public. Screening of newborns for a variety of treatable genetic conditions has been a successful public health measure to achieve early recognition and prompt intervention (Wilson and Jungner, 1968; Khoury et al., 2003). Criteria for evaluating whether newborn screening is indicated for a given disease include the following: the disease is serious and not evident by physical examination in the nursery; the disease is treatable; early treatment offers a better outcome; and incidence and test availability make screening cost-effective. Several inherited immunodeficiencies could potentially meet these criteria. For example, failure to recognize SCID leads to devastating or even fatal infections. Although the true incidence is not known, SCID is estimated to occur in 1 in 50,000 to 1 in 100,000 births, within the range of some metabolic disorders currently widely included in state newborn screening panels (Chan and Puck, 2005). Development of an inexpensive, sensitive screening test that could be performed on the dried blood filters already collected from all infants would be required. One test under consideration for SCID is quantitation by PCR of the presence of T cell receptor excision circles (TRECs), formed in maturing thymocytes as a byproduct of T cell receptor rearrangement (Douek et al., 1998). In contrast to dried blood spots of healthy infants, the original blood spots collected from infants subsequently diagnosed with SCID were negative for TRECs in a pilot study, as were blood spots made from SCID infants at the time of their diagnosis (Chan and Puck, 2005).

References

Allen RC, Nachtman, RG, Rosenblatt HM, Belmont JW. Application of carrier testing to genetic counseling for X-linked agammaglobulinemia. Am J Hum Genet 54:25–35, 1994.

American Society of Human Genetics Board of Directors and The American College of Medical Genetics Board of Directors. ASHG/ACMG report: points to consider: ethical legal and psychosocial implications of genetic testing in children and adolescents. Am J Hum Genet 57:1233–1241, 1995.

Anderson-Cohen M, Holland SM, Kuhns DB, Fleisher TA, Ding L, Brenner S, Malech HL, Roesler J. Severe phenotype of chronic granulomatous disease presenting in a female with a de novo mutation in gp91-phox and a nonfamilial, extremely skewed X chromosome inactivation. Clin Immunol 109:308–317, 2003.

Ao A, Handyside A, Winston RM. Preimplantation genetic diagnosis of cystic fibrosis (δ F508). Eur J Obstet Gynecol Reprod Biol 65:7–10, 1996.

Ausubel FM, Brent R, Kingston RE, Moore DD, Seidman JG, Smith JA, Struhl K, eds. Current Protocols in Molecular Biology. New York: John Wiley and Sons, 1994.

Beutler E, Blume KG, Kaplan JC, Lohr GW, Ramot B, Valentine WN. International committee for standardization in haematology: recommended screening test for glucose-6-phosphate dehydrogenase (G6PD) deficiency. Br J Haematol 43:465, 1979.

Botstein D, White RL, Skolnick M, Davis RW. Construction of a genetic linkage map in man using restriction fragment length polymorphisms. Am J Hum Genet 32:314–331, 1980.

Centers for Disease Control. Regulations for implementing the Clinical Laboratory Improvement Amendments of 1988: a summary. MMWR 41(RR-2), 1992. Available online at http://www.cdc.gov/mmwr/preview/mmwrhtml/00016177.htm

Chan K, Puck JM. Development of population-based newborn screening for severe combined immunodeficiency. J Allergy Clin Immunol 115:391–398, 2005.

Clarke A (Chair) and Members of the working party of the Clinical Genetics Society (UK). The genetic testing of children. J Med Genet 31:785–797, 1994.

Conley ME, Larche M, Bonagura VR, Lawton AR, Buckley RH, et al. Hyper IgM syndrome associated with defective CD40-mediated B cell activation. J Clin Invest 94:1404–1409, 1994.

Conley ME, Lavoie A, Briggs C, Guerra C, Puck JM. Non-random X chromosome inactivation in B cells from carriers of X-linked severe combined immunodeficiency. Proc Natl Acad Sci USA 85:3090–3094, 1988.

Conley ME, Puck JM. Carrier detection in typical and atypical X-linked agammaglobulinemia. J Pediatr 112:688–694, 1988.

Cooper DN, Krawczak M. Human Gene Mutation. Oxford: Bios Scientific Publishers, 1995.

Douek DC, McFarland RD, Keiser PH, Gage EA, Massey JM, Haynes BF, Polis MA, Haase AT, Feinberg MB, Sullivan JL, Jamieson BD, Zack JA, Picker LJ, Koup RA. Changes in thymic function with age and during the treatment of HIV infection. Nature 396:690–695, 1998.

Drayna D, White R. The genetic map of the human X chromosome. Science 230:753–758, 1985.

Erlich HA, ed. PCR Technology. New York: Freeman, 1992.

Everett CM, Wood NW. Trinucleotide repeats and neurodegenerative disease. Brain 127:2385–2405, 2004.

Fearon ER, Winkelstein JA, Civin CI, Pardoll DM, Vogelstein B. Carrier detection in X-linked agammaglobulinemia by analysis of X chromosome inactivation. N Engl J Med 316:427–431, 1987.

Flake AW, Almeida-Porada G, Puck JM, Roncarolo M-G, Evans MI, Johnson MP, Abella EM, Harrison DD, Zanjani ED. Treatment of X-linked SCID by the in utero transplantation of CD34-enriched bone marrow. N Engl J Med 355:1806–1810, 1996.

Flake AW, Zanjani ED. In utero hematopoietic stem cell transplantation. A status report. JAMA 278:932–937, 1997.

Gabriel SB, Schaffner SF, Nguyen H, Moore JM, Roy J, Blumenstiel B, Higgins J, DeFelice M, Lochner A, Faggart M, Liu-Cordero SN, Rotimi C, Adeyemo A, Cooper R, Ward R, Lander ES, Daly MJ, Altshuler D. The structure of haplotype blocks in the human genome. Science 296:2225–2229, 2002.

Hacia JG, Brody LC, Chee MS, Fodor SP, Collins FS. Detection of heterozygous mutations in BRCA1 using high-density oligonucleotide arrays and two-colour fluorescence analysis. Nat Genet 14:441–447, 1996.

Haldane JBS. The rate of spontaneous mutation of a human gene. J Genet 31:317–326, 1935.

Holgate ST. Asthma genetics: waiting to exhale. Nat Genet 15:227–229, 1997.

Hyashi K, Yandell DW. How sensitive is PCR-SSCP? Hum Mut 2:338–346, 1993.

The International HapMap Consortium. A haplotype map of the human genome. Nature 437:1299–1320, 2005.

Jirapongsananuruk O, Malech HL, Kuhns DB, Niemela JE, Brown MR, Anderson-Cohen M, Fleisher TA. Diagnostic paradigm for evaluation of male patients with chronic granulomatous disease, based on the dihydrorhodamine 123 assay. J Allergy Clin Immunol 111:374–370, 2002.

Kan YW. Development of DNA analysis for human diseases. Sickle cell anemia and thalassemia as a paradigm. JAMA 267:1532–1536, 1992.

Khoury MJ, McCabe LL, McCabe ERB. Population screening in the age of genomic medicine. N Engl J Med 348:50–58, 2003.

Lau YL, Levinski RJ. Prenatal diagnosis and carrier detection in primary immunodeficiency disorders. Arch Dis Child 63:758–764, 1988.

Li L, Moshous D, Zhou Y, Wang J, Xie G, Salido E, Hu D, de Villartay J-P, Cowan MJ. A founder mutation in Artemis, an SNM1-like protein, causes SCID in Athabascan-speaking Native Americans. J Immunol 168:6323–6329, 2002.

Litt M, Luty JA. A hypervariable microsatellite revealed by in vitro amplification of a dinucleotide repeat within the cardiac muscle actin gene. Am J Hum Genet 44:397–401, 1989.

Luzzatto L, Mehta A. Glucose 6-phosphate dehydrogenase deficiency. In: Scriver CR, Beaudet AL, Sly WS, Valle D, eds. The Metabolic and Molecular Basis of Inherited Disease, 7th ed. New York: McGraw-Hill, pp. 3367–3398, 1995.

Lyon MF. X-chromosome inactivation in mammals. Adv Teratol 1:25–54, 1966.

Naumova AK, Plenge RM, Bird LM, Leppert M, Morgan K, Willard HF, Sapienza C. Heritability of X chromosome-inactivation phenotype in a large family. Am J Hum Genet 58:1111–1119, 1996.

Orita M, Iwahana H, Kanazawa H, Hayashi K, Sekiya T. Detection of polymorphisms of human DNA by gel electrophoresis as single-strand conformation polymorphisms. Proc Natl Acad Sci USA 86:2766–2270, 1989.

Orkin SH. Molecular genetics of chronic granulomatous disease. Annu Rev Immunol 7:277–307, 1989.

Prchal JT, Carroll AJ, Prchal JF, Crist WM, Skalka HW, Gealy WJ, Harley J, Malluh A. Wiskott-Aldrich syndrome: cellular impairments and their implication for carrier detection. Blood 56:1048–1054, 1980.

Puck JM, Krauss C, Puck SM, Buckley R, Conley ME. Prenatal test for X-linked severe combined immunodeficiency by analysis of maternal X-chromosome inactivation and linkage analysis. N Engl J Med 322:1063–1066, 1990a.

Puck JM, Middelton LA, Pepper AE. Carrier and prenatal diagnosis of X-linked severe combined immunodeficiency: mutation detection methods and utilization. Hum Genet 99:628–633, 1997a.

Puck JM, Nussbaum RL, Conley ME. Carrier detection in X-linked severe combined immunodeficiency based on patterns of X chromosome inactivation. J Clin Invest 79:1395–1400, 1987.

Puck JM, Pepper AE, Henthorn PS, Candotti F, Isakov J, Whitwam T, Conley ME, Fischer RE, Rosenblatt HM, Small TN, Buckley RH. Mutation analysis of IL2RG in human X-linked severe combined immunodeficiency. Blood 89:1968–1977, 1997b.

Puck JM, Siminovitch KA, Poncz M, Greenberg CR, Rottem M, Conley ME. Atypical presentation of Wiskott-Aldrich syndrome: diagnosis in two un-related males based on studies of maternal T cell X-chromosome inactivation. Blood 75:173–178, 1990b.

Puck JM, Stewart CC, Nussbaum, RL. Maximum likelihood analysis of T-cell X chromosome inactivation: normal women vs. carriers of X-linked severe combined immunodeficiency. Am J Hum Genet 50:742–748, 1992.

Puck JM, Willard HF. X inactivation in females with X-linked disease. N Engl J Med 338:325–328, 1998.

Ram KT, Barker DF, Puck JM. Dinucleotide repeat polymorphism at the DXS441 locus. Nucl Acids Res 20:1428, 1992.

Richards CS, Bradley LA, Amos J, Allitto B, Grody WW, Maddalena A, McGinnis MJ, Prior TW, Popovich BW, Watson MS, Palomaki GE. Standards and guidelines for CFTR mutation testing. Genet Med 4:379–391, 2002.

Rowley PT, Loader S, Levenkron JC. Issues in genetic testing: cystic fibrosis carrier population screening: a review. Genet Testing 1:53–59, 1997.

Sachidanandam R, Weissman D, Schmidt SC, Kakol JM, Marth G, Sherry S, Mullikin JC, et al., for International SMP Map Working Group. A map of human genome sequence variation containing 1.42 million single nucleotide polymorphisms. Nature 409:928–933, 2001.

Sambrook J, Fritsch EF, Maniatis T. Molecular Cloning, 2nd ed. Cold Spring Harbor, NY: Cold Spring Harbor Laboratory Press, 1989.

Sarkar G, Yoon H-S, Sommer SS. Dideoxy fingerprinting (ddF): a rapid and efficient screen for the presence of mutations. Genomics 13:441–443, 1992.

Sheffield VC, Beck JS, Kwitek AE, Sandstrom DW, Stone EM. The sensitivity of single-strand conformation polymorphism analysis for the detection of single base substitutions. Genomics 16:325–332, 1993.

Southern EM. Detection of specific sequences among DNA fragments separated by gel electrophoresis. J Mol Biol 98:503–517, 1975.

Struewing JP, Hartge P, Wacholder S, Baker SM, Berlin M, McAdams M, Timmerman MM, Brody LC, Tucker MA. The risk of cancer associated with specific mutations of BRCA1 and BRCA2 among Ashkenazi Jews. N Engl J Med 336:1401–1408, 1997.

Vetrie D, Vorechovsky I, Sideras P, Holland J, Davies A, Flinter F, Hammarström L, Kinnon C, Levinsky R, Bobrow M, Smith CIE, Bentley DR. The gene involved in X-linked agammaglobulinaemia is a member of the src family of protein-tyrosine kinases. Nature 361:226–233, 1993.

Weber JL, May PE. Abundant class of human DNA polymorphisms which can be typed using the polymerase chain reaction. Am J Hum Genet 44:388–396, 1989.

Wengler GS, Allen RC, Parolini, Smith H, Conley ME. Nonrandom X chromosome inactivation in natural killer cells from obligate carriers of X-linked severe combined immunodeficiency. J Immunol 150:700–704, 1993.

Wilson JMG, Jungner G. Principles and practice of screening for disease. Public Health Papers (Geneva: WHO) 34:11–63, 1968.

Worton RG. Duchenne muscular dystrophy: gene and gene product; mechanism of mutation in the gene. J Inherit Metab Dis 15:539–550, 1992.

Zielenski J, Tsui LC. Cystic fibrosis: genotypic and phenotypic variations. Annu Rev Genet 29:777–807, 1995.

45

Immunodeficiency Information Services

JOUNI VÄLIAHO, CRINA SAMARGHITEAN, HILKKA PIIRILÄ,
MARIANNE PUSA, and MAUNO VIHINEN

Primary immunodeficiencies (PIDs) are a group of over 100 mainly rare disorders (Fischer, 2001; Vihinen et al., 2001) affecting the immune system. Although a lot of information is available on the Internet, it is scattered throughout cyberspace, especially data on rare diseases like immunodeficiencies. Therefore, a navigation starting point and knowledge service are very much needed. We have compiled all major data on immunodeficiencies into a server, the Immunodeficiency Resource (IDR), which contains thousands of useful and interesting links in addition to our own pages (Väliaho et al., 2000, 2002). Fact files for each disease function as the core of the IDR.

Over 3700 mutations have been discovered in unrelated families with PIDs (Vihinen et al., 2001) (Table 45.1). During the last few years many genes affected in PIDs have been cloned and analyzed (Chapter 1), and mutations have been identified from a number of patients, giving clues to disease mechanisms. In order to handle the ever-growing amount of information, immunodeficiency mutation databases (IDbases) have been established for a large number of diseases (Lappalainen et al., 1997; Vihinen et al., 2001). These registries make it possible to carry out detailed mutation studies.

We also maintain a directory of laboratories performing genetic and clinical analysis for patients with immunodeficiency. Because immunodeficiencies are such rare disorders, there are not many laboratories carrying out genetic testing for patients. The IDdiagnostics server is directed primarily at physicians and other health care professionals to enable them to find a laboratory where they can order the genetic and/or clinical diagnostics. In addition to providing contact information, the registry aims to promote the appropriate use of genetic services in patient care and increase the general awareness of immunodeficiency disorders, efforts important to fast and reliable diagnosis and proper treatment.

Immunodeficiency Resource

Although the Internet contains billions of pages of information, it is often difficult to find that specific piece of knowledge one is looking for. The IDR is maintained in order to collect and distribute all the essential information and links related to immunodeficiencies (Väliaho et al., 2000, 2002). The IDR aims to provide comprehensive, integrated knowledge on immunodeficiencies in an easily accessible format and offer data for clinical, biochemical, genetic, structural, and computational analysis.

The IDR is a compendium of information on immunodeficiencies available online via the Internet (http://bioinf.uta.fi/idr/) The service contains several introductory texts. From the IDR one can find classification and diagnostic criteria on immunodeficiencies (Conley et al., 1999). There is a plenty of genome-related information available, including that on immunodeficiency-related genes and their locus on the genome, reference sequences on three levels (genome, RNA, and protein), and markers, etc.

Validation of the information on the IDR is of prime importance. The service is maintained with the assistance of regional experts and expert curators and all data are validated. Each disease has its own curators, who are established scientists and experts on this particular field and who go through all the data submitted to the IDR. Nurse (INGID) and patient societies (IPOPI) are also included (see Table 45.2). The IDR offers tens of thousands of validated links to other sites, which are periodically automatically checked.

The IDR also contains articles, instructional resources, and analysis tools, as well as advanced-search capabilities. Extensive cross-referencing and links to other services are available. It is possible to search for any text string or multiple strings with Boolean logic search facility across IDR pages. The IDR pages

Table 45.1. Immunodeficiency Mutation Databases

Database	Immunodeficiency	OMIM	Internet Address of Database	Public Cases	Reference
ADAbase	Adenosine deaminase deficiency	608958	http://bioinf.uta.fi/ADAbase/	60	
AICDAbase	Non-X-linked hyper-IgM syndrome	605257	http://bioinf.uta.fi/AICDAbase/	46	
AIREbase	Autoimmune polyendocrinopathy with candidiasis and ectodermal dystrophy (APECEC)	607358	http://bioinf.uta.fi/AIREbase/	132	
AP3B1base	Hermansky-Pudlak syndrome 2	603401	http://bioinf.uta.fi/AP3B1base/	4	
AP3B1	Hermansky-Pudlak syndrome 2	603401	http://albinismdb.med.umn.edu/hps2mut.htm	4	
ATbase	Ataxia-telangiectasia	607585	http://www.cbt.ki.se/ATbase/	47	
ATM	Ataxia-telangiectasia	607585	http://www.benaroyaresearch.org/bri_investigators/atm.htm	621	Concannon et al., 1997
BLMbase	Bloom syndrome	604610	http://bioinf.uta.fi/BLMbase/	33	Rong et al., 2000
BLNKbase	BLNK deficiency	604515	http://bioinf.uta.fi/BLNKbase/	1	
BTKbase	X-linked agammaglobulinemia (XLA)	300300	http://bioinf.uta.fi/BTKbase/	956	Vihinen et al., 1995, 1996, 1999
C1QAbase	C1QA deficiency	120550	http://bioinf.uta.fi/C1QAbase/	6	
C1QGbase	C1QG deficiency	120575	http://bioinf.uta.fi/C1QGbase/	3	
C1Sbase	C1s deficiency	120580	http://bioinf.uta.fi/C1Sbase/	3	
C2base	C2 deficiency	217000	http://bioinf.uta.fi/C2base/	3	
C3base	C3 deficiency	120700	http://bioinf.uta.fi/C3base/	4	
C5base	C5 deficiency	120900	http://bioinf.uta.fi/C5base/	4	
C6base	C6 deficiency	217050	http://bioinf.uta.fi/C6base/	13	
C7base	C7 deficiency	217070	http://bioinf.uta.fi/C7base/	14	
C8Bbase	C8B deficiency	120960	http://bioinf.uta.fi/C8Bbase/	59	
C9base	C9 deficiency	120940	http://bioinf.uta.fi/C9base/	14	
CARD15	Blau syndrome and Crohn disease	605956	http://fmf.igh.cnrs.fr/infevers/	79	
CASP10base	Autoimmune lymphoproliferative syndrome, type II	601762	http://bioinf.uta.fi/CASP10base/	2	
CASP10	Autoimmune lymphoproliferative syndrome, type II	601762	http://research.nhgri.nih.gov/ALPS/alpsII_mut.shtml	2	
CASP8 base	Caspase 8 deficiency	601763	http://bioinf.uta.fi/CASP8base/	2	
CD3Dbase	Autosomal recessive CD3δ deficiency	186790	http://bioinf.uta.fi/CD3Dbase/	3	
CD3Ebase	Autosomal recessive CD3ε deficiency	186830	http://bioinf.uta.fi/CD3Ebase/	1	
CD3Gbase	Autosomal recessive CD3γ deficiency	186740	http://bioinf.uta.fi/CD3Gbase/	3	
CD40Lbase	X-linked hyper-IgM syndrome (XHIM)	300386	http://bioinf.uta.fi/CD40Lbase/	135	Notarangelo et al., 1996
CD59base	CD59 deficiency	107271	http://bioinf.uta.fi/CD59base/	1	
CD79Abase	Igα deficiency	112205	http://bioinf.uta.fi/CD79Abase/	1	
CD8Abase	CD8 deficiency	186910	http://bioinf.uta.fi/CD8Abase/	3	
CEBPEbase	Neutrophil-specific granule deficiency	600749	http://bioinf.uta.fi/CEBPEbase/	2	
CHS1base	Chediak-Higashi syndrome	606897	http://bioinf.uta.fi/CHS1base/	32	
CHS1	Chediak-Higashi syndrome	606897	http://albinismdb.med.umn.edu/chs1mut.html	15	
CIAS1	Familial cold autoinflammatory syndrome, Muckle-Wells syndrome, and chronic infantile neurological cutaneous and articular syndrome	606416	http://fmf.igh.cnrs.fr/infevers/	47	
CXCR4base	WHIM syndrome	162643	http://bioinf.uta.fi/CXCR4base/	17	
CYBAbase	Autosomal recessive p22phox deficiency	608508	http://bioinf.uta.fi/CYBAbase/	33	
CYBBbase	X-linked chronic granulomatous disease (XCGD)	300481	http://bioinf.uta.fi/CYBBbase/	484	Roos et al., 1996; Heyworth et al., 2001
DCLRE1Cbase	Artemis deficiency	605988	http://bioinf.uta.fi/DCLRE1Cbase/	17	
DFbase	Factor D deficiency	134350	http://bioinf.uta.fi/DFbase/	5	
DKC1base	Hoyeraal-Hreidarsson syndrome	300126	http://bioinf.uta.fi/DKC1base/	9	

(continued)

Table 45.1. (continued)

Database	Immunodeficiency	OMIM	Internet Address of Database	Public Cases	Reference
DNMT3Bbase	ICF syndrome	602900	http://bioinf.uta.fi/DNMT3Bbase/	14	Lappalainen et al., 2002
ELA2base	Cyclic neutropenia and severe congenital neutropenias	130130	http://bioinf.uta.fi/ELA2base/	129	
EVER1base	Epidermodysplasia verruciformis	605828	http://bioinf.uta.fi/EVER1base/	7	
EVER2base	Epidermodysplasia verruciformis	605829	http://bioinf.uta.fi/EVER2base/	5	
FANCA	Fanconi anemia complementation group A	607139	http://www.rockefeller.edu/fanconi/mutate/	121	Levran et al., 1997
FANCC	Fanconi anemia complementation group C	227645	http://www.rockefeller.edu/fanconi/mutate/	10	Gilio et al., 1997
FANCD2	Fanconi anemia complementation group D2	227646	http://www.rockefeller.edu/fanconi/mutate/	5	
FANCE	Fanconi anemia complementation group E	600901	http://www.rockefeller.edu/fanconi/mutate/	3	
FANCF	Fanconi anemia complementation group F	603467	http://www.rockefeller.edu/fanconi/mutate/	5	
FANCG	Fanconi anemia complementation group G	602956	http://www.rockefeller.edu/fanconi/mutate/	24	Auerbach et al., 2003
FCGR1Abase	CD64 deficiency	146760	http://bioinf.uta.fi/FCGR1Abase/	4	
FCGR3Abase	Natural killer cell deficiency	146740	http://bioinf.uta.fi/FCGR3Abase/	3	
FOXN1base	T cell immunodeficiency, congenital alopecia, and nail dystrophy	600838	http://bioinf.uta.fi/FOXN1base/	2	
FOXP3base	Immunodysregulation, polyendocrinopathy, and enteropathy, X-linked (IPEX)	300292	http://bioinf.uta.fi/FOXP3base/	12	
GFI1base	Severe congenital neutropenia and nonimmune chronic idiopathic neutropenia of adults	600871	http://bioinf.uta.fi/GFI1base/	4	
HF1base	Factor H deficiency	134370	http://bioinf.uta.fi/HF1base/	25	
ICOSbase	ICOS deficiency	604558	http://bioinf.uta.fi/ICOSbase/	4	
IFbase	Factor I deficiency	217030	http://bioinf.uta.fi/IFbase/	6	
IFNGR1base	IFN-γ1-receptor deficiency	107470	http://bioinf.uta.fi/IFNGR1base/	49	
IFNGR2base	IFN-γ2-receptor deficiency	147569	http://bioinf.uta.fi/IFNGR2base/	4	
IGHMbase	μ heavy-chain deficiency	147020	http://bioinf.uta.fi/IGHMbase/	4	
IGLL1base	λ5 surrogate light-chain deficiency	146770	http://bioinf.uta.fi/IGLL1base/	1	
IKBKGbase	NEMO deficiency	300248	http://bioinf.uta.fi/IKBKGbase/	19	
IL12Bbase	Interleukin-12 (IL-12) p40 deficiency	161561	http://bioinf.uta.fi/IL12Bbase/	11	
IL12RB1base	Interleukin-12 receptor β1 deficiency	601604	http://bioinf.uta.fi/IL12RB1base/	9	
IL2RAbase	IL2RA deficiency	147730	http://bioinf.uta.fi/IL2RAbase/	1	
IL2RGbase	X-linked severe combined immunodeficiency (XSCID)	308380	http://research.nhgri.nih.gov/apps/scid	264	Puck et al., 1996
IL7Rbase	Interleukin-7 receptor α deficiency	146661	http://bioinf.uta.fi/IL7Rbase/	5	
IRAK4base	IRAK4 deficiency	606883	http://bioinf.uta.fi/IRAK4base/	4	
ITGB2base	Leucocyte adhesion deficiency I (LAD-I)	600065	http://bioinf.uta.fi/ITGB2base/	42	
JAK3base	Autosomal recessive severe combined JAK3 deficiency	600173	http://bioinf.uta.fi/JAK3base/	16	Vihinen et al., 2000; Notarangelo et al., 2001
LIG1base	DNA ligase I deficiency	126391	http://bioinf.uta.fi/LIG1base/	1	
LIG4base	LIG4 syndrome	601837	http://bioinf.uta.fi/LIG4base/	4	
MASP2base	MASP-2 deficiency	605102	http://bioinf.uta.fi/MASP2base/	1	
MEFV	Familial Mediterranean fever	608107	http://fmf.igh.cnrs.fr/infevers/	78	
MHC2TAbase	MHCII transactivating protein deficiency	600005	http://bioinf.uta.fi/MHC2TAbase/	8	
MLPHbase	Griscelli syndrome, type 3 (GS3)	606526	http://bioinf.uta.fi/MLPHbase/	1	
MPObase	Myeloperoxidase deficiency	606989	http://bioinf.uta.fi/MPObase/	38	
MRE11Abase	Ataxia-telangiectasia–like disorder (ATLD)	600814	http://bioinf.uta.fi/MRE11Abase/	6	
MVK	Hyper-IgD syndrome and periodic fever	251170	http://fmf.igh.cnrs.fr/infevers/	47	
MYO5Abase	Griscelli syndrome, type 1 (GS1)	160777	http://bioinf.uta.fi/MYO5Abase/	2	

(continued)

Base	Disease	OMIM	URL	No.	Reference
NCF1base	Autosomal recessive p47phox deficiency	608512	http://bioinf.uta.fi/NCF1base/	33	
NCF2base	Autosomal recessive p67phox deficiency	608515	http://bioinf.uta.fi/NCF2base/	11	
NFKBIAbase	Autosomal dominant anhidrotic ectodermal dysplasia and T cell immunodeficiency	164008	http://bioinf.uta.fi/NFKBIAbase/	1	
NPbase	PNP deficiency	164050	http://bioinf.uta.fi/NPbase/	11	
PFCbase	Properdin deficiency	300383	http://bioinf.uta.fi/PFCbase/	36	
PRF1base	Familiar hemophagocytic lymphohistiocytosis, type II (FHL2)	170280	http://bioinf.uta.fi/PRF1base/	61	
PSTPIP1	Pyogenic sterile arthritis, pyoderma gangrenosum, and acne syndrome	606347	http://fmf.igh.cnrs.fr/infevers/	2	
PTPRCbase	CD45 deficiency	151460	http://bioinf.uta.fi/PTPRCbase/	2	
RAB27Abase	Griscelli syndrome, type 2 (GS2)	603868	http://bioinf.uta.fi/RAB27Abase/	27	
RAC2base	Neutrophil immunodeficiency syndrome	602049	http://bioinf.uta.fi/RAC2base/	1	
RAG1base	Autosomal recessive severe combined RAG1 deficiency	179615	http://bioinf.uta.fi/RAG1base/	39	Villa et al., 2001
RAG2base	Autosomal recessive severe combined RAG2 deficiency	179616	http://bioinf.uta.fi/RAG2base/	16	Villa et al., 2001
RFX5base	MHCII promoter X box regulatory factor 5 deficiency	601863	http://bioinf.uta.fi/RFX5base/	8	
RFXANKbase	Ankyrin repeat containing regulatory factor X–associated protein deficiency	603200	http://bioinf.uta.fi/RFXANKbase/	28	
RFXAPbase	Regulatory factor X–associated protein deficiency	601861	http://bioinf.uta.fi/RFXAPbase/	7	
SERPING1base	Hereditary angioedema	606860	http://bioinf.uta.fi/SERPING1base/	183	
SH2D1Abase	X-linked lymphoproliferative syndrome (XLP)	300490	http://bioinf.uta.fi/SH2D1Abase/	101	Lappalainen et al., 2000
SLC35C1base	Leukosyte adhesion deficiency II (LAD-II)	605881	http://bioinf.uta.fi/SLC35C1base/	4	
SMARCAL1base	Schimke immuno-osseous dysplasia	606622	http://bioinf.uta.fi/SMARCAL1base/	19	
SPINK5base	Netherton syndrome	605010	http://bioinf.uta.fi/SPINK5base/	53	
STAT1base	STAT1 deficiency	600555	http://bioinf.uta.fi/STAT1base/	4	
STAT5Bbase	Growth hormone insensitivity with immunodeficiency	604260	http://bioinf.uta.fi/STAT5Bbase/	1	
TAP1base	TAP1 deficiency	170260	http://bioinf.uta.fi/TAP1base/	2	
TAP2base	TAP2 deficiency	170261	http://bioinf.uta.fi/TAP2base/	3	
TAZbase	Barth syndrome	300394	http://bioinf.uta.fi/TAZbase/	65	
TCIRG1base	Autosomal recessive osteopetrosis	604592	http://bioinf.uta.fi/TCIRG1base/	38	
TCN2base	Transcobalamin II deficiency	275350	http://bioinf.uta.fi/TCN2base/	6	
TNFRSF1A	Tumor necrosis factor receptor–associated periodic syndrome	191190	http://fmf.igh.cnrs.fr/infevers/	52	
TNFRSF5base	CD40 deficiency	109535	http://bioinf.uta.fi/TNFRSF5base/	4	
TNFRSF6	Autoimmune lymphoproliferative syndrome, type 1A	134637	http://research.nhgri.nih.gov/ALPS/alps1a_mut.shtml	69	
TNFSF6base	Autoimmune lymphoproliferative syndrome, type 1B	134638	http://bioinf.uta.fi/TNFSF6base/	1	
UNC13Dbase	Familial hemophagocytic lymphohistiocytosis 3	608897	http://bioinf.uta.fi/UNC13Dbase/	10	
UNGbase	UNG deficiency (hyper-IgM syndrome, type 5)	191525	http://bioinf.uta.fi/UNGbase/	3	
WASbase	Wiskott-Aldrich syndrome (WAS)	300392	http://bioinf.uta.fi/WASbase/	27	
WASPbase	Wiskott-Aldrich syndrome and X-linked thrombocytopenia	300392	http://homepage.mac.com/kohsukeimai/wasp/WASPbase.html	441	
ZAP70base	Autosomal recessive severe combined ZAP-70 deficiency	176947	http://bioinf.uta.fi/ZAP70base/	14	

ICF, immunodeficiency, centromeric instability, facial anomalies; ICOS, inducible costimulator; PNP, purine nucleoside phosphorylase; UNG, uracil-N-glycosylase; WHIM, warts, hypogammaglobulinemia, immunodeficiency, myelokathexis.

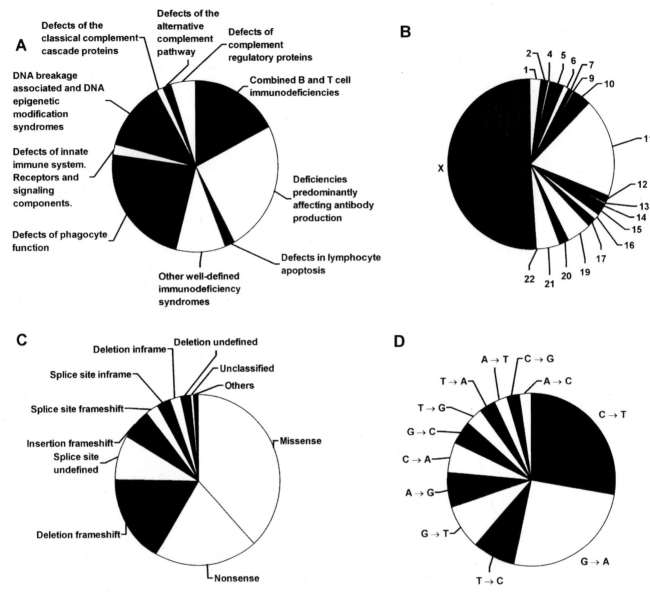

Figure 45.1. Distribution of number of patients having known immunodeficiency-causing mutations. (A) Distribution of patients in different immunodeficiency categories. (B) Distribution of mutations of patient chromosomes. (C) Distribution of mutation types. (D) Distribution of single nucleotide changes in immunodeficiency-causing mutations.

Table 45.2. Internet Sites Related to Primary Immunodeficiencies

Abbreviation	URL	Group or Society Name
ESID	http://www.esid.org/	European Society for Immunodeficiencies
IDF	http://www.primaryimmune.org/	Immune Deficiency Foundation (USA)
INGID	http://www.ingid.org/	International Nursing Group for Immunodeficiencies
IPOPI	http://www.ipopi.org/	International Patient Organization of Primary Immunodeficiencies
JMF	http://www.jmfworld.com/	Jeffrey Model Foundation
NPI	http://www.info4pi.org/	National Primary Immunodeficiency Resource Center (USA)
PAGID	http://www.clinimmsoc.org/pagid/	Pan American Group for Immunodeficiencies
PIA	http://www.pia.org.uk/	Primary Immunodeficiency Association (U.K.)
USIDNET	http://www.usidnet.org/	U.S. Immunodeficiency Network

General information		
Disease	X-linked agammaglobulinemia	
	Alternative names:	• XLA • Bruton type agammaglobulinemia • X-linked hypogammaglobulinemia
Description	Defects in the Bruton tyrosine kinase (BTK) gene cause agammaglobulinemia. Agammaglobulinemia is an X-linked immunodeficiency characterized by failure to produce mature B lymphocyte cells and associated with a failure of Ig heavy chain rearrangement.	
Classification	• Deficiencies Predominantly Affecting Antibody Production • Agammaglobulinemia	
OMIM	300300 Bruton agammaglobulinemia tyrosine kinase, BTK	
Cross references	Related immunodeficiencies • IDR factfile for X-linked hypogammaglobulinemia with growth hormone deficiency • IDR factfile for BLNK deficiency • IDR factfile for Igα deficiency • IDR factfile for λ heavy-chain deficiency • IDR factfile for λ5 surrogate light-chain deficiency	
Incidence	1/200,000	

Clinical information		
Description	Most patients with XLA develop recurrent bacterial infections, particularly otitis, sinusitis and pneumonia, in the first two years of life. The most common organisms are S. pneumoniae and H. influenzae. The serum IgG is usually less than 200 mg/dl and the IgG and IgA are generally less than 20 mg/dl. Approximately 20% of patients present with a dramatic, overwhelming infection, often with neutropenia. Another 10–15% have higher concentrations of serum immunoglobulin than expected or are not recognized to have immunodeficiency until after 5 years of age.	
Diagnosis	ESID/PAGID recommendations by IDR Additional information: • Patient and Family Handbook For The Primary Immune Deficiency Diseases by IDF • X-Linked Agammaglobulinemia by The Jeffrey Model Foundation (JMF)	
Diagnostic laboratories	Clinical:	• ORPHANET
	Genetic:	• IDdiagnostics • EDDNAL • GeneTests
Therapeutic options	• IDF patient/family handbook • X-Linked Agammaglobulinemia by The Jeffrey Model Foundation (JMF)	
Research programs, clinical trials	• The Jeffrey Model Foundation • Human Genome and Multifactor Diseases by Anna Villa at the Institute of Advanced Biomedical Technologies • Lois A. Steiner at Yale University, USA • Regulation of B cell Development and V(D)J Recombination by Christopher Roman • Molecular Mechanisms of DNA Recombination by Kevin Horn • David Schatz at Howard Hughes Medical Institute	

Genetic information		
Gene name	BTK	
Alias(es)	• AGMX1 • AT • ATK (Agammaglobulinemia tyrosine kinase) • BPK (B cell progenitor kinase) • IMD1 • PSCTK1 • XLA • Bruton agammaglobulinemia tyrosine kinase • Tyrosine-protein kinase BTK (Bruton's tyrosine kinase)	
Reference sequences	DNA: U78027 (EMBL), cDNA: X58957 (EMBL), Protein: Q06187 (SWISSPROT), other sequences	
Chromosomal location	Xq21.3–q22	
Maps	• BTK (Map View)	
Markers	• stSG89 • stSG50199 • WIAF-1356-STS • stWXD2763	
Other gene-based resources	• Ensembl ENSG00000010671 • GenAtlas BTK • GeneCard BTK • UniGene 159494 • LocusLink 695 • euGenes 695 • GDB 120542 • GeneLynx 2742 • SOURCE 159494	
Animal models	Mouse:	• MGD Btk • euGenes Btk1r1 (-/-)
	D. melanogaster:	• tbase Btk29A
	C. elegans:	• euGenes F26E4.5
Protein	Structures (PDB):	• 1BTK, PH domain and BTK motif from Bruton's tyrosine kinase, NMR, 42 structures • 1AWW, SH3 domain from Bruton's tyrosine kinase, NMR • 1AWX, SH3 domain from Bruton's tyrosine kinase, NMR, minimized average structure • 1B55, PH domain from Bruton's tyrosine kinase in complex with inositol 1,3,4,5-tetrakisphosphate • 1BWN, PH domain and BTK motif from Bruton's tyrosine kinase mutant E41K in complex with Ins(1,3,4,5)P4
	Domains:	Pleckstrin homology domain 1-138 — • Pfam PF00169, PH • InterPro IPR001849, PH • SMART SM00233, PH • PROSITE PS50003, PH DOMAIN
		Tec homology domain 139-215 — • PRINTS PR00402, TECBTKDOMAIN
		Src homology 3 domain 215-280 — • Pfam PF00018, SH3 • SH3, Smart • InterPro IPR001452, SH3 • PRINTS PR00452, SH3DOMAIN • ProDom PD000066, SH3 • SMART SM00326, SH3 • PROSITE PS50002, SH3
		Src homology 2 domain 281-377 — • Pfam PF00017, SH2 • SH2, Smart • InterPro IPR000980, SH2 • ProDom PD000093, SH2 • SMART SM00252, SH2 • PROSITE PS50001, SH2
		Tyrosine kinase domain 378-659 — • Pfam PF00069, pkinase • TwrKc, Smart • InterPro IPR001245, Tyr_pkinase • PRINTS PR00109, TYRKINASE • SMART SM00219, TyrKc
	Motifs:	BTK motif 139-165 — • InterPro IPR001562, BTK • Pfam PF00779, BTK • SMART SM00107, BTK
		ATP nucleotide phosphate-binding region: 408-416
		Atp binding site 430-430
	Resources:	• PIR S28912, • InterPro IPR000719, Euk_pkinase • ProDom PD000001, Euk_pkinase • PROSITE PS00107, PROTEIN_KINASE_ATP • PROSITE PS00109, PROTEIN_KINASE_TYR • PROSITE PS00011, PROTEIN_KINASE_DOM

Expression pattern (According to SOURCE)	Tissue	Expression (%)	Clones
	pheochromocytoma	22.49	1:1560
	leukocyte	15.62	4:8982
	lymph	9.26	17:64395
	b-cells	8.49	4:16533
	tonsil, enriched for germinal center b-cells	6.72	7:36522
	lung metastatic chondrosarcoma	5.44	1:6448
	corresponding non cancerous liver tissue	5.04	2:13909
	mixed	4.65	8:60341
	bone marrow	3.53	2:19854
	human skeletal muscle	3.26	1:10746

Variations/Mutations	• BTKbase, Mutation registry for X-linked agammaglobulinemia • HGMD, The human gene mutation database • BTKbase, Polymorphisms/Variations • dbSNP, Single nucleotide polymorphism	

Other resources		
Publications	• Pubmed search for X-linked agammaglobulinemia	
Societies	General:	• International Patient Organization for Primary Immunodeficiencies (IPOPI) • Immune Deficiency Foundation (IDF) • March of Dimes Birth Defects Foundation • NIH/National Institute of Allergy and Infectious Diseases • European Society for Immunodeficiencies (ESID)
Other information sources	• X-Linked Agammaglobulinemia by The Jeffrey Model Foundation • Primary Immunodeficiency by The Doctor's Medical Library • Bruton disease in Pediatric Database (PEDBASE) • X-Linked Agammaglobulinemia by The Immune Deficiency Foundation, Illinois Chapter	

are extensively hyperlinked to an immunology glossary that contains descriptions of over 1000 immunological terms.

The IDR immunology section lists collections of immunology-related data sources including lectures on immunology and immunodeficiencies. The pages also contain information about animal models and knockouts of immunodeficiency-related genes. There are several societies related to immunodeficiency research, care, and patients (see Table 45.2). Immunology societies, nurse societies, and patient organizations as well as patient pages include further links to other interest groups. Patient pages are usually more personal and often contain patient histories as well as personal experience of the diseases. Immunology laboratories contain a list of home pages of laboratories that are active in many fields of immunodeficiency research, including diagnosis, treatment, and basic research on areas such as genetic analysis, protein structure determination, and signal transduction. PubMed search is possible directly by individual disease or gene. Links to immunodeficiency-related genomic DNA and amino acid sequences as well as three-dimensional structures of proteins are also available.

The disease- and gene-specific information is stored in fact files that are eXtensible Markup Language (XML) based, making it easy to distribute IDR to different platforms, such as PCs, personal digital assistants (PDAs), and Wireless Application Protocol (WAP)-compliant devices (such as mobile phones). The fact files are central means of distributing and collecting information (Fig. 45.2). For this purpose we have developed Inherited Disease Markup Language (IDML), which is an XML-based tag set providing a standard method of exchanging genetic and clinical data along with general disease description, diagnostic information, and links to other related resources (Väliaho et al., 2005).

The IDR is continuously updated and new features will be added to provide a comprehensive navigation point for anyone interested in these disorders. Currently, we are working on classification of the links to provide validated, selected, and focused information for different user groups, from physicians and nurses to research scientists, as well as for patients, their families, and the general public.

Immunodeficiency Mutation Databases (IDbases)

Many immunodeficiency-related genes have been identified, as have a large number of disease-causing mutations in them. Frequently it is only the gene test that enables the final diagnosis. Mutation data have been collected into databases along with patient-related clinical information. This compilation allows the discovery of statistically relevant trends from large data sets. The first immunodeficiency mutation database, the BTKbase, was started in 1994 (Vihinen et al., 1995, 1999; Lindvall et al., 2005) for X-linked agammaglobulinemia (XLA) (Fig. 45.2); subsequently, more than 90 registries have been released (Table 45.1).

The European Society for Immunodeficiencies (ESID) has collected information on immunodeficiency patients into a large registry. The ESID database was established in 1992 and contains clinical information on more than 10000 patients (Abedi et al., 2000). The registry lists different immunodeficiency disorders, immunoglobulin values, and therapies as well as family histories of patients. To increase accessibility of the data, the

Figure 45.2. Example of an IDR fact file. The fact files form an XML-based database for immunodeficiency-related information providing basic knowledge on diseases and affected genes.

patient registry has recently undergoing a major revision and reorganization. A new, online-based database has been set up that is accessible via standard Internet browsers (http://www.esid.org/). A clinical data management system that fulfills a number of central needs, all of which are relevant to a modern approach to a multicenter clinical research database system, is being developed.

The new online PID database will greatly increase data accessibility to 24 hours a day, making a standard Internet browser and a valid login and password the only prerequisites for access. Moreover, the system will be very flexible and will enable follow-up of patients and increase the amount of collected data via automated data entry. Tools will also be developed to allow shared analysis of research data between new European PID database and the existing public mutation database hosted at Tampere University.

Currently there are more than 90 immunodeficiency mutation databases maintained mainly at the University of Tampere's Institute of Medical Technology (IMT) Bioinformatics (Table 45.1). Mutation data submissions from the community are instrumental for keeping the databases up-to-date. Scientists analyzing mutations are encouraged to submit their data by either contacting the

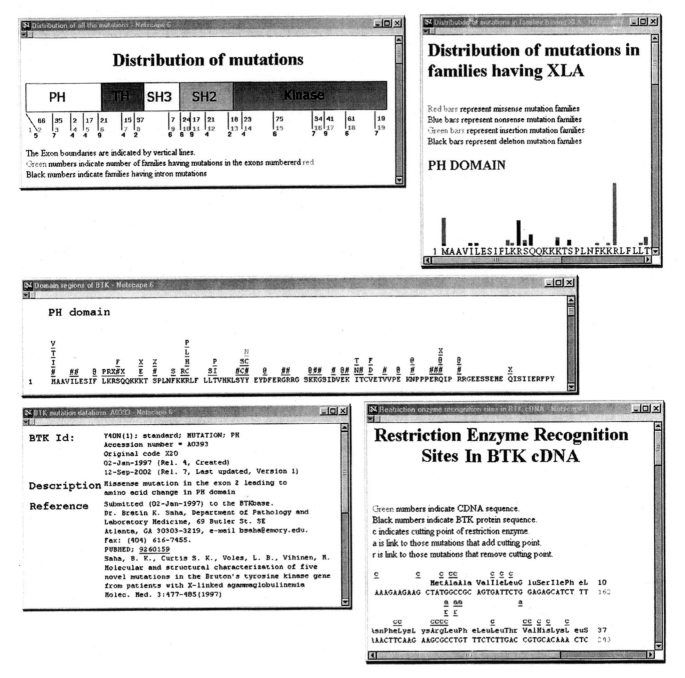

Figure 45.3. Montage of pages in BTKbase. Some main features of the BTKbase. Top left: Distribution of mutations in the BTK exons and introns. Top right: Distribution of mutations in families with X-linked agammaglobulinemia (XLA). Middle: Mutations causing XLA in the PH domain. Mutations above the sequence cause either severe (classical) or moderate XLA, whereas those below the sequence cause clinically mild disease. Bottom left: Short description of a mutation entry. Bottom right: Restriction enzyme recognition sites in the cDNA of BTK.

curators or using the Web submission option available on the homepages of databases. Many of the IDbases contain plenty of information in addition to the actual relevant mutation, making these registries valuable for physicians and scientists from a variety of different fields. The IMT Bioinformatics-maintained databases are also accessible via mobile devices by use of BioWAP (http://bioinf.uta.fi/) service (Riikonen et al., 2001, 2002).

All data in the IDbases are arranged according to concepts applied to sequence databases. Lines are organized into logical groups: first are the lines necessary for identification of the entry, accompanied by a description of the mutation in English. These are succeeded by reference lines and lines that formally characterize the mutation. The remaining lines describe various parameters from patients. The entries are linked to other data sources, such as sequence databanks, PubMed, OMIM (On-line Mendelian Inheritance in Man, 1998), and SwissProt. The databases also provide direct access to the sequence retrieval system search engine for potential further analysis and comparison to other registries (Etzold et al., 1993).

It is vital that representation of the information in the databases be standardized. We have developed a program suite, MUTbase (Riikonen and Vihinen, 1999), which provides interactive and quality-controlled submission of information to our mutation databases. It is a system for collecting, maintaining, and analyzing the data of disease-causing mutations. The MUTbase system generates new information from the raw data, part of which is added to the entries and the other part written on numerous interactive Web pages.

Several Web pages indicate the type of mutation and their distribution in the protein domains as well as that in the exons or introns of the gene (Fig. 45.3). The pages are interactive, providing access to patient and mutation information. The localization of mutations on the gene and the protein can be analyzed on the pages containing sequence information. Interactive graphic pages show the number of disorder-related families having different mutation types at each residue. Mutations are also listed according to mutation types. In addition to the disease-causing mutations, polymorphisms or variations are also included in separate files.

The IDbases may provide new insights into both genotype–phenotype correlations in patients and protein structure–function relationships for the encoded proteins and DNA-level phenomena (Vihinen and Durandy, 2005). These registries have a variety of users, including physicians and research scientists from various fields. The databases have been used to retrieve retrospective and prospective information on clinical presentation, immunologic phenotype, long-term prognosis, and efficacy of available therapeutic options. The information may be essential to developing new treatments including drug design.

Immunodeficiency Diagnostics Registry (IDdiagnostics)

The diagnosis of immunodeficiencies can be daunting because similar symptoms may be caused by several disorders (Samarghitean et al., 2004). A further complication is that many immunodeficiencies are rare. Early and reliable diagnosis is often crucial for efficient treatment of these diseases. Delayed diagnosis and management of immunodeficiency disorders can lead to severe and irreversible complications, even resulting in the death of the patient. Early or possibly prenatal molecular diagnosis allows enough time for the most suitable management and selection of treatment, which is crucial for the survival of the patient.

CLINICAL TESTS FOR IMMUNODEFICIENCIES

Contact Address:
Name:
Institution:
Address:
Telephone:
Fax:
E-mail:
http:
Please fill the form and send to:
Prof. Mauno Vihinen, Institute of Medical Technology,
FI-33014 University of Tampere, Finland
Fax : +358-3-35517710
e-mail: mauno.vihinen@uta.fi
or use electronic form at:
http://bioinf.uta.fi/cgi-bin/submit/IDClini.cgi

1 IMMUNE STATUS

1.1 Complete Blood Count
- ☐ Red Blood Cells (RBC)
- ☐ White Blood Cells (WBC)
  - ○ Neutrophils
  - ○ Lymphocytes
  - ○ Eosinophils
  - ○ Monocytes
  - ○ Basophils
- ☐ Platelets

1.2 Quantitative Serum Immunoglobulins
- ☐ IgG
- ☐ IgG1
- ☐ IgG2
- ☐ IgG3
- ☐ IgG4
- ☐ IgA
- ☐ IgA1
- ☐ IgA2
- ☐ IgM
- ☐ IgE
- ☐ IgD
- ☐ Immunoglobulin (κ, λ) light chains
- ☐ Detection of monoclonal / oligoclonal components of immunoglobulins

1.3 Enumeration of Blood Cell Populations and Evaluation of Functional Molecules - Flow Cytometry (absolute counts are requested)

1.3.1 T cell subsets
- ☐ Total T cells
- ☐ CD3/CD4+
- ☐ CD3/CD8+
- ☐ CD4
- ☐ CD8
- ☐ CD4/CD45RA+ in CD4
- ☐ CD4/CD45RO+ in CD4
- ☐ CD3/ TCR α/β
- ☐ CD3/TCR γ/δ
- ☐ CD3⁺CD4⁻CD8⁻
- ☐ CD3⁺CD4⁻CD8⁻

- ☐ Poliomyelitis
- ☐ Varicella-zoster
- ☐ Other antiviral antibodies, please specify

2.1.3 Antibodies to neoantigens
- ☐ Keyhole limpet hemocyanin (KLH)
- ☐ Bacteriophage Φ X174

2.2 Cell Function

2.2.1 Study of in vitro lymphocyte activation and proliferation by flow cytometry upon stimulation with mitogens or antigens
- ☐ Surface activation markers/molecules on T cells
- ☐ CD69
- ☐ CD25
- ☐ CD71
- ☐ HLA-DR
- ☐ CD45RO
- ☐ CD45RA
- ☐ CD154 (CD40 ligand)
- ☐ IL-12 receptor
- ☐ Cell (intra-cellular detection) cytokine production
- ☐ Blastogenesis (forward light scatter FS/side light scatter SS)
- ☐ Cell proliferation (DNA content, BrDU incorporation)
- ☐ Cell proliferation (tritiated thymidine incorporation)

2.2.2 In vitro studies of phagocytic cell metabolism
- ☐ Oxidative burst (oxidation of dihydrorodamina-123 DHR stimulation with PMA or with E.coli) by flow cytometry
- ☐ Phagocytosis of (fluoresceinated) E. coli by flow cytometry
- ☐ Nitroblue tetrazolium (NBT) test
- ☐ Glucose metabolism
- ☐ Oxygen consumption
- ☐ Glucose monophosphate shunt activity
- ☐ Chemiluminescence

2.2.3 In vitro studies of phagocytic cell chemotaxis
- ☐ Chemotaxis under agarose
- ☐ Chemotaxis across a membrane filter (e.g., Boyden chamber)

3. COMMENTS AND ADDITIONAL TESTS

1.3.2 B cells
- ☐ CD19
- ☐ CD20
- ☐ CD19/κ
- ☐ CD19/λ

1.3.3 NK cells
- ☐ CD16/CD56 (CD3 negative)
- ☐ CD8CD56
- ☐ CD3CD16
- ☐ CD3⁺CD16⁺CD56⁺

1.3.4 HLA-DR on monocytes
- ☐ HLA-DR/CD14

1.3.5 ex vivo Activation markers
- ☐ CD69
- ☐ CD3/HLA-DR (activated T cells)
- ☐ CD3/CD25 (activated T cells)
- ☐ CD3CD69
- ☐ CD19/CD23 (activated B cells)

1.3.6 Adhesion molecules
- ☐ CD18 on leukocytes
- ☐ Sialyl Lewis X (on phagocytes)
- ☐ CD11a (LFA1c)
- ☐ CD11b (MO1, CR3)
- ☐ CD11c

1.3.7 Functional molecules
- ☐ CD132 (common γ chain of IL's receptors)
- ☐ IFNγ receptor 1 (CD 119)
- ☐ Btk
- ☐ IL-4
- ☐ IL-5
- ☐ IL-12R
- ☐ IL7RA
- ☐ WASP

1.3.8 MHC class I and MHC class II on leukocytes
- ☐ by flow cytometry (using common MAbs)
- ☐ HLA class I (monomorphic epitopes of loci A, B, C)
- ☐ HLA class II (DR or DP⁺DQ⁺DR antigens)

1.3.9 Identification of TCR clonality
- ☐ by flow cytometry
- ☐ by PCR

2   STUDIES OF FUNCTION

2.1 Antibody Response

2.1.1 Natural antibodies (titer)
- ☐ anti-A isohemagglutinin (IgM)
- ☐ anti-B isohemagglutinin (IgM)

2.1.2 Antibodies to vaccination or exposure antigens (total IgG and IgG subclass specific)
- ☐ Diphteria
- ☐ Tetanus
- ☐ Hepatitis B
- ☐ Rubella
- ☐ Haemophilus influenzae b (Hib)
- ☐ Pneumococcal polysaccharide
- ☐ Measles
- ☐ Mumps

2.3 Enzyme assays
- ☐ Adenosine deaminase (ADA)
- ☐ Purine nucleoside phosphorylase (PNP)
- ☐ Glucose-6-phosphate dehydrogenase (G6PD)
- ☐ Glutathione peroxidase (GSH-Px)
- ☐ Myeloperoxidase (MPO)

2.4 Complement function
- ☐ CH50 (Hemolytic activity, classical pathway)
- ☐ AH50 (Hemolytic activity, alternate pathway)
- ☐ Function of C1 esterase inhibitor
- ☐ Assay of components
  - ○ C1
  - ○ C1 esterase inhibitor
  - ○ C2
  - ○ C3
  - ○ C4
  - ○ C5
  - ○ C6
  - ○ C7
  - ○ C8
  - ○ C9
  - ○ B
  - ○ D
  - ○ Properdin
  - ○ Other, please specify

2.5 Apoptosis assays
- ☐ Fas/Fas-ligand (flow cytometry, other)
- ☐ BCL-1
- ☐ Caspase expression
- ☐ Cells with reduced DNA content (fluorescent DNA stain with cell permeabilization, flow cytometry)
- ☐ Strand breaks in cell DNA (TdT incorporation of fluorescence labelled nucleotides, e.g., TUNEL, flow cytometry)
- ☐ Translocated phosphatidylserine on cell membrane (adsorption of Annexin V, flow cytometry)
- ☐ functional assays of apoptosis

2.6 Other diagnostic tests
- ☐ Sweat Cl⁻
- ☐ α1-antitrypsin
- ☐ Uric acid (serum)
- ☐ α -fetoprotein

Figure 45.4. The IDdiagnostics Clinical Tests submission form. A submission page for IDdiagnostics Clinical Tests, also available at http://bioinf.uta.fi/cgi-bin/submit/IDClini.cgi.

Data submission to IDdiagnostics registry

Please fill in one form per disease or use the electronic submission available at
http://bioinf.uta.fi/IDdiagnostics/ and send to Prof. Mauno Vihinen, Institute of Medical Technology,
FI-33014 University of Tampere, Finland or fax to +358-3-35517710

Contact address:
Name:
Address:

Telephone: **Fax:**
E-mail:
HTTP:

Disease/gene:
- Adenosine deaminase deficiency/*ADA*
- Artemis deficiency/*DLCRE1C*
- APO-1 ligand/Fas ligand defects/*TNFSF6*
- Apoptosis mediator APO-1/Fas defects/*TNFRSF6*
- Ataxia-telangiectasia/*ATM*
- Autoimmune polyendocrinopathy with candidiasis and ectodermal dystrophy (APECED)/*AIRE*
- Autosomal recessive CGD p22^{phox}/*CYBA*
- Autosomal recessive CGD p47^{phox}/*NCF1*
- Autosomal recessive CGD p67^{phox}/*NCF2*
- Bloom syndrome/*BLM*
- Cartilage-hair hypoplasia/*RMRP*
- Chediak-Higashi syndrome /*CHS1*
- Chronic granulomatous disease/*CYBB*
- CIITA, MHCII transactivating protein deficiency/*MHC2TA*
- CD40 deficiency/*TNFRSF5*
- CD45 deficiency/*PTPRC*
- CD59 or protectin deficiency/*CD59*
- CD3ε deficiency/*CD3E*
- CD3γ deficiency/*CD3G*
- CD8α deficiency/*CD8A*
- C9 deficiency/*C9*
- C4 binding protein αdeficiency/C4BPA
- C4 binding protein βdeficiency/C4BPB
- Cyclic neutropenia/*ELA2*
- Decay-accelerating factor (CD55)deficiency/*DAF*
- DiGeorge-anomaly/*DGCR*
- Factor B deficiency/*BF*
- Factor I deficiency/*IF*
- Factor III deficiency/*HF1*
- Glucose 6-phosphate dehydrogenase
- Glycogen storage disease 1b/*G6PT* deficiency/*G6PD*
- Griscelli syndrome/*MYO5A*
- Hereditary angioedema/*C1NH*
- JAK3 deficiency/*JAK3*
- IFN γ1-receptor deficiency/*IFNGR1*
- IFN γ2-receptor deficiency/*IFNGR2*
- IFN-γ R alpha chain deficiency

- κ light-chain deficiency/*IGKC*
- λ5 surrogate light-chain deficiency/*IGLL1*
- γ1 isotype deficiency/*IGHG1*
- γ2 isotype deficiency/*IGHG2*
- Other, specify:

- IL-2 receptor α-chain deficiency/*IL2RA*
- Immunodeficiency, polyendocrinopathy, enetropathy, enteropathy, X-linked /*IPEX*
- Interleukin-12 (IL-12) p40 deficiency/*IL12B*
- Interleukin-12 receptor β1 deficiency/*IL12RB1*
- Leukocyte adhesion deficiency 1/*ITGB2*
- Manose-binding lectin deficiency/*MBL*
- MHC class II transactivator deficiency
- Myeloperoxidase deficiency/*MPO*
- Nijmegen-breakage syndrome/*NBS1*
- Partial γ3 isotype deficiency/*IGHG3*
- Properdin factor deficiency/*PFC*
- Purine nucleoside phosphorylase deficiency/*NP*
- RAG1 deficiency/*RAG1*
- RAG2 deficiency/*RAG2*
- Regulatory factor X 5 deficiency/ *RFX5*
- RFXAP, Regulatory factor X-associated protein deficiency/*RFXAP*
- RFXANK, Ankyrin repeat containing regulatory factor X-associated protein deficiency/*RFXANK*
- Severe congenital neutropenias, including Kostmann syndrome/*CSF3R*
- TAP 2 peptide transporter deficiency
- ZAP70 deficiency/*ZAP70*
- Wiskott-Aldrich syndrome/*WAS*
- X-linked agammaglobulinemia/*BTK*
- X-linked hyper-IgM syndrome /*TNFSF5*
- X-linked chronic granulomatous disease/*CYBB*
- X-linked lymphoproliferative syndrome(Duncan disease)/*SH2D1A*
- X-linked severe combined immunodeficiency/*IL2RG*
- X-linked hyper-IgM syndrome and hypohydrotic ectodermal dysplasia/*IKBKG*
- μ heavy-chain deficiency/*IGHM*
- κ light-chain deficiency/*IGKC*
- λ5 surrogate light-chain deficiency/*IGLL1*

- γ4 isotype deficiency/*IGHG4*
- α1 isotype deficiency/*IGHA1*
- α2 isotype deficiency/*IGHA2*
- ε isotype deficiency/*IGHE*

Method:
- Direct sequencing
- SSCP
- PTT
- DGGE
- CCM
- EMC
- DHPLC
- Dideoxy finger printing
- FISH
- Heteroduplex analysis
- Other, specify:

How often analysis is performed?

Turnaround time?

How many samples of this disease analysed/year

Price and currency

Figure 45.5. The IDdiagnostics Genetic Tests submission form. A submission page for IDdiagnostics Genetic Tests, available at http://bioinf.uta.fi/cgi-bin/IDdiagnostics/IDdiag.cgi.

The definitive diagnosis of immunodeficiency disorders depends on genetic and clinical tests, as the physical signs may be nonspecific, very discreet, or absent. In many cases the diagnosis has to be based on the analysis of genetic defect(s). Because of the rareness of the diseases there are generally not many laboratories analyzing a particular disease. The IDdiagnostics registry contains two databases, genetic and clinical, that are collected to provide a service for those trying to find quickly the nearest and/or most suitable laboratory conducting immunodeficiency testing. It consists of a list of laboratories performing genetic and clinical testing for patients with inherited immunodeficiencies.

Contact addresses for laboratories performing diagnoses are provided in the IDdiagnostics registry along with the assay method(s) used. Mutation detection can be done by several methods. Many laboratories use direct sequencing, whereas others rely on fast screening methods followed by sequencing. Only with sequencing is it possible to analyze all the mutations, as most of the immunodeficiency-related genes are so large that primary scanning for the gene defect within an exon or intron can be more cost- and time-effective. Because the IDs are rare disorders, only large centers may have enough samples to run certain analyses on a constant basis. To get an idea of the time required to receive diagnostic details, the frequency with which the samples are run, and the number of samples studied annually, data are provided in the gene test laboratories database. The cost of analyses varies according to the method used, the type of laboratory, and the research interest in a particular disease. More common diseases are analyzed routinely. Laboratories can have special requirements for samples and their handling. These data are also available through the IDdiagnostics service. Physicians should consult the laboratories before sending any samples to learn about conditions, shipment details, and expected time for the test.

The IDdiagnostics database provides search facilities that allow users to run text-based search queries. Gene test laboratories can be searched by disease name (also alternative names), gene symbol, OMIM code, laboratory, laboratory location, and free text. Similar searches are available for clinical laboratories. A search engine makes it easy to find laboratories for certain disease(s), methods, and/or geographic locations. Physicians should contact the laboratory before sending in any samples as the standards vary across laboratories. The cost of the analysis also varies greatly, depending on whether testing is carried out for commercial or research purposes. Further information and submission pages for both genetic and clinical testing can be found at http://bioinf.uta.fi/IDdiagnostics/ and in Figures 45.4 and 45.5. The preferred method is Web submission. Laboratories carrying out testing are encouraged to fill out the form and send it to the database curators.

Conclusions

The IDR, IDbases, and IDdiagnostics have been developed over several years. They all have increasing numbers of users (e.g., there were about 158,000 requests sent to the IDR from 100 countries in the year 2005). This expanded use demonstrates that the Web is an effective way to deliver complex and updated information to the medical community. It also demonstrates the feasibility of IDML language to organize and distribute complex data and knowledge bases interlinked with other services on the Internet.

These services are aimed at collecting and distributing relevant information about immunodeficiency disorders in a systematized manner, starting with mutation data and ending with clinical information. They will serve as useful, fast, and easy instruments for physicians, nurses, researchers, and patients and their families in their fight against these diseases. All three registries are also an important instrument in the education of physicians and in providing health-care authorities information on the incidence of immunodeficiency disorders, the need for early diagnosis, updated diagnostic criteria, and the availability of different treatments and centers.

Acknowledgments

Financial support from the European Union Program on Rare Diseases, the Finnish Academy, and the Medical Research Fund of Tampere University Hospital is gratefully acknowledged.

References

Abedi MR, Morgan G, Goii H, Paganelli R, Matamoros N, Hammarström L. Report from the ESID registry of Primary Immunodeficiencies, 2000. Available at http://www.esid.org/.

Auerbach AD, Greenbaum J, Pujara K, Batish SD, Bitencourt MA, Kokemohr I, Schneider H, Lobitzc S, Pasquini R, Giampietro PF, Hanenberg H, Levran O. Spectrum of sequence variation in the *FANCG* gene: an International Fanconi Anemia Registry (IFAR) study. Hum Mutat 21:158–168, 2003.

Concannon P, Gatti RA. Diversity of *ATM* gene mutations detected in patients with ataxia-telangiectasia. Hum Mutat 10:100–107, 1997.

Conley ME, Notarangelo LD, Etzioni A. Diagnostic criteria for primary immunodeficiencies. Clin Immunol 93:190–197, 1999.

Etzold T, Argos P. SRS—an indexing and retrieval tool for flat file data libraries. Comput Appl Biosci 9:49–57, 1993.

Fischer A. Primary immunodeficiency diseases: an experimental model for molecular medicine. Lancet 357:1863–1869, 2001.

Gillio AP, Verlander PC, Batish SD, Giampietro PF, Auerbach AD. Phenotypic consequences of mutations in the Fanconi anemia *FAC* gene: an international Fanconi anemia registry study. Blood 90:105–110, 1997.

Heyworth PG, Curnutte JT, Rae L, Noack D, Roos D, van Koppen E, Cross AR. Hematologically important mutations: X-linked chronic granulomatous disease. Blood Cells Mol Dis 27:16–26, 2001.

Lappalainen I, Giliani S, Franceschini R, Bonnefoy JY, Duckett C, Notarangelo LD, Vihinen M. Structural basis for SH2D1A mutations in X-linked lymphoproliferative disease. Biochem Biophys Res Commun 269:124–130, 2000.

Lappalainen I, Ollila J, Smith CIE, Vihinen M. Registries of immunodeficiency patients and mutations. Hum Mutat 10:261–267, 1997.

Lappalainen I, Vihinen M. Structural basis of ICF-causing mutations in the methyltransferase domain of DNMT3B. Protein Eng 15:1005–1014, 2002.

Levran O, Erlich T, Magdalena N, Gregory JJ, Batish SD, Verlander PC, Auerbach AD. Sequence variation in the Fanconi anemia gene *FAA*. Proc Natl Acad Sci USA 94:13051–13056, 1997.

Lindvall J, Blomberg KEM, Väliaho J, Vargas L, Heinonen JE, Berglöf A, Mohamaed Aj, Nore BF, Vihinen M, Smith CIE. Bruton tyrosine kinase—cell biology, sequence conservation, mutation spectrum, siRNA modifications and expression profiling. Immunol Rev 176:2005.

Notarangelo LD, Mella P, Jones A, de Saint Basile G, Savoldi G, Cranston T, Vihinen M, Schumacher RF. Mutations in severe combined immune deficiency (SCID) due to JAK3 deficiency. Hum Mutat 18:255–263, 2001.

Notarangelo LD, Peitsch MC, Abrahamsen TG, Bachelot C, Bordigoni P, Cant AJ, Chapel H, Clementi M, Deacock S, de Saint Basile G, Duse M, Espanol T, Etzioni A, Fasth A, Fischer A, Giliani S, Gomez L, Hammarström L, Jones A, Kanariou M, Kinnon C, Klemola T, Kroczek RA, Levy J, Matamoros N, Monafo V, Paolucci P, Sanal O, Smith CIE, Thompson RA, Tovo P, Villa A, Vihinen M, Vossen J, Zegers BJM. CD40Lbase: a database of CD40L gene mutations causing X-linked hyper-IgM syndrome. Immunol Today 17:511–516, 1996.

Puck JM, de Saint Basile G, Schwarz K, Fugmann S, Fischer RE. IL2RGbase: a database of γc-chain defects causing human X-SCID. Immunol Today 17:507–511, 1996.

Riikonen P, Boberg J, Salakoski T, Vihinen M. BioWAP mobile Internet service for bioinformatics. Bioinformatics 17:855–856, 2001.

Riikonen P, Boberg J, Salakoski T, Vihinen M. Mobile access to biological databases on the Internet. IEEE Trans Biomed Eng 49:1477–1479, 2002.

Riikonen P, Vihinen M. MUTbase: maintenance and analysis of distributed mutation databases. Bioinformatics 15:852–859, 1999.

Rong SB, Väliaho J, Vihinen M. Structural basis of Bloom syndrome (BS) causing mutations in the BLM helicase domain. Mol Med 6:155–164, 2000.

Roos D, Curnutte JT, Hossle JP, Lau YL, Ariga T, Nunoi H, Dinauer MC, Gahr M, Segal AW, Newburger PE, Giacca M, Keep NH, van Zwieten R. X-CGDbase: a database of X-CGD-causing mutations. Immunol Today 17: 517–521, 1996.

Samarghitean C, Väliaho J, Vihinen M. Online registry of genetic and clinical immunodeficiency diagnostic laboratories, ID diagnostics. J Clin Immunol 24:53–61, 2004.

Väliaho J, Pusa M, Ylinen T, Vihinen M. IDR. The immunodeficiency resource. Nucl Acids Res 30:232–234, 2002.

Väliaho J, Riikonen P, Vihinen M. Novel data servers for immunodeficiencies. Immunol Rev 178:177–185, 2000.

Väliaho J, Riikonen P, Vihinen M. Biomedical data description with XML. Distribution of immunodeficiency fact files—from Web to WAP. BMC Medical Informatics and Decision Making 5:21, 2005.

Vihinen M, Arredondo-Vega FX, Casanova J-L, Etzioni A, Giliani S, Hammarström L, Heyworth PG, Hershfield MS, Hsu AP, Lappalainen I, Lähdesmäki A, Notarangelo LD, Puck JF, Reith W, Roos D, Schumacher RF, Schwarz K, Vezzoni P, Villa A, Väliaho J, Smith CIE. Primary immunodeficiency mutation databases. Adv Genet 43:103–188, 2001.

Vihinen M, Cooper MD, de Saint Basile G, Fischer A, Good RA, Hendriks RW, Kinnon C, Kwan SP, Litman GW, Notarangelo LD, Ochs HD, Rosen FS, Vetrie D, Webster ADB, Zegers BJM, Smith CIE. BTKbase: a database of XLA-causing mutations. Immunol Today 16:460–465, 1995.

Vihinen M, Durandy A. Primary immunodeficiencies: genotype-phenotype correlations. In: Falus A, ed. Immunogenomics and Human Disease. New York: John Wiley and Sons, pp. 443–460, 2005.

Vihinen M, Iwata T, Kinnon C, Kwan S-P, Ochs HD, Vorechovsky I, Smith, CIE. BTKbase, mutation database for X-linked agammaglobulinemia. Nucleic Acids Res 24:160–165, 1996.

Vihinen M, Kwan SP, Lester T, Ochs HD, Resnick I, Väliaho J, Conley E, Smith CIE. Mutations of the human *BTK* gene coding for Bruton tyrosine kinase in X-linked agammaglobulinemia. Hum Mutat 13:280–285, 1999.

Vihinen M, Villa A, Mella P, Schumacher RF, Savoldi G, O'Shea JJ, Candotti F, Notarangelo LD. Molecular modeling of the Jak3 kinase domains and structural basis for severe combined immunodeficiency. Clin Immunol 96: 108–118, 2000.

Villa A, Sobacchi C, Notarangelo LD, Bozzi F, Abinun M, Abrahamsen TG, Arkwright PD, Baniyash M, Brooks EG, Conley ME, Cortes P, Duse M, Fasth A, Filipovich AM, Infante AJ, Jones A, Mazzolari E, Müller SM, Pasic S, Rechavi G, Sacco MG, Santagata S, Schroeder ML, Seger R, Strina D, Ugazio A, Väliaho J, Vihinen M, Vogler LB, Ochs H, Vezzoni P, Friedrich W, Schwarz K. V(D)J recombination defects in lymphocytes due to *RAG* mutations: severe immunodeficiency with a spectrum of clinical presentations. Blood 97:81–88, 2001.

46

Conventional Therapy of Primary Immunodeficiency Diseases

E. RICHARD STIEHM and HELEN M. CHAPEL

Long-term care of patients with primary immunodeficiencies is aimed at prevention of infections and their long-term sequelae as well as treatment of breakthrough infections. The extent of both the protection required and the appropriate prophylaxis depends on the nature of the immune deficiency. For this reason, this chapter is divided into two sections: the first describes general measures applicable to all forms of immune deficiency, and the second details specific measures for patients with individual diseases.

The management of all forms of immunodeficiency disease requires interaction between generalists and specialists with experience and expertise in primary immune deficiencies. This usually requires a team of a primary care pediatrician or internist and an immunologist with assistance and advice from other specialists (e.g., dermatologists, pulmonologists, gastroenterologists, and radiologists) as necessary, since it is important that patients continue to have the benefit of optimal diagnostic procedures and new drugs for all organ-based complications they may develop.

For example, patients with bronchiectasis following repeated bronchial sepsis need not only regular monitoring with pulmonary function tests and computed tomography (CT) scans but also access to chest physiotherapists, and those with asthma require the latest and most effective bronchodilators. In the same way that the immune system is multi-organ, the failure of this system manifests diverse complications requiring organ-based specialist medical care.

General Considerations

Treatment

Because many patients with immunodeficiency will have a normal life span on immunoglobulin (Ig) or other therapy, their parents and relatives must avoid making the patient an emotional cripple through overprotection. A child should be encouraged to be outdoors, play with other children in small groups, attend nursery and regular school, and participate in sports and other extracurricular activities. The aim is to teach such children to live in a near-normal fashion with their disease, in much the same way as a diabetic child taking insulin would. Adolescents and even adults need advice about the importance of regular exercise (especially to improve bronchiectasis). They should not smoke, inhale second-hand smoke, or use illegal drugs. Like tobacco, marijuana is a pulmonary irritant and should be avoided.

Patients with immunodeficiency require extraordinary amounts of care to maintain general health and nutrition, prevent emotional problems related to their illness, and manage their numerous infectious episodes. This regimen applies equally to adults and children. Usually, no special dietary limitations are necessary; the aim is to provide a well-rounded, nutritious diet. Patients with immunodeficiency should be protected from unnecessary exposure to infection. They should sleep in their own beds, preferably with rooms of their own, and keep away from individuals with obvious serious respiratory or other infections.

Nutrition and Gastrointestinal Functions

The height and weight of children with immunodeficiency should be documented at 3- to 6-month intervals with a standard growth chart. Adults should be weighed regularly as well. A falling off of growth or an absolute weight loss is an ominous feature of immunodeficiency and suggests that infections are not under good control or that other medical conditions (e.g., hypothyroidism, chronic diarrhea, malignancy) are present. Chronic antibiotic therapy may decrease appetite and cause diarrhea. Febrile episodes with severe chronic infections will decrease appetite, increase metabolic demands, and result in slow growth.

Nutritional assessment including a calorie count may be indicated, and a dietary supplement might be tried. A multivitamin and mineral supplement is also advisable.

If there is noninfectious chronic diarrhea, a search for malabsorption, food intolerance, and hypovitaminosis is indicated. Symptoms of night blindness, proximal weakness, ataxia, or tremor should raise suspicions of secondary deficiencies of fat-soluble vitamins that are reversible on treatment (Aukrust et al., 2000). Coeliac disease may not necessarily present with frank malabsorption or even diarrhea; weight loss alone should lead to investigation of the gastrointestinal tract. However, it is important to remember that partial villous atrophy is common and due not just to coeliac disease. There should be a careful search for microbial agents, inflammatory bowel disease, and structural abnormalities of the gastrointestinal tract.

Many immunodeficiencies are associated with autoimmune or viral hepatitis and past or present use of intravenous immunoglobulin (IVIG) may result in hepatitis C (Centers for Disease Control, 1994). Liver function tests should be done at yearly intervals, although more regularly (3 to 6 months) in those receiving immunoglobulin therapy since early treatment of hepatitis C has been shown to be more effective (Chapel et al., 2001).

Respiratory and Pulmonary Problems

Sinusitis, bronchitis, and recurrent pneumonia are common in patients with most forms of immunodeficiency and are often the chief cause of morbidity and mortality (Hermananski and Webster, 1993). Sinusitis must be suspected if the patient has one of the following: purulent nasal discharge, frontal headaches, chronic nasal obstruction, postnasal drip, a decreased gag reflex, or unexplained coughing or wheezing. A microbial diagnosis including fungal cultures should be sought. Waters view sinus films are of value, particularly in youngsters, but a CT scan of the sinuses is used for definitive diagnosis. Treatment consists of prolonged courses of antibiotics, nasal decongestants, and nasal steroids. Nasal polyps should be surgically removed. Surgical sinus drainage is sometimes indicated if long-term antibiotics are not curative.

Many patients with a significant immunodeficiency develop pneumonia at one time or another and must be treated promptly. Vigorous exercise including team sports should be encouraged. A chronic cough due to bronchiectasis or wheezing is cause for special concern; attempts to detect structural damage or reversible airways disease are essential. Under such circumstances, pulmonary function tests are conducted, including the response to bronchodilator therapy. If bronchiectasis is found on CT scan, regular physiotherapy should be instigated. If the patient has antibody deficiency, a trial of a higher-dose IVIG (400–800 mg/kg) might be used and has been shown to improve pulmonary function (Bernatowska et al., 1987; Roifman et al., 1987; Eijkhout et al., 2001). If the patient is old enough, routine pulmonary function testing at 6-month or yearly intervals is recommended for all but the mildest immunodeficiency syndromes.

Patients who develop pulmonary infiltrations not responsive to antibiotics should undergo bronchoalveolar lavage or lung biopsy for an exact microbiologic diagnosis. Lung biopsy may reveal nonmicrobial granulomatous disease (Mechanic et al., 1997); Viallard et al., 1998; (Wislez et al., 2000), lymphoid interstitial pneumonitis (LIP) (Davies et al., 2000), or even frank lymphoma.

Immunodeficient individuals with chronic lung disease should be started on a program of pulmonary therapy including postural drainage, the use of a flutter devise to loosen secretions, and inhaled bronchodilators or other agents (Atrovent, cromolyn, an-

tibiotics). It is particularly important to identify patients likely to develop chronic lung disease early so that periodic assessment of pulmonary function, management of sinus disease, and vigorous treatment of early pulmonary infections can be undertaken. Pneumatoceles and abscesses must be treated surgically. Some patients with phagocytic deficiency also have IgE-mediated allergies and benefit from inhaled corticosteroids and oral antihistamines.

Skin Problems

Patients with immunodeficiency often have cutaneous abnormalities (telangiectasia, molluscum contagiosum, warts, eczema, etc.). The most common cutaneous complication is chronic skin infection, particularly in the hyper-IgE immunodeficiency syndrome and in certain T cell deficiencies such as mucocutaneous candidiasis. Most of these patients require local and systemic antibiotics, usually prophylactically.

Chronic eczema is a common problem in the immunocompetent population but this may be more severe or become infected in the immunodeficient patient. It is a cardinal feature of Wiskott-Aldrich syndrome (see Chapter 31). Local steroids, tacrolimus ointment, and antipruritic medications are the mainstays of therapy. If there is cracking, weeping, or regional lymphadenopathy, antibiotics, either local or systemic, should be used. Clarithromycin is particularly well tolerated in chronic eczema. Severe warts are not uncommon (Barnett et al., 1983) and may be the indicator of a rare syndrome, warts, hypogammaglobulinemia, infection, myelokathexis (WHIM) (see Chapter 23), and are often refractory to usual methods of control. Some success has been achieved with increased doses of immunoglobulin.

Aloplecia or vitiligo are also relatively common in antibody deficient adults with common variable immunodeficiency (CVID); both of these distressing conditions are untreatable. Subcutaneous granulomata (as well as pulmonary and gastrointestinal granulomata) are not uncommon in CVID. There are several reports suggesting that these granulomas respond to anti–tumor necrosis factor (TNF) therapy with etanercept (Smith and Skelton, 2001; Lin et al., 2006) or infliximab (Hatab et al., 2005; Thatayatikom et al., 2005).

Vaccines

A review of immunization strategies in special clinical circumstances is provided in the "Rod Book" (American Academy of Pediatrics, 2000), Live attenuated vaccines including smallpox, poliomyelitis, measles, mumps, rubella, bacillus Calmette-Guérin (BCG), and varicella should be avoided in all severe antibody or cellular immunodeficiencies because of the risk of vaccine-induced infection. The evidence from HIV-infected children suggests that it is safe to give live virus vaccines to those with CD4 counts above $200 \times 10^9/l$. These vaccines have also been given without sequelae to patients with selective IgA deficiency, mucocutaneous candidiasis with intact cellular immunity to other antigens, and phagocytic and complement immunodeficiencies and to children fully reconstituted following bone marrow transplantation.

Paralytic poliomyelitis, chronic encephalitis, and prolonged poliovirus shedding from the gastrointestinal tract together are recognized complications of attenuated live poliomyelitis vaccination in immunodeficiency (Wyatt, 1973). Parents, siblings, and other household members should be given inactivated poliomyelitis vaccine because of the risk of spread to the patient of live vaccine-strain virus.

Other routine vaccines should be given to patients with adequate antibody immunity, including a yearly influenza vaccine. We also administer killed vaccines to patients with partial antibody deficiencies (e.g., IgG subclass deficiency, ataxia-telangiectasia). The antibody response to these vaccines can be used to assess their B cell function. Many such patients have a short-lived antibody response that subsequently decreases in 6–12 months. Vaccines (except for attenuated poliovirus) should also be given to family members of patients with immunodeficiency. Individuals with a propensity to lower or upper respiratory infection and some antibody function should be given pneumococcal polysaccharide vaccine. For patients with intact cellular immunity, periodic tuberculin testing may be indicated, particularly if steroid therapy is anticipated.

Antibiotics and Antivirals

Antibiotics are life saving in the treatment of infectious episodes of patients with immunodeficiency. The choice and dosage of antibiotics for specific infections are identical to those used in normal subjects but it is essential that treatment be started early. Culture specimens may be obtained prior to therapy; these will be especially important if the infection does not respond promptly to the initial antibiotic chosen.

Patients should be overtreated for infectious episodes, even if this necessitates frequent or chronic use of antibiotics and occasional unnecessary hospitalizations. If the infection does not respond promptly to antibiotics, the physician should consider the possibility of fungal, mycobacterial, viral, or protozoal (*Pneumocystis carinii* also named *jiraveci*) infection. Invasive procedures such as bronchoalveolar lavage or biopsy may be necessary.

Antiviral therapy can be used effectively in many immunodeficiencies. Exposure to influenza or early symptomatic influenza infection can be managed with amantadine or ramatidine or the neuraminidase inhibitor drugs zanamivir and oseltamivir. Severe herpes simplex infection, chickenpox, or herpes zoster should be treated with acyclovir. Ribavirin aerosols have been used in the treatment of respiratory syncytial virus and parainfluenza viral infections occurring in severe immunodeficiencies (McIntosh et al., 1984). Acyclovir can also be used in the incubation period to modify or prevent chickenpox (Asano et al., 1993). Topical cidofovir has been used successfully to treat severe molluscum contagiosum (Davies et al., 1999).

Antibiotics should be given prophylactically with each dental or surgical procedure. Amoxicillin and gentamycin can be given intravenously 1 hour before and 8 and 18 hours after major surgery, or 3 days of oral broad-spectrum antibiotics can be used for less serious manipulation (e.g., dental procedures).

Antimicrobial Prophylaxis

Continuous prophylactic antibiotics often are of benefit in immunodeficiencies. They are especially useful in disorders characterized by rapid, overwhelming infections (e.g., complement deficiencies or in Wiskott-Aldrich syndrome if splenectomized or not receiving immunoglobulin therapy). They can also be used in patients with antibody deficiencies, especially in those with structural damage, when recurrent infections occur despite optimal immunoglobulin therapy, and in phagocytic disorders in which no other form of therapy is available. In these instances, penicillin, ampicillin, or dicloxacillin given orally, 0.5–1.0 g/day in divided doses, is recommended. Alternatively, azithromycin given once daily (5 mg/kg, maximum 250 mg/day) for 3 consecutive days every 2 weeks may be effective. In those rare babies with significantly delayed maturation of antibody production

Table 46.1. Recommendations for Prophylaxis Against *Pneumocystis carinii* in HIV and Primary Immunodeficiency on the Basis of CD4 Lymphocyte Count

Age	CD4 count
<12 months	<1500 cells/l
12–23 months	<750 cells/l
2–5 years	<500 cells/l
>5 years	<200 cells/l
Adults	<200 cells/l

Patients with a CD4 count <25% of total lymphocytes
Past history of *Pneumocystis carinii* infecion
Patients with X-linked hyper-IgM syndrome (CD40L mutations)
All patients with severe combined immunodeficiency

associated with recurrent bacterial infections, temporary prophylaxis may be used until the immune system has matured.

Pneumocystis carinii pneumonia (PCP) prophylaxis is recommended for children with significant primary and secondary cellular (T cell) immunodeficiencies (Centers for Disease Control, 1991) (see Table 46.1). Prophylaxis consists of trimethoprim-sulfamethoxazole (TMP/SMX), 160 mg/M^2 of body surface per day of the TMP and 750 mg/M^2 per day of SMX given orally in divided doses twice per day three times per week, with frequent checks of the leukocyte count. Alternative drugs for PCP prophylaxis include pentamidine, dapsone, and atovaquone.

Immunoglobulin Therapy

Two types of human immunoglobulin formulation are available for therapeutic use: intravenous immunoglobulin (IVIG) and the concentrated liquid products (IMIG, SCIG), occasionally used for intramuscular use but now mostly used for subcutaneous infusions. The route of administration depends on the dose needed to keep the patient free of infection and patient preference. Immunoglobulin therapy is indicated only for those patients with proven antibody deficiency (see Table 46.2). Immunoglobulin is not of value in the treatment of cellular, phagocytic, or complement immunodeficiencies, and it is of only limited value in combined antibody and cellu-

Table 46.2. Primary Immunodeficiencies in Which Human Intravenous or Subcutaneous Immunoglobulin May Be Beneficial

Antibody Deficiencies

X-linked and autosomal agammaglobulinemia (Chapters 21, 22)
Common variable immunodeficiency, including deficiencies of ICOS, Baff receptor, CD19, and TACI (Chapter 23)
Hyper-IgM syndromes (both X-linked and autosomal recessive forms, Chapters 19, 20)
Transient hypogammaglobulinemia of infancy (in selected cases)
IgG subclass deficiency, with or without IgA deficiency (in selected cases)
Antibody deficiency with normal serum immunoglobulins

Combined Deficiencies

Severe combined immunodeficiencies (all types prior to BMT and after BMT, if reconstitution of B cells has failed, Chapters 9–16)
Wiskott-Aldrich syndrome (if associated with severe immunodeficiency)
Ataxia-telangiectasia (if antibody deficiency, Chapter 29)
Short-limbed dwarfism or cartilage hair hypoplasia
Bare lymphocyte syndromes (Chapters 17, 18)
X-linked lymphoproliferative syndrome (possible benefit) (Chapter 32)
22q11 deletion syndromes (if severe antibody deficiency) (Chapter 33)

BMT, bone marrow transplantation; ICOS, inducible costimulator.

Table 46.3. Preparation of Intravenous Immunoglobulin from Cohn Fraction II*

1. Physical removal of aggregates by ultracentrifugation or gel filtration
2. Treatment with proteolytic enzymes
3. Treatment with chemicals that reduce sulfhydryl bonds, followed by alkylation of the free SH bonds
4. Addition of disaccharides as stabilizing agent
5. Incubation at low pH

*These methods are used to eliminate high–molecular weight complexes.

lar immunodeficiencies, though used routinely prior to bone marrow transplantation (BMT) and also in those BMT recipients in whom only the T cell system is reconstituted.

Immunoglobulin of either type is extracted from plasma pooled from 10,000–50,000 donors; the individual donor units are first screened for hepatitis B and C viruses and HIV (see below). After the cryoprecipitate is removed, cold ethanol (Cohn) fractionation of the resultant precipitate is used in several steps to concentrate the immunoglobulin and remove other serum proteins and live organisms, thus providing a sterile product (see Table 46.3). It contains a wide spectrum of antibodies to viral and bacterial antigens.

Immunoglobulin is >95% IgG, but trace quantities of IgM and IgA are present. The IgM and IgA globulins are therapeutically insignificant because of their short half-lives (less than 7 days) and their low concentrations in the immunoglobulin preparation. Immunoglobulin contains all IgG subclasses and multiple IgG allotypes (Gm and Km types). It is then treated by solvent-detergent or other chemicals, by pasteurization or nanofiltration for viral inactivation or virus removal, and brought to a 16.5% concentration for subcutaneous or intramuscular use.

Intravenous immunoglobulin therapy

IVIG is the most widely used treatment for several primary and secondary immunodeficiency syndromes (Table 46.2) (Stiehm, 1977). It is prepared from Cohn fraction II by eliminating high–molecular weight complexes and their resultant anticomplementary activity. Over 20 IVIG preparations have been used worldwide, and because of patent laws, all are slightly different and may therefore have minimally different risks. In practice, all of these preparations offer acceptable serum half-lives (18–25 days), contain all IgG subclasses, have minimal anticomplementary activity, have a good and diverse antibody content, and are negative for hepatitis B surface antigen (HBsAg), hepatitis C virus (HCV), and HIV.

There are several advantages to the administration of immunoglobulin by the intravenous route (see Table 46.4). Dosage,

Table 46.4. Advantages and Disadvantages of Intravenous Immunoglobulin

Advantages

Ease of administering large doses
More rapid action
No loss in tissues from proteolysis
Avoidance of painful intramuscular injections

Disadvantages

Requires venous access
Long duration of infusion
Occasional serious side effects

methods of administration, and adverse reactions are discussed in the section specifically devoted to antibody deficiencies.

Subcutaneous immunoglobulin therapy

Immunoglobulin for subcutaneous (SCIG) (and intramuscular) use is a sterile 16.5% (165 mg/ml) solution preferably without preservative. Immunoglobulin preparations for intramuscular injection in the United States may have thimerosal as a preservative and are therefore unsuitable for subcutaneous or higher dosage intramuscular use. An exception is Gamastan (Talecris), formulated as a 16% preparation without preservative, licensed in the United States for single intramuscular dose, but also used for subcutaneous infusion. Additional immunoglobulin preparations suitable for subcutaneous infusion are now available (Vivaglobin, ZLB-Behring).

Since there is no further modification step, the final product contains large molecular-weight complexes that are strongly anticomplementary and probably account for the occasional systemic reactions to 16% immunoglobulin if inadvertently injected intravenously; intravenous injections are contraindicated.

Slow subcutaneous infusion of IVIG at a concentration of 10%–12% has been given in the United States without adverse events (Welch and Stiehm, 1983; Stiehm et al., 1998). Dosage, methods of administration, and adverse reactions are discussed in the section devoted to antibody deficiencies.

Intramuscular immunoglobulin therapy

Intramuscular immunoglobulin therapy with the 16% product was used exclusively for the treatment of antibody deficiency up through the early 1980s, when IVIG was introduced. The recommended dose was 100 mg/kg per month, based on studies of the British Medical Research Council (1969). Treatment was given weekly at a dose of 25 mg/kg because of the large volumes needed (50 ml/month for a 70 kg adult).

Intramuscular injections are painful and have occasionally resulted in sterile abscesses at the site of injections. Adverse events were relatively uncommon, other than the local reactions. Occasional anaphylactic reactions have been reported, as well as one case of acrodynia in the United States from the mercury preservative (Matheson et al., 1980).

Presently, only an occasional patient is treated by this route because the amount of immunoglobulin that can be administered intramuscularly is limited and serious breakthrough infections may still occur.

Hepatitis C–Contaminated Intravenous Immunoglobulin

Hepatitis C virus has been transmitted through a number of IVIG lots (Lever et al., 1984; Ochs et al., 1985; Bjorkander et al., 1988; Williams et al., 1989; Bjoro et al., 1994; Centers for Disease Control, 1994; Schiff, 1994; Yap et al., 1994; Yu et al., 1995; Christie et al., 1997; Razvi et al., 2001). It has not been transmitted through commercial immunoglobulin made for intramuscular use even when given in large doses subcutaneously. SCIG preparations produced in recent years undergo testing for HCV by polymerase chain reaction (PCR) and viral inactivation steps.

The most recent outbreak of hepatitis C (Centers for Disease Control, 1994; Schiff et al., 1994; Yu et al., 1995; Healey et al., 1996; Christie et al., 1997; Razvi et al., 2001) followed the exclusion of plasma containing antibodies to HCV. Because HCV does not induce the production of detectable antibodies for up to 6 months after exposure in immunocompetent individuals (the open-window period), unchallenged virus from a few viremic donors may have contaminated a limited number of batches (Yu et al., 1995). Over 200 patients worldwide became infected (Centers for Disease Control, 1994; Schiff, 1994; Yu et al., 1995; Healey et al., 1996; Christie et al., 1997). The Gammagard/Polygam preparations involved in the outbreak were replaced with Gammagard-SD and Polygam-SD, whose manufacture now include a solvent-detergent treatment to inactivate HCV and other membrane-enveloped viruses.

In a previous outbreak, Bjoro et al. (1994) reported that immunocompromised patients had a severe and rapidly progressive course of hepatitis C infection, and the responses to interferon (IFN) were poor. However, this was a study of patients with chronic infection of undefined length and unknown or mixed genotypes of HCV.

The 1993/1994 outbreak in the United Kingdom and United States provided a unique opportunity to study the long-term rate of progression of HCV and responses to therapy in patients with known onset of infection and a single genotype, genotype 1a (Christie et al., 1997; Razvi et al., 2000; Chapel et al., 2001). With early (acute phase) high-dose IFN-α therapy, over half the patients cleared the virus and remain clear at 5 years (Chapel et al., 2001). Razvi et al. (2001) reported that 16 of 58 (27%) immunodeficient patients who developed HCV infection from IVIG resolved their infection; this rate of recovery was the same as that in IFN-α-treated patients and those receiving no therapy.

There have been no further reports of HCV infections transmitted by IVIG since 1994. Manufacturers of IVIG are now required to show that the virus inactivation processes are relevant to human disease. They have substantiated the antiviral efficacy of low pH and pepsin treatment and other procedures to inactivate HCV and other viruses including solvent-detergent, caprylate precipitation, heat treatment, and nanofiltration. Each of the various methods has been validated to be effective, but none can guarantee the total absence of known infectious virus, let alone unknown or new viruses.

No cases of HIV transmission have been identified with IVIG administration (Henin et al., 1988; Schiff, 1994) because of the efficient inactivation or partitioning of retroviruses by cold ethanol fractionation.

Prion Disease and Intravenous Immunoglobulin

Several IVIG lots derived from plasma obtained from donors subsequently found to be at risk for Creutzfeld-Jakob disease (CJD) have been recalled, although no cases of CJD or variant CJD (vCDJ) associated with mad cow disease transmitted by IVIG have been reported to date. Tests to identify prions in serum are being developed.

Vigilance is needed in this area, and the International Union of Immunological Societies (IUIS) Committee for Primary Immunodeficiency Diseases encourages early referral to the Edinburgh Surveillance Unit of immunoglobulin recipients, especially those on long-term, repeated therapy, if they develop unexplained neurological or psychiatric symptoms. Ziegner et al. (2002) have reported unexplained neurodegeneration in 14 immunodeficient patients treated with IVIG in the United States and Europe, although none of these patients has proven to have prion disease.

Currently, British plasma and that from individuals who have lived in Great Britain for more than 3 months between 1980 and 1996 or who have stayed in Europe for an accumulative time of more than 5 years since 1980 are excluded from use for immunoglobulin production in the United States.

Special High-Titered Immune Globulins

Following chickenpox or herpes zoster exposure of the immunodeficient child, varicella-zoster immune globulin (VZIG) may be given to prevent chickenpox. Alternatively, or in combination, oral acyclovir can be used. For antibody-deficient children receiving regular IVIG infusions at monthly intervals, VZIG is not usually given because IVIG contains antibody to varicella/zoster virus. Even if not prevented, varicella infections are markedly attenuated by IVIG.

RSV-IG (RespiGam), licensed in 1996 in the United States, was a high-titered human IVIG that prevented or modified respiratory syncytial virus (RSV) infections in high-risk infants such as ex-prematures and infants with bronchopulmonary dysplasia (Groothuis et al., 1993) during the respiratory virus season (November–April). RSV-IG was also recommended in the United States for patients with severe primary or secondary immunodeficiencies who were under the age of 2, and was used in infants under age 2 with combined immunodeficiency who were undergoing stem cell transplantation. RespiGam was replaced in 2003 with monthly intramuscular injections of the RSV monoclonal antibody palivizumab (Synagis, 15 mg/kg), along with regular IVIG infusion.

RSV-specific antibody has been used for treatment of infants with life-threatening RSV infections, in combination with ribavirin. Proof of efficacy in treatment protocols is lacking, however.

The prophylactic use of other high-titered immunoglobulins such as tetanus immunoglobulin (TIG) and hepatitis B immunoglobulin (HBIG) following exposure to these agents is particularly important in the unimmunized immunodeficient patient.

Corticosteroids

Corticosteroids are occasionally necessary in patients with immunodeficiency for such problems as asthma, lymphoid interstitial pneumonitis, and obstructive gastrointestinal or genitourinary tract lesions of chronic granulomatous disease, hemolytic anemia, anaphylactic reactions, or graft-versus-host disease. Short-term courses are well tolerated; if chronic or high-dose corticosteroid therapy is used, PCP prophylaxis should be considered. We have used inhaled corticosteroids in children with chronic granulomatous disease and local steroids for eczema in Wiskott-Aldrich syndrome and other immunodeficiencies without complications.

Prolonged high-dose corticosteroids will severely depress the lymphocyte count, including that of T and B cell subpopulations, in normal children, Lymphoproliferative and antibody responses usually remain intact (Lack et al., 1996).

Prenatal and Neonatal Management

If a previous sibling has had a severe T cell immunodeficiency and the mother is again pregnant, a number of options must be considered and prior planning is imperative. Fetal blood sampling is possible by 18–20 weeks gestation and can be used for the study and identification of cellular elements. If the molecular defect is known through gene analysis of affected family members, prenatal diagnosis can be performed by analyzing fetal DNA obtained by means of choriovillous biopsy (CVS) or by collecting amniocytes.

Cesarean section may be performed if a difficult labor is anticipated; however, it is not routinely indicated. Cesarean section prior to labor is recommended when neonatal thrombocytopenia is anticipated, such as in Wiskott-Aldrich syndrome, to prevent a cerebral bleed during labor. At birth, cord blood should be obtained for blood count, immunoglobulin assays, B and T cell enumeration, phytohemagglutinin (PHA) stimulation, and human leukocyte antigen (HLA) typing to detect maternal chimerism. The rest of the cord blood may also be cryopreserved for possible future gene therapy.

Newborns suspected to have combined immunodeficiency should remain in a protective environment with reverse isolation or in an isolator with food and liquid sterilized until his or her immunologic status is clarified or definitive treatment completed. A chest X-ray for thymic size should be done as soon as possible; an absent thymic shadow in an unstressed newborn is highly suggestive of a T cell immunodeficiency. Gastrointestinal sterilization (with nonabsorbable antibiotics) and PCP prophylaxis (with TMP-SMX) should be considered for patients with severe T cell immunodeficiency. PCP prophylaxis is indicated for young infants (after age 6 weeks) with suspected cellular immunodeficiency and CD4 cells <1500 cells/μl^3, which is less than the fifth percentile for that age-group (Stiehm et al., 2004).

The importance of an early diagnosis and treatment of primary immune deficiency to prevent death or long-term complications cannot be overemphasized. However, prevention of immunodeficiency is limited. In the main, it is only applicable to those with a previous affected pregnancy or positive family history. These considerations are of particular importance in countries where consanguineous marriages are common. Measures include providing genetic counseling to a family at risk, arranging for prenatal diagnosis, and, in certain circumstances, termination of pregnancy.

Prenatal diagnosis is of value if early treatment, therapeutic abortion, or cesarian section are possibilities. In utero tissue typing of the fetus is sometimes of value to identify a potential matched related or unrelated donor, or an umbilical cord transplant donor (Vowels et al., 1993). In utero haploidentical BMT has been accomplished (Flake et al., 1996; Bartolome et al., 2002).

Family Studies

Immunoglobulin and complement levels should be obtained in the immediate family of all patients with antibody or complement deficiencies to determine a familial pattern. If other family members have suggestive histories, they should also be studied. Newborn siblings of an affected patient are followed carefully from birth for manifestations of a similar disorder. In disorders in which procedures are available for heterozygosity testing, the parents, siblings, and children of the affected subject can be tested.

Support Groups

Participation in support groups (listed at end of this chapter) provides essential information and help for patients and their families with schooling, insurance, access to medical care, etc. Medical and nursing teams can provide only limited resources to help families cope with the social, economic, emotional, and psychologic issues that these diseases impose on families. Other patients and families can offer a perspective and mutual support not obtainable from medical personnel.

Antibody Deficiencies

In patients with severe symptomatic antibody deficiency (see Table 46.2), such as X-linked agammaglobulinemia, common

variable immunodeficiency, and the hyper-IgM syndromes, human immunoglobulin replacement therapy is the mainstay of therapy.

Immunoglobulin Therapy

Like the well-controlled diabetic on insulin therapy, many patients on regular immunoglobulin replacement are able to live symptom-free. However, some immunodeficient subjects given immunoglobulin remain chronically ill or undergo a progressive downhill course. Often these patients have immunologic or hematologic deficits other than antibody deficiency or have developed chronic lung or gastrointestinal disease. Patients with IgG subclass deficiency, transient hypogammaglobulinemia of infancy, and selective IgA deficiency should not be treated with immunoglobulin unless there is documented failure to produce specific antibodies following immunization.

Intravenous immunoglobulin

Dosage. Several studies indicate that larger doses of IVIG (400–800 mg/kg) are superior to lower doses (100–200 mg/kg per month) in terms of subjective improvement, reduced hospitalization rates, improved chest X-rays or CT scans, normalization of pulmonary function, and decreased incidence of major or minor infections (Montanaro and Pirofsky, 1984; Ochs et al., 1984; Bernatowska et al., 1987; Roifman et al., 1987; Garbett et al., 1989; Liese et al., 1992; Haeney, 1994; Stiehm, 1997). The aim of IVIG therapy is to maintain the serum IgG concentration at a sufficient level to keep the patient free of infection, usually at a trough level of IgG that is within the normal range or at least 400 mg/dl above the pretreatment baseline level.

A common practice is to start IVIG at 400 mg/kg at monthly intervals but give additional doses at the onset of therapy to raise the IgG level quickly. After initiation of IVIG, the trough level of IgG increases over several months as the tissue spaces become saturated with immunoglobulin. After 3 months the preinfusion IgG level is assessed and the dose adjusted (Stiehm, 1997). A few patients with chronic lung disease, vasculitis, rheumatic complaints, chronic diarrhea and protein-losing enteropathy, or failure to thrive may require a higher dose (e.g., 0.8–1.0 g/kg per month) to control disease manifestations (Roifman et al., 1987; Eijkhout et al., 2001).

Administration of intravenous immunoglobulin. IVIG administration requires venous access, which is sometimes a problem in small children. The use of EMLA cream, a local analgesic, applied to the infusion site 1 hour prior to starting the infusion, or a more rapidly acting spray, makes venipuncture much more acceptable to young children.

Close monitoring is initially required, especially during the first two infusions, when close to half of adult patients, particularly those with CVID, develop fever, chills, muscle ache, or nausea. However, adverse reactions are infrequent when IVIG is given regularly and at adequate doses, provided the correct rates for infusions are observed and the patients are not infused during a breakthrough infection (Brennan et al., 1995).

In Europe and the United States, IVIG infusions have been shown to be sufficiently safe to enable some patients (adults and children) to receive infusions at home with the help of either a home infusion service or a responsible adult family member or by self-infusion. Self-infusion without another informed adult in the house is discouraged. In one study, the number of adverse reactions in selected patients was 0.1%, and universally the reactions were mild (Brennan et al., 1995). Nurses, parents, or patients who perform home infusions must be taught to recognize and treat adverse reactions, and their competency documented.

In patients who have received infusions without adverse events, self- or parent administration at home can be accomplished at great cost savings (Ashida and Saxon, 1986; Sorensen et al., 1987; Kobayashi et al., 1990). Until recently, when subcutaneous infusion was introduced, this type of therapy was used by 75% of patients in the United Kingdom and some parts of Europe. In the United States, however, most IVIG infusions, with some exceptions, are performed in a clinic setting or by professional home infusion personnel.

Typically, an IVIG infusion requires 2–4 hours to administer. The initial rate is 0.5 mg/kg/min (0.01 ml/kg/min of the 5% product) and this can be doubled at 20- to 30-minute intervals if there are no side effects, to a maximal rate of 2 to 3 mg/kg/minute (0.04–0.06 ml/kg/minute). Adverse events tend to be associated with rapid infusion rates in patients with concurrent acute infections or previously untreated patients, or when significant time between infusions has transpired (>4-week intervals). On the other hand, if infusions are given more frequently, for example, every 2 weeks, the rate of adverse events is very low indeed.

Side effects of intravenous immunoglobulin therapy. Typical reactions associated with infusions include headaches, nausea and vomiting, flushing, chills, myalgia, arthralgia, and abdominal pain (Ochs et al., 1980; Duhem et al., 1994, Stiehm, 1997). Occasionally, chest tightness, hives, and anaphylactoid reactions can occur. Very rarely, severe, life-threatening anaphylactic reactions may be triggered.

Immediate minor reactions can be avoided or diminished by slowing the infusion rate. Patients with minor side effects such as headaches, shaking chills, nausea and vomiting, or myalgia/arthralgia can be treated (and for subsequent infusions pretreated) with oral acetaminophenon or a nonsteroidal anti-inflammatory drug and antihistamines. Severe reactions are treated with parenteral epinephrine, antihistamines, and corticosteroids.

If a severe reaction is anticipated, in addition to oral acetaminophen and antihistamines, hydrocortisone (6 mg/kg, maximum 100 mg) can also be given intravenously 1 hour before infusion. These drugs can be repeated after 3 or 4 hours if the infusion is not finished. Occasionally, switching to a different IVIG product may alleviate reactions.

Serious late but very rare adverse reactions are almost always confined to high-dose usage of IVIG in immunomodulating doses (Duhem et al., 1994). These include aseptic meningitis (Kato et al., 1988; Vera-Ramirez et al., 1992), thrombosis and disseminated intravascular coagulation (Woodruff et al., 1986; Comenzo et al., 1992), renal (Miller et al., 1992) and pulmonary (Rault et al., 1991) insufficiency, and hemolytic anemia (Brox et al., 1987).

IVIG is contraindicated in patients who have had an anaphylactic reaction to IVIG or other blood products. IVIG is initially given with great caution in patients who have IgG subclass deficiencies with IgA deficiency and/or anti-IgA antibodies (Burks et al., 1986), as these patients may be at higher risk of a serious reaction.

Certain brands of IVIG may be more reactogenic. In one study of Kawasaki disease, the two IVIG brands used were equivalent therapeutically, but one had a 12-fold (2% vs. 25%) increase in side effects (Rosenfeld et al., 1995).

A few investigators have given high concentrations (9%–12% solutions) infused rapidly over a period of 20–40 minutes. This rapid rate can be tolerated by some but not all patients (Schiff

et al., 1991). This dosage should be administered only by experienced personnel equipped to manage serious adverse reactions.

Subcutaneous immune globulin

Subcutaneous infusion of immunoglobulin (SCIG) has been developed as an alternative to IVIG. The monthly dose is the same as that for IVIG, starting typically at 0.4 g/kg per month, in divided doses every week. Initially, SCIG was given as a 16% formulation by slow subcutaneous infusion at a rate of 0.05 to 0.2 ml/kg/hour or 1–10 ml/hour, using a syringe driver as a pump (Berger et al., 1980). Because of contamination of an early IVIG product with HCV in Scandinavia and the availability of SCIG at costs lower than that of IVIG preparations, subcutaneous infusion of a 16% preparation became the predominant mode of immunoglobulin prophylaxis in northern Europe (Gardulf et al., 1991).

Rapid ("express") SCIG infusions at up to 40 ml/hour are well tolerated (Gardulf et al., 1995, 2001; Hansen et al., 2002). Because the technique of inserting a 23- or 25-gauge needle subcutaneously is simple and severe side effects are not encountered, the injections are self-administered into the abdominal wall and/or thighs by use of a battery-powered pump. The injections are well tolerated with minimal local reactions (pain or redness), and rarely do systemic reactions occur (Gardulf et al., 1991, 1995; Abrahamsen et al., 1996; Chapel et al., 2000; Berger, 2004; Gardulf et al., 2006; Ochs et al., 2006).

Because subcutaneous infusions are well tolerated and not associated with serious adverse events, there are no strict guidelines on how to initiate subcutaneous infusions. The following techniques have been used in several centers and accepted by most patients. The preparations best suited for subcutaneous infusion are those with 16% IgG and without preservatives. This type of preparation is licensed for intramuscular injections in the United States, under the trade name Gamastan. ZLB Behring has recently released its 16% IgG preparation (Vivagloblin) after extensive testing (Gardulf et al., 2006; Ochs et al., 2006) in Europe and the United States.

The standard dose is 100 to 150 mg/kg/week, approximately 45–60 ml of a 16% solution for a 70 kg patient. The infusion sites are most often the four abdominal quadrants and alternatively the lateral thighs and the lateral aspect of the upper arms. For administration, 23- to 25-gauge butterfly steel needles are preferred. Depending on the thickness of the subcutaneous tissue, the needle can be bent at the base 0° to 90° and secured with tape. If more than 20 ml is needed, a "Y" tubing or "triple" tubing allows simultaneous infusion at two or three sites. A simple syringe driving pump (e.g., Autosyringe AS-3B or Graseby MS16) can be used to deliver quantities of between 10 and 50 ml. Infusion of not more than 15 to 25 ml per site is recommended. Most patients infuse 20 ml per site over a 1-hour interval and are highly satisfied (Nicolay et al., 2006).

Patients switched from IVIG to subcutaneous infusion should receive their first dose within 1 week after the last IVIG infusion. Newly diagnosed patients who have not been treated with any form of immunoglobulin replacement can be started directly on subcutaneous treatment by loading with several daily doses of immunoglobulin (Berger, 2004). Ugazio et al. (1982) and Waniewski et al. (1993) have demonstrated that administration of five daily subcutaneous infusions (at 100 mg/kg each) can bring patients very rapidly to an apparent steady state that is then maintained by weekly subcutaneous infusions. Local anesthetic such as EMLA cream is widely used, especially in pediatric patients.

In infants and small children, subcutaneous infusions of 2 to 3 ml per site can be given directly without a pump over a 2- to

5-minute period. Depending on the size of the child, one or two subcutaneous injections per week may be sufficient. Daily direct injections without a pump are preferred by some adult patients so as to avoid the use of a pump. For a 70 kg patient, the daily volume of 16% SCIG would be approximately 6 ml, or 2 × 3 ml per site.

A multicenter comparison of the efficacy and safety of IVIG vs. SCIG replacement therapy showed no significant differences in rates of breakthrough infections or adverse reactions (Chapel et al., 2000). Two recent multicenter studies that included both pediatric and adult patients in a comparison of hospital-based IVIG to home-based SCIG therapy demonstrated that home-based SCIG therapy improved several important aspects of quality of life and provided patients and their families with greater independence and better control of aspects of treatment and daily life (Gardulf et al., 2004; Nicolay et al., 2006). Subcutaneous administration of immunoglobulin by infusion from a small pump or by direct injection is safe and easy to learn and represents an alternative to IVIG treatment regimens.

Intravenous immunoglobulin for treatment of enterovirus encephalitis and polymyositis

Chronic meningoencephalitis and polymyositis or fasciitis due to disseminated enterovirus infection (usually ECHOvirus) may occur in patients with X-linked agammaglobulinemia (XLA) (Wilfert et al., 1977; Mease et al., 1981; Erlendsson et al., 1985; Johnson et al., 1985; Lederman and Winklestein, 1985; Prentice et al., 1985; Crennan et al., 1986; McKinney et al., 1987; Schmugge et al., 1999; Quartier et al., 2000) and to a lesser extent in patients with CD40L deficiency (Cunningham et al., 1999) or CVID. Polymerase chain reaction may be required for establishing the diagnosis (Chesky et al., 2000). Since the introduction of IVIG, the incidence of disseminated enteroviral infections has dropped dramatically, but it still may occur in some patients receiving adequate doses of IVIG (Rotbart, 1990; Misbah et al., 1992) or in children prior to a diagnosis of XLA.

Treatment with high-dose IVIG may modify the severity of infection and improve survival (Mease et al., 1981; Erlendsson et al., 1985; Prentice et al., 1985; Quartier et al., 2000), but failure of high-dose IVIG has been reported (Johnson et al., 1985; Crennan et al., 1986). The response to IVIG may depend on the titer of neutralizing antibodies in the preparation against the specific echovirus (Mease et al., 1981). A review of published reports (Stiehm and Keller, 2004) indicates that more affected patients treated with IVIG survived than those given intramuscular immunoglobulin or immune plasma; of those who did not receive IVIG, none survived. The use of intraventricular infusion of IVIG contributed to the eradication of the virus in some patients but not in others. Patients originally responding appropriately to high-dose IVIG may relapse later (Mease et al., 1985; H.D. Ochs, personal observation).

Intravenous immunoglobulin for treatment of other viral infections

IVIG has been advocated for the treatment of chronic Epstein-Barr virus (EBV) infection. In uncontrolled studies, selected patients have shown clinical improvement (Tobi and Straus, 1985; Finberg, 1988). It has been suggested that IVIG be used prophylactically in EBV-seronegative infants and children known to have inherited a mutated *SH2D1A*, the gene responsible for X-linked lymphoproliferative syndrome (XLP) (see Chapter 32) to prevent EBV infection. One EBV-seronegative college student

known to have inherited the disorder died from overwhelming EBV infection despite monthly IVIG infusions (Okano et al., 1991). IVIG is still used prophylactically in XLP by some investigators and data on the success or failure are being collected by means of disease-specific registries and databases (Valiaho et al., 2000). To collect meaningful data, it is particularly important to ascertain the underlying molecular diagnosis and to differentiate XLP (see Chapter 32) from CVID (see Chapter 23) (Morra et al., 2001), X-linked hyper-IgM syndrome (see Chapter 19), and XLA (see Chapter 21).

High-dose IVIG (500 mg/kg/daily) may be of value in the treatment of immunodeficient patients with other viral diseases, including cytomegalovirus (CMV) infection, parvovirus-induced pure red cell aplasia (Kurtzman et al., 1989; Seyama et al., 1998), and respiratory virus infections such as parainfluenza or adenovirus (Stiehm et al., 1986). RSV-IG with high-titer antibody (replaced by the monoclonal anti-RSV preparation Synagis in 2003) may be used on a monthly basis to prevent RSV infection in young immunodeficient subjects (vide supra).

Oral immunoglobulin (150–300 mg/kg body weight) has been used in a few patients with antibody deficiency to stop enteroviral shedding following inadvertent poliomyelitis immunization (Losonsky et al., 1985) or to treat rotavirus infections (Barnes et al., 1982).

Other Therapies

A subset of patients with antibody deficiencies have concomitant and usually transient neutropenia (e.g., X-linked hyper-IgM syndrome, XLA). High-dose IVIG (2 g/kg) may reverse persistent and clinically significant neutropenia and should be tried first. In patients with X-linked hyper-IgM syndrome, granulocyte colony–stimulating factor (G-CSF) therapy may be required (see Chapter 19).

Continuous or intermittent antibiotic therapy may be necessary to keep some antibody-deficient patients free of infection or to prevent progression of chronic simopulmonary disease and bronchiectasis. We use full therapeutic doses of a set of antibiotics, including cephalosporin, ampicillin, clarithromycin, or TMP-SMX, which are rotated at 2-week or monthly intervals.

It is important to correct avitaminosis with replacement vitamins, especially the fat-soluble vitamins A, D, and E, by injection if they are not absorbed orally (Aukrust et al., 2000).

Most attempts to stimulate antibody synthesis by immunologic-enhancing agents have been unsuccessful. Of particular interest is the use of PEG-IL-2, an experimental preparation of interleukin-2 (IL-2) conjugated to polyethylene glycol (PEG) (Cunningham-Rundles et al., 1994). In one study, PEG-IL-2 was given to 15 CVID patients (Cunningham-Rundles et al., 2001). After 6 to 12 months of therapy, in vitro proliferative responses improved and antibody responses to a neoantigen developed (in 4 of 8 patients tested), but clinical benefit was minimal. Isolated successes have been reported with cimetidine (White and Ballow, 1985) and retinoic acid (Saxon et al., 1993). Blys (also known as BAFF), a cell surface molecule that activates B cells, looks promising in animal experiments, but robust clinical trials have not been initiated.

In antibody deficiency associated with drug treatment (e.g., IgA deficiency following phenytoin use or hypogammaglobulinemia following gold therapy), discontinuation of the drug may result in reversal of the disease. In some cases, however, the antibody deficiency persists indefinitely (Snowden et al., 1996; Cunningham-Rundles, 2004).

Cellular Immunodeficiencies

Precautions

Patients with a predominant T cell deficiency need preventive measures to avoid infective complications before attempting curative immunotherapy. As in antibody deficiencies, immunization with live attenuated vaccines is contraindicated. Progressive polio-encephalitis, measles encephalitis, and mumps encephalitis have been recorded in T cell–immunodeficient patients following routine childhood immunization. Additionally, siblings and other close contacts should be immunized with inactivated polio vaccine (which is used exclusively in most developed countries) because live virus may be transmitted to the patient.

Special care must be taken in administering blood products. Blood or blood cell components given to patients with primary (or secondary) T cell immunodeficiencies should be CMV negative and must be irradiated with 2700 rads (27 gys) to prevent graft-vs.-host reaction. Radiation of blood products is a simple procedure and can be accomplished rapidly in most blood banks.

Tonsillectomy and adenoidectomy are rarely indicated. Splenectomy is contraindicated, except in unusual circumstances, because the removal of an important immune organ and the creation of a de facto phagocytic defect in addition to the already existing immunodeficiency may result in sudden, overwhelming sepsis. Broad-spectrum prophylactic antibiotics may be of value in patients with recurrent or chronic bacterial disease.

Prophylactic Antimicrobial Therapy

Patients with a significant T cell deficiency are at risk for PCP. Those over age 5 years with CD4 counts <200/µl are candidates for PCP prophylaxis, and for those patients less than age 5, PCP prophylaxis should be considered at higher CD4 count levels (Stiehm et al., 2004) (see Table 46.1).

Continuous antifungal medications such as oral nystatin, ketoconazole, fluconazole, itraconazole, and caspofungin (Cancidas) are used to prevent or treat chronic candidiasis and other fungal infections.

All patients with severe combined immunodeficiency require prophylactic treatment with IVIG prior to stem cell transplantation because their B cells, if present, will either be nonfunctional or lack costimulation by T cells. Even if the T cell defect is relatively mild (as in X-linked hyper-IgM syndrome), the patient may have severely impaired B cell function and should be evaluated for abnormal antibody production. If it is deficient, IVIG therapy is indicated (Table 46.2). The dose of IVIG is similar to that discussed earlier for antibody deficiency.

Varicella-zoster immune globulin (VZIG) and/or acyclovir following chickenpox exposure and amantidine or ramatidine following influenza virus exposure may prevent or diminish the severity of infections.

Other Treatment

In patients with lymphopenia due to gastrointestinal lymphocyte loss as part of severe protein-losing enteropathy or lymphangiectasia of the gut not amenable to medical or surgical treatment, oral medium-chain triglycerides may be of value.

Endocrine abnormalities may be associated with T cell deficiency, notably hypoparathyroidism in DiGeorge anomaly and chronic mucocutaneous candidiasis, and hypothyroidism and hypoadrenalism in ataxia-telangiectasia and chronic mucocutaneous candidiasis. These should be treated appropriately, although correction of the endocrinopathies will not affect the T cell deficiency.

Restoration of immunity, short of transplantation, is rarely feasible in T cell immunodeficiencies. Immunomodulating agents such as thymic hormones, levamisole, and transfer factor have not been of proven benefit despite isolated reports of success.

An exception is the treatment of adenosine deaminase (ADA) deficiency (see Chapter 12) with PEG-ADA, given once or twice weekly at a dose of 30 U/kg. Close monitoring of plasma ADA levels and lymphocyte adenosine deoxyribonucleotides (dAXD) is required to assess the patient's response to therapy (Hershfield, 1995). Clinical and immunologic improvement are observed in most patients and include restoration of antibody responses and in vitro lymphocyte proliferation. PEG-ADA treatment is of particular value for patients who are too sick to undergo transplantation or who lack an HLA-matched bone marrow donor. A few patients have developed an antibody to PEG-ADA in association with increasing resistance to enzyme therapy. This complication was reversed by increasing the dose of enzyme and by a short course of corticosteroids and high-dose IVIG (Chaffee et al., 1992).

In the rare condition of multiple carboxylase deficiency, often associated with candidiasis and severe viral and bacterial infections, substitution with the coenzyme biotin given orally at a dose of 1–40 mg/day completely corrects the symptoms (Ochs et al., 2004).

Cytokine Therapy

The role of IL-2 substitution in individuals with poorly described T cell deficiencies has been explored. A few patients with phenotypic severe combined immunodeficiency were reported to have a defect of IL-2 synthesis with intact IL-2 receptors. IL-2 therapy resulted in temporary restoration of some cellular immunity in a patient with defective IL-2 synthesis (Pahwa et al., 1989). Other patients with T cell defects have been treated with IL-2 and appear to have achieved some improvement of in vitro T cell function (Flomenberg et al., 1983), but controlled studies are lacking. Cunningham-Rundles et al. (1999) used PEG-IL-2 in a single patient with idiopathic CD4 lymphopenia and attained a favorable clinical and laboratory response.

Interferon-γ therapy is of unproven efficacy in most T cell immunodeficiencies but has some theoretical value in the treatment of Griscelli syndrome, natural killer (NK) cell deficiency, and bare lymphocyte major histocompatibility complex (MHC) class I deficiency in that it may replace deficient production, enhance NK cytotoxicity, or increase expression of HLA class I antigens. High-dose IFN-γ therapy is of benefit in the treatment of patients with a partial IFN-γ receptor deficiency or in patients with IL-12 or IL-12 receptor defects. (Jouanguy et al., 1997; Holland, 2000) (see Chapter 28).

G-CSF is of value in certain T cell deficiencies where there is an associated neutropenia (e.g., X-linked hyper IgM syndrome). It is also useful in patients who have recently undergone stem cell transplantation for immunodeficiency disorders to hasten granulocyte recovery (see Chapter 47).

Stem Cell Transplantation and Gene Therapy

The treatment of choice, since it may be curative, is hematopoietic stem cell transplantation from a matched or partially matched donor using bone marrow, peripheral blood, or cord blood as the source of stem cells (see Chapter 47). More recently, gene therapy has been successfully performed in patients with common γ-chain deficiency (X-linked severe combined immunodeficiency) and with ADA deficiency (see Chapter 48).

Phagocytic Immunodeficiencies

General Care

Patients with phagocytic immunodeficiencies including chronic granulomatous disease (CGD) (see Chapter 37), leukocyte adhesion defects (LAD 1, 2, and 3) (see Chapter 38), and hyper-IgE syndrome (see Chapter 34) are particularly susceptible to cutaneous soft tissue infections and generally do well on continuous antimicrobial therapy, particularly TMP-SMX. Most patients with hyper-IgE syndrome need chronic antistaphylococcal treatment such as oral cloxacillin or dicloxacillin and antifungal therapy such as fluconazole or itraconazole. Those with demonstrable antibody deficiency improve on immunoglobulin therapy. Severe cutaneous infections in these patients are treated with intravenous and/or local antibiotics, and often in combination with local steroid therapy.

Patients with neutropenia or defects of cell adhesion and movement are particularly susceptible to periodontitis and oral ulcerations. Good oral hygiene must be stressed, and an antibacterial mouthwash (Peridex) should be used on a regular basis. Prophylactic antifungal drugs should be given if thrush or esophageal candidiasis has occurred. G-CSF can be used for most forms of persisting or cyclic neutropenia (see Chapter 39).

Chronic Granulomatous Disease

General treatment

In addition to prophylactic antibiotics, particularly TMP-SMX, vigorous treatment of each infectious episode is of crucial importance (see Chapter 37). Leukocyte transfusions may be of value in severe refractory infections such as hepatic abscesses or osteomyelitis (Yomtovian et al., 1981), but surgical therapy is required in most instances. Systemic corticosteroid therapy has been used successfully to reverse the gastrointestinal or genitourinary obstructive lesions that are a frequent complication in CGD (Chin et al., 1987). Multiple short courses of high-dose oral steroids may be necessary.

Interferon-γ prophylaxis

A randomized, double-blind study showed that recombinant human IFN-γ reduced the frequency and severity of infectious episodes in CGD patients (International Chronic Granulomatous Disease Cooperative Study Group, 1991). This was particularly true for a subgroup of CGD patients that did not receive adequate antibiotic prophylaxis and as a result had a significant reduction of the number of infective episodes compared with those receiving placebo. In fact, the frequency of infections fell to that of the group receiving antibiotics alone. The infections that did occur in IFN-γ-treated CGD patients were less severe, requiring fewer days of hospitalization and parenteral antibiotic treatment. The most frequent reactions to IFN-γ injections were flu-like symptoms, headache, myalgia, and mild fever, usually effectively prevented by acetaminophen.

In patients receiving either placebo or IFN-γ, no differences in NADPH oxidative response, bacterial killing, or cytochrome b_{558} levels were noted. This finding suggests that nonoxidase biologic responses may contribute to enhanced resistance in patients treated with IFN-γ (Klebanoff et al., 1992; Malmvall and Follin, 1993). The minimal toxicity and significant clinical effectiveness

have led to the recommendation to treat CGD patients of all inheritance patterns in the United States with IFN-γ, 50 μg/M² body surface, administered subcutaneously three times each week. In Europe, prophylaxis with TMP-SMX and antifungals remains the cornerstone of therapy in adults and older boys (see Chapter 37).

Transplantation

Bone marrow transplantation has been successful in CGD patients (Seger et al., 2002). A recent report of 10 patients (5 adults and 5 children) in whom nonmyeloablative conditioning combined with T cell depletion was performed indicated success in 8 of 10 transplants and a 70% survival rate at almost 2 years (Horwitz et al., 2001). Early transplantation before major infection occurs is associated with improved survival. Clinical trials of gene therapy are under way with early promising results (R. Seger, personal communication).

Leukocyte Adhesion Defects

The severe mouth ulcers and periodontal disease observed in patients with CD11/CD18 deficiency (LAD1) and in those with defective fucose transport (LAD2) necessitate good oral hygiene (see Chapter 38). Continuous antimicrobial therapy may be necessary to prevent cutaneous and deep-seated infections. Daily white blood cell transfusions for 1 or more weeks may be needed to treat severe, life-threatening infections.

De Ugarte et al. (2002) have used GM-CSF formulated for local application to treat nonhealing wounds in leukocyte adhesion defects and other granulocyte abnormalities (e.g., chronic granulomatous disease, glycogen storage disease type Ib).

Bone marrow transplantation is readily accomplished in patients with this disorder because the adhesion molecules that LAD1 patients lack contribute to graft rejection (Le Deist et al., 1989).

Hyper-IgE Syndrome

Continuous antimicrobial therapy is usually necessary to keep these patients' cutaneous and deep-seated abscesses under control (Buckley, 2004). Prompt treatment of infections, notably sinusitis and bronchitis, and in many cases continuous prophylactic treatment with antibiotics, may prevent acute pneumonia, lung abscesses, and pneumatocele formation (see Chapter 34).

No specific immunotherapeutic regimen has been successful (Roberts and Stiehm, 1996). Interferon-γ and IVIG reduce the IgE level but are without proven clinical benefit. Transfer factor, cimetidine, and ascorbic acid have been used without clinical benefit. Levamisole was inferior to placebo in a controlled, double-blind study (Donabedian et al., 1982). Isotretonin was used in a single case without proven benefit.

Glycogen Storage Type 1b

These patients have neutropenia, functional defects of neutrophil function, and recurrent infections including sinusitis, pneumonia, and septicemia. Continuous therapy with TMP-SMX has been recommended and GM-CSF or G-CSF may be beneficial (Hurst et al., 1993).

Chediak-Higashi Syndrome

Although vitamin C corrects some of the defects in vitro, its use in patients with Chediak-Higashi syndrome has not been effective

(Gallin et al., 1979). Affected patients have an in vitro defect of NK cell function, amenable to IFN-γ correction, but its use in vivo has not been documented. Bone marrow transplantation has been successful in these patients (see Chapter 40).

Complement Deficiencies

General Treatment

No specific treatment is available for most complement deficiencies (Sullivan and Winkelstein, 2004). Careful management, however, can improve the health and survival of affected patients (see Chapter 42). Complement-deficient patients, notably those with C2, C3, C5, C6, C7, C8, properdin, factor H, or factor I deficiencies, should be treated promptly with antibiotics at the first onset of fever. An antipneumococcal drug has to be included in the case of C2 deficiency, and an antineisserial drug should be used if the deficiency is of a late-acting component or involves properdin. Long-term penicillin therapy should be considered when meningococcal disease is endemic and for patients with a history of previous severe infections (Potter et al., 1990).

The patient and close household contacts should be immunized against *Streptococcus pneumoniae*, *Haemophilus influenzae*, and *Neisseria meningitides*. Repeat vaccinations (every 3–5 years) may be necessary if titers diminish to nonprotective levels. The use of the new conjugated pneumococcal vaccines is recommended, although with caution, in view of the reduced number of serotypes included in Prevnar.

A deficiency of an early-acting component predisposes to collagen-vascular disease, which should be treated appropriately. Carriers of C2 deficiency may also have a propensity to develop autoimmune diseases. Other family members should be studied in the case of any genetic complement deficiency, and genetic counseling can be offered as indicated.

Specific Treatment

An exception to the rule that no specific therapy for complement deficiencies exists is hereditary angioedema (HAE), an autosomal recessive disorder associated with deficiency or abnormal function of C1 inhibitor (C1INH). The therapy of HAE involves (1) the treatment of acute attacks and (2) prophylaxis of recurrent attacks.

Management of an acute episode of angioedema must be tailored to the extent of the problem. Laryngeal swelling or disabling abdominal pain requires intervention. The most effective therapy is C1INH concentrate given as an intravenous infusion, which is effective within 30 to 60 minutes. C1INH concentrate has not been approved by the U.S. Food and Drug Administration but is presently being clinically evaluated in the United States. Therefore, attenuated androgens are the most common specific treatment of an acute attack. Because androgens do not begin to have an effect until 24 to 48 hours, patients with serious symptoms have to be carefully monitored in a hospital to ensure that the angioedema does not progress.

Patients with a history of laryngeal obstruction or serious gastrointestinal involvement are candidates for long-term prevention of attacks. Impeded androgens such as Danazol, Stanozolol, and Oxandrolone are frequently used to increase serum concentrations of the normal C1INH by increasing transcription of the wild-type C1INH gene. Danazol is typically prescribed at a dose of 50 to 600 mg/day, Stanozolol at 1 to 10 mg/day, and Oxandrolone at 2.5 to 20 mg/day in adult patients. The goal of this prophylactic therapy is to maintain the C1INH functional level at approximately 50% of normal. Long-term therapy in adults is possible, but patients have to be monitored for adverse reactions including abnormal liver function tests, microscopic hematuria, and weight gain. Attenuated androgens should not be used in children with open epiphysis on a long-term basis. However, intermittent treatment is acceptable. Regular plasma infusions could theoretically be used to replace a missing complement component, especially C3 or C4. However, the short half-life of these proteins, the low levels in normal plasma, and the possibility of developing an antibody response to the missing complement component make such an effort futile.

Concluding Remarks

General care of the immunodeficient patient requires close monitoring of growth, nutrition, personal hygiene and habits, living conditions, school and work situations, and psychologic adjustment to the disease. The most important aspect of the care of an immunodeficient patient is to prevent, recognize, and vigorously treat infectious episodes. Associated disorders such as anemia, thrombocytopenia, respiratory or gastrointestinal problems, and autoimmune and inflammatory disorders are managed by conventional therapy. Avoidance of live-virus vaccines, unirradiated blood, and CMV antibody–positive blood is crucial for living with some of these illnesses. PCP prophylaxis is necessary in T cell immunodeficiency.

Specific therapies that are effective include immunoglobulin replacement therapy in patients with antibody deficiency, PEG-ADA injections for ADA deficiency, and IFN-γ for CGD and for deficiencies of IL-12 and IL-12 receptor, and partial deficiencies of the IFN-γ receptors. Other cytokines, including G-CSF and GM-CSF, and possibly IL-2 are of value in certain selected disorders. Stem cell transplantation has been pioneered in patients with primary immunodeficiency and continues to be a life-saving procedure for patients with many of these disorders. Minimal conditioning ("mini-transplants") is being increasingly performed in selected syndromes as a safe alternative to bone marrow transplantation and full conditioning. Progress in our understanding of the molecular basis of these disorders has paved the way for gene therapy, which is promising and at the same time a challenge.

References

Abrahamsen TG, Sandersen H, Bustnes A. Home therapy with subcutaneous immunoglobulin infusions in children with congenital immunodeficiencies. Pediatrics 98:1127–1131, 1996.
American Academy of Pediatrics. Immunization in special clinical circumstances. In: Pickering LK, ed. 2000 Red Book Report of the Committee on Infectious Diseases, 25th ed. Elk Grove Village, IL: American Academy of Pediatrics, pp. 54–61, 2000.
Asano Y, Yoshikawa T, Suga S, Kobayashi I, Nakashima T, Yazaki T, Ozaki T, Yamada A, Imanishi J. Postexposure prophylaxis of varicella in family contact by oral acyclovir. Pediatrics 92:219–222, 1993.
Ashida ER, Saxon A. Home intravenous immunoglobulin infusion by self-infusion. J Clin Immunol 6:306–309, 1986.
Aukrust P, Muller F, Ueland T, Svardal AM, Berge RK, Froland S. Decreased vitamin A levels in common variable immunodeficiency: vitamin A supplementation in vivo enhances immunoglobulin production and downregulates inflammatory responses Eur J Clin Invest 30:252–259, 2000.
Barnes GL, Doyle LW, Hewson PH, Knoches AM, McLellan JR, Kitchen WH, Bishop RF. A randomized trial of oral gammaglobulin in low-birth-weight infants infected with rotavirus. Lancet 1:1371–1373, 1982.
Barnett N, Mak H, Winkelstein JA. Extensive verrucosis in primary immunodeficiency diseases. Arch Dermatol 119:5–7, 1983.
Bartolome J, Porta F, Lafranchi A, Rodriguez-Molina JJ, Cela E, Cantalejo A, Fernandez-Cruz E, Gomez-Pineda A, Ugazio AG, Notarangelo LD,

Gil J. B cell function after haploidentical in utero bone marrow transplantation in a patient with severe combined immunodeficiency. Bone Marrow Transplant 229:625–628, 2002.

Berger M. Subcutaneous immunoglobulin replacement in primary immunodeficiencies. Clin Immunol 112:1–7, 2004.

Berger M, Cupps, TR, Fauci A, Immunoglobulin replacement therapy by slow subcutaneous infusion. Ann Intern Med 93:55–56, 1980.

Bernatowska E, Madalinski K, Janowicz W, Weremowicz R, Gutkowski P, Wolf HM, Eibl MM. Results of a prospective controlled two-dose crossover study with intravenous immunoglobulin and comparison (retrospective) with plasma treatment. Clin Immunol Immunopathol 43:153–162, 1987.

Bjorkander J, Cunningham-Rundles C, Lundin P, Olsson R, Soderstrom R, Hanson LA. Intravenous immunoglobulin prophylaxis causing liver damage in 16 of 77 patients with hypogammaglobulinemia or IgG subclass deficiency. Am J Med 84:107–111, 1988.

Bjoro K, Frland SS, Yun Z, Samdal HH, Haaland T. Hepatitis C infection in patients with primary hypogammaglobulinemia after treatment with contaminated immune globulin. N Engl J Med 331:1607–1611, 1994.

Brennan VM, Cochrane S, Fletcher C, Hendy D, Powell P. Surveillance of adverse reactions in patients self-infusing intravenous immunoglobulin at home. J Clin Immunol 15:116–119, 1995.

Brox AG, Cournoyer D, Sternbach M, Spurll G. Hemolytic anemia following intravenous immunoglobulin administration. Am J Med 83:633–635, 1987.

Buckley RH. The hyper IgE syndrome. In: Stiehm ER, Ochs HD, Winkelstein JA, eds. Immunologic Disorders in Infants and Childen, 5th ed. Philadelphia: WB Saunders, pp. 545–551, 2004.

Burks AW, Sampson HA, Buckley RH. Anaphylactic reactions after gamma globulin administration in patients with hypogammaglobulinemia. N Engl J Med 314:560–564, 1986.

Centers for Disease Control. Guidelines for prophylaxis against *Pneumocystis carinii* pneumonia for children infected with human immunodeficiency virus. MMWR Morb Mortal Wkly Rep 40:1–11, 1991.

Centers for Disease Control. Outbreak of hepatitis C associated with intravenous immunoglobulin administration: United States Oct 1993–June 1994. MMWR Morb Mortal Wkly Rep 43:505–509, 1994.

Chaffee S, Mary A, Stiehm ER, Girault D, Fischer A, Hershfield MS. IgG antibody response to polyethylene glycol–modified adenosine deaminase in patients with adenosine deaminase deficiency. J Clin Invest 89:1643–1651, 1992.

Chapel HM, Christie JM, Peach V, Chapman RW. Five-year follow-up of patients with primary antibody deficiencies following an outbreak of acute hepatitis C. Clin Immunol 99:320–324, 2001.

Chapel HM, Spickett GP, Ericson D, Engl W, Eibl MM, Bjorkander J. The comparison of the efficacy and safety of intravenous versus subcutaneous immunoglobulin replacement therapy. J Clin Immunol 20:94–100, 2000.

Chesky M, Scalco R, Failace L, Read S, Jobim LF. Polymerase chain reaction for the laboratory diagnosis of aseptic meningitis and encephalitis. Arq Neuropsiquiatr 58:836–842, 2000.

Chin TW, Stiehm ER, Falloon J, Gallin J. Corticosteroids in the treatment of obstructive lesions of chronic granulomatous disease. J Pediatr 111:349–352, 1987.

Christie JM, Healey CJ, Watson J, Wong VS, Duddridge M, Snowden N, Rosenberg WM, Fleming KA, Chapel H, Chapman RW. Clinical outcome of hypogammaglobulinaemic patients following outbreak of acute hepatitis C: 2-year follow-up. Clin Exp Immunol 110:4–8, 1997.

Comenzo RL, Malachowski ME, Meissner HC, Fulton DR, Berkman EM. Immune hemolysis, disseminated intravascular coagulation, and serum sickness after large doses of immune globulin given intravenously for Kawasaki disease. J Pediatr 120:926–928, 1992.

Crennan JM, Van Scoy RE, McKenna CH, Smith TF. Echovirus polymyositis in patients with hypogammaglobulinemia: failure of high-dose intravenous gammaglobulin therapy and review of the literature. Am J Med 81:35–42, 1986.

Cunningham CK, Bonville CA, Ochs HD, Seyama K, John PA, Rotbart HA, Weiner LB. Enteroviral meningoencephalitis as a complication of X-linked hyper IgM syndrome. J-Pediatr 134:584–588, 1999.

Cunningham-Rundles C. Selective IgA deficiency. In: Stiehm ER, Ochs HD, Winklestein JA, eds. Immunologic Disorders in Infants and Children, 5th ed. Philadelphia: WB Saunders, pp. 427–446, 2004.

Cunningham-Rundles C, Bodian C, Ochs, HD, Martin S, Reiter-Wong M Zhou Z. Long-term low-dose IL-2 enhances immune function in common variable immunodeficiency. Clin Immunol 100:181–190, 2001.

Cunningham-Rundles C, Kazbay K, Hassett J, Zhou Z, Mayer L. Enhanced humoral immunity in common variable immunodeficiency after long-term treatment with polyethylene glycol–conjugated interleukin-2. N Engl J Med 331:918–921, 1994.

Cunningham-Rundles C, Murray HW, Smith JP. Treatment of idiopathic CD4 lymphocytopenia with IL-2. Clin Exp Immunol 116:322–325, 1999.

Davies CW, Juniper MC, Gray W, Gleeson FV, Chapel HM, Davies RJ. Lymphoid interstitial pneumonitis associated with common variable hypogammaglobulinaemia treated with cyclosporin A. Thorax 55:88–90, 2000.

Davies EG, Thrasher A, Lacey K, Karper J. Topical cidofovir for severe molluscum contagiosum. Lancet 353:2042, 1999.

De Ugarte DA, Roberts RL, Lerdluedeeporn P, Stiehm ER, Atkinson JB. Treatment of chronic wounds by local delivery of granulocyte-macrophage colony-stimulating factor in patients with neutrophil dysfunction. Pediatr Surg Int 18:517–520, 2002.

Donabedian H, Alling DW, Gallin JI. Levamisole is inferior to placebo in the hyperimmunoglobulin E recurrent infection (Job's) syndrome. N Engl J Med 307:290–292, 1982.

Duhem C, Dicato MA, Ries F. Side-effects of intravenous immune globulins. Clin Exp Immunol 97:79–83, 1994.

Eijkhout HW, van Der Meer JW, Kallenberg CG, Weening RS, van Dissel JT, Sanders LA, Strengers PF, Nienhuis H, Schellekens PT, for the Inter-University Working Party for the Study of Immune Deficiencies. The effect of two different dosages of intravenous immunoglobulin on the incidence of recurrent infections in patients with primary hypogammaglobulinemia. A randomized, double-blind, multicenter crossover trial. Ann Intern Med 135:165–174, 2001.

Erlendsson K, Swartz T, Dwyer JM. Successful reversal of echovirus encephalitis in X-linked hypogammaglobulinemia by intraventricular administration of immunoglobulin. N Engl J Med 312:351–353, 1985.

Finberg RW. Immunology of infection. Immunol Allergy Clin North Am 8: 137–144, 1988.

Flake AW, Roncarolo MG, Puck JM, Almeida-Porada G, Evans MI, Johnson MP, Abella EM, Harrison DD, Zanjani ED. Treatment of X-linked severe combined immunodeficiency by in utero transplantation of paternal bone marrow. N Engl J Med 335:1806–1810, 1996.

Flomenberg N, Welte K, Mertelsmann R, Kernan N, Ciobanu N, Venuta S, Feldman S, Kruger G, Kirkpatrick D, Dupont B, O'Reilly R. Immunologic effects of interleukin-2 in primary immunodeficiency diseases. J Immunol 130:2644–2650, 1983.

Gallin JL, Ellin RJ, Hubert RT, Fauci AS, Kaliner MA, Wolf SM. Efficacy of ascorbic acid in Chediak-Higashi syndrome (CHS): studies in humans and mice. Blood 53:226–234, 1979.

Garbett ND, Currie DC, Cole PJ. Comparison of the clinical efficacy and safety of an intramuscular and an intravenous immunoglobulin preparation for replacement therapy in idiopathic adult onset panhypogammablobulinaemia. J Clin Exp Immunol 76:1–7, 1989.

Gardulf A, Andersen V, Bjorkander J, Ericson D, Froland SS, Gustafson R, Hammarstrom L, Jacobsen MB, Jonsson E, Moller G, Nystrom T, Soeberg V, Smith CIE. Subcutaneous immunoglobulin replacement in patients with primary antibody deficiencies: safety and costs. Lancet 345: 365–369, 1995.

Gardulf A, Andersson E, Lindqvist M, Hansen S, Gustafson R. Rapid subcutaneous IgG replacement therapy at home for pregnant immunodeficient women. J Clin Immunol 21:150–154, 2001.

Gardulf A, Hammarstrom L, Smith CIE. Home treatment of hypogammaglobulinemia with subcutaneous gammaglobulin by rapid infusion. Lancet 338:162–166, 1991.

Gardulf A, Nicolay U, Math D, Asensio O, Bernatowska E, Böck A, Costa-Carvalho BT, Granert C, Haag S, Hernandez D, Kiessling P, Kus J, Matamoros N, Niehues T, Schmidt S, Schulze I, Borte M. Children and adults with primary antibody deficiencies gain quality of life by subcutaneous IgG self-infusions at home. J Allergy Clin Immunol 114:936–942, 2004.

Gardulf A, Nicolay U, Asensio O, Bernatowska E, Böck A, Costa Carvalho B, Granert C, Haag S, Hernandez D, Kiessling P, Kus J, Pons J, Niehues T, Schmidt S, Schulze I, Borte M. Rapid subcutaneous IgG replacement therapy is effective and safe in children and adults with primary Immunodeficiencies—A prospective, multi-national study. J Clin Immunol 2006, in press.

Groothuis JR, Simoes EAF, Levin MJ, Hall CB, Long CE, Rodriguez WJ, Arrobio J, Meissner HC, Fulton DR, Welliver RC, Tristram DA, Siber GR, Prince GA, Raden MV, Hemming VG. Prophylactic administration of respiratory syncytial virus immune globulin to high-risk infants and young children. N Engl J Med 329:1524–1530, 1993.

Haeney M. Intravenous immune globulin in primary immunodeficiency. Clin Exp Immunol 9:11–15, 1994.

Hansen S, Gustafson R, Smith CI, Gardulf A. Express subcutaneous IgG infusions: decreased time of delivery with maintained safety. Clin Immunol 104:237–241, 2002.

Hatab AZ, Ballas Z. Caseating granulomatous disease in common variable immunodeficiency treated with infliximab. J Allergy Clin Immunol 116: 1161–1162, 2005.

Healey CJ, Sabharwal NK, Daub J, Davidson F, Yap PL, Fleming KA, Chapman RW, Simmonds P, Chapel H. Outbreak of acute hepatitis C following the use of anti-hepatitis C virus–screened intravenous immunoglobulin therapy. Gastroenterology 110:1120–1126, 1996.

Henin Y, Marechal V, Barre-Sinoussi F, Chermann JC, Morgenthaler JJ. Inactivation and partition of HIV during Kistler and Nitschmann fractionation of human blood plasma. Vox Sang 54:78–83, 1988.

Hermaszewski RA, Webster ABD. Primary hypogammaglobulinaemia: a survey of clinical manifestations and complications. Q J Med 86:31–42, 1993.

Hershfield MS. PEG-ADA replacement therapy for adenosine deaminase deficiency: an update after 8.5 years. Clin Immunol Immunopathol 76: S228–S232, 1995.

Holland SM. Treatment of infections in the patient with Mendelian susceptibility to mycobacterial infection. Microbes Infect 2:1579–1590, 2000.

Horwitz ME, Barrett AJ, Brown MR, Carter CS, Childs R, Gallin JI, Holland SM, Linton GF, Miller JA, Leitman SF, Read EJ, Malech HL. Treatment of chronic granulomatous disease with nonmyeloablative conditioned T-cell–depleted hematopoietic allograft. N Engl J Med 344:881–884, 2001.

Hurst D, Kilpatrick L, Becker J, Lipani J, Kleman K, Perine S, Douglas SD. Recombinant human GM-CSF treatment of neutropenia in glycogen storage disease 1b. Am J Pediatr Hematol Oncol 15:71–76, 1993.

International Chronic Granulomatous Disease Cooperative Study Group. A controlled trial of interferon gamma to prevent infection in chronic granulomatous disease. N Engl J Med 324:509–516, 1991.

Johnson PR Jr, Edwards KM, Wright PF. Failure of intraventricular gamma globulin to eradicate echovirus encephalitis in a patient with X-linked agammaglobulinemia. N Engl J Med 313:1546–1547, 1985.

Jouanguy E, Lamhamedi-Cherradi S, Altare F, Fondaneche MC, Tuerlinckx B, Blanche S, Emile JF, Gaillard JL, Schreiber R, Levin M, Fischer A, Hivroz C, Casanova JL. Partial interferon-γ receptor 1 deficiency in a child with tuberculoid bacillus Calmette-Guérin infection and a sibling with clinical tuberculosis. J Clin Invest 100:2658–2664, 1997.

Kato E, Shindo S, Eto Y, Hashimoto N, Yamamoto M, Sakata Y, Hiyoshi Y. Administration of immune globulin associated with aseptic meningitis. JAMA 259:3267–3271, 1988.

Klebanoff SJ, Olszowski S, Van Voorhis WC, Ledbetter JA, Waltersdorph AM, Schlechte KG. Effects of gamma-interferon on human neutrophils: protection from deterioration on storage. Blood 80:225–234, 1992.

Kobayashi RH, Kobayashi AD, Lee N, Fischer S, Ochs HD. Home self-administration of intravenous immunoglobulin in children. Pediatrics 85: 705–709, 1990.

Kurtzman G, Frickhofen N, Kimball J, Jenkins DW, Wienhuis AW, Young NS. Pure red-cell aplasia of 10 years duration due to persistent parvovirus B19 infection and its cure with immunoglobulin therapy. N Engl J Med 321:519–521, 1989.

Lack G, Ochs HD, Gelfand EW. Humoral immunity in steroid-dependent children with asthma and hypogammaglobulinemia. J Pediatr 129:898–903, 1996.

Le Deist F, Blanche H, Keable H, Gaud C, Pham H, Descamp-Latscha B, Wahn V, Griscelli C, Fischer A. Successful HLA nonidentical bone marrow transplantation in three patients with the leukocyte adhesion deficiency. Blood 74:512–516, 1989.

Lederman HM, Winkelstein JA. X-linked agammaglobulinemia: an analysis of 96 patients. Medicine 64:145–146, 1985.

Lever AM, Webster ADB, Brown D, Thomas HC. Non-A, non-B hepatitis occurring in agammaglobulinaemic patients after intravenous immunoglobulin. Lancet 2:1062–1064, 1984.

Liese JG, Wintergerst U, Tympner KD, Belohradsky B. High- vs. low-dose immunoglobulin therapy in the long-term treatment of X-linked agammaglobulinemia. Am J Dis Child 146:335–339, 1992.

Lin JH, Liebhaber M, Roberts RL, Dyer Z, Stiehm ER. Etanercept treatment of cutaneous granulomas in common variable immunodeficiency. J Allergy Clin Immunol 2006, in press.

Losonsky GA, Johnson JP, Winkelstein JA, Yolken RH. Oral administration of human serum immunoglobulin in immunodeficient patients with viral gastroenteritis. J Clin Invest 76:2362–2367, 1985.

Malmvall BE, Follin P. Successful interferon-gamma therapy in a chronic granulomatous disease (CGD) patient suffering from Staphylococcus aureus hepatic abscess and invasive Candida albicans infection. Scand J Infect Dis 25:61–66, 1993.

Matheson DS, Clarkson TW, Gelfand EW. Mercury toxicity (acrodynia) induced by long-term injection of gamma globulin. J Pediatr 97:153–155, 1980.

McIntosh K, Kurachek SC, Cairns LM, Burns JC, Goodspeed B. Treatment of respiratory viral infection in an immunodeficient infant with ribavirin aerosol. Am J Dis Child 138:305–308, 1984.

McKinney RE Jr, Katz SL, Wilfert CM. Chronic enteroviral meningoencephalitis in agammaglobulinemic patients. Rev Infect Dis 9:334–356, 1987.

Mease PJY, Ochs HD, Corey L, Dragavon J, Wedgwood RJ. Echovirus encephalitis/myositis in X-linked agammaglobulinemia (letter). N Engl J Med 313:758, 1985.

Mease PJ, Ochs HD, Wedgwood RJ. Successful treatment of echovirus meningoencephalitis and myositis fasciitis with intravenous immune globulin therapy in a patient with X-linked agammaglobulinemia. N Engl J Med 304:1278–1281, 1981.

Mechanic LJ, Dikman S, Cunningham-Rundles C. Granulomatous disease in common variable immunodeficiency. Ann Intern Med 127:613–617, 1997.

Medical Research Council Working Party. Hypogammaglobulinemia in the United Kingdom. Lancet 1:163–169, 1969.

Miller FW, Leitman SF, Plotz PH. High-dose intravenous immune globulin and acute renal failure. N Engl J Med 327:1032–1033, 1992.

Misbah SA, Spickett GP, Ryba PC, Hockaday JM, Kroll JS, Sherwood C, Kurtz JB, Moxon ER, Chapel HM. Chronic enteroviral meningoencephalitis in agammaglobulinemia: case report and literature review. J Clin Immunol 12:266–270, 1992.

Montanaro A, Pirofsky B. Prolonged interval high-dose intravenous immunoglobulin in patients with primary immunodeficiency states. Am J Med 76:67–72, 1984.

Morra M, Silander O, Calpe S, Choi M, Oettgen H, Myers L, Etzioni A, Buckley R, Terhorst C. Alterations of the X-linked lymphoproliferative disease gene SH2D1A in common variable immunodeficiency syndrome. Blood 98:1321–1325, 2001.

Nicolay U, Kiessling P, Berger M, Gupta S, Yel L, Roifman CM, Gardulf A, Eichmann F, Haag S, Massion C, Ochs HD. Health-related quality of life and treatment satisfaction in North American patients with primary immunedeficiency diseases receiving subcutaneous IgG self-infusions at home. J Clin Immunol. 26:65–72, 2006.

Ochs HD, Buckley RH, Pirofsky B, Fischer SH, Rousell RH, Anderson CJ, Wedgwood RJ. Safety and patient acceptability of intravenous immune globulin in 10% maltose. Lancet 2:1158–1159, 1980.

Ochs HD, Fischer SH, Virant FS, Lee ML, Kingdon HS, Wedgwood RJ. Non-A non-B hepatitis and intravenous immunoglobulin. Lancet 1:404–405, 1985.

Ochs HD, Fischer SH, Wedgwood RJ, Wara DW, Cowan MJ, Ammann AJ, Saxon A, Budinger MD, Allred RU, Rousell RH. Comparison of high-dose and low-dose immunoglobulin therapy in patients with primary immunodeficiency diseases. Am J Med 76:78–82, 1984.

Ochs HD, Gupta S, Kiessling P, Nicolay U, Math D, Berger M, and the Subcutaneous IgG Study Group. Safety and efficacy of self-administered subcutaneous immunoglobulin in patients with primary immunodeficiency diseases. J Clin Immunol 2006, in Press.

Ochs HD, Nelson DL, Stiehm ER. Other well-defined immunodeficiency syndromes. In: Stiehm ER, Ochs HD, Winkelstein JA, eds. Immunologic Disorders in Infants and Children, 5th ed. Philadelphia: Elsevier Saunders, pp. 505–516, 2004.

Okano M, Bashir RM, Davis JR, Purtilo DT. Detection of primary Epstein-Barr virus infection in a patient with X-linked lymphoproliferative disease receiving immunoglobulin prophylaxis. Am J Hematol 36:294–296, 1991.

Pahwa R, Chatila T, Pahwa S, Paradise C, Day NK, Geha R, Schwartz SA, Slade H, Oyaizu N, Good RA. Recombinant interleukin-2 therapy in severe combined immunodeficiency disease. Proc Natl Acad Sciences USA 86:5069–5073, 1989.

Potter PC, Frasch CE, van der Sande WJM, Cooper RC, Patel Y, Orren A. Prophylaxis against Neisseria meningitidis infections and antibody response in patients with deficiency of the sixth component of complement. J Infect Dis 161:932–937, 1990.

Prentice RL, Dalgleish AG, Gatenby PA, Loblay RH, Wade S, Kappagoda N, Basten A. Central nervous system echovirus infection in Bruton's X-linked hypogammaglobulinemia. Aust NZ J Med 15:443–445, 1985.

Quartier P, Foray S, Casanova JL, Hau-Rainsard I, Blanche S, Fischer A. Enteroviral meningoencephalitis in X-linked agammaglobulinemia: intensive immunoglobulin therapy and sequential viral detection in cerebrospinal fluid by polymerase chain reaction. Pediatr Infect Dis J 119:1106–1108, 2000.

Rault R, Piraino B, Johnston JR, Oral A. Pulmonary and renal toxicity of intravenous immunoglobulin. Clin Nephrol 36:83–86, 1991.

Razvi S, Schneider L, Jonas MM, Cunningham-Rundles C. Outcome of intravenous immunoglobulin-transmitted hepatitis C virus (HCV) infections in primary immunodeficiency. Clin Immunol 101:284–288, 2001.

Roberts RL, Stiehm ER. Hyperimmunoglobulin E syndrome (Job's syndrome). In: Lictenstein LM, Fauci AS, eds. Current Therapy in Allergy, Immunology and Rheumatology, 5th ed. St Louis: Mosby-Year Book, pp. 354–357, 1996.

Roifman CM, Levison H, Gelfand EW. High-dose versus low-dose intravenous immunoglobulin in hypogammaglobulinaemia and chronic lung disease. Lancet 1:1075–1077, 1987.

Rosenfeld EA, Shulman ST, Corydon KE, Mason W, Takahashi M, Kuroda C. Comparative safety and efficacy of two immune globulin products in Kawasaki disease. J Pediatr 126:1000–1003, 1995.

Rotbart HA. Diagnosis of enteroviral meningitis with the polymerase chain reaction. J Pediatr 117:85–89, 1990.

Saxon A, Keld B, Braun J, Dotson A, Sidell N. Long-term administration of 13-cis retinoic acid in common variable immunodeficiency: circulating interleukin-6 levels, B-cell surface molecule display, and in vitro and in vivo B-cell antibody production. Immunology 80:477–487, 1993.

Schiff RI. Transmission of viral infections through intravenous immune globulin. N Engl J Med 331:1649–1650, 1994.

Schiff RI, Sedlak D, Buckley RH. Rapid infusion of sandoglobulin in patients with primary humoral immunodeficiency. J Allergy Clin Immunol 88:61–67, 1991.

Schmugge M, Lauener R, Seger RA, Gungor T, Bossart W. Chronic enteroviral meningo-encephalitis in X-linked agammaglobulinaemia: favourable response to anti-enteroviral treatment. Eur J Pediatr 158:1010–1011, 1999.

Seger RA, Gungor T, Belohradsky BH, Blanche S, Bordigoni P, Di Bartolomeo P, Flood T, Landais P, Muller S, Ozsahin H, Passwell JH, Porta F, Slavin S, Wulffraat N, Zintl F, Nagler A, Cant A, Fischer A. Treatment of chronic granulomatous disease with myeloablative conditioning and an unmodified hemopoietic allograft: a survey of the European experience, 1985–2000. Blood 100:4344–4350, 2002.

Seyama K, Kobayashi R, Hasle H, Apter AJ, Rutledge JC, Rosen D, Ochs HD. Parvovirus B19-induced anemia as the presenting manifestation of X-linked hyper-IgM syndrome. J Infect Dis 178:318–324, 1998.

Smith KJ, Skelton H. Common variable immunodeficiency treated with a recombinant human IgG, tumour necrosis factor-alpha receptor fusion protein. Br J Dermatol 144:597–600, 2001.

Snowden N, Dietch DM, Teh LS, Hilton RC, Haeney MR. Antibody deficiency associated with gold treatment: natural history and management in 22 patients. Ann Rheum Dis 55:616–621, 1996.

Sorensen RU, Kallick MD, Berger M. Home treatment of antibody deficiency syndromes with intravenous immunoglcbulin. J Allergy Clin Immunol 80:810–815, 1987.

Stiehm ER. Human intravenous immunoglobulin in primary and secondary antibody deficiencies. Pediatr Infect Dis 16:696–707, 1997.

Stiehm ER, Casillas AM, Finkelstein JZ, Gallagher KT, Groncy PM, Kobayashi RH, Oleske JM, Roberts RL, Sandberg ET, Wakim ME. Slow subcutaneous human intravenous immunoglobulin in the treatment of antibody immunodeficiency: use of an old method with a new product. J. Allergy Clin Immunol 101:848–849, 1998.

Stiehm ER, Chin TW, Haas A, Peerless AG. Infectious complications of the primary immunodeficiencies. Clin Immunol Immunopathol 40:69–86, 1986.

Stiehm ER, Keller MA. Passive immunity. In: Feigen RD, Cherry JD, Demmler GJ, Kaplan SL, eds. Textbook of Pediatric Infectious diseases, 5th ed. Philadelphia: Elsevier Saunders, pp. 3182–3220, 2004.

Stiehm ER, Ochs HD, Winkelstein JA. Immunodeficiency disorders: general considerations. In: Stiehm ER, Ochs HD, Winkelstein JA, eds. Immunologic Disorders in Infants and Children, 5th ed. Philadelphia: Elsevier Saunders, pp. 289–355, 2004.

Sullivan KE, Winkelstein JA. Deficiencies of the complement system. In: Stiehm ER, Ochs HD, Winkelstein JA, eds. Immunologic Disorders in Infants and Children, 5th ed. Philadelphia: Elsevier Saunders, pp. 652–684, 2004.

Thatayatikom A, Thatayatikom S, White AJ. Infliximab treatment for severe granulomatous disease in common variable immunodeficiency: a case report and review of the literature. Ann Allergy Asthma Immunol 95: 293–300, 2005.

Tobi M, Straus SE. Chronic Epstein-Barr virus disease: a workshop held by the National Institute of Allergy and Infectious Diseases. Ann Intern Med 103:951–953, 1985.

Ugazio AG, Duse M, Re R, Mangili G, Burgio GR. Subcutaneous infusion of gammaglobulins in management of agammaglobulinaemia. Lancet 1: 226, 1982.

Valiaho J, Riikonen P, Vihinen M. Novel immunodeficiency data servers. Immunol Rev 178:177–185, 2000.

Vera-Ramirez M, Charlet M, Parry GJ. Recurrent aseptic meningitis complicating intravenous immunoglobulin therapy for chronic inflammatory demyelinating polyradiculoneuropathy. Neurology 42:1636–1637, 1992.

Viallard JF, Pellegrin JL, Moreau JF. Granulomatous disease in common variable immunodeficiency. Ann Intern Med 128:781–782, 1998.

Vowels MR, Lam-Po-Tang R, Berdoukas V, Ford D, Thierry D, Purtilo D, Gluckman E. Brief report: correction of X-linked lymphoproliferative disease by transplantation of cord-blood stem cells. N Engl J Med 329: 1623–1625, 1993.

Waniewski J, Gardulf A, Hammarstrom L. Bioavailability of γ-globulin after subcutaneous infusions in patients with common variable immunodeficiency. J Clin Immunol 14:90–97, 1993.

Welch MJ, Stiehm ER. Slow subcutaneous immunoglobulin therapy in a patient with reactions to intramuscular immunoglobulin. J Clin Immunol 3: 285–286, 1983.

White WB, Ballow M. Modulation of suppressor-cell activity by cimetidine in patients with common variable hypogammaglobulinemia. N Engl J Med 312:198–202, 1985.

Wilfert CM, Buckley RH, Mohanakumar T, Griffith JF, Katz SL, Whisnant JK, Eggleston PA, Moore M, Treadwell E, Oxman MN, Rosen FS. Persistent and fatal central-nervous-system ECHO virus infections in patients with agammaglobulinemia. N Engl J Med 296:1485–1489, 1977.

Wislez M, Sibony M, Naccache JM, Liote H, Carette MF, Oksenhendler E, Cadranel J. Organizing pneumonia related to common variable immunodeficiency. Case report and literature review. Respiration 67:467–470, 2000.

Williams PE, Yap PL, Gillon J, Crawford RJ, Urbaniak SJ, Galea G. Transmission of non-A or non-B hepatitis by pH4-treated intravenous immunoglobulin. Vox Sang 57:15–18, 1989.

Woodruff RK, Grigg AP, Firkin FL, Smith IL. Fatal thrombotic events during treatment of autoimmune thrombocytopenia with intravenous immunoglobulin in elderly patients. Lancet 2:217–219, 1986.

Wyatt HV. Poliomyelitis in hypogammaglobulinemics. J Infect Dis 128: 802–806, 1973.

Yap PL, McOmish F, Webster ADB, Hammarstrom L, Smith CIE, Bjorkander J, Ochs HD, Fischer SH, Quinti I, Simmonds P. Hepatitis C virus transmission by intravenous immunoglobulin. J Hepatol 21:455–460, 1994.

Yu MW, Mason BL, Guo ZP, Tankersley DL, Nedjar S, Mitchell FD, Biswas RM. Hepatitis C transmission associated with intravenous immunoglobulins. Lancet 345:1173–1174, 1995.

Yomtovian R, Abramson J, Quie PG. Granulocyte transfusion therapy in chronic granulomatous disease: report of a patient and review of the literature. Transfusion 21:739–743, 1981.

Ziegner UH, Kobayashi RH, Cunningham-Rundles C, Espanol T, Fasth A, Huttenlocher A, Krogstad P, Marthinsen L, Notarangelo LD, Pasic S, Rieger CH, Rudge P, Sankar R, Shigeoka AO, Stiehm ER, Sullivan KE, Webster AD, Ochs HD. Progressive neurodegeneration in patients with primary immunodeficiency disease on IVIG treatment. Clin Immunol 102:19–24, 2002.

Useful Web sites and Support Groups

Ataxia-Telangiectasia Children's Project. 6685 S. Military Trail, Deerfield Beach, FL 33442. www.atcp.org.

International Patient Organisation for Primary Immunodeficiencies. www. ipopi.org

Jeffrey Modell Foundation. 43 W. 47th Street, New York, NY 10036. http:// www.jmfworld.com/

National Immune Deficiency Foundation. 25 W. Chesapeake Avenue, Suite 206, Towson, MD 21204. http://www.primaryimmune.org/

National Organization for Rare Disorders. PO Box 8922, New Fairfield, CT 06812–8923. www.rarediseases.org.

Primary Immunodeficiency Association. PIA, 12 Caxton Way, London.

47

Bone Marrow Transplantation for Primary Immunodeficiency Diseases

REBECCA H. BUCKLEY and ALAIN FISCHER

Bone marrow transplantation was first attempted in the 1950s as a treatment for aplastic anemia. Except in identical twins (Pillow et al., 1966), however this therapy was unsuccessful until the late 1960s when the human major histocompatibility complex (MHC) was discovered (Amos and Bach, 1968). Shortly after that, immune function was successfully restored in two patients with fatal primary immunodeficiency diseases by transplants of unfractionated human leukocyte antigen (HLA)-identical allogeneic bone marrow. One patient had severe combined immunodeficiency (SCID) (Gatti et al., 1968) and the other had Wiskott-Aldrich syndrome (WAS) (Bach et al., 1968). The correction of these two conditions, as well as the later correction of many other forms of immunodeficiency by bone marrow transplantation (Friedrich, 1996; Buckley et al., 1999; Antoine et al., 2003), implied that the defects in most such conditions are intrinsic to cells of one or more hematopoietic lineages and that they are not due to failure of the microenvironment to support the growth and development of those cells.

The Principle of Bone Marrow Transplantation

In the early 1950s it was observed that the hematopoietic systems of lethally irradiated animals could be reconstituted by bone marrow cells (Lorenz et al., 1952). This was shown to be due to the presence of self-replicating cells in normal bone marrow that can given rise to erythrocytes, granulocytes, cells of the monocyte–macrophage lineage, megakaryocytes, and immunocompetent T and B cells (Brenner et al., 1993; Wu et al., 1967, 1968). Marrow transplantation has, therefore, been used in attempts to replace defective, absent, or malignant cells of the recipient with normal replicating hematopoietic and immunocompetent cells. Unfractionated bone marrow transplantation offers little

risk to the donor, as it involves removal of a tissue that is readily regenerated. Bone marrow cells are usually obtained by aspiration from multiple sites along the iliac crests, the sternum, or (in children) from the upper one-third of the tibia, while the donor is under general anesthesia (Thomas et al., 1975; Martin et al., 1987). The aspirate is placed in heparinized tissue culture medium and then passed through metal screens to remove bone spicules. If T cell depletion is necessary, the marrow is processed to remove T cells; nucleated marrow cells are then enumerated and the cells are given intravenously to the recipient.

Special Considerations in Bone Marrow Transplantation for Primary Immunodeficiency Diseases

Primary Goal: Immune Reconstitution

Unlike the situation in patients with malignancies or global bone marrow failure, the goal of bone marrow transplantation in patients with primary immunodeficiency is to provide normal cells of hematopoietic origin to correct underlying genetic deficits in the immune system. In SCID, no immunosuppression is needed because these patients lack T cells and are thus unable to reject a graft (Buckley, 2004). In other forms of primary immunodeficiency, however, there is usually enough T cell function to cause rejection. Therefore, immunosuppressive agents must be used. Drugs commonly used to ensure the acceptance of solid organ grafts have deleterious effects on the very cells one is trying to engraft in patients with genetically determined immunodeficiency. Thus, chemotherapy must be given *prior* to infusion of the marrow to avoid injury to the donor cells.

High Susceptibility to Graft-versus-Host Disease

In further contrast to the situation in solid organ transplantation, successful marrow engraftment until recently required HLA identity (at least for HLA class II determinants) between donor and recipient, primarily because of extreme susceptibility of marrow transplant recipients to graft-versus-host disease (GVHD). This is particularly problematic for patients with SCID and complete DiGeorge syndrome, who are highly susceptible to GVHD from T cells in transfused blood products even before transplantation because they cannot reject foreign T cells. Previously, this situation meant that an HLA-identical sibling donor was needed, and the likelihood that any given sibling will be a match is only 25%. However, one of the most important advances in the treatment of primary immunodeficiency diseases over the past two decades has been the development of methods to avoid GVHD by T cell depletion and thus to enable transplantation of half-matched (haploidentical) parental stem cells (Buckley et al., 1999; Antoine et al., 2003; Buckley, 2004).

The Problem of Ongoing Infections

Because infants and children with primary immunodeficiency often become infected with opportunistic infectious agents before a diagnosis has been made, such organisms cause particular problems from the standpoint of urgency of need for transplantation and in limiting the ability to use chemotherapeutic conditioning agents. This is particularly true for infections with viruses such as cytomegalovirus (CMV), Epstein-Barr virus (EBV), adenoviruses, and parainfluenza viruses, for which no effective antibiotic is available (Buckley, 2004).

Persistence of Transplacentally Acquired Maternal T Cells

Leukocytes from the mother often enter the fetal circulation during pregnancy; fetuses with SCID have no capacity to reject such cells. Therefore, persistence of maternal T cells in the infant's circulation is frequent. These maternal T cells are usually unable to respond normally to mitogens and fail to correct the infant's underlying immunodeficiency. They may or may not cause clinical signs of GVHD, such as eczema or splenomegaly. They can, however, create special problems (or benefits) when bone marrow transplantation is performed for SCID infants. If a donor other than the mother is used and no pretransplant chemotherapeutic conditioning is used, there is always the potential complication of a graft-versus-graft (GVG) reaction. If unfractionated HLA-identical sibling marrow is infused, this can lead to rejection of the maternal T cells, with or without a clinical GVG reaction (Friedman et al., 1991). By contrast, if a T cell–depleted haploidentical graft is given from the father without pretransplant conditioning, rejection of the paternal graft can occur, again with or without a clinical GVG reaction. On the other hand, if T cell–depleted haploidentical stem cells are given from the mother without pretransplant conditioning, immune reconstitution is often accelerated (Barrett et al., 1988), again with or without GVHD. GVHD that does occur in this setting usually requires either no treatment or only transient use of steroids.

Conditioning Regimens Are Not Always Needed

In contrast to the situation in patients with malignancy or marrow aplasia, it has been repeatedly shown that infants with SCID or with complete DiGeorge syndrome who have absent T cell function do not require pretransplant immunosuppression for successful bone marrow transplantation because they are unable to reject grafts (Buckley et al., 1999; Myers et al., 2002; Buckley, 2004). Some transplant centers have recommended conditioning for SCID patients with high numbers of natural killer (NK) cells because these patients are recognized as having a poorer outcome (Antoine et al., 2003). However, the underlying molecular defect, and not the NK cells may be the problem, as SCID infants with interleukin-7 receptor α (IL-7Rα) deficiency with high numbers of B and NK cells accept these grafts readily without conditioning (Buckley, 2004). Patients with most non-SCID types of primary immunodeficiency need to be preconditioned with chemotherapeutic agents to prevent graft rejection (see below) (Parkman, 1991a).

Post-transplant Graft-versus-Host Disease Prophylaxis Is Not Always Needed

As is the case for pretransplant conditioning, post-transplantation prophylaxis against GVHD is not always needed for bone marrow transplantation for primary immunodeficiency. This is particularly true for patients with SCID who are not given pretransplant conditioning, since conditioning enhances the likelihood that GVHD will occur (see below).

Sources of Stem Cells for Bone Marrow Transplantation and Donor Selection

The various potential sources of stem cells are listed in Table 47.1. All types of SCID and many other forms of primary immunodeficiency can be cured by bone marrow transplantation (Friedrich, 1996; Haddad et al., 1998; Antoine et al., 2003; Buckley, 2004).

Unfractionated HLA-Identical Bone Marrow or Peripheral Blood

If a patient with SCID or another form of primary immunodeficiency is fortunate enough to have an HLA-identical sibling, unfractionated bone marrow cells can be given, and this is the treatment of choice. In most cases, both T cell and B cell immunity have been fully reconstituted by such matched transplants, with evidence of function detected as early as 2 weeks following transplantation. Patients with SCID have required far fewer unfractionated nucleated marrow cells for successful immune reconstitution than the number needed to treat leukemic or aplastic patients; as few as 4×10^6 cells/kg of recipient body weight have

Table 47.1. Sources of Stem Cells for Transplantation

HLA-identical sibling marrow
Haploidentical parental marrow
  T cell–depleted by soy lectin/SRBC
  T cell–depleted by monoclonal antibodies
  T cell–depleted by CD34/CD133 positive selection
Matched unrelated adult marrow
  Unfractionated
  T cell depleted by CD34/CD133 positive selection
Unfractionated related or unrelated cord blood

SRBC, sheep red blood cells.

resulted in immunologic reconstitution (Friedrich, 1996). However, there is some evidence that higher numbers of stem cells result in better immune reconstitution (Buckley et al., 1999). Unfractionated marrow cells will also become engrafted in HLA-disparate SCID recipients who lack cellular immunity, but fatal GVHD can be anticipated because unfractionated marrow cell suspensions contain mature T cells in addition to stem cells.

T Cell–Depleted Haploidentical Bone Marrow Transplantation

If a SCID infant has no HLA-identical family members, the treatment of choice then becomes a T cell–depleted haploidentical marrow stem cell transplant from a half-matched family member. Following the leads from his own work in mice (Reisner et al., 1978) and from Muller-Ruchholtz et al.'s (1976) work in rats, Reisner et al. (1983) demonstrated in the early 1980s that removal of most mature T cells from half-matched parental marrow allowed successful immune reconstitution of human infants with SCID by the remaining cells without subsequent GVHD. Since that time, this principle has been successfully applied many times in the treatment of SCID (but not as successfully in other primary immunodeficiency diseases) (Table 47.2) (Buckley et al., 1986, 1999; Fischer et al., 1986a; O'Reilly et al., 1986; Moen et al., 1987; Wijnaendts et al., 1989; Dror et al., 1993; Stephan et al., 1993; Giri et al., 1994; Antoine et al., 2003). One condition in which this type of transplant is expected to have no benefit is the complete DiGeorge syndrome, where T cell-depleted marrow cells are ineffective because there is no thymus to "educate" the donor stem cells. The successful outcome after unfractionated HLA-identical marrow transplants into complete DiGeorge patients is due to the adoptive transfer of mature T and B cells that were educated in the donor's thymus (Goldsobel et al., 1987). The option of using a haploidentical donor, however, virtually ensures that all infants with SCID can have a related donor. Usually a mother or father (rather than a sibling) is the donor, since the volume of marrow donation required is much larger for this type of transplant. Because a high percentage of SCID infants have persistence of transplacentally transferred maternal T cells, the mother is often a better donor than the father, unless there are health issues that preclude use of the mother (e.g., if she is pregnant or positive for HIV or hepatitis antigen).

In Utero Bone Marrow Transplants

Availability of early prenatal diagnosis for several primary immunodeficiencies offers the option of in utero treatment. Two infants with γ_c-deficient SCID who were diagnosed in utero received CD34+ paternal stem cells intraperitoneally during the first half of gestation, and immune function developed in both postnatally (Flake et al., 1996; Wengler et al., 1996). In both instances, however, invasive procedures were performed on these fetuses on more than one occasion, there was the potential of a GVG reaction because of the likely presence of transplacentally transferred maternal T cells, and if either GVG or GVHD had occurred, there was no way of detecting it. Thus fetal wastage is a risk of this approach. Previous experience with in utero transplants was not very successful (Touraine,1996). Benefits of in

Table 47.2. Type of Immunodeficiency According to Donor Origin and Human Leukocyte Antigen (HLA) Matching

| Immunodeficiency | n (% of Category) | Related Donor | | | Unrelated |
		Genotypically HLA identical	Phenotypically HLA identical	HLA Mismatched	
SCID: Total	*475*	*104*	*49*	*294*	*28*
Reticular dysgenesis	12 (3%)	2	1	8	1
ADA deficiency	51 (11%)	19	2	26	4
Low T and low B cell count	137 (29%)	32	23	77	5
Low T cell count	217 (46%)	39	15	154	9
Other	58 (12%)	12	8	29	9
Non-SCID: Total	*444*	*148*	*40*	*176*	*80*
Wiskott-Aldrich syndrome	103 (23%)	33	5	45	20
T cell deficiencies					
Omenn syndrome	43 (10%)	9	6	20	8
PNP deficiency	4 (1%)	2	1	1	0
HLA class II deficiency	52 (12%)	17	10	22	3
CD40 ligand deficiency	11 (2%)	3	0	0	8
Other T cell immunodeficiency	76 (17%)	19	4	36	17
Phagocytic cell disorders					
Agranulocytosis	5 (1%)	3	0	2	0
Chronic granulomatous disease	17 (4%)	12	0	0	4
Leukocyte adhesion deficiency	26 (6%)	8	2	14	1
Hemophagocytic syndromes					
Familial lymphohistiocytosis	62 (14%)	19	4	29	10
Chediak-Higashi syndrome	20 (4%)	10	4	2	4
XLP (Purtillo)	2 (1%)	0	0	0	2
Griscelli disease	6 (1%)	3	1	1	1
Other	17 (4%)	8	3	4	2

ADA, adenosine deaminase; PNP, purine nucleoside phosphorylase; SCID, severe combined immunodeficiency; XLP, X-linked lymphoproliferative syndrome.
Source: Antoine et al., *Lancet* 361:553–560, 2003, with permission.

utero transplantation over immediate postnatal transplantation in settings where parents do not wish pregnancy termination have to be carefully assessed. In utero bone marrow transplantation obviously reduces the risks of infectious complications. On the other hand, early postnatal haploidentical bone marrow transplantation in SCID has been found to be successful in more than 97% of cases (Buckley et al., 1999; Myers et al., 2002; Buckley, 2004), making it difficult to justify the risk to the fetus of in utero transplantation.

It is likely that haploidentical bone marrow stem cell transplantation performed in utero later than 12 weeks of gestation will not be possible in conditions other than SCID, since development of the fetal T cells in those conditions will be an obstacle for engraftment.

Methods of T Cell Depletion

By far the best preventive approach to GVHD is the removal of mature T cells from the donor marrow.

Soybean lectin, sheep erythrocyte agglutination

The most successful method for rigorous T cell depletion involves agglutination of most mature marrow cells with soybean lectin, followed by sedimentation of these clumped cells and subsequent removal of T cells by sheep erythrocyte rosetting and density-gradient centrifugation (Reisner et al., 1983; Schiff et al., 1987). For an adequate yield of stem cells, it is necessary to collect approximately 1 liter of bone marrow from the donor. This is usually not a problem, since a parent is usually used as the donor, and the donations are made under general anesthesia. After soy lectin agglutination, there are still numerous T cells in the nonagglutinated fraction (Schiff et al., 1987). To remove T cells, two steps of sheep erythrocyte rosette depletion are required. The final cell preparation, representing <5%–10% of the initial number of nucleated marrow cells, consists of immature myeloid cells and stem cells, contains few if any lymphocytes, and is phytohemagglutinin (PHA) and mixed leukocyte culture (MLC) nonresponsive. (Schiff et al., 1987). This method, unlike CD34 selection, leaves all other immature marrow cells (including CD34-negative stem cells) available in the cell suspension for use in the transplant.

Some investigators have used sheep erythrocyte rosette-depletion alone to remove T cells from the donor marrow (Fischer et al., 1986a). Because different centers have used different numbers of rosette depletions and different methods of modifying the sheep red cells, there have been varying degrees of effectiveness of this approach to remove post-thymic T cells.

Monoclonal antibody and complement lysis

Another method of depleting post-thymic T cells from donor marrow is incubation with monoclonal antibodies to human T cells plus a source of complement (Reinherz et al., 1982; Filipovich et al., 1984; Waldmann et al., 1984; Morgan et al., 1986). Antibodies employed for this purpose have included T12, Leu 1, CT-2, and Campath-1 (Hale et al., 1988; Hale and Waldmann, 1994). T cell depletion by antibody and complement is not as effective as the above approach, possibly because of modulation of T cell antigens from the surface of the T cells, which then escape destruction. As a consequence, somewhat more frequent and severe GVHD has been observed.

CD34+ cell selection by affinity columns

Probably the most common method of T cell depletion employed in most transplant centers today is the use of commercially avail-

able antibody affinity columns that positively select for CD34+ cells (Handgretinger et al., 2001; Gordon et al., 2002). In this method, all other cells are discarded. In the earlier version of these columns there was a problem with trapping of T cells, such that an additional T cell depletion step was necessary to avoid GVHD. Reportedly, newer versions result in greater purity of CD34+ cells (Schumm et al., 1999). However, success with this type of T cell depletion may not be as great as with methods that just remove T cells, possibly because fewer cells are usually given. In addition, CD34− negative stem cells are discarded, along with other cells that could be important in promoting immune reconstitution, such as dendritic cells. Recently, the pentaspan molecule CD133 has been judged to be a marker of primitive hematopoietic progenitors. Lang et al. (2004) evaluated a CD133-based selection method in 10 pediatric patients given stem cells from matched unrelated ($n = 2$) or mismatched-related donors ($n = 8$). Engraftment occurred in all patients (sustained primary, $n = 8$; after reconditioning, $n = 2$). No primary acute GVHD of a magnitude greater than grade II or chronic GVHD was observed.

Unfractionated, Matched Unrelated Adult Marrow

Most patients with primary immunodeficiency will not have an HLA-identical donor. T cell–depleted marrow transplants are not as effective for non-SCID primary immunodeficiency conditions in which pretransplant conditioning is required (see below). Therefore, an alternate source of stem cells will have to be selected if immune reconstitution is to be possible, such as a matched unrelated marrow donor (MUD). The problem with both matched unrelated adult bone marrow donors and unrelated cord blood donors is that, because humans are an outbred population, the matching can never be perfect (Tiercy et al., 2000). Minor locus histocompatibility antigen differences are also much more likely to be present than in the related donor setting, resulting in a high probability of GVHD. Another drawback with the use of MUD adult donors is that it takes approximately 4 months (6 weeks to 12 months) to identify an unrelated adult donor.

Cord Blood

One rich source of hematopoietic stem cells for transplantation is unfractionated cord blood (Wagner et al., 1995). Part of the rationale for using cord blood is that the incidence and severity of GVHD appears to be lower with MUD cord blood than with MUD adult unfractionated marrow transplants, even with one to two HLA antigen mismatches (Barker and Wagner, 2002; Wagner et al., 2002). In addition, it generally takes less time to locate a cord blood unit than an adult donor. Several successes with cord blood transplantation from HLA identical siblings have been reported, notably in patients with genetic disorders—including immunodeficiencies (Vowels et al., 1993; Wagner et al., 1995, 2002; Stary et al., 1996; Barker and Wagner, 2002; Grewal et al., 2003). The graft failure rate could be increased, however. Affecting the success rate of cord blood transplants is the number of nucleated cells present in the unit, especially the number of CD34+ cells. It has been shown that at least 1.7×10^5 CD34+ cells/kg recipient body weight are needed (Wagner et al., 2002). In addition, there is a much longer period of thrombocytopenia following cord blood transplants than that after HLA-identical unfractionated marrow transplants (Thomson et al., 2000).

Most of the current protocols for cord blood transplantation call for pretransplant conditioning, regardless of the underlying diagnosis of the patient. If a patient with primary immunodeficiency is already infected, particularly in the case of SCID, these drugs increase risk for demise. Successful umbilical cord transplantation has, however, been achieved in SCID without pretransplant conditioning, even in an infant with NK cells (Toren et al., 1999). More importantly, GVHD prophylaxis is routinely given after transplants from either unrelated adults or cord blood donors and, in the case of cord blood transplants, this is continued for at least 9 months. The conditioning and GVHD prophylaxis both contribute to a long period of immune impairment post-transplantation, which is self-defeating if the goal of transplantation is immune reconstitution.

Usefulness of Computerized Bone Marrow Donor Banks

In 1989, the Italian Bone Marrow Donor Registry was established to facilitate donor search and marrow procurement for patients lacking an HLA-identical donor (Dini et al., 1996), and in 1992 the National Marrow Donor Program was established in the United States. Several similar registries have been established elsewhere. All are listed in the Bone Marrow Donors World Wide (BMDWW) directory, which includes more than 9,000,000 donors in its latest edition. These registries are quite useful if (1) the transplant is not an emergency and (2) if the patient has relatively common HLA antigens. It is often difficult to find donors for patients belonging to certain racial and ethnic groups, however, and the expense involved in conducting such a search is high (Tiercy et al., 2000). In addition to the above registries, a cord blood bank has been established in the United States.

Graft Rejection and Graft-versus-Host Disease

Unlike solid organ transplantation, allogeneic bone marrow transplantation is complicated not only by the possibility of graft rejection by the recipient but also by the potential of immune cells in the transplanted marrow to reject the recipient, causing GVHD.

Prevention of Graft Rejection

As noted above, immunosuppressive and myeloablative agents used to prevent graft rejection must be given prior to infusion of marrow cells so as to avoid injury to the donor cells. In transplant recipients who have the potential to reject grafts, factors influencing the likelihood of engraftment of donor marrow cells are (1) the degree of immunocompetence of the recipient; (2) the degree of MHC disparity between donor and recipient; (3) the degree of presensitization of the recipient to the histocompatibility antigens of the donor; (4) the number of marrow cells administered; (5) the type of conditioning regimen given the recipient; and (6) whether or not T cell depletion techniques are used. Initially, total body irradiation (TBI) was used to prepare non-SCID immunodeficiency patients for bone marrow transplantation. It was later recognized that TBI could be safely replaced by busulphan at dosages (16 to 20 mg/kg total) that did not produce comparable adverse late effects (Blazar et al., 1985), because preparation of the recipient need only be directed at immunosuppression and "spacing"—i.e., making room in the marrow for donor cells. It was also found that such doses of busulfan were sufficient for young patients (below the age of 2 to 4 years), despite the reduced bioavailabilitiy of busulphan in this age group (Blazar et al., 1985; Vassal et al., 1993). There is now general consensus on the use of busulphan at 2 or 4 mg/kg daily for 4 days, together with cyclophosphamide at 50 mg/kg daily for 4 days, with or without anti-thymocyte globulin (ATG), as a conditioning regimen for patients with non-SCID immunodeficiency to be treated by HLA-identical bone marrow transplantation (Parkman, 1991a). However, studies have demonstrated a high variability of busulphan disposition among young children (by a factor of 6) (Vassal et al., 1993). These results demonstrate the need for an individual, close adjustment of busulphan in infants and young children. The development of an intravenous form of busulfan has helped to reduce this problem immensely; much better control of dosing is possible by the intravenous route and the drug can be given once or twice a day (Fernandez et al., 2002; Bostrom et al., 2003; Dalle et al., 2003). The above agents may be insufficient for chemoablation in young patients with phagocytic cell disorders. Alternatively, other myeloablative drugs can be used, such as thiotepa (Przepiorka et al., 1994).

Nonmyeloablative Bone Marrow Transplantation

For patients with preexisting organ damage, there is significant morbidity and mortality from traditional conditioning regimens employing busulfan and cyclophosphamide or TBI. Therefore, there has been increasing interest in developing conditioning regimens that are less toxic (Nagler et al., 1999; Barta et al., 2001; Feinstein et al., 2001; Horwitz et al., 2001; Pulsipher and Woolfrey, 2001; Woolfrey et al., 2001; Gaspar et al., 2002; Mielcarek et al., 2002). Either total lymphoid irradiation or a combination of nucleoside analogs and anti-lymphocyte antibody preparations can be used to attain less toxicity. Although these regimens are significantly less cytotoxic than high-dose alkylating agents and TBI, they are profoundly immunosuppressive. Opportunistic infections such as the reactivation of CMV remain clinical obstacles when nonmyeloablative stem cell transplants are performed using these agents, especially in elderly and previously immunosuppressed patients. GVHD prophylaxis with cyclosporine and methotrexate, with added mycophenolate mofetil in some cases, has been necessary because GVHD is common following nonmyeloablative transplantation.

Use of Campath 1 Monoclonal Antibody In Vivo

It has become common practice to include the in vivo administration of alemtuzumab (anti-CD52, Campath 1) in reduced intensity or conventional pretransplant ablation protocols for patients with malignancies who are receiving peripheral blood stem cell transplants; the antibody is then also continued post-transplantation as prophylaxis against GVHD (Chakrabarti et al., 2004). While this approach has been effective in controlling GVHD and improving engraftment in the cancer transplant setting, it has also been associated with a much longer period of immunodeficiency post-transplantation (Chakrabarti et al., 2004) and with the development of lethal lymphoproliferative disease (Snyder et al., 2004). Therefore, this approach would appear to be counterproductive in transplants done with the goal of achieving immune reconstitution in immunodeficient patients.

Graft-versus-Host Disease

GVHD is the major barrier to widespread successful application of bone marrow transplantation for the correction of many different diseases (Glucksberg et al., 1974; Martin et al., 1987; Deeg and Henslee-Downey, 1990; Ferrara and Deeg, 1991; Parkman, 1991b). Acute GVHD begins 6 or more days post-transplantation (or post-transfusion in the case of nonirradiated blood products) (Anderson and Weinstein, 1990) with high, unrelenting fever, a morbilliform maculopapular erythematous rash, and severe diarrhea (Glucksberg et al., 1974). The rash becomes progressively confluent and may involve the entire body surface; it is both pruritic and painful and eventually leads to marked exfoliation. Eosinophilia and lymphocytosis develop, followed shortly by hepatosplenomegaly, abnormal liver function tests, and elevation in blood conjugated bilirubin levels. Watery diarrhea occurs and may become voluminous and bloody as the disease progresses. Nausea, vomiting, and severe, cramping abdominal pain occur as a consequence of the gastrointestinal involvement, which is also accompanied by a protein-losing enteropathy. The latter condition contributes to marked generalized edema ("third spacing") seen in more severe, acute GVHD. The most severe forms of acute GVHD are also characterized by bone marrow aplasia, marked susceptibility to infection (Gratama et al., 1987; Parkman,1991b; Skinner et al., 1986), and death in a high proportion of cases.

Staging

Staging of GVHD is based on severity and on the number of organ systems involved (Glucksberg et al., 1974). The four categories generally defined are as follows:

Grade 1: 1+ to 2+ skin rash without gut involvement and with no more than 1+ liver involvement
Grade 2: 1+ to 3+ skin rash with either 1+ to 2+ gastrointestinal involvement or 1+ to 2+ liver involvement or both
Grade 3: 2+ to 4+ skin rash with 2+ to 4+ gastrointestinal involvement with or without 2+ to 4+ liver involvement. Decrease in performance status and fever also characterize Grades 2 and 3.
Grade 4: The pattern and severity of GVHD are similar to those in Grade 3 with extreme constitutional symptoms.

Chronic Graft-versus-Host disease

If the patient does not succumb and the acute GVHD persists, it is termed chronic after 100 days. Chronic GVHD may evolve from acute GVHD or may develop in the absence of or after resolution of acute GVHD. It occurs in 45%–70% of conditioned patients receiving HLA-matched bone marrow transplants from unrelated donors (Martin et al., 1987; Weisdorf et al., 1990; Parkman, 1991b). Skin lesions of chronic GVHD resemble scleroderma, with hyperkeratosis, reticular hyperpigmentation, atrophy with ulceration, and fibrosis and limitation of joint movement. Other manifestations include the sicca syndrome, disordered immunoregulation, as evidenced by autoantibody and immune complex formation and poly- and monoclonal hyperimmunoglobulinemia (Noel et al., 1978; Graze and Gale, 1979), idiopathic interstitial pneumonitis, and frequent infections (Skinner et al., 1986; Parkman, 1991b).

Pathogenesis

Graft-versus-host disease is almost invariable in the case of HLA class II antigen differences between the donor and recipient, because the immunocompetent donor T cells recognize the foreign transplantation antigens of the recipient. In the case of HLA-identical marrow transplants, GVHD is likely due to responses by donor T cells (Theobald et al., 1992; Schwarer et al., 1993) to recipient minor locus histocompatibility or Y chromosome–associated transplantation antigens, since a significantly higher

incidence of GVHD occurs in male patients given unfractionated MHC-matched female marrows than in patients receiving MHC-matched and sex-matched marrows (Bortin and Rimm, 1977; Martin et al., 1987; Ferrara and Deeg, 1991; Parkman, 1991b). However, female marrow transplanted into male recipients does not appear to be a problem in the case of T cell–depleted grafts (Buckley et al., 1999; Buckley, 2004). GVHD is usually mild and self-limited in SCID hosts who receive unfractionated HLA-identical marrow, because there is no need for them to receive pretransplant immunosuppression (Parkman, 1991b). However, in 60% of recipients given pretransplant irradiation or immunosuppressive drugs, GVHD is moderate to severe despite HLA identity, and it is fatal in 15%–20% (Glucksberg et al., 1974; Martin et al., 1987; Deeg and Henslee-Downey, 1990). The severity of GVHD increases with the recipient's age (Parkman, 1991b; Storb et al., 1986), the use of HLA-matched unrelated donors, and, if a related donor is not HLA-identical, the degree of genetic disparity.

Prevention of Graft-versus-Host disease

The best approach to GVHD is prevention. As already noted, removal of T cells from the donor marrow or blood is the most effective means of preventing GVHD. For patients undergoing unfractionated HLA-identical marrow transplants and receiving pretransplant chemotherapy to prevent rejection, GVHD prophylaxis is necessary. GVHD prophylaxis ordinarily consists of a short course of methotrexate (15 mg/M^2 on the first day post-transplantation and 10 mg/M^2 on the third, sixth, and eleventh days), together with daily cyclosporine given for 6 months, as has been used in other transplant settings (Storb et al., 1986; Martin et al., 1987; Parkman, 1991b). Recently, studies have indicated that the addition of mycophenylate mofitil to this regimen improves the prevention of GVHD (Wang et al., 2002). Acute GVHD greater than grade II is 24% for patients in the European registry for immunodeficiencies. In addition, for unfractionated, unrelated matched cord blood transplantation, high doses of methylprednisolone are given from the time of transplantation until approximately 6 months post-transplantation.

Treatment of Graft-versus-Host disease

The above-mentioned agents have not prevented GVHD entirely, and they can delay and/or suppress the development of immune function. However, once severe GVHD has become established, it is extremely difficult to treat. Many regimens have been employed to mitigate GVHD in both MHC-incompatible and MHC-compatible bone marrow transplants. Anti-thymocyte globulin, steroids, cyclosporine, mycophenylate mofitil, and murine monoclonal antibodies directed against human T cell surface antigens have ameliorated GVHD in some cases, but fatal GVHD has still occurred in others even though treated (Martin et al., 1987; Deeg and Henslee-Downey, 1990; Parkman, 1991b). Anticytokine and anticytokine receptor antibodies have also been employed to mitigate GVHD (Deeg and Henslee-Downey, 1990); the most useful of these has been antibody to the IL-2 receptor α chain (anti-CD25) (Srinivasan et al., 2004).

Sequelae of Pretransplant Chemotherapy for Bone Marrow Transplantation

Veno-occlusive Disease

Veno-occlusive disease (VOD) is a major cause of mortality following conditioning regimens employing cytoreductive agents that damage the hepatic vascular endothelium (McDonald et al., 1985; Eltumi et al., 1993). Distinguishing VOD from other causes of liver damage can be difficult after bone marrow transplantation, particularly when thrombocytopenia poses an unacceptable risk for diagnostic percutaneous liver biopsy in the early post-transplant period. Most often the diagnosis has been made on clinical criteria; however, serum concentrations of the aminopropeptide of type III procollagen (PIIINP) above a standard deviation (SD) score of 8 have been predictive of VOD and are also useful in the diagnosis and monitoring of this condition (Eltumi et al., 1993). In addition to hepatic damage caused by chemotherapeutic agents for pretransplant conditioning, such agents can also result in considerable pulmonary toxicity post-transplantation, leading to prolonged oxygen dependency. Often this problem is difficult to distinguish from infectious pulmonary complications post-transplantation, such as CMV pneumonia.

Growth Retardation and Hormonal Disturbances

Growth retardation and hormonal disturbances frequently occur in children who have received pretransplant conditioning and who are long-term survivors (Clement-De Boers et al., 1996). However, the effect on height is not very great unless TBI is used. Hormonal disturbances leading to delayed puberty and sterility can be due either to TBI or to the effects of alkylating chemotherapy (cyclophosphamide). Elevated levels of follicle-stimulating hormone are found in those so affected.

Immune Reconstitution after Bone Marrow Transplantation

Bone Marrow Transplantation for Severe Combined Immunodeficiency

Bone marrow transplantation has been more widely applied and more successful in infants with SCID than in any other primary immunodeficiency (Friedrich, 1996; Buckley et al., 1999; Antoine et al., 2003; Buckley, 2004). Since the first such transplant was done, more than 800 patients with SCID worldwide have received transplants of HLA-identical or haploidentical bone marrow or of unrelated marrow or cord stem cells (Haddad et al., 1998; Antoine et al., 2003; R.H. Buckley, personal survey). In a recent report from the European Group for Blood and Marrow Transplantation and the European Society for Immunodeficiency, 475 infants with SCID were reviewed who had received bone marrow transplants from 1968 to 1999 (Table 47.2). One hundred fifty-three had received marrow from a genotypically or phenotypically HLA–identical relative and 77% survived, whereas 294 had received T cell–depleted haploidentical related transplants and only 54% survived (Antoine et al., 2003) (Fig. 47.1). Previously published survival rates for SCID patients transplanted at the two largest centers in Europe, Hopital Necker in Paris (Stephan et al., 1993) and the University of Ulm (Friedrich et al., 1993), were very similar—i.e., 80% for HLA-identical unfractionated marrow recipients and approximately 55% for recipients of haploidentical, T cell–depleted marrow. Similar survival statistics have also been reported by SCID transplant centers in the

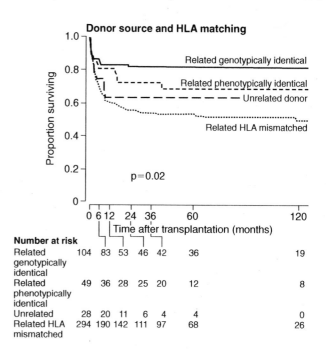

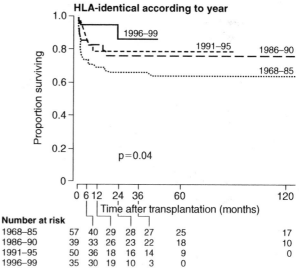

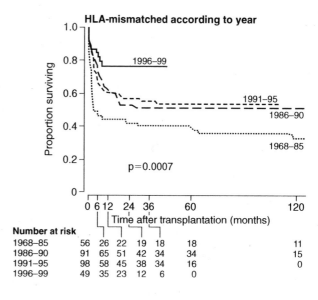

Figure 47.1. Cumulative probability of survival in SCID patients according to donor source (related or unrelated donor), HLA matching, and year of transplantation. (From Antoine et al., *Lancet* 361:553–560, 2003, with permission.)

United States (O'Reilly et al., 1986; O'Reilly, 1991; Dror et al., 1993). Even though the survival rate has been less with haploidentical donors, this is still a major accomplishment, because SCID is 100% fatal without marrow transplantation or, in the case of enzyme-deficient SCIDs, without enzyme-replacement therapy. However, the latter is helpful for only a small percentage of SCIDs, as adenosine deaminase (ADA) deficiency accounts for only approximately 16% of SCID cases (Stephan et al., 1993; Buckley et al., 1997; Buckley, 2004). Only 28 patients with SCID were reported in the European series as having received MUD transplants, and 63% were still surviving (Antoine et al., 2003). MUD transplant survival was somewhat better in a series from Brescia, Italy, and Toronto, Canada (Grunebaum et al., 2006).

One of the most significant findings from the European investigation was that there has been steady improvement over time in the survival rates of both HLA-identical and haploidentical marrow transplants in SCID recipients (Fig. 47.1), most likely because of more effective prevention or treatment of complications, notably infections and GVHD related to transplantation. Unfortunately, there is currently no similar comprehensive published summary for this time period for the overall experience in the United States.

Over the past 24 years, Buckley and associates have transplanted 152 infants with SCID, and 118 of these (78%) are currently surviving, for up to >24 years (Buckley, 2004). No pretransplant conditioning was given to any of these SCID patients prior to the marrow transplants. Only 16 of these 152 SCID patients had HLA-identical donors; all of them are surviving with functioning grafts. One hundred thirty-six patients received half-matched stem cells prepared by the T cell depletion technique in which soy lectin is followed by sheep red blood cell (SRBC) rosetting (Reisner et al., 1983; Schiff et al., 1987), without any pretransplant conditioning or GVHD prophylaxis. One hundred and two, or 75%, of these patients have survived. Most of the 34 deaths occurred from opportunistic viral infections—CMV in 6 patients, EBV/lymphoma in 3, enterovirus and adenovirus in 2 each, and parainfluenza and herpes simplex in 1 each. One patient died of multiple brain infarcts and another died of an unrelated mitochondrial defect.

Survival was clearly superior in those SCID infants transplanted soon after birth. Of 44 patients transplanted in the first 3.5 months of life, 42, or 95%, have survived (Fig. 47.2) (Buckley et al., 1999; Myers et al., 2002; Buckley, 2004). Unfortunately, although SCID could be diagnosed routinely at birth, there is no newborn screening. Consequently, most patients are diagnosed later, after they have developed serious infections.

Four of Buckley's SCID patients who received non–HLA-identical marrow were subsequently given matched, unrelated cord blood transplants because of resistance to engraftment of half-matched parental stem cells or for other reasons. One was a male infant with X-linked SCID (X-SCID) who engrafted T cell–depleted marrow from his IgA-deficient mother and, after immune function appeared, developed severe autoimmune cytopenias requiring long-term immunosuppressive agents. He then developed an mycobacterium avium complex (MAI) infection and was subsequently given a matched, unrelated cord blood transplant after chemotherapy to ablate his mother's graft; but unfortunately he died of CMV pneumonia. The second patient was a Jak3-deficient female SCID infant who became chimeric with T cell–depleted paternal marrow, but did not achieve adequate T cell function, even following a booster transplant from her father 10 months later. She was then given a successful MUD cord blood transplant after chemotherapy to ablate her father's

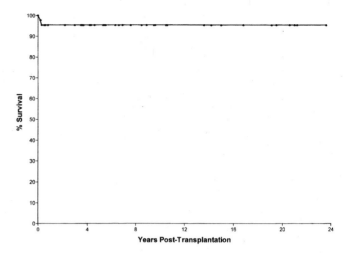

Figure 47.2. Kaplan-Meier survival curve for 44 consecutive infants with severe combined immunodeficiency (SCID) who received bone marrow transplants at R.H. Buckley's institution from HLA-identical ($n = 5$) or haploidentical ($n = 39$) donors before they were 3.5 months of age without pretransplantation chemoablation or post-transplantation graft-versus-host disease (GVHD) prophylaxis. Forty-two (95%) infants survived for periods of 2 months to 24 years after transplantation. The two deaths occurred from cytomegalovirus and EBV infections.

graft, and she is still surviving. Another X-SCID patient was given a cord blood transplant along with pretransplant ATG, but no post-transplant GVHD prophylaxis; and this patient developed grade 4 GVHD. The fourth patient, who had SCID of unknown molecular type, died of VOD after receiving pretransplant chemotherapy and a MUD cord blood transplant.

Problems Encountered with T Cell–Depleted Haploidentical Transplants

The period of vulnerability to infection is longer for recipients of T cell–depleted marrow than that for recipients of unfractionated HLA-identical marrow because of the 90–120 days required for donor stem cells to develop into T cells in the thymus and the fact that there are no adoptively transferred donor T cells. The occurrence of B cell lymphoproliferative disease is also a significant problem with this type of transplantation, whereas it does not occur in recipients of unfractionated HLA-identical marrow (Trigg et al., 1985; Filipovich et al., 1994; Levine, 1994). Most of these cases have been EBV positive (Shearer et al., 1985) and most have been in recipients of marrow T cell–depleted by monoclonal antibody. Again, the long period before development of normal T cell function is thought to be related to the propensity to develop such tumors.

Other problems encountered following haploidentical T cell–depleted transplants include resistance to engraftment and frequent failure to obtain engraftment of donor B cells or to develop B cell function. The latter is a particular problem in γĉ-deficient and Jak3-deficient SCID. Buckley has attempted to overcome both of the latter two problems by "booster" transplants, performed in 33 (24%) of the 152 patients previously discussed; 21 of these are currently surviving. Twenty-four patients received T cell–depleted booster transplants from the same parental donor without pre-booster conditioning; 8 (33%) of these patients died of opportunistic viral infections. Nine patients received T cell–depleted booster transplants from the other parent, again without conditioning; 4 (44%) died of infection. Immune function improved or normalized in a majority who received the booster transplants.

Kinetics of Development of Immune Function

The time to development of immune function following haploidentical stem cell grafts is quite different from that after unfractionated HLA-identical marrow. In contrast to the rapid development of immune function within 2 weeks after the latter type of grafts, lymphocytes with mature T cell phenotypes and functions fail to appear in significant numbers until 3–4 months after transplantation of T cell–depleted marrow (Fig. 47.3) (Buckley et al., 1986; Moen et al., 1987; Wijnaendts et al., 1989; Dror et al., 1993). This result holds true even if pretransplant conditioning is given (Friedrich et al., 1993) or if T cell–depleted, HLA-identical sibling marrow is used (R.H. Buckley, unpublished results). Thus, regardless of whether the donor is HLA-identical or haploidentical, it takes between 90 and 120 days for stem cells in T cell–depleted marrow to mature into

functioning T cells in SCID infants. The reason for this delay is not known, but presumably this is how long it takes for thymic maturation of stem cells to occur. This period of time is not unlike that in intrauterine life, in which PHA responsive T cells do not appear until around 12 weeks of gestation. The first function to develop after transplantation is NK cell function (in those molecular types in which this function is missing). Shortly after NK cells, T cell function appears, simultaneously with the development of phenotypically normal T cells (Fig. 47.3). Karyotype studies reveal that such T cells are always 100% of donor origin (Buckley et al., 1999). Thus, the tiny, architecturally abnormal epithelial thymi of patients with all forms of SCID treated thus far appear to have the ability to cause normal stem cells to become phenotypically and functionally normal T cells (Patel et al., 2000).

B cell function develops much more slowly, averaging 2 to 2.5 years for normalization in some patients; others fail to develop B cell function altogether, despite normal T cell function (Buckley et al., 1986, 1999; Moen et al., 1987; Wijnaendts et al., 1989; Dror

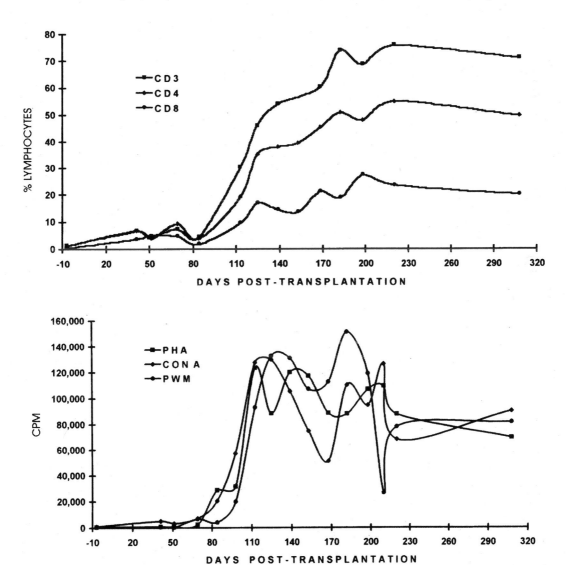

Figure 47.3. Results of sequential immunologic studies in a male infant with Jak3-deficient SCID before and after transplantation of T cell–depleted haploidentical maternal marrow stem cells, displaying (A) T cell phenotypes and (B) T cell responses to mitogens. T cell phenotypes and function appeared simultaneously, but not until more than 90 days post-transplantation. All dividing T cells in (B) were of female karyotype. Con A, concanavalin A; PHA, phytohemagglutinin; PWM, pokeweed mitogen.

et al., 1993; Giri et al., 1994; Buckley, 2004). Genetic analyses of the cells from such chimeric patients have revealed that all T cells are of donor origin, whereas the B cells, antigen-presenting cells, neutrophils, platelets, and red cells remain of recipient origin in a large majority of cases unless pretransplant conditioning is given (Buckley et al., 1986; Schouten et al., 1988; Friedrich et al., 1993; Vossen et al., 1993; van Leeuwen et al., 1994; Brady et al., 1996). Even following pretransplant conditioning, B cell engraftment and/or B cell function are not guaranteed. Indeed, in a careful evaluation of post–transplantation B cell function in SCID patients treated at a single center, B cell function was no better in those who had received pretransplant chemotherapy than in those who had not; however, the conditioning used was not fully myeloablative (Haddad et al., 1999). These observations suggest that the thymic microenvironment of most infants with SCID is capable of differentiating half-matched normal stem cells to become mature and functioning T lymphocytes that can cooperate effectively with host B cells for antibody production (Buckley, 2004). Thus, the genetic defect in SCID appears not to involve the thymus, except to the extent that it is small and morphologically abnormal because of a lack of interaction with normal developing thymocytes.

Bone Marrow Transplantation for Immunodeficiencies Other than Severe Combined Immunodeficiency

Allogeneic bone marrow transplantation has been found effective in conferring improved immune function to at least 21 distinct immunodeficiencies other than SCID (Tables 47.3 and 47.4) (Fischer et al., 1986b, 1990, 1994; Le Deist et al., 1989; Friedrich, 1996; Buckley and Fischer, 1999). A recent publication from the European Group for Blood and Marrow Transplantation and the European Society for Immunodeficiency (covering 37 centers in 18 countries) reported on the outcomes of 444 patients with these various forms of immunodeficiencies who had been transplanted from 1968 to 1999 (Antoine et al., 2003).

Indications

Indications for bone marrow transplantation in non-SCID primary immunodeficiency obviously depend on a critical assessment of life expectancy as well as quality of life in a given setting. Disease prognosis alone is not usually sufficient to lead to such a decision.

Table 47.3. Immunodeficiencies of the Lymphoid System That Are Curable by Allogeneic Bone Marrow Transplantation

Adenosine deaminase deficiency
Purine nucleoside phosphorylase deficiency
X-linked SCID (γ_c deficiency)
AR SCID with B cells (IL-7Rα, Jak-3, CD3δ, and CD3ϵ deficiencies)
AR SCID without B cells (Rag1/Rag2 and Artemis deficiencies)
Omenn syndrome
Reticular dysgenesis
Defective T cell activation (including ZAP-70 deficiency, calcium flux deficiency, and cytokine production deficiency)
HLA class II expression deficiency
Cartilage-hair hypoplasia
Wiskott-Aldrich syndrome
X-linked hyper-IgM syndrome (CD40 ligand deficiency)
X-linked lymphoproliferative syndrome (SH2D1A deficiency)
Lymphoproliferative syndrome with Fas (CD95 deficiency)

AR, autosomal recessive inheritance.

Table 47.4. Immunodeficiences of the Phagocytic System That Are Curable by Allogeneic Bone Marrow Transplantation

Chronic granulomatous diseases (X-linked and AR)
Leukocyte adhesion deficiency, type I
Chediak-Higashi syndrome
Immunodeficiency with partial albinism (Griscelli disease)
Familial hemophagocytic lymphohistiocytosis
Interferon-γ receptor deficiencies
Severe congenital neutropenia and other neutropenias (cyclic neutropenia, Shwachmann syndrome)

AR, autosomal recessive.

Age, past clinical history and sequelae of illnesses (chronic viral infection, immunosuppressive treatment required for control of autoimmunity, organ dysfunction), clinical course of previously affected family members, gene mutation determination when available, context of medical care (distance from specialized centers), and psychological assessment of the child and the family are some of the many factors to be taken into consideration when attempting to decide for or against bone marrow transplantation.

As greater experience with bone marrow transplantation has been gained, many of the factors leading to increased mortality and morbidity have decreased with time. It is not appropriate to assess the risks associated with bone marrow transplantation in the 1990s on the basis of results reported in the early 1980s. For instance, in Europe, the rate of success in bone marrow transplants performed from October 1985 up to March 1991 was 81.5% vs. 52% before October 1985 (Antoine et al., 2003). A specific example is seen in the case of the chronic granulomatous diseases, where recent comparisons of conservative treatment vs. bone marrow transplantation are leading to a possible change in attitude toward this treatment (see below). These remarks emphasize the need for careful updating of bone marrow transplantation registries to aid the medical community in decision making for treatment of this and other primary immunodeficiency diseases. Younger age at the time of bone marrow transplantation is associated with excellent outcome, and progress has been made in recent years, particularly in infection prevention with intravenous immunoglobulin [IVIG] and antiviral drugs (Antoine et al., 2003).

Bone Marrow Transplantation in Non-SCID Immunodeficiencies

Bone marrow transplantation has not been as uniformly effective in the treatment of patients with non-SCID T cell immunodeficiencies such as phagocyte disorders, as it has in SCID (Fig. 47.4). Such patients have somewhat less severe immune dysfunction than those with SCID, and this enables them to reject marrow grafts. However, a number of transplants with HLA-identical sibling marrow, matched unrelated adult marrow, peripheral blood stem cells, or cord blood have been successful after chemoablation (Tables 47.2 and 47.5). Following the improved results with T cell–depleted, HLA-haploidentical bone marrow transplantation for the treatment of SCID, this approach was tried for the treatment of other lethal immunodeficiency diseases. However, unlike the situation in SCID, there are relatively few reports of successful HLA-haploidentical bone marrow transplantation in non-SCID immunodeficiencies because of a high incidence of graft rejection (up to 75%) and of infectious complications (Fischer et al., 1986b, 1991). Delay in the development of T and B cell function (6 to 40 months) causes significant infectious

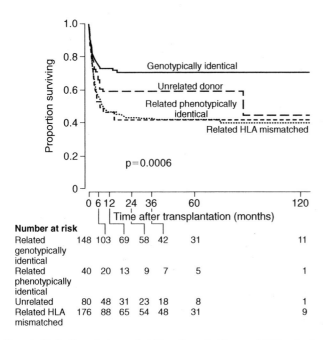

Figure 47.4. Cumulative probability of survival in non-SCID patients, according to donor source (related or unrelated donor) and HLA matching (From Antoine et al., *Lancet* 361:553–560, 2003, with permission.)

complications that remain a major concern in recipients of T cell–depleted, HLA-haploidentical transplants. For example, 16 of 71 patients who underwent two or three HLA antigen–incompatible, T cell–depleted bone marrow transplantations for immunodeficiencies (excluding SCID) had EBV-induced B lymphocyte proliferative syndromes, and 10 of them died from this complication (Fischer et al., 1994). Lymphoproliferative disease was particularly frequent in Wiskott-Aldrich patients who underwent HLA haploidentical bone marrow transplantation. In a European survey, 39% of such patients (compared with 12% of patients with combined immunodeficiency and 3% of those with SCID) developed a lymphoproliferative disorder after HLA haploidentical marrow transplantation (European Bone Marrow Transplantation/European Society of Immunodeficiency Diseases Registry, unpublished data). This result may have been caused by poor T cell control of EBV replication. Because of these outcomes, the preferred bone marrow donors in this group of patients are HLA-matched siblings. If this is not possible, a search for a matched unrelated donor should be undertaken.

Table 47.5. Three-year Survival in Non-SCID Patients According to Primary Disease and Donor–Recipient Compatibility

Disorder	Genotypically Identical HSCT		Related, HLA-Mismatched HSCT	
	n	% Survival (95% CI)	n	% Survival (95% CI)
Phagocytic cell disorders	23	70 (49–91)	14	69 (44–95)
Wiskott-Aldrich syndrome	32	81 (67–94)	43	45 (30–60)*
Hemophagocytic syndrome	32	68 (48–87)	28	49 (30–67)
T cell deficiency	47	63 (50–77)	72	35 (24–46)

CI, confidence interval; HSCT, hematopoietic stem cell transplantation.

*$p < 0.001$, for difference between genotypically identical and related, mismatched transplants.

Source: Antoine et al., *Lancet* 361:553–560, 2003, with permission.

Matched Unrelated Donors

More recently, success has been obtained in non-SCID immunodeficiency diseases by bone marrow tranplants from matched unrelated donors (MUD) (Ash et al., 1990; Kernan et al., 1993). In a survey of MUD transplantation, Kernan et al. (1993) indicated that the success rate of bone marrow transplantation for patients with inborn errors was 50%. Filipovich et al. (1992) reported successful MUD bone marrow transplantation in six of eight SCID recipients, two of two patients with WAS, and two of two patients with Chediak-Higashi syndrome. Some success using HLA partially incompatible, unrelated donor marrow has also been reported, especially when the degree of incompatibility was restricted to one HLA antigen and provided that marrow was T cell depleted (Ash et al., 1990; Filipovich et al., 1992). Perhaps the greatest success has been in WAS (see below) (Filipovich et al., 2001).

Wiskott-Aldrich Syndrome

This defect (see Chapter 31) is the second most common primary immunodeficiency for which bone marrow transplantation has been applied. After only partial correction by the first bone marrow transplant given a WAS patient in 1968 (Bach et al., 1968) full correction was achieved in other WAS patients in 1978 by use of a more effective conditioning regimen (Parkman et al., 1978). HLA-identical bone marrow transplantation has thus far been successful in 85%–90% of WAS patients who had an HLA-identical sibling donor (Tables 47.2 and 47.5) (Brochstein et al., 1991; Ozsahin et al., 1996).

Rumelhart et al. (1990) reported success with haploidentical transplants in three of four WAS patients, while Brochstein et al. (1991) reported success in only one of six with the same condition. In general, however, T cell–depleted haploidentical marrow transplants have not been very successful in WAS. Because of this result, MUD bone marrow, peripheral blood, and cord blood transplants have been carried out in a significant number of WAS patients (Lenarsky et al., 1993; Miano et al., 1998; Knutsen et al., 2003). In a report from the International Bone Marrow Transplant Registry, 170 patients with WAS had been transplanted, and the 5-year probability of survival (95% confidence interval) for all subjects was 70% (63%–77%) (Filipovich et al., 2001). Probabilities differed by donor type: 87% (74%–93%) with HLA-identical sibling donors, 52% (37%–65%) with other related donors, and 71% (58%–80%) with MUD (p = 0.0006). Boys who had received a MUD transplant before age 5 had survival rates similar to those receiving HLA-identical sibling transplants.

All aspects of WAS are corrected by marrow transplantation, including the eczema, autoimmunity, and risk of lymphomas. This outcome indicates that these disease complications are related to the immunodeficiency. Similarly, thrombocytopenia and the bleeding tendency have disappeared after successful bone marrow transplantation. Bone marrow, peripheral blood stem cell, or cord blood transplantation is recommended for patients with WAS and should be performed as early in life as possible. While the ideal donor is an HLA-identical sibling, it is clear that matched unrelated marrow, peripheral blood stem cells, or cord blood transplants can be effective if given to patients under the age of 5 years.

The poor results with T cell–depleted HLA haploidentical bone marrow transplants in WAS stress the need for careful evaluation of whether even to attempt an HLA haploidentical bone marrow transplantation in WAS patients who lack both

HLA-identical related and unrelated donors (Fischer et al., 1994). Mullen et al. (1993) stressed that splenectomized WAS patients can survive at least until adulthood. Nevertheless, WAS patients who develop refractory thrombctyopenia and/or severe autoimmune manifestations could be considered for HLA haploidentical bone marrow transplantation.

Omenn Syndrome

Forty-five patients with Omenn syndrome have been reported in the literature (Fischer et al., 1994; Gomez et al., 1995; Lanfranchi et al., 2000; Loechelt et al., 1995) or to one of the authors (R.H.B.) as having received marrow transplants since 1968, and 23, or 51%, were alive at the time of this writing. As with the other non-SCID defects, however, the greatest success was in patients with HLA-identical sibling transplants, 9 out of 12 (75%) of whom were still surviving, whereas only 11 of 27 (41%) haploidentical marrow and 3 of 6 (50%) MUD marrow recipients were alive.

X-Linked Hyper-IgM Syndrome (CD40 Ligand Deficiency)

X-linked hyper-IgM syndrome (XHIM; see Chapter 19) was for a long time considered to be a pure B cell immunodeficiency because of the observed defective production of IgG, IgA, and IgE. Following the discovery that deficiency in CD40 ligand expression on activated T cells caused the disease, it was better appreciated that many XHIM patients suffered from consequences of T cell deficiency as well, including opportunistic infections caused by microorganisms such as *Pneumocystis carinii*, *Toxoplasma*, and *Cryptosporidia*. The last organism induces in many patients chronic cholangitis, leading to cirrhosis. A recent survey has shown that the likelihood of survival of patients with XHIM to adulthood is <25% (Levy et al., 1997). It is unclear how additional genetic or environmental factors significantly modify the disease prognosis.

Bone marrow or cord blood transplantation are the only curative treatments for XHIM; transplantation has been carried out thus far in only 56 patients, 40 of whom were surviving at the time of this writing (Duplantier et al., 2001; Fasth, 1993; Thomas et al., 1995a; Scholl et al., 1998; Khawaja et al., 2001; Ziegner et al., 2001; Leone et al., 2002; Gennery et al., 2004; Jacobsohn et al., 2004). Early bone marrow transplantation is recommended if an HLA-identical donor is available. Non–X-linked forms of the hyper-IgM syndrome do not share the same poor outcome. Therefore, there is currently no indication for bone marrow transplantation in non–X-linked hyper-IgM patients, except possibly in those who lack CD40.

X-linked Lymphoproliferative Syndrome

This syndrome (see Chapter 32) is caused by mutations in the *SH2D1A* gene at Xp28 that encodes the SLAM-associated protein (SAP) necessary for control of SLAM signaling and for NK cell function. Patients with this condition are typically well until they contract EBV infections. However following EBV exposure they die of fulminating EBV infection, develop lymphoma, or develop a condition clinically indistinguishable from CVID. No patient has been reported alive beyond the age of 38 years; most have died before the age of 20 (Sullivan and Woda, 1989). Following a first unsuccessful attempt, several patients have been cured by either bone marrow or cord blood transplantation (Vowels et al., 1993; Williams et al., 1993; Pracher et al., 1994; Gross

et al., 1996; Ziegner et al., 2001). Diagnosis of the condition prior to EBV infection is difficult, since, in the absence of a family history, there is no clear biological marker of the disease. However, if there is a family history, mutation analysis can be carried out in potentially affected males so that transplantation can be carried out before an EBV infection occurs (Morra et al., 2001) (see Chapter 32).

Other Predominant T Cell Immunodeficiencies

Other T cell immunodeficiency syndromes for which transplantation with stem cells from various sources have been used include reticular dysgenesis (9 of 11 surviving) (De Santes et al., 1996; Knutsen and Wall, 1999); purine nucleoside phosphorylase (PNP) deficiency (6 of 12 surviving) (Broome et al., 1996; Carpenter et al., 1996; Classen et al., 2001; Baguette et al., 2002) cartilage-hair hypoplasia (4 of 7 surviving) (Berthet et al., 1996); IL-2 deficiency (2 of 2 surviving) (Berthet et al., 1994); common variable immunodeficiency (CVID) (none of 4 surviving); defective binding of nuclear factor of activated T cells (1 of 1 surviving) (Feske et al., 1996); chronic mucocutaneous candidiasis (1 not surviving); ataxia-telangiectasia (none of 4 surviving); and Fas (CD95) deficiency (1 of 1 surviving) (Benkerrou et al., 1997).

Buckley and associates have also transplanted 58 patients with non-SCID immunodeficiency, with the following survival rates: 11 of 26 with CID (42%); 5 of 7 with leukocyte adhesion deficiency (LAD) (71%); 2 of 2 with Chediak-Higashi syndrome (100%); 3 of 3 with chronic granulomatous disease (CGD) (100%); 2 of 2 with ZAP-70 deficiency (100%); 4 of 7 with Omenn syndrome (57%); 2 of 4 with PNP deficiency (50%); 1 of 2 with WAS (50%); 2 of 2 with XHIM (100%); 1 of 2 with IFN-γR2 deficiency; and 0 of 1 with Griscelli syndrome.

Without bone marrow transplantation, survival to adulthood is rare in most of these conditions (Berthet et al., 1994; Fischer et al., 1994; Antoine et al., 2003). When bone marrow transplantation is performed, death is often related to complications of prior viral infection or organ failure. Patients with immunodeficiencies less pronounced than SCID may survive for several years. However, many harbor latent or subclinical infections, such as with facultative intracellular microorganisms, and these infections are exacerbated following myeloablative and immunosuppressive conditioning regimens. Early diagnosis of non-SCID immunodeficiencies should permit bone marrow transplantation as early as possible, if a suitable donor is available, to offer maximal likelihood of survival and immunoreconstitution. Indeed, in a European survey, transplants performed before the age of 2 years gave a 79% success rate vs. 48% over 4 years of age (Fischer et al., 1994).

Gaspar and associates at Great Ormand Street, United Kingdom, have reported on the outcomes of their treatment of 21 patients with a variety of different immunodeficiencies using four different nonmyeloablative conditioning regimens: (1) fludarabine/melphalan/ATG or Campath 1H ($n = 16$), (2) fludarabine/cyclophosphamide/Campath 1H ($n = 1$), (3) TBI/CyA/MMF ($n = 1$), and (4) fludarabine/melphalan/busulphan/ATG ($n = 3$) (Gaspar et al., 2002). In 13 cases, matched ($n = 9$) and 1 antigen (Ag) mismatched ($n = 4$) unrelated donors were used, and in 8 cases transplants from matched siblings ($n = 4$), an Ag mismatched sibling ($n = 1$), a matched parent ($n = 1$), and haploidentical parents ($n = 3$) were performed. At a median post-transplantation follow-up of 13 months, 19 of 21 (90%) patients were still alive. Despite using T cell–replete grafts and unrelated donor grafts in the majority of these patients, no significant organ disease was evident. Immune reconstitution in terms of CD3$^+$ and CD4$^+$ T cell recovery and function was reported to be equivalent to that of a historical cohort (Gaspar et al., 2002).

Major Histocompatibility Complex Class II Deficiency

Bone marrow transplantation for HLA class II deficiency disease (Chapter 17) deserves specific comments. In the absence of immune reconstitution, patients lacking HLA class II molecule expression suffer from recurrent infections, including frequent, devastating cryptosporidial infections and viral infections of the CNS. Life expectancy is 5 years on average, with no improvement in recent years, despite supportive care with parenteral nutrition and antibiotic therapy. Bone marrow transplantation can cure the disease, provided it is performed before complications leading to severe organ failure develop (Klein et al., 1993). The relatively low overall success rate of transplantation in HLA class II antigen deficiency, compared with that of some other forms of immunodeficiency (i.e., only a 54% survival rate following HLA-identical transplantation), may reflect the considerable heterogeneity in clinical presentation of these disorders and in age at transplantation. Two interesting observations have been made on long-term survivors of successful transplants (Klein et al., 1995); (1) persistence of a relative CD4 T cell lymphopenia, possibly due to a lack of HLA class II molecules on thymic epithelial cells, even though the donor-derived CD4$^+$ T cells are functional; and (2) absence of detrimental consequences secondary to defective expression of HLA class II molecules on nonhematopoietic cells. Finally, heterogeneity of the disease, because of the existence of at least four different disease genes, prevents making a clear-cut prognosis.

Phagocytic Cell Disorders

A number of the inherited phagocytic cell disorders remain lethal, either because of the severity of infections in the absence of alternative therapy, or because of the onset of specific complications, such as the acute phase of the Chediak-Higashi syndrome.

Chronic Granulomatous Disease

Most CGD patients can survive to adulthood, because prophylaxis with trimethoprim/sulfamethoxazole, itraconazole, and/or interferon-γ (IFN-γ) (International Chronic Granulomatous Disease Cooperative Study Group, 1991) has considerably reduced the incidence of life-threatening infections (see Chapter 37). It is estimated, however, that the risk of severe aspergillosis remains at 1 in every 100 patients per year, with a death rate of 30%. Also, some CGD patients develop other debilitating complications, such as granulomas of the lung, esophagus, bladder, or colon, requiring long-term steroid therapy. Therefore, it was recommended some years ago that bone marrow transplantation be considered as a therapeutic option in CGD patients who have developed severe complications and who have an HLA-matched donor (Kamani et al., 1988).

Seger et al. (2002) have reviewed the outcomes of 27 transplantations for CGD, from 1985 to 2000, reported to the European Bone Marrow Transplant Registry for primary immunodeficiencies. Twenty-five of the transplant recipients were children who had received bone marrow transplants from HLA-identical sibling donors. The 23 children who received myeloablative condi-

tioning were fully engrafted with donor cells, whereas only 2 of 4 patients who had received myelosuppressive regimens were fully engrafted. Overall survival was 23 of 27, with 22 of 23 cured of CGD (median follow-up, 2 years). Survival was especially good in patients without infection at the moment of transplantation (18 of 18). Preexisting infections and inflammatory lesions had cleared in all survivors, except in one patient who had autologous reconstitution. Myeloablative conditioning followed by transplantation of unmodified hemopoietic stem cells, if performed at the first signs of a severe course of the disease, is a valid therapeutic option for children with CGD who have an HLA-identical donor (Table 47.5) (Seger et al., 2002). Buckley has also had recent success in curing three young patients with CGD with HLA-identical sibling, unfractionated bone marrow transplants following full myeloablative conditioning. Thus, as with other immunodeficiency syndromes with predictable serious complications, in CGD, HLA-matched stem cell transplantation is best if carried out early in life before such complications arise and is recommended.

Nonmyeloablative bone marrow transplantation has also been used for patients with CGD when HLA-identical sibling donors were available (Nagler et al., 1999; Horwitz et al., 2001). The conditioning regimens used were fludarabine, busulfan, and ATG in one case (Nagler et al., 1999) and cyclophosphamide, fludarabine, and ATG in 10 cases (Horwitz et al., 2001); 7 of the 11 patients were surviving at this writing with mixed chimerism and good health. However, in view of the success with full myeloablative conditioning, there appears to be little indication for this approach (Seger et al., 2002).

Leukocyte Adhesion Deficiency, Type I

Leukocyte adhesion deficiency, type I (LAD1) is a rare disease characterized by defective expression of the β$_2$ integrin subunit shared by the leukocyte adhesion proteins (see Chapter 38). Its complete absence leads to the severe phenotype of LAD, which predisposes to severe bacterial infections, often causing death within the first years of life. HLA-identical bone marrow transplantation is the treatment of choice for this condition. Aggressive conditioning, including the use of etoposide or thiotepa, may be required for appropriate marrow ablation (Fischer et al., 1994). Results of allogeneic bone marrow transplantation have been quite satisfactory.

Chediak-Higashi Syndrome, Pigmentary Dilution (Griscelli) Syndrome, and Familial Hemophagocytic Lymphohistiocytosis

HLA-identical bone marrow transplantation can cure the hematological manifestations of Chediak-Higashi syndrome (Haddad et al., 1995) (Chapter 40) and of immunodeficiency with partial albinism (Griscelli syndrome) (Schneider et al., 1990) (Chapter 41).

As in the above two conditions, bone marrow transplantation can cure the hematological manifestations of familial hemophagocytic lymphohistiocytosis (FHL) (Blanche et al., 1991; Henter et al., 2002) (Chapter 41). In these instances, bone marrow transplantation prevents relapse of lymphohistiocytic activity. It is worth noting that mixed chimerism is sufficient to achieve disease control (Landman-Parker et al., 1993). This result indicates that an abnormal regulatory process, rather than a malignant process, underlies these conditions. Use of TBI is not necessary, and a combination of busulphan and cyclophosphamide appears both a safe and efficient conditioning regimen for these diseases. Optimal control of the acute phase before bone marrow transplantation appears to be of crucial importance to avoid graft rejection and/or major toxic complications such as VOD after bone marrow transplantation. ATG treatment given immediately prior to cytoreduction is sufficient to achieve remission. Attention should also be paid, however, to ongoing CNS disease. Exclusion of the diagnosis of FHL in siblings of FHL patients is extremely difficult, since no pre-symptomatic disease markers are available. Siblings who were 5 and 8 years of age have been found affected after they had donated marrow for their younger affected siblings (Blanche et al., 1991; G. Morgan, personal communication).

Severe Congenital Neutropenias

The prognosis of severe congenital neutropenias (SCN) has been considerably modified by the use of granulocyte–colony stimulating factor (G-CSF). Injections of G-CSF enable almost all of these patients to have near-normal granulocyte counts and thus few or no infections so that they can enjoy good health (Dale et al., 1993). In a proportion of these patients, however, myelodysplasia and overt leukemia have developed. It is possible that the malignancies are associated with the presence of acquired clonal heterozygous mutations of the G-CSF receptor (Dong et al., 1995). Therefore, detection of such a mutation in marrow cells of a patient with SCN could be a good marker to indicate a need for bone marrow transplantation, provided that there is a matched donor (Rappeport et al., 1980).

Cytokine Receptor Deficiencies

It is also possible that patients with severe idiopathic mycobacterial infections, some of them caused by deficiencies in the IFN-γ receptor (see Chapter 18), could benefit from allogeneic bone marrow transplantation (Jouanguy et al., 1996; Newport et al., 1996). Unfortunately, with one or two exceptions (Reuter et al., 2002; R.H. Buckley, unpublished results), the experience to date has been not very successful, for reasons that are unclear.

Long-term Outcome

Similar to the case with all types of transplants in infants with SCID (Fig. 47.1), the long-term (10-year) outcome of HLA-identical bone marrow transplantation for most forms of primary immunodeficiency appears reasonably satisfactory. Correction of the underlying deficiency is sustained, despite frequent mixed chimerism in the absence of TBI usage. Sequelae are generally limited to consequences of the primary disease. Chronic GVHD is of limited frequency (<10%) in these young patients (Fischer et al., 1986b).

Overcoming Resistance to Engraftment and Prevention of Graft Rejection

In the mid-1980s, one of the authors (A.F.) was surprised by the consecutive success of three HLA haploidentical bone marrow transplants for patients with the severe phenotype of LAD following pretransplant conditioning (Le Deist et al., 1989). These data have since been confirmed in nine patients with the severe phenotype of LAD who received SRBC–T cell–depleted, HLA haploidentical bone marrow following pretransplant conditioning. Engraftment occurred in all and seven are alive with partial

or full correction of their LAD (Thomas et al., 1995b). This is in sharp contrast to the engraftment rate of T cell–depleted haploidentical marrow transplanted under the same conditions in other immunodeficiency patients (excluding SCID), for whom the engraftment rate was 26% (Fischer et al., 1986b). Therefore, it was postulated that the defective expression of the LFA-1 molecule on graft rejection effector cells (cytotoxic T cells and NK cells) impaired cell contact with donor marrow cells and thereby permitted engraftment, as shown in a murine model (van Dijken et al., 1990). This finding led to the pretransplant infusion of a monoclonal anti-LFA-1 (anti-CD11a) antibody to inhibit LFA-1–ligand interactions in humans undergoing T cell–depleted haploidentical marrow transplantation (Fischer et al., 1991). Patients with functional T cell immunodeficiencies (including HLA class II deficiency) have a poor prognosis (median survival 5 years) in the absence of bone marrow transplantation (Klein et al., 1993; Berthet et al., 1994). In a multicenter trial, it was found that a 10-day course of 0.2 mg/kg of antibody per day reduced the graft failure rate from 74% to 28% following transplantation of T cell–depleted marrow into patients with various non-SCID forms of immunodeficiency and into some with osteopetrosis (Fischer et al., 1991). No late rejection occurred. Acute GVHD was observed in 35.5% of cases, and chronic GVHD occurred in 12.9%. The survival rate with a functioning graft was 47% in 42 patients (median follow-up, 50 months), instead of 20% in similar patients who did not receive anti-LFA-1. An update of these data showed a 74% engraftment rate, with 45% long-term survival in 38 immunodeficient patients who were treated with anti LFA-1, while engraftment occurred in only 37.5% and survival in 20.8% of 24 patients not given anti-LFA-1 (Fischer et al., 1994).

Surprisingly, recipients of closely matched related (phenotypically identical or one HLA antigen mismatched) marrow were found in a recent survey not to have a better outcome than those of two or three HLA antigen mismatched related marrow (Fischer et al., 1994). These results may be related to the low number of patients (n = 22) in this group (Fischer et al., 1994). The simultaneous infusion of another anti-adhesion antibody (anti-CD2), as performed in 43 patients, resulted in an engraftment rate of 80% without additional toxicity, with 55% survival. By using this strategy, five of nine patients with FHL have been cured by SRBC-rosetted T cell–depleted haploidentical bone marrow transplantation (Jabado et al., 1996). Unfortunately, at this writing anti-LFA-1 antibody is no longer available for clinical use. Apart from LAD (see above), HLA haploidentical bone marrow transplantation for patients with phagocytic cell disorders remains highly investigational, given the high risk of failure.

Other approaches aimed at selectively inhibiting graft rejection have been developed experimentally and could be of potential benefit. Anti-CD4 and anti-CD8 antibody infusions promote engraftment of H-2 incompatible marrow in mice (Cobbold et al., 1986). Selective T cell subset depletion of marrow might prevent complications such as EBV-induced B lymphocyte proliferative disorders (Cavazzana-Calvo et al., 1994).

Another approach to enhancing the rate of engraftment has been to transplant a higher number of hematopoietic stem cells than has been traditionally used. The theoretical possibility exists that higher numbers of CD34$^+$ stem cells could accelerate the development of T cell function. Aversa et al. (1994) reported success with this approach in adults with leukemia by infusion of 3- to 10-fold more CD34$^+$ cells (derived from donor peripheral blood after mobilization with G-CSF) than would have been possible with marrow transplantation alone. A very high rate of engraftment was achieved, with only limited GVHD. Handgretinger et al. (2001) transplanted 39 children, 6 of whom had primary immunodeficiencies, with high-dose (20.7 ± 9.8 × 10⁶ kg), affinity-purified CD34⁺, rigorously T cell–depleted, G-CSF-mobilized, peripheral blood haploidentical parental stem cells. In 32 patients, no GVHD was seen despite the fact that no GVHD prophylaxis was given. Only 15 of the patients survived; 13 died of malignancy relapse. However, this method may have little added benefit in immunodeficient patients, who are mostly young children, since a relatively high number of CD34⁺ cells/kg of the recipient is already infused with T cell–depleted, haploidentical marrow transplants. It is also possible that addition of cytokines such as IL-7 could contribute to improved engraftment (Bolotin et al., 1997).

Future of Bone Marrow Transplantation in the Treatment of Primary Immunodeficiency

It is abundantly clear that allogeneic bone marrow transplantation can provide a cure for many children with life-threatening immunodeficiency diseases. Until gene therapy is perfected, bone marrow transplantation will remain the standard of care for such conditions. Thus far, bone marrow transplantation seems to be associated with acceptable long-term sequelae, although outcome beyond a follow-up of 30 years is not yet known. There is evidence of waning thymic output in some SCID marrow recipients in the second decade post-transplantation (Patel et al., 2000), and some long-term survivors have had extensive lesions of verruca vulgaris (Laffort et al., 2004). Except in the case of SCID, major problems still exist for the many patients who lack an HLA-identical sibling. Stem cell and lymphocyte manipulation may provide better success in the future, while alternative therapies might be developed for more diseases. Better assessment of genetic mutations associated with diseases, as well as individual genetic and environmental cofactors, should also lead to a better delineation of which child should be transplanted.

References

Amos DB, Bach FH. Phenotypic expressions of the major histocompatibility locus in man (HL-A): leukocyte antigens and mixed leukocyte culture reactivity. J Exp Med 128:623–637, 1968.

Anderson KC, Weinstein HJ. Transfusion-associated graft-versus-host disease. N Engl J Med 323:315–321, 1990.

Antoine C, Muller S, Cant A, Cavazzana-Calvo M, Veys P, Vossen J, Fasth A, Heilman C, Wulffraat N, Seger R, Blanche S, Friedrich W, Abinun M, Davies G, Bredius R, Schulz A, Landais P, Fischer A. Long-term survival and transplantation of haemopoietic stem cells for immunodeficiencies: report of the European experience 1968–99. Lancet 361:553–560, 2003.

Ash RC, Casper JT, Chitambar CR, Hansen R, Bunin N, Truitt RL, Lawton C, Murray K, Hunter J, Baxter-Lowe LA, Gottschall JL, Oldham K, Anderson T, Camitta B, Menitove J. Successful allogeneic transplantation of T cell depleted bone marrow from closely HLA-matched unrelated donors. N Engl J Med 322:485–494, 1990.

Aversa F, Tabilio A, Terenzi A, Velardi A, Falzetti F, Giannoni C, Iacucci R, Zei T, Martelli MP, Gambelunghe C, Rossetti M, Caputo P, Latini P, Aristei C, Raymondi C, Reisner Y, Martelli MF. Successful engraftment of T cell depleted haploidentical "three-loci" incompatible transplants in leukemia patients by addition of recombinant human granulocyte colony-stimulating factor-mobilized peripheral blood progenitor cells to bone marrow inoculum. Blood 84:3948–3955, 1994.

Bach FH, Albertini RJ, Joo P, Anderson JL, Bortin MD. Bone marrow transplantation in a patient with the Wiskott-Aldrich syndrome. Lancet 2:1364–1366, 1968.

Baguette C, Vermylen C, Brichard B, Louis J, Dahan K, Vincent MF, Cornu G. Persistent developmental delay despite successful bone marrow transplantation for purine nucleoside phosphorylase deficiency. J Pediatr Hematol Oncol 24:69–71, 2002.

Barker JN, Wagner JE. Umbilical cord blood transplantation: current state of the art. Curr Opin Oncol 14:160–164, 2002.

Barrett MJ, Buckley RH, Schiff SE, Kidd PC, Ward FE. Accelerated development of immunity following transplantation of maternal marrow stem cells into infants with severe combined immunodeficiency and transplacentally acquired lymphoid chimerism. Clin Exp Immunol 72:118–123, 1988.

Barta A, Denes R, Masszi T, Remenyi P, Batai A, Torbagyi E, Sipos A, Lengyel L, Jakab K, Gyodi E, Reti M, Foldi J, Paldi-Haris P, Avalos M, Paloczi K, Fekete S, Torok J, Hoffer I, Jakab J, Varadi G, Kelemen E, Petranyi G. Remarkably reduced transplant-related complications by dibromomannitol non-myeloablative conditioning before allogeneic bone marrow transplantation in chronic myeloid leukemia. Acta Haematol 105:64–70, 2001.

Benkerrou M, Le Deist F, De Villartay JP, Caillat-Zucman S, Rieux-Laucat F, Jabado N, Cavazzana-Calvo M, Fischer A. Correction of Fas (CD95) deficiency by haploidentical bone marrow transplantation. Eur J Immunol 27:2043–2047, 1997.

Berthet F, Le Deist F, Duliege AM, Griscelli C, Fischer A. Clinical consequences and treatment of primary immunodeficiency syndromes characterized by functional T and B lymphocyte anomalies (combined immune deficiency). Pediatrics 93:265–270, 1994.

Berthet F, Siegrist CA, Ozsahin H, Tuchschmid P, Eich G, Superti-Furga A, Seger RA. Bone marrow transplantation in cartilage-hair hypoplasia: correction of the immunodeficiency but not of the chondrodysplasia. Eur J Pediatr 155:286–290, 1996.

Blanche S, Caniglia M, Girault D, Landman J, Griscelli C, Fischer A. Treatment of hemophagocytic lymphohistiocytosis with chemotherapy and bone marrow transplantation: a single-center study of 22 cases. Blood 78:51–54, 1991.

Blazar DR, Ramsay NKC, Kersey JH, Krivit W, Arthur DC, Filipovich AH. Pretransplant conditioning with busulfan (Myleran) and cyclophosphamide for nonmalignant diseases. Assessment of engraftment following histocompatible allogeneic bone marrow transplantation. Transplantation 39:597, 1985.

Bolotin E, Nolta J, Smith S, Dao M, Weinberg K. Effective immune reconstitution in mice after co-tranplantation of bone marrow and marrow stroma transduced with the IL-7 gene: gene therapy for post-BMT immune deficiency. J Allergy Clin Immunol 99S:100, 1997.

Bortin MM, Rimm AA. Severe combined immunodeficiency disease. Characterization of the disease and results of transplantation. JAMA 238:591–600, 1977.

Bostrom B, Enockson K, Johnson A, Bruns A, Blazar B. Plasma pharmacokinetics of high-dose oral busulfan in children and adults undergoing bone marrow transplantation. Pediatr Transplant 7(Suppl 3):12–18, 2003.

Brady KA, Cowan MJ, Leavitt AD. Circulating red cells usually remain of host origin after bone marrow transplantation for severe combined immunodeficiency. Transfusion 36:314–317, 1996.

Brenner MK, Rill DR, Holladay MS, Heslop HE, Moen RC, Buschle M, Krance RA, Santana VM, Anderson WF, Ihle JN. Gene marking to determine whether autologous marrow infusion restores long-term haemopoiesis in cancer patients. Lancet 342:1134–1137, 1993.

Brochstein J, Gillio AP, Ruggerio M. Marrow transplantation from HLA-identical or haploidentical donors for correction of Wiskott-Aldrich syndrome. J Pediatr 119:907–912, 1991.

Broome CB, Graham ML, Saulsbury FT, Hershfield MS, Buckley RH. Correction of purine nucleoside phosphorylase deficiency by transplantation of allogeneic bone marrow from a sibling. J Pediatr 128:373–376, 1996.

Buckley RH. Molecular defects in human severe combined immunodeficiency and approaches to immune reconstitution. Annu Rev Immunol 55:625–656, 2004.

Buckley RH, Fischer A. Bone marrow transplantation for primary immunodeficiency diseases. In: Ochs HD, Smith CIE, Puck JM, eds. Primary Immunodeficiency Diseases: A Molecular and Genetic Approach, 1st ed. New York: Oxford University Press, pp. 459–475, 1999.

Buckley RH, Schiff SE, Sampson HA, Schiff RI, Markert ML, Knutsen AP, Hershfield MS, Huang AT, Mickey GH, Ward FE. Development of immunity in human severe primary T cell deficiency following haploidentical bone marrow stem cell transplantation. J Immunol 136:2398–2407, 1986.

Buckley RH, Schiff RI, Schiff SE, Markert ML, Williams LW, Harville TO, Roberts JL, Puck JM. Human severe combined immunodeficiency (SCID): genetic, phenotypic and functional diversity in 108 infants. J Pediatr 130:378–387, 1997.

Buckley RH, Schiff SE, Schiff RI, Markert L, Williams LW, Roberts JL, Myers LA, Ward FE. Hematopoietic stem cell transplantation for the treatment of severe combined immunodeficiency. N Engl J Med 340:508–516, 1999.

Carpenter PA, Ziegler JB, Vowels MR. Late diagnosis and correction of purine nucleoside phosphorylase deficiency with allogeneic bone marrow transplantation. Bone Marrow Transplant 17:121–124, 1996.

Cavazzana-Calvo M, Stephan JL, Sarnacki S, Chevret S, Fromont C, de Coene C, Le Deist F, Guy-Grand D, Fischer A. Attenuation of graft-versus-host disease and graft rejection by ex vivo immunotoxin elimination of alloreactive T cells in an H-2 haplotype disparate mouse combination. Blood 83:288–298, 1994.

Chakrabarti S, Hale G, Waldmann H. Alemtuzumab (Campath-1H) in allogeneic stem cell transplantation: where do we go from here? Transplant Proc 36:1225–1227, 2004.

Classen CF, Schulz AS, Sigl-Kraetzig M, Hoffmann GF, Simmonds HA, Fairbanks L, Debatin KM, Friedrich W. Successful HLA-identical bone marrow transplantation in a patient with PNP deficiency using busulfan and fludarabine for conditioning. Bone Marrow Transplant 28:93–96, 2001.

Clement-De Boers A, Oostdijk W, Van Weel-Sipman MH, Van den Broeck J, Wit JM, Vossen JM. Final height and hormonal function after bone marrow transplantation in children. J Pediatr 129:544–550, 1996.

Cobbold SP, Martin G, Qin S, Waldmann H. Monoclonal antibodies to promote marrow engraftment and tissue graft tolerance. Nature 323:164–166, 1986.

Dale DC, Bonilla MA, Davis MW, Nakanishi AM, Hammond WP, Kurtzberg J, Wang W, Jakubowski A, Winton E, Lalezari P, Robinson W, Glaspy JA, Emerson S, Gabrilove J, Vincent M, Boxer LA. A randomized controlled phase III trial of recombinant human granulocyte colony-stimulating factor (filgrastim) for treatment of severe chronic neutropenia. Blood 81:2496–2502, 1993.

Dalle JH, Wall D, Theoret Y, Duval M, Shaw L, Larocque D, Taylor C, Gardiner J, Vachon MF, Champagne MA. Intravenous busulfan for allogeneic hematopoietic stem cell transplantation in infants: clinical and pharmacokinetic results. Bone Marrow Transplant 32:647–651, 2003.

Deeg HJ, Henslee-Downey PJ. Management of acute graft-versus-host disease. Bone Marrow Transplant 6:1–8, 1990.

De Santes KB, Lai SS, Cowan MJ. Haploidentical bone marrow transplants for two patients with reticular dysgenesis. Bone Marrow Transplant 17:1171–1173, 1996.

Dini G, Lanino E, Lamparelli T, Barbanti M, Sacchi N, Carcassi C, Locatelli F, Porta F, Rosti G, Alessandrino EP, Aversa F, Marenco P, Guidi S, Uderzo C, Amoroso A, di Bartolomeo P, Garbarino L, La Nasa G, Rossetti F, Miniero R, Soligo D, Manfredini L, Bacigalupo A. Unrelated donor marrow transplantation: initial experience of the Italian bone marrow transplant group (GITMO). Bone Marrow Transplant 17:55–62, 1996.

Dong F, Brynes RK, Tidow N, Welte K, Lowenberg B, Touw IP. Mutations in the gene for the granulocyte colony-stimulating factor receptor in patients with acute myeloid leukemia preceded by severe congenital neutropenia. N Engl J Med 333:487–493, 1995.

Dror Y, Gallagher R, Wara DW, Colombe BW, Merino A, Benkerrou M, Cowan MJ. Immune reconstitution in severe combined immunodeficiency disease after lectin-treated, T cell–depleted haplocompatible bone marrow transplantation. Blood 81:2021–2030, 1993.

Duplantier JE, Seyama K, Day NK, Hitchcock R, Nelson RP, Jr., Ochs HD, Haraguchi S, Klemperer MR, Good RA. Immunologic reconstitution following bone marrow transplantation for X-linked hyper IgM syndrome. Clin Immunol 98:313–318, 2001.

Eltumi M, Trivedi P, Hobbs JR, Portmann B, Cheeseman P, Downie C, Risteli J, Risteli L, Mowat AP. Monitoring of veno-occlusive disease after bone marrow transplantation by serum aminopropeptide of type III procollagen. Lancet 342:518–521, 1993.

Fasth A. Bone marrow transplantation for hyper-IgM syndrome. Immunodeficiency 4:323, 1993.

Feinstein L, Sandmaier B, Maloney D, McSweeney PA, Maris M, Flowers C, Radich J, Little MT, Nash RA, Chauncey T, Woolfrey A, Georges G, Kiem HP, Zaucha JM, Blume KG, Shizuru J, Niederwieser D, Storb R. Nonmyeloablative hematopoietic cell transplantation. Replacing high-dose cytotoxic therapy by the graft-versus-tumor effect. Ann NY Acad Sci 938:328–337, 2001.

Fernandez HF, Tran HT, Albrecht F, Lennon S, Caldera H, Goodman MS. Evaluation of safety and pharmacokinetics of administering intravenous busulfan in a twice-daily or daily schedule to patients with advanced hematologic malignant disease undergoing stem cell transplantation. Biol Blood Marrow Transplant 8:486–492, 2002.

Ferrara JL, Deeg HJ. Graft-versus-host disease. N Engl J Med 324:667–674, 1991.

Feske S, Muller JM, Graf D, Kroczek RA, Drager R, Niemeyer C, Baeuerle PA, Peter HH, Schlesier M. Severe combined immunodeficiency due to defective binding of the nuclear factor of activated T cells in T lymphocytes of two male siblings. Eur J Immunol 26:2119–2126, 1996.

Filipovich AH, Mathur A, Kamat D, Kersey JH, Shapiro RS. Lymphoproliferative disorders and other tumors complicating immunodeficiencies. Immunodeficiency 5:91–112, 1994.

Filipovich AH, Shapiro RS, Ramsay NK, Kim T, Blazar B, Kersey J, McGlave P. Unrelated donor bone marrow transplantation for correction of lethal congenital immunodeficiencies. Blood 80:270–276, 1992.

Filipovich AH, Stone JV, Tomany SC, Ireland M, Kollman C, Pelz CJ, Casper JT, Cowan MJ, Edwards JR, Fasth A, Gale RP, Junker A, Kamani NR, Loechelt BJ, Pietryga DW, Ringden O, Vowels M, Hegland J, Williams AV, Klein JP, Sobocinski KA, Rowlings PA, Horowitz MM. Impact of donor type on outcome of bone marrow transplantation for Wiskott-Aldrich syndrome: collaborative study of the International Bone Marrow Transplant Registry and the National Marrow Donor Program. Blood 97:1598–1603, 2001.

Filipovich AH, Vallera DA, Youle RJ, Quinones RR, Neville DM Jr, Kersey JH. Ex-vivo treatment of donor bone marrow with anti-T-cell immunotoxins for prevention of graft-versus-host disease. Lancet 1:469–472, 1984.

Fischer A, Durandy A, De Villartay JP, Vilmer E, Le Deist F, Gerota I, Griscelli C. HLA-haploidentical bone marrow transplantation for severe combined immunodeficiency using E rosette fractionation and cyclosporine. Blood 67:444–449, 1986a.

Fischer A, Friedrich W, Fasth A, Blanche S, Le Deist F, Girault D, Veber F, Vossen J, Lopez M, Griscelli C. Reduction of graft failure by a monoclonal antibody (anti-LFA-1 CD11a) after HLA nonidentical bone marrow transplantation in children with immunodeficiencies, osteopetrosis and Fanconi's anemia: a European Group for Immunodeficiency/European Group for Bone Marrow Transplantation report. Blood 77:249–256, 1991.

Fischer A, Griscelli C, Friedrich W, Kubanek B, Levinsky R, Morgan G, Vossen J, Wagemaker G, Landais P. Bone marrow transplantation for immunodeficiencies and osteopetrosis: European survey, 1968–1985. Lancet 2:1080–1084, 1986b.

Fischer A, Landais P, Friedrich W, Gerritsen B, Fasth A, Porta F, Vellodi A, Benkerrou M, Jais JP, Cavazzana-Calvo M, Souillet G, Bordigoni P, Morgan G, Van Dijken P, Vossen J, Locatelli F, di Bartolomeo P. Bone marrow transplantation (BMT) in Europe for primary immunodeficiencies other than severe combined immunodeficiency: a report from the European Group for BMT and the European Group for Immunodeficiency. Blood 83:1149–1154, 1994.

Fischer A, Landais P, Friedrich W, Morgan G, Gerritsen B, Fasth A, Porta F, Griscelli C, Goldman SF, Levinsky R. European experience of bone marrow transplantation for severe combined immunodeficiency. Lancet 336:850–854, 1990.

Flake AW, Roncarolo MG, Puck JM, Almeida-Porada G, Evans MI, Johnson MP, Abella EM, Harrison DD, Zanjani ED. Treatment of X-linked severe combined immunodeficiency by in utero transplantation of paternal bone marrow. N Engl J Med 335:1806–1810, 1996.

Friedman NJ, Schiff SE, Ward FE, Schiff RI, Buckley RH. Graft-versus-graft and graft-versus-host reactions after HLA-identical bone marrow transplantation in a patient with severe combined immunodeficiency with transplacentally acquired lymphoid chimerism. Pediatr Allergy Immunol 2:111–116, 1991.

Friedrich W. Bone marrow transplantation in immunodeficiency diseases. Ann Med 28:115–119, 1996.

Friedrich W, Knobloch C, Greher J, Hartmann W, Peter HH, Goldmann SF, Kleihauer E. Bone marrow transplantation in severe combined immunodeficiency: potential and current limitations. Immunodeficiency 4:315–322, 1993.

Gaspar HB, Amrolia P, Hassan A, Webb D, Jones A, Sturt N, Vergani G, Pagliuca A, Mufti G, Hadzic N, Davies G, Veys P. Non-myeloablative stem cell transplantation for congenital immunodeficiencies. Recent Results Cancer Res 159:134–142, 2002.

Gatti RA, Meuwissen HJ, Allen HD, Hong R, Good RA. Immunological reconstitution of sex-linked lymphopenic immunological deficiency. Lancet 2:1366–1369, 1968.

Gennery AR, Khawaja K, Veys P, Bredius RG, Notarangelo LD, Mazzolari E, Fischer A, Landais P, Cavazzana-Calvo M, Friedrich W, Fasth A, Wulffraat NM, Matthes-Martin S, Bensoussan D, Bordigoni P, Lange A, Pagliuca A, Andolina M, Cant AJ, Davies EG. Treatment of CD40 ligand deficiency by hematopoietic stem cell transplantation: a survey of the European experience, 1993–2002. Blood 103:1152–1157, 2004.

Giri N, Vowels M, Ziegler JB, Ford D, Lam-Po-Tang R. HLA non-identical T-cell-depleted bone marrow transplantation for primary immunodeficiency diseases. Aust NZ J Med 24:26–30, 1994.

Glucksberg H, Storb R, Fefer A, Buckner CD, Neiman PE, Clift RA, Lerner KG, Thomas ED. Clinical manifestations of graft-versus-host disease in human recipients of marrow from HLA-matched sibling donors. Transplantation 18:295–304, 1974.

Goldsobel AB, Haas A, Stiehm ER. Bone marrow transplantation in DiGeorge syndrome. J Pediatr 111:40–44, 1987.

Gomez L, Le Deist F, Blanche S, Cavazzana-Calvo M, Griscelli C, Fischer A. Treatment of Omenn syndrome by bone marrow transplantation. J Pediatr 127:76–81, 1995.

Gordon PR, Leimig T, Mueller I, Babarin-Dorner A, Holladay MA, Houston J, Kerst G, Geiger T, Handgretinger R. A large-scale method for T cell depletion: towards graft engineering of mobilized peripheral blood stem cells. Bone Marrow Transplant 30:69–74, 2002.

Gratama JW, Zwaan FE, Stijnen T, Weijers TF, Weiland HT, D'Amaro J, Hekker AC, The TH, de Gast GC, Vossen JM. Herpes-virus immunity and acute graft-versus-host disease. Lancet 1:471–474, 1987.

Graze PR, Gale RP. Chronic graft-versus-host disease: a syndrome of disordered immunity. Am J Med 66:611–620, 1979.

Grewal SS, Barker JN, Davies SM, Wagner JE. Unrelated donor hematopoietic cell transplantation: marrow or umbilical cord blood? Blood 101: 4233–4244, 2003.

Gross TG, Filipovich AH, Conley ME, Pracher E, Schmiegelow K, Verdirame JD, Vowels M, Williams LL, Seemayer TA. Cure of X-linked lymphoproliferative disease (XLP) with allogeneic hematopoietic stem cell transplantation (HSCT): report from the XLP registry. Bone Marrow Transplant 17:741–744, 1996.

Grunebaum E, Mazzolari E, Porta F, Dallera D, Atkinson A, Reid B, Notarangelo LD, Roifman CM. Bone marrow transplantation for severe combined immunodeficiency. JAMA 295:508–516, 2006.

Haddad E, Le Deist F, Aucouturier P, Cavazzana-Calvo M, Blanche S, Basile GD, Fischer A. Long-term chimerism and B-cell function after bone marrow transplantation in patients with severe combined immunodeficiency with B cells: a single-center study of 22 patients. Blood 94:2923–2930, 1999.

Haddad E, Landais P, Friedrich W, Gerritsen B, Cavazzana-Calvo M, Morgan G, Bertrand Y, Fasth A, Porta F, Cant A, Espanol T, Muller S, Veys P, Vossen J, Fischer A. Long-term immune reconstitution and outcome after HLA-nonidentical T cell–depleted bone marrow transplantation for severe combined immunodeficiency: a European retrospective study of 116 patients. Blood 91:3646–3653, 1998.

Haddad E, Le Deist F, Blanche S, Benkerrou M, Rohrlich P, Vilmer E, Griscelli C, Fischer A. Treatment of Chediak-Higashi syndrome by allogenic bone marrow transplantation: report of 10 cases. Blood 85:3328–3333, 1995.

Hale G, Cobbold S, Waldmann H. T cell depletion with CAMPATH-1 in allogeneic bone marrow transplantation. Transplantation 45:753–759, 1988.

Hale G, Waldmann H. Control of graft-versus-host disease and graft rejection by T cell depletion of donor and recipient with Campath-1 antibodies. Results of matched sibling transplants for malignant diseases. Bone Marrow Transplant 13:597–611, 1994.

Handgretinger R, Klingebiel T, Lang P, Schumm M, Neu S, Geiselhart A, Bader P, Schlegel PG, Greil J, Stachel D, Herzog RJ, Niethammer D. Megadose transplantation of purified peripheral blood CD34+ progenitor cells from HLA-mismatched parental donors in children. Bone Marrow Transplant 27:777–783, 2001.

Henter JI, Samuelsson-Horne A, Arico M, Egeler RM, Elinder G, Filipovich AH, Gadner H, Imashuku S, Komp D, Ladisch S, Webb D, Janka G. Treatment of hemophagocytic lymphohistiocytosis with HLH-94 immunochemotherapy and bone marrow transplantation. Blood 100:2367–2373, 2002.

Horwitz ME, Barrett AJ, Brown MR, Carter CS, Childs R, Gallin JI, Holland SM, Linton GF, Miller JA, Leitman SF, Read EJ, Malech HL. Treatment of chronic granulomatous disease with nonmyeloablative conditioning and a T-cell-depleted hematopoietic allograft. N Engl J Med 344:881–888, 2001.

The International Chronic Granulomatous Disease Cooperative Study Group. A controlled trial of interferon gamma to prevent infection in chronic granulomatous disease. N Engl J Med 324(8):509–516, 2001.

Jabado N, Le Deist F, Cant A, De Graeff-Meeders ER, Fasth A, Morgan G, Vellodi A, Hale G, Bujan W, Thomas C, Cavazzana-Calvo M, Wijdenes J, Fischer A. Bone marrow transplantation from genetically HLA-nonidentical donors in children with fatal inherited disorders excluding severe combined immunodeficiencies: use of two monoclonal antibodies to prevent graft rejection. Pediatrics 98:420–428, 1996.

Jacobsohn DA, Emerick KM, Scholl P, Melin-Aldana H, O'Gorman M, Duerst R, Kletzel M. Nonmyeloablative hematopoietic stem cell transplant for X-linked hyper-immunoglobulin M syndrome with cholangiopathy. Pediatrics 113:e122–e127, 2004.

Jouanguy E, Altare F, Lamhamedi S, Revy P, Emile JF, Newport M, Levin M, Blanche S, Seboun E, Fischer A, Casanova JL. Interferon-gamma-receptor deficiency in an infant with fatal bacille Calmette-Guérin infection. N Engl J Med 335:1956–1961, 1996.

Kamani N, August CS, Campbell DE, Hassan NF, Douglas SD. Marrow transplantation in chronic granulomatous disease: an update, with 6-year follow up. J Pediatr 113:697–700, 1988.

Kernan NA, Bartsch G, Ash RC, Beatty PG, Champlin R, Filipovich A, Gajewski J, Hansen JA, Henslee-Downey J, McCullough J, McGlave P, Perkins HA, Phillips GL, Sanders J, Stroncek D, Thomas ED, Blume KG. Analysis of 462 transplantations from unrelated donors facilitated by the National Marrow Donor Program. N Engl J Med 328:593–602, 1993.

Khawaja K, Gennery AR, Flood TJ, Abinun M, Cant AJ. Bone marrow transplantation for CD40 ligand deficiency: a single centre experience. Arch Dis Child 84:508–511, 2001.

Klein C, Cavazzana-Calvo M, Le Deist F, Jabado N, Benkerrou M, Blanche S, Lisowska-Grospierre B, Griscelli C, Fischer A. Bone marrow transplantation in major histocompatibility complex class II deficency: a single center study of 19 patients. Blood 85:580–587, 1995.

Klein C, Lisowska-Grospierre B, LeDeist F, Fischer A, Griscelli C. Major histocompatibility complex class II deficiency: clinical manifestations, immunologic features, and outcome. J Pediatr 123:921–928, 1993.

Knutsen AP, Steffen M, Wassmer K, Wall DA. Umbilical cord blood transplantation in Wiskott Aldrich syndrome. J Pediatr 142:519–523, 2003.

Knutsen AP, Wall DA. Kinetics of T-cell development of umbilical cord blood transplantation in severe T-cell immunodeficiency disorders. J Allergy Clin Immunol 103:823–832, 1999.

Laffort C, Le Deist F, Favre M, Caillat-Zucman S, Radford-Weiss I, Debre M, Fraitag S, Blanche S, Cavazzana-Calvo M, de Saint BG, De Villartay JP, Giliani S, Orth G, Casanova JL, Bodemer C, Fischer A. Severe cutaneous papillomavirus disease after haemopoietic stem-cell transplantation in patients with severe combined immune deficiency caused by common gammac cytokine receptor subunit or JAK-3 deficiency. Lancet 363:2051–2054, 2004.

Landman-Parker J, Le Deist F, Blaise A, Brison O, Fischer A. Partial engraftment of donor bone marrow cells associated with long-term remission of haemophagocytic lymphohistiocytosis. Br J Haematol 85:37–41, 1993.

Lanfranchi A, Verardi R, Tettoni K, Neva A, Mazzolari E, Pennacchio M, Pasic S, Ugazio AG, Albertini A, Porta F. Haploidentical peripheral blood and marrow stem cell transplantation in nine cases of primary immunodeficiency. Haematologica 85:41–46, 2000.

Lang P, Bader P, Schumm M, Feuchtinger T, Einsele H, Fuhrer M, Weinstock C, Handgretinger R, Kuci S, Martin D, Niethammer D, Greil J. Transplantation of a combination of CD133+ and CD34+ selected progenitor cells from alternative donors. Br J Haematol 124:72–79, 2004.

Le Deist F, Blanche S, Keable H, Gaud C, Pham H, Descamp-Latscha B, Wahn V, Griscelli C, Fischer A. Successful HLA nonidentical bone marrow transplantation in three patients with the leukocyte adhesion deficiency. Blood 74:512–516, 1989.

Lenarsky C, Weinberg K, Kohn DB, Parkman R. Unrelated donor bone marrow transplantation for Wiskott-Aldrich syndrome. Bone Marrow Transplant 12:145–147, 1993.

Leone V, Tommasini A, Andolina M, Runti G, De Vonderweid U, Campello C, Notarangelo LD, Ventura A. Elective bone marrow transplantation in a child with X-linked hyper-IgM syndrome presenting with acute respiratory distress syndrome. Bone Marrow Transplant 30:49–52, 2002.

Levine AM. Lymphoma complicating immunodeficiency disorders. Ann Oncol 5:S29–S35, 1994.

Levy J, Espanol-Boren T, Thomas C, Fischer A, Tovo P, Bordigoni P, Resnick I, Fasth A, Baer M, Gomes L, Sanders EAM, Tabone M, Plantaz D, Etzioni A, Monafo V, Abinun M, Hammarstrom L, Abrabamsen T, Jones A, Finn A, Klemola T, DeVries E, Sanal O, Peitsch M, Notarangelo LD. Clinical spectrum of X-linked hyper IgM syndrome. J Pediatr 131:47–54, 1997.

Loechelt BJ, Shapiro RS, Jyonouchi H, Filipovich AH. Mismatched bone marrow transplantation for Omenn syndrome: a variant of severe combined immunodeficiency. Bone Marrow Transplant 16:381–385, 1995.

Lorenz E, Cogdon C, Uphoff D. Modification of acute radiation injury in mice and guinea pigs by bone marrow injection. Radiology 58:863–877, 1952.

Martin PJ, Hansen JA, Storb R, Thomas ED. Human marrow transplantation: an immunological perspective. Adv Immunol 40:379–438, 1987.

McDonald GB, Sharma P, Matthews DE, Shulman HM, Thomas ED. The clinical course of 53 patients with venocclusive disease of the liver after marrow transplantation. Transplantation 39:603–608, 1985.

Miano M, Porta F, Locatelli F, Miniero R, La Nasa G, di Bartolomeo P, Giardini C, Messina C, Balduzzi A, Testi AM, Garbarino L, Lanino E, Crescenzi F, Zecca M, Dini G. Unrelated donor marrow transplantation for inborn errors. Bone Marrow Transplant 21(Suppl 2):S37–S41, 1998.

Mielcarek M, Sandmaier BM, Maloney DG, Maris M, McSweeney PA, Woolfrey A, Chauncey T, Feinstein L, Niederwieser D, Blume KG, Forman S, Torok-Storb B, Storb R. Nonmyeloablative hematopoietic cell transplantation: status quo and future perspectives. J Clin Immunol 22: 70–74, 2002.

Moen RC, Horowitz SD, Sondel PM, Borcherding WR, Trigg ME, Billing R, Hong R. Immunologic reconstitution after haploidentical bone marrow transplantation for immune deficiency disorders: treatment of bone marrow cells with monoclonal antibody CT-2 and complement. Blood 70: 664–669, 1987.

Morgan G, Linch DC, Knott LT, Davies EG, Sieff C, Chessells JM, Hale G, Waldmann H, Levinsky RJ. Successful haploidentical mismatched bone marrow transplantation in severe combined immunodeficiency: T cell removal using CAMPATH-I monoclonal antibody and E-rosetting. Br J Haematol 62:421–430, 1986.

Morra M, Silander O, Calpe-Flores S, Choi MSK, Oettgen H, Myers LA, Buckley RH. Alterations of the X-linked lymphoproliferative disease gene SH2DIA in common variable immunodeficiency syndrome. Blood 98:1321–1325, 2001.

Mullen CA, Anderson KD, Blaese RM. Splenectomy and/or bone marrow transplantation in the management of the Wiskott-Aldrich syndrome: long-term follow-up of 62 cases. Blood 82:2961–2966, 1993.

Muller-Ruchholtz W, Wottge HU, Muller-Hermelink HK. Bone marrow transplantation in rats across strong histocompatibility barriers by selective elimination of lymphoid cells in donor marrow. Transplant Proc 8: 537–541, 1976.

Myers LA, Patel DD, Puck JM, Buckley RH. Hematopoietic stem cell transplantation for severe combined immunodeficiency in the neonatal period leads to superior thymic output and improved survival. Blood 99:872–878, 2002.

Nagler A, Ackerstein A, Kapelushnik J, Or R, Naparstek E, Slavin S. Donor lymphocyte infusion post–non-myeloablative allogeneic peripheral blood stem cell transplantation for chronic granulomatous disease. Bone Marrow Transplant 24:339–342, 1999.

Newport MJ, Huxley CM, Huston S, Hawrylowicz CM, Oostra BA, Williamson R, Levin M. A mutation in the interferon-gamma-receptor gene and susceptibility to mycobacterial infection. N Engl J Med 335: 1941–1949, 1996.

Noel DR, Witherspoon RP, Storb R, Atkinson K, Doney K, Mickelson EM, Ochs HD, Warren RP, Weiden PL, Thomas ED. Does graft-versus-host disease influence the tempo of immunologic recovery after allogeneic human marrow transplantation? An observation on 56 long-term survivors. Blood 51:1087–1105, 1978.

O'Reilly RJ. Bone marrow transplants in patients lacking an HLA-matched sibling donor. Pediatr Ann 20(12):682–690, 1991.

O'Reilly RJ, Brochstein J, Collins N, Keever C, Kapoor N, Kirkpatrick D, Kernan N, Dupont B, Burns J, Reisner Y. Evaluation of HLA-haplotype disparate parental marrow grafts depleted of T lymphocytes by differential agglutination with a soybean lectin and E-rosette depletion for the treatment of severe combined immunodeficiency. Vox Sang 51:81–86, 1986.

Ozsahin H, Le Deist F, Benkerrou M, Cavazzana-Calvo M, Gomez L, Griscelli C, Blanchi S, Fischer A. Bone marrow transplantation in 26 patients with Wiskott-Aldrich syndrome from a single center. J Pediatr 129: 238–244, 1996.

Parkman R. Bone marrow transplantation for genetic diseases. Pediatr Ann 20:677–681, 1991a.

Parkman R. Human graft-versus-host disease. Immunodef Rev 2:253–264, 1991b.

Parkman R, Rappeport J, Geha R, Belli J, Cassady R, Levey R, Nathan DG, Rosen FS. Complete correction of the Wiskott-Aldrich syndrome by allogenic bone-marrow transplantation. N Engl J Med 298:921–927, 1978.

Patel DD, Gooding ME, Parrott RE, Curtis KM, Haynes BF, Buckley RH. Thymic function after hematopoietic stem-cell transplantation for the treatment of severe combined immunodeficiency. N Engl J Med 342: 1325–1332, 2000.

Pillow RP, Epstein RB, Buckner CD, Giblett ER, Thomas ED. Treatment of bone marrow failure by isogeneic marrow infusion. N Engl J Med 275: 94–97, 1966.

Pracher E, Panzer-Grumayer ER, Zoubek A, Peters C, Gadner H. Successful bone marrow transplantation in a boy with X-linked lymphoproliferative syndrome and acute severe infectious mononucleosis. Bone Marrow Transplant 13:655–658, 1994.

Przepiorka D, Ippoliti C, Giralt S, van Beisen K, Mehra R, Deisseroth AB, Andersson B, Luna M, Cork A, Lee M, Estey E, Andreeff M, Champlin R. A phase I–II study of high dose thiotepa, busulfan and cyclophosphamide as a preparative regimen for allogeneic marrow transplantation. Bone Marrow Transplant 14:449–453, 1994.

Pulsipher MA, Woolfrey A. Nonmyeloablative transplantation in children. Current status and future prospects. Hematol Oncol Clin North Am 15: 809–834, vii–viii, 2001.

Rappeport JM, Parkman R, Newburger P, Camitta BM, Chusid MJ. Correction of infantile agranulocytosis (Kostmann's syndrome) by allogeneic bone marrow transplantation. Am J Med 68:605–609, 1980.

Reinherz EL, Geha R, Rappeport JM, Wilson M, Penta AC, Hussey RE, Fitzgerald KA, Daley JF, Levine H, Rosen FS, Schlossman SF. Reconstitution after transplantation with T-lymphocyte–depleted HLA haplotype-mismatched bone marrow for severe combined immunodeficiency. Proc Natl Acad Sci USA 79:6047–6051, 1982.

Reisner Y, Itzicovitch L, Meshorer A, Sharon N. Hematopoietic stem cell transplantation using mouse bone marrow and spleen cells fractionated by lectins. Proc Nat Acad Sci USA 75:2933–2936, 1978.

Reisner Y, Kapoor N, Kirkpatrick D, Pollack MS, Cunningham-Rundles S, Dupont B, Hodes MZ, Good RA, O'Reilly RJ. Transplantation for severe combined immunodeficiency with HLA-A, B, D, DR incompatible parental marrow cells fractionated by soybean agglutinin and sheep red blood cells. Blood 61:341–348, 1983.

Reuter U, Roesler J, Thiede C, Schulz A, Classen CF, Oelschlagel U, Debatin KM, Friedrich W. Correction of complete interferon-γ receptor 1 deficiency by bone marrow transplantation. Blood 100:4234–4235, 2002.

Rumelhart SL, Trigg ME, Horowitz SD, Hong R. Monoclonal antibody T-cell-depleted HLA-haploidentical bone marrow transplantation for Wiskott-Aldrich syndrome. Blood 75:1031–1035, 1990.

Schiff SE, Kurtzberg J, Buckley RH. Studies of human bone marrow treated with soybean lectin and sheep erythrocytes: stepwise analysis of cell morphology, phenotype and function. Clin Exp Immunol 68:685–693, 1987.

Schneider LC, Berman RS, Shea CR, Perez-Atayde AR, Weinstein H, Geha RS. Bone marrow transplantation (BMT) for the syndrome of pigmentary dilution and lymphohistiocytosis (Griscelli's syndrome). J Clin Immunol 10:146–153, 1990.

Scholl PR, O'Gorman MR, Pachman LM, Haut P, Kletzel M. Correction of neutropenia and hypogammaglobulinemia in X-linked hyper-IgM syndrome by allogeneic bone marrow transplantation. Bone Marrow Transplant 22:1215–1218, 1998.

Schouten HC, Sizoo W, van't Veer MB, Hagenbeek A, Lowenberg B. Incomplete chimerism in erythroid, myeloid and B lymphocyte lineage after T cell depleted allogeneic bone marrow transplantation. Bone Marrow Transplant 3:407–412, 1988.

Schumm M, Lang P, Taylor G, Kuci S, Klingebiel T, Buhring HJ, Geiselhart A, Niethammer D, Handgretinger R. Isolation of highly purified autologous and allogeneic peripheral CD34+ cells using the CliniMACS device. J Hematother 8:209–218, 1999.

Schwarer AP, Jiang YZ, Brookes PA, Barrett AJ, Batchelor JR, Goldman JM, Lechler RI. Frequency of anti-recipient alloreactive helper T-cell precursors in donor blood and graft-versus-host disease after HLA-identical sibling bone marrow transplantation. Lancet 341:203–205, 1993.

Seger RA, Gungor T, Belohradsky BH, Blanche S, Bordigoni P, di Bartolomeo P, Flood T, Landais P, Muller S, Ozsahin H, Passwell JH, Porta F, Slavin S, Wulffraat N, Zintl F, Nagler A, Cant A, Fischer A. Treatment of chronic granulomatous disease with myeloablative conditioning and an unmodified hemopoietic allograft: a survey of the European experience, 1985–2000. Blood 100:4344–4350, 2002.

Shearer WT, Ritz J, Finegold MJ, Guerra IC, Rosenblatt HM, Lewis DE, Pollack MS, Taber LH, Sumaya CV, Grumet FC, Cleary ML, Warnke R, Sklar J. Epstein-Barr virus–associated B-cell proliferations of diverse clonal origins after bone marrow transplantation in a 12-year-old patient with severe combined immunodeficiency. N Engl J Med 312:1151–1159, 1985.

Skinner J, Finlay JL, Sondel PM, Trigg ME. Infectious complications in pediatric patients undergoing transplantation with T lymphocyte–depleted bone marrow. Pediatr Infect Dis 5:319–324, 1986.

Snyder MJ, Stenzel TT, Buckley PJ, Lagoo AS, Rizzieri DA, Gasparetto C, Vredenburgh JJ, Chao NJ, Gong JZ. Posttransplant lymphoproliferative disorder following nonmyeloablative allogeneic stem cell transplantation. Am J Surg Pathol 28:794–800, 2004.

Srinivasan R, Chakrabarti S, Walsh T, Igarashi T, Takahashi Y, Kleiner D, Donohue T, Shalabi R, Carvallo C, Barrett AJ, Geller N, Childs R. Improved survival in steroid-refractory acute graft versus host disease after non-myeloablative allogeneic transplantation using a daclizumab-based strategy with comprehensive infection prophylaxis. Br J Haematol 124: 777–786, 2004.

Stary J, Bartunkova J, Kobylka P, Vavra V, Hrusak O, Calda P, Kral V, Svorc K. Successful HLA-identical sibling cord blood transplantation in a 6-year-old boy with leukocyte adhesion deficiency syndrome. Bone Marrow Transplant 18:249–252, 1996.

Stephan JL, Vlekova V, Le Deist F, Blanche S, Donadieu J, de Saint-Basile G, Durandy A, Griscelli C, Fischer A. Severe combined immunodeficiency: a retrospective single-center study of clinical presentation and outcome in 117 cases. J Pediatr 123:564–572, 1993.

Storb R, Deeg HJ, Whitehead J, Appelbaum F, Beatty P, Bensinger W, Buckner CD, Clift R, Doney K, Farewell V, Hansen J, Hill R, Lum L, Martin P, McGuffin R, Sanders J, Stewart P, Sullivan K, Witherspoon R, Yee G, Thomas ED. Methotrexate and cyclosporine compared with cyclosporine alone for prophylaxis of acute graft versus host disease after marrow transplantation for leukemia. N Engl J Med 314:729–735, 1986.

Sullivan JL, Woda BA. X-linked lymphoproliferative syndrome. Immunodef Rev 1:325–347, 1989.

Theobald M, Nierle T, Bunjes D, Arnold R, Heimpel H. Host-specific interleukin-2-secreting donor T-cell precursors as predictors of acute graft-versus-host disease in bone marrow transplantation between HLA-identical siblings. N Engl J Med 327:1613–1617, 1992.

Thomas C, de Saint Basile G, Le Deist F, Theophile D, Benkerrou M, Haddad E, Blanche S, Fischer A. Brief report: correction of X-linked hyper-IgM syndrome by allogeneic bone marrow transplantation. N Engl J Med 333:426–429, 1995a.

Thomas C, Le Deist F, Cavazzana-Calvo M, Benkerrou M, Haddad E, Blanche S, Hartmann W, Friedrich W, Fischer A. Results of allogeneic bone marrow transplantation in patients with leukocyte adhesion deficiency. Blood 86:1629–1635, 1995b.

Thomas ED, Storb R, Clift RA, Fefer A, Johnson L, Neiman PE, Lerner KG, Glucksberg H, Buckner CD. Bone marrow transplantation. N Engl J Med 292:823–843, 1975.

Thomson BG, Robertson KA, Gowan D, Heilman D, Broxmeyer HE, Emanuel D, Kotylo P, Brahmi Z, Smith FO. Analysis of engraftment, graft-versus-host disease, and immune recovery following unrelated donor cord blood transplantation. Blood 96:2703–2711, 2000.

Tiercy JM, Bujan-Lose M, Chapuis B, Gratwohl A, Gmur J, Seger R, Kern M, Morell A, Roosnek E. Bone marrow transplantation with unrelated donors: what is the probability of identifying an HLA-A/B/Cw/DRB1/B3/B5/DQB1-matched donor? Bone Marrow Transplant 26:437–441, 2000.

Toren A, Nagler A, Amariglio N, Neumann Y, Golan H, Bilori B, Kaplinsky C, Mandel M, Biniaminov M, Levanon M, Rosenthal E, Davidson J, Brok-Simoni F, Rechavi G. Successful human umbilical cord blood stem cell transplantation without conditioning in severe combined immune deficiency. Bone Marrow Transplant 23:405–408, 1999.

Touraine JL. Treatment of human fetuses and induction of immunological tolerance in humans by in utero transplantation of stem cells into fetal recipients. Acta Haematol 96:115–119, 1996.

Trigg ME, Billing R, Sondel PM, Exten R, Hong R, Bozdech MJ, Horowitz SD, Finley JL, Moen R, Longo W, Erickson C, Peterson A. Clinical trial depleting T lymphocytes from donor marrow for matched and mismatched allogeneic bone marrow transplants. Cancer Treat Rep 69:377–386, 1985.

van Dijken PJ, Ghayur T, Mauch P, Down J, Burakoff SJ, Ferrara JL. Evidence that anti-LFA-1 in vivo improves engraftment and survival after allogeneic bone marrow transplantation. Transplantation 49:882–886, 1990.

van Leeuwen JE, van Tol MJ, Joosten AM, Schellekens PT, van den Bergh RL, Waaijer JL, Oudeman-Gruber NJ, van der Weijden-Ragas CP, Roos MT, Gerritsen RJ, Van Den Berg H, Haraldsson A, Khan PM, Vossen JM. Relationship between patterns of engraftment in peripheral blood and immune reconstitution after allogeneic bone marrow transplantation for (severe) combined immunodeficiency. Blood 84:3936–3947, 1994.

Vassal G, Fischer A, Challine D, Boland I, Ledheist F, Lemerle S, Vilmer E, Rahimy C, Souillet G, Gluckman E, Michel G, Deroussent A, Gouyette A. Busulfan disposition below the age of three: alteration in children with lysosomal storage disease. Blood 82:1030–1034, 1993.

Vossen JM, van Leeuwen JE, van Tol MJ, Joosten AM, Van Den Berg H, Gerritsen EJ, Haraldsson A, Khan PM. Chimerism and immune reconstitution following allogeneic bone marrow transplantation for severe combined immunodeficiency disease. Immunodeficiency 4:311–313, 1993.

Vowels MR, Tang RL, Berdoukas V, Ford D, Thierry D, Purtilo D, Gluckman E. Brief report: correction of X-linked lymphoproliferative disease by transplantation of cord-blood stem cells. N Engl J Med 329:1623–1625, 1993.

Wagner JE, Barker JN, DeFor TE, Baker KS, Blazar BR, Eide C, Goldman A, Kersey J, Krivit W, MacMillan ML, Orchard PJ, Peters C, Weisdorf DJ, Ramsay NK, Davies SM. Transplantation of unrelated donor umbilical cord blood in 102 patients with malignant and nonmalignant diseases: influence of CD34 cell dose and HLA disparity on treatment-related mortality and survival. Blood 100:1611–1618, 2002.

Wagner JE, Kernan NA, Steinbuch M, Broxmeyer HE, Gluckman E. Allogeneic sibling umbilical-cord-blood transplantation in children with malignant and non-malignant disease. Lancet 346:214–219, 1995.

Waldmann H, Polliak A, Hale G, Or R, Cividalli G, Weiss L, Weshler Z, Samuel S, Manor D, Brautbar C, Rachmilewitz EA, Slavin S. Elimination of graft-versus-host disease by in vitro depletion of alloreactive lymphocytes with a monoclonal rat anti-human lymphocyte antibody (CAMPATH-1). Lancet 2:483–486, 1984.

Wang J, Song X, Zhang W, Tong S, Hou J, Chen L, Lou J, Li H, Ding X, Min B. [Combination of mycophenolate mofetil with cyclosporine A and methotrexate for the prophylaxes of acute graft versus host disease in allogeneic peripheral stem cell transplantation]. Zhonghua Yi Xue Za Zhi 82:507–510, 2002.

Weisdorf D, Haake R, Blazar B, Miller W, McGlave P, Ramsay N, Kersey J, Filipovich A. Treatment of moderate/severe acute graft-versus-host disease after allogeneic bone marrow transplantation: an analysis of clinical risk features and outcome. Blood 75:1024–1030, 1990.

Wengler GS, Lanfranchi A, Frusca T, Verardi R, Neva A, Brugnoni D, Giliani S, Fiorini M, Mella P, Guandalini F, Mazzolari E, Pecorelli S, Notarangelo LD, Porta F, Ugazio AG. In-utero transplantation of parental CD34 haematopoietic progenitor cells in a patient with X-linked severe combined immunodeficiency (SCIDX1). Lancet 348:1484–1487, 1996.

Wijnaendts L, LeDeist F, Griscelli C, Fischer A. Development of immunologic functions after bone marrow transplantation in 33 patients with severe combined immunodeficiency. Blood 74:2212–2219, 1989.

Williams LL, Rooney CM, Conley ME, Brenner MK, Krance RA, Heslop HE. Correction of Duncan's syndrome by allogeneic bone marrow transplantation. Lancet 342:587–588, 1993.

Woolfrey A, Pulsipher MA, Storb R. Nonmyeloablative hematopoietic cell transplant for treatment of immune deficiency. Curr Opin Pediatr 13:539–545, 2001.

Wu AM, Till JE, Siminovitch L, McCulloch EA. A cytological study of the capacity for differentiation of normal hemopoietic colony-forming cells. J Cell Physiol 69:177–184, 1967.

Wu AM, Till JE, Siminovitch L, McCulloch EA. Cytological evidence for a relationship between normal hematopoietic colony-forming cells and cells of the lymphoid system. J Exp Med 127:455–464, 1968.

Ziegner UH, Ochs HD, Schanen C, Feig SA, Seyama K, Futatani T, Gross T, Wakim M, Roberts RL, Rawlings DJ, Dovat S, Fraser JK, Stiehm ER. Unrelated umbilical cord stem cell transplantation for X-linked immunodeficiencies. J Pediatr 138:570–573, 2001.

48

Gene Therapy

FABIO CANDOTTI and ALAIN FISCHER

As currently practiced, gene therapy can be defined as the transfer of exogenous genes to somatic cells of a patient in order to correct an inherited or acquired gene defect, or to introduce a new function or trait. In the last 15 years, gene therapy has moved from the speculative stage to clinical applications as clinical gene transfer protocols have been applied to inherited genetic defects, malignancies, and infectious diseases. Primary immunodeficiciency diseases (PIDs), especially severe combined immunodeficiency (SCID) disorders, have played a major role in this process as they have provided a proving ground for the first therapeutic applications (Blaese et al., 1995) as well as the first evidence that gene therapy can be curative (Cavazzana-Calvo et al., 2000; Hacein-Bey-Abina et al., 2002). Several advantageous characteristics have made PIDs attractive candidate diseases for gene therapy. First, PIDs are often curable by allogeneic hematopoietic stem cell transplantation (HSCT), which translates into the possibility that they should also be treatable with procedures combining ex vivo manipulation and reinfusion of autologous, gene-corrected hematopoietic stem cells. Second, the target cells reside in the bone marrow, a readily accessible tissue, which makes them amenable to harvest for ex vivo gene transfer, the procedure that currently offers the best success. In addition, the regulation of genes responsible for many PIDs (i.e., adenosine deaminase deficiency, chronic granulomatous disease, X-linked severe combined immunodeficiency, leukocyte adhesion deficiency) appears relatively simple and, while currently available technology does not allow reproducing the physiological control mechanisms of gene expression, the available gene transfer vectors are more than adequate to provide expression of these genes at levels required for clinical benefit. Finally, for several PIDs, gene-corrected progenitors and mature cells have a survival advantage over the unmodified, affected cell populations. This selective survival translates into the very advanta-

geous circumstance that even low gene transfer efficiency can have therapeutic effects.

Because of the extensive recent progress in the molecular and biological characterization of PIDs, several PIDs also fulfill the general prerequisites for any gene therapy approach that are based on the comprehensive knowledge of the molecular and cellular basis of the candidate disease. In general, the sequence of the cDNA of the gene responsible for the disease represents one critical piece of information for preliminary experiments of corrective gene transfer; however, the elucidation of the genomic organization and the characteristics of the promoting element(s) are also of great practical importance. Moreover, the specific function(s) and regulatory mechanisms of expression of the gene of interest should be understood, and the potential deleterious effects of overexpression investigated. Where possible, the safety and efficacy of gene transfer protocols should be tested in animal models, either naturally occurring or experimentally generated. Finally, it is fundamental to verify that the correction of the genetic defect can induce the restoration of gene function(s) in affected cells.

The complete and careful consideration of these issues is critical for development of new gene therapy strategies and should help in defining the answer for the ethical dilemma that is proposed whenever the traditional treatment for the candidate disease is already highly successful, but not completely curative.

Performing gene therapy for PIDs involves a series of specific difficulties. As mentioned, the ultimate target of corrective gene transfer for PIDs is the hematopoietic stem cell (HSC). Targeting the HSC is an exceptionally challenging task for several reasons. First, cells with the characteristics of true hematopoietic progenitors are extremely infrequent in hematopoietic tissues and have thus far eluded all attempts to define their specific cellular phenotype, making their collection and enrichment laborious and

Table 48.1. Present Status and Challenges of Gene Therapy Approaches for Primary Immunodeficiency Diseases

Disease	Efficacy of BMT	Potential Target Cells for Gene Transfer	Status of Corrective Gene Transfer Studies	Challenges	Available Animal Model
ADA-SCID	Good (HLA-identical)	BM, CB, T	Ongoing clinical trials	Adequacy of immune repertoire in T cell–directed protocols	muKO
CGD	Good (HLA-identical)	BM, CB	Ongoing clinical trial	No selective advantage	muKO
LAD1	Good	BM, CB	Preclinical	Tissue specific gene expression, no selective advantage	muKO
X-SCID	Good	BM, CB	Ongoing clinical trials	Definition of risk of insertional oncogenesis	dog, muKO
JAK3-SCID	Good	BM, CB	Ongoing clinical trial	Definition of risk of insertional oncogenesis	muKO
PNP deficiency	Poor*	BM, CB, T	Approved clinical trial	Adequacy of immune repertoire in T cell–directed protocols	muKO
ZAP70-SCID	Good*	BM, CB	Preclinical	Lineage/differentiation stage restricted expression	muKO
MHC class II deficiency	Poor	BM, CB	Preclinical	Regulated gene expression	muKO
X-HIM	Fair	BM, CB, T	Preclinical	Regulated gene expression, no selective advantage	muKO
XLA	Limited experience	BM, CB	Preclinical	Restricted gene expression	Xid mouse, muKO
RAG-2	Good	BM, CB	Preclinical	Preclinical	muKO
WAS	Good	BM, CB	Preclinical	High levels of gene expression seem necessary	muKO
CD3γ deficiency	Irrelevant**	BM, CB, T	Preclinical	Regulated gene expression	muKO
BS	Good	BM, CB, T	Preclinical	Regulated gene expression	muKO

BM, bone marrow progenitors; CB, cord blood progenitors; muKO, murine knockout model; T, peripheral T lymphocytes.
*Very few cases reported, **Mild phenotype.

inefficient. In addition, HSC are mostly quiescent and therefore resistent to the insertion of genetic material by viral vectors requiring active cell division. Extensive studies have been dedicated to the identification of "ex-vivo" culture conditions that could stimulate HSC to proliferate, thus making them susceptible to gene integration, without inducing differentiation and loss of long-term repopulating ability. In addition to the original cytokines and growth factors such as interleukin (IL)-3, IL-6, and stem cell factor (SCF), new molecules and culture supports such as thrombopoietin, Flt-3 ligand, and fibronectin (Hanenberg et al., 1996; Dao et al., 1997; Piacibello et al., 1997, 1999; Zandstra et al., 1997; Kohn, 1999). Have been demonstrated to be of primary importance to this goal. Research efforts have resulted in a major improvement in our ability to efficiently introduce genes into HSC in large animal models (Kiem et al., 1998; Tisdale et al., 1998). However, the current levels of gene transfer may still not be adequate for achieving therapeutic effects in hematopoietic diseases in which corrected cells do not have a strong selective advantage over the mutated ones (e.g., thalassemias or sickle cell disease). On the other hand, progress has resulted in successful clinical protocols for X-linked SCID and adenosine deaminase (ADA) deficiency (Cavazzana-Calvo et al., 2000; Aiuti et al., 2002a; Hacein-Bey-Abina et al., 2002), thus providing the basis for future clinical applications for other PIDs.

Another obstacle to gene therapy for PIDs is that several of the causative genes that have been identified have expression restricted to specific hematopoietic elements or particular cellular phases of cell development (see Table 48.1). In the gene transfer vectors currently available for clinical use, the gene of interest is under the transcriptional control of strong viral promoters and is therefore expected to give rise to unregulated expression of the gene in transduced HSCs and all deriving cell lineages. This strong, ubiquitous promoter activity raises the concern that constitutive expression of an ectopic gene could have detrimental

consequences on the differentiation and/or function of targeted populations. The necessity of tissue-specific and/or precise regulation of gene expression represents a formidable challenge for the development of future gene therapies. Theoretically, the use of gene-specific promoting and/or enhancing elements could be exploited to obtain physiologically regulated expression of the therapeutic gene; alternatively, inducible or repressible systems could also be used to modulate gene expression.

Finally, patients with inherited disorders of immunity may present with complete lack of expression of the affected gene(s) or show detectable levels of nonfunctional (mutated) gene product(s). It is not obvious which one of these two possibilities represents the better scenario for successful gene therapy. In the case of subjects carrying "null" mutations, there is the possibility that the newly expressed molecule could induce an immune response resulting in the elimination of the transduced, therapeutic cell populations. In the presence of mutations allowing for the expression of an inactive gene product, by contrast, the mutated molecules could manifest dominant negative effects in the presence of the correct protein(s), generating the necessity of obtaining very high levels of expression of the transgene to achieve therapeutic effects.

Methods for Gene Transfer

A variety of systems have been developed for gene transfer and expression in mammalian cells. In the case of inherited genetic errors, the choice of a gene delivery system is dictated by the need for persistent expression of the therapeutic gene. This can be most readily achieved if the exogenous genetic material is stably integrated into the host cell genome, thus ensuring the transmission of the transferred gene to the progeny of that cell during normal mitotic cell division. In the absence of integration, the inserted gene will be diluted out as the cell divides and thus the

MoMuLV

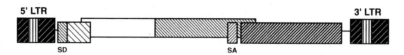

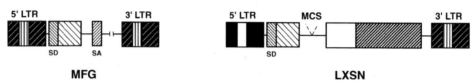

MFG   **LXSN**

Figure 48.1. Schematic representation of the Moloney leukemia virus (MoMuLV) and MoMuLV-based LXSN (Miller and Rosman, 1989) and MFG (Dranoff et al., 1993) retroviral vectors. The organization of Mo-MuLV *gag, pol,* and *env* genes, as well as of splice donor (SD) and acceptor (SA) sites, packaging signal sequence (ψ), and long tandem repeats (LTRs) are represented. The of MoMuLV *gag, pol,* and *env* sequences are deleted to obtain the backbone of retroviral vectors. The MFG cassette is an example of "splicing vector" and maintains both splice donor and acceptor sites of the MoMuLV *env* coding sequence, thus mimicking the natural pattern of viral mRNA splicing. In the LXSN cassette and the MoMuLV 5′ LTR is replaced with the homologous region from the Moloney murine sarcoma virus (MoMuSV). MCS, multiple cloning site; *neo,* neomycin resistance gene; SV40p, SV40 early promoter region.

therapeutic effects will ultimately be lost. Gene transfer vectors based on integrating viral systems such as murine oncoretroviruses, lentiviruses, and adeno-associated viruses represent efficient tools for stable gene expression. Of these, only vectors derived from murine oncoretroviruses have been used to date in clinical applications of gene therapy for PIDs.

Vectors Based on Retroviruses

Retroviral vectors, the most commonly used gene transfer systems in human gene therapy, are gene transfer constructs that reproduce the replication and integration mechanisms of retroviruses. The Moloney murine leukemia virus (MoMLV) of the mammalian type C retroviruses is the most extensively studied retrovirus model (Miller, 1992), although other viruses from this group have also been exploited. More recently, vectors based on the two other major groups of retroviruses, lentiviruses and spumaviruses, have also been extensively studied.

MoMLV vectors

A complete, wild-type MoMLV particle is composed of two copies of the viral RNA contained within a protein capsid and an external phospholipid envelope. Important enzymes, such as the retroviral reverse transcriptase, integrase, and protease, are also packaged within the virion.

The retrovirus life cycle is constituted by (1) binding of the retroviral envelope to a specific receptor on the cell membrane followed by internalization of the viral capsid; (2) un-coating and reverse transcription of viral genomic RNA to produce double-stranded viral DNA; (3) migration of this DNA through the cytoplasm to the nucleus; and (4) integration of the proviral DNA into the host cell genome. Integration occurs, however, only if the targeted cells are actively proliferating, presumably because nuclear membranes must be disrupted for nuclear DNA transport. After reverse transcription, the viral genome (provirus) consists of 8.3 kb of double-stranded DNA containing the *gag, pol,* and *env* genes flanked by the viral long terminal repeats

(LTR). The *gag* and *env* genes encode the structural proteins of viral core and envelope, respectively, while the reverse transcriptase, integrase, and protease are derived from the *pol* region. The two identical LTRs contain sequences promoting and enhancing transcription, as well as a polyadenylation signal (polyA). Between the 5′ LTR and the *gag* gene is a region of the genome termed ψ containing the encapsidation sequence that is necessary for efficient packaging of newly produced viral genomic RNA into the capsid structure (Temin, 1984).

To obtain viral vectors incapable of replicating in transduced cells, the genes encoding viral proteins are deleted and replaced with selectable markers and/or multiple cloning sites for the insertion of experimental genes (see Fig. 48.1). To obtain complete and infectious viral particles, "packaging" cell lines have been developed that express the *gag, pol,* and *env* genes products, but are unable to encapsidate the viral genomic RNA because of mutations or deletions in their ψ region. However, these cells allow packaging of the genome of retroviral vectors in which the ψ region is conserved (see Fig. 48.2).

Several packaging cell lines are now available. They are characterized by different host ranges, in turn determined by the specificity of their *env* genes. Among these, the PG13 (Miller et al., 1991) and the FlyRD18 (Cosset et al., 1995) packaging lines incorporate the gibbon-ape leukemia virus (GALV) and the cat endogenous virus (CEV) envelope proteins, respectively. In hematopoietic cells and progenitors, the expression levels of receptors for GALV and CEV are higher than that of the receptor for the Moloney envelope. In some cases, receptors can be metabolically up-regulated (Bunnell et al., 1995). These characteristics make packaging cells effective tools for diseases potentially treatable by gene transfer into peripheral blood elements or hematopoietic stem cells (Kiem et al., 1998; Kelly et al., 2000).

Another packaging system is based on the incorporation of the vesicular-stomatitis virus envelope protein G (VSV-G) into the virions of MoMLV-derived vectors. The particles carrying VSV-G have the advantage of a broader host range compared to virions encapsidated into the amphotropic envelope protein, and

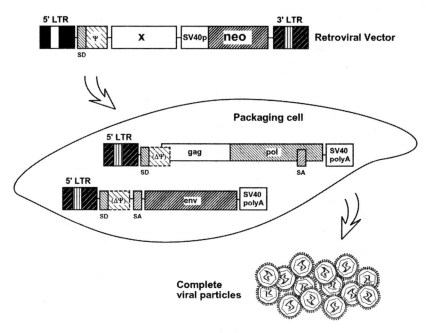

Figure 48.2. Production of retroviral vector supernatants. The retroviral construct is transfected into the packaging cell line that contains the "helper" MoMuLV modified genomes. The *gag, pol,* and *env* genes provide the necessary viral proteins, whereas deletions of the packaging signal sequences prevent the encapsidation of the helper genomic RNA into virions. The retroviral vector, however, contains the complete packaging signal and generates RNA molecules that can be efficiently encapsidated. Finally, infectious viral particles containing the recombinant retroviral vector can be obtained in the culture supernatant.

allow the generation of concentrated, high-titer retroviral vector preparations (Rebel et al., 1999).

In vitro gene transfer is usually achieved by single or repeated exposure of the target cells to retroviral supernatants. Alternative procedures involving cocultivation of retroviral producer and target cells can increase gene transfer efficiency, but pose significant hurdles to development of clinical protocols.

Advantages of retroviral vectors for gene transfer include the broad range of infectable cell types and the efficient gene integration that can be achieved with dividing cells. Retroviral-based vectors, however, also present drawbacks. The maximum amount of DNA that these vectors can accommodate is ~8 kb, a size that prevents the transfer of large genomic sequences. Furthermore, retroviral vector integration into the host cell genome raises a twofold problem. First, the levels of gene expression can drastically vary from cell to cell depending on the particular site of proviral integration. These *position effects* are thought to depend on the basal chromatin structure at the integration site and can completely silence transgene expression in some cases while augmenting expression in others. Clearly, for many genes a tightly regulated range of expression is required, and this wide variability is not acceptable. Second, the integration events could theoretically disrupt critical nearby genetic sequences leading either to cell death or to activation of oncogenes, resulting in malignancy. The risk of insertional oncogenesis is unfortunately real, as recently indicated by the development of leukemia-like disorders in subjects receiving retroviral-mediated gene transfer as a treatment for X-linked severe combined immunodeficiency (XSCID) (Hacein-Bey-Abina et al., 2003a, 2003b).

Lentiviral vectors

Gene transfer vectors based on lentiviruses including human immunodeficiency virus type 1 (HIV-1) may have advantages over retroviral vectors for transduction into quiescent lymphocytes and hematopoietic stem cells. The genome of HIV-1 is more complex than that of other retroviruses. In addition to the structural *gag, pol,* and *env* genes, it also contains two regulatory genes, *tat* and *rev,* and four additional transcripts, *vif, vpr, vpu,* and *nef,* which encode accessory proteins critical for viral replication and pathogenesis.

In contrast to type C retroviruses like MoMLV the lentiviruses' replicative cycle is independent of cell division and dissolution of the nuclear envelope during cell mitosis. Lentivirus vectors are therefore potentially able to integrate into the genome of nondividing host cells. A number of gene transfer systems based on HIV-1, HIV-2, and nonprimate lentiviruses, such as equine infectious anemia virus (EIAV) and feline immunodeficiency virus (FIV), have been described (Naldini et al., 1996b; Reiser et al., 1996; Arya et al., 1998; Olsen, 1998; Poeschla et al., 1998a, 1998b; Uchida et al., 1998). Naldini et al. (1996a) first developed an HIV-1-based gene transfer system in which replication-defective viral particles were obtained by pseudotyping the HIV-1 core—that is, packaging it into the heterologous envelope of the Moloney leukemia virus or the VSV-G-protein. This strategy not only increased the safety of the system by excluding the HIV envelope but also broadened the tropism of the vectors to allow transduction of many cell types. Several groups have confirmed that lentiviral vectors can efficiently transduce nondividing cells in experimental conditions (Naldini et al., 1996a; Kafri et al., 1997; Miyoshi et al., 1997, 1999; Zufferey et al., 1997; Poeschla et al., 1998a, 1998b; Uchida et al., 1998; Case et al., 1999). Therefore, these vectors have the potential to become useful tools for gene therapy of diseases affecting tissues composed of quiescent or postmitotic cells, such neuronal and retinal cells, hepatocytes, myocytes, and lymphohematopoietic cells.

However, clinical applications await resolution of biosafety concerns, particularly in the case of vectors derived from HIV-1, a highly pathogenic human virus. Unwanted recombination events during vector production could generate replication-competent viruses. If this occurred, patients receiving gene therapy could be at risk for infection by an HIV-like virus. In addition, treated patients carrying integrated HIV sequences might subsequently come in contact with wild-type HIV, in which case recombination between virus sequences in vivo could mobilize the gene therapy vector, leading to spread of a new virus to additional patient cells or even to infection of individuals in contact with the patient. Already, the newer systems use nonoverlapping split-genome packaging constructs and self-inactivating vector cassettes to decrease these risks (Dull et al., 1998; Miyoshi et al., 1998; Zufferey et al., 1998).

Recent mapping studies of lentiviral vector integration sites seem to indicate, however, that these vectors may have less tendency to target dangerous transcription start sites than vectors based on MoMLV (Wu et al., 2003; Hematti et al., 2004), thus suggesting that these vectors may be less prone to induce insertional oncogenesis.

In addition to questions about safety, further discussion is warranted to identify suitable genetic diseases for initial gene therapy clinical trials using lentiviral vectors.

Foamy virus vectors

Foamy viruses (FV) are nonpathogenic retroviruses commonly found in mammals. In contrast to other retroviruses, reverse transcription in FV occurs during virion formation, and infectious viral particles therefore contain DNA genomes. This characteristic may improve transduction of quiescent cells, in which inefficient reverse transcription can prevent transduction by oncoviral or lentiviral vectors. This and other favorable characteristics, including broad tropism, large genome size (>13 kb), and lack of pathogenicity, have stimulated their development as gene transfer vectors. The FV genome contains the *gag, pol,* and *env* genes, but also three additional genes (*bel1, bel2, bel3*) located between *env* and the 3′ LTR and expressed from an internal viral promoter. The *bel1* gene encodes for Tas, a transcriptional transactivator of the FV LTR and internal promoter. In the absence of Tas, the FV LTR is silent. The function of the *bel2* and *bel3* genes is unknown. The FV Gag protein contains a functional nuclear localization signal, raising the possibility that nuclear entry of FV genomes is independent of mitosis (Rethwilm, 1995).

In the last 5 years, replication-defective FV vectors have been generated and perfected. The initial version of the vectors carried deletions that abolish *bel1* expression and contain expression cassettes (composed on an internal promoter and the gene of interest) within the two FV LTRs. More recent constructs have reduced the FV sequences to a minimum, making abundant space (>9 kb) for a transgene (Russell and Miller, 1996; Wu et al., 1998; Wu and Mergia, 1999; Park et al., 2002; Trobridge et al., 2002).Transient expression systems or packaging cells provide the structural and regulatory FV gene products and allow for production of complete, infectious viral particles (Russell and Miller, 1996; Wu and Mergia, 1999; Trobridge et al., 2002). The virions are stable, are not inactivated by human serum (Russell and Miller, 1996), and can be concentrated by ultracentrifugation to titers of ~10^7 (Trobridge et al., 2002).

FV vectors have been shown to efficiently enter quiescent cells where functional vector genomes survive until the cells are stimulated to divide, suggesting that, similar to HIV vectors, a stable intracellular transduction intermediate is formed (Russell and Miller, 1996; Mergia et al., 2001). This property may account for the ability of FV vectors to efficiently transduce hematopoietic cells, including murine and human pluripotent hematopoietic stem cells (Vassilopoulos et al., 2001; Josephson et al., 2002; Trobridge et al., 2002; Zucali et al., 2002). Such findings suggest that they will be useful for clinical gene transfer applications.

Vectors Based on Adeno-Associated Viruses

Adeno-associated viruses (AAV) integrate their DNA into the host cell genome and are not pathogenic for humans (Berns, 1995). These important characteristics have made them a very appealing

model for the development of gene transfer systems. AAV are a subfamily of single-stranded DNA parvoviruses that requires the presence of a coinfecting helper virus (from the adenovirus, herpes, or vaccinia virus families) to undergo a complete infectious cycle leading to virus replication and cellular lysis (Berns, 1995). In absence of a coinfecting helper virus, wild-type AAV undergo chromosomal integration (with a specific tendency to target human chromosome 19) and may persist in latent phase for extended periods of time (Cheung et al., 1980; Kotin et al., 1990).

The human AAV serotype 2 presents two major genes (*rep* and *cap*) flanked by viral inverted terminal repeats (ITRs). The *rep* gene is responsible for a series of critical steps of the AAV life cycle, including DNA replication and accumulation, while the *cap* gene products are necessary for AAV encapsidation. The ITR sequences have been shown to be essential for AAV chromosomal integration as well as for viral DNA replication and packaging (Srivastava et al., 1983).

Gene transfer vectors based on AAV are produced by deleting the *rep* and *cap* genes and replacing them with a transcriptional unit consisting of the promoter plus experimental gene of interest (Samulski et al., 1989). Complete recombinant AAV particles are then obtained by cotransfection of the plasmid containing the foreign gene with a helper plasmid providing the expression in *trans* of *rep* and *cap* genes onto cells infected with helper adenovirus. Being based on a transient expression method, the AAV packaging system can only provide a limited supply of viral vector. For this reason, stable AAV producer cell lines are under development (Flotte et al., 1995).

AAV vectors have been tested for a variety of gene transfer application, both in vitro and in vivo. Evidence emerging from these studies indicates that recombinant AAV vectors may either persist in an episomal stage or integrate in the host cell genome. In contrast to wild-type AAV infections, however, integration of AAV-based vectors seems to take place only at very high multiplicity of infection, and is not directed to chromosome 19 (Flotte et al., 1994; Halbert et al., 1995).

Even more limited than retroviral vectors, AAV constructs cannot accommodate more than 4.7 kb of foreign DNA in between the ITRs. The major advantages of AAV vectors for gene transfer are their nonpathogenic nature and their ability to transfer and express genes into nondividing cells (Podsakoff et al., 1994). However, AAV vector–mediated gene expression can be demonstrated in the absence of integration (Flotte et al., 1994), and the reliability of DNA insertion using these vectors in the absence of cell replication is not fully proven (Russell et al., 1994).

AAV vectors can infect hematopoietic tissues and have been tested in preclinical studies for the treatment of hemoglobinopathies (Walsh et al., 1992; Goodman et al., 1994; Miller et al., 1994). More recent data obtained using highly purified recombinant AAV stocks seem to indicate that these vectors can transduce primitive human hematopoietic cells efficiently, but only transiently. Clinical trials will be needed to determine the real potential of AAV-based gene transfer into human hematopoietic stem cells (Nathwani et al., 2000).

Results of Gene Therapy Trials for Immunodeficiencies

Adenosine Deaminase Deficiency

Genetic defects resulting in loss or severe reduction of ADA (MIM *608958, #102700; EC 3.5.4.4) result in extreme reduction of lymphocyte numbers and impairment of immune functions

(Hirschhorn, 1993; Markert, 1994) (see Chapter 12). Complete ADA deficiency causes SCID, or ADA-SCID.

In the mid-1980s, ADA deficiency was identified as the initial candidate disorder for trials of gene therapy because of a combination of favorable characteristics. The organization of the ADA gene and cDNA were well known, and ADA gene function and regulation had been defined (Orkin et al., 1983; Valerio et al., 1983; Wiginton et al., 1983). A wide array of enzyme concentrations ranging from 10% of normal to about 50 times the normal mean was known to be compatible with normal immunity (Valentine et al., 1977; Daddona et al., 1983). This situation provided an ideal scenario where the expression of the transferred gene was not required to be tissue-specific, nor tightly regulated. In addition, the experience from allogeneic bone marrow transplantation (BMT) experiments suggested that normal ADA expressing cells had a selective advantage over the ADA-deficient bone marrow progenitors, thus potentially eliminating the need for myeloablation preceding the infusion of the patient gene-corrected HSCs. Finally, the fact that some BMT patients achieving engraftment of only donor T cells were shown to have full reconstitution of lymphocyte functions provided the rationale for the correction and reinfusion of patient mature T lymphocytes as an alternative, and technically less complex, gene therapy approach than HSC gene transfer.

The first clinical gene therapy protocol for ADA deficiency was begun September 14, 1990, at the United States (U.S.) National Institutes of Health (NIH). It enrolled two ADA-deficient girls with persisting signs of immunodeficiency despite the institution and regular administration of polyethylene glycol-ADA (PEG-ADA) replacement therapy. This protocol involved apheresis of the patient's peripheral blood and culture of peripheral blood mononuclear cells with IL-2 and anti-CD3 antibody to stimulate intense proliferation of the small number of T lymphocytes from the patient's circulation. Once actively proliferating, cells were exposed to supernatants containing retroviral vectors carrying the human ADA cDNA, and expanded ~100-fold before being reinfused into the patient (Blaese, 1990). Over a 2-year period, both patients underwent a series of treatments with the intention to target, and thus correct, a large proportion of each patient's T cell repertoire. Both children improved or developed de novo several aspects of humoral and cellular immune function, including production of IgM in vitro upon stimulation of cultured cells with pokeweed mitogen (PWM), in vivo antibody responses to vaccines against *Hemophilus influenza B* (HIB) and tetanus toxoid, titers of isohemoagglutinin antibodies, T cell counts, cutaneous delayed-type hypersensitivity (DTH) to various antigens, T cell production of IL-2 after stimulation with tetanus toxoid and influenza A virus, and in vitro cytolytic T cell–specific activity against allogeneic cells and influenza A virus–infected autologous cells. All of these immune responses were absent or barely detectable before gene therapy (Blaese et al., 1995).

Ten years after the last cell infusion, ~20% of circulating T cells from the first patient still contained the ADA vector and expressed the transgene, whereas <0.1% of T cells from the second patient had detectable vector sequences. Both patients continue to receive weekly injections of PEG-ADA, although at a reduced dose. Even as the dose of PEG-ADA was lowered by ~50%–60%, numbers of peripheral blood CD3$^+$ T cells remained in the normal range for 7 years, but more recently showed signs of decline. Proliferative responses to mitogens and recall antigens have remained at the lower range for healthy controls in both patients.

The marked difference between the two patients in the achieved level of gene marking and ADA expression appears to be the result of several factors. In vitro proliferation of cells from the second patient was poor, limiting the transduction efficiency. In addition, this patient developed a persistent immune response against the retroviral envelope and the lipoprotein components of the fetal calf serum used to culture the cells, and these responses may have induced immune-mediated elimination of infused cells (Tuschong et al., 2002; Muul et al., 2003).

The long-term clinical benefit of this first gene therapy trial is difficult to evaluate because of the concomitant administration of PEG-ADA. Nevertheless, several unique pieces of information could be drawn from this study, including the apparent safety of administering genetically modified autologous T cells, the long persistence (>12 years) of such cells in vivo, and the long-term transgene expression that can be obtained in vivo by the Moloney retroviral promoter (Muul et al., 2003). In addition, the results of this trial point out that immune responses, even in immunodeficient patients, can confound the outcome of gene therapy experiments in unpredicted ways (Tuschong et al., 2002; Muul et al., 2003).

Following protocol and vector preparations identical to those used in the NIH trial, in August 1995, Dr. Sakiyama and colleagues from Hokkaido University School of Medicine, in Sapporo, treated a Japanese ADA-SCID patient with 11 infusions of genetically modified autologous T lymphocytes over a period of 20 months. Periodic analysis of peripheral blood lymphocytes showed transduction frequencies of 10%–20% (Egashira et al., 1998; Onodera et al., 1998), accompanied by gradual increases of ADA enzyme activity in the patient's circulating T cells to levels comparable to those of a heterozygous carrier. Evidence of improvement of the patient's immune function after gene therapy included increased T lymphocyte counts and DTH responses, appearance of isohemagglutinins, increase in serum immune globulin levels, and specific antibody production (Egashira et al., 1998; Onodera et al., 1998; Kawamura et al., 1999). Similar to the first patient in the NIH trial, follow-up studies demonstrated long-term persistence of transduced, polyclonal T cells (Misaki et al., 2001).

A second gene therapy clinical trial for ADA deficiency was begun in 1992 in Milan, Italy. Bordignon and coworkers used two distinguishable forms of the same retroviral vector to transduce separately the lymphocytes and bone marrow cells from two ADA-deficient patients who had shown a progressive decline of efficacy of PEG-ADA therapy. This study involved the in vitro culture, retroviral transduction, and reinfusion of patients' lymphocytes and bone marrow cells in an attempt to define the specific contribution of gene-corrected mature T lymphocytes and bone marrow progenitors to long-term immune reconstitution (Bordignon et al., 1993). The two patients were treated with intravenous infusions of autologous transduced cells over a period of 9 to 24 months, during which PEG-ADA dosage was decreased. Normalization of lymphocyte counts and isohemoagglutinins titers, restoration antigen-specific antibody production, and mitogen- and antigen-specific T cell proliferation were observed in both patients. At the molecular level, both forms of the integrated provirus were individually detectable in the patients' peripheral lymphocytes, with the clear long-term predominance of the construct used to transduce bone marrow cells. Of particular interest, vector-derived ADA activity was detectable in bone marrow cells, peripheral lymphocytes, and also mature granulocytes and erythrocytes, indicating that the correction of bone marrow progenitors was stably transferred to their progeny of multiple lineages (Bordignon et al., 1995).

Similar to the U.S. previous study, the clinical impact of gene therapy in these patients was difficult to assess because of concomitant administration of PEG-ADA, which, on the one hand, might have contributed to the immunological improvement but, on the other, may also have abolished any selective advantage of genetically engineered cells over the defective cell populations in ADA-deficient patients. One of the patients treated in Italy with multiple infusions of transduced peripheral blood lymphocytes offered the opportunity to evaluate the latter hypothesis directly when complications attributed to the PEG-ADA treatment developed that justified the discontinuation of the enzyme injections. Withdrawal of PEG-ADA led to a selective growth advantage of gene-transduced, ADA-expressing circulating T lymphocytes that, from a prevalence of ~3%, eventually reached nearly 100%. Absolute CD3[+] T cell counts also rose to levels significantly higher than those observed during PEG-ADA treatment, and intracellular ADA activity increased to levels of approximately 50% of that of normal individuals. These findings were accompanied by full restoration of T cell function that had been inadequate during PEG-ADA treatment. The increase of lymphocyte ADA activity, however, was not sufficient to achieve systemic detoxification; red blood cell deoxyribonucleotides (dAXP) increased to levels substantially higher than those observed in ADA-deficient patients treated with HSCT (Aiuti et al., 2002b). These findings suggest that even high numbers of genetically corrected lymphocytes were insufficient for achieving full, lasting metabolic correction of ADA deficiency and justified additional attempts by the same investigators at correcting the HSC as a more efficacious approach for gene therapy of this disease.

Recently, these efforts have resulted in the first clear evidence that gene therapy following a low-intensity conditioning regimen can result in clinical benefit for ADA deficiency when administered in the absence of PEG-ADA treatment. Reasoning that an initial developmental advantage was important for the transduced HSC, the Italian investigators decided to create space in the bone marrow by administering a low dose of busulfan (2 mg/kg per day for 2 days before infusion of gene-corrected cells) to four ADA-deficient patients before the infusion of gene-corrected cells. The degree of myelosuppression was mild in patients 2 and 4, but resulted in short-term neutropenia and more prolonged thrombocytopenia and neutropenia in patients 1 and 3, respectively. All patients showed an increase in peripheral blood lymphocyte counts that reached normal values in patients 1 and 3. Development of gene-corrected T, B, and natural killer (NK) cells and restoration of in vitro proliferative responses to mitogens and antigens was observed in all patients, as was improvement of serum immunoglobulin levels and production of specific antibodies following vaccination. Moreover, the biochemical abnormalities characteristic of ADA-deficient patients (low intracellular ADA activity and accumulation of toxic adenosine metabolites) were corrected. The presence of the retroviral ADA gene in myeloid cells (megakaryocytes, erythroid cells, and granulocytes) ranged between 0.1% and 10% and correlated with the dose of infused gene-corrected CD34[+] cells and the patient's response to the myelosuppressive agent. All patients were well, at home more than a year after treatment (Aiuti et al., 2002a). Because in addition to receiving chemotherapy these patients also were not given PEG-ADA, it remained to be established what circumstance had an impact on the outcome of the procedure.

The very exciting, successful results described above marked a clear difference from those obtained from previous clinical gene transfer attempts into the HSC of ADA-deficient patients that were carried out in the mid 1990s in the U.S. and Europe with neither chemotherapy nor withholding of PEG-ADA. One of these trials had been initiated by Kohn and collaborators in 1993 at the Childrens Hospital Los Angeles. Notably, this was the first gene therapy protocol using umbilical cord blood CD34[+] hematopoietic progenitors, a cell source very rich in HSC. Three newborns were enrolled in this protocol, which involved separation of CD34[+] progenitors from the cord blood immediately after birth, repeated retroviral transductions with the normal ADA cDNA, and intravenous infusions into the patients on their fourth day of life. PEG-ADA treatment was also instituted and maintained in all three patients. Patients' peripheral and bone marrow hemopoietic cell populations were analyzed over time to determine the efficacy of the engraftment of ADA-transduced CD34[+] progenitors and their contribution to the patients' hematopoiesis. Serial molecular studies demonstrated that integrated vector sequences were detectable in bone marrow–derived CD34[+] cells, granulocyte-macrophage colony forming units (CFU-GM), and both the mononuclear and polymorphonuclear mature leukocyte populations of all three infants (Kohn et al., 1995).

Four years after the infusion of gene-corrected cells, 1%–10% of circulating T lymphocytes contained the transduced gene, whereas only 0.01%–0.1% of other hematopoietic elements were vector positive. After PEG-ADA treatment was stopped in the patient carrying the highest percentage of gene-corrected T lymphocytes (~10%), the proliferative response to tetanus toxoid was lost, as were most of the circulating B and NK cells. Reduction of total numbers of CD3[+] and CD4[+] T lymphocytes was also observed; however the percentage of circulating T cells containing the transduced ADA gene increased to 30%–100% and lymphocyte proliferation response to phytohemagglutin (PHA) was retained. These findings and the development of an upper respiratory tract infection induced the investigators to reinstate PEG-ADA therapy, leading to restoration of clinical and laboratory findings to pre-withdrawal levels. The low levels of ADA gene marking and expression did not justify the suspension of PEG-ADA treatment in the other patients (Kohn et al., 1998).

These observations supported the notion that ADA gene-corrected T cells have a selective survival advantage over unmodified lymphocytes. However, the trial also demonstrated that the level of transduced progenitors (particularly for B and NK cells) was not sufficiently high to guarantee sustained, adequate immune function in the absence of enzyme replacement. A possible contributing reason for these findings was that the expression of ADA afforded by the LASN vector in HSCs was not adequate to allow differentiation and function of large numbers of mature lymphocytes. Based on this last hypothesis a two-site trial using ADA vectors with higher expression capabilities was started in 2001 at Children Hospital Los Angeles and the NIH with the aim of comparing the relative efficacy of two different vectors in vivo after transduction in bone marrow CD34[+] cells. In this trial, patients were maintained on PEG-ADA treatment. The initial results of this trial indicate that long-term marking was achieved in two of four treated patients. However, the level of marking was low, and the patients did not show immunological improvement (Candotti et al., 2003).

An additional French and British pilot trial of gene therapy for ADA deficiency in 1993 involved retroviral transduction of HSCs isolated from bone marrow (Hoogerbrugge et al., 1996). Three ADA-deficient children were enrolled. The results were disappointing because vector-containing cells were detectable by polymerase chain reaction (PCR) 6 months after the treatment in the bone marrow of only one patient, and no signal was detected in the peripheral blood of any of the three children. No clinical improvement was observed in these patients. On the basis of their preclinical results in the *Rhesus* model, the authors theorized a need for preemptive myeloablation to obtain efficient engraftment of gene-corrected stem cells in ADA deficiency. Interestingly, the recent results from Italy described above (Aiuti et al., 2002a) are in line with this hypothesis.

In summary, while BMT from an HLA-identical sibling remains the therapy of choice for ADA deficiency, the results obtained by the pioneer and current clinical trials indicate that gene therapy approaches can be effective and to date maintain a record of safety. At present, however, it is not clear whether the selective advantage of gene-corrected cells is sufficient to provide immune reconstitution in the absence of preparative chemotherapy. A clinical trial in Japan enrolled two patients in 2003 to receive gene-corrected CD34$^+$ bone marrow cells after discontinuation of PEG-ADA, but without chemotherapy. This trial will likely provide insights into the relative importantce of chemotherapy and PEG-ADA withdrawal (Otsu et al., 2005). This and other ongoing efforts are expected to advance gene therapy for ADA deficiency to phase II and III trials to obtain definitive conclusions as to the efficacy of this therapy.

Chronic Granulomatous Disease

Genetic defects involving both gp91^{phox} and p22^{phox}, as well as in p47^{phox} and p67^{phox} have been identified in chronic granulomatous disease (CGD) patients who, because of impaired superoxide production in phagocytic cells, usually present early in life with abscesses and/or granulomas in the skin, liver, lungs, or bone resulting from catalase-positive bacteria and fungal pathogens (see Chapter 37). Current management of CGD patients includes antibiotic prophylaxis, administration of interferon-γ (IFN-γ), and allogeneic HSC transplantation (Lekstrom-Himes and Gallin, 2000). For several patients, however, available therapeutic options remain unsatisfactory. Cloning of the genes encoding all the elements of the NAPDH oxidase system (Forehand and Johnston, 1994; Roos, 1994) has allowed gene therapy strategies to be developed.

Several groups have demonstrated the feasibility of viral vector gene transfer in reconstituting the respiratory burst activity of B cell lines and monocytes from CGD patients (Thrasher et al., 1992, 1995a, 1995b; Sekhsaria et al., 1993; Li et al., 1994). The ultimate target for gene correction of CGD, however, is the HSC because of the very limited life span and the reduced proliferative state of mature phagocytes.

In vitro preclinical studies have demonstrated that CD34$^+$ hematopoietic progenitors derived from peripheral blood after G-CSF mobilization and genetically corrected by retroviral-mediated gene transfer showed restoration of superoxide production when induced to differentiate into mature monocytes and neutrophils (Sekhsaria et al., 1993; Li et al., 1994; Porter et al., 1996; Weil et al., 1997; Becker et al., 1998). In addition, in vivo restoration of respiratory burst in p47^{phox} and gp91^{phox} knockout mice has been demonstrated, following gene correction of bone marrow cells with retroviral vectors (Bjorgvinsdottir et al., 1997; Mardiney et al., 1997). On the basis of these encouraging results, Malech and coworkers at the NIH initiated a phase I clinical study for gene therapy of the autosomal recessive form of CGD due to defective expression of the NAPDH complex p47^{phox} subunit. Five CGD patients were subjected to pharmacological mobilization of CD34$^+$ hematopoietic progenitors that were then collected from the peripheral blood by apheresis. Enriched CD34$^+$ cells were transduced in vitro using a retroviral

vector expressing cDNA encoding p47^{phox}. The transduced cells were then reinfused into the patients. Appearance of NAPDH oxidase activity in PMA-stimulated peripheral blood granulocytes was followed in each subject over time. At variable intervals between 15 and 32 days after infusion of transduced progenitors, all patients showed oxidase-positive granulocytes, with maximum percentages ranging between 0.004% and 0.05%. Presence of the transduced gene in the DNA of peripheral blood lymphocytes was confirmed by PCR. Oxydase-positive cells were detected for a minimum of 79 and a maximum of 172 days (Malech et al., 1996). Although silencing of the transduced gene has not been excluded, these findings are most consistent with loss of the transduced cells and with the possibility that lineage-committed progenitors, rather than true self-renewing HSC, were the primary transduction target in this study.

More recently, the same research group has conducted a second clinical trial aimed at correction of the more common X-linked form of CGD (X-CGD), caused by mutation of the gp91^{phox} subunit of NAPDH oxidase. Using a high-titer retroviral vector and improved transduction procedures, three X-CGD patients each received two infusions of gp91^{phox}-transduced CD34$^+$ cells. Preliminary results indicated that levels of NAPDH-positive neutrophils were markedly higher than those observed in the previous trial and ranged from 0.2% to 0.06% at 3–4 weeks after treatment (Malech et al., 1998).

Similar results were obtained by Dinauer et al. in another phase I trial for X-CGD at the University of Indiana Medical School, although the results observed at this center have not been formally reported yet.

The results of these phase I clinical gene transfer studies for CGD suggest the following considerations. Because of the lack of a strong selective advantage of gene-corrected populations in this disease, significant levels of HSC transduction and engraftment or conditioning chemotherapy will likely be needed to obtain clinical benefit. More efficient methods of gene transfer are being developed based on lentiviral vectors (Saulnier et al., 2000; Roesler et al., 2002). Alternatively, in vivo selection of gene-corrected cells could be engineered by the addition of drug resistance markers such as the multidrug resistance (MDR) or dihydrofolate reductase (DHFR) genes to gene transfer vectors. Studies of these approaches in animal models are ongoing and are likely to provide clear indication on the prospects of future success of gene therapy for CGD.

Marrow conditioning prior to reinfusion of transduced cells is being evaluated by several groups in the U.S., England, and Germany to help achieve higher levels of engraftment of corrected stem/progenitor cells. In January 2004, a new trial in Germany by Grez and collaborators used a retroviral vector to target G-CSF-mobilized CD34$^+$ progenitor cells of two patients with X-linked CGD. Before infusion of gene-corrected cells, patients were given intravenous busulfan (4 mg/kg for 2 consecutive days), which resulted in transitory myelodepression from which patients recovered by day 30 after treatment. Preliminary results of a 6-month follow-up have shown significant levels of gene marking and therapeutic levels of NAPDH oxydase activity (Ott et al., 2004). These results are encouraging, although long-term evaluation is needed to support definitive efficacy and safety of this approach.

Leukocyte Adhesion Deficiency Type 1

Leukocyte adhesion deficiency type 1 (LAD1) is an inherited defect of leukocyte functions caused by absence or reduced levels of expression of the common β$_2$-integrin subunit (CD18) (Harlan,

1993). In LAD1 granulocytes fail to migrate into inflamed tissues to exert their phagocytic functions. Affected patients initially present retarded separation of the umbilical cord and subsequently develop recurrent severe bacterial and fungal infections (Fischer et al., 1988; Etzioni, 1994) (see Chapter 38). Allogeneic BMT from an HLA-matched related donor has been curative for this disease. The insertion of normal cDNA into the HSC of a patient may therefore lead to correction of this disease phenotype, and studies using viral vectors have demonstrated in vitro functional reconstitution of CD18 molecules in transduced LAD1 lymphocytes (Hibbs et al., 1990; Wilson et al., 1990; Bauer et al., 1995).

The expression of CD18 is limited to myeloid cells and lymphocytes; however, functional adhesion complexes require dimerization of CD18 molecules with other subunits (CD11a, CD11b, or CD11c) also expressed only by the same cell types. Expression of CD18 in other lineages derived from gene-corrected HSCs and not normally expressing CD18 should therefore not result in unregulated and unwanted expression of complete adhesion complexes.

Similarly to CGD, because of the short life span of myeloid cells, the target for corrective gene transfer of LAD1 is necessarily the HSC. Retroviral vectors have been used to reconstitute CD18 expression in granulocytes that differentiate in vitro from gene-corrected CD34+ cells (Bauer et al., 1998; Yorifuji et al., 1993). Following these studies, a clinical protocol for gene therapy of LAD1 at the University of Washington in Seattle used retroviral-mediated correction of G-CSF-mobilized peripheral blood CD34+ cells in two LAD1 patients (Bauer and Hickstein, 2000). Peripheral blood CD34+ cells were obtained after mobilization with G-CSF and exposed to a retroviral vector expressing CD18 before being reinfused into the patients. One month after the infusion of transduced CD34+ cells, both patients showed low percentages (0.03%–0.04%) of CD18+ myeloid cells, and in one patient there was some evidence of functional correction, as CD18+ myeloid cells were demonstrated to migrate into a site of inflammation. Unfortunately, gene-corrected cells were not detectable beyond 2 months after treatment (Bauer and Hickstein, 2000).

Allogeneic HSC transplantation studies in a canine model of LAD1 have shown that very low levels of donor CD18+ neutrophils (<500/μl) were sufficient to reverse the disease phenotype (Bauer et al., 2004). However, no selective survival advantage of gene-corrected myeloid cells is expected in LAD1. As with CGD, strategies involving preparative myeloablation, engineered vectors to confer in vivo selection, and the use of more efficient vectors will likely be required to improve the outcome of future gene therapy trials for LAD1.

X-linked Severe Combined Immunodeficiency

The X-linked recessive form of severe combined immunodeficiency (XSCID) is caused by mutations of the common γ chain (γc) of the receptors for IL-2, IL-4, IL-7, IL-9, IL-15, and IL-21 (Noguchi et al., 1993; Puck et al., 1993). Affected males present combined impairment of T and B cell immunity, despite the presence of B cells in normal or even elevated numbers (see Chapter 9). Allogeneic BMT can be curative for these patients, and it generally shows good success in terms of survival (Antoine et al., 2003; Buckley, 2004) (see Chapter 47). However, especially in the case haploidentical donors, transplanted patients often achieve only partial chimerism of hematopoietic lineages with persistence of autologous B lymphocytes and poor humoral immune function that requires continuous replacement therapy

with immunoglobulins (Antoine et al., 2003). Such unsatisfactory results have prompted the development of gene therapy approaches for XSCID.

In preclinical studies, several groups of investigators have shown that retroviral-mediated transfer of γc into B lymphoblastoid cell lines derived from XSCID patients could correct a series of cellular defects, including γc membrane expression, IL-2 high affinity binding and internalization, ligand binding-mediated phosphorylation of JAK3 and JAK1 tyrosine kinases, and IL-2-induced cell proliferation (Candotti et al., 1996; Hacein-Bey et al., 1996; Taylor et al., 1996b). More importantly, normal development of mature T lymphocytes and NK cells could be demonstrated from gene-corrected XSCID stem cells in vitro (Hacein-Bey et al., 1998; Cavazzana-Calvo et al., 1996; Tsai et al.,). In addition, in vivo experiments in mouse models of XSCID have shown safety and efficacy of γc gene transfer in bone marrow stem cells with reconstitution of lymphoid development and function in these animals (Lo et al., 1999; Otsu et al., 2000, 2001; Soudais et al., 2000; Aviles Mendoza et al., 2001).

These results formed the basis for the first clinical gene transfer protocol for XSCID that was launched in 1999 in Paris, France. This trial involved retroviral γc gene transfer into CD34+ bone marrow cells harvested from XSCID patients who lacked HLA-identical bone marrow donors and has enrolled 11 patients to date. The results observed in typical XSCID patients have shown that as soon as 60–90 days after the infusion of gene-corrected cells, T lymphocytes expressing γc appeared in the circulation and reached normal values within 4 to 8 months in eight patients (Cavazzana-Calvo et al., 2000; Hacein-Bey-Abina et al., 2002, 2003b). Most importantly, these T lymphocytes were polyclonal and functionally competent as demonstrated by normal responses to stimulation with mitogens and specific antigens. In contrast to the T lymphocytes, the NK cell counts declined to values lower than normal after an initial significant rise during which restoration of NK cell function could be demonstrated. In addition, despite the fact that less than 1% of the patients' B cells carried the γc transgene, close to normal serum levels of IgM and IgG were demonstrated in three patients who developed specific antibody responses to tetanus and diphtheria toxins, as well to as poliovirus vaccines. Not surprisingly, based on the predicted lack of selective advantage in myeloid lineages, only 0.01%–1% of the patients' monocytes and granulocytes showed evidence of genetic correction (Sun et al., 1997; Cavazzana-Calvo et al., 2001; Hacein-Bey-Abina et al., 2002).

The first series of 5 patients clearly demonstrated that γc gene transfer can restore the immune system in XSCID patients (Hacein-Bey-Abina et al., 2002). Although the restoration was incomplete with regard to the numbers of gene-corrected B and NK cells, the effects of the treatment were sufficient to provide protective immunity and to allow the patients to return home and lead a normal life. Similar results were obtained in 5 out of 6 additional patients enrolled in the trial. The failure of the treatment in 2 of the total 11 patients treated in Paris was attributed to the specific clinical conditions of these two patients, who had chronic infections that may have affected the engraftment of gene-corrected cells (Hacein-Bey-Abina et al., 2002). In addition, one of these two patients was an atypical patient of 15 years of age at the time of treatment, raising the possibility that loss of thymic function may have contributed to the failure of the procedure in this case.

Late in 2002, two patients who had been treated with gene therapy about 3 years earlier presented with uncontrolled clonal proliferation of mature (TCRγδ⁺ or TCRαβ⁺) T lymphocytes. The malignant behavior of such proliferation required conventional treatment for T-cell acute lymphoblastic leukemia to be administered that in one case was followed by matched unrelated bone marrow transplantation.

In both cases, the adverse event was the result of insertional oncogenesis due to the aberrant expression of the *LMO2* gene (LIM domain only-2; OMIM 180385) induced by the integration of the γ_c retroviral vector in the proximity of the *LMO2* regulatory region (Hacein-Bey-Abina et al., 2003a, 2003b). LMO2 is a cysteine-rich proetin required for normal hematopoiesis. LMO2 is activated in childhood acute T cell leukemias by chromosomal translocation and its deregulated expression in transgenic mice promotes high incidence of T cell tumors (Larson et al., 1994). Although our understanding of the mechanism underlying the development of LMO2-mediated lymphoproliferation remains incomplete, it appears plausible that the enhancer activity of the retroviral vector promoter was responsible for the activation of the LMO2 promoter and consequent deregulated *LMO2* gene expression. Vigorous cell proliferation of LMO2-expressing cells due to the selective advantage conferred to them by the concomitant expression of the γ_c gene may have provided a "second hit" needed for the onset of the overt malignancy.

Whether the leukemic transformation observed in these patients can be therefore attributed to a specific cooperation between γ_c and LMO2 in the context of a strong selective advantage conferred by the genetic correction remains to be established, but it is obviously of critical importance, as it could change the assessment of the risk that similar events may occur after retroviral-mediated gene transfer into HSC for other diseases. It is worth noting that the patients who developed LMO2-associated T cell leukemias were the youngest enrolled in the trial and had received the highest numbers of gene-corrected cells/kg body weight (Hacein-Bey-Abina et al., 2003a, 2003b). Specific biological characteristics of hematopoietic stem cells obtained at a very young age may be conducive to insertional mutagenesis through mechanisms that are still unknown. These serious adverse events have had major repercussions on the field of gene therapy. It is clear that a complete reassessment of the risks of gene therapy for XSCID and of the validity of previous safety studies in animal models is warranted to provide an understanding of how to proceed with an approach that has provided clear clinical benefit, but also unintended severe complications.

Despite aggressive therapy, one of the two patients who developed lymphoproliferation died, while the other remains in continuous remission >2 years after the diagnosis of leukemia and treatment with conventional chemotherapy. In January 2005, a third case of uncontrolled T cell proliferation was observed. Characterization of this last case is under way at this writing (http://afssaps.sante.fr/htm/10/filcoprs/indco.htm).

In July 2001, a second gene therapy trial for XSCID was started by Thrasher et al. at the Great Ormond Street Hospital in London. The protocol design was similar to the French trial with the exception of culture conditions (lower concentration of IL-3 and use of serum-free medium) and the use of a vector pseudotyped with a gibbon-ape-leukaemiavirus (GALV) envelope. Data published on the first 4 enrolled children, 4 to 33 months of age at treatment, indicated that all patients showed substantial clinical improvements and immunological reconstitution. The latter included recovery of T cell numbers (up to normal in 2 of 4 patients), normal T cell–proliferative responses, and a polyclonal TcR Vβ repertoire. Improvement of humoral immunity was also observed that allowed discontinuation of prophylactic immunoglobulin replacement treatment in 2 patients. With a follow-up of 2 to 4 years, none of the patients has manifested serious adverse events (Gaspar et al., 2004). Altogether, these data confirm the successful correction of immunity obtained in the French trial and corroborate the notion that gene therapy can be curative for XSCID.

One additional trial was begun at the NIH in 2003 with the aim of offering a rescue treatment option for older XSCID patients who had failed previous haploidentical BMT treatment. In this trial, the target cells were G-CSF-mobilized peripheral blood CD34⁺ cells. Three patients have been enrolled and preliminary results on the first subject (11 years old) were published in abstract form (Chinen et al., 2004). Administration of gene-corrected cells was followed by amelioration of clinical features, including resolution of chronic diarrhea, rashes, and alopecia, although no increase in T cell numbers was observed. Gene marking could be detected in T and B lymphocytes as well as NK cells at 6 months after treatment (Chinen et al., 2004). Additional follow-up will determine the potential of this strategy and provide important information on the prospects of gene therapy in older X-SCID patients in whom reduced thymopoiesis may pose an obstacle to the success of the procedure.

JAK3 Deficiency

The JAK3 member of the Janus family of protein tyrosine kinases is a lymphoid tissue-specific tyrosine kinase (Kawamura et al., 1994) involved in the signal transduction pathway of several cytokines, including IL-2, IL-4, IL-7, IL-9, IL-15, and IL-21 (Johnston et al., 1995; Asao et al., 2001; Habib et al., 2002). Patients with mutations of JAK3 usually present with autosomal recessive SCID (Macchi et al., 1995; Russell et al., 1995; Candotti et al., 1997; Notarangelo et al., 2001) with clinical characteristics virtually identical to those presented by XSCID patients, except that JAK3 deficiency is found in both male and female patients (see Chapter 10).

Because of the clear similarities between the effects of γ_c and JAK3 genetic defects, the theoretical possibilities for gene therapy are analogous. Retrovirally mediated gene correction has reconstituted IL-2 and IL-4 responses in JAK3-deficient cell lines (Candotti et al., 1996; Oakes et al., 1996), leading to the hypothesis that the gene correction of HSC may be a useful therapy for JAK3-deficient patients. Preclinical in vivo studies have demonstrated the feasibility of retroviral-mediated gene correction of JAK3 deficiency in murine models using irradiated adult recipients and nonirradiated newborn animals (Bunting et al., 1998, 1999, 2000). Of note, an in vivo selective advantage of transduced cells over untransduced JAK3-deficient counterparts was demonstrated for lymphoid lineages, a finding suggesting that similar treatment procedures as those used in the gene therapy trial for XSCID could lead to successful results in JAK3 deficiency. On the basis of these results, Sorrentino et al. at the St. Jude Children's Research Hospital in Memphis attempted the genetic correction of bone marrow CD34⁺ cells of a JAK3-deficient patient who had failed HSCT. Infusion of retrovirally transduced cells was attempted twice in this patient, but resulted in only low levels of marking without improvement in immunological status. The reasons for unsatisfactory outcome are not clear, and it is hoped that further investigations in this and additional patients will clarify prospects for gene therapy for JAK3 SCID.

Preclinical Experiments of Gene Therapy for Other Immunodeficiencies

Purine Nucleoside Phosphorylase Deficiency

In most cases, the immunologic disorder associated with genetic deficit of purine nucleoside phosphorylase (PNP; EC 2.4.2.1) is restricted to the T cell compartment, whereas B cell functions are generally normal (see Chapter 12). Enzyme replacement therapy, by means of irradiated red blood cells transfusions (Rich et al., 1980), has not been definitively proven beneficial for PNP deficiency, and allogeneic HLA-matched HSCT is the current therapy of choice, although reports indicating its success in patients with PNP deficiency are limited.

The lack of PNP activity leads to the block of the same purine salvage pathway that is affected by the genetic deficit of ADA. Since the biochemical defects of ADA and PNP deficiency are similar, the prospect for successful gene therapy of PNP deficiency also seems likely.

In preclinical studies using retroviral-mediated gene transfer, in vitro reconstitution of PNP activity in T lymphocytes derived from PNP-deficient subjects has been described (Nelson et al., 1995). These results suggested that T cells could potentially be used as vehicles for therapeutic PNP gene expression, and a clinical protocol testing this hypothesis has been proposed. Contrary to ADA-SCID, no enzyme replacement treatment is available for this disease. PNP-deficient patients are usually lymphopenic and, for this reason, the possibility remains that PNP-deficient patients will not have a sufficiently developed peripheral T cell repertoire to achieve meaningful immune reconstitution with T lymphocyte–directed gene therapy. The correction of the gene defect at the level of HSC seems a better strategy.

ZAP-70 Deficiency

Mutations affecting the expression of ZAP-70 protein tyrosine kinase are a rare cause of autosomal recessive SCID characterized by absence of mature circulating $CD8^+$ T lymphocytes and T cell antigen receptor (TCR) signal transduction defects in peripheral $CD4^+$ T cells (Arpaia et al., 1994; Chan et al., 1994; Elder et al., 1994) (see Chapter 14). Since ZAP-70-deficient patients have been successfully treated by allogeneic HSCT, this disease is another candidate for stem cell gene correction. The presence of circulating T lymphocytes in these patients has allowed the establishment of HTLV-1-transformed T cell lines that have been used as targets for corrective gene transfer to study the feasibility of a gene therapy approach for this disease. Upon retroviral-mediated gene transduction of the normal ZAP-70 cDNA into T cells from a ZAP-deficient patient, ZAP-70 kinase was expressed that was appropriately tyrosine phosphorylated upon TCR engagement. More importantly, reconstitution of in vitro kinase activity of the transduced ZAP-70 and normalization of calcium mobilization after TCR stimulation in gene-corrected cells was demonstrated (Taylor et al., 1996a). More recently, Steinberg and coworkers transferred the ZAP-70 cDNA into primary T lymphocytes from ZAP-70 deficient patients. Upon gene correction, several biological functions were restored in these T cells, including TCR signaling, Ras-mitogen-activated proten kinase (MAPK) activation, and IL-2 secretion. In addition and importantly, selective growth advantage of gene corrected cells was observed after in vitro culture of transduced cells (Steinberg et al., 2000), suggesting that the genetic correction of few HSCs and/or lymphoid progenitor cells may generate significant num-

bers of corrected T lymphocytes and restoration of T cell immunodeficiency.

Because of the normally restricted expression of the ZAP-70 protein to specific lymphoid lineages, evaluation of potential deleterious effects of the ectopic expression of ZAP-70 in cell types normally not expressing this protein is a concern. However, gene correction of bone marrow cells of ZAP knockout mice using a retroviral vector expressing the human ZAP-70 gene resulted in the development of mature, polyclonal, and functional T lymphocytes, while expression of the retroviral transgene in B cells did not affect their function (Otsu et al., 2002). Altogether, these data indicate that retroviral-mediated transfer of the ZAP-70 gene may prove to have a therapeutic benefit for patients with ZAP-70 deficiency.

Major Histocompatibility Complex Class II Deficiency

Deficit of expression of MHC class II molecules can be caused by defects of any of four different MHC class II–specific transcription factors—CIITA, RFX5, RFXAP, and RFXANK. MHC class II deficiency is characterized by severe immunodeficiency with low numbers of $CD4^+$ lymphocytes (see Chapter 17). Allogeneic HSCT is potentially curative, but its success rate is very low (Huss et al., 1995; Klein et al., 1995). Alternative forms of therapy are therefore needed, and HSC-directed gene therapy could be beneficial for these patients. Exploring this possibility, Bradley et al. (1997) showed that retrovirus-mediated gene transfer of the CIITA factor could restore expression of MHC class II in B lymphoblastoid lines and peripheral blood cells from an MHC class II–deficient patient. Recently, lentiviral vectors that may prove useful for future gene therapy applications have been described that express each of the four MHC class II–specific transcription factors (Matheux et al., 2002). A cautionary note, however, comes from reports indicating that ectopic expression of MHC class II genes can result in pathological hyperactivity of $CD4^+$ lymphocytes (Bottazzo et al., 1986). Since expression of MHC class II molecules is regulated in such cell types as T lymphocytes, fibroblasts, and endothelial cells, it will be important to determine if tissue-specific expression of the therapeutic gene will be needed for clinical gene therapy.

Immunodeficiency with Hyper-IgM

The X-linked hyper-IgM syndrome (XHIM) is another rare PID caused by genetic mutations in the CD40 ligand molecule (CD40L) expressed on activated $CD4^+$ T lymphocytes (see Chapter 19). XHIM patients lack functional CD40L on their T cells and have profound impairment of T cell–B cell interactions. A detailed follow-up of XHIM patients has made it clear that the immunoglobulin substitution used as treatment does not provide an adequate long-term solution to the severe infectious episodes suffered by these boys. Allogeneic HSCT is therefore now considered definitive treatment for this disease, and XHIM is also a potential candidate for gene therapy.

Unfortunately, however, CD40L expression is highly regulated, with expression restricted to activated $CD4^+$ lymphocytes, thus introducing the need for regulated gene transfer systems. The necessity of strictly regulating the CD40L expression in gene-corrected cells was stressed by Brown et al., who performed transplantation of retrovirally gene-corrected bone marrow or thymic cells into CD40L knockout mice. Humoral and cellular immune responses to influenza virus were partially or fully restored by this treatment; however, more than 60% of the treated mice developed lymphoproliferative disease in the form of prelymphoma of T-lymphoblastic lymphoma. T cell proliferation was most likely due to enhanced positive selection driven by the costitutive expression of CD40L on developing thymocytes (Brown et al., 1998). Gene transfer systems allowing effective regulation of CD40L will therefore have to be developed before gene correction can be proposed for the treatment of humans with XHIGM. One such approach by Tahara et al. aimed at preserving physiological regulation of CD40L by using spliceosome-mediated RNA *trans*-splicing. Bone marrow from CD40L knockout mice was transduced with a lentiviral vector encoding a pre–*trans*-splicing molecule containing wild-type CD40L exons 2–5 and transplanted into lethally irradiated recipient animals. Corrected CD40L mRNA, regulated CD40L expression in CD4+ T cells, antigen-specific IgG1 responses, and attenuation of *Pneumocystis carinii* pneumonia were observed in treated mice in the absence of lymphoproliferative complications (Tahara et al., 2004). Although this strategy seems promising, further studies are needed to establish whether the efficacy of RNA *trans*-splicing will be adequate to correct the human phenotype.

Soluble CD40L is available and could represent an alternative form of therapy for XHIGM. If proven beneficial, administration of autologous cells or "pseudo-organs" engineered to produce CD40L that are easily removable could become a more controllable option.

X-Linked Agammaglobulinemia

Bruton's disease, or X-linked agammaglobulinemia (XLA), is a genetic disorder of B lymphocyte differentiation that results in the absence of mature circulating B cells and undetectable serum immune globulins of all isotypes (Conley et al., 1994; Smith et al., 1994) (see Chapter 21). The molecular defect of XLA has been identified in mutations the gene encoding Bruton's tyrosine kinase (*BTK*) (Tsukada et al., 1993; Vetrie et al., 1993), normally expressed by developing B and myeloid cells, but not plasma cells or T cells. The current management of XLA is to administer immunoglobulin, which is generally efficacious in preventing infections. This treatment, however, is expensive, inconvenient, and, in some cases, insufficient to avoid lethal infections.

XLA patients therefore could benefit from development of gene therapy. The generation of retroviral vectors expressing *BTK* has been attempted since the mid-1990s, but several laboratories failed to produce high-titer retroviral-producing cell lines. These difficulties were explained by the demonstration that expression of *BTK* can mediate apoptosis (Islam et al., 2000). Thus high levels of *BTK* expression in target cells may induce toxic effects, and vector selection could be critical for the development of successful gene therapy for XLA. Progress in vector design and production has made possible preclinical experiments of genetic correction in the X-linked immunodeficiency (Xid) mouse, in which *btk* is mutated. Preliminary results show that gene transfer into *Xid* bone marrow cells can reconstitute B cell development and production of IgM and IgG3 antibodies (Conley et al., 2000; Yu et al., 2000). In addition, BTK-expressing B cell progenitors were found to have a selective advantage over BTK-negative progenitors (Rohrer and Conley, 1999). Mice deficient in both Btk and the related kinase Tec have been corrected by retroviral-mediated gene therapy with a human *BTK* vector (Yu et al., 2004). Treated mice showed restoration of both primary and peripheral B-lineage development, correction of serum IgM and IgG3 levels, and restoration of T-independent immunity and B cell–proliferative responses. Together, these data support the concept of therapeutic *BTK* gene transfer and hold promise for future gene therapy for XLA.

RAG-2 Deficiency

Patients with mutations of the recombination activating genes *RAG1* or *RAG2* suffer from a from of SCID characterized by the lack of both T and B lymphocytes. HSCT is currently the only curative treatment, which, however, is only partially successful in the absence of an HLA-identical familial donor. Exploring the potential of gene therapy for this disease is therefore justified. Recently, Rag-2-deficient mice were used to test a retroviral-mediated gene therapy approach. Genetic correction and transplantation of HSC into Rag-2 knockout mice could provide long-term correction of the immunologic deficiency in treated animals. T cell and B cell development was accompanied by diverse T cell repertoire, normal proliferative responses to mitogens and alloantigens, and humoral responses to antigenic challenge. A selective advantage for transduced lymphoid cells was demonstrated by comparative provirus quantification in of RAG-2 lymphoid and myeloid cells, while there was no evidence of toxicity due to constitutive expression (Yates et al., 2002). Altogether, these preliminary experiments demonstrate the feasibility of gene therapy for RAG-2 deficiency and encourage the further development of preclinical protocols for this disease.

Wiskott-Aldrich Syndrome

The Wiskott-Aldrich syndrome (WAS) is characterized by eczema, thrombocytopenia, recurrent infections, autoimmune disorders, and a high incidence of lymphomas (Fischer, 1993; Sullivan et al., 1994). The breadth and severity of WAS symptoms make management of this disease a complex problem (Mullen et al., 1993). The WAS gene encodes a highly proline-rich protein, WASP (Derry et al., 1994), that has been implicated in actin organization in the cytoskeleton (see Chapter 31). The unsatisfactory results of haplodentical BMT in WAS patients (Antoine et al., 2003) justify efforts to test the safety and efficacy of gene therapy for this disease.

Studies in WAS lymphoblastoid B cell lines (Candotti et al., 1999; Huang et al., 2000) as well as T cell lines and primary T lymphocytes (Dupre et al., 2002; Wada et al., 2002; Strom et al., 2003) have shown that retroviral-mediated gene transfer can correct the phenotype of WAS cells. More recent experiments have shown that *WASP* gene transfer using lentiviral vectors can provide functional correction of WAS patients' T cells with higher efficacy (Dupre et al., 2004). More importantly, in vivo models of gene therapy using knockout mice have shown that T cell numbers and responses can be improved in animals treated with both retroviral and lentiviral *WASP* gene transfer, albeit at reduced levels compared to wild-type animals (Strom et al., 2002; Klein et al., 2003; Charrier et al., 2004). Interestingly, competitive repopulation experiments have also documented a selective advantage of wild-type over WASP knockout cells, thus suggesting that gene-corrected lymphocytes could similarly have a selective advantage over unmodified populations after gene therapy. These observations are in line with the reports of somatic reversion of *WASP* mutations in T lymphocyte progenitors of WAS patients; somatic reversion resulted in significant numbers of WASP-expressing circulating T lymphocytes that had selective survival advantage in vivo over WASP-negative cells (Wada et al., 2001, 2003, 2004).

CD3γ Deficiency

The T cell antigen receptor (TcR) is constituted by a glycoprotein heterodimeric complex containing TcRα and TcRβ, or TcRγ and TcRδ chains that associate with the CD3 complex composed of CD3γ, CD3δ, CD3ε, and CD3ζ (or CD3η) polypeptides. Selective defects of the expression of CD3γ have been reported in humans, resulting in only partial disorders of cellular immunity (Arnaiz-Villena et al., 1992) (see Chapter 16). Because of the presence of circulating T lymphocytes in these patients, a T lymphocyte–directed gene therapy approach could be developed. Retroviral-mediated expression of CD3γ in mutant Jurkat T cells resulted in normalization of IL-2 production after TCR/CD3 engagement and TCR/CD3 down-modulation in response to phorbol myristate acetate (Sun et al., 1997). Similarly, CD3γ introduction into peripheral blood T lymphocytes from CD3γ-deficient patients corrected the TCR/CD3 expression and down-regulation defects, but unfortunately also induced constitutive IL-2 synthesis, causing death of nontransduced T lymphocytes. CD3γ gene transfer into post-thymic lymphocytes therefore can become detrimental to the host, and regulated expression will be necessary if gene therapy is to be developed this disease.

X-Linked Lymphoproliferative Syndrome

Mutations or deletions in *SH2D1A*, or *SAP*, gene result in the X-linked lymphoproliferative disease (XLP), a combined immunodeficiency associated with severe or fatal outcome after EBV infection (see Chapter 32). The SAP protein is primarily expressed in T and NK cells (Parolini et al., 2000; Czar et al., 2001; Wu et al., 2001). Among T lymphocytes, cytotoxic T cells (CTL$_8$) play a crucial role in the immune response to EBV. CTL from XLP patients are characterized by reduced IFN-γ production in response to EBV-mediated stimulation and decreased cytotoxic activity against autologous lymphocytoid cell lines. These defects were restored using retroviral-mediated *SAP* gene transfer, thus opening the way to approaches for corrective gene transfer into CTL as potential form of therapy for this disease (Sharifi et al., 2004).

Conclusions

Primary immunodeficiency diseases fully meet the definition of "experiments of nature" as proposed by Garrod in 1924: they provide unique examples of what are the real consequences of genetic defects in humans, thus shedding light on the physiological role of the missing gene product(s) (Garrod, 1924). For this important characteristic, the highly heterogeneous group of extremely rare PID diseases has been the focus of extensive clinical and molecular studies, and has often been the object of innovative therapeutic approaches.

The first demonstration that allogeneic HSCT could be successfully applied to clinical practice was reported in 1968 following the treatment of children with XSCID and WAS (Bach et al., 1968; Gatti et al., 1968); similarly, successful enzyme replacement therapy was first achieved in a case of ADA deficient SCID (Pahwa et al., 1989). Finally, XSCID was also the first disease to be successfully treated by gene therapy (Cavazzana-Calvo et al., 2000). With the first clear clinical benefits, the first serious potential complications of gene therapy have unfortunately also become evident (Hacein-Bey-Abina et al., 2003b) and sparked a revision of the assessment of risks and benefits that will be critical for future development of gene therapy approaches for all PIDs and other genetic disorders.

As HSCT has subsequently emerged as an essential form of treatment for a wide variety of clinical applications, it is likely that the experience acquired from the pioneering gene therapy experiments for immunodeficient patients will constitute a guide for developing and applying gene therapy strategies to an increasing number of congenital and acquired genetic conditions in which conventional therapies have failed or are not a satisfactory long-term option.

References

Aiuti A, Slavin S, Aker M, Ficara F, Deola S, Mortellaro A, Morecki S, Andolfi G, Tabucchi A, Carlucci F, Marinello E, Cattaneo F, Vai S, Servida P, Miniero R, Roncarolo MG, Bordignon C. Correction of ADA-SCPI by stem cell gene therapy combined with nonmyeloablative conditioning. Science 296:2410–2413, 2002a.

Aiuti A, Vai S, Mortellaro A, Casorati G, Ficara F, Andolfi G, Ferrari G, Tabucchi A, Carlucci F, Ochs HD, Notarangelo LD, Roncarolo MG, Bordignon C. Immune reconstitution in ADA-SCPI after PBL gene therapy and discontinuation of enzyme replacement. Nat Med 8:423–425, 2002b.

Antoine C, Muller S, Cant A, Cavazzana-Calvo M, Veys P, Vossen J, Fasth A, Heilmann C, Wulffraat N, Seger R, Blanche S, Friedrich W, Abinun M, Davies G, Bredius R, Schulz A, Landais P, Fischer A. Long-term survival and transplantation of haemopoietic stem cells for immunodeficiencies: report of the European experience 1968–99. Lancet 361:553–560, 2003.

Arnaiz-Villena A, Timon M, Corell A, Perez-Aciego P, Martin-Villa JM, Regueiro JR. Brief report: primary immunodeficiency caused by mutations in the gene encoding the CD3-γ subunit of the T-lymphocyte receptor. N Engl J Med 327:529–533, 1992.

Arpaia E, Shahar M, Dadi H, Cohen A, Roifman CM. Defective T cell receptor signaling and CD8+ thymic selection in humans lacking ZAP-70 kinase. Cell 76:947–958, 1994.

Arya SK, Zamani M, Kundra P. Human immunodeficiency virus type 2 lentivirus vectors for gene transfer: expression and potential for helper virus-free packaging. Hum Gene Ther 9:1371–1380, 1998.

Asao H, Okuyama C, Kumaki S, Ishii N, Tsuchiya S, Foster D, Sugamura K. Cutting edge: the common γ-chain is an indispensable subunit of the IL-21 receptor complex. J Immunol 167:1–5, 2001.

Aviles Mendoza GJ, Seidel NE, Otsu M, Anderson SM, Simon-Stoos K, Herrera A, Hoogstraten-Miller S, Malech HL, Candotti F, Puck JM, Bodine DM. Comparison of five retrovirus vectors containing the human IL-2 receptor γ chain gene for their ability to restore T and B lymphocytes in the X-linked severe combined immunodeficiency mouse model. Mol Ther 3:565–573, 2001.

Bach FH, Albertini RJ, Joo P, Anderson JL, Bortin MM. Bone-marrow transplantation in a patient with the Wiskott-Aldrich syndrome. Lancet 2: 1364–1366, 1968.

Bauer TR Jr, Creevy KE, Gu YC, Tuschong LM, Donahue RE, Metzger ME, Embree LJ, Burkholder T, Bacher JD, Romines C, Thomas ML 3rd, Colenda L, Hickstein DD. Very low levels of donor CD18+ neutrophils following allogeneic hematopoietic stem cell transplantation reverse the disease phenotype in canine leukocyte adhesion deficiency. Blood 103: 3582–3589, 2004.

Bauer TR, Hickstein DD. Gene therapy for leukocyte adhesion deficiency. Curr Opin Mol Ther 2:383–388, 2000.

Bauer TR Jr, Miller AD, Hickstein DD. Improved transfer of the leukocyte integrin CD18 subunit into hematopoietic cell lines by using retroviral vectors having a gibbon ape leukemia virus envelope. Blood 86:2379–2387, 1995.

Bauer TR, Schwartz BR, Conrad Liles W, Ochs HD, Hickstein DD. Retroviral-mediated gene transfer of the leukocyte integrin CD18 into peripheral blood CD34+ cells derived from a patient with leukocyte adhesion deficiency type 1. Blood 91:1520–1526, 1998.

Becker S, Wasser S, Hauses M, Hossle JP, Ott MG, Dinauer MC, Ganser A, Hoelzer D, Seger R, Grez M. Correction of respiratory burst activity in X-linked chronic granulomatous cells to therapeutically relevant levels after gene transfer into bone marrow CD34+ cells. Hum Gene Ther 9: 1561–1570, 1998.

Berns KI. Parvoviridae: the viruses and their replication. In: Fields BN, Knipe DM, Howley PM, eds. Virology. Philadelphia: Lippincott-Raven, pp. 2173–2197, 1995.

Bjorgvinsdottir H, Ding C, Pech N, Gifford MA, Li LL, Dinauer MC. Retroviral-mediated gene transfer of gp91phox into bone marrow cells rescues defect in host defense against *Aspergillus fumigatus* in murine X-linked chronic granulomatous disease. Blood 89:41–48, 1997.

Blaese RM. The ADA human gene therapy clinical protocol. Hum Gene Ther 1:327–362, 1990.

Blaese RM, Culver KW, Miller AD, Carter CS, Fleisher T, Clerici M, Shearer G, Chang L, Chiang Y, Tolstoshev P, Greenblatt JJ, Rosenberg SA, Klein H, Berger M, Mullen CA, Ramsey WJ, Muul L, Morgan RA, Anderson WF. T lymphocyte-directed gene therapy for ADA-SCPI: initial trial results after 4 years. Science 270:475–480, 1995.

Bordignon C, Mavilio F, Ferrari G, Servida P, Ugazio AG, Notarangelo LD, Gilboa E, Rossini S, O'Reilly RJ, Smith CA, Gillio AP, Anderson WF, Blaese RM, Moen RC, Eglitis MA. Transfer of the ADA gene into bone marrow cells and peripheral blood lymphocytes for the treatment of patients affected by ADA-deficient SCPI. Hum Gene Ther 4:513–520, 1993.

Bordignon C, Notarangelo LD, Nobili N, Ferrari G, Casorati G, Panina P, Mazzolari E, Maggioni D, Rossi C, Servida P, Ugazio AG, Mavilio F. Gene therapy in peripheral blood lymphocytes and bone marrow for ADA-immunodeficient patients. Science 270:470–475, 1995.

Bottazzo GF, Todd I, Mirakian R, Belfiore A, Pujol-Borrell R. Organ-specific autoimmunity: a 1986 overview. Immunol Rev 94:137–169, 1986.

Bradley MB, Fernandez JM, Ungers G, Diaz-Barrientos TA, Steimle V, Mach B, O'Reilly R, Lee JS. Correction of defective expression in MHC class II deficiency (bare lymphocyte syndrome) cells by retroviral transduction of CIITA. J Immunol 159:1086–1095, 1997.

Brown MP, Topham DJ, Sangster MY, Zhao J, Flynn KJ, Surman SL, Woodland DL, Doherty PC, Farr AG, Pattengale PK, Brenner MK. Thymic lymphoproliferative disease after successful correction of CD40 ligand deficiency by gene transfer in mice. Nat Med 4:1253–1260, 1998.

Buckley RH. Molecular defects in human severe combined immunodeficiency and approaches to immune reconstitution. Annu Rev Immunol 22: 625–655, 2004.

Bunnell BA, Muul LM, Donahue RE, Blaese RM, Morgan RA. High-efficiency retroviral-mediated gene transfer into human and nonhuman primate peripheral blood lymphocytes. Proc Natl Acad Sci USA 92:7739–7743, 1995.

Bunting KD, Flynn KJ, Riberdy JM, Doherty PC, Sorrentino BP. Virus-specific immunity after gene therapy in a murine model of severe combined immunodeficiency. Proc Natl Acad Sci USA 96:232–237, 1999.

Bunting KD, Lu T, Kelly PF, Sorrentino BP. Self-selection by genetically modified committed lymphocyte precursors reverses the phenotype of JAK3-deficient mice without myeloablation. Hum Gene Ther 11:2353–2364, 2000.

Bunting KD, Sangster MY, Ihle JN, Sorrentino BP. Restoration of lymphocyte function in Janus kinase 3–deficient mice by retroviral-mediated gene transfer. Nat Med 4:58–64, 1998.

Candotti F, Facchetti F, Blanzuoli L, Stewart DM, Nelson DL, Blaese RM. Retrovirus-mediated WASP gene transfer corrects defective actin polymerization in B cell lines from Wiskott-Aldrich syndrome patients carrying 'null' mutations. Gene Ther 6:1170–1174, 1999.

Candotti F, Johnston JA, Puck JM, Sugamura K, O'Shea JJ, Blaese RM. Retroviral-mediated gene correction for X-linked severe combined immunodeficiency. Blood 87:3097–3102, 1996.

Candotti F, Oakes SA, Johnston JA, Giliani S, Schumacher RF, Mella P, Fiorini M, Ugazio AG, Badolato R, Notarangelo LD, Bozzi F, Macchi P, Strina D, Vezzoni P, Blaese RM, O'Shea JJ, Villa A. Structural and functional basis for JAK3-deficient severe combined immunodeficiency. Blood 90:3996–4003, 1997.

Candotti F, Podsakoff G, Schurman SH, Muul LM, Engel BC, Carbonaro DA, Jagadeesh GJ, Hematti P, Tuschong LM, Carter CS, Ramsey WJ, Choi C, Smogorzewska M, Hershfield MS, Read EJ, Tisdale JF, Dunbar CE, Kohn DB. Corrective gene transfer into bone marrow CD34+ cells for adenosine deaminase (ADA) deficiency: results in four patients after one year of follow-up. Mol Ther 7:S448–S449, 2003.

Case SS, Price MA, Jordan CT, Yu XJ, Wang L, Bauer G, Haas DL, Xu D, Stripecke R, Naldini L, Kohn DB, Crooks GM. Stable transduction of quiescent CD34(+)CD38(−) human hematopoietic cells by HIV-1-based lentiviral vectors. Proc Natl Acad Sci USA 96:2988–2993, 1999.

Cavazzana-Calvo M, Hacein-Bay S, de Saint Basile G, De Coene F, Selz F, Le Deist F, Fischer A. Role of interleukin-2 (IL-2), IL-7, and IL-15 in natural killer cell differentiation from cord blood hematopoietic progenitor cells and from gc transduced severe combined immunodeficiency X1 bone marrow cells. Blood 88:3901–3909, 1996.

Cavazzana-Calvo M, Hacein-Bey S, de Saint Basile G, Gross F, Yvon E, Nusbaum P, Selz F, Hue C, Certain S, Casanova JL, Bousso P, Le Deist F, Fischer A. Gene therapy of human severe combined immunodeficiency (SCPI)-X1 disease. Science 288:669–672, 2000.

Cavazzana-Calvo M, Hacein-Bey S, Yates F, de Villartay JP, Le Deist F, Fischer A. Gene therapy of severe combined immunodeficiencies. J Gene Med 3:201–206, 2001.

Chan AC, Kadlecek TA, Elder ME, Filipovich AH, Kuo WL, Iwashima M, Parslow TG, Weiss A. ZAP-70 deficiency in an autosomal recessive form of severe combined immunodeficiency. Science 264:1599–1601, 1994.

Charrier S, Stockholm D, Seye K, Opolon P, Taveau M, Gross DA, Bucher-Laurent S, Delenda C, Vainchenker W, Danos O, Galy A. A lentiviral vector encoding the human Wiskott-Aldrich syndrome protein corrects immune and cytoskeletal defects in WASP knockout mice. Gene Ther 16:16, 2004.

Cheung AK, Hoggan MD, Hauswirth WW, Berns KI. Integration of the adeno-associated virus genome into cellular DNA in latently infected human Detroit 6 cells. J Virol 33:739–748, 1980.

Chinen J, Puck JM, Davis J, Linton GF, Whiting-Theobald NL, Woltz PC, Bucley RH, Malech HL. Ex vivo gene therapy of a preadolescent with X-linked severe combined immunodeficiency. Blood 104: Abstract 410, 2004.

Conley ME, Parolini O, Rohrer J, Campana D. X-linked agammaglobulinemia: new approaches to old questions based on the identification of the defective gene. Immunol Rev 138:5–21, 1994.

Conley ME, Rohrer J, Rapalus L, Boylin EC, Minegishi Y. Defects in early B-cell development: comparing the consequences of abnormalities in pre-BCR signaling in the human and the mouse. Immunol Rev 178:75–90, 2000.

Cosset FL, Takeuchi Y, Battini JL, Weiss RA, Collins MK. High-titer packaging cells producing recombinant retroviruses resistant to human serum. J Virol 69:7430–7436, 1995.

Czar MJ, Kersh EN, Mijares LA, Lanier G, Lewis J, Yap G, Chen A, Sher A, Duckett CS, Ahmed R, Schwartzberg PL. Altered lymphocyte responses and cytokine production in mice deficient in the X-linked lymphoproliferative disease gene *SH2D1A/DSHP/SAP*. Proc Natl Acad Sci USA 98: 7449–7454, 2001.

Daddona PE, Mitchell BS, Meuwissen HJ, Davidson BL, Wilson JM, Koller CA. Adenosine deaminase deficiency with normal immune function. An acidic enzyme mutation. J Clin Invest 72:483–492, 1983.

Dao MA, Hannum CH, Kohn DB, Nolta JA. FLT3 ligand preserves the ability of human CD34+ progenitors to sustain long-term hematopoiesis in immune-deficient mice after ex vivo retroviral-mediated transduction. Blood 89:446–456, 1997.

Derry JM, Ochs HD, Francke U. Isolation of a novel gene mutated in Wiskott-Aldrich syndrome. Cell 78:635–644, 1994.

Dranoff G, Jaffee E, Lazenby A, Golumbek P, Levitsky H, Brose K, Jackson V, Hamada H, Pardoll D, Mulligan RC. Vaccination with irradiated tumor cells engineered to secrete murine granulocyte-macrophage colony-stimulating factor stimulates potent, specific, and long-lasting anti-tumor immunity. Proc Natl Acad Sci USA 90:3539–3543, 1993.

Dull T, Zufferey R, Kelly M, Mandel RJ, Nguyen M, Trono D, Naldini L. A third-generation lentivirus vector with a conditional packaging system. J Virol 72:8463–8471, 1998.

Dupre L, Aiuti A, Trifari S, Martino S, Saracco P, Bordignon C, Roncarolo MG. Wiskott-Aldrich syndrome protein regulates lipid raft dynamics during immunological synapse formation. Immunity 17:157–166, 2002.

Dupre L, Trifari S, Follenzi A, Marangoni F, Lain de Lera T, Bernad A, Martino S, Tsuchiya S, Bordignon C, Naldini L, Aiuti A, Roncarolo MG. Lentiviral vector-mediated gene transfer in T cells from Wiskott-Aldrich syndrome patients leads to functional correction. Mol Ther 10:903–915, 2004.

Egashira M, Ariga T, Kawamura N, Miyoshi O, Niikawa N, Sakiyama Y. Visible integration of the adenosine deaminase (ADA) gene into the recipient genome after gene therapy. Am J Med Genet 75:314–317, 1998.

Elder ME, Lin D, Clever J, Chan AC, Hope TJ, Weiss A, Parslow TG. Human severe combined immunodeficiency due to a defect in ZAP-70, a T cell tyrosine kinase. Science 264:1596–1599, 1994.

Etzioni A. Adhesion molecule deficiencies and their clinical significance. Cell Adhes Commun 2:257–260, 1994.

Fischer A. Primary T-cell immunodeficiencies. Curr Opin Immunol 5:569–578, 1993.

Fischer A, Lisowska-Grospierre B, Anderson DC, Springer TA. Leukocyte adhesion deficiency: molecular basis and functional consequences. Immunodefic Rev 1:39–54, 1988.

Flotte TR, Afione SA, Zeitlin PL. Adeno-associated virus vector gene expression occurs in nondividing cells in the absence of vector DNA integration. Am J Respir Cell Mol Biol 11:517–521, 1994.

Flotte TR, Barraza-Ortiz X, Solow R, Afione SA, Carter BJ, Guggino WB. An improved system for packaging recombinant adeno-associated virus vectors capable of in vivo transduction. Gene Ther 2:29–37, 1995.

Forehand JR, Johnston RB Jr. Chronic granulomatous disease: newly defined molecular abnormalities explain disease variability and normal phagocyte physiology. Curr Opin Pediatr 6:668–675, 1994.

Garrod AE. The Harveian oration on the debt of science to medicine. BMJ 2:747–752, 1924.

Gaspar HB, Parsley KL, Howe S, King D, Gilmour KC, Sinclair J, Brouns G, Schmidt M, Von Kalle C, Barington T, Jakobsen MA, Christensen HO, Al Ghonaium A, White HN, Smith JL, Levinsky RJ, Ali RR, Kinnon C, Thrasher AJ. Gene therapy of X-linked severe combined immunodeficiency by use of a pseudotyped gammaretroviral vector. Lancet 364: 2181–2187, 2004.

Gatti RA, Meuwissen HJ, Allen HD, Hong R, Good RA. Immunological reconstitution of sex-linked lymphopenic immunological deficiency. Lancet 2:1366–1369, 1968.

Goodman S, Xiao X, Donahue RE, Moulton A, Miller J, Walsh C, Young NS, Samulski RJ, Nienhuis AW. Recombinant adeno-associated virus–mediated gene transfer into hematopoietic progenitor cells. Blood 84:1492–1500, 1994.

Habib T, Senadheera S, Weinberg K, Kaushansky K. The common γ chain (γc) is a required signaling component of the IL-21 receptor and supports IL-21-induced cell proliferation via JAK3. Biochemistry 41:8725–8731, 2002.

Hacein-Bey S, Basile GD, Lemerle J, Fischer A, Cavazzana-Calvo M. Gammac gene transfer in the presence of stem cell factor, FLT-3L, interleukin-7 (IL-7), IL-1, and IL-15 cytokines restores T-cell differentiation from γc(-) X-linked severe combined immunodeficiency hematopoietic progenitor cells in murine fetal thymic organ cultures. Blood 92:4090–4097, 1998.

Hacein-Bey S, Cavazzana-Calvo M, Le Deist F, Dautry-Varsat A, Hivroz C, Rivière I, Danos O, Heard JM, Sugamura K, Fischer A, De Saint Basile G. Gamma-c gene transfer into SCPI X1 patients' B-cell lines restores normal high-affinity interleukin-2 receptor expression and function. Blood 87:3108–3116, 1996.

Hacein-Bey-Abina S, Le Deist F, Carlier F, Bouneaud C, Hue C, De Villartay JP, Thrasher AJ, Wulffraat N, Sorensen R, Dupuis-Girod S, Fischer A, Davies EG, Kuis W, Leiva L, Cavazzana-Calvo M. Sustained correction of X-linked severe combined immunodeficiency by ex vivo gene therapy. N Engl J Med 346:1185–1193, 2002.

Hacein-Bey-Abina S, von Kalle C, Schmidt M, Le Deist F, Wulffraat N, McIntyre E, Radford I, Villeval JL, Fraser CC, Cavazzana-Calvo M, Fischer A. A serious adverse event after successful gene therapy for X-linked severe combined immunodeficiency. N Engl J Med 348:255–256, 2003a.

Hacein-Bey-Abina S, von Kalle C, Schmidt M, McCormack MP, Wulffraat N, Leboulch P, Lim A, Osborne CS, Pawliuk R, Morillon E, Sorensen R, Forster A, Fraser P, Cohen JI, de Saint Basile G, Alexander I, Wintergerst U, Frebourg T, Aurias A, Stoppa-Lyonnet D, Romana S, Radford-Weiss I, Gross F, Valensi F, Delabesse E, Macintyre E, Sigaux F, Soulier J, Leiva LE, Wissler M, Prinz C, Rabbitts TH, Le Deist F, Fischer A, Cavazzana-Calvo M. LMO2-associated clonal T cell proliferation in two patients after gene therapy for SCPI-X1. Science 302:415–419, 2003b.

Halbert CL, Alexander IE, Wolgamot GM, Miller AD. Adeno-associated virus vectors transduce primary cells much less efficiently than immortalized cells. J Virol 69:1473–1479, 1995.

Hanenberg H, Xiao XL, Dilloo D, Hashino K, Kato I, Williams DA. Colocalization of retrovirus and target cells on specific fibronectin fragments increases genetic transduction of mammalian cells. Nat Med 2:876–882, 1996.

Harlan JM. Leukocyte adhesion deficiency syndrome: insights into the molecular basis of leukocyte emigration. Clin Immunol Immunopathol 67: S16–S24, 1993.

Hematti P, Hong BK, Ferguson C, Adler R, Hanawa H, Sellers S, Holt IE, Eckfeldt CE, Sharma Y, Schmidt M, von Kalle C, Persons DA, Billings EM, Verfaillie CM, Nienhuis AW, Wolfsberg TG, Dunbar CE, Calmels B. Distinct genomic integration of MLV and SIV vectors in primate hematopoietic stem and progenitor cells. PLoS Biol 2:e423, 2004.

Hibbs ML, Wardlaw AJ, Stacker SA, Anderson DC, Lee A, Roberts TM, Springer TA. Transfection of cells from patients with leukocyte adhesion deficiency with an integrin beta subunit (CD18) restores lymphocyte function–associated antigen-1 expression and function. J Clin Invest 85: 674–681, 1990.

Hirschhorn R. Overview of biochemical abnormalities and molecular genetics of adenosine deaminase deficiency. Pediatr Res 33:S35–41, 1993.

Hoogerbrugge PM, van Beusechem VW, Fischer A, Debree M, Le Deist F, Perignon JL, Morgan G, Gaspar B, Fairbanks LD, Skeoch CH, Moseley A, Harvey M, Levinsky RJ, Valerio D. Bone marrow gene transfer in three patients with adenosine deaminase deficiency. Gene Ther 3:179–183, 1996.

Huang MM, Tsuboi S, Wong A, Yu XJ, Oh-Eda M, Derry JM, Francke U, Fukuda M, Weinberg KI, Kohn DB. Expression of human Wiskott-Aldrich syndrome protein in patients' cells leads to partial correction of a phenotypic abnormality of cell surface glycoproteins. Gene Ther 7:314–320, 2000.

Huss R, Nepom GT, Deeg HJ. Defective CD4+ T-lymphocyte reconstitution in major histocompatibility complex class II–deficient transplant models. Blood 85:3354–3356, 1995.

Islam TC, Branden LJ, Kohn DB, Islam KB, Smith CIE. BTK mediated apoptosis, a possible mechanism for failure to generate high titer retroviral producer clones. J Gene Ther 2:204–209, 2000.

Johnston JA, Bacon CM, Finbloom DS, Rees RC, Kaplan D, Shibuya K, Ortaldo JR, Gupta S, Chen YQ, Giri JD, et al. Tyrosine phosphorylation and activation of STAT5, STAT3, and Janus kinases by interleukins 2 and 15. Proc Natl Acad Sci USA 92:8705–8709, 1995.

Josephson NC, Vassilopoulos G, Trobridge GD, Priestley GV, Wood BL, Papayannopoulou T, Russell DW. Transduction of human NOD/SCPI-repopulating cells with both lymphoid and myeloid potential by foamy virus vectors. Proc Natl Acad Sci USA 99:8295–8300, 2002.

Kafri T, Blomer U, Peterson DA, Gage FH, Verma IM. Sustained expression of genes delivered directly into liver and muscle by lentiviral vectors. Nat Genet 17:314–317, 1997.

Kawamura M, McVicar DW, Johnston JA, Blake TB, Chen YQ, Lal BK, Lloyd AR, Kelvin DJ, Staples JE, Ortaldo JR, O'Shea JJ. Molecular cloning of L-JAK, a Janus family protein-tyrosine kinase expressed in natural killer cells and activated leukocytes. Proc Natl Acad Sci USA 91: 6374–6378, 1994.

Kawamura N, Ariga T, Ohtsu M, Kobayashi I, Yamada M, Tame A, Furuta H, Okano M, Egashira M, Niikawa N, Kobayashi K, Sakiyama Y. In vivo kinetics of transduced cells in peripheral T cell–directed gene therapy: role of CD8+ cells in improved immunological function in an adenosine deaminase (ADA)-SCPI patient. J Immunol 163:2256–2261, 1999.

Kelly PF, Vandergriff J, Nathwani A, Nienhuis AW, Vanin EF. Highly efficient gene transfer into cord blood nonobese diabetic/severe combined immunodeficiency repopulating cells by oncoretroviral vector particles pseudotyped with the feline endogenous retrovirus (RD114) envelope protein. Blood 96:1206–1214, 2000.

Kiem HP, Andrews RG, Morris J, Peterson L, Heyward S, Allen JM, Rasko JEJ, Potter J, Miller AD. Improved gene transfer into baboon marrow repopulating cells using recombinant human fibronectin fragment CH-296 in combination with interleukin-6, stem cell factor, FLT-3 ligand, and megakaryocyte growth and development factor. Blood 92:1878–1886, 1998.

Klein C, Cavazzana-Calvo M, Le Deist F, Jabado N, Benkerrou M, Blanche S, Lisowska-Grospierre B, Griscelli C, Fischer A. Bone marrow transplantation in major histocompatibility complex class II deficiency: a single-center study of 19 patients. Blood 85:580–587, 1995.

Klein C, Nguyen D, Liu CH, Mizoguchi A, Bhan AK, Miki H, Takenawa T, Rosen FS, Alt FW, Mulligan RC, Snapper SB. Gene therapy for Wiskott-Aldrich syndrome: rescue of T-cell signaling and amelioration of colitis upon transplantation of retrovirally transduced hematopoietic stem cells in mice. Blood 101:2159–2166, 2003.

Kohn DB. Gene therapy using hematopoietic stem cells. Curr Opin Mol Ther 1:437–442, 1999.

Kohn DB, Hershfield MS, Carbonaro D, Shigeoka A, Brooks J, Smogorzewska EM, Barsky LW, Chan R, Burotto F, Annett G, Nolta JA, Crooks G, Kapoor N, Elder M, Wara D, Bowen T, Madsen E, Snyder FF, Bastian J, Muul L, Blaese RM, Weinberg K, Parkman R. T lymphocytes with a normal ADA gene accumulate after transplantation of transduced autologous umbilical cord blood CD34+ cells in ADA-deficient SCPI neonates. Nat Med 4:775–780, 1998.

Kohn DB, Weinberg KI, Nolta JA, Heiss LN, Lenarsky C, Crooks GM, Hanley ME, Annett G, Brooks JS, el-Khoureiy A, Lawrence K, Wells S, Moen RC, Bastian J, Williams-Herman DE, Elder M, Wara D, Bowen T, Hershfield MS, Mullen CA, Blaese RM, Parkman R. Engraftment of gene-modified umbilical cord blood cells in neonates with adenosine deaminase deficiency. Nat Med 1:1017–1023, 1995.

Kotin RM, Siniscalco M, Samulski RJ, Zhu XD, Hunter L, Laughlin CA, McLaughlin S, Muzyczka N, Rocchi M, Berns KI. Site-specific integration by adeno-associated virus. Proc Natl Acad Sci USA 87:2211–2215, 1990.

Larson RC, Fisch P, Larson TA, Lavenir I, Langford T, King G, Rabbitts TH. T cell tumours of disparate phenotype in mice transgenic for Rbtn-2. Oncogene 9:3675–3681, 1994.

Lekstrom-Himes JA, Gallin JI. Immunodeficiency diseases caused by defects in phagocytes. N Engl J Med 343:1703–1714, 2000.

Li F, Linton GF, Sekhsaria S, Whiting-Theobald N, Katkin JP, Gallin JI, Malech HL. CD34+ peripheral blood progenitors as a target for genetic correction of the two flavocytochrome b558 defective forms of chronic granulomatous disease. Blood 84:53–58, 1994.

Lo M, Bloom ML, Imada K, Berg M, Bollenbacher JM, Bloom ET, Kelsall BL, Leonard WJ. Restoration of lymphoid populations in a murine model of X-linked severe combined immunodeficiency by a gene-therapy approach. Blood 94:3027–3036, 1999.

Macchi P, Villa A, Giliani S, Sacco MG, Frattini A, Porta F, Ugazio AG, Johnston JA, Candotti F, O'Shea JJ, Vezzoni P, Notarangelo LD. Mutations of Jak-3 gene in patients with autosomal severe combined immune deficiency (SCPI). Nature 377:65–68, 1995.

Malech HL, Horwitz ME, Linton GF, Theobald-Whiting N, Brown MR, Farrell CJ, Butz RE, Carter CS, DeCarlo E, Miller JA, Van Epps DE, Read EJ, Fleisher TA. Extended production of oxidase normal neutrophils in X-linked chronic granulomatous disease (CGD) following gene therapy with gp91(phox) transduced CD34+ cells. Blood 92:690A, 1998.

Malech HL, Sekhsaria S, Whiting-Theobald N, Linton GL, Vowells SJ, Li F, Miller JA, Holland SM, Leitman SF, Carter CS, Read EJ, Butz R, Wannebo C, Fleisher TA, Deans RJ, Spratt SK, Maack CA, Rokovich JA, Cohen LK, Maples PB, Gallin JI. Prolonged detection of oxidase-positive neutrophils in the peripheral blood of five patients following a single cycle of gene therapy for chronic granulomatous disease. Blood 88:486a, 1996.

Mardiney MR, Jackson SH, Spratt SK, Li F, Holland SM, Malech HL. Enhanced host defense after gene transfer in the murine p47phox-deficient model of chronic granulomatous disease. Blood 89:2268–2275, 1997.

Markert ML. Molecular basis of adenosine deaminase deficiency. Immunodeficiency 5:141–157, 1994.

Matheux F, Ikinciogullari A, Zapata DA, Barras E, Zufferey M, Dogu F, Regueiro JR, Reith W, Villard J. Direct genetic correction as a new method for diagnosis and molecular characterization of MHC class II deficiency. Mol Ther 6:824–829, 2002.

Mergia A, Chari S, Kolson DL, Goodenow MM, Ciccarone T. The efficiency of simian foamy virus vector type-1 (SFV-1) in nondividing cells and in human PBLs. Virology 280:243–252, 2001.

Miller AD. Retroviral vectors. Curr Top Microbiol Immunol 158:1–24, 1992.

Miller AD, Garcia JV, von Suhr N, Lynch CM, Wilson C, Eiden MV. Construction and properties of retrovirus packaging cells based on gibbon ape leukemia virus. J Virol 65:2220–2224, 1991.

Miller AD, Rosman GJ. Improved retroviral vectors for gene transfer and expression. Biotechniques 7:980–990, 1989.

Miller JL, Donahue RE, Sellers SE, Samulski RJ, Young NS, Nienhuis AW. Recombinant adeno-associated virus (rAAV)-mediated expression of a human γ-globin gene in human progenitor-derived erythroid cells. Proc Natl Acad Sci USA 91:10183–10187, 1994.

Misaki Y, Ezaki I, Ariga T, Kawamura N, Sakiyama Y, Yamamoto K. Gene-transferred oligoclonal T cells predominantly persist in peripheral blood from an adenosine deaminase-deficient patient during gene therapy. Mol Ther 3:24–27, 2001.

Miyoshi H, Blomer U, Takahashi M, Gage FH, Verma IM. Development of a self-inactivating lentivirus vector. J Virol 72:8150–8157, 1998.

Miyoshi H, Smith KA, Mosier DE, Verma IM, Torbett BE. Transduction of human CD34+ cells that mediate long-term engraftment of NOD/SCPI mice by HIV vectors. Science 283:682–686, 1999.

Miyoshi H, Takahashi M, Gage FH, Verma IM. Stable and efficient gene transfer into the retina using an HIV-based lentiviral vector. Proc Natl Acad Sci USA 94:10319–10323, 1997.

Mullen CA, Anderson KD, Blaese RM. Splenectomy and/or bone marrow transplantation in the management of the Wiskott-Aldrich syndrome: long-term follow-up of 62 cases. Blood 82:2961–2966, 1993.

Muul LM, Tuschong LM, Soenen SL, Jagadeesh GJ, Ramsey WJ, Long Z, Carter CS, Garabedian EK, Alleyne M, Brown M, Bernstein W, Schurman SH, Fleisher TA, Leitman SF, Dunbar CE, Blaese RM, Candotti F. Persistence and expression of the adenosine deaminase gene for 12 years and immune reaction to gene transfer components: long-term results of the first clinical gene therapy trial. Blood 101:2563–2569, 2003.

Naldini L, Blomer U, Gage FH, Trono D, Verma IM. Efficient transfer, integration, and sustained long-term expression of the transgene in adult rat brains injected with a lentiviral vector. Proc Natl Acad Sci USA 93:11382–11388, 1996a.

Naldini L, Blomer P, Gallay P, Ory D, Mulligan R, Gage FH, Verma IM, Trono D. In vivo gene delivery and stable transduction of nondividing cells by a lentiviral vector. Science 273:263–267, 1996b.

Nathwani AC, Hanawa H, Vandergriff J, Kelly P, Vanin EF, Nienhuis AW. Efficient gene transfer into human cord blood CD34+ cells and the CD34+CD38− subset using highly purified recombinant adeno-associated viral vector preparations that are free of helper virus and wild-type AAV. Gene Ther 7:183–195, 2000.

Nelson DM, Butters KA, Markert ML, Reinsmoen NL, McIvor RS. Correction of proliferative responses in purine nucleoside phosphorylase (PNP)-deficient T lymphocytes by retroviral-mediated PNP gene transfer and expression. J Immunol 154:3006–3014, 1995.

Noguchi M, Yi H, Rosenblatt HM, Filipovich AH, Adelstein S, Modi WS, McBride OW, Leonard WJ. Interleukin-2 receptor gamma chain mutation results in X-linked severe combined immunodeficiency in humans. Cell 73:147–157, 1993.

Notarangelo LD, Mella P, Jones A, de Saint Basile G, Savoldi G, Cranston T, Vihinen M, Schumacher RF. Mutations in severe combined immune deficiency (SCPI) due to JAK3 deficiency. Hum Mutat 18:255–263, 2001.

Oakes SA, Candotti F, Johnston JA, Chen YQ, Ryan JJ, Taylor N, Liu X, Hennighausen L, Notarangelo LD, Paul WE, Blaese RM, O'Shea JJ. Signaling via IL-2 and IL-4 in JAK3-deficient severe combined immunodeficiency lymphocytes: JAK3-dependent and independent pathways. Immunity 5:605–615, 1996.

Olsen JC. Gene transfer vectors derived from equine infectious anemia virus. Gene Ther 5:1481–1487, 1998.

Onodera M, Ariga T, Kawamura N, Kobayashi I, Ohtsu M, Yamada M, Tame A, Furuta H, Okano M, Matsumoto S, Kotani H, McGarrity GJ, Blaese RM, Sakiyama Y. Successful peripheral T lymphocyte–directed gene transfer for a patient with severe combined immune deficiency due to adenosine deaminase deficiency. Blood 91:30–36, 1998.

Orkin SH, Daddona PE, Shewach DS, Markham AF, Bruns GA, Goff SC, Kelley WN. Molecular cloning of human adenosine deaminase gene sequences. J Biol Chem 258:12753–12756, 1983.

Otsu M, Anderson SM, Bodine DM, Puck JM, O'Shea JJ, Candotti F. Lymphoid development and function in X-linked severe combined immunodeficiency mice after stem cell gene therapy. Mol Ther 1:145–153, 2000.

Otsu M, Ariga T, Maeyama Y, Yoshida I, Nakajima S, Kida M, Toita N, Hatano N, Kawamura N, Okano M, Kobayashi R, Tatsuzawa O, Onodera M, Candotti F, Kobayashi K, Sakiyama Y. A clinical trial in Japan of retroviral-mediated gene transfer to bone marrow CD34+ cells as a treatment of adenosine deaminase (ADA)-deficiency. Mol Ther 2005.

Otsu M, Steinberg M, Ferrand C, Merida P, Rebouissou C, Tiberghien P, Taylor N, Candotti F, Noraz N. Reconstitution of lymphoid development and function in ZAP-70-deficient mice following gene transfer into bone marrow cells. Blood 100:1248–1256, 2002.

Otsu M, Sugamura K, Candotti F. Lack of dominant-negative effects of a truncated gamma(c) on retroviral-mediated gene correction of immunodeficient mice. Blood 97:1618–1624, 2001.

Ott GM, Stein S, Koehl U, Kunkel H, Siler U, Schilz A, Kuhlcke K, Schmidt M, von Kalle C, Hassan M, Hoelzer D, Seger R, Grez M. Gene therapy for X-linked chronic granulomatous disease. In: Proceedings of the XI Meeting of the European Society for Immunodeficiencies, p. 97, 2004.

Pahwa R, Chatila T, Pahwa S, Paradise C, Day NK, Geha R, Schwartz SA, Slade H, Oyaizu N, Good RA. Recombinant interleukin 2 therapy in severe combined immunodeficiency disease. Proc Natl Acad Sci USA 86:5069–5073, 1989.

Park J, Nadeau PE, Mergia A. A minimal genome simian foamy virus type 1 vector system with efficient gene transfer. Virology 302:236–244, 2002.

Parolini S, Bottino C, Falco M, Augugliaro R, Giliani S, Franceschini R, Ochs HD, Wolf H, Bonnefoy JY, Biassoni R, Moretta L, Notarangelo LD, Moretta A. X-linked lymphoproliferative disease. 2B4 molecules displaying inhibitory rather than activating function are responsible for the inability of natural killer cells to kill Epstein-Barr virus-infected cells. J Exp Med 192:337–346, 2000.

Piacibello W, Sanavio F, Garetto L, Severino A, Bergandi D, Ferrario J, Fagioli F, Berger M, Aglietta M. Extensive amplification and self-renewal of human primitive hematopoietic stem cells from cord blood. Blood 89:2644–2653, 1997.

Piacibello W, Sanavio F, Severino A, Dane A, Gammaitoni L, Fagioli F, Perissinotto E, Cavalloni G, Kollet O, Lapidot T, Aglietta M. Engraftment in nonobese diabetic severe combined immunodeficient mice of human CD34(+) cord blood cells after ex vivo expansion: evidence for the amplification and self-renewal of repopulating stem cells. Blood 93:3736–3749, 1999.

Podsakoff G, Wong KK Jr, Chatterjee S. Efficient gene transfer into nondividing cells by adeno-associated virus-based vectors. J Virol 68:5656–5666, 1994.

Poeschla E, Gilbert J, Li X, Huang S, Ho A, Wong-Staal F. Identification of a human immunodeficiency virus type 2 (HIV-2) encapsidation determinant and transduction of nondividing human cells by HIV-2-based lentivirus vectors. J Virol 72:6527–6536, 1998a.

Poeschla EM, Wong-Staal F, Looney DJ. Efficient transduction of nondividing human cells by feline immunodeficiency virus lentiviral vectors. Nat Med 4:354–357, 1998b.

Porter CD, Parkar MH, Collins MKL, Levinsky RJ, Kinnon C. Efficient retroviral transduction of human bone marrow progenitor and long-term culture-initiating cells: partial reconstitution of cells from patients with X-linked chronic granulomatous disease by gp91-phox expression. Blood 87:3722–3730, 1996.

Puck JM, Deschenes SM, Porter JC, Dutra AS, Brown CJ, Willard HF, Henthorn PS. The interleukin-2 receptor gamma chain maps to Xq13.1 and is mutated in X-linked severe combined immunodeficiency, SCPIX1. Hum Mol Genet 2:1099–1104, 1993.

Rebel VI, Tanaka M, Lee JS, Hartnett S, Pulsipher M, Nathan DG, Mulligan RC, Sieff CA. One-day ex vivo culture allows effective gene transfer into human nonobese diabetic/severe combined immune-deficient repopulating cells using high-titer vesicular stomatitis virus G protein pseudotyped retrovirus. Blood 93:2217–2224, 1999.

Reiser J, Harmison G, Kluepfel-Stahl S, Brady RO, Karlsson S, Schubert M. Transduction of nondividing cells using pseudotyped defective high-titer HIV type 1 particles. Proc Natl Acad Sci USA 93:15266–15271, 1996.

Rethwilm A. Regulation of foamy virus gene expression. Curr Top Microbiol Immunol 193:1–24, 1995.

Rich KC, Majias E, Fox IH. Purine nucleoside phosphorylase deficiency: improved metabolic and immunologic function with erythrocyte transfusions. N Engl J Med 303:973–977, 1980.

Roesler J, Brenner S, Bukovsky AA, Whiting-Theobald N, Dull T, Kelly M, Civin CI, Malech HL. Third-generation, self-inactivating gp91(phox) lentivector corrects the oxidase defect in NOD/SCPI mouse-repopulating peripheral blood-mobilized CD34+ cells from patients with X-linked chronic granulomatous disease. Blood 100:4381–4390, 2002.

Rohrer J, Conley ME. Correction of X-linked immunodeficient mice by competitive reconstitution with limiting numbers of normal bone marrow cells. Blood 94:3358–3365, 1999.

Roos D. The genetic basis of chronic granulomatous disease. Immunol Rev 138:121–157, 1994.

Russell DW, Miller AD. Foamy virus vectors. J Virol 70:217–222, 1996.

Russell DW, Miller AD, Alexander IE. Adeno-associated virus vectors preferentially transduce cells in S phase. Proc Natl Acad Sci USA 91:8915–8919, 1994.

Russell SM, Tayebi N, Nakajima H, Riedy MC, Roberts JL, Aman MJ, Migone TS, Noguchi M, Markert ML, Buckley RH, O'Shea JJ, Leonard WJ. Mutation of Jak3 in a patient with SCPI: essential role of Jak3 in lymphoid development. Science 270:797–800, 1995.

Samulski RJ, Chang LS, Shenk T. Helper-free stocks of recombinant adeno-associated viruses: normal integration does not require viral gene expression. J Virol 63:3822–3828, 1989.

Saulnier SO, Steinhoff D, Dinauer MC, Zufferey R, Trono D, Seger RA, Hossle JP. Lentivirus-mediated gene transfer of gp91phox corrects chronic granulomatous disease (CGD) phenotype in human X-CGD cells. J Gene Med 2:317–325, 2000.

Sekhsaria S, Gallin JI, Linton GF, Mallory RM, Mulligan RC, Malech HL. Peripheral blood progenitors as a target for genetic correction of p47phox-deficient chronic granulomatous disease. Proc Natl Acad Sci USA 90:7446–7450, 1993.

Sharifi R, Sinclair JC, Gilmour KC, Arkwright PD, Kinnon C, Thrasher AJ, Gaspar HB. SAP mediates specific cytotoxic T-cell functions in X-linked lymphoproliferative disease. Blood 103:3821–3827, 2004.

Smith CI, Islam KB, Vorechovsky I, Olerup O, Wallin E, Rabbani H, Baskin B, Hammarstrom L. X-linked agammaglobulinemia and other immunoglobulin deficiencies. Immunol Rev 138:159–183, 1994.

Soudais C, Shiho T, Sharara LI, Guy-Grand D, Taniguchi T, Fischer A, Di Santo JP. Stable and functional lymphoid reconstitution of common cytokine receptor gamma chain deficient mice by retroviral-mediated gene transfer. Blood 95:3071–3077, 2000.

Srivastava A, Lusby EW, Berns KI. Nucleotide sequence and organization of the adeno-associated virus 2 genome. J Virol 45:555–564, 1983.

Steinberg M, Swainson L, Schwarz K, Boyer M, Friedrich W, Yssel H, Taylor N, Noraz N. Retrovirus-mediated transduction of primary ZAP-70-deficient human T cells results in the selective growth advantage of gene-corrected cells: implications for gene therapy. Gene Ther 7:1392–1400, 2000.

Strom TS, Li X, Cunningham JM, Nienhuis AW. Correction of the murine Wiskott-Aldrich syndrome phenotype by hematopoietic stem cell transplantation. Blood 99:4626–4628, 2002.

Strom TS, Turner SJ, Andreansky S, Liu H, Doherty PC, Srivastava DK, Cunningham JM, Nienhuis AW. Defects in T-cell–mediated immunity to influenza virus in murine Wiskott-Aldrich syndrome are corrected by oncoretroviral vector–mediated gene transfer into repopulating hematopoietic cells. Blood 102:3108–3116, 2003.

Sullivan KE, Mullen CA, Blaese RM, Winkelstein JA. A multiinstitutional survey of the Wiskott-Aldrich syndrome. J Pediatr 125:876–885, 1994.

Sun JY, Pacheco-Castro A, Borroto A, Alarcon B, Alvarez-Zapata D, Regueiro JR. Construction of retroviral vectors carrying human CD3 gamma cDNA and reconstitution of CD3 gamma expression and T cell receptor surface expression and function in a CD3 gamma-deficient mutant T cell line. Hum Gene Ther 8:1041–1048, 1997.

Tahara, M, Pergolizzi RG, Kobayashi H, Krause A, Luettich K, Lesser ML, Crystal RG. Trans-splicing repair of CD40 ligand deficiency results in naturally regulated correction of a mouse model of hyper-IgM X-linked immunodeficiency. Nat Med 10:835–841, 2004.

Taylor N, Bacon KB, Smith S, Jahn T, Kadlecek TA, Uribe L, Kohn DB, Gelfand EW, Weiss A, Weinberg K. Reconstitution of T cell receptor signaling in ZAP-70-deficient cells by retroviral transduction of the ZAP-70 gene. J Exp Med 184:2031–2036, 1996a.

Taylor N, Uribe L, Smith S, Jahn T, Kohn DB, Weinberg K. Correction of interleukin-2 receptor function in X-SCPI lymphoblastoid cells by retrovirally mediated transfer of the gamma-c gene. Blood 87:3103–3107, 1996b.

Temin HM. The Biology of RNA-Tumor Viruses. New York: MSS Information Corp., 1984.

Thrasher A, Chetty M, Casimir C, Segal AW. Restoration of superoxide generation to a chronic granulomatous disease–derived B-cell line by retrovirus mediated gene transfer. Blood 80:1125–1129, 1992.

Thrasher AJ, Casimir CM, Kinnon C, Morgan G, Segal AW, Levinsky RJ. Gene transfer to primary chronic granulomatous disease monocytes. Lancet 346:92–93, 1995a.

Thrasher AJ, de Alwis M, Casimir CM, Kinnon C, Page K, Lebkowski J, Segal AW, Levinsky RJ. Functional reconstitution of the NADPH-oxidase by adeno-associated virus gene transfer. Blood 86:761–765, 1995b.

Tisdale JF, Hanazono Y, Sellers SE, Agricola BA, Metzger ME, Donahue RE, Dunbar CE. Ex vivo expansion of genetically marked rhesus peripheral blood progenitor cells results in diminished long-term repopulating ability. Blood 92:1131–1141, 1998.

Trobridge G, Josephson N, Vassilopoulos G, Mac J, Russell DW. Improved foamy virus vectors with minimal viral sequences. Mol Ther 6:321–328, 2002.

Tsai EJ, Malech HL, Kirby MR, Hsu AP, Seidel NE, Porada CD, Zanjani ED, Bodine DM, Puck JM. Retroviral transduction of IL2RG into CD34(+) cells from X-linked severe combined immunodeficiency patients permits human T- and B-cell development in sheep chimeras. Blood 100:72–79, 2002.

Tsukada S, Saffran DC, Rawlings DJ, Parolini O, Allen RC, Klisak I, Sparkes RS, Kubagawa H, Mohandas T, Quan S, Belmont JW, Cooper MD, Conley ME, Witte ON. Deficient expression of a B cell cytoplasmic tyrosine kinase in human X-linked agammaglobulinemia. Cell 72:279–290, 1993.

Tuschong L, Soenen SL, Blaese RM, Candotti F, Muul LM. Immune response to fetal calf serum by two adenosine deaminase-deficient patients after T cell gene therapy. Hum Gene Ther 13:1605–1610, 2002.

Uchida N, Sutton RE, Friera AM, He D, Reitsma MJ, Chang WC, Veres G, Scollay R, Weissman IL. HIV, but not murine leukemia virus, vectors mediate high efficiency gene transfer into freshly isolated G0/G1 human hematopoietic stem cells. Proc Natl Acad Sci USA 95:11939–11944, 1998.

Valentine WN, Paglia DE, Tartaglia AP, Gilsanz F. Hereditary hemolytic anemia with increased red cell adenosine deaminase (45- to 70-fold) and decreased adenosine triphosphate. Science 195:783–785, 1977.

Valerio D, Duyvesteyn MG, Meera Khan P, Geurts van Kessel A, de Waard A, van der Eb AJ. Isolation of cDNA clones for human adenosine deaminase. Gene 25:231–240, 1983.

Vassilopoulos G, Trobridge G, Josephson NC, Russell DW. Gene transfer into murine hematopoietic stem cells with helper-free foamy virus vectors. Blood 98:604–609, 2001.

Vetrie D, Vorechovsky I, Sideras P, Holland J, Davies A, Flinter F, Hammarstrom L, Kinnon C, Levinsky R, Bobrow M, Smith CIE, Bentley DR. The gene involved in X-linked agammaglobulinaemia is a member of the src family of protein-tyrosine kinases. Nature 361:226–233, 1993.

Wada T, Jagadeesh GJ, Nelson DL, Candotti F. Retrovirus-mediated WASP gene transfer corrects Wiskott-Aldrich syndrome T-cell dysfunction. Hum Gene Ther 13:1039–1046, 2002.

Wada T, Konno A, Schurman SH, Garabedian EK, Anderson SM, Kirby M, Nelson DL, Candotti F. Second-site mutation in the Wiskott-Aldrich syndrome (WAS) protein gene causes somatic mosaicism in two WAS siblings. J Clin Invest 111:1389–1397, 2003.

Wada T, Schurman SH, Jagadeesh GJ, Garabedian EK, Nelson DL, Candotti F. Multiple patients with revertant mosaicism in a single Wiskott-Aldrich syndrome family. Blood 104:1270–1272, 2004.

Wada T, Schurman SH, Otsu M, Garabedian EK, Ochs HD, Nelson DL, Candotti F. Somatic mosaicism in Wiskott-Aldrich syndrome suggests in vivo reversion by a DNA slippage mechanism. Proc Natl Acad Sci USA 98:8697–8702, 2001.

Walsh CE, Liu JM, Xiao X, Young NS, Nienhuis AW, Samulski RJ. Regulated high level expression of a human gamma-globin gene introduced into erythroid cells by an adeno-associated virus vector. Proc Natl Acad Sci USA 89:7257–7261, 1992.

Weil WM, Linton GF, Whiting-Theobald N, Vowells SJ, Rafferty SP, Li F, Malech HL. Genetic correction of p67phox deficient chronic granulomatous disease using peripheral blood progenitor cells as a target for retrovirus mediated gene transfer. Blood 89:1754–1761, 1997.

Wiginton DA, Adrian GS, Friedman RL, Suttle DP, Hutton JJ. Cloning of cDNA sequences of human adenosine deaminase. Proc Natl Acad Sci USA 80:7481–7485, 1983.

Wilson JM, Ping AJ, Krauss JC, Mayo-Bond L, Rogers CE, Anderson, DC, Todd RF. Correction of CD18-deficient lymphocytes by retrovirus-mediated gene transfer. Science 248:1413–1416, 1990.

Wu C, Nguyen KB, Pien GC, Wang N, Gullo C, Howie D, Sosa MR, Edwards MJ, Borrow P, Satoskar AR, Sharpe AH, Biron CA, Terhorst C. SAP controls T cell responses to virus and terminal differentiation of TH2 cells. Nat Immunol 2:410–414, 2001.

Wu M, Chari S, Yanchis T, Mergia A. cis-Acting sequences required for simian foamy virus type 1 vectors. J Virol 72:3451–3454, 1998.

Wu M, Mergia A. Packaging cell lines for simian foamy virus type 1 vectors. J Virol 73:4498–4501, 1999.

Wu X, Li Y, Crise B, Burgess SM. Transcription start regions in the human genome are favored targets for MLV integration. Science 300:1749–1751, 2003.

Yates F, Malassis-Seris M, Stockholm D, Bouneaud C, Larousserie F, Noguiez-Hellin P, Danos O, Kohn DB, Fischer A, de Villartay JP, Cavazzana-Calvo M. Gene therapy of RAG-2$^{-/-}$ mice: sustained correction of the immunodeficiency. Blood 100:3942–3949, 2002.

Yorifuji T, Wilson RW, Beaudet AL. Retroviral mediated expression of CD18 in normal and deficient human bone marrow progenitor cells. Hum Mol Genet 2:1443–1448, 1993.

Yu PW, Tabuchi RS, Kato RM, Astrakhan A, Humblet-Baron S, Kipp K, Chae K, Ellmeier W, Witte, ON, Rawlings DJ. Sustained correction of B-cell development and function in a murine model of X-linked agammaglobulinemia (XLA) using retroviral-mediated gene transfer. Blood 104:1281–1290, 2004.

Yu PW, Tabuchi RS, Kato RM, Dang VK, Lansigan E, Hernandez R, Witte ON, Rawlings DJ. Correction of X-linked immunodeficiency by retroviral mediated transfer of Bruton's tyrosine kinase. Blood 96:896, 2000.

Zandstra PW, Conneally E, Petzer AL, Piret JM, Eaves CJ. Cytokine manipulation of primitive human hematopoietic cell self-renewal. Proc Natl Acad Sci USA 94:4698–4703, 1997.

Zucali JR, Ciccarone T, Kelley V, Park J, Johnson CM, Mergia A. Transduction of umbilical cord blood CD34+ NOD/SCPI-repopulating cells by simian foamy virus type 1 (SFV-1) vector. Virology 302:229–235, 2002.

Zufferey R, Dull T, Mandel RJ, Bukovsky A, Quiroz D, Naldini L, Trono D. (1998) Self-inactivating lentivirus vector for safe and efficient in vivo gene delivery. J Virol 72:9873–9880, 1998.

Zufferey R, Nagy D, Mandel RJ, Naldini L, Trono D. Multiply attenuated lentiviral vector achieves efficient gene delivery in vivo. Nat Biotechnol 15:871–875, 1997.

Index

Note: Page numbers followed by the letter f refer to figures and those followed by t refer to tables.